DIAGNOSTIC PATHOLOGY
GENITOURINARY

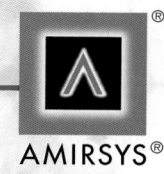
AMIRSYS®

DIAGNOSTIC PATHOLOGY
GENITOURINARY

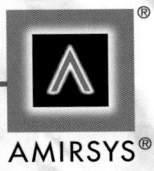

Mahul B. Amin, MD
Professor and Chairman
Department of Pathology and Laboratory Medicine
Cedars-Sinai Medical Center
Los Angeles, CA

Jesse K. McKenney, MD
Assistant Professor
Departments of Pathology and Urology
Director of Urologic Pathology
Stanford University Medical Center
Stanford, CA

Satish K. Tickoo, MD
Attending Pathologist
Department of Pathology
Memorial Sloan-Kettering Cancer Center
New York, NY

Gladell P. Paner, MD
Assistant Professor
Departments of Pathology and Urology
Director of Immunohistochemistry Laboratory
Loyola University Medical Center
Maywood, IL

Steven S. Shen, MD, PhD
Department of Pathology
The Methodist Hospital
Associate Professor of Pathology and Lab Medicine
Weill Medical College of Cornell University
Houston, TX

Elsa F. Velazquez, MD
Assistant Professor of Pathology
Brigham and Women's Hospital
Harvard Medical School
Boston, MA
Currently: Associate Dermatopathologist
Caris Dx a division of Caris Life Sciences
Newton, MA

Antonio L. Cubilla, MD
Professor of Pathology
Universidad Nacional de Asunción
Instituto de Patología e Investigación
Asunción, Paraguay

Jae Y. Ro, MD, PhD
Director of Surgical Pathology
Department of Pathology
The Methodist Hospital
Professor of Pathology and Laboratory Medicine
Weill Medical College of Cornell University
Houston, TX

Victor E. Reuter, MD
Attending Pathologist and Vice-Chairman
Department of Pathology
Memorial Sloan-Kettering Cancer Center
Professor of Pathology
Weill Medical College of Cornell University
New York, NY

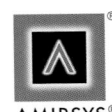

AMIRSYS®

Names you know. Content you trust.®

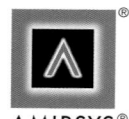

AMIRSYS®
Names you know. Content you trust.®

First Edition

© 2010 Amirsys, Inc.

Compilation © 2010 Amirsys Publishing, Inc.

Printed in Canada by Friesens, Altona, Manitoba, Canada

ISBN: 978-1-931884-28-0

Notice and Disclaimer

Library of Congress Cataloging-in-Publication Data

Diagnostic pathology. Genitourinary / [edited by] Mahul B. Amin.
   p. ; cm.
 Other title: Genitourinary
 Includes bibliographical references and index.
 ISBN 978-1-931884-28-0
 1. Genitourinary organs--Diseases--Diagnosis. I. Amin, Mahul B. II. Title: Genitourinary.
 [DNLM: 1. Male Urogenital Diseases--diagnosis. 2. Male Urogenital Diseases--pathology. 3. Kidney Neoplasms--diagnosis. 4. Kidney Neoplasms--pathology. WJ 140 D536 2010]
 RC874.D52 2010
 616.6'075--dc22
              2010003295

"To my wonderful family, Ushma, Anmol, and Aneri, for their everlasting warmth, love, and support;
My late parents, who constantly motivated and inspired me to excel and serve;
My residents and fellows, who support and challenge me to push the envelope of urologic pathology;
My consultees, for sharing their difficult cases, which serve as a nidus for my educational and research efforts;
My clinical and scientific colleagues, urologists, oncologists, and radiation oncologists, who constantly push me to try to be a better surgical pathologist; and
My patients, who continually help engage me in a process of life-long learning and serve as a vivid and constant reminder that there is a lot more to be done for them."

Acknowledgments
"I gratefully acknowledge the assistance of visiting physician scholars to Cedars Sinai (Dr. Ghee Yong Kwon, Korea; Dr. Nalan Nese, Turkey; and Dr. Anniah Chandrakanth, Canada) for going through my teaching files and helping to obtain innumerable pictures for this book, and the assistance of Dolores Ramirez, my Executive Administrative Assistant, for her efficient project management that kept this large initiative on track."
MBA

"To my family, Amy, Madeleine, Hannah Jane, and Ennis."
JKM

"To Roma and Sharang, for their patience and tolerance."
SKT

"To my wife Agnes, my son Gabriel, and my parents Bernardo and Adelfa, to whom I'm forever indebted for their love and unwavering support."
GPP

"To my wife Jing-Fang, my children Kevin and Megan for their love."
SSS

"To my family."
EFV

"To my wife Jungsil Ro, MD, and my mentor Alberto G. Ayala, MD, for their invaluable comments, guidance, and support!"
JYR

"To all my colleagues and fellows who have taught me so much."
VER

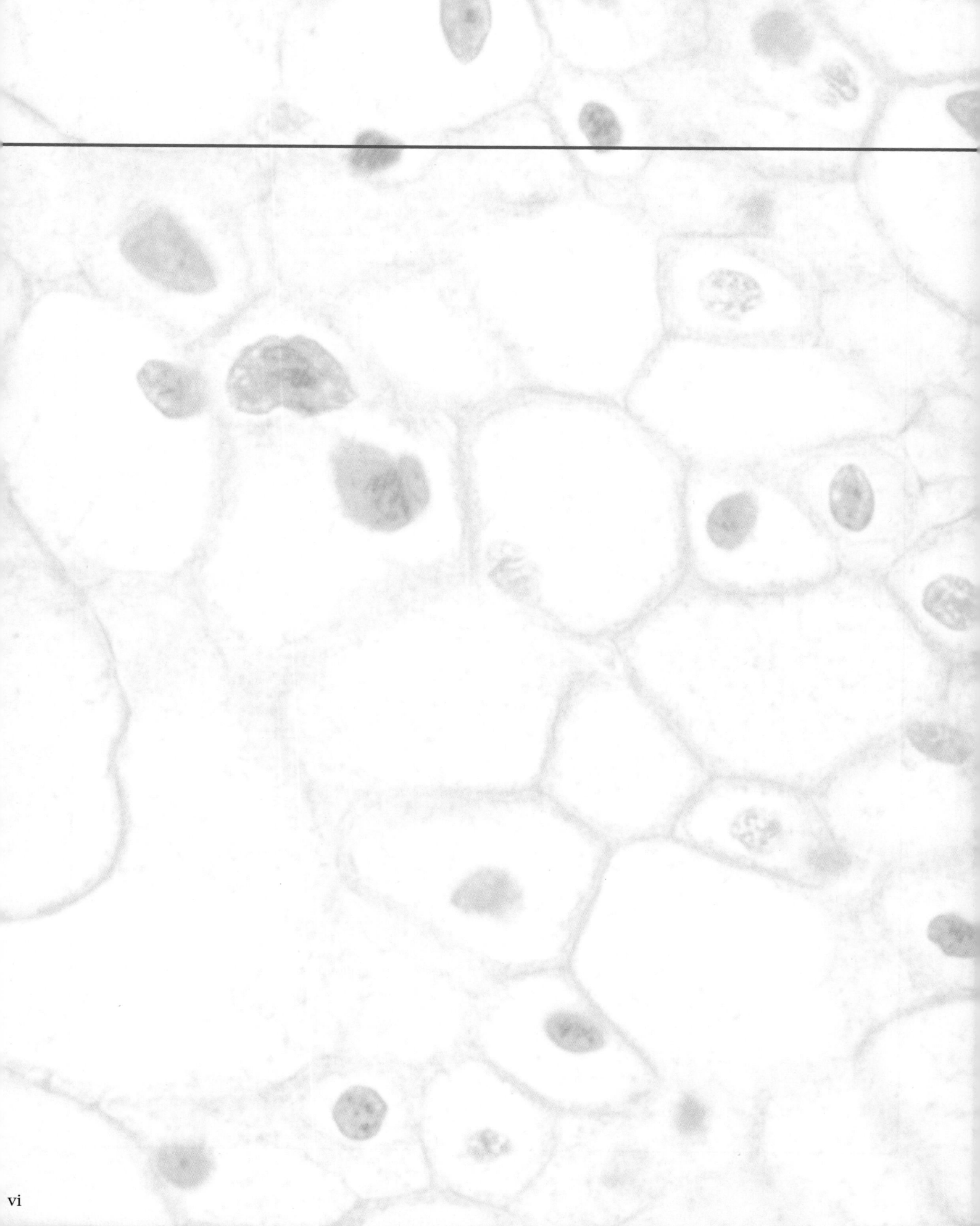

vi

DIAGNOSTIC PATHOLOGY
GENITOURINARY

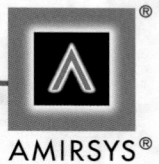

Amirsys, creators of the highly acclaimed radiology series Diagnostic Imaging, proudly introduces its new Diagnostic Pathology series, designed as easy-to-use reference texts for the busy practicing surgical pathologist. Written by world-renowned experts, the series will consist of 15 titles in all the crucial diagnostic areas of surgical pathology.

The second book in this series, *Diagnostic Pathology: Genitourinary*, contains approximately 1,000 pages of comprehensive, yet concise, descriptions of more than 170 specific diagnoses. Amirsys's pioneering bulleted format distills pertinent information to the essentials. Each chapter has the same organization providing an easy-to-read reference for making rapid, efficient, and accurate diagnoses in a busy surgical pathology practice. A highlighted Key Facts box provides the essential features of each diagnosis. Detailed sections on Terminology, Etiology/Pathogenesis, Clinical Issues, Macroscopic and Microscopic Findings, and the all important Differential Diagnoses follow so you can find the information you need in the exact same place every time.

Most importantly, every diagnosis features numerous high-quality images, including gross pathology, H&E and immunohistochemical stains, correlative radiographic images, and richly colored graphics, all of which are fully annotated to maximize their illustrative potential.

We believe that this lavishly illustrated series, with its up-to-date information and practical focus, will become the core of your reference collection. Enjoy!

Elizabeth H. Hammond, MD
Executive Editor, Pathology
Amirsys, Inc.

Anne G. Osborn, MD
Chairman and Chief Executive Officer
Amirsys Publishing, Inc.

PREFACE

Urologic pathology cases constitute a significant proportion of any routine surgical pathology practice. In terms of estimated new cases annually in males in the United States, carcinoma of the prostate is the most common noncutaneous malignancy, and carcinomas of the urinary bladder, and kidney and renal pelvis, are the 4th and 7th most common. In recent years, there has been a large body of work to further the clinicopathologic aspects of these and other urologic cancers, and updated knowledge is critical to the seminal role the surgical pathologist plays in the diagnosis and management of these patients.

Diagnostic Pathology: Genitourinary is intended to be a succinct user-friendly, "1-stop" diagnostic compendium for the busy practicing pathologist, as well as residents and fellows in training. A combination of pithy factual bulleted text along with rich and diverse illustrations help the pathologist to arrive at the correct diagnosis, consider key differential diagnostic possibilities, employ contemporary and judicious ancillary studies as appropriate, with reporting guidelines that enable generation of a complete and accurate surgical pathology report. The numerous illustrations depict not only the classic but also uncommon morphologic presentations; all of these are accompanied by figure legends with educational points that enhance the text. Not only is there wide coverage of more common entities, but there is ample coverage of the not so common to esoteric entities such as pediatric renal tumors, MiTF/TFE family of translocation-associated carcinomas, basaloid and adenoid cystic carcinoma of the prostate, sex cord stromal tumors of the testis, adenocarcinoma of the rete testis, and pseudohyperplastic squamous cell carcinoma and carcinoma cuniculatum of the penis.

The book is organized in 5 sections: Kidney Tumors and Tumor-like Conditions, Urinary Bladder, Prostate Gland and Seminal Vesicles, Testis and Paratesticular Structures, and Penis and Scrotum. At the end of each section, the protocol for reporting resected specimens is provided, as are differential diagnostic-based comprehensive immunohistochemical tables and panels. As the field of urologic pathology continues to evolve in the era of personalized medicine, it is likely that the list of companion diagnostic, prognostic, and predictive markers will increase exponentially. The eBook version of this book will undergo regular updates, making *Diagnostic Pathology: Genitourinary*, what we hope to be, a dynamic and valuable practice resource.

Mahul B. Amin, MD
Professor and Chairman
Department of Pathology and Laboratory Medicine
Cedars-Sinai Medical Center
Los Angeles, CA

ACKNOWLEDGMENTS

Text Editing

Ashley R. Renlund, MA

Kellie J. Heap

Arthur G. Gelsinger, MA

Katherine Riser, MA

Image Editing

Jeffrey J. Marmorstone

Danny C. La

Medical Text Editing

Karen Moser, MD

Illustrations

Laura C. Sesto, MA

Richard Coombs, MS

Lane R. Bennion, MS

Art Direction and Design

Laura C. Sesto, MA

Assistant Editor

Dave L. Chance, MA

Production Lead

Melissa A. Hoopes

AJCC stage grouping and TNM staging tables are derived from Edge SE, Byrd DR, Carducci MA, Compton CA, eds. AJCC Cancer Staging Manual. 7th ed. New York, NY: Springer, 2010. They are used with permission from Springer Science and Business Media LLC, www.springerlink.com.

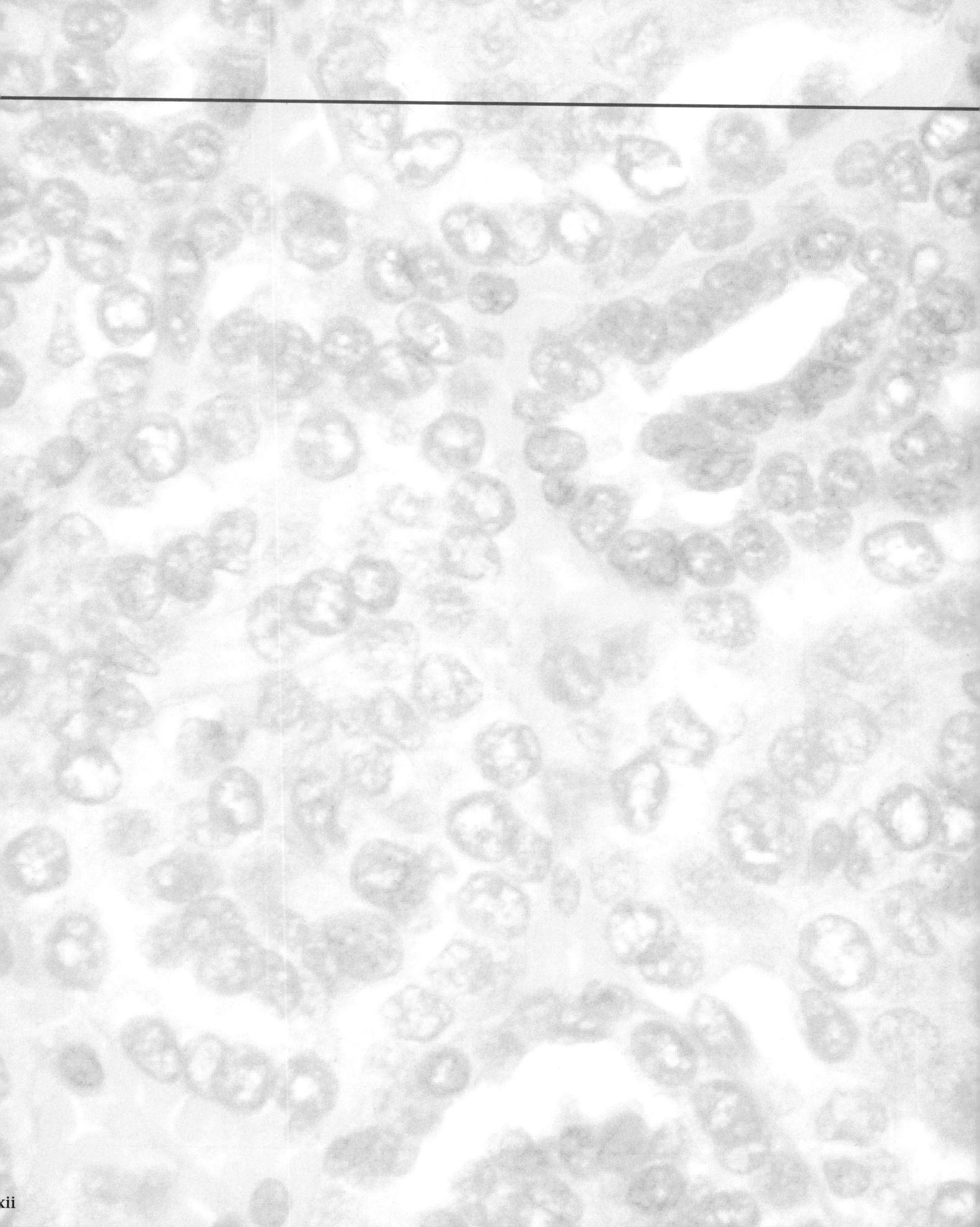

SECTIONS

Kidney Tumors and Tumor-like Conditions

Urinary Bladder

Prostate Gland and Seminal Vesicle

Testis and Paratesticular Structures

Penis and Scrotum

TABLE OF CONTENTS

SECTION 4
Testis and Paratesticular Structures

Introduction and Overview

Nonneoplastic Lesions

Germ Cell Tumors

SECTION 5
Penis and Scrotum

Introduction and Overview

Nonneoplastic Lesions

Primary Preneoplastic and Neoplastic Lesions

Metastatic Tumors

Protocol for the Examination of Specimens from Patients with Primary Carcinoma of the Penis

Immunohistochemical Profiles for Tumors Involving the Penis

SECTION 6
Antibody Cross Reference

DIAGNOSTIC PATHOLOGY
GENITOURINARY

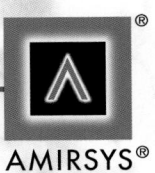

Kidney Tumors and Tumor-like Conditions

CLASSIFICATION OF KIDNEY TUMORS & TUMOR-LIKE LESIONS

NONNEOPLASTIC LESIONS

Tumor-like Lesions
- Xanthogranulomatous pyelonephritis
- Renal malakoplakia
- Inflammatory myofibroblastic lesion/tumor
- Perirenal and sinus cysts

NEOPLASMS

Kidney Tumors in Children
- Nephroblastic tumors
  - Nephroblastoma (Wilms tumor)
    - Favorable histology
    - Anaplasia (diffuse or focal)
  - Nephrogenic rests and nephroblastomatosis
  - Cystic partially differentiated nephroblastoma
  - Cystic nephroma
- Congenital mesoblastic nephroma
  - Classic
  - Cellular
  - Mixed
- Clear cell sarcoma
- Malignant rhabdoid tumor
- Renal cell tumors
  - MiTF/TFE family translocation-associated carcinoma
  - Renal medullary carcinoma
  - Papillary renal cell carcinoma
  - Clear cell renal cell carcinoma
- Metanephric tumors
  - Metanephric adenoma
  - Metanephric adenofibroma
  - Metanephric stromal tumor
- Rare tumors
  - Ossifying renal tumor of infancy

Kidney Tumors in Adults
- Benign epithelial tumors
  - Renal oncocytoma
  - Papillary adenoma
- Metanephric tumors
  - Metanephric adenoma
  - Metanephric adenofibroma
  - Metanephric stromal tumor
  - Metanephric adenosarcoma
- Renal cell carcinoma
  - Clear cell renal cell carcinoma
    - Multilocular cystic renal cell carcinoma
  - Papillary renal cell carcinoma
    - Type 1
    - Type 2
    - Oncocytic variant
    - Sarcomatoid
  - Chromophobe renal cell carcinoma
    - Classic
    - Eosinophilic variant
    - Sarcomatoid
  - Collecting duct carcinoma
  - Renal medullary carcinoma
  - Tubulocystic carcinoma
  - MiTF/TFE family translocation-associated carcinoma
    - Xp11.2 with *TFE3* gene fusion
    - t(6;11) with *TFEB* gene fusion
  - Mucinous tubular and spindle cell carcinoma
  - Thyroid-like follicular carcinoma of kidney
  - Clear cell papillary renal cell carcinoma
  - Renal cell carcinoma, unclassified
  - Tumors associated with end-stage kidney disease
    - Acquired cystic disease-associated renal cell carcinoma
    - Clear cell papillary renal cell carcinoma
    - Papillary renal cell carcinoma
    - Clear cell renal cell carcinoma
    - Chromophobe renal cell carcinoma
    - Collecting duct carcinoma
    - Renal oncocytoma
- Urothelial carcinoma of renal pelvis
- Other neoplasms of renal pelvis: Epithelial
  - Inverted papilloma
  - Nephrogenic adenoma/metaplasia
  - Villous adenoma
  - Squamous cell carcinoma
  - Adenocarcinoma
  - Micropapillary carcinoma
  - Lymphoepithelioma-like carcinoma
  - Small cell carcinoma
  - Others
- Other neoplasms of renal pelvis: Nonepithelial
  - Fibroepithelial polyp
  - Hemangioma
  - Leiomyoma
  - Leiomyosarcoma
  - Rhabdomyosarcoma
  - Others
- 2nd tumors
  - Post neuroblastoma
  - Post transplant
  - Post chemotherapy

Mesenchymal Tumors: Benign
- Angiomyolipoma
- Medullary fibroma (renomedullary interstitial tumor)
- Leiomyoma
- Lipoma
- Hemangioma
- Lymphangioma
- Others

Mesenchymal Tumors: Malignant or Potentially Malignant
- Epithelioid angiomyolipoma (PEComa)
- Solitary fibrous tumor
- Hemangiopericytoma
- Leiomyosarcoma
- Synovial sarcoma
- Liposarcoma
- Fibrosarcoma
- Malignant fibrous histiocytoma
- Rhabdomyosarcoma
- Angiosarcoma
- Osteosarcoma
- Others

CLASSIFICATION OF KIDNEY TUMORS & TUMOR-LIKE LESIONS

Rare Tumors with Epithelial &/or Parenchymal Differentiation
- Juxtaglomerular cell tumor (reninoma)
- Nephroblastoma and other "pediatric-type" renal tumors
- Renal epithelial and stromal tumor
  - Mixed epithelial and stromal tumor
  - Cystic nephroma

Neuroendocrine/Neural Tumors
- Renal carcinoid tumor
- Small cell carcinoma
- Large cell neuroendocrine carcinoma
- Ewing/primitive neuroectodermal tumor
- Paraganglioma
- Intrarenal schwannoma
- Pheochromocytoma
- Neuroblastoma

Hematopoietic Tumors
- Lymphoma
- Leukemia
- Plasmacytoma/multiple myeloma
- Post-transplantation lymphoproliferative lesions

Tumors Associated with Familial Syndromes
- von Hippel-Lindau syndrome: Clear cell renal cell carcinoma
- Hereditary papillary renal carcinoma syndrome: Papillary renal cell carcinoma, type 1
- Birt-Hogg-Dubé syndrome
  - Chromophobe renal cell carcinoma
  - Renal oncocytoma
  - Hybrid tumors
  - Others
- Hereditary leiomyomatosis and renal cell carcinoma syndrome (HLRCC)
  - Type 2-like papillary renal cell carcinoma
  - Others
- Tuberous sclerosis syndrome
  - Angiomyolipoma
  - Clear cell renal cell carcinoma
  - Others, including unusual unclassified renal cell carcinoma

Metastatic Tumors
- Prostate
- Lung
- Colon
- Female genital organs
- Salivary gland
- Others

Others
- Renal-adrenal fusion
- Intracortical adrenal rests
- Intrarenal adrenal cortical neoplasms

INTRODUCTION TO KIDNEY TUMORS

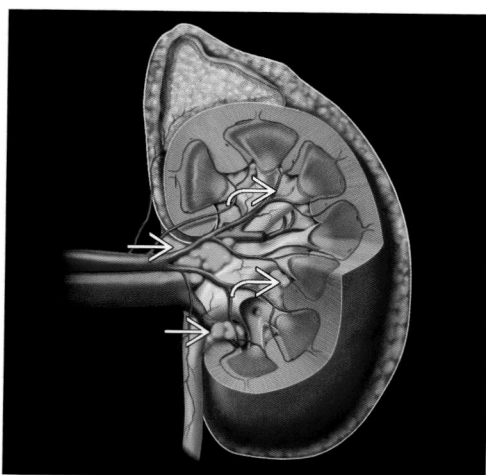

The relationship of renal sinus soft tissues with renal parenchyma is depicted. Sinus fat invasion (pT3a) may occur not only at the medial aspect of kidney ➡, but also in the deeper "intrarenal" component of the sinus ➡.

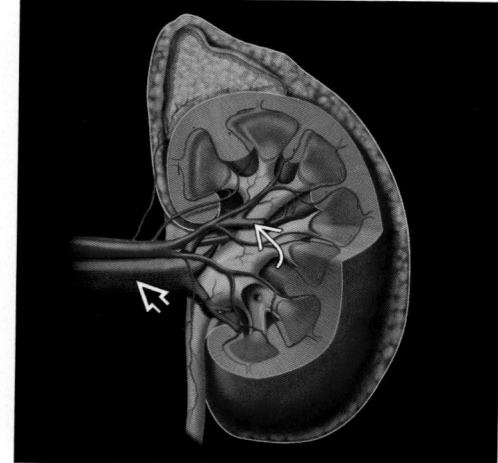

This graphic shows the arrangement of renal vessels in the renal sinus. AJCC/TNM staging regards the invasion of the renal vein branches in the renal sinus ➡ as equivalent to the main renal vein ➡ invasion.

TERMINOLOGY

Abbreviations
- Renal cell carcinoma (RCC), urothelial carcinoma (UC)

EPIDEMIOLOGY

Incidence
- RCC accounts for approximately 2% of all cancers
  - In 2009, there were estimated 57,760 new cases of kidney and renal pelvic cancer in USA
    - In UK, more than 6,500 cases are reported per year
- Incidence of RCC has increased substantially over the last 2 decades
  - Increased incidence, at least in part, is a result of improved diagnostic techniques
  - Most cases of RCC in larger medical centers are now incidentally detected, mostly on radiologic investigations for unrelated conditions
- Compared to renal cortical tumors, carcinomas of renal pelvis and ureter are relatively uncommon
  - They constitute 0.1% and 0.07% of all cancers in men and women, respectively, in North America
    - Account for 4-5% of all urothelial tumors
    - Majority (> 90%) of these tumors are usual urothelial (transitional cell) carcinomas
    - The rest are tumors with aberrant histologies, squamous cell carcinomas being the most common of these

Ethnicity Relationship
- Incidence varies among countries, with highest rates in North America and Scandinavia
- In USA, incidence is equal among whites and blacks

Gender
- RCCs and urothelial carcinomas of renal pelvis occur 2x more frequently in men than in women

Natural History
- Renal cell tumors
  - In USA, close to 13,000 deaths due to RCC are reported each year
  - Worldwide, the disease results in > 100,000 deaths every year
  - Up to 30% of patients with RCC present with metastatic disease, and recurrence develops in 40% of patients treated for localized tumor
  - 5-year survival rates historically are approximately 40%; median overall survival in patients with metastasis is approximately 12 months
    - Recently, targeted therapies against various pathway molecules active in RCC have shown promising results
- Renal pelvic and ureteric tumors
  - 5-year survival
    - > 99% for Ta
    - 91% for T1
    - 72% for T2
    - 40% for T3
    - 16% for patients with metastasis

Age Range
- RCC and UC of upper tract show wide age spectrum
  - However, peak incidence in 6th and 7th decades of life

CLINICAL IMPLICATIONS

Anatomic Considerations: Renal Cell Tumors
- Gerota fascia (renal fascia)
  - Layer of connective tissue encapsulating perirenal fat, and the kidney and adrenal within it
    - Anterior to this fascia is anterior pararenal space, which contains pancreas, transverse colon, and parts of duodenum
    - Surgeons typically remove the kidney along with its Gerota fascia

- Microscopically, Gerota fascia does not have any distinctive features, other than ill-defined, somewhat compressed connective tissue
  - For practical purposes, tumors present at soft tissue margins of specimen are considered to invade Gerota fascia (pT4)
- Protrusion vs. perinephric fat invasion
  - RCC frequently shows exophytic, often mushroom-like component protruding into perirenal fat
    - It is usually capped by well-defined smooth fibrous capsule
    - Unless tumor shows irregular extensions, incomplete pseudocapsule, or single cells invading fat, not regarded as extracapsular extension (pT3a)
- Renal sinus
  - It constitutes extrarenal soft tissue lateral to imaginary vertical line joining medial-most aspects of upper and lower renal poles
  - Contains adipose tissue, lymphatics, veins, arteries, nerves, and pelvicalyceal system
  - Extends deep into kidney, while surrounding calyces ("intrarenal portion of sinus")
  - Invasion of sinus fat or sinus veins may occur around pelvis or deep within "intrarenal portion of sinus" (pT3a)
  - Unlike that in the rest of the organ, the kidney lacks a renal capsule in sinus
- Renal sinus vein and fat invasion
  - According to AJCC/TNM staging, sinus fat or extrarenal fat invasion assigned same pT stage (pT3a)
  - Similarly, invasion of muscular branches of renal vein in renal sinus and main renal vein invasion also assigned same pT stage (pT3a)
  - Careful evaluation reveals sinus fat or vein invasion in overwhelming majority of tumors > 7 cm in diameter
    - Smaller tumors located close to renal sinus also frequently show sinus vein or fat invasion
  - Current AJCC/TNM staging designates tumors > 10 cm confined to kidney as pT2b
    - However, probability of such large tumors limited to kidney is low and warrants close gross evaluation and adequate sampling to rule out extrarenal extension
  - Microscopic presence of large tumor masses in sinus veins, in spite of not being mentioned in gross description, usually suggests inadequate gross evaluation
    - Presence of intravenous tumor masses on microscopy may be considered equivalent to gross venous involvement not picked up on grossing
  - Sinus fat invasion may occur as direct tumor extension into fat or tumor present in veins penetrating through vessel wall
    - Some authors believe that penetration out of venous walls is main mechanism of sinus fat invasion

Anatomic Considerations: Renal Pelvic and Ureteric Tumors

- Renal papillae are directly covered by urothelium, without underlying muscularis
  - Early invasion in area of renal papilla directly involves renal parenchyma (pT3)
  - On the other hand, invasion in pelvicalyceal system away from renal parenchyma often results in lower pT stage (pT1 or pT2)
- Ureter does not contain muscularis mucosae, and muscularis (propria) often extends close to urothelium
  - Therefore, invasion in ureter more readily involves muscularis propria (pT2)

Intraoperative (Frozen Section) Evaluation: Main Indications

- To determine whether the tumor is a renal cortical neoplasm or urothelial carcinoma of pelvicalyceal system
  - Distinction particularly important when partial nephrectomies are being contemplated
    - For urothelial carcinoma, partial or even total nephrectomy is usually not adequate or acceptable option
    - Standard surgical procedure for urothelial carcinoma is nephroureterectomy, ± resection of bladder cuff
    - For renal cortical neoplasms, no further intraoperative action may be needed
    - Specific intraoperative subtyping of cortical tumors is not required/necessary, as surgical management is not dependent on specific tumor type
- To evaluate surgical margins, particularly in partial nephrectomies
  - Positive "frozen section" margins will often lead to additional surgical resection for cortical tumors

Staging Issues: Renal Cortical Tumors

- Renal cortical tumors confined to kidney assigned stages pT1 or pT2 by AJCC/WHO
  - Specific maximum size of primary tumors reported as important prognostic factor in many studies, but not always on multivariate analysis
    - Size as a continuous variable more often shown to have impact on clinical outcome
    - However, specific size limits are considered useful for purposes of management and clinical trial protocols
    - Therefore, specific sizes used in TNM staging
- Soft tissue or vascular spread beyond kidney (pT3) recognized as major prognostic factor
  - Before the 6th edition of TNM/AJCC staging system (2002), no mention was made of renal sinus fat or renal vein branch invasion
  - Multiple recent studies report prognostic significance of renal sinus fat or muscular branches of renal vein invasion
    - Currently, sinus fat and muscular renal sinus vein invasion equated with perinephric fat and

main renal vein invasion, respectively, for staging purposes
- Adrenal gland invasion
  - Involvement of ipsilateral adrenal gland by direct spread occurs in about 5% of cases
    - In current AJCC/TNM staging system, it is regarded as stage pT4
  - Discontinuous involvement of adrenal gland is considered as a metastasis
    - Current staging system regards it as stage M1
    - Therefore, careful sampling and identification of direct spread is crucial

Staging Issues: Renal Pelvic and Ureteric Tumors

- Noninvasive papillary tumors in upper tract may have prominent endophytic or inverted growth
  - Such tumors pushing into wall or sinus fat without invasion may raise the question of invasion
  - Uniform, broad tumor fronds and lack of stromal reaction argue against invasion
  - Generous sampling and careful search for small irregular foci of invasion is imperative in such cases
- Extension of tumor into renal tubules is akin to urothelial carcinoma in situ involving Brunn nests
  - Such extensions may mimic renal parenchymal invasion
  - Tubular tumor spread is in situ process, whereas parenchymal invasion is considered pT3 disease
  - Unlike true stromal invasion, tumor extension into tubules maintains tubular configuration and often only partially involves tubules
  - True invasion of renal parenchyma shows irregular destructive growth that is often associated with desmoplastic response

Specimen Handling Issues: Radical and Total Nephrectomy Specimens for Renal Cortical Tumors

- Inking entire external surface often not required
  - However, inking must be performed in cases with apparent extrarenal involvement on gross evaluation or on external surface overlying bulge of renal tumor
- Specimen should be bisected in sagittal plane into anterior and posterior halves
  - Traditionally, specimens have been cut from lateral border toward hilum
  - Opening the renal vein and bisecting outward through the vein may be a better option
    - This approach more often identifies gross sinus vein invasion
  - Bivalving is best performed without perinephric fat being disturbed, particularly in areas where tumor bulge may be palpable
  - Tumor is usually adequately displayed by this procedure, showing its relationship to renal parenchyma, renal sinus, pelvis, and sinus vessels

Specimen Handling Issues: Partial Nephrectomy Specimens for Renal Cortical Tumors

- Inking of parenchymal resection margin is a must
- Inking external surface is usually not required but should be performed in cases with apparent extrarenal involvement or bulging on gross evaluation
- Specimen should be bisected in sagittal plane into anterior and posterior halves
  - Dissection may be done from lateral border toward the hilum but should be from medial to lateral if large vessels are noted in the hilum

Sections to be Submitted for Renal Cortical Tumors

- At least 1 block/cm of primary tumor
- Appropriate/variable number of blocks to identify extension into perirenal fat
- At least 2-3 blocks from tumor–renal sinus interface
- 1 block from renal vein, renal artery, and ureter margins
- Multiple blocks from identifiable or suspected venous or collecting system invasion
- At least 1 block from tumor-kidney interface
- 1 block from adrenal gland if away from tumor or multiple blocks if close to tumor
- All identified lymph nodes
- Blocks from all identifiable other renal abnormalities
- At least 1 block from macroscopically normal renal parenchyma, away from tumor

Specimen Handling Issues: Nephroureterectomy and Segmental Ureterectomy Specimens for Urothelial Tumors

- Inherently friable papillary tumors are prone to fragmentation and displacement, precluding accurate staging in some cases
  - Therefore, fixation prior to prosecting essential to prevent such artifacts
- Sampling should document the relationship of tumor to adjacent renal parenchyma, renal sinus fat, nearest soft tissue margin, and ureter
- Margins include radial hilar soft tissue margin; bladder cuff or ureteral; Gerota fascia margins

Grading Issues: Renal Cortical Tumors

- Multiple grading schemes have been proposed
  - Fuhrman grading system most commonly used at present
- Fuhrman grading system useful in clear cell and some other cortical carcinomas
  - Utility in papillary and chromophobe RCC not substantiated in most studies
    - Therefore, multiple studies are ongoing or have reported to assess better grading systems in these 2 entities
  - No role in grading of renal oncocytomas because of benign clinical behavior in all tumors
- Fuhrman Grading System

○ Grade 1: Nuclei round and uniform, nucleoli inconspicuous or absent
○ Grade 2: Nuclei slightly irregular, nucleoli identifiable
○ Grade 3: Nuclei very irregular, nucleoli large and prominent
○ Grade 4: Nuclei bizarre and multilobated, nucleoli large and prominent

Grading Issues: Renal Pelvic and Ureteric Tumors

- Grading system for urothelial tumors is identical to that for urinary bladder neoplasms
- Urothelial tumors classified and graded as
  ○ Urothelial (transitional cell) papilloma
  ○ Inverted papilloma
  ○ Papillary urothelial neoplasm of low malignant potential (PUNLMP)
  ○ Urothelial carcinoma, low grade
  ○ Urothelial carcinoma, high grade
- Urothelial carcinomas of upper tract more often high grade compared to urinary bladder carcinomas
  ○ PUNLMP is extremely uncommon in upper urinary tract
- Adenocarcinoma and squamous cell carcinoma graded as
  ○ G1: Well differentiated
  ○ G2: Moderately differentiated
  ○ G3: Poorly differentiated

Management

- Renal cortical tumors
  ○ Partial, total, or radical nephrectomy is mainstay of treatment options
    ▪ Surgical resection of primary tumor is often performed to decrease tumor load even in patients with metastatic disease
  ○ In situ tumor ablations are becoming more common recently, particularly for smaller tumors
  ○ Traditionally, immunotherapy using IL-2 and interferons was treatment of choice in metastatic settings; chemotherapy not effective in most RCCs
    ▪ 5-year survivals only approximately 20% with these therapeutic approaches
  ○ Targeted therapies against molecules of multiple pathways active in renal cancer have become treatment of choice in recent years, with promising results
    ▪ Besides their use in metastatic RCC, these therapies are currently also being evaluated in adjuvant setting in some high-risk tumors
- Renal pelvic and ureteric tumors
  ○ Nephroureterectomy ± bladder cuff is most commonly used therapeutic option
  ○ Segmental ureterectomy often performed for tumors in distal ureter
  ○ Various chemotherapies, similar to those in bladder tumors, used for metastatic tumors
    ▪ Recently, targeted therapies against molecules of multiple pathways active in urothelial cancer are also being implemented

Prognostic Factors

- Renal cell carcinoma
  ○ Some of established factors influencing clinical outcome in RCC include
    ▪ Primary tumor stage, size, distant/nodal metastases, histologic subtype, nuclear grade (in clear cell RCC), sarcomatoid features, tumor necrosis
    ▪ Performance status, presence or absence of systemic symptoms, thrombocytosis, anemia, elevated ESR, elevated C-reactive protein, etc.
  ○ Molecular factors, including CA9, HIF-1-α, CXCR3, CXCR4, B7-H1, PTEN, Ki-67, survivin, vitamin D receptors, etc., reported to influence prognosis
    ▪ The role of none of these is established yet
- Renal pelvic and ureteric tumors
  ○ Tumor stage is most important and, on multivariate analyses in multiple studies, the only prognostic factor
    ▪ On univariate analyses, age, tumor site, grade, nontransitional cell histologies, and multiple molecular factors reported to be associated with prognosis

SELECTED REFERENCES

1. Aubert S et al: MUC1, a new hypoxia inducible factor target gene, is an actor in clear renal cell carcinoma tumor progression. Cancer Res. 69(14):5707-15, 2009
2. Delahunt B: Advances and controversies in grading and staging of renal cell carcinoma. Mod Pathol. 22 Suppl 2:S24-36, 2009
3. Hagemann IS et al: A retrospective comparison of 2 methods of intraoperative margin evaluation during partial nephrectomy. J Urol. 181(2):500-5, 2009
4. Jain P et al: Renal cell carcinoma: Impact of mode of detection on its pathological characteristics. Indian J Urol. 25(4):479-82, 2009
5. Jemal A et al: Cancer statistics, 2009. CA Cancer J Clin. 59(4):225-49, 2009
6. Lam JS et al: Staging of renal cell carcinoma: Current concepts. Indian J Urol. 25(4):446-54, 2009
7. Luo JH et al: Analysis of long-term survival in patients with localized renal cell carcinoma: laparoscopic versus open radical nephrectomy. World J Urol. Epub ahead of print, 2009
8. Osunkoya AO et al: Diagnostic biomarkers for renal cell carcinoma: selection using novel bioinformatics systems for microarray data analysis. Hum Pathol. 40(12):1671-8, 2009
9. Sorbellini M et al: Renal Cell Carcinoma and Prognostic Factors Predictive of Survival. Ann Surg Oncol. Epub ahead of print, 2009
10. Sunela KL et al: Prognostic factors and long-term survival in renal cell cancer patients. Scand J Urol Nephrol. 43(6):454-60, 2009
11. Gupta R et al: Neoplasms of the upper urinary tract: a review with focus on urothelial carcinoma of the pelvicalyceal system and aspects related to its diagnosis and reporting. Adv Anat Pathol. 15(3):127-39, 2008
12. Lane BR et al: Prognostic models and algorithms in renal cell carcinoma. Urol Clin North Am. 35(4):613-25; vii, 2008
13. Kirkali Z et al: What does the urologist expect from the pathologist (and what can the pathologists give) in reporting on adult kidney tumour specimens? Eur Urol. 51(5):1194-201, 2007

INTRODUCTION TO KIDNEY TUMORS

Primary Tumor (pT) Staging for Renal Cell Tumors (2010)

TNM		Definitions
pT1		Tumor 7 cm or less in greatest dimension, limited to kidney
	pT1a	Tumor 4 cm or less in greatest dimension, limited to kidney
	pT1b	Tumor > 4 cm but ≤ 7 cm in greatest dimension, limited to kidney
pT2		Tumor > 7 cm in greatest dimension, limited to kidney
	pT2a	Tumor > 7 cm but ≤ 10 cm in greatest dimension, limited to kidney
	pT2b	Tumor > 10 cm, limited to kidney
pT3		Tumor extends into major veins or perinephric tissues but not into ipsilateral adrenal gland and not beyond Gerota fascia
	pT3a	Tumor grossly extends into renal vein or its segmental (muscle containing) branches, or tumor invades perirenal &/or renal sinus fat but not beyond Gerota fascia
	pT3b	Tumor grossly extends into vena cava below diaphragm
	pT3c	Tumor grossly extends into vena cava above diaphragm or invades wall of vena cava
pT4		Tumor invades beyond Gerota fascia (including contiguous extension into ipsilateral adrenal gland)

Primary Tumor (pT) Staging for Renal Pelvic and Ureteral Tumors

TNM	Definitions
pT0	No evidence of primary tumor
pTa	Papillary noninvasive carcinoma
pTis	Flat carcinoma in situ
pT1	Tumor invades subepithelial connective tissue (lamina propria)
pT2	Tumor invades muscularis propria
pT3	Tumor invades beyond muscularis into peripelvic or periureteral fat or renal parenchyma
pT4	Tumor invades adjacent organs or through kidney into perinephric fat

Used with the permission of the American Joint Committee on Cancer (AJCC), Chicago, Illinois. The original source for this material is the AJCC Cancer Staging Manual, Seventh Edition (2010) published by Springer Science and Business Media LLC, www.springerlink.com.

14. Berdjis N et al: Impact of resection margin status after nephron-sparing surgery for renal cell carcinoma. BJU Int. 97(6):1208-10, 2006
15. Che M et al: Handling and reporting of tumor-containing kidney specimens. Clin Lab Med. 25(2):417-32, 2005
16. Fleming S et al: Best Practice No 180. Nephrectomy for renal tumour; dissection guide and dataset. J Clin Pathol. 58(1):7-14, 2005
17. Algaba F et al: Handling and pathology reporting of renal tumor specimens. Eur Urol. 45(4):437-43, 2004
18. Kubinski DJ et al: Utility of frozen section analysis of resection margins during partial nephrectomy. Urology. 64(1):31-4, 2004
19. Olgac S et al: Urothelial carcinoma of the renal pelvis: a clinicopathologic study of 130 cases. Am J Surg Pathol. 28(12):1545-52, 2004
20. Amin MB et al: Updated protocol for the examination of specimens from patients with carcinoma of the urinary bladder, ureter, and renal pelvis. Arch Pathol Lab Med. 127(10):1263-79, 2003
21. Farrow G et al: Protocol for the examination of specimens from patients with carcinomas of renal tubular origin, exclusive of Wilms tumor and tumors of urothelial origin: a basis for checklists. Cancer Committee, College of American Pathologists. Arch Pathol Lab Med. 123(1):23-7, 1999
22. Guinan P et al: Renal pelvic cancer: a review of 611 patients treated in Illinois 1975-1985. Cancer Incidence and End Results Committee. Urology. 40(5):393-9, 1992

Diagrammatic and Microscopic Features

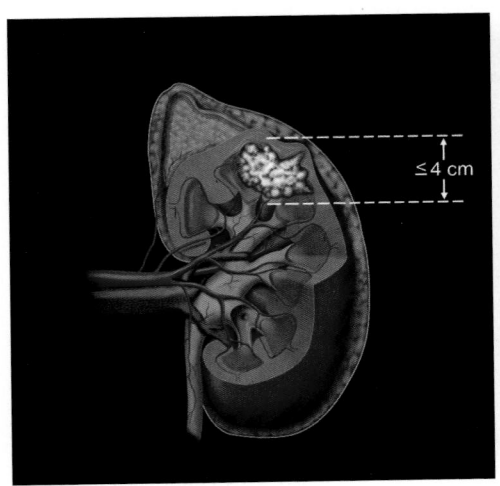

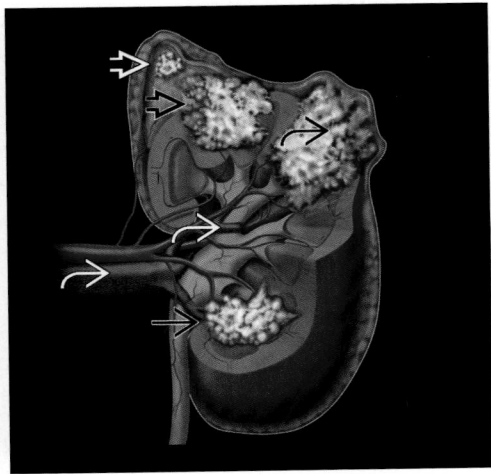

(Left) Renal cell tumors confined to the kidney and 7 cm or less in diameter are assigned stage pT1 (up to 4 cm, pT1a; 4-7 cm, pT1b). Tumors > 7 cm and confined to the kidney are regarded pT2. *(Right)* The size criterion does not apply to tumors with extrarenal extension. Tumors with renal sinus ⇨ or perirenal ⇗ fat or renal vascular ⤵ invasion are all assigned stage pT3a. Tumors directly invading the adrenal ⇛ are considered pT4, and those with discontinuous adrenal invasion ⮊ as pM1.

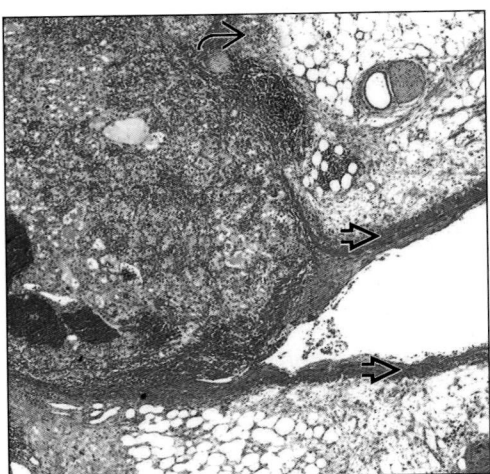

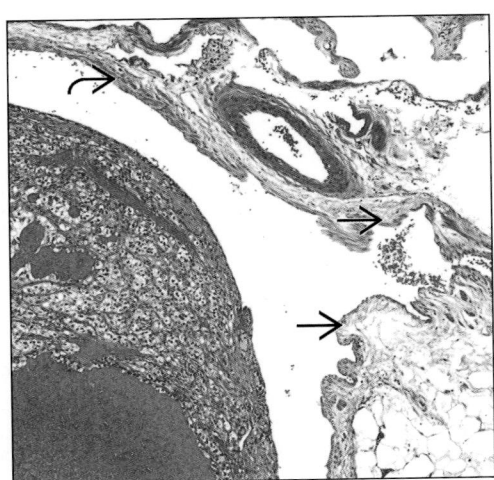

(Left) Invasion of muscular renal vein branches ⇛ in the renal sinus is equated with renal vein invasion (pT3a), making it imperative to thoroughly sample tumor-sinus interface. Renal sinus fat invasion may occur as direct tumor extension or by the invasion of tumor through the walls of the sinus veins ⇗. *(Right)* The muscle layer ⇛ is often discontinuous ⇨ even in the largest of the veins in the renal sinus. AJCC/TNM staging system does not address the issue of this anatomic variation.

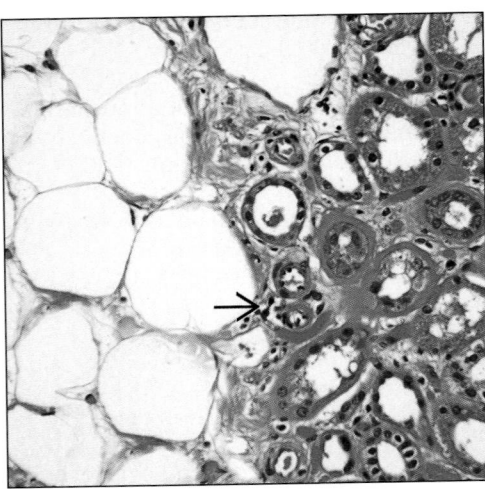

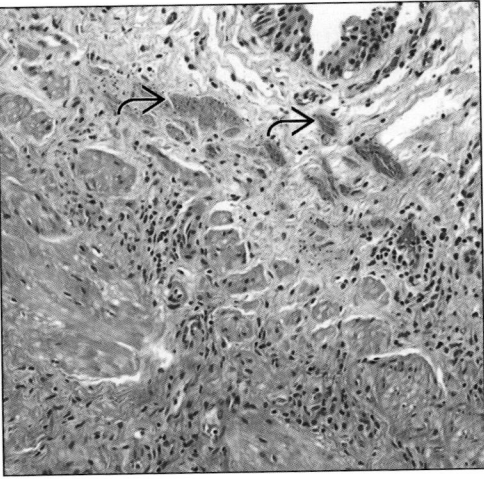

(Left) The renal capsule is lacking in the renal sinus, and the tubules may be in direct contact ⇨ with sinus fat. This may result in an easy approach for RCCs to invade the sinus fat, although such invasion frequently occurs by penetration through the walls by intravenous tumors. *(Right)* The ureter lacks muscularis mucosae, and muscularis propria often extends close to the surface urothelium ⇗. Therefore, invasive ureteric tumors often show muscularis propria invasion (pT2).

1

FAMILIAL CANCER SYNDROMES

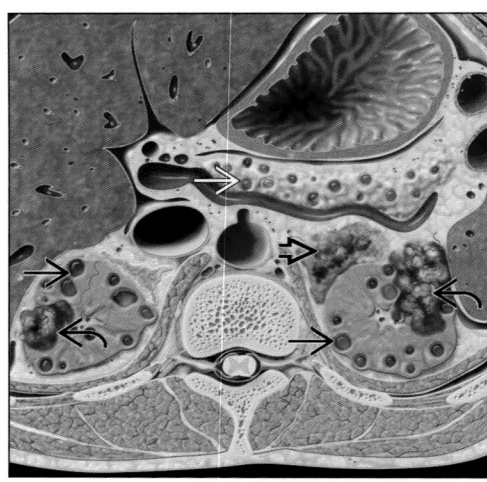

Graphic representation of abdominal lesions in von Hippel-Lindau syndrome shows bilateral, multiple renal cysts ⮕, renal tumors ⮕, pancreatic cysts ⮕, and adrenal pheochromocytoma ⮕.

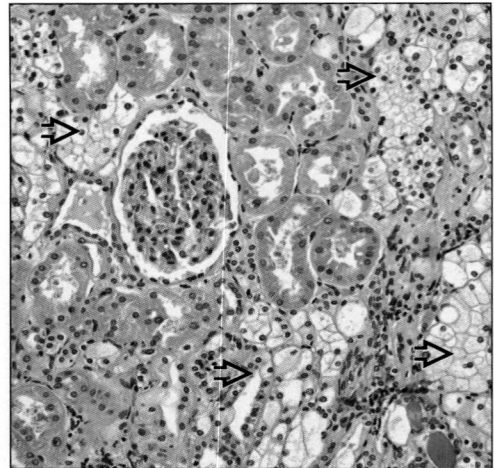

Besides the larger, macroscopic clear cell renal cell carcinomas, VHL kidneys often show numerous microscopic aggregates or tumorlets of clear cells, frequently with irregular outlines ⮕.

TERMINOLOGY

Abbreviations
- von Hippel-Lindau (VHL) syndrome
- Hereditary papillary renal carcinoma (HPRC) syndrome
- Birt-Hogg-Dubé (BHD) syndrome
- Hereditary leiomyomatosis and renal cell carcinoma (HLRCC) syndrome
- Tuberous sclerosis (TS) syndrome

SYNDROMES

General Considerations
- In all forms of inherited renal neoplasms, tumors are usually diagnosed at earlier age and are more likely to be multifocal and bilateral
  - At present, only exception to multifocality and bilaterality appears to be HLRCC syndrome
- Because of consistent defects within tumor groups, genetic profiles of inherited neoplasms are relatively easier to study
  - Knowledge thus gained may be applied in similar, more common sporadic tumors
    - This has resulted in better understanding of genetic mechanisms involved in various sporadic tumor subtypes
    - Most targeted therapies currently in use/under investigation have been direct consequence of this better understanding of tumor genetics

SYNDROMIC RENAL TUMORS

von Hippel-Lindau Syndrome
- Autosomal dominant syndrome, characterized by
  - Retinal hemangioblastomas
  - Clear cell renal cell carcinomas (RCC) and multiple renal cysts

- Cerebellar and spinal hemangioblastomas
- Pheochromocytomas
- Pancreatic cysts and endocrine pancreatic tumors
- Endolymphatic sac tumors of ear
- Epididymal cystadenomas
- VHL, unlike most other familial renal cancer syndromes, shows high degree of genetic penetrance
- Estimated incidence: 1/36,000-1/45,500
- Syndrome is associated with alterations in tumor suppressor *VHL* gene
  - Gene located at chromosome 3p25
  - Inactivated by various mutations, loss of heterozygosity (LOH), hypermethylations, or alterations in *VHL* modifier genes
  - In VHL syndrome, germline mutation present in 1 allele of *VHL* gene
    - Clinical manifestations of disease result when mutations/silencing occur in other wild-type allele
- *VHL* gene product pVHL essential for proteosomic degradation of hypoxia-inducible factor-1α (HIF-1α)
  - Absence of functional pVHL results in overexpression of HIF-1α
  - Activated HIF-1 heterodimers localize to nucleus and regulate transcription of multiple genes by binding to hypoxia-responsive elements (HRE); activated targets include
    - Vascular endothelial and platelet-derived growth factors (VEGF and PDGF) and receptors
    - Glucose transporter protein-1 (GLUT1)
    - Erythropoietin
    - Carbonic anhydrase-IX (CA9)
    - Transforming growth factor-alpha (TGF-α)
    - C-X-C chemokine receptor type 4 (CXCR4)
    - C-mesenchymal-epithelial transition factor (c-MET)
  - Many of these factors associated with angiogenesis, tumorigenesis, and tumor metastasis

FAMILIAL CANCER SYNDROMES

- Depending on whether pheochromocytomas are present or not, VHL disease can be divided into 2 major types
  - Type 1 is not associated with pheochromocytomas
    - It involves "loss of function" mutations, including deletion, microinsertion, and nonsense mutations
  - Type 2 has high risk for pheochromocytomas and is divided into 3 subtypes
    - Type 2A, associated with low risk for RCC
    - Type 2B, associated with high risk for RCC
    - Type 2C, with pheochromocytomas only
    - Mutations that predispose to type 2 VHL are mainly of missense type that result in conformationally altered pVHL
    - These mutant pVHLs still may be able to retain some of their functions or may gain other novel functions
- Renal lesions in VHL syndrome include multiple bilateral benign cysts, atypical cysts, cystic RCCs, and solid RCCs
- Kidneys are usually of normal size and weight, chiefly because most cysts and RCCs are small
- Renal cysts
  - Cysts are usually few (3–30 in number; mean: 7.8 per kidney), usually small (almost all < 1.5 cm, mean size: 0.7 cm)
  - Cysts may be unilocular or multilocular
  - They are almost entirely lined by clear cells; focal or predominant granular cytoplasm is rarely present
    - Cysts are designated as benign cysts (1 layer of clear cells without atypia) or atypical cysts (2 or 3 cells thick ± atypia)
    - Focal proliferations more than 3 cells thick are regarded as cystic RCCs
  - Increased vascularity is often seen around cysts
- Clear cell renal cell carcinoma
  - Mean age for development of renal carcinoma: 37 years (range: 16-67)
  - By age 70, chance of kidney cancer is 70%
  - Retinal and CNS hemangioblastomas usually manifest at earlier mean ages (25 and 30 years)
    - Renal lesions are earlier manifestation in only 7%
  - In spite of relatively few patients developing metastasis, metastatic RCC is leading cause of death from VHL
  - In addition to macroscopically identifiable tumors, numerous microscopic nodules of clear cells seen in VHL kidneys
    - Some nodules well circumscribed
    - Others present as aggregates of clear cells, with irregular outlines
    - Clusters and sheets of clear cells appearing to percolate between nephrons also common
  - Screening for renal tumors in VHL patients recommended after age 10
- Management of renal tumors
  - Current strategies advocate conservative management for all genetic, multifocal, bilateral tumors
    - Nephron-sparing surgery/tumor ablation strategy is used with intent to remove all solid and semicystic lesions from kidney

- Procedure is usually delayed until tumors grow beyond 3 cm in size
    - During follow-up, as new tumors develop, repeat procedures are performed
    - Main intent of this approach is to preserve renal function as much and as long as possible
  - Targeted therapies currently being investigated to potentially reduce tumor burden of even localized tumors in VHL

Hereditary Papillary Renal Carcinoma Syndrome

- Autosomal dominant syndrome, with incomplete penetrance, characterized by
  - Multiple, bilateral papillary renal cell carcinomas
    - Hundreds to thousands of tumors known to occur in each kidney
- Syndrome is associated with activating mutations of c-MET proto-oncogene
  - Gene is located at chromosome 7q31
  - Hepatocyte growth factor (a.k.a. scatter factor) acts as ligand for MET trans-member tyrosine kinase protein
  - Normally, binding to hepatocyte growth factor activates MET tyrosine kinase protein
    - Tyrosine phosphorylation induces proliferation and differentiation of epithelial and endothelial cells, cell branching, and invasion
- c-MET mutations result in ligand-independent constitutive activation of MET tyrosine kinase
  - Activated tyrosine kinase then binds to and activates several signal transducers and adaptors, such as
    - Phosphatidylinositol 3 kinase (PI3K)
    - pp60src
    - Growth factor receptor-bound protein 2 (Grb2)
    - GRB2-associated binding protein 1 (Gab1)
  - This constitutive activation results in tumorigenesis
- Renal tumors associated with syndromic c-MET mutations are all type 1 papillary RCC
  - Tumors show papillary or tubulo-papillary architecture, similar to type 1 sporadic carcinomas
  - Foamy macrophages and calcifications commonly present
- Tumors often manifest at relatively late age (50 to 70 years)
  - Recently, early onset form of disease has also been described
- Low genetic penetrance is supported by relatively low proportion of cases demonstrating syndrome manifestations
  - Approximately 50% of members of affected families develop disease
- Tumors are multifocal and bilateral
- No extrarenal manifestations of HPRC are known at present

Birt-Hogg-Dubé Syndrome

- Autosomal dominant syndrome with incomplete penetrance, characterized by
  - Renal tumors

○ Cutaneous lesions (fibrofolliculomas, trichodiscomas, and acrochordons)
○ Pulmonary cysts, spontaneous pneumothorax, bronchiectasis, and bronchospasm
○ Colonic neoplasms
○ Medullary thyroid carcinoma
○ Lipomas
• Syndrome involves mutations in *BHD* gene
  ○ *BHD* gene maps to chromosome 17p12-q11.2
  ○ Gene codes for folliculin protein
  ○ Multiple mutations, including germline and somatic, have been reported in *BHD* gene
  ○ Usually, germline mutation in 1 allele is inherited, followed by somatic-type mutation in the other allele that may result in tumorigenesis
    ▪ This supports the role of *BHD* as a tumor suppressor gene
  ○ Renal tumors in BHD syndrome usually have oncocytic cytoplasm
    ▪ Most common tumor type displays hybrid features of renal oncocytoma and chromophobe RCC
    ▪ Characteristically, many oncocytic tumors show scattered clusters of cells with clear cytoplasm
    ▪ Pure chromophobe RCC and renal oncocytomas are other common tumor types
    ▪ Other types of renal cell carcinoma are also seen, including clear cell and papillary RCC
  ○ Renal oncocytosis is evident in surrounding renal parenchyma in large proportion of cases
  ○ Morphologic spectrum of renal oncocytosis includes
    ▪ Numerous microscopic oncocytic nodules: May have features of chromophobe RCC, oncocytoma, or even hybrid tumors
    ▪ Cysts lined by oncocytic cells
    ▪ Oncocytic changes in nonneoplastic renal tubules
    ▪ Clusters and sheets of oncocytic cells percolating between nonneoplastic nephrons
  ○ Skin tumors usually appear before renal manifestations
    ▪ Renal tumors are usually diagnosed in 6th decade of life (range: 31-73 years)
    ▪ Skin lesions often appear in 3rd decade
  ○ Renal tumors occur in 15-27% of patients with this syndrome
  ○ Loss of heterozygosity at *BHD* locus and promoter methylation have been reported in rare sporadic RCC of various histologic subtypes
    ▪ Wide spectrum of renal tumor morphologies also seen in BHD syndrome
    ▪ These observations suggests that *BHD* may play role in tumorigenesis across spectrum of RCC, regardless of histologic subtype

Hereditary Leiomyomatosis and Renal Cell Cancer Syndrome

• Autosomal dominant syndrome, characterized by
  ○ Leiomyomas of skin and uterus
  ○ Occasional leiomyosarcoma of uterus
  ○ Renal carcinomas
• Genetic basis is germline inactivating mutations in fumarate hydratase (*FH*) gene

○ *FH* gene is located at 1q42.3-q43
○ Gene encodes for the enzyme fumarate hydratase
  ▪ Fumarate hydratase is required to convert fumarate to malate in Krebs (tricarboxylic acid) cycle
○ Germline mutations in *FH* gene are accompanied by mutations or deletions of wild-type *FH* allele in tumors
○ Most common germline mutations are missense mutations, although truncation and whole gene deletion may be present
○ Loss of FH function results in increased levels of fumarate in cell
  ▪ Increased fumarate acts as competitive inhibitor of prolyl hydroxylase domain-containing proteins or PHDs (EGLN, HPH)
  ▪ Inhibition of these proteins prevents hydroxylation of HIF-1
  ▪ This results in its overexpression and transcription of multiple downstream products
• Renal tumors in HLRCC syndrome
  ○ Aggressive type of renal carcinoma
    ▪ Often regarded as type 2 papillary or collecting duct RCC in the past
  ○ Renal tumors are often solitary and unilateral, unlike most syndromic tumors
  ○ Penetrance for RCC lower than for cutaneous and uterine manifestations, with only 20–35% of patients developing RCC
  ○ Most patients develop cutaneous leiomyomas
  ○ In women, most will have uterine leiomyomas at young age
    ▪ Some cases have had hysterectomy prior to diagnosis of HLRCC
    ▪ Uterine leiomyomas often cellular and with some atypical features
    ▪ No specific features described in cutaneous leiomyomas at present
• Renal carcinoma shows variable, but often prominent, papillary architecture
  ○ Because of papillary architecture, tumors were considered as type 2 papillary RCC in recent past
  ○ Other common patterns in tumor include, solid alveolar, tubular/glandular, and sheet-like
  ○ Desmoplasia and multinodularity are also common
    ▪ Cystic features even more frequent
  ○ Tumor cells are large and usually with abundant eosinophilic cytoplasm
  ○ Rarely, focal clear cell change also observed
  ○ Most diagnostic and consistent feature of tumors is large nuclei with very prominent orangeophilic or eosinophilic nucleoli, surrounded by clear halo
    ▪ Appearance somewhat resembles Cytomegalovirus (CMV) inclusions
  ○ Possibility of HLRCC tumor should always be considered if these features present in kidney tumor in proper clinical and immunohistochemical setting
  ○ Immunostain for CK7 is often negative, or only very focally positive
  ○ Stains for mucin and ULEX-1 negative

FAMILIAL CANCER SYNDROMES

- Because of papillary features, multinodularity, and desmoplasia, many tumors resemble collecting duct carcinoma
  - Immunostaining patterns, along with nucleolar features, distinguish the tumor from collecting duct carcinoma
- Metastases often present at time of diagnosis; common metastatic sites include
  - Regional lymph nodes
  - Lungs
  - Liver
- Average age at diagnosis of renal tumor was 36 and 46 years in 2 different studies (range: 24-75 years)
- Currently, no specific therapy against metastatic tumors is available
  - Drugs affecting Krebs cycle molecules are being investigated at this stage

Tuberous Sclerosis Syndrome

- Autosomal dominant syndrome, characterized by tumors or tumor-like lesions in multiple sites, including
  - Lymphangioleiomyomatosis of lung
  - Clear cell "sugar" tumors of lung, pancreas, and uterus
  - PEComas of other viscera and soft tissues
  - Cardiac rhabdomyomas
  - Subependymomas and giant cell astrocytomas
  - Retinal hamartomas
  - Angiomyolipomas of kidney and other organs
- Associated with inactivating mutations in tumor suppressor genes, tuberous sclerosis complex (*TSC1* and *TSC2*)
  - *TSC1* localized to chromosome 9q34, and *TSC2* to 16p13.3
  - Prevalence of mutations in *TSC1* and *TSC2* are roughly equal
    - In sporadic angiomyolipomas, mutations in *TSC2* more frequent
  - Proteins encoded by *TSC1* (hamartin) and *TSC2* genes (tuberin) function as complex to negatively regulate mTOR signaling
  - Negative regulation done through activation of Ras homologue expressed in brain (*Rheb*)
    - *Rheb*-specific GTPase is located downstream of tuberin
    - Altered *TSC* gene functions generate excessive Rheb-GTP
    - This leads to increased activated mTOR, activator of multiple protein synthesis pathways and possible tumorigenesis
  - Activated mTOR pathway markers overexpressed in AML and related tumors
- Approximately 70% of all patients diagnosed with tuberous sclerosis have new, spontaneous mutations
  - Such patients will lack family history
- Most common renal manifestation is angiomyolipoma (AML)
  - In contrast to sporadic AMLs, patients with TS have multiple, bilateral lesions
    - Many of these lesions are small and detected only in surgical specimens
  - Involvement of multiple organs is common

- AMLs often show typical triphasic histology
  - However, any variant histology, as seen in sporadic tumors, may be present
  - Some believe that epithelioid AMLs are more likely to occur in TS than in sporadic settings
  - However, many recent studies do not confirm this hypothesis
  - Rare cases of epithelioid AMLs and malignant perivascular epithelioid cell (PEC)omas with metastatic disease have been described
- Multifocality, bilaterality, and involvement of other organs often present
  - Multiple, bilateral tumors and multiple organ involvement are hallmark of tuberous sclerosis
- Other reported tumors include
  - Clear cell RCC
  - RCCs with unusual histology including
    - High-grade tumors with clear cell cytology and prominent papillary architecture
    - Tumors with variable architecture, but high-grade pleomorphic nuclei and prominent eosinophilic cytoplasm
- Renal cysts, usually lined by large atypical cells with prominent eosinophilic cytoplasm, also common
- For metastatic malignant AMLs, no specific therapeutic options available until recently
- Currently, randomized control trials of mTOR inhibitors for treatment of renal, lung, and brain manifestations of *TSC1* and *TSC2* in progress
  - Rare responses to mTOR inhibitors reported in malignant PEComas

Other Rare Familial Tumor Syndromes

- **Hyperparathyroidism-jaw tumor syndrome**
  - Characterized by
    - Hyperparathyroidism and parathyroid tumors
    - Fibroosseous tumors of jaw
  - Renal lesions include
    - Renal cysts
    - Hamartomas
    - Renal cell carcinomas
    - Wilms tumors
  - Mutations involve *HRPT2* gene located at 1q21-32
    - Gene encodes for parafibromin protein
    - Parafibromin normally interacts with PAF1 and RNA polymerase II, both critical mediators of transcription elongation
- **Familial oncocytoma syndrome**
  - Many of these are now known to belong to Birt-Hogg-Dubé (BHD) syndrome families
- Constitutional chromosome 3 translocations syndrome
  - Diagnostic criteria for syndromic renal tumors require presence of RCC in member of family with constitutional chromosome 3 translocation
  - Tumors are often multifocal and bilateral
    - Histologically, tumors are clear cell renal cell carcinomas
  - Association with other systemic manifestations not identified to date
  - Multiple breakpoints and defined translocations reported

FAMILIAL CANCER SYNDROMES

Genetic and Pathological Features in Hereditary Renal Tumor Syndromes

Syndrome	Gene Involved	Gene Product	Pathways Involved	Renal Tumors	Other Associations
von Hippel-Lindau	*VHL* (3p25)	pVHL	Hypoxia-inducible factor (HIF)	Clear cell renal cell carcinoma	Renal cysts, CNS and retinal hemangioblastoma, pheochromocytoma, pancreatic cysts/endocrine pancreatic tumors
Hereditary papillary renal carcinoma	*c-MET* (7q31)	MET tyrosine kinase	MET/hepatocyte growth factor	Papillary renal cell carcinoma, type 1	None
Birt-Hogg-Dubé	*BHD* (17p12)	Folliculin	Mammalian target of rapamycin (mTOR)	Oncocytic tumors (hybrid, chromophobe, oncocytoma), other renal cell carcinomas	Cutaneous lesions, lung cysts, pneumothorax, colonic neoplasms, lipomas
Hereditary leiomyomatosis and renal cell cancer	Fumarate hydratase (1q42.3-q43)	Fumarate hydratase	HIF	High-grade carcinomas with papillary, tubular, solid architecture	Leiomyomas of skin and uterus
Tuberous sclerosis	Tuberous sclerosis complex *(TSC)1* (9q34) and *2* (16p13.3)	Hamartin and tuberin	mTOR	Angiomyolipomas, renal cell carcinoma	Lymphangioleiomyomatosis of lung, clear cell "sugar" tumors of lung, pancreas, and uterus, PEComas of other viscera and soft tissues, subependymomas, and giant cell astrocytomas

- These breakpoints and translocations involve both short and long arms of chromosome 3
- **Familial papillary thyroid carcinoma–papillary renal neoplasia**
  - Link between papillary RCC and germline genetic abnormalities related to familial papillary thyroid carcinoma suspected
    - However, link is not confirmed yet

Familial Pediatric Renal Tumor Syndromes

- WAGR syndrome, characterized by
  - **W**ilms tumor, **A**niridia, **G**enitourinary malformations, mental **R**etardation
- Denys-Drash syndrome, characterized by
  - Wilms tumor, mesangial sclerosis, pseudohermaphroditism
- Beckwith-Wiedemann syndrome, characterized by
  - Wilms tumor, hemihypertrophy, macroglossia, omphalocele, visceromegaly
- Familial nephroblastoma
- Trisomy 18, Perlman syndrome, Bloom syndrome, Frasier syndrome, Klippel-Trenaunay syndrome

SELECTED REFERENCES

1. Linehan WM et al: Hereditary kidney cancer: unique opportunity for disease-based therapy. Cancer. 115(10 Suppl):2252-61, 2009
2. Sampson JR: Therapeutic targeting of mTOR in tuberous sclerosis. Biochem Soc Trans. 37(Pt 1):259-64, 2009
3. Hansel DE et al: Molecular genetics of hereditary renal cancer: new genes and diagnostic and therapeutic opportunities. Expert Rev Anticancer Ther. 8(6):895-905, 2008
4. Stewart L et al: Association of germline mutations in the fumarate hydratase gene and uterine fibroids in women with hereditary leiomyomatosis and renal cell cancer. Arch Dermatol. 144(12):1584-92, 2008
5. Tickoo SK et al: Pathologic features of renal cortical tumors. Urol Clin North Am. 35(4):551-61; v, 2008
6. Merino MJ et al: The morphologic spectrum of kidney tumors in hereditary leiomyomatosis and renal cell carcinoma (HLRCC) syndrome. Am J Surg Pathol. 31(10):1578-85, 2007
7. Toro JR et al: Lung cysts, spontaneous pneumothorax, and genetic associations in 89 families with Birt-Hogg-Dubé syndrome. Am J Respir Crit Care Med. 175(10):1044-53, 2007
8. Sudarshan S et al: Genetic basis of cancer of the kidney. Semin Oncol. 33(5):544-51, 2006
9. Cohen D et al: Molecular genetics of familial renal cell carcinoma syndromes. Clin Lab Med. 25(2):259-77, 2005
10. Dharmawardana PG et al: Hereditary papillary renal carcinoma type I. Curr Mol Med. 4(8):855-68, 2004
11. Khoo SK et al: Inactivation of BHD in sporadic renal tumors. Cancer Res. 63(15):4583-7, 2003
12. Truong LD et al: Renal cystic neoplasms and renal neoplasms associated with cystic renal diseases: pathogenetic and molecular links. Adv Anat Pathol. 10(3):135-59, 2003
13. Pavlovich CP et al: Renal tumors in the Birt-Hogg-Dubé syndrome. Am J Surg Pathol. 26(12):1542-52, 2002
14. Takahashi M et al: Familial adult renal neoplasia. J Med Genet. 39(1):1-5, 2002
15. Herring JC et al: Parenchymal sparing surgery in patients with hereditary renal cell carcinoma: 10-year experience. J Urol. 165(3):777-81, 2001
16. Lindor NM et al: Papillary renal cell carcinoma: analysis of germline mutations in the MET proto-oncogene in a clinic-based population. Genet Test. 5(2):101-6, 2001
17. Poston CD et al: Characterization of the renal pathology of a familial form of renal cell carcinoma associated with von Hippel-Lindau disease: clinical and molecular genetic implications. J Urol. 153(1):22-6, 1995
18. Zbar B et al: Hereditary papillary renal cell carcinoma: clinical studies in 10 families. J Urol. 153(3 Pt 2):907-12, 1995

FAMILIAL CANCER SYNDROMES

Microscopic and Gross Features

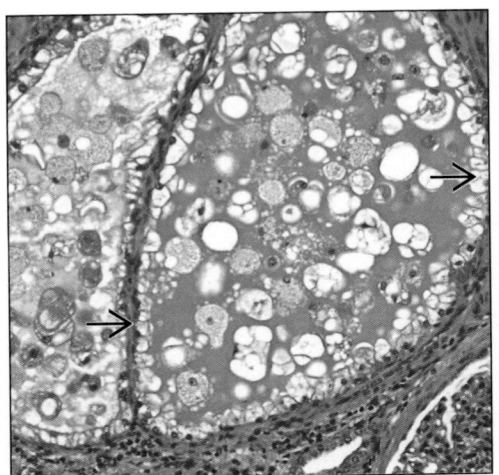
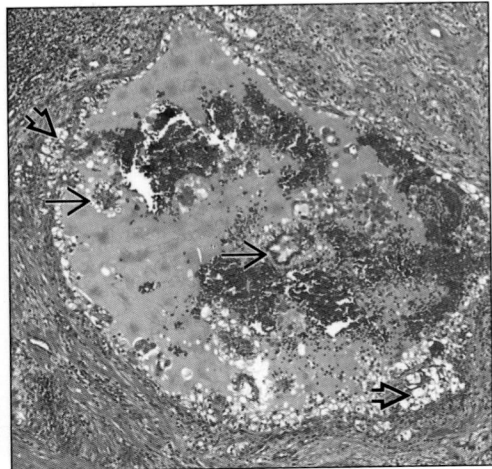

(Left) Multiple, but usually not numerous, cysts are also present in VHL kidneys. These are often lined entirely by cells with clear cytoplasm ➡. Cysts with a single layer of lining cells are termed "benign" cysts in such kidneys. *(Right)* Cysts that have mildly proliferative lining (up to 3 layers thick) ⮊ are regarded as "atypical" cysts in VHL, irrespective of cytologic atypia. Focal papillations ➡ may be seen in such cysts. The average number of cysts in VHL kidneys is 8.

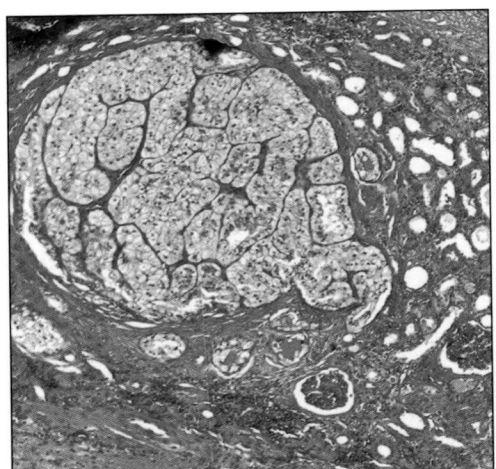
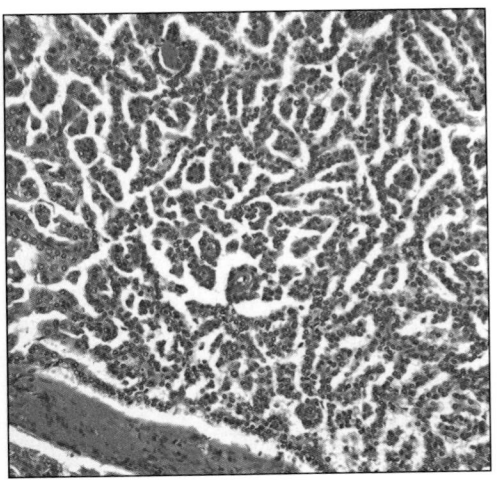

(Left) This H&E image of a VHL kidney shows a microscopic clear cell renal cell carcinoma that appears well circumscribed. *(Right)* In hereditary papillary renal carcinoma syndrome, numerous type 1 papillary RCCs are seen in the kidney. They are morphologically and immunohistochemically similar to those seen in sporadic settings. The carcinomas in HPRC usually manifest later in life (> 50 years of age), although rarely they may be appear earlier in some families.

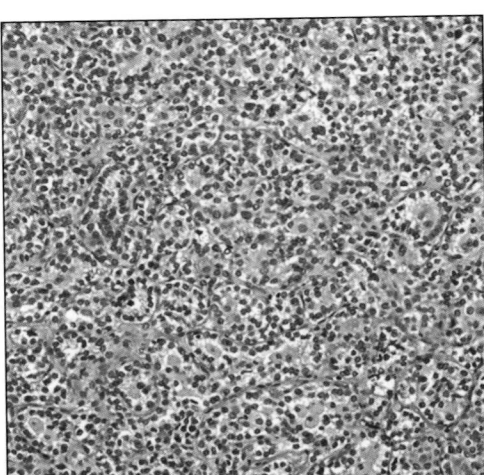
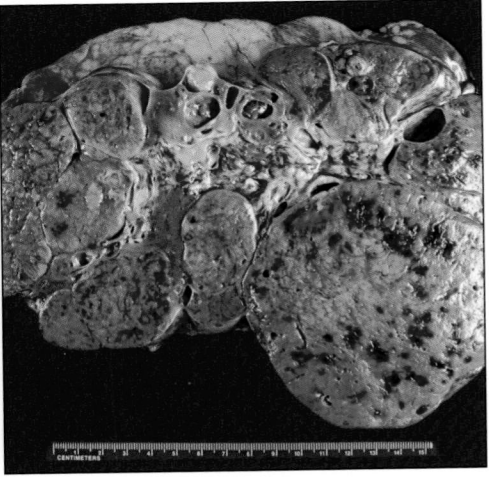

(Left) The papillary RCCs in HPRC syndrome have either papillary or tubulo-papillary architecture. Foamy macrophages are also common, similar to that in nonfamilial type 1 tumors. *(Right)* The cut surface of a nephrectomy specimen from a case of Birt-Hogg-Dubé (BHD) syndrome shows the renal parenchyma studded with multiple solid tumors. The tumors have a yellow-brown appearance, indicative of an oncocytic cells component.

FAMILIAL CANCER SYNDROMES

Microscopic Features

(Left) *This whole-mount image from a BHD kidney shows 3 different tumor types. The largest ⇒ is an oncocytic tumor, the smaller ➡ with papillary features, and the smallest ⇒ with clear cell features. Combination of different tumor subtypes is not uncommon in BHD.* **(Right)** *The most common tumor in BHD shows hybrid features of renal oncocytoma and chromophobe RCC. A typical and common feature in oncocytic tumors is the focal presence of cells with cytoplasmic clearing ➡.*

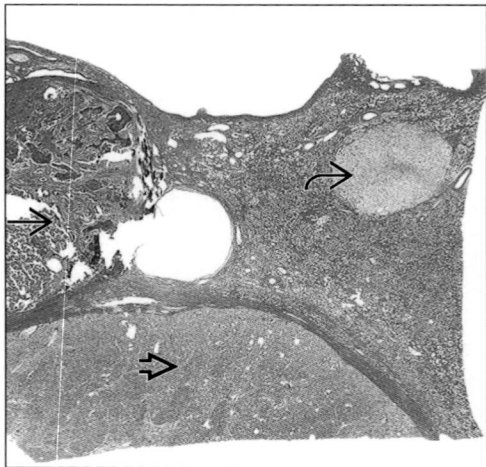
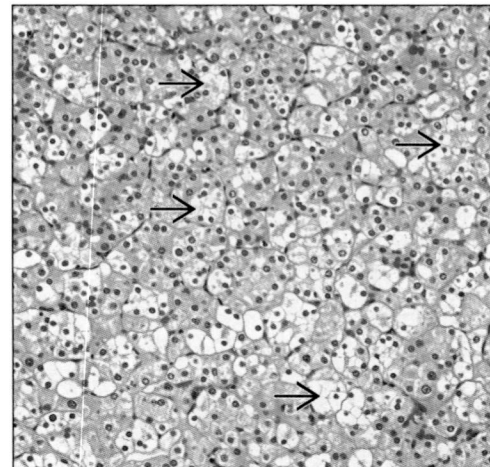

(Left) *The kidneys in BHD syndrome often show background oncocytosis. Numerous microscopic oncocytic nodules ⇒, oncocytic cysts, and oncocytic tubules percolating between the residual nephrons are often present in these kidneys.* **(Right)** *This photomicrograph from the kidney in a case of BHD syndrome shows sheets of oncocytic cells present between nonneoplastic tubules ➡. The presence of oncocytosis in a nephrectomy specimen should always raise the suspicion of BHD syndrome.*

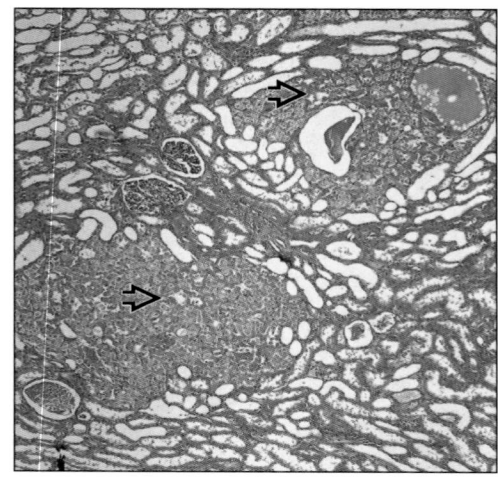
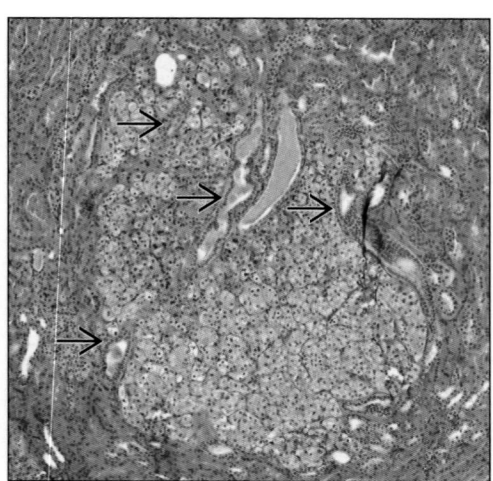

(Left) *The renal tumors in hereditary leiomyomatosis and renal cell cancer syndrome often show variable papillary architecture. However, other architectural patterns, including tubular, solid, cystic and solid alveolar, are often admixed. These tumors were considered as papillary RCC, type 2 in the past.* **(Right)** *In HLRCC, the tumor is almost entirely composed of cells with eosinophilic cytoplasm. Occasionally, focal cytoplasmic clarity ➡ may be also present.*

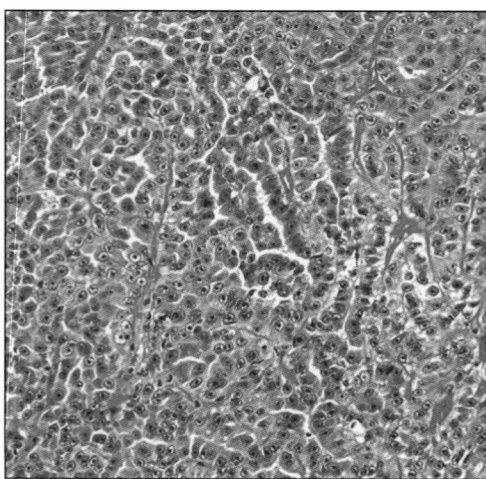
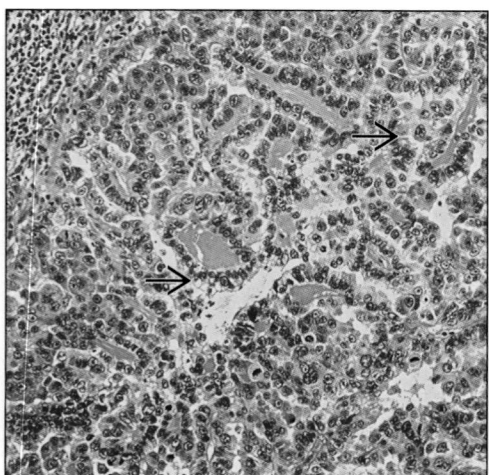

FAMILIAL CANCER SYNDROMES

Microscopic Features

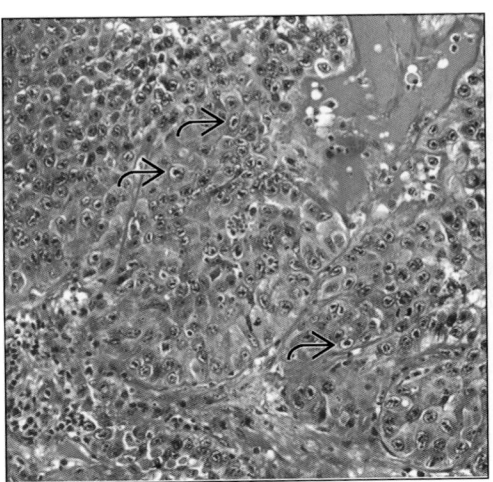
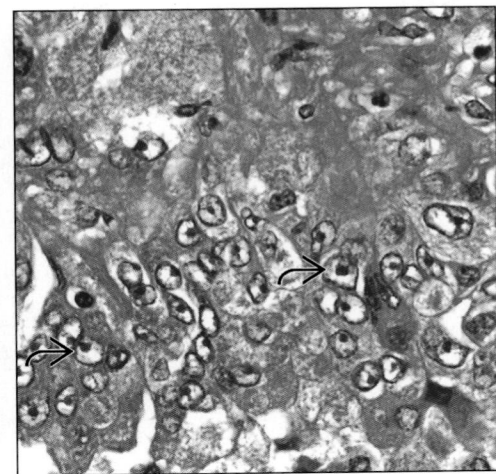

(Left) The most characteristic feature of the HLRCC tumor is presence of large nuclei with very prominent orangeophilic or eosinophilic nucleoli, surrounded by a clear halo ➔. *(Right)* Large nuclei with prominent nucleoli, surrounded by clear halos ➔ are somewhat reminiscent of a Cytomegalovirus inclusion in HLRCC renal cancers. Such nuclear features in a renal tumor with mixed papillary and other architectures should always raise the possibility of HLRCC syndrome.

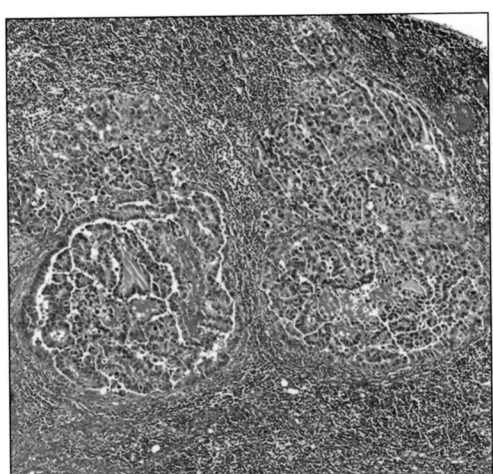
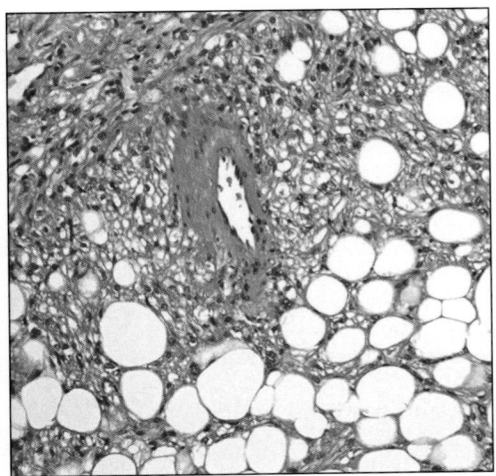

(Left) This image shows a metastatic HLRCC carcinoma in a lymph node. The carcinomas in HLRCC show aggressive morphologic features, and patients often present with metastatic disease. Unlike other familial tumors, bilateral tumors have not yet been described in HLRCC. *(Right)* Angiomyolipoma (AML) in tuberous sclerosis syndrome shows the typical triphasic morphology. Tumors are often multifocal and bilateral. The cell of origin is believed to be the epithelioid perivascular cell.

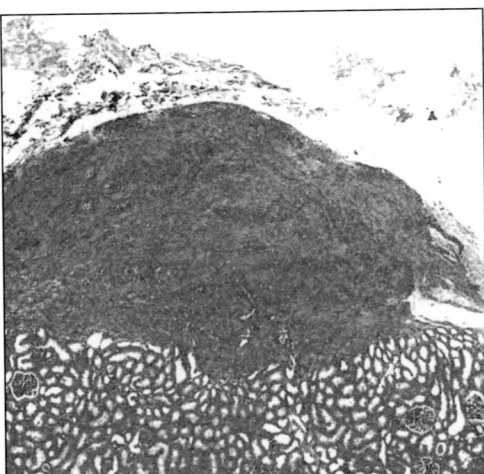
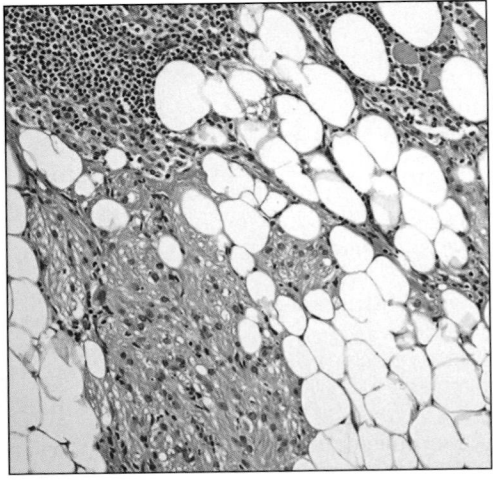

(Left) This leiomyomatous AML from a case of tuberous sclerosis (TS) syndrome is arising from the renal capsule ("capsuloma"). All morphologic variants of the tumor may be seen in TS. Some believe that epithelioid AMLs are more likely to arise in TS, but other studies do not substantiate this. *(Right)* Hematoxylin & eosin shows AML involving a lymph node. Multifocality and involvement of multiple organs by AMLs is a hallmark of tuberous sclerosis syndrome and by itself not indicative of malignancy.

XANTHOGRANULOMATOUS PYELONEPHRITIS/RENAL MALAKOPLAKIA

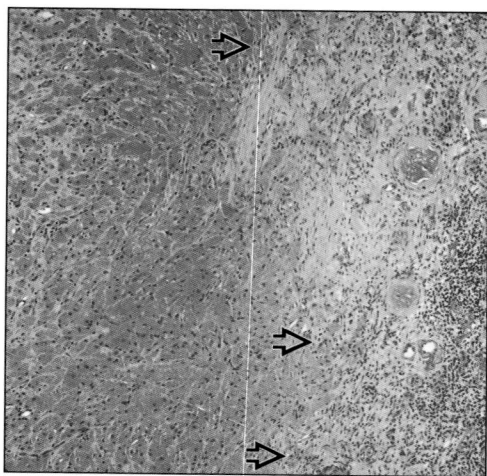

Periodic acid-Schiff stained section shows the irregular outline ⊳ of sheets of histiocytes without any capsule or circumscription in a case of mass-forming xanthogranulomatous pyelonephritis.

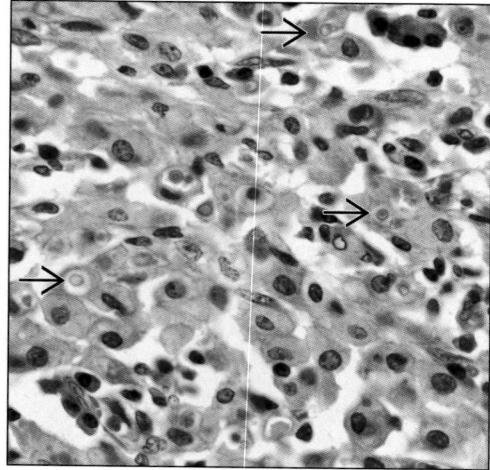

Hematoxylin & eosin stained section shows the typical features of renal malakoplakia. Sheets of histiocytes are seen, many containing the characteristic Michaelis-Gutmann bodies →.

TERMINOLOGY

Abbreviations

- Xanthogranulomatous pyelonephritis (XGP)
- Renal malakoplakia (RMP)

Definitions

- XGP: Subacute and chronic pelvicalyceal and renal parenchymal inflammatory mass-like lesion predominantly composed of histiocytes
- RMP: Renal inflammatory mass-like lesion showing histiocytes with abundant eosinophilic cytoplasm and containing Michaelis-Gutmann bodies
  - Term derived from Greek words malakos (soft) and plakos (plaque)
- XGP and RMP morphologically, and possibly causally, closely related

ETIOLOGY/PATHOGENESIS

Infectious Agents

- Gram-negative bacteria are most often associated with both disorders
  - *Escherichia coli* is found in most cases
  - *Proteus*, *Klebsiella*, and *Pseudomonas* other less common pathogens
  - Very occasional cases associated with *Mycobacterium tuberculosis*, *Shigella*, *Paracoccidioides*, *Rhodococcus*, *Yersinia enterocolitica*, *Staphylococcus aureus*, and *Enterobacter*
- XGP: Consistently associated with obstruction, calculi, and recurrent urinary tract infections
- RMP: Believed to be due to defective macrophage lysosomal digestion of phagocytosed bacteria (particularly coliforms)
- Decreased levels of intracellular cyclic guanosine monophosphate (cGMP) might be cause of defective phagocytosis in RMP
  - Inadequate elimination leads to accumulation of partially digested bacteria/bacterial glycolipids
  - Deposition of calcium and iron occurs on residual bacterial glycolipid in monocytes or macrophages, forming Michaelis-Gutmann bodies
- Patients with XGP usually have underlying systemic disease
  - e.g., systemic lupus erythematosus, diabetes mellitus, myotonic dystrophy, or chronic active hepatitis

CLINICAL ISSUES

Epidemiology

- Incidence
  - XGP present in approximately 20% of specimens in which nephrectomy is performed for chronic pyelonephritic renal disease
  - RMP very uncommon; mostly as case reports
- Age
  - Typically, patients are in their 40s or 50s
    - Both entities have been described in children and in older people (range: 4 weeks to 84 years)
- Gender
  - Both XGP and RMP affect females more than males

Presentation

- Most patients are symptomatic
  - Common presenting symptoms include fever, flank or abdominal pain, anorexia, weight loss, lower urinary tract symptoms, and gross hematuria
  - Other rare presentations of RMP
    - Acute renal failure with bilateral disease
    - End-stage renal disease
    - Unilateral diffuse renal enlargement

Treatment

- Most patients receive antibiotics before nephrectomy

XANTHOGRANULOMATOUS PYELONEPHRITIS/RENAL MALAKOPLAKIA

Key Facts

Terminology
- Xanthogranulomatous pyelonephritis (XGP), renal malakoplakia (RMP)
- XGP: Subacute and chronic pelvicalyceal and renal parenchymal inflammatory mass-like lesion predominantly composed of histiocytes
- RMP: Renal inflammatory mass-like lesion showing histiocytes with abundant eosinophilic cytoplasm and containing Michaelis-Gutmann bodies
- XGP and RMP morphologically and possibly causally closely related

Etiology/Pathogenesis
- Gram-negative bacteria are most often associated with both disorders
- XGP, consistently associated with obstruction, calculi, and recurrent urinary tract infections

- RMP believed to be due to defective macrophage lysosomal digestion of phagocytosed bacteria (particularly coliforms)

Clinical Issues
- Both XGP and RMP affect more females than males

Microscopic Pathology
- XGP: Aggregates of foamy histiocytes forming small clusters below urothelium to large, destructive, nodular lesions
- RMP: Dominant feature is aggregates of histiocytes with eosinophilic cytoplasm (von Hansemann histiocytes)
- Some histiocytes contain targetoid, calcific, basophilic inclusions (Michaelis-Gutmann bodies)
  - Most characteristic feature of RMP

- Improving immunodeficient states and use of bethanechol chloride (urecholine) are medical treatment options for RMP
  - Urecholine: Cholinergic agonist that improves bactericidal activity of monocytes against *E. coli*
- Disease often only diagnosed in nephrectomy specimens in both XGP and RMP
  - Partial nephrectomy may be option for segmental XGP and localized RMP, if diagnosed before surgery

Prognosis
- If unilateral or localized, usually cured by surgery
  - But, primary cause of urinary tract obstruction may need to be addressed in XGP
- Immunodeficient state in RMP needs to be improved to prevent recurrences in genitourinary or other organ systems

MACROSCOPIC FEATURES

General Features
- Changes may be diffuse, segmental, or focal
- Pelvicalyceal system is usually outlined by thick bands of often friable, partially necrotic yellow tissue
- Irregular yellow masses, usually centered on renal medulla
  - Masses are ill defined and at least partly necrotic
- Hydronephrosis or pyonephrosis is common accompanying feature
- Renal calculi, often staghorn type, very frequently associated, particularly in XGP

MICROSCOPIC PATHOLOGY

Histologic Features
- Xanthomatous pyelonephritis
  - Foamy histiocytes with abundant clear cytoplasm as small clusters below urothelium to large, destructive, nodular lesions
    - Lesions may involve pelvicalyceal tissues with secondary involvement of renal parenchyma

- Histiocytes with eosinophilic cytoplasm may be present but usually not prominent finding
  - Admixed polymorphous inflammation with presence of lymphocytes, plasma cells, and neutrophils
    - Microabscesses almost always present
  - Variable number of multinucleated histiocytic giant cells often observed
  - Background of chronic pyelonephritis, characterized by
    - Often patchy or segmental, renal tubular atrophy, fibrosis, chronic inflammation, and tubular dilatation
  - Extension of process to ureter &/or perirenal fat is commonly present
- Malakoplakia
  - Dominant feature is aggregates of histiocytes with eosinophilic cytoplasm (von Hansemann histiocytes)
    - Cytoplasm often PAS(+)
  - Some histiocytes contain concentrically lamellar or targetoid, basophilic, often calcified inclusions (Michaelis-Gutmann bodies)
    - Usually equal to size of surrounding nuclei
    - Michaelis-Gutmann bodies are most characteristic feature of RMP
  - Often accompanied by mixed inflammatory infiltrate, including lymphocytes, plasma cells, and neutrophils
  - Variable number of multinucleated histiocytic giant cells frequently observed
  - Prussian blue (iron), PAS, and von Kossa stains may be needed to visualize Michaelis-Gutmann bodies, when rare
  - Microscopically, malakoplakia evolves through 3 phases
  - Early (prediagnostic) phase
    - Characterized by plasma cells and von Hansemann histiocytes in edematous stroma, with absent Michaelis-Gutmann bodies
  - Classic phase

XANTHOGRANULOMATOUS PYELONEPHRITIS/RENAL MALAKOPLAKIA

- Shows histiocytes containing easily identifiable Michaelis-Gutmann bodies and few lymphocytes and plasma cells
  - Fibrosing phase
    - Shows fibroblasts and collagen interspersed between foci of histiocytes, with occasional Michaelis-Gutmann bodies
- Both XGP and RMP are often destructive, and associated with variable degrees of fibrosis
- Both lesions usually are multifocal, with irregular outlines, without pseudocapsule

Predominant Pattern/Injury Type
- Inflammatory

Predominant Cell/Compartment Type
- Histiocyte/macrophage

Ultrastructure
- Bacilliform microorganisms, either intact or in different stages of disintegration within phagolysosomes in macrophages in RMP

DIFFERENTIAL DIAGNOSIS

Clear Cell Renal Cell Carcinoma
- Cells arranged in nests, alveoli, tubules, and cysts
- Presence of brisk inflammatory infiltrate intimately admixed with sheets of clear cells should raise possibility of XGP over renal cell carcinoma
  - Inflammatory infiltrate in renal cell carcinoma tends to be absent or focal
  - If and when inflammation is prominent, it usually extends between nests and alveoli
- Intricate, branching vascular septations surrounding groups of cells
- Nuclei are round or oval, or with nuclear membrane irregularities in carcinoma
  - Chromatin usually dark and granular
- In XGP and RMP, nuclear chromatin is usually pale (as is usual for histiocytes)
  - In addition, nuclear membranes often show angulations
- Immunohistochemistry rarely required but is invariably decisive in differentiation
  - Cytokeratins and EMA/MUC1 positive in carcinoma
  - Histiocytic markers positive in XGP and RMP

DIAGNOSTIC CHECKLIST

Pathologic Interpretation Pearls
- XGP and RMP are pseudotumorous lesions that closely mimic malignancy clinically, radiographically, and pathologically
- Main differential diagnostic consideration for XGP is clear cell RCC with associated extensive inflammation
- Carcinoma with clear cell cytology is usually of lower grade
  - Typical intricately branching vasculature is particularly prominent in such lower grade tumors

SELECTED REFERENCES

1. Guzzo TJ et al: Xanthogranulomatous pyelonephritis: presentation and management in the era of laparoscopy. BJU Int. Epub ahead of print, 2009
2. Hussein N et al: Xanthogranulomatous pyelonephritis in pediatric patients: effect of surgical approach. Urology. 73(6):1247-50, 2009
3. Ho CI et al: Xanthogranulomatous pyelonephritis successfully treated with antibiotics only. J Chin Med Assoc. 71(12):643-5, 2008
4. Joshi AA et al: Laparoscopic nephrectomy for xanthogranulomatous pyelonephritis in childhood: the way forward. J Pediatr Urol. 4(3):203-5, 2008
5. Korkes F et al: Xanthogranulomatous pyelonephritis: clinical experience with 41 cases. Urology. 71(2):178-80, 2008
6. Bartoli F et al: Xanthogranulomatous pyelonephritis is associated with higher tissue expression of monocyte chemotactic protein-1. Eur J Pediatr Surg. 17(5):365-9, 2007
7. Yiğiter M et al: Renal parenchymal malacoplakia: a different stage of xanthogranulomatous pyelonephritis? J Pediatr Surg. 42(7):E35-8, 2007
8. Zugor V et al: Xanthogranulomatous pyelonephritis in childhood: a critical analysis of 10 cases and of the literature. Urology. 70(1):157-60, 2007
9. Hegde S et al: End stage renal disease due to bilateral renal malakoplakia. Arch Dis Child. 89(1):78-9, 2004
10. Kajbafzadeh A et al: Renal malakoplakia simulating neoplasm in a child: successful medical management. Urol J. 1(3):218-20, 2004
11. Tam VK et al: Renal parenchymal malacoplakia: a rare cause of ARF with a review of recent literature. Am J Kidney Dis. 41(6):E13-7, 2003
12. Tamboli P et al: Benign tumors and tumor-like lesions of the adult kidney. Part II: Benign mesenchymal and mixed neoplasms, and tumor-like lesions. Adv Anat Pathol. 7(1):47-66, 2000
13. Zia-ul-Miraj M et al: Xanthogranulomatous pyelonephritis presenting as a pseudotumor in a 2-month-old boy. J Pediatr Surg. 35(8):1256-8, 2000
14. Gregg CR et al: Xanthogranulomatous pyelonephritis. Curr Clin Top Infect Dis. 19:287-304, 1999
15. Evans NL et al: Renal malacoplakia: an important consideration in the differential diagnosis of renal masses in the presence of Escherichia coli infection. Br J Radiol. 71(850):1083-5, 1998
16. Marteinsson VT et al: Focal xanthogranulomatous pyelonephritis presenting as renal tumour in children. Case report with a review of the literature. Scand J Urol Nephrol. 30(3):235-9, 1996
17. August C et al: Renal parenchymal malakoplakia: ultrastructural findings in different stages of morphogenesis. Ultrastruct Pathol. 18(5):483-91, 1994
18. Levy M et al: Xanthogranulomatous pyelonephritis in children. Etiology, pathogenesis, clinical and radiologic features, and management. Clin Pediatr (Phila). 33(6):360-6, 1994
19. Dobyan DC et al: Renal malacoplakia reappraised. Am J Kidney Dis. 22(2):243-52, 1993
20. Mittal BV et al: Xanthogranulomatous pyelonephritis-- (a clinicopathological study of 15 cases). J Postgrad Med. 35(4):209-14, 1989

XANTHOGRANULOMATOUS PYELONEPHRITIS/RENAL MALAKOPLAKIA

Gross and Microscopic Features

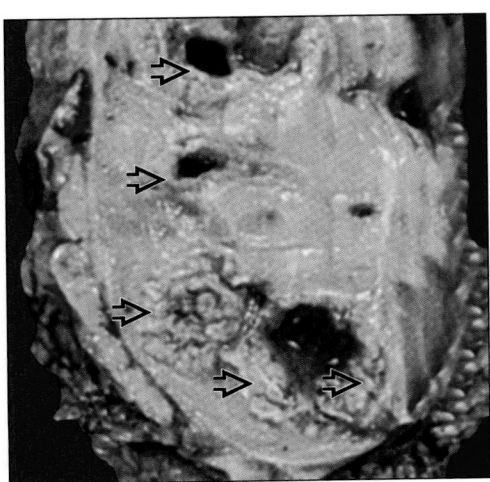
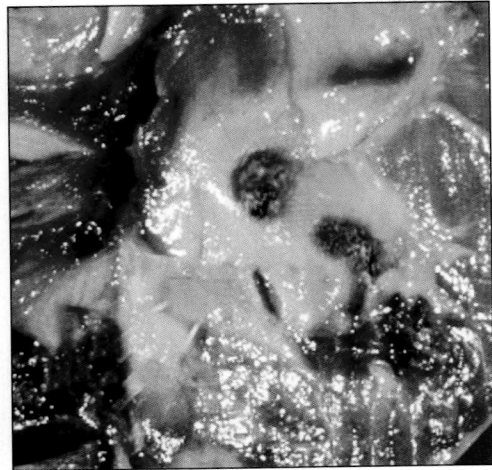

(Left) Gross photograph depicts the characteristic appearance of xanthogranulomatous pyelonephritis. The dilated calyces are surrounded by an irregular band of yellow, necrotic material ➡. The yellow coloration is reflective of lipid-containing (foamy) histiocytes in the lesion. *(Right)* While XGP is usually diffuse, some cases may show only segmental or focal involvement. Such nondiffuse appearance is usually because of the involvement of individual calyces alone.

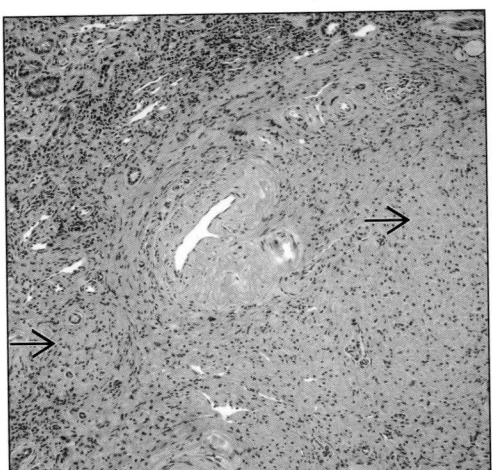
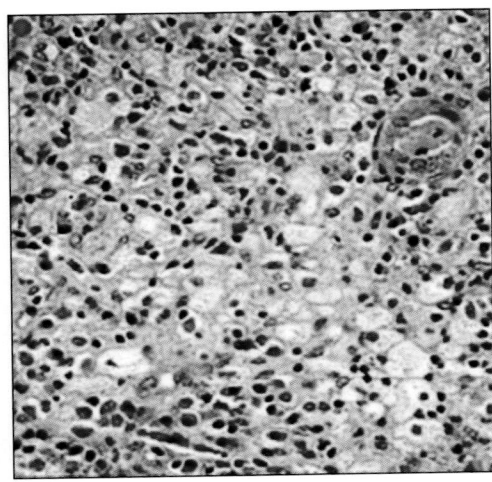

(Left) Hematoxylin & eosin stained section shows a nonencapsulated mass-like lesion. Although it appears circumscribed in this image, multifocal appearance ➡ of the lesions should alert to the possibility of xanthogranulomatous pyelonephritis. *(Right)* This XGP shows morphology that may raise the possibility of a RCC. The intimate admixture of inflammatory cells with the clear cells, as well as histiocytic cytologic features of these clear cells, argues for a nonneoplastic diagnosis.

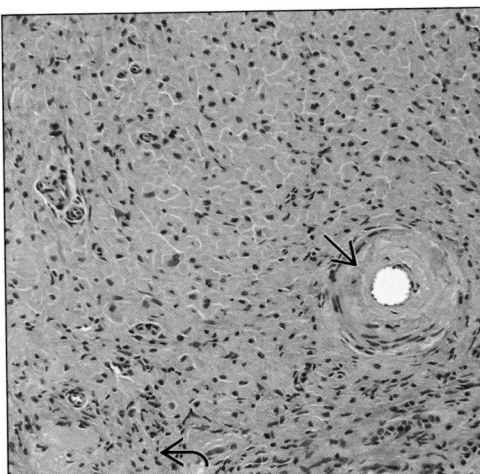
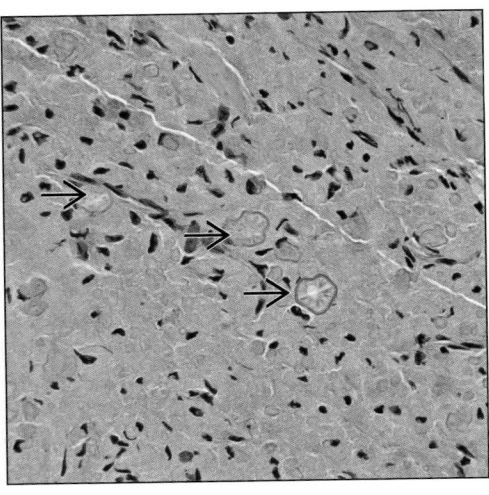

(Left) Sheets of histiocytes devoid of circumscription, with finger-like projections ➡, and entrapped medium-sized arteries ➡ go against the diagnosis of RCC. Close evaluation of cytology reveals absence of distinct epithelial features, pale nuclear chromatin, and angulations of nuclear membranes in XGP. *(Right)* This image of XGP shows a collection of histiocytes with focal calcification ➡. Calcifications suggest a longstanding process and are not specific of either XGP or RMP.

1

XANTHOGRANULOMATOUS PYELONEPHRITIS/RENAL MALAKOPLAKIA

Microscopic Features and Ancillary Techniques

(Left) Most XGP cases show mixed inflammatory infiltrate, including lymphocytes, plasma cells, and neutrophils. Polymorphous inflammatory infiltrate is common in both xanthogranulomatous pyelonephritis and malakoplakia. **(Right)** Periodic acid-Schiff stain shows diffuse positivity in the lesional cells. The histiocytic nuclei usually show uniform pale chromatin, unlike that in carcinoma, which has hyperchromatic and often irregular nuclei.

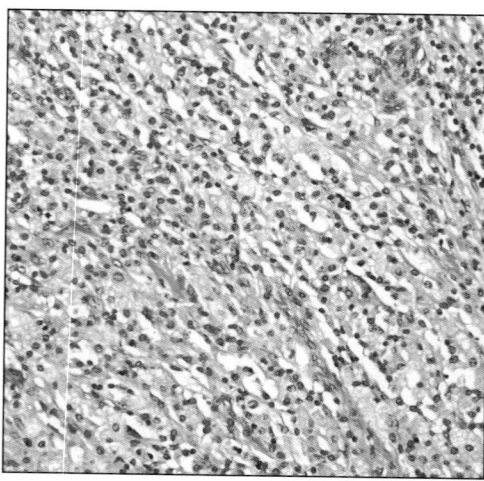
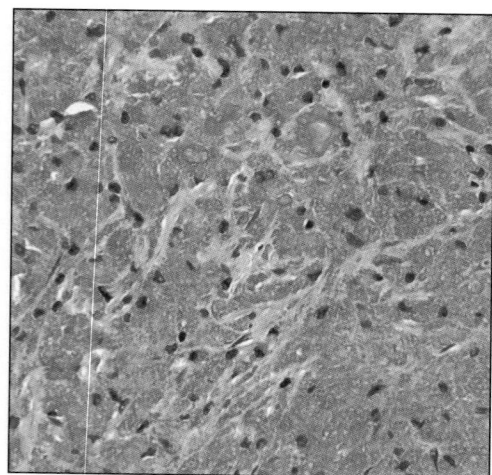

(Left) Periodic acid-Schiff shows a collection of histiocytes in a cortical cyst. The presence of sheets of histiocytes in renal parenchyma is not always diagnostic of XGP or malakoplakia. By definition, the diagnosis requires involvement of the pelvicalyceal system. **(Right)** While the histiocytic nature of the clear cells in XGP is quite apparent on H&E in most cases, sometimes immunohistochemistry may be needed. CD68 ➡ and CD163 histiocytic markers diffusely stain these cells.

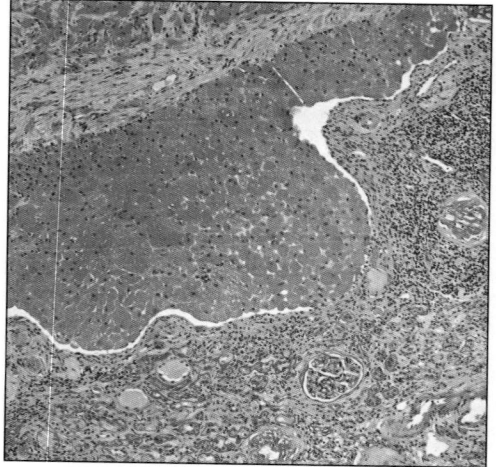
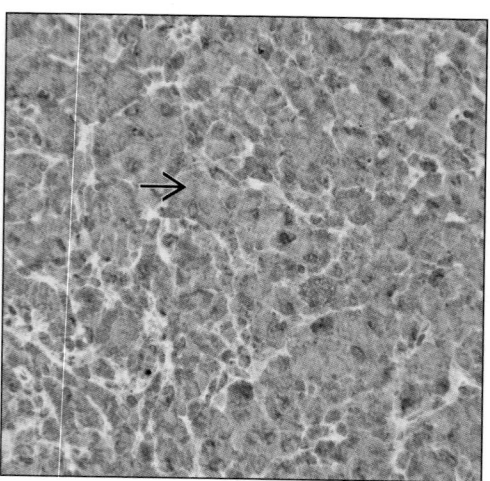

(Left) Low-power view of renal malakoplakia shows that the lesion has its epicenter in the pelvicalyceal system ➡. **(Right)** As seen at higher magnification, the histiocytic proliferation surrounds and invades the urothelial lining ➡ in renal malakoplakia. Both XGP and RMP involve the pelvicalyceal system, the lining of which is usually markedly roughened and irregular on gross evaluation. On microscopic examination, most of the lining appears ulcerated or reactive.

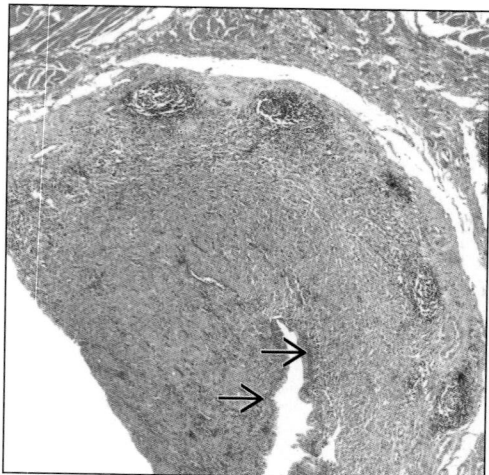
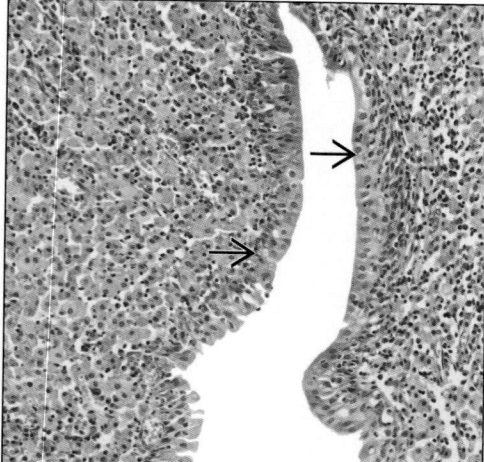

Microscopic Features and Ancillary Techniques

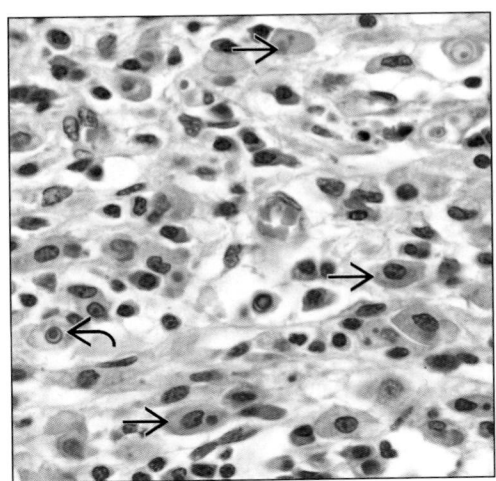

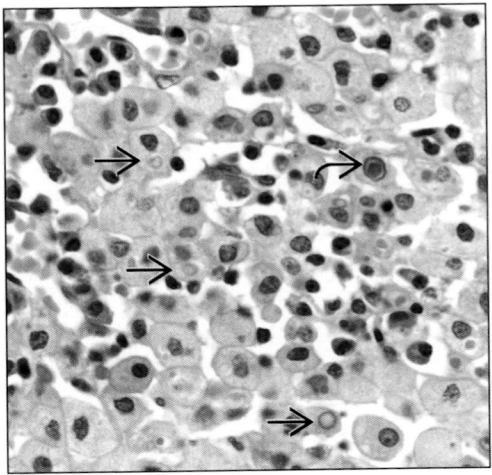

(Left) This image of renal malakoplakia shows the typical morphology of von Hanseman histiocytes. Unlike the foamy, clear macrophages in XGP, the histiocytes in malakoplakia have predominantly eosinophilic cytoplasm ➡. A classical Michaelis-Gutmann body is present in 1 of the histiocytes ➡. (Right) This image of RMP shows multiple Michaelis-Gutmann bodies in the histiocytes ➡. Characteristically, these appear as concentrically lamellar or targetoid, basophilic structures ➡.

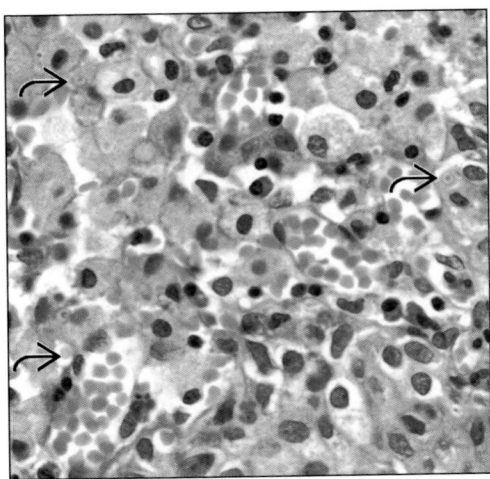

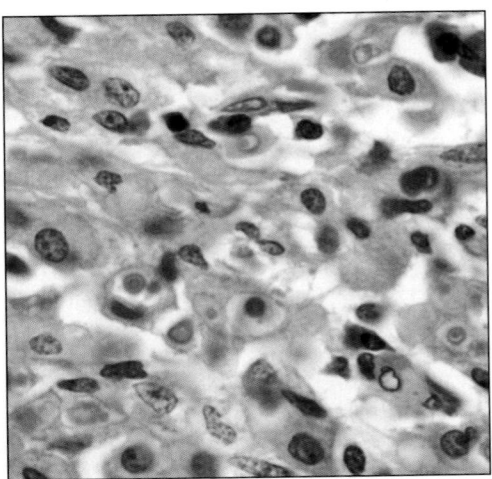

(Left) This image demonstrates the classic phase of malakoplakia. Sheets of histiocytes are admixed with relatively few plasma cells and lymphocytes in this phase. Michaelis-Gutmann bodies are abundant ➡. In the early (pre-diagnostic) phase, Michaelis-Gutmann bodies may be absent or very difficult to find. (Right) A high magnification view of RMP shows the typical nuclear features of histiocytes, including pale chromatin and nuclear membrane irregularities.

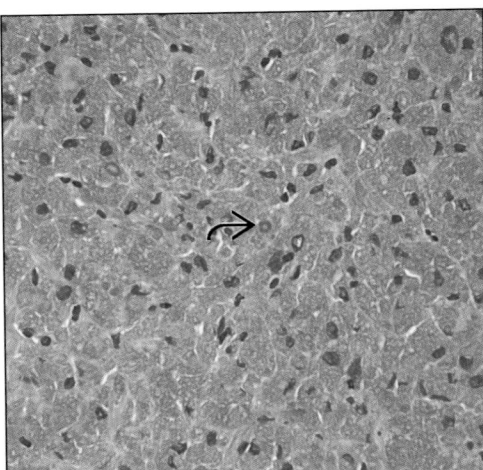

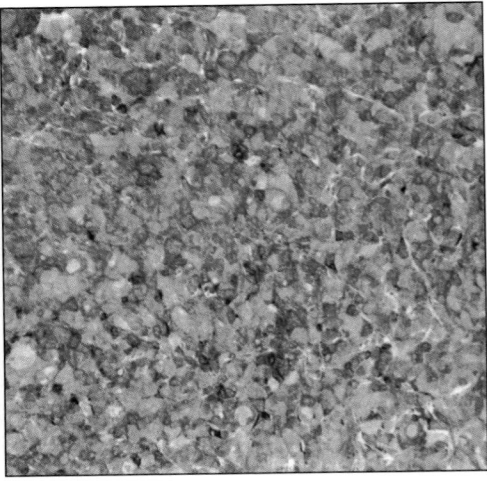

(Left) Periodic acid-Schiff (seen here), von Kossa, or iron stains highlight the Michaelis-Gutmann bodies ➡ and may be needed in cases with paucity of such bodies. Note the diffuse granular cytoplasmic stain in the histiocytes, which may be seen in both XGP and RMP. (Right) As in XGP, CD68 shows diffuse positivity in malakoplakia. Immunohistochemical staining is only rarely needed to make the diagnosis of XGP or RMP in nephrectomy specimens but is often useful in needle biopsies.

PAPILLARY ADENOMA

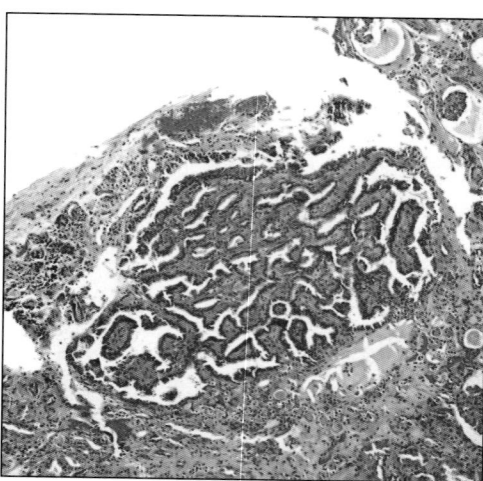

Papillary adenomas show papillary &/or tubular architectural features, similar to that seen in larger papillary renal cell carcinomas. By definition, these are 5 mm or less in maximum diameter.

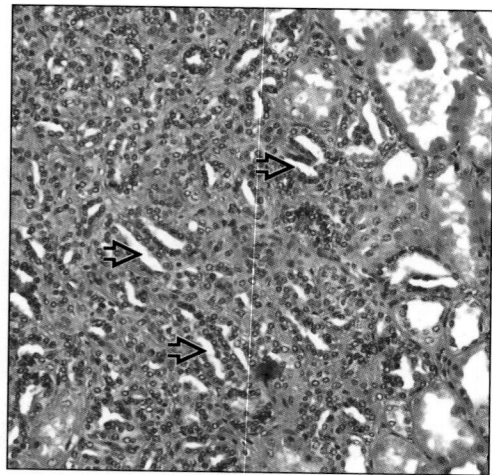

In spite of the nomenclature of "papillary" adenoma, many of these minute tumorous lesions show variable, but sometimes predominant or exclusive, tubular architecture ⊡.

TERMINOLOGY

Synonyms
- Chromophil adenoma, renal cortical adenoma

Definitions
- Small epithelial proliferations with papillary, tubular, or tubulo-papillary configuration; ≤ 5 mm

ETIOLOGY/PATHOGENESIS

Genetic Features
- Trisomy 7 and 17, and loss of Y chromosome very frequently observed
  - Such changes also frequent in papillary RCC
- In addition to gains of chromosomes 7, 17 and loss of Y chromosome, gains of chromosomes 12, 16, and 20 also frequently present
  - Progressive gains of these specific chromosomes do not appear to correlate with transition from adenoma to papillary carcinoma
- Frequent association with papillary RCC has raised the question of adenomas representing intrarenal metastases from papillary RCC
  - Loss of heterozygosity assays on multiple tumors in each kidney have shown discordant allelic loss patterns between tumors
    - Thus, likelihood of adenomas representing intrarenal metastases from papillary RCC is very low

CLINICAL ISSUES

Epidemiology
- Incidence
  - 7-40% in autopsy studies
    - Frequency increases with age (10% < 40 years old vs. 40% > 70 years old)
  - Higher incidence in patients with chronic renal disease, particularly acquired cystic disease of kidney
    - Incidence > 30% in acquired cystic disease of kidney
  - Reported incidence of 7% in nephrectomy specimens resected for other tumors
    - Actual incidence is likely higher because of retrospective nature of study that did not specifically target to find papillary adenomas

Presentation
- Incidental finding in kidneys removed for larger tumors or other causes, and at autopsy
- More often seen in kidneys harboring papillary RCC, compared to other types of renal tumors
  - > 25% of kidneys with papillary RCC also show papillary adenomas
  - Adenomas more likely to be multifocal in kidneys with papillary RCC, compared to other tumor subtypes
- When papillary adenomas bilateral and multifocal (numerous), called "renal adenomatosis"

Treatment
- Surgical approaches
  - Determined by the other presenting lesions (tumor or nontumorous condition)

Prognosis
- Considered to be putative precursor of papillary RCC
  - However, marked differences in incidences of papillary adenomas vs. papillary RCC raises some doubts about this presumption

MACROSCOPIC FEATURES

General Features
- Larger lesions may be apparent grossly
  - Appear as well-circumscribed grayish-white to yellow nodules

PAPILLARY ADENOMA

Key Facts

Terminology
- Small epithelial proliferations with papillary, tubular, or tubulo-papillary configuration; ≤ 5 mm

Etiology/Pathogenesis
- Trisomy 7 and 17, and loss of Y chromosome very frequently observed

Clinical Issues
- Incidence of 7-40% in autopsy studies
- Higher incidence in patients with chronic renal disease, particularly acquired cystic disease of kidney
- Reported incidence of 7% in nephrectomy specimens resected for other tumors
- More often seen in kidneys harboring papillary RCC, compared to other types of renal tumors

Macroscopic Features
- Appear as well-circumscribed grayish-white to yellow nodules
- By definition, all tumors are 5 mm or less in diameter

Microscopic Pathology
- Resembles papillary RCC (usually type 1)
- Have papillary, tubular, or tubulopapillary architecture; usually with low-grade nuclei

Ancillary Tests
- Most are CK7 and AMACR positive; CD10 often shows luminal staining pattern

Top Differential Diagnoses
- Papillary renal cell carcinoma

○ Most are sub-capsular in location in renal cortex

Size
- By definition, all tumors are 5 mm or less in diameter

MICROSCOPIC PATHOLOGY

Histologic Features
- Resembles papillary RCC, usually type 1
- Cytoplasm is often amphophilic/basophilic and scant
  ○ Rare tumors have more abundant eosinophilic cytoplasm
  ○ Rare tumors may have cytoplasmic clarity, similar to that seen in some papillary RCCs
    ■ In such cases, cells are not optically transparent but show fine and scant cytoplasmic granularity
- Have papillary, tubular, or tubulopapillary architecture
- Usually with low-grade nuclei
  ○ Rare tumors may have nuclei with prominent nucleoli
    ■ Because of higher nuclear grade, such tumors may not be regarded papillary adenomas by some
- Foam cells and calcification may be present
- Most tumors do not show a capsule and are in direct contact with surrounding renal parenchyma
  ○ Larger tumors may bear capsules that are usually ill-formed and thin
- Very small examples may consist of only very few neoplastic tubules clustered together
- Lesions with clear cell carcinoma-like features, even if < 5 mm, are not considered adenomas

Predominant Cell/Compartment Type
- Epithelial

ANCILLARY TESTS

Immunohistochemistry
- Similar to papillary RCC
  ○ Most are CK7 and AMACR positive

○ CD10 often shows luminal or inverted cup-like staining pattern

DIFFERENTIAL DIAGNOSIS

Papillary Renal Cell Carcinoma
- Size is sole definitive distinguishing criterion
  ○ Additionally, papillary RCC, unlike most papillary adenomas, usually have well-formed pseudocapsule

DIAGNOSTIC CHECKLIST

Pathologic Interpretation Pearls
- By definition (WHO), upper limit of size acceptable in papillary adenomas is 5 mm
  ○ However, metastatic potential for lesions measuring even up to 1 cm and containing low-grade nuclei is also virtually nonexistent

SELECTED REFERENCES

1. Wang KL et al: Renal papillary adenoma--a putative precursor of papillary renal cell carcinoma. Hum Pathol. 38(2):239-46, 2007
2. Jones TD et al: Molecular genetic evidence for the independent origin of multifocal papillary tumors in patients with papillary renal cell carcinomas. Clin Cancer Res. 11(20):7226-33, 2005
3. Kiyoshima K et al: Multicentric papillary renal cell carcinoma associated with renal adenomatosis. Pathol Int. 54(4):266-72, 2004
4. Brunelli M et al: Gains of chromosomes 7, 17, 12, 16, and 20 and loss of Y occur early in the evolution of papillary renal cell neoplasia: a fluorescent in situ hybridization study. Mod Pathol. 16(10):1053-9, 2003
5. Grignon DJ et al: Papillary and metanephric adenomas of the kidney. Semin Diagn Pathol. 15(1):41-53, 1998
6. Kovacs G: High frequency of papillary renal-cell tumours in end-stage kidneys--is there a molecular genetic explanation? Nephrol Dial Transplant. 10(5):593-6, 1995

PAPILLARY ADENOMA

Microscopic Features

(Left) The definitional criterion of up to 5 mm size for papillary adenoma by WHO is arbitrary, as almost all small tumors, even up to 10 mm in size, have shown a benign outcome. This photomicrograph depicts a papillary neoplasm that was 8 mm in size. **(Right)** Most papillary adenomas are well circumscribed and nonencapsulated. However, irregular extensions ⇗ into surrounding parenchyma are not uncommon. Notice the prominent tubular architecture in this example.

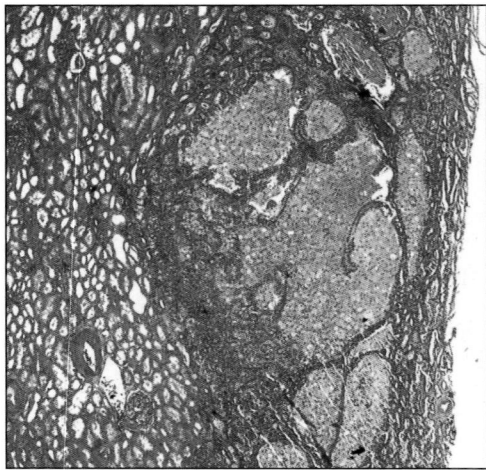 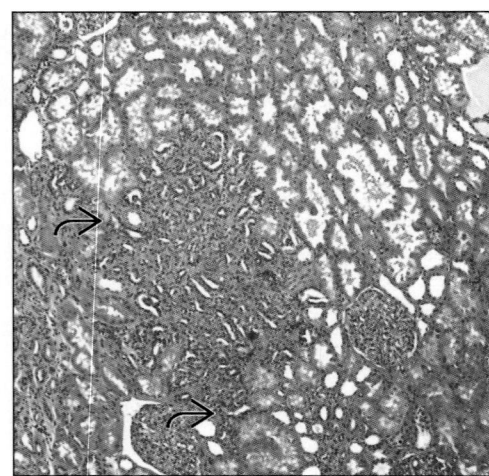

(Left) While most papillary adenomas are similar to minute type 1 papillary carcinomas, rare examples, as depicted here, have prominent eosinophilic cytoplasm ⇒, larger nuclei, and prominent nucleoli. **(Right)** Occasional papillary adenomas show cytoplasmic clarity ⇒, similar to that seen rarely in some papillary renal cell carcinomas. However, the cytoplasm is not optically transparent and shows fine and irregular cytoplasmic granularity.

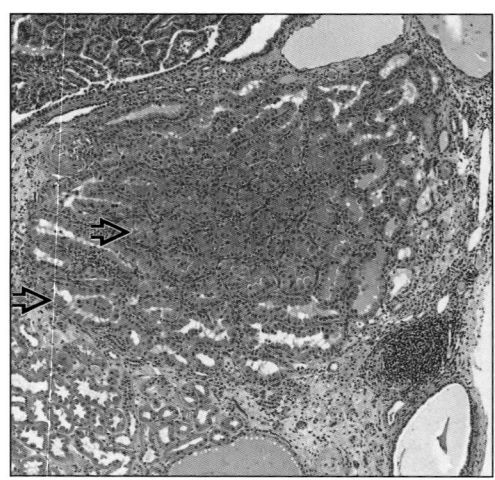 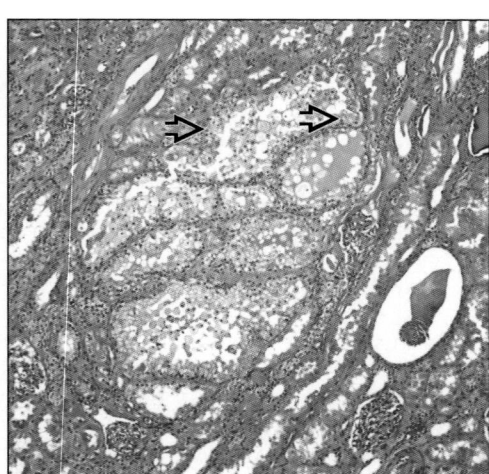

(Left) This example of papillary adenoma shows mild spindling ⇒ of the tumor cells. This feature is also noted in some type 1 papillary RCCs. Spindling in papillary adenomas, as in low-grade papillary carcinomas, does not have any biological implications. **(Right)** This minute papillary adenoma consists of a collection of only 3 neoplastic tubules. Notice the combined papillary ⇒ and tubular ⇗ architecture of the lesion, a frequent finding in most papillary adenomas.

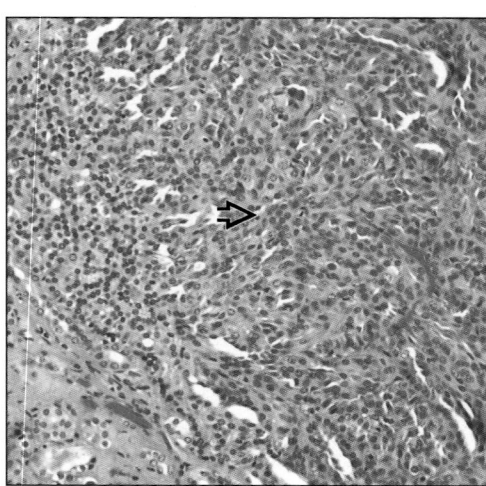 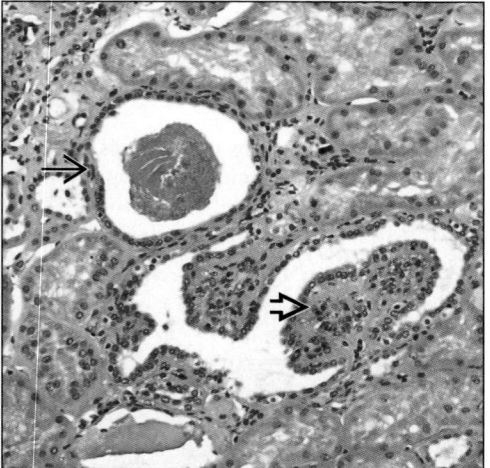

Microscopic and Immunohistochemistry Features

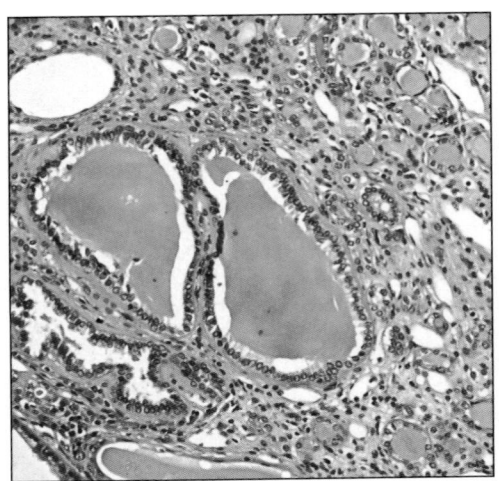

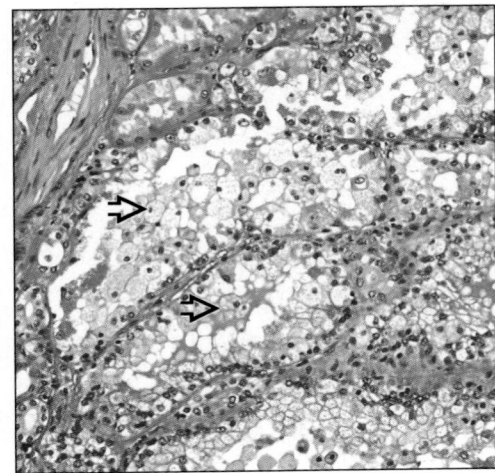

(Left) This minute papillary adenoma is composed of neoplastic tubules only. The incidence of adenomas progressively increases with age. In autopsy studies, incidence ranges from < 10% before 40 years of age to 40% in people > 70. *(Right)* This image shows a papillary adenoma with cytoplasmic clarity and abundant foamy macrophages ⮕. Psammomatous calcifications may be observed. In contrast to papillary RCC, a fibrous capsule is absent in most adenomas.

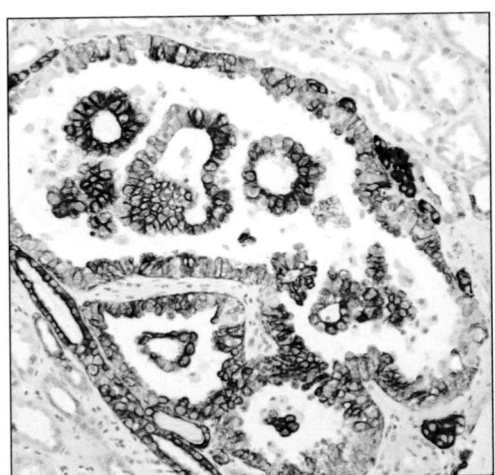

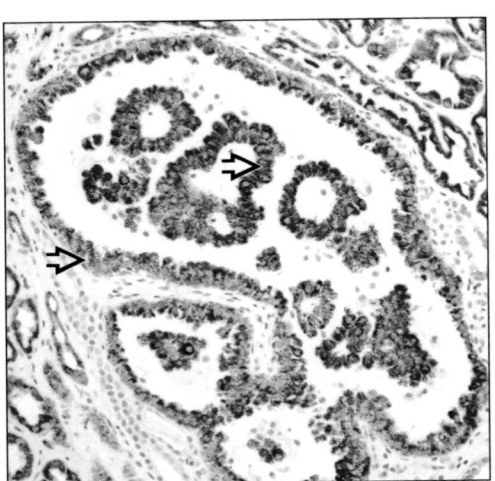

(Left) The image shows a minute papillary adenoma with diffuse positivity for CK7. As is usual in papillary renal cell carcinoma, particularly type 1, almost all papillary adenomas show such diffuse immunoreactivity for CK7. *(Right)* Most papillary adenomas also stain diffusely and strongly for AMACR. Similar to papillary RCC, the positivity is in the form of diffuse, cytoplasmic, granular staining ⮕.

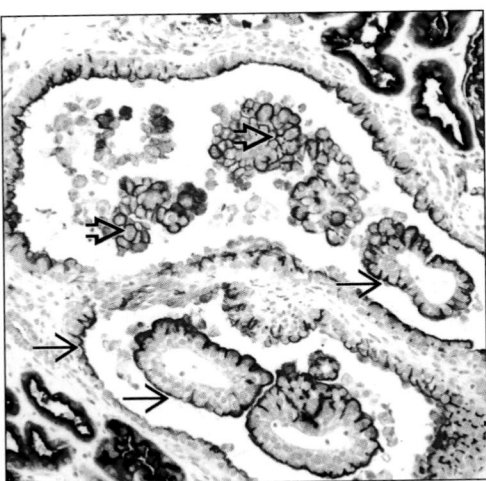

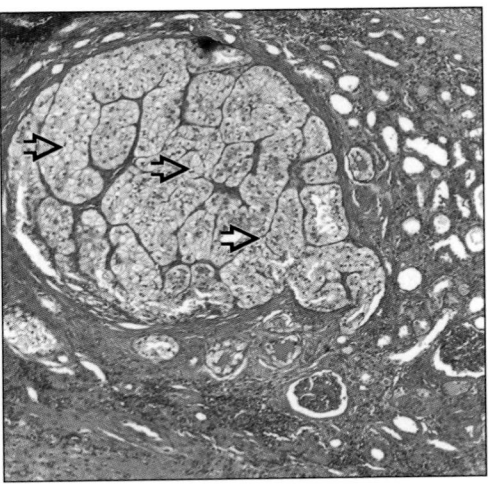

(Left) This image shows a papillary adenoma with positive immunoreactivity for CD10. The positivity is membrane-predominant. While it focally stains the membranes on all sides of the cell (box-like pattern) ⮕, in most of the lesion only a luminal or inverted cup-like pattern ⮕ is present, similar to that in most papillary RCCs. *(Right)* Microscopic lesions with features of clear cell ⮕ or other subtypes of renal cell carcinoma are not designated as adenomas, even when < 5 mm in size.

RENAL ONCOCYTOMA

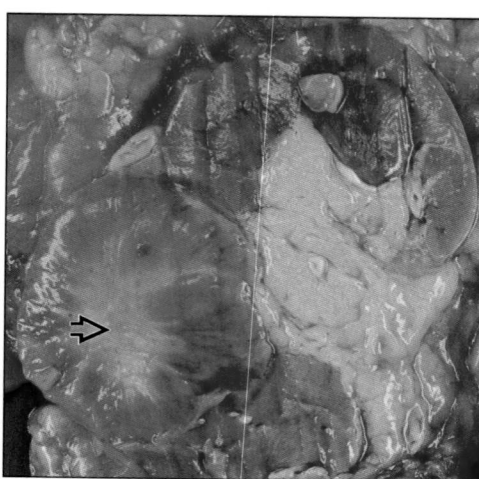

Renal oncocytoma is typically well circumscribed with tan-brown cut surface. A central scar ⊃ is present in about 30% of the tumors. Such scars may also be seen in other low-grade slow-growing tumors.

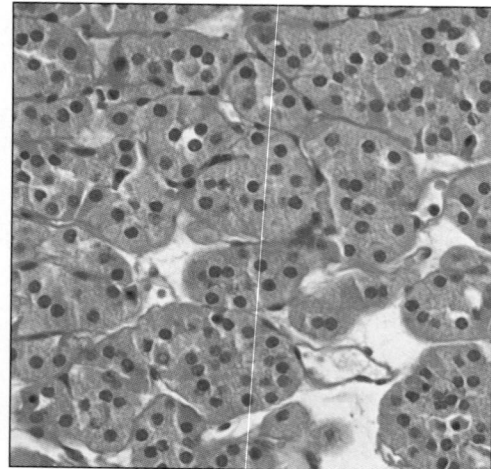

The typical histologic features of renal oncocytoma include solid nests of cells with oncocytic cytoplasm and uniform, round nuclei, in a background of variable, but often loose, stroma.

TERMINOLOGY

Definitions
- Benign, oncocytic renal neoplasms with prominent or exclusive nested architecture and uniform round nuclei

ETIOLOGY/PATHOGENESIS

Molecular Abnormalities
- Loss of chromosomes Y and 1
- Chromosome 11q13 alterations, including translocations
  - 11q13 alterations often involving *CCDN1* gene, with overexpression of gene product cyclin-D1
- Mitochondrial DNA (*mtDNA*) mutations, particularly with losses of genes for respiratory chain complex I
- Many tumors with normal karyotype and no known FISH abnormalities
- Rare familial cases described; later, many of these found to have Birt-Hogg-Dubé syndrome

CLINICAL ISSUES

Epidemiology
- Incidence
  - 6-9% of renal tumors
- Age
  - Mean: 62 years (range: 32-89 years)
- Gender
  - M:F = 2:1

Presentation
- Usually asymptomatic, detected on radiologic investigations for unrelated symptoms

Prognosis
- Benign

MACROSCOPIC FEATURES

General Features
- Well-circumscribed, nonencapsulated, usually solitary mass; sometimes multifocal (17%) and bilateral (4%)
- Mahogany brown to yellow-tan color
- Central stellate scar in up to 1/3 of cases; usually in larger tumors
- Uncommon features: Gross cysts, extension into perinephric fat, or vascular invasion

Size
- Mean: 4.4 cm (range: 0.6-15 cm)

MICROSCOPIC PATHOLOGY

Histologic Features
- Architecture: Typically solid nests, but micro- and macrocysts or tubules also common
  - Closely packed nests sometimes imparting solid appearance
  - Nest separated by distinct reticulum framework
- Cells with deeply eosinophilic, granular cytoplasm
  - Nuclei uniform and round, with vesicular chromatin and frequently prominent central nucleoli
  - Cytoplasmic clearing rare, usually restricted to areas of scarring
  - Sometimes cells at periphery of nests, "oncoblasts," have scant cytoplasm
- Occasional isolated or groups of cells with marked degenerative-appearing hyperchromasia and pleomorphism
- Stroma hypocellular, often hyalinized
- Some tumors with perinephric fat (20%) or vascular (5%) invasion

Predominant Pattern/Injury Type
- Neoplastic

RENAL ONCOCYTOMA

Key Facts

Etiology/Pathogenesis
- Loss of chromosomes Y and 1; Ch 11q13 alterations
- Many tumors with normal karyotype

Clinical Issues
- Benign

Macroscopic Features
- Well circumscribed, nonencapsulated
- Mahogany brown to yellow-tan color
- Central stellate scar: 33%

Microscopic Pathology
- Architecture: Typically solid nests, but micro- and macrocysts or tubules also common
- Abundant granular eosinophilic cytoplasm; uniform, round nuclei with vesicular chromatin and frequently prominent central nucleoli

- CD117 positive; CK7 usually negative, occasionally focal positive; claudin-7 negative or focal positive
- Occasional isolated cells or groups of cells with marked degenerative-appearing hyperchromasia and pleomorphism

Ancillary Tests
- EM: Cytoplasm packed with mitochondria
- Round nucleus; cytoplasm packed with mitochondria mostly showing lamellar cristae

Top Differential Diagnoses
- Chromophobe RCC (eosinophilic variant)
- Clear cell RCC (eosinophilic variant)
- Epithelioid (oncocytoma-like) AML
- RCC, unclassified (oncocytic, low-grade type)

Predominant Cell/Compartment Type
- Oncocytic

ANCILLARY TESTS

Immunohistochemistry
- CD117 and Ksp-cadherin positive; CK7 usually negative to occasionally focal positive; claudin-7 negative or focal positive

Electron Microscopy
- Round nucleus
- Cytoplasm packed with mitochondria mostly showing lamellar cristae

DIFFERENTIAL DIAGNOSIS

Chromophobe RCC (Eosinophilic Variant)
- Nuclear irregularities, with perinuclear halos; variety of growth patterns, including solid and broad alveoli
- CK7 is often diffusely positive; microvesicles and mitochondria with tubulovesicular cristae on EM

Clear Cell RCC (Eosinophilic Variant)
- Fine arborizing vascularity; nuclear atypia, chromatin irregularities
- CA9 and CD10, diffuse membranous positivity

Epithelioid (Oncocytoma-like) Angiomyolipoma
- Nuclear pleomorphism is common
- Smooth muscle and adipose component
- Melanocytic markers HMB-45 and Melan-A(MART-1) are positive

RCC, Unclassified (Low-Grade, Oncocytic Type)
- Nuclear pleomorphism, easily identifiable mitotic figures, atypical mitoses

SELECTED REFERENCES

1. Sukov WR et al: CCND1 rearrangements and cyclin D1 overexpression in renal oncocytomas: frequency, clinicopathologic features, and utility in differentiation from chromophobe renal cell carcinoma. Hum Pathol. Epub ahead of print, 2009
2. Picken MM et al: Analysis of chromosome 1p abnormalities in renal oncocytomas by loss of heterozygosity studies: correlation with conventional cytogenetics and fluorescence in situ hybridization. Am J Clin Pathol. 129(3):377-82, 2008
3. Tickoo SK et al: Pathologic features of renal cortical tumors. Urol Clin North Am. 35(4):551-61; v, 2008
4. Hornsby CD et al: Claudin-7 immunohistochemistry in renal tumors: a candidate marker for chromophobe renal cell carcinoma identified by gene expression profiling. Arch Pathol Lab Med. 131(10):1541-6, 2007
5. Rohan S et al: Gene expression profiling separates chromophobe renal cell carcinoma from oncocytoma and identifies vesicular transport and cell junction proteins as differentially expressed genes. Clin Cancer Res. 12(23):6937-45, 2006
6. Skinnider BF et al: An immunohistochemical approach to the differential diagnosis of renal tumors. Semin Diagn Pathol. 22(1):51-68, 2005
7. Amin MB et al: Prognostic impact of histologic subtyping of adult renal epithelial neoplasms: an experience of 405 cases. Am J Surg Pathol. 26(3):281-91, 2002
8. Tickoo SK et al: Ultrastructural observations on mitochondria and microvesicles in renal oncocytoma, chromophobe renal cell carcinoma, and eosinophilic variant of conventional (clear cell) renal cell carcinoma. Am J Surg Pathol. 24(9):1247-56, 2000
9. Reuter VE: Renal tumors exhibiting granular cytoplasm. Semin Diagn Pathol. 16(2):135-45, 1999
10. Füzesi L et al: Cytogenetic analysis of 11 renal oncocytomas: further evidence of structural rearrangements of 11q13 as a characteristic chromosomal anomaly. Cancer Genet Cytogenet. 107(1):1-6, 1998
11. Tickoo SK et al: Discriminant nuclear features of renal oncocytoma and chromophobe renal cell carcinoma. Analysis of their potential utility in the differential diagnosis. Am J Clin Pathol. 110(6):782-7, 1998
12. Amin MB et al: Renal oncocytoma: a reappraisal of morphologic features with clinicopathologic findings in 80 cases. Am J Surg Pathol. 21(1):1-12, 1997

RENAL ONCOCYTOMA

Microscopic Features

(Left) Although renal oncocytomas, both grossly and on microscopic evaluation, are well-circumscribed, they usually lack a pseudocapsule. In this hematoxylin and eosin image, notice the advancing edge of the tumor ⬇ that is in direct contact with the surrounding nephrons. *(Right)* Microcystic &/or tubular architecture is quite common in renal oncocytoma and usually exists in combination with other more common architectural patterns, including solid nests and acini.

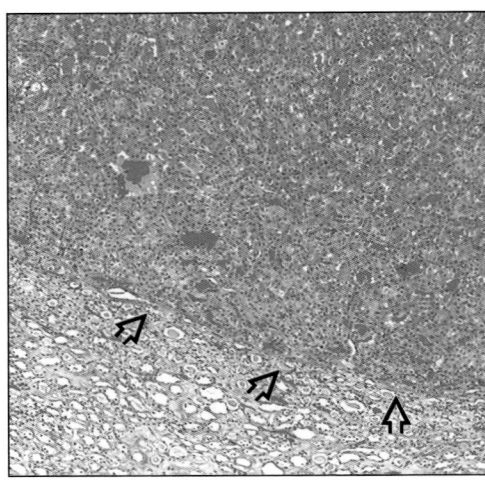
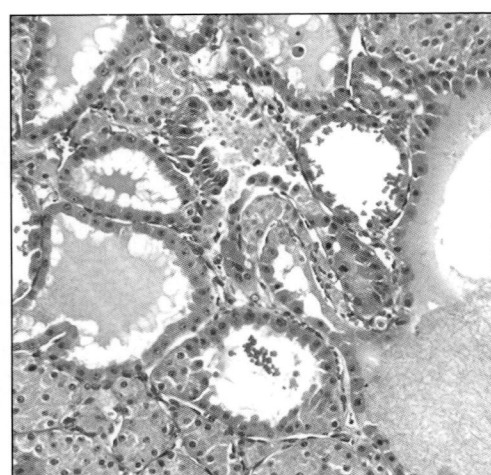

(Left) Some renal oncocytomas may show extensive or exclusive tubulo-cystic architecture and may superficially mimic tubulocystic carcinoma. Nuclear features are helpful, as the nuclei are typically round and uniform with evenly distributed chromatin, in renal oncocytoma. Tubulocystic carcinoma has high-grade nuclei with significant, diffuse nuclear membrane irregularities. *(Right)* In some oncocytomas, tightly packed nests and trabeculae may result in an apparent solid architecture.

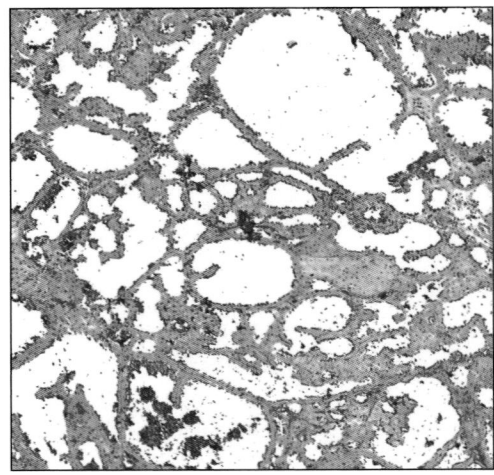
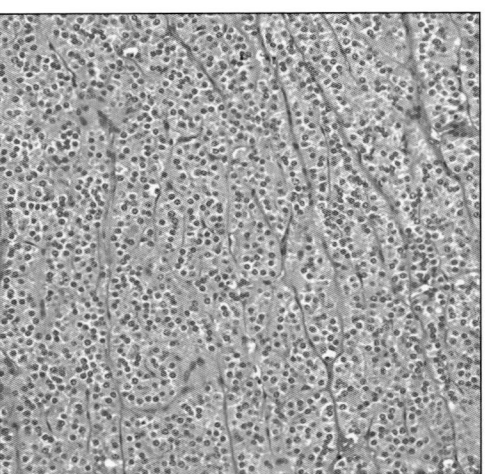

(Left) Typically the nests of cells, arranged in discrete islands or interconnected archipeligenous pattern, are separated by loose ⬇ stroma in most cases of renal oncocytoma. *(Right)* In some renal oncocytomas, variable proportions of the stroma may be fibrotic and hyalinized ⬇. Fibrotic stroma is particularly evident in the grossly identifiable scars in the tumor but may be present only as a microscopic finding. In rare cases, the stroma may be entirely fibrotic.

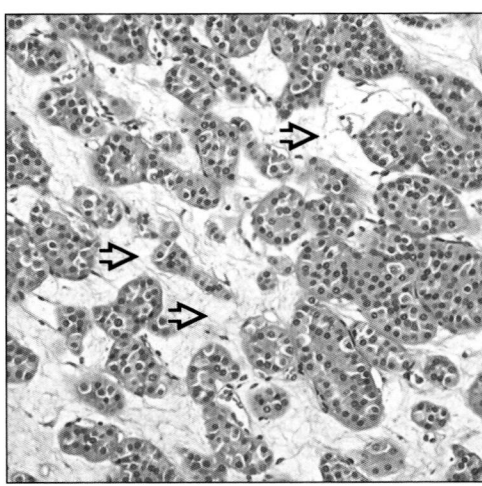
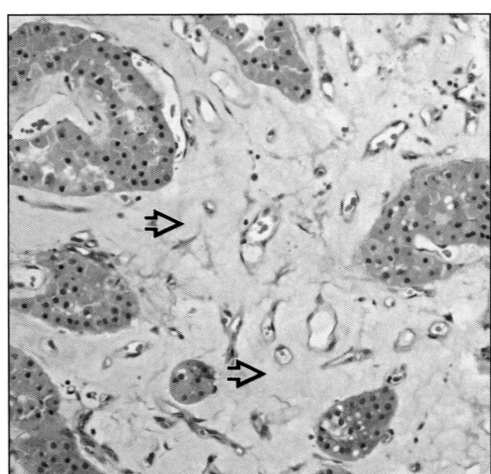

RENAL ONCOCYTOMA

Microscopic Features

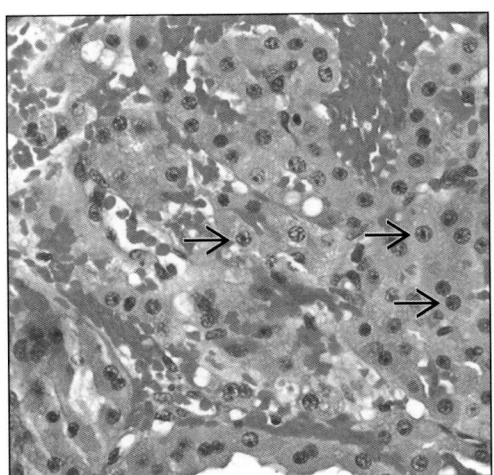

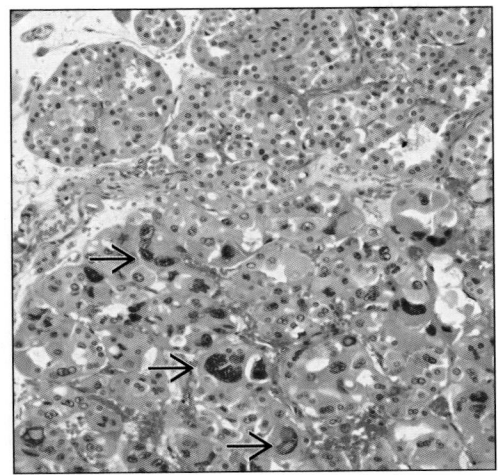

(Left) Uniformity of the shape and size of the nuclei is a prerequisite for rendering the diagnosis of renal oncocytoma in an oncocytic renal tumor. A significant proportion of renal oncocytomas possess prominent nucleoli ➡. *(Right)* Foci with marked nuclear hyperchromasia and pleomorphism ➡ are quite common in renal oncocytoma. Such nuclear atypia is believed to be a degenerative phenomenon, showing no proliferative activity on Ki-67 immunostaining.

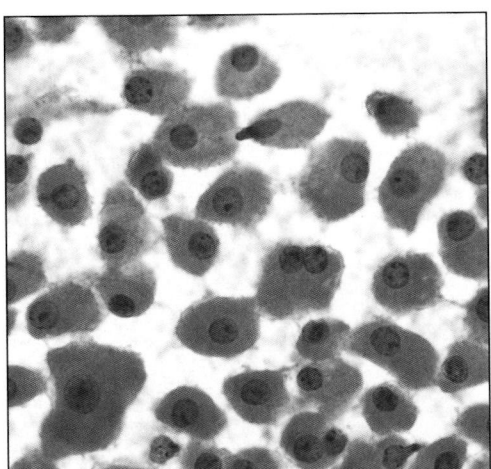

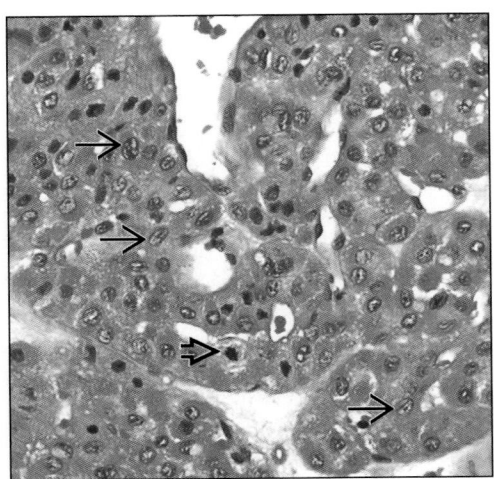

(Left) A cytology preparation of renal oncocytoma highlights the uniformity of the nuclei with prominent nucleoli. Cytoplasm is consistently finely granular and richly eosinophilic. *(Right)* Other than the markedly pleomorphic foci, only minimal background nuclear atypia is acceptable in renal oncocytoma. Diffuse nuclear irregularities and variation in nuclear size and shape ➡ and frequent mitoses ➡ are not the features of renal oncocytoma and suggest an alternative diagnosis.

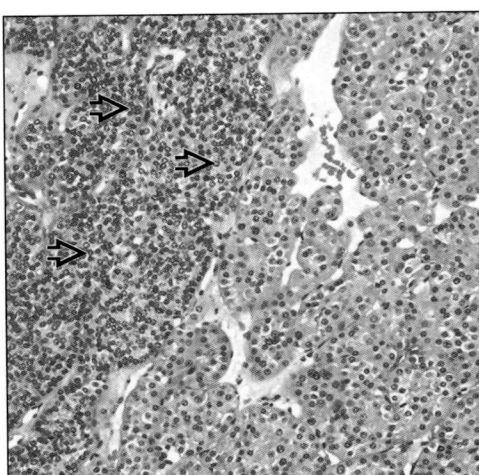

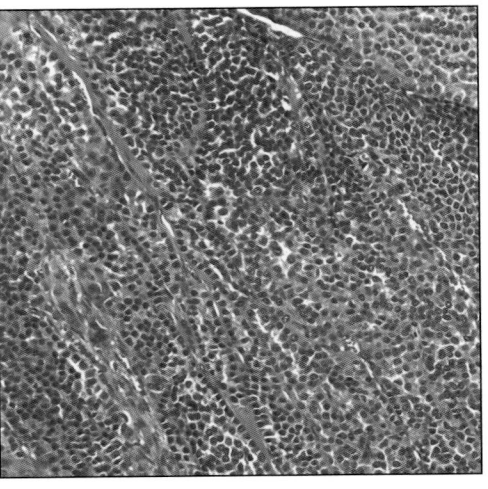

(Left) Many renal oncocytomas show collections of darker appearing cells, the so-called oncoblasts ➡. These cells possess scant cytoplasm, but nuclear details are somewhat similar to those in the larger oncocytic cells. *(Right)* Rarely, renal oncocytomas may show prominent or even predominant oncoblast-like areas, and such cases have been designated as small cell variants of renal oncocytoma by some. Some oncocytomas may show extensive degenerative (symplastic) atypia.

Microscopic Features and Ancillary Techniques

(Left) Focal, clear cells may be observed in and around the areas of scarring in renal oncocytomas ⇨. Otherwise, cells with clear cytoplasm are not seen in oncocytoma. Tumors with such clear cytoplasm in other areas should raise the possibility of alternative diagnoses, including Birt-Hogg-Dubé syndrome, in which focal clear cells in oncocytic tumors are common. *(Right)* Tubules and microcysts in oncocytomas frequently show the presence of fresh blood in the lumina.

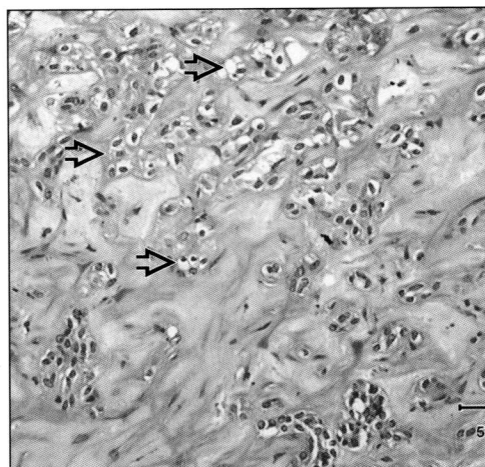
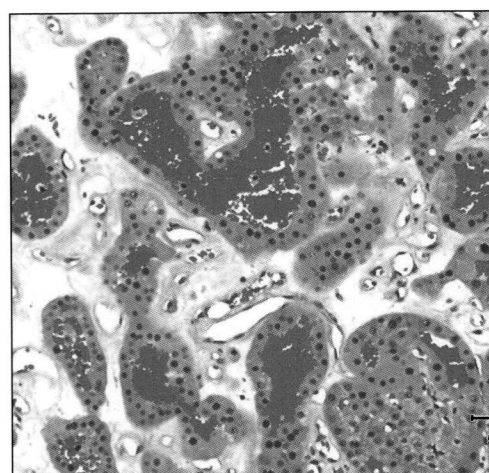

(Left) Diffuse, cytoplasmic positivity for CD117 is typically present in most oncocytomas. This may help in cases where the differentiation from eosinophilic clear cell RCC is difficult on H&E sections. *(Right)* Negative or only very focal positivity ⇨ for CK7 in renal oncocytoma may be helpful in the differential diagnosis from eosinophilic variant of chromophobe RCC. Heavy emphasis on CK7 alone in the distinction from chromophobe RCC is not advisable.

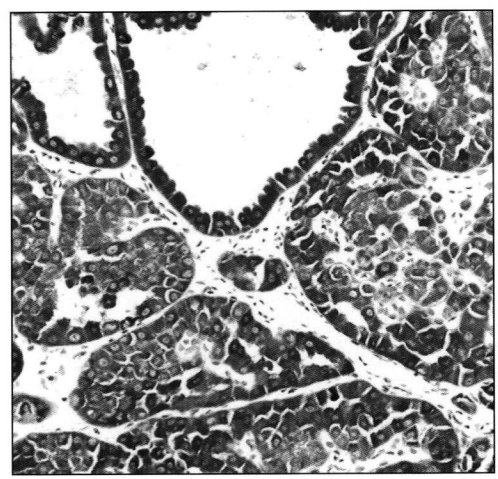
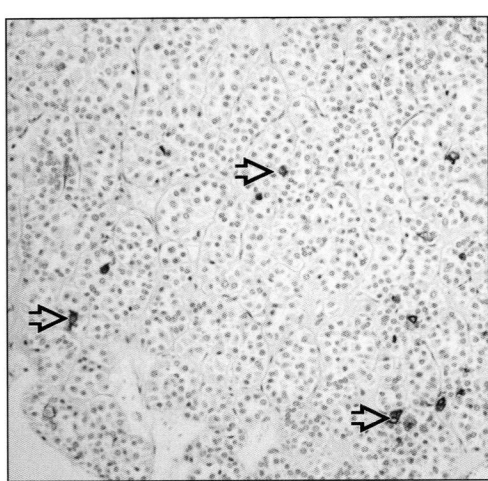

(Left) Diffuse CK7 positivity is often seen limited to the clear cell areas in and around scars ⇨ of renal oncocytomas. On the other hand, CK7 positivity in chromophobe RCC is often more diffuse, not limited to the areas of scarring. *(Right)* While vimentin usually does not label the tumor cells ⇨ in renal oncocytoma, rare cases may show focal to more diffuse staining. CD10 and monoclonal RCC are usually negative in renal oncocytoma.

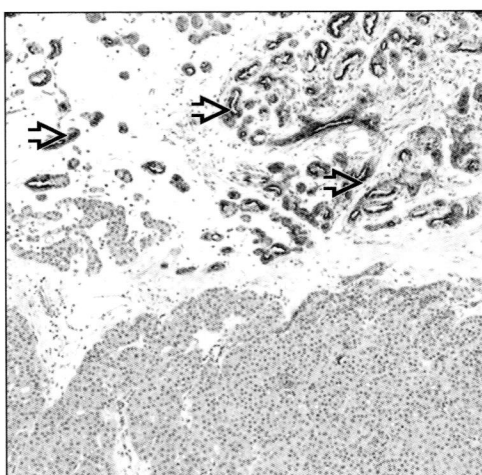
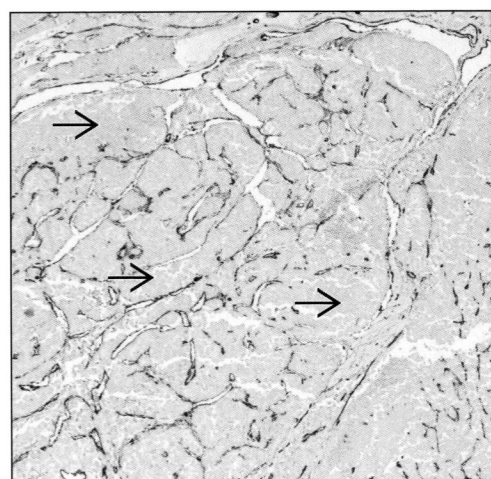

Variant Microscopic Features

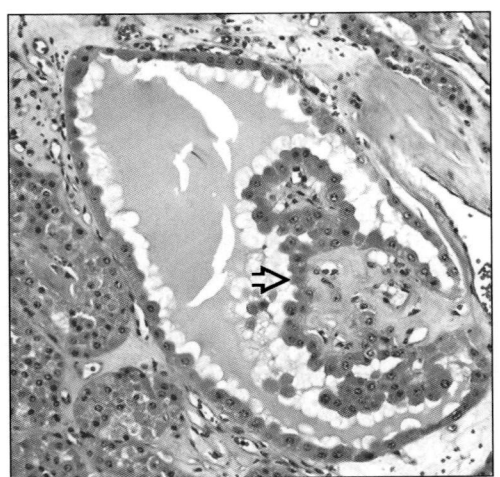

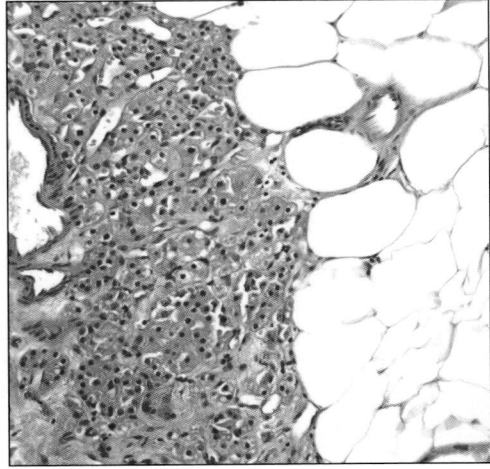

(Left) Focal papillations ⊳, particularly within the cysts, are occasionally present in renal oncocytoma. However, prominent papillary architecture is not a feature of the tumor. (Right) Up to 20% of renal oncocytomas show extension into perinephric fat. Usually, no desmoplastic response is present in these areas. Presence of neoplastic cells in fat in a tumor with features otherwise typical of renal oncocytoma does not merit histologic grading or pathologic staging.

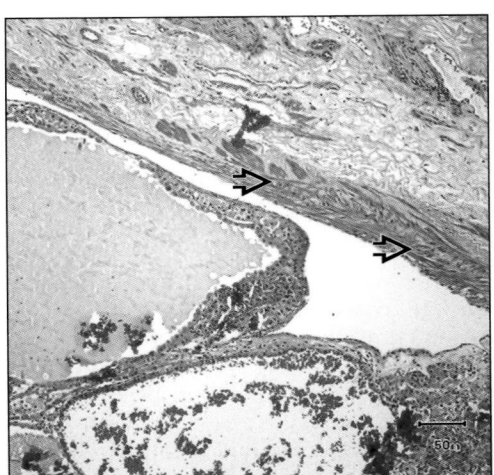

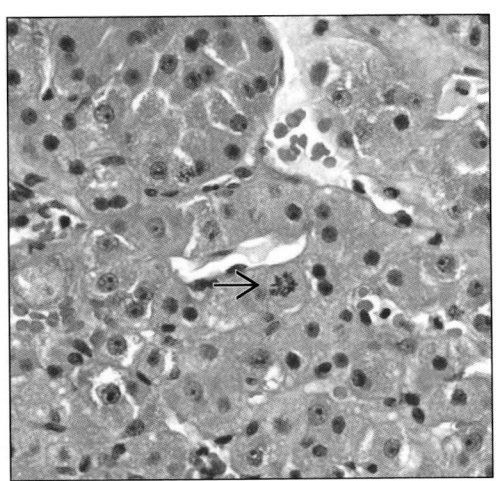

(Left) Vascular invasion, including that of large muscle-bearing vessels ⊳, may be present in less than 5% of cases. Neither the vascular invasion nor extrarenal extension influences the benign nature of otherwise typical oncocytoma. (Right) Very rare mitotic figures ➡ may be seen in occasional renal oncocytoma. However, in the presence of easy-to-identify or brisk, particularly atypical, mitotic activity, it is prudent to consider alternate diagnoses.

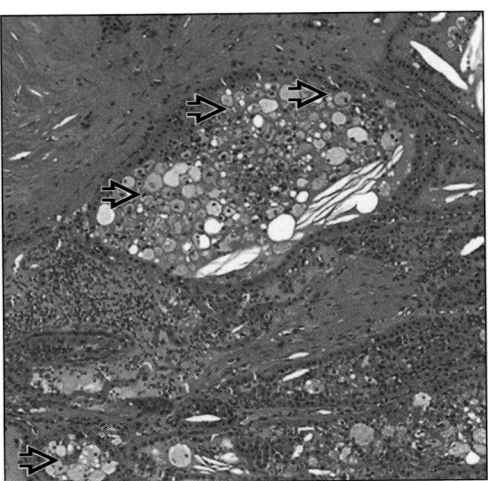

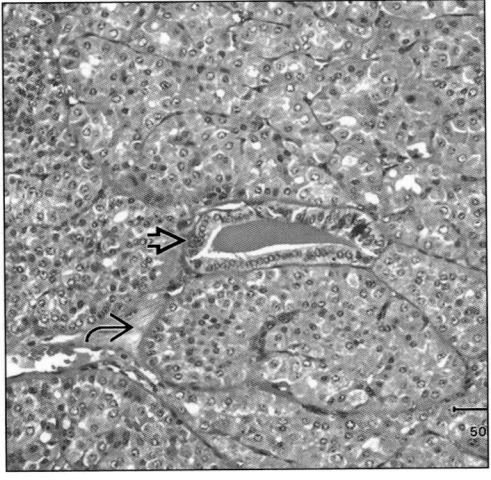

(Left) Focal intratumoral foamy macrophages ⊳ may be observed in rare cases of renal oncocytoma. These may be associated with prior fine needle aspiration biopsy. (Right) Entrapped renal tubules are frequently seen in renal oncocytomas ⊳. These are often concentrated at the periphery but may appear deep inside the tumor, often within intratumoral fibrous septations ➡. These entrapped tubules may be the source of rare papillary adenomas described within renal oncocytomas.

CLEAR CELL RENAL CELL CARCINOMA

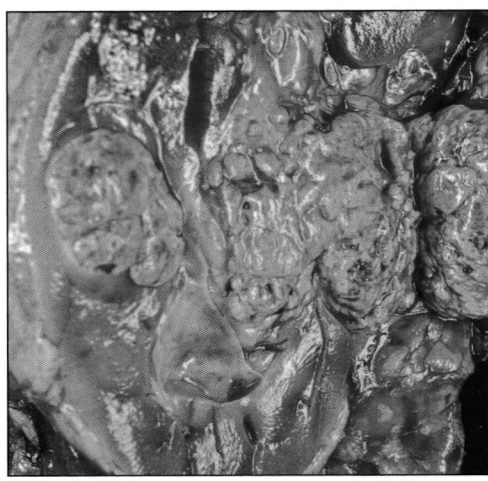

A clear cell renal cell carcinoma typically shows a golden-yellow cut surface. This gross appearance is a reflection of abundant intracytoplasmic lipid in these tumors.

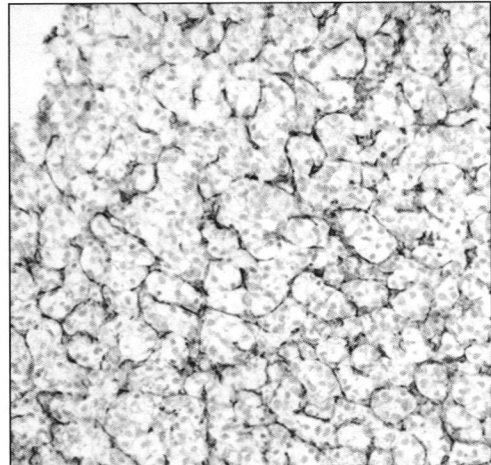

Intricately branching fibrovascular septations that surround the tumor cell nests, highlighted here by CD31 immunostain, are diagnostically the most important characteristic of CC-RCC.

TERMINOLOGY

Abbreviations
- Clear cell renal cell carcinoma (CC-RCC)

Synonyms
- Conventional (clear cell) renal cell carcinoma

ETIOLOGY/PATHOGENESIS

Mutations in VHL Gene (3p25-26) or Chromosome 3p Losses
- Present in virtually all cases of von Hippel-Lindau (VHL) syndrome
- Somatic mutations/losses/promoter hypermethylation in > 80% of sporadic CC-RCC

Hypoxia-Inducible Factor (HIF) and von Hippel-Lindau Pathways
- Normal von Hippel-Lindau gene product, pVHL, required to target and degrade hydroxylated HIF-1 in normoxemic states
- In states of hypoxia (as in ischemic/perinecrotic areas in any tumor), or when pVHL is absent or abnormal (as in all VHL cases and most sporadic CC-RCC), HIF1-α escapes degradation
- Overexpressed HIF1-α activates a number of downstream molecules, including
  - Vascular endothelial growth factor (VEGF)
  - Glucose transporter 1 (GLUT1)
  - Carbonic anhydrase IX (CA9)
  - Epidermal and platelet derived growth factors (EDGF, PDGF)
  - Many of these factors believed to have role in tumor initiation and progression in CC-RCC

CLINICAL ISSUES

Presentation
- Currently, most cases asymptomatic; diagnosed as result of radiologic investigations for unrelated symptoms
- Classical triad of hematuria, mass lesion, and pain present in < 30% of cases

Treatment
- Surgical approaches
  - Nephrectomy still most common mode of management in clinically localized disease
  - Partial nephrectomy becoming standard of care in many cases (> 70% of cases in some institutions)
  - Total or radical nephrectomies associated with long-term higher incidence of deteriorating renal function compared to partial nephrectomies
  - Partial nephrectomy replacing more radical procedures in overwhelming majority, including centrally occurring tumors and tumors > 4 cm
- Drugs
  - Response to chemotherapy &/or radiation for advanced disease is unsatisfactory
  - Immunotherapies, including interleukins and cytokines, were major therapeutic options in metastatic disease until recently, with only limited positive responses
  - Targeted therapies against HIF and mammalian target of rapamycin (mTOR) pathway markers have recently shown promising clinical responses
  - Targeted therapies more now being investigated as adjuvant therapies for high-risk, locally advanced, nonmetastatic tumors

Prognosis
- Most aggressive subtype among common subtypes of renal cell carcinoma
- Overall 5- and 10-year survival of 75 and 62%, respectively

CLEAR CELL RENAL CELL CARCINOMA

Key Facts

Clinical Issues
- Currently, most cases are asymptomatic; diagnosed as result of radiologic investigations for unrelated symptoms
- Nephrectomy still most common mode of management in clinically localized disease
- Partial nephrectomy becoming standard of care in many cases
- Targeted therapies against HIF and mTOR pathway markers have had promising clinical responses in recent past
- Most aggressive subtype among common subtypes of renal cell carcinoma
- Overall 5- and 10-year survival of 75% and 62%, respectively

Macroscopic Features
- Cut surface typically golden-yellow (due to presence of intracytoplasmic lipid); areas of necrosis, fibrosis, cystic change, hemorrhage are quite common

Microscopic Pathology
- Cells arranged in nests, micro or macro-cysts, or solid sheets, surrounded by intricate, branching fibrovascular septations
- Areas with granular/eosinophilic cytoplasm usually higher grade

Diagnostic Checklist
- Intricate, branching vasculature most important pathologic feature; clear cell cytology may not be present in all cases

---

- Most important indicators of prognosis include pathologic stage, nuclear grade, sarcomatoid features, and Memorial Sloan Kettering Cancer Center clinical status

MACROSCOPIC FEATURES

Size
- 1-24 cm

Gross Features
- May be well circumscribed but usually unencapsulated
- Cut surface typically golden-yellow (due to presence of intracytoplasmic lipid); areas of necrosis, fibrosis, cystic change, hemorrhage are quite common
- Tumors may be variegated in appearance with variable degrees of aforementioned features
- Cystic change may vary from focal to extensive multicystic
- In high-grade/sarcomatoid areas, solid gray, tannish-white to fleshy-appearing cut surface
- Most tumors limited to renal parenchyma
  - Larger tumors, particularly those > 7 cm, often involve renal sinus veins and sinus fat
    - Careful sampling of sinus essential to demonstrate sinus fat or muscular segmental branches of renal vein invasion

MICROSCOPIC PATHOLOGY

Histologic Features
- Cells arranged in nests, solid alveoli, tubules, micro- or macro cysts, or solid sheets, surrounded by intricate, branching fibrovascular septations
- Typical vascularity retained in most cases except in high-grade solid or sarcomatoid areas
- Lower grade areas usually with clear cell (optically transparent) cytology; related to abundant intracytoplasmic glycogen and fat
- Areas with granular/eosinophilic cytoplasm usually higher grade

- Fuhrman nuclear grade of tumor highly associated with biologic behavior
  - Nuclear grade assigned according to highest grade in tumor, even if focal
  - Tumors with sarcomatoid areas are assigned grade 4
- Focal papillary architecture acceptable; most often related to tumor cell dropout and pseudopapillary architecture; rare cases with focal true papillations
  - Prominent papillation should raise possibility of alternative diagnoses including translocation-associated, clear cell papillary, or unclassified RCC
- Some tumors may have prominent cell borders superficially resembling chromophobe RCC

Predominant Pattern/Injury Type
- Alveolar

Predominant Cell/Compartment Type
- Epithelial

ANCILLARY TESTS

Immunohistochemistry
- PAN-CK(AE1/AE3), EMA/MUC1, and vimentin are positive
- CD10, RCC, pax-2, pax-8, and CA9 are positive
  - CA9 often positive even in high-grade and sarcomatoid areas
- CK7, AMACR, CD117, and Ksp-cadherin are negative

DIFFERENTIAL DIAGNOSIS

Papillary Renal Cell Carcinoma
- Prominent papillary architecture
- Foamy histiocytes within fibrovascular stalks and stroma, and hemosiderin deposition
- IHC: Usually CK7 and AMACR diffusely positive; CA9 negative to focal perinecrotic/papillary tip positive

Translocation-Associated RCC
- Usually combination of prominent papillary architecture and clear cell cytology

CLEAR CELL RENAL CELL CARCINOMA

- High nuclear grade
- IHC: Cytokeratins and EMA/MUC1 negative to focally positive; strong and diffuse nuclear immunoreactivity for TFE3 or TFEB

Clear Cell Papillary RCC
- Prominent papillary architecture with exclusive clear cell cytology
- Usually low nuclear grade
- Nuclei arranged in linear manner away from basement membrane
- IHC: CK7 and CA9 diffusely positive; AMACR negative; CD10 usually negative

Epithelioid Angiomyolipoma
- Usually high nuclear grade even in areas with clear cell cytology; multilobulated/multinucleated polymorphous cells often present
- Vasculature usually not as intricate or branching as in CC-RCC
- Often associated, at least focally, with typical angiomyolipoma areas, or focal fat &/or dysmorphic vessels
- IHC: Cytokeratin/EMA/MUC1 negative; HMB-45/ Melan-A(MART-1)/MITF positive

Chromophobe RCC
- Characteristic nuclear and cytoplasmic features
- Plant cell appearance and koilocytoid atypia
- Fibrovascular septations most often incomplete
- 2 cell populations (eosinophilic and clear cell) in predictable arrangement
- IHC: CK7 and CD117 usually positive; CA9 negative

Adrenal Cortical Tumors
- Correlation with imaging findings is crucial
- Clear cells with "bubbly" cytoplasm
- IHC: EMA/MUC1 and cytokeratins negative; inhibin, Melan-A(MART-1) positive

DIAGNOSTIC CHECKLIST

Clinically Relevant Pathologic Features
- Currently, tumors invading renal sinus or perinephric fat assigned the same pT stage
- Similarly, tumors invading segmental (muscle-containing) branches of renal vein assigned the same pT stage as renal vein invasion

Pathologic Interpretation Pearls
- Intricate, branching vasculature most important pathologic feature
  - Clear cell cytology not present in all cases; therefore, not essential to diagnosis

SELECTED REFERENCES

1. Bertini R et al: Renal sinus fat invasion in pT3a clear cell renal cell carcinoma affects outcomes of patients without nodal involvement or distant metastases. J Urol. 181(5):2027-32, 2009
2. Nese N et al: Renal cell carcinoma: assessment of key pathologic prognostic parameters and patient characteristics in 47,909 cases using the National Cancer Data Base. Ann Diagn Pathol. 13(1):1-8, 2009
3. Ozcan A et al: PAX-2 in the diagnosis of primary renal tumors: immunohistochemical comparison with renal cell carcinoma marker antigen and kidney-specific cadherin. Am J Clin Pathol. 131(3):393-404, 2009
4. Rini BI et al: Renal cell carcinoma. Lancet. 373(9669):1119-32, 2009
5. Simmons MN et al: Laparoscopic radical versus partial nephrectomy for tumors >4 cm: intermediate-term oncologic and functional outcomes. Urology. 73(5):1077-82; discussion 1082, 2009
6. Thompson RH et al: Contemporary use of partial nephrectomy at a tertiary care center in the United States. J Urol. 181(3):993-7, 2009
7. Al-Ahmadie HA et al: Carbonic anhydrase IX expression in clear cell renal cell carcinoma: an immunohistochemical study comparing 2 antibodies. Am J Surg Pathol. 32(3):377-82, 2008
8. Hutson TE et al: Targeted therapies for metastatic renal cell carcinoma: an overview of toxicity and dosing strategies. Oncologist. 13(10):1084-96, 2008
9. Molina AM et al: Current algorithms and prognostic factors in the treatment of metastatic renal cell carcinoma. Clin Genitourin Cancer. 6(3):s7-s13, 2008
10. Pfaffenroth EC et al: Genetic basis for kidney cancer: opportunity for disease-specific approaches to therapy. Expert Opin Biol Ther. 8(6):779-90, 2008
11. Tickoo SK et al: Pathologic features of renal cortical tumors. Urol Clin North Am. 35(4):551-61; v, 2008
12. Thompson RH et al: Patients with pT1 renal cell carcinoma who die from disease after nephrectomy may have unrecognized renal sinus fat invasion. Am J Surg Pathol. 31(7):1089-93, 2007
13. Tickoo SK et al: Immunohistochemical expression of hypoxia inducible factor-1alpha and its downstream molecules in sarcomatoid renal cell carcinoma. J Urol. 177(4):1258-63, 2007
14. Bonsib SM: Renal lymphatics, and lymphatic involvement in sinus vein invasive (pT3b) clear cell renal cell carcinoma: a study of 40 cases. Mod Pathol. 19(5):746-53, 2006
15. Reuter VE: The pathology of renal epithelial neoplasms. Semin Oncol. 33(5):534-43, 2006
16. Bonsib SM: T2 clear cell renal cell carcinoma is a rare entity: a study of 120 clear cell renal cell carcinomas. J Urol. 174(4 Pt 1):1199-202; discussion 1202, 2005
17. Skinnider BF et al: An immunohistochemical approach to the differential diagnosis of renal tumors. Semin Diagn Pathol. 22(1):51-68, 2005
18. Bonsib SM: The renal sinus is the principal invasive pathway: a prospective study of 100 renal cell carcinomas. Am J Surg Pathol. 28(12):1594-600, 2004
19. Cheville JC et al: Comparisons of outcome and prognostic features among histologic subtypes of renal cell carcinoma. Am J Surg Pathol. 27(5):612-24, 2003
20. Amin MB et al: Prognostic impact of histologic subtyping of adult renal epithelial neoplasms: an experience of 405 cases. Am J Surg Pathol. 26(3):281-91, 2002

CLEAR CELL RENAL CELL CARCINOMA

Gross Features

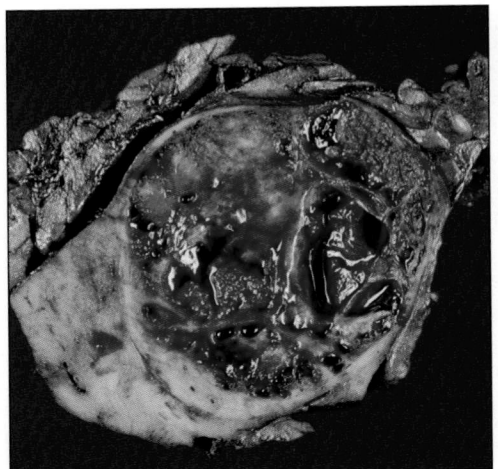

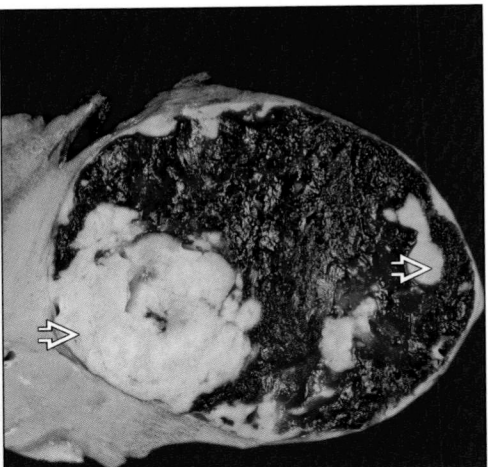

(Left) This gross photograph shows a cystic, necrotic, and hemorrhagic cut surface of a clear cell RCC. Gross necrosis, hemorrhage, and cystic changes are frequently observed in these tumors. *(Right)* Gross photograph of another tumor shows extensive hemorrhage. Note the characteristic golden-yellow appearance ⊞ of the nonhemorrhagic area. Sampling should target interfaces between the tumor and kidney, tumor and pelvicaliceal system/renal sinus, and tumor and perinephric fat.

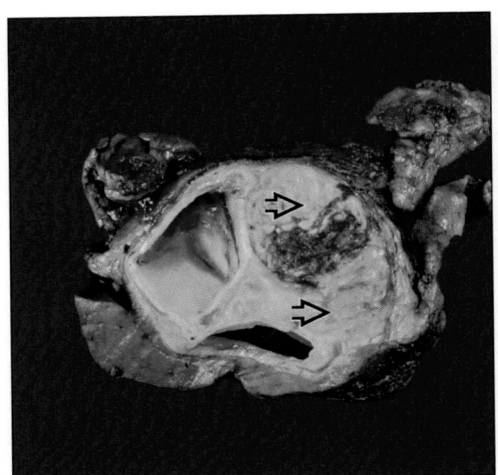

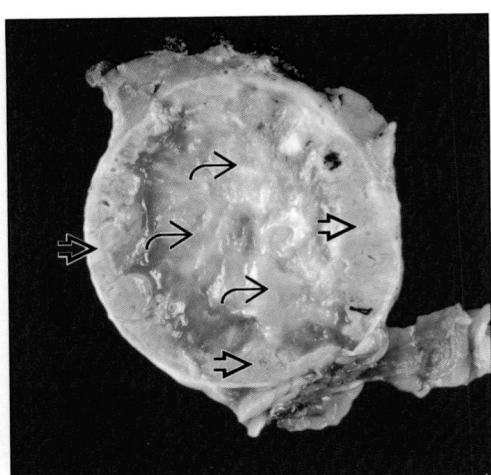

(Left) Gross photograph of another clear cell RCC shows a markedly cystic cut surface. The solid areas in the tumor reveal the characteristic golden-yellow appearance ⊞. *(Right)* This gross photograph shows a large central scar ⊞ in a clear cell renal cell carcinoma, surrounded by a rim of viable tumor ⊞. Central scar can be seen in a number of slow-growing renal tumors, including clear cell renal cell carcinoma, renal oncocytoma, and chromophobe RCC.

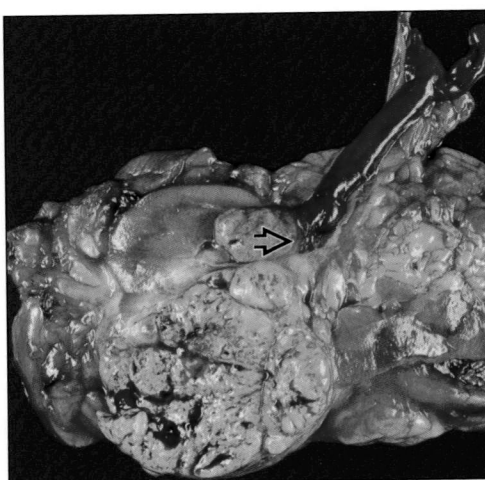

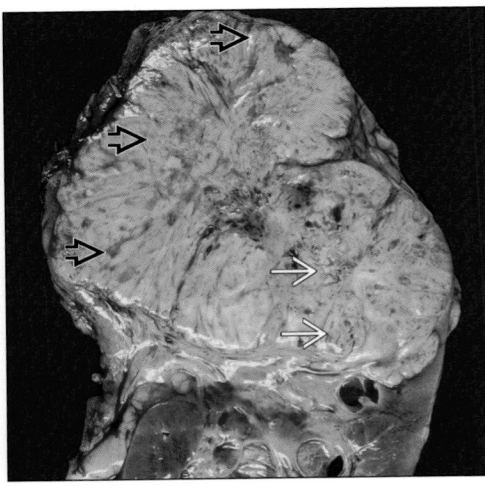

(Left) Gross photograph of this clear cell RCC shows a tumor extending into the renal vein ⊞. *(Right)* Gross photograph shows a clear cell RCC with large sarcomatoid areas. Compared to the golden-yellow cut surface in the lower grade ⊞ epithelial areas, the sarcomatoid ⊞ areas show a pale tan to fleshy appearance. Sampling of areas with grossly different appearance, particularly fleshy and gray-tan, is a key to identifying sarcomatoid and higher grade areas in a tumor.

CLEAR CELL RENAL CELL CARCINOMA

Microscopic Features

(Left) Hematoxylin & eosin shows a prototypic example of clear cell renal cell carcinoma, Fuhrman nuclear grade 1, with nests of clear cells surrounded by intricately branching vascular septae. *(Right)* This tumor shows Fuhrman grade 2 nuclei. The delicate, prominent interconnecting vascular framework, as seen here, is identified in most clear cell renal cell carcinomas. This characteristic vascular pattern is lost only in the very high-grade and sarcomatoid areas.

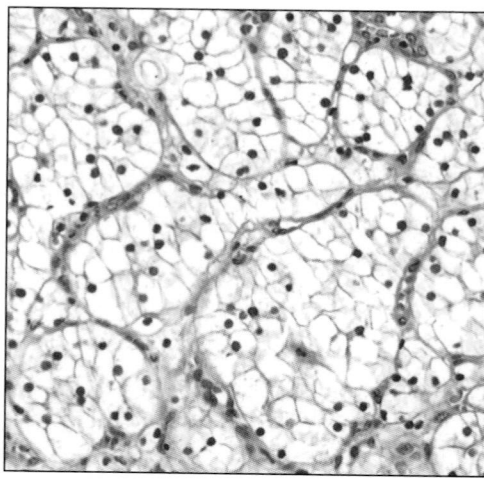 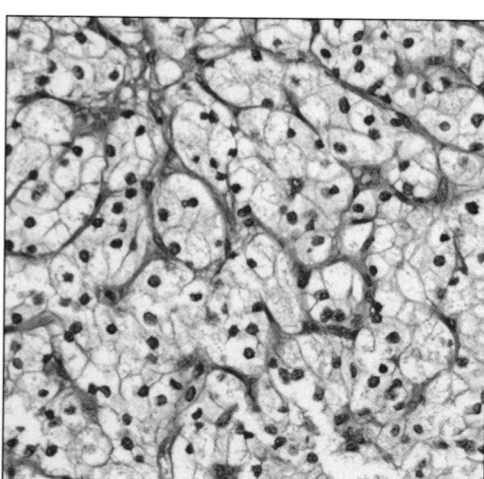

(Left) Hematoxylin & eosin stained section shows a clear cell renal cell carcinoma with grade 3 nuclei. Note the eosinophilic cytoplasm in some of the the cells. Some clear cell RCCs may have predominantly or even exclusively eosinophilic cytoplasm. *(Right)* A nuclear grade 4 clear cell RCC shows multilobulated and hyperchromatic nuclei ➔. Some cells contain multiple nuclei ➔. Grade heterogeneity is common, and the tumor is graded by the highest grade, even if focal.

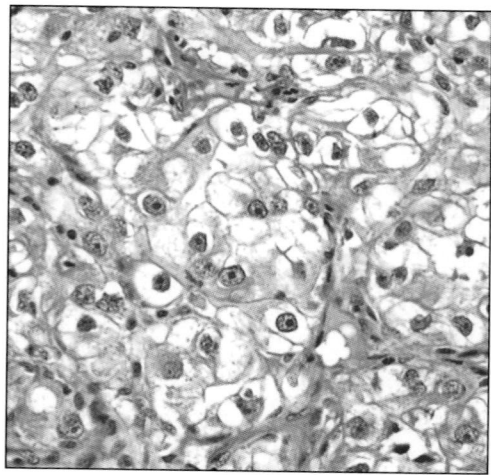 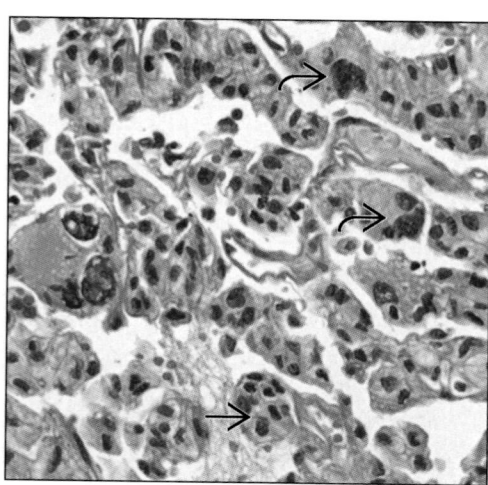

(Left) Many tumors show a combination of cells with clear and eosinophilic cytoplasm, either intimately admixed or as separate, discrete foci. Note the higher nuclear grade in the cells with eosinophilic cytoplasm, a finding that is quite common in clear cell RCC. *(Right)* This photomicrograph shows a high-grade clear cell renal cell carcinoma with rhabdoid cytology. Although the tumor cells are arranged in broad sheets and alveoli, the typical vascular pattern is retained ➔.

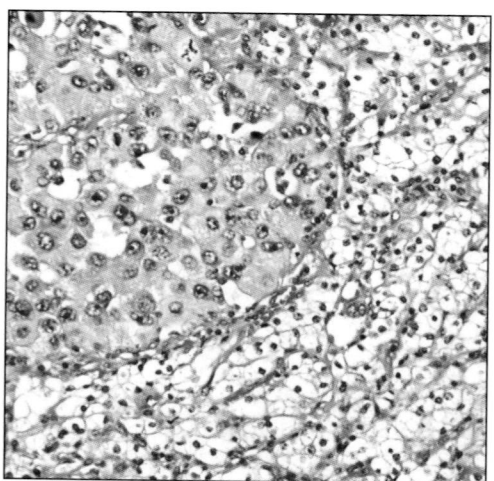 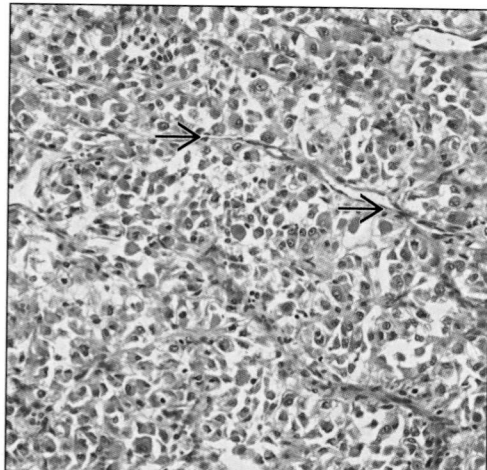

Microscopic Features and Ancillary Techniques

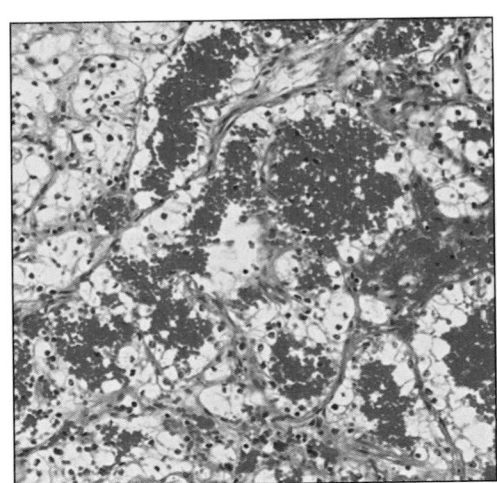
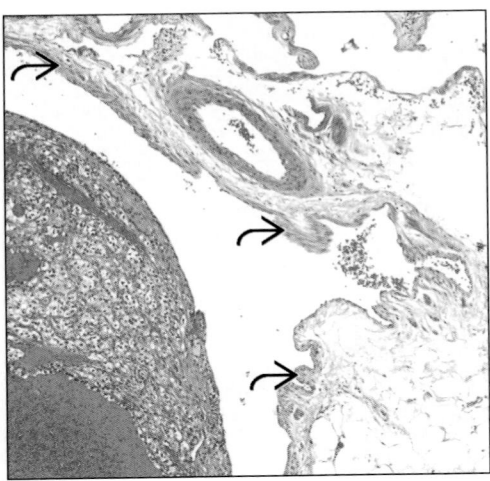

(Left) Clear cell renal cell carcinoma frequently shows fresh hemorrhage into the glandular lumina. This feature is also often retained in the metastatic sites. *(Right)* This image shows the tumor invading a muscle-containing branch of renal vein ➔ in the renal sinus. Such a finding is now considered equivalent to renal vein invasion for pT staging purposes. Careful sampling of renal sinus, even when the tumor grossly appears away from it, is essential to identify this feature.

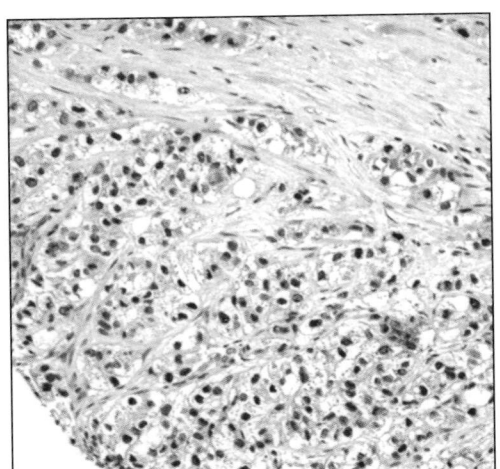
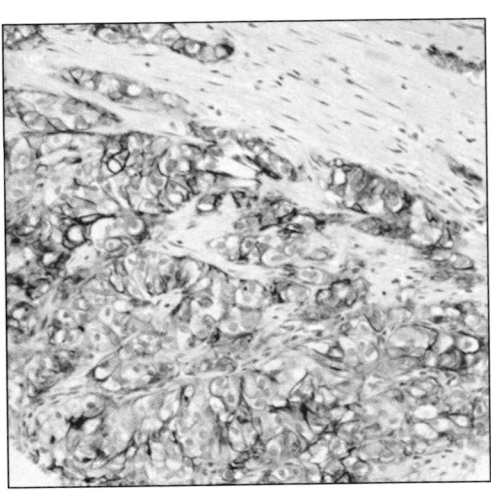

(Left) Immunohistochemical staining shows diffuse nuclear immunoreactivity for HIF-1 α in clear cell RCC. Diffuse overexpression of HIF in CC-RCC is a consequence of the absence/mutation of VHL gene in most of these tumors. *(Right)* Diffuse, membrane-predominant immunostaining for CA9 is present in more than 90% of CC-RCC. CA9 is a downstream molecule for HIF, and like HIF, diffuse overexpression indicates defective/absent VHL.

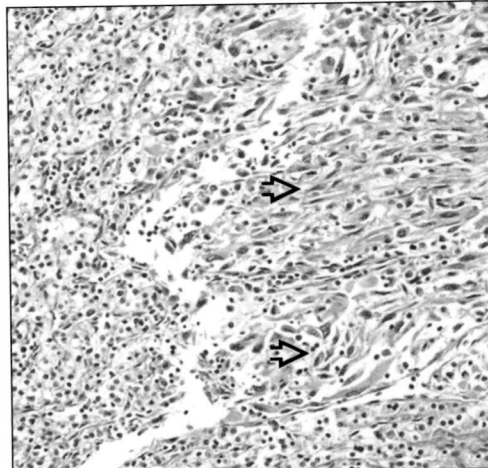
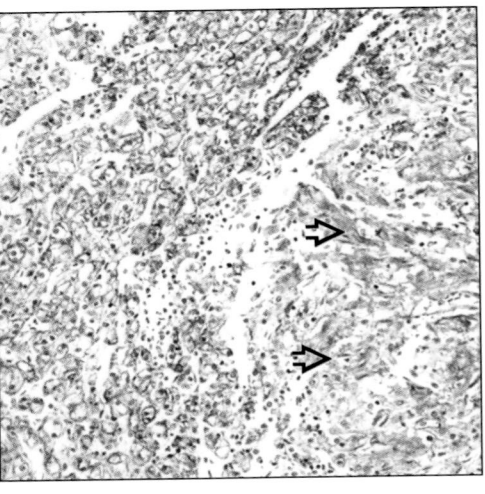

(Left) Sarcomatoid features ➔ in clear cell RCC portend an aggressive clinical behavior. All tumors with sarcomatoid areas are considered high grade (grade 4). *(Right)* Diffuse immunohistochemical positivity for CA9 is often retained in the spindle cell/ sarcomatoid components of clear cell renal cell carcinoma ➔. This is unlike the staining pattern with most other antibodies, which generally show decreased or absent staining in the high-grade or sarcomatoid areas.

Microscopic Features and Ancillary Techniques

(Left) Immunohistochemical staining for CD10 typically shows diffuse membranous positivity. Any other pattern of staining (e.g., in metastasis of unknown primary) should not be considered characteristic of clear cell RCC. *(Right)* However, CD10 positivity generally tends to be lost or become focal and weaker in higher grade ⊡ compared to lower grade areas ➔. A combination of markers CA9, CD10, RCC, pax-2, and vimentin is helpful, particularly in a metastatic setting.

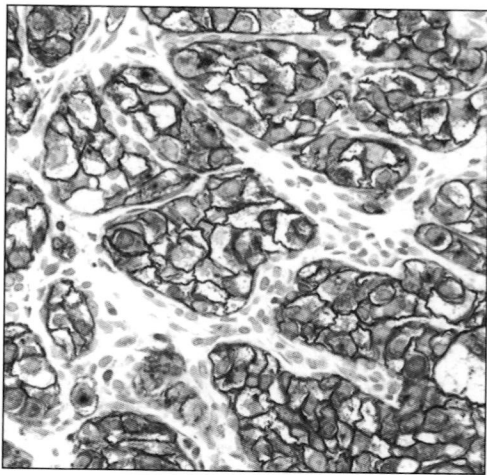
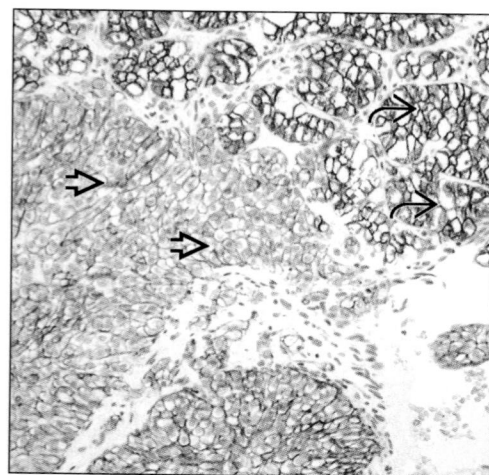

(Left) Staining for vimentin is usually positive in clear cell RCC. However, the diffuse positivity, as depicted here, is seen in less than 2/3 of tumors. Vimentin is more often positive in high-grade tumors and sarcomatoid areas in a tumor. *(Right)* This image shows microscopic tumor necrosis ⊡ in a clear cell RCC. Microscopic tumor necrosis is usually associated with high-grade tumors and has been considered by some to be an independent prognostic indicator in clear cell RCC.

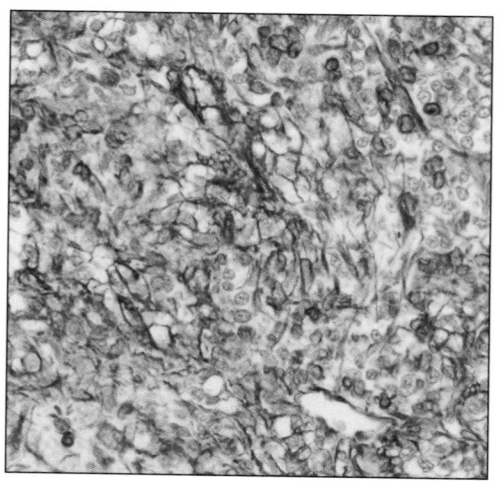
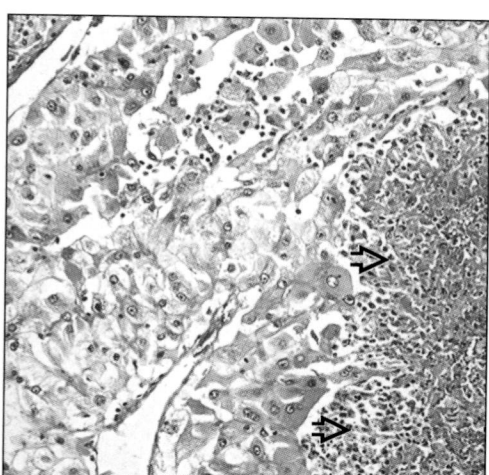

(Left) This clear cell RCC shows a markedly myxoid/chondroid background. Such features are uncommon but acceptable in clear cell RCC if transitions to a more typical appearance can be identified. *(Right)* Cytoplasmic hyaline globules ⊡ may sometimes be seen in clear cell RCC carcinoma. These most likely represent ubiquitinized proteins. CC-RCC can show a variety of unusual morphologic features. In such cases, transitions to a more classic appearances should always be looked for.

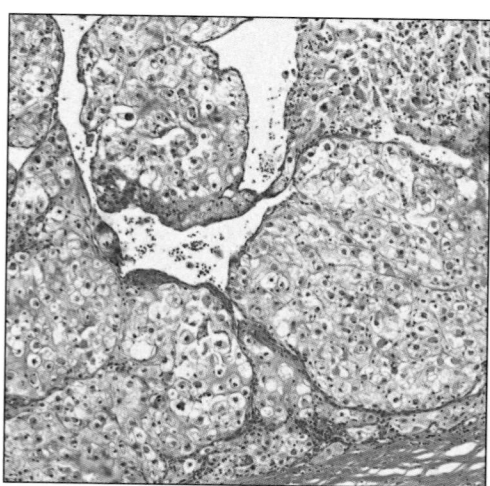
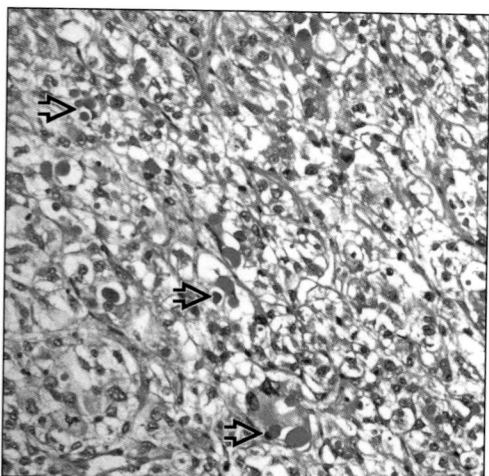

Microscopic Features of Metastases

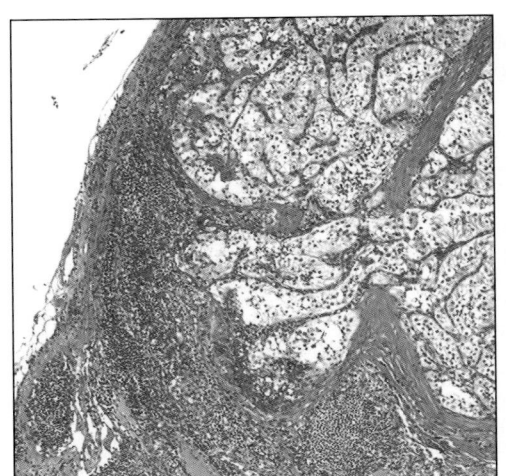

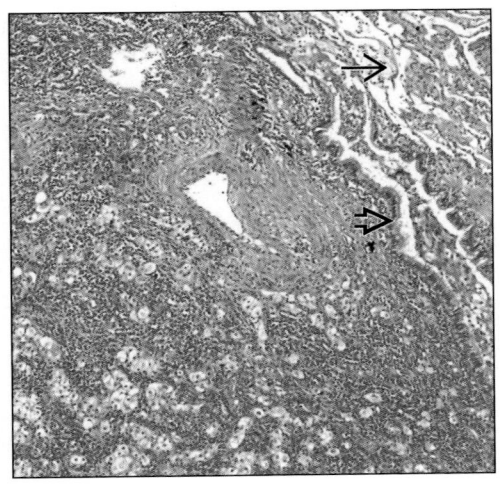

(Left) The image shows a clear cell RCC metastatic to a regional lymph node. Clinical history or imaging findings of renal mass are helpful if metastasis is the primary presentation. A combination of CA9, CD10, RCC, pax-2 and pax-8, and vimentin is a useful immunohistochemical panel. *(Right)* Clear cell renal cell carcinoma frequently metastasizes to the lungs. Notice the background alveolar parenchyma ➡ and bronchial tissue ➡ in the image.

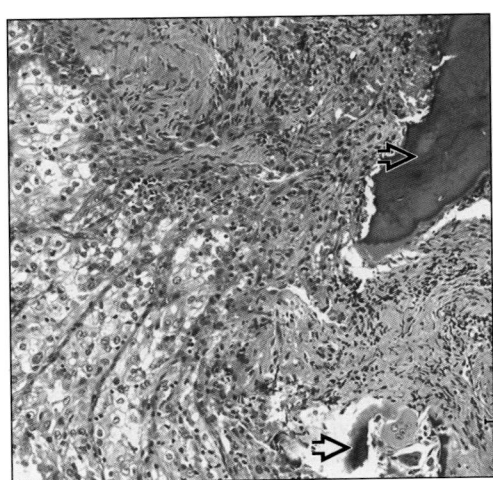

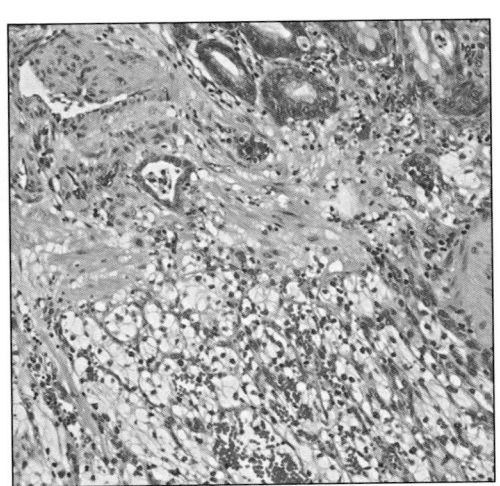

(Left) Besides the lymph nodes, lungs and bone are the most common sites of metastases from clear cell RCC. Distorted bony trabeculae ➡ are identified in this image. *(Right)* This image shows a gastric metastasis from CC-RCC. Clear cell RCC shows a remarkable predilection of metastasizing to unusual sites, and metastases may occur many years after the primary diagnosis. Renal cell carcinoma should always be in the differential diagnosis of an unusual clear cell tumor at any site.

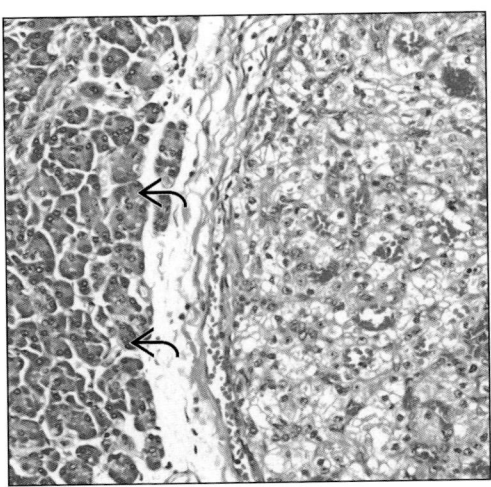

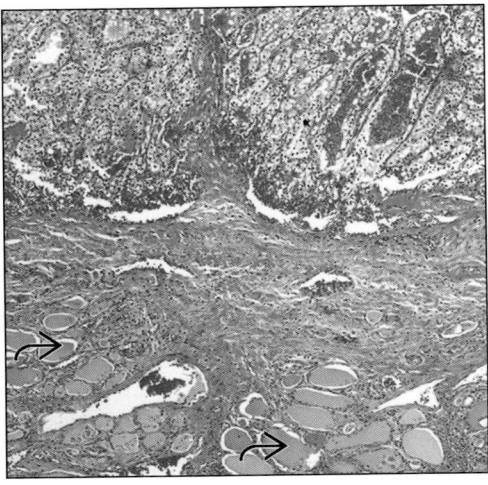

(Left) Hematoxylin and eosin shows clear cell renal cell carcinoma metastatic to the pancreas. Note the native pancreatic parenchyma (acini) ➡. *(Right)* This image shows clear cell RCC metastatic to the thyroid gland. The residual thyroid tissue is seen in the lower half of the figure ➡. CC-RCC is only 1 of the differential diagnostic possibilities in a metastasis of unknown primary, as many other neoplasms can have clear cytoplasm.

MULTILOCULAR CYSTIC RENAL CELL CARCINOMA

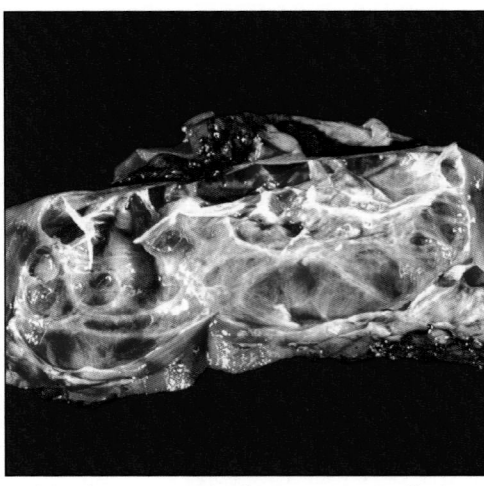

Multilocular cystic renal cell carcinoma typically shows a well-circumscribed tumor almost entirely composed of cysts with thin walls, a prominent fibrous capsule, and no solid expansile areas.

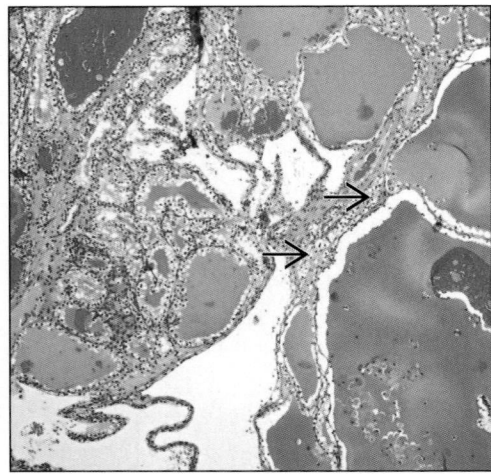

Microscopic evaluation reveals a tumor entirely composed of variably sized cysts, lined by clear cells with low nuclear grade, and thin septations showing clusters of cells with clear cytoplasm ⇒.

TERMINOLOGY

Abbreviations
- Multilocular cystic renal cell carcinoma (MC-RCC)

Definitions
- Renal cortical neoplasm composed of numerous clear cell-lined cysts with small clusters of clear cells in tumor septae
  - Solid, grossly recognizable component of clear cell RCC should be considered inconsistent with the diagnosis

ETIOLOGY/PATHOGENESIS

Genetic Features
- No detailed published studies based on evaluation of a large number of cases available
- Results of 1 study, published as an abstract, indicate presence of VHL alterations similar to that in clear cell RCC
  - These results are considered as evidence in support of its classification as variant of clear cell renal cell carcinoma

CLINICAL ISSUES

Epidemiology
- Incidence
  - 2 most recent large studies on combined 76 cases suggest that these constitute approximately 4% of all clear cell RCCs
    - Although this incidence may not be representative of true clinical practice
  - Overall, ~ 160 cases reported in literature
- Age
  - Range of mean age: 46-53 years in different studies (overall range: 30-80)

- Gender
  - M:F = 1.2-2.1:1

Presentation
- Up to 90% cases (range: 51-90%) discovered incidentally on radiologic evaluation for non-tumor-related conditions
- Unifocal and unilateral, with only rare exceptions

Prognosis
- On mean follow-up > 6.5 years, no recurrences or metastases described
- > 80% cases with stage pT1 disease at presentation
  - Very rare cases with stage pT3 disease, and even those with benign outcome
  - Because of such outcomes, redesignation as multilocular cystic renal cell neoplasm of low malignant potential has been suggested by some

MACROSCOPIC FEATURES

General Features
- Well-circumscribed, almost always with fibrous pseudocapsule
- Multicystic cut surface with marked variation in size of cysts
  - Cysts have smooth lining
  - May contain serous or bloody fluid, or blood clots
- Septations are usually quite thin
- No solid or expansile masses are present in tumor
- Calcifications in septae may occasionally be observed

Size
- Size quite variable; range: 1-14 cm (mean: 4.9)

MICROSCOPIC PATHOLOGY

Histologic Features
- Multilocular cysts with thin fibrous septa

MULTILOCULAR CYSTIC RENAL CELL CARCINOMA

Key Facts

Terminology

- Multilocular cystic renal cell carcinoma (MC-RCC)
- Renal cortical neoplasm composed of numerous clear cell-lined cysts with small clusters of clear cells in tumor septae

Clinical Issues

- On mean follow-up of > 6.5 years, no recurrences or metastases described
- > 80% cases with stage pT1 disease at presentation

Macroscopic Features

- Well circumscribed, almost always with fibrous pseudocapsule
- Multicystic cut surface with marked variation in size of cysts
- No solid or expansile masses are present in the tumor

Microscopic Pathology

- Cyst lining usually consisting of 1 or several layers of neoplastic cells, although in many areas, epithelial lining may be absent
- Clusters of tumor cells with clear cytoplasm always present within fibrous septa or in adjacent pseudocapsule
- No expansile or solid masses of tumor are evident

Top Differential Diagnoses

- Cystic nephroma
- Benign multiloculated renal cortical cysts
- Cystic partially differentiated nephroblastoma
- Cystic clear cell papillary renal cell carcinoma

- Cyst lining usually consisting of 1 or several layers of neoplastic cells, although in many areas, epithelial lining may be absent
- Tumor cells with clear cytoplasm and Fuhrman grade 1 or 2 nuclei
- Clusters of tumor cells with clear cytoplasm always present within fibrous septa or in adjacent pseudocapsule
  - Such collections of cells are a definitional requirement
- No expansile or solid masses of tumor are evident
- Occasionally, foamy macrophages may also line cyst wall
- Lining tumor cells may exhibit focal papillary tufting

Predominant Pattern/Injury Type

- Cystic

Predominant Cell/Compartment Type

- Clear

DIFFERENTIAL DIAGNOSIS

Cystic Nephroma

- Multiloculated cysts, often lined by flat to cuboidal or "hobnailed" cells; rarely with clear cell cytology; no clear cell nests in septa
- ER and PR(+); ovarian-type stroma commonly present

Benign Multiloculated Renal Cortical Cysts

- Multiloculated cysts, usually lined by flat to cuboidal, nonclear cells; no clear cell nests in septa

Cystic Partially Differentiated Nephroblastoma

- Clusters of blastemal or primitive epithelial elements present in septae
- Primarily a lesion of children

Cystic Clear Cell Papillary Renal Cell Carcinoma

- Rarely, predominantly cystic

- Predominant papillary and tubular architectural pattern
  - Nuclei typically arranged away from basement membrane
  - Cells commonly have clear cytoplasm

SELECTED REFERENCES

1. Radopoulos D et al: Solitary multilocular cystic renal cell carcinoma in adults: diagnostic problems, pathological features and treatment. Scand J Urol Nephrol. 43(1):84-7, 2009
2. Gong K et al: Multilocular cystic renal cell carcinoma: an experience of clinical management for 31 cases. J Cancer Res Clin Oncol. 134(4):433-7, 2008
3. Halat SK et al: Multilocular cystic renal cell carcinoma. J Urol. 177(1):343, 2007
4. Suzigan S et al: Multilocular cystic renal cell carcinoma : a report of 45 cases of a kidney tumor of low malignant potential. Am J Clin Pathol. 125(2):217-22, 2006
5. Grignon DJ et al: VHL gene mutations in multilocular cystic renal cell carcinoma: evidence in support of its classification as a type of clear cell renal cell carcinoma. Mod Pathol. 17(1):154A, 2004
6. Imura J et al: Multilocular cystic renal cell carcinoma: a clinicopathological, immuno- and lectin histochemical study of nine cases. APMIS. 112(3):183-91, 2004
7. Bloom TL et al: Multilocular cystic renal cell carcinoma with osseous metaplasia in a 25-year-old woman. Urology. 61(2):462, 2003
8. Nassir A et al: Multilocular cystic renal cell carcinoma: a series of 12 cases and review of the literature. Urology. 60(3):421-7, 2002
9. Eble JN et al: Extensively cystic renal neoplasms: cystic nephroma, cystic partially differentiated nephroblastoma, multilocular cystic renal cell carcinoma, and cystic hamartoma of renal pelvis. Semin Diagn Pathol. 15(1):2-20, 1998
10. Murad T et al: Multilocular cystic renal cell carcinoma. Am J Clin Pathol. 95(5):633-7, 1991

MULTILOCULAR CYSTIC RENAL CELL CARCINOMA

Microscopic Features

(Left) All multilocular renal cell carcinomas have a variably prominent fibrous pseudocapsule ➲ delineating them from the surrounding renal parenchyma. Occasionally, the capsule may also contain clusters of tumor cells with clear cytology. *(Right)* By definition, multilocular cystic renal cell carcinoma always shows the presence of clusters of clear cells ➲ within the fibrous septations. Notice that these clear cells do not alter the smooth profiles of the septae.

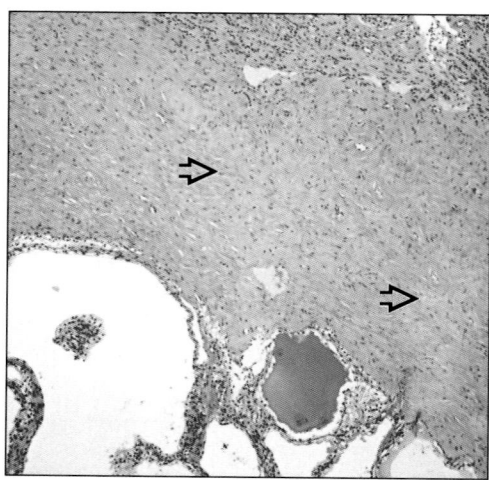
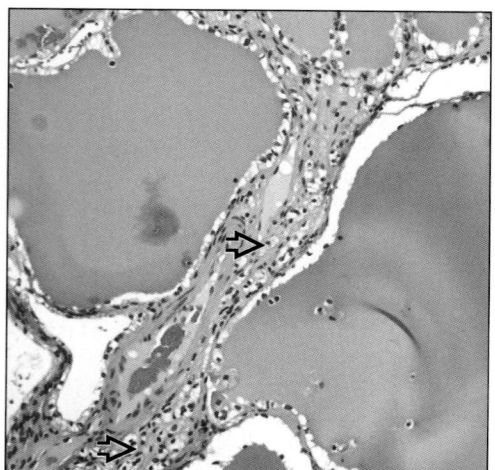

(Left) The cysts in multilocular cystic renal cell carcinoma are of variable size and shape. Many tumors are composed of relatively small cysts. Such tumors may appear somewhat solid on gross evaluation. *(Right)* Other multilocular cystic renal cell carcinomas may be almost entirely composed of large cysts. Grossly, such tumors will show spongy to predominantly macrocystic features, often filled with serous or hemorrhagic fluid, and occasionally clotted blood.

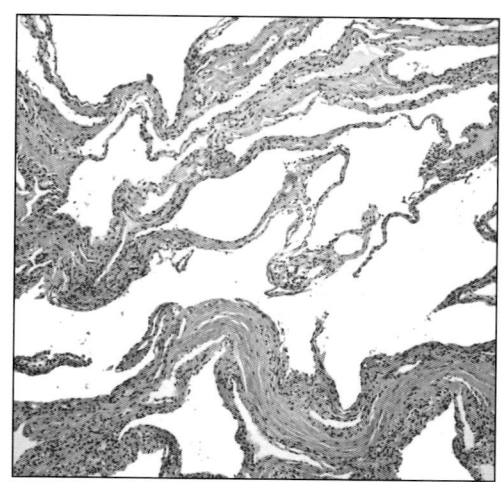
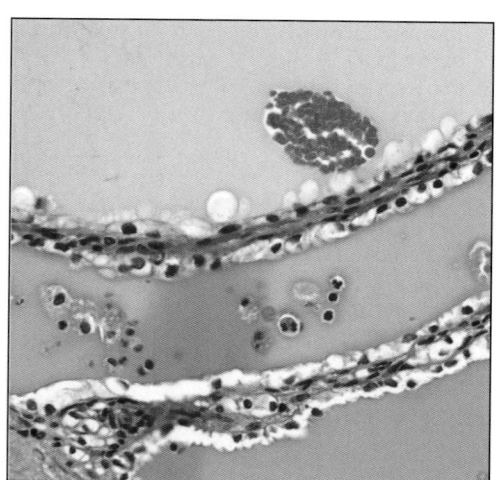

(Left) Rarely, multilocular cystic RCC may be composed of only a few cysts. Careful sampling and microscopic evaluation often reveals clusters of clear cells within fibrous septations or capsule ➲. Because of the compression artifacts in such clusters, the use of epithelial markers may be needed to confirm the diagnosis. *(Right)* Hematoxylin & eosin shows clear cell RCC with multicystic growth. Expansile nodule of clear cells in a cystic tumor essentially excludes the designation of multilocular RCC.

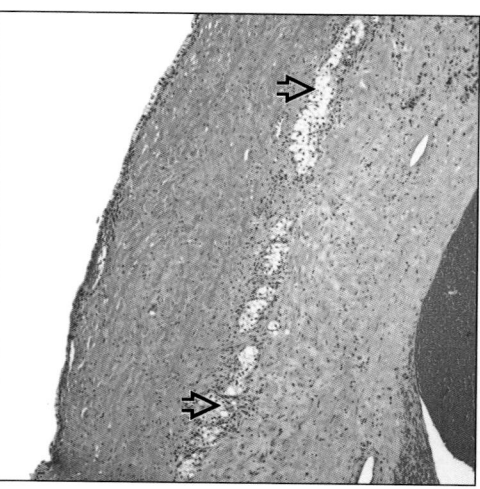
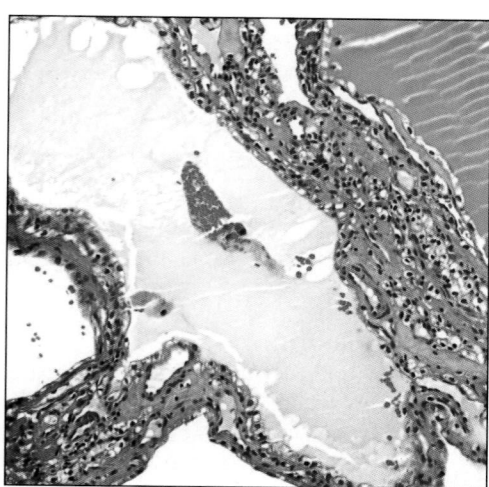

Differential Diagnosis and Immunohistochemistry Features

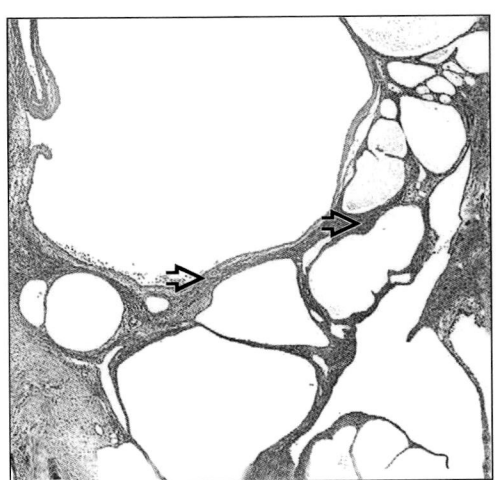

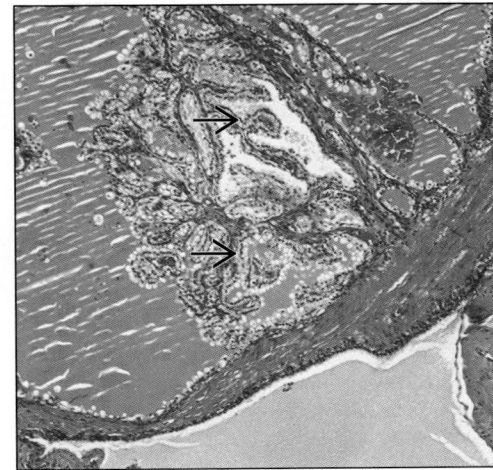

(Left) Cystic nephroma is a close differential diagnostic consideration for multilocular cystic RCC. These tumors often have cellular spindle cell histology ⇒ in the septae. Immunostains for ER and PR are positive. *(Right)* Clear cell papillary RCC with cystic features is another close differential diagnostic consideration for multilocular cystic RCC. The papillary proliferations in the former typically show a linear arrangement of nuclei away from basement membrane ➡.

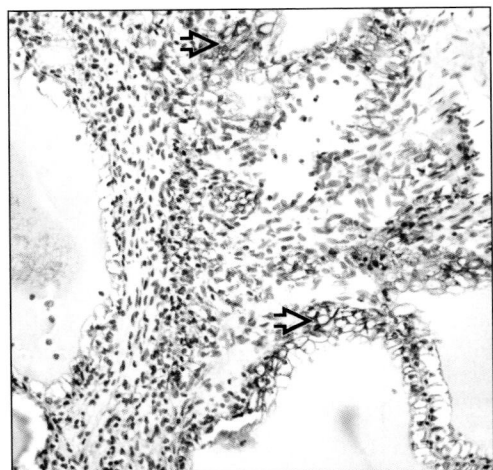

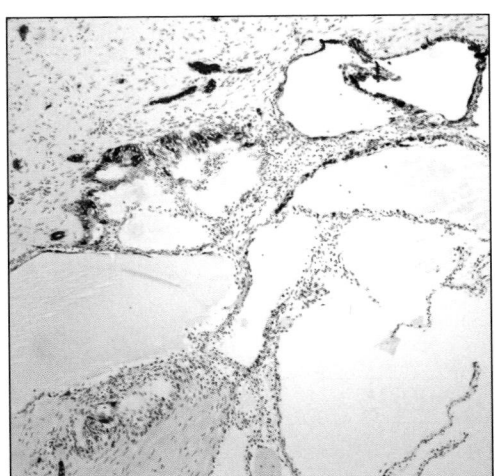

(Left) Multilocular cystic renal cell carcinomas show diffuse membranous positivity ⇒ for CA9, similar to that seen in clear cell renal cell carcinoma. *(Right)* Most multilocular cystic RCC show positivity for CK7, highlighting the differential diagnostic consideration of clear cell papillary RCC. However, the positivity is often patchy, similar to that in clear cell RCCs with cystic features. CK7 is positive in almost all cells in clear cell papillary RCC.

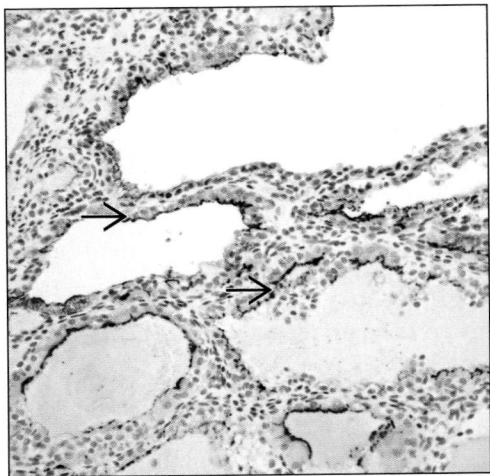

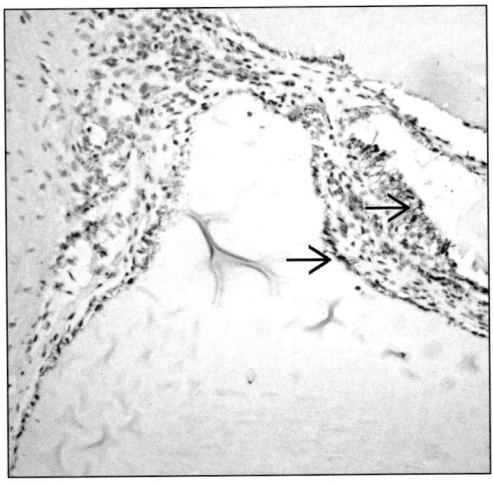

(Left) CD10 immunoreactivity is frequent in multilocular cystic RCC. In most cases it is patchy and luminal ➡, unlike the diffuse membranous reactivity seen in most clear cell RCCs. *(Right)* Similar to typical clear cell and unlike clear cell papillary RCC, staining with HMCK(34βE12) is either negative or focally positive ➡ in multilocular cystic RCC. Thus the relationship of multilocular cystic RCC with clear cell RCC and clear cell papillary RCC remains indeterminate.

PAPILLARY RENAL CELL CARCINOMA

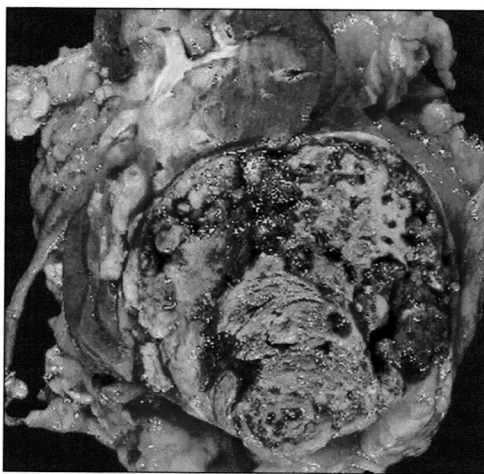

Gross photograph of a papillary RCC shows an encapsulated mass with a necrotic and hemorrhagic cut surface. Among the common renal cell tumors, papillary RCC is the most likely to have a capsule.

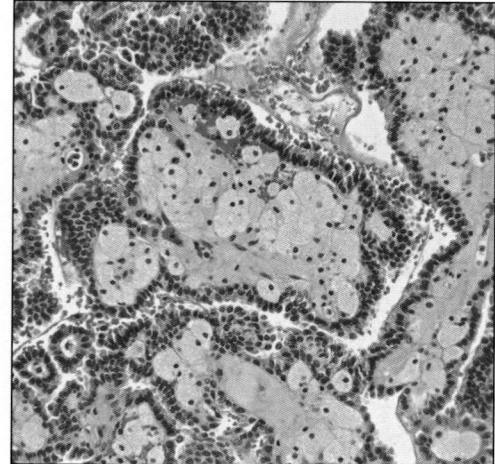

This photomicrograph shows the typical features of a papillary RCC, with prominent papillae and abundant foamy macrophages in the papillary cores. The lining cells are amphophilic and cuboidal.

TERMINOLOGY

Abbreviations
- Papillary renal cell carcinoma (PRCC)

Synonyms
- Chromophilic renal cell carcinoma

Definitions
- 2nd most common subtype of renal cell carcinoma, usually showing predominant or exclusive papillary architecture, frequently with well-formed tumor capsule

ETIOLOGY/PATHOGENESIS

Molecular Characteristics
- Majority of sporadic PRCCs are characterized by trisomy of chromosomes 7 and 17, as well as loss of chromosome Y
- Trisomies of chromosomes 12, 16, and 20 and loss of heterozygosity at 9p13 are observed in some cases
  - Some investigators suggest that tumors with trisomy 7/17 alone are likely to have benign behavior
    - Whereas those with additional genetic abnormalities behave aggressively
- More gains of 7p and 17p by CGH reported by some in type 1, compared to type 2 tumors
- Activating mutations of *MET* oncogene, located at 7q31, present in all cases of hereditary papillary renal carcinoma syndrome
  - Similar mutations observed in approximately 13% sporadic papillary RCCs

CLINICAL ISSUES

Epidemiology
- Incidence
  - Comprise 11-15% of renal cell neoplasms

- Age
  - Ranges from 3rd to 8th decades of life with peak incidence in 6th and 7th decades
  - Similar to other renal cell tumors
- Gender
  - Reported M:F = 1.8:1-4:1

Presentation
- > 50% of cases present as incidental masses, detected on radiologic investigation for unrelated conditions
- Reported size ranges from 1-18 cm (median: 6.4 cm)
  - However, downward size migration seen in modern times due to incidental discovery on imaging
- Although majority of patients have unilateral tumors, PRCC is more often bilateral and multifocal compared to other common renal cell tumors

Treatment
- Surgical approaches
  - Partial nephrectomy is preferred option
    - Total or radical nephrectomy rarely performed now at some institutions even for tumors > 4 cm in size
- Drugs
  - Resistance to systemic therapy characterizes patients with metastatic papillary RCC
  - Targeted therapies against VEGF tyrosine kinases (e.g., sunitinib) in metastatic PRCC with clinical responses in occasional case
    - Similar targeted therapies are focus of attention in multiple ongoing clinical trials
  - Targeting *MET* signaling pathway is another therapeutic approach under active investigation

Prognosis
- Overall, 5- and 10-year survivals better than clear cell RCC, and possibly worse than chromophobe RCC
  - However, some studies show no significant prognostic differences between PRCC and chromophobe RCC

PAPILLARY RENAL CELL CARCINOMA

Key Facts

Terminology

- Papillary renal cell carcinoma (PRCC)
- 2nd most common subtype of renal cell carcinoma, usually showing predominant or exclusive papillary architecture, frequently with well-formed tumor capsule

Etiology/Pathogenesis

- Majority of sporadic PRCCs are characterized by trisomy of chromosomes 7 and 17, as well as loss of chromosome Y

Clinical Issues

- Although majority of patients with unilateral tumors, PRCC is more often bilateral and multifocal compared to other common renal cell tumors

Macroscopic Features

- Often surrounded by fibrous pseudocapsule on gross evaluation
- Most exhibit variegated cut surface

Microscopic Pathology

- Majority of PRCCs exhibit broad morphologic spectrum, including papillary, tubular, and solid patterns
- Areas containing papillary architecture seen in most cases
- Cores of papillae are mostly loose and fibrovascular, often containing variable amount of foamy macrophages
- WHO divides papillary RCC into type 1 and type 2

MACROSCOPIC FEATURES

General Features

- Well-circumscribed mass
- Often surrounded by fibrous pseudocapsule on gross evaluation
  - Of all common renal cell tumor types, papillary renal cell carcinoma is most likely to be surrounded by fibrous pseudocapsule
- Most exhibit variegated cut surface
  - Color is related to microscopic findings
    - Tumors with abundant foamy macrophages, tan to yellow
    - Tumors with intratumoral hemorrhage, dark tan to brown
- Grossly visible areas of necrosis, hemorrhage, and cystic change very common, present in 32-70% of tumors
  - Some tumors almost entirely necrotic
- Multifocality is present in > 45% of cases
  - In some, this is reported to be only a microscopic finding
    - Many such microscopic tumors may be considered papillary adenomas now

MICROSCOPIC PATHOLOGY

Histologic Features

- Majority of PRCCs exhibit broad morphologic spectrum, including papillary, tubular, and solid patterns
  - Papillary patterns include
    - Classic papillary with discrete papillary fronds lined by neoplastic cells with central fibrovascular core
    - Papillary-trabecular with delicate, elongated papillations arranged in parallel fashion
    - Papillary-solid with closely packed papillae, sometimes masking their true growth pattern
  - Areas containing papillary architecture seen in most cases

  - However, > 50% show variable proportion of "solid," tubular, &/or glomeruloid growth patterns
    - Glomeruloid growth pattern composed of tubular structures with intraluminal tufting of tumor cells
    - Cells lining tubules are cuboidal with scant to moderate amphophilic cytoplasm
    - Cells tufting into lumen with abundant eosinophilic cytoplasm and usually higher-grade nuclei
  - Rarely, sarcomatoid growth may be seen and is sign of aggressive disease
- Cores of papillae are mostly loose and fibrovascular, often containing variable number of foamy macrophages
  - However, variations in morphology of cores are not uncommon, and may include
    - Cores with no macrophages
    - Cores with branching papillae
    - Some papillae with no distinct cores, as in tumors with micropapillary features
    - Marked hyalinization of cores
    - Variable degree of edema, sometimes leading to fluid-filled, grape-like polypoid structures
- WHO divides papillary RCC into 2 types
  - Type 1 with papillae covered by smaller cells with scant, amphophilic cytoplasm
  - Type 2 with larger tumor cells, often with higher nuclear grade, eosinophilic cytoplasm, and nuclear pseudostratification
  - Type 1 tumors more often positive for CK7 than type 2 PRCC
  - Reportedly worse prognosis in type 2 compared to type 1 tumors
  - Trisomies 7 and 17 more often reported in type 1 than type 2 PRCC
  - *MET* gene mutations only present in type 1 PRCC
  - Many tumors that are not PRCC and have prominent papillary architecture are more often mistakenly regarded as type 2 PRCC
- Psammoma bodies, hemosiderin-laden macrophages, hemosiderin deposition within tumor cells are often seen in PRCC

PAPILLARY RENAL CELL CARCINOMA

- WHO classification system does not address issue of PRCC with mixture of type 1 and type 2 morphologic features
  - Combination of features of both types not uncommon
    - In older literature, such tumors designated as "duophilic"
  - Recently, tumors with oncocytic cytoplasm with low-grade nonoverlapping nuclei described as "oncocytic" PRCC
    - Immunohistochemically CK7 positive
    - Show trisomies 7 and 17
    - Show biologic behavior similar to type 1 PRCC
    - Features suggest that eosinophilic PRCC with low-grade nuclei are molecularly and biologically similar to type 1 tumors
  - Molecular evaluation also suggests modified classification of PRCC
    - Type 1: Similar to type 1 of WHO
    - Type 2A: Tumors with eosinophilic cytoplasm but low-grade nuclei
    - Type 2B: Tumors with mixture of type 1 and type 2A features
    - Type 2C: Tumors with high-grade nuclei; tumors often with topoisomerase II-α overexpression
  - Nuclear grading
    - Many believe Fuhrman grading system is well suited for PRCC
    - Others disagree and do not use Fuhrman grading scheme in PRCC
    - Others recently proposed only assessment of nucleolar prominence in most pleomorphic foci rather than Fuhrman grade

Predominant Pattern/Injury Type

- Neoplastic

Predominant Cell/Compartment Type

- Epithelial

ANCILLARY TESTS

Immunohistochemistry

- Diffuse positivity for CK7 very frequent
  - More often in type 1 than type 2 tumors
- AMACR diffusely positive, with cytoplasmic granular staining
- CD10 often positive, usually with luminal membranous staining
- CA9 either negative or focally positive
  - Positivity usually limited to papillary tips or perinecrotic areas
- RCC and pax-2 positive

DIFFERENTIAL DIAGNOSIS

Clear Cell RCC Exhibiting Papillary or Pseudopapillary Growth

- Focal papillary architecture may be seen in clear cell RCC

- Usually result of cell drop-off in areas away from feeding vessels
  - This usually creates pseudopapillary appearance
  - Adequate sampling and presence of typical cytoarchitectural features of clear cell RCC in other areas should clarify issue
  - Prominent psammoma bodies and hemosiderin deposition within tumor cells are not present in clear cell RCC
  - Any fibrovascular cores would be unusual in clear cell RCC and, if present, would be focal
  - Clear cells in clear cell RCC usually have optically transparent, completely clear cytoplasm
    - In papillary RCC, clear-appearing cells usually with variable granularity and often fine hemosiderin
  - CK7 and AMACR immunoreactivity usually (-) or very focal in clear cell RCC
  - CA9 shows diffuse membranous reactivity in majority of clear cell RCCs

Collecting Duct Carcinoma (CDC)

- Has variable amount of papillary growth pattern
- Is centered in medulla
- Invariably widely infiltrative and pseudocapsule, if present, is focal
- Virtually always high grade
- Associated with pronounced desmoplastic stroma
- Shows prominent multinodular growth pattern and glandular and sheet-like architecture
- Intracytoplasmic and luminal mucin, often focal, common feature
- Often reactive for CEA, PNA, soybean agglutin, ULEX-1, Ulex europaeus, and HMCK(34βE12)
  - CK7 may be expressed in both tumors
- Cytogenetic studies may be needed to solve difficult diagnostic problems

MiTF/TFE Family Translocation-associated Renal Carcinomas (TFE Carcinoma)

- More common in young patients
- Rarely multifocal
- Admixture of solid, nested, and papillary growth
- Usually with high nuclear grade and often with cells showing voluminous cytoplasm
  - Cytoplasm varies from clear to eosinophilic
- (-) or only focally (+) for cytokeratins and EMA/MUC1
  - Characteristically exhibit nuclear immunoreactivity for TFE3 or TFEB, depending on the translocation

Hereditary Leiomyomatosis RCC (HLRCC)-Related Renal Carcinoma

- Tumors show variable, but often prominent, papillary architecture
  - Considered to be type 2 PRCCs in the past
- Other architectural patterns, including glandular, alveolar, and solid are often present
- Usually CK7 negative
- History of leiomyomas, both uterine and others, is common
- Most characteristic morphologic feature is very prominent nucleoli with perinucleolar halos

PAPILLARY RENAL CELL CARCINOMA

- Molecular evidence of fumarate hydratase (*FH*) gene alterations

Clear Cell Papillary RCC (CC-PRCC)

- Clear cell cytology with almost exclusive clear cell cytology
- Usually have low nuclear grade
- Variable amount of papillary and tubular architecture and cystic change
- Most characteristic feature: Nuclei aligned in linear fashion away from basal aspect of cells
- Almost 100% cells stain diffusely with CK7
- Stains diffusely (+) for CA9
- (-) AMACR and CD10 (most often) staining
- At least focal staining for HMCK(34βE12)

Metanephric Adenoma

- Vs. solid-architecture PRCC
  - Metanephric adenoma mostly without pseudocapsule
  - Most important feature in PRCC
    - PRCC has more abundant cytoplasm, along with prominent nucleoli
    - These nuclear features are not acceptable in metanephric adenoma
- CK7 and AMACR immunostaining usually (-) or only focally (+) in metanephric adenoma
  - (+) in PRCC
- CD57 and WT1 usually (+) in metanephric adenoma
  - (-) in PRCC

Mucinous Tubular Spindle Cell Carcinoma (MTSCC)

- Vs. PRCC with low-grade spindle cell areas
  - One of the more difficult differential diagnoses
  - Luminal surfaces in MSTCC are regular and smooth
    - Glands and papillae in such PRCCs often with very irregular luminal outlines
- Myxoid or mucinous stroma in MTSCC; not present in PRCC
- Molecular analysis shows trisomies of chromosomes 7 and 17 and loss of Y chromosomes in this variant of PRCC
  - Such features not found in MTSCC

Other Tumors with Papillary Architecture

- Papillary urothelial carcinoma of pelvicalyceal system
  - Papillae lined by transitional epithelium; usually CK7, CK20, HMCK(34βE12), and p63(+)
- Chromophobe RCC with papillary architecture
  - Papillations focal; raisinoid nuclei with perinuclear halos; accompanying other architectural patterns almost always present
- Juxtaglomerular cell tumor with papillary architecture
  - Tumor cells with uniform round nuclei; papillary lining CK(+), rest of cells CK(-)

DIAGNOSTIC CHECKLIST

Pathologic Interpretation Pearls

- Many renal cell tumors besides papillary RCC show variable, often prominent, papillary architecture

- Prominent multinodular growth pattern and more than focal desmoplasia are not usual features in papillary RCC, including type 2 PRCC
- Alternative diagnosis in nonclassic cases should always be considered, and diagnosis should be based on overall cytoarchitectural features

SELECTED REFERENCES

1. Chowdhury S et al: Recent advances in the systemic treatment of metastatic papillary renal cancer. Expert Rev Anticancer Ther. 9(3):373-9, 2009
2. Giubellino A et al: Targeting the Met signaling pathway in renal cancer. Expert Rev Anticancer Ther. 9(6):785-93, 2009
3. Klatte T et al: Cytogenetic and molecular tumor profiling for type 1 and type 2 papillary renal cell carcinoma. Clin Cancer Res. 15(4):1162-9, 2009
4. Linehan WM: Genetic basis of bilateral renal cancer: implications for evaluation and management. J Clin Oncol. 27(23):3731-3, 2009
5. Okoń K et al: Renal papillary carcinoma classification into subtypes may be reproduced by nuclear morphometry. Anal Quant Cytol Histol. 31(2):109-17, 2009
6. Rosner I et al: The clinical implications of the genetics of renal cell carcinoma. Urol Oncol. 27(2):131-6, 2009
7. Suh JH et al: Clinicopathologic features of renal cell carcinoma in young adults: a comparison study with renal cell carcinoma in older patients. Int J Clin Exp Pathol. 2(5):489-93, 2009
8. Vikram R et al: Papillary renal cell carcinoma: radiologic-pathologic correlation and spectrum of disease. Radiographics. 29(3):741-54; discussion 755-7, 2009
9. Choueiri TK et al: Efficacy of sunitinib and sorafenib in metastatic papillary and chromophobe renal cell carcinoma. J Clin Oncol. 26(1):127-31, 2008
10. Kunju LP et al: Papillary renal cell carcinoma with oncocytic cells and nonoverlapping low grade nuclei: expanding the morphologic spectrum with emphasis on clinicopathologic, immunohistochemical and molecular features. Hum Pathol. 39(1):96-101, 2008
11. Tickoo SK et al: Pathologic features of renal cortical tumors. Urol Clin North Am. 35(4):551-61; v, 2008
12. Hes O et al: Oncocytic papillary renal cell carcinoma: a clinicopathologic, immunohistochemical, ultrastructural, and interphase cytogenetic study of 12 cases. Ann Diagn Pathol. 10(3):133-9, 2006
13. Ronnen EA et al: Treatment outcome for metastatic papillary renal cell carcinoma patients. Cancer. 107(11):2617-21, 2006
14. Skinnider BF et al: An immunohistochemical approach to the differential diagnosis of renal tumors. Semin Diagn Pathol. 22(1):51-68, 2005
15. Yang XJ et al: A molecular classification of papillary renal cell carcinoma. Cancer Res. 65(13):5628-37, 2005

PAPILLARY RENAL CELL CARCINOMA

Gross and Microscopic Features

(Left) This PRCC shows a homogeneous tan cut surface. The appearance of the cut surface is reflective of the microscopic features, indicating relative lack of necrosis and paucity of lipid-laden macrophages in this case. Solid, homogeneous-appearing PRCC are frequently type 1 tumors. (Right) This papillary renal cell carcinoma shows a prominent yellow cut surface. Yellow color is indicative of prominent lipid-laden (foamy) macrophages in the tumor.

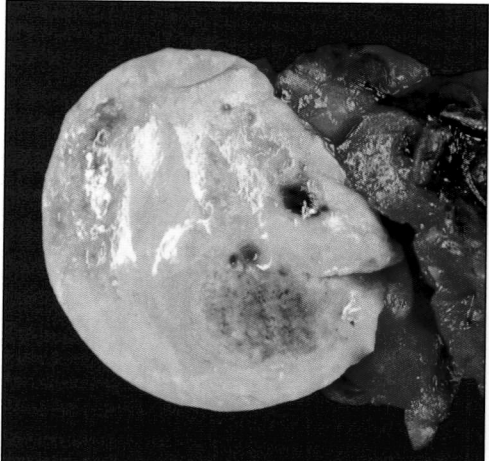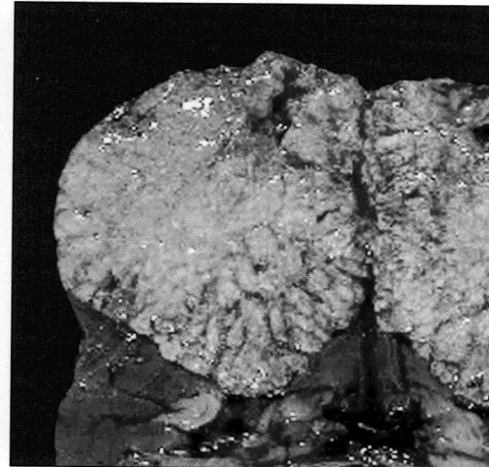

(Left) This kidney shows at least 5 PRCCs ➡. Among the more common tumors, PRCC is most likely to show multifocality in addition to encapsulation or circumscription. Each tumor may have a different gross appearance depending on the amount of necrosis and foam cells. The largest mass shows extensive necrosis ⮕. (Right) As is usually evident on gross appearance, many PRCCs show a prominent capsule on microscopy. The capsule is often lined by epithelial cells of the tumor ➡.

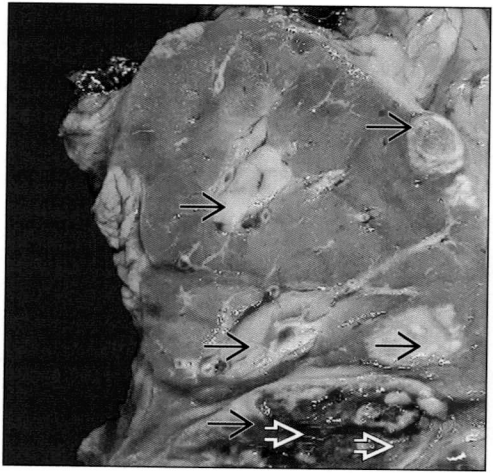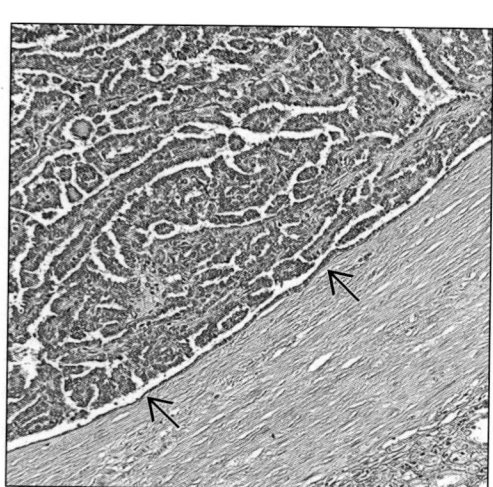

(Left) This image of a papillary RCC shows no encapsulation, and the tumor front is in direct contact with surrounding nephrons ⮕. Absent or discontinuous pseudocapsule is uncommon in papillary RCC, and this is usually, but not always, associated with smaller tumors. (Right) This hematoxylin & eosin stained section of papillary renal cell carcinoma shows discrete papillary fronds lined by neoplastic cells and with central fibrovascular cores.

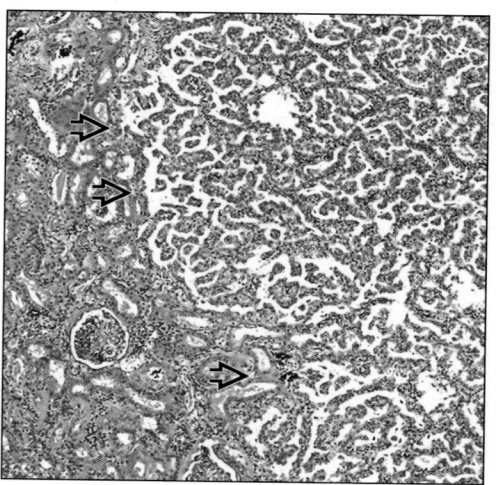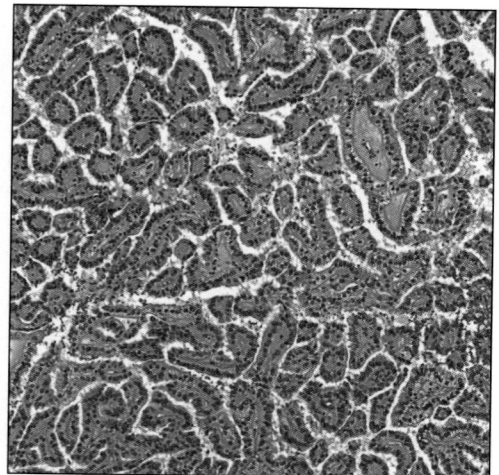

PAPILLARY RENAL CELL CARCINOMA

Microscopic Features

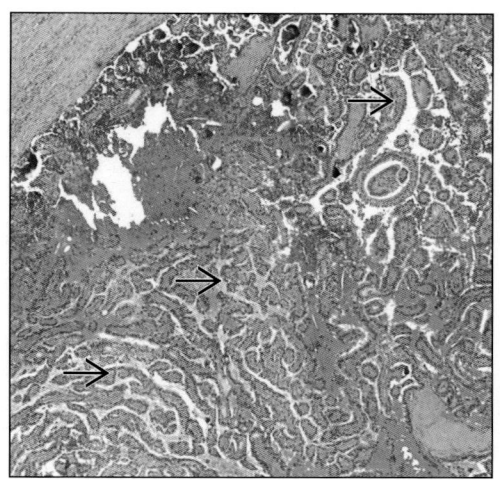

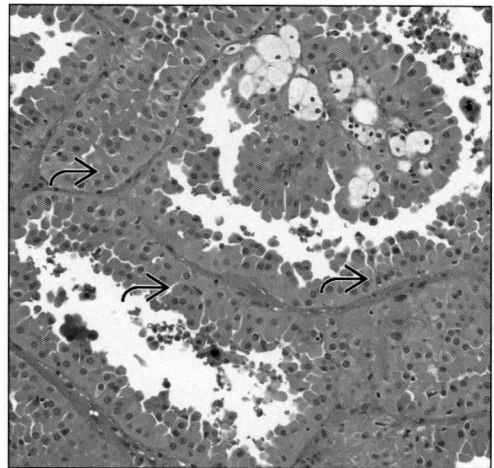

(Left) The papillae may be lined by smaller cells with scant, amphophilic cytoplasm ➡. Papillary RCC with these features are regarded as type 1, according to WHO. (Right) Type 2 papillary renal cell carcinoma shows larger tumor cells, often with higher nuclear grade, eosinophilic cytoplasm, and nuclear pseudostratification ➡. Differences in the molecular profiles and biological behaviors between type 1 and type 2 tumors have been reported in multiple studies.

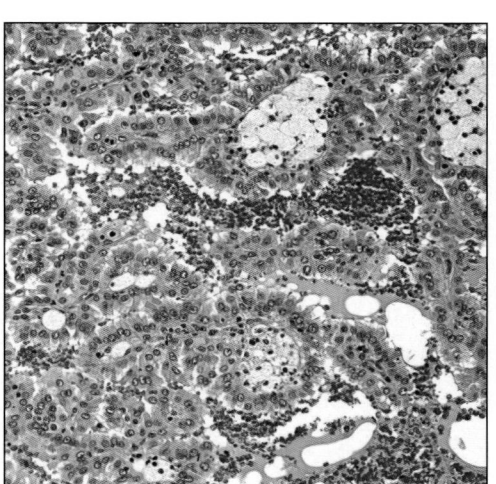

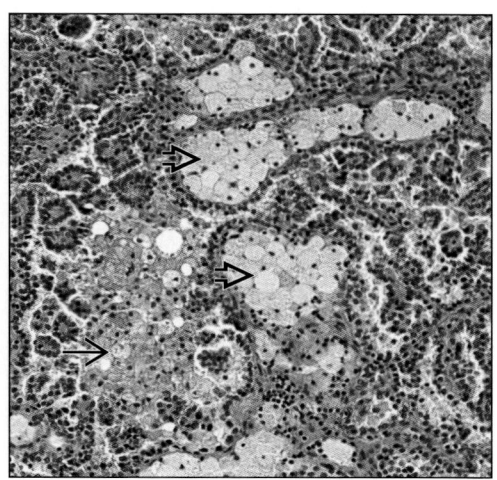

(Left) Foamy macrophages are usually more prominent in tumors with low-grade cytology and may be scant or absent in tumors composed of high-grade eosinophilic epithelial cells. (Right) The cores of the papillae in papillary renal cell carcinoma commonly show variable amounts of foamy macrophages ➡. Occasionally, the foam cells may also be observed in the spaces between papillae ➡. Predominant areas of foam cells in the interstitium may raise concern for a clear cell RCC.

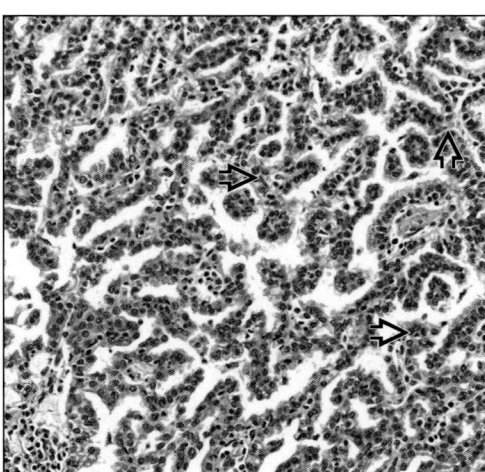

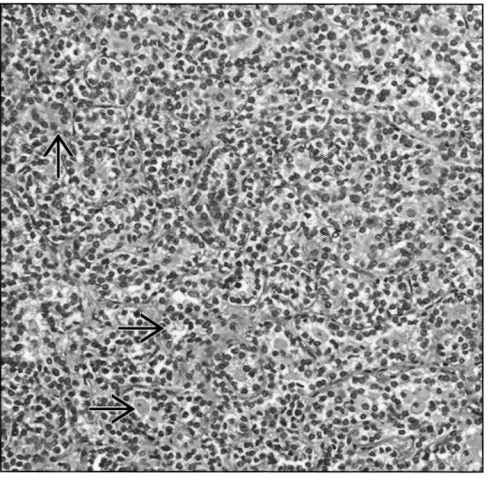

(Left) PRCC showing branching papillae ➡ is not a rare finding. Some have suggested the term "micropapillary variant" when fibrovascular cores are absent. (Right) PRCC shows tightly packed papillae, resulting in a "solid" appearance. Also note multiple tubular structures ➡ in the image. Many of these tubules represent cross-sectional profiles of papillae. When the papillae are arranged in long parallel arrays, a papillary-trabecular appearance may be appreciated.

Microscopic Features and Ancillary Techniques

(Left) Glomeruloid architecture may be seen in PRCC. While this finding may be focal, some tumors are entirely composed of glomeruloid structures arranged back to back. (Right) The glomeruloid structures in PRCC consist of tubules with intraluminal tufting of tumor cells. In this case, the cells lining the tubules ⊟ are cuboidal with scant, amphophilic cytoplasm, while the tufting cells are larger with abundant, often eosinophilic cytoplasm, and display prominent nucleoli ⊟.

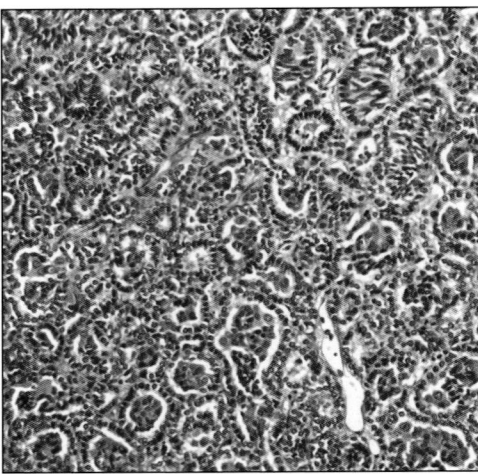 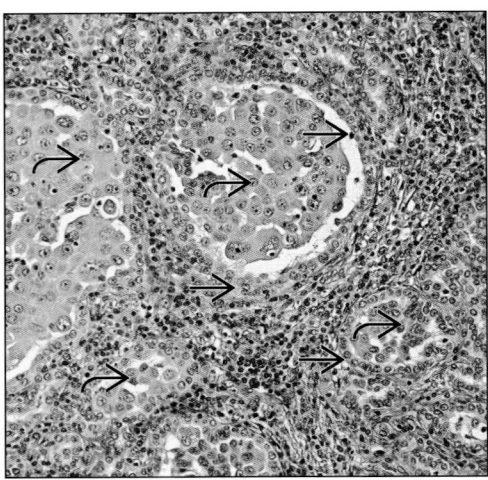

(Left) Type 2 PRCC usually shows a paucity of foamy macrophages. Tumoral-cell hemosiderin is more common in these tumors than type 1 tumors. They also show absence of MET gene mutations and are less commonly CK7 positive than type 1 cases. (Right) Some PRCCs show an admixture of type 1 ⊟ and type 2 ⊟ areas. The WHO classification system does not address the issue of tumors with such combined histologies, and it is not necessary in pathology reports to subclassify PRCC.

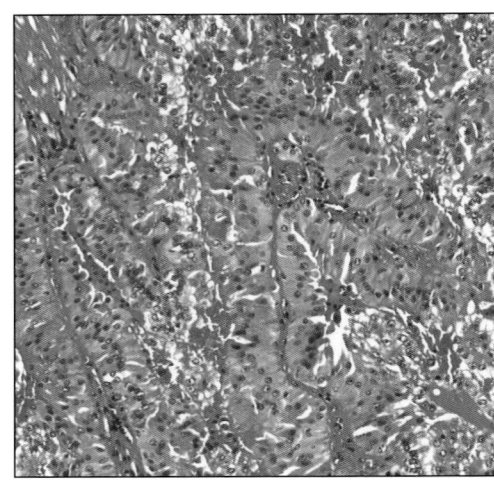 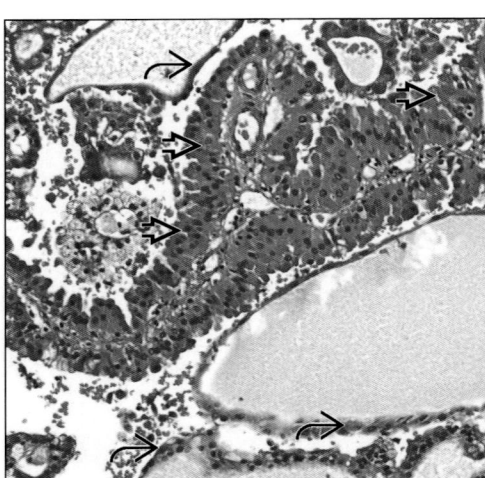

(Left) One of the other common findings in PRCC is the presence of hemosiderin in the macrophages as well as tumor cells ⊟. While this finding may be seen in tumors with type 1 histology, it is more common in tumors with abundant eosinophilic cytoplasm. (Right) Perl iron stain confirms hemosiderin in the tumor cells ⊟ as well as in the macrophages ⊟ between the papillae. Hale colloidal iron may also show intense staining with hemosiderin.

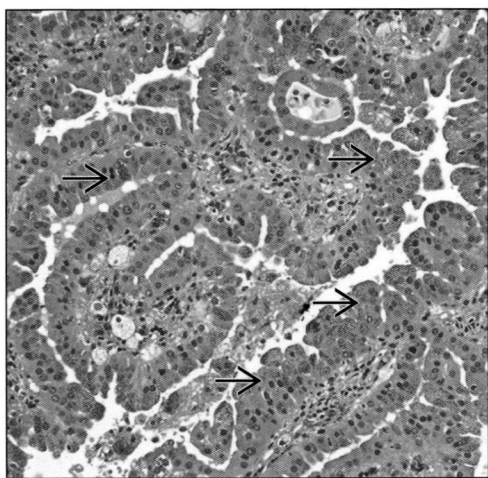 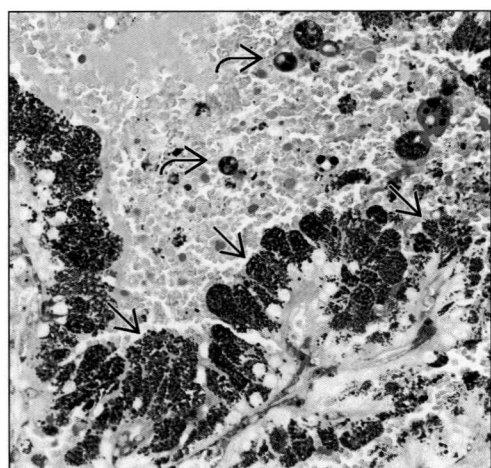

PAPILLARY RENAL CELL CARCINOMA

Microscopic and Immunohistochemical Features

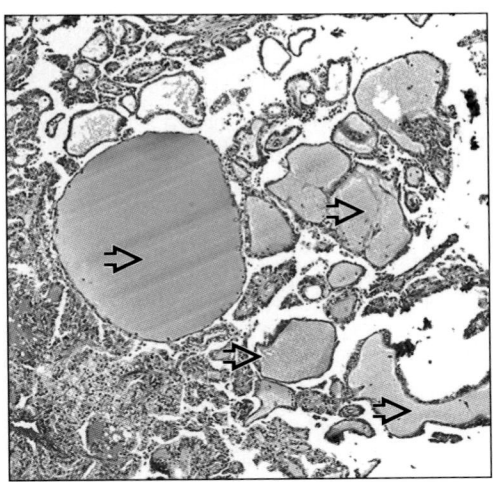

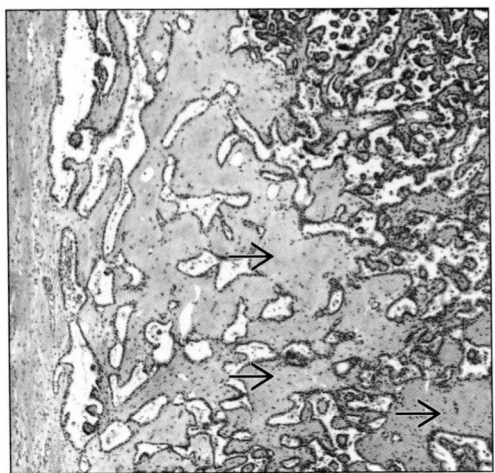

(Left) Hematoxylin & eosin of PRCC shows papillary cores with marked edema ⊟. Variable degrees of edematous fluid collection within the cores is sometimes present and occasionally may lead to grape-like, polypoid structures. *(Right)* Hematoxylin & eosin stained section shows expanded but hyalinized papillary cores ⊡ in a papillary renal cell carcinoma. This pattern of sclerotic appearance in cores is relatively uncommon and is usually only seen in type 1 papillary RCC.

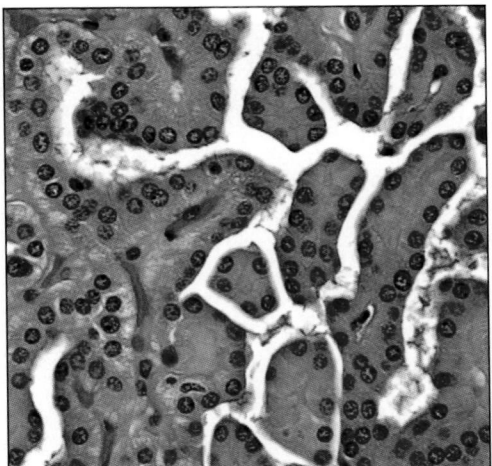

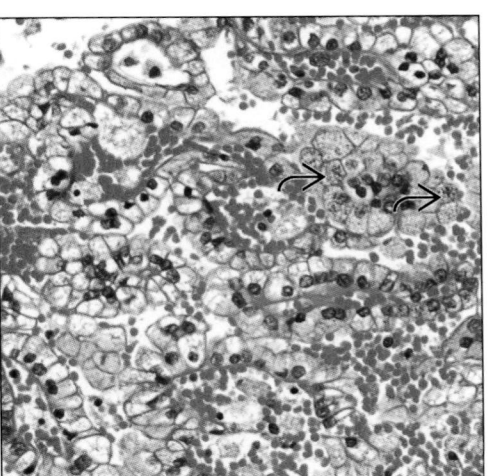

(Left) "Oncocytic" PRCC, such as this, with abundant pink cytoplasm may be considered as type 2 tumors by some. Such tumors with oncocytic cells and nonoverlapping low-grade nuclei have similar CK7 positivity & clinical outcome to type 1 RCC. The absence of pseudostratification & the finely granular cytoplasm argue against type 2 PRCC. *(Right)* Some PRCC show variable or often prominent "clear cell" areas. These clear-appearing cells often contain finely granular hemosiderin ⊡.

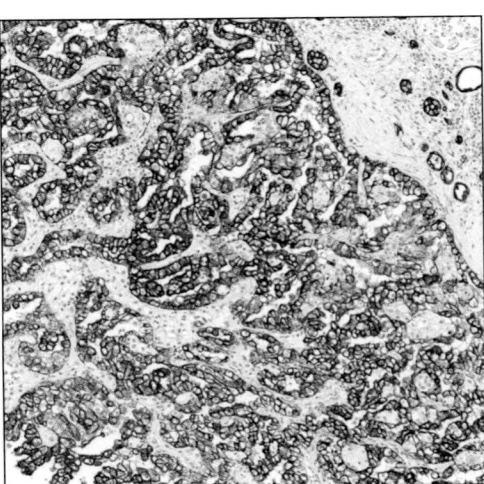

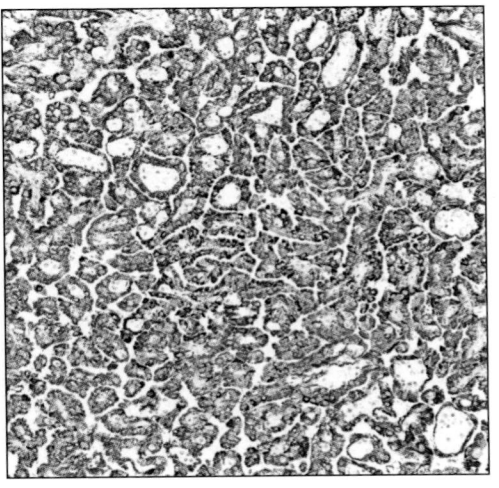

(Left) CK7 shows diffuse, cytoplasmic, & membranous positivity in PRCC. Such diffuse staining is more often seen in tumors with type 1, rather than type 2, features. Other positive markers include RCC, pax-2, & CD10. *(Right)* AMACR stain shows diffuse & strong positivity in PRCC. AMACR immunoreactivity is characterized by granular positivity in the cytoplasm. Coexpression of CK7 & AMACR is supportive of a PRCC diagnosis over other tumors, which may have papillary architecture.

Microscopic and Immunohistochemical Features

(Left) Similar to clear cell RCC, papillary RCC also shows diffuse, membrane-predominant immunoreactivity for CD10. However, the pattern of positivity is usually different. CD10 highlights the luminal aspects of the cells in PRCC ➔, whereas it usually stains all the cell membranes in clear cell RCC in a box-like fashion. *(Right)* Unlike clear cell RCC, PRCC is usually negative for immunostaining with CA9. Less often, it may show focal positivity in the papillary tips ➔.

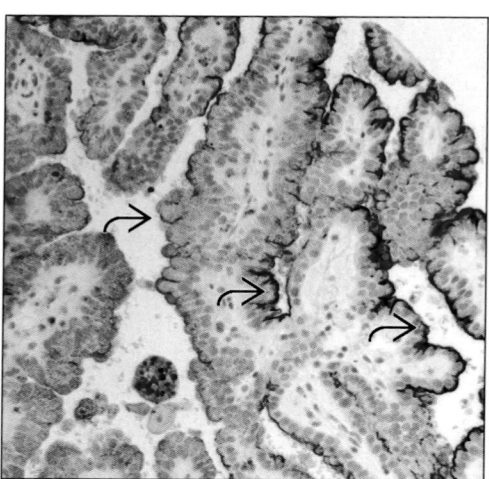
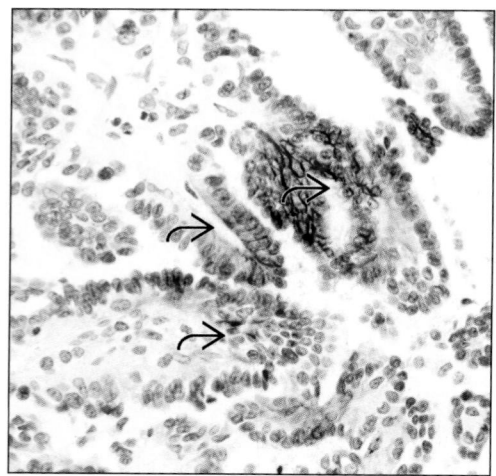

(Left) In addition to staining the papillary tips, CA9 often shows focal reactivity ➔ around foci of necrosis ➔. This pattern of staining reflects hypoxic areas and is related to overexpressed HIF. *(Right)* Rarely, PRCC may show low-grade spindle cell foci ➔ and mimic mucinous tubular spindle cell carcinoma. Usually the glands in such tumors have irregular, "shaggy" lumina ➔, and lack stromal mucin. Such tumors also show trisomies 7 and 17, as is usual in PRCC.

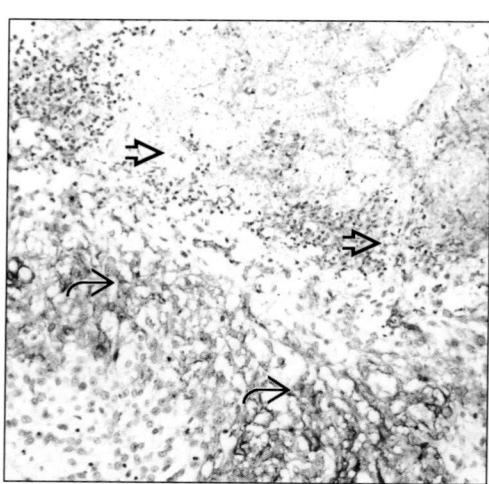
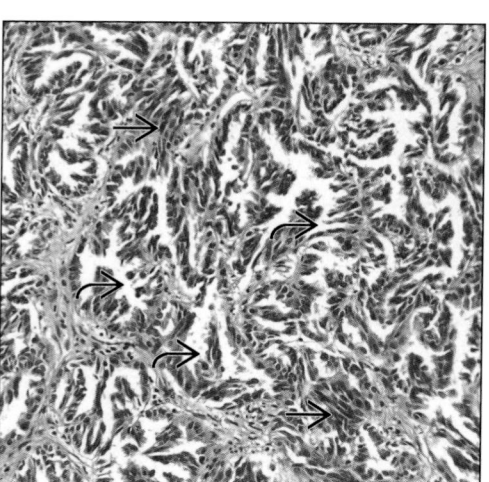

(Left) Image of hematoxylin & eosin stained section shows a PRCC with sarcomatoid features ➔. Sarcomatoid areas always show high-grade cytology. Presence of sarcomatoid areas in PRCC, as in other tumor types, predicts an aggressive behavior. *(Right)* This image shows PRCC metastatic to the lung. PRCC proportionately more often metastasizes to lymph nodes than other sites, compared to clear cell RCC, although this belief has been challenged more recently by some.

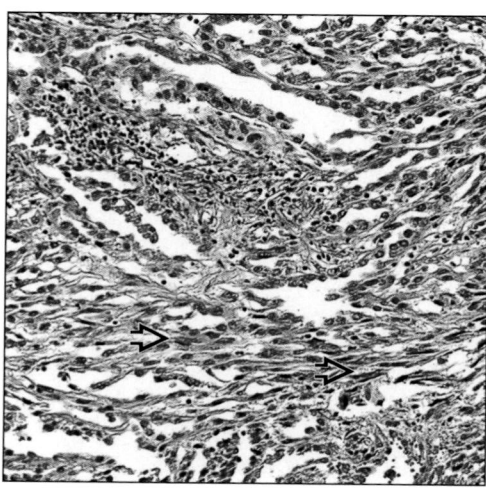
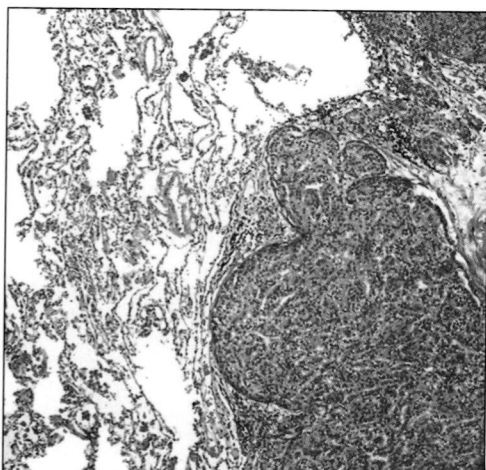

PAPILLARY RENAL CELL CARCINOMA

Differential Diagnosis

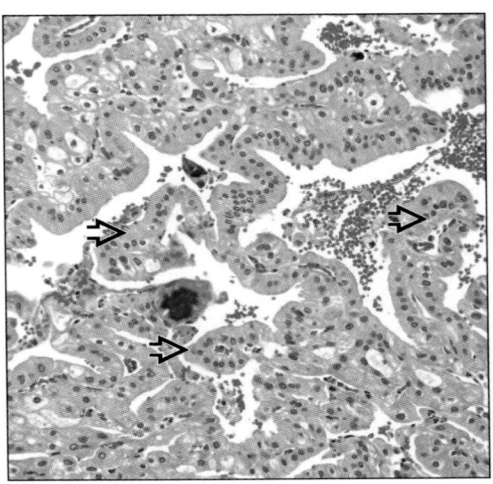

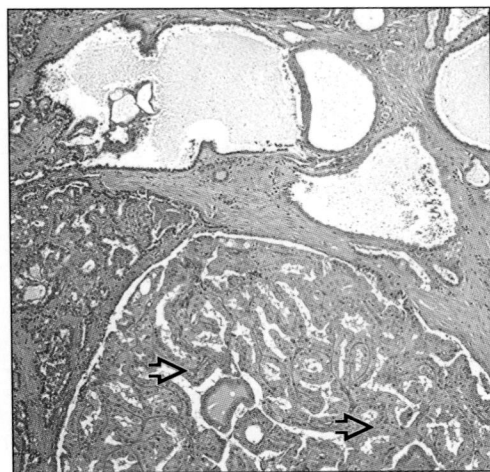

(Left) *Papillary architecture alone is not diagnostic of PRCC. Variable papillary architecture may be seen in many other tumors. This image shows focal papillations ⊳ in an otherwise typical chromophobe RCC.* **(Right)** *Collecting duct carcinoma (CDC) is often misdiagnosed as type 2 PRCC. Multinodular growth pattern, prominent stromal desmoplasia, solid sheet-like areas, glands and cysts, in spite of variable papillary architecture ⊳, favor the diagnosis of a CDC.*

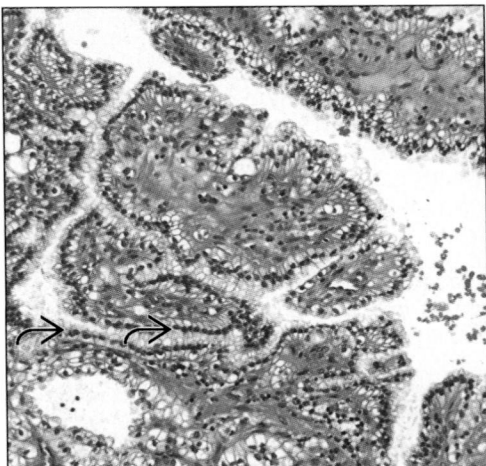

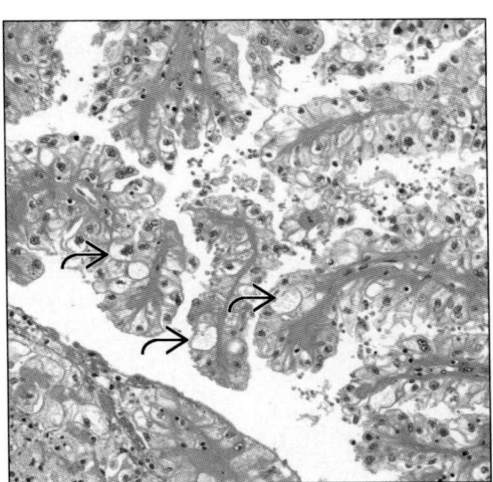

(Left) *Clear cell papillary-RCC also shows prominent papillary architecture. It has almost exclusive clear cell cytology and nuclei aligned in a linear fashion away from the basal aspect ⇗. They are AMACR(-) and CA9 diffusely(+).* **(Right)** *TFE RCCs often show prominent papillary architecture. However, they usually have clear cells, show high nuclear grade, and some cells with voluminous cytoplasm ⇗. Epithelial markers are usually negative, and the age of the patient is important.*

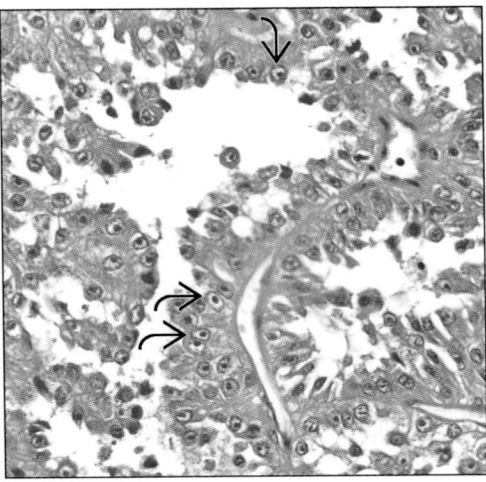

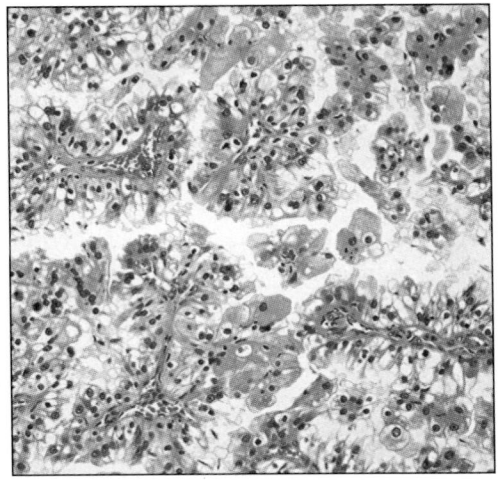

(Left) *HLRCC-related RCC usually shows features of type 2 PRCC. Other nonpapillary patterns are also common. The characteristic feature is the presence of prominent nucleoli with perinucleolar halos ⇗. They are usually CK7 negative.* **(Right)** *Some tumors with exclusive papillary architecture show features suggestive of TFE renal carcinoma, including keratin negativity. Sometimes TFE3 or TFEB positivity is not demonstrable. Such tumors are best regarded as RCC, unclassified.*

CHROMOPHOBE RENAL CELL CARCINOMA

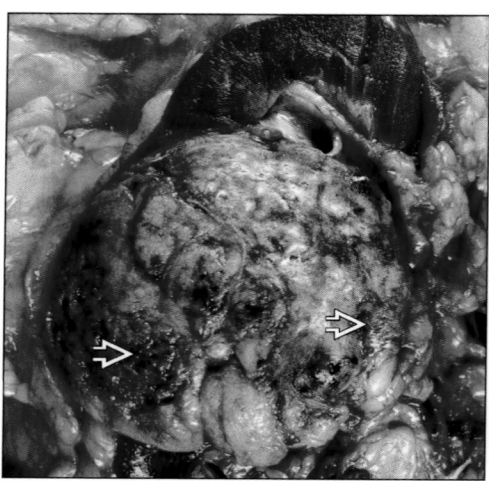

Chromophobe renal cell carcinoma is typically well circumscribed, with tan-gray, multilobulated cut surface. Hemorrhage and necrosis ⊟ are grossly identified in more than a quarter of the cases.

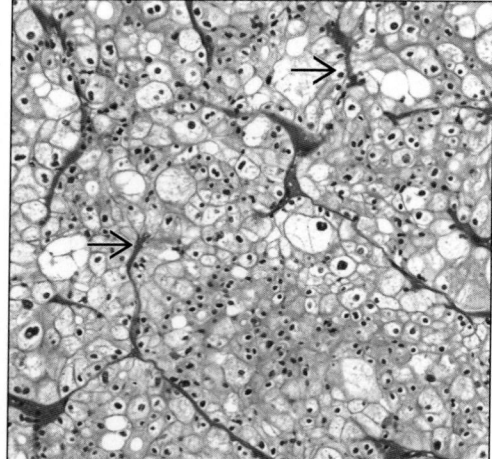

Typically, a chromophobe renal cell carcinoma shows solid sheets of clear and eosinophilic cells, separated by thin and incomplete ⊟ vascular septations that do not completely encircle cell nests.

TERMINOLOGY

Abbreviations
- Chromophobe renal cell carcinoma (Ch-RCC)

Definitions
- 3rd most common subtype of renal cell carcinoma
  - Characterized by large pale and smaller eosinophilic tumor cells in variable proportions, with wrinkled nuclei and perinuclear halos

ETIOLOGY/PATHOGENESIS

Genetic Features
- Ch-RCC typically shows combined chromosomal losses usually affecting chromosomes 1, 6, 10, 13, 17, 21, and Y
  - Loss of multiple chromosomes leads to almost consistently present hypodiploidy
- Abnormalities in mitochondrial DNA may be observed, but their specificity remains controversial
- Recently, gene expression profiling has shown up-regulation of a number of genes encoding proteins integrated to membranes
  - Many of these up-regulated gene products are related to vesicle-mediated transport

Cell of Origin
- Ch-RCC are thought to arise from intercalated cells of renal cortex, similar to renal oncocytomas

CLINICAL ISSUES

Epidemiology
- Incidence
  - Comprise 6-11% of renal epithelial tumors
- Age
  - Mean: 58 years (range: 26-62 years)
- Gender

  - M:F = 1.5:1

Presentation
- Usually present as unilateral renal mass
- Overwhelming majority are asymptomatic, with incidentally detected tumors following investigations for unrelated symptoms
- < 1/3 present with palpable mass
  - Hematuria is presenting symptom in rare cases

Treatment
- Surgical approaches
  - Partial nephrectomy surgical treatment of choice, whenever feasible
- Drugs
  - No specific chemotherapeutic agent consistently effective in metastatic cases
  - Recently, targeted therapies against vascular growth factor tyrosine kinase receptors and mTOR pathway molecules have shown some rare responses

Prognosis
- Prognosis of Ch-CRC better than papillary RCC in some studies and consistently better than clear cell RCC
- Overall, close to 95% survival rates at 5-year follow-ups
- Sarcomatoid features and perinephric extension frequently associated with aggressive clinical behavior
- Other important indicators correlating with adverse clinical outcome include
  - Pathologic tumor stage
  - Large tumor size
  - Tumor necrosis
- Overall, patients with metastatic Ch-RCC tend to do better than patients with metastasis from other common subtypes of RCC

CHROMOPHOBE RENAL CELL CARCINOMA

Key Facts

Terminology
- Chromophobe renal cell carcinoma (Ch-RCC)
- Characterized by large pale and smaller eosinophilic tumor cells in variable proportions, with wrinkled nuclei and perinuclear halos

Etiology/Pathogenesis
- Ch-RCC typically shows combined chromosomal losses usually affecting chromosomes 1, 6, 10, 13, 17, 21, and Y

Clinical Issues
- Prognosis of Ch-CRC much better than clear cell RCC, and also than papillary RCC in some studies
- Sarcomatoid features in tumor; most frequent association with aggressive clinical behavior

Microscopic Pathology
- Pattern of growth is predominantly solid, separated by thin, incomplete fibrovascular septa
- In "classic" type tumors, predominant cell type is that with a pale, somewhat clear-appearing cytoplasm
- In "eosinophilic" variants, predominance of tumor cells with densely eosinophilic, granular cytoplasm
- Most tumors show admixture of pale and eosinophilic cells
- Most characteristic histological feature: Hyperchromatic nuclei with irregular, wrinkled outlines ("raisinoid" nuclei)
- Another characteristic feature: Presence of perinuclear cytoplasmic clarity (perinuclear halos)
- Presence of cytoplasmic microvesicles is unique and consistent ultrastructural feature of Ch-RCC

IMAGE FINDINGS

Radiographic Findings
- Usually large, well-circumscribed, unicentric renal mass
- Often with features of hypovascularity
- May show central scar, similar to that seen in oncocytomas and large, low-grade clear cell RCC
  - Presence of radiographically detected central scar offers little diagnostic information except suggesting presence of slow-growing neoplasm

MACROSCOPIC FEATURES

General Features
- Characteristically, well circumscribed but not encapsulated
- Cut surface homogeneous beige or pale-tan; occasionally dark brown or mahogany
  - Gross appearance is reflection of microscopic cell types
    - More brown with increasing proportion of cells with eosinophilic cytoplasm
- Central scar is present in approximately 15% of tumors
- Gross hemorrhage and necrosis present in 25-30%
  - Cystic change less common
- Multifocality in < 10%
- Gross involvement of renal vein seen in small number of cases
- Up to 1/3 of patients may exhibit perirenal adipose tissue invasion

Size
- Mean: ~ 9 cm (range: 2-23 cm)
  - Largest among common subtypes of renal cell carcinoma
    - Mean tumor size progressively decreasing now because of earlier incidental detection on radiologic investigations for unrelated causes
    - Mean size in past 10-15 years has decreased to much smaller than 9 cm

MICROSCOPIC PATHOLOGY

Key Descriptors
- Predominant Pattern/Injury Type
  - Neoplastic
- Predominant Cell/Compartment Type
  - Epithelial
- Histologic Features
  - Pattern of growth is predominantly solid, separated by thin, incomplete fibrovascular septa
  - Some tumors with variable nested, broad alveolar, solid, cystic, tubular, trabecular, or even papillary/pseudopapillary patterns
    - Nested/alveolar pattern usually associated with eosinophilic variants
  - Small percentage exhibit sarcomatoid pattern of growth
    - Probably the subtype with proportionately most frequent sarcomatoid differentiation among all RCCs
  - Microscopic foci of necrosis present in 15-25% of cases
  - In classic type tumors, predominant cell type is that with pale, somewhat clear-appearing cytoplasm
    - Unlike clear cell RCC, cytoplasm is not optically entirely clear but somewhat translucent and finely reticulated
    - Cytoplasm has frothy/microvesiculated appearance
    - Some larger cells with more voluminous clear to foamy ("hydropic") cytoplasm often present among other "clear" cells
  - In eosinophilic variants, predominance of tumor cells with densely eosinophilic, granular cytoplasm
    - Cells with eosinophilic cytoplasm predominate in 30-40% of tumors
  - Most tumors show admixture of pale and eosinophilic cells

- Both cell types may be juxtaposed to one another without specific patterns, or
- Both cell types may have special spatial arrangement with eosinophilic cell in center and clear cells at periphery
  ○ Hyperchromatic nuclei with irregular, wrinkled outlines ("raisinoid" nuclei) is most characteristic feature
    - Proportion of such nuclei variable from case to case
    - Wrinkled nuclei more prevalent in classic types than eosinophilic variants
  ○ Another characteristic feature is presence of perinuclear cytoplasmic clarity (perinuclear halos)
    - While usually prominent, perinuclear halos may be only focal in some eosinophilic variants, and require careful search in such cases
  ○ Binucleated cells present in virtually all cases
  ○ Cell membranes usually appear prominent
    - Most cytoplasmic organelles are displaced to periphery of cytoplasm by abundant microvesicles in these tumors
    - This leads to impression of thick cell membranes, somewhat resembling thick cell walls in plant cells
  ○ Foci with bizarre, hyperchromatic, degenerate atypia similar to those in renal oncocytoma are common, and may be prominent in rare cases
  ○ Mitotic activity is uncommon in Ch-RCC but may be prominent in sarcomatoid and some epithelial tumors
  ○ Because of consistent presence of hyperchromatic, wrinkled, pleomorphic nuclei, Fuhrman nuclear grading is not appropriate for Ch-RCC
    - Currently, attempts are ongoing for clinically more relevant type-specific grading system

ANCILLARY TESTS

Histochemistry
- Colloidal iron stain
  ○ Variable granular or reticular and diffuse cytoplasmic staining with Hale colloidal iron in majority of cases
  ○ Difficult stain to perform well with consistency and is highly laboratory-dependent
    - Focal, weak, or luminal-type staining may be seen in some cases with predominance of eosinophilic cells
    - Value limited in difficult cases

Immunohistochemistry
- CK7 shows diffuse expression in > 75% Ch-RCC typically showing membranous accentuation
  ○ In eosinophilic variants, however, positivity is often less diffuse
  ○ Occasionally, may be present only in few clusters of cells
- CD117 and Ksp-cadherin are diffusely positive in overwhelming majority
- Most cases also show positivity with MOC-31, claudin-7, and EpCAM/BER-EP4/CD326

- CA9 is negative, or only focally positive in perinecrotic areas
- CD10 is usually negative but may show focal positivity in some cases

Electron Microscopy
- Cytoplasmic microvesicles are unique and consistent ultrastructural feature of Ch-RCC
  - These vesicles lack affinity for H&E stain, imparting cells with "clear" cytoplasmic appearance on light microscopy
  - Their origin is uncertain but may be related to defective mitochondriogenesis
  - Microvesicles often concentrated in perinuclear location, corresponding to perinuclear halos on light microscopy
- Abundant mitochondria present in cells with eosinophilic cytoplasm
- Mitochondria often show tubulocystic cristae

DIFFERENTIAL DIAGNOSIS

Renal Oncocytoma
- Eosinophilic variant of Ch-RCC closely mimics renal oncocytoma, particularly in cases with solid and nested growth patterns
- Separation of the 2 is essential, as renal oncocytoma is benign tumor
- Distinction is primarily histomorphological
- Nuclei in renal oncocytoma are round and uniform
  ○ Lack nuclear membrane irregularities that are always present, at least focally, in Ch-RCC
- Perinuclear halos are absent in renal oncocytomas
- Immunohistochemistry may help
  ○ CK7(-) or shows rare single cell positivity in oncocytoma
  ○ Other markers claimed to help in this distinction (EpCAM/BER-EP4/CD326, pax-2, claudin-7, MOC-31, MAl1, and S1001A)
    - Not proven helpful in difficult cases yet
  ○ Presence of microvesicles in Ch-RCC on ultrastructural evaluation is most distinctive feature
  ○ Cytogenetic investigations excluding combined multiple chromosomal losses, typical of Ch-RCC, may be helpful
    - Recently recognized differences in gene expression profiling may prove valuable in future

Clear Cell Renal Cell Carcinoma
- Both classic and eosinophilic variants need separation from clear cell RCC
  ○ Distinction less difficult than its separation from renal oncocytoma
- Separation is essential because of relatively indolent clinical behavior of Ch-RCC
- Cytoplasm in clear cells of clear cell RCC usually optically transparent; cytoplasmic clarity due to lipid and glycogen
  ○ In Ch-RCC, cytoplasm is not entirely optically clear in "clear" cells but is finely reticulated or irregularly granulated due to presence of microvesicles
- Clear cell RCC shows intricate, branching vasculature

- Clear cell RCC may show foci with perinuclear clearing, but this is not a prominent feature
- Immunohistochemical stains show diffuse membranous reactivity for CA9 and CD10, but negativity for CK7 in most cases
- Ultrastructurally, clear cell RCC lacks prominent microvesicles and tubulovesicular cristae in mitochondria
- 3p losses and *VHL* gene alterations in clear cell RCC will prove conclusive in very rare cases where genetic evaluation may be needed

Renal Cell Carcinoma, Unclassified (Low-Grade Oncocytic Type)

- Usually shows solid nests/alveoli with oncocytoma-like architecture, similar to some Ch-RCCs
- Tumors demonstrate nuclear pleomorphism and mitotic index beyond that acceptable for oncocytoma
- Do not show nuclear wrinkling and perinuclear halos as seen in Ch-RCC, eosinophilic variant
- Immunophenotypic differences, if any on consistent basis, have not been studied well
- Term "hybrid oncocytic tumor" used by some authors to express overlap with, but also to separate it from, oncocytoma, which has benign outcome

Epithelioid Angiomyolipoma (Oncocytoma-Like)

- Nuclear pleomorphism is usually significant
- Perinuclear halos are not observed
- Focal presence of fat cells &/or dysmorphic vessels is quite common
- Tumors negative for cytokeratin and CK7
  - Positive for melanocytic markers HMB-45 and Melan-A(MART-1)

DIAGNOSTIC CHECKLIST

Pathologic Interpretation Pearls

- Renal cell tumors with clear cell cytoplasm may raise differential diagnostic possibilities of Ch-RCC and clear cell RCC
- Solid acinar growth pattern with clear cytoplasm is more indicative of clear cell RCC
  - Ch-RCC with clear cells is more likely to show sheet-like architecture
- Intricate arborizing vascular pattern and optically clear cytoplasm is feature of clear cell RCC
  - Ch-RCC with clear cells almost always shows incomplete septae that do not completely surround cell nests or alveoli
  - Cytoplasm is not completely clear in Ch-RCC; it shows fine reticulations or irregularly clustered granules
- Tumors with pink cytoplasm and nested/solid alveolar growth often raise possibility of onocytoma, Ch-RCC (eosinophilic), or unclassified RCC/hybrid tumors
- Uniform nuclei throughout tumor, with exception of markedly pleomorphic symplastic foci, are indicative of oncocytoma

- Nuclear irregularities may be present in Ch-RCC or RCC, unclassified
  - It is important to look for foci with perinuclear halos to make diagnosis of Ch-RCC
    - If such foci are absent and there is no intra-tumoral fat/dysmorphic vessels, it is prudent to consider tumor as unclassified RCC

SELECTED REFERENCES

1. Kauffman EC et al: Differential expression of KAI1 metastasis suppressor protein in renal cell tumor histological subtypes. J Urol. 181(5):2305-11, 2009
2. Yusenko MV et al: Gene expression profiling of chromophobe renal cell carcinomas and renal oncocytomas by Affymetrix GeneChip using pooled and individual tumours. Int J Biol Sci. 5(6):517-27, 2009
3. Amin MB et al: Chromophobe renal cell carcinoma: histomorphologic characteristics and evaluation of conventional pathologic prognostic parameters in 145 cases. Am J Surg Pathol. 32(12):1822-34, 2008
4. Choueiri TK et al: Efficacy of sunitinib and sorafenib in metastatic papillary and chromophobe renal cell carcinoma. J Clin Oncol. 26(1):127-31, 2008
5. Tickoo SK et al: Pathologic features of renal cortical tumors. Urol Clin North Am. 35(4):551-61; v, 2008
6. Delahunt B et al: Fuhrman grading is not appropriate for chromophobe renal cell carcinoma. Am J Surg Pathol. 31(6):957-60, 2007
7. Rohan S et al: Gene expression profiling separates chromophobe renal cell carcinoma from oncocytoma and identifies vesicular transport and cell junction proteins as differentially expressed genes. Clin Cancer Res. 12(23):6937-45, 2006
8. Brunelli M et al: Eosinophilic and classic chromophobe renal cell carcinomas have similar frequent losses of multiple chromosomes from among chromosomes 1, 2, 6, 10, and 17, and this pattern of genetic abnormality is not present in renal oncocytoma. Mod Pathol. 18(2):161-9, 2005
9. Cindolo L et al: Chromophobe renal cell carcinoma: comprehensive analysis of 104 cases from multicenter European database. Urology. 65(4):681-6, 2005
10. Sengupta S et al: Histologic coagulative tumor necrosis as a prognostic indicator of renal cell carcinoma aggressiveness. Cancer. 104(3):511-20, 2005
11. Beck SD et al: Effect of papillary and chromophobe cell type on disease-free survival after nephrectomy for renal cell carcinoma. Ann Surg Oncol. 11(1):71-7, 2004
12. Amin MB et al: Prognostic impact of histologic subtyping of adult renal epithelial neoplasms: an experience of 405 cases. Am J Surg Pathol. 26(3):281-91, 2002
13. Motzer RJ et al: Treatment outcome and survival associated with metastatic renal cell carcinoma of non-clear-cell histology. J Clin Oncol. 20(9):2376-81, 2002
14. Tickoo SK et al: Ultrastructural observations on mitochondria and microvesicles in renal oncocytoma, chromophobe renal cell carcinoma, and eosinophilic variant of conventional (clear cell) renal cell carcinoma. Am J Surg Pathol. 24(9):1247-56, 2000
15. Tickoo SK et al: Colloidal iron staining in renal epithelial neoplasms, including chromophobe renal cell carcinoma: emphasis on technique and patterns of staining. Am J Surg Pathol. 22(4):419-24, 1998
16. Tickoo SK et al: Discriminant nuclear features of renal oncocytoma and chromophobe renal cell carcinoma. Analysis of their potential utility in the differential diagnosis. Am J Clin Pathol. 110(6):782-7, 1998

CHROMOPHOBE RENAL CELL CARCINOMA

Gross and Microscopic Features

(Left) Gross features in Ch-RCC are usually a reflection of the microscopic features of the tumor. This tumor shows a tan to fleshy cut surface, indicating paucity of eosinophilic cells and high likelihood of sarcomatoid features in the tumor. *(Right)* The brown cut surface of this Ch-RCC suggests prominence of cells with eosinophilic cytoplasm in this tumor. Such an appearance raises the possibility of a renal oncocytoma. This tumor was an eosinophilic variant of Ch-RCC.

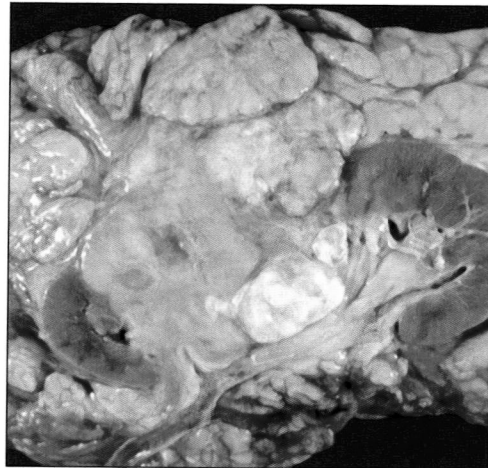
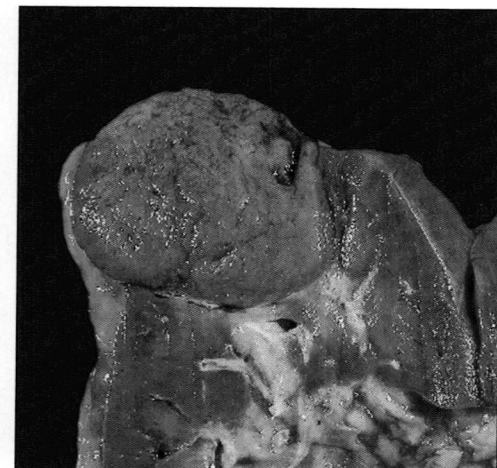

(Left) A macroscopic central scar ⊵ is observed in approximately 15% of Ch-RCCs. Such a scar is indicative of a slowly growing tumor and is also seen in a number of renal oncocytomas and low-grade clear cell renal cell carcinomas. *(Right)* The cells in a chromophobe RCC usually show a mixture of clear ⊡ and eosinophilic ⊡ features, often with spatial localization. Here the clear cells are concentrated along the septae, with most of the eosinophilic cells distal to septations.

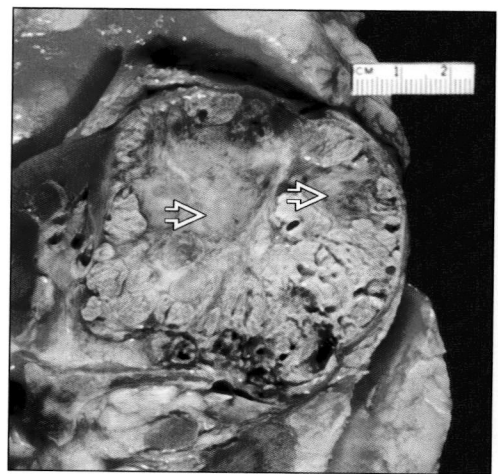
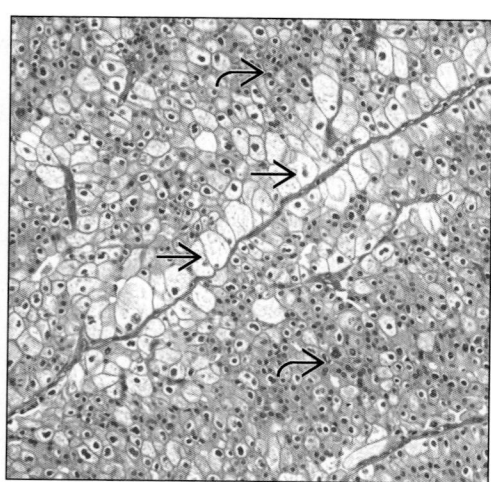

(Left) Some tumors are almost entirely composed of cells with eosinophilic cytoplasm and are regarded as eosinophilic variants. The architectural pattern in eosinophilic variants is often entirely acinar. Eosinophilic variants constitute approximately 30-40% of all Ch-RCCs. *(Right)* In some Ch-RCCs, the eosinophilic and clear cells are intimately admixed without any particular organization. This image also shows multiple microcalcifications ⊵ in the tumor, not an uncommon finding.

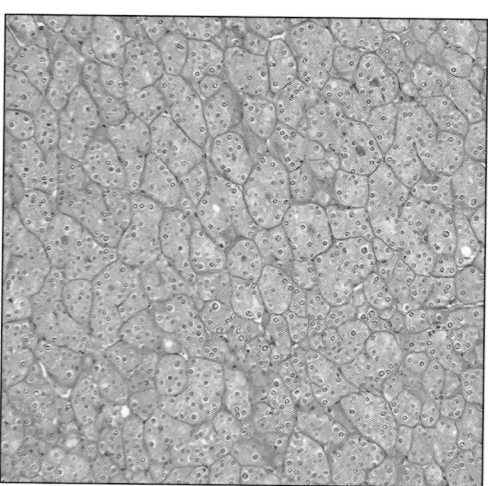
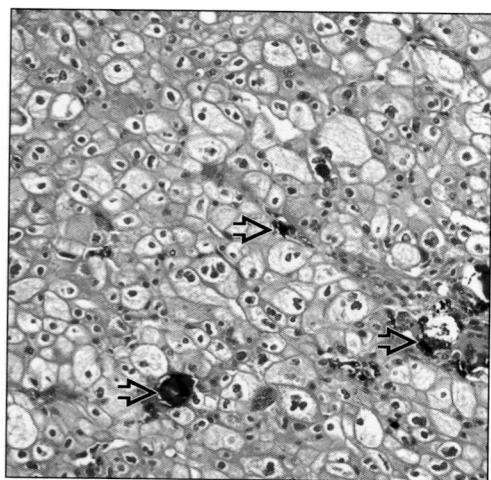

Microscopic Features

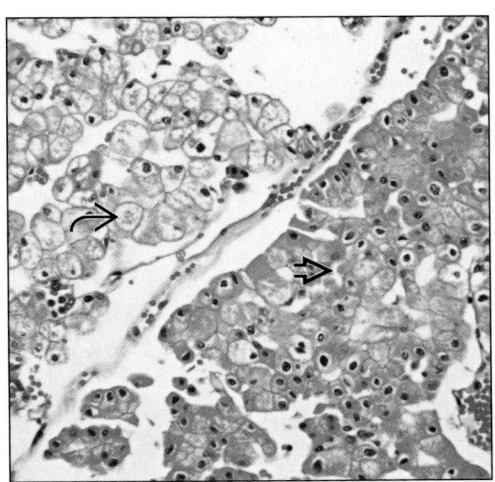
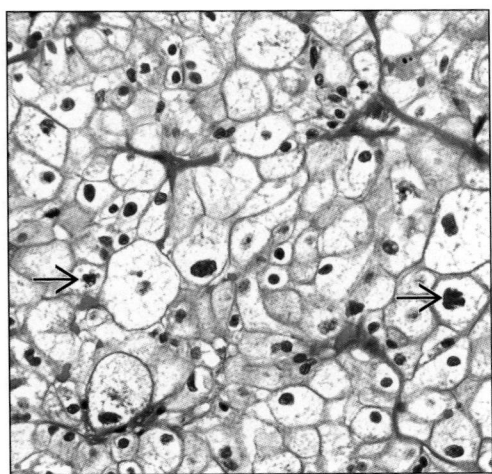

(Left) Occasionally, Ch-RCC shows well-defined foci with either pure eosinophilic ➯ or clear cells ➯ adjacent to each other. In spite of cytologic differences, both the classic and eosinophilic variants show similar cytogenetic, and to a great extent, immunophenotypic profiles. (Right) The nuclei in Ch-RCC are typically hyperchromatic, with markedly irregular nuclear membranes ➯. Cytoplasmic clarity is due to the presence of numerous microvesicles that do not stain with H&E.

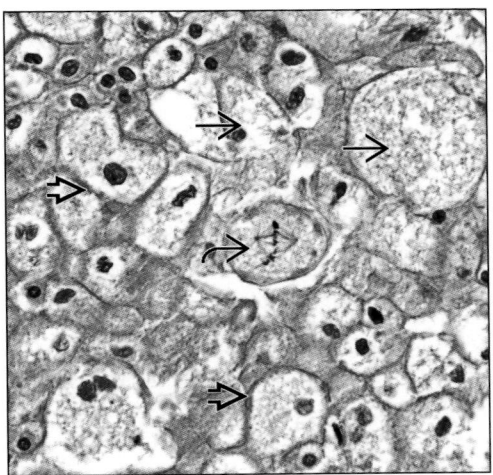
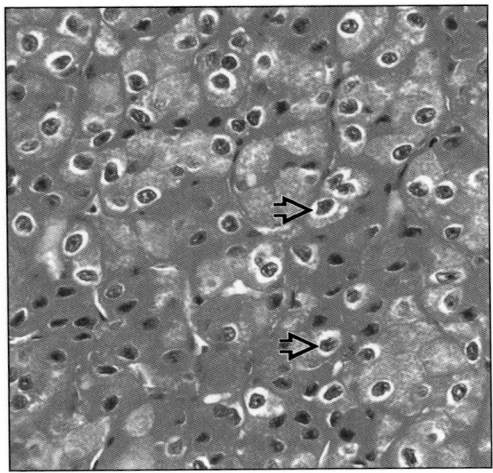

(Left) The "clear" cells in Ch-RCC are not optically clear and show reticular/ irregularly granular cytoplasm. Many clear cells appear ballooned-out and "hydropic" ➯. Also note a mitotic figure ➯ here. The apparent thick, plant-like ➯ cell wall appearance is a result of abundant microvesicles pushing the organelles to the periphery. (Right) Perinuclear halos ➯ around irregular, "raisinoid" nuclei seen in this eosinophilic variant is the most diagnostic feature of Ch-RCC.

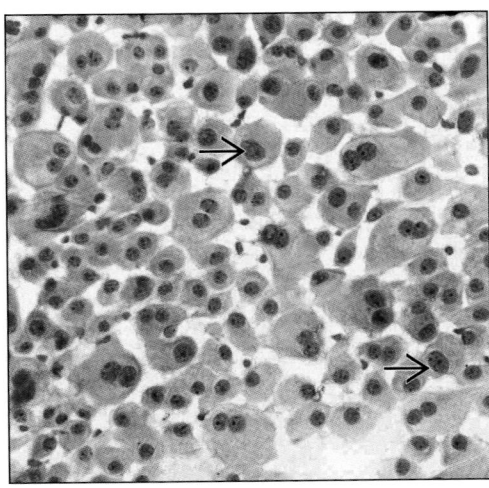
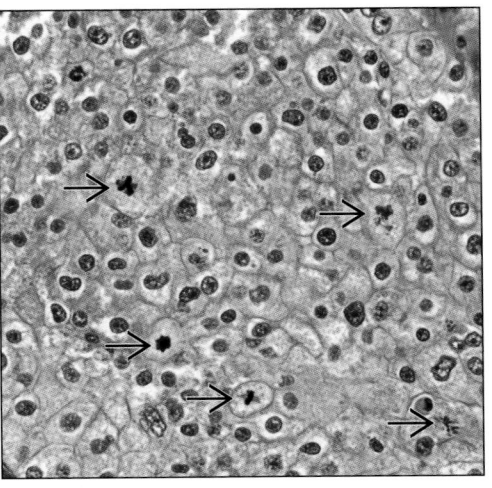

(Left) Cytologic preparations often do not show the perinuclear halos, but significant nuclear atypia and minimal paleness of perinuclear cytoplasm ➯ is quite characteristic. (Right) Other than in tumors with sarcomatoid differentiation, mitotic figures are unusual in Ch-RCC. However, rare cases with pure epithelial histology may also show brisk mitotic activity ➯. Because of the rarity of this finding, its clinical significance has not been studied well and remains undetermined.

CHROMOPHOBE RENAL CELL CARCINOMA

Microscopic Features and Ancillary Techniques

(Left) Approximately 15% or more chromophobe RCCs show microscopic foci of tumor necrosis ⊳. Even in tumors without sarcomatoid features, microscopic tumor necrosis in Ch-RCC has been shown to be associated with aggressive clinical behavior in multiple studies. *(Right)* This hematoxylin & eosin image of a Ch-RCC shows an area with markedly pleomorphic, hyperchromatic, and polyploid nuclei ⊳. Such degenerate-appearing foci are not as common as in oncocytomas but are not rare.

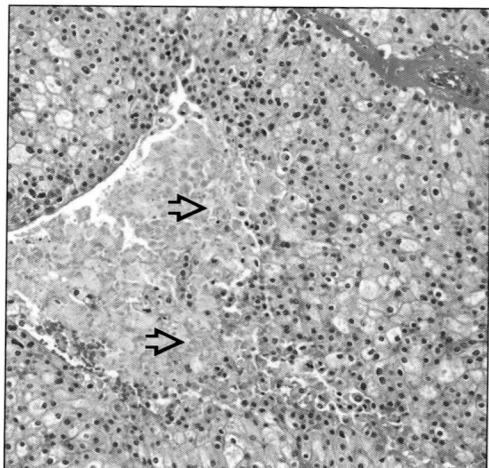
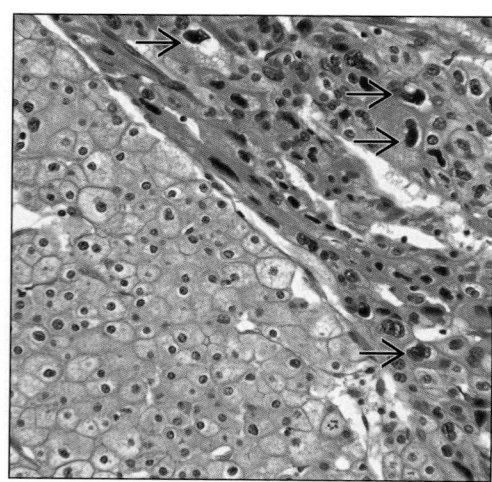

(Left) Hale colloidal iron stain often shows diffuse, reticular cytoplasmic staining in Ch-RCC. However, the stain is fastidious and laboratory-dependent. *(Right)* Numerous cytoplasmic microvesicles are the ultrastructural hallmark of Ch-RCC ⊳. Their predominant localization in perinuclear areas results in the light microscopic perinuclear halos. Displacement of other organelles to the cell periphery by abundant microvesicles leads to the apparently prominent cell membranes.

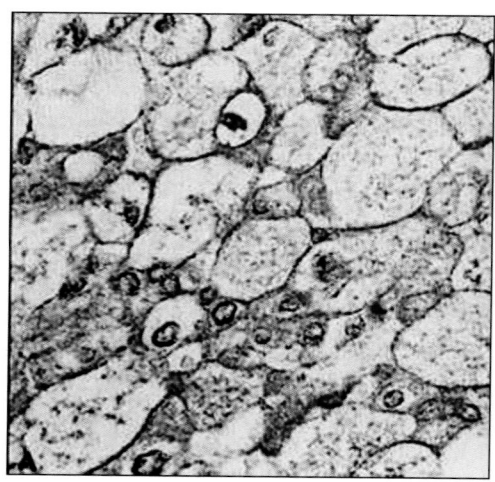
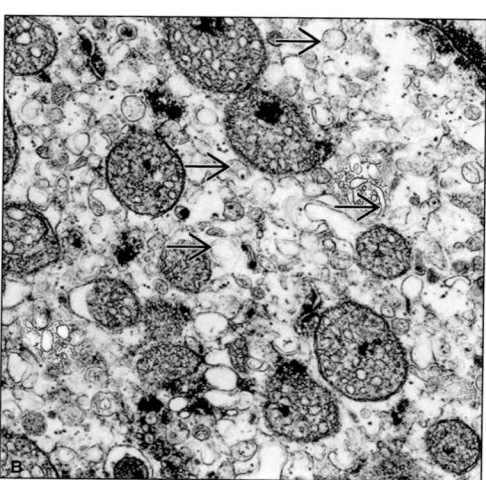

(Left) CK7 often shows diffuse membrane-predominant positivity in chromophobe RCC, a pattern different from that in renal oncocytoma. CK7 is either negative or usually only stains rare single cells in renal oncocytoma. *(Right)* CD117 stains both chromophobe-RCC and renal oncocytoma in a diffuse fashion, usually with membrane accentuation in Ch-RCC. The diffuse positivity may help in distinguishing these tumors from eosinophilic variants of clear cell RCC. Vimentin is negative.

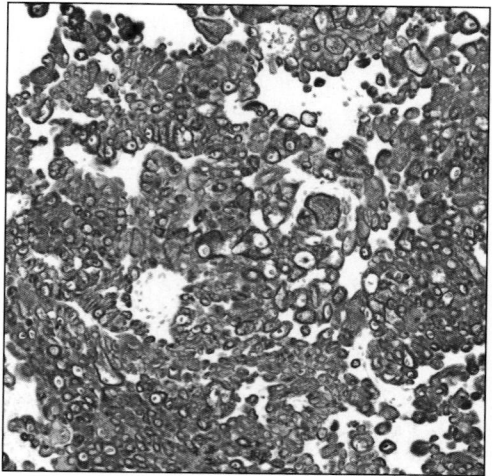
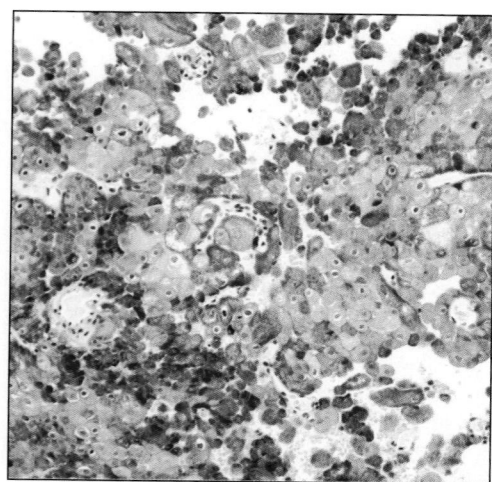

CHROMOPHOBE RENAL CELL CARCINOMA

Microscopic, Including Variant, Features

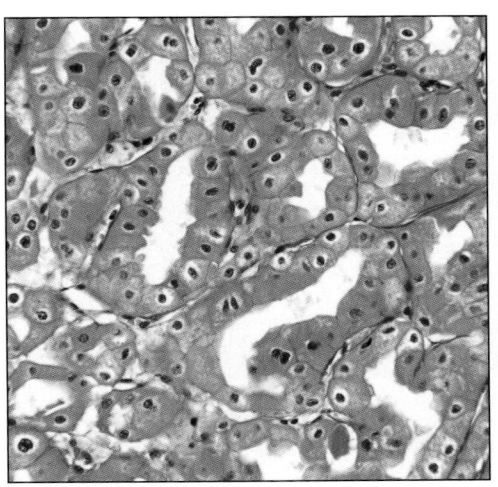

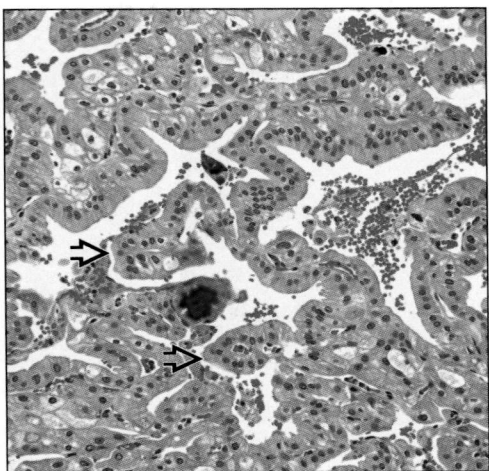

(Left) In addition to the more common sheet-like architecture, separated by incomplete septations or solid acinar growth pattern, other architectural patterns are not uncommon in Ch-RCC. This image shows a predominant tubular growth pattern in a Ch-RCC. Notice the nuclear and cytoplasmic features typical of eosinophilic variant of Ch-RCC are retained. (Right) Focal papillations ⊅ may be present in some chromophobe RCCs and are often seen in areas with tubulocystic architecture.

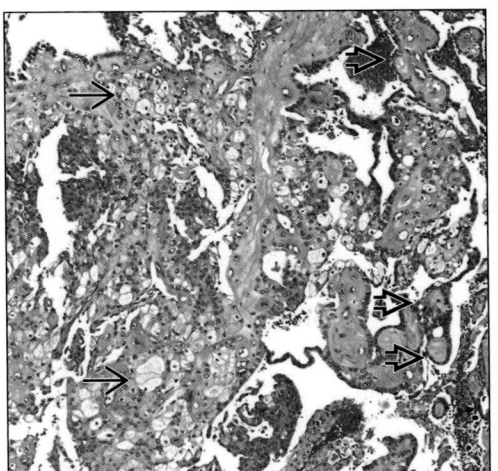

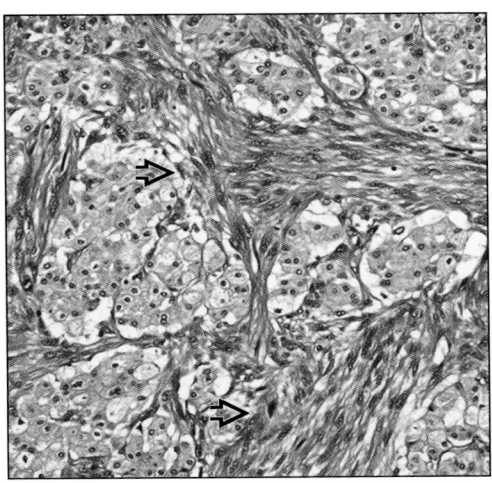

(Left) In some Ch-RCCs, degenerative changes and cell drop-out may lead to prominent cystic and pseudopapillary architecture ⊅. However, areas with usual typical morphologic features are almost invariably easy to find ⊅. (Right) Sarcomatoid features in Ch-RCC are predictive of aggressive tumor behavior, as in other subtypes of RCC. Sarcomatoid areas in Ch-RCC generally appear abrupt ⊅, in direct contact with epithelial nests, and usually without any apparent transitions.

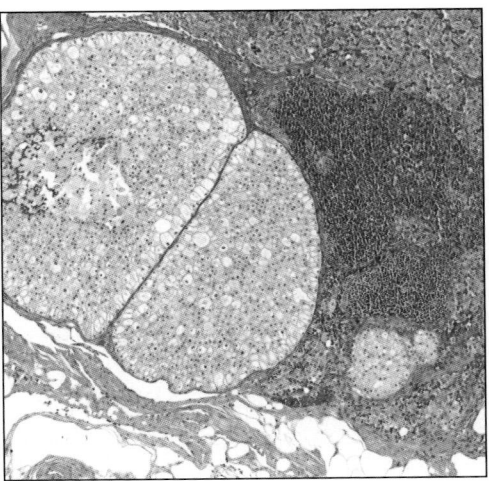

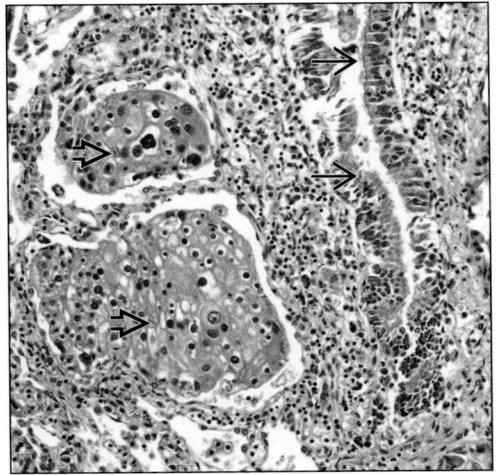

(Left) Stage for stage, Ch-RCC has better prognosis than clear cell RCC, and possibly papillary RCC. Metastases most often involve the regional lymph nodes, as shown here. (Right) This image shows a Ch-RCC metastatic to the lung ⊅. Notice the adjacent benign bronchial epithelium ⊐ and alveolar parenchyma. The overall survival with metastatic Ch-RCC seems to be better than that with other metastatic nonclear cell renal cell carcinomas, supporting its more indolent nature.

COLLECTING DUCT CARCINOMA

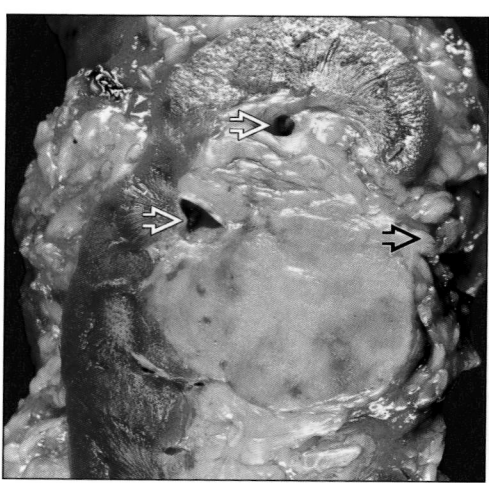

This example of CDC centered in the renal medullary region of a kidney shows a somewhat homogeneous cut surface. Extension into sinus fat ⊅ and pelvicalyceal system ⇨ are common.

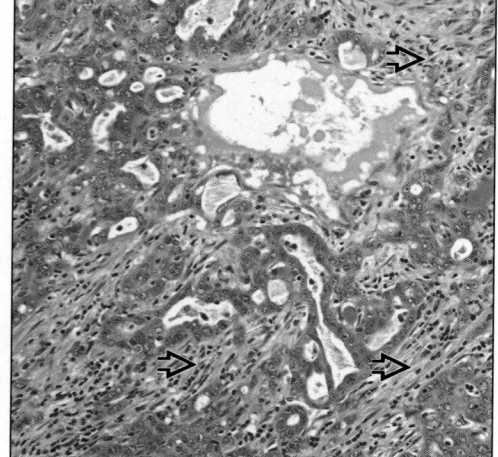

Microscopically, collecting duct carcinoma is a high-grade adenocarcinoma that may show variable architectural patterns. Multinodularity and abundant stromal desmoplasia ⊅ are characteristic.

TERMINOLOGY

Abbreviations
- Collecting duct carcinoma (CDC)

Synonyms
- Carcinoma of collecting ducts of Bellini

Definitions
- Rare, high-grade renal cell carcinoma, likely arising from cells of collecting ducts of renal medulla
  - Diagnostic features still evolving, with characteristic but not entirely specific morphologic and immunophenotypic features

ETIOLOGY/PATHOGENESIS

Genetic Features
- Monosomies of chromosomes 1, 6, 14, 15, and 22 consistently observed in the few tumors tested
- Loss of heterozygosity (LOH) of multiple chromosomal arms, including 1q, 6p, 8p, 13q, and 21q present in most cases
  - Minimal area of deletion located at 1q32.1-32.2 also identified
- Amplification of *HER2* present in some cases
- Trisomies of 7 and 17 (typical of papillary RCC) are absent
- Chromosome 3 losses (typical of clear cell RCC) not present

CLINICAL ISSUES

Epidemiology
- Incidence
  - Constitute < 1% of malignant renal cell tumors
  - Until recently, largest series in literature included a mere 12 cases

  - Recent nationwide survey study from Japan was able to include 81 cases in their report
- Age
  - Occurs over wide range of 13-83 years
    - Mean age is close to 50 years in different studies

Site
- Predominantly centered in medulla of kidney
  - In larger tumors, site of origin difficult to determine

Presentation
- Hematuria
- Palpable flank mass, pain, and weight loss
- Symptoms related to metastases
- Unlike what is usual in more common RCC subtypes, approximately 2/3 cases symptomatic at presentation

Treatment
- Currently, surgical excision and urothelial carcinoma-like chemotherapeutic options commonly followed
  - Responses to any therapy very limited and of short duration
  - Recently, targeted therapies against tyrosine kinase receptors of VEGF-related molecules have shown some promise

Prognosis
- Unfavorable outcomes very common
  - Approximately 1/2 of patients die of disease within 2 years
- Frequently metastatic at presentation, commonly with multiple organ involvement, including
  - Lymph nodes (44%)
  - Various viscera (32%), with lungs being most common site (17%)
  - Bones (16%) with both osteolytic and osteoblastic lesions

COLLECTING DUCT CARCINOMA

Key Facts

Terminology
- Collecting duct carcinoma (CDC)
- Rare, high-grade renal cell carcinoma likely arising from cells of collecting ducts of renal medulla
- Diagnostic features still evolving, with characteristic but not entirely specific, morphologic and immunophenotypic features
- Collecting duct carcinoma (CDC)

Clinical Issues
- Occurs over wide range (13-83 years) but mostly in patients 50 or younger
- Predominantly centered in medulla of kidney
- 1/2 of patients dead of disease within 2 years

Microscopic Pathology
- Primarily high-grade adenocarcinoma

- Variable architectural patterns, usually in various combinations, including tubular, papillary, solid, cribriform
- Typically with multinodular growth pattern, desmoplastic stroma, and intratumoral inflammatory infiltrate

Ancillary Tests
- Often stain positive with lectins, ULEX-1, PNA, and soybean agglutinin

Top Differential Diagnoses
- Papillary renal cell carcinoma
- Urothelial carcinoma with glandular features
- Metastatic carcinoma
- Other tumors, including renal medullary carcinoma and HLRCC syndrome tumors

MACROSCOPIC FEATURES

General Features
- Predominantly located in medulla, but larger tumors often involve cortex secondarily
- Classically, gray-pale with invasive borders
- Typically has multinodular growth pattern
- Areas of necrosis, hemorrhage, and cystic change are frequently present
- Grossly, majority of tumors invade renal sinus and perinephric fat
- Well-circumscribed tumors with purely cystic appearance previously considered low-grade CDC
  - Currently, such tumors regarded as separate entity, "tubulocystic carcinoma"
  - Whether these represent distinct tumor entities or variations in morphologic spectrum of CDC is not clear at present
    - Some CDCs with otherwise typical high-grade features also show variable amount of tubulocystic areas

Size
- 1-15 cm (median: 6 cm)

MICROSCOPIC PATHOLOGY

Key Descriptors
- Predominant Pattern/Injury Type
  - Neoplastic
- Predominant Cell/Compartment Type
  - Epithelial
- Histologic Features
  - Primarily high-grade adenocarcinoma
  - Variable architectural patterns, usually in various combinations
    - Including tubular, solid tubular/acinar, papillary, solid sheet-like, cribriform, and (rarely) diffuse signet ring cell-like
  - Like other RCCs, CDCs may also show sarcomatoid features

  - Biologic significance of such features not as dramatic as in other RCCs, as usual CDC by itself is very aggressive tumor
  - Multinodular growth pattern with marked desmoplastic stroma and intratumoral inflammatory infiltrate, including microabscesses
  - Surrounding renal collecting ducts often show dysplastic cytologic features
  - High-grade cytology, often with marked nuclear pleomorphism and brisk mitotic activity
  - Sometimes cytoplasmic mucin may be seen, highlighted by Alcian blue or mucicarmine stain
- Lymphatic/Vascular Invasion
  - Present in majority of cases
- Lymph Nodes
  - Metastases to regional nodes frequent in CDC

ANCILLARY TESTS

Immunohistochemistry
- Generally positive for
  - HMCK(34βE12), EMA/MUC1, CK7, CEA
- Often stain positive with lectins, ULEX-1, PNA, and soybean agglutinin
- Usually negative for
  - CD10, AMACR, E-cadherin, pax-2, and CA9

DIFFERENTIAL DIAGNOSIS

Papillary Renal Cell Carcinoma
- Usually well circumscribed; stromal desmoplasia rare
- Papillary cores often contain foamy macrophages
- Usually CK7 and AMACR positive; HMCK(34βE12) and lectin stains negative

Urothelial Carcinoma (UC) with Glandular Features
- Often with intrapelvic papillary or flat in situ carcinoma component
- Presence of squamous morphology and sheets or other typical patterns of urothelial carcinoma

1

COLLECTING DUCT CARCINOMA

Comparative Features Between Collecting Duct Carcinoma and Its Close Differential Diagnoses

Feature	Collecting Duct Carcinoma	Papillary Renal Cell Carcinoma	Urothelial Carcinoma
Tumor circumscription/ encapsulation	Not present	Most often present	Not present
Papillary architecture	Often present	Most often present	Often present
Multinodular growth pattern	Almost always	Usually not seen	May be present
Stromal desmoplasia	Almost always, prominent	Extremely uncommon, focal at the most	Frequently present in invasive tumors
Intratumoral inflammatory cell infiltrate	Almost always	Very rare	May be present, particularly in tumors with anaplastic features
Foam cells in papillary cores	Not present	Most often present	Not present
Immunohistochemistry			
CK7	Usually positive, diffuse to focal	Usually positive, diffuse in type 1 to focal or absent in some type 2 tumors	Usually diffuse; rarely focal to absent
CK20	Negative to rarely focally positive	Negative	Often positive
HMCK(34βE12)	Often (but not always) positive	Negative	Positive in most cases
ULEX-1 and other lectins	Often (but not always) positive	Negative	Frequently positive

Metastatic Carcinoma
- History of a primary tumor
- Most often bilateral
- Ulex europaeus and PNA staining depends on type of primary (e.g., enteric tumors may be positive); other tumor specific characteristics also helpful

Renal Cell Carcinoma, Unclassified
- Morphologic features of CDC may be shared by many other high-grade tumors, and CDC may show marked variability in morphology
  - In such situations, dependence on immunoprofile, even though not highly specific, is prudent
  - In the absence of typical immunophenotype, such tumors should be considered RCC, unclassified

Other Tumors
- Renal medullary carcinoma, considered a variant of CDC by some
  - Typically with sickle cell trait, and presence of sickled red cells in specimen
- Hereditary leiomyomatosis renal cell cancer (HLRCC) syndrome tumors
  - Presence of prominent nucleoli and perinucleolar halos characteristic

DIAGNOSTIC CHECKLIST

Pathologic Interpretation Pearls
- Stromal desmoplasia, multinodular growth pattern, intratumoral inflammation, and renal tubular dysplasia common to both CDC and UC
- Immunophenotyping may also not be helpful in their separation
  - Finding of in situ urothelial component is only reliable differentiating feature
  - Adequate sampling of urothelium, including that of urothelium away from tumor mass, is therefore an absolute requirement
- Collecting duct carcinomas with prominent papillary architecture are often misdiagnosed as papillary RCC, type 2
  - In papillary tumors with other architectural patterns, desmoplasia, and multinodularity, possibility of CDC must always be considered

SELECTED REFERENCES

1. Choueiri TK et al: Sunitinib in renal-cell carcinoma: expanded indications. Lancet Oncol. 10(8):740, 2009
2. Srigley JR et al: Uncommon and recently described renal carcinomas. Mod Pathol. 22 Suppl 2:S2-S23, 2009
3. Wright JL et al: Effect of Collecting Duct Histology on Renal Cell Cancer Outcome. J Urol. Epub ahead of print, 2009
4. Kobayashi N et al: Collecting duct carcinoma of the kidney: an immunohistochemical evaluation of the use of antibodies for differential diagnosis. Hum Pathol. 39(9):1350-9, 2008
5. Tokuda N et al: Collecting duct (Bellini duct) renal cell carcinoma: a nationwide survey in Japan. J Urol. 176(1):40-3; discussion 43, 2006
6. Polascik TJ et al: Molecular genetics and histopathologic features of adult distal nephron tumors. Urology. 60(6):941-6, 2002
7. Srigley JR et al: Collecting duct carcinoma of kidney. Semin Diagn Pathol. 15(1):54-67, 1998
8. MacLennan GT et al: Low-grade collecting duct carcinoma of the kidney: report of 13 cases of low-grade mucinous tubulocystic renal carcinoma of possible collecting duct origin. Urology. 50(5):679-84, 1997
9. Polascik TJ et al: Distal nephron renal tumors: microsatellite allelotype. Cancer Res. 56(8):1892-5, 1996
10. Steiner G et al: High-density mapping of chromosomal arm 1q in renal collecting duct carcinoma: region of minimal deletion at 1q32.1-32.2. Cancer Res. 56(21):5044-6, 1996
11. Fleming S et al: Collecting duct carcinoma of the kidney. Histopathology. 10(11):1131-41, 1986

COLLECTING DUCT CARCINOMA

Gross and Microscopic Features

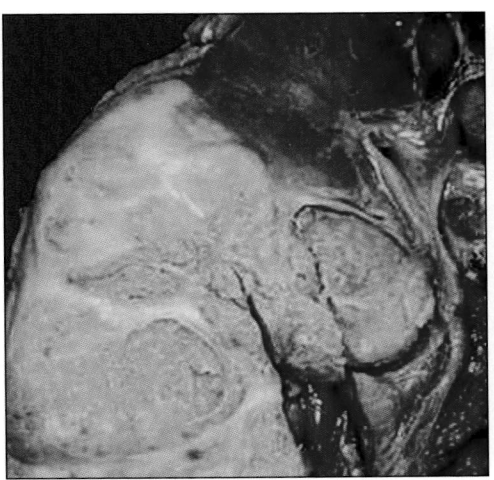
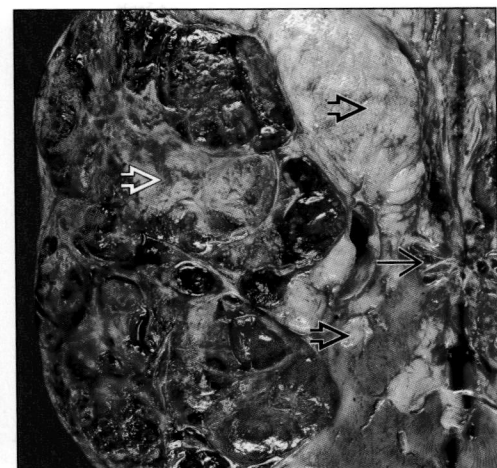

(Left) This image shows the typical gross features of a collecting duct carcinoma. It is a renal medulla-centered tumor with multinodular growth pattern. The boundaries of the tumor are often ill defined due to infiltrative tumor front. *(Right)* Gross and microscopic variability is frequent in collecting duct carcinoma. This multinodular tumor shows a combination of solid, tan ➡, and hemorrhagic necrotic ➡ areas. Note the invasion of the renal sinus fat ➡, a frequent finding.

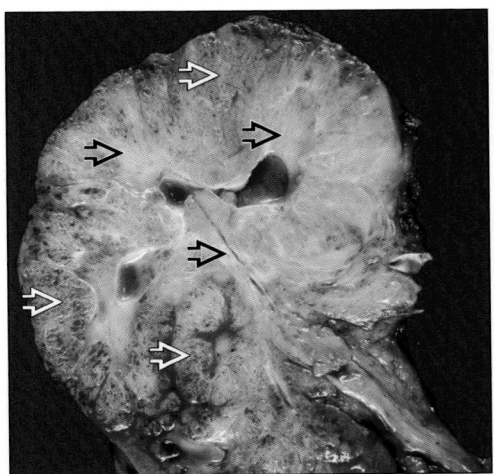
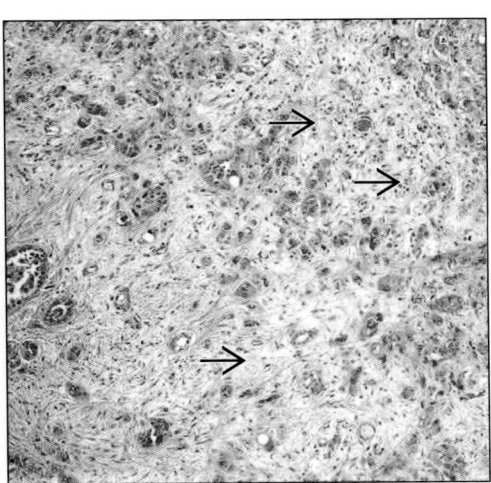

(Left) This CDC shows fleshy solid areas of sarcomatoid differentiation ➡. The epithelial component in this tumor reveals a fine, sieve-like microcystic growth pattern ➡. In large tumors, it may be difficult to ascertain whether the tumor is centered in the renal medulla. *(Right)* Among the most consistent features of CDC is the high-grade glandular infiltrative pattern with desmoplasia ➡. Similar desmoplasia may be seen in renal parenchyma involved by invasive urothelial carcinoma.

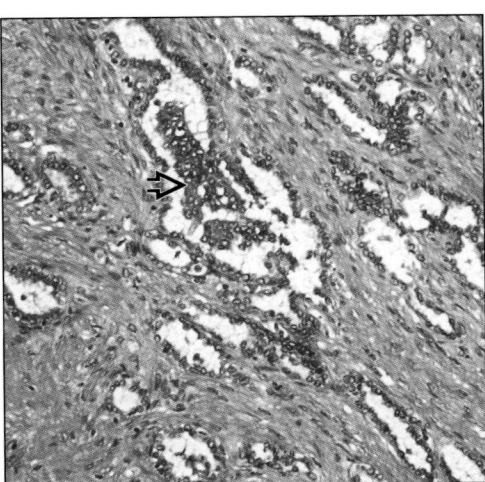
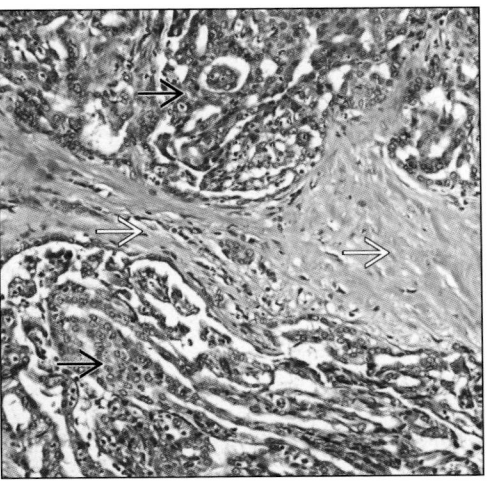

(Left) A combination of architectural patterns is the rule in CDC, with rare exceptions. This tumor shows a predominantly tubular architecture with focal papillations ➡. *(Right)* Some CDCs show variable, and occasionally extensive, papillary architecture. However, high-grade cytology ➡, marked stromal desmoplasia ➡, and multinodular growth pattern are maintained, and these features should differentiate such tumors from type 2 papillary renal cell carcinoma.

COLLECTING DUCT CARCINOMA

Microscopic Features

(Left) Collecting duct carcinomas are essentially high-grade adenocarcinomas. However, solid areas ⊵, as depicted in this photomicrograph, are not uncommon. Such architecture makes distinction from invasive urothelial carcinoma difficult in some cases. *(Right)* Some cases of CDC may have a prominent solid tubular architecture, with tubules surrounded by basement membrane-like material ⊡. Extensive sampling of urothelium is a must to exclude urothelial carcinoma.

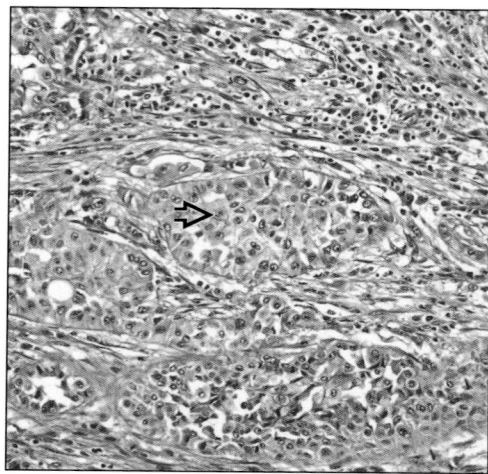
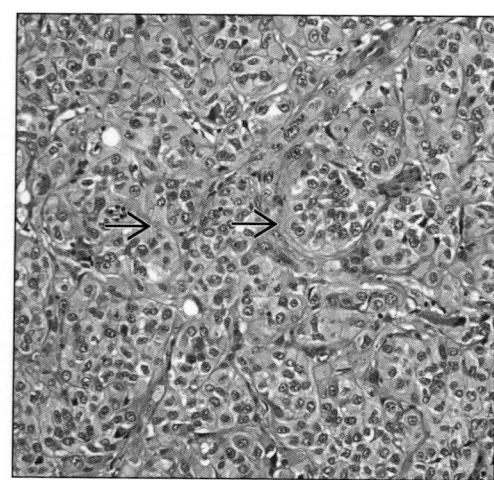

(Left) Like other renal cancers, CDC may show sarcomatoid differentiation ⊵. This finding may not portend a more aggressive clinical behavior, as the tumor is inherently clinically aggressive. *(Right)* The presence of tubular dysplasia in the areas surrounding the tumor is a helpful feature ⊵. However, tubular dysplasia may also be observed in urothelial carcinomas of renal pelvis and occasionally in papillary RCC. Thus, this finding should not be considered specific of CDC.

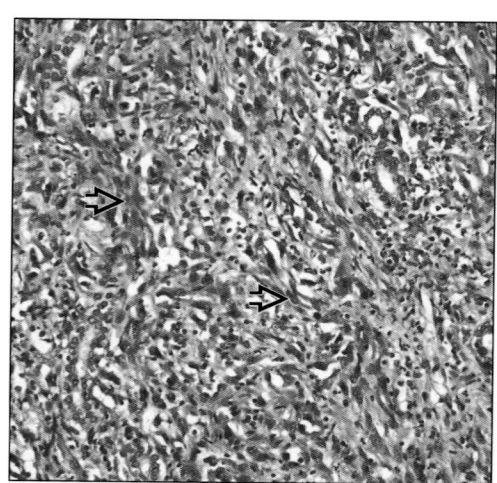
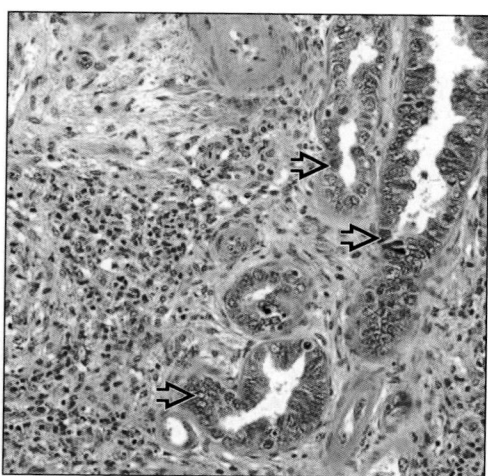

(Left) This photomicrograph shows angiolymphatic invasion in a case of collecting duct carcinoma. The vast majority of collecting duct carcinomas show angiolymphatic invasion and metastasis at presentation. *(Right)* Renal sinus ⊵ and perinephric fat invasion are also very frequent in cases of CDC. Also note the small vessel tumor invasion ⊡ in this photomicrograph. Presentation with pT1 or pT2 stages is uncommon in CDC. Metastatic carcinoma is also a common differential diagnosis.

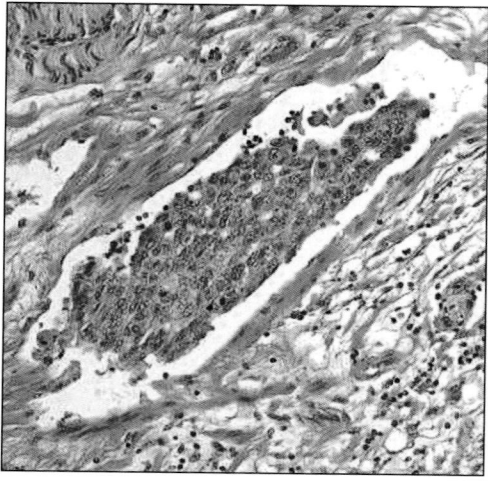
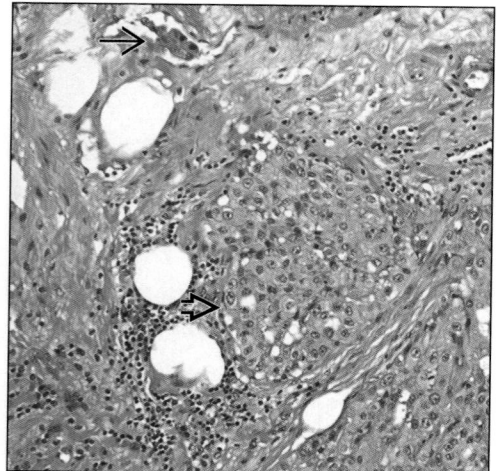

1

COLLECTING DUCT CARCINOMA

Microscopic and IHC Features and Differential Diagnoses

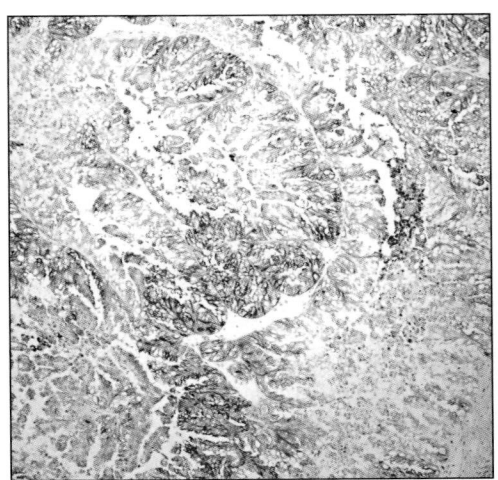

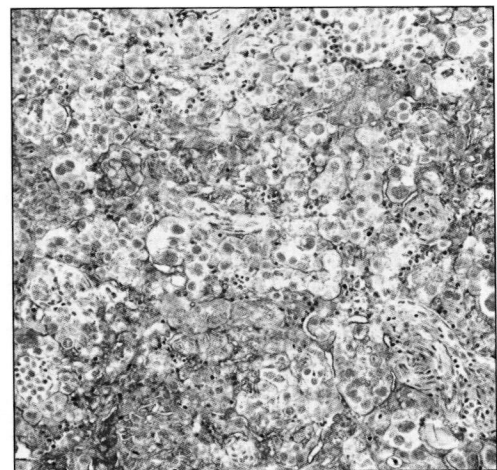

(Left) While HMCK(34βE12) immunostaining is often positive in CDC, the positivity may be quite focal or entirely absent in some cases. In general, immunohistochemical staining patterns are often not reliable in the distinction of CDC from urothelial carcinoma invading the renal parenchyma. (Right) ULEX-1 often stains positive in CDC. However, some tumors completely lack staining. ULEX-1 may also stain other renal tumors related to the distal nephron and urothelial carcinoma.

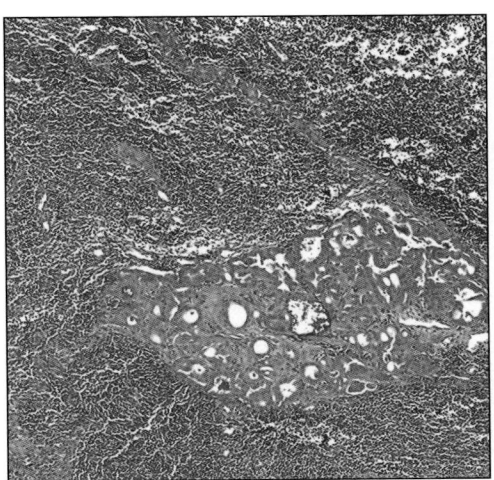

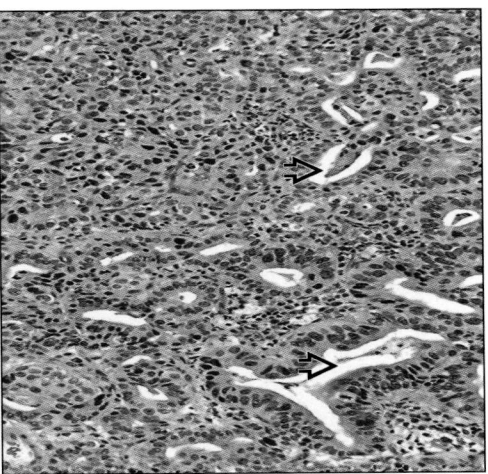

(Left) This image shows CDC metastatic to a regional lymph node. Regional nodal metastases are present in approximately 1/2 of cases of CDC. Visceral and bone metastases are also common, and the bone metastases are often osteoblastic. (Right) The distinction of urothelial carcinoma with glandular differentiation ⊳ invading renal parenchyma from CDC may be difficult, and the most definitive distinguishing feature is the presence of in situ carcinoma in the pelvicalyceal system.

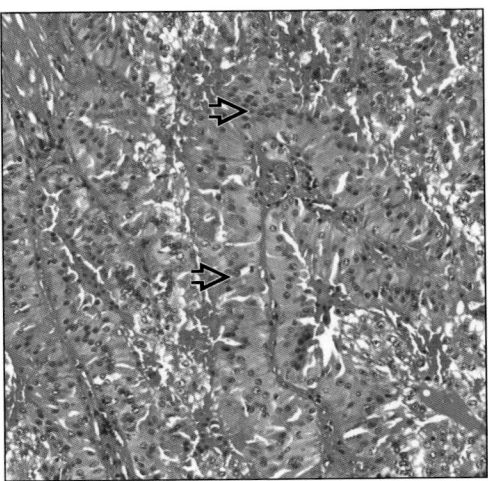

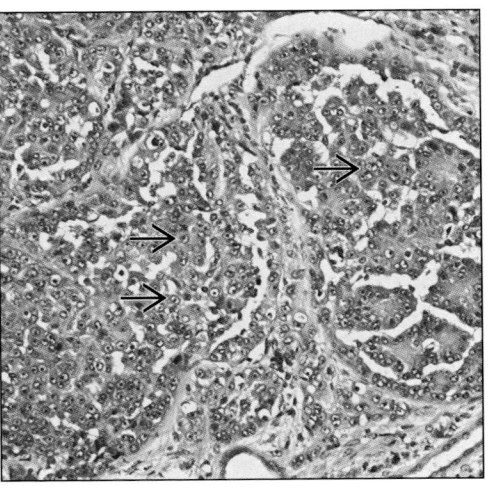

(Left) CDC with prominent papillary architecture is often misdiagnosed as papillary RCC ⊳. Predominantly papillary tumors that show multinodularity and prominent stromal desmoplasia are more likely to be CDC. A fibrous capsule is a helpful feature for papillary RCC. (Right) Renal tumors in the recently recognized hereditary leiomyomatosis and renal cell cancer syndrome also show many similarities with CDC. However, these show very prominent nucleoli with perinucleolar halos ⊳.

RENAL MEDULLARY CARCINOMA

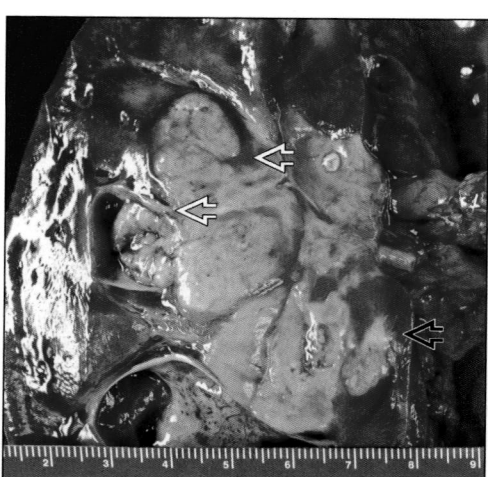

The photograph demonstrates the gross appearance of a renal medullary carcinoma. The tumors, particularly the smaller ones, are renal medulla based, with infiltrative borders ⮕. Here, it also invades the renal pelvis ⮕.

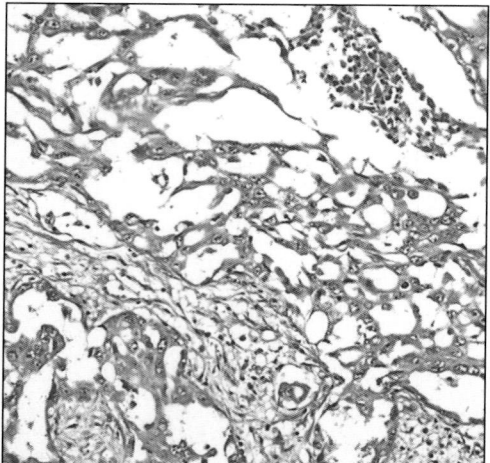

Renal medullary carcinoma often shows a mixture of architectural patterns, reticular and cribriform patterns being the most common. The tumor invariably shows high nuclear grade.

TERMINOLOGY

Abbreviations
- Renal medullary carcinoma (RMC)

Synonyms
- Medullary renal cell carcinoma (RCC)

Definitions
- Distinctive clinicopathologic entity occurring almost exclusively in patients with sickle cell trait
  - Rare cases in patients with hemoglobin SC disease and very occasionally in sickle cell disease (SS)

ETIOLOGY/PATHOGENESIS

Sickle Cell Hemoglobinopathies
- Presence of HbS in virtually all cases, suggesting some cause-effect relationship between hemoglobinopathy and this tumor
  - Exact mechanism unknown; role of tissue hypoxia and hypoxia-inducible factor (HIF) in tumorigenesis or tumor viability/tumor progression is suggested

INI1(hSNF5/BAF47)
- Loss of immunohistochemical nuclear expression of SNF5 (INI1) protein, similar to pediatric rhabdoid tumor of kidney, is consistent finding
  - Molecular mechanism, i.e., mutations/loss of gene or others, for this absent SNF5 expression is not known

ABL-BCR Amplifications
- Amplification of both *ABL* and *BCR* genes described in few cases
- *ABL-BCR* translocation described in 1 case but not in 3 others tested

Relationship to Collecting Duct Carcinoma
- Some consider RMC to be a particularly aggressive form of collecting duct carcinoma

CLINICAL ISSUES

Epidemiology
- Incidence
  - Very uncommon tumor
- Age
  - Range: 5-39 years; only occasionally in older patients
- Gender
  - Predominantly male, especially in patients < 25 years old
- Ethnicity
  - Mostly African-American; occasionally of Mediterranean ancestry, rarely others

Presentation
- Often with hematuria or flank pain, and many presenting with symptoms related to metastases

Laboratory Tests
- Most with sickle cell trait (Hb-AS) or Hb-SC on hemoglobin electrophoresis
- Rarely with homozygous sickle cell anemia (Hb-SS)

Prognosis
- Biologic behavior very aggressive; mean survival approximately 4 months; most cases with metastases at presentation

MACROSCOPIC FEATURES

General Features
- Medullary-based, gray-white cut surface, infiltrative borders often with extension into perihilar fat

RENAL MEDULLARY CARCINOMA

Key Facts

Terminology
- Distinctive clinicopathologic entity in patients with sickle cell hemoglobinopathies

Etiology/Pathogenesis
- Presence of HbS in virtually all cases suggesting some cause-effect relationship between hemoglobinopathy and this tumor
- Loss of immunohistochemical nuclear expression of INI1 (SNF5) protein, similar to pediatric rhabdoid tumor of kidney, is consistent finding

Clinical Issues
- Usually male and African-American
- Medullary region of kidney
- Patients with sickle cell trait (Hb-AS), Hb-SC, and rarely Hb-SS

- Very aggressive tumor with metastases at presentation in almost all, and mean survival of 4 months

Macroscopic Features
- Gray-white, possessing infiltrative borders and extending into perihilar fat

Microscopic Pathology
- Reticular, cribriform, solid, tubular, or adenoid cystic-like growth patterns
- Marked desmoplastic stroma and intratumoral inflammatory infiltrate, usually neutrophilic
- Sickled RBCs frequently observed, both within tumor and surrounding parenchymal vessels

Top Differential Diagnoses
- Collecting duct carcinoma
- Urothelial carcinoma

- Satellite nodules in adjacent parenchyma frequently observed
  - Often representing tumor emboli in large vessels

MICROSCOPIC PATHOLOGY

Histologic Features
- Most common architectural features: Reticular or cribriform glands
  - Other patterns include yolk sac-like, glandular, solid nests, and tubules; undifferentiated sheet-like or adenoid cystic-like
- Stroma almost always fibrotic or desmoplastic, and intratumoral inflammatory infiltrate, mostly neutrophils, is very frequent
- Tumor margins always infiltrative
- Cytoplasmic mucin is commonly observed
- Cytology usually high grade, with moderate to marked nuclear atypia
  - Occasional cases with rhabdoid features
- Sickled RBCs frequently observed, both within tumor and surrounding renal parenchymal vessels
- Often with high pT and pN stage and satellite tumor nodules due to very frequent vascular spread

Predominant Pattern/Injury Type
- Neoplastic

Predominant Cell/Compartment Type
- Epithelial

DIFFERENTIAL DIAGNOSIS

Collecting Duct Carcinoma
- Medullary carcinoma believed by some to be particularly virulent variant of collecting duct carcinoma
- No hemoglobinopathy
- Usually HMCK(34βE12) positive

Urothelial Carcinoma
- Intrapelvicalyceal papillary component or in situ urothelial carcinoma

SELECTED REFERENCES

1. Cheng JX et al: Renal medullary carcinoma: rhabdoid features and the absence of INI1 expression as markers of aggressive behavior. Mod Pathol. 21(6):647-52, 2008
2. Tickoo SK et al: Pathologic features of renal cortical tumors. Urol Clin North Am. 35(4):551-61; v, 2008
3. Hakimi AA et al: Renal medullary carcinoma: the Bronx experience. Urology. 70(5):878-82, 2007
4. Bell MD: Response to paclitaxel, gemcitabine, and cisplatin in renal medullary carcinoma. Pediatr Blood Cancer. 47(2):228, 2006
5. Ronnen EA et al: Medullary renal cell carcinoma and response to therapy with bortezomib. J Clin Oncol. 24(9):e14, 2006
6. Simpson L et al: Renal medullary carcinoma and ABL gene amplification. J Urol. 173(6):1883-8, 2005
7. Strouse JJ et al: Significant responses to platinum-based chemotherapy in renal medullary carcinoma. Pediatr Blood Cancer. 44(4):407-11, 2005
8. Yang XJ et al: Gene expression profiling of renal medullary carcinoma: potential clinical relevance. Cancer. 100(5):976-85, 2004
9. Swartz MA et al: Renal medullary carcinoma: clinical, pathologic, immunohistochemical, and genetic analysis with pathogenetic implications. Urology. 60(6):1083-9, 2002
10. Wesche WA et al: Renal medullary carcinoma: a potential sickle cell nephropathy of children and adolescents. Pediatr Pathol Lab Med. 18(1):97-113, 1998
11. Herring JC et al: Renal medullary carcinoma: a recently described highly aggressive renal tumor in young black patients. J Urol. 157(6):2246-7, 1997
12. Avery RA et al: Renal medullary carcinoma: clinical and therapeutic aspects of a newly described tumor. Cancer. 78(1):128-32, 1996
13. Davis CJ Jr et al: Renal medullary carcinoma. The seventh sickle cell nephropathy. Am J Surg Pathol. 19(1):1-11, 1995

RENAL MEDULLARY CARCINOMA

Microscopic Features

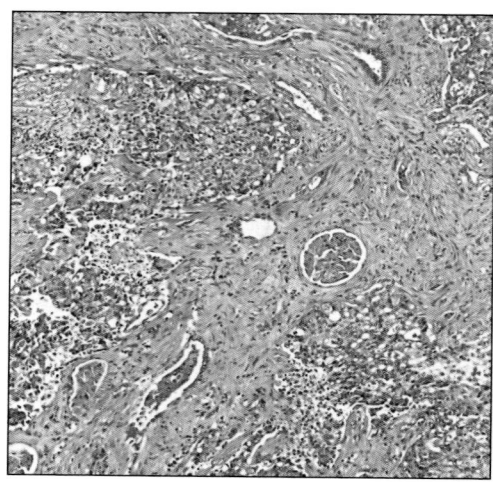
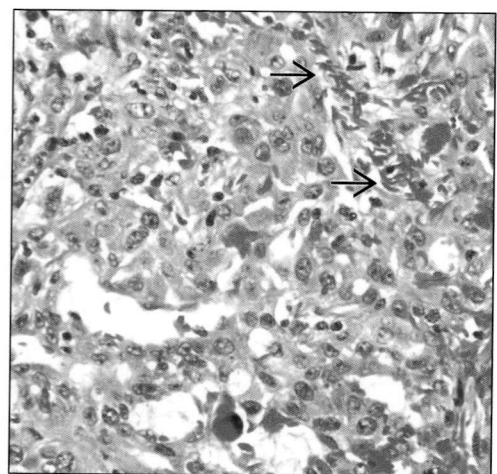

(Left) Renal medullary carcinoma frequently shows a multinodular growth pattern, extensive desmoplasia, multinodularity and satellite nodules away from the main tumor mass. *(Right)* One of the characteristic features of renal medullary carcinoma is the presence of sickled red blood cells ⊡. Such cells are seen both within the tumor and in the nonneoplastic renal parenchyma. Many times the RBCs appear clustered and agglutinated within small capillaries.

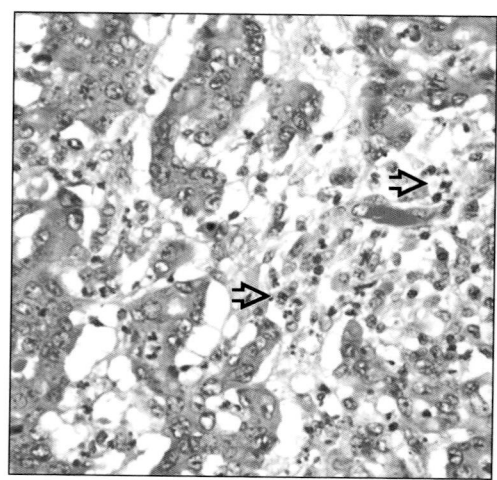
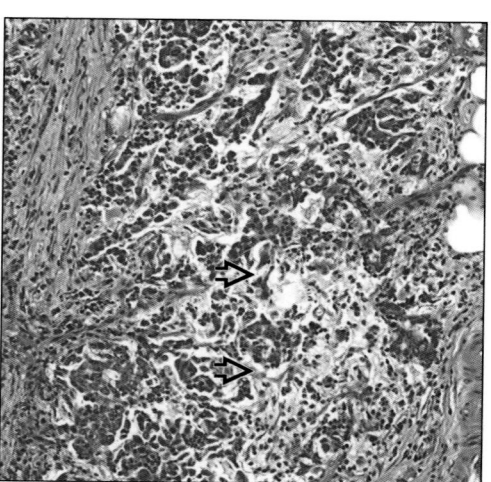

(Left) The photomicrograph shows a renal medullary carcinoma with prominent inflammatory infiltrate within the tumor ⊡. Intratumoral inflammatory infiltrate, often neutrophils, but sometimes predominantly lympho-plasmacytic, is very common in these tumors. *(Right)* Many renal medullary carcinomas show areas that bear superficial resemblance to yolk sac tumor ⊡. It is not unusual for renal medullary carcinomas to show a combination of growth patterns within the same tumor.

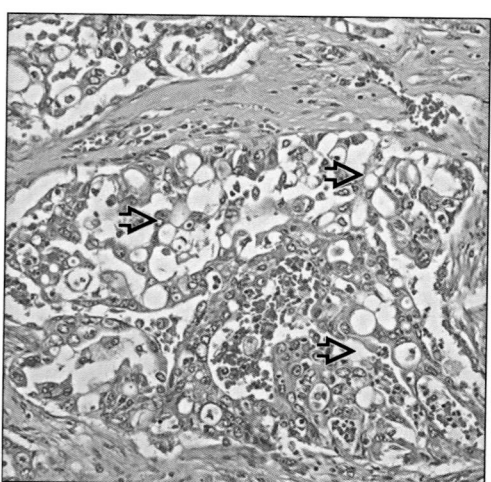
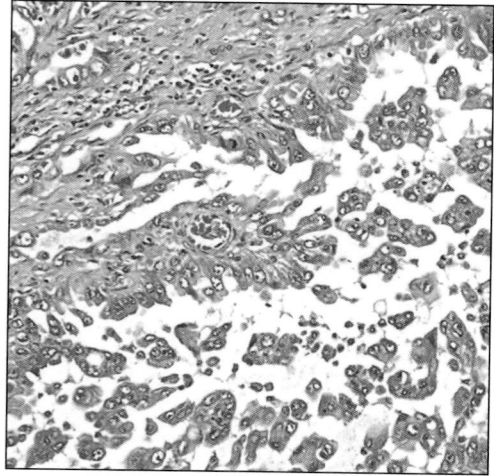

(Left) This hematoxylin & eosin image shows cribriform architecture ⊡ in a renal medullary carcinoma. Cribriform architecture with small lumina may sometimes give an impression of adenoid cystic carcinoma-like areas. *(Right)* This intermediate magnification view of a renal medullary carcinoma shows a micropapillary architecture in the tumor. Papillary and micropapillary features are often present focally, usually in combination with other architectural patterns.

Microscopic Features

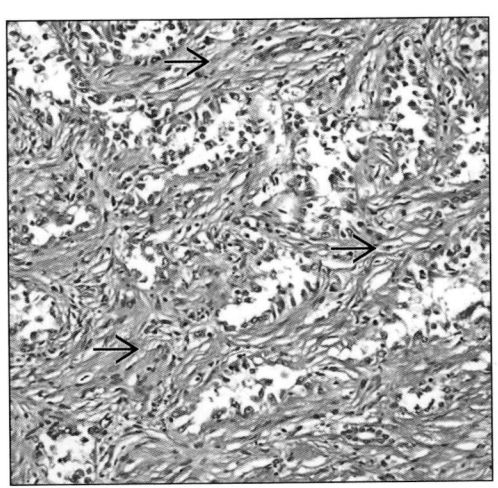

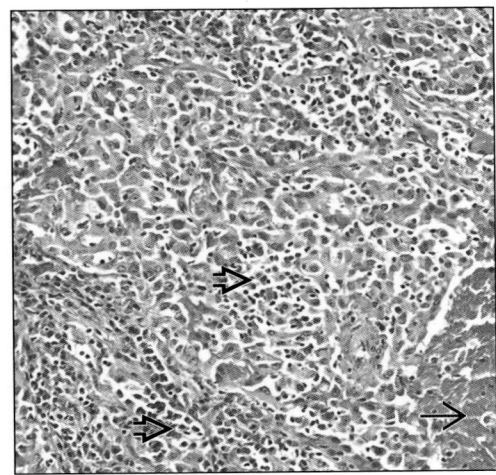

(Left) This renal medullary carcinoma shows a prominent tubular architecture. Some tumors may be predominantly tubular. Irrespective of the architectural patterns, stromal desmoplasia ⊟ is a consistent finding. *(Right)* Solid growth pattern in renal medullary carcinoma is also common and is usually associated with other growth patterns within the same tumor. Notice the intratumoral inflammatory infiltrate ⊟ and agglutinated red blood cells ⊟, both consistent features in RMC.

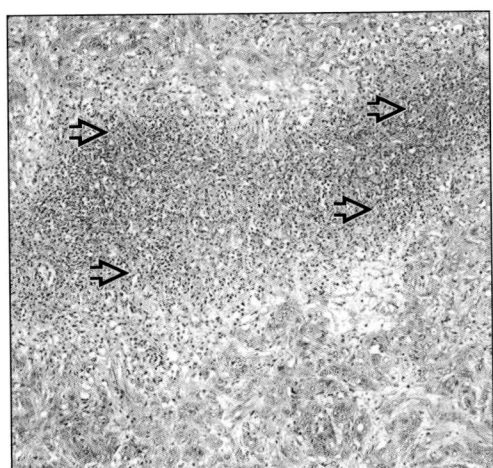

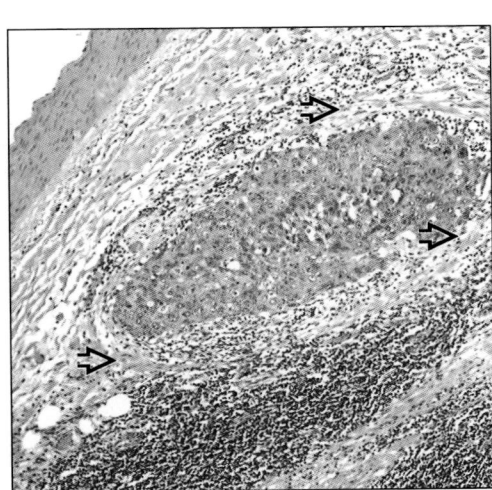

(Left) Microscopic foci of tumor necrosis ⊟ are frequent in renal medullary carcinoma. The cytologic features of this aggressive tumor are always high grade. *(Right)* Similarly, vascular invasion, including that of large muscular ⊟ vessels, is also very common in renal medullary carcinoma. This feature, along with the high nuclear grade and extensively infiltrative margins, are in keeping with high metastatic potential for this tumor.

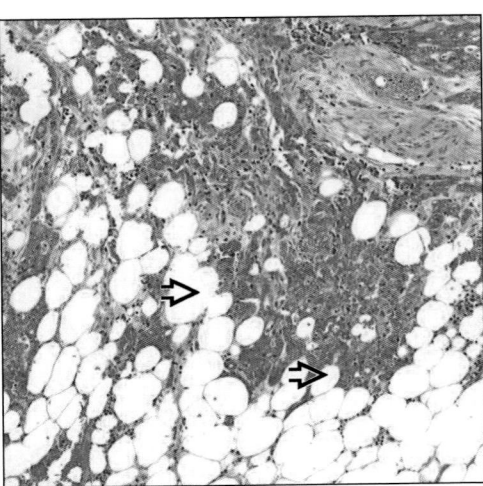

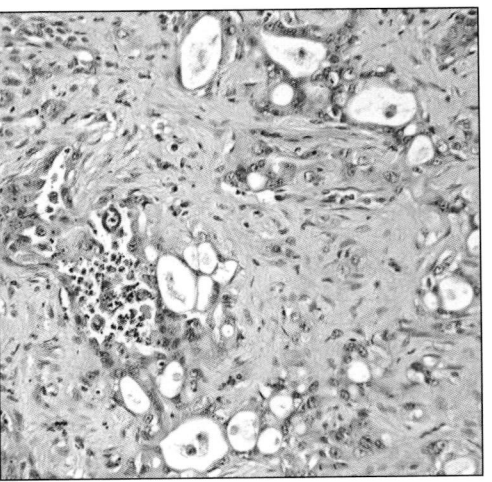

(Left) Renal medullary carcinoma characteristically shows high pT stage and frequently invades perinephric fat ⊟. *(Right)* Stromal desmoplasia with stromal hyalinization is the norm in renal medullary carcinoma. Other tumors in the kidney that demonstrate this feature almost consistently include collecting duct carcinoma, invasive urothelial carcinoma, metastatic carcinoma to the kidney, and unclassified high-grade renal cell carcinoma, NOS.

RENAL MEDULLARY CARCINOMA

Microscopic and Ancillary Features

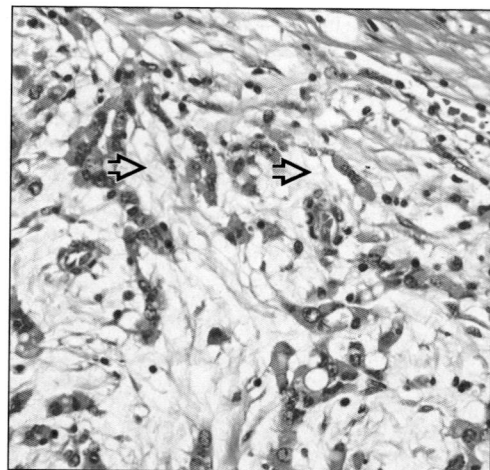 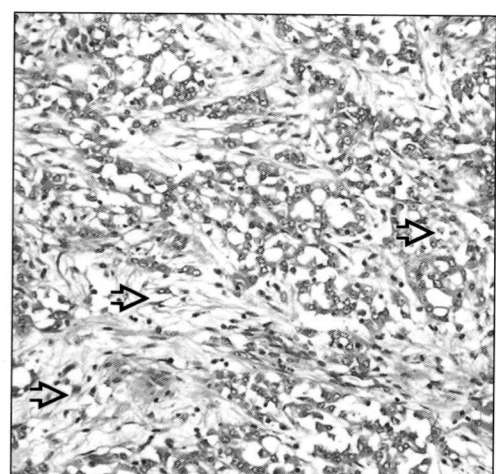

(Left) This photomicrograph shows a RMC with loose and myxoid stroma ⇨. Such a stroma may give a superficial resemblance to yolk-sac tumor in some cases. *(Right)* On the other hand, the stroma can also be quite cellular ⇨ and desmoplastic in RMC. Urothelial carcinomas may also have prominent desmoplastic stromal response. That tumor usually also shows an in situ urothelial component in the pelvicalyceal system and frequently has solid, glandular, &/or squamous differentiation.

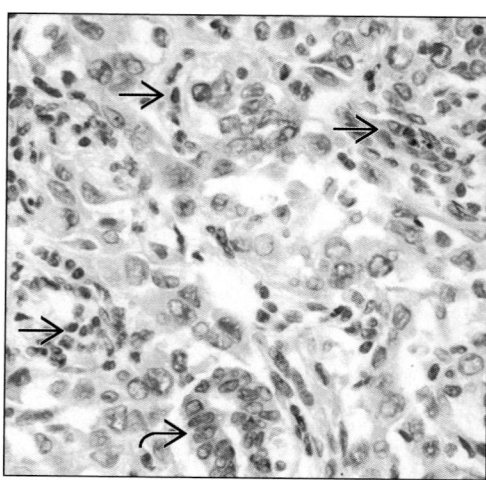 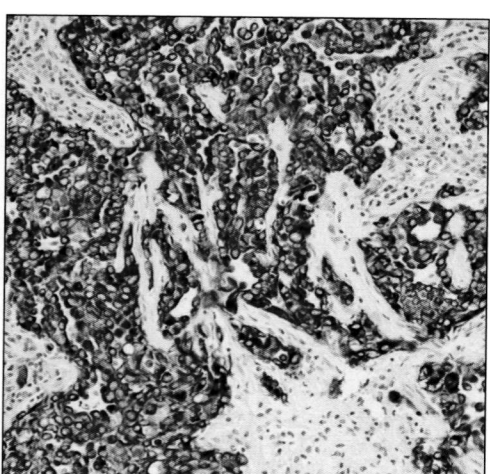

(Left) Renal medullary carcinomas consistently lack immunohistochemical nuclear reactivity for SNF5(INI1), similar to that seen in renal rhabdoid tumor. Notice the retained reactivity in the stromal cells and lymphocytes ⇨, as well as a benign renal tubule ⇨. *(Right)* Immunohistochemical staining with CK7 usually shows a diffuse and strong immunoreactivity in renal medullary carcinomas.

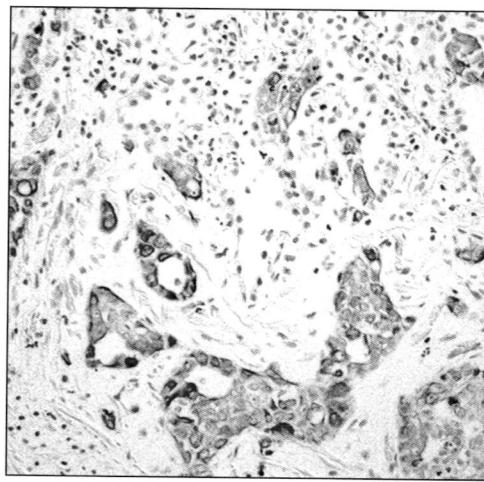 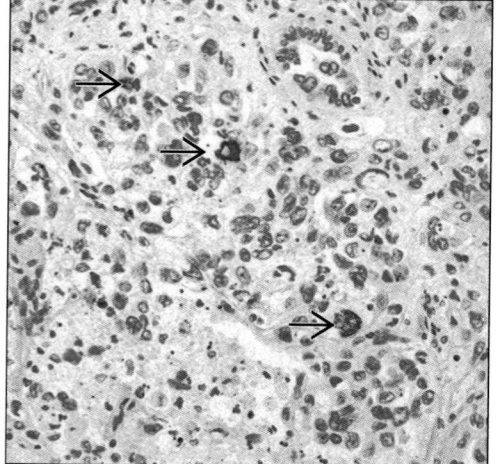

(Left) Immunostaining for CK20 is also often focally to more diffusely positive in RMC. Thus, immunostaining profiles for CK7 and CK20 can usually not distinguish renal medullary carcinoma from urothelial carcinoma. *(Right)* On the other hand, staining for HMCK(34βE12) is either negative or very focal ⇨ in RMC. Lack of reactivity for HMCK(34βE12) has been considered by some as a feature suggesting that RMC is unrelated to collecting duct carcinoma.

RENAL MEDULLARY CARCINOMA

Microscopic and Ancillary Features

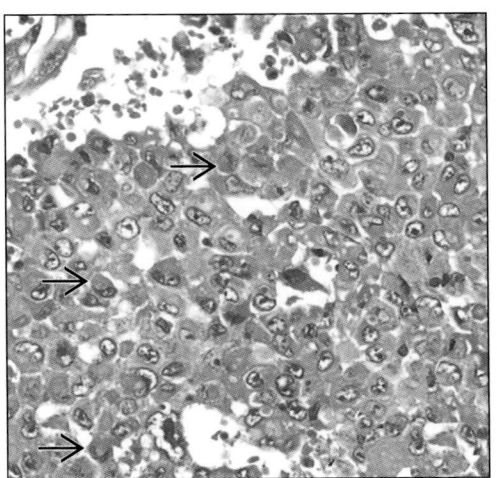
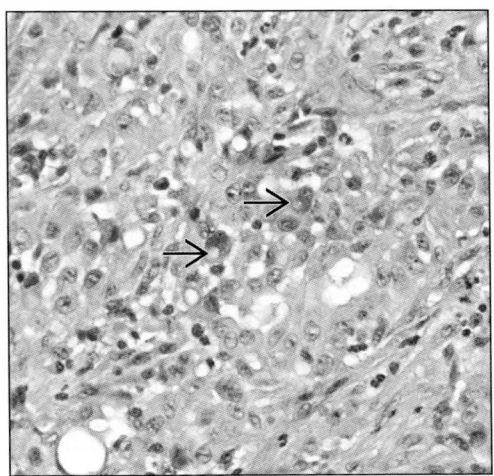

(Left) This photomicrograph shows a RMC with solid architecture. Sometimes the solid areas may show rhabdoid features ➡, raising the possibility of a rhabdoid tumor of the kidney. The negative nuclear reactivity for SNF5 in both may further compound the confusion. However, other areas of the tumor will usually show more classic morphology. Diffuse staining for CK7 may also help. *(Right)* RMC often shows focal intracellular mucin ➡, highlighted by mucicarmine stain.

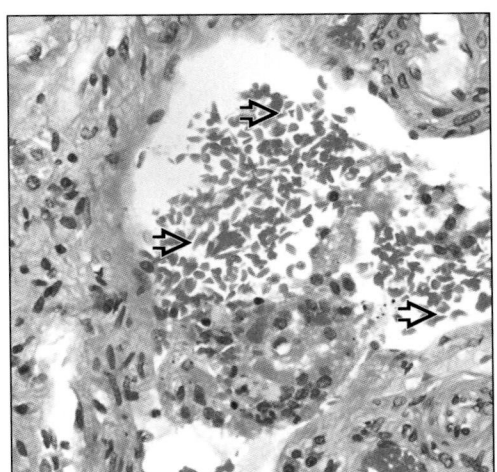
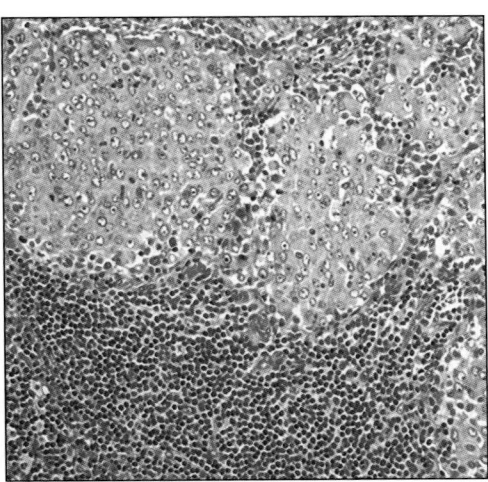

(Left) Crenated or sickled red blood cells both within the tumor and in the benign parenchymal vasculature ➡ is an almost consistent finding in renal medullary carcinoma. *(Right)* This hematoxylin & eosin image shows a renal medullary carcinoma metastatic to a regional lymph node. Most cases of renal medullary carcinoma show metastatic disease at presentation, and in many, it is the metastasis that brings the presence of a renal tumor into focus.

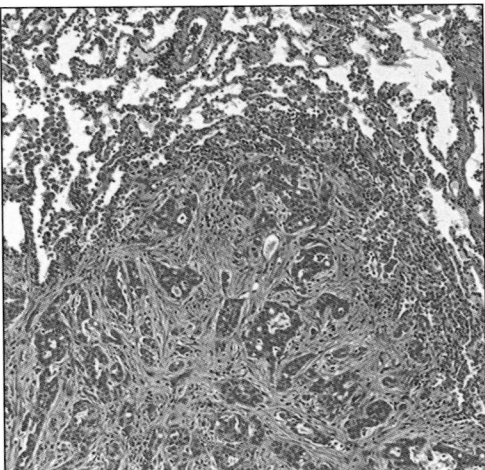
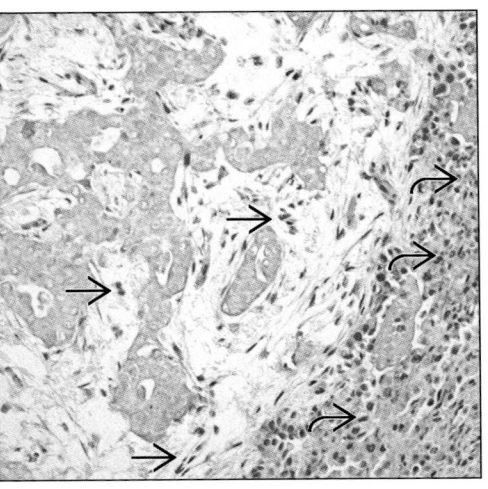

(Left) This hematoxylin & eosin image shows renal medullary carcinoma metastatic to the lung. The presence of crenated/ sickled red cells in a metastatic focus, and in the surrounding tissues, may bring to notice the presence of the hemoglobinopathy for the 1st time in some cases. *(Right)* SNF5(INI1) nuclear staining is absent in metastases from renal medullary carcinoma. Notice the preserved nuclear positivity in the tumor stroma ➡ and surrounding lung parenchyma ➡.

MITF/TFE FAMILY TRANSLOCATION-ASSOCIATED CARCINOMA

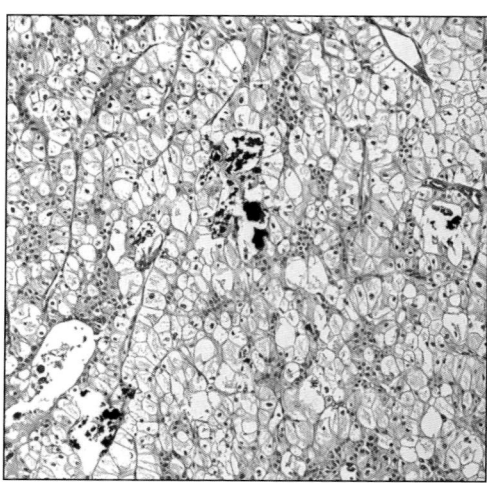

Photomicrograph of a TFE3 renal carcinoma shows nests of clear cells separated by delicate vasculature. Voluminous cytoplasm and psammomatous calcifications are quite typical.

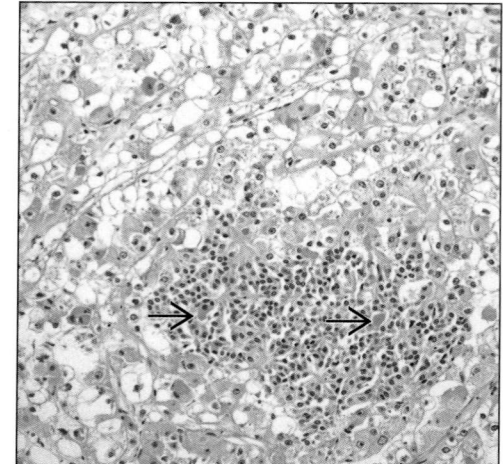

Typical microscopic features of TFEB renal carcinoma include sheets of cells separated by vascular septations and 2 cell types with the smaller cells surrounding hyaline material ➡.

TERMINOLOGY

Abbreviations

- Microphthalmia-associated transcription factor (*MiTF*), transcription factor binding to IGHM enhancer 3 (*TFE3*), transcription factor EB (*TFEB*) translocation-associated carcinoma

Synonyms

- Translocation-associated carcinoma, Xp11.2 and t(6;11) renal carcinomas, *TFE3* (Xp11.2) and *TFEB* [t(6;11)] carcinomas

Definitions

- Renal carcinomas characterized and defined by translocations involving MiTF/TFE family genes (*TFE3* or *TFEB*), with fusions to different genes at a number of different chromosomal locations, including
  - 17q25 (*ASPL*), 1q21 (*PRCC*), 1p34 (*PSF*), Xq12 (*nonO*), 17q23 (*CLTC*), 17q25 (*RCC17*), 3q23 (unknown), 11q12 (*alpha*)

ETIOLOGY/PATHOGENESIS

Molecular Abnormalities

- *TFE3*, *TFEB*, *TFEC*, and *MiTF* are members of MiTF-TFE family of basic helix-loop-helix zipper (bHLH-Zip) factors that bind DNA as homo- and heterodimers
- Members of this family believed to be involved in developmental and cellular processes in various cell types
  - *MiTF* in maturation of melanocytes of neural crest origin, retinal pigment epithelium, and bone marrow-derived mast cells and osteoclasts
  - *TFEB* in placental vascularization
  - *TFE3* in transforming growth factor β (TGF-b)-activated signal transduction and B-cell activation, as well as cooperation with *MiTF* and *TFEC* in osteoclast development

- *TFE3* gene localized to chromosome Xp11.2
- Reported chromosomal translocations and corresponding gene fusion identified in *TFE3* carcinomas
  - Alveolar soft part sarcoma chromosome region, candidate 1 gene (*ASPSCR1* or *ASPL*)-TFE3; t(X;17)(p11.2;q25)
    - *ASPL* (a.k.a. *ASPSCR1* or *PRCC2*) is novel gene of unknown function
    - Translocation similar to that in alveolar soft part sarcoma (ASPS)
    - However, translocation balanced in TFE3 renal carcinoma, unlike the unbalanced translocation (loss of some genetic material) in ASPS
  - Papillary renal cell carcinoma (translocation-associated) gene (*PRCC*)-TFE3; t(X;1)(p11.2;q21)
    - *PRCC* is novel gene encoding major subunit of clathrin, a multimeric cytoplasmic organelle protein
  - PTB-associated splicing factor gene (*PSF*)-TFE3; t(X;1)(p11.2;p34)
  - *NonO*-TFE3; Inv(X)(p11;q12)
    - *PSF* and *nonO* are splicing factor genes
  - Clathrin heavy chain 1 gene (*CLTC*)-TFE3; t(X;17)(p11.2;q23)
    - *CLTC* encodes a major subunit of clathrin
  - *RCC17*-TFE3; t(X;17)(p11.2;q25.3)
  - Unknown gene-*TFE3*; t(X;3)(p11;q23)
  - Different *TFE3* gene fusions consistently lead to overexpression of fusion protein relative to native TFE3, such that protein becomes detectable by immunohistochemical assay
- *TFEB* gene localized to chromosome 6p21
  - *TFEB* gene fused to *alpha* gene, an intron-less gene of unknown function on chromosome 11q12
    - Translocation fuses *alpha* gene with 1st intron of *TFEB* transcription factor gene
  - *Alpha-TFEB* fusion gene results in dysregulated expression of normal full-length TFEB protein detectable by immunohistochemistry

MITF/TFE FAMILY TRANSLOCATION-ASSOCIATED CARCINOMA

Key Facts

Terminology

- Renal carcinomas characterized, and defined, by translocations involving MiTF/TFE family genes (*TFE3* or *TFEB*) and with fusions to different, mostly well-characterized genes at a number of different chromosomal locations, including
  - 17q25 (*ASPL*), 1q21 (*PRCC*), 1p34 (*PSF*), Xq12 (*nonO*), 17q23 (*CLTC*), 17q25 (*RCC17*), 3q23 (unknown), 11q12 (*alpha*)

Clinical Issues

- Uncommon, but constitute a large proportion of renal cell carcinomas in pediatric age groups
- TFE3 renal carcinomas among children, particularly ASPL-TFE3 carcinomas, usually present at advanced stage

- Clinical course more aggressive in adults, with multiple reported deaths due to disease

Microscopic Pathology

- Carcinoma with high nuclear grade, prominent papillary &/or solid alveolar growth patterns, and composed of clear cells is most distinctive histopathologic appearance in Xp11 tumors
  - However, presence of cells with granular eosinophilic cytoplasm is not uncommon

Ancillary Tests

- These carcinomas are negative or only focally positive for epithelial markers and vimentin
- TFE3 and TFEB are highly sensitive and specific immunohistochemical markers for TFE3 and TFEB renal carcinomas

Post-Chemotherapy

- Approximately 10-15% of cases in children with prior exposure to chemotherapy
  - Exposure usually during 1st and 2nd decades of life for other childhood malignancies or SLE
  - Interval between chemotherapy and development of renal carcinoma ranges between 2-13 years
  - Exact mechanism for post-chemotherapy development of these tumors not known
  - Possible contributing factor
    - Relatively increased proliferation in growing pediatric kidney rendering it more sensitive to mutagenic effects of chemotherapeutic agents

CLINICAL ISSUES

Epidemiology

- Incidence
  - Renal cell carcinomas account for < 5% of pediatric renal neoplasms
    - Although uncommon, translocation-associated renal carcinomas constitute large proportion of renal cell carcinomas in pediatric age group
  - Few cases described in adults, with the oldest in a 78-year-old man
    - However, in a large recent consecutive series from Japan, comprised 1.6% of all RCCs in adults and 15% of RCCs in patients < 45 years of age
    - Because of marked differences in number of RCCs in adults and children, absolute total number of cases in adults likely greater than in children
- Gender
  - As more cases are being reported, there seems to be no definite sex bias

Presentation

- Pediatric and young adult patients are usually symptomatic at presentation, and only a few cases are incidentally discovered
- Most common symptom is hematuria, followed by abdominal mass, abdominal pain, and weight loss

- Rare atypical presentations in adults include heavily calcified renal mass, outflow obstruction with consequent pyelonephritis, misdiagnosis as renal cyst or nephrolithiasis

Treatment

- Optimal treatment approach remains to be determined
- Reported cases have been managed similarly to conventional renal cell carcinoma

Prognosis

- TFE3 renal carcinomas among children, particularly ASPL-TFE3 carcinomas, usually present at advanced stage
  - In spite of high stage at presentation, including lymph node metastasis, based on relatively short follow-up, clinical behavior usually not aggressive
- Among the relatively small number of reported cases in adults, clinical course more aggressive, with multiple reported deaths due to disease
- Sites of metastasis include lymph nodes, lung, liver, spine, and adrenal gland
- All reported cases of TFEB renal carcinoma have been organ-confined tumors, and none has recurred or metastasized
  - However, clinical follow-up information limited

MACROSCOPIC FEATURES

General Features

- Mostly well circumscribed but nonencapsulated
  - Some tumors with irregular infiltrative outlines, with perirenal and renal sinus extensions
  - Rarely, pseudocapsule is present, and it may show calcifications
- Cut surface tan-yellow, often showing hemorrhage and necrosis; similar to clear cell renal cell carcinoma

Size

- 2.7-21 cm, reported mean = 6.8 cm

MITF/TFE FAMILY TRANSLOCATION-ASSOCIATED CARCINOMA

MICROSCOPIC PATHOLOGY

Histologic Features

- While morphologic features often correlate with translocation type, significant morphologic overlap between different translocation groups
- Carcinoma with high nuclear grade, prominent papillary &/or solid alveolar growth patterns, and composed of clear cells is most distinctive histopathologic appearance in Xp11 tumors
- However, presence of cells with granular eosinophilic cytoplasm is not uncommon
- Histology of Xp11 translocation carcinomas with specific chromosomal translocations often have characteristic features
  - ASPL-TFE3 carcinoma usually shows
    - Cells with voluminous, clear to eosinophilic cytoplasm; discrete cell borders; vesicular nuclear chromatin; and prominent nucleoli
    - Tumor cells often are discohesive, which leads to alveolar and pseudopapillary architecture
    - True papillary formations are also not uncommon and rarely may be predominant architectural pattern
    - Psammoma bodies are almost universal and sometimes extensive; usually form upon characteristic hyaline nodules
  - PRCC-TFE3 carcinoma typically shows
    - Less abundant cytoplasm
    - Few psammoma bodies and hyaline nodules
    - More nested and compact architecture
    - Some nests with central lumina forming acinar pattern
    - Papillary architecture is common; present either merging with or sharply defined from the acinar areas
    - Usually, but not always, lower nuclear grade than *ASPL-TFE3* tumors
- Unusual histologic features
  - Biphasic population of larger clear cells and smaller cells clustered around nodular hyaline material similar to t(6;11) translocation renal cell carcinoma
  - Pleomorphic giant cells
  - Focal "hobnailed" pattern
  - Fascicles of neoplastic spindle cells
- Morphologic features of other Xp11 translocation carcinomas (PSF-TFE3, nonO-TFE3, CLTC-TFE3) not well defined because of few reported cases
- Alpha-TFEB carcinomas with t(6;11)(p21;q12) usually with
  - Nests, sheets, and tubules of cells separated by thin vascular septae
  - Papillary architecture is uncommon but may be focally to extensively present in some tumors
  - Most tumor cells with abundant clear cytoplasm, well-defined cell borders, and round nuclei
    - Nuclei usually uniform but often with prominent nucleoli
  - Some tumors with variable proportion of granular eosinophilic cytoplasm

  - Usually minor subpopulation of smaller cells with high nuclear/cytoplasmic ratio and dense nuclear chromatin
    - Typically clustered around nodules of hyaline basement membrane material
    - Hyaline material may not be present in some of the smaller cell areas or may be entirely absent
  - Similar, biphasic morphology may rarely also be seen in Xp11 (TFE3) carcinomas

Predominant Pattern/Injury Type

- Neoplastic

Predominant Cell/Compartment Type

- Epithelial

ANCILLARY TESTS

Immunohistochemistry

- Unlike common RCCs, these carcinomas are negative or only focally positive for cytokeratins and epithelial membrane antigen (EMA/MUC1)
- Vimentin is usually negative but may be weakly and focally positive
- CD10, RCC antigen, AMACR, and E-cadherin are usually positive in TFE3 carcinomas
- CD10 and RCC antigen are usually absent or only focally positive in TFEB tumors
- TFE3 is highly sensitive and specific marker for Xp11 translocation-associated carcinomas
  - Diffuse nuclear labeling reported to have sensitivity of 97.5% and specificity of 99.6%
  - ASPS also shows diffuse and strong nuclear reactivity
  - Very rare cases of adrenal cortical carcinoma reported to be positive
  - Other renal cell tumors and large number of nonrenal tumors tested have been negative
- TFEB is highly sensitive and specific marker for 6;11 translocation-associated carcinomas
  - Lymphocytes sometimes may show weak nuclear reactivity
- Melanocytic markers Melan-A(MART-1) and HMB-45 frequently positive in TFEB carcinoma
- Melan-A(MART-1) and HMB-45 rarely expressed in TFE3 tumors, particularly those with *PSF–TFE3* and *CLTC–TFE3* fusions

Electron Microscopy

- TFE3 renal carcinomas
  - Evidence of epithelial differentiation present varying from cell junctions, well-formed glandular lumens containing microvilli, and basement membranes
  - Intracytoplasmic fat and glycogen are present, similar to conventional renal cell carcinoma
  - In PRCC-TFE3 carcinoma, intracisternal microtubules similar to those in melanoma are sometimes present
  - In ASPL-TFE3 carcinoma, abundant electron-dense granules similar in size and shape to those seen in alveolar soft part sarcoma are present

- Rare instance of well-formed rhomboid crystals characteristic of alveolar soft part sarcoma reported
- TFEB renal carcinomas
  - Polygonal cells rich in mitochondria, with scattered membrane-bound granules and varying amount of glycogen
  - Occasional cell junctions; true desmosomes not prominent
  - Distinctive extracellular pools of duplicated basement membrane material surrounded by smaller tumor cells
  - Multilamellar appearance of basement membrane material at higher magnification

DIFFERENTIAL DIAGNOSIS

Clear Cell Renal Cell Carcinoma

- High-grade clear cell carcinoma with large solid alveoli vs. ASPL-TFE3 carcinoma
  - Transition to more typical lower grade, smaller acinar growth pattern is often present
  - Cells with voluminous cytoplasm are uncommon
  - Psammomatous calcifications are rarely, if ever, seen
  - Immunostains for PAN-CK(AE1/AE3), Cam5.2, and EMA/MUC1 are positive, and AMACR and TFE3 are negative
- Clear cell carcinoma vs. TFEB renal carcinoma
  - Clear cell carcinoma lacks biphasic pattern of large epithelioid cells and clusters of smaller cells
  - Immunostains for PAN-CK(AE1/AE3), Cam5.2, EMA/MUC1, CD10, and vimentin are usually diffusely positive
  - TFEB is negative

Papillary Renal Cell Carcinoma

- Foamy macrophages are frequent in papillary cores
- PAN-CK(AE1/AE3), Cam5.2, CK7, and AMACR are positive
- TFE3 and TFEB are negative

Clear Cell-Papillary Renal Cell Carcinoma

- Nuclei are low grade and arranged in linear pattern away from basement membrane
- Tumors are often cystic
- On immunostaining, these are CK7, CA9, and HMCK(34βE12) positive
- AMACR and CD10 mostly negative

DIAGNOSTIC CHECKLIST

Pathologic Interpretation Pearls

- Renal tumors with clear cell cytology with voluminous cytoplasm should always raise differential diagnostic consideration of translocation-associated carcinoma
  - Possibility is particularly high in younger patients
  - Level of suspicion should be higher in cases
    - Not showing areas typical of lower grade clear cell renal cell carcinoma morphology
    - Show any papillary architecture

- Immunohistochemical staining for epithelial markers (cytokeratins and EMA/MUC1) in such cases must be performed
  - Negative or only focal positivity of these stains further strengthens possibility of translocation-associated carcinoma
- Tumors resembling high-grade clear cell renal cell carcinoma, but showing prominent psammomatous calcifications, also require exclusion of translocation-associated renal carcinoma
  - Psammomatous calcifications, particularly when numerous, very unusual finding in clear cell renal cell carcinoma

SELECTED REFERENCES

1. Komai Y et al: Adult Xp11 translocation renal cell carcinoma diagnosed by cytogenetics and immunohistochemistry. Clin Cancer Res. 15(4):1170-6, 2009
2. Camparo P et al: Renal translocation carcinomas: clinicopathologic, immunohistochemical, and gene expression profiling analysis of 31 cases with a review of the literature. Am J Surg Pathol. 32(5):656-70, 2008
3. Geller JI et al: Translocation renal cell carcinoma: lack of negative impact due to lymph node spread. Cancer. 112(7):1607-16, 2008
4. Argani P et al: Xp11 translocation renal cell carcinoma in adults: expanded clinical, pathologic, and genetic spectrum. Am J Surg Pathol. 31(8):1149-60, 2007
5. Argani P et al: Translocation carcinomas of the kidney after chemotherapy in childhood. J Clin Oncol. 24(10):1529-34, 2006
6. Argani P et al: Renal carcinomas with the t(6;11)(p21;q12): clinicopathologic features and demonstration of the specific alpha-TFEB gene fusion by immunohistochemistry, RT-PCR, and DNA PCR. Am J Surg Pathol. 29(2):230-40, 2005
7. Argani P et al: Primary renal neoplasms with the ASPL-TFE3 gene fusion of alveolar soft part sarcoma: a distinctive tumor entity previously included among renal cell carcinomas of children and adolescents. Am J Pathol. 159(1):179-92, 2001
8. Weterman MJ et al: Nuclear localization and transactivating capacities of the papillary renal cell carcinoma-associated TFE3 and PRCC (fusion) proteins. Oncogene. 19(1):69-74, 2000
9. Sidhar SK et al: The t(X;1)(p11.2;q21.2) translocation in papillary renal cell carcinoma fuses a novel gene PRCC to the TFE3 transcription factor gene. Hum Mol Genet. 5(9):1333-8, 1996
10. Suijkerbuijk RF et al: Identification of a yeast artificial chromosome that spans the human papillary renal cell carcinoma-associated t(X;1) breakpoint in Xp11.2. Cancer Genet Cytogenet. 71(2):164-9, 1993
11. Tomlinson GE et al: Cytogenetics of a renal cell carcinoma in a 17-month-old child. Evidence for Xp11.2 as a recurring breakpoint. Cancer Genet Cytogenet. 57(1):11-7, 1991
12. de Jong B et al: Cytogenetics of a renal adenocarcinoma in a 2-year-old child. Cancer Genet Cytogenet. 21(2):165-9, 1986

MITF/TFE FAMILY TRANSLOCATION-ASSOCIATED CARCINOMA

Gross and Microscopic Features

(Left) Typical gross appearance of a TFE3 renal carcinoma that shows a well-circumscribed tumor with tan-yellow cut surface. Many tumors, however, show invasion into perinephric fat ⮞. *(Right)* Well-circumscription of a TFE3 renal carcinoma is shown. Most MiTF renal carcinomas are well circumscribed, without a distinct tumor capsule. However, satellite nodules into the surrounding parenchyma are quite common. Some TFE3 carcinomas show a pseudocapsule ⮞, often with calcifications.

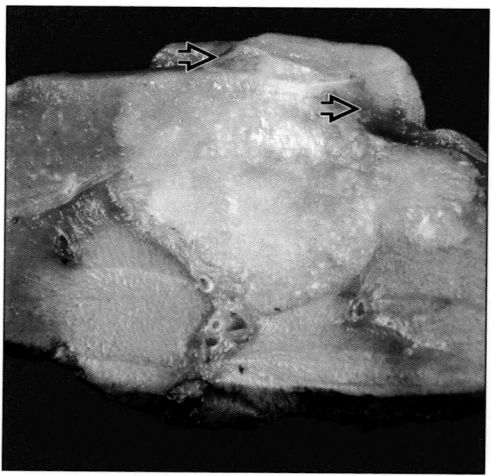
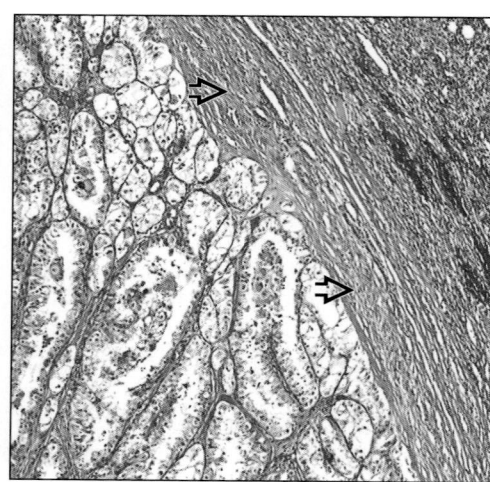

(Left) Hematoxylin & eosin stain shows characteristic light microscopic features of a TFE3 renal carcinoma. The presence of numerous psammomatous calcifications ➡ in a tumor resembling high-grade clear cell RCC should always be investigated for a TFE carcinoma. *(Right)* Solid alveolar architectural pattern in a TFE3 carcinoma, as seen here, is quite common, and the thin branching septations may raise the possibility of a high-grade clear cell renal cell carcinoma.

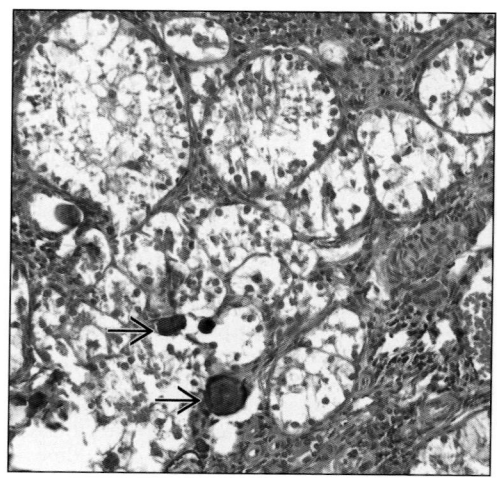
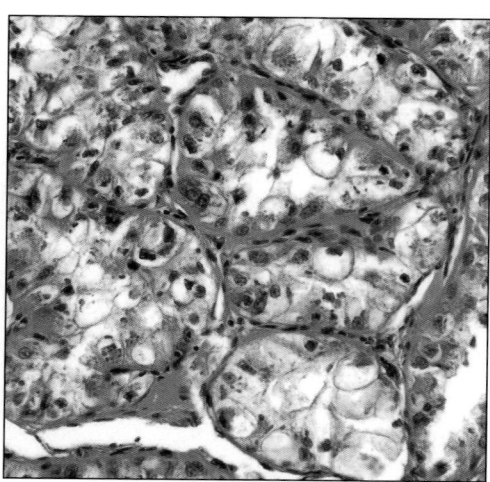

(Left) Papillary architecture in TFE3 renal carcinoma is quite common. Clear cell cytology with papillary architecture ➡, psammomatous calcifications ⤴, and cells with voluminous cytoplasm ⮞ strongly point toward the diagnosis of a TFE3 carcinoma, rather than a clear cell RCC. *(Right)* A high magnification view of TFE3 carcinoma with papillary architecture shows voluminous clear cytoplasm and high-grade nuclei. Intracytoplasmic hyaline globules ➡ are also occasionally seen.

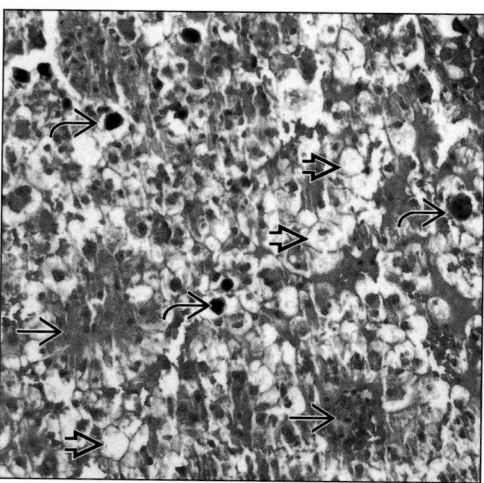
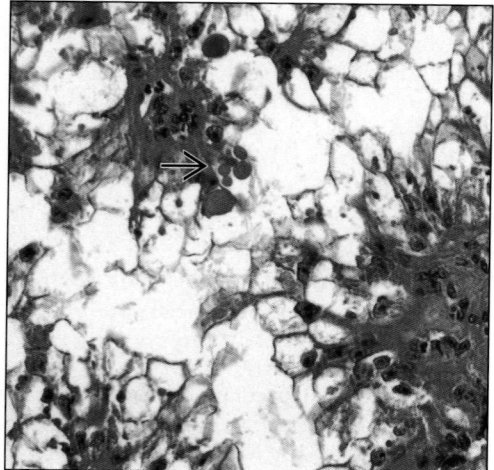

MITF/TFE FAMILY TRANSLOCATION-ASSOCIATED CARCINOMA

Microscopic and Ancillary Features

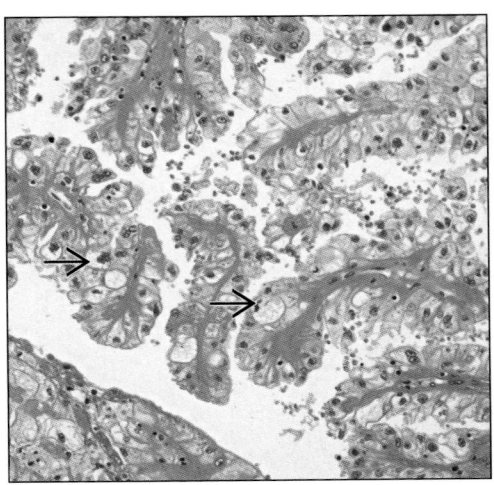

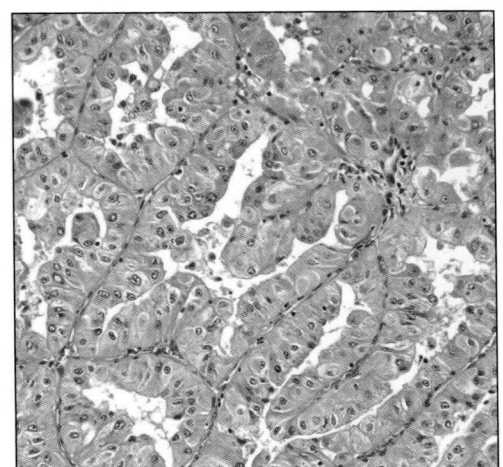

(Left) Most TFE3 tumors may show pseudopapillary architecture with discohesive solid acini, but true papillary architecture is not uncommon. The voluminous cytoplasm in some of the cells ➡ is a prominent pointer toward translocation-associated carcinoma. *(Right)* While clear cell cytology is common in TFE3 carcinomas, some tumors may show prominent to predominant, and, rarely, almost exclusive cytoplasmic eosinophilia.

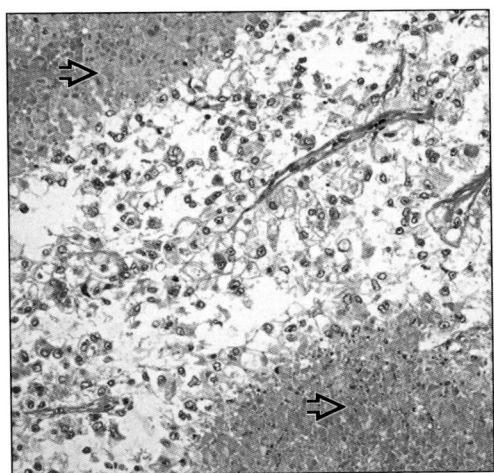

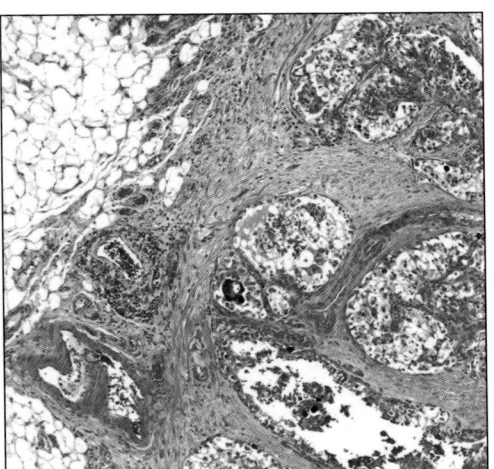

(Left) Coagulative tumor necrosis ➡ and hemorrhage are commonly observed in TFE renal carcinoma. These findings are often noted even in gross specimens. This photomicrograph is a reflection of such commonly observed gross findings. *(Right)* This photomicrograph shows perinephric fat invasion in a TFE3 carcinoma. TFE3 renal carcinomas often present at high tumor stage. However, compared to the adults, high stage does not necessarily predict aggressive outcome in children.

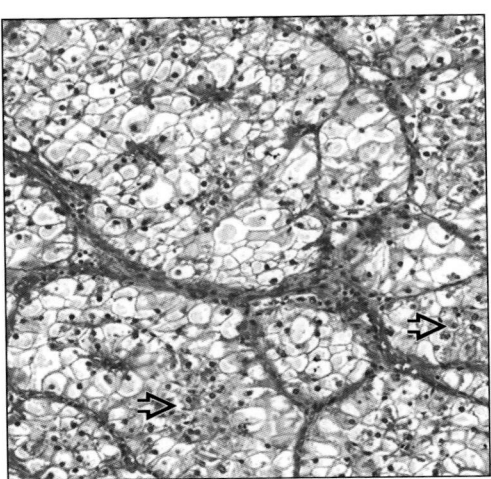

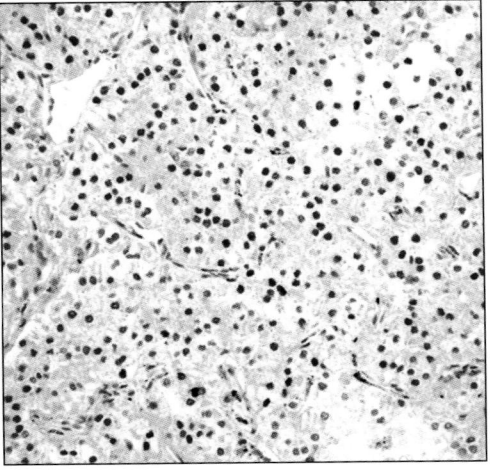

(Left) Solid alveolar growth pattern is not uncommon in TFE3 renal carcinoma. The solid alveoli may show central cell discohesion ➡ and morphologically mimic alveolar soft part sarcoma. Such a growth pattern is commonly associated with ASPL-TFE3 gene fusion. *(Right)* This image depicts TFE3 immunohistochemical staining in a ASPL-TFE3 carcinoma. Diffuse and strong nuclear positivity for TFE3 is characteristic of all types of Xp11 renal carcinomas, irrespective of the fusion gene partner.

MITF/TFE FAMILY TRANSLOCATION-ASSOCIATED CARCINOMA

Microscopic and Ancillary Features

(Left) This TFE3 renal carcinoma depicts prominent papillary architecture. Papillary architecture with prominent clear cell and high-grade cytology should always raise the differential diagnostic possibility of a translocation-associated renal carcinoma. *(Right)* TFE3 immunoreactivity is seen in a TFE3 renal carcinoma with prominent papillary architecture. Diffuse TFE3 positivity is highly specific and sensitive for TFE3 carcinoma; it correlates very well with Xp11.2 (TFE3 gene) translocation.

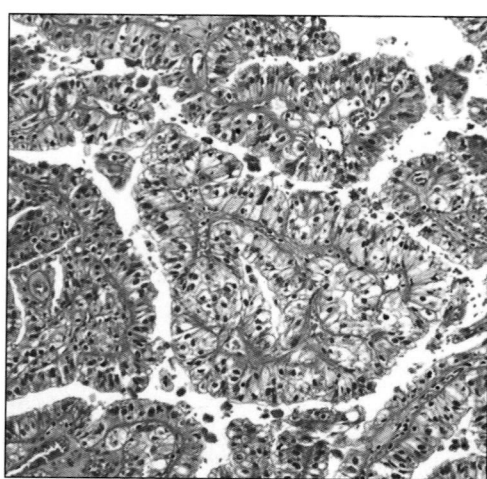
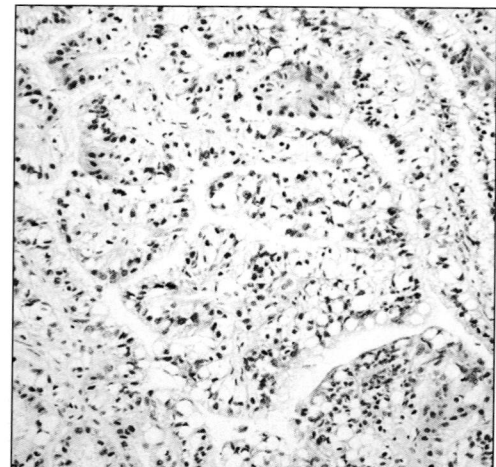

(Left) Immunostaining for PAN-CK(AE1/AE3) in TFE3 carcinoma is usually negative. *(Right)* Unlike other renal tumors, translocation-associated renal carcinomas are negative or only focally and weakly positive for cytokeratins and EMA/MUC1. Tumors with clear cells, voluminous cytoplasm, with or without papillary architecture, and lacking staining for epithelial markers strongly point toward TFE3 renal carcinoma. Note the positive internal control ⇨.

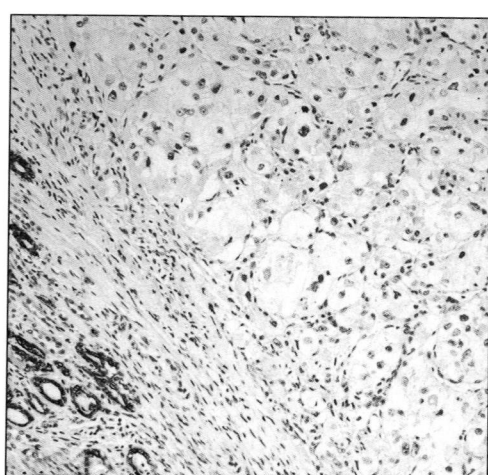
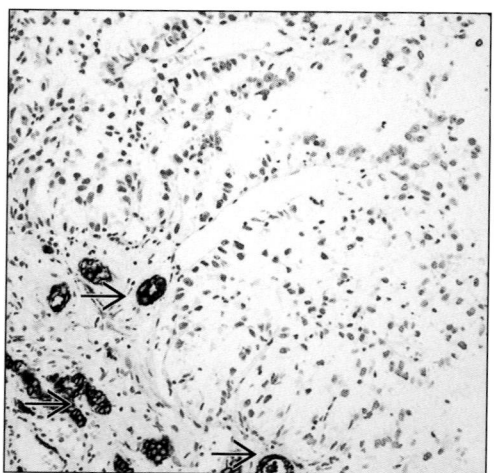

(Left) Vimentin immunostain shows rare tumor cells positive in a TFE3 renal carcinoma. Note the diffuse and strong positivity in the fibrovascular septa ⇨. Diffuse and strong positivity for vimentin is rare in MiTF/TFE family translocation-associated carcinomas. *(Right)* AMACR usually shows diffuse positivity in translocation-associated carcinomas. Negativity for CK7 and diffuse positivity for AMACR can help in differentiating these tumors from both the clear cell and papillary RCC.

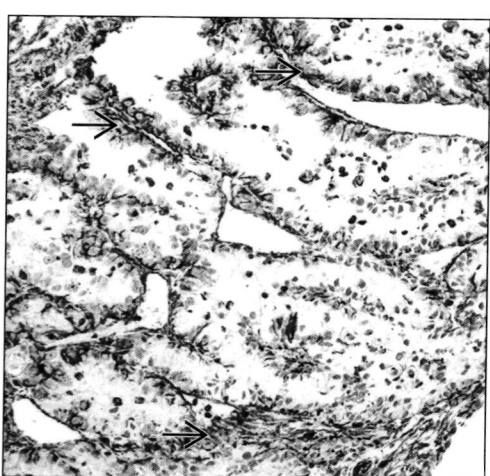
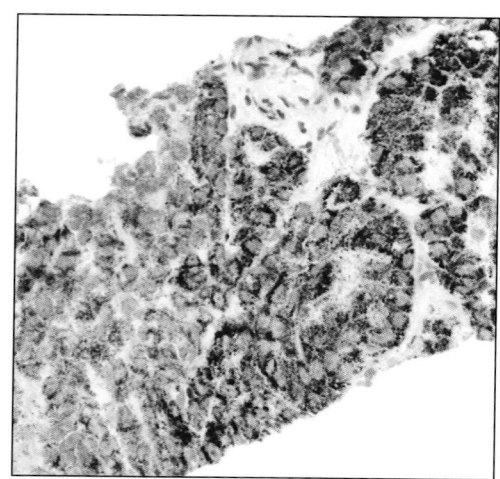

1

MITF/TFE FAMILY TRANSLOCATION-ASSOCIATED CARCINOMA

Microscopic and Ancillary Features

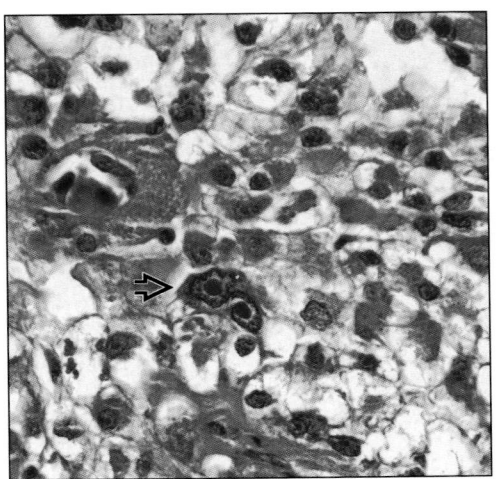
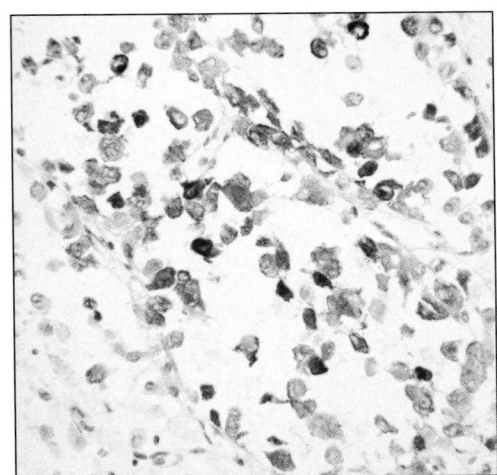

(Left) Some translocation-associated renal carcinomas, particularly those in adults, may occasionally show marked focal cytologic atypia ⇨ and presence of pleomorphic giant cells. (Right) While melanocytic markers HMB-45 and Melan-A(MART-1) are frequently positive in TFEB renal carcinomas, rare cases of TFE3 tumors may also show focal positivity, particularly those with PSF-TFE3 and CLTC-TFE3 fusions. This image depicts HMB-45 positivity in a TFE3 renal carcinoma.

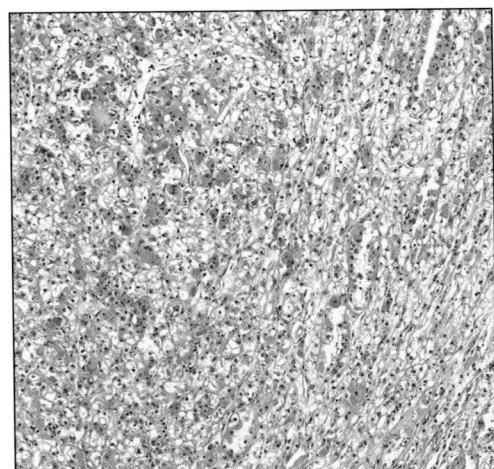
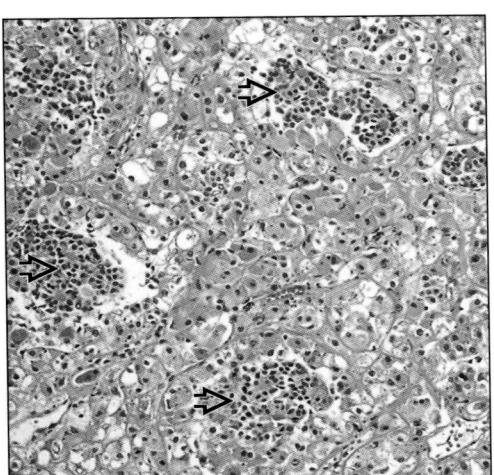

(Left) A low magnification view of a TFEB [t(6;11)] renal carcinoma shows nests, sheets, and tubules of cells, predominantly with clear cytoplasm, separated by thin vascular septae. (Right) However, the most characteristic feature of TFEB renal carcinoma is a biphasic morphology. Dispersed among the larger cells are clusters and islands of smaller cells ⇨ with high nuclear/cytoplasmic ratio and somewhat denser-appearing nuclear chromatin.

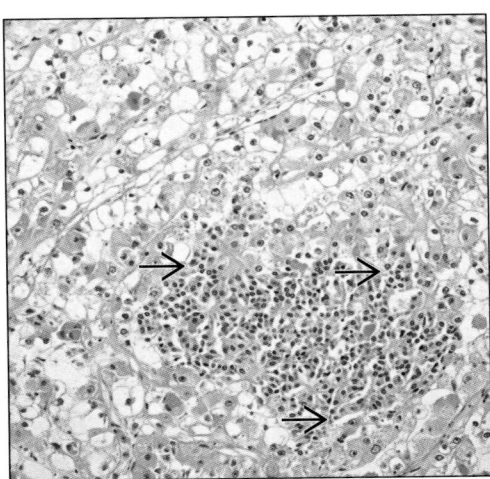
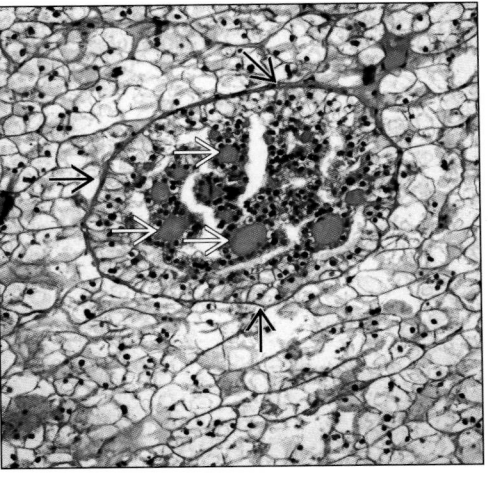

(Left) The collections of smaller cell population in TFEB tumors may show irregular outlines ⇨ but may be sharply delimited in some instances. (Right) This smaller cell population in a TFEB renal carcinoma is present within the confines of a tubular structure ⇨ lined by larger epithelioid cells similar to rest of the tumor. The smaller cells are arranged around small nodules of hyaline material ⇨ that is ultrastructurally shown to be basement membrane material.

Microscopic and Ancillary Features

(Left) While the nodules of basement membrane material within the smaller cell clusters are typically abundant in a given tumor, in some cases such hyaline nodules may be quite rare and difficult to find. *(Right)* Focal calcification is seen in a t(6;11) renal carcinoma ➢. Compared to the TFE3 tumors, psammomatous calcifications in TFEB carcinomas are quite rare and may be completely absent.

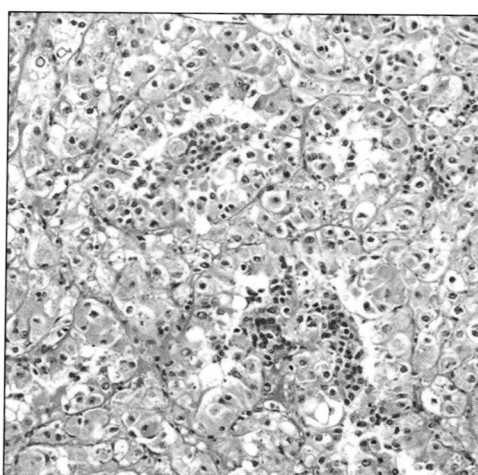
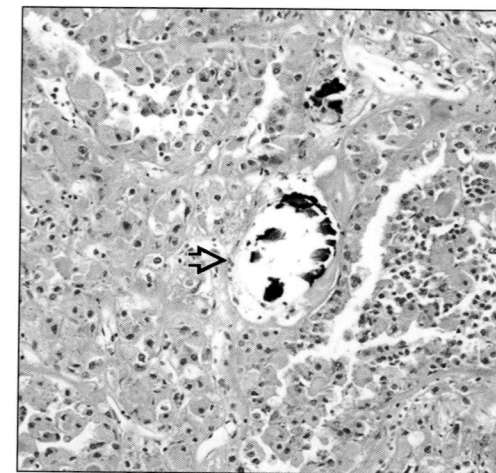

(Left) While most tumors show an admixture of cells with clear and eosinophilic cytoplasm, some TFEB tumors are predominantly or almost exclusively composed of cells with eosinophilic cytoplasm. Most tumors do not show significant nuclear pleomorphism, but the presence of prominent nucleoli ➔ is not uncommon. *(Right)* Focal papillations are seen in many of the TFEB renal carcinomas, but prominent papillary architecture may be observed in some cases.

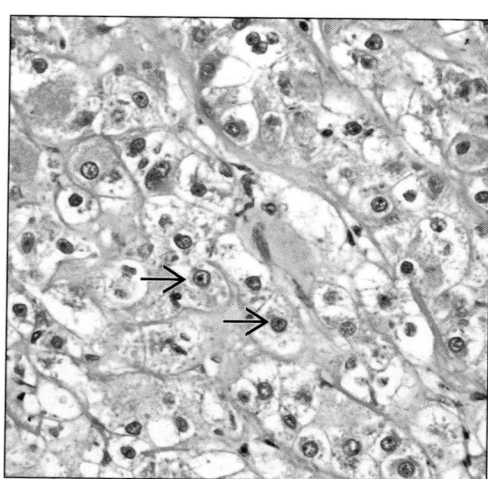
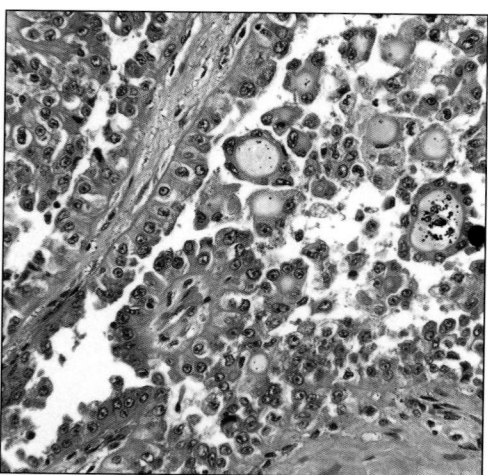

(Left) This TFEB renal carcinoma has focal papillations ➢ in a background of a predominantly nested growth pattern. *(Right)* TFEB immunostaining shows diffuse nuclear positivity in a TFEB renal carcinoma. As with TFE3 immunostain in Xp11.2 carcinomas, TFEB immunostain is highly specific for t(6;11) tumors. Both these antibodies show no cross-reactivity with each other. TFEB immunostain may also show focal nuclear staining in some lymphocytes.

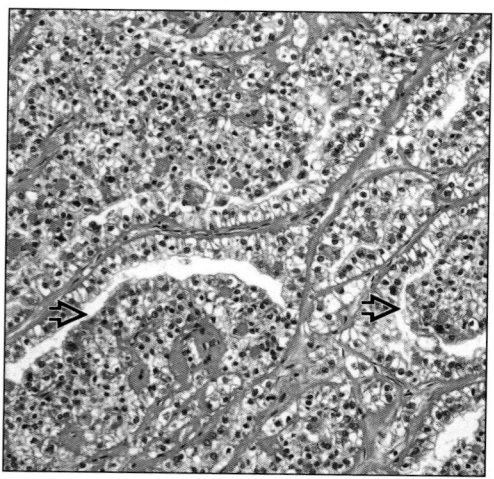
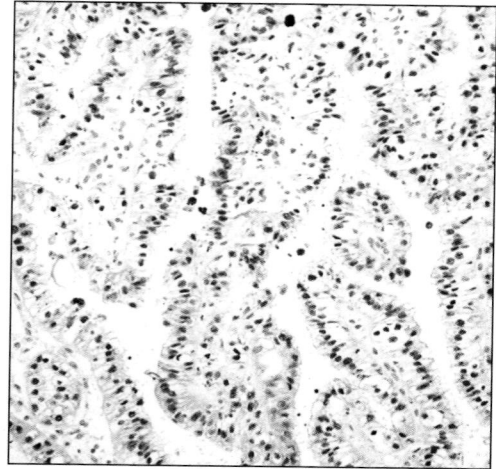

Microscopic and Ancillary Features

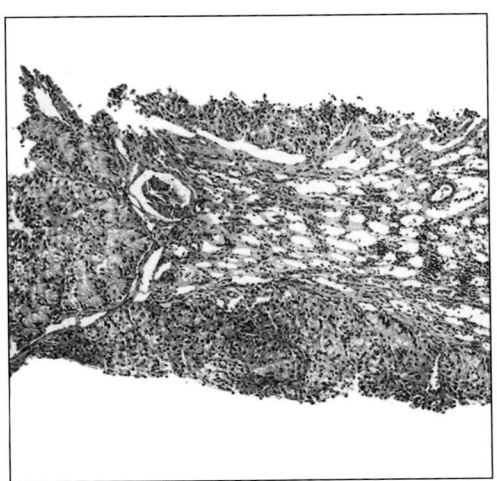 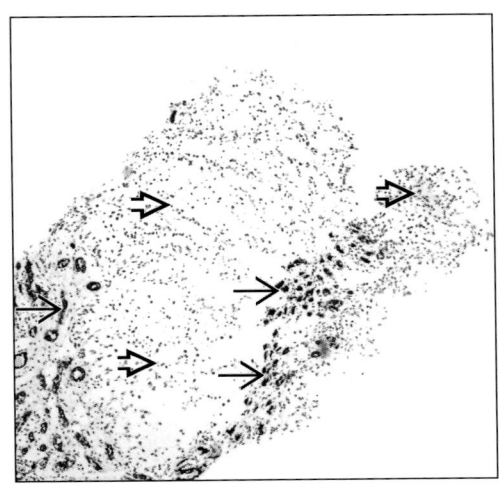

(Left) Solid nests, variable papillary architecture, clear cell cytology, and voluminous cytoplasm in a renal tumor should alert one to the possibility of a translocation-associated carcinoma. Attention to these findings may lead to accurate diagnosis even on needle biopsies of the kidney. *(Right)* The suspicion of TFE carcinoma is further strengthened by the absence of immunoreactivity ⊵ for epithelial markers (PAN-CK[AE1/AE3] in this instance), with appropriate internal control ⊳.

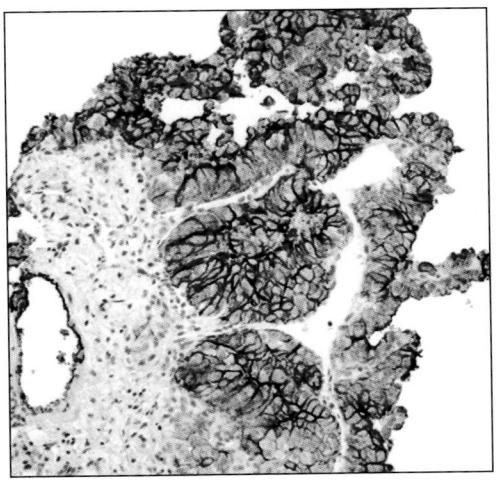 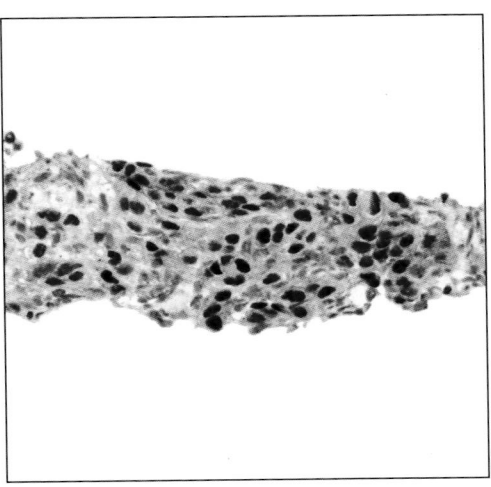

(Left) CD10 usually shows diffuse positivity in TFE3 renal carcinomas. However, the staining is usually weak and more focal in TFEB tumors. *(Right)* TFE3 immunoreactivity is observed in a needle core biopsy of a renal mass in a 35-year-old man. Although the lack of staining for cytokeratins (including CK7) and diffuse positivity for AMACR and CD10 increase the morphologic suspicion of a TFE carcinoma, only diffuse nuclear reactivity with the TFE antibodies will confirm the diagnosis.

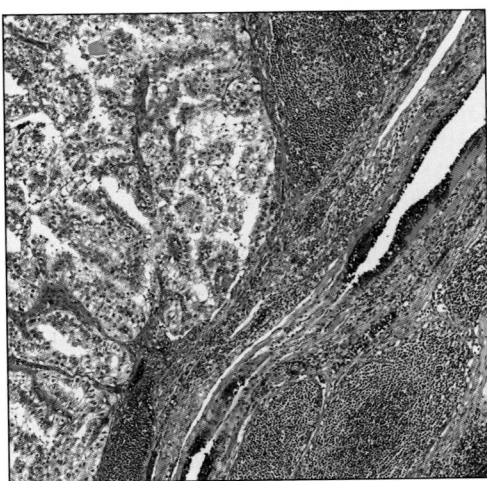 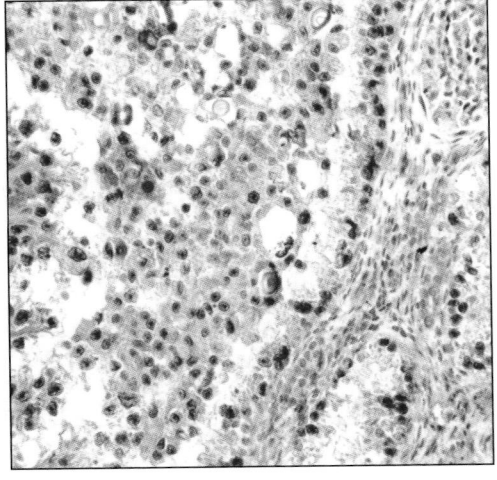

(Left) This image shows a TFE3 renal carcinoma metastatic to a lymph node. Metastatic sites include lymph nodes, lung, liver, spine, and adrenal gland. Lymph node metastases are quite common, both in children and adults. Children with lymph node metastases, however, maintain a favorable prognosis (at least in the short term), whereas the same does not hold true in adults with metastases. *(Right)* Diffuse nuclear immunoreactivity for TFE3 in a metastatic lymph node mass confirms the diagnosis.

MUCINOUS TUBULAR AND SPINDLE CELL CARCINOMA

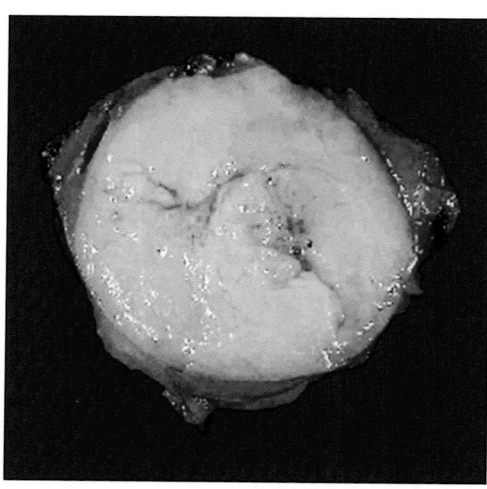

Gross photograph of mucinous tubular and spindle cell carcinoma shows a well-circumscribed mass with typical homogeneous tan-white, glistening cut surface. Some tumors may possess a distinct capsule.

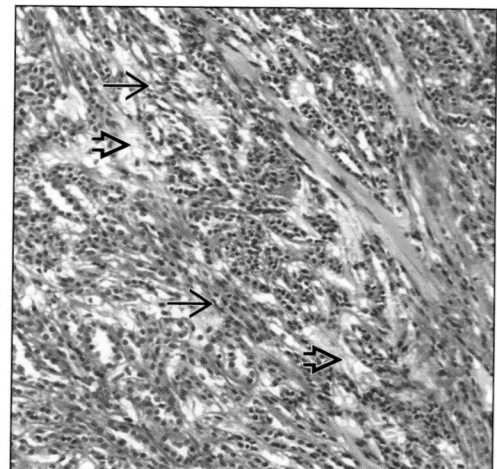

Typical microscopic appearance of MTSCC shows variably shaped tubules, low-grade spindle cell areas ➡, and stromal mucin ▷. Any of these 3 features may be focal or rare in some tumors.

TERMINOLOGY

Abbreviations
- Mucinous tubular and spindle cell carcinoma (MTSCC)

Definitions
- Recently recognized low-grade biphasic neoplasm with epithelial and spindle cell components usually associated with favorable prognosis

ETIOLOGY/PATHOGENESIS

Molecular Abnormalities
- Loss of Chr 1, 4q, 6, 8p, 11q, 13, 14, and 15
- Gains of 11q, 16q, 17, and 20q
- No trisomies 7 and 17

CLINICAL ISSUES

Epidemiology
- Incidence
  - Approximately 100 cases described in the literature
- Age
  - 17-78 years (average = 53 years)
- Gender
  - Female preponderance (M:F = 1:4)

Presentation
- Majority are asymptomatic and discovered incidentally on radiological evaluation for other conditions

Prognosis
- Mostly show indolent behavior
  - Rare reported cases with local lymph node metastasis
  - Very occasional cases with sarcomatoid differentiation have been reported

MACROSCOPIC FEATURES

General Features
- Tumor is usually well circumscribed, occasionally encapsulated, and may be centered in medulla
  - Gray-white to tan or yellow, often glistening, cut surface
  - Hemorrhage or necrosis is unusual, except in sarcomatoid areas

Size
- 2-18 cm (mean = 4.2 cm)

MICROSCOPIC PATHOLOGY

Histologic Features
- Architectural details
  - Tubules with slit-like luminal spaces, many with branching
    - Some tubules may be small and more rounded
  - Low-grade spindle cell areas with nuclei similar to epithelial areas
  - Presence of variable amounts of basophilic extracellular mucin
  - Focal papillations are common
- Cytologic details
  - Cells with cuboidal to low-columnar cytology lining tubules
  - Usually scant cytoplasm with relatively uniform nuclei usually bearing inconspicuous nucleoli
- Uncommon morphologic features include
  - Predominant spindle cell or epithelial components, very scant mucin, focal clear cell or eosinophilic cytology, foamy macrophages, multifocal papillary areas, or sarcomatoid/high-grade epithelial areas
- Tumors often contain background of inflammatory infiltrate

MUCINOUS TUBULAR AND SPINDLE CELL CARCINOMA

Key Facts

Terminology
- Low-grade biphasic carcinoma usually associated with favorable prognosis

Etiology/Pathogenesis
- Loss of Chr 1, 4q, 6, 8p, 11q, 13, 14, and 15
- Gains of 11q, 16q, 17, and 20q

Clinical Issues
- M:F = 1:4
- Majority are discovered incidentally
- Indolent fashion with less aggressive biologic behavior

Macroscopic Features
- Well-circumscribed mass
- Gray-white to tan or yellow cut surface

Microscopic Pathology
- Tightly packed elongated, often branching, tubules
- Basophilic extracellular mucin separating tubules
- Variable spindled cell appearance
  - Low-grade spindle cell areas with nuclei similar to epithelial areas
- Low nuclear grade

Ancillary Tests
- IHC results: Significant overlap with papillary renal cell carcinoma
- EM: Resemble loop of Henle

Top Differential Diagnoses
- Papillary renal cell carcinoma
  - Often show prominent papillary architecture and foam cells, lack mucin

Predominant Pattern/Injury Type
- Neoplastic

Predominant Cell/Compartment Type
- Epithelial, biphasic or mixed

ANCILLARY TESTS

Immunohistochemistry
- Significant overlap with papillary renal cell carcinoma
  - Usually CK7, AMACR positive; CD10 often negative or focal

DIFFERENTIAL DIAGNOSIS

Papillary Renal Cell Carcinoma
- Usual type, including sarcomatoid differentiation
  - Predominant papillary architecture
  - Necrosis and hemorrhage common
  - Frequently prominent foamy macrophages and psammoma bodies
  - Absent stromal mucin
  - Presence of trisomy Chr 7 and Chr 17; loss of Chr Y
- With low-grade spindle cell foci
  - Absent stromal mucin
  - Presence of trisomy of Chr 7 and Chr 17
  - Male sex
  - More commonly CD10 positive

DIAGNOSTIC CHECKLIST

Pathologic Interpretation Pearls
- Key reason to be aware of MTSCC is to avoid mistaking it for sarcomatoid papillary carcinoma
- Immunohistochemical stains cannot differentiate MTSCC from papillary RCC
- Close attention to morphologic features is essential and useful in most instances
- In rare difficult cases, molecular evaluation will be decisive in this distinction

- Sarcomatoid change may very rarely occur in MTSCC

SELECTED REFERENCES

1. Dhillon J et al: Mucinous tubular and spindle cell carcinoma of the kidney with sarcomatoid change. Am J Surg Pathol. 33(1):44-9, 2009
2. Argani P et al: Papillary renal cell carcinoma with low-grade spindle cell foci: a mimic of mucinous tubular and spindle cell carcinoma. Am J Surg Pathol. 32(9):1353-9, 2008
3. Kuroda N et al: Mucinous tubular and spindle cell carcinoma with Fuhrman nuclear grade 3: a histological, immunohistochemical, ultrastructural and FISH study. Histol Histopathol. 23(12):1517-23, 2008
4. Brandal P et al: Genomic aberrations in mucinous tubular and spindle cell renal cell carcinomas. Mod Pathol. 19(2):186-94, 2006
5. Cossu-Rocca P et al: Renal mucinous tubular and spindle carcinoma lacks the gains of chromosomes 7 and 17 and losses of chromosome Y that are prevalent in papillary renal cell carcinoma. Mod Pathol. 19(4):488-93, 2006
6. Fine SW et al: Expanding the histologic spectrum of mucinous tubular and spindle cell carcinoma of the kidney. Am J Surg Pathol. 30(12):1554-60, 2006
7. Kuroda N et al: Frequent expression of neuroendocrine markers in mucinous tubular and spindle cell carcinoma of the kidney. Histol Histopathol. 21(1):7-10, 2006
8. Paner GP et al: Immunohistochemical analysis of mucinous tubular and spindle cell carcinoma and papillary renal cell carcinoma of the kidney: significant immunophenotypic overlap warrants diagnostic caution. Am J Surg Pathol. 30(1):13-9, 2006
9. Ferlicot S et al: Mucinous tubular and spindle cell carcinoma: a report of 15 cases and a review of the literature. Virchows Arch. 447(6):978-83, 2005
10. Kuroda N et al: Review of mucinous tubular and spindle-cell carcinoma of the kidney with a focus on clinical and pathobiological aspects. Histol Histopathol. 20(1):221-4, 2005
11. Eble JN: Mucinous tubular and spindle cell carcinoma and post-neuroblastoma carcinoma: newly recognised entities in the renal cell carcinoma family. Pathology. 35(6):499-504, 2003

MUCINOUS TUBULAR AND SPINDLE CELL CARCINOMA

Microscopic Features

(Left) Most, but not all, mucinous tubular and spindle cell carcinoma are well circumscribed, and/or partly encapsulated ⊟, similar to most of the papillary RCC. Myxoid stroma in a predominantly long tubular pattern is seen. *(Right)* Mucinous tubular and spindle cell carcinoma may sometimes be nonencapsulated and show somewhat irregular tumor borders. The tumor front in some of such tumors appears multi-nodular ⊟ and may be associated with lymphoid aggregates ⇥.

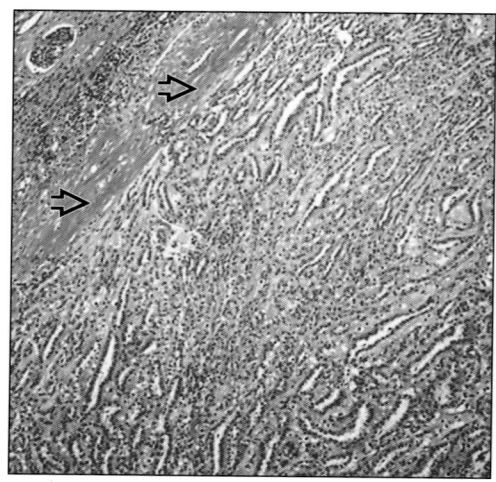
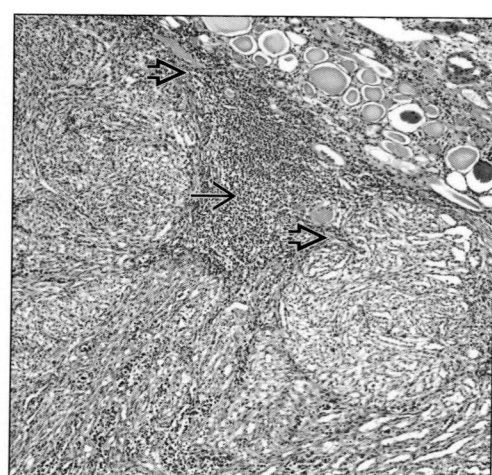

(Left) The banal-appearing spindle cells ⊟ appear to be intimately admixed with the tubular component. The juxtaposition or the imperceptible blending of these 2 features is typical. *(Right)* Most of the tubules show narrow slit-like lumina ⊟. Other tubules may be small and have more rounded contours ⇥. The cells lining the tubules are low-columnar or cuboidal, with uniform, low-grade, round nuclei. Nuclear pleomorphism is very uncommon but may be present in very rare cases.

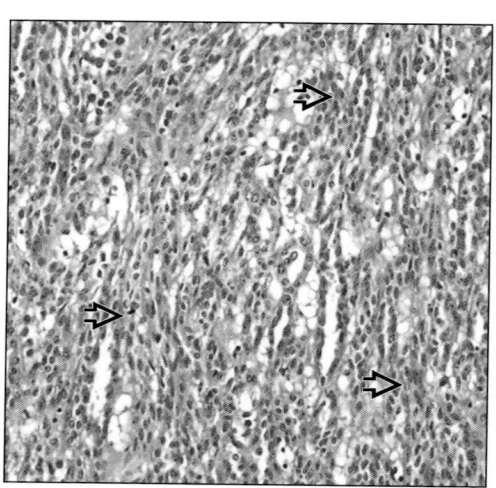
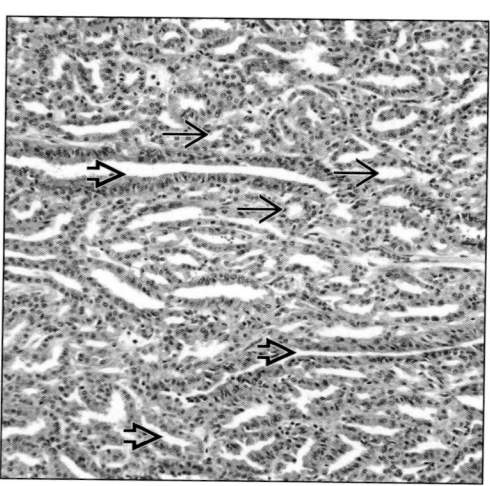

(Left) Extensive tubular branching is shown here. While the tubules show some branching in most cases, in some mucinous tubular and spindle cell carcinomas this branching is exquisite and may be associated with marked interconnecting tubular architecture ⊟. In such areas, the myxoid background may be quite prominent ⇥. *(Right)* In some areas, the tubules may be short and round, bearing superficial resemblance to those seen in metanephric adenoma or solid papillary RCC.

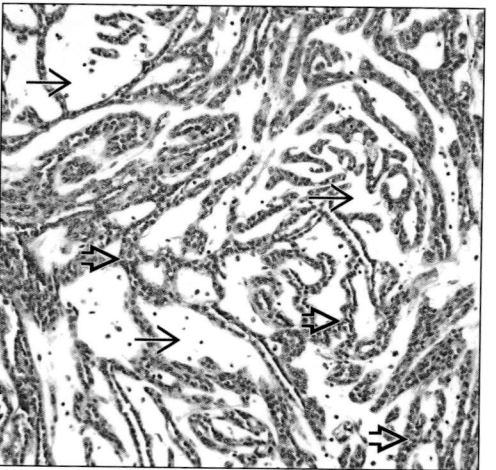
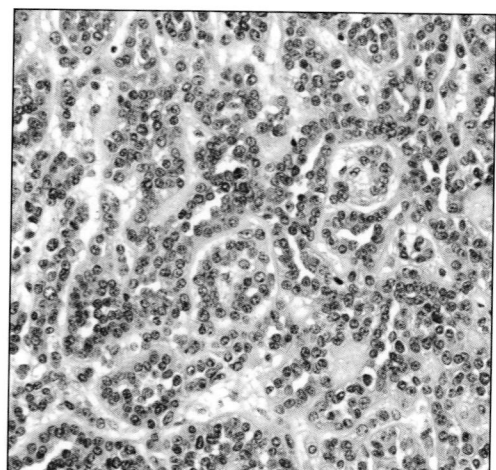

Microscopic Features

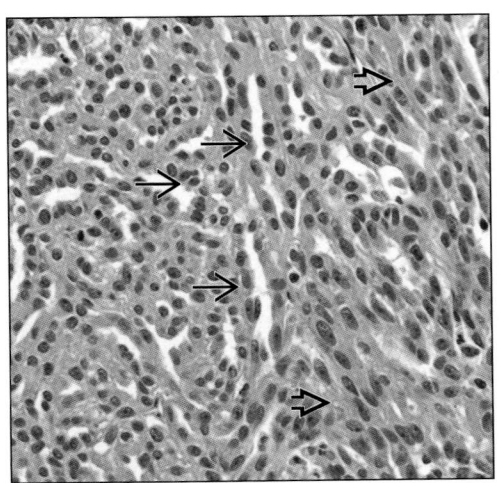

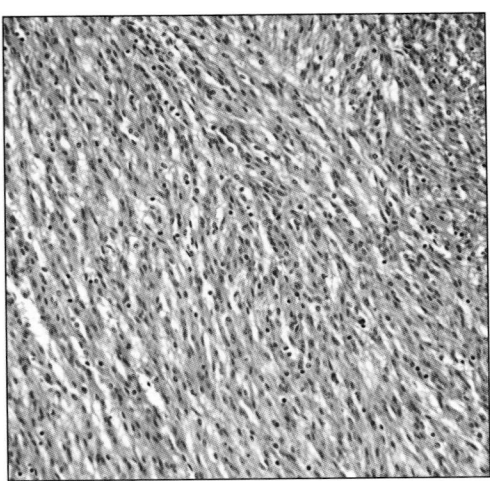

(Left) The spindle cells often appear to emerge from the epithelial component and show low-grade nuclear features ▷, morphologically almost identical to the nuclei in the epithelial component ➡. (Right) Some mucinous tubular and spindle cell carcinomas show marked paucity of epithelial component. Such spindle cell predominant tumors may be mistaken for a sarcoma, but the cytologic features are low grade, and some epithelial component is invariably seen on careful search.

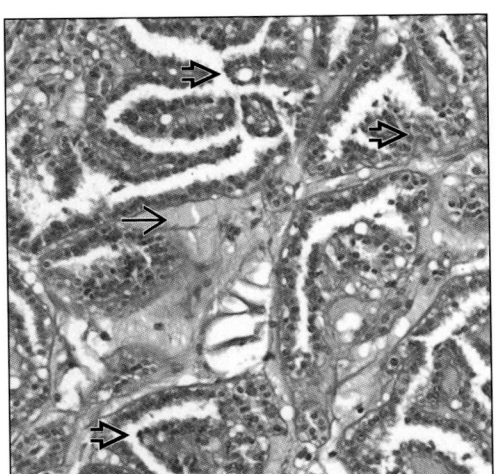

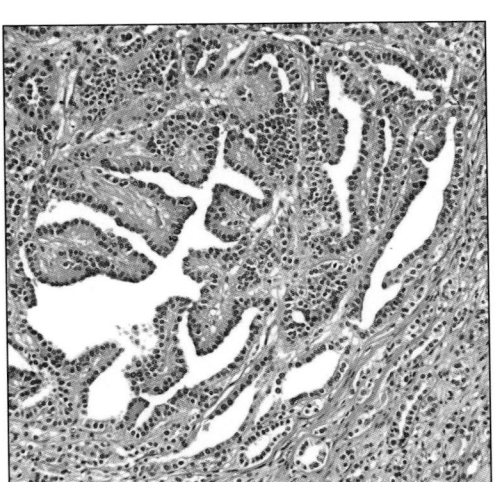

(Left) While the epithelial component in MTSCC predominantly consists of elongated, sometimes branching, or more rounded tubules, focal ill-defined papillations are not uncommon ▷. The typical mucinous stroma ➡ is seen. (Right) Some tumors show well-formed papillae, and in rare cases papillary formations may be multifocal and prominent. Presence of other typical tubules, low-grade spindle cell areas, and mucinous background easily points toward the proper diagnosis.

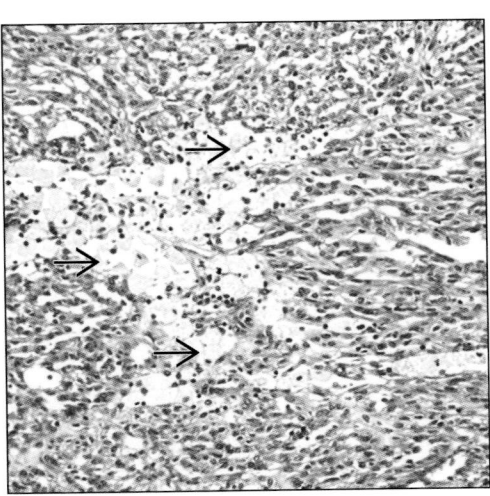

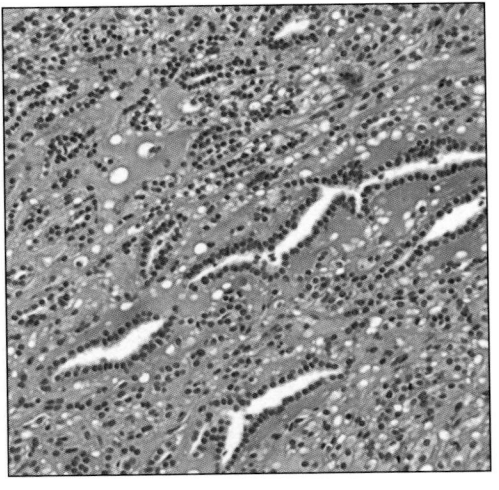

(Left) Occasionally the tumors may show focal, to rarely more diffuse foamy macrophages ➡, raising the differential diagnostic possibility of papillary RCC. However, unlike papillary RCC, the foam cells are usually randomly distributed and not always related to papillary cores in MTSCC. (Right) Some MTSCC show extensive mucinous background. Rare cases may contain very scant amount of stromal mucin. Low-grade nuclear features and typical tubular morphology are retained.

MUCINOUS TUBULAR AND SPINDLE CELL CARCINOMA

Variant Microscopic Features

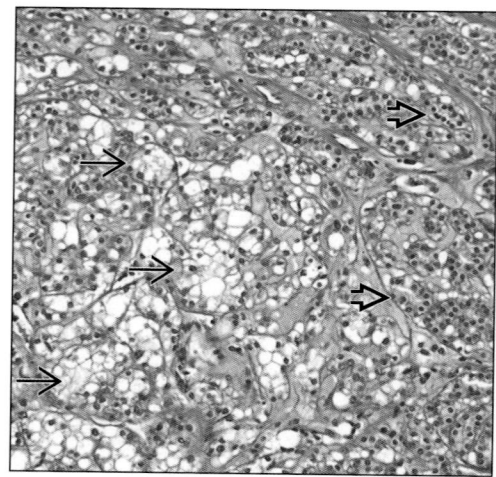
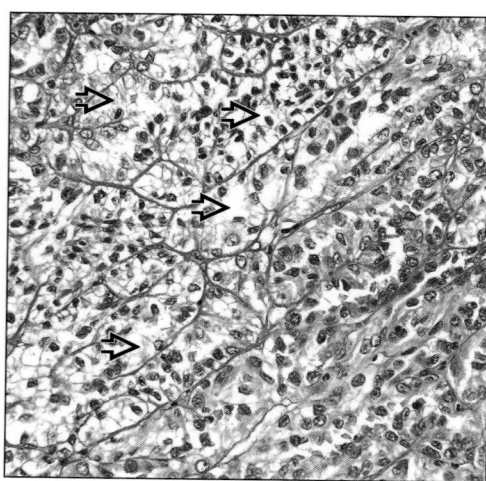

(Left) Typically, the tubular cells in MTSCC are cuboidal in shape, with a small amount of amphophilic cytoplasm ➪. Rarely, foci with more abundant and clear cytoplasm may also be observed ➡, and such cells are often closely associated with the other more typical cell types. **(Right)** In very occasional cases, tubules with clear cell cytoplasm may be clustered together ➪, forming small, usually ill-defined nodular areas. Appreciation of the 3 diagnostic features is important.

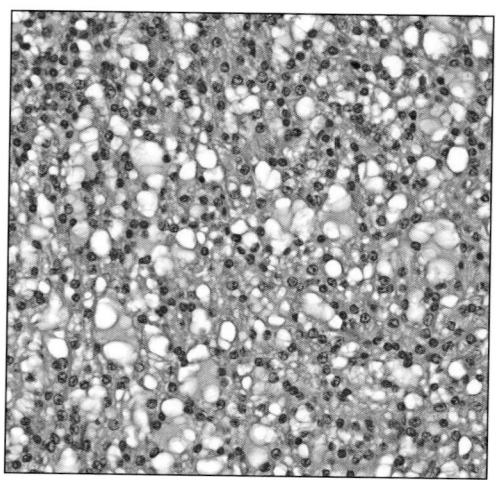
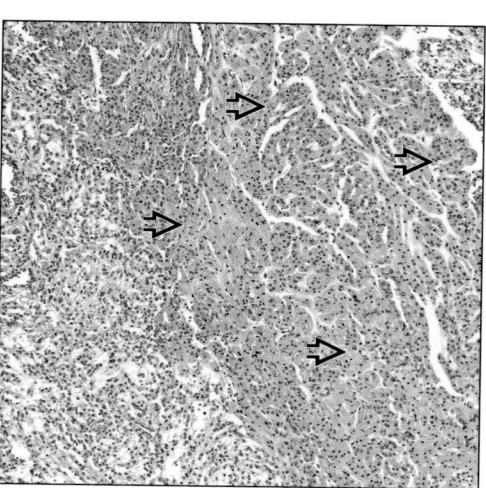

(Left) In some cases, the stromal mucin shows prominent vacuolization that may lead to a mistaken belief of the presence of clear and signet ring cells. **(Right)** Focal cytoplasmic eosinophilia is not uncommon in mucinous tubular and spindle cell carcinoma. In some tumors, sheets and ill-formed nodules of cells with oncocytic cytology ➪ may also be seen. Like papillary RCC, MTSCC may show multiple cell types, and this has no bearing on the classification or prognosis of the tumor.

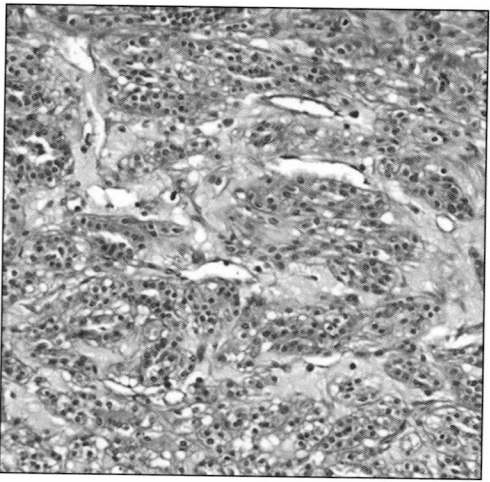
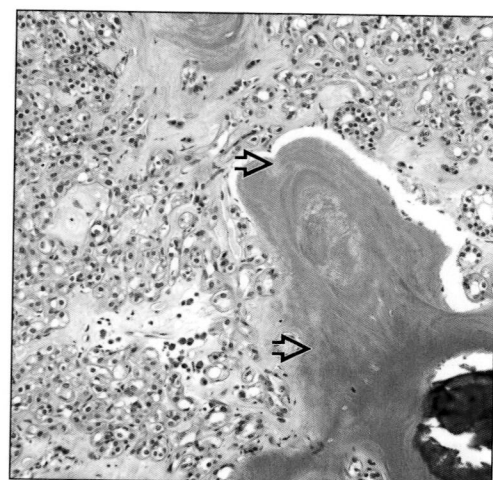

(Left) This mucinous tubular and spindle cell carcinoma shows prominent cytoplasmic eosinophilia. Usually the cytoplasmic eosinophilia is focal but may be diffuse and predominant feature in some rare tumors. **(Right)** Focal calcifications are not uncommon in MTSCC. Rare cases, however, may show foci of bone formation ➪. Dystrophic ossification in a tumor is generally believed to be evidence for a slow-growing tumor, which appears to reflect on the known biology of these tumors.

Variant Features and Ancillary Techniques

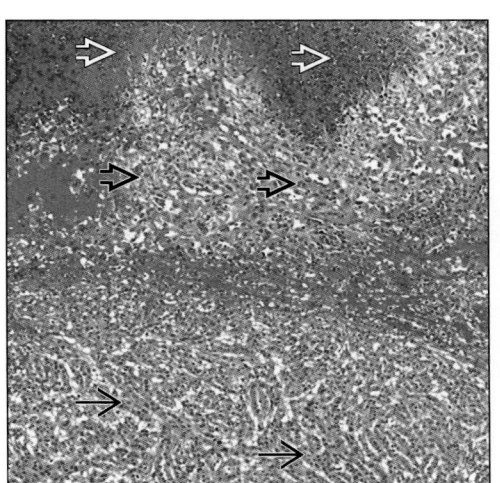

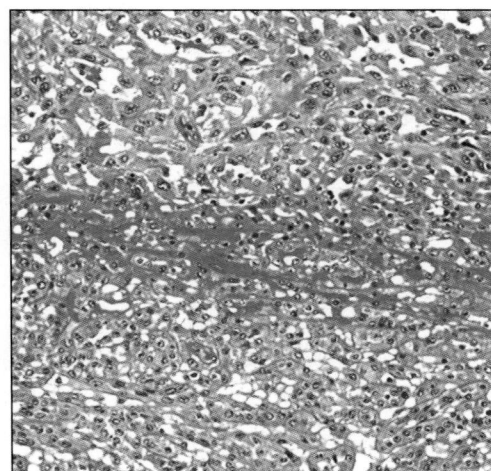

(Left) This MTSCC ⊠ shows sarcomatoid features ⊠ with a large area of necrosis ⊠. Compared to the usual low-grade MTSCC, tumors with sarcomatoid features usually show infiltrative borders and gross necrosis. (Right) Unlike the low-grade spindle cell elements that are common in MTSCC, true sarcomatoid areas are high-grade, mitotically active, and may show areas of necrosis. True sarcomatoid features are extremely uncommon in mucinous tubular and spindle cell tumors.

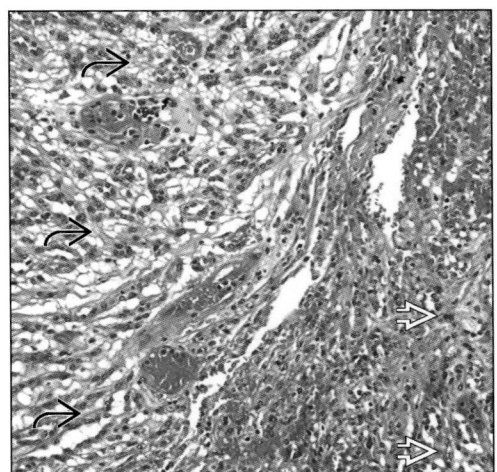

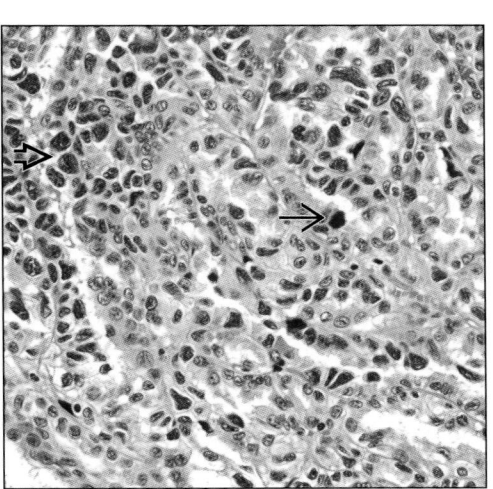

(Left) Similar to the high-grade sarcomatoid areas in rare tumors, occasional cases of otherwise typical MTSCC ⊠ may also show high-grade epithelial areas ⊠. (Right) This image of a mucinous tubular and spindle cell carcinoma shows significant nuclear atypia, including pleomorphism ⊠ and brisk mitotic activity ⊠ in the epithelial component of the tumor. Appreciation of other typical features of these tumors are necessary in such rare cases.

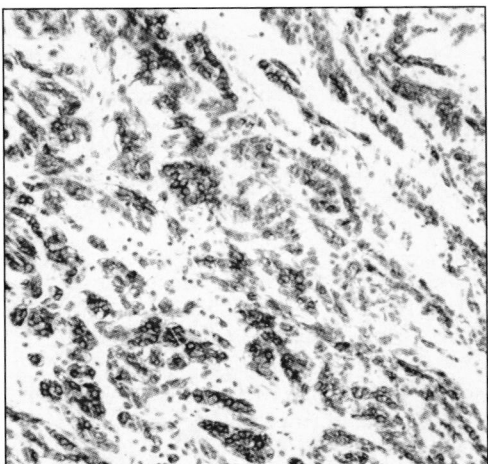

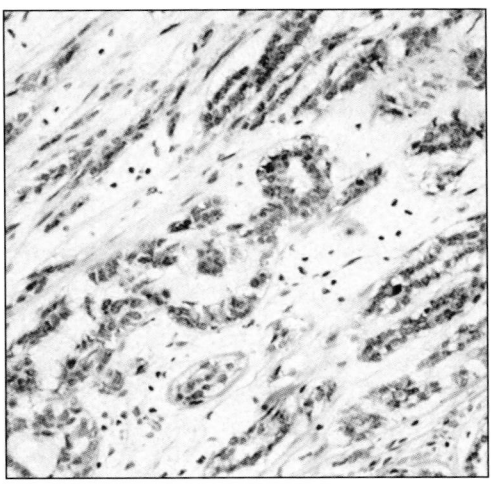

(Left) Similar to papillary RCC, CK7 is diffusely positive in MTSCC, staining both the epithelial and spindle cell components. (Right) Immunostaining with AMACR is usually diffusely positive in both the epithelial and spindle cell components. Thus CK7 and AMACR do not help in the differentiation between MTSCC and papillary renal cell carcinoma. Careful attention to the presence of a low-grade spindle cell morphology and myxoid features may be more helpful in this distinction.

TUBULOCYSTIC CARCINOMA

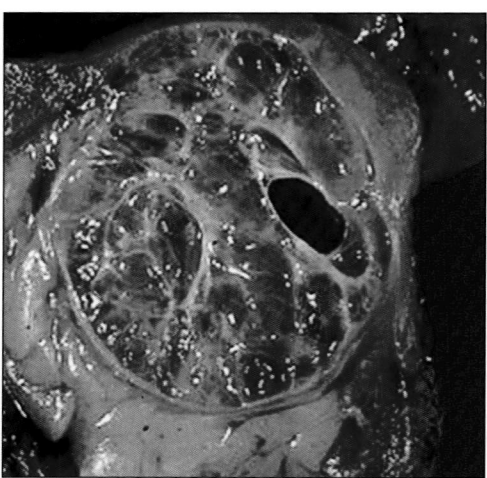

Gross photograph demonstrates a well-circumscribed tumor with a spongy cut surface and variable sized cysts, the typical gross appearance of a tubulocystic carcinoma.

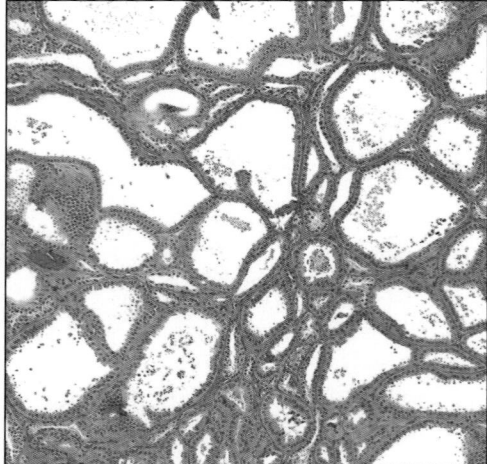

A low-power view of tubulocystic carcinoma shows variably sized tubules and cysts, lined by a single layer of epithelium.

TERMINOLOGY

Abbreviations
- Tubulocystic carcinoma (TC) of kidney

Definitions
- Well-circumscribed renal cell carcinoma (RCC) with pure tubular and cystic architectural growth
  - Cysts and tubules lined by single layer of atypical cells with abundant eosinophilic cytoplasm and variable "hobnail" appearance

ETIOLOGY/PATHOGENESIS

Historic Perspective
- Initially described in 1956 by Masson and designated as Bellinien epithelioma
- Examples illustrated in 3rd AFIP fascicle as collecting duct carcinoma (CDC), subsequently designated low-grade CDC
  - This group also contained some cases now regarded as mucinous tubular and spindle cell carcinoma
- Recently considered as distinct entity
  - Exact relationship with collecting duct carcinoma still unclear
    - Particularly because areas with TC-like morphology are occasionally observed in otherwise typical CDCs

Molecular Abnormalities
- Unique molecular signature distinct from clear cell and chromophobe RCC reported in Affymetrix X3P oligonucleotide microanalysis
  - Overexpression of genes related to
    - Amino acid metabolism
    - Cell cycle
  - Underexpression of many biopolymer metabolism genes

- Based on a single case, using clustering analysis, molecular signature also reported to be closely related to papillary RCC
- No published large molecular study analyzing relationship to, or distinction from, collecting duct carcinoma

CLINICAL ISSUES

Epidemiology
- Incidence
  - Uncommon; < 60 cases reported in literature
- Age
  - 34-94 years (mean: 60 years)
- Gender
  - Strong male preponderance; M:F = 7:1 or greater

Presentation
- Majority asymptomatic, incidentally discovered radiologically; occasionally abdominal fullness, flank pain, or hematuria

Treatment
- Usually amenable to surgical treatment due to low tumor stage at presentation
- Single reported case of metastatic disease treated with multikinase inhibitor sunitinib as adjuvant with documented clinical and radiographic regression

Prognosis
- Tumor with relatively less aggressive clinical behavior
  - Overwhelming majority with stage pT1 at presentation; possible contributing factor for favorable prognosis
  - < 10% reported with stage pT3 disease
- Disease progression, including local recurrence and metastasis to lymph nodes, bone, and liver in approximately 10% of cases

TUBULOCYSTIC CARCINOMA

Key Facts

Terminology
- Tubulocystic carcinoma (TC) of kidney
  - Well-circumscribed carcinoma with pure tubular and cystic architectural growth
  - Cysts and tubules lined by single layer of atypical cells with abundant eosinophilic cytoplasm and variable "hobnailed" appearance

Clinical Issues
- Uncommon; < 60 cases reported in literature
- Considered potentially of low malignant behavior
- Strong male preponderance; M:F = 7:1 or greater

Macroscopic Features
- Well-circumscribed tumors with spongy "bubble wrap" appearance

Microscopic Pathology
- Composed of small to intermediate-sized tubules admixed with cystically dilated tubules, dispersed evenly in frequently fibrotic stroma
- Tubule and cyst lining composed of single layer of flat, "hobnail," or cuboidal to columnar cells
- Cellular stratification and papillations very focal and uncommon

Ancillary Tests
- Majority are positive for CK7, CK19, parvalbumin, CD10, AMACR, and Ksp-cadherin

Top Differential Diagnoses
- Collecting duct carcinoma with TC-like areas
- Other adult renal epithelial tumors with predominant tubules and cysts

MACROSCOPIC FEATURES

General Features
- Well-circumscribed, usually unifocal, spongy "bubble wrap" appearance with multiple variable-sized cysts containing clear serous fluid

Size
- Range: 0.2-17 cm (mean: 4.2 cm)

MICROSCOPIC PATHOLOGY

Histologic Features
- Well-circumscribed tumor with small to intermediate-sized and cystically dilated tubules
- Tubule and cyst lining composed of single layer of flat, "hobnail," or cuboidal to columnar cells
  - Cellular stratification and papillations very focal and uncommon
- Cells with abundant eosinophilic cytoplasm and large nuclei, often with irregular nuclear membranes and prominent nucleoli
- Mitotic activity and tumor necrosis rare to absent
- Intervening stroma between tubules and cysts usually fibrotic

Predominant Pattern/Injury Type
- Neoplastic

Predominant Cell/Compartment Type
- Granular

ANCILLARY TESTS

Immunohistochemistry
- Majority positive for CK7, AMACR (racemase), CD10, and Ksp-cadherin
  - Occasional tumors immunoreactive with HMCK(34βE12)

Electron Microscopy
- Abundant microvilli (like proximal renal tubules) or sparse microvilli and cytoplasmic interdigitations (similar to intercalated cells of collecting duct)

DIFFERENTIAL DIAGNOSIS

Collecting Duct Carcinoma with TC-like Areas
- Multinodular growth pattern with extensive desmoplasia; solid, papillary, and glandular areas common; frequent intratumoral inflammation

Other Adult Renal Epithelial Tumors with Predominant Tubules and Cysts
- Focal or prominent area with tubules and cysts; lining cells and background typical of primary histologic subtype

SELECTED REFERENCES

1. Amin MB et al: Tubulocystic carcinoma of the kidney: clinicopathologic analysis of 31 cases of a distinctive rare subtype of renal cell carcinoma. Am J Surg Pathol. 33(3):384-92, 2009
2. Mego M et al: Sunitinib in the treatment of tubulocystic carcinoma of the kidney. A case report. Ann Oncol. 19(9):1655-6, 2008
3. Yang XJ et al: Tubulocystic carcinoma of the kidney: clinicopathologic and molecular characterization. Am J Surg Pathol. 32(2):177-87, 2008
4. Azoulay S et al: Tubulocystic carcinoma of the kidney: a new entity among renal tumors. Virchows Arch. 451(5):905-9, 2007
5. MacLennan GT et al: Tubulocystic carcinoma, mucinous tubular and spindle cell carcinoma, and other recently described rare renal tumors. Clin Lab Med. 25(2):393-416, 2005
6. MacLennan GT et al: Low-grade collecting duct carcinoma of the kidney: report of 13 cases of low-grade mucinous tubulocystic renal carcinoma of possible collecting duct origin. Urology. 50(5):679-84, 1997

TUBULOCYSTIC CARCINOMA

Microscopic Features

(Left) A low magnification view of a tubulocystic carcinoma that shows the typical well circumscription ⤵ of the tumor. Notice that the tumor border is directly in contact with the adjacent renal parenchyma. A pseudocapsule is typically not present in TC.
(Right) Tubulocystic carcinoma is entirely composed of evenly distributed tubules and cysts of variable size, separated by fibrous-appearing stroma ➡. The low-power impression is that of a relatively low-grade neoplastic process.

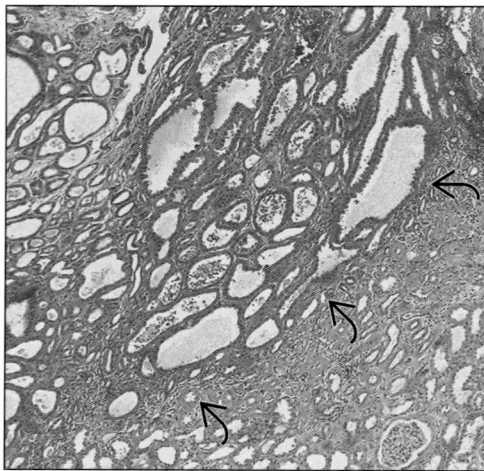
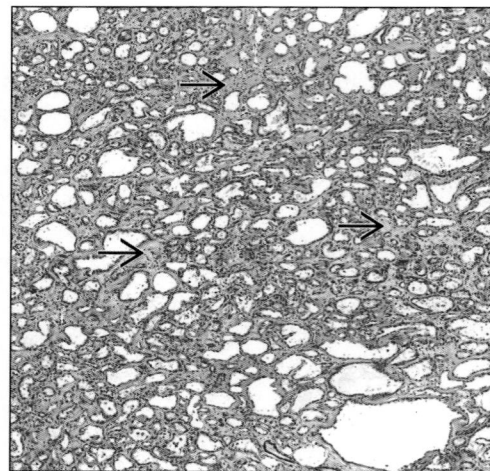

(Left) A characteristic feature of TC is the presence of fibrous to hyalinized stroma ➡ that separates cysts and tubules. Multilocular cystic renal cell carcinoma shows a similar architecture, but the lining cells in that tumor are clear, and nests of clear cells are present within the septae.
(Right) The lining cells in TC may be focally to sometimes predominantly columnar. Nuclear pseudostratification is focal, at most, and the nuclei are high grade.

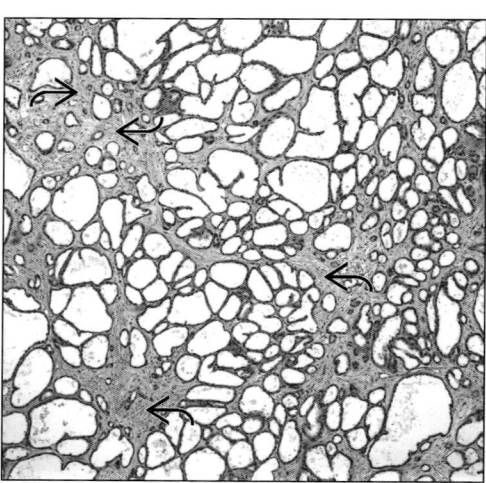
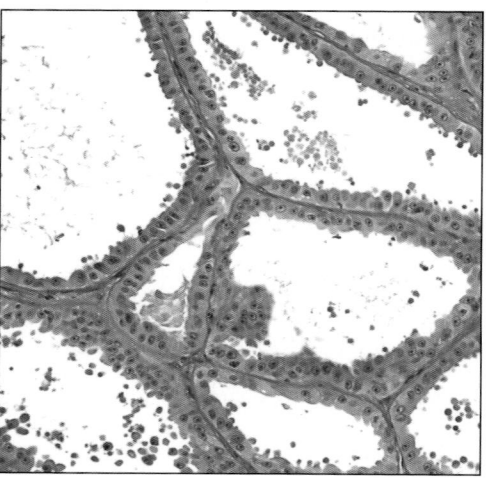

(Left) The cells in TC typically show abundant eosinophilic cytoplasm ⇨. Very focal areas may show cytoplasmic clarity in some cases. Focal pseudostratification may be the result of tangential sectioning. Sometimes incomplete septations may appear hanging free in the cyst lumina ➡. (Right) The nuclei in tubulocystic carcinoma are typically large and show irregular nuclear chromatin distribution and prominent nucleoli. Most tumors also show areas with "hobnail" appearance ⇨.

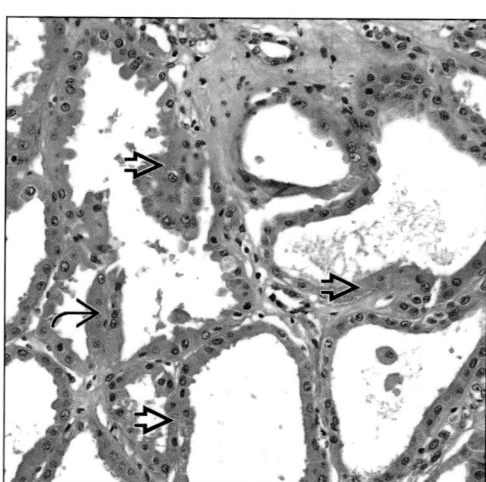
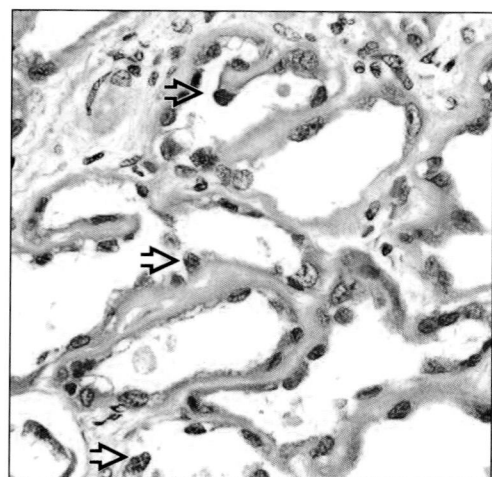

1

TUBULOCYSTIC CARCINOMA

Microscopic Features and Differential Diagnosis

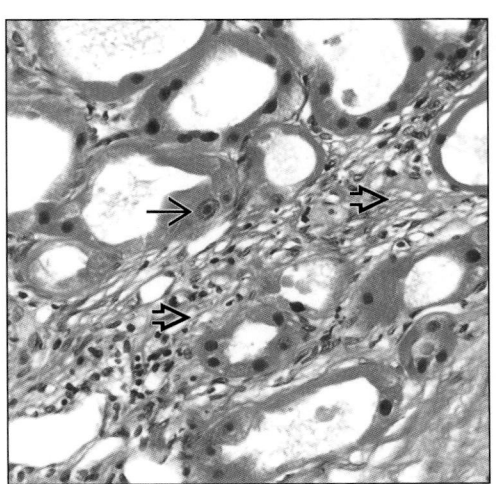

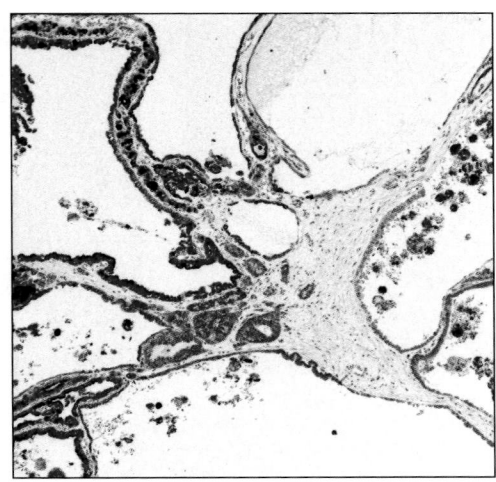

(Left) This high-magnification view of a tubulocystic carcinoma shows the characteristic features of the tumor: Cells with eosinophilic cytoplasm, large nuclei with prominent nucleoli ➡, and fibrotic stroma ⮊. In contrast to oncocytoma, the nuclei show irregular outlines and often variable chromatin distribution. *(Right)* Immunostaining for CK7 is often positive in TC but may be patchy or weak in some cases. Other positive markers include AMACR (diffuse and strong).

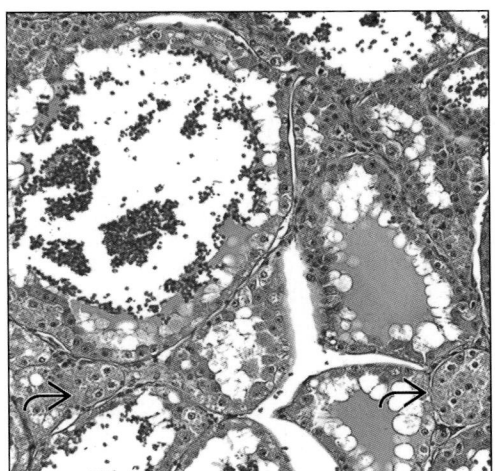

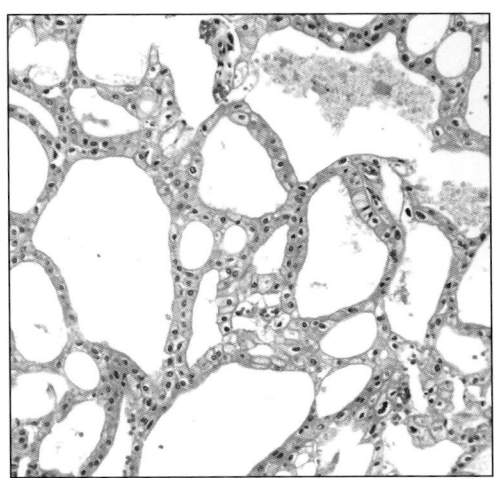

(Left) A close differential diagnosis of TC is renal oncocytoma with prominent tubular and cystic areas (as seen here). Oncocytoma has uniform round nuclei, a variable number of solid tumor nests ➡, and frequently loose stroma. It lacks AMACR and CK7 positivity. *(Right)* Although this chromophobe RCC has cystic areas architecturally resembling a tubulocystic carcinoma, its cytologic features (binucleation, koilocytoid atypia, and 2 cell types) would suggest the correct diagnosis.

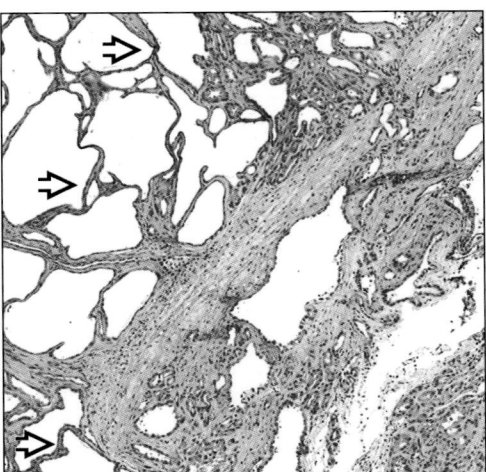

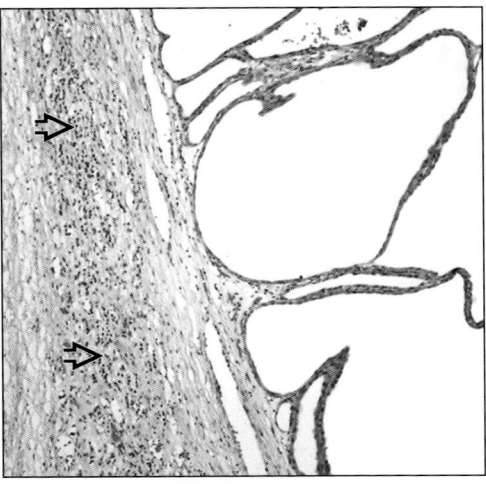

(Left) Tubulocystic carcinoma-like areas ⮊ may be seen in otherwise typical collecting duct carcinoma. However, TC lacks the multinodular growth pattern, desmoplasia, and the solid and papillary architecture that is typical of collecting duct carcinoma. *(Right)* This image shows TC-like metastasis to the adrenal gland ⮊ from a CDC that contained TC-like areas in the primary. Because of such features in some CDCs, the exact relationship of TC with CDC still remains to be determined.

THYROID-LIKE FOLLICULAR CARCINOMA OF THE KIDNEY

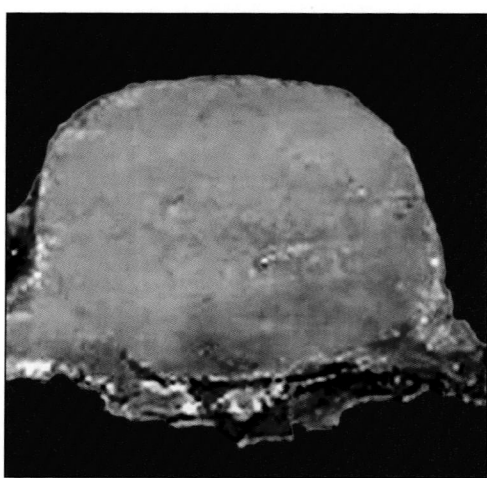

Thyroid-like follicular carcinoma that shows a well-circumscribed tumor with homogeneous, tan-brown cut surface, typical for this tumor. The tan-brown color resembles thyroid parenchyma.

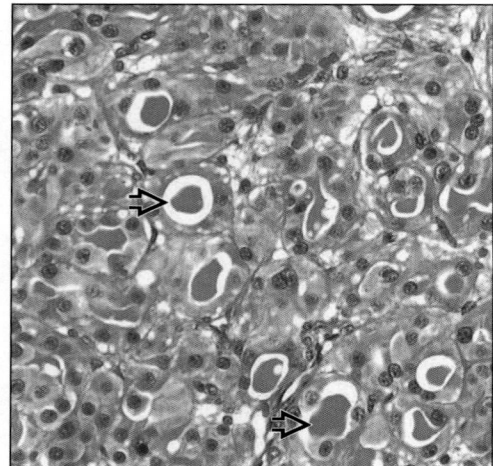

The characteristic histologic features of thyroid-like follicular carcinoma of the kidney include a prominent micro- or macrofollicular architecture with colloid-like material ➢ in the follicles.

TERMINOLOGY

Abbreviations
- Thyroid-like follicular carcinoma of the kidney (TLFC-K)

Definitions
- Recently described primary renal cell carcinoma closely mimicking well-differentiated thyroid follicular neoplasms

ETIOLOGY/PATHOGENESIS

Genetic Features
- Gene expression profiling comparing with clear cell and chromophobe RCC showed overexpressed 135 and underexpressed 46 genes
  - Overexpression of multiple cell cycle regulatory genes observed
- Multiple losses involving chromosomes 1p, 3, 9p, 9q, 12, 17, and X, and gains involving 7q, 8q, 12, 16, 17p, 17q, 19q, 20, 21q, and Xp described in case reports

CLINICAL ISSUES

Epidemiology
- Incidence
  - Extremely uncommon
    - < 10 cases described
- Age
  - Range: 29-83 years

Presentation
- Most incidentally discovered during radiologic work-up for other medical conditions

Prognosis
- Based on the few cases described, possibly renal cell carcinoma of low malignant potential

- Only 1 case known to have regional lymph node metastasis at presentation
- No known deaths due to disease

MACROSCOPIC FEATURES

General Features
- Well circumscribed
- Unifocal tumor
- Homogeneous, tan-brown to dark brown cut surface
  - Necrosis or hemorrhage quite uncommon

Size
- 1.9-11.8 cm (mean: 2.8 cm)

MICROSCOPIC PATHOLOGY

Histologic Features
- Well circumscribed
  - Distinct fibrous capsule of variable thickness present in all cases
- All described tumors organ confined
  - Only 2 tumors reported to be > 7 cm in size
    - All others with pathologic tumor stage 1 (pT1)
- Prominent follicular architecture composed of microfollicles and macrofollicles
  - Follicles filled with inspissated colloid-like material
  - Occasionally the colloid is focally calcified
- Patchy intratumoral lymphoid aggregates
  - Some tumors with germinal center formation
- Clear cell change or spindle cells not observed
  - Focal papillary architecture described in 1 case
- Necrosis or lymphovascular invasion usually absent
- Follicles lined by cells with moderate amount of amphophilic to eosinophilic cytoplasm
  - Nuclei mostly round and rarely oval, with uniform chromatin
    - Mild nuclear membrane irregularities often present

THYROID-LIKE FOLLICULAR CARCINOMA OF THE KIDNEY

Key Facts

Terminology

- Thyroid-like follicular carcinoma of the kidney (TLFC-K)
- Recently described primary renal cell carcinoma closely mimicking well-differentiated thyroid follicular neoplasms

Clinical Issues

- Extremely uncommon; < 10 cases described
- Based on the few cases described, possibly renal cell carcinoma of low malignant potential
- Only 1 case known to have regional lymph node metastasis at presentation

Macroscopic Features

- Well circumscribed
- Homogeneous, tan-brown to dark brown cut surface

- Size: 1.9-11.8 cm (mean: 2.8 cm)

Microscopic Pathology

- Well circumscribed with distinct fibrous capsule
- Prominent follicular architecture composed of microfollicles and macrofollicles
- Clear cell change or spindle cells not observed
- Follicles lined by cells with moderate amount of amphophilic to eosinophilic cytoplasm
- Tumors lack histologic features seen in papillary carcinoma of thyroid, including prominent papillations, nuclear clearing, inclusions or grooves
- Mostly negative for CK7

Top Differential Diagnoses

- Metastatic thyroid carcinoma

- o Nucleoli inconspicuous
- o Nuclear features similar to Fuhrman nuclear grade 2
- o Rare mitotic figures may be present
- o Tumors lack histologic features typical in papillary carcinoma of thyroid, including
  - Prominent papillations
  - Nuclear clearing
  - Pseudoinclusions or grooves

ANCILLARY TESTS

Immunohistochemistry

- Typically negative for CK7
  - o Rare cases may be positive for CK7
- Usually, but not always, negative for pax-2, RCC, CD10, WT1, Ksp-cadherin, AMACR, vimentin, CD56, and CD57
- All cases negative for thyroglobulin and TTF-1

DIFFERENTIAL DIAGNOSIS

Metastatic Thyroid Carcinoma

- Rare event, although more reported cases than primary thyroid-like follicular carcinoma of kidney described
- About 1/2 of metastatic cases from thyroid carcinoma have architectural &/or nuclear features of papillary thyroid carcinoma
  - o Others follicular, morphologically similar to thyroid-like follicular carcinoma of the kidney
- Most metastatic thyroid carcinoma cases present with disseminated metastatic disease, in addition to renal involvement
- All reported cases of metastatic thyroid carcinoma with immunoreactivity for thyroid markers
  - o Including thyroglobulin &/or TTF-1
- All cases with confirmed thyroid neoplasms

DIAGNOSTIC CHECKLIST

Pathologic Interpretation Pearls

- Before accepting diagnosis of primary thyroid-like follicular carcinoma of kidney, possibility of metastatic thyroid carcinoma must be excluded
- In addition to clinical history, immunostaining for thyroglobulin and TTF-1 are pre-requisites for rendering this diagnosis
- Focal thyroid-like follicular histology may be seen in several renal tumors, including oncocytoma

SELECTED REFERENCES

1. Amin MB et al: Primary thyroid-like follicular carcinoma of the kidney: report of 6 cases of a histologically distinctive adult renal epithelial neoplasm. Am J Surg Pathol. 33(3):393-400, 2009
2. Insabato L et al: Primary thyroid and thyroid-like follicular carcinoma of the kidney versus solitary metastatic carcinoma of the thyroid: a vexing issue. Virchows Arch. 454(6):717-8, 2009
3. Sterlacci W et al: Primary thyroid-like renal tumor or renal metastasis from the thyroid? Virchows Arch. 455(1):97-8, 2009
4. Gupta R et al: Metastatic papillary carcinoma of thyroid masquerading as a renal tumour. J Clin Pathol. 61(1):143, 2008
5. Sterlacci W et al: Thyroid follicular carcinoma-like renal tumor: a case report with morphologic, immunophenotypic, cytogenetic, and scintigraphic studies. Virchows Arch. 2008 Jan;452(1):91-5. Epub 2007 Aug 18. Erratum in: Virchows Arch. 452(4):471, 2008
6. von Falck C et al: Renal metastases from follicular thyroid cancer on SPECT/CT. Clin Nucl Med. 32(9):751-2, 2007
7. Jung SJ et al: Thyroid follicular carcinoma-like tumor of kidney: a case report with morphologic, immunohistochemical, and genetic analysis. Am J Surg Pathol. 30(3):411-5, 2006
8. Kumar A et al: Adrenal and renal metastases from follicular thyroid cancer. Br J Radiol. 78(935):1038-41, 2005
9. Liou MJ et al: Renal metastasis from papillary thyroid microcarcinoma. Acta Otolaryngol. 125(4):438-42, 2005
10. Angell SK et al: Primary thyroidlike carcinoma of the kidney. Urology. 48(4):632-5, 1996

THYROID-LIKE FOLLICULAR CARCINOMA OF THE KIDNEY

Microscopic Features

(Left) Thyroid-like follicular carcinoma is well circumscribed, with a well-defined fibrous capsule ▷. However, the thickness of the capsule is quite variable. *(Right)* Microscopic features of a thyroid-like follicular carcinoma of the kidney are reminiscent of a follicular carcinoma of the thyroid. Based on the relative incidences, the probability of a tumor with such histologic features representing a metastasis from thyroid is at least equal to, if not greater than, a renal primary.

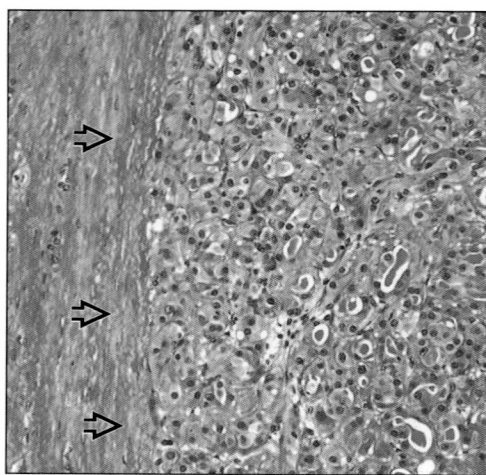
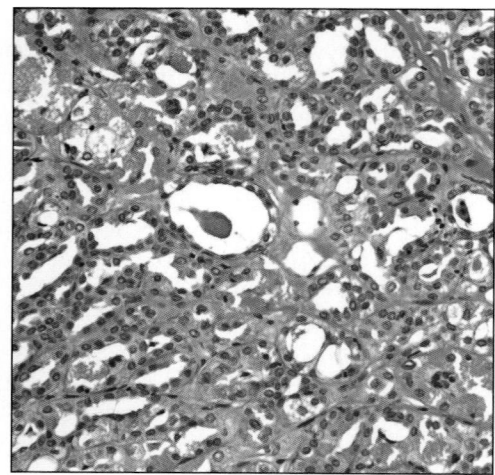

(Left) Thyroid-like follicular carcinomas of the kidney often show a microfollicular architectural pattern. Many of the microfollicles contain inspissated colloid-like material ▷. *(Right)* Some thyroid-like follicular carcinomas of the kidney have a prominent macrofollicular pattern ▷. The colloid-like material in such follicles usually appears less dense and is often retracted away from the lining cells. Occasionally, this colloid-like material may show calcifications ▷.

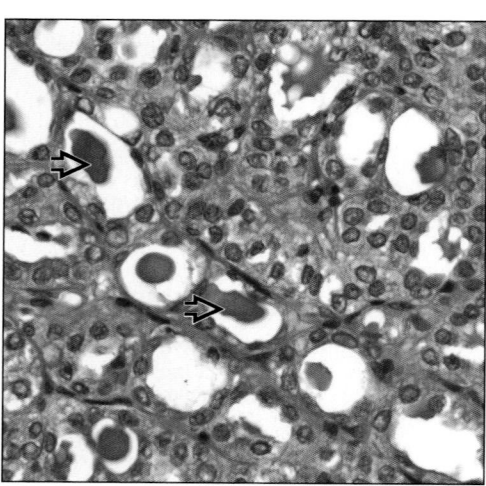
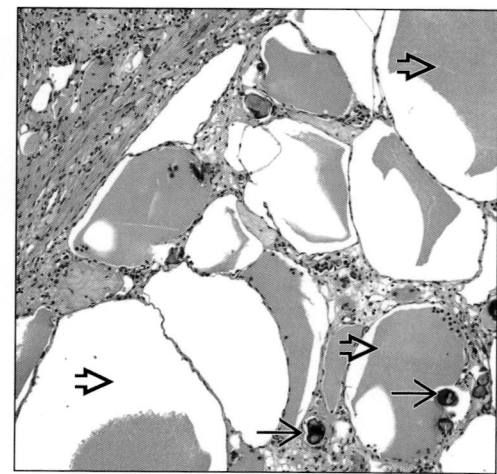

(Left) Marked lymphocytic infiltration ▷ may occasionally be observed in thyroid-like follicular carcinoma of the kidney. The infiltrate is often present as prominent intratumoral collections but may sometimes be seen predominantly surrounding the tumor. *(Right)* Occasionally, the lymphoid infiltration in thyroid-like follicular carcinomas of the kidney may show prominent lymphoid follicle formation ▷. Also, note the complex follicular architecture ▷ in this tumor.

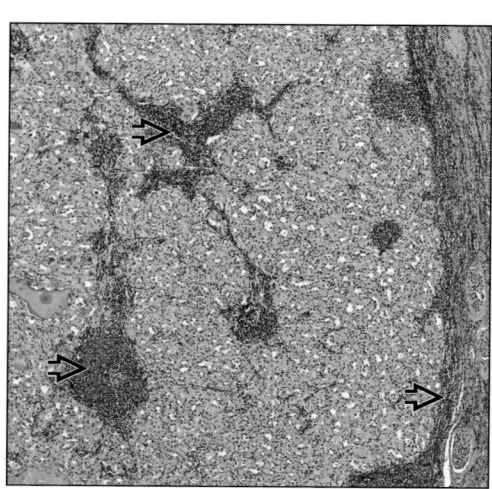
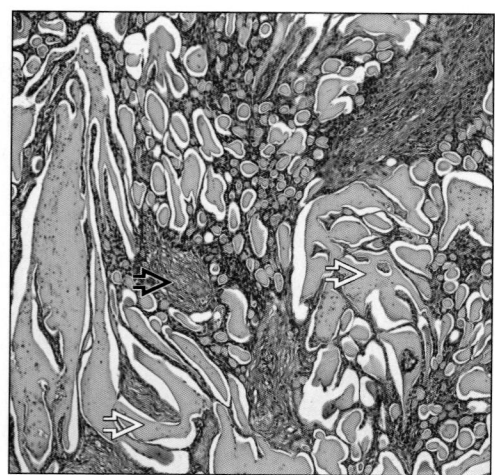

THYROID-LIKE FOLLICULAR CARCINOMA OF THE KIDNEY

Microscopic and Immunohistochemical Features

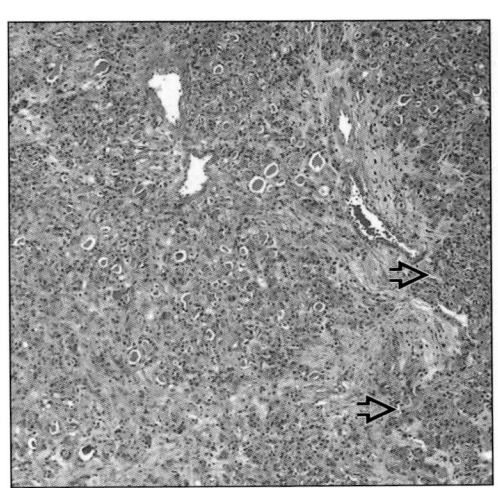

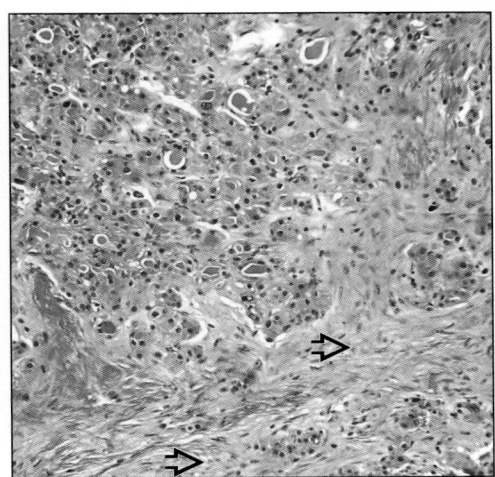

(Left) While follicular architecture is the most characteristic and defining feature of the tumor, rarely more solid and irregular nests ⇒ may be focally present in thyroid-like follicular carcinomas. *(Right)* Rare cases of thyroid-like follicular carcinoma may show irregular areas with desmoplasia inside the tumor ⇒. However, all tumors are well circumscribed and encapsulated and do not show an invasive or desmoplastic front into the adjacent renal parenchyma.

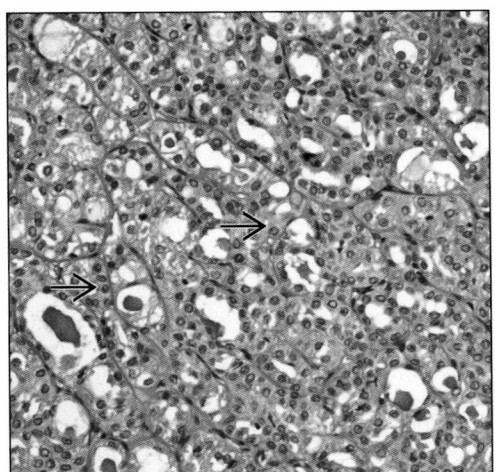

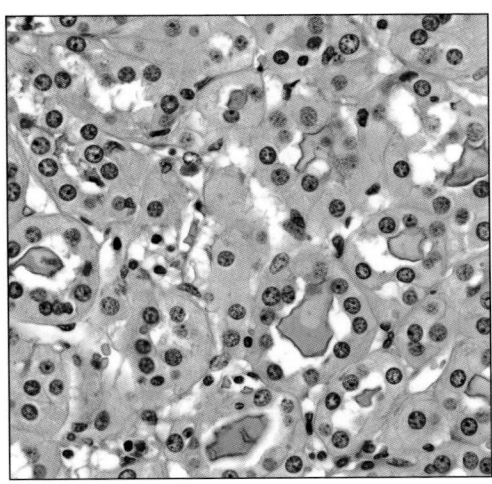

(Left) The cells lining the follicles ⇒ in thyroid-like follicular carcinoma of the kidney show a moderate amount of amphophilic to eosinophilic cytoplasm. The nuclei are round and rarely oval, with uniform chromatin pattern. Mitotic activity is rare, and necrosis and vascular invasion are very uncommon. *(Right)* Unlike the typical nuclear features in papillary thyroid carcinoma, the nuclei in thyroid-like follicular carcinomas usually lack grooves, inclusions, and clearing of chromatin.

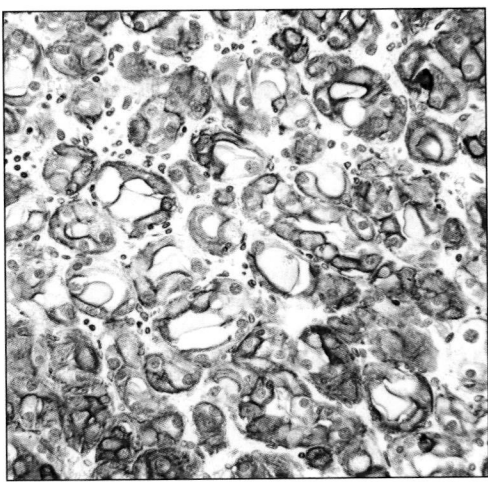

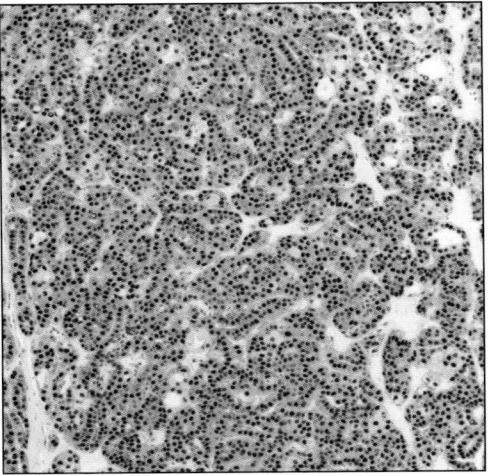

(Left) Immunohistochemical staining shows consistent, diffuse reactivity for pan-keratins, including PAN-CK(AE1/AE3), in thyroid-like follicular carcinomas of the kidney. All tumors are negative for thyroglobulin and TTF-1. *(Right)* Thyroid-like follicular carcinoma with diffuse nuclear positivity for pax-2. Most of these tumors are negative for CK7, pax-2, CD10, AMACR, and vimentin. Negativity for thyroglobulin and TTF-1 are more important in confirming the diagnosis of a tumor as a renal primary.

ACQUIRED CYSTIC DISEASE-ASSOCIATED RENAL CELL CARCINOMA

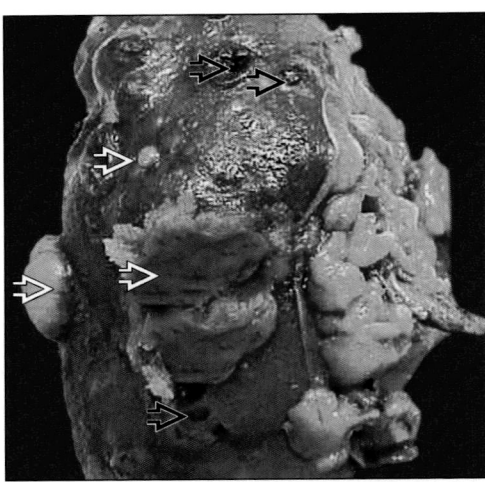

Gross photograph shows multiple cysts ⊳ and solid tumors ⊳ in an end-stage kidney. Unless almost totally occupied by large tumors, such kidneys are often small in size.

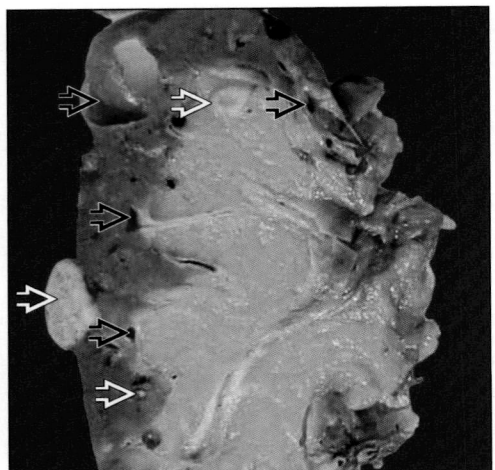

Multiple cysts ⊳ and solid tumors ⊳ are identified in the cut surface of this specimen. The marked cortical thinning and blunting of the papillae are hallmarks of an end-stage kidney.

TERMINOLOGY

Abbreviations

- Acquired cystic disease-associated renal cell carcinoma (ACD-associated RCC)

Definitions

- Most common subtype of renal cell carcinoma occurring in end-stage kidneys, specifically those with acquired cystic disease
- Tumor composed of cells with eosinophilic cytoplasm, cribriform/sieve-like appearance, and oxalate crystals in setting of end-stage kidney disease

ETIOLOGY/PATHOGENESIS

Role of Dialysis and End-Stage Renal Disease

- Acquired cystic kidney disease (ACKD) usually (but not always) seen in patients on dialysis
  - Incidence of cystic disease progressively higher with longer durations of dialysis
    - 10-20% for dialysis up to 3 years
    - 40-60% at 5 years
    - > 90% at 10 years or more
- Type of dialysis, hemodialysis or peritoneal, is not important
- Causes of increased tumorigenesis in end-stage and ACKD are possibly multifactorial, and include
  - Depressed cellular and humoral immunity in renal failure
  - Impaired antioxidant defense and increased synthesis of reactive oxygen species
  - Release of free radicals with resultant DNA damage, mutations, and cancer
  - Use of immunosuppressive medications
  - Oxalate crystal-induced tubular proliferative activity

CLINICAL ISSUES

Epidemiology

- Incidence
  - Incidence of renal tumors up to 100x greater in patients with end-stage kidney disease, particularly ACKD, compared with that in general population
    - Overall incidence of renal cancer 3-7% in end-stage kidneys
  - Previously, papillary RCC believed to be most common RCC subtype in end-stage kidneys
  - In reality, ACD-associated RCC is most common subtype of RCC in end-stage kidneys
    - ACD-associated RCC accounts for dominant mass in 36% of end-stage kidneys overall and 46% of end-stage kidneys with acquired cystic disease
    - ACD-associated RCC also most common tumor type among other, often multiple, small tumor nodules dispersed within end-stage kidneys
  - Other subtypes commonly occurring in both cystic and noncystic end-stage kidneys include
    - Clear cell papillary RCC
    - Papillary RCC
    - Clear cell RCC
    - Chromophobe RCC
    - Rare cases of collecting duct carcinoma, renal oncocytoma, "renal capsuloma" also described

Presentation

- ACD-associated RCC is seen exclusively in end-stage kidneys with acquired cystic disease
- Most cases diagnosed incidentally on radiologic follow-up in patients with chronic renal disease

Prognosis

- Most tumors with nonaggressive biologic behavior
  - Likely because diagnosed at small size with low pT stage

ACQUIRED CYSTIC DISEASE-ASSOCIATED RENAL CELL CARCINOMA

Key Facts

Terminology

- Most common subtype of renal cell carcinoma occurring in end-stage kidneys, specifically with acquired cystic disease

Etiology/Pathogenesis

- ACD-associated RCC mostly (but not always) seen in patients on dialysis
- Overall, incidence of renal cancer markedly increased (3-7%) in patients with end-stage kidneys
- Most common subtype of RCC in end-stage kidneys
- Other subtypes commonly occurring in both cystic and noncystic end-stage kidneys include clear cell papillary, papillary, clear cell, and chromophobe renal cell carcinoma

Microscopic Pathology

- Acinar, solid alveolar, solid sheet-like, micro- or macrocystic, and papillary architecture in various combinations
- Intra- and intercytoplasmic microscopic lumina ("holes"), imparting cribriform/sieve-like appearance
- Presence of intratumoral oxalate crystals in majority of tumors
- Most cells large with abundant eosinophilic cytoplasm and prominent nucleoli

Diagnostic Checklist

- Presence of multiple small lumina/sieve-like, cribriform architecture and intratumoral oxalate crystals diagnostic
- Variable proportions of papillary architecture and clear cell cytology

---

- Usual small size because of constant care due to medical condition and resultant earlier radiologic detection
- Very few with aggressive features, including pT3 stage or sarcomatoid change
- Rare deaths due to tumor reported; only in those with sarcomatoid features and metastatic disease

MACROSCOPIC FEATURES

Background Kidney

- Usually with numerous cysts
- Frequently small, shrunken, and granular

Tumors

- Often multifocal and bilateral
- Carcinomas usually well circumscribed, many appearing to arise within cysts
- Larger tumors with thick fibrous capsule, often with foci of calcification

MICROSCOPIC PATHOLOGY

Histologic Features

- Acinar, solid alveolar, solid sheet-like, micro- or macrocystic, and papillary architecture in various combinations and proportions
- Intra- and intercytoplasmic microscopic lumina ("holes"), imparting cribriform/sieve-like appearance
- Presence of intratumoral oxalate crystals in majority of tumors
  o Only tumor type in end-stage kidneys consistently displaying intratumoral oxalate crystals
- Most tumor cells are large with abundant eosinophilic cytoplasm and prominent nucleoli
  o Foci with clear cytoplasm are also seen
- Rare cases of ACD-associated RCCs with sarcomatoid features
  o Aggressive behavior observed in some cases with sarcomatoid features, including
    ▪ Widespread metastases

- Death due to disease

Cytologic Features

- Clusters of cells with papillary configuration
- Cells polygonal to columnar with abundant eosinophilic granular cytoplasm and round, centrally located nuclei
  o Finely granular nuclear chromatin
  o Prominent central nucleoli
- Differentiation from type 2 papillary renal cell carcinoma difficult on cytologic basis

Lymph Nodes

- Rare cases with metastasis reported

Predominant Pattern/Injury Type

- Neoplastic

Predominant Cell/Compartment Type

- Epithelial

Pathology of Background Kidney

- Numerous cysts in renal parenchyma, some multiloculated, some occurring in clusters
  o Cyst lining often resembles cells of ACD-associated RCC
    ▪ Large cells with granular, pink cytoplasm and prominent nucleoli
    ▪ Focal proliferation, sometimes with papillary architecture may be present
  o Other cysts with cuboidal to low-columnar lining, occasionally with papillary infoldings
  o Sometimes groups of cysts clustered together
  o Cysts lined by large eosinophilic cells with immunophenotype similar to ACD-associated RCC
    ▪ AMACR positive; CK7 negative
  o Cysts lined by cuboidal cells with amphophilic or clear cytoplasm and small nuclei with different immunophenotype
    ▪ AMACR and CK7 positive

1

ACQUIRED CYSTIC DISEASE-ASSOCIATED RENAL CELL CARCINOMA

ANCILLARY TESTS

Immunohistochemistry
- Diffusely positive for AMACR
- Negative/very focally positive for CK7
- Also positive for CD10, RCC, and GST-α

Cytogenetics
- ACD-associated RCC lacks trisomies 7 and 17, or 3p losses
  - Gains of chromosomes 1, 2, 6, and 10 reported in some cases
    - Genotype is quite different from that of papillary and clear cell RCC
  - Rare cases with loss of chromosome 7 or 17
  - Recently, in a larger study using FISH and CGH, shown to have combined gains of multiple chromosomes, including
    - Chromosomes 3, 7, 16, and Y

DIFFERENTIAL DIAGNOSIS

Papillary Renal Cell Carcinoma
- Lacks "holes" and sieve-like areas
- Intratumoral oxalate crystals extremely uncommon
- Usually show abundant foamy macrophages in cores of papillae
- Typically CK7 and AMACR positive by immunohistochemistry
- Often with trisomies/polysomies 7 and 17

Clear Cell Renal Cell Carcinoma
- Arborizing, branching vascular septations are distinctive
- Lacks "holes" and sieve-like areas, and intratumoral oxalate crystals
- Mostly negative for CK7 and negative/only focally positive for AMACR
  - Diffuse membranous positivity for CA9 and CD10 characteristic for clear cell renal cell carcinoma

DIAGNOSTIC CHECKLIST

Pathologic Interpretation Pearls
- Papillary architecture in ACD-associated RCC may suggest diagnosis of papillary renal cell carcinoma
- Similarly, clear cell cytology may raise possibility of clear cell renal cell carcinoma
- However, in background of acquired cystic disease, attention to morphologic features in entire tumor is essential for correct diagnosis
- Presence of multiple small lumina/sieve-like, cribriform architecture and intratumoral oxalate crystals diagnostic
- Diffuse AMACR positivity with CK7 negativity characteristic

SELECTED REFERENCES

1. Pan CC et al: Immunohistochemical and molecular genetic profiling of acquired cystic disease-associated renal cell carcinoma. Histopathology. 55(2):145-53, 2009
2. Srigley JR et al: Uncommon and recently described renal carcinomas. Mod Pathol. 22 Suppl 2:S2-S23, 2009
3. Hes O et al: End-stage kidney disease: gains of chromosomes 7 and 17 and loss of Y chromosome in non-neoplastic tissue. Virchows Arch. 453(4):313-9, 2008
4. Kuroda N et al: Sarcomatoid acquired cystic disease-associated renal cell carcinoma. Histol Histopathol. 23(11):1327-31, 2008
5. Inoue H et al: Somatic mutations of the von Hippel-Lindau disease gene in renal carcinomas occurring in patients with long-term dialysis. Nephrol Dial Transplant. 22(7):2052-5, 2007
6. Ito K et al: Laparoscopic radical nephrectomy in ACDK-associated renal cell carcinoma accompanied by duplicated IVC: a case report. Hinyokika Kiyo. 53(12):875-8, 2007
7. Schwarz A et al: Renal cell carcinoma in transplant recipients with acquired cystic kidney disease. Clin J Am Soc Nephrol. 2(4):750-6, 2007
8. Cossu-Rocca P et al: Acquired cystic disease-associated renal tumors: an immunohistochemical and fluorescence in situ hybridization study. Mod Pathol. 19(6):780-7, 2006
9. Kojima Y et al: Renal cell carcinoma in dialysis patients: a single center experience. Int J Urol. 13(8):1045-8, 2006
10. Petrolla AA et al: Renal cell carcinoma associated with end stage renal disease. J Urol. 176(1):345, 2006
11. Tickoo SK et al: Spectrum of epithelial neoplasms in end-stage renal disease: an experience from 66 tumor-bearing kidneys with emphasis on histologic patterns distinct from those in sporadic adult renal neoplasia. Am J Surg Pathol. 30(2):141-53, 2006
12. Sule N et al: Calcium oxalate deposition in renal cell carcinoma associated with acquired cystic kidney disease: a comprehensive study. Am J Surg Pathol. 29(4):443-51, 2005
13. Cheuk W et al: Atypical epithelial proliferations in acquired renal cystic disease harbor cytogenetic aberrations. Hum Pathol. 33(7):761-5, 2002
14. Denton MD et al: Prevalence of renal cell carcinoma in patients with ESRD pre-transplantation: a pathologic analysis. Kidney Int. 61(6):2201-9, 2002
15. Koul HK et al: COM crystals activate the p38 mitogen-activated protein kinase signal transduction pathway in renal epithelial cells. J Biol Chem. 277(39):36845-52, 2002
16. Umekawa T et al: Oxalate ions and calcium oxalate crystals stimulate MCP-1 expression by renal epithelial cells. Kidney Int. 61(1):105-12, 2002
17. Gronwald J et al: Chromosomal abnormalities in renal cell neoplasms associated with acquired renal cystic disease. A series studied by comparative genomic hybridization and fluorescence in situ hybridization. J Pathol. 187(3):308-12, 1999
18. Dry SM et al: Extensive calcium oxalate crystal deposition in papillary renal cell carcinoma: report of two cases. Arch Pathol Lab Med. 122(3):260-1, 1998
19. Hammes MS et al: Calcium oxalate monohydrate crystals stimulate gene expression in renal epithelial cells. Kidney Int. 48(2):501-9, 1995

ACQUIRED CYSTIC DISEASE-ASSOCIATED RENAL CELL CARCINOMA

Microscopic Features

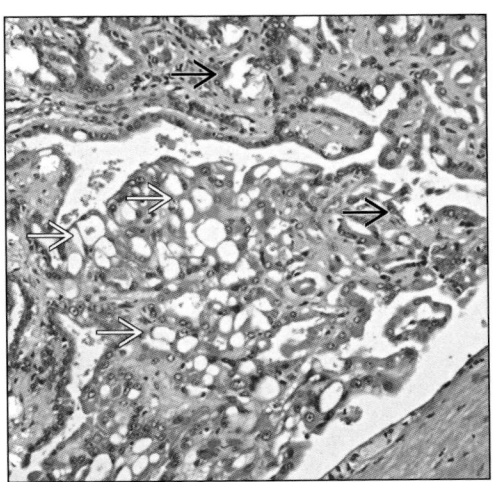

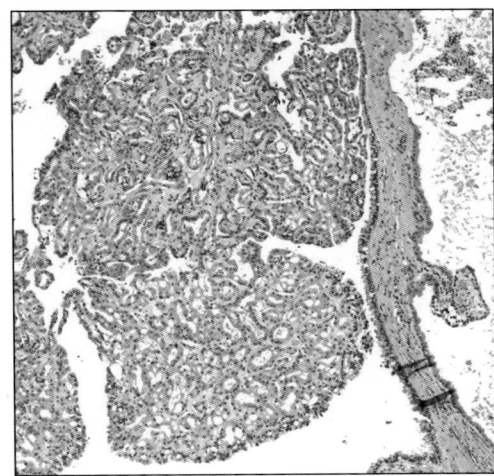

(Left) Typical microscopic appearance of ACD-associated RCC shows papillary and tubular architecture, small lumina ("holes") ➡, large cells with eosinophilic cytoplasm, and intratumoral oxalate crystals ➡. *(Right)* ACD-associated RCC are often seen arising from the wall of a cyst, and many such tumors may have prominent papillary architecture. Because of architectural similarity, such tumors in the past may have been considered papillary renal cell carcinoma by some.

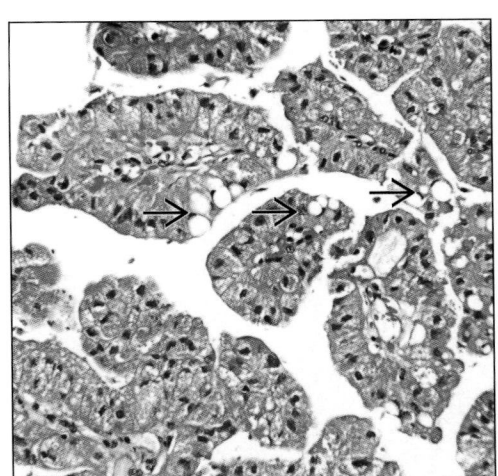

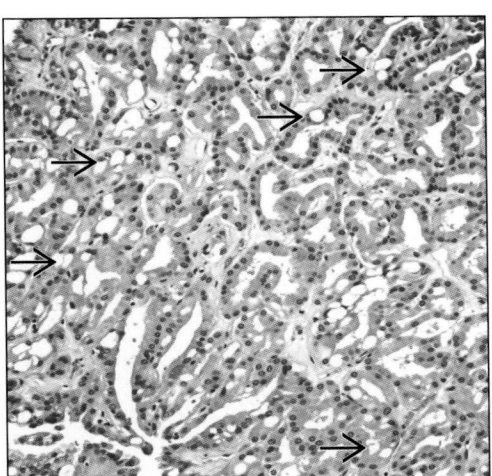

(Left) This photomicrograph shows prominent papillary architecture in an ACD-associated RCC. Differential diagnostic considerations in tumors with prominent papillary architecture include papillary RCC. However, papillary RCC does not show the cytoplasmic lumina ➡ as seen here. *(Right)* This hematoxylin & eosin section highlights predominant tubular features in an ACD-associated RCC. The small intra- and intercellular lumina ➡ are easily identified.

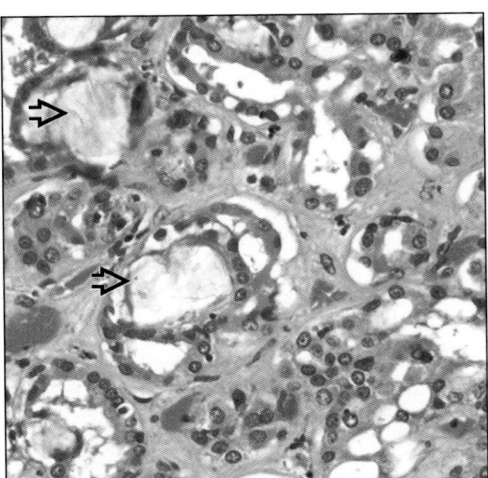

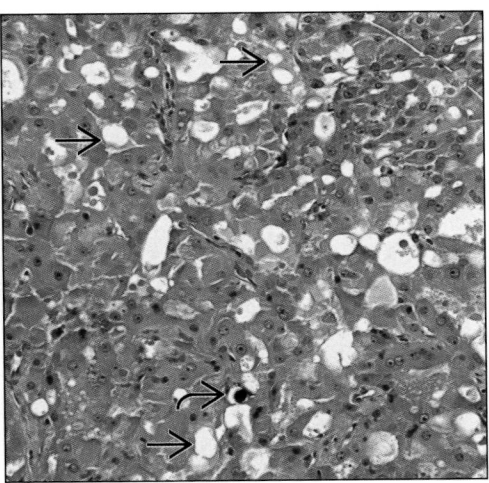

(Left) ACD-associated RCC almost invariably shows cells containing abundant eosinophilic cytoplasm. The oxalate crystals are also easily identifiable ➡ even without using polarized light. *(Right)* Typical cytologic features of ACD-associated RCC include cells with abundant eosinophilic cytoplasm and large nuclei with prominent nucleoli. Notice the prominent inter- and intracellular lumina ➡, a characteristic feature of the tumor. Presence of calcifications ➡ is also common.

ACQUIRED CYSTIC DISEASE-ASSOCIATED RENAL CELL CARCINOMA

Microscopic and Immunohistochemical Features

(Left) Focal areas with clear cell cytology are not uncommon in ACD-associated RCC ➡. Such areas frequently raise the possibility of clear cell RCC, and may be 1 of the reasons for the reported high incidence of clear cell RCC in end-stage kidneys. *(Right)* This higher magnification view highlights clear cell cytology in an ACD-associated RCC. Predominance of such areas in a tumor may lead to the misdiagnosis of clear cell RCC. Careful evaluation of the rest of the tumor is required.

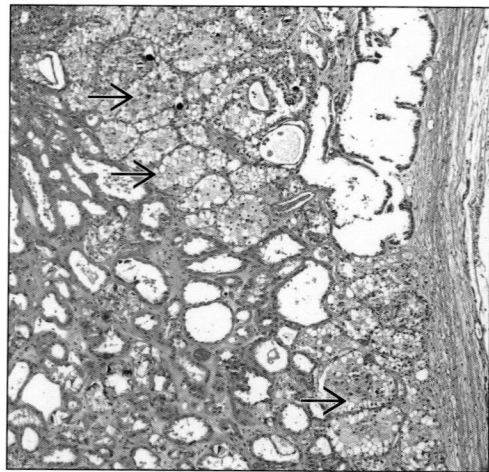 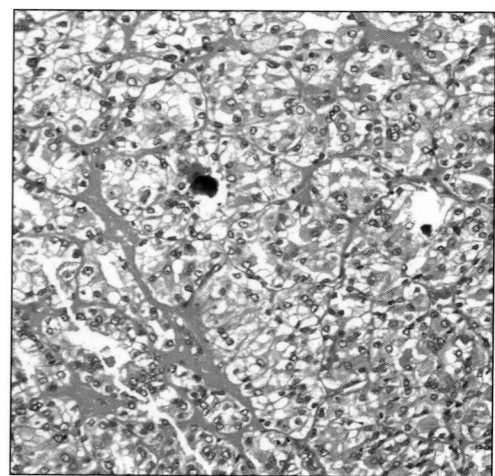

(Left) A higher magnification view shows the characteristic lumina imparting a cribriform/sieve-like appearance to the tumor. Such lumina are present, at least focally, in all architectural and cytological patterns of ACD-associated RCC. *(Right)* Diffuse AMACR positivity, similar to that which may be seen in papillary RCC, is typical. Variable levels of positivity for AMACR are observed even in areas that show clear cell cytology in ACD-associated RCC.

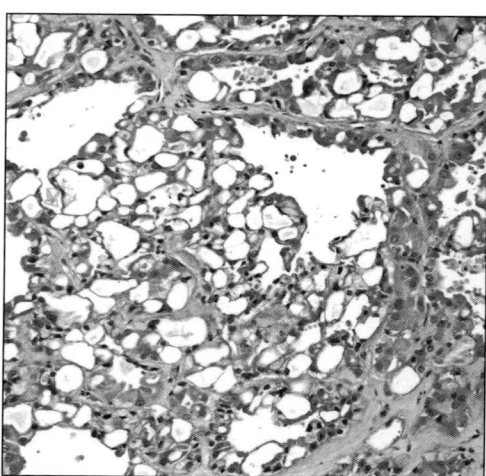 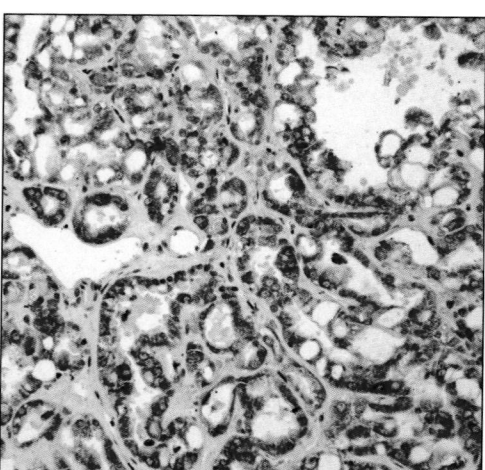

(Left) Cystic and tubular architecture in ACD-associated RCC is quite common. Most tumors show a combination of architectural patterns. *(Right)* In spite of prominent papillary architecture in some cases, immunoreactivity for CK7 is absent or very focal ➡ in ACD-associated RCC. This staining pattern is unlike what is common in papillary RCC, and in association with morphologic features, is quite important in differentiating these tumors from papillary RCC.

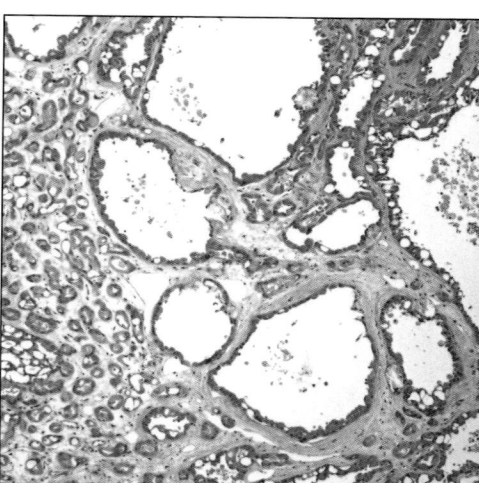 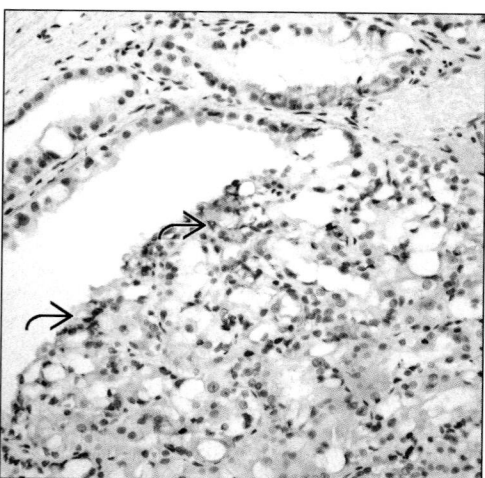

ACQUIRED CYSTIC DISEASE-ASSOCIATED RENAL CELL CARCINOMA

Microscopic and Immunohistochemical Features

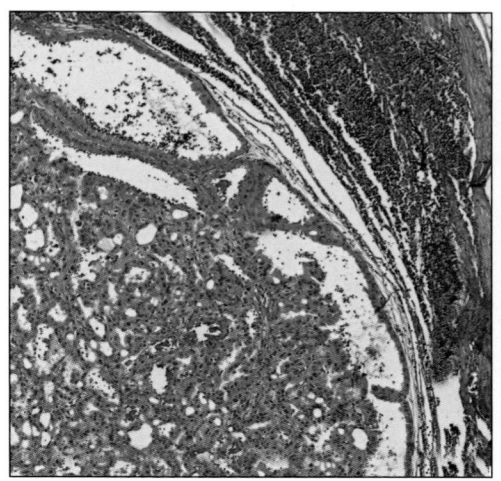
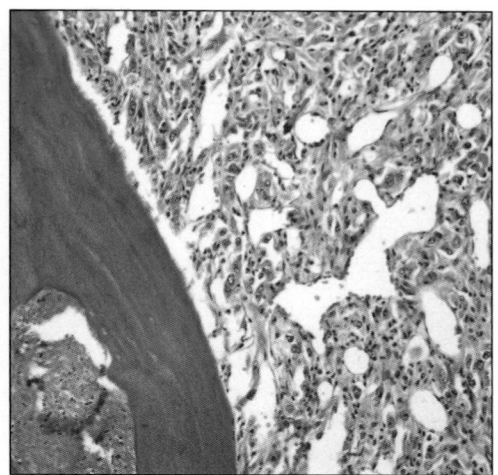

(Left) This hematoxylin & eosin section shows a metastasis to a lymph node. Metastasis is rarely reported in ACD-associated RCC, and in most cases, the metastasis is reported in regional lymph nodes. (Right) This microphotograph shows ACD-associated RCC metastasis to bone. Metastases and other evidence of aggressive behavior, while uncommon, are not infrequent. In addition to lymph nodes and bones, metastases have been reported in unusual sites, including myocardium.

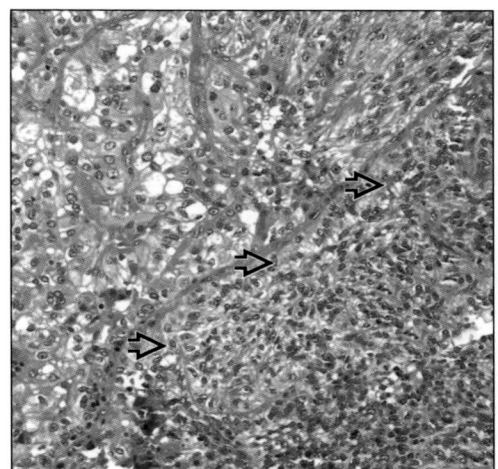
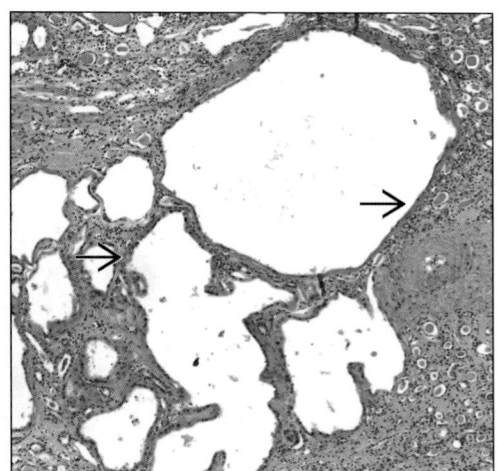

(Left) An ACD-associated RCC shows sarcomatoid ⊅ features. Sarcomatoid differentiation is very rare in this tumor. However, tumors with such features show aggressive biological behavior and have resulted in deaths with widespread metastases. (Right) This photomicrograph shows clustered cysts in the surrounding renal parenchyma. Such cysts are often lined by large pink cells ⊒, morphologically similar to the cells of acquired cystic disease-associated RCC.

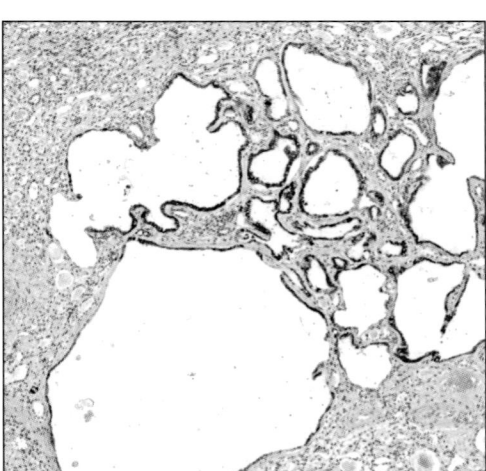
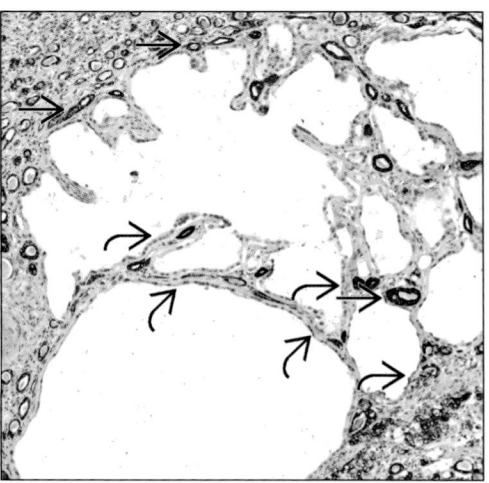

(Left) The eosinophilic cells lining the cysts in the surrounding renal parenchyma often show an immunohistochemical profile that is similar to that of ACD-associated RCC. This AMACR preparation shows diffuse AMACR positivity in the clustered cysts. (Right) Similarly, such clustered cysts in the surrounding renal parenchyma often do not stain for CK7 ⊅. Notice the strong and diffuse positivity in the surrounding renal tubules ⊒.

1

CLEAR CELL PAPILLARY RENAL CELL CARCINOMA

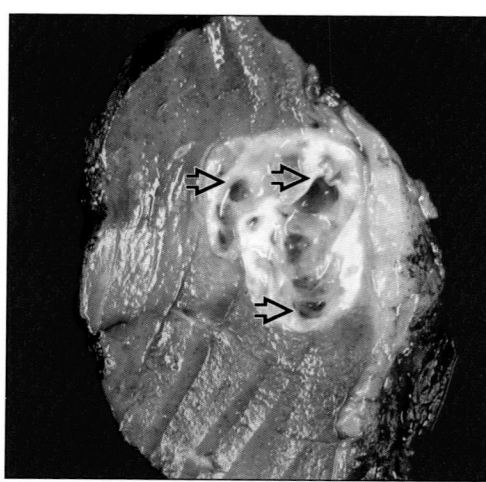

Most clear cell papillary renal cell carcinomas of the kidney are prominently or predominantly cystic ➡. The tumors are often small in size and well circumscribed with a well-defined capsule.

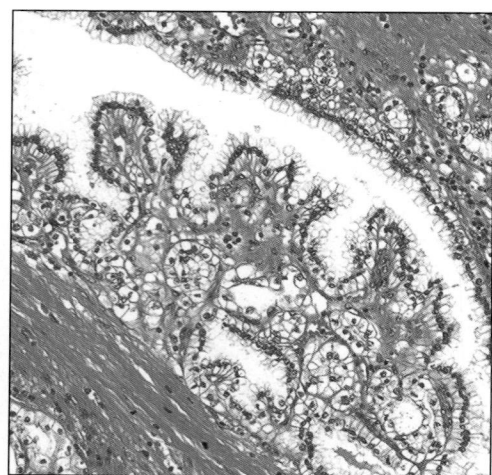

This photomicrograph shows the typical light microscopic features of CC-PRCC. There is a papillary proliferation in a cyst with clear cell cytology. The nuclei are aligned away from the basal aspect.

TERMINOLOGY

Abbreviations
• Clear cell papillary renal cell carcinoma (CC-PRCC)

Definitions
• Carcinoma with exclusive clear cell cytology, low nuclear grade, papillary and tubular/acinar architecture, and nuclei in linear arrangement away from basal aspect of cells

ETIOLOGY/PATHOGENESIS

End-Stage Kidneys
• Initially reported in end-stage renal disease, with reported caveat that these are also seen in non-end-stage setting ± without impaired renal function

Molecular Features
• No 3p25.3 losses
• No *VHL* gene mutations
• No trisomies of chromosome 7 or losses of Y
  ○ 1 case reported to have trisomy 17

CLINICAL ISSUES

Presentation
• Initially reported in setting of end-stage renal disease, ± acquired cystic disease
• Are also seen in non-end-stage setting
• Unicentric, and occasionally multicentric, at presentation
• Most tumors small, pT1 stage
  ○ Only rarely invading perinephric fat, pT3a
• No lymph node or other metastases reported to date

Treatment
• Surgical approaches

○ Due to size and nonaggressive radiologic appearance, usually partial nephrectomy

Prognosis
• Biologically likely to be indolent tumor

MACROSCOPIC FEATURES

General Features
• Well circumscribed
  ○ Usually encapsulated
  ○ Capsule variable in thickness
• Variably, but often prominently, cystic

Size
• Usually small
  ○ Mean size: 2.5 cm; largest described tumor: 5 cm in size

MICROSCOPIC PATHOLOGY

Histologic Features
• Well circumscribed, often encapsulated
  ○ Capsule variable in thickness
  ○ Some cases with prominent myoid metaplasia of thick capsule with extensions into tumor mass
• Usually cystic
  ○ However, some tumors are predominantly solid with very few cystic areas
• Usually prominent papillary architecture
  ○ Some cases with tightly packed papillae giving rise to solid appearance
• Tubular/acinar features are also common
• Some tumors with tightly packed, very small "collapsed" acini, giving the tumor solid sheet-like appearance
  ○ Tumors with "collapsed" acini, variable tubular architecture, myoid metaplasia, and diffuse CK7 positivity are considered by some to be separate

CLEAR CELL PAPILLARY RENAL CELL CARCINOMA

Key Facts

Terminology
- Carcinoma with exclusive clear cell cytology, low nuclear grade, papillary and tubular/acinar architecture, and nuclei in linear arrangement away from basal aspect of cells

Etiology/Pathogenesis
- No 3p25.3 losses
- No *VHL* gene mutations
- No trisomies of chromosome 7 or losses of Y

Clinical Issues
- Most tumors small, pT1stage
- No lymph node or other metastases reported (as of now)
- Biologically likely to be indolent tumor

Microscopic Pathology
- Usually cystic
- Usually prominent papillary architecture
- Almost all cells with clear cytoplasm
- Nuclei, almost always low grade
- Nuclei arranged in linear alignment, away from basal aspect of cells, usually in center of cytoplasm or more apical
- CK7(+), CA9(+), HMCK(34βE12)(+), CD10(-) or focally (+), AMACR(-)

Top Differential Diagnoses
- Clear cell renal cell carcinoma
- Papillary renal cell carcinoma
- Translocation-associated renal carcinoma

---

tumor entities (renal angiomyoadenomatous tumor/ RCC with diffuse CK7 immunoreactivity)
  - Such features maybe seen in otherwise typical clear cell papillary RCC
    - Therefore, no reason to consider these as separate tumors
    - Logical to accept these within the spectrum of clear cell papillary RCC
- Foamy macrophages and tumor necrosis invariably absent
- Almost all cells have clear cytoplasm
  - Except in solid "collapsed" acinar areas
    - Scanty cytoplasm in these areas makes cells appear somewhat amphophilic
- Nuclei almost always low grade (equivalent to Fuhrman grade 2)
- Most characteristic feature is arrangement of nuclei
  - Nuclei in linear arrangement, away from basal aspect of cells, usually in center of cytoplasm or more apical

ANCILLARY TESTS

Immunohistochemistry
- CK7: Diffusely and strongly positive (almost always 100% of cells)
- CA9: Diffusely positive
- HMCK(34βE12): Often diffusely positive
- AMACR: Negative
- CD10: Negative or very focally positive

DIFFERENTIAL DIAGNOSIS

Clear Cell Renal Cell Carcinoma
- Papillary areas uncommon
- Random nuclear arrangement in cytoplasm
- Usually strongly CD10 immunoreactive with diffuse membranous positivity; CK7(-)

Papillary Renal Cell Carcinoma
- Optically transparent clear cytoplasm not seen; clear cells if present, finely bubbly, granular, and focal
- Foamy macrophages, areas of necrosis very common
- IHC: CK7(+), AMACR(+), and CA9([-] or focally [+])

Translocation-Associated Renal Carcinoma
- Predominantly clear cell histology is rare
  - Often accompanied by cells with eosinophilic cytoplasm
- Usually high nuclear grade
- Cytokeratins and EMA/MUC1 usually (-) or very focally (+)
- TFE (TFE3 or TFEB) immunostains are positive depending on cytogenetic profile

SELECTED REFERENCES

1. Michal M et al: Difference between RAT and clear cell papillary renal cell carcinoma/clear renal cell carcinoma. Virchows Arch. 454(6):719, 2009
2. Michal M et al: Renal angiomyoadenomatous tumor: morphologic, immunohistochemical, and molecular genetic study of a distinct entity. Virchows Arch. 454(1):89-99, 2009
3. Srigley JR et al: Uncommon and recently described renal carcinomas. Mod Pathol. 22 Suppl 2:S2-S23, 2009
4. Verine J: Renal angiomyoadenomatous tumor: morphologic, immunohistochemical, and molecular genetic study of a distinct entity. Virchows Arch. 454(4):479-80, 2009
5. Gobbo S et al: Clear cell papillary renal cell carcinoma: a distinct histopathologic and molecular genetic entity. Am J Surg Pathol. 32(8):1239-45, 2008
6. Mai KT et al: Sporadic clear cell renal cell carcinoma with diffuse cytokeratin 7 immunoreactivity. Pathology. 40(5):481-6, 2008
7. Tickoo SK et al: Pathologic features of renal cortical tumors. Urol Clin North Am. 35(4):551-61; v, 2008
8. Tickoo SK et al: Spectrum of epithelial neoplasms in end-stage renal disease: an experience from 66 tumor-bearing kidneys with emphasis on histologic patterns distinct from those in sporadic adult renal neoplasia. Am J Surg Pathol. 30(2):141-53, 2006

Gross and Microscopic Features

(Left) Some clear cell papillary renal cell carcinomas show a combination of solid and cystic appearance with a spongy cut surface. Irregular scars ⇨ may occasionally be seen in the center of the lesion. *(Right)* Some tumors appear more solid. Notice the prominent capsule ➡. This is a typical finding in clear cell papillary RCC. CC-PRCC shares this gross feature with papillary renal cell carcinoma. On the other hand, it lacks necrosis, a common finding in papillary RCC.

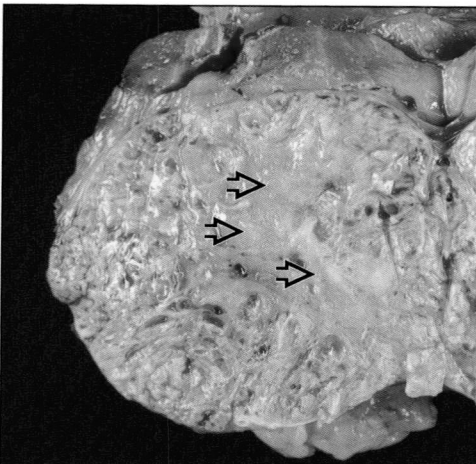 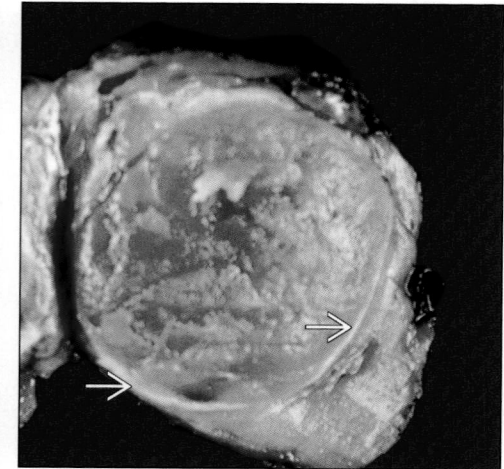

(Left) Hematoxylin & eosin stained section shows a thick fibrous capsule in a CC-PRCC ⇨. The tumor is composed of elongated tubules and tightly packed papillae. *(Right)* A clear cell papillary renal cell carcinoma shows papillary ⇨ and solid tubular ➡ architectural patterns. The cytoplasm is predominantly clear, and the nuclei are arranged toward the luminal aspect. The presence of prominent clear cell cytology distinguishes this tumor from a papillary renal cell carcinoma.

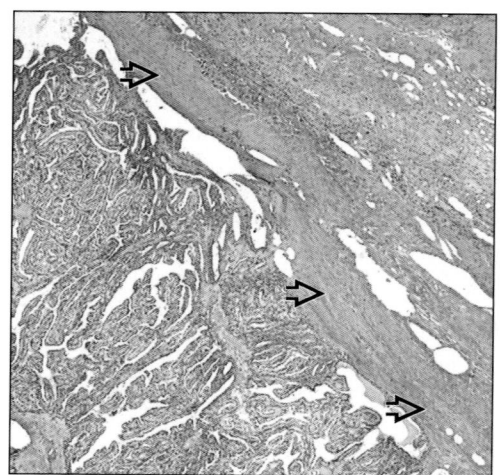 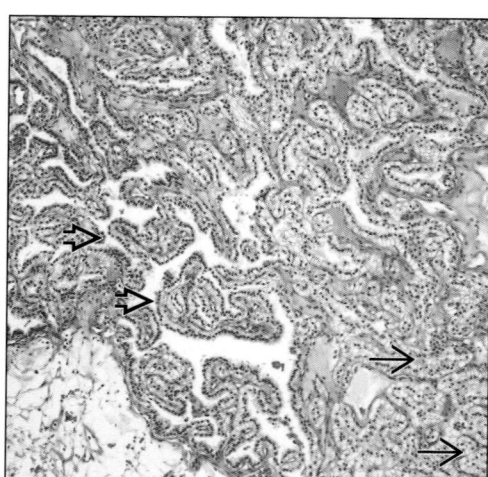

(Left) Most CC-PRCC contain a prominent cystic component. In such areas, as seen here, the walls of the cysts show papillary proliferations lined by cells with clear cytoplasm. The nuclei are aligned in a single layer, away from the basal aspect of the cells ⇨. *(Right)* Section from a noncystic component of the tumor shows more solid areas with tightly packed papillae. Papillary architecture and clear cells are constant and diagnostic features of this subtype of renal cell carcinoma.

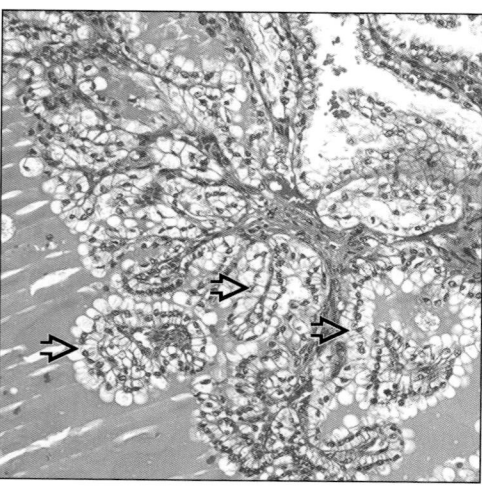 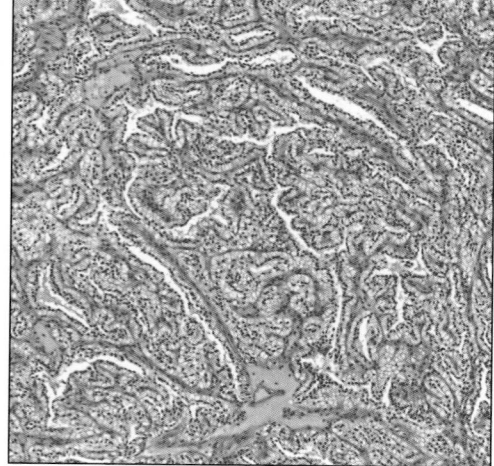

CLEAR CELL PAPILLARY RENAL CELL CARCINOMA

Microscopic Features

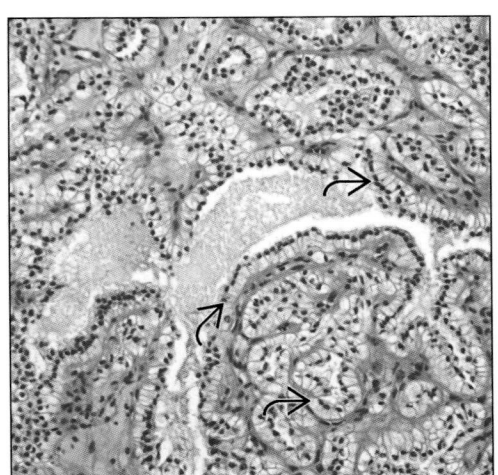

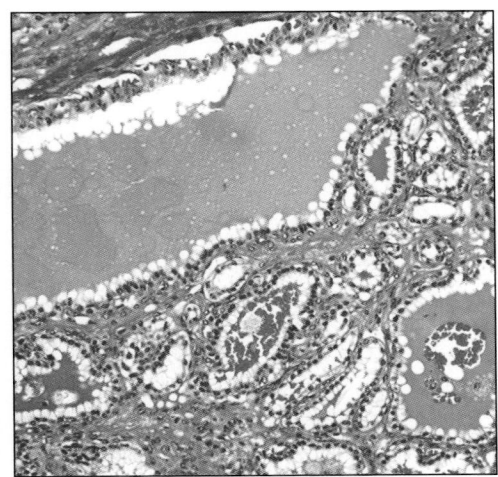

(Left) Whether cystic, solid, or papillary, the most characteristic feature is the linear alignment of the nuclei away from the basal aspects of the cells ⮕. *(Right)* Some tumors show prominent tubular and cystic architecture. The tubules often contain eosinophilic secretions or hemorrhage. In these areas, the tumor may resemble a clear cell RCC. Distinction between these 2 subtypes of renal cell carcinoma is based on the recognition of distinct delicate vasculature in clear cell RCC.

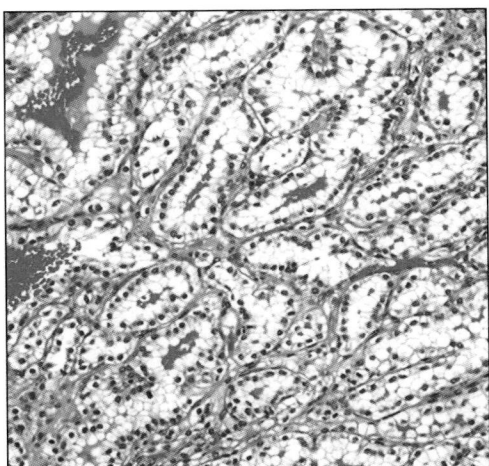

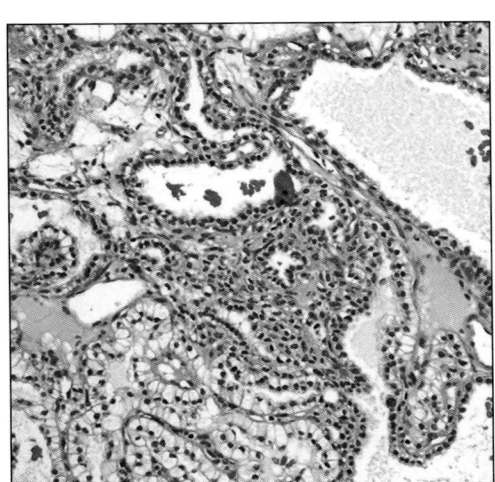

(Left) In spite of the prominent tubular pattern, the characteristic nuclear arrangement is retained. Because of this architectural pattern, the tumor may be mistaken for a clear cell RCC. *(Right)* Clear cell papillary RCC frequently shows a combination of architectural patterns, including papillary, tubular, cystic, and solid. Translocation-associated renal carcinomas share similar diversity of architectural features with clear cell papillary RCC.

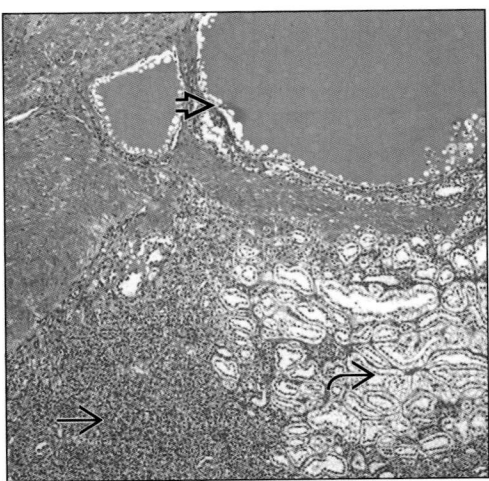

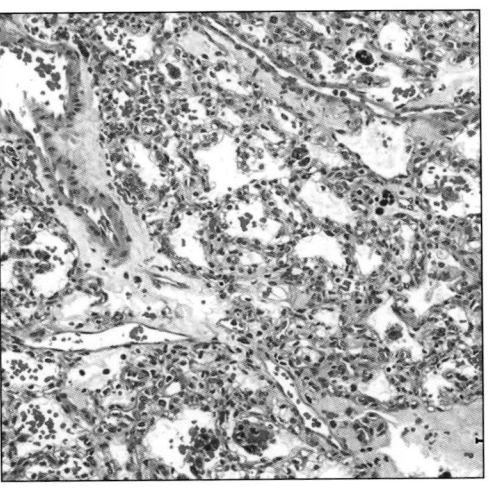

(Left) A combination of architectural patterns are often seen in clear cell papillary RCC. In this section, the tumor shows mixed cystic ⮕, tubular ⮕, and solid collapsed acinar ⮕ architectural patterns. *(Right)* Although the nuclear arrangement in a linear array and away from the basement membrane is typical, there may be foci in otherwise typical tumors in which the nuclei, particularly in some tubular areas, may not be aligned in a linear manner.

CLEAR CELL PAPILLARY RENAL CELL CARCINOMA

Microscopic and Immunohistochemical Features

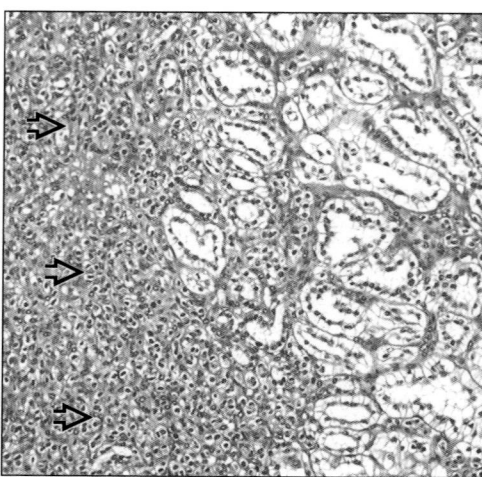 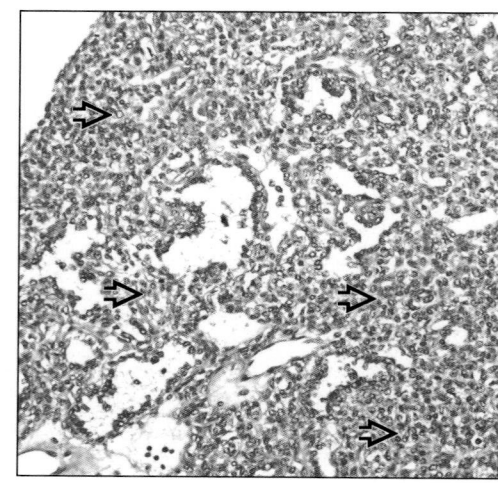

(Left) While the term angiomyoadenomatous tumor has been proposed for similar lesions with myoid metaplasia, features in the tumor that are otherwise typical for clear cell papillary RCC, including solid acinar pattern ⊋, do not support a separate designation. (Right) Some CC-PRCC may show multiple areas of collapsed tightly packed acinar growth pattern ⊋. Such areas in a needle biopsy may be mistaken for clear cell RCC. Immunohistochemistry may be of value in such settings.

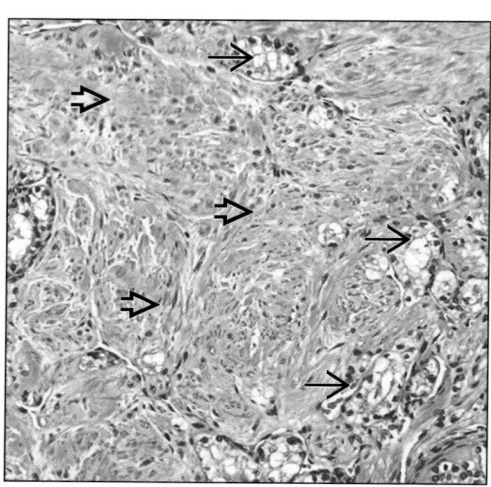 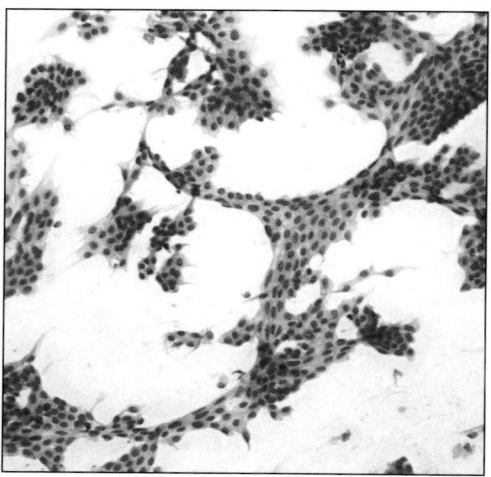

(Left) The presence of a tumor capsule is a distinctive feature of clear cell papillary RCC. It may occasionally be quite thick, as also seen in other slow-growing renal tumors, and may show myoid metaplasia ⊋. Occasionally this smooth muscle proliferation may entrap epithelial nests →. (Right) Cytologic smears from clear cell papillary RCC show papillary fragments that may raise the diagnostic possibility of a type 1 papillary RCC.

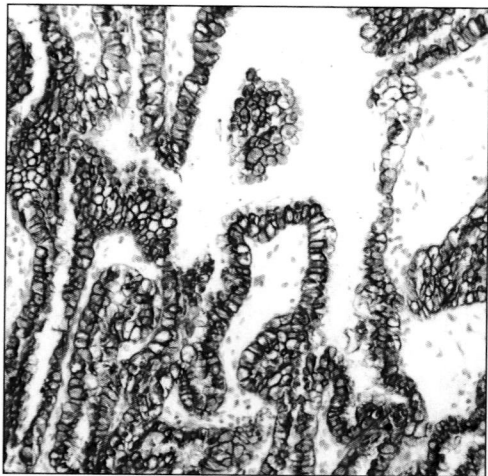 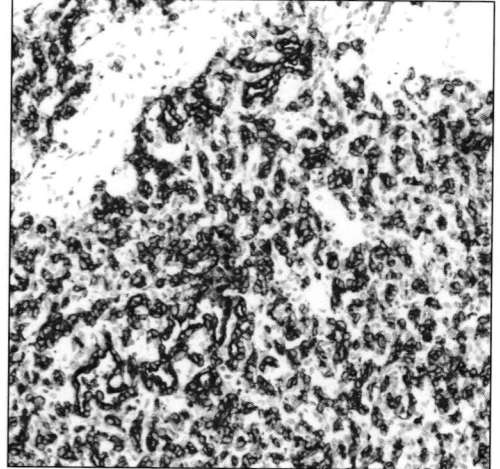

(Left) Although the histologic features are relatively classic, immunohistochemistry may be particularly helpful in needle biopsies. CC-PRCC shows diffuse and intense positivity (in almost 100% of the cells) for CK7 and is 1 of the most characteristic features of the tumor. (Right) Similar to the papillary and tubular areas, CK7 shows diffuse and strong immunoreactivity in the collapsed tightly packed acinar areas as well. This is quite unlike what is observed in clear cell RCC.

CLEAR CELL PAPILLARY RENAL CELL CARCINOMA

Immunohistochemical Features

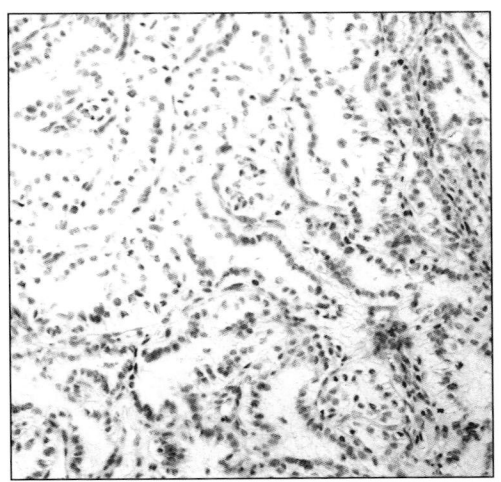

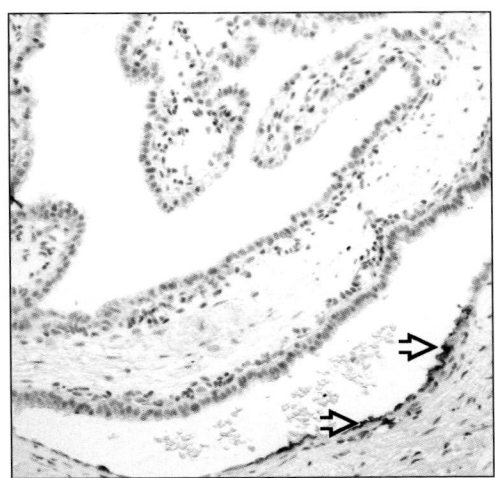

(Left) Clear cell papillary RCC, like papillary RCC, is strongly positive for CK7. However, unlike papillary RCC, clear cell papillary RCC is negative for AMACR, as shown here, or at the most, very focally positive. *(Right)* In contrast to clear cell RCC, CD10 is usually negative or only focally positive ⊟ in clear cell papillary RCC. Cytogenetically, these tumors are also distinct from clear cell RCC and papillary RCC.

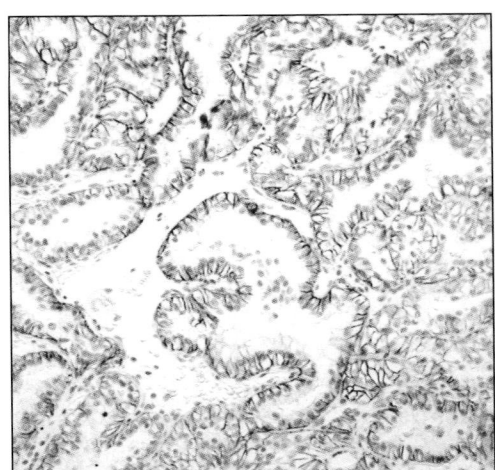

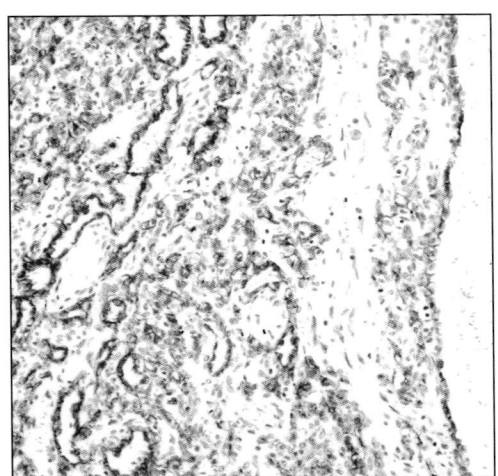

(Left) CA9 also marks the tumor in a diffuse membranous staining pattern. This immunoreactivity overlaps with that of clear cell RCC, which is typically negative for CK7. *(Right)* CA9 immunoreactivity in tightly packed acinar areas is shown adjacent to more prominent cystic change.

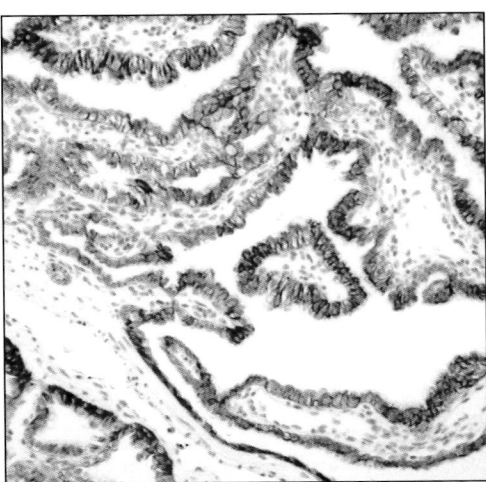

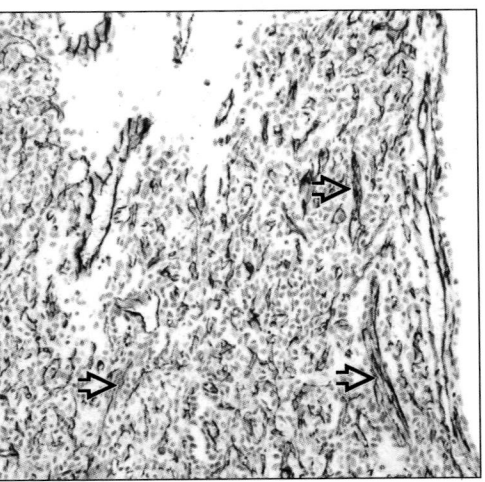

(Left) Another interesting aspect of clear cell papillary RCC is the diffuse immunoreactivity for HMCK(34βE12) in a distinct subset of tumors. In general, expression of this marker is limited in the more common subtypes of RCC. *(Right)* Clear cell papillary RCC shows morphologic overlap with clear cell RCC in areas with closely packed small tubules. This is exaggerated by the presence of delicate supporting vasculature by CD31 ⊟, as shown here.

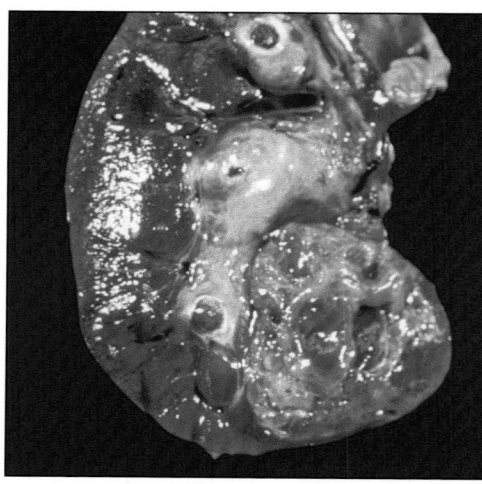

This post-chemotherapy renal cell carcinoma has oncocytoid features similar to neuroblastoma-associated renal carcinoma. Such tumors may develop after therapy for other tumors, as well.

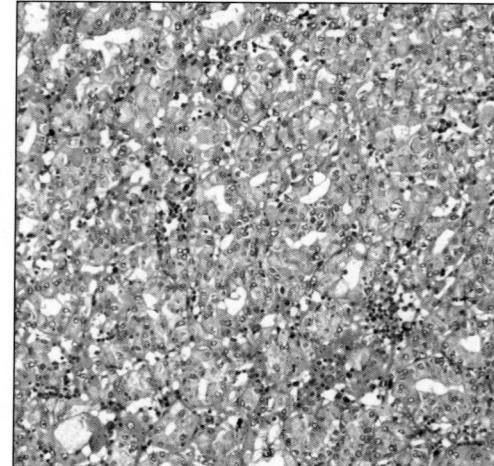

Typical features of a neuroblastoma-associated renal carcinoma include solid sheet-like architecture, with cells showing abundant oncocytic cytoplasm and nuclei with prominent nucleoli.

TERMINOLOGY

Definitions

- Renal cell tumors that develop following earlier renal or nonrenal tumor or other treated nonneoplastic autoimmune conditions
  - Most of these tumors develop after prior chemotherapy
  - Rare tumors occur spontaneously and without any chemotherapy

ETIOLOGY/PATHOGENESIS

Prior Tumors

- Best recognized prior tumor is neuroblastoma
  - 2nd tumors in most cases have developed after chemotherapy for high-stage neuroblastoma
    - Suggests possible role for chemotherapy-induced chromosomal instability
  - Rare tumors have presented synchronously or without receiving any chemotherapy
    - Suggesting possible underlying genetic susceptibility as a factor, rather than chemotherapy, at least in some cases
- Rare 2nd tumors also reported in cases with prior Wilms tumor
  - Many of these, in addition to receiving chemotherapy, have also received radiation
- Another entity, recognized to be associated with chemotherapy, is TFE-translocation-associated renal carcinoma
  - Prior conditions requiring chemotherapy have included leukemias, Wilms tumor, or nonneoplastic diseases like SLE and Hurler syndrome
  - In these cases, cytotoxic chemotherapy is proposed to predispose for development of 2nd tumors
- Chemotherapy also implicated in very rare cases reported after therapy for other tumor types, including leiomyosarcoma

Genetic Features

- Few post-neuroblastoma tumors tested have often been aneuploid, with multiple allelic imbalances in different chromosomes
  - Many tumors with 14q31 and 20q13 abnormalities
- Translocation-associated renal carcinomas with spectrum of fusions, similar to cases with no prior history of therapy, including
  - *ASPL-TFE3*, *α-TFEB*, and *PRCC-TFE3* fusions

CLINICAL ISSUES

Epidemiology

- Incidence
  - Following childhood cancer, incidence of 2nd cancer in survivors is higher than in general population
    - Incidence is about 1%, 3%, and > 8%, without any therapy, with chemo- or radiotherapy alone, and with both together, respectively
    - Last incidence is roughly 20x greater than in general population
  - Majority of 2nd tumors are leukemias, melanoma, soft tissue and bone sarcoma, thyroid, breast, and brain tumors
  - 2nd tumors involving kidney are quite rare
    - Approximately 20 cases post-neuroblastoma and less than 10 cases post-Wilms tumor reported in literature
    - However, approximately 15% of cases with translocation-associated renal carcinoma have history of prior cytotoxic chemotherapy
    - Tumors post-chemotherapy for other tumors only reported as single cases or small case series
- Age
  - Patients with neuroblastoma-associated and post-chemotherapy TFE carcinomas

Key Facts

Terminology

- Renal cell tumors that develop following earlier renal or nonrenal tumor or other treated nonneoplastic autoimmune conditions
- Most of these tumors develop after prior chemotherapy

Etiology/Pathogenesis

- Best recognized prior tumor is neuroblastoma
- Rare 2nd tumors also reported in cases with prior Wilms tumor
- Another entity recognized to be associated with chemotherapy is TFE renal carcinoma

Microscopic Pathology

- Initially described to be characteristic for specific tumor-associated 2nd tumors

  - However, similar morphologic features are seen in 2nd tumors developing after variety of 1st tumors
  - Morphologically different 2nd tumors can also develop following same 1st tumor
- Most post-neuroblastoma carcinomas with eosinophilic and focally reticular cytoplasm, with solid and papillary architecture
  - More recently, tumors with more variable cytoarchitectural features also described
  - Rare cases confirmed to be MiTF/TFE family translocation-associated carcinomas in post-neuroblastoma setting
- Rare carcinomas reported after therapy for other tumors similar to neuroblastoma-associated carcinoma

---

- Younger; range: 2-35 years; mean interval between prior tumor and RCC: 7 years (range: A few months to 13 years)
  - Patients with renal tumors post-Wilms tumor
    - Older; range: 34-50 years; reported intervals after prior therapy: Often > 30 years

Prognosis

- RCC associated with neuroblastoma
  - > 25% of cases reported to develop metastases
  - Sites of metastases have been lymph nodes, liver, adrenal, thyroid, and bone
- Post-chemotherapy TFE renal carcinoma
  - In children, often present at advanced stage
    - Some cases have shown unusually aggressive behavior and proven fatal

MICROSCOPIC PATHOLOGY

Histologic Features

- Initially, characteristic 2nd tumors were described after specific primary tumor
  - Subsequently, great overlap in morphology of 2nd tumors, as well as associated primary tumors was described
- Most post-neuroblastoma carcinomas have eosinophilic and focally reticular cytoplasm with solid and papillary architecture
  - More recently, tumors with more variable cytoarchitectural features have been described
    - Some of these have papillary or clear cell RCC-like features
    - Rare cases confirmed to be MiTF/TFE family translocation-associated carcinomas in post-neuroblastoma setting
- Translocation-associated renal carcinomas post-chemotherapy have been both TFEB and TFE3 tumors
- Tumors developing after therapy for Wilms tumor have predominantly been reported as clear cell, and rarely papillary RCC, and oncocytomas

  - However, these tumors have not been systematically investigated for TFE translocations; 1 case reported to be TFE carcinoma
- Rare carcinomas reported after therapy for other tumors similar to neuroblastoma-associated carcinoma

DIAGNOSTIC CHECKLIST

Pathologic Interpretation Pearls

- 2nd tumors of similar morphologic phenotype may develop after variety of initial tumor types
- 2nd tumors of different morphologies may also develop after specific initial tumor type
- 2nd renal tumor should always be considered in renal tumors with unclassified morphology

SELECTED REFERENCES

1. Shnorhavorian M et al: Genitourinary long-term outcomes for childhood cancer survivors. Curr Urol Rep. 10(2):134-7, 2009
2. Dhall D et al: Pediatric renal cell carcinoma with oncocytoid features occurring in a child after chemotherapy for cardiac leiomyosarcoma. Urology. 70(1):178, 2007
3. Rais-Bahrami S et al: Xp11 translocation renal cell carcinoma: delayed but massive and lethal metastases of a chemotherapy-associated secondary malignancy. Urology. 70(1):178, 2007
4. Argani P et al: Translocation carcinomas of the kidney after chemotherapy in childhood. J Clin Oncol. 24(10):1529-34, 2006
5. Bassal M et al: Risk of selected subsequent carcinomas in survivors of childhood cancer: a report from the Childhood Cancer Survivor Study. J Clin Oncol. 24(3):476-83, 2006
6. Cherullo EE et al: Renal neoplasms in adult survivors of childhood Wilms tumor. J Urol. 165(6 Pt 1):2013-6; discussion 2016-7, 2001
7. Medeiros LJ et al: Oncocytoid renal cell carcinoma after neuroblastoma: a report of four cases of a distinct clinicopathologic entity. Am J Surg Pathol. 23(7):772-80, 1999

Microscopic Features

(**Left**) Neuroblastoma is the most well known, but relatively uncommon, tumor associated with the development of 2nd renal tumors. Neuroblastoma-associated renal carcinoma is recognized as a distinct tumor entity by the WHO. (**Right**) Neuroblastoma-associated renal carcinoma is typically composed of large oncocytic cells, with large, mildly pleomorphic nuclei with prominent nucleoli ➡. Rare dispersed cells may have somewhat clear, bubbly cytoplasm ➡.

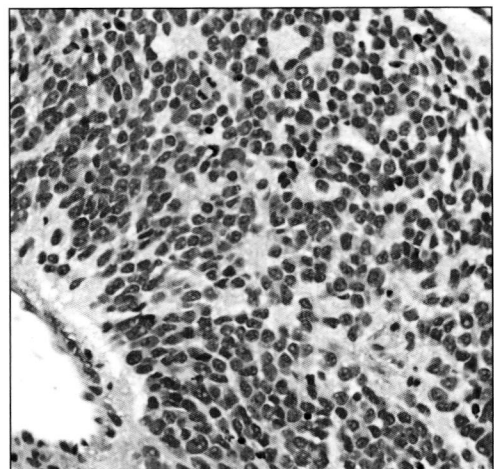
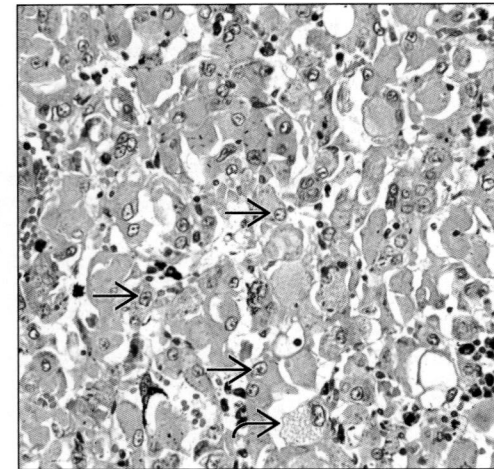

(**Left**) Morphologic features similar to neuroblastoma-associated renal carcinoma may also be seen in 2nd tumors developing after other neoplasms. This tumor arose in the kidney of a child previously treated for leiomyosarcoma. Notice focal papillations ➡, a finding frequent in post-neuroblastoma carcinomas. (**Right**) Tumors with a variety of histologic features are now known to arise following neuroblastoma, including those with papillary architecture and clear cell cytology.

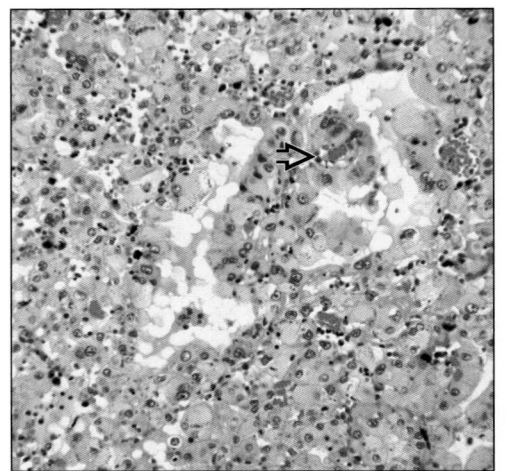
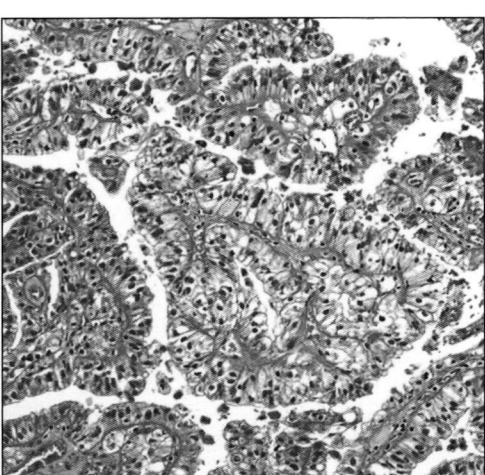

(**Left**) Although most 2nd tumors with clear cell &/or papillary features arising after neuroblastoma have not been studied for TFE translocations, these translocations have been confirmed in some tumors. Post-neuroblastoma carcinomas may have typical morphologic features of TFE family translocation-associated renal carcinomas. (**Right**) Neuroblastoma-associated TFE carcinomas may show morphologic features of TFE3 or TFEB (as seen here) carcinomas, and immunostaining is confirmatory.

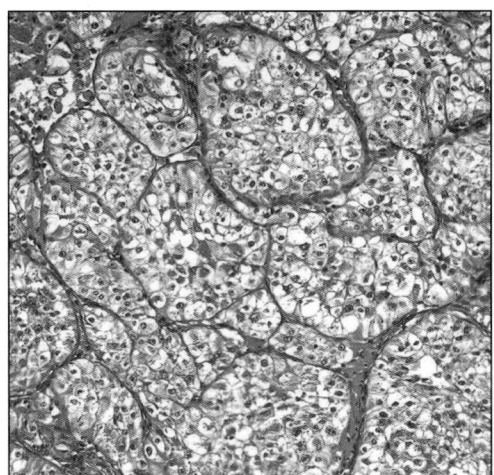
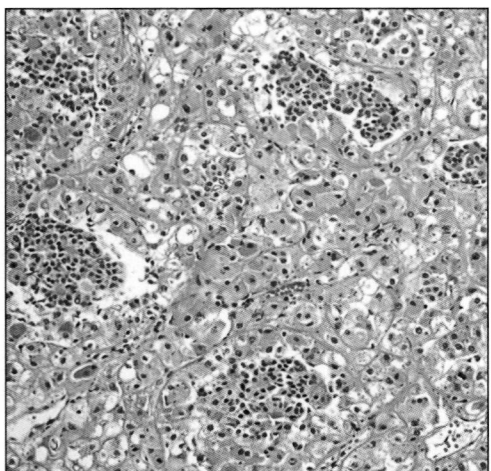

SECOND TUMORS

Microscopic Features

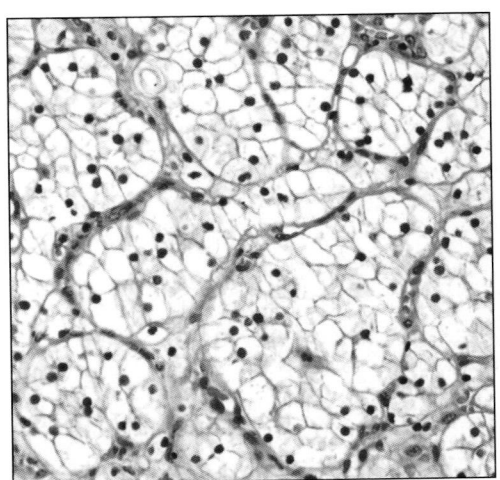

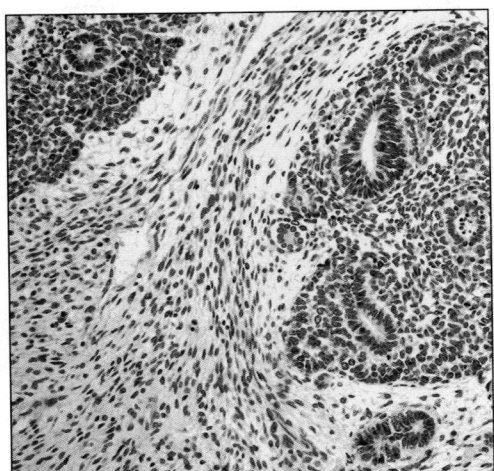

(Left) A number of post-neuroblastoma 2nd tumors are regarded as clear cell RCC. However, many tumors with clear cell features in children are TFE carcinomas. Also, most post-neuroblastoma 2nd tumors arise in children. Some of these tumors are proven to be TFE carcinomas, making it prudent to investigate all post-neuroblastoma tumors with clear cell/papillary features for TFE translocations. *(Right)* Some 2nd tumors are known to arise following Wilms tumor (shown here).

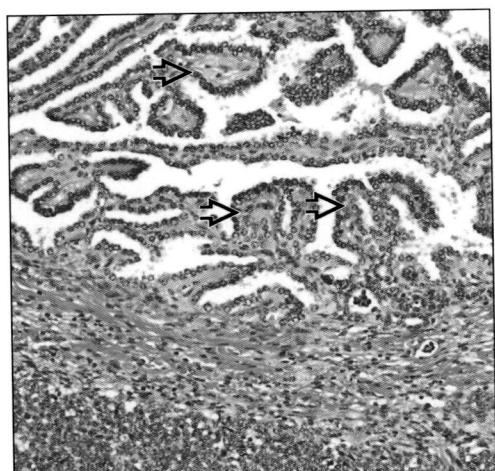

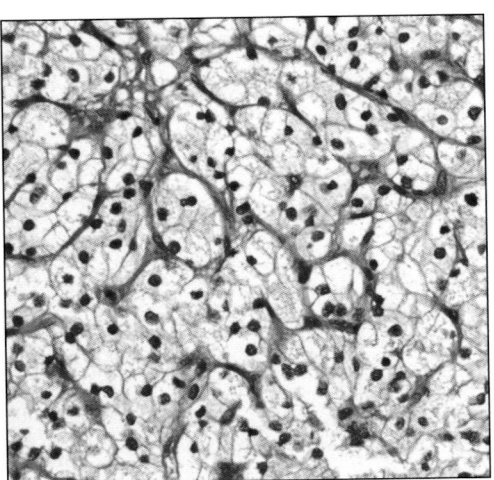

(Left) Wilms tumors after chemotherapy often show large areas with differentiating epithelium, particularly with papillary architecture ➢. These areas, taken out of context, may closely resemble papillary RCC. Such synchronous epithelial differentiation likely does not play a big role in 2nd tumors arising after Wilms tumor, as most 2nd tumors arise many years, often > 30, after a Wilms tumor. *(Right)* Most post-Wilms tumor 2nd tumors have been called clear cell RCC.

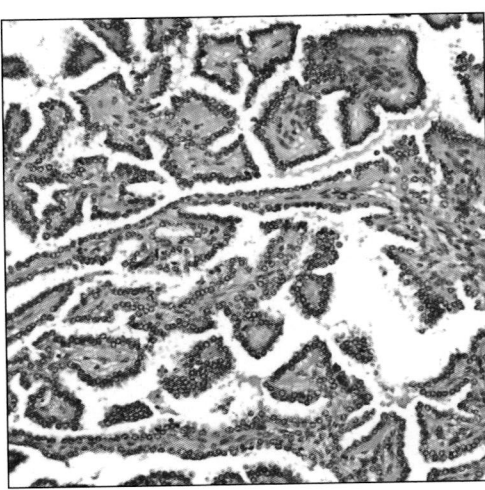

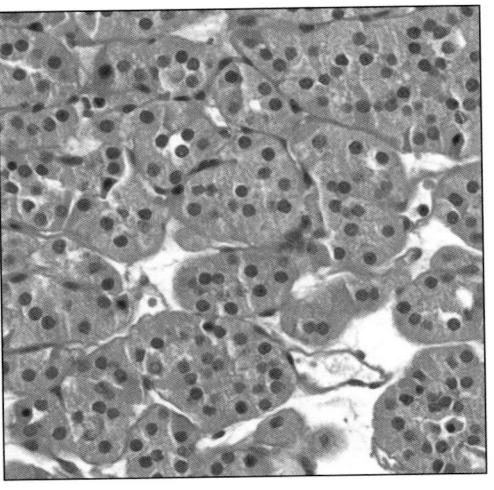

(Left) Occasionally, papillary renal cell carcinoma has also been reported as the 2nd tumor following a Wilms tumor. One case of post-Wilms TFE carcinoma has been reported and the frequency is likely to be higher if more tumors are tested, as 15% of translocation-associated carcinomas arise following chemotherapy. *(Right)* Very occasional oncocytic tumors, described as renal oncocytomas, have also been reported in the post-Wilms tumor setting.

RENAL CELL CARCINOMA, UNCLASSIFIED

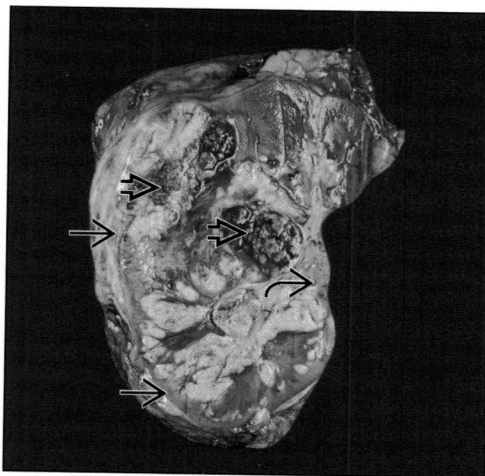

Some renal cell carcinomas, unclassified, show grossly apparent aggressive features, including large size, infiltrative borders ➡, sinus fat invasion ➡, areas of hemorrhage, and necrosis ➡.

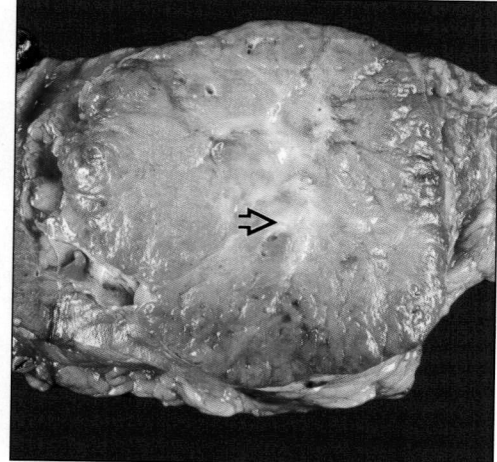

Other RCC, unclassified, may have gross features that do not suggest aggressive behavior. They are well circumscribed, lack gross vascular/fat invasion, or necrosis. Central scar ➡ in some suggests slow growth.

TERMINOLOGY

Abbreviations
- Renal cell carcinoma, unclassified (RCC-U)

Definitions
- Renal cell carcinomas that do not readily fit into 1 of the usual distinctive categories
  - Features that place renal carcinoma in the category include
    - Combination of features of more than 1 recognized subtype or unrecognized cell types
    - Sarcomatoid morphology without identifiable epithelial component or mixture of spindle cell and unrecognized epithelial cell type
  - By definition, category does not include only high-grade, aggressive tumors
    - Some low-grade, indolent tumors are also a part of this category, including some with cytoplasmic eosinophilia (oncocytoma-like features)

ETIOLOGY/PATHOGENESIS

Category Of Unknown Pathogenesis
- Since these are tumors of a variety of cell types, distinct from other well-recognized renal cell tumors, no definite pathogenetic mechanisms or molecular features are known

CLINICAL ISSUES

Main Advantages for Creating the Category
- RCC, unclassified category prevents forcible inclusion of unusual tumors into common subtypes
  - This averts dilution of well-known clinicopathologic features of recognized subtypes of renal cell tumors
- Accumulation of tumors in unclassified category, and gaining more experience with them, enables us to
  - Extract groups of tumors with similar features from the category
  - Reclassify them as distinct entities, as more experience and data becomes available
- Examples of success of such an approach include some now-well-recognized tumors, including
  - Mucinous tubular and spindle cell, clear cell papillary, acquired cystic disease-associated and translocation-associated RCCs
  - Epithelioid angiomyolipoma (PEComa)

Presentation
- Largely depends on histomorphologic features of tumor
  - High-grade, morphologically aggressive-appearing tumors often present with high pT stage
    - > 30% have regional lymph node metastasis and > 50% distant metastasis
  - There are no large studies that have included all, including the low-grade indolent, tumor types
    - Low-grade tumors, particularly those with oncocytic features, often detected incidentally

Treatment
- High-grade, aggressive-type tumors have been treated with surgery and a variety of chemotherapeutic/immunotherapeutic agents
- In low-grade, indolent tumors, usually surgical resection, particularly partial nephrectomy, is performed

Prognosis
- Depends on tumor type, pathologic stage, and metastatic status
  - In recent large study on aggressive tumor types, > 50% of patients were dead of disease on mean follow-up of 1.9 years (range: 0.1-13 years)
  - In lower-grade indolent tumors, only anecdotal incidence of metastasis has been observed

RENAL CELL CARCINOMA, UNCLASSIFIED

Key Facts

Terminology
- Renal cell carcinoma, unclassified (RCC-U)
- Renal cell carcinomas that do not readily fit into 1 of the more usual categories of renal carcinomas
- By definition, category does not include only high-grade, aggressive tumors
  - Some low-grade, indolent tumors are also a part of this category, including some with cytoplasmic eosinophilia (oncocytoma-like features)

Clinical Issues
- RCC, unclassified category prevents inclusion of unusual tumors into common subtypes
- Accumulation of tumors in unclassified category, and gaining more experience with them, enables us to extract groups of tumors with similar features from the category

- These may then be reclassified as distinct entities
- Prognosis depends on tumor type, pathologic stage, and metastatic status

Microscopic Pathology
- High-grade tumors may have sheet-like, rhabdoid, large solid-alveolar, papillary, unusual tubulo-papillary, glandular or sarcomatoid architecture
  - Most of these have Fuhrman grade 3 or 4 features
- Some tumors have cytoarchitectural features closely resembling renal oncocytoma

Top Differential Diagnoses
- Collecting duct carcinoma
- Renal oncocytoma/chromophobe renal cell carcinoma, eosinophilic variant
- Metastatic carcinoma

MACROSCOPIC FEATURES

General Features
- Tumors with aggressive morphologic features are usually large and often multinodular
  - Cut surface is variable, usually tan-white
    - Areas of hemorrhage and necrosis often present
  - Gross extension into veins &/or perinephric and sinus fat are common
- Tumors with nonaggressive morphologic features are of variable size and often organ-confined
  - Many of these have tan-brown or brown cut surface that suggests eosinophilic cell microscopic features
  - Others may have tan or pink cut surface, sometimes with granular appearance and texture, similar to that in some papillary RCCs
  - Central scar may be present, which is usually indicative of slow-growing tumor

MICROSCOPIC PATHOLOGY

Histologic Features
- Variety of cytoarchitectural features may be noted within same tumor or between different tumors
- High-grade tumors may have sheet-like, rhabdoid, large solid-alveolar, papillary, unusual tubulo-papillary, glandular, or sarcomatoid architecture
  - Most of these tumors show high-grade nuclear features (Fuhrman grade 3 or 4)
  - Tumor necrosis, brisk mitotic activity, small vessel invasion, and extrarenal and renal vein invasion are common
  - Cytoplasm may be variably amphophilic, basophilic, clear, or eosinophilic
- Some tumors have cytoarchitectural features closely resembling renal oncocytoma
  - Cell nests and alveoli similar to renal oncocytoma may be present
    - However, many oncocytic, low-grade, unclassified RCCs have more solid architecture

- Some others may have variable papillary, along with solid, architecture
- Nuclei are more pleomorphic than in oncocytoma, often with more than occasional mitotic figures
- Perinuclear halos, similar to that in chromophobe RCC, are not present
- Tumor necrosis is rarely, and only focally, present

DIFFERENTIAL DIAGNOSIS

Collecting Duct Carcinoma (CDC)
- Rigid, consistent, and well-established morphologic features are not established in CDC, hence distinction may be difficult
- It is essentially a high-grade adenocarcinoma, based in renal medulla
- Immunoreactivity for ULEX-1 and other lectins favors diagnosis of CDC

Renal Oncocytoma/Chromophobe Renal Cell Carcinoma, Eosinophilic Variant
- Renal oncocytoma has uniform round nuclei and often nested growth pattern
- Immunostains are usually positive for CD117; CK7 shows only focal positivity
- Chromophobe RCC shows perinuclear halos

Metastatic Carcinoma
- Clinical history, multifocal, interstitial growth

SELECTED REFERENCES

1. Karakiewicz PI et al: Unclassified renal cell carcinoma: an analysis of 85 cases. BJU Int. 100(4):802-8, 2007
2. Reuter VE: The pathology of renal epithelial neoplasms. Semin Oncol. 33(5):534-43, 2006
3. Amin MB et al: Prognostic impact of histologic subtyping of adult renal epithelial neoplasms: an experience of 405 cases. Am J Surg Pathol. 26(3):281-91, 2002
4. Zisman A et al: Unclassified renal cell carcinoma: clinical features and prognostic impact of a new histological subtype. J Urol. 168(3):950-5, 2002

Microscopic Features

(Left) This photomicrograph shows a renal cell carcinoma, unclassified with high-grade nuclear features, loose sheet-like architecture, and somewhat rhabdoid ⮕ cytology. *(Right)* Another RCC, unclassified, shows a cribriform and papillary architecture. This tumor also shows high-grade cytologic features. Some publications on RCC, unclassified, have included only high-grade, aggressive tumors in their studies. Expectedly, these report a poor prognosis for such tumors.

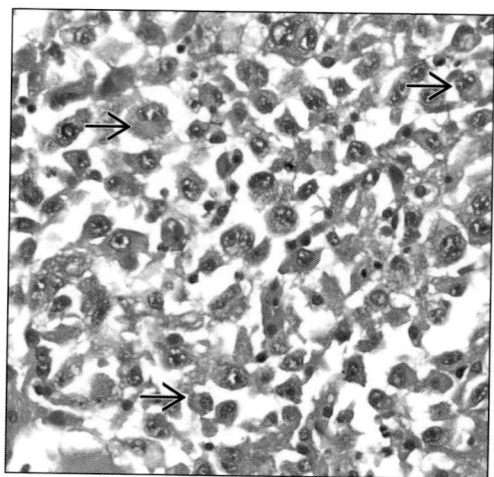
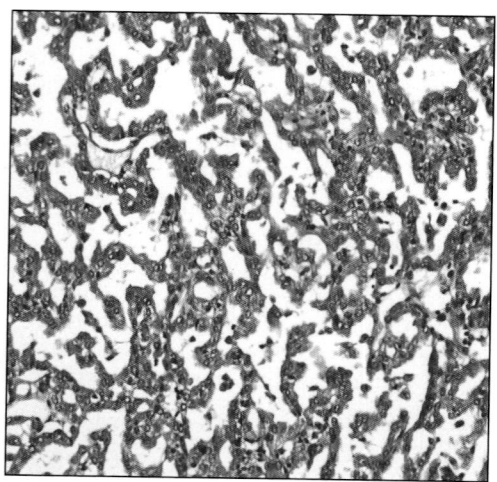

(Left) This RCC, unclassified, shows a predominantly sarcomatoid histology. Renal tumors with the absence or presence of unrecognizable epithelial components are included in the unclassified category after specific sarcomas are ruled out. Similar to other renal carcinomas with sarcomatoid differentiation, the tumors generally have a poor clinical outcome. *(Right)* This tumor has an irregular tumor front ⮕, which is a typical feature in clinically aggressive high-grade RCC, unclassified.

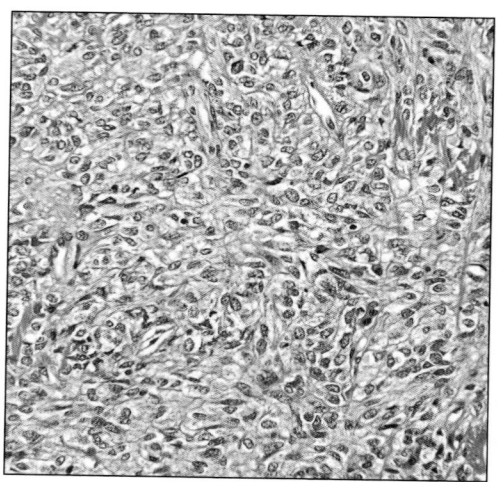
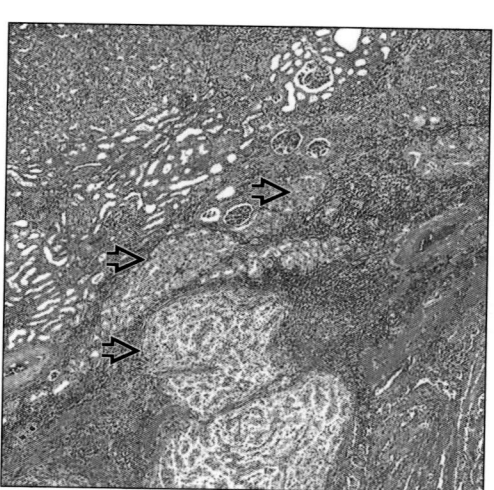

(Left) This photomicrograph depicts a renal cell carcinoma, unclassified, that has a morphologically less aggressive, oncocytic appearance, and superficially resembles a renal oncocytoma. Although nuclear features are not truly low-grade, these tumors usually have an indolent clinical behavior. *(Right)* Many such oncocytic renal cell carcinomas, unclassified, show sheet-like architectural pattern, at least focally. Only anecdotal cases of metastasis from such tumors exist.

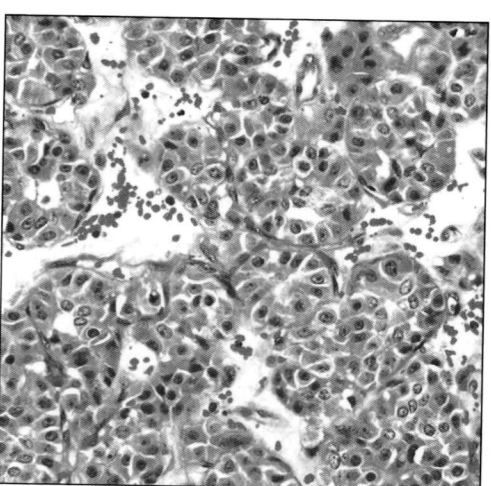
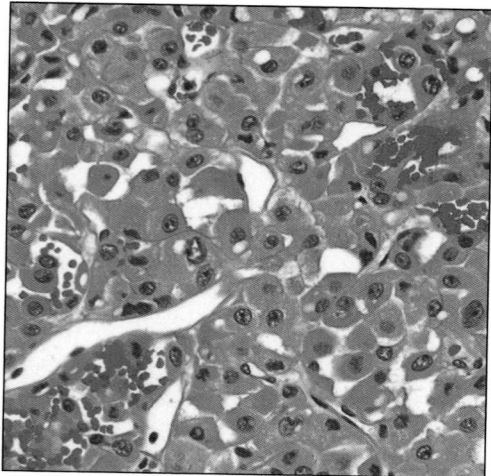

Microscopic and Immunohistochemical Features

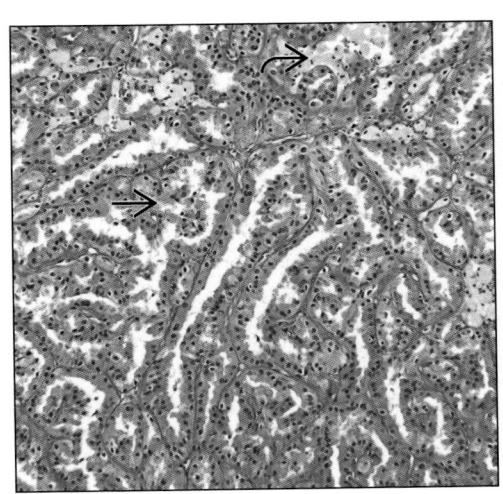

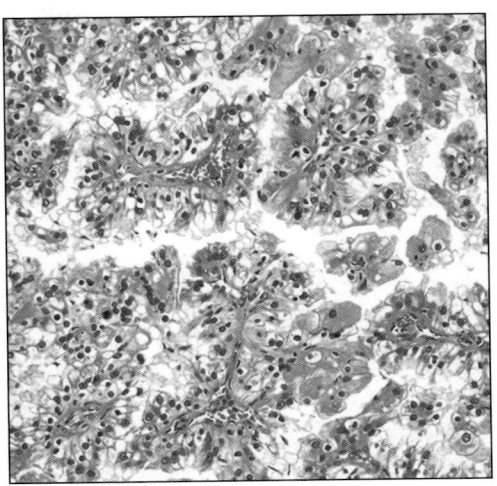

(Left) Rare low-grade oncocytic RCC, unclassified, may show areas with papillary architecture ⮕ and even foamy macrophages ⮕. However, prominent solid, tubular &/or cystic features preclude their classification as papillary RCC. *(Right)* This RCC, unclassified, shows combination of prominent papillary architecture and clear and eosinophilic cell cytology. Such features will often raise the possibility of translocation-associated RCC, particularly if keratins are only focally positive.

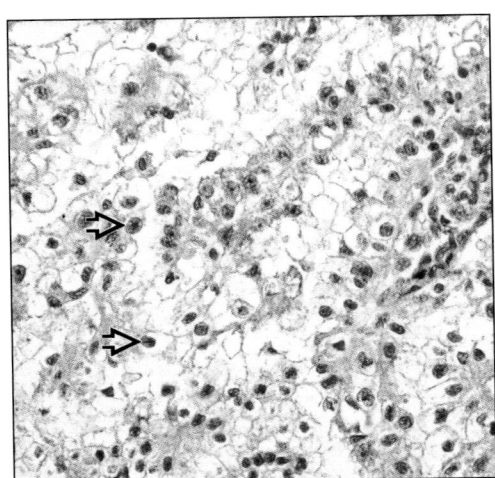

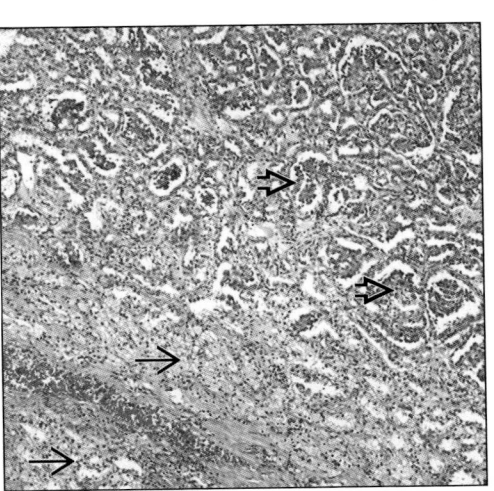

(Left) This renal tumor with papillary architecture & predominant clear cell cytology was only focally (+) for cytokeratins & EMA/MUC1, mandating immunostaining for TFE3 & TFEB. However, both TFE3 & TFEB showed no nuclear immunoreactivity ⮕, leading to categorizing this tumor as RCC, unclassified. *(Right)* Renal tumors with a combination of more than 1 type of the usual subtypes are also considered RCC, unclassified. Note papillary ⮕ and clear cell ⮕ features.

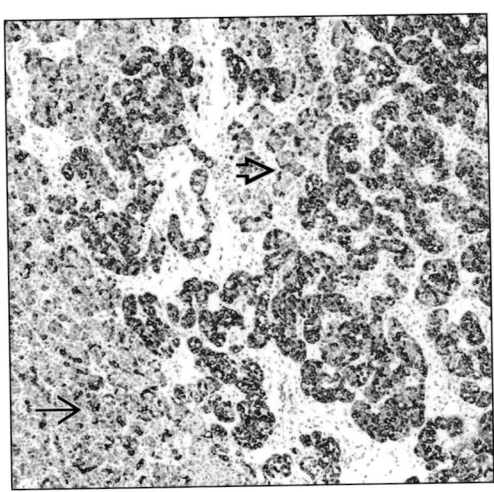

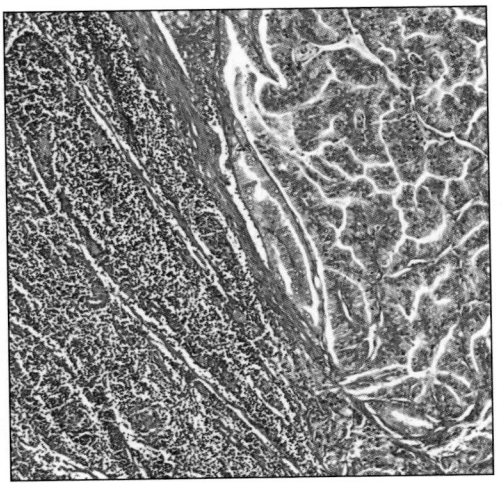

(Left) Immunostain for CK7 in this RCC, unclassified, with combination of papillary ⮕ and clear cell-like ⮕ features, shows strong and diffuse immunoreactivity in both components. This staining pattern would be unusual in clear cell RCC. Histologic evidence of morphologic transitions and unusual immunopatterns help in excluding the possibility of collision tumors. *(Right)* This image shows RCC, unclassified, metastatic to a lymph node, a common finding in high-grade tumors.

UROTHELIAL CARCINOMA OF THE RENAL PELVIS

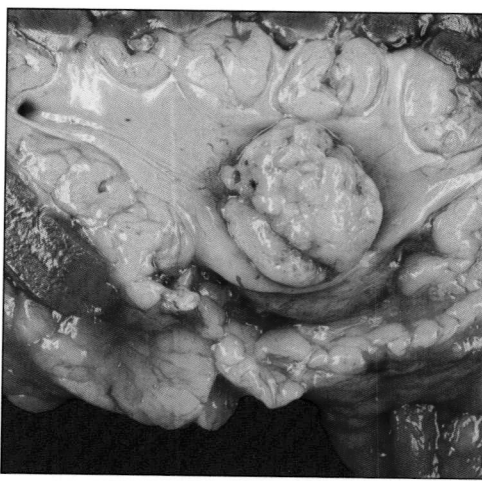

This gross specimen of a urothelial papillary carcinoma of the renal pelvis shows a polypoid lesion with solid, smooth surface, indicative of a histologically high-grade tumor.

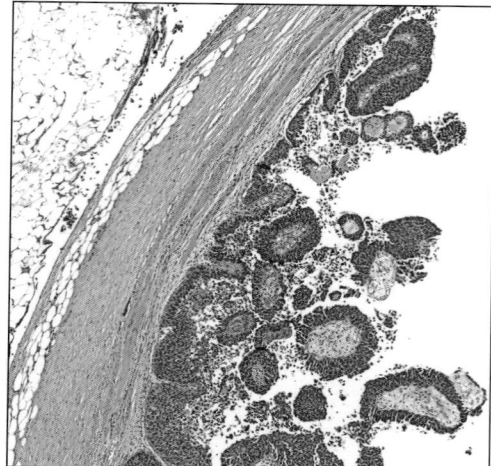

Hematoxylin & eosin image shows the typical histologic features of a papillary urothelial carcinoma. At this magnification, the tumor shows discrete papillae, without any evidence of invasion.

TERMINOLOGY

Abbreviations
- Urothelial carcinoma of renal pelvis (UCP)

Definitions
- Malignant neoplasm of urothelial (transitional cell) origin involving renal pelvicalyceal system

ETIOLOGY/PATHOGENESIS

Risk Factors
- Tobacco smoking is important risk factor
  - Lifetime risk increases with increased consumption and intensity of smoking
- Long-term use of analgesics, especially phenacetin, is also implicated as independent risk factor
  - Increases risk of renal pelvis tumors 4–8x in men and 10–13x in women
  - With decrease in usage of phenacetin, it is a less significant risk factor
- Other risk factors include Balkan nephropathy and occupational exposures
  - Petrochemicals, plastic materials, coal, asphalt, tar, and thorium-containing contrast media
- History of previous lower urinary tract carcinoma is also well-known predisposing factor
  - > 2/3 have prior, concurrent, or subsequent bladder carcinoma

Molecular Features
- Similar to that of urothelial carcinomas of bladder
- Deletions of part or all of chromosome 9; common event in urothelial carcinoma
  - Occurs early in tumorigenesis
    - Present in most cases of urothelial carcinoma, both papillary and nonpapillary
- Fibroblastic growth factor receptor 3 (FGFR3) gene mutations
  - Occur in > 80% of noninvasive papillary urothelial carcinomas (stage Ta)
  - Also found in 20% of lamina propria invasive (stage T1) and 15% of muscle invasive tumors
  - No such mutations in carcinoma in situ
- Relative incidences of FGFR3 mutations suggest that noninvasive papillary tumors do progress, although infrequently
  - Papillary tumors appear to progress along pathway that is different than carcinoma in situ (CIS) in most cases
  - Tumors with FGFR3 mutations have lower risk for recurrence than those without
- Increased gene expression of HRAS is found in CIS and high-grade tumors
  - Often associated with allelic loss of p53, which might contribute to its upregulation
  - Mutations in p53 are found at high rate in CIS (> 70% cases)
- Microsatellite instability and loss of mismatch repair proteins MSH2, MLH1, or MSH6 present in upper urinary tract tumors
  - Seen in up to 20-30% tumors of upper urinary tract
    - Incidence in upper tract is many times more common than in bladder tumors
  - More commonly observed in females or patients with low tumor stage, grade, or inverted tumor growth pattern
  - Upper urinary tract tumors form 3rd most common tumor with microsatellite instability
    - Colon and endometrium are 2 most common sites within hereditary nonpolyposis colorectal cancer (HNPCC) related tumors

CLINICAL ISSUES

Epidemiology
- Incidence
  - 4-5% of all urothelial tumors

UROTHELIAL CARCINOMA OF THE RENAL PELVIS

Key Facts

Terminology
- Malignant neoplasm of urothelial (transitional cell) origin involving renal pelvicalyceal system
- Urothelial carcinoma of renal pelvis (UCP)

Etiology/Pathogenesis
- Tobacco smoking is important risk factor
- Long-term use of analgesics, especially phenacetin, also implicated as independent risk factor

Clinical Issues
- 4-5% of all urothelial tumors
- Pathologic stage is single most important prognostic factor for urothelial carcinomas of upper urinary tract

Macroscopic Features
- Either predominantly papillary or polypoid, or infiltrative mass with thickening of pelvic wall

Microscopic Pathology
- Papillary urothelial neoplasms of low malignant potential (PUNLMP) extremely uncommon in upper tract
- Low-grade carcinoma relatively less common, compared to that in bladder
- Overall lymph node involvement reported to be approximately 10%

Top Differential Diagnoses
- Collecting duct carcinoma (CDC)/RCC, unclassified
- Metastatic carcinoma

- o Most common type of tumor in pelvicalyceal (90%) location
- Age
  - o Mean: 67-70 years (range: 34-93 years)
- Gender
  - o More common in males; M:F = 1.7-2:1

Presentation
- Flank pain
- Hematuria

Treatment
- Surgical approaches
  - o Nephroureterectomy, ± removal of bladder cuff in high-grade or high-stage lesions
  - o Segmental ureterectomy coupled with ureteral reimplantation in distal uretal tumors, generally of lower grade and stage
  - o Renal-sparing surgery, including segmental ureterectomy and endoscopic therapy

Prognosis
- Pathologic stage is single most important prognostic factor for urothelial carcinomas of upper urinary tract
- On univariate analysis, significant prognostic indicators include
  - o Size
  - o Tumor grade
  - o Pathologic stage
    - pTa: Papillary noninvasive carcinoma
    - pT1: Tumor invades subepithelial connective tissue
    - pT2: Tumor invades muscularis
    - pT3: Tumor invades (for renal pelvis): Beyond muscularis in peripelvic fat/renal parenchyma; (for ureter): Beyond muscularis in periureteric fat
    - pT4: Tumor invades adjacent organs or through kidney to perinephric fat
  - o Lymphovascular invasion
- However, on multivariate analysis, stage is only significant prognostic factor for survival

- o Based on multiple studies, 5-year survivals > 99% for pTa, 91% for pT1, 72% for pT2, 40% for pT3, and 16% for patients with metastasis

IMAGE FINDINGS

Radiographic Findings
- Filling defect, obstructive mass associated with hydronephrosis, hydroureter, renal stones

MACROSCOPIC FEATURES

General Features
- Either predominantly papillary or polypoid, or infiltrative mass with thickening of pelvic wall
  - o Tumors that primarily appear as papillary or polypoid
    - May expand and fill pelvicalyceal system
    - Tend to be noninvasive or are associated with limited invasion
    - Systematic sampling after fixation and maintaining relationship to underlying structures important for accurate staging
  - o Infiltrative mass may sometimes extensively involve renal parenchyma, mimicking primary renal parenchymal tumor
    - Occasionally may arise from minor calyx and grossly appear cortical in location
  - o Equivocal radiographic localization may warrant intraoperative assessment of urothelial vs. renal parenchymal origin
    - Surgical approaches quite different in these 2 situations
    - Radical nephroureterectomy for urothelial vs. partial, total, or radical nephrectomy for renal cortical tumors

UROTHELIAL CARCINOMA OF THE RENAL PELVIS

MICROSCOPIC PATHOLOGY

Histologic Features

- Histopathological features of upper tract urothelial tumors similar to those in urinary bladder
- However, papillary urothelial neoplasms of low malignant potential (PUNLMP) extremely uncommon in upper tract
- Low-grade carcinoma relatively less common, compared to that in bladder
- High-grade tumors are most common and invasion should be diligently looked for, if not obvious
- Histopathologic diversity with morphologic variants/aberrant differentiations similar to that in bladder
- Variant morphologies seen, among others, include
  - Micropapillary variant
  - Lymphoepithelioma-like carcinoma
  - Squamous differentiation and squamous cell carcinoma
  - Sarcomatoid differentiation
  - Signet ring or plasmacytoid features
  - Small cell carcinomatous features
- Renal parenchymal invasion requires destructive invasive beyond renal tubules
  - Tumors often extend inside kidney within tubules
    - May, at times, form grossly identified expansile nodules
    - For staging purposes of renal parenchymal invasion, tumor cells have to invade out of well-defined tubular structures

Lymph Nodes

- Overall lymph node involvement reported to be approximately 10%
  - Reported incidence is not based on cases where lymph nodes were removed at time of nephroureterectomy
  - Rates of lymph node metastasis close to 25% among cases where lymph nodes were removed at surgery

Predominant Pattern/Injury Type

- Neoplastic

Predominant Cell/Compartment Type

- Epithelial, transitional

ANCILLARY TESTS

Immunohistochemistry

- CK7 diffusely positive
- HMCK and p63 often strongly and diffusely positive
- CK20 at least focally positive in approximately 1/2 to 2/3 of cases

DIFFERENTIAL DIAGNOSIS

Collecting Duct Carcinoma (CDC)/RCC, Unclassified

- Highly infiltrative neoplasm extensively involving renal parenchyma may mimic high-grade RCC, undifferentiated, or CDC

- Features in favor of urothelial carcinoma include carcinoma in situ or papillary tumor involving pelvicalyceal system
  - Predominantly nested or solid architecture with variable squamous or glandular differentiation also favors urothelial carcinoma
- CDC is primarily high-grade adenocarcinoma, usually with glandular architecture
- Immunohistochemical staining may not be useful in distinction
  - CDC often positive for CK7, HMCK(34βE12), and occasionally CK20
  - Role of CK20 in distinction not known at present
  - Unclassified RCC may show variable immunophenotype, as it likely is not a uniform single entity

Metastatic Carcinoma

- Features that would favor metastatic carcinoma over urothelial carcinoma include
  - Known history of nonurothelial carcinoma
  - Histology not conforming to any known subtypes of RCC or typical urothelial carcinoma
  - Extensive interstitial growth
  - Multifocality both grossly and microscopically
  - Extensive vascular-lymphatic invasion
  - Immunophenotype, matching tumor in primary site and is different from that in urothelial carcinomas

DIAGNOSTIC CHECKLIST

Pathologic Interpretation Pearls

- Collecting duct and urothelial carcinomas, both may show extensive desmoplasia in renal parenchyma
- Morphologic and immunophenotypic features may not be absolutely reliable to distinguish these 2 entities
- Adequate sampling of urothelial mucosa to identify urothelial carcinoma in situ is a must to definitively diagnose urothelial carcinoma

SELECTED REFERENCES

1. Amin MB: Histological variants of urothelial carcinoma: diagnostic, therapeutic and prognostic implications. Mod Pathol. 22 Suppl 2:S96-S118, 2009
2. Colin P et al: Environmental factors involved in carcinogenesis of urothelial cell carcinomas of the upper urinary tract. BJU Int. Epub ahead of print, 2009
3. Ferriero M et al: Re: Lymphovascular invasion predicts poor outcome of urothelial carcinoma of the renal pelvis after nephroureterectomy. BJU Int. 103(8):1143, 2009
4. Margulis V et al: Outcomes of radical nephroureterectomy: a series from the Upper Tract Urothelial Carcinoma Collaboration. Cancer. 115(6):1224-33, 2009
5. Gupta R et al: Neoplasms of the upper urinary tract: a review with focus on urothelial carcinoma of the pelvicalyceal system and aspects related to its diagnosis and reporting. Adv Anat Pathol. 15(3):127-39, 2008
6. Olgac S et al: Urothelial carcinoma of the renal pelvis: a clinicopathologic study of 130 cases. Am J Surg Pathol. 28(12):1545-52, 2004

UROTHELIAL CARCINOMA OF THE RENAL PELVIS

Gross and Microscopic Features

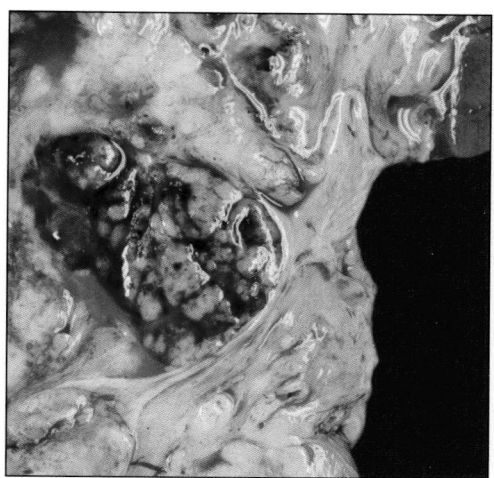

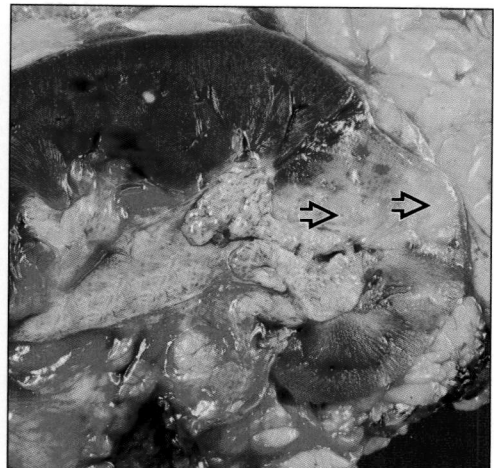

(Left) Two distinctive growth patterns are seen in UC. This photograph illustrates a polypoid, exophytic pattern. Such tumors may fill the pelvicalyceal system, often without gross evidence of invasion. Microscopic determination of invasion is often complicated by autolytic and degenerative changes, and therefore requires adequate fixation before prosecting. (Right) This pattern is predominantly invasive, with extensive invasion of the full thickness of renal parenchyma ⊳.

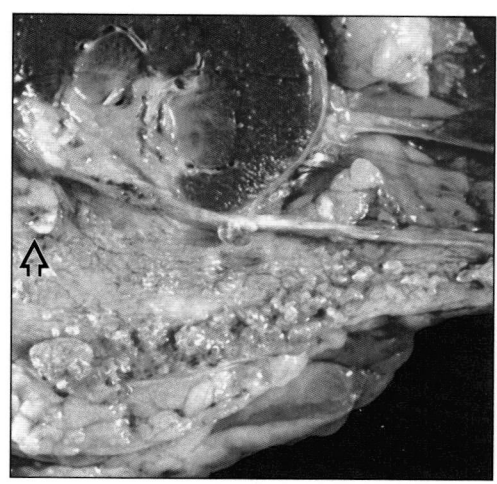

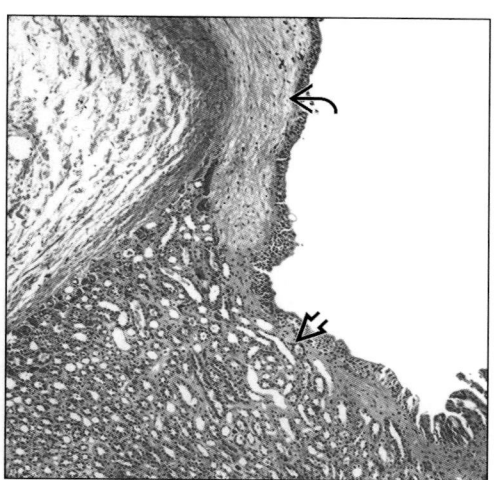

(Left) As in bladder, UC of upper urinary tract often shows multifocality. This specimen photograph depicts numerous papillary tumors involving the uretero-pelvic junction ⊳ and ureter. (Right) A low magnification image of a renal papilla ⊳ and adjacent calyx ⊳ demonstrates some staging issues in UC of pelvicalyceal system. Invasion in the area of papilla may involve the renal parenchyma (pT3), while invasion away from renal parenchyma may result in a lower pT stage (pT2).

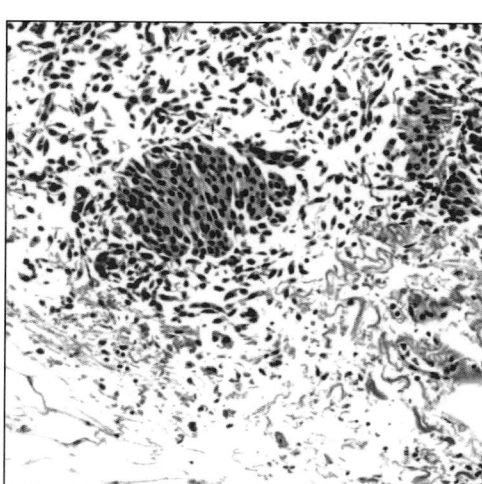

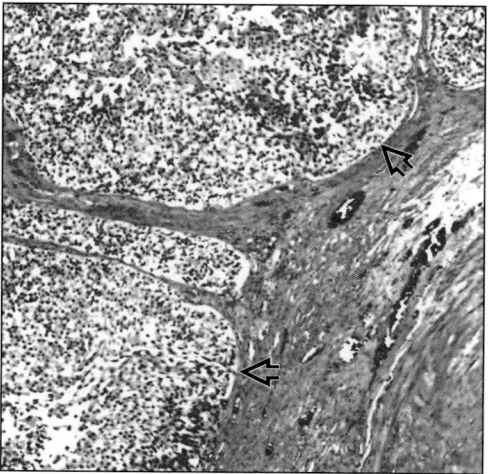

(Left) Inherently friable papillary tumors are prone to fragmentation and displacement, precluding accurate staging in some cases. Fixation prior to prosecting may prevent such artifacts. (Right) Inverted pattern of growth in papillary urothelial carcinomas may cause difficulty in staging. The uniform, broad tumor fronds ⊳ and the lack of stromal reaction argue against invasion. Careful search for small irregular foci of invasion is imperative in such cases as is generous sampling.

Microscopic Features

(Left) This image shows an exophytic, papillary urothelial carcinoma in the renal pelvis. Tumors with prominent papillary architecture are often bulky and may fill the pelvicalyceal system, often showing limited or no invasion. *(Right)* Papillary tumors may show morphology of a low-grade UC ➡. However, high-grade carcinomas are more frequent in the upper urinary tract. Papillary urothelial neoplasms of low malignant potential (PUNLMP) are very infrequent in this location.

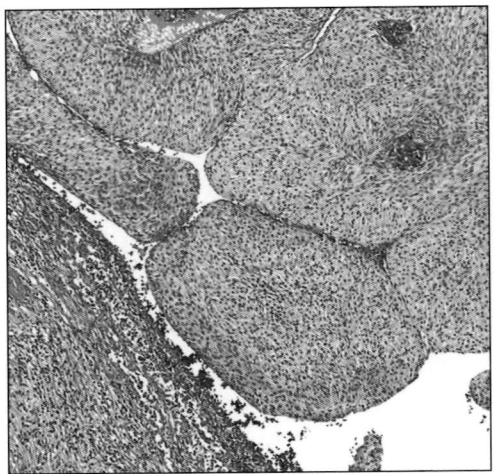
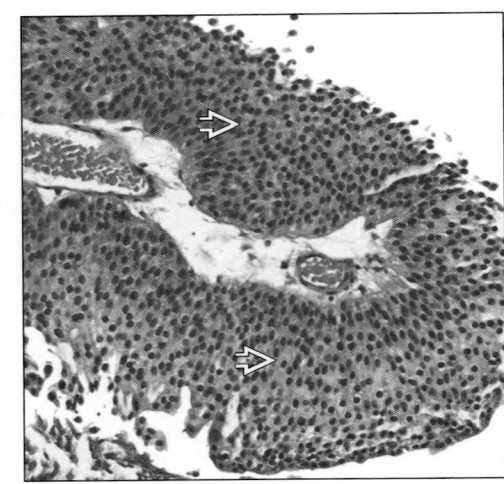

(Left) This papillary UC shows a combination of low- ➡ and high-grade ➡ features. Similar to bladder tumors, carcinomas with a combination of tumor grades are graded according to the highest grade in the lesion. *(Right)* This image shows a scanner view of a papillary UC involving the ureter. It completely fills the ureteral lumen. Carcinoma in the ureter is morphologically similar to those in the renal pelvis.

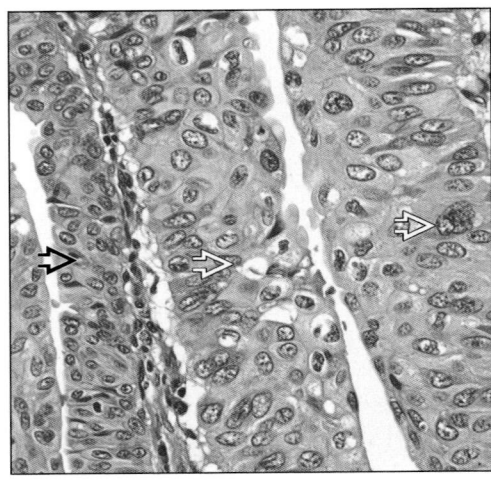
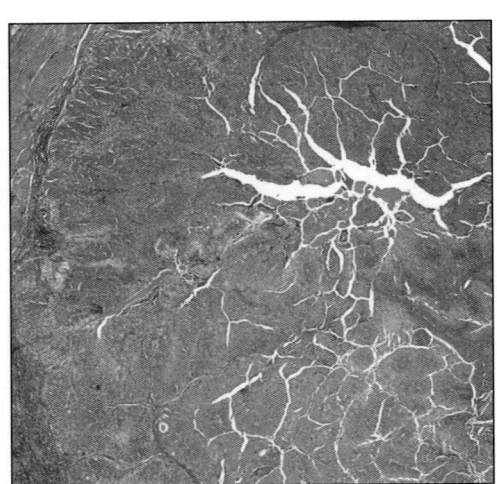

(Left) High-grade UC of the pelvis with a smooth surface and prominent inverted growth pattern ➡, which is not indicative of invasion. Invasive islands usually have irregular outline and illicit stromal response, except in the nested variant. *(Right)* This photomicrograph shows urothelial carcinoma in situ of the pelvicalyceal system. Unlike the papillary tumors, flat in situ tumors are often associated with invasive disease in the upper urothelial tract similar to that in bladder.

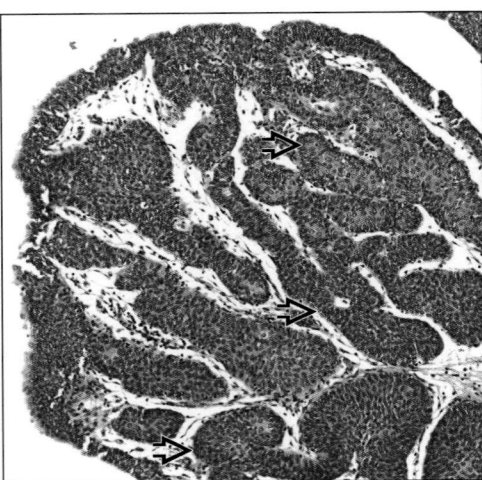
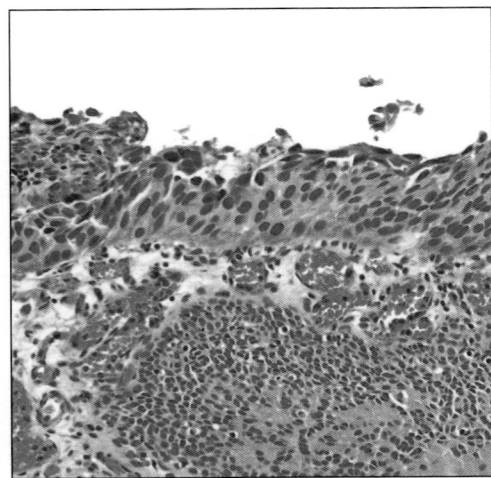

1

UROTHELIAL CARCINOMA OF THE RENAL PELVIS

Microscopic Features

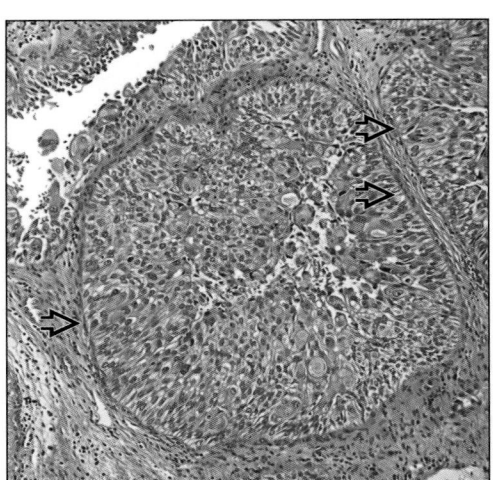

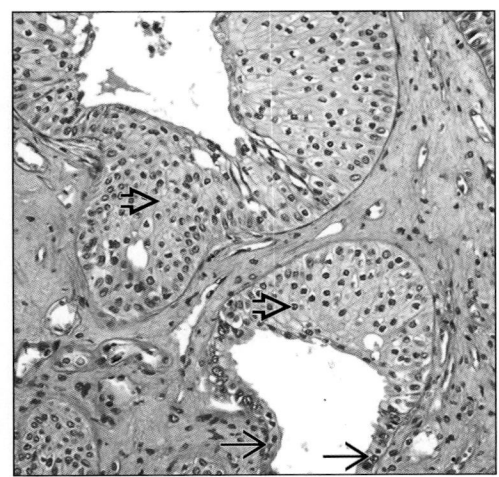

(Left) An important staging issue among papillary UC is the invasion of renal parenchyma. The tumor commonly involves and may expand renal tubules ⊵. (Right) Urothelial carcinomas with in situ disease often show an invasive component. However, extension within renal tubules ⊵ does not qualify as renal parenchymal invasion. This is akin to prostatic duct involvement in bladder carcinomas. The residual renal tubular cells ⊐ are seen in this image.

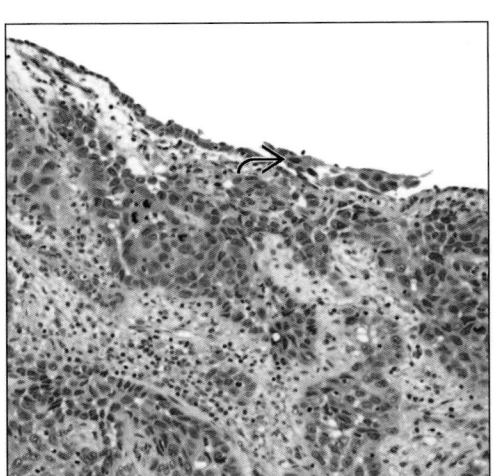

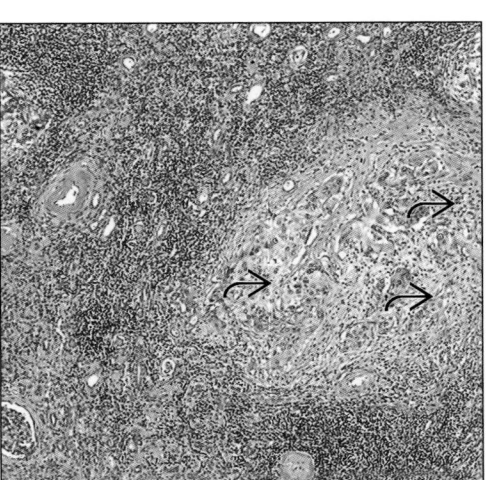

(Left) Tumors with flat in situ disease, similar to that in the bladder ⊐, not only morphologically but also at the molecular level, show significant differences from the predominantly papillary tumors of the upper urinary tract. (Right) Renal parenchymal invasion requires the presence of tumor nests with irregular outlines or invasive single cells. Stromal response ⊐ is usually prominent.

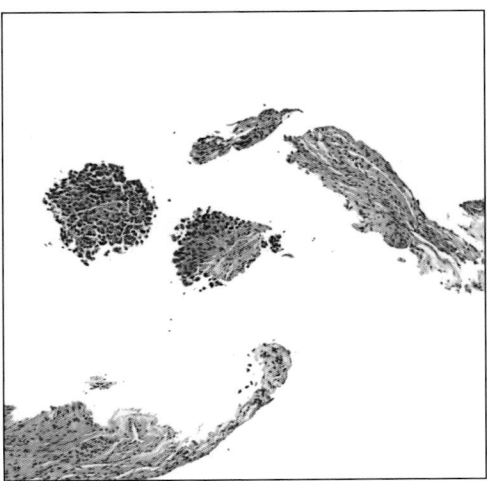

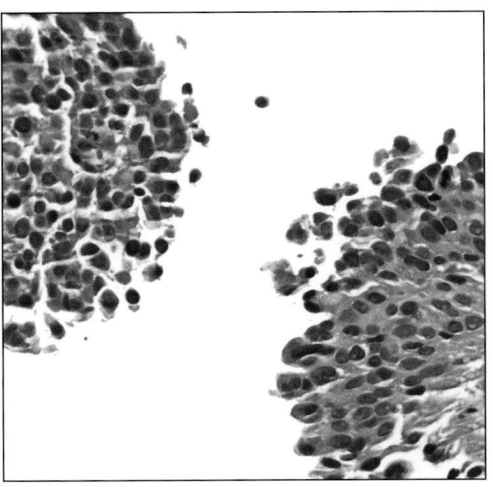

(Left) H&E shows a ureteroscopic biopsy from a renal pelvic tumor. Since such biopsies often yield limited material, the pathologist's role is primarily to document a urothelial tumor. Grade and invasion status must be reported but may vary in the resection. (Right) Biopsy from renal pelvic tumor shows a high-grade UC. Determination of invasion is often precluded by limited material from such biopsies but that usually does not influence further management, i.e., nephroureterectomy.

Microscopic Features with Variants

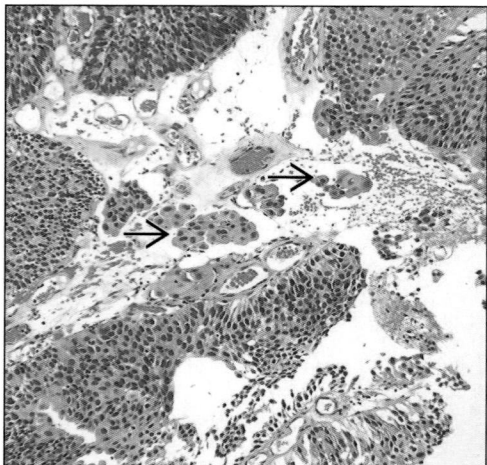
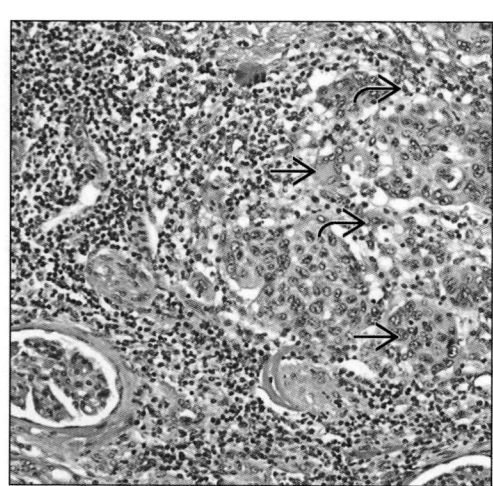

(Left) Only 18% of renal pelvic UC show lamina propria invasion ⇨ alone (pT1), a much lower incidence than in the bladder. *(Right)* Renal parenchymal invasive tumor shows irregular cell nests ⇨ along with fibroinflammatory stromal response ⇨. Predominantly invasive tumors in the upper tract share most genetic features with bladder tumors. A significant difference is the higher incidence of association with microsatellite instability in pelvic tumors.

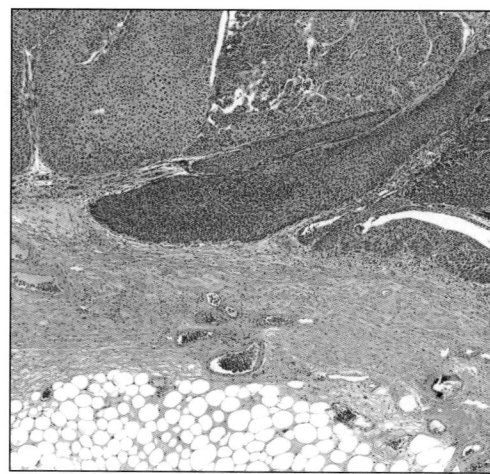
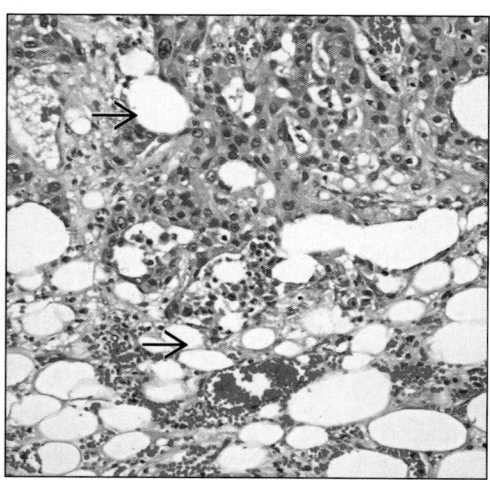

(Left) While 3/4 of patients with bladder carcinoma 1st present with superficial (pTis, pTa, pT1) disease, superficial disease in the upper urothelial tract is much less common. Approximately 1/2 of cases with renal pelvic tumors show pT3 or higher stage disease at presentation. *(Right)* This image shows a tumor invading renal sinus fat ⇨. Tumors invading the perirenal fat or renal parenchyma are both regarded pT3 tumors and seem to have similar clinical outcomes.

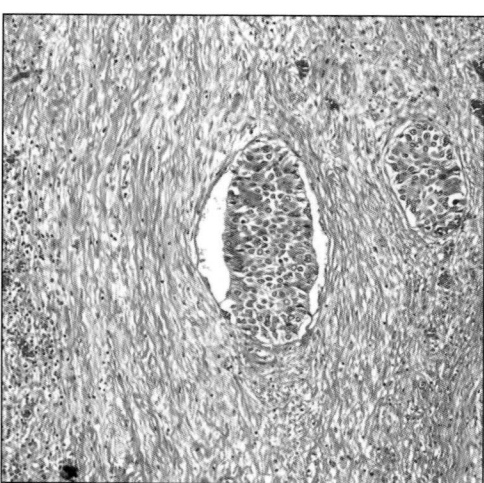
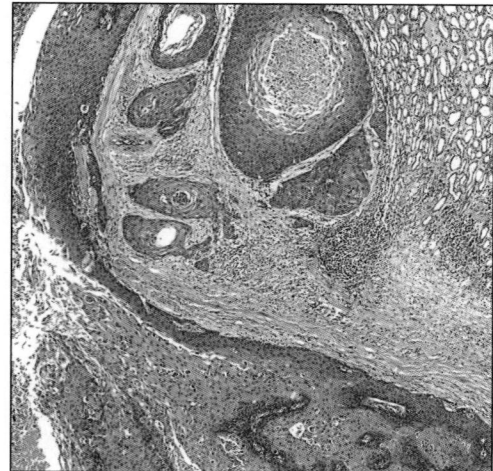

(Left) Vascular invasion may be an adverse prognostic indicator in renal pelvic carcinomas. Multiple studies have reaffirmed its clinical significance on univariate analysis. However, tumor stage appears to be the only significant variable associated with outcome on multivariate analysis, in multiple studies. *(Right)* A number of variant histologies of UCs may be seen in the upper tract, similar to those in bladder. This image shows a squamous cell carcinoma of the urothelium.

UROTHELIAL CARCINOMA OF THE RENAL PELVIS

Microscopic Features and Differential Diagnosis

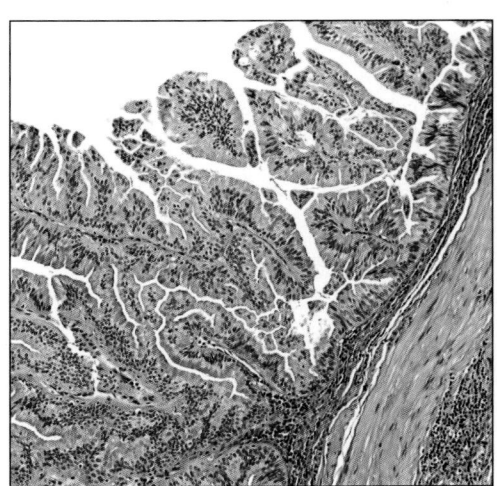

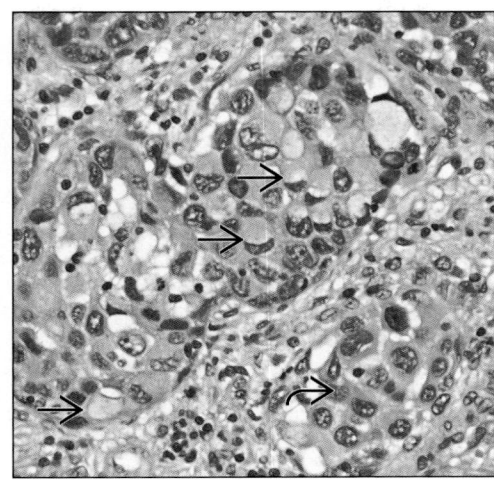

(Left) This image shows a villous adenoma-like variant of UC. In the presence of a variant histology, ruling out a metastasis from other sources is essential. The presence of an in situ component usually, but not always, favors a urothelial origin. *(Right)* This high-grade carcinoma shows signet ring cell differentiation in some of the tumor cells ➡. The typical urothelial (transitional cell) morphology ➘ in the adjacent tumor islands supports an urothelial origin.

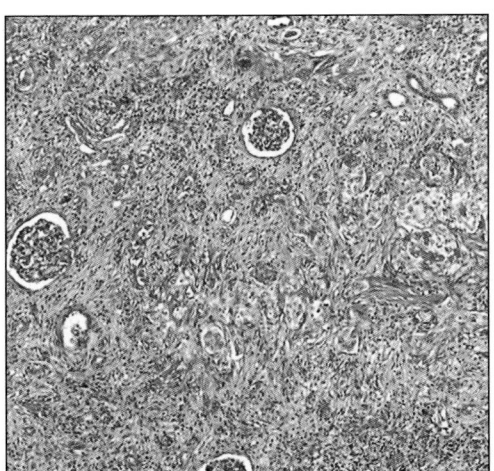

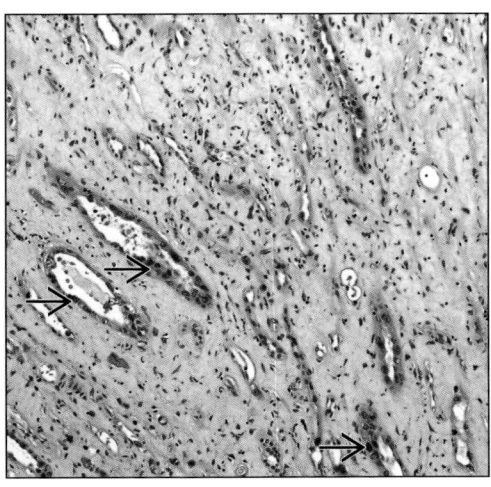

(Left) UC with extensive stromal invasion and desmoplasia may mimic collecting duct carcinoma. Solid nests and squamoid features favor UC, but definitive diagnosis requires the presence of in situ carcinoma in the pelvis. *(Right)* Renal tubules away from the tumor may show dysplasia of tubular lining ➡. This feature is also seen in collecting duct carcinoma and occasionally in papillary RCC. Therefore, this feature cannot be considered specific for any entity.

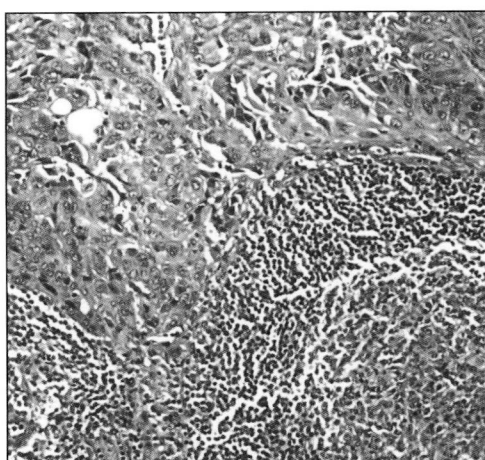

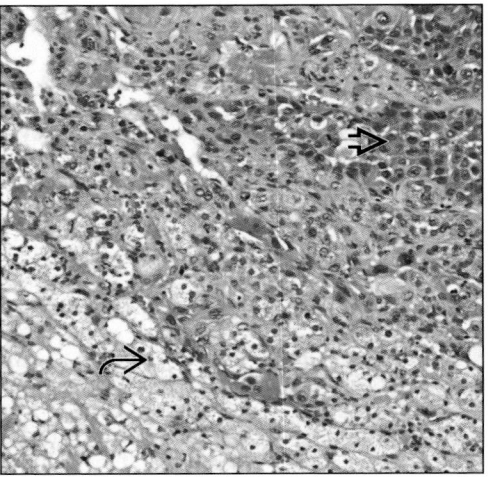

(Left) This image shows UC metastatic to a regional lymph node. Overall incidence of lymph node metastasis is reported to be approximately 10%. However, some studies report 25% incidence in cases where lymph node dissection was part of the surgery. *(Right)* Hematoxylin & eosin shows a renal pelvic urothelial carcinoma ➘ metastatic to adrenal gland. Note the adrenal cortical cells ➘ in the left-hand corner of the image. Metastatic disease is often widespread.

OTHER TUMORS AND TUMOR-LIKE LESIONS OF THE RENAL PELVIS

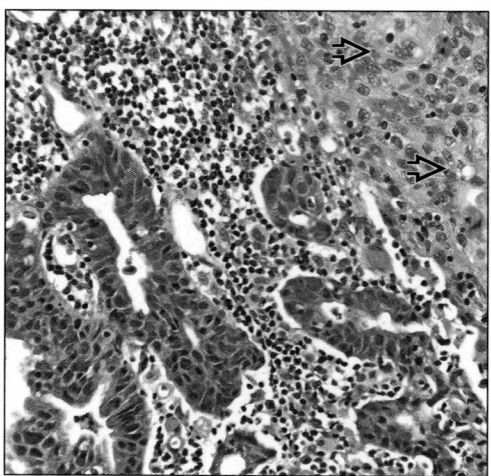

All aberrant morphologies of urothelial carcinoma seen in the bladder may be seen in the upper tract. Adenocarcinomas may be pure but often appear in association with a urothelial component ⊵.

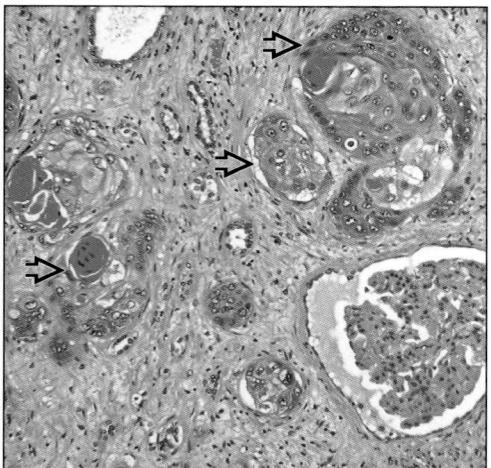

Squamous cell carcinoma, seen here invading the renal parenchyma ⊵, is the 2nd most common carcinoma in the pelvis. Most cases occur as aberrant differentiation in UC, but pure forms may be seen.

TERMINOLOGY

Definitions
- Neoplasms other than usual urothelial carcinoma involving upper urinary tract

ETIOLOGY/PATHOGENESIS

Nephrolithiasis and Repeated Infections
- Squamous cell carcinoma and adenocarcinoma often occur in background of nephrolithiasis
  - Reported incidence of coexisting calculus disease in squamous cell carcinoma of renal pelvis varies from 18-100%
    - Squamous cell carcinoma is often associated with squamous metaplasia of urothelium
  - Adenocarcinoma is usually associated with intestinal metaplasia, which is regarded as putative precursor of adenocarcinoma

Bladder Cancer
- Most cases of renal pelvic urothelial (transitional cell) carcinoma are associated with prior, concurrent, or subsequent bladder carcinoma
- However, for nontransitional cell carcinomas of upper tract, such association is not observed

CLINICAL ISSUES

Epidemiology
- Incidence
  - Most carcinomas with nontransitional cell features in pelvis coexist with usual urothelial (transitional cell) carcinomas of pelvis
  - Pure nonurothelial carcinomas of renal pelvis are very rare
    - Squamous cell carcinoma is 2nd most common carcinoma of renal pelvis
      - Incidence of 10% of renal pelvic cases is reported in older study; likely includes urothelial carcinomas with squamous differentiation
      - More recent studies report a combined incidence of < 1% for squamous cell carcinomas and adenocarcinomas of renal pelvis
      - All other types of carcinoma in the literature exist as case reports or small case series
  - Benign epithelial, mesenchymal, and other tumors are also very rare
    - Fibroepithelial polyps, although more common in adults, are most common benign polypoid ureteric tumors in children
- Age
  - Carcinomas: Range 41-87 years (mean: 66)
  - Fibroepithelial polyps: Range 7-73 years (mean: 40)
  - Inverted papillomas: Range 19-89 years (mean: 64)
  - Primitive neuroectodermal tumors: Mostly young adults/adolescents; range 10-60 years (mean: 27)
  - Other tumors: Variable, mostly older adults

Presentation
- Flank pain &/or hematuria common presentations
- Ureteral or pelvi-ureteric junction obstruction with resultant hydronephrosis also not uncommon
- Episodic colicky pain, especially in tumors of ureter

Treatment
- Surgical approaches
  - Usually nephroureterectomy performed for carcinomas of pelvis or proximal-most ureter
  - Malignant tumors of more distal ureters may be amenable to ureterectomy
  - Polypoid smaller benign tumors, particularly fibroepithelial polyps, may be resected endoscopically

Prognosis
- Most pure nontransitional cell, as well as urothelial carcinomas with divergent/aberrant differentiation, are high-grade and high-stage tumors

OTHER TUMORS AND TUMOR-LIKE LESIONS OF THE RENAL PELVIS

Key Facts

Terminology
- Neoplasms other than usual urothelial carcinoma involving upper urinary tract

Clinical Issues
- Most carcinomas with nontransitional cell features in pelvis exist in association with usual urothelial (transitional cell) carcinomas
- Pure nonurothelial carcinomas of pelvis are very rare

Microscopic Pathology
- Inverted papilloma with endophytic interconnected trabeculae and cords of urothelium, extensively invaginating from surface into lamina propria
- Nephrogenic metaplasia/adenoma shows multiple architectural patterns, including papillary, tubular/glandular, cystic, single cells, and sheet-like

- ○ Typically, thick basement membrane/hyalinized sheath surrounds epithelium
- Squamous cell carcinoma usually accompanied by extensive squamous metaplasia of urothelium and squamous cell carcinoma in situ
- Adenocarcinoma shows various phenotypes, including glandular NOS, enteric, micropapillary, signet ring/plasmacytoid, mucinous
- Benign nonepithelial tumors include fibroepithelial polyp, inflammatory myofibroblastic tumor, hemangioma, angiomyolipoma, leiomyoma, neurofibroma

Top Differential Diagnoses
- Metastatic tumors
- Urothelial carcinoma with inverted growth pattern

- Most patients with pT3 or pT4 tumors die of disease, and 5-year survivals are extremely uncommon
- Some of benign tumors may cause obstruction and resultant hydronephrosis, with related complications

MACROSCOPIC FEATURES

General Features
- Carcinomas
  - ○ Usually large bulky tumors, filling pelvicalyceal system, usually with renal parenchymal and renal sinus soft tissue invasion
- Fibroepithelial polyps, hemangiomas, squamous papillomas, and nephrogenic adenomas
  - ○ Mostly polypoid lesions in pelvis or ureter
  - ○ Size usually small (mean: 2 cm; mostly 0.5-4 cm in maximum diameter); rare tumors are much larger
- Inverted papillomas
  - ○ Smooth surfaced and often broad based, sessile and domed, rarely pedunculated
    - More common in ureter than pelvis
- Malignant mesenchymal tumors
  - ○ Often arising in perirenal and renal hilar soft tissues, and secondarily involving pelvicalyceal system and renal parenchyma

MICROSCOPIC PATHOLOGY

Histologic Features
- Benign epithelial tumors/lesions
  - ○ Inverted papilloma
    - Endophytic interconnected trabeculae and cords of urothelium, extensively invaginating from surface into lamina propria
    - Covered by flat-surfaced urothelium
    - Periphery of cords typically show palisading of basal nuclei
    - Tumor periphery is smooth and pushing, and no desmoplastic stromal reaction is present
    - Some cases show small glandular structures lined by metaplastic mucinous epithelium

  - ○ Nephrogenic metaplasia/adenoma
    - Shows wide spectrum of architectural patterns, with cases often showing mixed patterns
    - Architectural patterns include papillary, tubular/glandular, cystic, single cells, and sheet-like
    - Lining epithelial cells are cuboidal and single layered, or occasionally "hobnailed"
    - Cytoplasm varies from eosinophilic to clear; prominent nucleoli may be present
    - In single cell areas, cells may show minute lumina, and closely mimic blood vessels or signet ring cells
    - Typically, thick basement membrane/hyalinized sheath surrounds epithelium
    - Often associated with inflammatory infiltrate
  - ○ Villous adenoma
    - Similar to villous adenomas of colorectum
    - Biopsy-based diagnosis of villous adenoma should not be made, as adenocarcinoma in vicinity may be missed
    - Until thorough evaluation of completely excised resection specimen performed, terminology, such as "biopsy fragments with histology of at least villous adenoma," may be used
  - ○ Other rare benign epithelial lesions include squamous and urothelial papillomas
- Malignant epithelial tumors
  - ○ Squamous cell carcinoma
    - More common in renal pelvis than ureter; often associated with nephrolithiasis
    - Usually accompanied by extensive squamous metaplasia of urothelium and squamous cell carcinoma in situ
    - Often high stage, frequently with renal parenchymal invasion
  - ○ Adenocarcinoma
    - Variety of morphologic phenotypes seen, similar to that in bladder
    - Different morphologic forms include glandular NOS, enteric, signet ring, mucinous

- Often accompanied by glandular and intestinal metaplasia of surrounding urothelium, or occasionally by villous adenoma
- Usually high-stage tumors, often with renal parenchymal invasion
  - Other rare forms of carcinoma (Ca) include
    - Small cell and large cell neuroendocrine Ca, lymphoepithelioma-like Ca, sarcomatoid Ca, hepatoid Ca, rhabdoid Ca, and lipid-rich Ca
- Benign nonepithelial tumors/lesions
  - Fibroepithelial polyp
    - Usually solitary but sometimes multifocal
    - Consist of proliferation and expansion of subepithelial stromal cells with prominent vascularity, inflammatory infiltrate, and edema
    - Stromal cells usually loosely arranged but may have hypercellular, compact areas
    - Atypical and giant cell forms of stromal cells may be present
    - Mitotic activity uncommon, and proliferation index as judged by immunostaining is very low
    - Covering urothelium is benign; usually flat but may show papillary or polypoid fronds and may be ulcerated, hyperplastic, and reactive
  - Hemangioma
    - Usually solitary and polypoid but may be multifocal and dome-like
    - Often cavernous type but may be capillary or venous-type
    - Covered by benign, often ulcerated, urothelium
  - Other reported benign mesenchymal lesions include
    - Inflammatory myofibroblastic tumor, angiomyolipoma, leiomyoma, neurofibroma, hibernoma, and periureteric lipoma
- Malignant nonepithelial tumors
  - Leiomyosarcoma most common
  - Rhabdomyosarcoma, including botryoides type, angiosarcoma, fibrosarcoma, Ewing tumor, malignant peripheral nerve sheath tumor are other usual types
  - Sarcomatoid carcinoma always needs to be excluded in all malignant spindle cell neoplasms of ureter and pelvis

DIFFERENTIAL DIAGNOSIS

Metastatic Tumors

- Based on histologic features alone, distinction of primary squamous cell or adenocarcinoma from metastases is very difficult
- Immunohistochemical stains are usually not helpful
- Metastatic tumors are often multifocal and bilateral, lack in situ component, have interstitial growth, and usually show prominent vascular invasion
- Clinical history is often critical
- Both primary and metastatic small cell carcinomas share morphologic and immunohistochemical features
  - In particular, TTF-1 positivity may be seen in both
  - Presence of at least focal urothelial component strongly favors primary origin

Urothelial Carcinoma with Inverted Growth

- Distinction from inverted papilloma is critical
- Presence of following features favors urothelial carcinoma with inverted growth pattern
  - Significant cytologic atypia, noncircumscribed growth pattern, prominent mitotic activity beyond basal layers, and desmoplastic stromal response

DIAGNOSTIC CHECKLIST

Pathologic Interpretation Pearls

- For all unusual renal pelvic carcinomas, clinical history is a must to exclude metastasis
- Immunohistochemistry often not useful in this distinction

SELECTED REFERENCES

1. Childs MA et al: Fibroepithelial polyps of the ureter: a single-institutional experience. J Endourol. 23(9):1415-9, 2009
2. Guo CC et al: Micropapillary variant of urothelial carcinoma in the upper urinary tract: a clinicopathologic study of 11 cases. Arch Pathol Lab Med. 133(1):62-6, 2009
3. La Rosa S et al: Primary small cell neuroendocrine carcinoma of the kidney: morphological, immunohistochemical, ultrastructural, and cytogenetic study of a case and review of the literature. Endocr Pathol. 20(1):24-34, 2009
4. Volkmer BG et al: Upper urinary tract recurrence after radical cystectomy for bladder cancer--who is at risk? J Urol. 182(6):2632-7, 2009
5. Gupta R et al: Neoplasms of the upper urinary tract: a review with focus on urothelial carcinoma of the pelvicalyceal system and aspects related to its diagnosis and reporting. Adv Anat Pathol. 15(3):127-39, 2008
6. Holmäng S et al: Squamous cell carcinoma of the renal pelvis and ureter: incidence, symptoms, treatment and outcome. J Urol. 178(1):51-6, 2007
7. Tamas EF et al: Lymphoepithelioma-like carcinoma of the urinary tract: a clinicopathological study of 30 pure and mixed cases. Mod Pathol. 20(8):828-34, 2007
8. Frickmann H et al: [Villous adenoma of the renal pelvis and ureter.] Urologe A. 45(11):1435-7, 2006
9. Perez-Montiel D et al: High-grade urothelial carcinoma of the renal pelvis: clinicopathologic study of 108 cases with emphasis on unusual morphologic variants. Mod Pathol. 19(4):494-503, 2006
10. Darras J et al: Synchronous inverted papilloma of bladder and renal pelvis. Urology. 65(4):798, 2005
11. Kapusta LR et al: Inflammatory myofibroblastic tumors of the kidney: a clinicopathologic and immunohistochemical study of 12 cases. Am J Surg Pathol. 27(5):658-66, 2003
12. Raghavendran M et al: Stones associated renal pelvic malignancies. Indian J Cancer. 40(3):108-12, 2003
13. Nowak MA et al: Benign fibroepithelial polyps of the renal pelvis. Arch Pathol Lab Med. 123(9):850-2, 1999
14. Ford TF et al: Adenomatous metaplasia (nephrogenic adenoma) of urothelium. An analysis of 70 cases. Br J Urol. 57(4):427-33, 1985

OTHER TUMORS AND TUMOR-LIKE LESIONS OF THE RENAL PELVIS

Microscopic Features

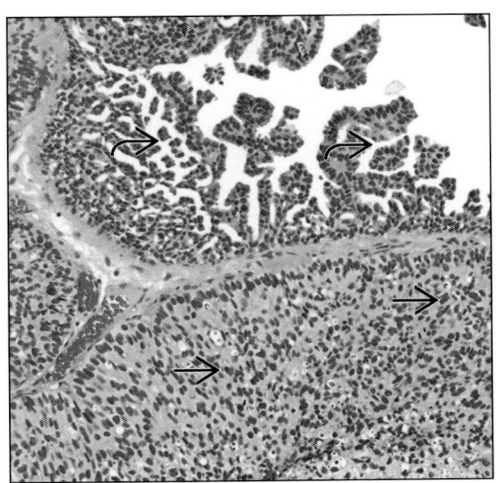

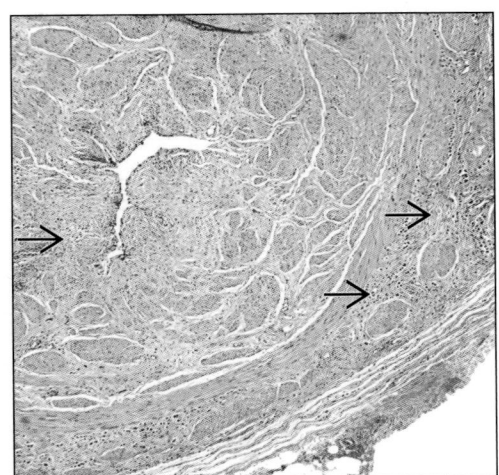

(Left) As in the bladder, a variety of morphologic types of adenocarcinoma may be seen in the upper urinary tract. This image shows a micropapillary in situ component ⊇ in otherwise typical urothelial carcinoma ⊇. Pure invasive micropapillary carcinomas may also be noted and are usually high stage. *(Right)* This image depicts the diffuse growth pattern of a carcinoma with plasmacytoid urothelial carcinoma and signet ring cell ⊇ features in the ureter.

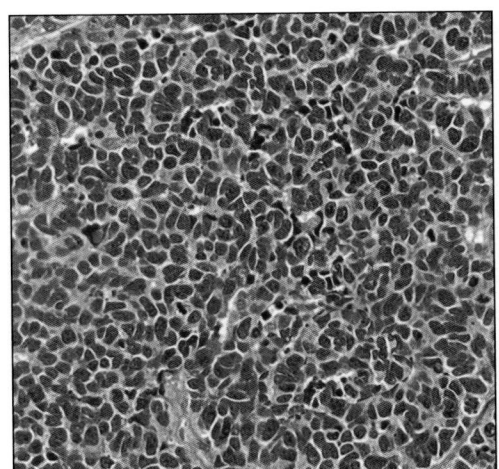

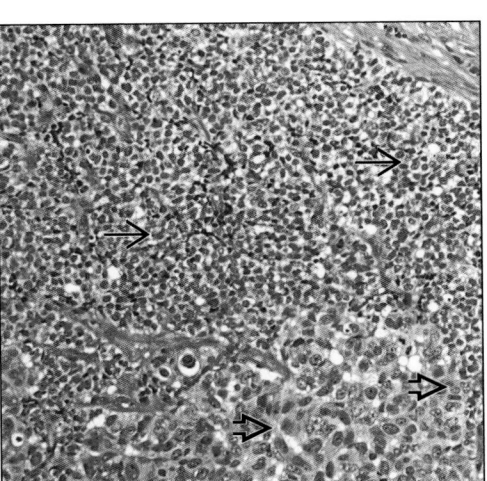

(Left) Pure small cell carcinomas, although quite rare, may be seen in the renal pelvis. At both the morphological and immunophenotypic levels, they are similar to small cell carcinomas of the lung and other sites. Thus, immunostains, including TTF-1, do not discriminate between primary and metastatic tumors. *(Right)* In most cases, small cell carcinoma of the renal pelvis exists as aberrant, and often focal, differentiation ⊇ in an otherwise typical urothelial carcinoma ⊇.

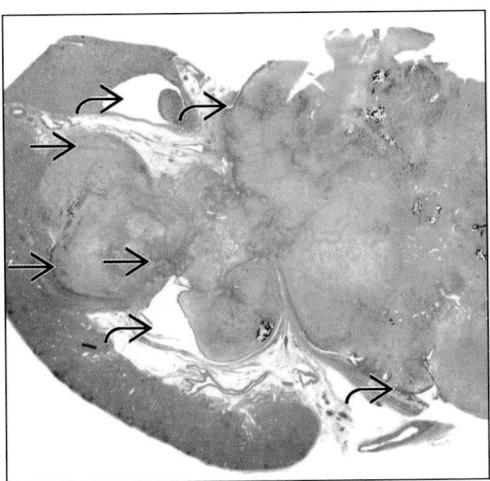

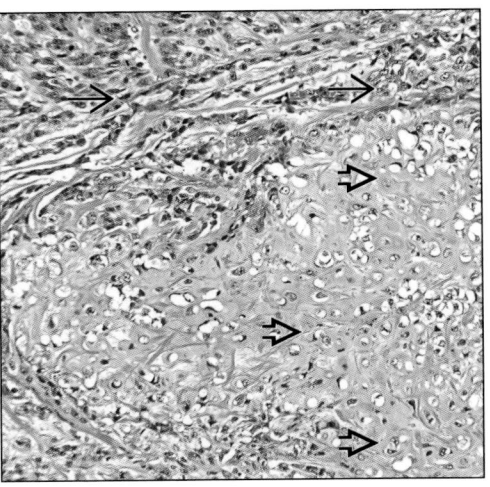

(Left) This whole-mount shows a very large exophytic tumor mass, completely filling a markedly dilated ⊇ pelvicalyceal system. The blue areas ⊇ in the tumor are suggestive of chondromatous differentiation. Sarcomatoid carcinoma and sarcomas may present with large bulky intraluminal masses. *(Right)* The renal pelvic tumor shows chondrosarcomatous ⊇ differentiation. In all sarcomatous tumors of the pelvis, the possibility of sarcomatoid carcinoma ⊇ must always be excluded.

Gross and Microscopic Features

(Left) Lymphoepithelioma-like carcinomas are extremely rare in the renal pelvis. Like their bladder counterparts, they are not associated with Epstein-Barr (EB) virus in the kidney, although the morphologic features are similar to EB virus-associated nasopharyngeal tumors. *(Right)* Fibroepithelial polyps are polypoid masses in the ureter, pelvi-ureteric junction, or pelvis with fibrotic and white ➡ cores. The covering mucosa may be flat but often shows polypoid or papillary excrescences ➜.

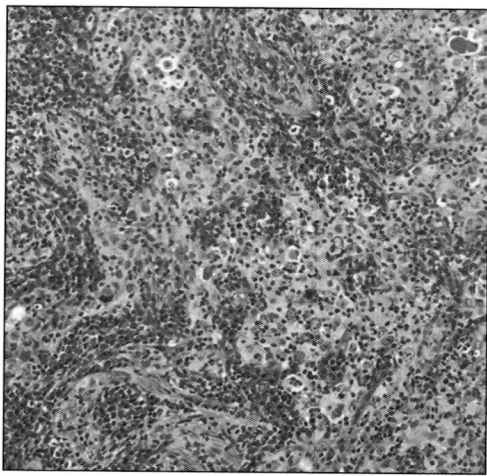
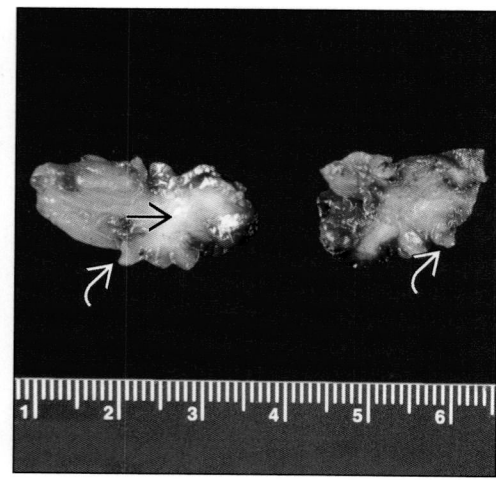

(Left) Fibroepithelial polyps are the most common benign lesions of the ureter in the pediatric population, although most occur in adults. They predominantly consist of proliferation and expansion of subepithelial stroma ➜, often accompanied by prominent vascularity and inflammatory infiltrate. *(Right)* The polypoid or papillary architecture in fibroepithelial polyps is primarily a result of stromal proliferation ➜. Overlying urothelium is benign and often unremarkable ➡.

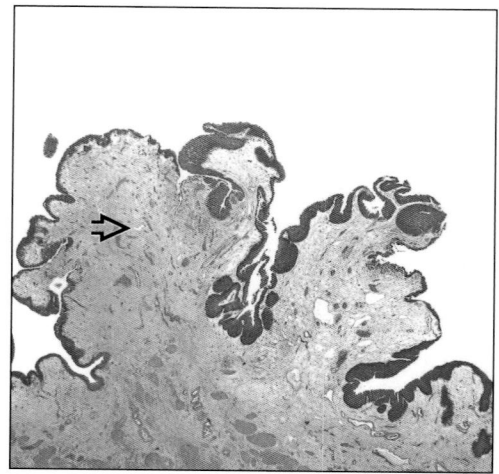
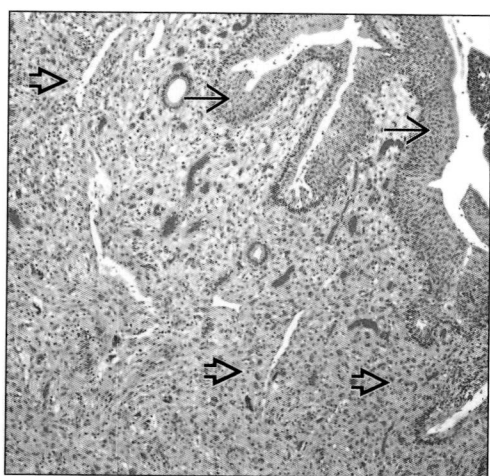

(Left) Compared to the bladder, nephrogenic metaplasia is relatively rare in the ureter or pelvis. Many lesions appear polypoid or papillary, raising the suspicion of a papillary neoplasm. Typically, the lining cells in nephrogenic metaplasia are cuboidal and single layered ➡. *(Right)* Nephrogenic metaplasia often shows a mixture of architectural patterns, including tubular ➡ and nested ➜, as seen here. Prominent basement membrane ➡ surrounding the epithelial nests is a characteristic feature.

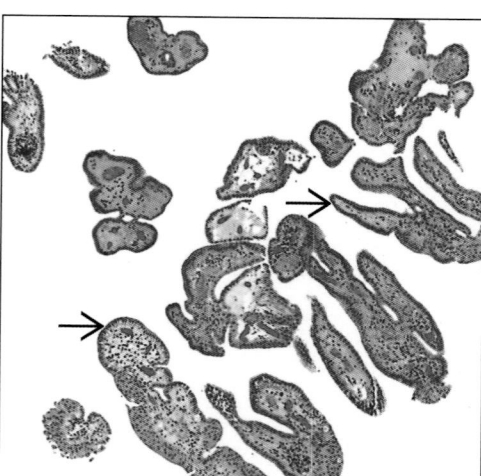
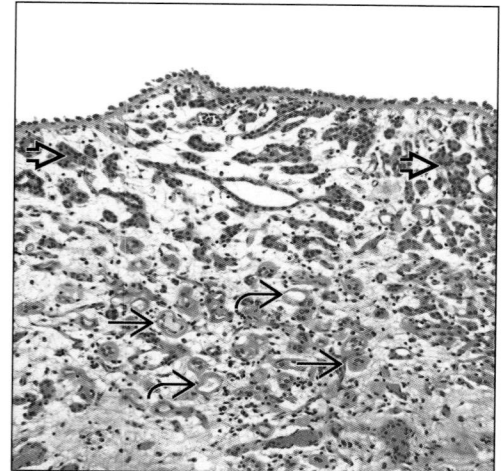

Microscopic and Immunohistochemical Features

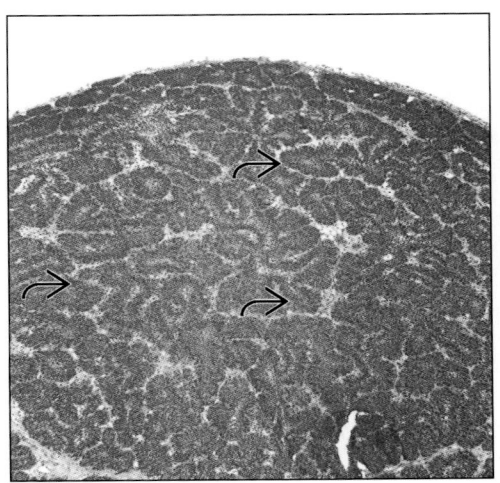

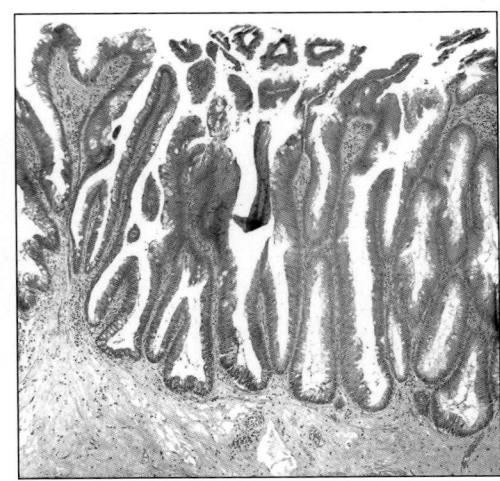

(Left) Inverted papilloma is rare in the upper urinary tract, with more tumors identified in the ureter than in the pelvis. It shows interconnecting cords/trabeculae invaginated into the lamina propria, with a flat surface urothelium. Periphery of cords typically show palisading of nuclei ⤳. *(Right)* Villous adenoma is morphologically identical to its more common colorectal counterpart. Prominent thin papillae, lined by mucin-producing columnar epithelium, is the hallmark.

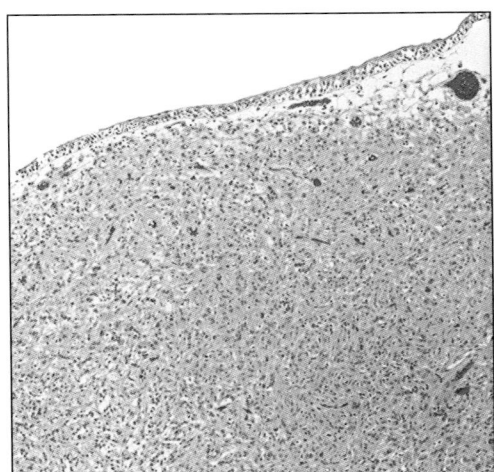

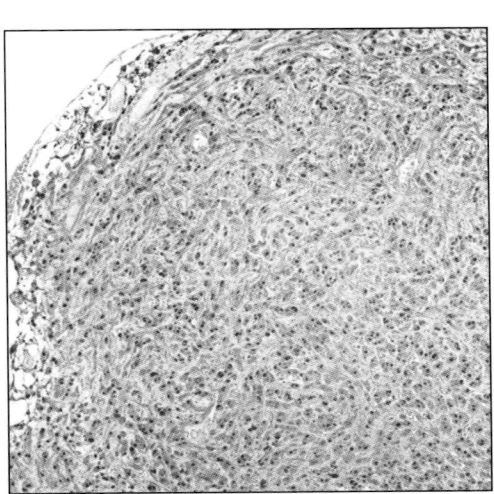

(Left) Benign mesenchymal tumors arising from or involving the pelvis are very uncommon. These include schwannoma (as shown here), hemangioma, lipoma, myxoma, and leiomyoma, among others. For any spindle cell neoplasm of the pelvis or ureter, the possibility of a sarcomatoid urothelial carcinoma must be excluded. *(Right)* This image shows diffuse cytoplasmic and nuclear positivity for S100 in the tumor cells, supporting the diagnosis of a schwannoma.

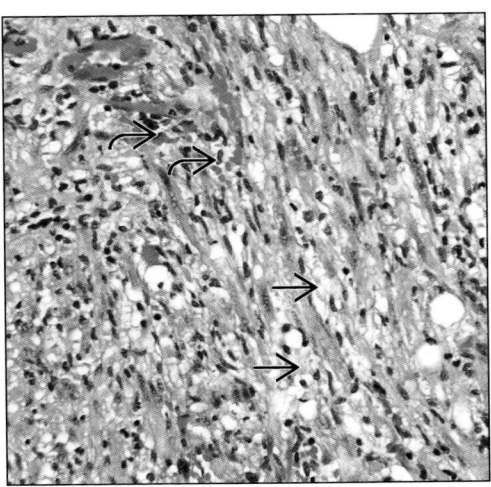

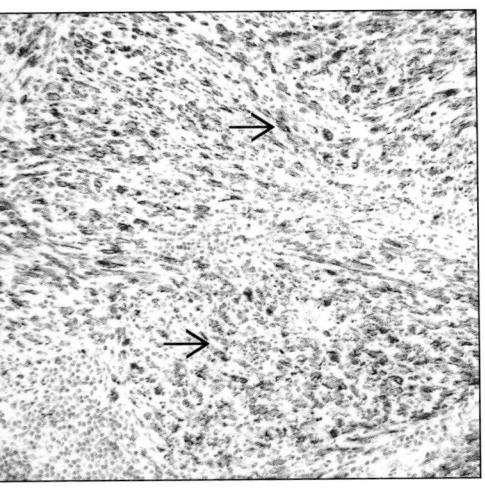

(Left) Inflammatory myofibroblastic tumor of the renal pelvis is rare and morphologically similar to lesions occurring at other sites, including the bladder. Notice alternating loose ➡ and hypercellular areas, with extravasated red blood cells ➡, typical of the lesion. *(Right)* Most of the inflammatory myofibroblastic tumors of the renal pelvis are reported in the pediatric age group. Rare reported cases at this site also show immunoreactivity ➡ for ALK1.

METANEPHRIC ADENOMA

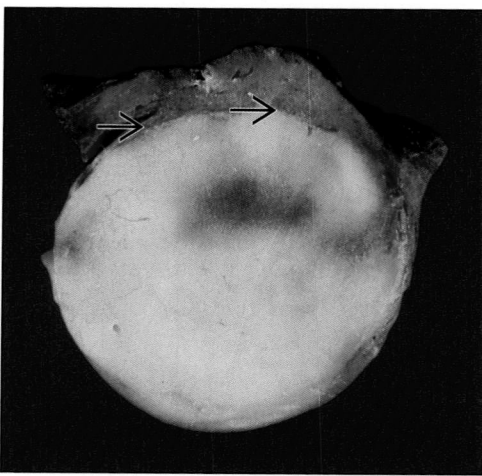

This gross image shows the typical gross features of a metanephric adenoma: A well-circumscribed tumor ⇒, without a capsule, and with a cut surface that is homogeneous and tan-yellow.

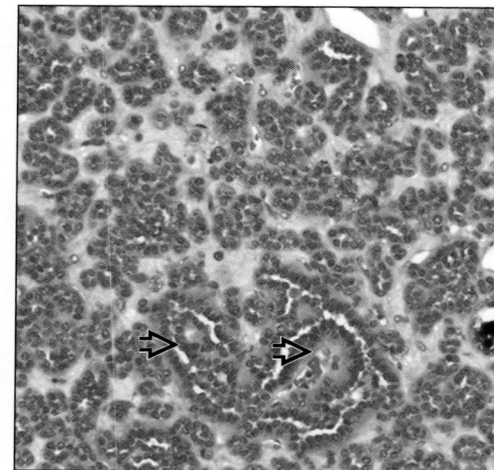

This microscopic image of a metanephric adenoma shows tubular and focally papillary ⇒ structures lined by cells with monotonous small nuclei without significant atypia and minimal cytoplasm.

TERMINOLOGY

Abbreviations
- Metanephric adenoma (MA)

Synonyms
- Embryonal adenoma, nephrogenic nephroma

Definitions
- Benign neoplasm composed of small primitive cells resembling early metanephric tubular differentiation
  - Part of spectrum of neoplasms that includes metanephric adenofibroma and metanephric stromal tumor

ETIOLOGY/PATHOGENESIS

Molecular Abnormalities
- Microsatellite allelotyping has shown potential tumor suppressor gene on chromosome 2p13 in 56% of informative cases
- No allelic changes in Wilms tumor (*WT*) gene region at chromosome 11p13 or in papillary renal cell tumor (*PRCC*) gene region at chromosome 17q21.32
- Prior reported trisomies 7 and 17 are possibly related to the study of solid PRCC misdiagnosed as MA

CLINICAL ISSUES

Epidemiology
- Age
  - 11 months to 83 years (mean: 41 years)
- Gender
  - Female predominance (M:F = 1:2)

Presentation
- > 50% of cases detected incidentally
  - Most symptomatic cases show abdominal or flank pain, hematuria, and palpable mass

- About 12% with symptoms related to polycythemia

Prognosis
- Benign course with no reported metastasis in tumors with typical morphology
  - Single case of lymph node metastasis reported in child was probably a Wilms tumor because of reported atypical high mitotic activity

IMAGE FINDINGS

General Features
- Calcifications seen in up to 43% of cases

MACROSCOPIC FEATURES

General Features
- Typically unilateral, solitary, well circumscribed, and well delineated
- Majority are unencapsulated, but discontinuous or continuous capsule present in some
- Cut surface solid tan-pink, gray to yellow, and partially cystic in 12% of cases
- Hemorrhage and necrosis are common
- Gross calcifications in up to 20%, including rare instances of entirely calcified tumor

Size
- Few mm to 20 cm; reported mean: 5.5 cm

MICROSCOPIC PATHOLOGY

Histologic Features
- Cellular tumor composed of crowded small acini of primitive blue cells in paucicellular intervening stroma, and often with elongated tubules
- Papillary component, including glomeruloid structures, fairly common

METANEPHRIC ADENOMA

Key Facts

Terminology
- Benign neoplasm composed of small primitive cells resembling early metanephric tubular differentiation
  - Part of spectrum of neoplasms that includes metanephric adenofibroma and metanephric stromal tumor

Etiology/Pathogenesis
- Microsatellite allelotyping has shown potential tumor suppressor gene on chromosome 2p13 in 56% of informative cases

Clinical Issues
- Age range 11 months to 83 years (reported mean: 41 years)
- Female preponderance (M:F = 1:2)
- About 12% with symptoms related to polycythemia

- Benign course with no reported metastasis

Microscopic Pathology
- Cellular tumor composed of crowded small acini of primitive blue cells in paucicellular intervening stroma
- Papillary component, including glomeruloid appearance, fairly common
- Tumor cells have minimal cytoplasm with uniform, round to ovoid nuclei, slightly larger than size of lymphocyte

Ancillary Tests
- Often positive for WT1 (diffuse nuclear), AMACR (cytoplasmic, granular), and CD57

- Cells have minimal cytoplasm with relatively uniform, round to ovoid nuclei bearing occasional folds
- Nucleoli are generally inconspicuous, and mitosis is rare to absent
- Chromatin distribution is uniform
- Rare cysts and blastemal-like sheet-like patterns
- Many tumors show regressive features, including hyalinization, calcifications often psammomatous, necrosis and hemorrhage, and dystrophic ossification

Predominant Pattern/Injury Type
- Neoplastic

ANCILLARY TESTS

Immunohistochemistry
- Often positive for WT1 (diffuse nuclear), AMACR (cytoplasmic, granular), pax-2, and CD57
- Usually negative for CK7 except in branching large tubules and papillary areas

Electron Microscopy
- Clusters of cells occasionally forming microlumen and surrounded by smooth, basal lamina matrix
- Junctional complexes at apical end of luminal lining cells with florid microvilli

DIFFERENTIAL DIAGNOSIS

Papillary Renal Cell Carcinoma
- PRCC type 1, solid variant and tubular predominant, is closest differential diagnosis
- Often multifocal and commonly with fibrous pseudocapsule
- Nuclei higher grade, often with more pleomorphism and prominent nucleoli
- Amount of cytoplasm usually exceeds minimal cytoplasm of MA
- Diffusely positive for AMACR, CK7, and EMA/MUC1; usually WT1 and CD57 negative
- Trisomy 7 and 17 and loss of Y chromosome

Epithelial Predominant Wilms Tumor
- Pseudocapsule usually present
- Nuclei are primitive-appearing, hyperchromatic, and pleomorphic
  - Mitotic activity is usually brisk
- Other components of Wilms tumor (stromal and blastemal) may be present
- Usually negative or only focally positive for CD57

DIAGNOSTIC CHECKLIST

Pathologic Interpretation Pearls
- Rare but distinctive benign renal tumor that may appear "alarming" at low-power microscopy due to "primitive" round blue cells or tubular appearance
- Attention to bland nuclear features without significant chromatin alteration or mitotic activity is key
- Scant cytoplasm is also the norm

SELECTED REFERENCES

1. Burger M et al: Metanephric adenoma of the kidney: a clinicopathological and molecular study of two cases. J Clin Pathol. 60(7):832-3, 2007
2. Argani P: Metanephric neoplasms: the hyperdifferentiated, benign end of the Wilms tumor spectrum? Clin Lab Med. 25(2):379-92, 2005
3. Muir TE et al: Metanephric adenoma, nephrogenic rests, and Wilms' tumor: a histologic and immunophenotypic comparison. Am J Surg Pathol. 25(10):1290-6, 2001
4. Pesti T et al: Mapping a tumor suppressor gene to chromosome 2p13 in metanephric adenoma by microsatellite allelotyping. Hum Pathol. 32(1):101-4, 2001
5. Davis CJ Jr et al: Metanephric adenoma. Clinicopathological study of fifty patients. Am J Surg Pathol. 19(10):1101-14, 1995
6. Jones EC et al: Metanephric adenoma of the kidney. A clinicopathological, immunohistochemical, flow cytometric, cytogenetic, and electron microscopic study of seven cases. Am J Surg Pathol. 19(6):615-26, 1995

METANEPHRIC ADENOMA

Gross and Microscopic Features

(Left) Most metanephric adenomas are solid and homogeneous. However, some tumors are variably cystic ⊳ with focal hemorrhage and necrosis in the cystic areas. *(Right)* This gross image shows a relatively uncommon gross appearance of metanephric adenoma. While cystic areas are often seen, extensive cyst formation, as seen here, is very rare. Microscopically, besides cystic degeneration, tumors with this change frequently show extensive sclerosis and prominent calcifications.

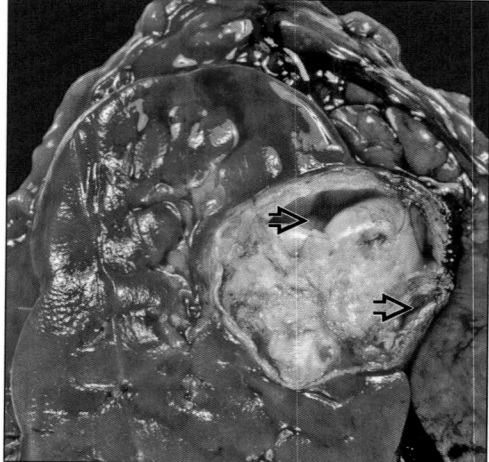
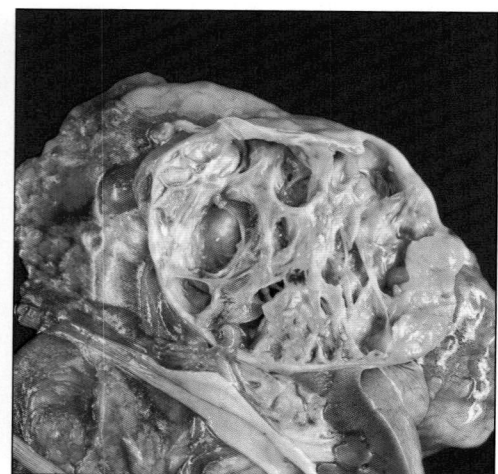

(Left) Metanephric adenomas are typically well circumscribed and most often (not always) without a capsule, with the tumor in direct contact with renal parenchyma ⊳. In such cases, there are usually no features of compression in the surrounding renal parenchyma. *(Right)* Rarely, MA may be surrounded by a variably well-formed fibrous capsule ⊳. In some of such cases, distinction from a papillary RCC might be difficult, and the diagnosis depends on careful morphologic evaluation.

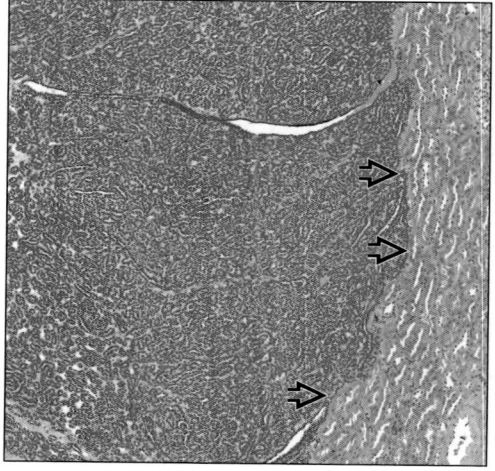
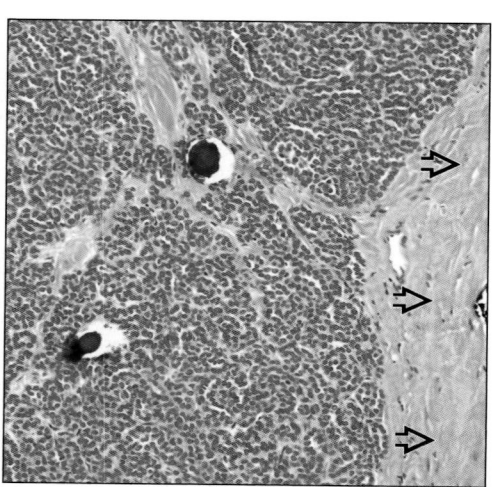

(Left) A low magnification evaluation of metanephric adenoma characteristically reveals tightly packed small tubules separated by a modest amount of stroma. The scant stroma is usually pauci-cellular. *(Right)* At low magnification, in addition to the small tubules, glomeruloid-formations ⊳ and elongated tubules with branching are also commonly observed in metanephric adenoma. Psammomatous calcifications ⊳ are quite common and may be diffuse and extensive in some tumors.

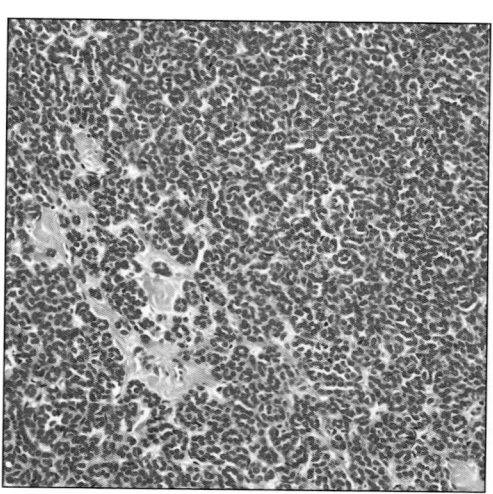
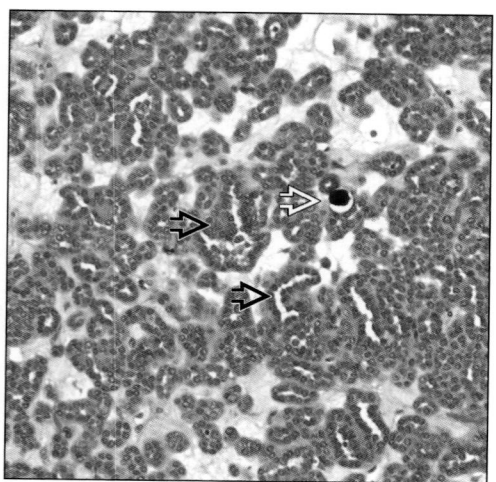

Microscopic Features

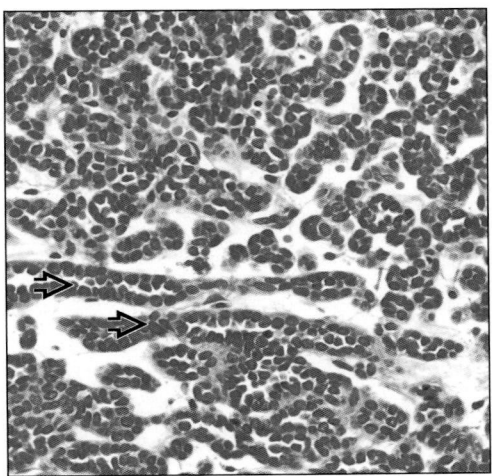

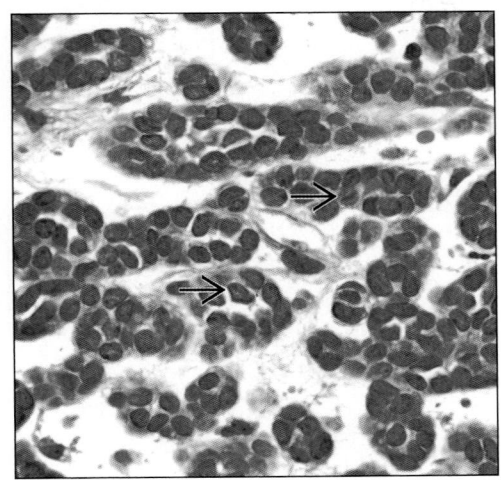

(Left) Elongated tubules ⊡ along with the small, round tubules are quite common in metanephric adenoma. At lower magnification, the small tubules may appear somewhat primitive and superficially resemble the cells and tubules of Wilms tumor. (Right) Careful evaluation and higher magnification assessment reveals the nuclei to be uniform, round-to-ovoid, often overlapping, and sometimes with central folds ⊡. Unlike blastema, nucleoli are inconspicuous, and mitotic figures are rare.

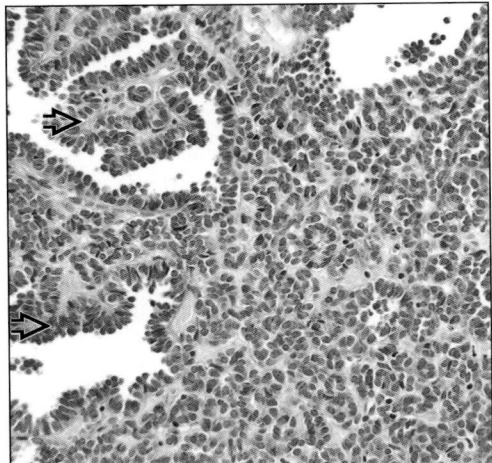

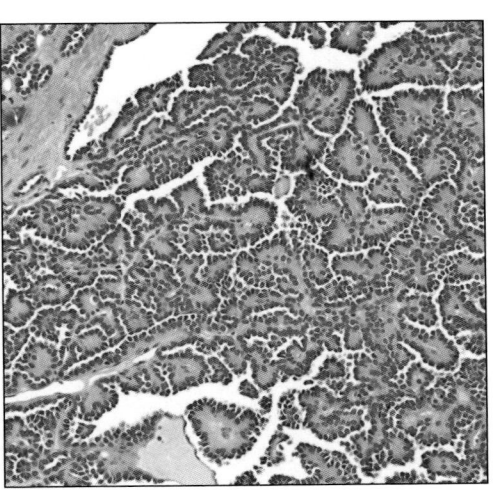

(Left) Focal papillations ⊡ are quite frequent in metanephric adenoma. (Right) Some MAs may have prominent papillary architecture. The small primitive tubules and usually focal papillations and glomerulations may raise the possibility of a Wilms tumor. The nuclear features, including the chromatin pattern and level of mitotic activity, are helpful in distinction from Wilms tumor. MAs lack significant cytoplasm, which helps in the distinction from papillary RCC.

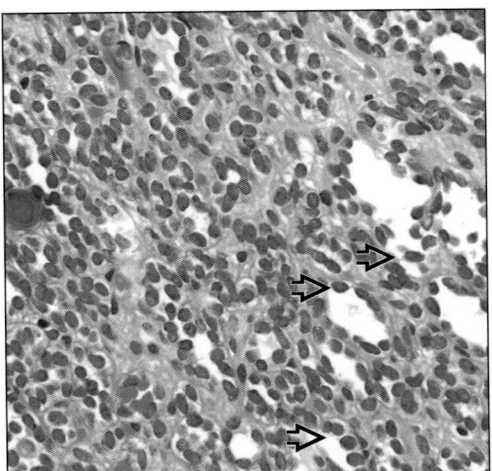

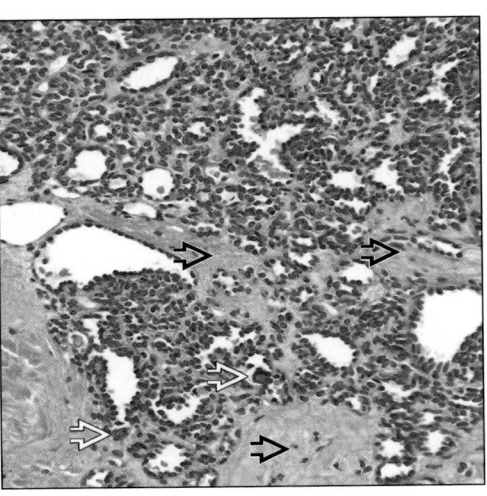

(Left) Some metanephric adenomas may show more mature-appearing tubules with "hobnailing" ⊡. This pattern is often focal, and the more common small primitive-appearing tubules are almost invariably present. (Right) Open tubular architecture is frequently associated with sclerosis ⊡ and calcifications, including psammomatous type ⊡. Although there is architectural variation, the nuclear features of MA are usually quite monomorphous and characteristic of this entity.

METANEPHRIC ADENOMA

Microscopic and Immunohistochemical Features

(Left) This image depicts a metanephric adenoma with extensive sclerosis. Rarely, metanephric adenomas show extensive degenerative changes. Such tumors are often grossly cystic, and on microscopic evaluation show dispersed tubules in a background of extensive sclerosis ⊘. Calcifications ⊟ are usually very prominent in these tumors. *(Right)* Sclerotic tumors also show a variable, usually prominent, cystic component. The cysts are lined by low-cuboidal cells ⊟ or may show no lining.

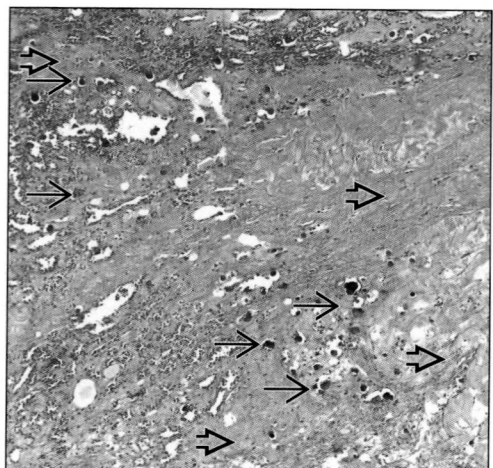
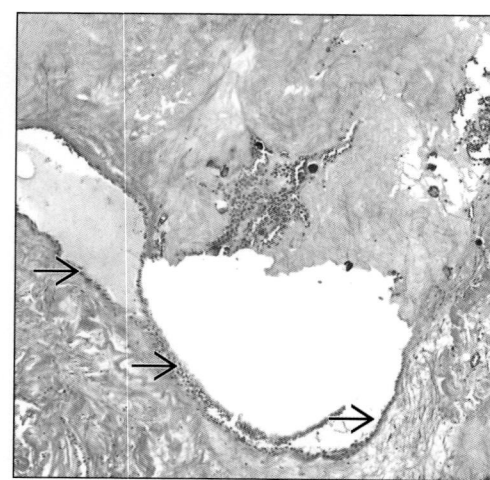

(Left) Immunohistochemical staining for CK7 is either negative or may show very focal ⊟ to patchy positivity in some metanephric adenomas. Note the diffuse positive staining in the surrounding renal tubules ⊘. *(Right)* MAs are usually negative for AMACR. However, approximately 10% may show focal to more diffuse positivity. Strong CK7 and AMACR positivity in the same tumor argues against the diagnosis of MA, and in appropriate morphologic context, favors a papillary RCC.

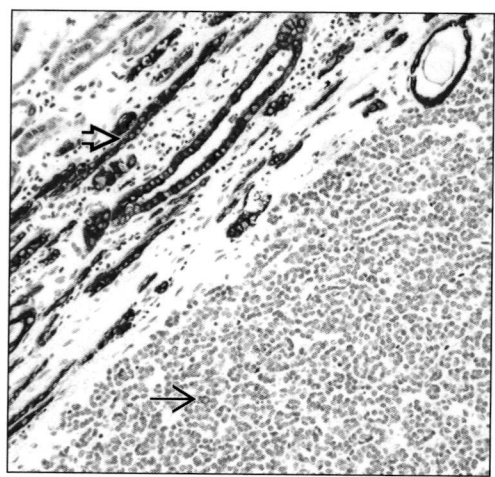
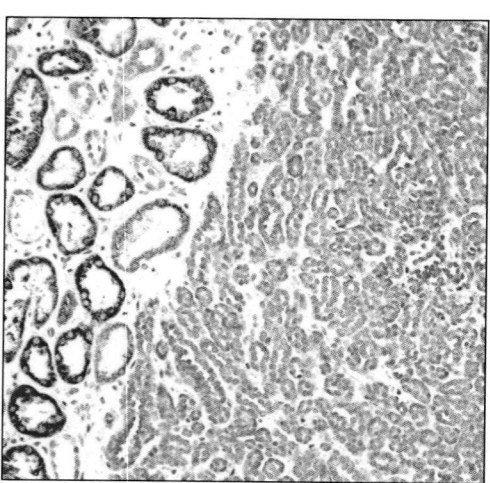

(Left) WT1 usually shows diffuse nuclear staining in metanephric adenoma. Thus, by itself, WT1 immunostaining cannot distinguish metanephric adenoma from a tubular Wilms tumor. *(Right)* CD57 is usually diffusely positive in MA, although focal positivity may be present in some cases of solid papillary RCC and tubular Wilms tumor, as well. Therefore, a panel that includes AMACR, CK7, WT1, and CD57 is useful in differentiating MA from these occasionally close morphologic mimics.

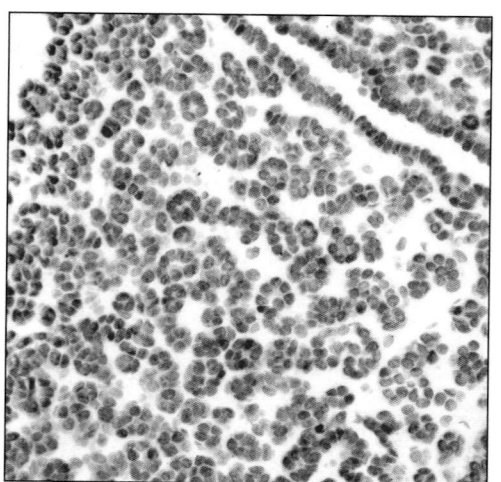
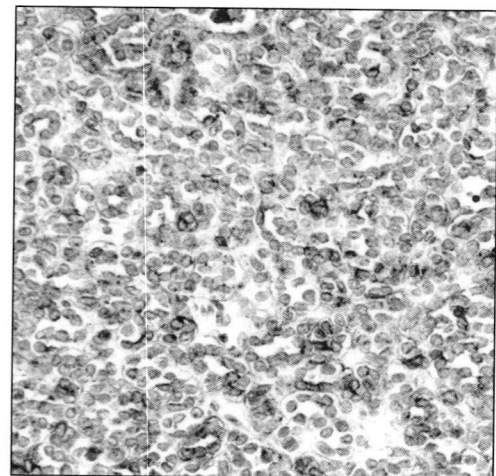

METANEPHRIC ADENOMA

Microscopic and Immunohistochemical Features

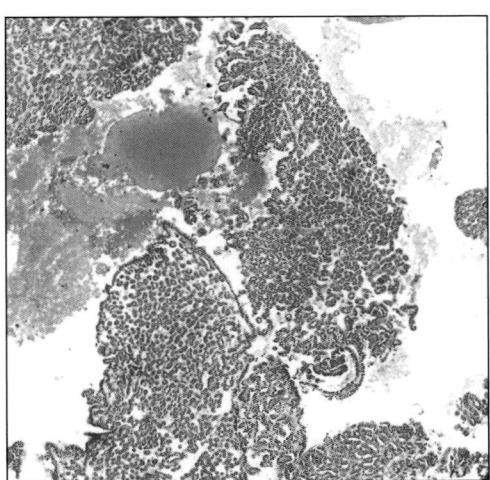
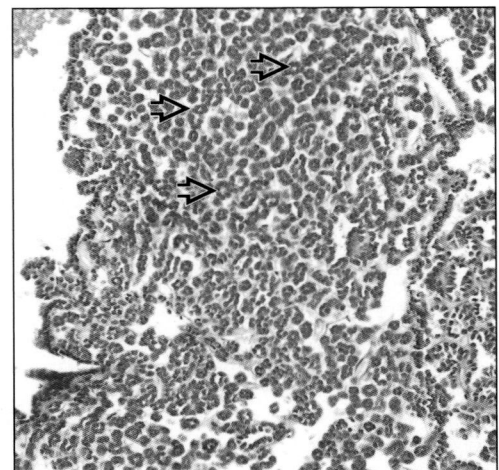

(Left) This needle core biopsy of the kidney shows a MA. Caution is warranted in making an outright diagnosis on a biopsy if the classic features are absent. *(Right)* A higher magnification details the typical small tubules ⊳, lined by monomorphic cells, with no nucleoli or significant mitotic activity. These morphologic features, even on limited material, are sufficiently diagnostic of a metanephric adenoma and may be supported by appropriate immunohistochemistry.

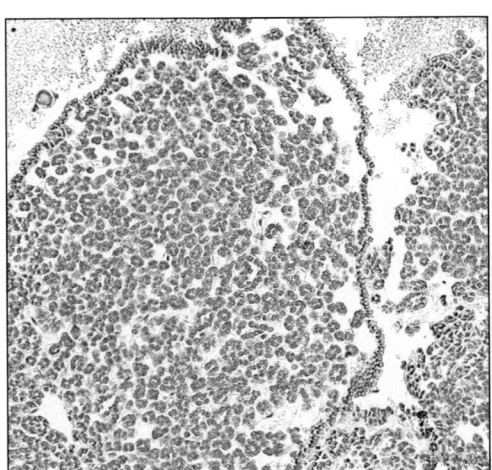
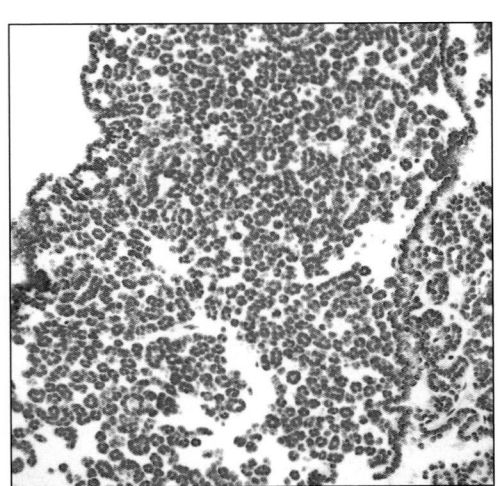

(Left) Immunohistochemical stain for AMACR on this needle core biopsy specimen is completely negative. *(Right)* Immunostain for CK7 is also completely negative in this tumor. While morphology is sufficiently diagnostic in most cases, in rare instances and if the pathologist has less experience with these tumors, a panel of immunostains may help distinguish metanephric adenoma from its mimics, which include solid, tubular papillary RCC and epithelial-predominant Wilms tumor.

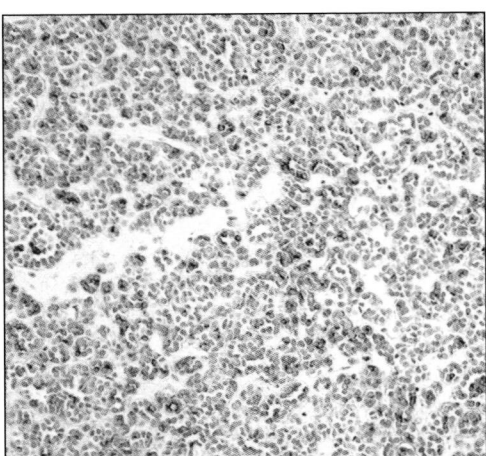
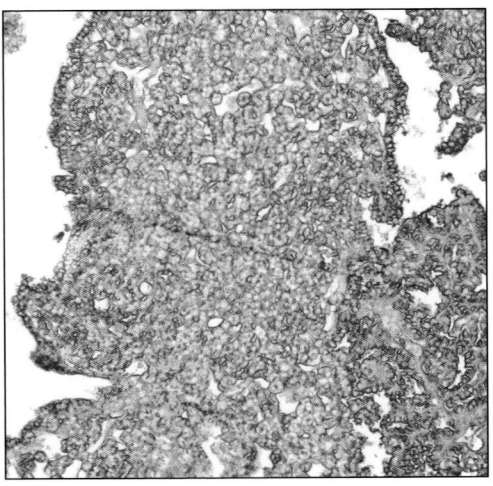

(Left) CD57 shows diffuse cytoplasmic positivity in a core biopsy of this tumor, a characteristic feature of MA. *(Right)* CD10 immunostain is usually focally to diffusely positive in MA. Quantitative results for CD10 do not help in the distinction from a papillary RCC, but the staining pattern in MA is different from membranous/luminal positivity in papillary RCC. The use of a judiciously constructed panel of markers may have greater diagnostic utility on small specimens like biopsies.

METANEPHRIC TUMORS OTHER THAN METANEPHRIC ADENOMA

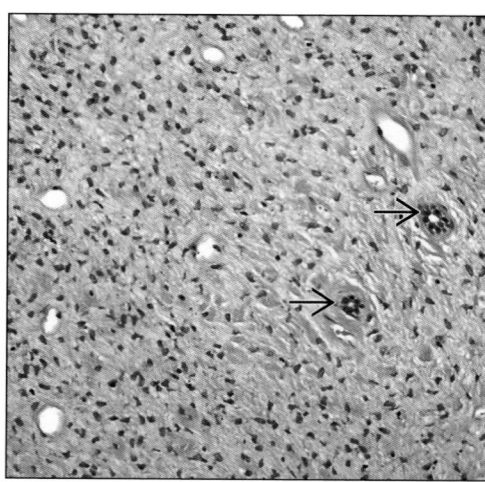

Metanephric stromal tumor is a benign, pediatric stromal neoplasm, usually with entrapped renal tubules ➡ and glomeruli. Most cases were previously misdiagnosed as congenital mesoblastic nephroma.

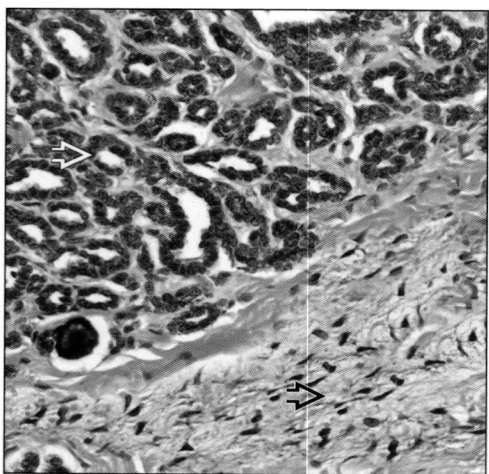

Metanephric adenofibroma shows a mixture of stromal elements similar to metanephric stromal tumor ➡ and primitive-appearing epithelial components ➡ similar to that in metanephric adenoma.

TERMINOLOGY

Abbreviations
- Metanephric stromal tumor (MST), metanephric adenofibroma (MAF)

Definitions
- Metanephric adenofibroma: Biphasic tumor composed of metanephric adenoma-like epithelial and MST-like stromal components
- Metanephric stromal tumor: Pure benign pediatric stromal tumor

ETIOLOGY/PATHOGENESIS

Relationship with Wilms Tumor
- Some believe metanephric tumors represent hyperdifferentiated Wilms tumors or intralobar nephrogenic rests (ILNR), due to
  - Presence of epithelial-predominant Wilms tumor-like areas in some MAF
  - Occurrence of ILNR in surrounding renal parenchyma in occasional case

CLINICAL ISSUES

Epidemiology
- Incidence
  - Both tumors very rare
    - < 70 MAFs reported in literature
    - MST < 1/10 as common as congenital mesoblastic nephroma, by itself a rare entity
- Age
  - MAF: Mean age = 72 months (range: 5 months to 36 years); MST: mean age = 2 years (range: 4 days to 15 years)
    - Only very rare cases of MST reported in adults
- Gender
  - MAF: M:F = 2:1; MST: Equally represented in both

Site
- Both usually based in renal medulla

Presentation
- Often asymptomatic and incidental findings
- Hypertension may be presentation in some, particularly MST, due to juxtaglomerular apparatus hyperplasia (JGAH)
- Hematuria may be another presenting symptom because of renal pelvis involvement
- Polycythemia, in some MAF

Treatment
- Surgical resection; adjuvant chemotherapy for MAFs that may be associated with Wilms tumor

Prognosis
- Both lesions with benign outcome, regardless of presence of epithelial features in MAF

MACROSCOPIC FEATURES

General Features
- Usually solitary, but rarely multifocal, particularly MST
- Predominantly solid, with variable cystic components, usually with indistinct tumor borders
- Usually yellow-tan to fibrous-appearing cut surface
- Hemorrhagic and necrotic areas very rare; when present, may be associated with Wilms tumor

Size
- Mean for both: 3.8 cm (range: 1.8-11 cm)

MICROSCOPIC PATHOLOGY

Histologic Features
- Stroma similar in both tumors

METANEPHRIC TUMORS OTHER THAN METANEPHRIC ADENOMA

Key Facts

Terminology
- Metanephric stromal tumor (MST), metanephric adenofibroma (MAF)
- Metanephric adenofibroma: Biphasic tumor composed of metanephric adenoma-like epithelial and MST-like stromal components
- Metanephric stromal tumor: Pure benign pediatric stromal tumor

Clinical Issues
- Both tumors very rare
- MAF: Mean age 72 months (range: 5 months to 36 years); MST: Mean age 2 years (range: 4 days to 15 years)
- Hypertension may be presentation in some, particularly MST, because of JGAH
- Polycythemia, in some metanephric adenofibromas

Macroscopic Features
- Hemorrhagic and necrotic areas very rare

Microscopic Pathology
- Stroma similar in both tumors
- MSTs often show JGA hyperplasia within entrapped glomeruli; this feature not seen in MAF
- Epithelium in MAF usually mitotically inactive metanephric adenoma-like, with other rarer variant features
- Stromal components immunoreactive for CD34, usually patchy

Top Differential Diagnoses
- MST vs. congenital mesoblastic nephroma (CMN), classical variant

---

- o Spindled to stellate cells with thin hyperchromatic nuclei and slender indistinct cytoplasmic extensions
- o Stroma surrounds and entraps renal tubules/blood vessels to form concentric "onion skin" rings or collarettes around these structures
- o More cellular, less myxoid spindle cell areas at periphery of collarettes yielding vaguely nodular architecture
- o Epithelioid transformation of medial smooth muscle of intratumoral arterioles (angiodysplasia of vessels)
- o Heterologous differentiation (glia or cartilage); glial tissue intimately associated with epithelium
- o MSTs often show JGAH within entrapped glomeruli; this feature not seen in MAF
- Epithelium in MAF described with 4 different patterns
- o Most common type with mitotically inactive metanephric adenoma-like features
- o Metanephric adenoma-like but with areas showing brisk mitotic activity (> 5/20 high power fields)
- o Composite metanephric adenoma/epithelial predominant Wilms tumor-like areas
- o Composite tumors with metanephric adenoma/ tubulopapillary carcinomatous areas

Predominant Pattern/Injury Type
- Neoplastic

Predominant Cell/Compartment Type
- Spindle and epithelioid

ANCILLARY TESTS

Immunohistochemistry
- Stromal components immunoreactive for CD34, often patchy; desmin, keratins, and S100 are negative, but glial foci label for GFAP and S100
- Epithelial components usually positive for keratins; AMACR usually negative

DIFFERENTIAL DIAGNOSIS

Congenital Mesoblastic Nephroma (CMN), Classical Variant
- Differentiation has to be made from MST
- CMN shows deeply infiltrative borders with entrapment of large clusters of native nephrons; MST is superficially infiltrative with entrapped single tubules or glomeruli
- MST shows angiodysplasia, concentric peritubular growth pattern, and JGAH
- CD34 positive in MST, and not in CMN

DIAGNOSTIC CHECKLIST

Pathologic Interpretation Pearls
- Stroma is similar in MST and MAF
  - o Exception: No JGAH seen in MAF
- MST need extensive sampling to exclude focal epithelial components of MAF
  - o From prognostic perspective, no significant differences between the 2

SELECTED REFERENCES

1. Argani P: Metanephric neoplasms: the hyperdifferentiated, benign end of the Wilms tumor spectrum? Clin Lab Med. 25(2):379-92, 2005
2. Bluebond-Langner R et al: Adult presentation of metanephric stromal tumor. J Urol. 168(4 Pt 1):1482-3, 2002
3. Arroyo MR et al: The spectrum of metanephric adenofibroma and related lesions: clinicopathologic study of 25 cases from the National Wilms Tumor Study Group Pathology Center. Am J Surg Pathol. 25(4):433-44, 2001
4. Palese MA et al: Metanephric stromal tumor: a rare benign pediatric renal mass. Urology. 58(3):462, 2001
5. Argani P et al: Metanephric stromal tumor: report of 31 cases of a distinctive pediatric renal neoplasm. Am J Surg Pathol. 24(7):917-26, 2000
6. Guzman E et al: Nephrogenic adenofibroma in a young child. Pathol Res Pract. 196(12):853-6, 2000

METANEPHRIC TUMORS OTHER THAN METANEPHRIC ADENOMA

Microscopic Features

(Left) Most metanephric stromal tumors show superficially invasive borders entrapping individual native tubules ⇨ and glomeruli. This is in contrast with mesoblastic nephromas that show extensive finger-like extensions, entrapping large collections of native renal nephrons. *(Right)* Most MST show vaguely nodular cellular patterns, primarily a result of loose, myxoid stroma surrounding the entrapped tubules ⇨ and blood vessels, separated by more dense stromal cellularity ➡.

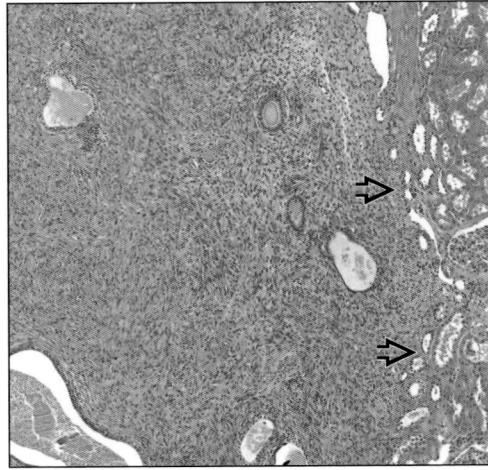
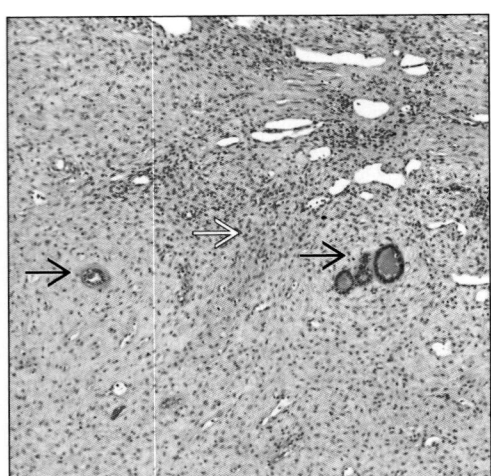

(Left) The stroma in both metanephric stromal tumors and metanephric adenofibromas show tumor vessels with epithelioid transformation of medial smooth muscle (so-called angiodysplasia) ⇨. This image also shows the typical myxoid stroma around the vessels ➡. *(Right)* Some metanephric stromal tumors, as well as MAFs, show a reverse cellular pattern, with the tubules ⇨ and vessels ⇨ surrounded by more cellular stroma, compared to less dense stroma in-between.

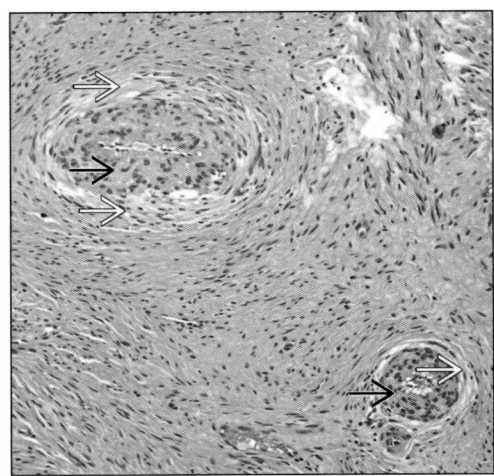
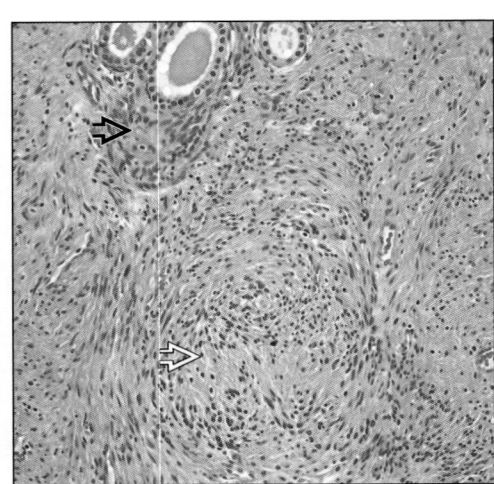

(Left) Myxoid stroma around this vessel with angiodysplastic features shows the typical concentric arrangement of the stromal cells. This often leads to what has been called an "onion skin" appearance. *(Right)* Many MSTs show marked hyperplasia of the juxtaglomerular cells ⇨ of the entrapped glomeruli. Note the residual, compressed residual glomerulus ⇨ at the top of the hyperplastic cells. Juxtaglomerular cell hyperplasia is not seen in metanephric adenofibromas.

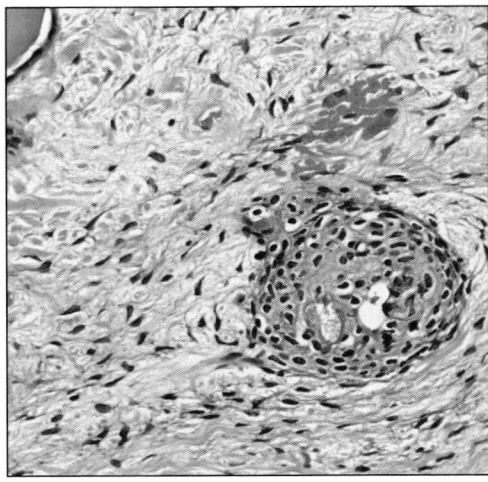
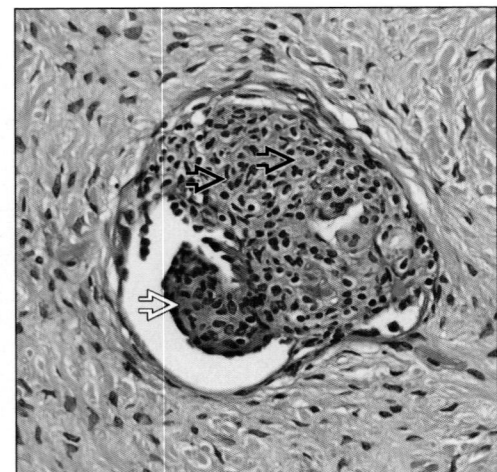

METANEPHRIC TUMORS OTHER THAN METANEPHRIC ADENOMA

Microscopic Features

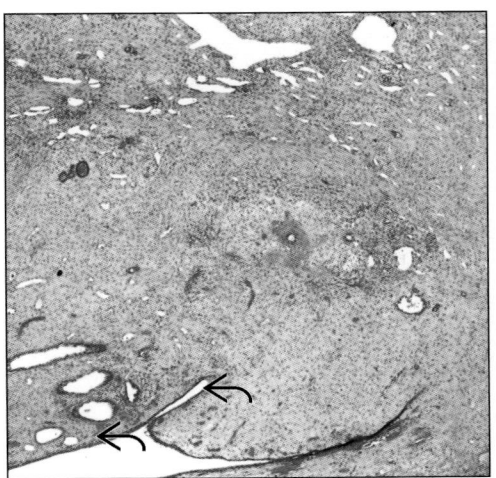

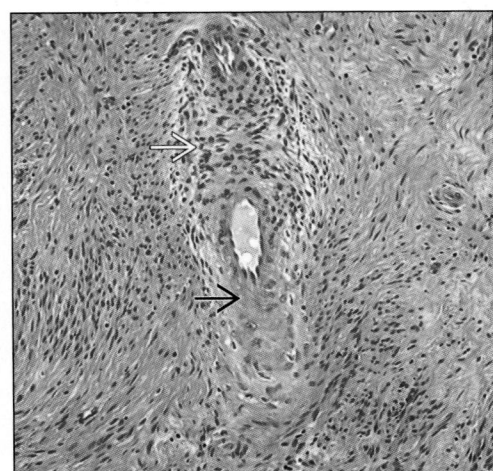

(Left) Most MST and MAF are medulla-centric and may invade the pelvicalyceal system ⊞. *(Right)* The stromal cells are spindled to stellate with thin hyperchromatic nuclei and indistinct cytoplasmic borders. Morphologically, these are not much different from the cells in classical variant of congenital mesoblastic nephroma, with which most metanephric stromal tumors were confused in the past. Note the angiodysplasia ⊞ and perivascular "onion skin" stromal pattern ➡.

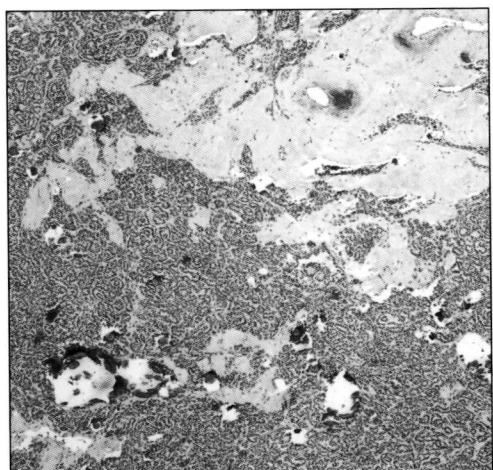

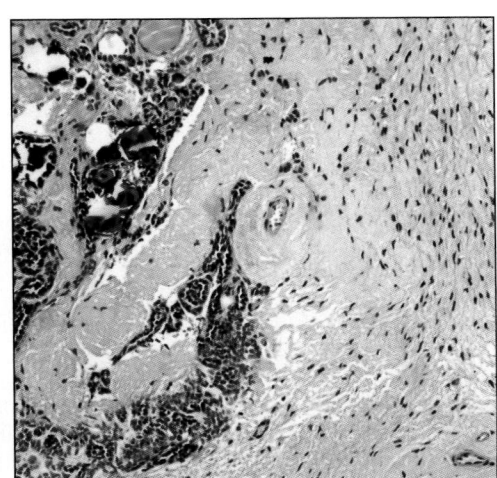

(Left) The epithelial component of a MAF may represent a metanephric adenoma, but for the presence of a small stromal component in this tumor. Conversely, some MAF may be predominantly stromal, with very minute epithelial foci. *(Right)* The epithelial component in MAF may closely resemble packed tubules in MA. However, some tumors may show brisk mitotic activity, or even epithelial-predominant Wilms tumor-like areas. Calcification may be a prominent feature.

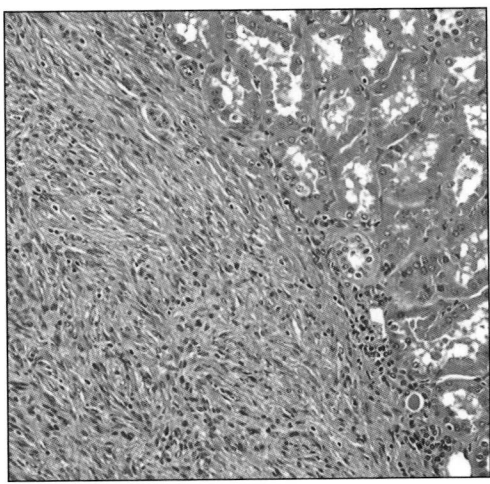

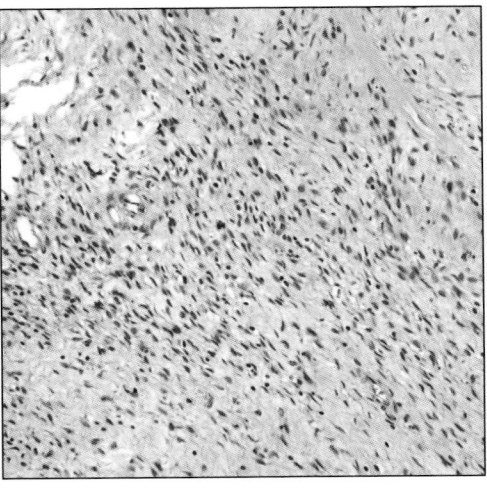

(Left) Although the stroma in both MST and MAF shows marked similarities, MAF lacks the juxtaglomerular cell hyperplasia, commonly seen in metanephric stromal tumors. The epithelial component in MAF remains the most distinctive feature between the two. *(Right)* Based on this photomicrograph alone that depicts the stroma in a metanephric tumor, it is not possible to discriminate between a MST and MAF because of the similarities between the two.

NEPHROGENIC RESTS

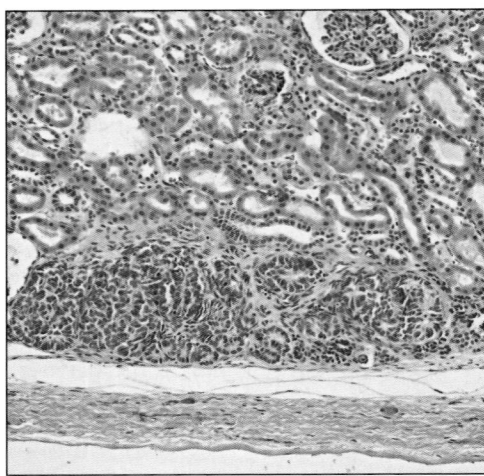

Perilobar nephrogenic rests are located at the periphery of the renal lobes, well delineated from adjacent nephrons, and composed of blastema and tubules without any significant stromal components.

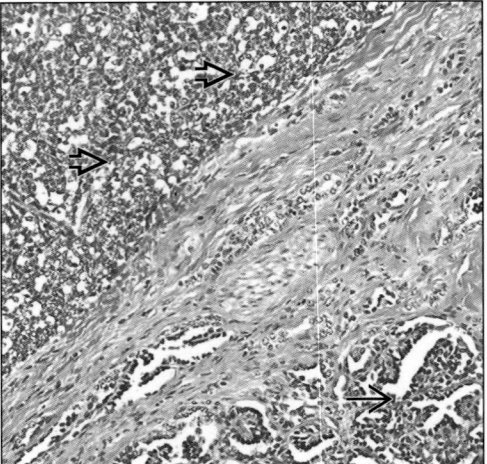

Interlobar cell rest is adjacent to a Wilms tumor ⊵. ILNRs ➡ are located within the renal lobes, have irregular outlines, and often show prominent stromal components.

TERMINOLOGY

Abbreviations
- Nephrogenic rest (NR), perilobar nephrogenic rest (PLNR), intralobar nephrogenic rest (ILNR)

Definitions
- Abnormally persistent nephrogenic cells associated with and capable of developing into nephroblastomas

ETIOLOGY/PATHOGENESIS

Molecular Alterations
- Like those in Wilms tumor (WT), alterations in *WT1* (11p13), *WT2* (11p15), and *WT3* (16q) genes are present in accompanying NRs
  - Mutations in *WT1* are present in ILNR
  - Insulin growth factor 2 loss of paternal imprinting (LOI) (in putative *WT2* gene region) in PLNR of all types (sclerosing, hyperplastic, etc.)

CLINICAL ISSUES

Epidemiology
- Incidence
  - Encountered in up to 40% of patients with WT; incidence > 95% in patients with bilateral tumors
  - Observed in 1% of infant autopsies; isolated intralobar NRs less common (1 in 1,000 autopsies)
- Age
  - Median at presentation: WT and ILNR = 18.5 months; WT and PLNR = 35.5 months
- Gender
  - WT and NR show equal sex distribution or slight female preponderance in the West, but significant male preponderance in Asia
- Ethnicity
  - PLNR somewhat more common than ILNR in West, but PLNR extremely uncommon in Asia

Treatment
- Hyperplastic rests difficult to distinguish from WT on biopsy; these and later forms treated similar to stage 1 WT (National Wilms Tumor Study Group [NWTS])
  - Treating hyperplastic rests prevents compression and damage to native kidney
  - Also, treating these diminishes targets for neoplastic transformation

Prognosis
- NRs in WT-bearing kidneys are associated with higher incidence of synchronous or metachronous WT in other kidney
  - Higher incidence of concurrent bilateral Wilms tumor in patients with NRs, particularly PLNR
  - Risk of metachronous WT 15x higher in children < 1 year of age with WT and NR (particularly PLNR) than those without NR
  - Identifying NR on nephrectomy for WT leads to increased frequency of ultrasonographic follow-up for child

MICROSCOPIC PATHOLOGY

Histologic Features
- Based primarily on location, classified as perilobar or intralobar types
- **Perilobar nephrogenic rests**
  - Usually multifocal, located at periphery of lobes and sharply demarcated from surrounding parenchyma
  - Consist predominantly of blastema and tubules, with scant stromal component
  - Associated WTs are usually also blastemal and tubular, lacking prominent stromal components
  - PLNR are believed to represent genesis late in embryonal state
- **Intralobar nephrogenic rests**

NEPHROGENIC RESTS

Key Facts

Terminology
- Abnormally persistent nephrogenic cells, capable of developing into nephroblastomas

Clinical Issues
- Encountered in up to 40% of patients with Wilms tumor and > 95% in patients with bilateral tumors
- Both PLNR and ILNR are observed in patients in Western countries, but PLNR are rarely, if ever, seen in Asian countries

Microscopic Pathology
- PLNR usually multifocal, located at periphery of renal lobes and sharply demarcated from surrounding renal parenchyma

- ILNR usually unifocal, localized within renal lobes, and poorly circumscribed with interdigitations into surrounding nephrons
- Dormant NR, small rests without evidence of proliferation
- Sclerosing and obsolete rests consist predominantly of tubules in fibrotic background
- Hyperplastic NR, showing signs of proliferation with abundant blastemal elements and increased size
- Neoplastic NR, arising within dormant, sclerosing, or hyperplastic rests
- Presence of pseudocapsule important in distinguishing hyperplastic or neoplastic (adenomatous) rest from nephroblastoma

Top Differential Diagnoses
- Papillary adenoma

- Usually unifocal, localized within renal lobes, not in periphery, and poorly circumscribed with interdigitations into surrounding nephrons
  - Rests occurring in renal sinus and pelvicaliceal system are also considered ILNR
- Rich in stromal component
- Associated WTs, usually with heterologous components and rich in stroma (e.g., rhabdomyocytes)
- ILNR are believed to represent genesis very early in embryonal state
- PLNR and ILNR subclassified as
  - **Dormant**, small rests without evidence of proliferation
  - **Sclerosing**, consisting mainly of remnants of differentiated blastema (usually tubular) in background of varying amounts of fibrosis
    - **Obsolete** rests similar consisting predominantly of fibrosis with rare tubules
  - **Hyperplastic**, showing signs of proliferation with abundant blastemal elements and increased size
    - Usually grossly visible, showing significant proliferative activity, including prominent mitoses
    - Represents generalized hyperplasia in rest, with all cells in NR participating in proliferation
    - Due to proliferation of all cells within rest, shape is maintained
    - Differentiation from WT very difficult on limited material, such as biopsies, as lesional borders may not be well sampled
  - **Neoplastic**, arising within dormant, sclerosing, or hyperplastic rests
    - Usually spherical nodule, grossly visible
    - Believed to represent proliferation from single cell, therefore spherical with pushing borders compressing surrounding structures
    - No pseudocapsule present
  - Presence of pseudocapsule important in distinguishing hyperplastic or neoplastic (adenomatous) rest from nephroblastoma
  - Designation of **nephroblastomatosis** is used for multifocal and diffuse NRs

- Can be perilobar, interlobar, combined, or panlobar (replacing entire lobe)
- All or any stage of rests (dormant, hyperplastic, neoplastic) can be present
- There are no quantitative criteria to determine how many rests constitute nephroblastomatosis
- Present as thick cortical rind of hyperplastic nephrogenic tissue encasing kidney

DIFFERENTIAL DIAGNOSIS

Papillary Adenoma
- Frequently encountered in adults; shows mature epithelial component; lacks blastema

DIAGNOSTIC CHECKLIST

Pathologic Interpretation Pearls
- Intraoperative renal biopsies are often of limited utility in distinguishing between WT and mitotically active NR in small samples
  - Requires abundant tissue at periphery of lesion for distinction

SELECTED REFERENCES

1. Fukuzawa R et al: Molecular pathology and epidemiology of nephrogenic rests and Wilms tumors. J Pediatr Hematol Oncol. 29(9):589-94, 2007
2. Breslow NE et al: Age distributions, birth weights, nephrogenic rests, and heterogeneity in the pathogenesis of Wilms tumor. Pediatr Blood Cancer. 47(3):260-7, 2006
3. Hennigar RA et al: Clinicopathologic features of nephrogenic rests and nephroblastomatosis. Adv Anat Pathol. 8(5):276-89, 2001
4. Coppes MJ et al: Factors affecting the risk of contralateral Wilms tumor development: a report from the National Wilms Tumor Study Group. Cancer. 85(7):1616-25, 1999
5. Beckwith JB et al: Nephrogenic rests, nephroblastomatosis, and the pathogenesis of Wilms' tumor. Pediatr Pathol. 10(1-2):1-36, 1990

Microscopic Features

(Left) Low-magnification view shows a large intralobar nephrogenic rest ➡. Unlike PLNR, ILNR are usually single. Isolated ILNRs are much less common than PLNRs in pediatric autopsies. However, these are the predominant type of NR found in Asia. *(Right)* An interlobar nephrogenic rest shows the typical irregular outlines, interdigitating with surrounding nonneoplastic tubules and glomeruli ⍈. Note the prominent stromal component ➡ in the rest, a characteristic feature.

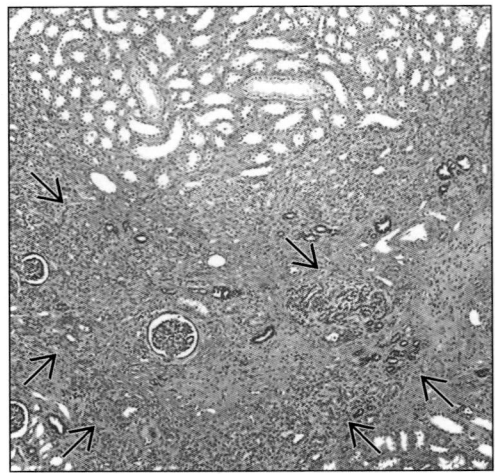
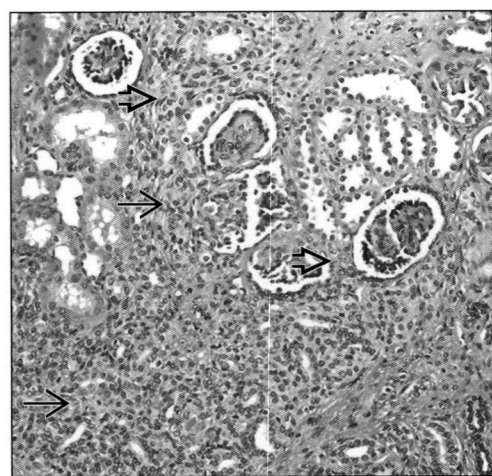

(Left) A dormant ⍈ and sclerosing ➡ PLNR is shown. Sclerosing NRs show variable proportion of fibrosis and usually consist of tubules separated by fibrous background. *(Right)* Multiple PLNRs show features in between dormant and hyperplastic. Dormant NR are defined as rests without proliferation, and hyperplastic as those with increased size and proliferative activity. However, these features represent a continuous spectrum rather than absolute static entities, as demonstrated by this image.

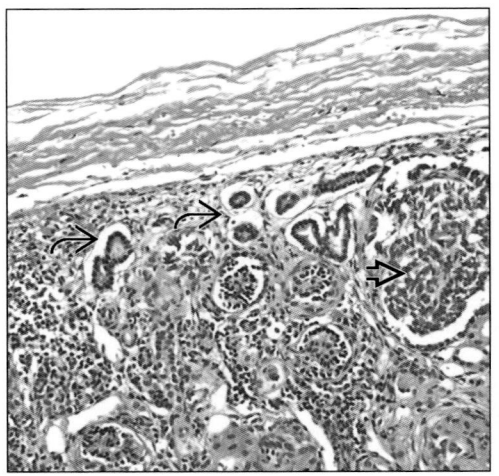
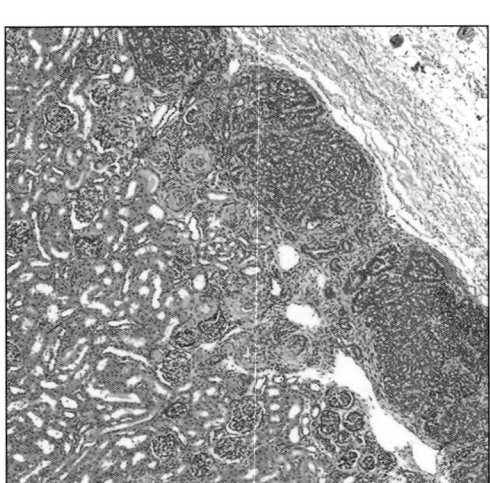

(Left) A hyperplastic PLNR, by definition, represents an enlarged, proliferating rest. Proliferation involves all cells in rest; therefore, the shape of the rest is preserved. *(Courtesy P. Argani, MD.)* *(Right)* This image shows a neoplastic nephrogenic rest, occurring in a post-chemotherapeutic setting. Neoplastic rests are believed to arise from the proliferation of a single cell; therefore, these are spherical and compress the surrounding NR remnants ⍈.

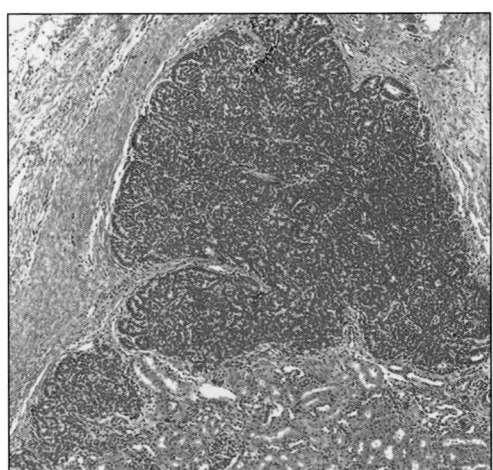
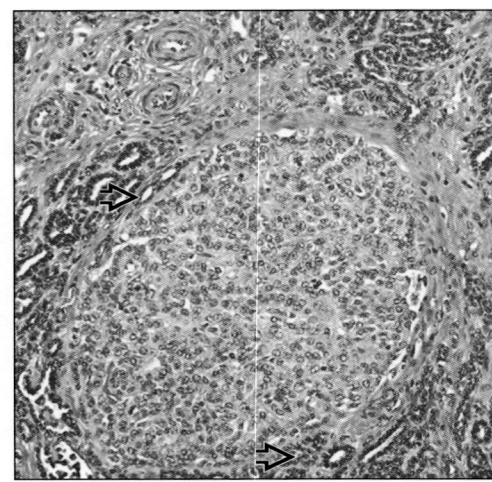

NEPHROGENIC RESTS

Microscopic Features

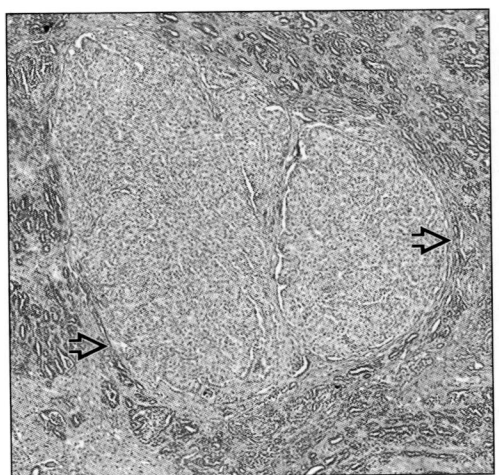

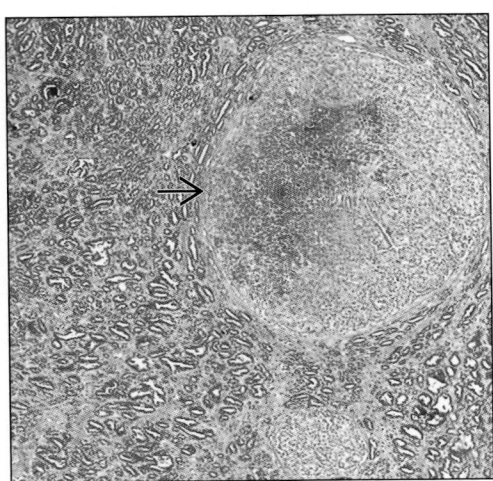

(Left) This image shows a post-chemotherapy neoplastic NR. Neoplastic rests are often grossly visible spherical nodules, compressing the surrounding residual NR ⊵. These, as well as hyperplastic rests, by definition lack a pseudocapsule. (Right) Neoplastic nephrogenic rests ⊟, in the spectrum of progression of NRs, precede the stage of what may be considered early nephroblastoma. The major difference is the lack of a pseudocapsule in neoplastic/adenomatous rests.

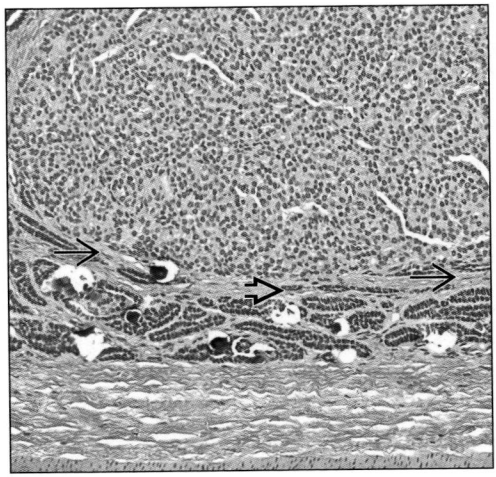

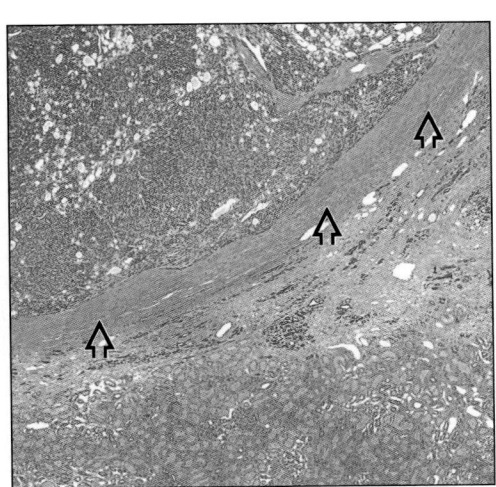

(Left) This image shows a post-chemotherapy nephrogenic nodule with compression of residual nephrogenic rest components ⊵ and early pseudocapsule formation ⊟. Such nodules may be considered adenomatous/neoplastic by some and early WT by others. (Right) Unlike all types of nephrogenic rests, Wilms tumor usually shows the presence of a pseudocapsule ⊵. Encapsulation is an important distinguishing feature that separates Wilms tumor from all forms of NRs.

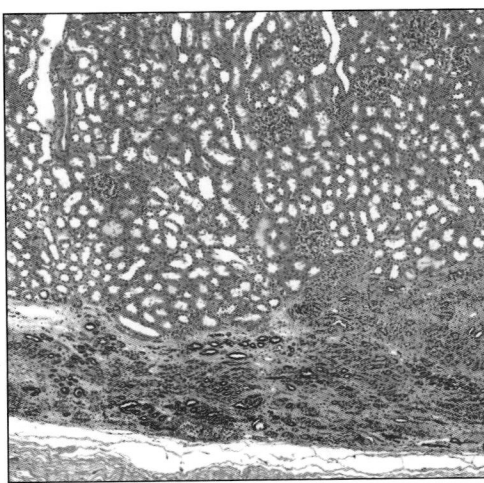

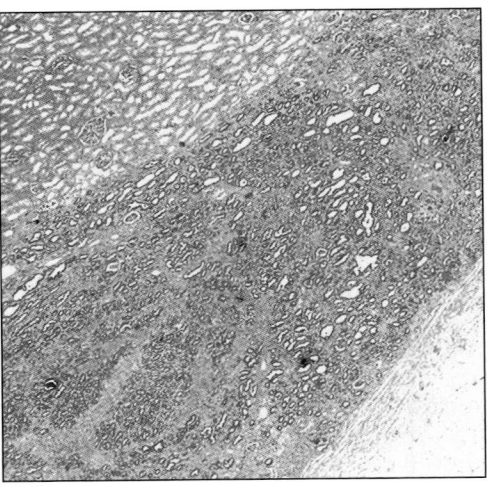

(Left) A low-magnification view of nephroblastomatosis, which is characterized by the presence of a thick cortical rind of hyperplastic nephrogenic tissue encasing the kidney. (Right) There are no quantitative criteria to determine how many rests would constitute nephroblastomatosis. However, diffuse radiologic thickening of renal cortex is typical of nephroblastomatosis. At morphologic levels, all or any stage of nephrogenic rests (dormant, hyperplastic, neoplastic) may be present.

NEPHROBLASTOMA (WILMS TUMOR)

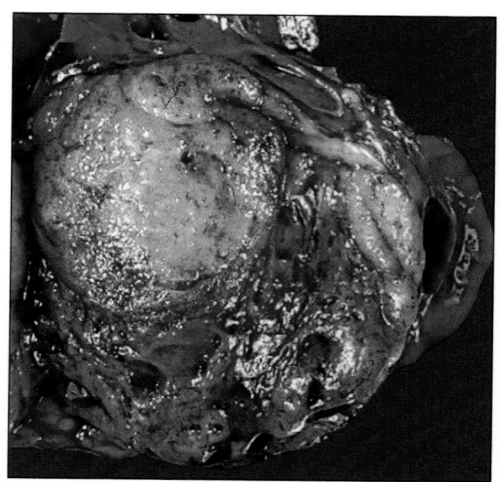

Gross appearance of a Wilms tumor shows a well-circumscribed soft, tan mass with encephaloid cut surface bulging from the native renal parenchyma. Examination of the renal sinus is important.

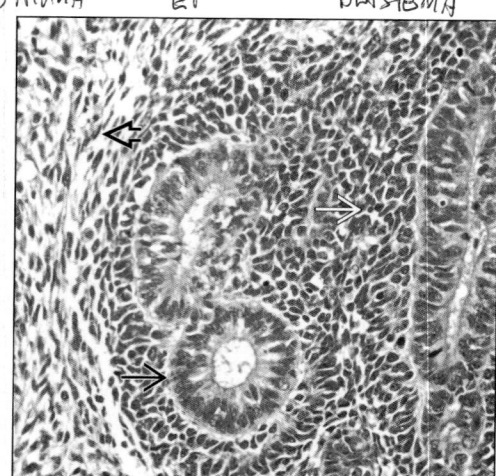

Typical triphasic morphology of Wilms tumor is shown with blastemal ➡, epithelial ➡, and stromal ➡ components. Tubular differentiation is the most common epithelial pattern in Wilms tumor.

TERMINOLOGY

Abbreviations
- Wilms Tumor (WT)

Synonyms
- Nephroblastoma

Definitions
- Malignant embryonal neoplasm derived from nephrogenic blastema cells often, but not always, showing multiphasic patterns of differentiation

ETIOLOGY/PATHOGENESIS

Developmental Anomaly
- Approximately 10% are associated with syndromic conditions, including
  - WAGR syndrome (Wilms tumor, Aniridia, Genitourinary malformations, mental Retardation)
  - Denys-Drash syndrome (Wilms tumor, mesangial sclerosis, pseudohermaphroditism)
  - Beckwith-Wiedemann syndrome (Wilms tumor, hemihypertrophy, macroglossia, omphalocele, visceromegaly)
  - Familial nephroblastoma
  - Others
    - Trisomy 18, Perlman syndrome, Bloom syndrome, Frasier syndrome, Klippel-Trenaunay syndrome

WT1 Gene Deletions or Point Mutations
- *WT1* gene is localized to chromosome 11p13
- *WT1* gene alterations are consistently present in WAGR and Denys-Drash syndromes
- Among sporadic nephroblastomas, deletions in focus are present in 1/3 and mutations in 10% of cases only
  - *WT1*-mutant tumors also show β-*catenin* (*CTNNB1*) mutations, activating Wnt signaling pathway

- Tumors with *WT1* mutations usually have stromal-prominent histology and presence of rhabdomyogenesis
  - Often associated with intralobar nephrogenic rests (ILNR)
- Such tumors common in both East Asians and Whites

WT2 Gene Alterations
- 11p15 is location for putative *WT2* gene
- 11p15 alterations are common in Beckwith-Wiedemann syndrome
  - Insulin growth factor 2 (*IGF2*) gene and closely related H19 locus located within *WT2* region
  - Normally, only paternal allele-specific *IGF2* expressed (imprinting), because of differential methylation status of *H19* in paternal and maternal alleles
- Loss of imprinting (LOI) of *IGF2* and hypermethylation of *H19*-related genes identified in 33-50% of Wilms tumors
- Tumors with LOI usually stroma poor
  - Often associated with perilobar nephrogenic rests (PLNR)
- Such tumors are rare in East Asians

Tumor-Specific LOH for Chromosomes 1p and 16q
- Loss of heterozygosity (LOH) for chromosomes 1p and 16q are present in a proportion of Wilms tumor with favorable histology
  - Such LOHs are indicator of significantly increased risk of aggressive behavior
    - Current COG treatment protocols recommend more aggressive treatment for favorable histology Wilms tumors with LOH

NEPHROBLASTOMA (WILMS TUMOR)

Key Facts

Terminology
- Malignant embryonal neoplasm derived from nephrogenic blastema cells often, but not always, showing multiphasic patterns of differentiation

Clinical Issues
- Peak incidence, 2-3 years; 98% of cases in children < 10 years of age
- In general, NWTS (now included in COG) advocates primary resection, followed by further therapy if required
- SIOP advocates pre-operative therapy followed by surgical resection; further therapy determined by the response to prior therapy
- Overall survival currently > 90%

- Most significant unfavorable factors include high stage at presentation and diffuse anaplasia (unfavorable histology)

Microscopic Pathology
- Most characteristic: Triphasic pattern consisting of undifferentiated blastema, and epithelial and stromal components
- Features of anaplasia include markedly increased (3x) tumor cell nuclei with hyperchromasia and multipolar mitotic figures
- Only diffuse anaplasia clinically/therapeutically important; therefore, differentiation from focal anaplasia essential
- Anaplasia correlates with resistance to chemotherapy, and with *p53* mutations in tumor

CLINICAL ISSUES

Epidemiology
- Incidence
  - 1/8,000 children
    - Approximately 85% of pediatric renal malignancies
- Age
  - Peak incidence: 2-3 years
    - 98% of cases in children < 10 years of age
    - Very uncommon in adults
    - Possibility of other uncommon tumor types needs to be excluded before accepting a tumor as Wilms in adults

Presentation
- Abdominal mass is most common presentation
  - Often detected by parents while bathing or clothing child
- Pain, hematuria, hypertension, acute abdominal crisis are other common presentations

Treatment
- In general, COG (which includes NWTS now) advocates primary resection; further therapy is determined by stage and "favorable" or "unfavorable" histology of resected tumor
  - Post-nephrectomy, stage I and favorable-histology stage II tumors given vincristine and dactinomycin (18 weeks)
  - Stage II tumors with LOH and stage III tumors given vincristine, dactinomycin, and doxorubicin (triple therapy) (24 weeks)
    - Stage III patients patients in addition receive radiotherapy
    - Stage III tumors demonstrating LOH receive standard triple therapy regimen plus cyclophosphamide and etoposide
  - Stage IV tumors given triple therapy (24 weeks) together with abdominal radiotherapy for local residual disease &/or whole-lung radiotherapy if lung metastases visualized on chest radiography

  - Patients with stage II to IV Wilms with diffuse anaplasia treated more aggressively
    - Cyclophosphamide/carboplatin/etoposide and vincristine/doxorubicin/cyclophosphamide (30 weeks) plus radiation therapy
    - Stage I tumors with diffuse anaplasia treated like nonanaplastic tumors
  - Adjuvant chemotherapy now avoided for young patients (< 2 years) with small (< 550 g nephrectomy weight) stage I favorable histology Wilms tumor
    - Pathologic evaluation of lymph nodes an essential requirement for this approach
- SIOP advocates pre-operative therapy followed by surgical resection; further therapy determined by response to prior therapy
  - Before resection, cases without metastasis receive vincristine and dactinomycin (4 weeks); those with metastases receive vincristine, dactinomycin, and doxorubicin (6 weeks)
  - Additional therapy given is based on residual tumor in nephrectomy specimen
    - Stage I residual disease: Additional vincristine and dactinomycin (4 weeks)
    - Stage II and III residual tumors: Adjuvant vincristine, dactinomycin, and doxorubicin (27 weeks)
    - Stage II with lymph node metastasis and all stage III patients: Additional radiotherapy
    - Children with stage IV Wilms tumor initially started on 3 drug regimen; those with incomplete remission switched to ifosfamide, carboplatin, etoposide, and doxorubicin

Prognosis
- In spite of differences in management, survivals are similar with both the NWTS and SIOP protocols
- Overall survival currently > 90%
- Most significant unfavorable factors include
  - High stage at presentation and diffuse anaplasia (unfavorable histology)
- Majority of pre-therapy Wilms tumors with blastemal predominance are very sensitive to therapy

NEPHROBLASTOMA (WILMS TUMOR)

○ Blastemal-type post-therapy tumors are considered resistant to chemotherapy and treated as anaplastic tumors in SIOP protocols

MACROSCOPIC FEATURES

General Features

- Most tumors are unicentric
  ○ 7% multicentric and 5% bilateral
- Usually sharply demarcated from surrounding renal parenchyma, and very often encapsulated
  ○ Cut surface often shows soft consistency and is uniformly pale gray or tan
  ○ Tumors with prominent stromal component are firm with whorled cut surface

Specimen Handling and Sections to be Submitted

- All pediatric renal tumor specimens must be weighed
  ○ Weight determines decisions about therapy in some cases, e.g., no chemotherapy in younger patients with stage I tumor and total kidney weight < 550 g
- Before opening specimen, perihilar and perirenal lymph nodes should be identified and sampled
  ○ Lack of pathologic evaluation of lymph nodes excludes some (otherwise qualifying) patients from "no-chemotherapy-required" approach
- In addition to inking entire surface of specimen, areas with suspected ruptures may be inked in colors different from rest
- After opening specimen and sampling its cut surface for tumor banking and other special studies, specimen should be fixed overnight
- Sampling from renal sinus and margins of resection are essential for adequate staging
- Most sections taken from tumor must include tumor-renal parenchyma interface, to evaluate tumor borders
- Documenting exact site from which each block is obtained is necessary
  ○ This is often critical for evaluating focal vs. diffuse anaplasia and for addressing staging issues in some cases

MICROSCOPIC PATHOLOGY

Histologic Features

- Most characteristic: Triphasic pattern consisting of undifferentiated blastema and epithelial and stromal components
  ○ Many tumors have only biphasic or monophasic features
- **Blastemal cells**: Small, closely packed, mitotically active cells with scant cytoplasm, overlapping nuclei, evenly distributed coarse chromatin, and usually small nucleoli
  ○ Tumors with diffuse blastemal pattern, often have infiltrative margins, unlike most other types of Wilms tumor
- **Epithelial components**: Ranging from primitive rosette-like tubules to well-formed maturing and mature tubules, ill-formed glomerular structures, variable papillary architecture
  ○ Mucinous or squamous differentiation may occasionally be present
    ▪ Tumors with extensive heterologous differentiation are designated "teratoid Wilms tumor" by some
- **Stromal component**: Nondescript spindle cells, smooth muscle, skeletal muscle, or fibroblastic differentiation
  ○ Occasionally, fat, cartilage, bone, ganglion cells, or neuroglia are also seen
- Most components in Wilms tumor correspond to structures at various stages of nephrogenesis
  ○ Rarely, mesenchymal elements are heterologous
    ▪ Heterologous elements may include mucinous, cartilaginous, neuroglial elements, etc.
- Post-chemotherapy nephroblastomas are subclassified into 3 prognostic groups
  ○ Further therapy depends on risk assessment (SIOP) and is divided into
    ▪ Tumors with low risk, intermediate risk, or high risk
  ○ Typical therapy-induced changes include coagulative tumor necrosis, fibrosis, foamy, &/or hemosiderin-laden macrophages
  ○ Post-therapy tumors are often regressive type or completely necrotic
    ▪ Complete necrosis is not seen in pre-therapy specimens
  ○ Tumors with at least 1/3 viable area typed according to predominant component in viable areas (> 2/3 of viable areas)
    ▪ Tumors with < 1/3 viable area are considered completely necrotic
    ▪ Tumors with < 2/3 of dominant histology in viable area are considered mixed type
  ○ Post-therapy blastemal-type tumor (blastemal component constituting more than 2/3rd of viable tumor [SIOP]) considered high-risk tumor
  ○ Tumors with regressive changes occupying > 2/3 of tumor considered regressive-type tumor
- Tumors with anaplasia are only type of nephroblastoma with "unfavorable" histology by NWTS/COG
  ○ Approximately 5% WTs show anaplasia
    ▪ Features of anaplasia include markedly enlarged tumor cell nuclei with hyperchromasia and multipolar mitotic figures
  ○ Anaplasia is rare before 2 years of age and involves 13% of tumors beyond age 5
  ○ Anaplasia correlates with resistance to chemotherapy and with *p53* mutations in tumor
  ○ Only diffuse anaplasia clinically/therapeutically important; therefore, differentiation from focal anaplasia essential
  ○ Anaplasia is considered focal when only present
    ▪ In single/multiple sharply localized regions
    ▪ Within primary intrarenal tumor, surrounded by nonanaplastic tumor
    ▪ With no severe nuclear unrest (pleomorphism and hyperchromasia) in rest of tumor

- **■** And is not present in intravascular tumor
- Tumor with anaplasia not meeting these criteria is classified as tumor with diffuse anaplasia

Lymphatic/Vascular Invasion

- Invasion of renal sinus veins or lymphatics considered stage II in both COG and SIOP staging systems
  - o Intrarenal vascular invasion does not upstage tumor

Predominant Pattern/Injury Type

- Neoplastic

Predominant Cell/Compartment Type

- Nephrogenic blastema

ANCILLARY TESTS

Immunohistochemistry

- Immunoreactive for WT1 protein
  - o Immunoreactivity usually limited to blastemal and epithelial elements; stroma negative
  - o Blastemal cells may label for desmin, but not other muscle markers like actin, myogenin, MYOD1
  - o Vimentin and cytokeratin negative or focal positive in blastema: Cytokeratin usually positive in epithelial components
    - **■** CK7 may also be positive in more differentiated epithelial cells
  - o pax-2 usually positive

DIFFERENTIAL DIAGNOSIS

Other Small Blue-Cell Tumors

- Differentiation from blastemal Wilms tumor
  - o Presence of nuclear molding, early tubular differentiation with organized nuclear alignment around early lumina is typical of blastema
    - **■** Presence of true tubular lumina always favors Wilms tumor
  - o Immunostains may be required in small biopsies to exclude other possibilities, including neuroblastoma, rhabdomyosarcoma, and PNET

Immature Teratoma

- Differentiation from Wilms tumor with extensive heterologous differentiation (so-called teratoid Wilms)
  - o Teratoma shows organized (organ-like) differentiation (e.g., ciliated epithelium with smooth muscle and cartilage, etc.)
  - o Wilms tumor is characterized by random juxtaposition of different tissue types
  - o Presence of nephrogenic blastema with true tubules and other nephrogenic patterns supports diagnosis of Wilms tumor

Metanephric Adenoma

- Differentiation from epithelial-predominant Wilms tumor
  - o Uniform, nonoverlapping nuclei with delicate chromatin and inconspicuous nucleoli and lack of mitotic figures in metanephric adenoma

- o Immunostain for WT1 may be negative or weak and focally positive in metanephric adenoma vs. usually strong and diffuse in Wilms tumor
- o CD57 is positive

Papillary Renal Cell Carcinoma (Type 1, Solid Glomeruloid Variant)

- Differentiation from epithelial-predominant Wilms tumor with papillary areas
  - o Papillary RCC often with foamy macrophages
  - o Glomeruloid tufts in tumor occasionally with higher-grade cytology, including more prominent nucleoli, compared to cells forming tubules
  - o AMACR and CK7 diffuse and strongly positive and WT1 usually negative in papillary RCC
    - **■** In Wilms tumor, AMACR negative, CK7 usually negative or focal positive, and WT1 diffuse and strong positive

DIAGNOSTIC CHECKLIST

Clinically Relevant Pathologic Features

- Gross appearance
  - o Most Wilms tumors, other than those with diffuse blastemal pattern, are well circumscribed
    - **■** It differentiates them radiologically and grossly from more aggressive pediatric tumors like rhabdoid tumor of kidney, as well as most mesoblastic nephromas

Pathologic Interpretation Pearls

- Reporting of presence or absence of anaplasia is 1 essential component of surgical pathology report on Wilms tumor
  - o Diffuse anaplasia, when present, is usually apparent in most tumor sections
  - o Anaplasia at any margin, or in extrarenal sites, is considered diffuse anaplasia
  - o Anaplasia present in random biopsy (although rarely performed) is considered diffuse anaplasia

SELECTED REFERENCES

1. Davidoff AM: Wilms' tumor. Curr Opin Pediatr. 21(3):357-64, 2009
2. Huang CC et al: Predicting relapse in favorable histology Wilms tumor using gene expression analysis: a report from the Renal Tumor Committee of the Children's Oncology Group. Clin Cancer Res. 15(5):1770-8, 2009
3. Vujanic GM et al: The pathology of Wilms' tumour (nephroblastoma): The International Society of Paediatric Oncology approach. J Clin Pathol. Epub ahead of print, 2009
4. Cerrato F et al: Different mechanisms cause imprinting defects at the IGF2/H19 locus in Beckwith-Wiedemann syndrome and Wilms' tumour. Hum Mol Genet. 17(10):1427-35, 2008
5. Sonn G et al: Management of Wilms tumor: current standard of care. Nat Clin Pract Urol. 5(10):551-60, 2008
6. Dome JS et al: Treatment of anaplastic histology Wilms' tumor: results from the fifth National Wilms' Tumor Study. J Clin Oncol. 24(15):2352-8, 2006

NEPHROBLASTOMA (WILMS TUMOR)

Staging of Pediatric Renal Tumors (Children's Oncology Group)

Stage	Main Pathologic Feature	Details of Pathologic Findings
I	Tumor limited to kidney and completely resected	Renal capsule intact
		No invasion of lymphatics or veins of renal sinus
		No prior biopsy
		No metastases
		Margins negative
II	Tumor extends beyond kidney but completely resected	Tumor penetrates renal capsule
		Tumor invades lymphatics or veins in renal sinus
		Tumor invades renal vein, but vein margin negative
		No metastases
		Margins negative
III	Residual tumor or nonhematogenous metastases confined to abdomen	Involves abdominal lymph nodes
		Peritoneal contamination or implants
		Tumor spillage of any degree occurring before or during surgery
		Gross residual tumor in abdomen
		Biopsy of tumor (including fine needle aspiration)
		Resection margin involved by tumor
IV	Hematogenous metastases or spread beyond abdomen	
V	Bilateral renal tumors	Tumor on each side to be staged separately and reported as substage on that side (e.g., stage V; substage III [right], substage I [left])

Revised SIOP Working Classification of Nephroblastoma after Neo-Adjuvant Therapy

Stage	Risk Level	Residual Tumor Type
I	Low-risk tumors	Cystic partially differentiated nephroblastoma
		Completely necrotic nephroblastoma
II	Intermediate-risk tumors	Nephroblastoma, epithelial type, stromal type, mixed type, or regressive type
		Nephroblastoma, focal anaplasia
III	High-risk tumors	Nephroblastoma, blastemal type
		Nephroblastoma, diffuse anaplasia

7. Grundy PE et al: Loss of heterozygosity for chromosomes 1p and 16q is an adverse prognostic factor in favorable-histology Wilms tumor: a report from the National Wilms Tumor Study Group. J Clin Oncol. 23(29):7312-21, 2005
8. Fukuzawa R et al: Epigenetic differences between Wilms' tumours in white and east-Asian children. Lancet. 363(9407):446-51, 2004
9. Vujanić GM et al: Revised International Society of Paediatric Oncology (SIOP) working classification of renal tumors of childhood. Med Pediatr Oncol. 38(2):79-82, 2002
10. Green DM et al: Treatment with nephrectomy only for small, stage I/favorable histology Wilms' tumor: a report from the National Wilms' Tumor Study Group. J Clin Oncol. 19(17):3719-24, 2001
11. Beckwith JB: National Wilms Tumor Study: an update for pathologists. Pediatr Dev Pathol. 1(1):79-84, 1998
12. Beckwith JB: Nephrogenic rests and the pathogenesis of Wilms tumor: developmental and clinical considerations. Am J Med Genet. 79(4):268-73, 1998
13. Faria P et al: Focal versus diffuse anaplasia in Wilms tumor--new definitions with prognostic significance: a report from the National Wilms Tumor Study Group. Am J Surg Pathol. 20(8):909-20, 1996
14. Green DM et al: Treatment outcomes in patients less than 2 years of age with small, stage I, favorable-histology Wilms' tumors: a report from the National Wilms' Tumor Study. J Clin Oncol. 11(1):91-5, 1993
15. Breslow N et al: Prognostic factors in nonmetastatic, favorable histology Wilms' tumor. Results of the Third National Wilms' Tumor Study. Cancer. 68(11):2345-53, 1991
16. Beckwith JB et al: Histopathology and prognosis of Wilms tumors: results from the First National Wilms' Tumor Study. Cancer. 41(5):1937-48, 1978

NEPHROBLASTOMA (WILMS TUMOR)

Microscopic Features

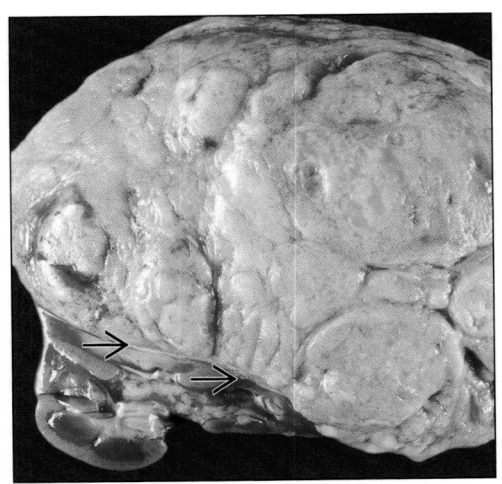

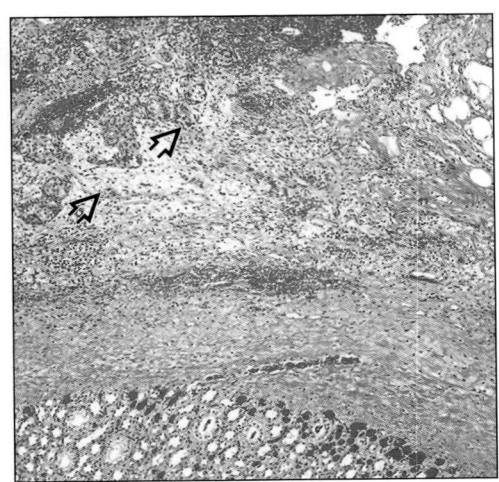

(Left) Most Wilms tumors are well delineated, often with a prominent capsule ➡. The only notable exception to well circumscription may be in a Wilms tumor with diffuse blastemal pattern. The capsule should not be stripped. (Right) Prior biopsies (including FNA) result in upstaging the tumors to stage III (COG) with the presumption that biopsies lead to tumor spillage ➡ as was seen in this case. Pre-resection or pre-chemotherapy biopsies of these tumors are not performed routinely.

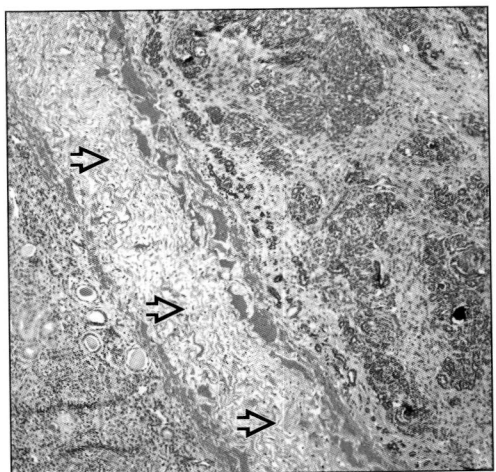

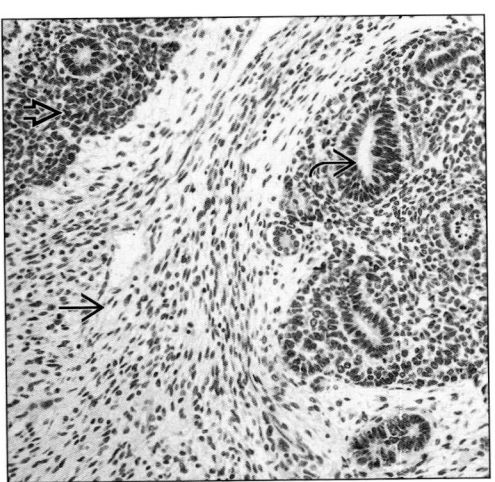

(Left) The usual well-circumscribed nature of a Wilms tumor with a prominent capsule ➡ is seen. Tumors with diffuse blastemal pattern, however, often show aggressive, infiltrative borders. (Right) Triphasic patterns (blastemal ➡, epithelial ➡, and stromal ➡) are characteristic of Wilms tumor but not essential. Some tumors may only be biphasic or monophasic. Within the epithelial and stromal components, considerable heterogeneity in histology may be present.

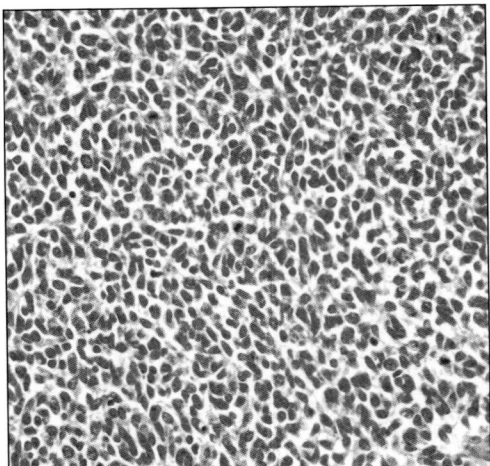

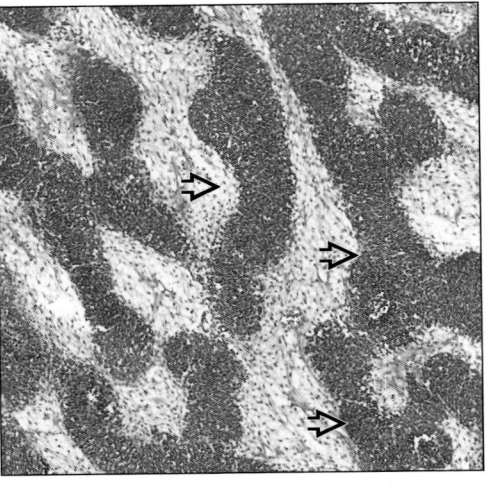

(Left) This image shows a blastemal pattern WT. Some tumors may be composed of noncohesive sheets of blastemal elements alone. This is known as WT with diffuse blastemal pattern and is considered an aggressive pattern in the tumor. However, most tumors with blastemal pattern are responsive to current therapeutic approaches. (Right) In addition to the diffuse pattern, blastemal patterns may show more organized, serpentine ➡, or nodular growth patterns with myxoid stroma.

NEPHROBLASTOMA (WILMS TUMOR)

Microscopic Features

(Left) In tumors with nodular growth pattern, the blastema consists of variable-sized nodules in a usually loose, myxoid mesenchymal background ⇗. Tumors with such organized blastemal patterns usually lack the invasive front seen in diffuse blastemal pattern tumors. *(Right)* Blastema consists of small, closely packed, mitotically active cells with scant cytoplasm, overlapping nuclei, evenly distributed coarse chromatin, and usually small nucleoli.

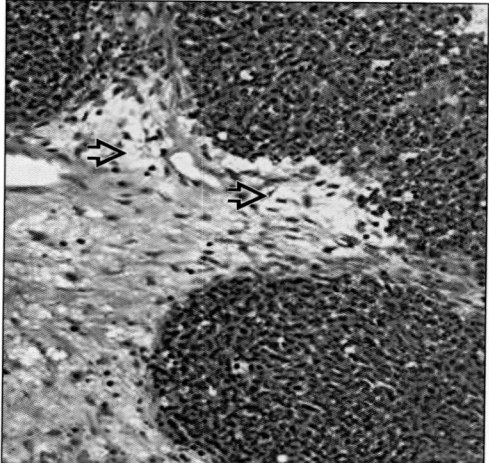
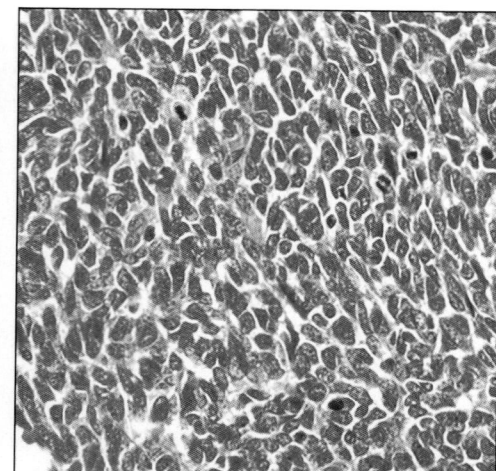

(Left) Epithelial areas in Wilms tumors most often show tubular differentiation of variable degrees, ranging from poorly developed tubular structures embedded in blastema to tubules showing well-formed lumina, usually lined by primitive and mitotically active cells. *(Right)* Glomerular differentiation in Wilms tumor may range from primitive or attempted glomerular formations ⇗ to almost mature glomeruli closely resembling those of normal kidneys.

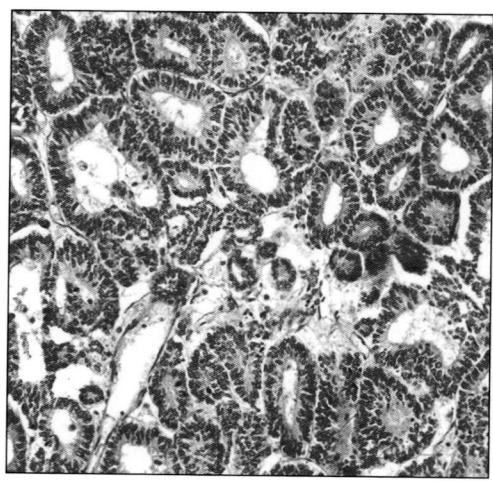
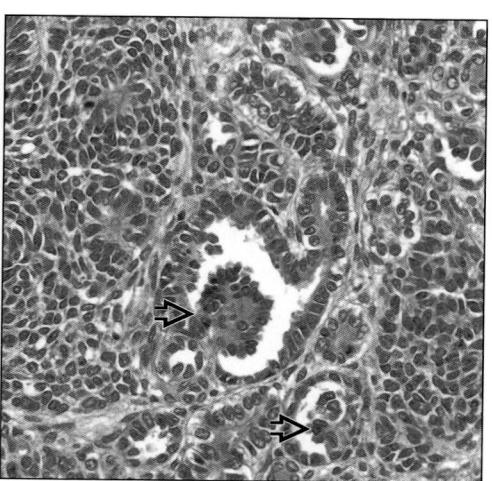

(Left) Papillary formations are also common in epithelial areas. Very often, the lining cells appear primitive ⇗, but differentiation to more mature cells may also be seen, particularly in patients who receive prior chemotherapy. *(Right)* Among the stromal components, rhabdomyoblastic differentiation ⇗ is quite common, and is the most frequent heterologous mesenchymal differentiation type in Wilms tumor. This differentiation is particularly common in cases receiving prior chemotherapy.

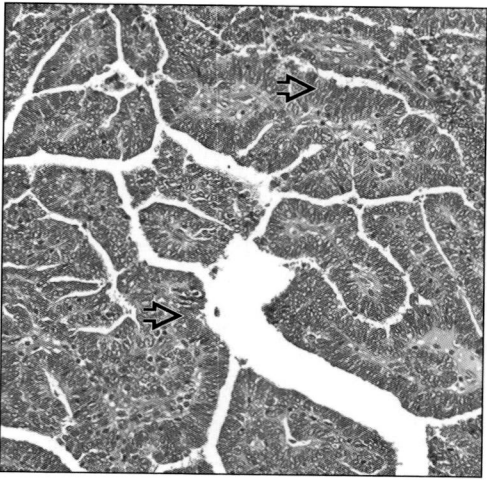
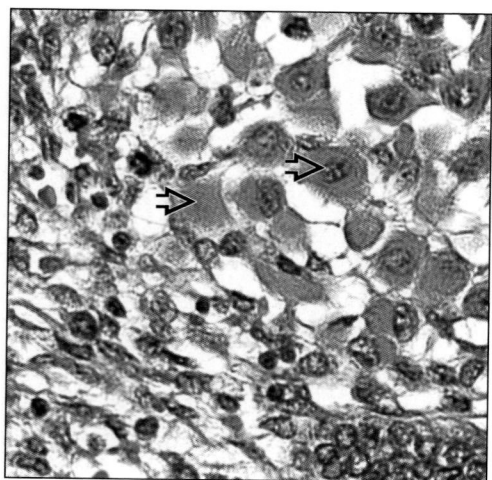

1

NEPHROBLASTOMA (WILMS TUMOR)

Microscopic Features

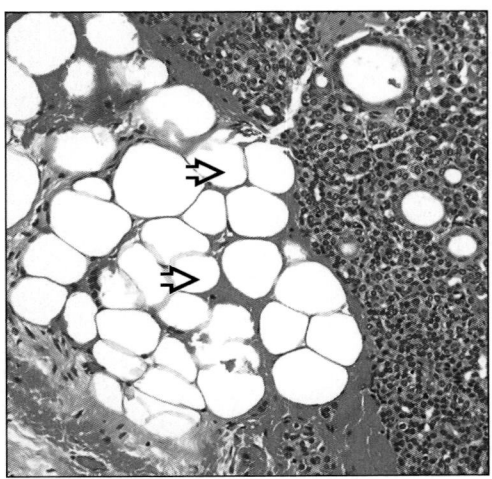

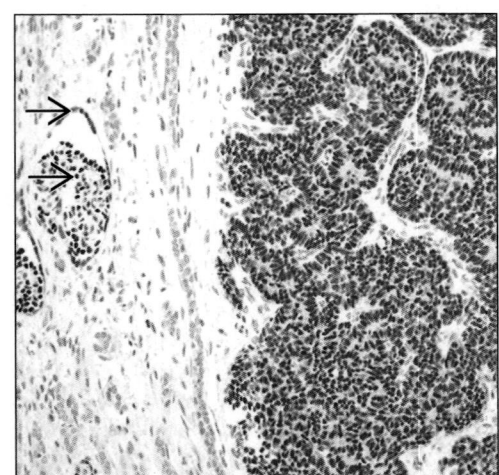

(Left) Undifferentiated, myxoid, fibroblastic, myofibroblastic, adipocytic ⊅, smooth muscle, cartilage, bone, and neuroglial type cells are the other stromal components that may be present in WT. *(Right)* WT1 staining usually shows diffuse nuclear positivity in the blastemal and epithelial areas of the tumor, with the stroma being negative. Note the positive reaction in the glomerular mesangium and Bowman capsule lining ⊅ that acts as an internal control for WT1.

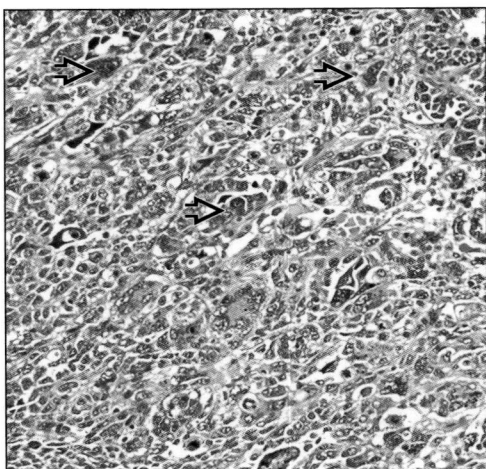

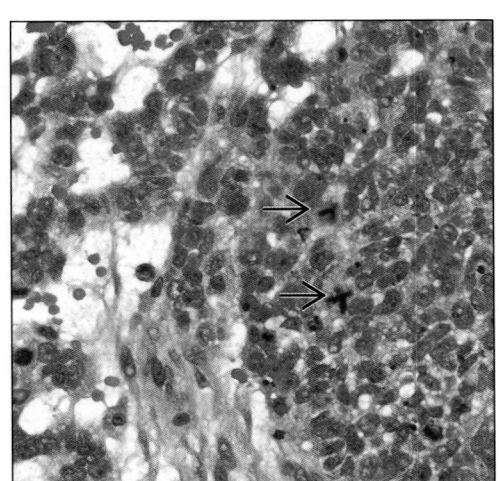

(Left) Tumors showing anaplasia are now considered the only tumor type with unfavorable histology. Features of anaplasia include markedly enlarged ⊅ tumor cell nuclei (3x in size compared to the rest of the tumor cells), hyperchromasia, and multipolar mitotic figures. *(Right)* Multipolar mitotic figures ⊅ are considered a diagnostic feature of anaplasia in Wilms tumor. Only diffuse, and not focal, anaplasia is used in making therapeutic decisions in Wilms tumor.

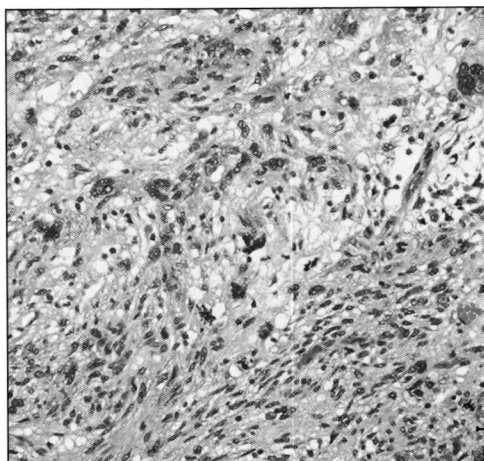

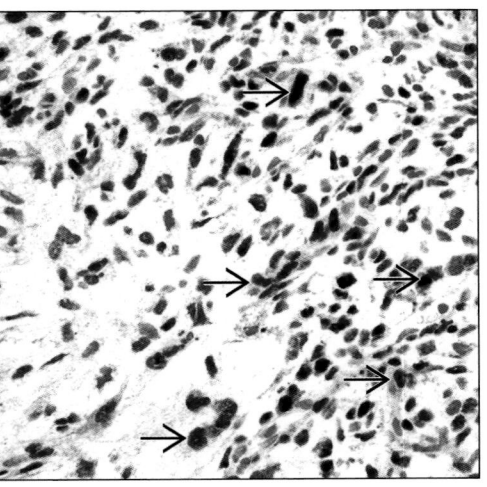

(Left) Anaplasia may be present in any or all the 3 components of Wilms tumor. This image shows anaplastic features in the mesenchymal element of a tumor. Focal vs. diffuse anaplasia essentially do not convey the relative amount but the distribution and location of anaplasia. *(Right)* Most anaplastic tumors show p53 gene mutations, corresponding to immunohistochemical overexpression ⊅ in majority of cases. p53 mutations have been associated with resistance to chemotherapy.

NEPHROBLASTOMA (WILMS TUMOR)

Gross and Microscopic Features, Post-Therapy

(Left) While NWTS/COG recommends pretherapy resection of most tumors, SIOP protocols (Europe) advocate chemotherapy before resection. Most post-therapy tumors show areas of necrosis and cystic change ⇨. Note the separate nonaffected tumor nodule in perinephric fat ➡. *(Right)* Another gross photograph of a post-therapy WT shows extensive necrosis ⇨. While focal necrosis is common, extensive or total necrosis is very uncommon in specimens without prior treatment.

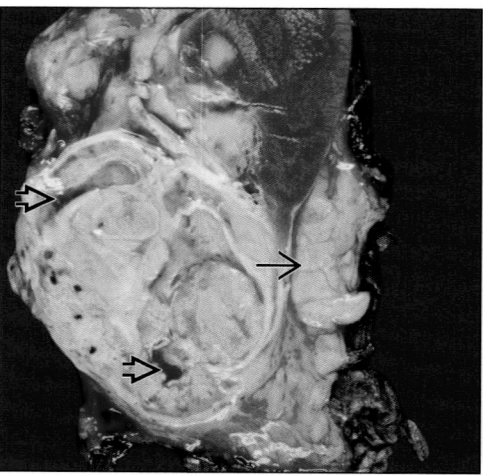
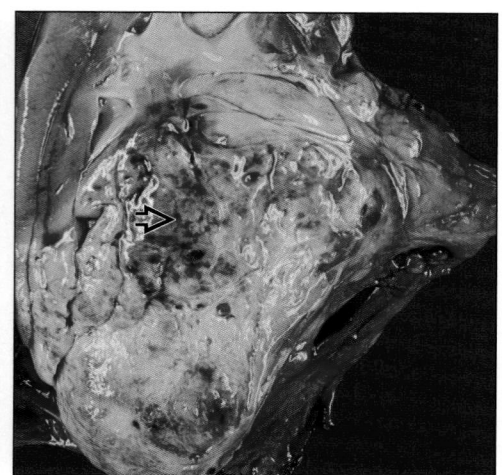

(Left) Post-therapy tumors often show large areas with foamy ⇨ or hemosiderin-laden macrophages. Rare, differentiated tubules may be present in such areas, and these are regarded as regressive changes ⇨. *(Right)* Coagulative-type necrosis is common in post-therapy Wilms tumor. While dying tumor cells with vaguely recognizable nuclear details ⇨ may help in the diagnosis of a WT, these areas with incompletely necrotic outlines are included among "completely necrotic" areas (SIOP).

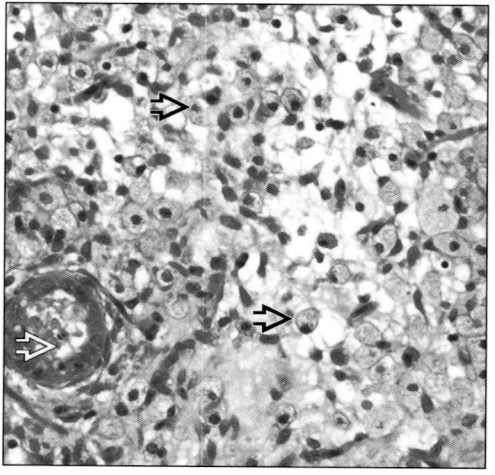
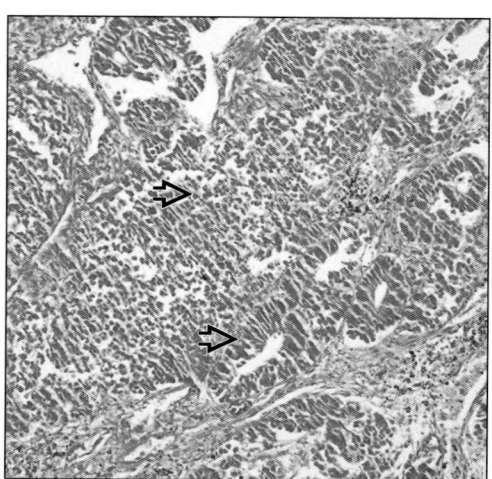

(Left) Extensive skeletal muscle differentiation is often seen in WT, particularly post-therapy. While tumors resected before therapy more often show blastemal or mixed (triphasic) phenotypes, post-chemotherapy WTs are mostly regressive type or completely necrotic. About 10% of post-therapy WTs are blastemal type. These are considered chemo resistant and, together with diffuse anaplasia tumors, are regarded as "high risk" by SIOP. *(Right)* Post-therapy WT often show necrosis ⇨ and squamous differentiation ⇨.

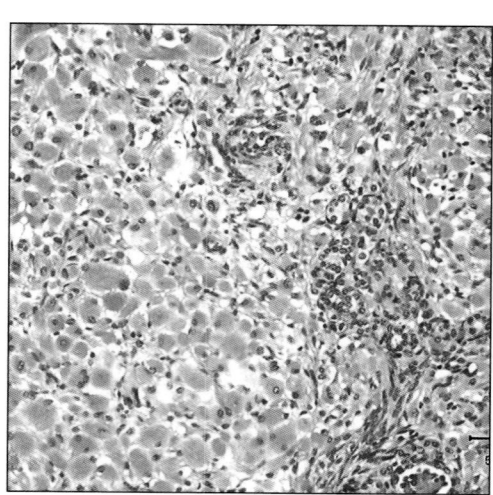
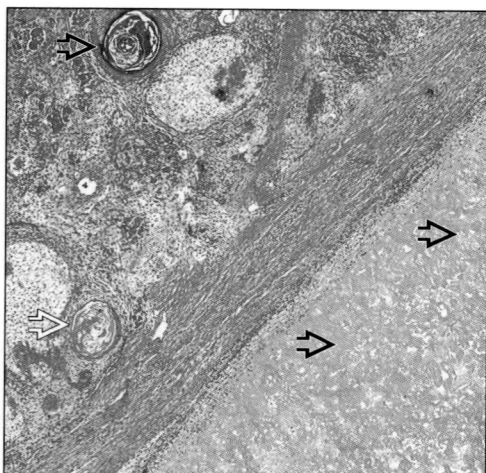

NEPHROBLASTOMA (WILMS TUMOR)

Microscopic Features, Post-Therapy and Metastases

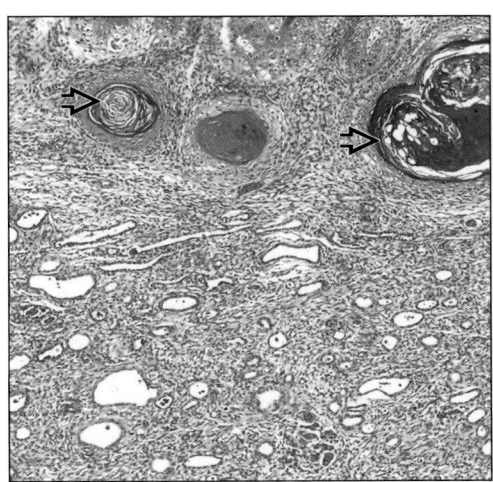

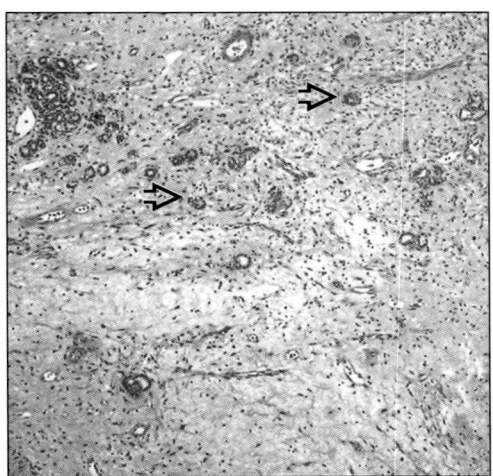

(Left) While squamous differentiation may be seen in pre-treatment cases, this is a more common feature in post-chemotherapy residual tumors ⮊. Tumors with such extensive features have been regarded as "teratoid" WT by some authors. *(Right)* A majority of post-therapy WT show extensive fibrosis. Relatively mature-appearing tubules in such a background are regarded as epithelial rests ⮊ and not considered in the classification of post-therapy tumors.

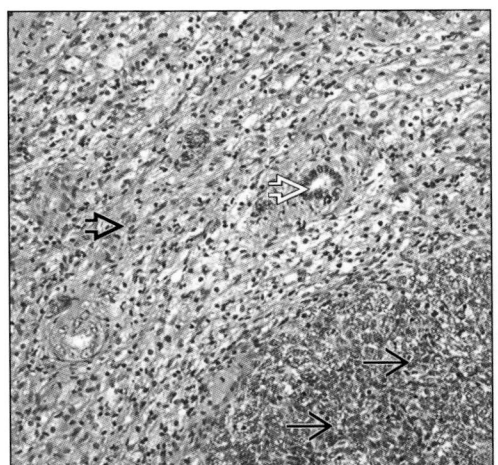

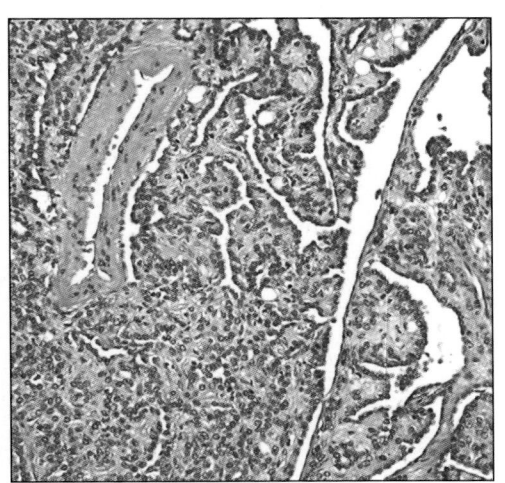

(Left) Post-therapy WT shows histiocytic response ⮊, few "cell rests" ⮊, and residual blastemal elements ⮊. SIOP requires determination of proportion of blastemal elements in the viable areas, for risk stratification and further therapy. *(Right)* Prominent papillary formations, appearing well differentiated, may be present in untreated cases of WT. However, these features are more common in post-therapy Wilms and may raise the possibility of a papillary renal cell carcinoma.

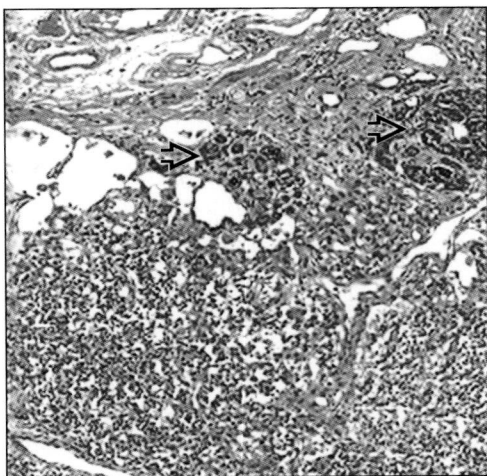

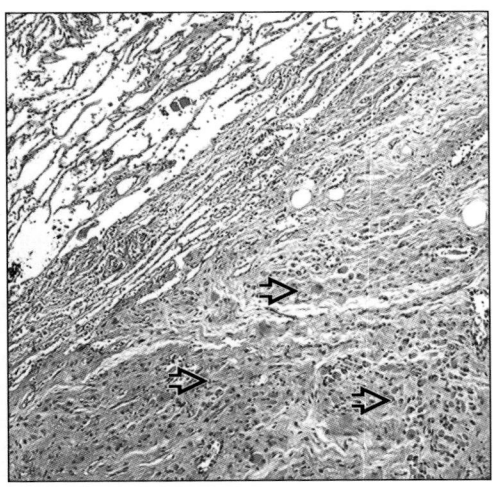

(Left) Wilms tumor mainly metastasizes to the "three Ls": Lymph nodes ⮊, liver, and lungs. Other sites of metastasis are rare. *(Right)* Lung is a common site of metastasis for Wilms tumor. In spite of the basic differences in therapeutic approaches between COG and SIOP, overlaps are not uncommon. Most stage IV diseases in COG are treated by chemotherapy, and post-therapy resection specimens often show regression or differentiation, e.g., rhabdomyoblasts ⮊.

CYSTIC PARTIALLY DIFFERENTIATED NEPHROBLASTOMA

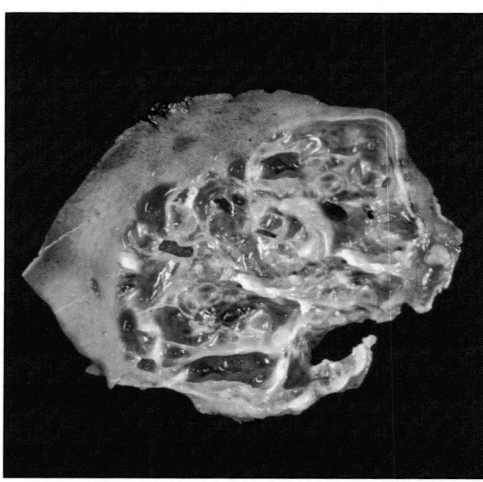

Multicystic tumor in pediatric kidneys may represent, among others, a cystic nephroma or cystic partially differentiated nephroblastoma. Gross distinction between the 2 is difficult.

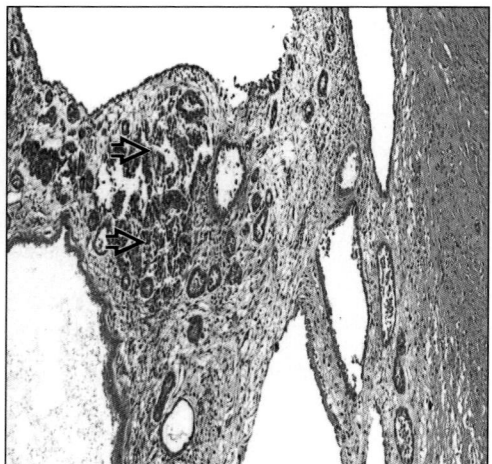

Immature blastemal or differentiating epithelial elements ⊳ within the septations of a multicystic tumor, without forming a nodular or mass-forming expansion, is diagnostic of CPDN.

TERMINOLOGY

Abbreviations
- Cystic partially differentiated nephroblastoma (CPDN)

Definitions
- Entirely multilocular cystic tumor, mostly occurring before 2 years of age
  - Tumor with thin septations showing clusters of blastemal cells admixed with their derivatives
  - No expansile masses altering smooth contours of septae
  - Luminal papillonodular protrusions are acceptable
    - Such tumors classified as papillonodular type of CPDN

CLINICAL ISSUES

Histology vs. Radiologic Evaluation
- Radiologic distinction of cystic nephroma (CN), CPDN, and cystic Wilms tumor (CWT) is quite difficult
  - CT shows well-defined expansile cystic masses
    - May also have solid enhancing areas
- Definitive discrimination between the 3 only possible on histologic evaluation
  - Distinction is essential for further therapy, since biologic behaviors are different
    - CN: Benign
    - CPDN: Usually nonaggressive clinical behavior; rare recurrences reported
    - CWT: Malignant

Treatment
- COG recommends primary resection
  - No further therapy in stage I tumors
  - Rare stage II or higher stage tumors receive chemotherapy
- SIOP recommends therapy before resection

  - Since radiological evaluation not definitive, pre-surgery chemotherapy quite common in Europe
  - Recently, some experts have questioned need of pre-surgery chemotherapy of cystic renal masses without any obvious solid components

Prognosis
- Only 2 cases with recurrence, both with incomplete resection or spillage during surgery

MACROSCOPIC FEATURES

General Features
- Often large (up to 18 cm) multicystic tumors
- No apparent solid areas

MICROSCOPIC PATHOLOGY

Histologic Features
- Multilocular cystic tumor
  - Cysts usually lined by flat or cuboidal epithelium
  - Cyst walls with blastemal clusters or their epithelial derivatives
    - Mesenchymal elements also common
  - Some tumors with papillary or papillonodular excrescences protruding into cyst lumina
  - No expansile masses that alter smooth shape of septae

DIFFERENTIAL DIAGNOSIS

Cystic Nephroma
- Tumor composed entirely of cysts and cyst septa without any solid expansile areas or mural nodules
- Septations with arbitrarily chosen thickness of < 5 mm
- No blastemal elements in the septae
- Unlike cystic nephromas of adults, pediatric CN without any ovarian-type stroma

CYSTIC PARTIALLY DIFFERENTIATED NEPHROBLASTOMA

Key Facts

Terminology

- Cystic partially differentiated nephroblastoma (CPDN)
  - Entirely multilocular cystic tumor, mostly occurring before 2 years of age
  - Tumor with thin septations showing clusters of blastemal cells admixed with their derivatives
  - No expansile masses altering smooth contours of septae

Clinical Issues

- Radiologic distinction of cystic nephroma (CN), CPDN, and cystic Wilms tumor (CWT) is quite difficult
  - Definitive discrimination between the 3 only possible on histologic evaluation
  - Distinction is essential for further therapy, since biologic behaviors are different

Cystic Wilms Tumor

- Variably cystic tumor with solid expansile blastemal, epithelial, &/or mesenchymal elements
- Often, but not always, seen after chemotherapy
  - Large areas of necrosis may be present, particularly in post-chemotherapy setting

Cystic Renal Dysplasia

- Usually diffuse and bilateral
  - May be localized and segmental
- Often associated with obstruction to urinary outflow
  - Ureter and pelvicalyceal system distorted and atretic
    - May be dilated, if obstruction distal to pelvi-ureteric junction
- Presence of "primitive ducts" lined by cuboidal to columnar epithelium, surrounded by cellular mesenchyme = histologic hallmark
- Larger cysts lined by more flat epithelium, surrounded by fibrotic stroma, also common
- Small islands of cartilage and occasionally smooth muscle stroma may be present
- Ducts and cysts usually separated by fibrous stroma with scattered glomeruli, sometimes appearing immature or cystic

Localized or Segmental Cystic Kidney Disease

- Gross and microscopic appearance of cysts similar to that in autosomal dominant polycystic kidney disease (ADPKD)

- Grossly, consists of clusters of spherical, thin-walled cysts
  - Cysts separated by areas of uninvolved kidney
- Cysts lined by cuboidal to flattened epithelium
- Cystic dilatation of Bowman capsule often present
  - Glomerulocystic change may be a predominant finding in infants
- Cysts often separated by noncystic, relatively normal renal parenchyma

SELECTED REFERENCES

1. van den Hoek J et al: Cystic nephroma, cystic partially differentiated nephroblastoma and cystic Wilms' tumor in children: a spectrum with therapeutic dilemmas. Urol Int. 82(1):65-70, 2009
2. Baker JM et al: Stage III cystic partially differentiated nephroblastoma recurring after nephrectomy and chemotherapy. Pediatr Blood Cancer. 50(1):129-31, 2008
3. Blakely ML et al: Outcome of children with cystic partially differentiated nephroblastoma treated with or without chemotherapy. J Pediatr Surg. 38(6):897-900, 2003
4. Rajangam K et al: Partial nephrectomy in cystic partially differentiated nephroblastoma. J Pediatr Surg. 35(3):510-2, 2000
5. Joshi VV et al: Pathologic delineation of the papillonodular type of cystic partially differentiated nephroblastoma. A review of 11 cases. Cancer. 66(7):1568-77, 1990

IMAGE GALLERY

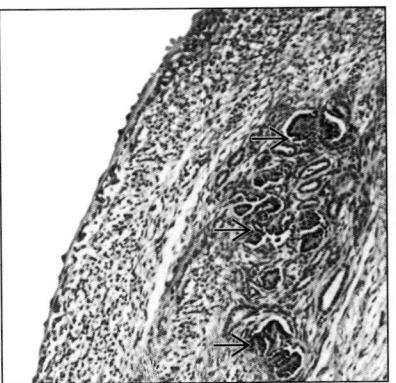 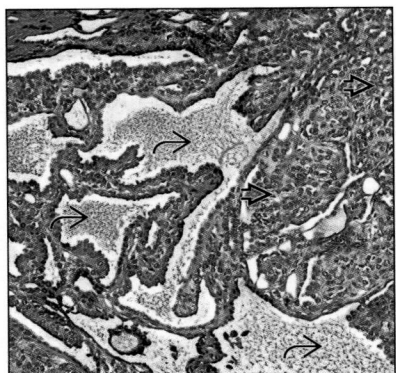 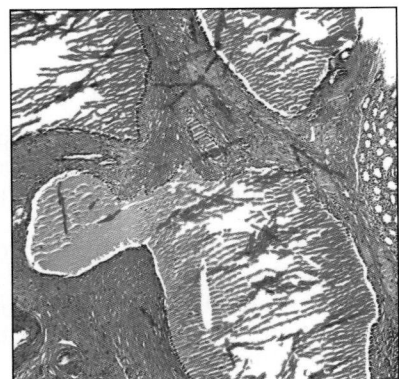

(Left) This image shows nests of differentiating epithelial ➔ as well as stromal components in the septum of a CPDN. The cell nests do not alter the smooth contours of the septae. *(Center)* This predominantly cystic ➔ tumor shows solid areas of differentiating blastema ➔. Such expansile areas preclude its consideration as a CPDN and are characteristic of cystic Wilms tumor. *(Right)* A multilocular cystic lesion with flat to cuboidal cyst lining and no nephrogenic elements in the septation is designated as cystic nephroma.

ANGIOMYOLIPOMA

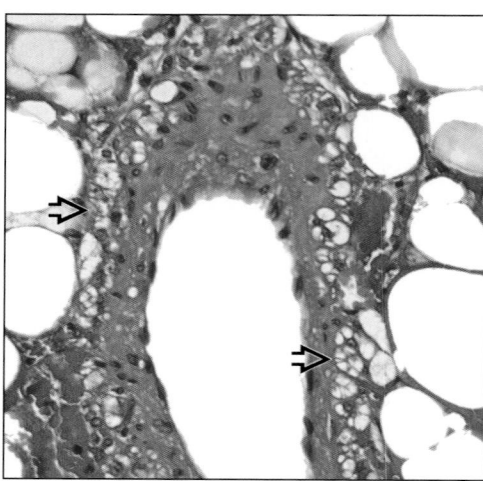

This hematoxylin & eosin section shows perivascular epithelioid cells (PEC) ➡. PEC is considered to be the cell of origin of AML and related tumors. However, no normal counterpart of PEC is known.

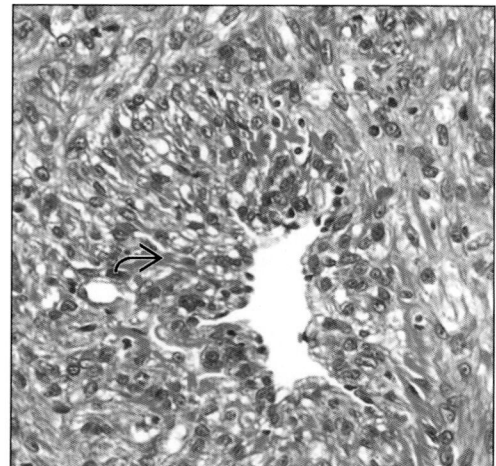

Smooth muscle cells are often seen originating from a vessel wall ➡. This typical finding helps in the accurate diagnosis in tumors with unusual histology (in "lipomatous" or "leiomyomatous" AML).

TERMINOLOGY

Abbreviations
- Angiomyolipoma (AML)

Definitions
- Mesenchymal tumor believed to originate from perivascular epithelioid cell (PEC)
- Closely related to other PEC-related group of tumors (e.g., lymphangioleiomyomatosis, clear cell "sugar" tumors of lung, pancreas, and uterus, PEComas, and cardiac rhabdomyomas)

ETIOLOGY/PATHOGENESIS

Tuberous Sclerosis Complex
- Approximately 55-75% patients with tuberous sclerosis develop renal AML
- Less than 50% of patients with renal AMLs have tuberous sclerosis
- Associated with genetic alterations in tuberous sclerosis genes, *TSC1* (9q34) and *TSC2* (16p13.3)
  - Sporadic AML more often show *TSC2* alterations

Mammalian Target of Rapamycin (mTOR) Pathway
- Proteins encoded by *TSC1* (hamartin) and *TSC2* genes (tuberin) function as a complex to negatively regulate mTOR signaling
  - Negative regulation done through activation of Ras homologue expressed in brain (*Rheb*)
    - *Rheb*: Specific GTPase is located downstream of tuberin
    - Altered *TSC* gene functions generate excessive *Rheb*-GTP
    - This leads to increased activated mTOR, an activator of multiple protein synthesis pathways and possible tumorigenesis
- Activated mTOR pathway markers overexpressed in AML and related tumors

CLINICAL ISSUES

Presentation
- Most sporadic cases diagnosed incidentally by radiological investigations for other conditions
- Multifocality and bilaterality is often associated with tuberous sclerosis
  - AMLs seen in patients with tuberous sclerosis also tend to manifest at younger age, are larger, and grow faster
- Presence of synchronous or metachronous involvement of other sites regarded as manifestation of multicentric disease rather than metastasis
- Small tumors usually asymptomatic
  - Larger tumors (usually > 4 cm) rarely present with hemorrhage and shock
    - Tumor size often increases in pregnancy and may increase risk of hemorrhage
  - Extreme multifocality occasionally associated with renal failure
- Classical fat-containing tumors often easily diagnosed on radiologic evaluation
- Tumors with scant fat or other uncommon features are difficult to diagnose radiologically
  - Rarely, intratumoral hemorrhage masks fat, hindering radiologic diagnosis

Treatment
- No treatment required in most asymptomatic, small, radiologically definite AMLs
  - Resection often delayed by surgeons until tumor attains size of 4 cm or greater

Prognosis
- Overwhelming majority with benign clinical behavior
- Retroperitoneal hemorrhage is rare complication that can be fatal

ANGIOMYOLIPOMA

Key Facts

Terminology

- Angiomyolipoma (AML)
- Mesenchymal tumors believed to originate from so-called perivascular epithelioid cell (PEC)
- Closely related to other PEC-related group of tumors (e.g., lymphangioleiomyomatosis, clear cell "sugar" tumors of lung, pancreas, and uterus, PEComas, and cardiac rhabdomyomas)

Etiology/Pathogenesis

- Approximately 55-75% patients of tuberous sclerosis with renal AML
- < 50% of AMLs in patients with tuberous sclerosis
- Associated with genetic alterations in tuberous sclerosis genes *TSC1* (9q34) and *TSC2* (16p13.3)

Clinical Issues

- Multifocality and bilaterality often associated with tuberous sclerosis
- Overwhelming majority with benign clinical behavior

Microscopic Pathology

- Typically contains adipose tissue, smooth muscle, and dystrophic vessels in variable proportions
- Uncommon types include predominantly lipomatous or leiomyomatous, lymphangioleiomyomatous, oncocytoma-like, sclerosing type, and angiomyolipoma with epithelial cysts
  - AMLs invariably positive for melanocytic markers (HMB-45, Melan-A[MART-1], MiTF)

  - Large tumor size important factor in this complication
- Rare aggressive behavior, particularly those with predominant epithelioid and other atypical features

IMAGE FINDINGS

CT Findings

- Unenhanced CT with thin sections usually permits specific diagnosis of renal AML by demonstrating presence of intratumoral fat
  - However, intratumoral fat not detectable reportedly in approximately 5% and possibly in many more of these tumors

MACROSCOPIC FEATURES

Key Findings

- Often well circumscribed but not encapsulated
- Mean size = 6 cm (range = 0.5-25 cm)
- Cut surface variable, reflecting relative proportion of fat, smooth muscle, or vessels in tumor

MICROSCOPIC PATHOLOGY

Histologic Features

- Typically contains adipose tissue, smooth muscle, and dystrophic vessels in variable proportions
  - Areas of mature adipose tissue are present in over 90% of tumors, at least focally
  - Smooth muscle component as fascicles of spindle cells or sheets of epithelioid cells with abundant eosinophilic granular cytoplasm
    - Tumors with prominent spindled smooth muscle frequently with thin-walled vessels showing hemangiopericytoma-like architecture
  - Smooth muscle cells often appear to originate and radiate from vessel walls
  - Thickened and hyalinized vessels with eccentric lumina seen in most cases

  - Mitotic activity very rare
- Uncommon types include predominantly lipomatous or leiomyomatous, lymphangioleiomyomatous, oncocytoma-like, and sclerosing type
- Smooth muscle predominant or exclusive tumors arising from renal capsule, so-called renal "capsulomas," often HMB-45 positive
  - Most experts believe that "capsulomas" are leiomyomatous AMLs
- AML with epithelial cysts (AMLEC), rare variant
  - Epithelial cysts lined by cuboidal to "hobnailed" cells
  - Layer of cellular, Müllerian-like stroma with prominent admixed chronic inflammation surrounding cysts in AML
  - Cysts believed to arise from trapped renal tubules by some and described as integral part of tumor by others
- Ultrastructural evaluation reveals
  - Spherical structures with internal lamellations, consistent with aberrant melanosomes
  - Rare type 2 premelanosomes
  - Rhomboid crystals in some cases

Lymphatic/Vascular Invasion

- Vascular invasion, including that of large renal sinus vessels, renal vein, or inferior vena cava may be present
  - No adverse influences on prognosis, if tumor otherwise typical

Lymph Nodes

- Regional lymph nodes occasionally contain angiomyolipomas
  - Considered tumor multicentricity
  - No such patients reported to die of disease progression

Predominant Pattern/Injury Type

- Triphasic

Predominant Cell/Compartment Type

- Mesenchymal, mixed

ANCILLARY TESTS

Immunohistochemistry

- Expression of melanocytic markers: HMB-45, Melan-A(MART-1), MiTF, tyrosinase
- More common in epithelioid cells
- Expression of smooth muscle markers (actin-sm and h-caldesmon)
- Negative immunoreactivity for epithelial markers (cytokeratin, EMA/MUC1), except in areas with cysts
- Periepithelial stroma in AMLEC: ER, PR, CD10 positive
- Immunohistochemistry is useful adjunct in tumors with unusual pattern, usually not necessary in triphasic tumors

DIFFERENTIAL DIAGNOSIS

Liposarcoma

- Mostly extrarenal, surrounding kidney
- Lack of dysmorphic vessels &/or smooth muscle component (unless a part of dedifferentiation)
- Negative staining for melanocytic markers (HMB-45, Melan-A[MART-1], MiTF)
  - Caution: Immunoreactivity in fat-predominant AML usually in very few cells
- Positive immunoreactivity for mdm2 and CDK4

Leiomyoma or Leiomyosarcoma

- Primary smooth muscle tumors are very rare in kidney
- No intratumoral fat or dysmorphic vessels are present even after careful search
- Melanocytic markers are negative

Renal Oncocytoma

- Cells usually arranged in nests and solid alveoli
- Uniform nuclei, with occasional foci of marked pleomorphism
- Presence of groups of smaller cells (oncoblasts)
- Positivity for epithelial markers and negative staining for melanocytic markers

DIAGNOSTIC CHECKLIST

Pathologic Interpretation Pearls

- Primary smooth muscle tumors of kidney are extremely rare
  - Smooth muscle-predominant AML should always be excluded before accepting such a diagnosis
  - Immunohistochemical staining for melanocytic markers of all primary smooth muscle tumors in kidney is reasonable and practical approach
- Lipomatous tumors lack large abnormal vessels
  - Fat-predominant AML to be excluded even if only rare dysmorphic vessels and focal spindle cells observed
    - Staining for melanocytic markers and careful evaluation for even focal positivity imperative in such lesions

SELECTED REFERENCES

1. Aydin H et al: Renal angiomyolipoma: clinicopathologic study of 194 cases with emphasis on the epithelioid histology and tuberous sclerosis association. Am J Surg Pathol. 33(2):289-97, 2009
2. Bonsib SM et al: Lymphatic differentiation in renal angiomyolipomas. Hum Pathol. 40(3):374-80, 2009
3. Boorjian SA et al: Hormone receptor expression in renal angiomyolipoma: clinicopathologic correlation. Urology. 72(4):927-32, 2008
4. Lane BR et al: Clinical correlates of renal angiomyolipoma subtypes in 209 patients: classic, fat poor, tuberous sclerosis associated and epithelioid. J Urol. 180(3):836-43, 2008
5. Matsuyama A et al: Sclerosing variant of epithelioid angiomyolipoma. Pathol Int. 58(5):306-10, 2008
6. Pan CC et al: Constant allelic alteration on chromosome 16p (TSC2 gene) in perivascular epithelioid cell tumour (PEComa): genetic evidence for the relationship of PEComa with angiomyolipoma. J Pathol. 214(3):387-93, 2008
7. Schade GR et al: Renal angiomyolipoma with intravascular extension into the inferior vena cava: a case report and review of the literature. Can J Urol. 15(2):4012-5, 2008
8. Seyam RM et al: Changing trends in presentation, diagnosis and management of renal angiomyolipoma: comparison of sporadic and tuberous sclerosis complex-associated forms. Urology. 72(5):1077-82, 2008
9. Kenerson H et al: Activation of the mTOR pathway in sporadic angiomyolipomas and other perivascular epithelioid cell neoplasms. Hum Pathol. 38(9):1361-71, 2007
10. Davis CJ et al: Cystic angiomyolipoma of the kidney: a clinicopathologic description of 11 cases. Mod Pathol. 19(5):669-74, 2006
11. Fine SW et al: Angiomyolipoma with epithelial cysts (AMLEC): a distinct cystic variant of angiomyolipoma. Am J Surg Pathol. 30(5):593-9, 2006
12. Kutikov A et al: Incidence of benign pathologic findings at partial nephrectomy for solitary renal mass presumed to be renal cell carcinoma on preoperative imaging. Urology. 68(4):737-40, 2006
13. Martignoni G et al: Oncocytoma-like angiomyolipoma. A clinicopathologic and immunohistochemical study of 2 cases. Arch Pathol Lab Med. 126(5):610-2, 2002
14. Zavala-Pompa A et al: Immunohistochemical study of microphthalmia transcription factor and tyrosinase in angiomyolipoma of the kidney, renal cell carcinoma, and renal and retroperitoneal sarcomas: comparative evaluation with traditional diagnostic markers. Am J Surg Pathol. 25(1):65-70, 2001
15. Eble JN: Angiomyolipoma of kidney. Semin Diagn Pathol. 15(1):21-40, 1998
16. Pea M et al: Perivascular epithelioid cell. Am J Surg Pathol. 20(9):1149-53, 1996
17. Zamboni G et al: Clear cell "sugar" tumor of the pancreas. A novel member of the family of lesions characterized by the presence of perivascular epithelioid cells. Am J Surg Pathol. 20(6):722-30, 1996
18. Henske EP et al: Loss of heterozygosity in the tuberous sclerosis (TSC2) region of chromosome band 16p13 occurs in sporadic as well as TSC-associated renal angiomyolipomas. Genes Chromosomes Cancer. 13(4):295-8, 1995
19. Bonetti F et al: Clear cell ("sugar") tumor of the lung is a lesion strictly related to angiomyolipoma--the concept of a family of lesions characterized by the presence of the perivascular epithelioid cells (PEC). Pathology. 26(3):230-6, 1994

ANGIOMYOLIPOMA

Gross and Microscopic Features

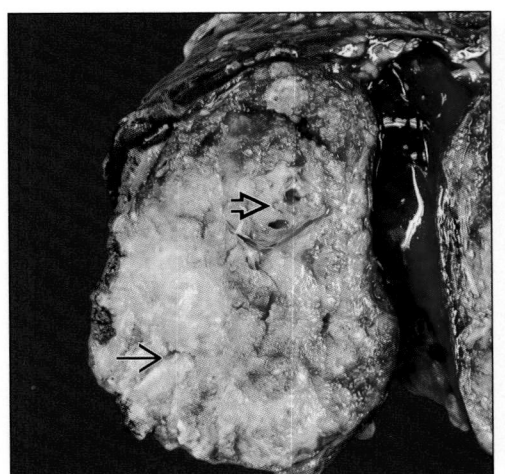

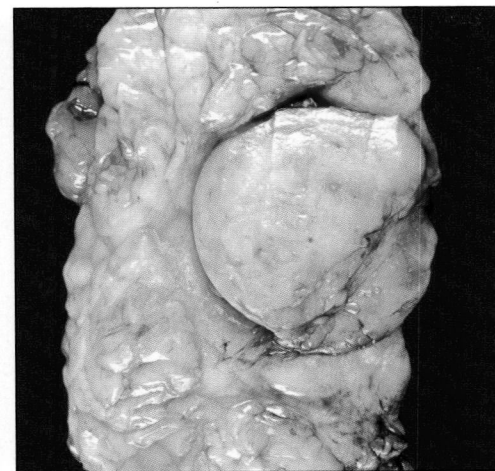

(Left) This typical angiomyolipoma with variegated gross appearance reflects fatty ⇨ and vascular ⇨ areas. Some tumors, composed predominantly of smooth muscle, may have a whorled appearance, reminiscent of uterine leiomyomas. *(Right)* This lipomatous angiomyolipoma was resected with a clinical diagnosis of liposarcoma. Generous sampling is essential, and recognition of abnormal blood vessels and perivascular epithelioid cells is necessary in such tumors.

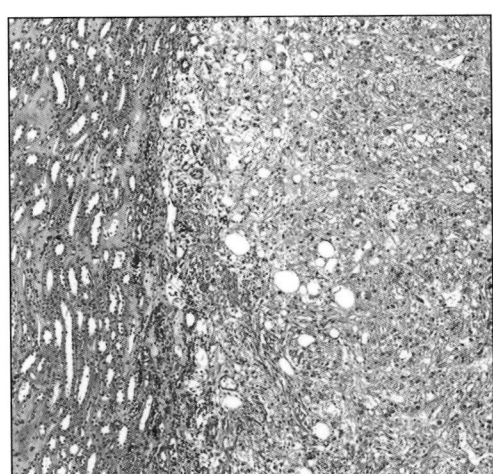

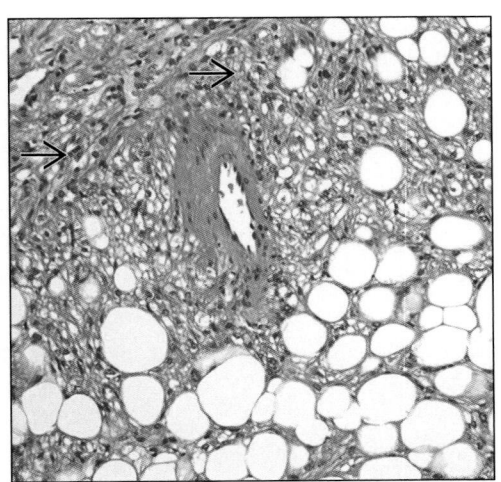

(Left) Angiomyolipomas are often well circumscribed but mostly lack a capsule. At this low-power magnification, a distinct adipocytic component is recognized. *(Right)* Hematoxylin & eosin stained section shows a typical triphasic angiomyolipoma composed of fat, spindled smooth muscle fascicles ⇨ and a dysmorphic blood vessel. The smooth muscle cells in this image have an epithelioid appearance and emanate from the vascular wall.

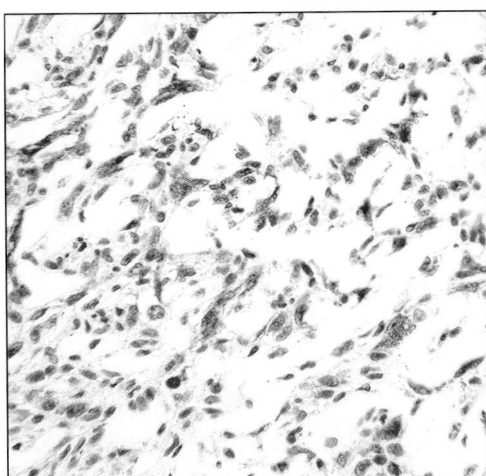

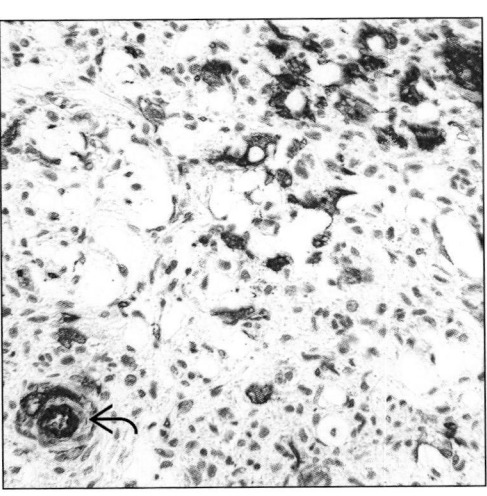

(Left) HMB-45 (seen here) &/or Melan-A(MART-1) immunostains are invariably positive in AML. The staining pattern may vary according to the cell type, but it is most prominent in epithelioid smooth muscle cells. *(Right)* Smooth muscle actin shows positivity in spindled and epithelioid smooth muscle cells. Note the positivity in a vessel wall ⇨ that acts as an internal control. HMB-45 and Melan-A(MART-1) show stronger expression in epithelioid areas, while actin-sm is positive in spindled cells.

ANGIOMYOLIPOMA

Microscopic Features

(Left) Dysmorphic vessels in angiomyolipoma show marked variation in the thickness and disorganization of the musculature of the vessel walls. *(Right)* Fat-predominant angiomyolipoma (lipomatous angiomyolipoma) shows an unusual vasculature; recognition of this feature, even when focal, should lead to the interpretation of the tumor as angiomyolipoma rather than a lipomatous tumor. Identification of other similar areas or further support by immunohistochemistry is helpful.

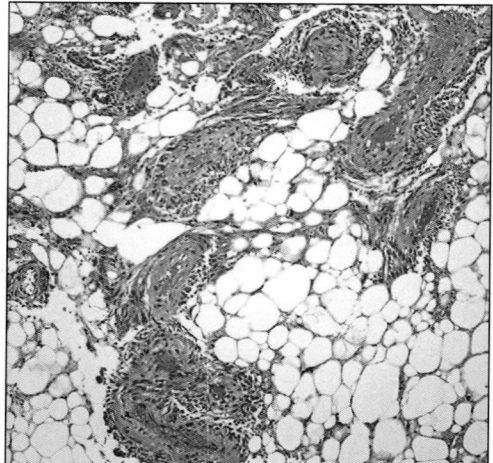 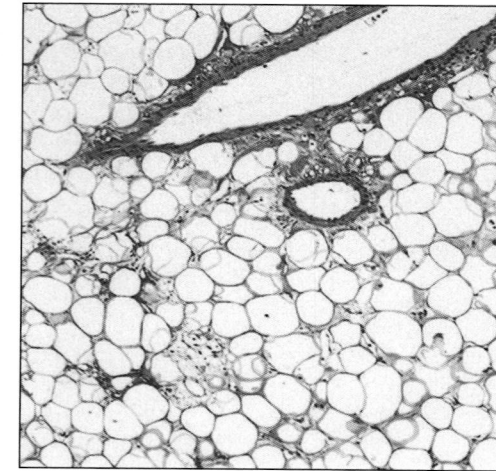

(Left) Fat-predominant angiomyolipoma with atypical lipocytes ⇨ may be mistaken for a liposarcoma. Atypical vasculature, sheets of spindle cell areas, and appropriate support by immunostains for melanocytic and smooth muscle markers will help in making the correct diagnosis of angiomyolipoma. *(Right)* HMB-45 shows positivity in a fat-predominant angiomyolipoma; the positivity is always focal in fatty areas, compared to more diffuse staining in epithelioid areas.

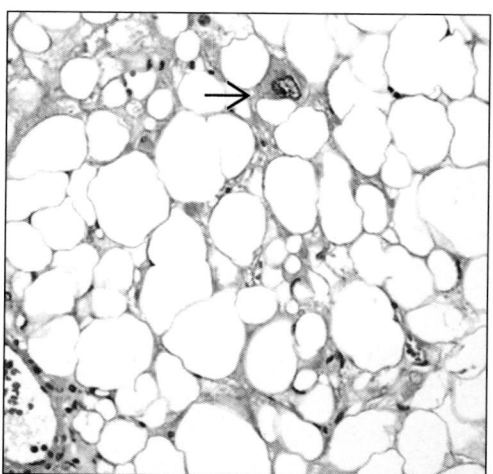 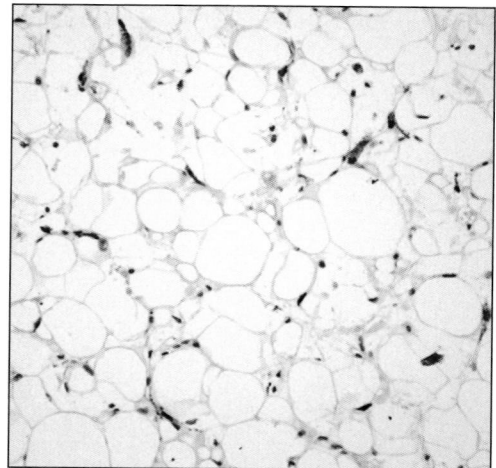

(Left) This hematoxylin & eosin stained-section shows a predominantly leiomyomatous angiomyolipoma. Primary smooth muscle tumors of the kidney are very rare. Careful search for lipocytes ⇨ should always be performed in such tumors. Staining for melanocytic markers may often be needed for the correct diagnosis. *(Right)* Immunohistochemical staining for HMB-45 is shown in a smooth-muscle predominant angiomyolipoma. Often, only very focal positivity may be observed.

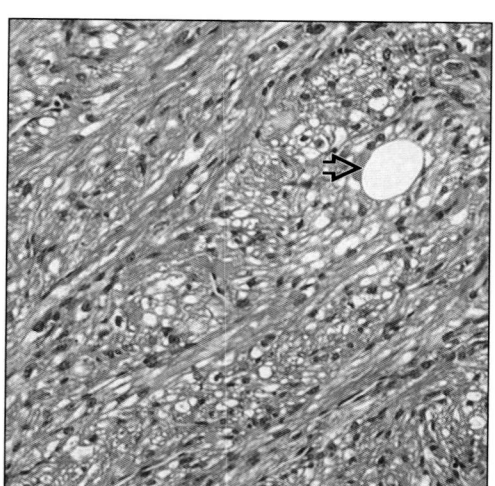 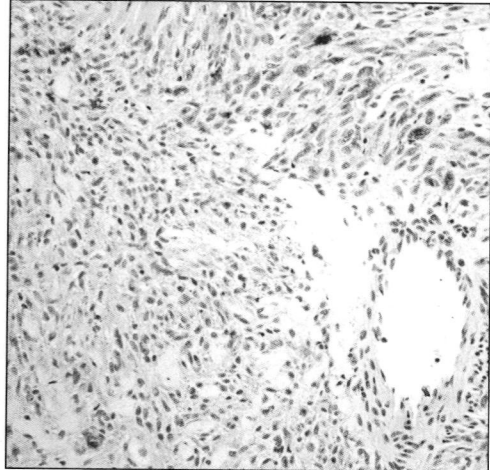

ANGIOMYOLIPOMA

Microscopic Features

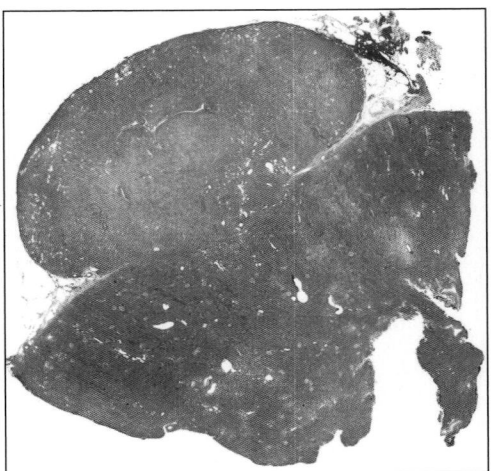
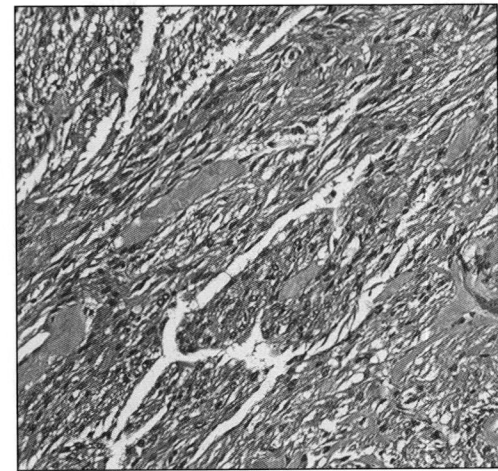

(Left) A hematoxylin & eosin-stained section shows a whole-mount of a leiomyomatous AML arising from renal capsule. Such tumors have been called renal "capsulomas" by some. Immunoexpression of melanocytic markers is confirmatory of AML. *(Right)* Smooth muscle predominant AML sometimes display a lymphangioleiomyomatous pattern. This pattern is often more conspicuous in pulmonary "PEC-associated" lesions in tuberous sclerosis.

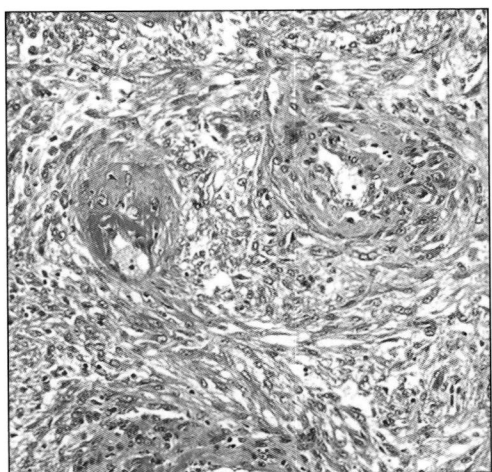
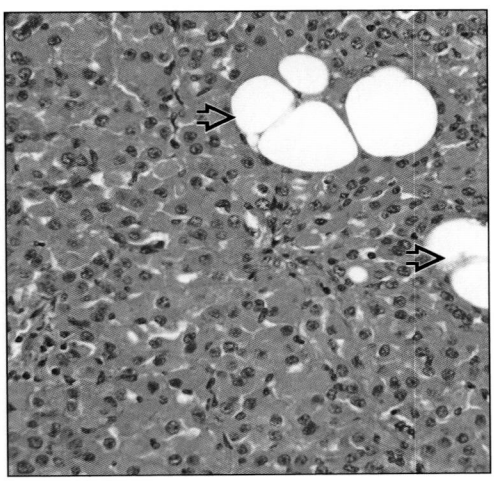

(Left) Spindled cells often appear to originate from the walls of dysmorphic vessels. This feature is characteristic of AML and helps suggest the diagnosis in a predominantly spindled cell tumor. *(Right)* Oncocytoma-like AML is a rare variant of AML. The presence of dysmorphic vessels, sclerosing areas, adipocytes ➡, & nuclear variability should point toward the appropriate diagnosis. These are also diffusely positive for HMB-45/Melan-A(MART-1) and negative for epithelial markers.

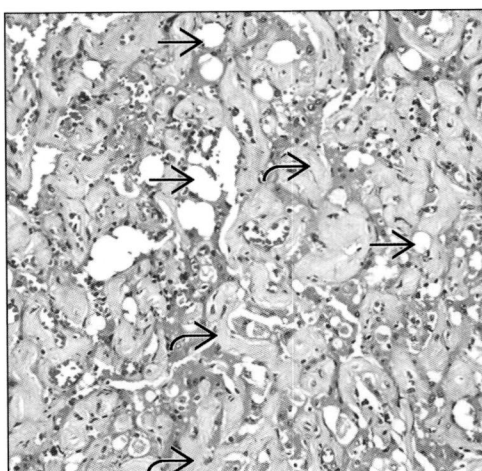
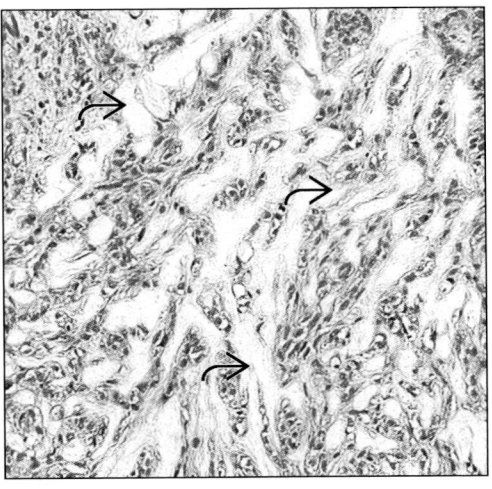

(Left) Angiomyolipoma with oncocytoma-like cytologic features. Note the scant adipocytes ➡ and sclerosing vessels ➡ that clearly point toward the diagnosis. *(Right)* Focal sclerosis is quite common in renal angiomyolipomas, but rare tumors may be exclusively of sclerosing type ➡. Such tumors have been designated as sclerosing angiomyolipoma. Immunohistochemistry is a useful diagnostic adjunct in angiomyolipomas with unusual histologic patterns.

ANGIOMYOLIPOMA

Microscopic Features

(Left) *Immunostain for actin-sm almost always shows diffuse positivity in sclerosing angiomyolipomas and leiomyomatous variants. Coexpression of smooth muscle markers with melanocytic markers is the immunohistochemical hallmark of PEC-related neoplasms, including angiomyolipoma.* **(Right)** *Angiomyolipoma with epithelial cysts (AMLEC) show cysts lined by cuboidal epithelium with eosinophilic cytoplasm ➯. Occasionally this cystic component may be conspicuous.*

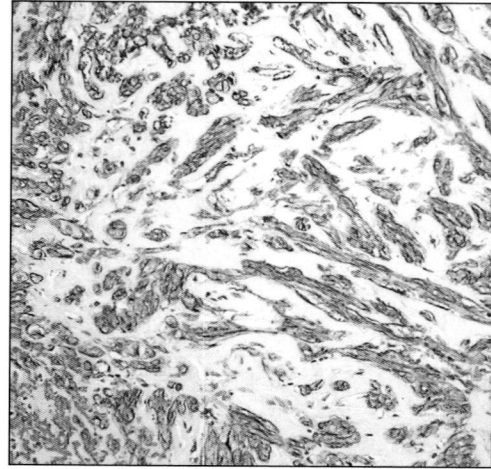
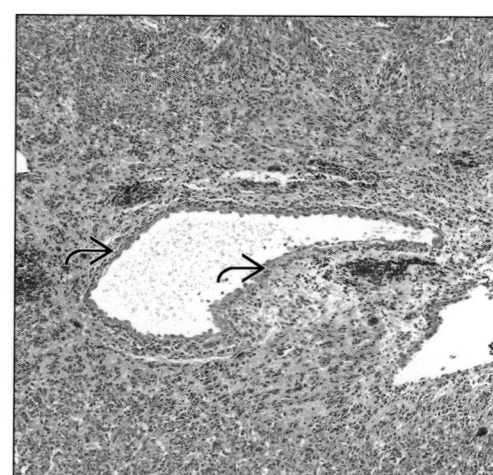

(Left) *The cysts in AMLEC are usually lined by cuboidal to "hobnailed" ➯ cells. Occasionally this cystic component may be striking, resulting in a multicystic gross appearance. The epithelial cysts may be the cell of origin of renal epithelial neoplasms rarely coexisting with and closely spatially related to angiomyolipomas.* **(Right)** *HMB-45 positivity in AMLEC reveals that the epithelial cells are negative for the marker and likely not an integral part of this PEC-related neoplasms.*

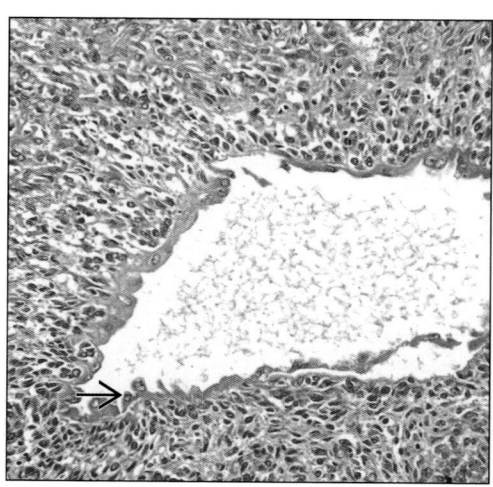
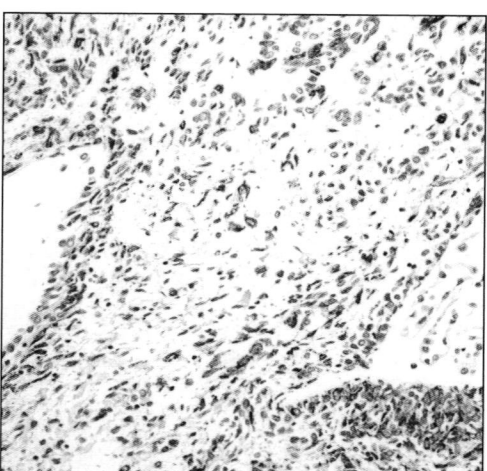

(Left) *The stroma around epithelial component in AMLEC is usually positive for CD10. This is in keeping with the light microscopic appearance of the spindle cells resembling cellular müllerian-like stroma.* **(Right)** *Nuclear positivity for progesterone receptor protein is also commonly present in the periepithelial stroma of AMLEC. This feature, as well as the cambium-like cellular stroma and bland spindled cells with prominent capillaries, suggests endometriotic-like stroma.*

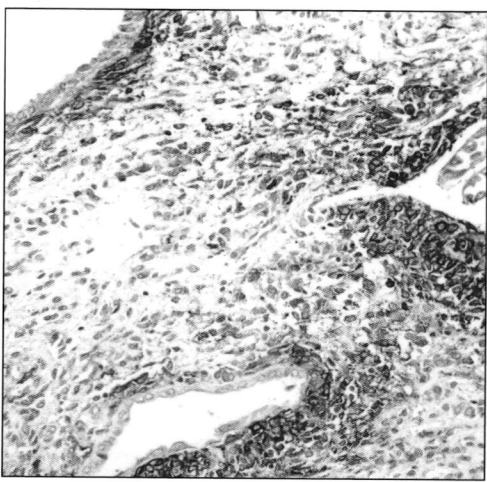
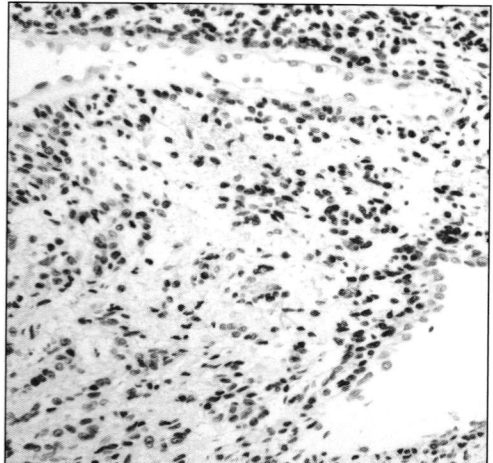

ANGIOMYOLIPOMA

Microscopic Features

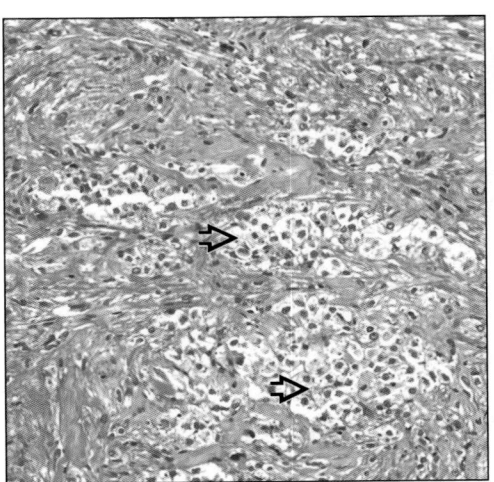 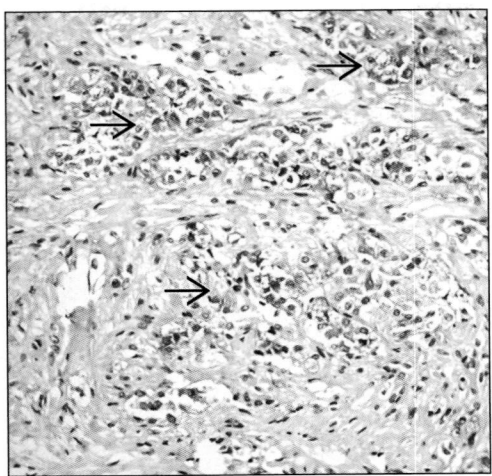

(Left) Occasionally, angiomyolipomas show variable areas with epithelioid features and clear cell cytology ⊵. When present, this finding is more commonly focal. Tumors with prominence of such areas have been designated as epithelioid angiomyolipomas. These epithelioid areas are negative for cytokeratin and usually show strong expression of melanocytic markers. (Right) HMB-45 positivity ⊳ in clear cell epithelioid foci within an otherwise typical angiomyolipoma is shown.

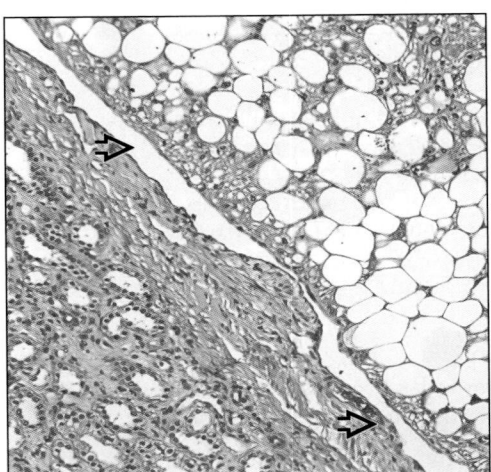 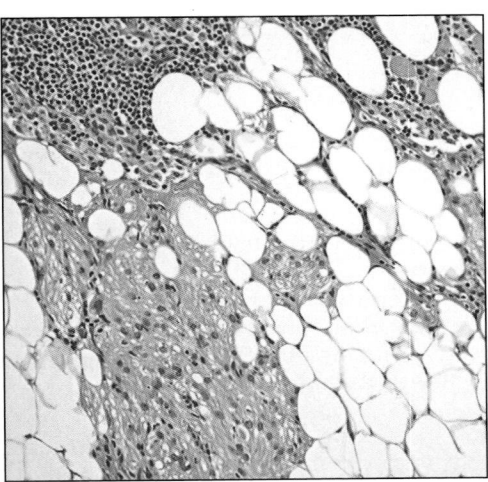

(Left) A large muscular vein ⊵ is involved by a typical triphasic neoplasm. Angiomyolipoma may show vascular invasion, rarely even involving the renal vein or inferior vena cava. This finding is not associated with aggressive tumoral behavior. (Right) Presence of angiomyolipoma in regional lymph nodes of a nephrectomy specimen with angiomyolipoma is not an indicator of metastatic disease or aggressive behavior but indicates multifocality.

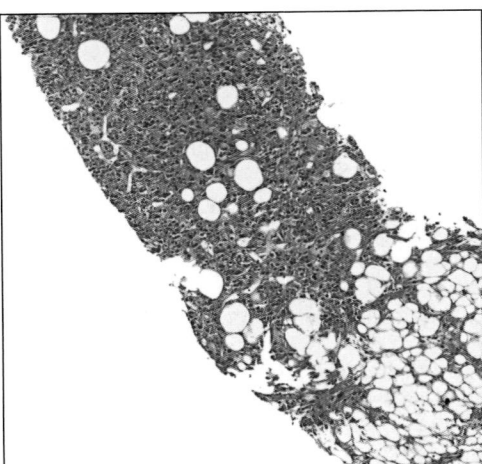 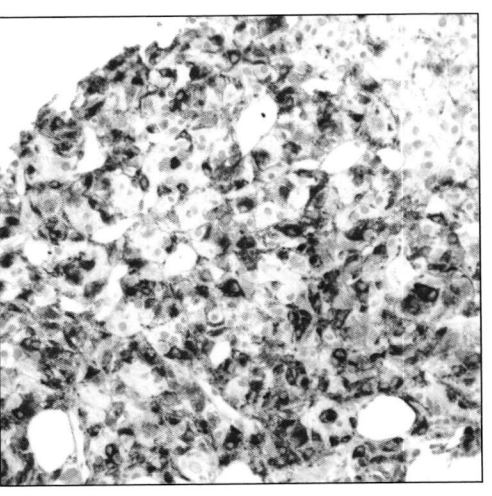

(Left) A definitive diagnosis of renal AML can easily be rendered on needle core biopsies for mass lesions, if the typical triphasic morphology is present. (Right) Immunohistochemical positivity for HMB-45 and lack of keratin expression confirms the diagnosis. In needle core biopsies with predominant epithelioid morphology and not resembling any of the known subtypes of RCC, a keratin stain may be very helpful; if negative, it supports an AML diagnosis.

EPITHELIOID ANGIOMYOLIPOMA

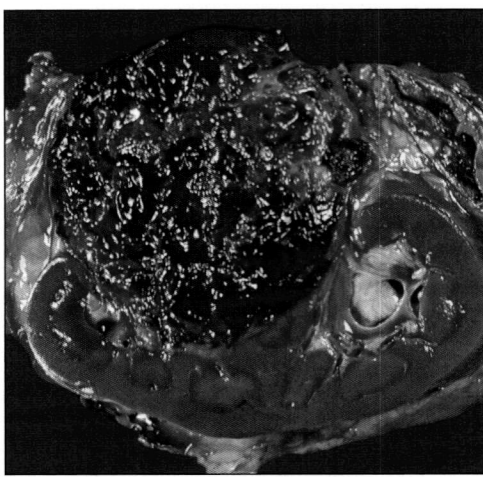

Epithelioid angiomyolipomas are usually large tumors that are mostly well circumscribed, frequently with extensive hemorrhage and necrosis. Some tumors may have a more homogeneous tan cut surface.

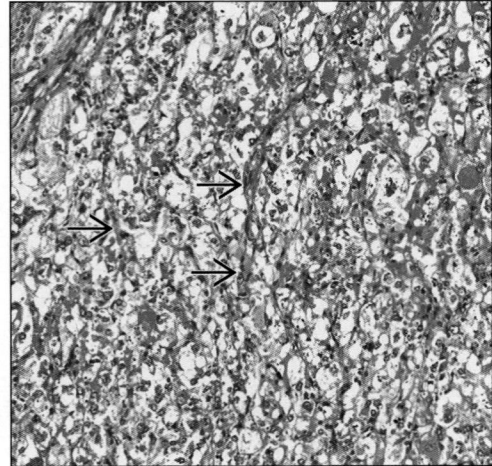

Microscopically, epithelioid AMLs may show nests, alveoli, and sheets of cells separated by thin vascular septae ⊟. Such architecture often leads to misdiagnosis as clear cell renal cell carcinoma.

TERMINOLOGY

Abbreviations
- Epithelioid angiomyolipoma (E-AML)

Synonyms
- Perivascular epithelioid cell (PEC)-oma (PEComa)

Definitions
- Mesenchymal tumor believed to originate from PEC with predominant epithelioid features
  - Closely related to usual (triphasic) AML
  - Percentage of tumor with epithelioid morphology that constitutes "predominant" is not established
  - Some tumors are morphologically similar to PEComas of soft tissues

ETIOLOGY/PATHOGENESIS

Tuberous Sclerosis Complex and mTOR Pathway
- Like typical AML, E-AML is associated with genetic alterations in tuberous sclerosis complex (TSC) genes, TSC1 (9q34) and TSC2 (16p13.3)
- Hamartin and tuberin proteins encoded by TSC1 and TSC2 genes, respectively, negatively regulate mTOR signaling
  - Alterations or absence of these proteins results in increased activated mammalian target of rapamycin (mTOR), possibly resulting in tumorigenesis
- AMLs in patients with TSC syndrome more often show epithelioid features (> 25%), compared to AML in those without TSC (7%)

TP53 Mutations
- TP53 mutations have been reported in some E-AML
  - However, more recent studies have not confirmed this finding

CLINICAL ISSUES

Epidemiology
- Incidence
  - In a large study with arbitrary cut-off of 10% epithelioid cells for designation of E-AML, 8% of all AMLs were E-AML
    - Most experts would require at least 50-80% epithelioid cells to be designated as E-AML
- Age
  - Mean age of presentation: 38 years (range: 14-70 years)

Presentation
- Mostly similar to that for usual angiomyolipoma
- Cases associated with tuberous sclerosis often present with
  - Larger tumors
  - Younger age at presentation
  - Multiple tumors, many of which include small usual angiomyolipomas
- Some tumors have metastases at presentation

Treatment
- Adjuvant therapy
  - mTOR pathway is shown to be activated in many tumors
    - Targeted therapies against mTOR have proven effective in some tumors
    - However, many tumors tend to regrow once therapy is stopped
    - More recently, some cases have been reported to be unresponsive to mTOR inhibitor sirolimus
  - Epidermal growth factor receptor (EGFR) inhibitor, gefitinib, has also recently been show to be useful in rare cases

Prognosis
- E-AMLs may have metastasis or recurrence and hence are considered potentially malignant

EPITHELIOID ANGIOMYOLIPOMA

Key Facts

Terminology
- Epithelioid angiomyolipoma (E-AML)
- Perivascular epithelioid cell (PEC)-oma (PEComa)

Clinical Issues
- In a large study with arbitrary cut-off of 10% epithelioid cells for designation of E-AML, 8% of all AMLs were E-AML
- Mammalian target of rapamycin (mTOR) pathway is shown to be activated in many tumors
- Many angiomyolipomas with metastases have epithelioid features and contain pleomorphic, multinucleated cells
- Overall true incidence of metastasis among all cases of E-AML is yet to be determined

Macroscopic Features
- Typically solid
- Often show hemorrhagic cut surface, with areas of necrosis and cystic change

Microscopic Pathology
- Cells arranged as cohesive nests, broad alveoli, and sheets separated by thin vascular septae
- Plump spindled and epithelioid cells arranged in diffuse sheets, with less prominent vascularity
- Cells with clear or eosinophilic cytoplasm
- Pleomorphic multinucleated cells

Top Differential Diagnoses
- Clear cell renal cell carcinoma
- Metastatic malignant melanoma

- Sites of metastases include
  - Liver (most common)
  - Lymph nodes
  - Lungs
  - Retroperitoneal organs and mesentery
  - Bones and other rare sites
- Overall true incidence of metastasis among all cases of E-AML is yet to be determined
  - Malignant potential is difficult to determine due to variable criteria to define E-AML, rarity of tumors, and lack of prolonged information on follow-up
  - In recent large study on AML, authors considered 15 cases as E-AML (designated such with > 10% epithelioid cells)
    - All of their E-AMLs showed benign outcomes
    - 2 of these E-AMLs had 100% epithelioid morphology
- Recent study of > 40 cases containing > 80% epithelioid cells reports
  - Rate of metastasis to be as high as > 45%
  - However, many cases in study represented cases received in consultation
    - Therefore, influence of referral bias in this study cannot be underestimated
- Reported adverse prognostic pathologic indicators include
  - Pure epithelioid histology
  - Large tumor size (> 7 cm)
  - Perirenal tumor extension
  - Frequent mitoses (> 2/10 high-power fields)
  - Combination of multiple adverse prognostic indicators compounds risk for malignant potential

MACROSCOPIC FEATURES

General Features
- Typically solid
- Most are well circumscribed but some with gross extrarenal extension
- Often show hemorrhagic cut surface
- Variable amounts of necrosis or cystic change frequent

MICROSCOPIC PATHOLOGY

Histologic Features
- Epithelioid features in tumors characterized by the following
- Architectural patterns
  - Cells arranged as cohesive nests, broad alveoli, and sheets separated by thin vascular septae
  - Plump spindled and epithelioid cells arranged in diffuse sheets, with less prominent vascularity (similar to many soft tissue PEComas)
  - Occasionally, with glomus tumor-like perivascular arrangement of cells with dilated vascular spaces
    - Such tumors may also contain branching, dilated vessels with hemangiopericytomatous pattern
- Cytologic features
  - Cells with clear cytoplasm
    - Frequently, these "clear cells" show dispersed, irregular intracytoplasmic granularity
    - Granularity is occasionally concentrated around nuclei, with periphery of cytoplasm appearing more clear
    - Cells are usually relatively uniform, with only mild nuclear variability
  - Cells with eosinophilic cytoplasm
    - Cells may be small to intermediate in size or may appear quite large with abundant cytoplasm
    - Cytoplasm often shows fine vacuolization
    - Nuclei are more pleomorphic and atypical compared to those in clear cells
    - Nuclear chromatin is vesicular, and nucleoli are often prominent
    - Intranuclear pseudoinclusions may be present
    - Rare cases have finely granular cytoplasm, resembling renal oncocytoma
  - Pleomorphic multinucleated cells
    - These cells usually have abundant, eosinophilic, and finely vacuolated cytoplasm
    - They bear multiple nuclei
    - Nuclei may either be similar to those in mononuclear eosinophilic cells

EPITHELIOID ANGIOMYOLIPOMA

- - Or these nuclei may be polyploid, multilobulated, and hyperchromatic
- Mitoses are commonly observed in E-AML
  - Most mitoses are typical
  - In rare cases, atypical mitoses may also be observed
  - In some cases, mitotic activity is quite brisk (> 5-8/10 high-power fields)
- Areas of tumor necrosis may be observed
- Vascular and extrarenal fat invasion, both perinephric and in renal sinus, are not uncommon

ANCILLARY TESTS

Immunohistochemistry
- Epithelioid cells in E-AML usually show strong and diffuse positivity for melanocytic markers and smooth muscle markers
  - HMB-45, MiTF, Melan-A(MART-1), tyrosinase: Positive; S100: Negative
  - Actin-sm is frequently positive, although focal in epithelioid tumors
- Epithelial markers, including EMA/MUC1 and various cytokeratins, are negative
- Recently, E-AML has been reported to display positivity for CD1a, a molecule typically expressed in Langerhans cell histiocytosis

DIFFERENTIAL DIAGNOSIS

Clear Cell Renal Cell Carcinoma
- E-AML are often mistaken for clear cell RCC because of
  - Presence of clear cell histology
  - Eosinophilic cells with solid nested/alveolar growth pattern
  - Cells with pleomorphic lobulated nuclei (feature commonly present in high-grade clear cell RCC)
- Clear cell RCC frequently show
  - Vascular septae that are usually very well formed with intricately branching enclosing nests of clear cells
- Careful examination of E-AML may often reveal focal presence of
  - Adipocytes &/or occasional dysmorphic vessels
- Immunostains for CA9, CD10, EMA/MUC1, and cytokeratins are usually positive in clear cell RCC
  - Stains for melanocytic markers, HMB-45, Melan-A(MART-1), and MiTF, and actin-sm are negative in clear cell RCC

Metastatic Malignant Melanoma
- Melanomas show spectrum of morphologic patterns and are positive for melanocytic markers, similar to E-AML
- They are most often positive for S100, which is very uncommon in E-AML
- Adipocytes and dysmorphic vessels are not seen in malignant melanoma
- Clinical history of primary melanoma may be useful
- Metastatic malignant melanoma may be multifocal

DIAGNOSTIC CHECKLIST

Pathologic Interpretation Pearls
- Many AMLs that have metastatic disease have epithelioid features
- E-AML may be tumor with aggressive biologic behavior
  - Percentage of cells with epithelioid features required to classify a tumor as E-AML is yet to be determined; > 50-80% of epithelioid histology is recommended
  - True incidence of metastatic potential remains unknown due to variable criteria and limited follow-up
  - Currently reported metastatic incidence (as high as 45-50%) is primarily based on case reports or consultation cases with possible referral bias
  - If one accepts incidence of metastasis as currently reported, E-AML would be among most malignant of all renal tumors
  - Thus, determination of overall biologic potential in E-AML will require a study of a large number of all cases diagnosed as E-AML
- High index of suspicion for E-AML is necessary before diagnosis of unclassified RCC is made
  - In needle biopsies, a PAN-CK(AE1/AE3) stain in the appropriate setting may be useful screening marker for this tumor

SELECTED REFERENCES

1. Aydin H et al: Renal angiomyolipoma: clinicopathologic study of 194 cases with emphasis on the epithelial histology and tuberous sclerosis association. Am J Surg Pathol. 33(2):289-97, 2009
2. Higa F et al: Malignant epithelioid angiomyolipoma in the kidney and liver of a patient with pulmonary lymphangioleiomyomatosis: lack of response to sirolimus. Intern Med. 48(20):1821-5, 2009
3. Kato I et al: Epithelioid angiomyolipoma of the kidney. Pathol Int. 59(1):38-43, 2009
4. Adachi Y et al: CD1a expression in PEComas. Pathol Int. 58(3):169-73, 2008
5. Bissler JJ et al: Sirolimus for angiomyolipoma in tuberous sclerosis complex or lymphangioleiomyomatosis. N Engl J Med. 358(2):140-51, 2008
6. Lane BR et al: Clinical correlates of renal angiomyolipoma subtypes in 209 patients: classic, fat poor, tuberous sclerosis associated and epithelioid. J Urol. 180(3):836-43, 2008
7. Pan CC et al: Constant allelic alteration on chromosome 16p (TSC2 gene) in perivascular epithelioid cell tumour (PEComa): genetic evidence for the relationship of PEComa with angiomyolipoma. J Pathol. 214(3):387-93, 2008

EPITHELIOID ANGIOMYOLIPOMA

Microscopic Features

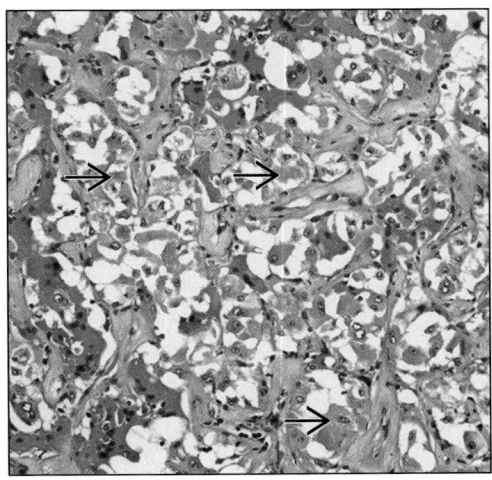
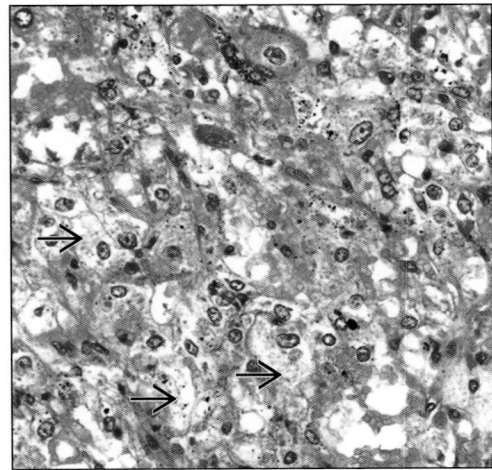

(Left) E-AML with predominant eosinophilic cytoplasm ➡, superficially resembling a RCC with abundant eosinophilic cytoplasm. The diagnosis rests on exclusion of the known subtypes of RCC and appropriate immunohistochemistry. (Right) The epithelioid cells in E-AML often show clear cytoplasm. Frequently, these clear cells show irregularly dispersed intracytoplasmic granules ➡. The granularity may be perinuclear, with the periphery of the cytoplasm appearing more clear.

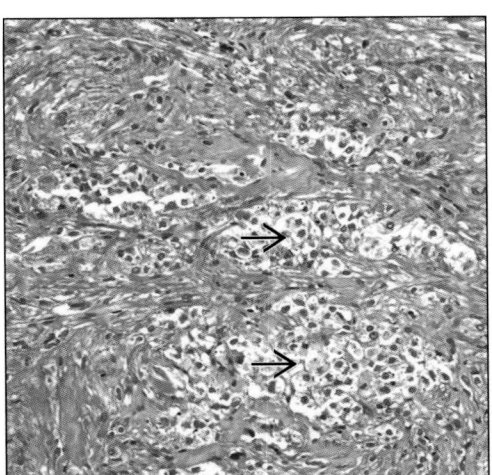
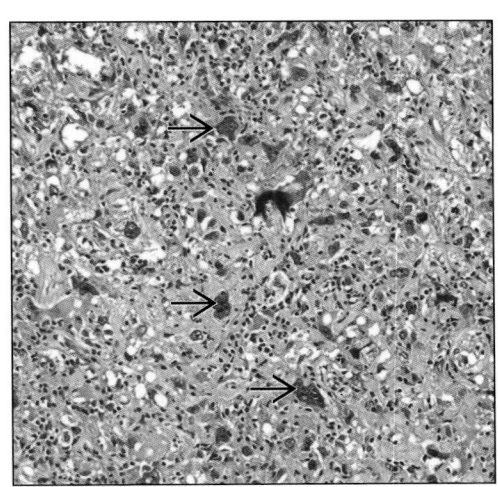

(Left) A major contentious issue is when to designate an AML as E-AML. Focal epithelioid areas ➡ are often present in otherwise typical AMLs. (Right) It is not uncommon to see multinucleated giant cells ➡ in E-AML. The presence of multinucleated giant cells in an epithelioid tumor should raise the possibility of an E-AML and prompt search for adipocytes or dysmorphic blood vessels. In the absence of the latter, immunohistochemistry is necessary.

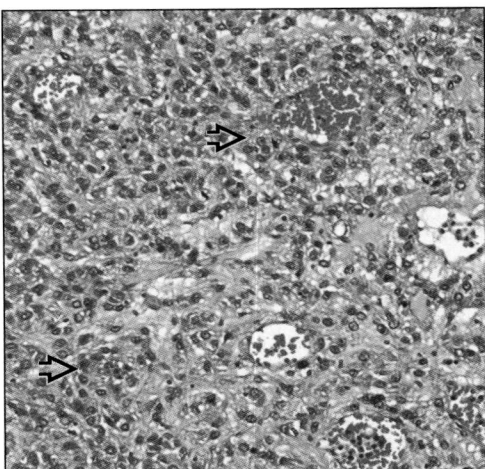
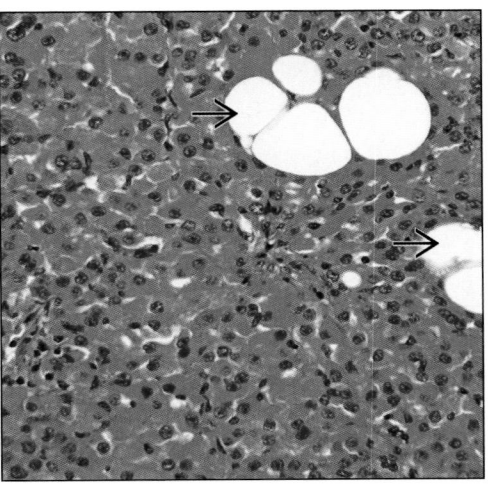

(Left) Occasional E-AMLs show prominent vascularity with plump epithelioid cells surrounding the vessels in a glomoid pattern ➡. Occasionally, the dilated vessels may be branching, showing a hemangiopericytomatous pattern. (Right) This angiomyolipoma with epithelioid features shows oncocytoma-like eosinophilic granularity. Careful microscopic search often leads to identification of at least focal features of typical AML, for example adipocytes ➡, as shown here.

EPITHELIOID ANGIOMYOLIPOMA

Microscopic and Immunohistochemical Features

(Left) Some E-AMLs show sheets of spindled and plump epithelioid cells. Although there is noticeable vascularity in the background, the branching is irregular and does not encircle nests of tumor. *(Right)* This photomicrograph depicts sheet-like growth pattern of plump epithelioid cells. Note the absence of prominent vascularity in this case. Intranuclear pseudoinclusions ➡ and prominent mitotic activity ➡ are also present; both are common features in epithelioid angiomyolipoma.

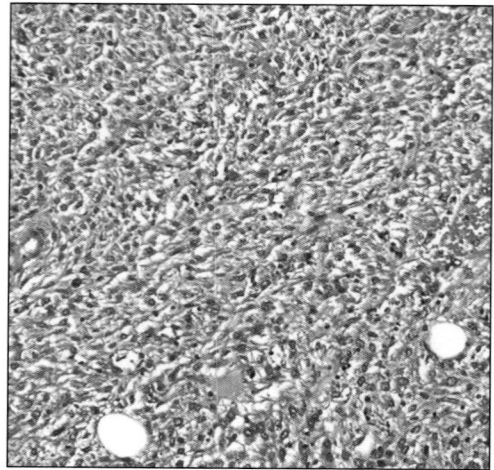
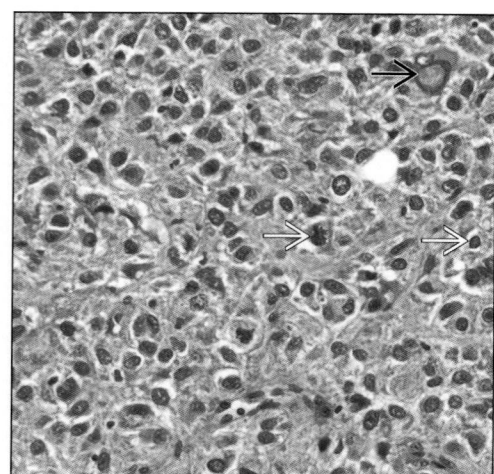

(Left) This epithelioid angiomyolipoma shows nested growth pattern, with prominent vascularity. In spite of the apparent clear cell features, the cells are not optically clear and show irregular cytoplasmic granularity. A large proportion of E-AMLs, even with very prominent epithelioid features, show the focal presence of adipocytes ➡ or dysmorphic vessels. *(Right)* This photomicrograph from an epithelioid angiomyolipoma shows the presence of focal, dysmorphic vessels ➡ in the tumor.

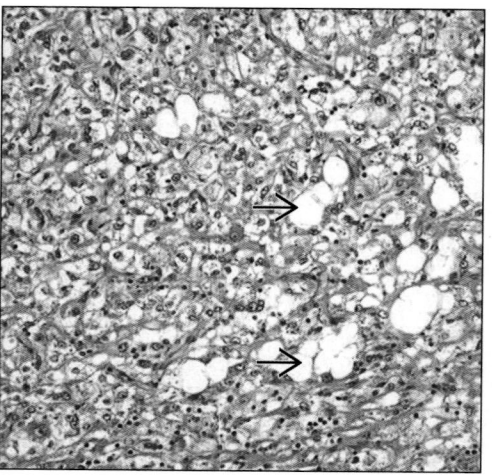
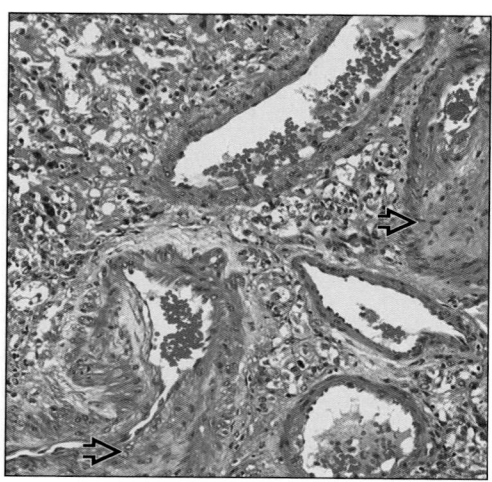

(Left) Epithelioid cells usually show diffuse and strong immunoreactivity for melanocytic markers like HMB-45 (as shown here) and Melan-A(MART-1). Besides careful attention to the histology, the tumor immunoprofile is the most distinctive feature distinguishing E-AML from RCC. *(Right)* This image shows diffuse cytoplasmic immunoreactivity for Melan-A in an E-AML. Because of the nested epithelioid cells and vascular pattern many E-AML were misdiagnosed as clear cell RCC in the past.

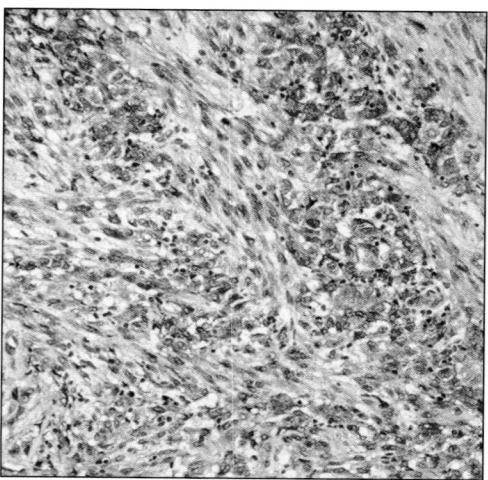
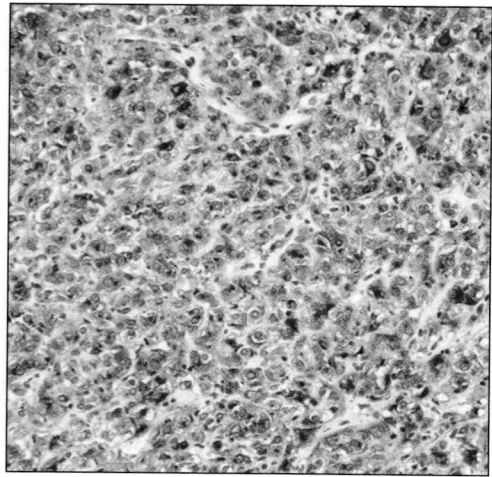

EPITHELIOID ANGIOMYOLIPOMA

Microscopic, IHC, and Differential Diagnostic Features

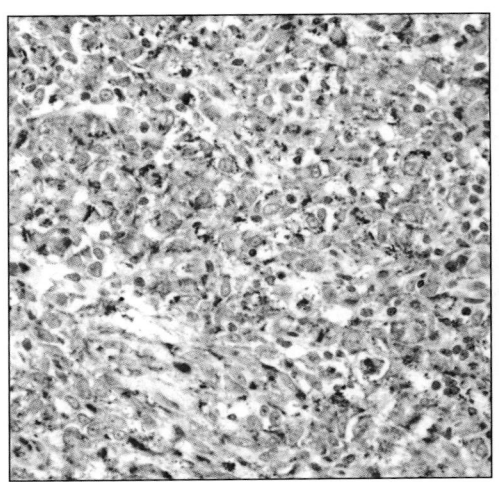

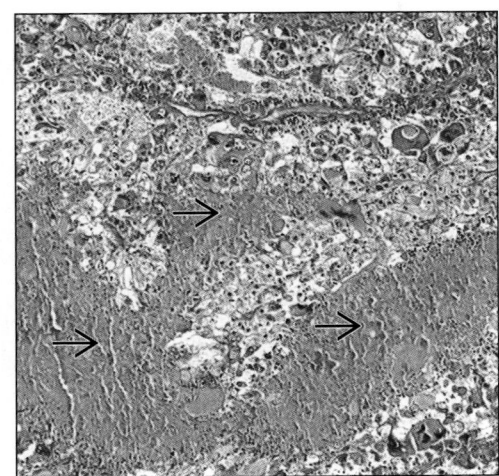

(Left) Phospho-S6 positivity in E-AML. Phospho-S6 is activated by mTOR, and over-expression of phospho-S6 is a strong indicator of an active mTOR pathway. This finding is considered a justification for using mTOR inhibitors in managing E-AML is shown. *(Right)* Tumor necrosis ➡ in E-AML. Cellular anaplasia, mitotic activity, necrosis, and extrarenal extension are more commonly associated with metastasis. All E-AMLs (predominant epithelioid histology) are considered potentially malignant.

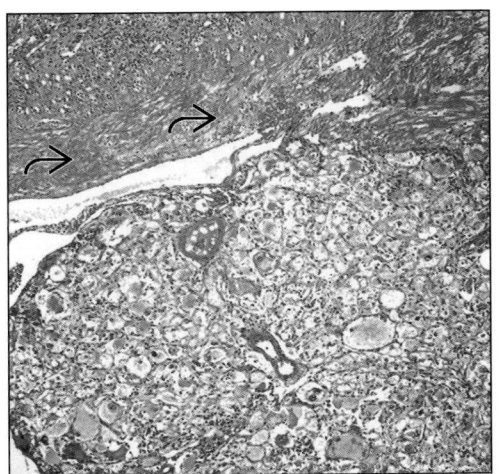

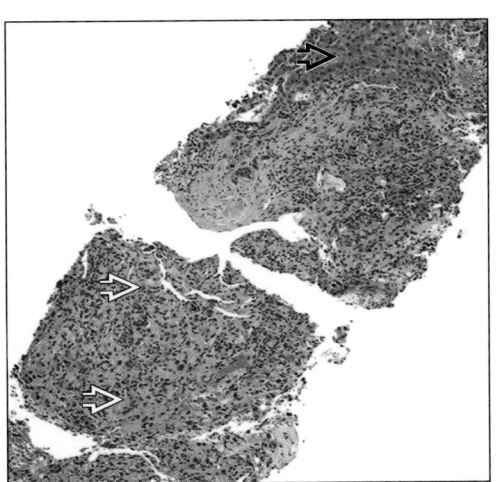

(Left) This epithelioid AML invades a large muscular branch of renal vein ➡ in the renal sinus. Along with large size (> 7 cm), tumor necrosis, and high mitotic index, vascular and perinephric fat invasion have been regarded as adverse prognostic markers in E-AML in some studies. *(Right)* This image from a needle core liver biopsy shows an epithelioid AML ➡ metastatic to liver ➡. Liver is the most common site for metastasis from E-AML, followed by lymph nodes and lungs.

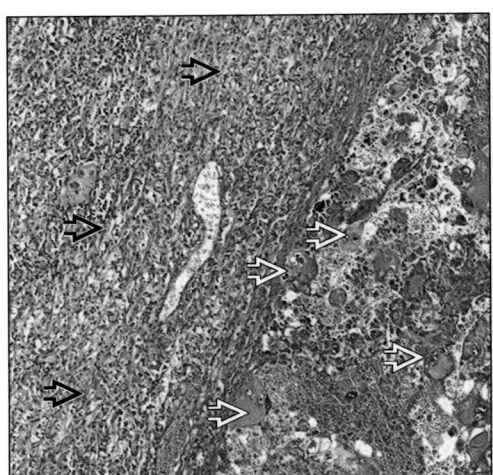

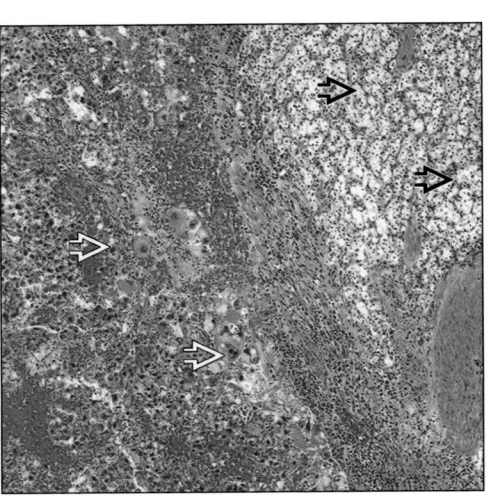

(Left) This E-AML shows a mixture of clear cell cytology ➡ with relatively low-grade nuclei and high-grade areas with eosinophilic cytoplasm and multinucleated tumor giant cells ➡. Such tumors may be confused with clear cell RCC. *(Right)* This clear cell RCC shows a low-grade area ➡ adjacent to a high-grade area with multinucleated tumor giant cells ➡. Presence of pleomorphic tumor giant cells in a clear cell tumor should always raise the differential possibility of an E-AML.

CONGENITAL MESOBLASTIC NEPHROMA

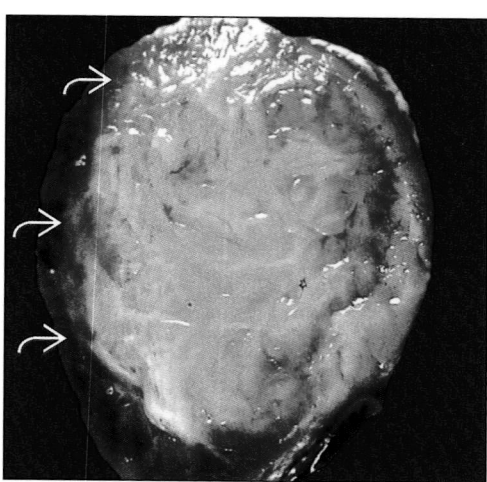

This gross picture of a classic congenital mesoblastic nephroma shows the characteristic tan-white, fibrous whorled and trabeculated cut surface. The tumor-kidney interface is ill defined ➡.

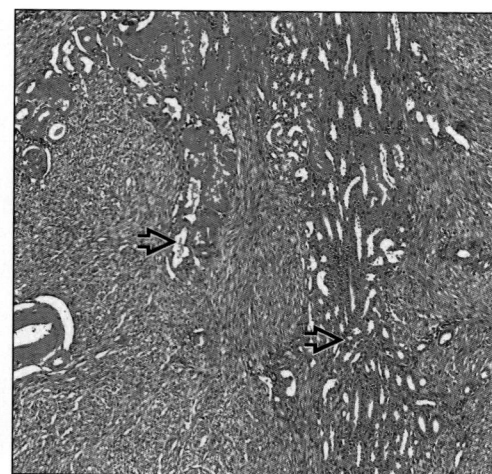

Classic mesoblastic nephroma typically shows finger-like peripheral extensions, infiltrating and entrapping surrounding nephrons ➡, and often invading the renal sinus soft tissues as well.

TERMINOLOGY

Abbreviations
- Congenital mesoblastic nephroma (CMN)

Definitions
- Most common renal neoplasm of infancy with spindle cell features, mimicking fibromatosis or infantile fibrosarcoma
- Tumors classified as adult mesoblastic nephroma in past are now classified as mixed epithelial stromal tumor

ETIOLOGY/PATHOGENESIS

Genetic Features
- Classic variant has no consistent genetic abnormality and may represent fibromatosis involving kidney
- Cellular variant has t(12;15)(p13;q25) chromosomal translocation resulting in *ETV6-NTRK3* gene fusion
  - Same translocation as seen in infantile fibrosarcoma; also recently reported in secretory carcinomas of breast
- No gene fusions demonstrated in mixed pattern
- Occasional association of CMN with Beckwith-Wiedemann syndrome

CLINICAL ISSUES

Epidemiology
- Age
  - Most common renal tumor of very young children
    - Most common renal tumor in 1st 3 months of life
    - > 90% of tumors occur with 1 year of age

Presentation
- Presents as abdominal mass; may be associated with polyhydramnios, premature delivery, and nonimmune hydrops

- Hypertension (due to renin production by entrapped renal elements) may be present

Treatment
- Surgical approaches
  - Because of marked infiltrative nature of classic type, partial nephrectomy may not be feasible option in many cases

Prognosis
- Majority cured with surgery with excellent outcome
  - Recurrences and metastases occur in ~ 5-10% of patients, risk factors for which are
    - Incomplete excision, cellularity, stage III or higher presentation, and involvement of intrarenal or sinus vessels

MACROSCOPIC FEATURES

General Features
- Solitary, unilateral
  - Classic CMN with characteristic whorled or trabeculated, gray-white cut surface and indistinct tumor-kidney interface
  - Cellular CMN often fleshy and with more circumscribed advancing edges
- Cysts, hemorrhage, and necrosis are common and have no prognostic significance
- Tumor tends to arise centrally within kidney and often involves renal sinus extensively

MICROSCOPIC PATHOLOGY

Histologic Features
- CMN divided into 3 types, based on histologic features
  - Classic type (24% of cases)
    - Shows intersecting bundles of spindle cells with minimal atypia and infrequent mitoses
    - Resembles fibromatosis

CONGENITAL MESOBLASTIC NEPHROMA

Key Facts

Terminology
- Congenital mesoblastic nephroma (CMN)
- Spindle cell neoplasm of kidney, composed of myofibroblasts
- Subtypes/variants: Classic, cellular, and mixed

Etiology/Pathogenesis
- Cellular variant has t(12;15)(p13;q25) chromosomal translocation resulting in *ETV6-NTRK3* gene fusion
  - Same translocation as seen in infantile fibrosarcoma
- Occasional association of CMN with Beckwith-Wiedemann syndrome

Clinical Issues
- Most common renal tumor of infancy

- Majority cured with surgery and have excellent outcome
- Increased risk of local recurrence with incomplete excision

Microscopic Pathology
- Classic variant (24% of cases): Intersecting bundles of spindle cells with minimal atypia and infrequent mitoses
- Cellular variant (66% of cases): Pushing border, dense cells, mitoses, and "sarcomatous" appearance

Top Differential Diagnoses
- Metanephric stromal tumor
- Clear cell sarcoma of kidney
- Wilms tumor (particularly post-therapy)
- Rhabdoid tumor of kidney

- Tumor infiltrates extensively into adjacent renal parenchyma and renal sinus structures
- Dysplastic renal tubules and islands of cartilage are often seen trapped within tumor
  - Cellular variant (66% of cases)
    - Shows pushing border, dense cellularity, and numerous mitoses
    - Morphologically, quite similar to infantile fibrosarcoma
  - Mixed (10-20% of cases)
    - Shows combination of both histologic patterns

Predominant Pattern/Injury Type
- Neoplastic, infiltrative

Predominant Cell/Compartment Type
- Myofibroblast

DIFFERENTIAL DIAGNOSIS

Metanephric Stromal Tumor
- May mimic classic CMN
- Usually does not present within 1st year of life
- Margins are not as infiltrative as in classic CMN
- Shows dysmorphic vessels, juxtaglomerular hyperplasia, and concentric spindle cell proliferation around vessels and tubules
- Stroma usually CD34 positive

Clear Cell Sarcoma of Kidney (CCSK)
- May mimic cellular CMN
- Cellular variant of CMN lacks "chicken wire" vascular pattern of CCSK
- CMN is positive for desmin &/or actin-sm and vimentin; CCSK is positive for vimentin only
- Presence of other patterns of CCSK (e.g., myxoid, sclerosing, epithelioid, palisading)

Wilms Tumor (WT)
- Most difficult differential is post-therapy Wilms with stromal-type residual tumor

- WT very rare in infants, especially those < 6 months old
- Extensive necrosis, seen in post-therapy WT, is not a feature of CMN
- WT shows compressed pseudocapsule in contrast to extensively infiltrating borders in CMN
- Presence of rhabdomyomatous differentiation, common in WT, does not occur in CMN

Rhabdoid Tumor of Kidney (RTK)
- Occasionally CMN may have unusually prominent nucleoli, raising suspicion of RTK
  - Immunohistochemical stain for SNF5(INI1) (positive nuclear staining in CMN and absent staining in RTK) is diagnostic

DIAGNOSTIC CHECKLIST

Pathologic Interpretation Pearls
- Vast majority of patients are < 1 year old, at which age other pediatric renal tumors are less common
- Cellular variant has sarcomatous appearance, but complete resection is often curative
- Surgical margins, especially medial margin, need careful evaluation

SELECTED REFERENCES

1. Bayindir P et al: Cellular mesoblastic nephroma (infantile renal fibrosarcoma): institutional review of the clinical, diagnostic imaging, and pathologic features of a distinctive neoplasm of infancy. Pediatr Radiol. 39(10):1066-74, 2009
2. van den Heuvel-Eibrink MM et al: Characteristics and survival of 750 children diagnosed with a renal tumor in the first seven months of life: A collaborative study by the SIOP/GPOH/SFOP, NWTSG, and UKCCSG Wilms tumor study groups. Pediatr Blood Cancer. 50(6):1130-4, 2008

CONGENITAL MESOBLASTIC NEPHROMA

Microscopic Features

(Left) This image of congenital mesoblastic nephroma depicts the low-grade cytologic features seen in the classic type. With its low cellularity, minimal nuclear pleomorphism, and low mitotic activity, histologically the classic type closely resembles fibromatosis. *(Right)* The classic type of congenital mesoblastic nephroma usually shows tongue-like extensions into the surrounding renal parenchyma and soft tissues, often entrapping these elements within its advancing edges ➡️.

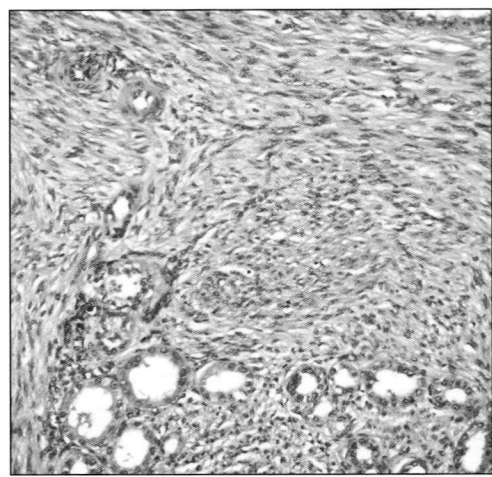
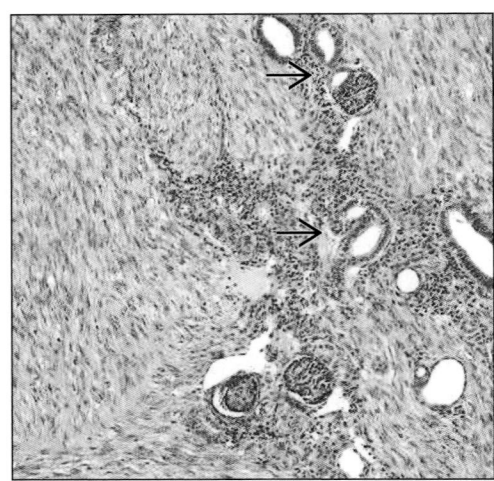

(Left) The adjacent kidney in classic CMN often shows dysplastic changes, including cartilage ➤, and often the dysplastic foci are included within the tumor edge. In spite of being termed classic, this type constitutes < 1/4 of all CMNs. *(Right)* Besides invading the sinus, classic CMN also extends into perinephric fat ➤. Because of the frequent and irregular extensions into the renal sinus and perinephric fat, partial nephrectomy is not a surgical option in most cases.

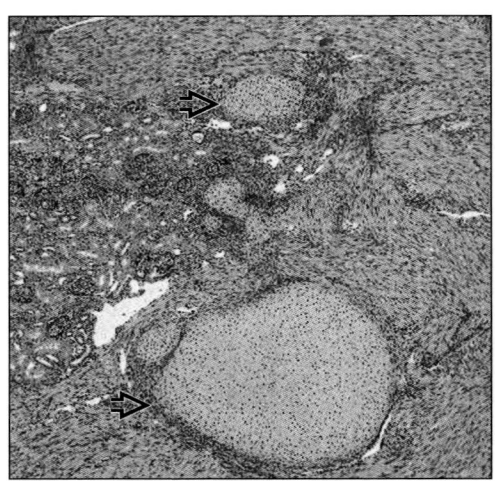
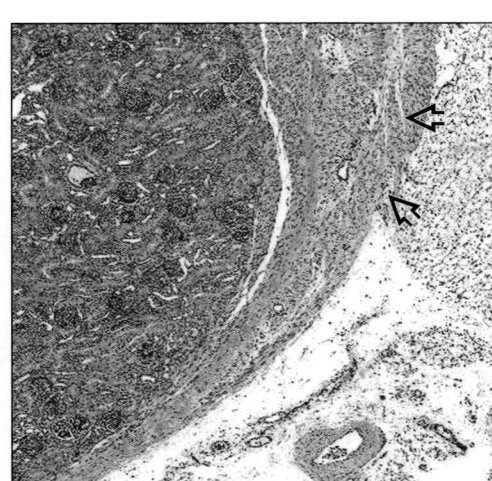

(Left) The cellular variant is the most frequent type of CMN. It shows fleshy gross features, along with high cellularity with abundant mitotic figures. Morphologically, as well as on a genetic basis, it exactly resembles infantile fibrosarcoma. *(Right)* The advancing edges of cellular congenital mesoblastic nephroma are pushing ➡️, rather than infiltrative. Because of these similarities, cellular CMN is considered by some to be infantile fibrosarcoma, centered in the renal hilum.

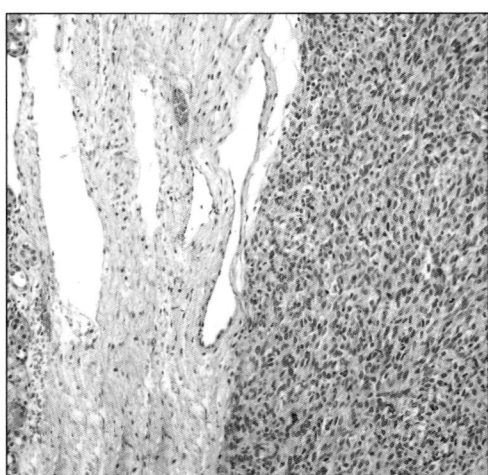
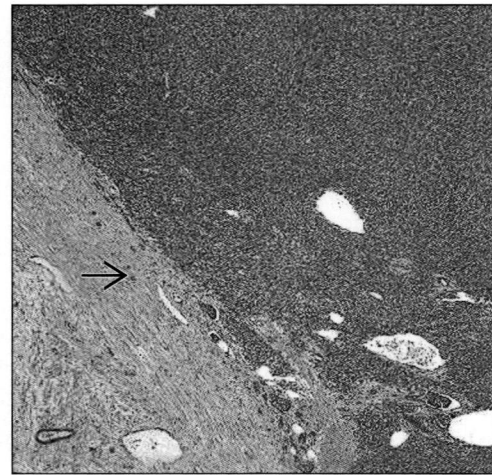

Microscopic Features and Differential Diagnoses

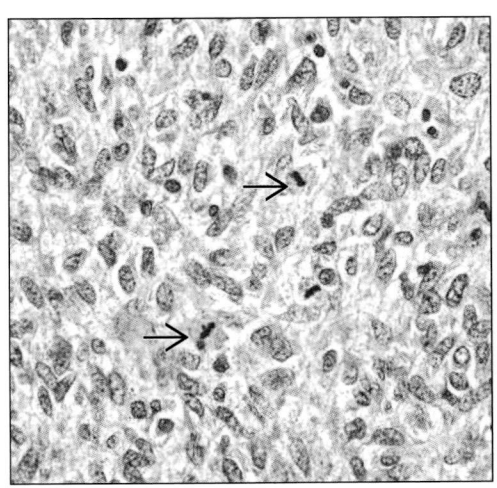

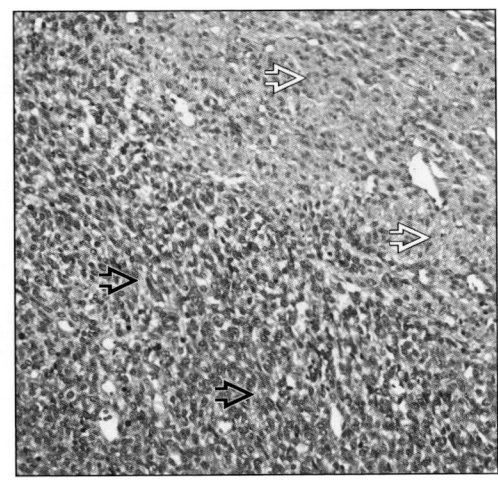

(Left) Mitotic figures ⇥ are quite frequent in cellular CMN. Recurrences and metastases occur in < 10% of patients with CMN, risk factors for which are incomplete excision, cellularity, stage III or higher tumors, and involvement of intrarenal or sinus vessels. *(Right)* A small but significant proportion of congenital mesoblastic nephromas show mixed histologic features, with cellular ⇥ and classic ⇥ areas often present side-by-side.

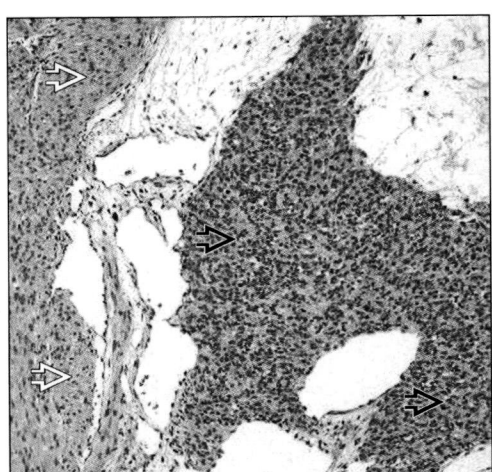

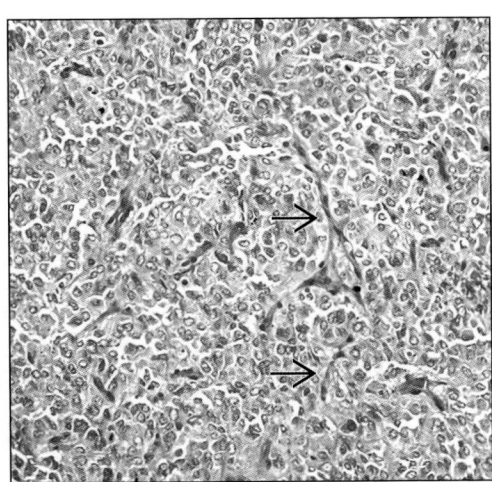

(Left) Although morphologically similar to the cellular CMN, the cellular areas ⇥ in mixed CMN, interestingly, do not show the ETV6-NTRK3 gene fusion, characteristic of all cellular CMN. This genetic characteristic is also absent in classic tumors and classic areas ⇥ of mixed CMN. *(Right)* Cellular, epithelioid areas in clear cell sarcoma of kidney may mimic a cellular CMN. However, the "chicken wire" vasculature ⇥ of CCSK is not seen in CMN and helps in this distinction.

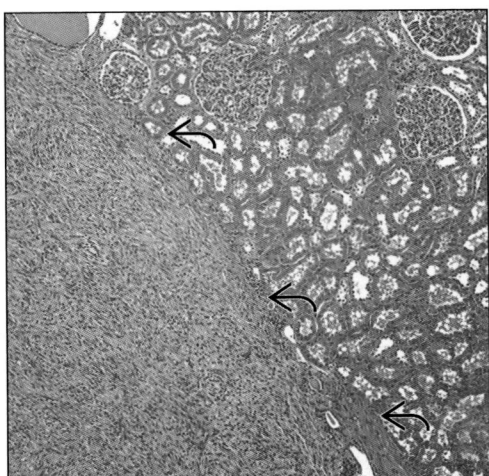

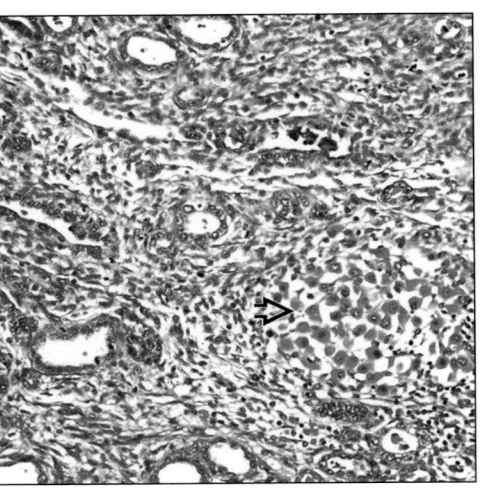

(Left) Metanephric stromal tumors (MST) may closely resemble classic CMN. Unlike CMN, MST has less infiltrative borders ⇥. Dysmorphic vessels, and onion skin-like concentric spindle cells around vessels and tubules in the latter also support an MST. *(Right)* Post-therapy stromal-type residual Wilms is often a problematic morphologic differential. CMN does not show the extensive necrosis seen in such WTs. Rhabdomyomatous features ⇥ are also not seen in CMN.

CLEAR CELL SARCOMA OF THE KIDNEY

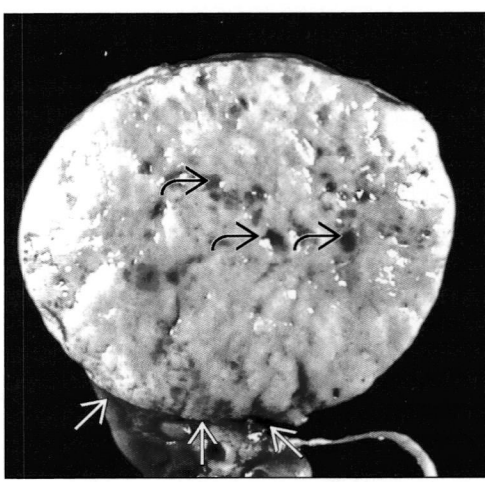

Typical gross features of a clear cell sarcoma include a large, well-circumscribed tumor ➡ with fleshy tan, mucoid cut surface, often with variably prominent cystic areas ➡.

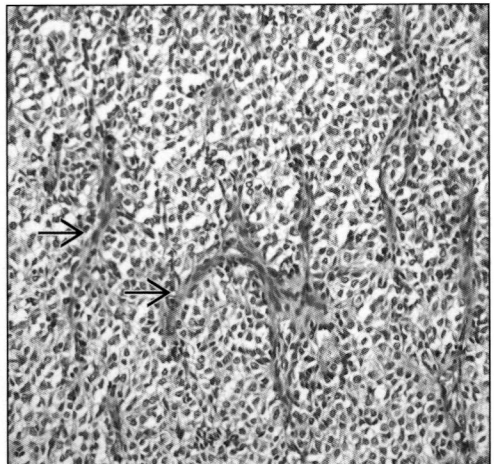

Characteristic features are seen in this classic pattern of clear cell sarcoma. Cords and nests of tumor cells are separated by branching vascular septa with "chicken wire" appearance ➡.

TERMINOLOGY

Abbreviations
- Clear cell sarcoma of kidney (CCSK)

Synonyms
- Bone-metastasizing renal tumor of childhood

Definitions
- Uncommon malignant renal neoplasm of childhood of uncertain histogenesis with aggressive clinical behavior

ETIOLOGY/PATHOGENESIS

Molecular Genetics
- Gene expression profiling has reported expression of neural markers, like nerve growth-factor receptor, and sonic hedgehog and Akt pathway markers
- Recently, nonrandom translocation t(10;17) and deletion 14q also described
  - 17p13 is locus of *p53* gene, but *p53* alterations seen only in anaplastic CCSK

CLINICAL ISSUES

Epidemiology
- Incidence
  - ~ 20 new cases/year in USA; comprise 3% of childhood renal tumors
- Age
  - 2 months to 14 years old; peak incidence: 2-3 years old
    - Congenital cases reported, and very rare cases also described in adults
- Gender
  - M:F = 2:1

Presentation
- Large unicentric renal mass
- Other common presentations include hematuria and hypertension

Treatment
- Combined therapeutic options
  - Unilateral nephrectomy, adjuvant chemotherapy with doxorubicin, dactinomycin, and vincristine (NWTS 4 regimen), and tumor bed radiation therapy
    - Addition of doxorubicin to drug regimen has shown definite improvement in outcome

Prognosis
- Aggressive clinical course
- Frequent metastases
  - Ipsilateral renal hilar lymph nodes most common site at presentation
  - Bones are most common sites of recurrence, followed closely by lung; other sites of relapse include abdomen/retroperitoneum
- Independent prognostic factors for survival
  - Treatment with doxorubicin
    - Improves outcome
  - Stage 1 disease (NWTS 5 criteria)
    - 98% overall survival rate
  - Patient age
    - Improved outcome in patients 2-4 years old
  - Presence of tumor necrosis
    - Adverse factor for survival; only histological prognostic variable

MACROSCOPIC FEATURES

General Features
- Unicentric renal mass, usually large in size
- Well circumscribed
- Often homogeneous, solid, tan-gray, glistening, gelatinous cut surface; often with cystic areas

CLEAR CELL SARCOMA OF THE KIDNEY

Key Facts

Terminology
- Clear cell sarcoma of kidney (CCSK)
- Uncommon malignant renal neoplasm of childhood of uncertain cell of origin with aggressive clinical behavior

Clinical Issues
- Treatment with doxorubicin shown to improve outcome
- Ipsilateral renal hilar lymph nodes most common site at presentation
- Bones are most common sites of recurrence
- Presence of tumor necrosis
  - Only histological prognostic variable

Microscopic Pathology
- Diagnosis primarily based on histologic criteria

- No diagnostic immunohistochemical or molecular features available at present
- Morphologic hallmark: Evenly distributed network of vascular septa, with branching "chicken wire" pattern

Ancillary Tests
- Immunostaining primarily useful for excluding other renal tumors
- No specific stains available for CCSK

Top Differential Diagnoses
- Blastema predominant Wilms tumor
- Mesoblastic nephroma

- Occasionally foci of hemorrhage and necrosis

Size
- Mean diameter: 11.3 cm (range: 2.3 cm to 24 cm)

MICROSCOPIC PATHOLOGY

Microscopic Features
- Diagnosis primarily based on histologic criteria; no specific immunohistochemical or molecular features available at present
- Classic pattern, present in 90% tumors at least focally
  - Almost evenly distributed network of vascular septa, with branching "chicken wire" pattern, similar to myxoid liposarcoma and oligodendroglioma
  - Septae divide tumor into nests and cords of polygonal cells with indistinct cell borders, nuclei showing finely granular chromatin, and inconspicuous nucleoli
  - Cells often surrounded by pale, mucopolysaccharide material, often creating illusion of clear cytoplasm
  - Necrosis: Only independent histologic factor for adverse prognosis
  - Entrapped renal tubules along periphery
- Variant patterns (listed in order of observed frequency)
  - Myxoid, sclerosing, cellular, epithelioid trabecular, palisading (Verocay body-like), spindle cell, storiform, anaplastic
    - Anaplasia defined by nuclear hyperchromasia, nuclear gigantism, and atypical mitoses
- Histologic variants do not affect prognosis

ANCILLARY TESTS

Immunohistochemistry
- Immunostaining primarily useful for excluding other renal tumors
  - No specific stains available for CCSK
- Tumor cells immunoreactive for vimentin and bcl-2
- Stains for epithelial markers consistently negative
- All CCSK are CD99 and WT1 negative

- Immunoreactivity for p53 consistently observed in anaplastic tumors only

DIFFERENTIAL DIAGNOSIS

Blastema Predominant Wilms Tumor
- Chromatin pattern coarse with molding; WT1 positive

Primitive Neuroectodermal Tumor
- CD99 and FLI-1 positive

Congenital Mesoblastic Nephroma, "Plump Cell" Pattern
- Spindled and polygonal cells with prominent nucleoli; actin positive

Malignant Rhabdoid Tumor
- Negative for SNF5(INI1)

DIAGNOSTIC CHECKLIST

Pathologic Interpretation Pearls
- Diagnosis of CCSK is primarily based on histologic criteria alone, but variant patterns make diagnosis difficult in some cases
- Diagnostic hallmark is evenly distributed network of vascular septa, with branching "chicken wire" pattern
- Attention to overall morphology and immunohistochemical stains usually help in excluding other differential diagnostic possibilities

SELECTED REFERENCES

1. Argani P et al: Clear cell sarcoma of the kidney: a review of 351 cases from the National Wilms Tumor Study Group Pathology Center. Am J Surg Pathol. 24(1):4-18, 2000
2. Amin MB et al: Clear cell sarcoma of kidney in an adolescent and in young adults: a report of four cases with ultrastructural, immunohistochemical, and DNA flow cytometric analysis. Am J Surg Pathol. 23(12):1455-63, 1999

CLEAR CELL SARCOMA OF THE KIDNEY

Microscopic Features

(Left) Despite the well-circumscribed gross and low-power, CCSK almost invariably has invasive fronts, with entrapped nephrons at the periphery of the tumor ➡. (Right) Occasionally, entrapped tubules may show embryonic-type metaplasia ➡, raising the suspicion of nephroblastoma. The lack of blastemal elements and the presence of typical vasculature with minimally pleomorphic, pale nuclei in the tumor should point toward the correct diagnosis of CCSK.

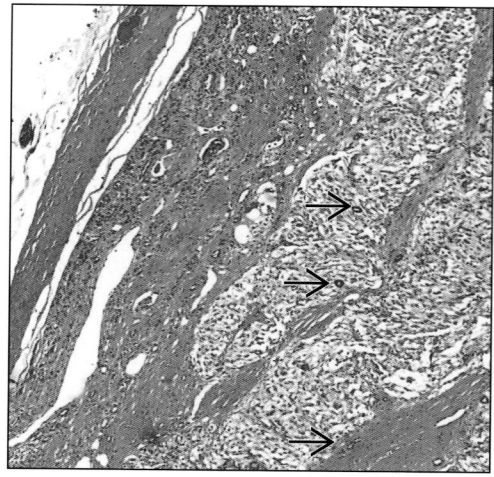
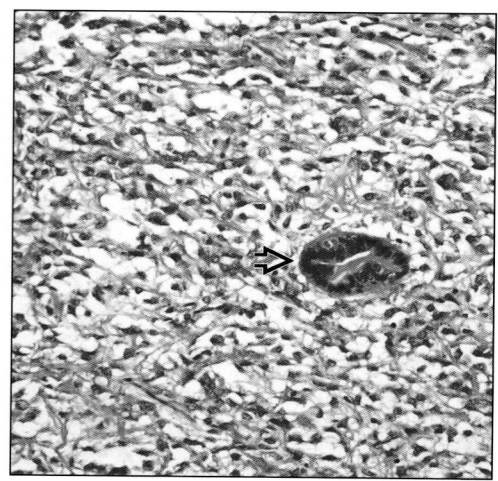

(Left) CCSK is shown with loosely spaced and discohesive cells attached to the delicate fibrovascular septae ➡. The tumor has a pseudoglandular pattern. (Right) Tumor cells in CCSK show vesicular nuclei and pale cytoplasm with indistinct cell borders, separated by delicate fibrovascular septae ➡. Tumor cells are often surrounded by pale, mucopolysaccharide material ➡, creating the illusion of clear cytoplasm, as well as the pale appearance of a glass slide held against light.

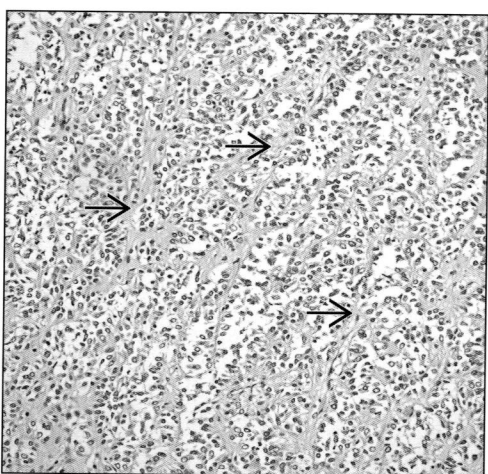
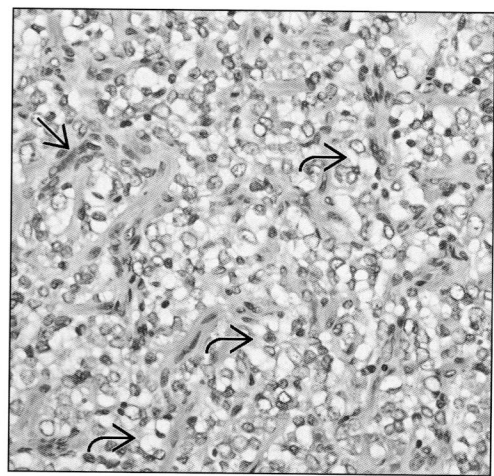

(Left) High magnification of classic pattern of CCSK shows tumor nuclei with vesicular, finely granular chromatin and inconspicuous nucleoli ➡. In well-fixed specimens, this chromatin pattern is the most helpful clue to the diagnosis. (Right) Diagnosis of CCSK is primarily based on morphologic criteria. The classic pattern is seen in more than 90% of cases, but variant morphologies may coexist in the same tumor. This spindle cell pattern may raise the differential of a mesoblastic nephroma.

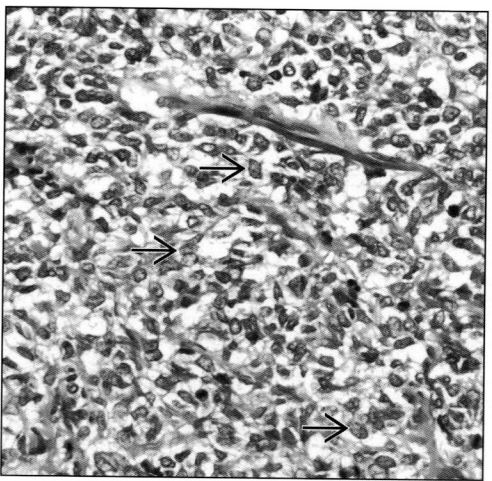
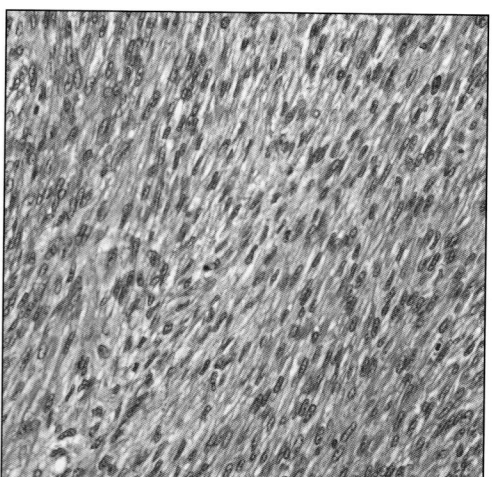

CLEAR CELL SARCOMA OF THE KIDNEY

Microscopic Features

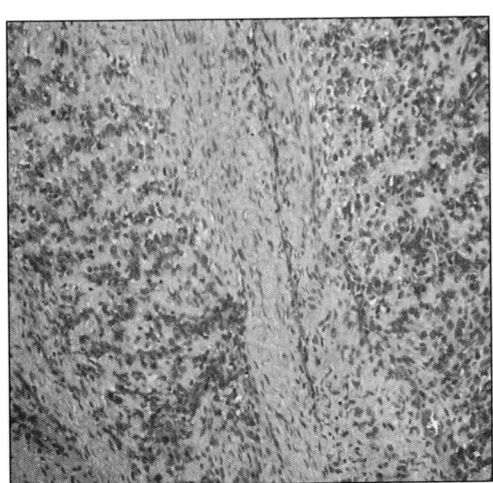

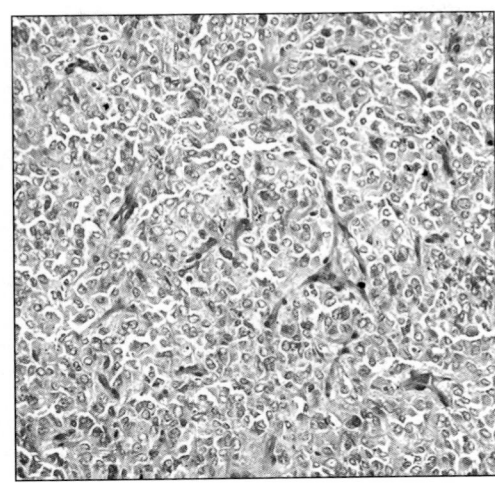

(Left) Palisading pattern may be rarely seen in CCSK, and in such areas, closely resembles schwannoma. Immunostain for S100 protein is invariably negative, excluding the possibility of a schwannoma. *(Right)* This image shows a CCSK with epithelioid features. The presence of well-defined cytoplasmic membranes and focal eosinophilic cytoplasm may raise suspicion of a rhabdoid tumor. Vesicular chromatin, lack of prominent nucleoli, and the vascular pattern point to the correct diagnosis.

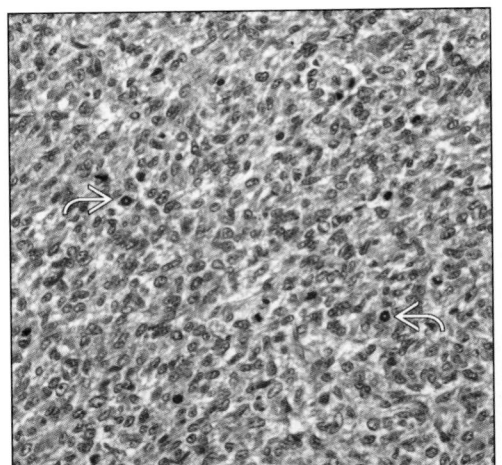

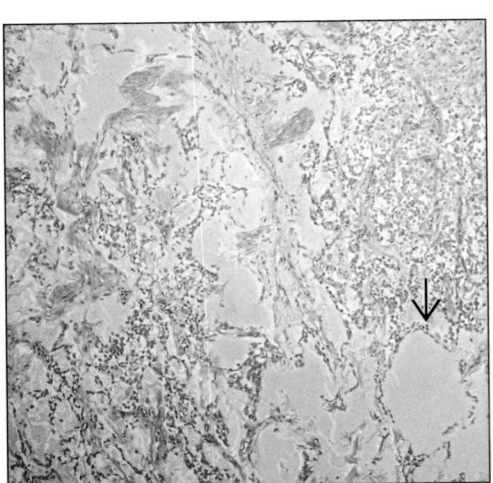

(Left) Some CCSK show areas of increased cellularity, nuclear hyperchromasia, mild pleomorphism, and mitotic figures ➡. Anaplasia in CCSK is defined by nuclear hyperchromasia, nuclear gigantism, and the presence of atypical mitoses. *(Right)* Medium-power view shows a CCSK with numerous prominent pseudocysts ➡ containing pools of amorphous-myxoid material. Other areas showing the more classical pattern, including the typical vasculature, are almost invariably present.

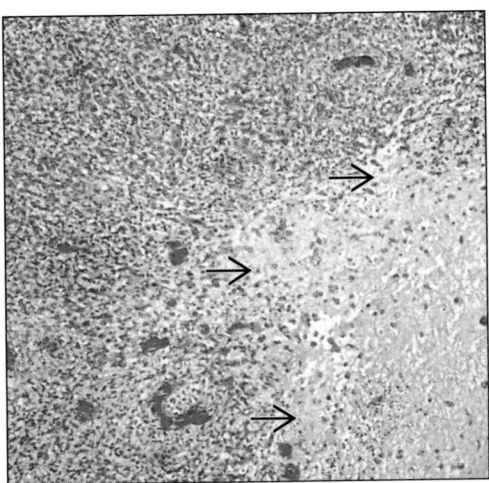

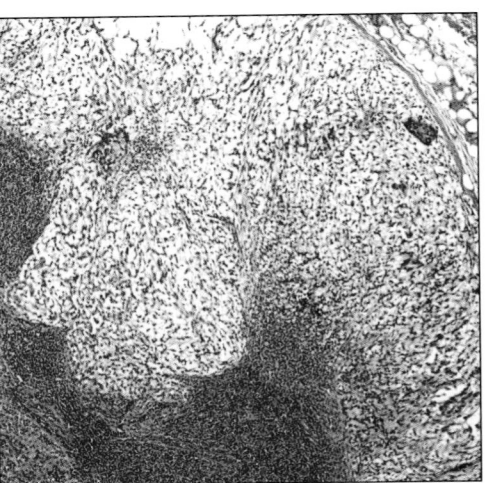

(Left) This clear cell sarcoma of the kidney shows an area of tumor necrosis ➡. Tumor necrosis is an adverse factor for survival and is the only histological prognostic variable in CCSK. *(Right)* This hematoxylin & eosin shows lymph node metastasis in clear cell sarcoma of the kidney. Ipsilateral renal hilar lymph nodes are the most common site of metastasis at presentation. In contrast, osseous metastases are the most common site of recurrence, followed closely by the lung.

MALIGNANT RHABDOID TUMOR

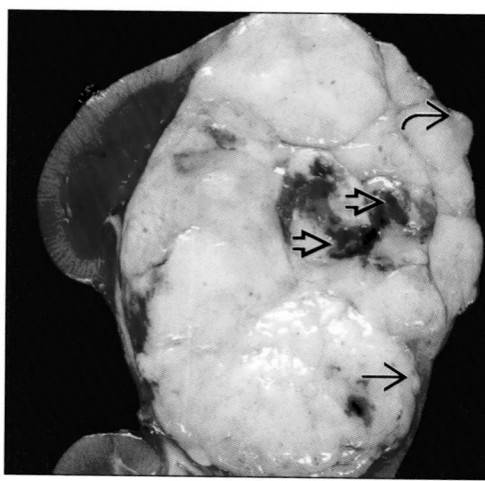

RTK is seen with necrosis ⊡, irregular invasive borders ⊡, and extension beyond renal parenchyma ⊡. Necrosis may be more extensive, and some tumors may be relatively small due to early dissemination.

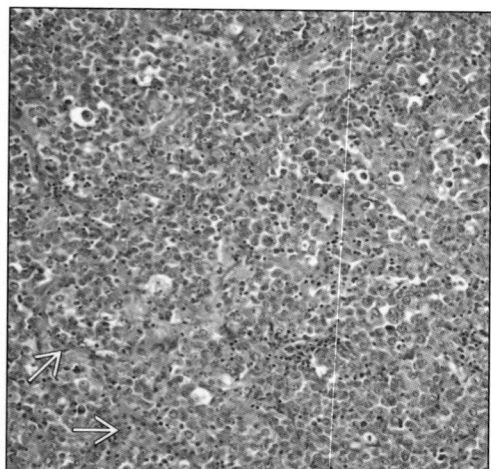

Sheets of loosely cohesive tumor cells with large nuclei and abundant eosinophilic cytoplasm are typical of RTK. A delicate network of fibrovascular septae ⊡ may also be appreciated.

TERMINOLOGY

Abbreviations
- Malignant rhabdoid tumor of kidney (RTK) ,

Definitions
- Highly malignant pediatric renal tumor with very poor prognosis and genetic abnormalities of *hSNF5/INI1* tumor suppressor gene on chromosome 22

ETIOLOGY/PATHOGENESIS

HSNF5/INI1 Tumor Suppressor Gene
- Biallelic inactivation of gene, located at 22q11.2; consistent feature of RTK
  - Usually associated with deletion of 1 copy with mutation in remaining copy
  - Gene believed to be important for chromatin remodeling

CLINICAL ISSUES

Epidemiology
- Incidence
  - Comprises approximately 2% of pediatric renal tumors
- Age
  - Mean age of presentation around 1 year
  - Predominantly affects younger children; 80% < 2 years old, 60% < 1 year old
    - Virtually nonexistent after 5 years of age
  - Overwhelming majority of stage IV renal tumors in 1st 7 months of life are RTK
- Gender
  - M:F = 1.5:1

Site
- Originally described in kidney; similar tumors later recognized in extrarenal sites, including
  - Central nervous system (atypical teratoid/rhabdoid tumor) and soft tissue

Presentation
- Abdominal mass; most common mode of presentation
- Hematuria &/or fever, other common symptoms
- Hypercalcemia
  - Some tumors may produce parathyroid hormone-related protein or prostaglandin E2
- High tumor stage at presentation
  - Up to 75% present with stage III, IV, or V disease
- Frequent metastases to lung, abdomen, liver, brain, and bone
- Tumors in kidney, CNS, or soft tissue may occur sporadically or as part of rhabdoid tumor predisposition syndrome
  - Germline mutations of *INI1* are common in patients with apparent sporadic tumors as well as in familial rhabdoid tumor predisposition syndrome

Treatment
- Combination of surgery, multiagent chemotherapy, and radiotherapy coupled with autologous stem cell transplantation offer the best results

Prognosis
- Extremely poor prognosis with aggressive behavior
  - Mortality rate > 80% within 2 years of diagnosis
- Increasing age at diagnosis with increasing survival
- Predictors of poorer prognosis include
  - Younger age at diagnosis, higher tumor stage, and presence of CNS lesions

MACROSCOPIC FEATURES

General Features
- Typically, large tumors with ill-defined borders
- Cut surface with areas of hemorrhage and necrosis

MALIGNANT RHABDOID TUMOR

Key Facts

Terminology
- Malignant rhabdoid tumor of kidney (RTK)
- Highly malignant pediatric renal tumor with very poor prognosis and genetic abnormalities of *hSNF5/INI1* tumor suppressor gene on chromosome 22

Etiology/Pathogenesis
- Biallelic inactivation of gene, located at 22q11.2; consistent feature of RTK

Clinical Issues
- Mean age of presentation: Around 1 year old
- Predominantly affects younger children; 80% < 2 years old, 60% < 1 year old
- Overwhelming majority of stage IV renal tumors in 1st 7 months of life are RTK
- High tumor stage at presentation

Macroscopic Features
- Well-circumscribed and unencapsulated
- Foci of hemorrhage and necrosis

Microscopic Pathology
- Sheets of monotonous, loosely cohesive, large ovoid to polygonal cells, with high nuclear grade
- Characteristic cytologic features: Vesicular chromatin, prominent eosinophilic nucleoli, and intracytoplasmic hyaline, pink inclusion, at least in some cells

Ancillary Tests
- SNF5(INI1) negative immunostaining considered specific
  - Reliable surrogate marker of *hSNF5/INI1* gene deletion or inactivating mutations

Size
- Range, 3-17 cm in diameter (mean: 9.6 cm), sometimes replacing entire kidney

MICROSCOPIC PATHOLOGY

Histologic Features
- Sheets of monotonous loosely cohesive large, ovoid to polygonal cells, with high nuclear grade
  - Extensively infiltrating the renal parenchyma
- Characteristic cytologic features: Vesicular chromatin, prominent eosinophilic nucleoli, and intracytoplasmic hyaline, pink inclusions (at least in some cells)
  - Inclusions are sometimes difficult to find; increased chances of finding these in perinecrotic regions
- Brisk mitotic activity and areas of necrosis frequent
- Vascular invasion and extrarenal extension common
- Variant histology may be present in some tumors, usually in association with typical areas
  - Sclerosing (most common), spindled, pseudopapillary and cystic, among others

Predominant Pattern/Injury Type
- Neoplastic

ANCILLARY TESTS

Immunohistochemistry
- Loss of nuclear staining for SNF5(INI1), very sensitive and highly specific for RTK, among pediatric renal tumors
- Nonspecific polyphenotypic patterns due to trapping of antibodies in hyaline inclusions
- Vimentin, keratin, and focal EMA/MUC1 positivity

Electron Microscopy
- Ultrastructurally, hyaline inclusions correspond to whorled intermediate filaments

DIFFERENTIAL DIAGNOSIS

Renal Medullary Carcinoma
- Older age, sickle cell trait, and occasionally glandular histology
- Loss of nuclear staining for SNF5(INI1), keratin typically strong

Cellular Mesoblastic Nephroma, "Plump Cell" Variant
- Spindle cell pattern and less invasive tumor periphery

Clear Cell Sarcoma of Kidney
- Lack prominent nucleoli

DIAGNOSTIC CHECKLIST

Pathologic Interpretation Pearls
- Large number of renal and extrarenal tumors may show pseudorhabdoid features
- Clear cell carcinoma and collecting duct carcinoma in adults may show focal or prominent rhabdoid change
- In addition to their specific morphologic and immunohistochemical features, nuclear immunoreactivity for SNF5(INI1) is retained in all such tumors

SELECTED REFERENCES

1. Kohashi K et al: Infrequent SMARCB1/INI1 gene alteration in epithelioid sarcoma: a useful tool in distinguishing epithelioid sarcoma from malignant rhabdoid tumor. Hum Pathol. 40(3):349-55, 2009
2. Vujanić GM et al: Rhabdoid tumour of the kidney: a clinicopathological study of 22 patients from the International Society of Paediatric Oncology (SIOP) nephroblastoma file. Histopathology. 28(4):333-40, 1996
3. Weeks DA et al: Rhabdoid tumor of kidney. A report of 111 cases from the National Wilms' Tumor Study Pathology Center. Am J Surg Pathol. 13(6):439-58, 1989

MALIGNANT RHABDOID TUMOR

Microscopic Features

(Left) Hematoxylin & eosin section shows the typical invasive border ⮕ in a malignant rhabdoid tumor of kidney. No encapsulation is present in these tumors. *(Right)* Hematoxylin & eosin shows a RTK with large areas of necrosis ⮕. Hemorrhage and necrosis, at both the gross and microscopic levels, are quite frequent in these tumors and support their aggressive nature. An important diagnostic feature is that cytoplasmic inclusions are more common around necrotic areas.

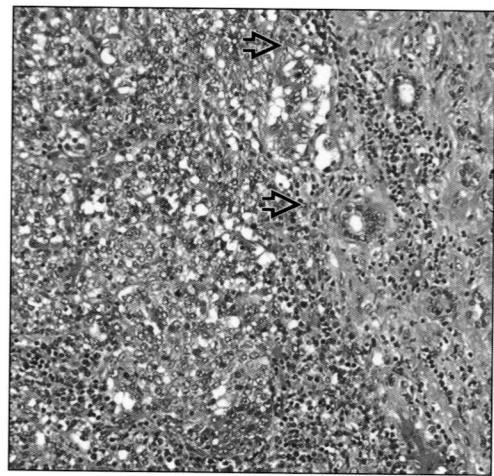
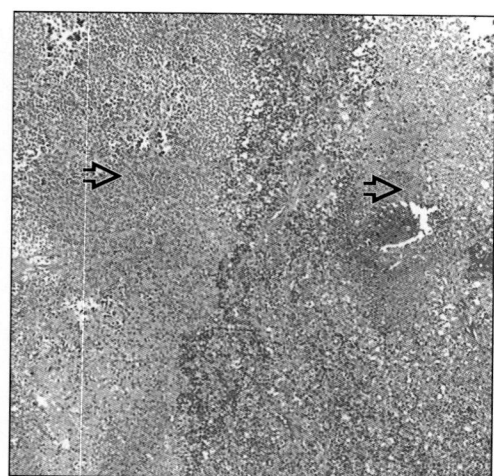

(Left) Besides overrunning the renal parenchyma, other features in malignant rhabdoid tumors that indicate an aggressive phenotype include a very high mitotic index. This photomicrograph depicts a prominent mitotic activity ⮕ in a malignant rhabdoid tumor. *(Right)* Vascular invasion ⮕ is usually extensive in malignant rhabdoid tumor of the kidney. Many tumors show both gross and microscopic invasion of the sinus vessels, as well as the renal vein.

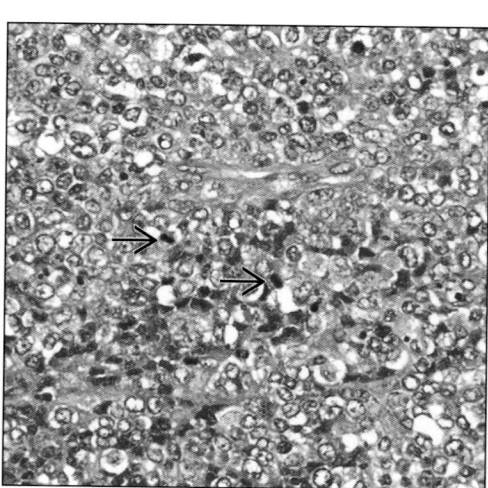
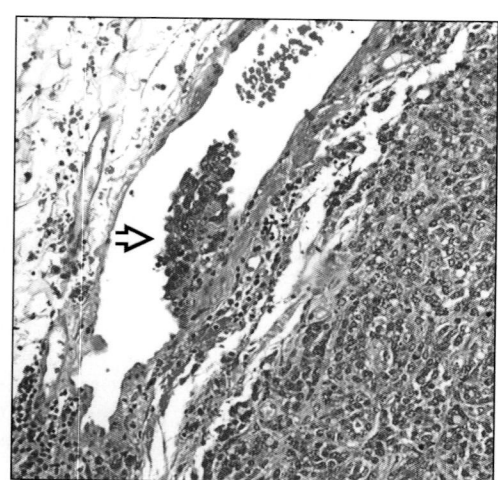

(Left) Malignant rhabdoid tumors of the kidney frequently extend beyond renal parenchyma. Sinus fat or perinephric fat invasion are quite common, as is invasion of the pelvicalyceal system ⮕. *(Right)* Medium-power view shows sheets of loosely cohesive tumor cells with eccentric nuclei and abundant eosinophilic cytoplasm in a malignant rhabdoid tumor of the kidney. The nuclei show vesicular chromatin and prominent nucleoli, easily identifiable at this magnification.

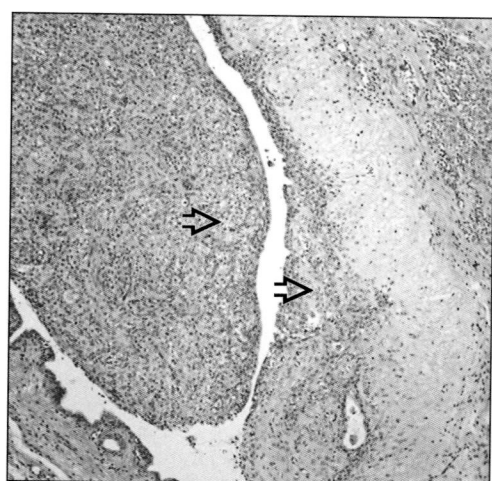
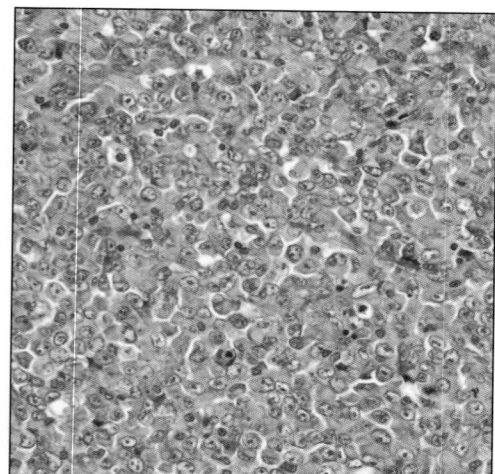

MALIGNANT RHABDOID TUMOR

Microscopic Features

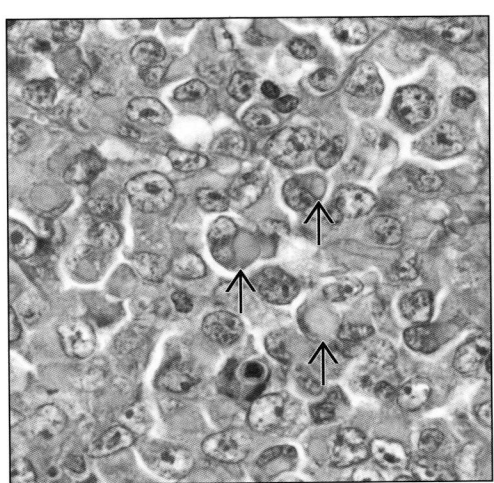
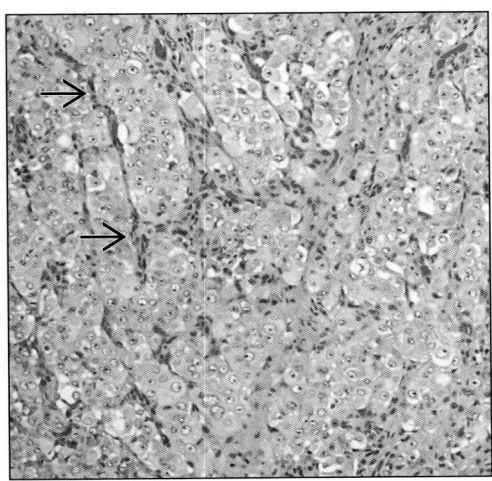

(Left) Malignant rhabdoid tumor of the kidney shows mononuclear cells with pleomorphic nuclei, vesicular chromatin, conspicuous nucleoli, and intracytoplasmic eosinophilic hyaline inclusions ➡. (Right) Some malignant rhabdoid tumors show a trabecular pattern of growth. Delicate fibrovascular septations separating the tumor trabeculae ➡ are also present here, and this may raise the suspicion of a clear cell sarcoma. The cytologic features are usually diagnostic.

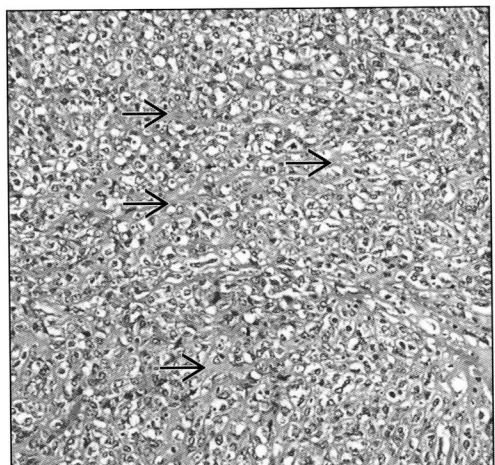
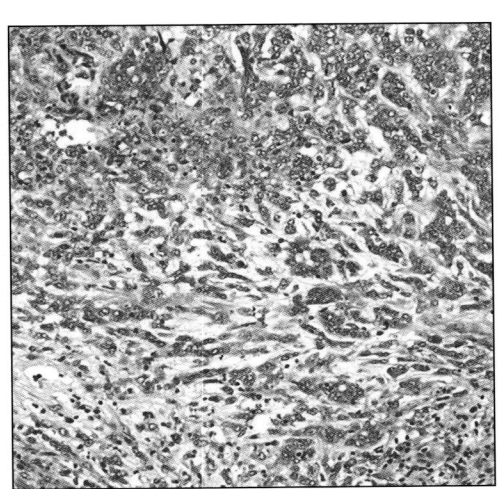

(Left) Some RTK show areas with abundant sclerosis ➡. This feature is more common in clear cell sarcoma of the kidney. Close attention to the cytologic features will help in arriving at the proper diagnosis. (Right) This hematoxylin & eosin image shows marked myxoid change in the stroma of a RTK. Marked variation in the histomorphologic patterns is not infrequent in rhabdoid tumors of the kidney, and the overall cytoarchitectural findings are essential for a proper diagnosis.

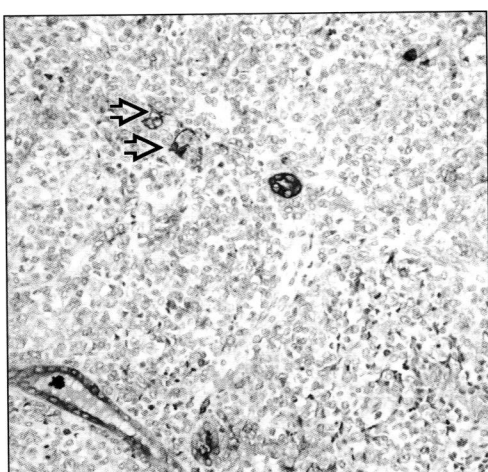
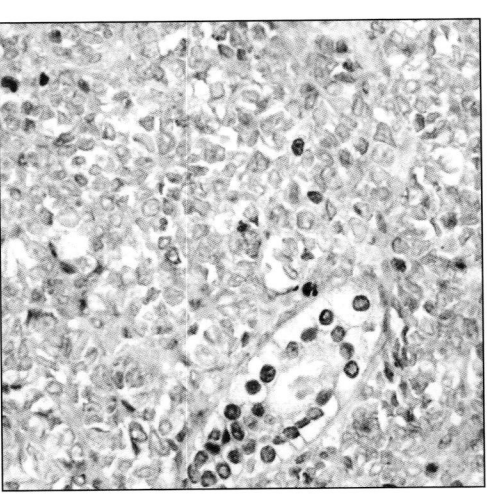

(Left) Immunostaining in RTK usually shows a polyphenotypic expression, due to nonspecific entrapment of the antibodies by the whorled structures in cytoplasmic inclusions. However, stains for EMA/MUC1 ➡ and vimentin are consistently positive. (Right) The most consistent and diagnostic immunostaining in rhabdoid and related CNS and soft tissue tumors is the loss of nuclear staining for SNF5. It is a reliable surrogate marker of hSNF5/INI1 gene deletions or inactivating mutations.

1

CYSTIC NEPHROMA/MIXED EPITHELIAL AND STROMAL TUMOR

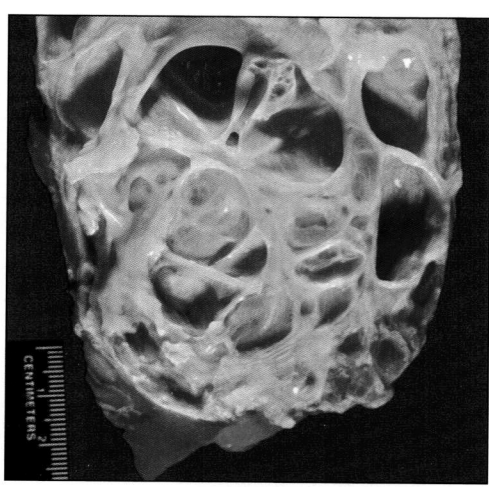

Gross photograph of a cystic nephroma shows an exclusively cystic, well-circumscribed tumor with no solid areas. Gross distinction from multilocular cystic RCC is not possible in such cases.

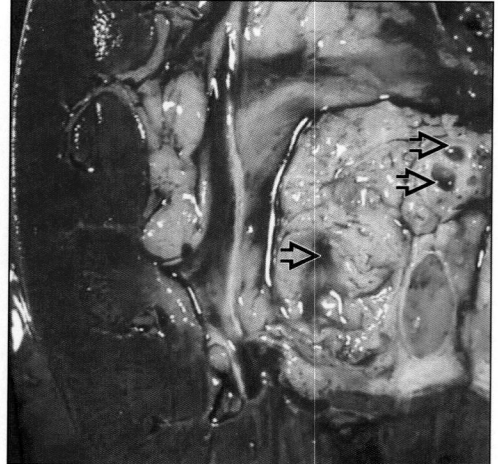

Gross appearance of a mixed epithelial and stromal tumor shows a predominantly solid morphology. Relatively few cysts ⇗ are apparent on gross evaluation.

TERMINOLOGY

Abbreviations
- Cystic nephroma (CN), mixed epithelial and stromal tumor (MEST)

Synonyms
- Renal epithelial and stromal tumor (REST)
- For MEST: Adult mesoblastic nephroma, cystic hamartoma of renal pelvis, leiomyomatous renal hamartoma, or solid and cystic biphasic tumor

Definitions
- Multicystic to solid and cystic, mostly benign, biphasic renal tumors that likely represent morphologic spectrum of same entity
- CN: Tumor composed entirely of cysts and cyst septae without any solid expansile areas or mural nodules
  - Septations with arbitrarily chosen thickness of less than 5 mm
- MEST: Tumors with variable amounts of solid components

ETIOLOGY/PATHOGENESIS

Role of Hormones
- Features that suggest role of steroid hormones in genesis and evolution of these tumors include
  - Marked female preponderance
  - Common history of long-term estrogen replacement in female patients
  - Long-term sex steroid exposure in male patients
  - Frequent expression of ER and PR in tumor mesenchymal component

Genetic Alterations
- Gene expression profiles of mRNA demonstrate that both CN and MEST share similar expression profiles
  - Highest differentially expressed gene, relative to other tumors and nonneoplastic parenchyma, is insulin-like growth factor 2
  - Lowest differential expression is of carbonic anhydrase 2 gene
- Single case of translocation t(1;19) in MEST also reported

CLINICAL ISSUES

Epidemiology
- Age
  - Mean age similar for both CN and MEST: Approximately 53 years (range: 34-78 years)
  - CN in pediatric age group considered to be fully differentiated nephroblastoma
    - Not related to tumors seen in adults
- Gender
  - CN: F:M approximately 8:1
  - MEST: Mostly in females with only rare reported cases in males

Presentation
- Incidentally detected kidney mass is most common clinical presentation
- Other described symptoms
  - Abdominal pain
  - Hematuria
  - Urinary tract infections

Prognosis
- All reported cases of typical CN and MEST have behaved in benign fashion following surgical excision
  - 1 reported case of MEST recurred locally 21 years after resection
- A few cases of malignant MEST reported in literature
  - Malignant phenotype observed in either epithelial or mesenchymal components

CYSTIC NEPHROMA/MIXED EPITHELIAL AND STROMAL TUMOR

Key Facts

Terminology
- Cystic nephroma (CN), mixed epithelial and stromal tumor (MEST)
- Multicystic to solid and cystic biphasic renal tumors that likely represent morphologic spectrum of same entity

Clinical Issues
- CN: F:M = approximately 8:1; MEST: Mostly in females with only rare reported cases in males
- Incidentally detected kidney mass is most common clinical presentation
- All reported cases of typical CN and MEST have behaved in benign fashion following surgical excision

Macroscopic Features
- CN: All tumors entirely cystic with no solid areas or expansile nodules
- MEST: Variably solid and cystic, sometimes with predominant solid component

Microscopic Pathology
- Stroma in both CN and MEST with varied histologic features
- Epithelial components in both CN and MEST with varied but similar features

Top Differential Diagnoses
- Multilocular cystic RCC, tubulocystic carcinoma, CPDN, mesoblastic nephroma (classical type), metanephric adenofibroma

---

- Morphologic features of malignancy include increased cellularity, cytologic atypia, prominent nucleoli, and high mitotic rate
  - Spindle cell NOS, synovial sarcoma, rhabdoid, rhabdomyosarcoma, and chondrosarcoma differentiation in malignant stromal components

MACROSCOPIC FEATURES

General Features
- Cystic nephroma
  - Tumors usually solitary; very rare bilateral cases reported
  - Most tumors well circumscribed and confined to kidney
  - Located mostly close to renal hilum but may involve cortex, particularly in larger tumors
  - All tumors entirely cystic with no solid areas or expansile nodules
    - Majority of cysts contain clear serous fluid, rarely hemorrhagic or purulent material
- Mixed epithelial and stromal tumor
  - Mostly solitary and unilateral, with rare bilateral cases
  - Most tumors well circumscribed and confined to kidney
    - Very few tumors with ill-defined, infiltrative borders
  - Located mostly close to renal hilum and renal pelvis but may involve cortex, particularly in larger tumors
  - Variably solid and cystic, sometimes with predominant solid component

Size
- Size range similar for both CN and MEST: 1.7-21 cm (mean: 6.5 cm)

MICROSCOPIC PATHOLOGY

Histologic Features
- Stroma in both CN and MEST show varied histologic features, including
  - Loose fibrous and edematous
  - Dense fibrous and sclerotic
  - Hypercellular spindled, NOS
  - Ovarian stroma-like
  - Smooth muscle type
- Prominent vasculature more common in MEST
- Calcifications and foamy histiocytes present in both CN and MEST
- Cells in epithelial components in both CN and MEST show varied features, including
  - Flat
  - Hobnailed
  - Cuboidal
  - Columnar
  - Urothelial-like
  - Clear cell
  - However, clear cell or urothelial-like cyst lining relatively uncommon in CN
- Prominent ovarian stroma, smaller cysts, complex branching glands, phyllodes gland pattern, and stromal luteinization more common in MEST than CN

Predominant Pattern/Injury Type
- Neoplastic

Predominant Cell/Compartment Type
- Epithelial, biphasic or mixed

ANCILLARY TESTS

Immunohistochemistry
- Stromal cells often positive for ER, PR, and less commonly for inhibin and calretinin, in both (but more often in MEST)

CYSTIC NEPHROMA/MIXED EPITHELIAL AND STROMAL TUMOR

Differentiating Features Between Adult and Pediatric Cystic Nephroma

Features	Cystic Nephroma in Adults	Cystic Nephroma in Children
Age at presentation	Usually > 30 years	Usually < 4 years
Male to Female ratio	1:8	2:1
Pathogenesis	Not related to Wilms tumor	Related to Wilms tumor; considered to represent fully differentiated Wilms tumor
Tumor stroma	Variable; may resemble ovarian-type stroma, ER and PR positive	Consists of myxoid to collagenous fibrous tissue

DIFFERENTIAL DIAGNOSIS

Multilocular Cystic Renal Cell Carcinoma

- Differentiation is required from CN and predominantly cystic MEST
  - Multilocular cystic RCC with cysts showing variable flattened lining or almost entirely larger cells with clear cytoplasm
  - Clusters or nests of clear cells are always present in septae
  - No cellular or ovarian-type stroma
  - Lining cells with a CA9, CD10, and often CK7 positive immunophenotype
  - No stromal immunoreactivity for ER and PR

Tubulocystic Carcinoma

- Tubulocystic carcinoma needs to be differentiated from CN and predominantly cystic MEST
  - Cells lining tubules and cysts in tubulocystic carcinoma have high-grade nuclei and abundant eosinophilic cytoplasm
  - Stroma usually dense fibrotic and desmoplastic
  - Septae often incomplete and free floating
  - No ER and PR positivity

Cystic Partially Differentiated Nephroblastoma (CPDN)

- CPDN needs to be differentiated from CN and predominantly cystic MEST
  - CPDN shows at least focal nephroblastematous tissue, such as blastema, immature stromal cells, and primitive epithelium in septae
  - Almost all patients < 24 months old

Mesoblastic Nephroma (Classical Type)

- Differential is with solid MEST
  - Classical mesoblastic nephroma shows finger-like extensions into surrounding renal parenchyma
  - Entrapped native tubules and glomeruli are often seen in mesoblastic nephroma
    - However, these are seen almost entirely in periphery of tumor
  - Mesoblastic nephroma shows no ER or PR positivity

Metanephric Adenofibroma

- Metanephric adenofibroma needs to be differentiated from solid MEST
  - Epithelial component of metanephric adenofibroma is typically composed of tightly packed small uniform acini
  - Epithelial component has embryonal appearance similar to metanephric adenoma
  - Stromal component in metanephric adenoma is ER and PR negative

SELECTED REFERENCES

1. Mohanty SK et al: Mixed epithelial and stromal tumors of the kidney: an overview. Arch Pathol Lab Med. 133(9):1483-6, 2009
2. Portier BP et al: Mixed epithelial and stromal tumor of the kidney. J Urol. 181(4):1879-80, 2009
3. Zhou M et al: Adult cystic nephroma and mixed epithelial and stromal tumor of the kidney are the same disease entity: molecular and histologic evidence. Am J Surg Pathol. 33(1):72-80, 2009
4. Colombo P et al: Non-hormone-induced mixed epithelial and stromal tumor of kidney in a man: description of a rare case. Urology. 71(1):168, 2008
5. Jung SJ et al: Mixed epithelial and stromal tumor of kidney with malignant transformation: report of two cases and review of literature. Hum Pathol. 39(3):463-8, 2008
6. Kuroda N et al: Carcinosarcoma arising in mixed epithelial and stromal tumor of the kidney. APMIS. 116(11):1013-5, 2008
7. Lane BR et al: Adult cystic nephroma and mixed epithelial and stromal tumor of the kidney: clinical, radiographic, and pathologic characteristics. Urology. 71(6):1142-8, 2008
8. Montironi R et al: Cystic nephroma and mixed epithelial and stromal tumour of the kidney: opposite ends of the spectrum of the same entity? Eur Urol. 54(6):1237-46, 2008
9. Mai KT et al: Mixed epithelial and stromal tumour (MEST) of the kidney: report of 14 cases with male and PEComatous variants and proposed histopathogenesis. Pathology. 39(2):235-40, 2007
10. Sukov WR et al: Malignant mixed epithelial and stromal tumor of the kidney with rhabdoid features: report of a case including immunohistochemical, molecular genetic studies and comparison to morphologically similar renal tumors. Hum Pathol. 38(9):1432-7, 2007
11. Turbiner J et al: Cystic nephroma and mixed epithelial and stromal tumor of kidney: a detailed clinicopathologic analysis of 34 cases and proposal for renal epithelial and stromal tumor (REST) as a unifying term. Am J Surg Pathol. 31(4):489-500, 2007
12. Antic T et al: Mixed epithelial and stromal tumor of the kidney and cystic nephroma share overlapping features: reappraisal of 15 lesions. Arch Pathol Lab Med. 130(1):80-5, 2006
13. Compérat E et al: Benign mixed epithelial and stromal tumor of the kidney (MEST) with cytogenetic alteration. Pathol Res Pract. 200(11-12):865-7, 2005
14. Mukhopadhyay S et al: Corpora albicantia-like bodies in cystic nephroma: yet another similarity to mixed epithelial stromal tumor of kidney. Int J Surg Pathol. 13(2):233, 2005

CYSTIC NEPHROMA/MIXED EPITHELIAL AND STROMAL TUMOR

Gross and Microscopic Features

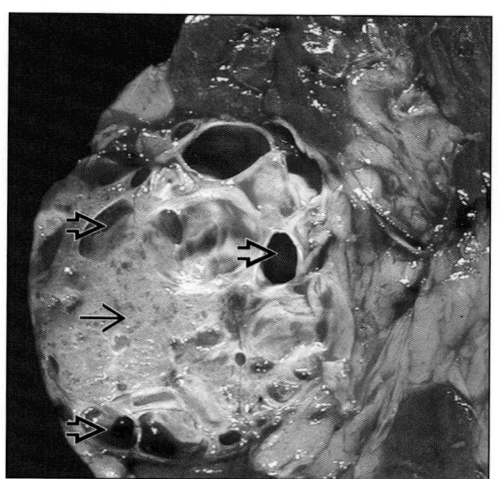
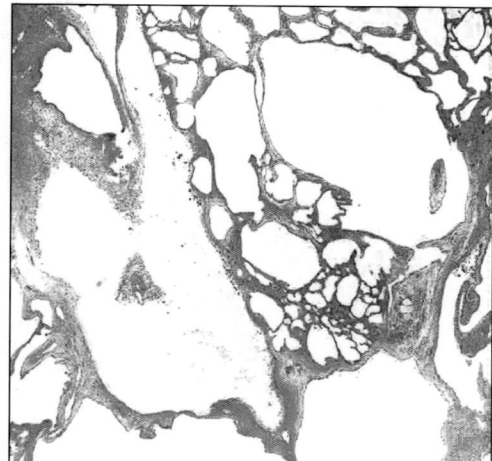

(Left) Some tumors, on both gross and microscopic evaluation, are difficult to classify as either CN or MEST. This tumor shows both prominent cystic areas ⇒ characteristic of CN, and solid regions →, more typical of MEST. The microscopic diagnosis may be influenced by variations in sampling in such a case. (Right) Microscopic image of a CN shows an exclusive cystic architecture, typical of the tumor. The cysts are discrete, without any apparent interconnections.

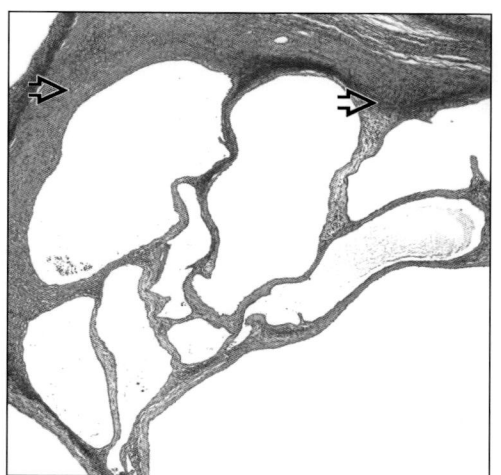
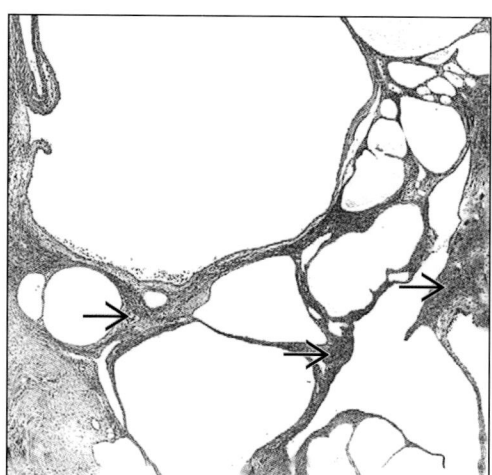

(Left) This hematoxylin & eosin image shows a cystic nephroma with slightly widened cellular septae ⇒. The lining is flattened without significant stratification. (Right) Hematoxylin & eosin image shows a cystic nephroma with septae composed of cellular ovarian-type stroma →. While such stroma may be present in cystic nephroma, it is a more common finding in mixed epithelial and stromal tumor. The ovarian stroma may show areas with luteinization and foam cells.

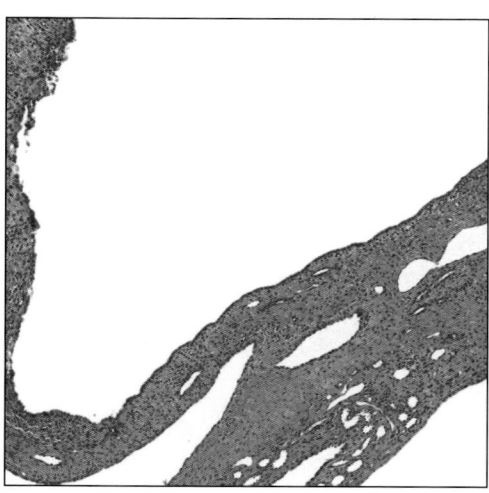
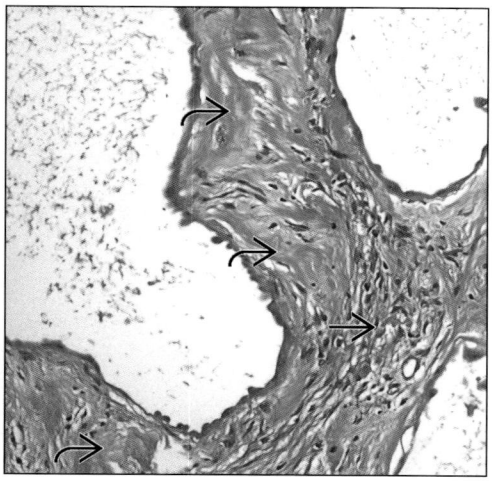

(Left) By definition, cystic nephroma does not show any solid areas or mural nodules. Septal thickness > 5 mm would place the tumor into the category of MEST. Even though these histologic criteria are arbitrary, these reiterate the morphologic overlap and close relationship between the two tumors. (Right) This hematoxylin & eosin image of a CN shows a combination of sclerotic ⇗ and cellular spindle cell → stroma. Mixture of stromal patterns is common in both CN and MEST.

1

189

CYSTIC NEPHROMA/MIXED EPITHELIAL AND STROMAL TUMOR

Microscopic Features

(Left) A lower power view depicts a minute-mixed epithelial and stromal tumor. Notice the well-circumscribed nature of the tumor, a relatively typical finding in cystic nephroma and MEST. Interspersed within a cellular stroma are benign epithelial elements ➡. *(Right)* Hematoxylin & eosin image of a mixed epithelial and stromal tumor shows multiple, variably sized tubules and cysts. Smaller cysts and complex branching glands are more common in MEST than in cystic nephroma.

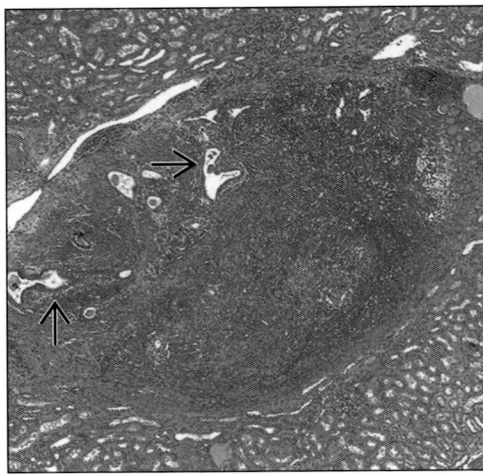
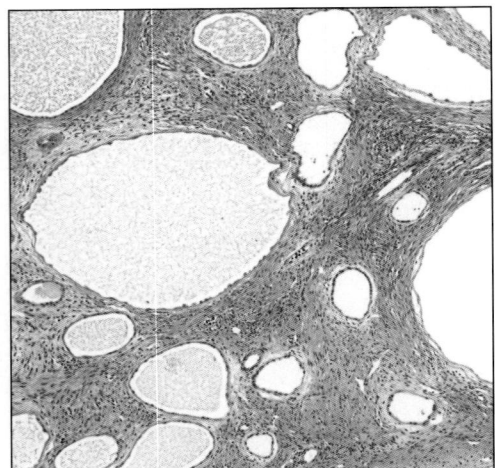

(Left) This hematoxylin & eosin image depicts cellular stroma in a MEST that resembles ovarian-type stroma. Cellular stroma is often immunoreactive for ER and PR in MEST, irrespective of its resemblance to ovarian stroma. *(Right)* Densely cellular ovarian-type stroma in a MEST is shown. Predominant occurrence in females, rare tumors in males on hormone therapy, and ER/PR positivity raises the strong possibility of the role of hormones in the pathogenesis of these tumors.

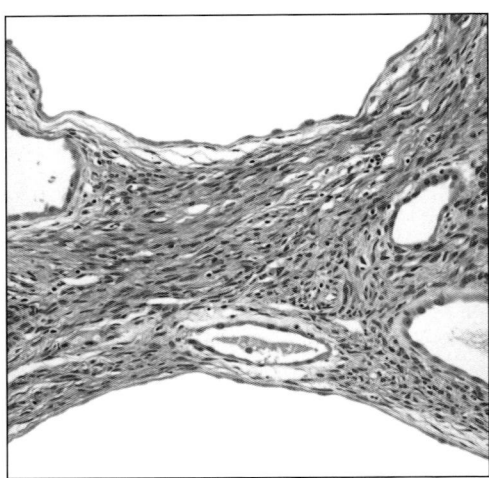
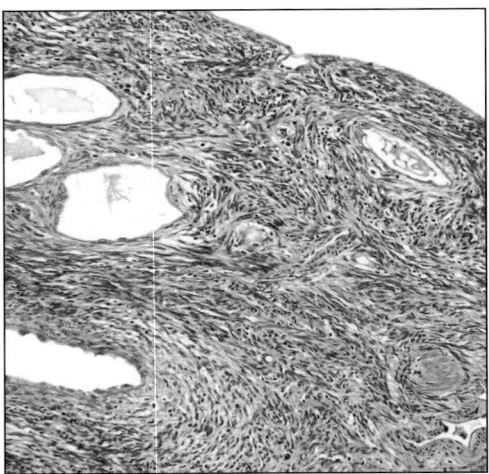

(Left) While the stroma is often nondescript or ovarian-type, some MESTs show prominent smooth muscle differentiation ➡ of the stroma. Not unexpectedly, such areas are strongly positive for actin-sm, actin-HHF-35, and desmin. The lining epithelium is "hobnailed" and pseudostratified. *(Right)* In addition to smooth muscle, the stroma in MEST may also show adipocytic differentiation. Usually such a finding is focal, but some tumors contain a prominent fatty component.

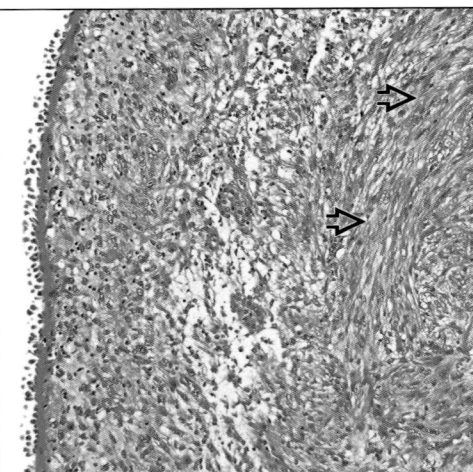
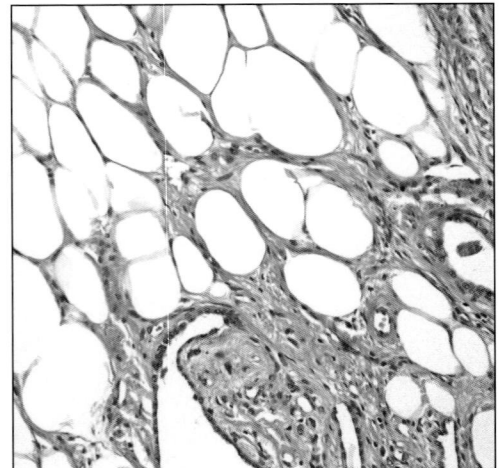

1

CYSTIC NEPHROMA/MIXED EPITHELIAL AND STROMAL TUMOR

Microscopic Features

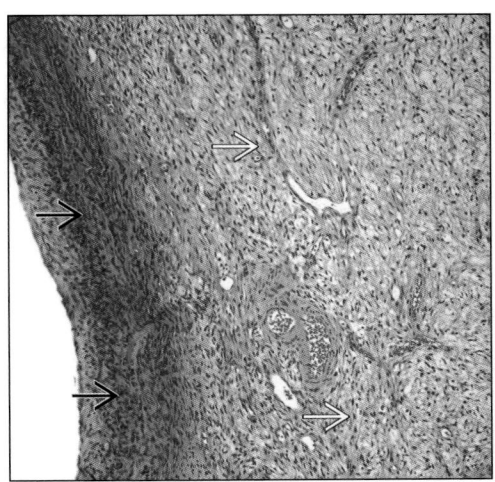

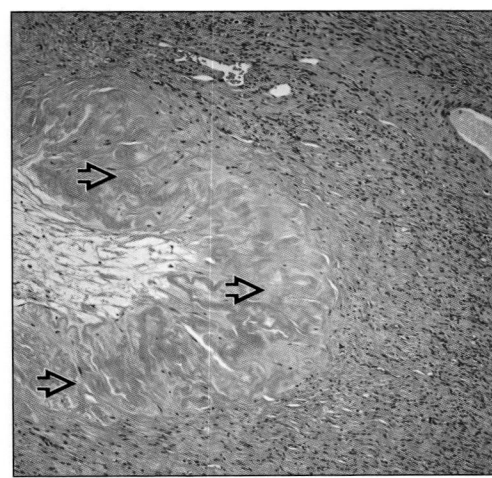

(Left) Some mixed epithelial and stromal tumors show a cambium-like condensed ovarian-type stroma underlying the epithelium. This image shows ovarian-type stroma ⮕ under the cyst lining, surrounded by more loose stroma ⮕ in the rest of the tumor. ER/PR reactivity is more likely in ovarian-type stroma but may be seen in other types of stroma. *(Right)* This hematoxylin & eosin image shows a corpus albicantia-like structure ⮕ in a background of ovarian-type stroma.

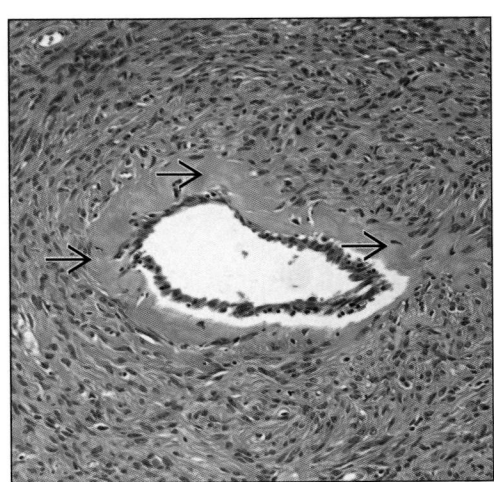

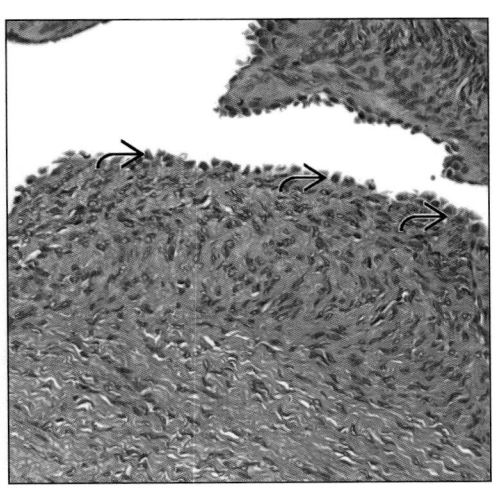

(Left) This photomicrograph depicts periepithelial hyalinization ⮕, supporting that the hyalinized structures are not similar to corpora albicantia of the ovary. In most cases, the pathogenesis of such structures cannot be determined, but in many cases these seem to result from hyalinization of vessels or epithelial structures. *(Right)* The epithelial cells in both CN and MEST share many features. This hematoxylin & eosin image illustrates "hobnailing" ⮕ of the lining epithelium in a MEST.

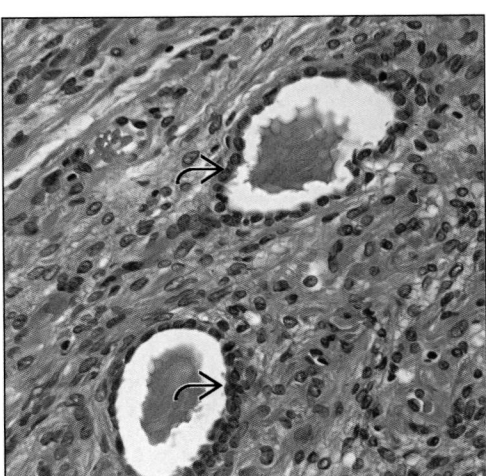

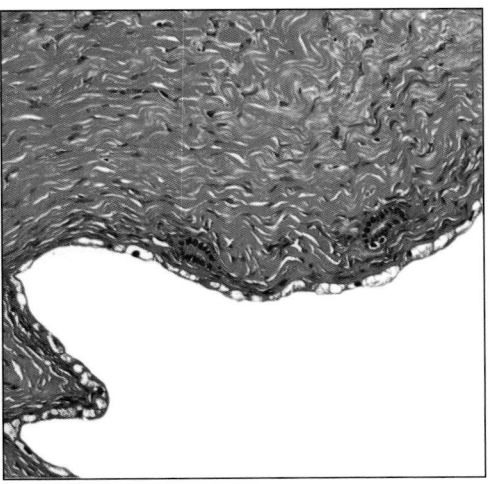

(Left) The cells in the epithelial component often are flat, "hobnailed," cuboidal, or columnar. This image shows cuboidal epithelial lining ⮕ in small cysts of MEST. There is no nuclear atypia or nucleolar prominence. *(Right)* Some CN and MEST show variable clear cell cytology. This may raise the possibility of a multilocular cystic RCC. However, many of these have ER/PR positive ovarian-type stroma, and lack solid nests of clear cells in the septae as seen multilocular cystic RCC.

CYSTIC NEPHROMA/MIXED EPITHELIAL AND STROMAL TUMOR

Microscopic Features

(Left) The stromal proliferation in mixed epithelial and stromal tumors may occasionally lead to leaf-like expanded (phyllodes-like) phenotype. Such proliferations would be inconsistent with the diagnosis of cystic nephroma. *(Right)* MESTs often show a complex branching glandular pattern and minute glands, a feature that is usually lacking in cystic nephromas. Occasionally the proliferation of small tubular structures resembles nephrogenic adenoma or prostatic epithelium.

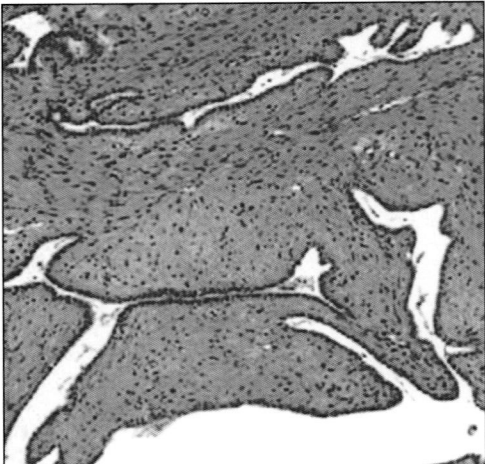
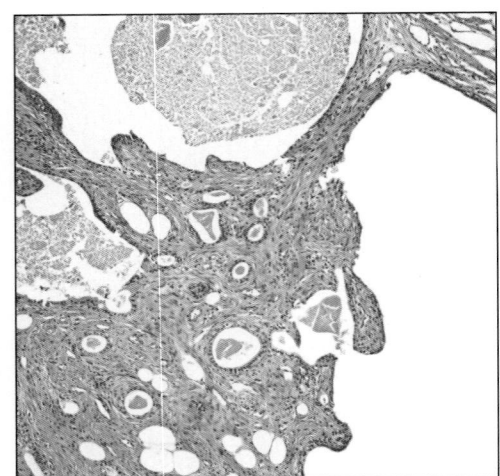

(Left) This hematoxylin & eosin image of a mixed epithelial and stromal tumor shows branching glandular structures. The stroma in this case is predominantly smooth muscle type. *(Right)* This image shows marked epithelial proliferation in a MEST. Due to lack of stromal invasion, this would qualify at least as a borderline tumor. Malignant transformation in MEST is quite rare but has been reported. Malignant transformation may occur in both epithelial and mesenchymal elements.

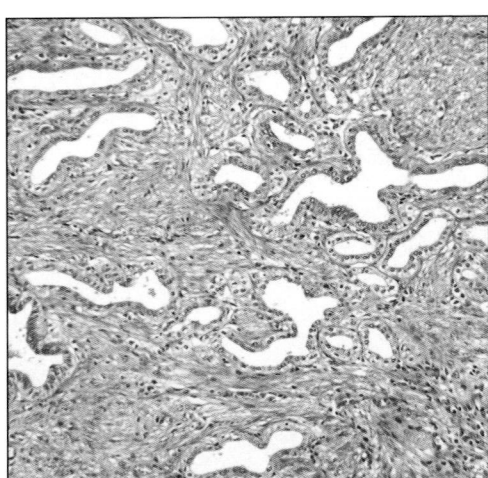
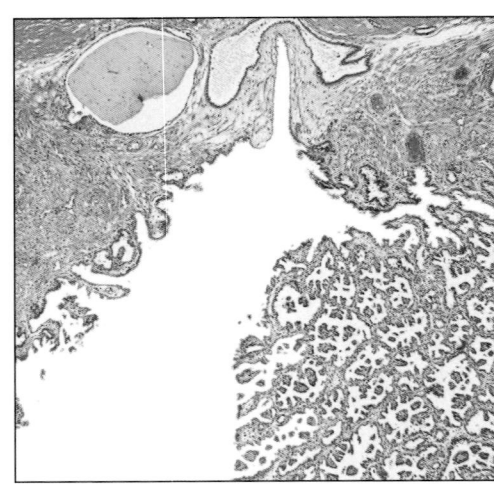

(Left) Although rare carcinomas arising in MEST are reported, most associated malignant tumors are sarcomas. This image shows a spindle cell sarcoma ⇨ arising within a MEST ➡. *(Right)* A higher magnification view of a sarcoma arising within a MEST shows marked hypercellularity, anaplastic features, and high mitotic activity ⇨ in the tumor. Sarcomas with rhabdoid, rhabdomyosarcomatous, and chondrosarcomatous differentiation have been described in mixed epithelial and stromal tumors.

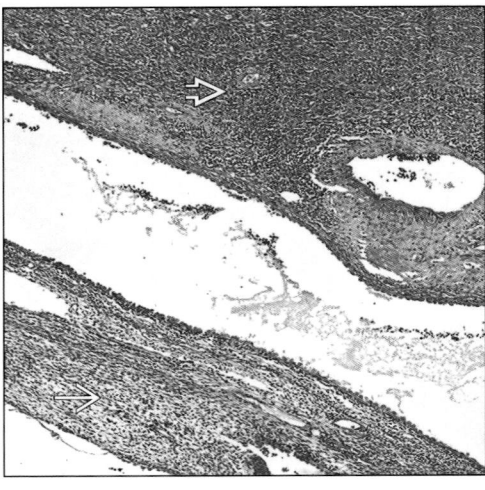
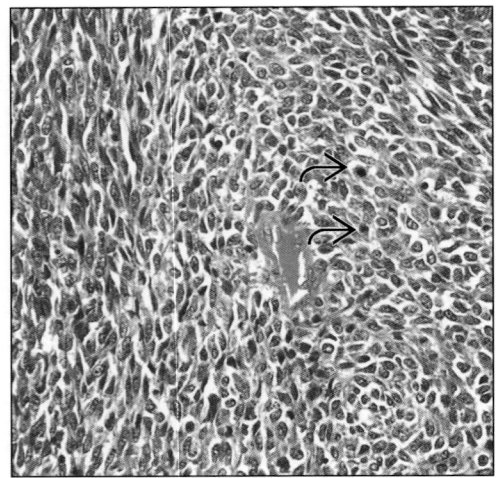

CYSTIC NEPHROMA/MIXED EPITHELIAL AND STROMAL TUMOR

Ancillary Studies and Differential Diagnosis

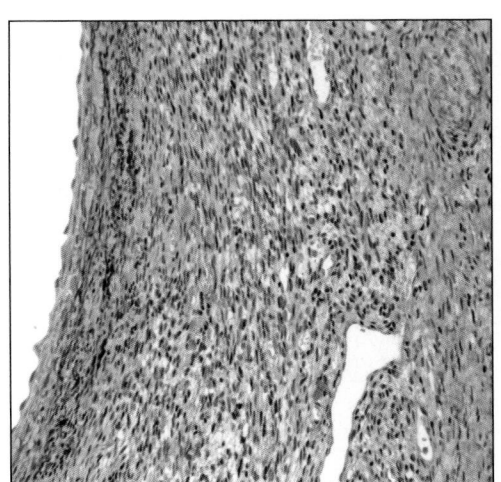
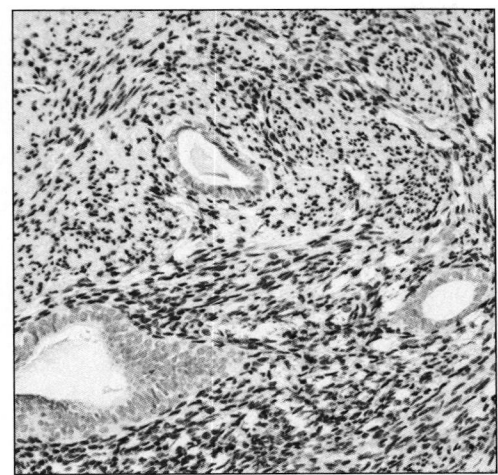

(Left) This image depicts immunohistochemical nuclear positivity for ER in an MEST. (Right) Similar to the ER receptors, PR receptors may also be expressed in both CN and MEST. While some consider such positivity as favoring specific origins for these tumors, others have shown that ER and PR immunoreactivity in renal stroma may be a metaplastic change that may be associated with obstruction and nonneoplastic cyst formation.

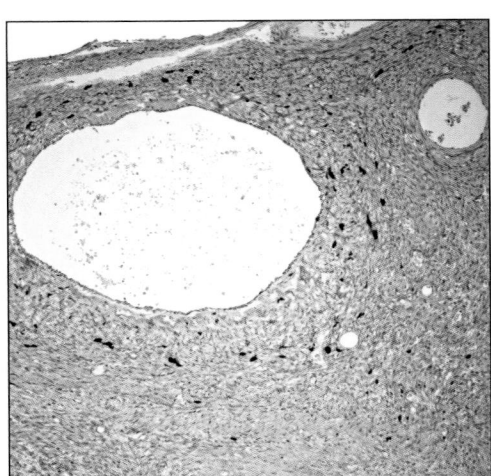
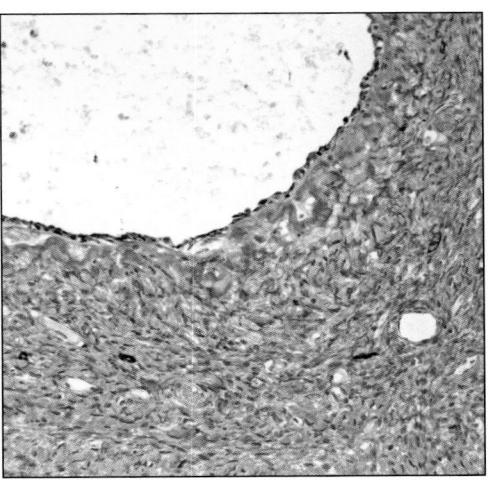

(Left) Some MESTs may show clusters or single cells with reactivity for calretinin, similar to ovarian stromal cells. Occasional cells may be luteinized, and these tend to be more intensely positive for sex cord stromal markers. (Right) Similarly, immunoreactivity for inhibin may be noted in some single or clusters of cells in mixed epithelial and stromal tumors. While this immunoreactivity raises the possibility of müllerian origin, the metaplastic nature cannot be completely excluded.

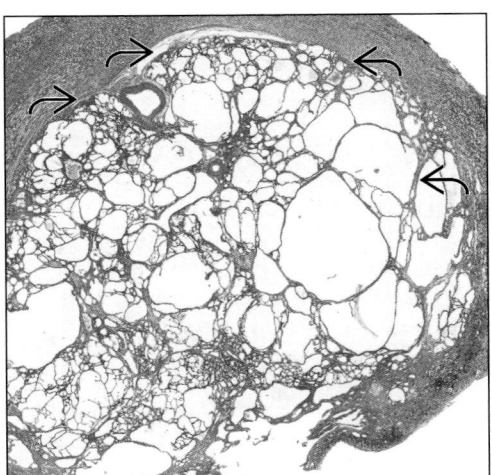
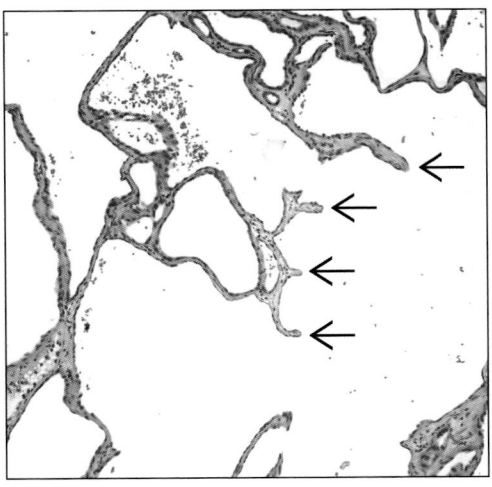

(Left) Tubulocystic carcinoma ⊅ at lower magnification may mimic a CN. However, evaluation at higher magnification reveals lining cells with abundant eosinophilic cytoplasm and prominent nucleoli. The stroma is often fibrotic and desmoplastic in tubulocystic carcinoma. (Right) Tubulocystic carcinoma also shows breaking or incomplete septae ⊅ floating free in the lumen of some of the cysts. In addition, it lacks immunoreactivity for ER and PR.

SYNOVIAL SARCOMA

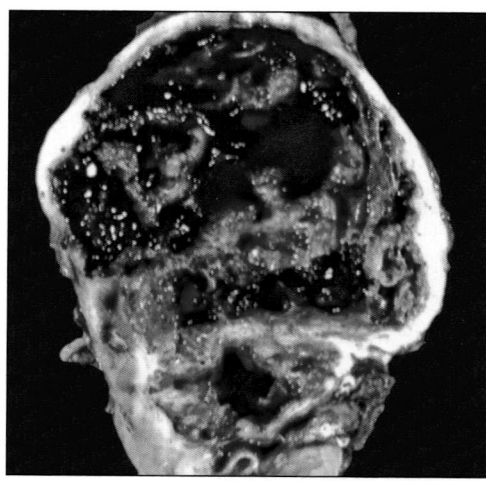

Primary renal synovial sarcoma shows the typical features of the tumor: Large size, extensive necrosis, cystic change, and hemorrhage. Cysts are grossly observed in 2/3 of the cases.

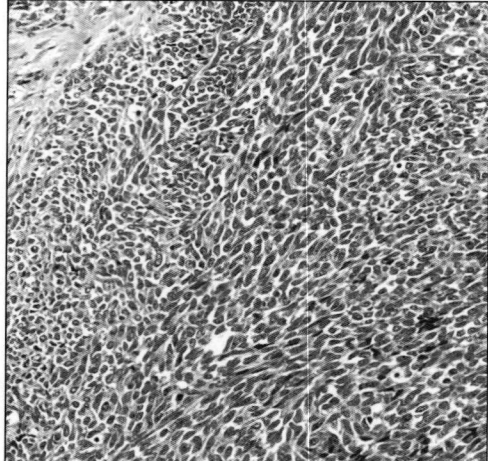

Hematoxylin & eosin image shows the typical interlacing short fascicles of spindle-shaped cells in a primary renal synovial sarcoma. Most renal synovial sarcomas are of the monophasic type.

TERMINOLOGY

Abbreviations
- Synovial sarcoma (SS)

Definitions
- Mesenchymal spindle cell tumor with rare epithelial differentiation characterized by specific chromosomal translocation t(X;18)(p11;q11)

ETIOLOGY/PATHOGENESIS

Molecular Features
- Primary renal synovial sarcoma shares characteristic SYT-SSX gene fusion with its more common soft tissue counterpart
  - Unlike predominance of SYT-SSX1 fusion in soft tissue SS, most reported renal SS have shown SYT-SSX2 gene fusion
    - SYT-SSX2 fusion correlates with monophasic histology in soft tissue
    - This may explain predominance of monophasic spindle cell morphology of SS in kidney

CLINICAL ISSUES

Epidemiology
- Incidence
  - Rare primary mesenchymal tumor; not more than 50 cases described
- Age
  - Range: 20-61 years (median: 35 years)
- Gender
  - Almost equal M:F incidence

Presentation
- Presentation is similar to that of other mass lesions
  - Cases may present with symptoms related to metastases

Treatment
- Managed with combination of surgery and adjuvant chemotherapy
  - Response rates to ifosphamide and doxorubicin-based chemotherapy ~ 24%

Prognosis
- Aggressive tumors
- Concurrent or subsequent metastases very frequent
  - Lung is most commonly reported site of metastasis
  - Other sites of metastasis include regional lymph nodes, liver, bones, and abdominal cavity soft tissues
    - 1 of few sarcomas with metastases to lymph nodes

MACROSCOPIC FEATURES

General Features
- Most tumors are large, necrotic, and grossly cystic
  - Approximately 2/3 show cysts on gross evaluation

Size
- 10-17 cm (mean: 11 cm)

MICROSCOPIC PATHOLOGY

Histologic Features
- Most renal synovial sarcomas show monophasic spindle cell histology
  - Highly cellular, composed of plump, embryonal-appearing spindle cells growing in short, intersecting fascicles
  - Cytoplasm is scant and ill defined
  - Nuclei are ovoid to fusiform with coarse chromatin and variable-sized nucleoli
  - Mitoses are frequent and extensive necrosis is common
  - Intratumoral cysts common (> 80% with cysts on microscopy)

SYNOVIAL SARCOMA

Key Facts

Terminology
- Synovial sarcoma (SS)
- Mesenchymal spindle cell tumor with rare epithelial differentiation characterized by specific chromosomal translocation t(X;18)(p11;q11)

Etiology/Pathogenesis
- Primary renal synovial sarcoma shares characteristic *SYT-SSX* gene fusion with its more common soft tissue counterpart

Clinical Issues
- Rare primary mesenchymal tumor; not more than 50 cases described
- Concurrent or subsequent metastases very frequent
- Lung is most commonly reported site of metastasis

Macroscopic Features
- Most of these tumors are large, necrotic, and cystic

Microscopic Pathology
- Most renal synovial sarcomas show monophasic spindle cell histology
- Intratumoral cysts common (> 80% with cysts on microscopy)

Ancillary Tests
- Frequently positive for bcl-2, CD99, and vimentin
- In some, focal or rare cell positivity for EMA/MUC1 and cytokeratins (EMA more often than cytokeratins)

Top Differential Diagnoses
- Primitive neuroectodermal tumor
- Blastemal Wilms tumor
- Cellular mesoblastic nephroma

- Cysts lined by mitotically inactive cells with extensive eosinophilic cytoplasm and often "hobnail" appearance
- Cysts believed to represent native, entrapped tubules obstructed by tumor, with cystic dilatation
- Because of such cysts, some primary renal SS have been classified as primitive sarcomas arising in cystic nephroma in past
  - True epithelial differentiation yielding biphasic synovial sarcoma may occur but is rare
  - Alternating hypocellular myxoid areas and prominent hemangiopericytomatous pattern
  - Angiolymphatic invasion frequently present

Predominant Pattern/Injury Type
- Spindled

Predominant Cell/Compartment Type
- Spindled

ANCILLARY TESTS

Immunohistochemistry
- Frequently positive for bcl-2, CD99, and vimentin
- Many cases completely negative for all epithelial markers
  - In some, focal or rare cell positivity for EMA/MUC1 and cytokeratins (EMA/MUC1 more often than cytokeratins)
- Negative for CD34 and muscle markers

DIFFERENTIAL DIAGNOSIS

Primitive Neuroectodermal Tumor
- Sheets and lobules of small round cells with scant cytoplasm
- Rosette formation is useful pointer to diagnosis
- Molecular evidence of *FLI1-EWS* fusion confirmatory

Blastemal Wilms Tumor
- Wilms tumor (WT) typically seen in patients < 5 years old; SS is tumor of older patients

- SS is usually a spindle cell neoplasm, except in cases of poorly differentiated subtype
- WT1 and pax-2 is positive in WT
- Demonstration of *SYT-SSX* gene fusion is diagnostic

Cellular Mesoblastic Nephroma (CMN)
- Tumor of very young children, mostly seen in 1st year of life
- Demonstration of *SYT-SSX* gene fusion is diagnostic of SS, whereas *ETV6-NTRK3* gene fusion is characteristic of CMN

Other Monophasic Sarcomas
- Malignant peripheral nerve sheath tumor, fibrosarcoma, leiomyosarcoma, malignant solitary fibrous tumor
- Appropriate immunohistochemical panel, including S100, CD34, actin-sm, desmin

DIAGNOSTIC CHECKLIST

Pathologic Interpretation Pearls
- Monophasic spindle cell sarcoma occurring in young patient should prompt consideration and work-up for synovial sarcoma
  - Renal cell carcinoma with sarcomatoid differentiation are rare in this age group

SELECTED REFERENCES

1. Divetia M et al: Synovial sarcoma of the kidney. Ann Diagn Pathol. 12(5):333-9, 2008
2. Vujanić GM et al: Anaplastic sarcoma of the kidney: a clinicopathologic study of 20 cases of a new entity with polyphenotypic features. Am J Surg Pathol. 31(10):1459-68, 2007
3. Argani P et al: Primary renal synovial sarcoma: molecular and morphologic delineation of an entity previously included among embryonal sarcomas of the kidney. Am J Surg Pathol. 24(8):1087-96, 2000

SYNOVIAL SARCOMA

Microscopic Features

(Left) Primary renal monophasic synovial sarcoma shows infiltrative borders, a characteristic feature of the tumor. The tumor often shows extrarenal extensions and vascular invasion, along with necrosis and high mitotic index. **(Right)** Hematoxylin & eosin image of a renal synovial sarcoma shows embryonal-appearing spindle cells with plump nuclei, coarse chromatin, scant cytoplasm, and indistinct cell borders. Note the prominent mitotic activity ➡ in the tumor.

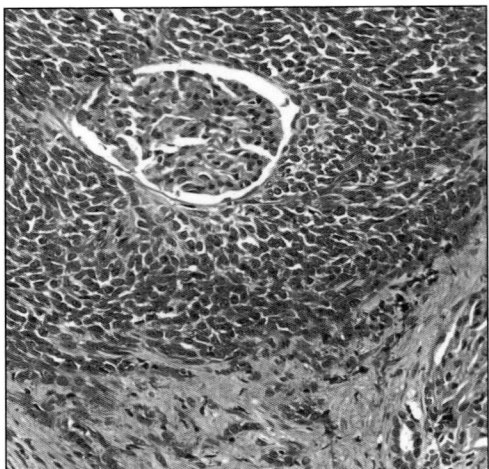
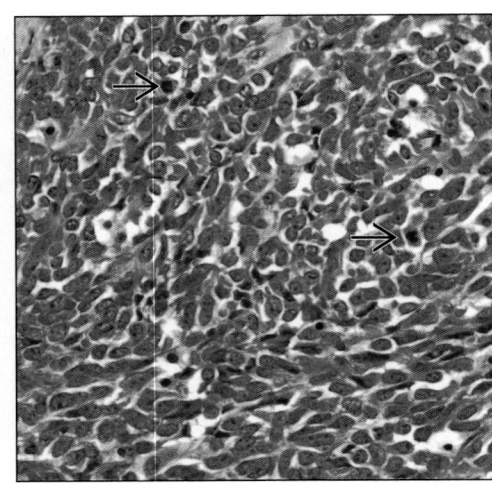

(Left) Hematoxylin & eosin image shows a cystic space ➡ surrounded by solid, highly cellular spindled tumor cells. Cysts are a characteristic feature in renal SS, being observed in > 65% of cases on gross evaluation and > 80% on light microscopy. The cysts are believed to represent entrapped and obstructed native tubules with cystic dilatation. **(Right)** The spindle cell component in the tumor is histologically similar to monophasic synovial sarcoma of soft tissue.

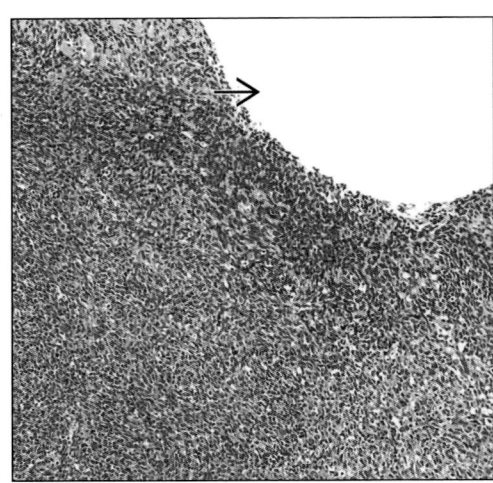
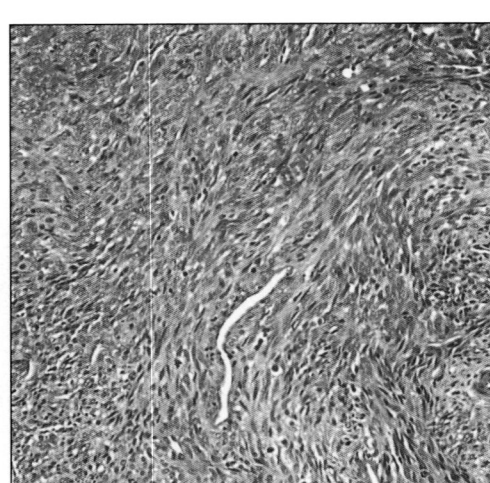

(Left) The cysts in renal SS are often lined by mitotically inactive, "hobnailed" eosinophilic cells ➡. The cysts are occasionally surrounded by ovarian-type stroma ➡, suggesting origin from cystic nephroma. Similar cases were considered embryonal sarcomas in the past. However, these tumors often show the typical SYT-SSX gene fusion of SS. **(Right)** This image shows renal sinus fat ➡ invasion by a synovial sarcoma. Extrarenal fat and vascular invasion are frequent in renal SS.

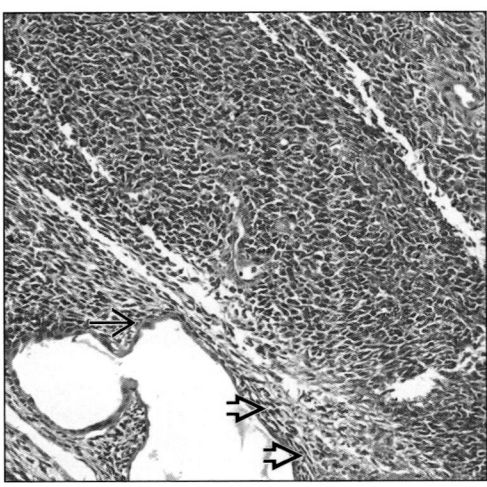
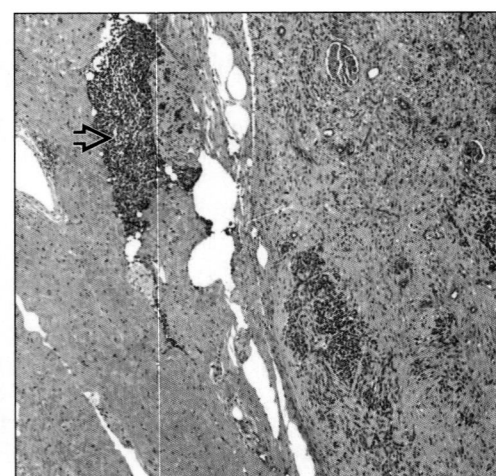

Microscopic and Immunohistochemical Features

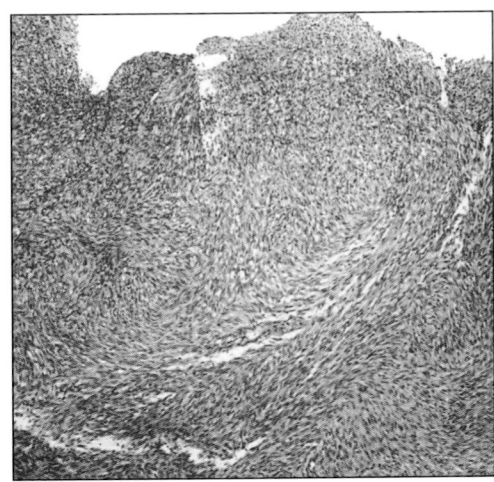

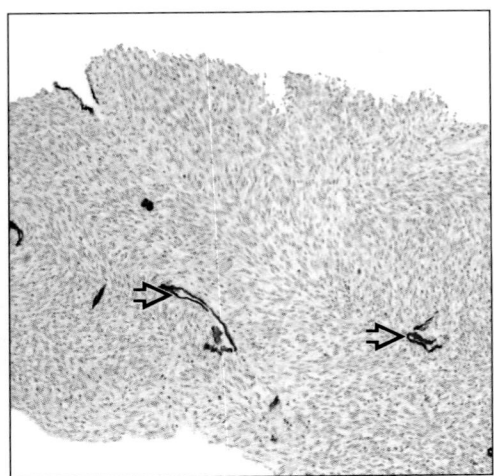

(Left) Presence of a spindle cell sarcoma in a renal core biopsy, particularly in a young adult, should always raise the differential diagnostic possibility of renal SS and mandates ancillary testing for appropriate classification. *(Right)* Immunostains may suggest the diagnosis of SS but are not consistent or specific. Molecular confirmation is usually required for diagnosis. SS are consistently CD34 negative. Positive staining in the tumor vasculature ⇨ acts as internal control.

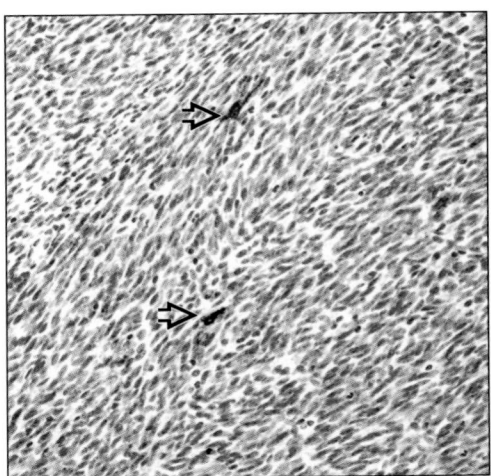

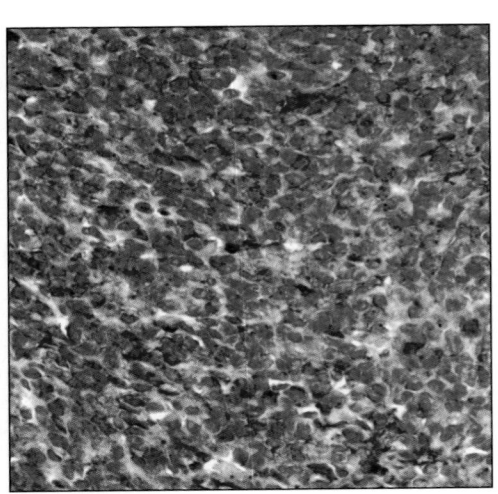

(Left) Epithelial markers are usually negative in the spindled cells of SS. However, focal and rare positivity may be present in some cases. EMA/MUC1 ⇨ is the most sensitive antibody in this regard. *(Right)* CD99 is frequently positive in renal SS, as in its extrarenal counterparts. However, unlike the diffuse, membranous positivity in renal primitive neuroectodermal tumors, the positivity is often focal and usually cytoplasmic. Bcl-2 also frequently stains synovial sarcomas.

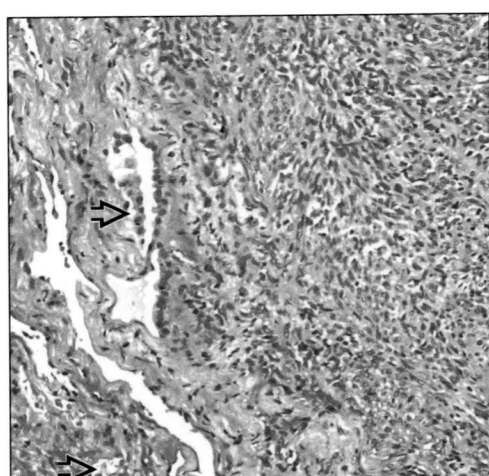

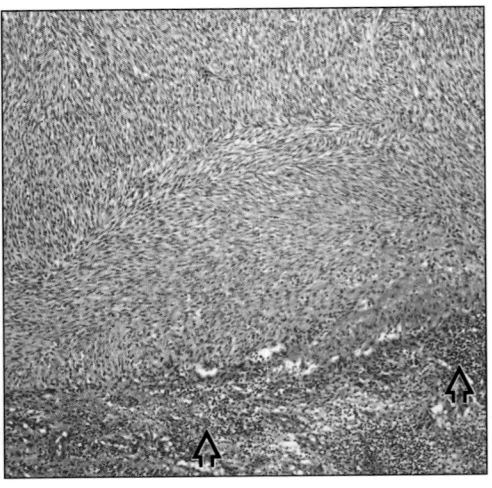

(Left) This image shows a renal SS metastatic to the lung ⇨. Most cases of renal SS have lung metastasis at presentation or develop them soon after the primary diagnosis. *(Right)* This photomicrograph shows a renal synovial sarcoma metastatic to a regional lymph node ⇨. Unlike most other sarcomas, synovial sarcoma, including that of renal origin, may sometimes show metastasis to the lymph nodes. However, lungs are the most common site of metastasis in renal SS.

CARCINOID

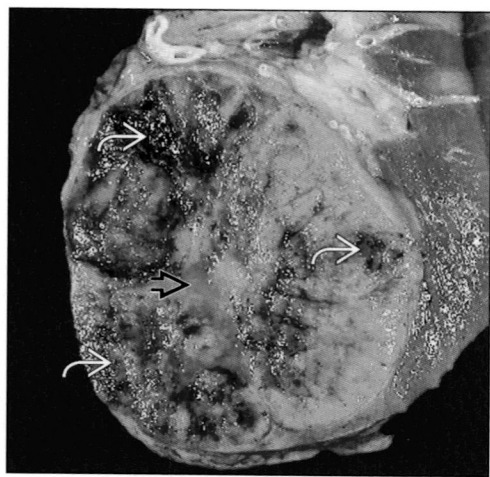

Primary renal carcinoid is a well-circumscribed tumor with homogeneous cut surface. Foci of hemorrhage ➤ are not uncommon, but necrosis is rare. A central scar ⊳ is present.

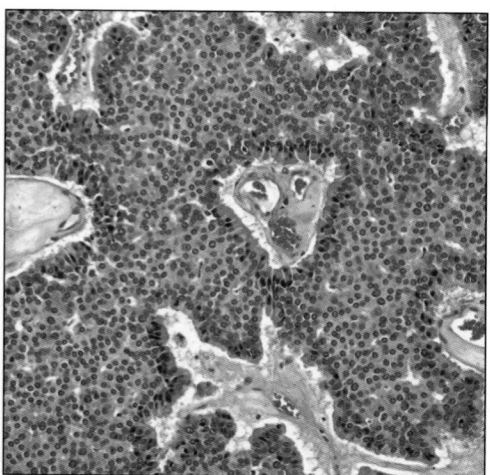

Renal carcinoid tumor is morphologically identical to that in extrarenal sites. This image shows sheets and trabeculae of cells with uniform and mostly round nuclear profiles.

TERMINOLOGY

Abbreviations
- Renal carcinoid tumor (RCT)

Definitions
- Well-differentiated primary neuroendocrine neoplasm arising within kidney

ETIOLOGY/PATHOGENESIS

Developmental Anomaly
- Up to 20% of primary renal carcinoids arise in "horseshoe" kidneys
  - Pathogenesis of this association not clear

Association With Renal Teratoma
- Rarely reported to arise in renal teratoma or "teratoid tumors," both extremely uncommon tumors in kidney

CLINICAL ISSUES

Epidemiology
- Incidence
  - Very rare tumor of kidney
    - Approximately 80 cases reported in literature
  - After the gonads, kidney is 2nd most common site for genitourinary carcinoids in both sexes
- Age
  - Range: 27-78 years (mean: 52 years)
    - Approximately 1/2 of cases < 50 years at diagnosis

Presentation
- Approximately 40% present with tumor-related symptoms, including back or flank pain, hematuria, or enlarging abdominal mass
- Clinical signs or symptoms of carcinoid syndrome are extremely uncommon

Treatment
- Surgical approaches
  - Nephron-sparing surgery for organ-confined tumors is preferred surgical approach
- Adjuvant therapy
  - Because of usual prolonged clinical course even in widely metastatic disease
    - Role of adjuvant therapies uncertain; effective therapies are unavailable
    - Value of anti-angiogenic targeted therapies in widely metastatic settings is currently suggested

Prognosis
- Regional lymph node metastasis often present in cases undergoing lymph node resection with nephrectomy
- Lung, liver, and bone are other reported metastatic sites
- Most patients with metastasis have protracted clinical course, with only rare reported deaths due to disease
- Reported adverse prognostic features include
  - Age ≥ 40 years
  - Tumor size ≥ 4 cm
  - Mitotic rate > 1/10 HPF
  - Metastasis at initial diagnosis

IMAGE FINDINGS

General Features
- Location
  - Anywhere in kidney; 1/4 in renal pelvis
- Somatostatin receptor scintigraphy (octreotide scan)
  - Adjunct value in staging and surveillance for recurrent or metastatic disease

MACROSCOPIC FEATURES

General Features
- Solitary tumor, usually well circumscribed

CARCINOID

Key Facts

Terminology
- Well-differentiated neuroendocrine neoplasm arising within kidney

Etiology/Pathogenesis
- Up to 20% of primary renal carcinoids arise in "horseshoe" kidneys

Clinical Issues
- Approximately 1/2 of cases < 50 years at diagnosis
- Clinical signs or symptoms of carcinoid syndrome extremely uncommon
- Regional lymph node metastasis often present in cases undergoing lymph node resection with nephrectomy
- Most patients with metastasis have protracted clinical course, with only rare reported deaths due to disease

Macroscopic Features
- Solitary tumor, usually well circumscribed
- Necrosis very uncommon

Microscopic Pathology
- Tumor-renal parenchymal junctions sharply defined in most cases, with focal infiltration in occasional case
- Morphologically similar to carcinoid tumors at other sites
- Invasion into perinephric fat was observed in > 40% cases in a recent study (largest to date)
- Often positive for metastasis to lymph nodes (> 1/3 of cases)

Top Differential Diagnoses
- Carcinoid tumor metastatic to kidney

- Solid homogeneous, yellow-tan, beige or red-brown cut surface
  - Focal hemorrhage, calcification, or cystic change not uncommon; necrosis quite rare
- Size range: 2-17 cm (mean: 6.4 cm)

MICROSCOPIC PATHOLOGY

Histologic Features
- Tumor-renal parenchymal junction sharply defined in most cases, with focal infiltration in occasional cases
- Most common architectural pattern is tightly packed cords and trabeculae with ribbon-like appearance
  - Intervening stroma may range from minimal to abundant and sclerotic to edematous
- Other growth patterns include solid sheets, solid nests, and presence of gland-like lumina
- Morphologically similar to carcinoid tumors at other sites
  - Uniform cells with round nuclei and moderate cytoplasm; nuclei occasionally elongated, mildly spindled or oval
  - Focal, mild to moderate nuclear pleomorphism
  - Nuclear chromatin is finely granular and dispersed ("salt and pepper") with inconspicuous nucleoli
  - Most tumors with < 2 mitoses/10 high-power fields (HPF); rarely, 3-4 or more mitoses/10 HPF
  - Focal hemorrhage and calcification present, but necrosis extremely uncommon
- Invasion into perinephric fat was observed in > 40% cases in a recent study (largest to date)
  - Vascular invasion very rare in primary renal carcinoids

Lymph Nodes
- Often positive for metastasis (> 1/3 of cases)

Predominant Pattern/Injury Type
- Small Islands/Nested
- Cords and ribbons

Predominant Cell/Compartment Type
- Neuroendocrine

DIFFERENTIAL DIAGNOSIS

Carcinoid Tumor Metastatic to Kidney
- Histologically, similar to primary tumors, but often multiple
- Presence of lymphovascular emboli favor metastasis

DIAGNOSTIC CHECKLIST

Pathologic Interpretation Pearls
- Possibility of metastasis from other sites needs to be excluded, particularly in multifocal tumors and tumors with vascular invasion

SELECTED REFERENCES

1. Kuroda N et al: Carcinoid tumor of the renal pelvis: consideration on the histogenesis. Pathol Int. 58(1):51-4, 2008
2. Hansel DE et al: Renal carcinoid tumor: a clinicopathologic study of 21 cases. Am J Surg Pathol. 31(10):1539-44, 2007
3. Lane BR et al: Renal neuroendocrine tumours: a clinicopathological study. BJU Int. 100(5):1030-5, 2007
4. Rodríguez-Covarrubias F et al: Carcinoid tumor arising in a horseshoe kidney. Int Urol Nephrol. 39(2):373-6, 2007
5. Yoo J et al: Primary carcinoid tumor arising in a mature teratoma of the kidney: a case report and review of the literature. Arch Pathol Lab Med. 126(8):979-81, 2002
6. McCaffrey JA et al: Carcinoid tumor of the kidney. The use of somatostatin receptor scintigraphy in diagnosis and management. Urol Oncol. 5(3):108-111, 2000
7. Krishnan B et al: Horseshoe kidney is associated with an increased relative risk of primary renal carcinoid tumor. J Urol. 157(6):2059-66, 1997
8. Raslan WF et al: Primary carcinoid of the kidney. Immunohistochemical and ultrastructural studies of five patients. Cancer. 72(9):2660-6, 1993

CARCINOID

Gross and Microscopic Features

(Left) This gross image shows a carcinoid tumor with multinodular growth pattern, intravascular tumor thrombi ➡, and large area of necrosis ➡. Such features are highly suggestive of a metastasis to the kidney, and merit thorough clinical investigations for such a possibility if a prior history is not known. *(Right)* Most primary renal carcinoids are well circumscribed. This image shows a tumor with a prominent capsule ➡, an unusual but not a very uncommon finding.

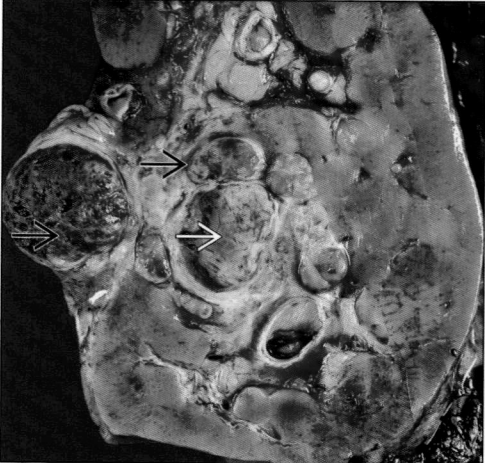
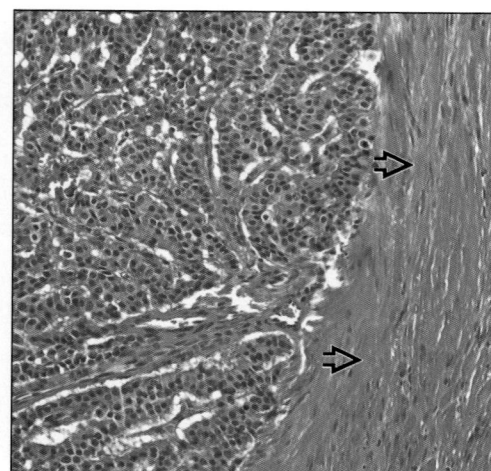

(Left) Rare primary RCTs may have an infiltrative margin, with irregular extensions between and surrounding the nontumorous nephrons. *(Right)* As is typical of extrarenal tumors, the nuclei in renal carcinoid tumors are relatively uniform and round. The nuclear chromatin is finely granular, showing "salt and pepper" appearance. Mitotic activity is usually low. Although not specifically used in the kidneys, carcinoid tumors are now designated as well-differentiated neuroendocrine tumors.

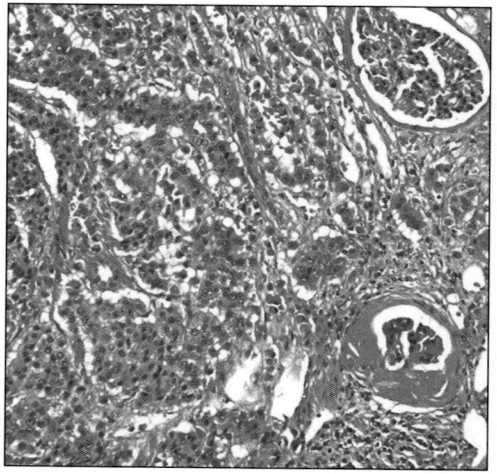
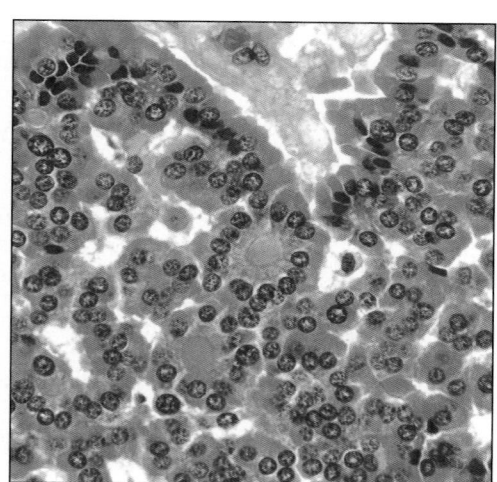

(Left) Ribbon-like ➡ and wider cords constitute the most common architectural pattern in renal carcinoid tumors. This may be associated with scant or abundant, usually hyalinized, stroma. *(Right)* Combination of architectural patterns is quite common in renal carcinoid tumors. This photomicrograph shows a tumor with mixture of cord-like ➡ and more solid ➡ growth patterns. Note the similarity in nuclear morphology and scant to moderate cytoplasm in both types of areas.

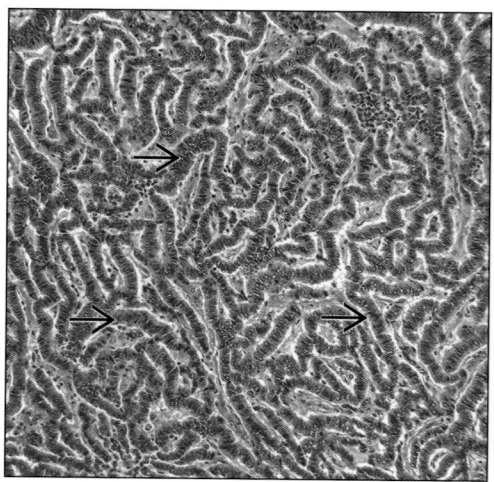
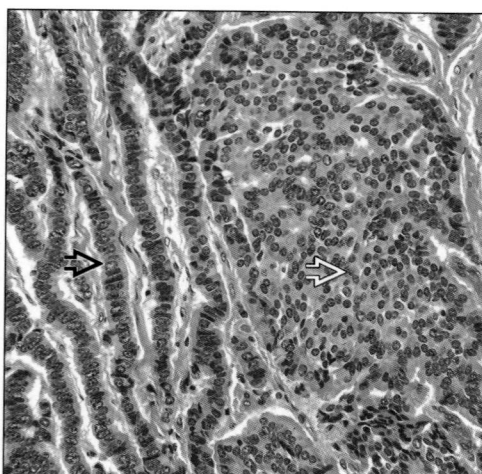

1

CARCINOID

Microscopic and Immunohistochemical Features

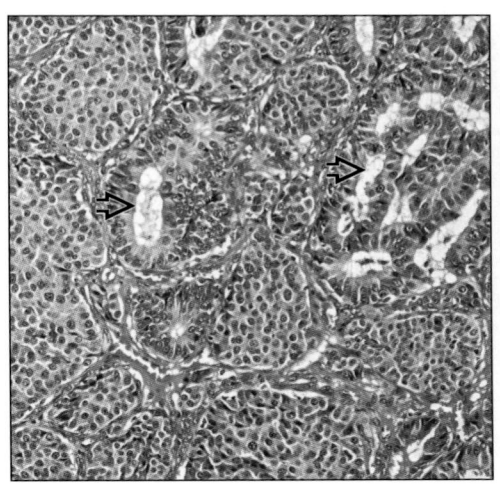
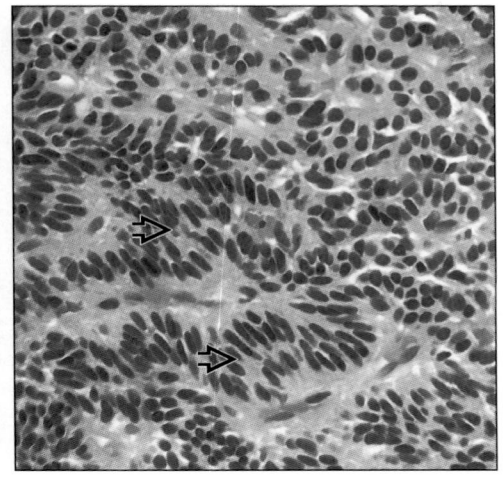

(Left) RCT, like its extrarenal counterpart, may show gland-like ➲ features. This raises the differential diagnostic possibility of a Wilms tumor. However, the solid areas do not show the characteristics of blastema, i.e., nuclear molding and high mitotic/apoptotic index. *(Right)* Occasionally, the nuclei may appear elongated ➲ and oval in renal carcinoid tumors, similar to what is seen in small cell carcinomas. However, no increased mitotic activity is present.

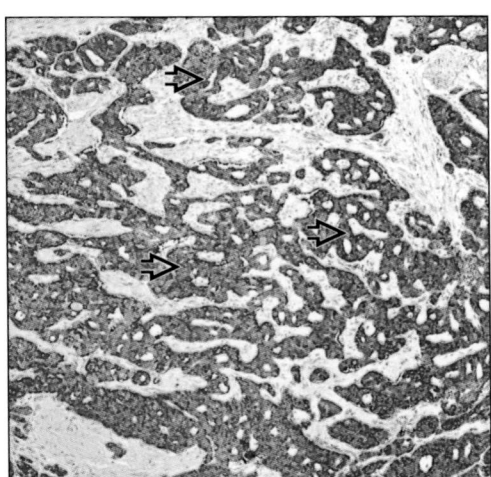
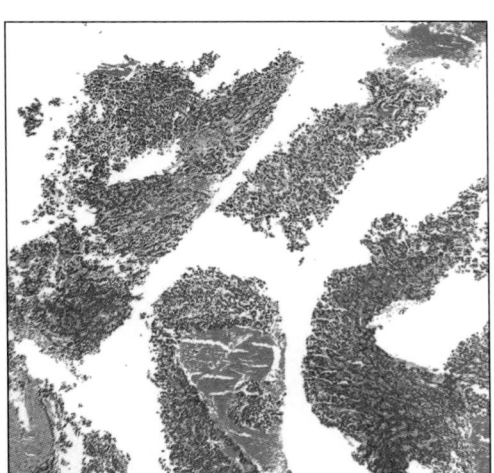

(Left) Immunostains for synaptophysin ➲ and chromogranin are usually positive in RCTs. CK7 may show focal positivity, but TTF-1 is usually negative. *(Right)* Based on the morphological and immunophenotypical features, the diagnosis of RCT can be rendered on needle core biopsies. Exclusion of the possibility of other small, blue round cell tumors requires negative staining for CD99, WT-1, muscle markers, and sometimes lymphoid markers.

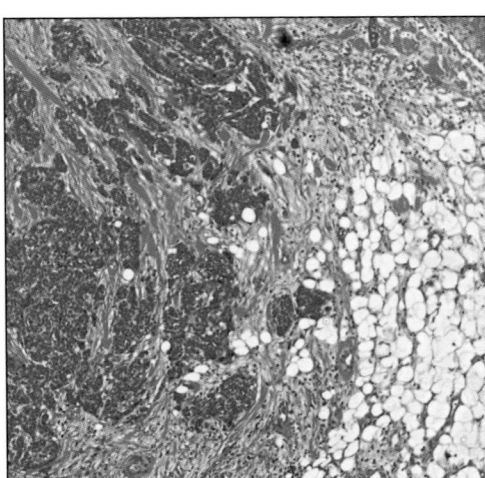
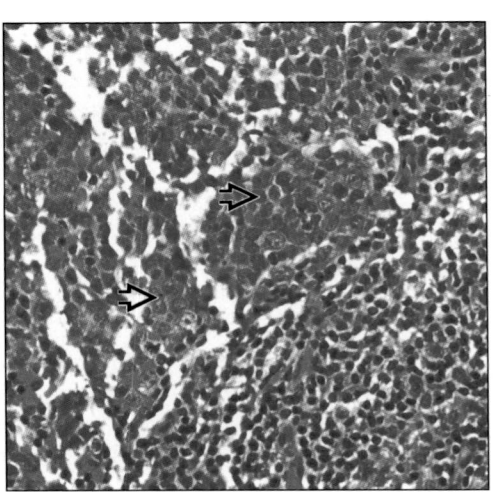

(Left) A large proportion of renal carcinoids show invasion of the perirenal fat (stage pT3a). Some, but not all, believe this to reflect a potentially more aggressive biologic behavior. *(Right)* This image shows renal carcinoid tumor ➲ metastatic to a regional lymph node. Metastasis to lymph nodes is quite common in renal carcinoids. However, most patients with metastasis, even when widespread, have protracted clinical course with only rare reported deaths due to disease.

PRIMITIVE NEUROECTODERMAL TUMOR

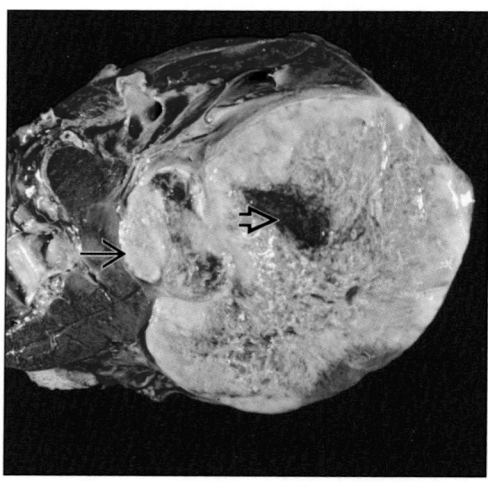

Primitive neuroectodermal tumors are usually large tumors with infiltrative borders, areas of necrosis ➡ and cystic change ⊅, multilobulated growth pattern, and tan-yellow cut surface.

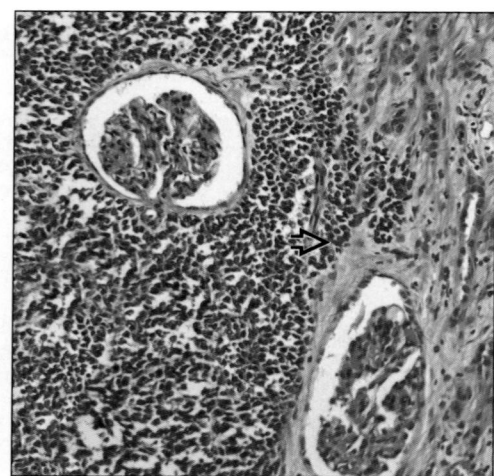

Renal PNET is morphologically similar to tumors in the bone and soft tissue and is characterized by small round blue cells. Tumor margins show irregular extensions ⊅ into surrounding kidney.

TERMINOLOGY

Abbreviations

- Primitive neuroectodermal tumor (PNET)

Definitions

- Aggressive small blue round cell tumor characterized by fusion of *EWS* gene with a gene from *ETS* (E-twenty six) family of transcription factors

ETIOLOGY/PATHOGENESIS

Molecular Features

- Similar to Ewing sarcoma (ES)/PNET of bone and soft tissue
  - Primary renal PNET also demonstrates characteristic *EWS-FLI1* gene fusion resulting from translocation t(11;22)(q24;q12)
- In bone and soft tissue, 70% of *EWS/FLI1* gene fusions involve fusion of *EWS* exon 7 and *FLI1* exon 6 (so-called type 1 fusion)
  - Nontype 1 gene fusions in ES/PNET of soft tissue are associated with poor outcome
- In renal PNET, only 1/2 have demonstrated type 1 fusion, while other 1/2 have variant fusions
  - Other than *FLI1*, genes of *ETS* family that may be fused with *EWS* include, *ERG, ETV1, E1AF, FEV, ZSG*
  - Increased predilection for variant gene fusions in renal cases may contribute to their more adverse prognosis

CLINICAL ISSUES

Epidemiology

- Incidence
  - Very uncommon; approximately 120 cases described in literature
- Age
  - Most common in young adults and adolescents; mean age: 27 years (range: 10-60 years)

Presentation

- Presenting symptoms include abdominal pain, hematuria, palpable mass, and rarely, night sweats

Prognosis

- Generally aggressive tumors often with poor clinical outcome, particularly in the past
- Multimodal therapy (surgery, chemotherapy, and radiation) is standard of care with improved outcomes recently reported
  - Median survival in patients with disease localized to kidney is up to 60 months
    - Compared to only 15 months in patients with regional nodal or distant metastatic disease

MACROSCOPIC FEATURES

General Features

- Tan to yellow, lobulated solid tumors, often extensively replacing normal renal parenchyma
- Hemorrhage, necrosis, and cystic changes common; gross renal vein and perinephric fat invasion frequent

Size

- Usually large, with mean diameter 16 cm (range: 7-21 cm)

MICROSCOPIC PATHOLOGY

Histologic Features

- Identical to their soft tissue counterparts
- Typically infiltrates surrounding renal parenchyma in broad sheets or finger-like projections
- Vaguely lobulated proliferations of primitive-appearing round cells with high nuclear to cytoplasmic ratio

PRIMITIVE NEUROECTODERMAL TUMOR

Key Facts

Terminology
- Primitive neuroectodermal tumor (PNET)

Etiology/Pathogenesis
- Nontype 1 gene fusions in ES/PNET of soft tissue are associated with poor outcome
- Ewing sarcoma (ES)/PNET family of tumors characterized by fusion of *EWS* with gene from *ETS* (E-twenty six) family of transcription factors

Clinical Issues
- Most common in young adults and adolescents

Macroscopic Features
- Usually large, with mean diameter 16 cm (range: 7-21 cm)

Microscopic Pathology
- Identical to their soft tissue counterparts
- Vaguely lobulated proliferations of primitive-appearing round cells with high nuclear to cytoplasmic ratio
- Occasionally with small amount of clear cytoplasm, and more vesicular nuclei showing small nucleoli
- Epithelial, myogenous, or cartilaginous differentiation not seen
- ES/PNET strongly and diffusely positive in membranous pattern for CD99; most, but not all, with FLI-1 nuclear positivity

Top Differential Diagnoses
- Blastemal Wilms tumor
- Other small blue round cell tumors

- ○ Occasionally with small amount of clear cytoplasm and more vesicular nuclei showing small nucleoli
- Mitotic figures easily identified, with occasional atypical mitoses
- Foci of necrosis common
- Rare cases with prominent Homer Wright rosettes
  - ○ Such rosettes different from early tubular differentiation of Wilms tumor
    - ■ True tubular differentiation as seen in Wilms tumor shows prominent lumens with rigid cytoplasmic luminal borders
- Epithelial, myogenous, or cartilaginous differentiation not seen
- Angiolymphatic invasion very common
- Frequent presence of glycogen (diastase-sensitive PAS positivity), particularly in cells with clear cytoplasm

Predominant Pattern/Injury Type
- Neoplastic

Predominant Cell/Compartment Type
- Neuroectodermal

ANCILLARY TESTS

Immunohistochemistry
- ES/PNET strongly and diffusely positive in membranous pattern for CD99; most, but not all, with FLI-1 nuclear positivity
- Focal positivity for cytokeratins in occasional tumors
- All tumors negative for desmin and other skeletal muscle markers and WT1

DIFFERENTIAL DIAGNOSIS

Blastemal Wilms Tumor
- Wilms tumor (WT) typically seen in patients < 5 years old; PNET is tumor of older patients
- PNETs usually have uniform morphology/architecture throughout tumor

- ○ Blastemal WT often show foci of other distinctive patterns of growth in some parts of neoplasm
- Nuclei of PNET are more evenly spaced than those of blastemal WT, and nuclear chromatin of PNET less coarse than that of WT
- > 95% of PNETs demonstrate complete membranous labeling for CD99, while WT is usually negative

Other Small Round Blue Cell Tumors
- Clear cell sarcoma of the kidney (CCSK) typically occurs in patients < 5 years old, and PNET more often in young adults
- Cellular CCSK almost always shows foci of other distinctive growth patterns
- > 95% of PNETs demonstrate complete membranous labeling for CD99, while CCSK and rhabdomyosarcomas are virtually always negative
- FLI-1 nuclear positivity in PNET and negative staining for MYOD1, myogenin may also help
- Neuroblastomas with more dense chromatin, nuclear molding, and often variable neuropil
- Molecular tests diagnostic in almost all difficult cases

DIAGNOSTIC CHECKLIST

Pathologic Interpretation Pearls
- Small blue round cell tumor in young adults is more likely to be PNET rather than Wilms tumor

SELECTED REFERENCES

1. Thyavihally YB et al: Primitive neuroectodermal tumor of the kidney: a single institute series of 16 patients. Urology. 71(2):292-6, 2008
2. Argani P et al: Recent advances in pediatric renal neoplasia. Adv Anat Pathol. 10(5):243-60, 2003
3. Jimenez RE et al: Primary Ewing's sarcoma/primitive neuroectodermal tumor of the kidney: a clinicopathologic and immunohistochemical analysis of 11 cases. Am J Surg Pathol. 26(3):320-7, 2002

PRIMITIVE NEUROECTODERMAL TUMOR

Gross and Microscopic Features

(Left) The typical multilobulated gross appearance is prominent in this specimen. As is common in renal primitive neuroectodermal tumors, this tumor almost completely replaces the renal parenchyma. Notice the extrarenal extension into perinephric fat ⇨ close to adrenal gland ⇨. *(Right)* Like blastemal WT, PNET also shows an infiltrative margin. However, the nuclear chromatin in PNET is pale compared to that in WT. WT also often shows variable growth patterns, unlike PNET.

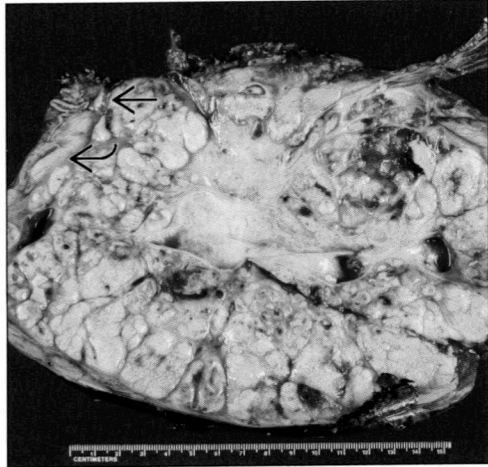
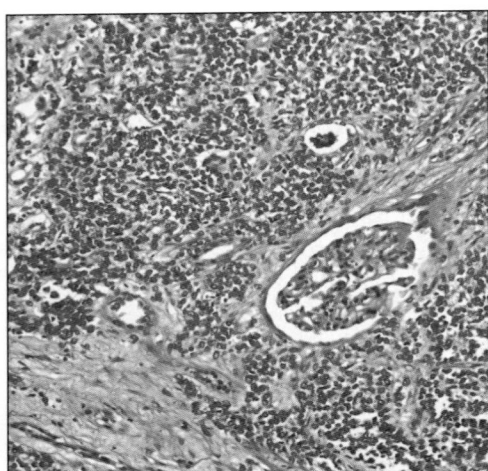

(Left) The chromatin pattern in PNET is relatively pale and often shows small nucleoli and focal moderate amount of pale cytoplasm, unlike most other small round blue cell tumors. *(Right)* A small round blue cell tumor in the kidney may raise the possibility of a Wilms tumor, neuroblastoma, and rhabdomyosarcoma, among other possibilities. Presence of pale chromatin, lack of tubular differentiation, neuropil and nuclear overlapping should raise the differential diagnostic possibility of PNET.

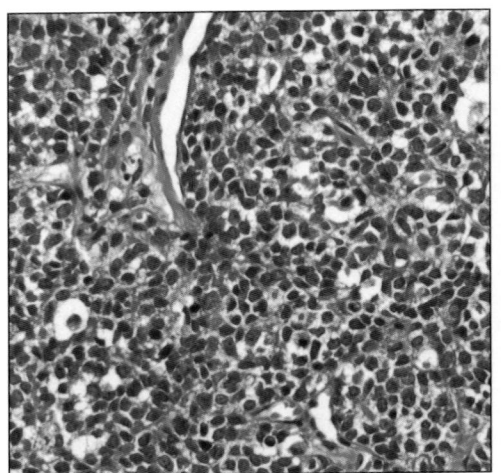
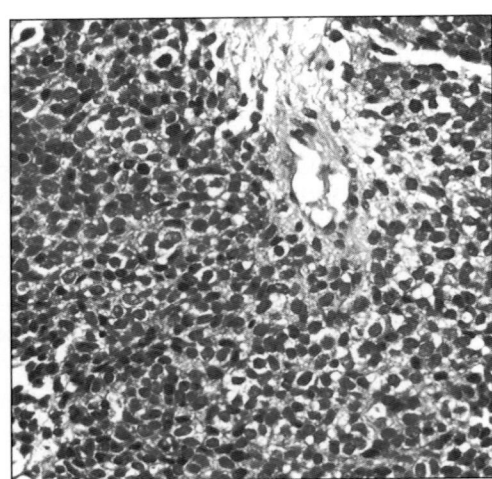

(Left) Similar to neuroblastoma, PNET may show Homer Wright rosettes characterized by tumor cells arranged around fibrillary material ⇨. However, nuclei in PNET show more open chromatin and lack neuropil that is often present in neuroblastoma. Diffuse membranous positivity for CD99, and often FLI-1, will clinch the diagnosis of PNET in most cases. *(Right)* PNETs often show at least focal presence of glycogen, as demonstrated here by diastase-sensitive PAS positivity ⇨.

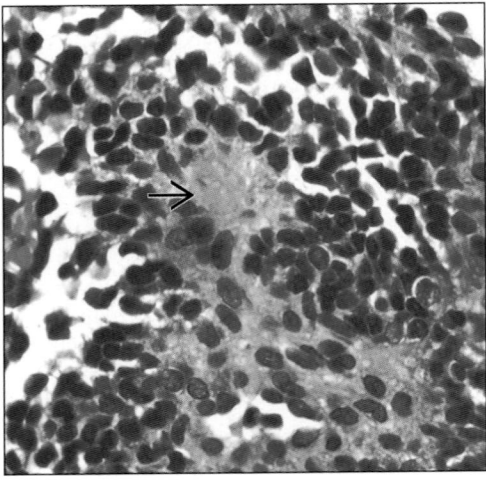
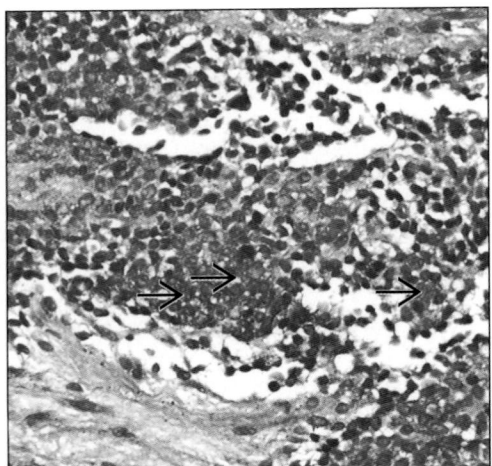

PRIMITIVE NEUROECTODERMAL TUMOR

Ancillary Techniques and Microscopic Features

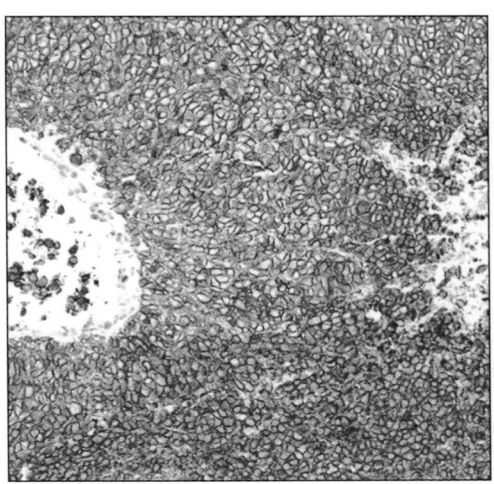

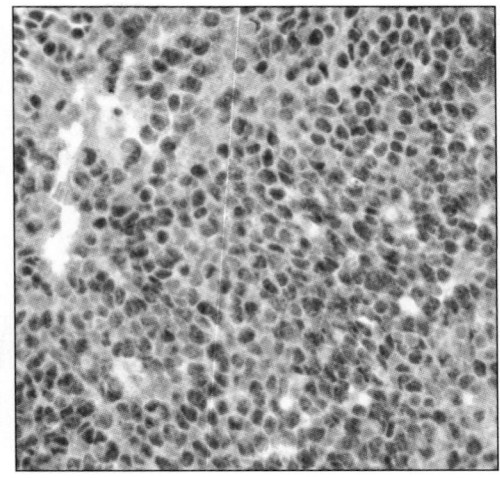

(Left) CD99 usually shows diffuse membranous reactivity in PNET. It is often difficult to diagnose renal PNET without such immunoreactivity. At the same time, it must be noted that CD99 positivity may be seen in other tumors, including T-lymphoblastic lymphoma, rhabdomyosarcoma, desmoplastic small round cell tumor, and sex cord-stromal tumors. (Right) FLI-1 shows strong and diffuse nuclear immunoreactivity in most, but not all, PNETs.

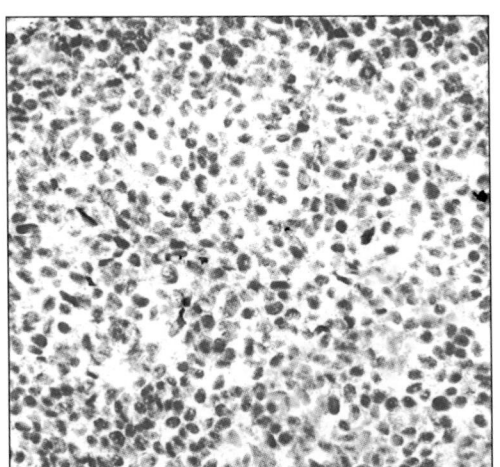

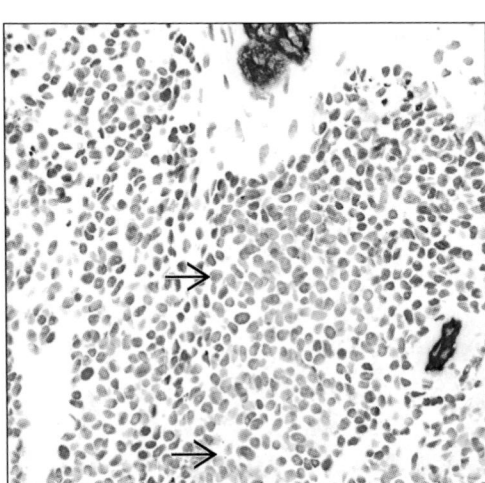

(Left) The possibility of embryonal rhabdomyosarcoma (RMS) may arise in renal tumors with small round blue cell morphology. While CD99 is diffusely positive in PNET, it may also stain some RMS. However, muscle markers MYOD1 and myogenin are always negative in PNET, as shown here. (Right) Stains for cytokeratins may be negative in PNET ➡. However, rare cases of renal PNET may show focal immunoreactivity for keratins, usually in a dot-like pattern.

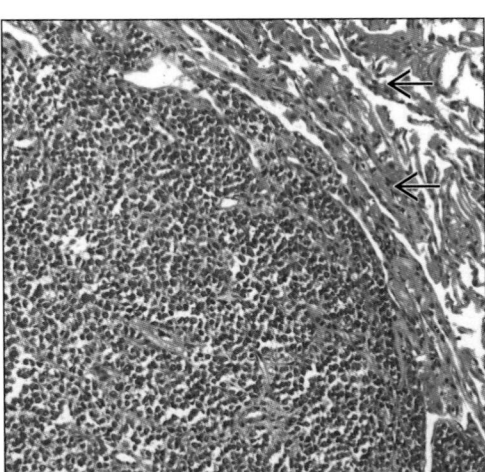

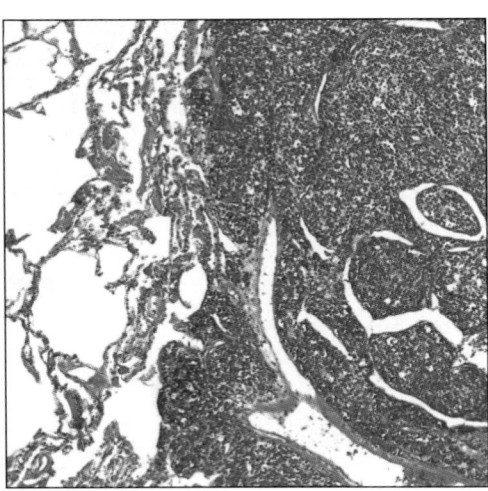

(Left) Most cases of renal PNET show metastasis at initial diagnosis or on follow-up. Lung is among the most common sites for metastasis ➡. (Right) This hematoxylin & eosin image shows renal PNET metastatic to the lung. Among PNETs of soft tissue, gene fusions other than EWS-FLI1 are often associated with a poor clinical outcome. In renal PNET, approximately 1/2 of cases show variant EWS fusions, and this may be a factor in the relatively poorer outcome in renal PNET.

HEMATOPOIETIC TUMORS

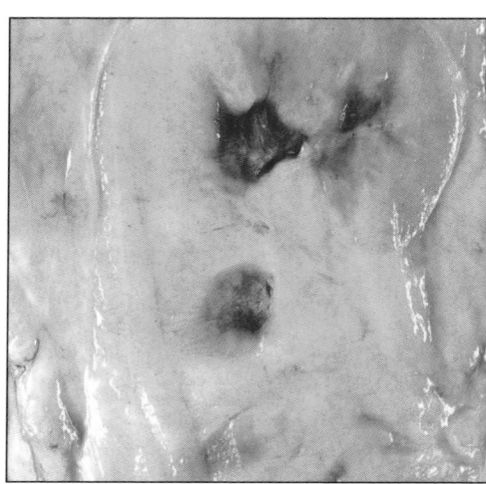

This gross photograph shows complete replacement of renal parenchyma by gray-tan, fleshy tumor. Such appearance of lymphoma/leukemia involving the kidney is more often seen in autopsy specimens.

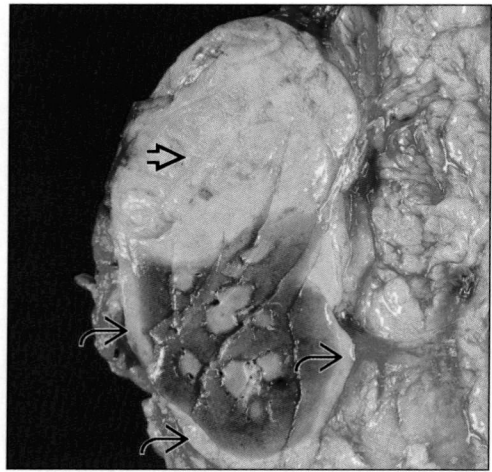

Nephrectomy specimens revealing hematological malignancies usually show mass lesions ⟹ that are often clinically misdiagnosed as cortical tumors. Note the sheath-like perirenal infiltration ⟹ here.

TERMINOLOGY

Abbreviations
- Diffuse large B-cell lymphoma (DLBCL), Burkitt lymphoma (BL), follicular lymphoma (FL), mantle cell lymphoma (MCL), mucosa-associated lymphoid tissue (MALT)

Definitions
- Lymphoid, myeloid, or other neoplastic proliferations infiltrating renal parenchyma
  - Most often, kidney is secondarily involved in systemic diseases but may be primary organ of involvement in rarer cases
  - Tumors seen in kidney include
    - Malignant lymphoma
    - Leukemia
    - Plasmacytoma/myeloma
    - Post-transplant lymphoproliferative disorders (PTLD)
    - Other very rare conditions, including Langerhans cell histiocytosis, Rosai-Dorfman disease, etc.

ETIOLOGY/PATHOGENESIS

Genetic Features
- **Diffuse large B-cell lymphoma**
  - In 30-40% cases of DLBCL, translocation of *BCL6* gene (located at 3q27) with various partners is present
    - Might contribute to tumorigenesis by blocking terminal lymphoid differentiation and providing resistance to apoptotic signals
  - Other alterations in some DLBCL include translocation of *BCL2* gene and translocation t(8;14) involving *MYC* gene
- **Burkitt lymphoma**
  - In > 80% cases translocation t(8;14)(q24;q32) is present

  - Juxtaposes *MYC* gene (located at 8q24) to immunoglobulin-heavy chain *(IGH)* locus (located at 14q32)
    - Occasionally *MYC* gene translocates to 1 of light chain loci
- **Follicular lymphoma**
  - Follicular lymphoma typically shows translocation t(14;18)(q32;q21), detected in approximately 85% of cases
  - It leads to juxtaposition of *BCL2* gene (located at 18q21) to *IGH* enhancer (located on chromosome 14)
    - Leads to constitutive overexpression of *BCL2* and impaired apoptotic signaling
- **Mantle cell lymphoma**
  - Typical cytogenetic aberration is translocation t(11;14)(q13;q32), detected in almost all cases
  - Translocation leads to juxtaposition of *CCND1* gene (located at 11q13) to *IGH* enhancer (located on chromosome 14)
    - Results in overexpression of its gene product cyclin D1, a key regulator of cell cycle and controller of G1/S-phase transition
- **Mucosa-associated lymphoid tissue lymphoma**
  - MALT lymphomas carry 1 of 4 known chromosomal translocations: t(11;18)(q21;q21), t(14;18)(q32;q21), t(3;14)(p14.1;q32), and t(1;14)(q22;q32)
    - Activate nuclear factor κ light chain enhancer of activated B cells (NF-κB) pathway, which has roles in multiple cellular responses
- **Leukemias**
  - Numerous nonrandom genetic alterations have been reported in different forms of leukemia
  - Many of these have diagnostic, biologic, and therapeutic implications
  - Some of better known alterations include
    - t(9;22), in chronic myelogenous leukemia (CML) and approximately 20-30% of adult patients with acute lymphoblastic leukemia (ALL) →

HEMATOPOIETIC TUMORS

Key Facts

Terminology
- Lymphoid, myeloid, or other neoplastic proliferations infiltrating renal parenchyma
- Most often, kidney is secondarily involved in systemic diseases but may be primary organ of involvement in rarer cases
- Tumors seen in kidney include
  - Malignant lymphoma, leukemia, plasmacytoma/myeloma
  - Post-transplant lymphoproliferative disorders (PTLD)
  - Other very rare conditions, including Langerhans cell histiocytosis, Rosai-Dorfman disease, etc.

Clinical Issues
- Lymphomas arising in urinary tract and male genital organs account for < 5% of extranodal lymphomas

- Secondary renal involvement is many times more common than primary renal hematopoietic malignancies

Macroscopic Features
- 2 gross growth patterns
  - Kidney completely replaced by homogeneous gray-white tumor tissue
  - Mass-forming lesion

Microscopic Pathology
- Most common growth pattern is interstitial
- Other tumors may have nodular growth pattern
- Rarely, tumor cells may be entirely or predominantly intravascular (intravascular lymphoma)

---

translocation between proto-oncogene c-ABL on chromosome 9 and *BCR* gene on chromosome 22
- t(15;17), in almost all patients with acute promyelocytic leukemia (APL); results in fusion of RARα gene on chromosome 17 with *PML* gene on chromosome 15
- Inv(16)/t(16;16), in a subgroup of patients with acute myeloid leukemia; results in fusion of *CBF*β gene at chromosome 16q22 with *MYH11* gene at chromosome 16p13
- t(8;21), in a subgroup of patients with acute myeloid leukemia; fuses *AML1 (RUNX1)* gene on chromosome 21 with *ETO* gene on chromosome 8
- Most (> 95%) B-lineage ALL (B-ALL) cases have *IG* gene rearrangements
- *TCR* genes are rearranged in most cases of T-lineage ALL (T-ALL)

Infectious Agents
- Post-transplant lymphoproliferative disorders are true Epstein-Barr virus (EBV)-driven tumors
  - Unlike malignancies occurring in immunocompetent individuals, where EBV is cofactor rather than driving influence
  - Number of factors that predispose transplant recipients to this EBV-driven PTLD include
    - Recipient EBV seronegativity at time of transplantation
    - Younger age at transplantation
    - Hepatitis C infection
    - Use of monoclonal antibodies OKT3 and antithymocyte globulin (ATG) as antirejection therapy
  - Most commonly seen after solid organ but occasionally also after stem cell transplantation

CLINICAL ISSUES

Epidemiology
- Incidence

- Lymphomas arising in urinary tract and male genital organs account for < 5% of extranodal lymphomas
- Genitourinary tract lymphomas most commonly occur in kidney
  - In recent large study, renal lymphomas constituted 60% of all genitourinary tract lymphomas
- Secondary renal involvement is many times more common than primary renal hematopoietic malignancies

Presentation
- Because multiorgan involvement, including kidneys, is usually clinically apparent, most secondary tumors are not biopsied/sampled
- Most renal hematopoietic malignancies presented to pathologists are either multiorgan tumors as autopsy specimens, or primary tumors
  - Primary renal hematopoietic malignancies diagnosed by pathologists often present with symptoms related to a mass lesion, including
    - Palpable mass, renal insufficiency, and hematuria
- Involvement may also be noted incidentally in specimens resected for other clinically apparent causes, such as
  - Nonhematopoietic tumors or nonfunctional kidneys

Treatment
- Lymphomas and leukemias are managed with type-dependent chemotherapeutic agents
- For PTLD, variety of therapeutic approaches used, including
  - Surgical resection and radiation therapy to localized disease
  - Reduction of immunosuppression if clinically feasible
  - Antiviral agents
  - Infusion of IL-2 activated autologous lymphocyte activated killer cells
  - More recently, humanized anti-CD20 mouse antibody, rituximab, has shown promising results in some cases

○ Cytotoxic chemotherapy is used in cases with EBV-derived lymphoma

Prognosis

- Prognosis for lymphomas is usually not promising
  ○ > 35% die of disease within 2 years of presentation
  ○ In a recent study, 12 of 16 patients with either primary or secondary renal lymphoma died with disease between 1-18 months
- With combination of available approaches, overwhelming majority of patients with PTLD show complete long-term remission of disease
  ○ Very rare deaths due to disease are now reported

MACROSCOPIC FEATURES

General Features

- 2 gross growth patterns
  ○ Kidney may be completely replaced by homogeneous gray-white tumor tissue
    ■ Such patterns, particularly when bilateral, are usually seen at autopsy
    ■ Kidney is diffusely enlarged, while its shape is generally maintained
  ○ Mass-like lesion
    ■ Tan-white single or multiple tumor nodules
    ■ Gross appearance similar to epithelial tumors of kidney

MICROSCOPIC PATHOLOGY

Histologic Features

- Most common growth pattern is interstitial
  ○ Sheets of tumor cells percolating between nephrons
- Other tumors may have nodular growth pattern
  ○ Tumor nodules completely replacing parenchyma, with rare nephrons embedded within tumor, particularly at periphery
- Rarely, tumor cells may be entirely or predominantly intravascular (intravascular lymphoma)
- A number of cases have been recently diagnosed on needle core biopsy specimens
- Subtypes of malignant lymphoma seen include
  ○ DLBCL, small cell lymphocytic lymphoma (SCLL), MCL, FL, BL, MALT lymphoma
    ■ Other subtypes of lymphoma very rarely seen
  ○ Immunophenotype is similar to that in extrarenal sites and is generally required to make specific diagnosis
- Post-transplantation lymphoproliferative disorder
  ○ May show any of 3 histologic forms or stages of development
    ■ Early or hyperplastic lesion with plasma cell hyperplasia, lesions resembling infectious mononucleosis, or atypical lymphoid hyperplasias
    ■ Polymorphic PTLD, with polymorphous infiltrate containing variable number of large atypical cells
    ■ Lymphomatous or monomorphic PTLD, with appearance of malignant lymphoma
    ■ Lymphomas are usually B-cell type

■ Unusual non-B-cell subtypes may also be seen in rare situations
○ Venules often show heavy infiltration by PTLD
○ Usually accompanied by presence of irregular, serpentine areas of coagulative necrosis in surrounding renal parenchyma
○ In situ hybridization for EBER is almost always positive in B-cell lymphomas developing early after transplant
○ PTLD developing after a few years post-transplant are often EBV negative
- Plasmacytoma
  ○ Primary plasmacytomas of kidney are very rare and show proliferation of mature to atypical plasma cells
    ■ They are all light chain-restricted, with either κ or λ phenotype on immunostaining or in situ hybridization
- Leukemias
  ○ Leukemic infiltrates often (approximately 50%) seen in autopsies on patients dying of leukemia
  ○ Primary leukemic involvement of kidney is extremely rare
    ■ Designated as granulocytic sarcoma
- Other hematopoietic malignancies
  ○ Occasional cases of Langerhans cell histiocytosis, Rosai-Dorfman disease, and reticulum cell tumors have been described
    ■ Morphologic and immunophenotypic features are similar to those in extrarenal sites

DIAGNOSTIC CHECKLIST

Pathologic Interpretation Pearls

- Multifocal and bilateral renal masses should raise concern for metastasis and malignant lymphoma
- Majority of renal hematopoietic tumors are B-cell lymphomas
  ○ However, entire range of hematopoietic malignancies may involve kidney
- Other than at autopsy, hematopoietic tumors may also be encountered by pathologists in nephrectomy specimens
  ○ In most such cases, these are often clinically misdiagnosed as parenchymal tumors

SELECTED REFERENCES

1. Kuo CC et al: Primary renal lymphoma. Br J Haematol. 144(5):628, 2009
2. Schniederjan SD et al: Lymphoid neoplasms of the urinary tract and male genital organs: a clinicopathological study of 40 cases. Mod Pathol. 22(8):1057-65, 2009
3. Garcia M et al: MALT lymphoma involving the kidney: a report of 10 cases and review of the literature. Am J Clin Pathol. 128(3):464-73, 2007

HEMATOPOIETIC TUMORS

Microscopic and Immunohistochemical Features

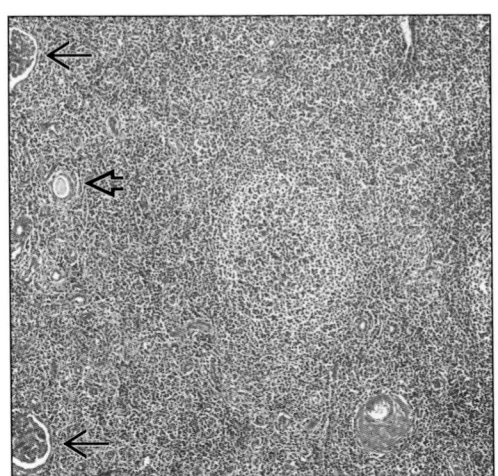
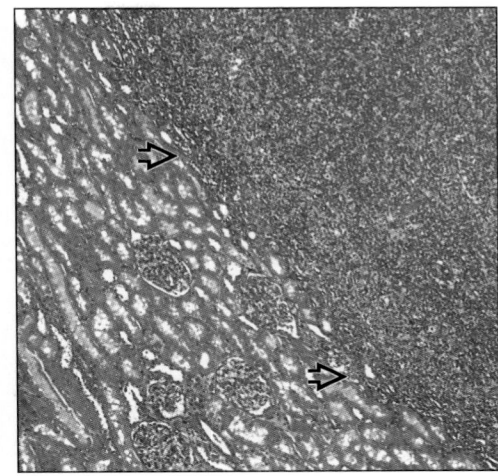

(Left) The most common architectural pattern in hematopoietic tumors involving the kidney is interstitial. Sheets of tumor cells infiltrate between residual glomeruli ➡ and tubules ⊵, although most of the nephrons are completely replaced. *(Right)* A less common architectural pattern in renal hematopoietic tumors is the sharply demarcated ⊵ nodular growth. Glomeruli and tubules may be entrapped within the tumor but usually only at the periphery of the tumor.

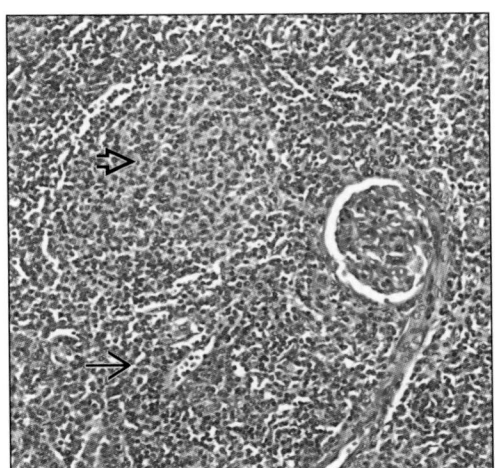
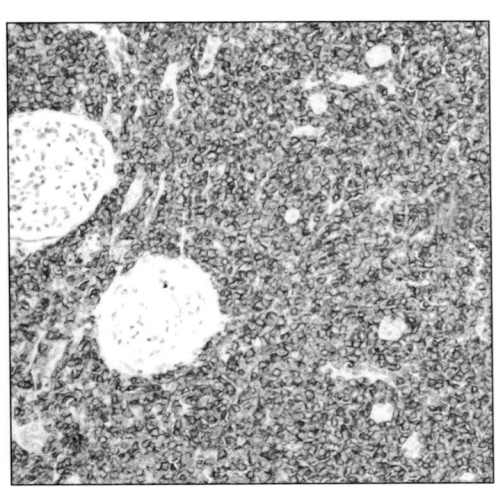

(Left) This image shows a lymphoid neoplastic proliferation with vague nodular ⊵ & diffuse ➡ growth patterns. Such growth patterns suggest a follicular lymphoma. However, the possibility of a MALT lymphoma needs to be excluded, & therefore, immunohistochemical confirmation is a must. *(Right)* CD20 immunostain shows diffuse positivity in this lymphoma, indicating that it is of B-cell origin. This, however, only excludes the possibility of a T-cell lymphoma.

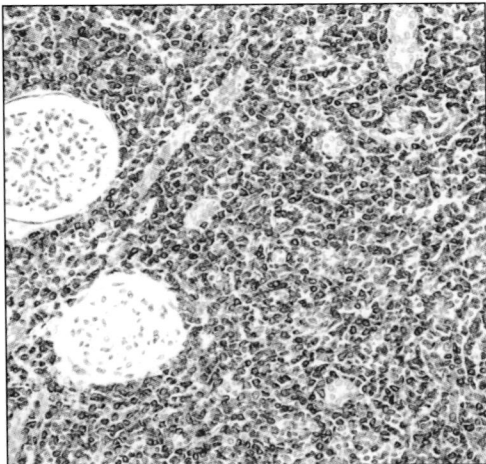
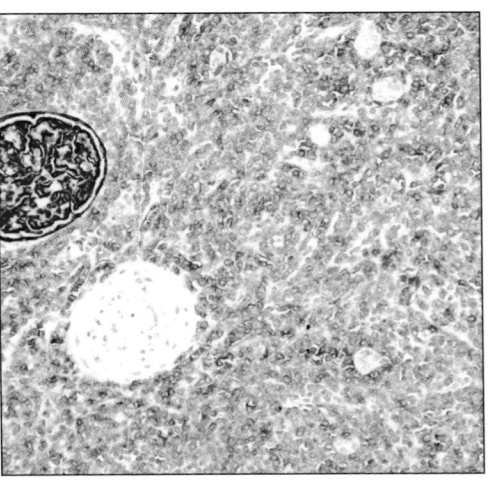

(Left) Diffuse bcl-2 immunoreactivity in this lymphoid tumor, along with the morphologic features, is highly suggestive of a follicular lymphoma. Diffuse large B-cell lymphomas are also often bcl-2 positive. Therefore morphologic as well as the expression of other immunohistochemical features are necessary for proper classification. *(Right)* Diffuse positivity for CD10, along with morphology and other immunostaining patterns, clinches the diagnosis of a follicular lymphoma in this case.

HEMATOPOIETIC TUMORS

Microscopic Features

(Left) This image from an autopsy specimen shows diffuse infiltration by large lymphoid cells ➡ admixed with many smaller cells. This case was diagnosed as diffuse T-cell/histiocyte rich large B-cell lymphoma based on the histology and immunophenotype. *(Right)* This malignant lymphoid neoplasm, in addition to the kidney, also invaded hepatic parenchyma ⊳. Morphologically, it is composed of large ➡ lymphoid cells with mixed cell infiltration, making specific typing difficult.

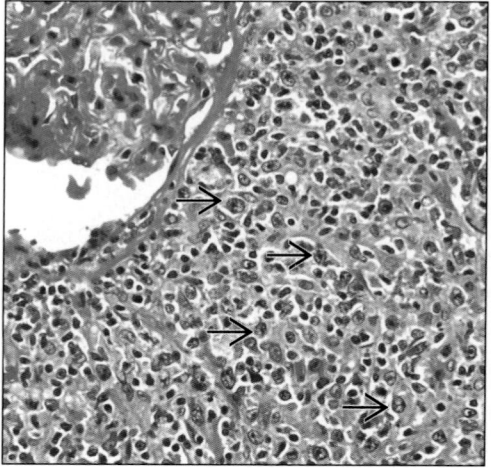
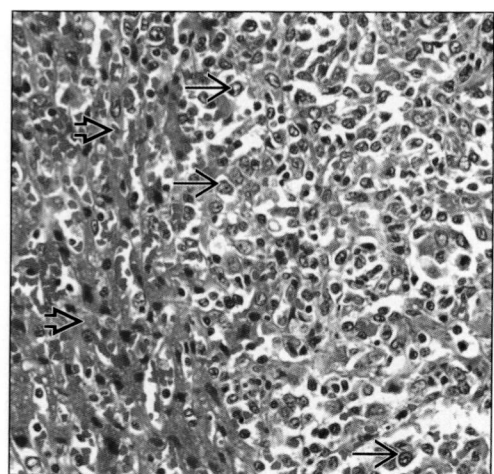

(Left) This malignant lymphoma shows diffuse infiltration of soft tissue ➡ around the adrenal gland ⊳. Secondary malignant lymphomas of the kidneys are more often bilateral than primary renal lymphomas. They are usually also associated with extensive systemic involvement. *(Right)* This image shows a post-transplant lymphoproliferative disorder, polymorphic type, involving the kidney. The infiltrate is polymorphous, but abundant, large atypical lymphoid cells ➡ are present.

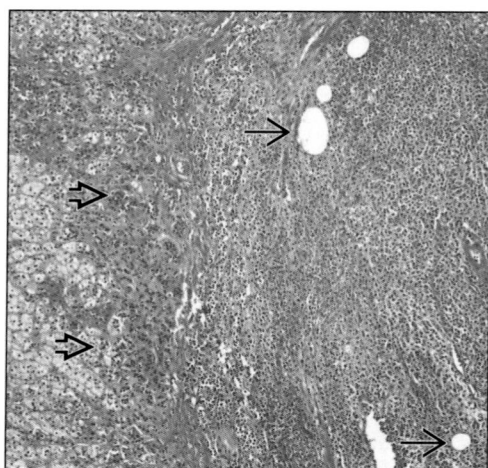
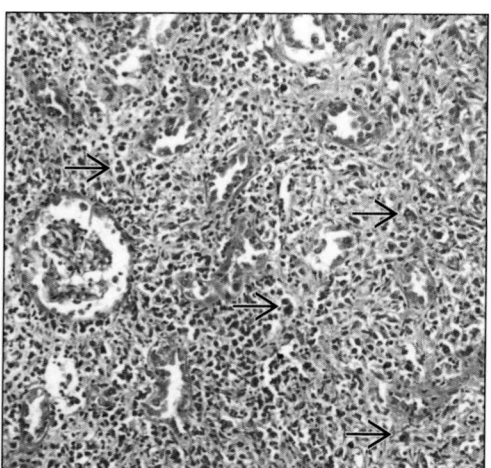

(Left) Post-transplant lymphoproliferative disorder besides the infiltrates, is characterized by serpentine, coagulative necrosis ⊳ of the renal parenchyma. Presence of such necrosis on needle biopsies should alert one to the possibility of PTLD, in appropriate settings. *(Right)* Typically, post-transplant lymphoproliferative disorder also shows venulitis ⊳, within or outside the lymphoid infiltrates. The arterioles are relatively spared ➡ by the process.

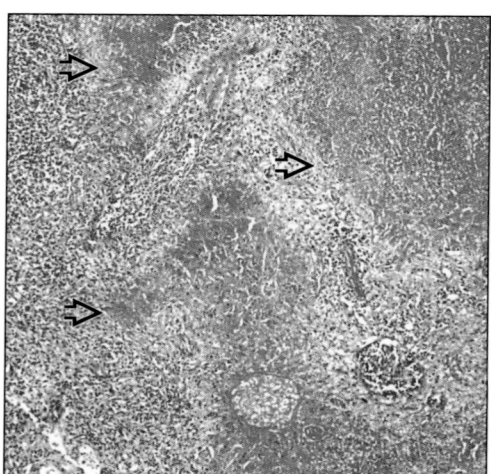
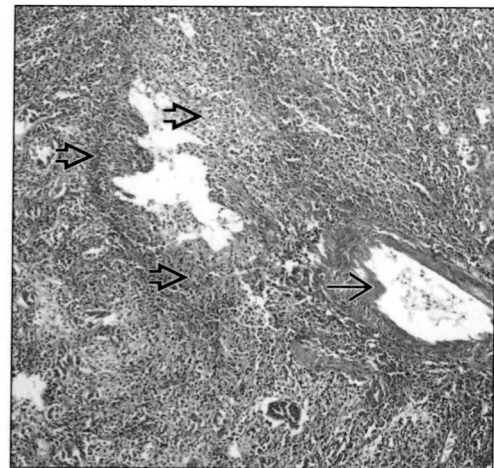

HEMATOPOIETIC TUMORS

Microscopic Features and Ancillary Techniques

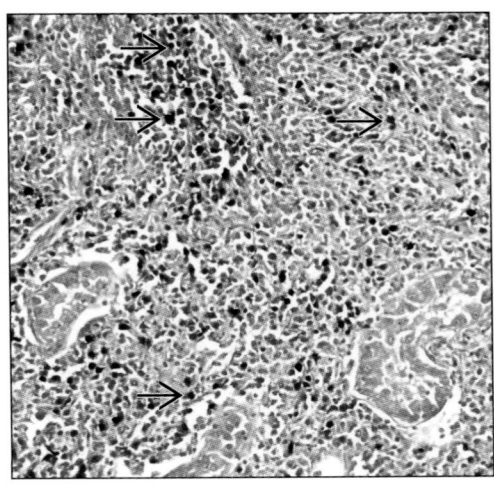

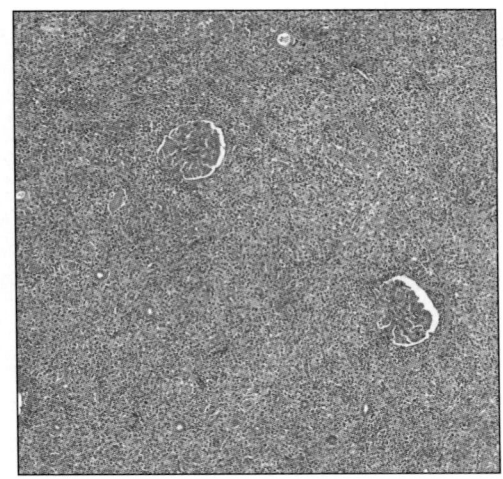

(Left) The atypical lymphoid cells in PTLD are almost always monoclonal B cells. Only rare T or other cell type neoplasias are described. The neoplastic B cells are almost always positive for EB virus (nuclear positivity ➡ demonstrated here by in situ hybridization for EBER). However, PTLD developing years after the transplant are usually EBV negative. *(Right)* Plasma cell neoplasms involving kidney are almost always secondary. Only very rare primary renal plasmacytomas are described.

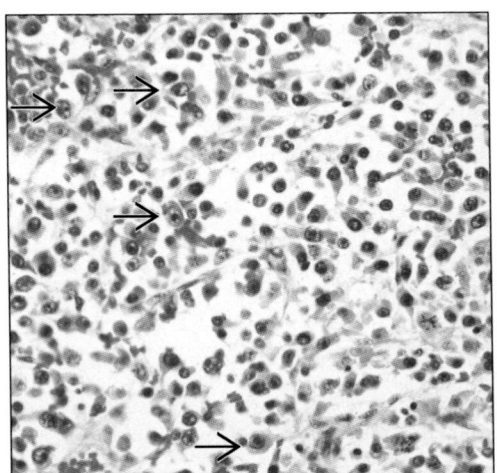

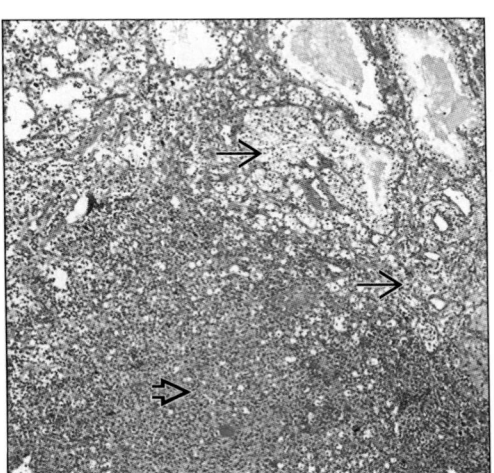

(Left) This image shows loose sheets of neoplastic plasma cells from a case of multiple myeloma involving the kidney. Many cells are atypical, with prominent nucleoli ➡, a common feature in plasma cell neoplasms. *(Right)* This image shows a Langerhans cell histiocytosis ➡ lesion, in close association with a clear cell RCC ➡. Some authors have suggested increased incidence of hematopoietic malignancies in cases with RCC, but other studies do not confirm such association.

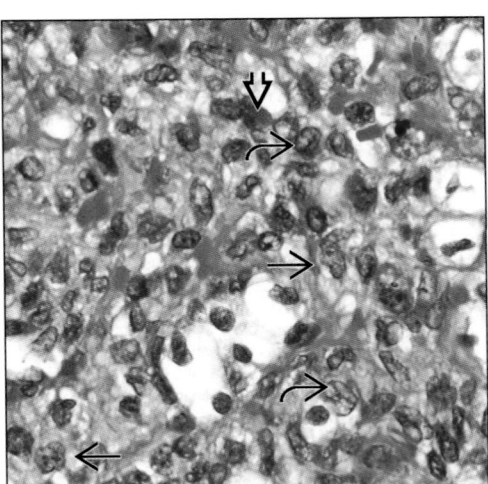

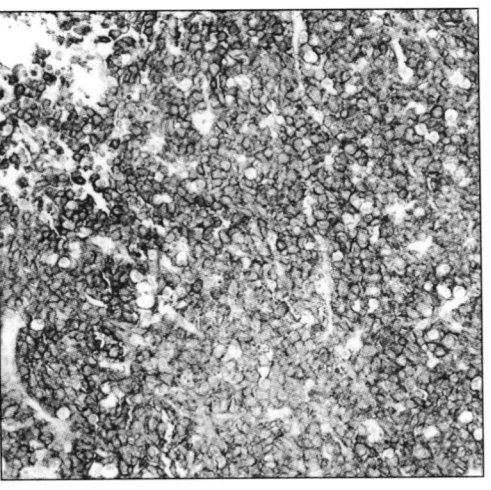

(Left) This higher magnification view depicts the typical nuclear features of Langerhans cell histiocytes in a tumor. These show pale chromatin, marked nuclear angulations ➡, and frequent grooves ➡. A rare eosinophil is also present ➡. *(Right)* This photomicrograph shows diffuse immunoreactivity for CD1a in a case of Langerhans cell histiocytosis involving the kidney. Such staining, along with the positivity for S100, is typical of the tumor.

JUXTAGLOMERULAR CELL TUMOR (RENINOMA)

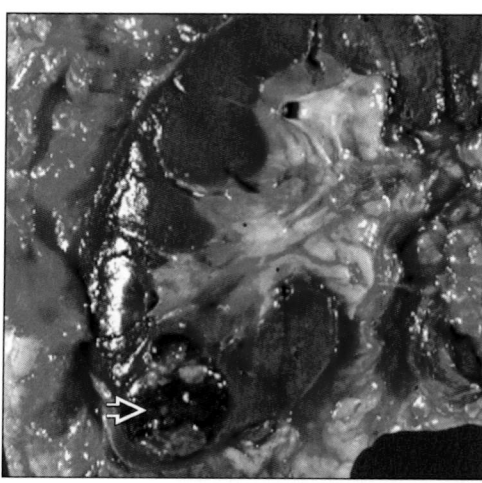

Juxtaglomerular cell tumors of the kidney are usually small, well-circumscribed tumors. Most tumors are less than 2-3 cm in size. The cut surface is often hemorrhagic ➡ and partially cystic.

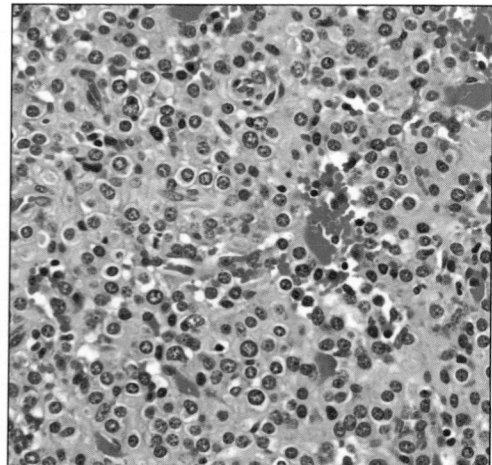

Juxtaglomerular cell tumors often show uniform cytology and resemble a glomus tumor. Most tumors are highly vascular and often show a hemangiopericytoma-like pattern.

TERMINOLOGY

Abbreviations
- Juxtaglomerular cell tumor (JGCT)

Synonyms
- Reninoma

Definitions
- Tumors derived from juxtaglomerular apparatus cells of the kidney, often characterized by
  - Association with hyperreninism, hypokalemia, and hyperaldosteronism
  - Hypertension that usually does not respond to medical antihypertensive therapy

ETIOLOGY/PATHOGENESIS

Hyperreninemia
- With rare exceptions of nonfunctional tumors, most patients have elevated serum renin levels
  - Renal vein catheterization and selective measurement of renin values often helps to lateralize small tumors

Genetic Features
- Loss of chromosomes 9 and 11, or LOHs of the same chromosomes, reported to be recurrent chromosomal abnormality
  - Involved genes not yet known

CLINICAL ISSUES

Epidemiology
- Incidence
  - Rare tumor, < 100 cases reported
- Age
  - Usually tumor of young adults (2nd-3rd decade)
    - However, age range of 6 to > 80 years (mean: 24)

- Gender
  - More often reported in females than males (1.5:1)

Presentation
- Hypertension
  - Most patients present with severe hypertension that shows no or only minimal response to medical therapies
    - Usually associated with hyperreninemia, hypokalemia, and hyperaldosteronism
  - Radiologically, no evidence of renal artery stenosis
  - All young patients with renal mass and hypertension need investigations to exclude JGCT
  - Surgical excision of tumor mostly alleviates hypertension
    - In rare cases, hypertension after nephrectomy due to secondary hypertensive angiopathy caused by tumor

Treatment
- Surgical approaches
  - Surgical removal of tumor, by partial or total nephrectomy, is currently best therapeutic option
  - Medical antihypertensive therapies only transiently effective at best

Prognosis
- Primarily tumor with benign outcome after resection
  - Rare cases with persistent, but usually less severe, post-nephrectomy hypertension
- Only 1 reported case with lung metastases

IMAGE FINDINGS

General Features
- Radiologic studies essential to rule out other causes of hypertension
- Renal arteriography helps to exclude renal artery stenosis
  - Also reveals hypovascular mass lesion in most cases

JUXTAGLOMERULAR CELL TUMOR (RENINOMA)

Key Facts

Terminology
- Tumors derived from juxtaglomerular apparatus cells of the kidney, often characterized by association with hyperreninism, hypokalemia, hyperaldosteronism, and hypertension

Clinical Issues
- Usually tumor of young adults
- Most present with severe hypertension showing no to minimal response to medical therapies
  - Surgical excision of tumor mostly alleviates hypertension
- Primarily tumor with benign outcome

Macroscopic Features
- Well-encapsulated, unilateral, solitary tumor
- Majority of tumors 2-3 cm in diameter

Microscopic Pathology
- Typically, glomoid appearance with sheets of uniform round to polygonal cells with clear to slightly eosinophilic cytoplasm
- Numerous capillaries, branching blood vessels, and sinusoids similar to those of hemangiopericytoma
- Tumors often contain dispersed lymphoplasmacytic infiltrates
- Diffuse (+) staining with antibodies to renin, vimentin, CD34, and CD117; variable positivity for actin-sm
- Ultrastructure reveals typical membrane-bound rhomboid crystals representing renin protogranules

Top Differential Diagnoses
- Glomus tumor
- Solitary fibrous tumor/hemangiopericytoma

MACROSCOPIC FEATURES

General Features
- Well-encapsulated, unilateral, solitary tumor
- Cut surface light tan to yellow, mostly solid, but often with variable, usually small, cysts

Size
- Majority of tumors 2-3 cm in diameter; however, tumors < 1 cm and > 6 cm also reported

MICROSCOPIC PATHOLOGY

Histologic Features
- Histologic appearance highly variable
  - Typically, glomoid appearance with sheets of uniform round to polygonal cells with clear to slightly eosinophilic cytoplasm
    - Cell borders usually distinct
  - Occasionally, sheets or irregular cords of polygonal to spindle cells with indistinct cell borders
  - Most with numerous capillaries, branching blood vessels, and sinusoids similar to those of hemangiopericytoma
  - Stroma is scanty, hyalinized, or myxoid
  - Tumors often contain dispersed lymphocytic infiltrates
  - Some tumors with entrapped tubules in periphery, sometimes hyperplastic and with papillary configuration
  - Rare cases with prominent papillary pattern; likely representing entrapped epithelium
  - Mitotic activity or necrosis uncommon

ANCILLARY TESTS

Immunohistochemistry
- Diffuse (+) staining with antibodies to renin, vimentin, CD34, and CD117; variable positivity for actin-sm

- Neuroendocrine markers and keratins (-); cytokeratins label entrapped tubules but not polygonal or spindle cells

Electron Microscopy
- Reveals typical membrane-bound rhomboid crystals representing renin protogranules

DIFFERENTIAL DIAGNOSIS

Glomus Tumor
- Marked morphologic overlap with JGCT, particularly in areas with glomoid features
- JGCT most often with history of hypertension
- CD34(-) or only focally (+) in glomus tumor; laminin shows pericellular positivity, and CD117(-)
- Glomus tumor lacks typical ultrastructural crystals

Solitary Fibrous Tumor/ Hemangiopericytoma
- Usually spindle cell neoplasms but may have round cell areas
- CD34(+) in both solitary fibrous tumor and JGCT
  - However, solitary fibrous tumor/hemangiopericytomas (+) for bcl-2 and CD99, and (-) for CD117 and renin

SELECTED REFERENCES

1. Capovilla M et al: Loss of chromosomes 9 and 11 may be recurrent chromosome imbalances in juxtaglomerular cell tumors. Hum Pathol. 39(3):459-62, 2008
2. Kim HJ et al: Juxtaglomerular cell tumor of kidney with CD34 and CD117 immunoreactivity: report of 5 cases. Arch Pathol Lab Med. 130(5):707-11, 2006
3. Duan X et al: Metastatic juxtaglomerular cell tumor in a 52-year-old man. Am J Surg Pathol. 28(8):1098-102, 2004
4. Endoh Y et al: Juxtaglomerular cell tumor of the kidney: report of a non-functioning variant. Pathol Int. 47(6):393-6, 1997
5. McVicar M et al: Hypertension secondary to renin-secreting juxtaglomerular cell tumor: case report and review of 38 cases. Pediatr Nephrol. 7(4):404-12, 1993

JUXTAGLOMERULAR CELL TUMOR (RENINOMA)

Microscopic Features

(Left) Most juxtaglomerular cell tumors are well circumscribed with a well-formed, fibrous capsule. Occasionally, the capsule may show focal discontinuity ⮥. Notice the marked lymphocytic infiltration in the tumor periphery in this case. *(Right)* Juxtaglomerular cell tumors often show relative uniformity of nuclear size and shape. Cells often contain a moderate amount of eosinophilic cytoplasm and cell membranes are usually prominent ➡, features similar to those in glomus tumors.

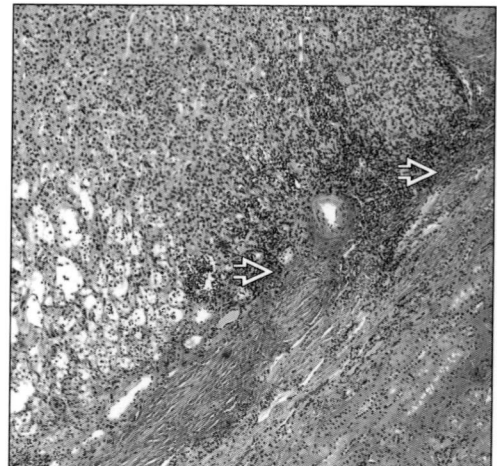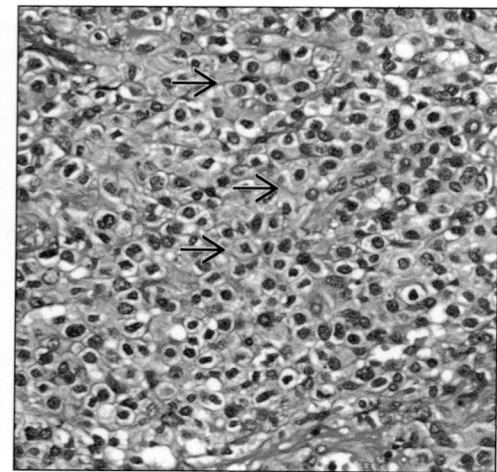

(Left) Most juxtaglomerular cell tumors are highly vascular. Some cases show dilated, thin-walled vascular channels ⮥ as a prominent vascular pattern in the tumor. Others may have a branching, antler-like vascularity, similar to that seen in hemangiopericytomas. *(Right)* A consistent feature in juxtaglomerular cell tumors is the presence of widely dispersed clusters of lymphocytic infiltrates. Usually, these clusters are small and resemble foci of extramedullary hematopoiesis.

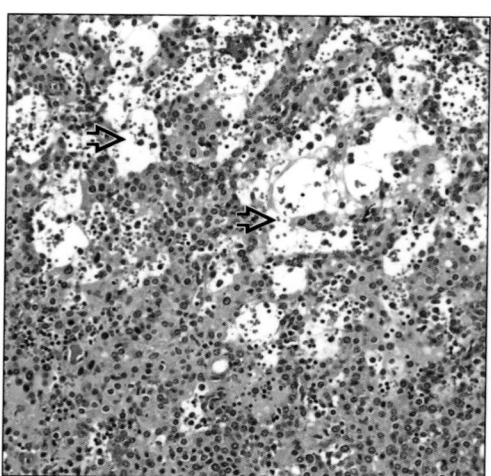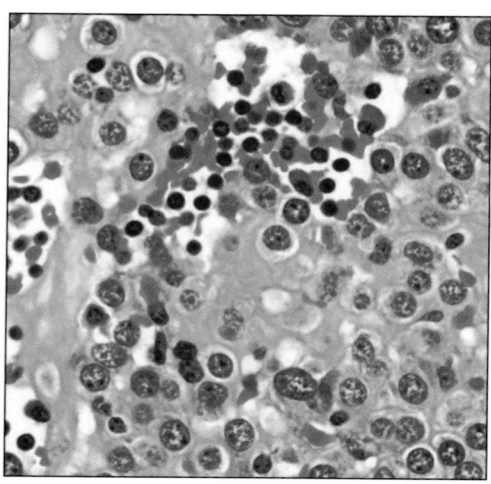

(Left) This photomicrograph shows a spindle cell phenotype in a juxtaglomerular cell tumor. This architectural feature is usually focal. The differential diagnosis with hemangiopericytoma is resolved by immunohistochemistry, including bcl-2 and CD99. *(Right)* This juxtaglomerular cell tumor with polygonal cells contains scant eosinophilic cytoplasm. The cells are in small clusters and may raise the possibility of a renal epithelial neoplasm. Cytokeratin stain is typically negative.

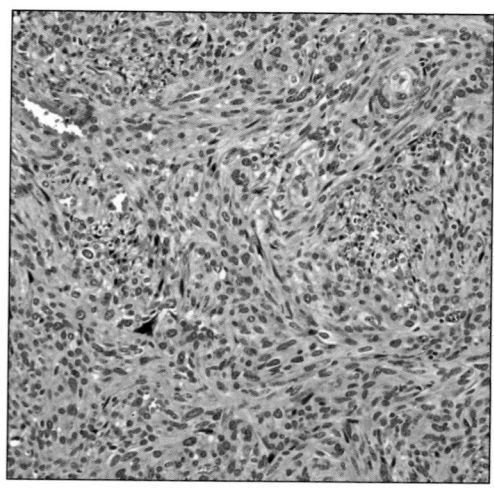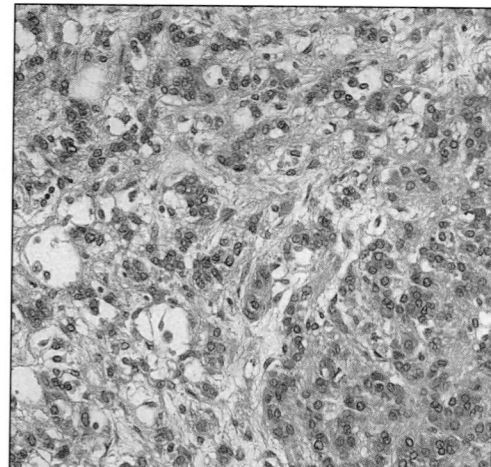

Microscopic and Immunohistochemical Features

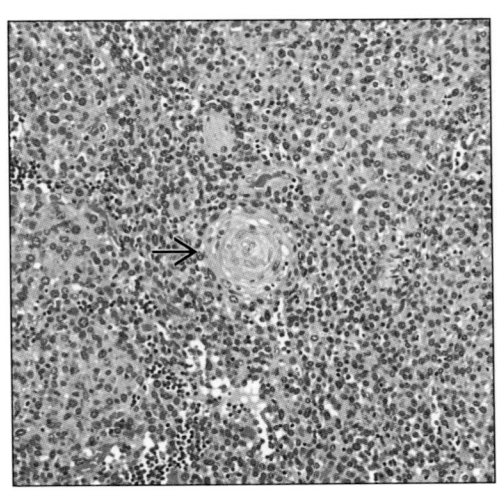

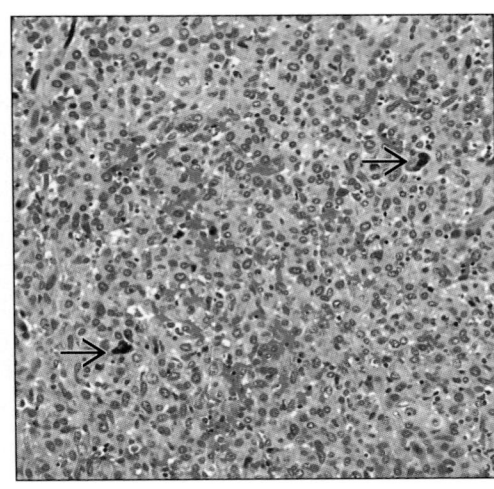

(Left) Typical cytoarchitectural features of a juxtaglomerular cell tumor. Note a medium-sized vessel with "onion skin" proliferation of medial smooth muscle ➡. Such vascular changes are quite common in the tumor and possibly represent the effect of marked hypertension. **(Right)** Focal, marked nuclear atypia ➡ in a JGCT. The presence of such focal endocrine-like, markedly atypical, polyploid, hyperchromatic nuclei is not uncommon in the tumor and has no bearing on prognosis.

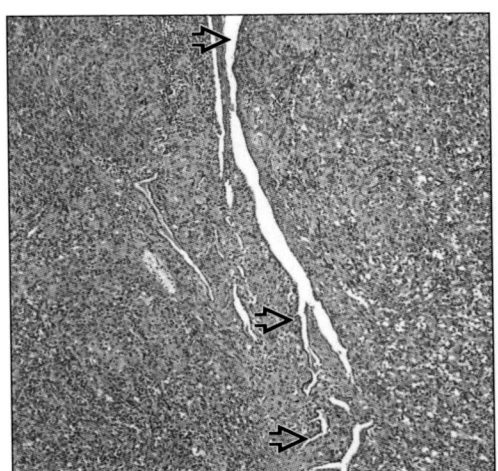

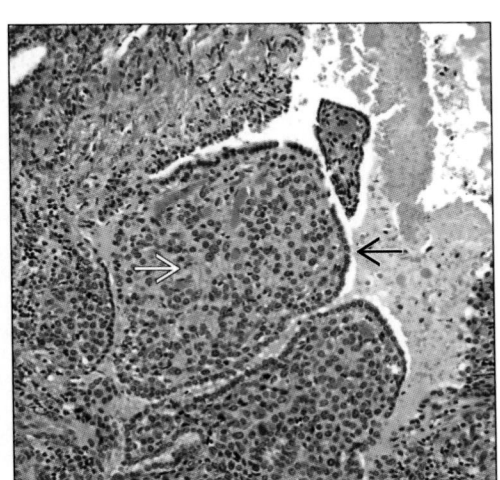

(Left) Many JGCTs show entrapped tubules ➡, particularly at the periphery of the tumor. Often, these tubules show a variety of proliferative and reactive changes. **(Right)** Among the morphologically more striking proliferative changes in the entrapped tubules in JGCTs is the papillary change. In this image, the tubular epithelium ➡ is seen along the rim of neoplastic cells ➡ forming the papillary structure. Tumors with markedly prominent papillary features have been described.

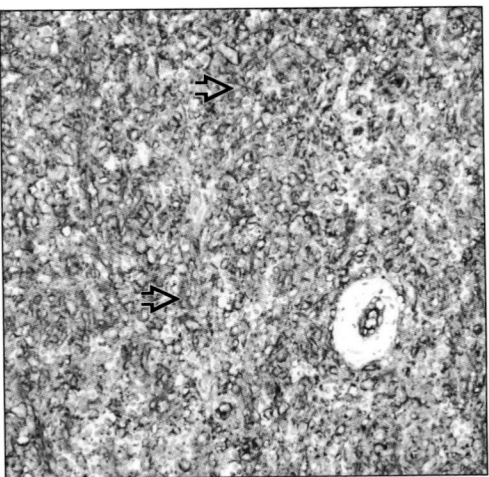

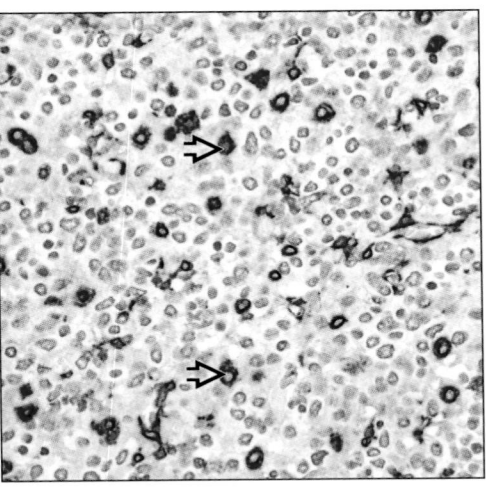

(Left) Diffuse immunohistochemical positivity for CD34 ➡ is present in most juxtaglomerular cell tumors. Immunoreactivity for CD117 is also present. However, many tumors show abundant mast cell infiltration, associated with lymphoplasmacytic infiltrates. Therefore, interpretation of the results with CD117 positivity requires adequate caution. **(Right)** Variable positivity ➡ for actin-sm is also frequently present in juxtaglomerular cell tumors.

RENOMEDULLARY INTERSTITIAL CELL TUMOR

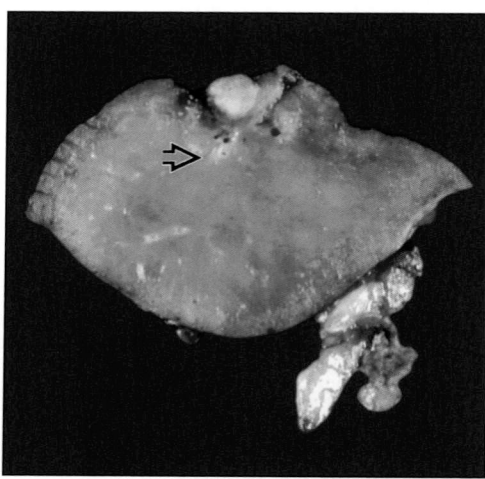

Renomedullary interstitial cell tumors are usually sub-centimeter white or tan nodules ⊳, mostly detected incidentally at autopsy or in nephrectomy specimens resected for other conditions.

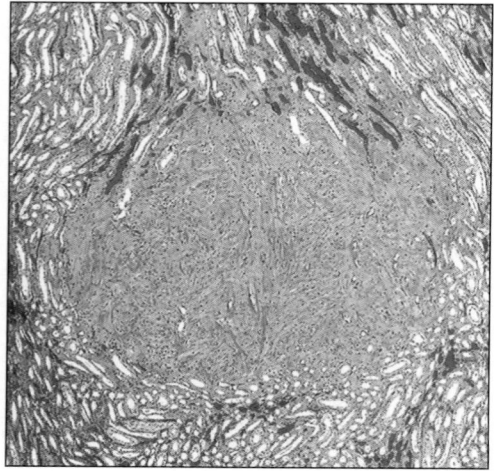

RMIC tumors are well-circumscribed nodules, invariably present in the renal medulla. These are the most common renal tumors, and thorough sampling of the kidneys reveals an incidence of > 40%.

TERMINOLOGY

Abbreviations
- Renomedullary interstitial cell tumor (RMICT)

Synonyms
- Medullary fibroma

Definitions
- Benign renal medullary neoplasm, arising from renomedullary interstitial cells

ETIOLOGY/PATHOGENESIS

Renal Medullary Interstitial Cell
- Renomedullary interstitial cells (RMIC) are located in inner renal medulla
  - These cells express receptors for multiple vasoactive peptides, including angiotensin II
  - RMIC plays important role in renin release and regulation of sodium excretion
    - These, in turn, maintain renal blood flow and normal blood pressure
- RMIC tumors are believed by many to develop in response to systemic hypertension
  - Others have found no such relationship between these tumors and systemic hypertension
- Recently, concomitant expression of COX-2, microsomal prostaglandin E synthase-1, and prostaglandin E2 (PGE2) receptor have been demonstrated in RMIC tumors
  - COX-2 activity is known to provide antiapoptotic protection of interstitial cells during osmotic stress
  - RMIC tumors show constitutive activation of COX-2
    - Results in increased PGE2 production and activation of PGE2 receptors
    - This activation is believed to act in autocrine manner, leading to tumoral proliferation of interstitial medullary cells

CLINICAL ISSUES

Epidemiology
- Incidence
  - Most common kidney tumor of adults
    - Incidence in autopsy series is 16-42%
    - Incidence increases with age
    - Very rare tumors are described in young patients; youngest reported in a 14 year old
    - Incidence is also related to relative thoroughness of sampling of tissue

Presentation
- Most often incidental finding in nephrectomies performed for other tumors or at autopsy
- Rare association between multiple RMICTs and systemic hypertension has been reported
- Very rarely, tumor may compress pelvicalyceal system, leading to hydronephrosis and urosepsis
- Occasional incidental finding in needle biopsy of kidney has also been described

Prognosis
- Benign tumors

MACROSCOPIC FEATURES

General Features
- Well-circumscribed, tan to white nodules within renal medulla
- Most measure < 5 mm in greatest dimension
  - Size usually ranges from 1-10 mm
  - Very occasionally, much larger masses (≥ 5 cm) also reported
    - Rare large tumor protrudes into renal pelvis
    - These large tumors obstruct pelvicalyceal system and may be associated with hydronephrosis

RENOMEDULLARY INTERSTITIAL CELL TUMOR

Key Facts

Terminology
- Benign renal medullary neoplasm, arising from renomedullary interstitial cells

Clinical Issues
- Most common kidney tumor of adults
- Most often, incidental finding in nephrectomies performed for other tumors or at autopsy
- Incidence in autopsy series varies from 16-42%
- Very rarely, tumor may compress pelvicalyceal system, leading to hydronephrosis and urosepsis

Macroscopic Features
- Most measure < 5 mm in greatest dimension
- Very occasional, much larger masses (≥ 5 cm) also reported

Microscopic Pathology
- Densely collagenized tumors with sparse spindle cells
  ○ Keloid-like collagenous bands may be present in such tumors
- Or variably cellular tumors usually with abundant spindle to stellate cells in myxoid stroma

Top Differential Diagnoses
- Mixed epithelial and stromal tumor (MEST)
  ○ Usually larger mass lesion and primary reason for nephrectomy
  ○ Epithelial component in MEST distributed throughout tumor, and stroma in MEST usually ER and PR positive

MICROSCOPIC PATHOLOGY

Histologic Features
- Stroma in RMICT may either be
  ○ Loose and myxoid, or
  ○ Densely collagenized, occasionally with keloid-like collagen
- Stromal cells may be scant and widely separated or hypercellular and tightly packed
  ○ Stromal cells are spindled or stellate
  ○ Nuclei show absent to minimal pleomorphism and regular chromatin
  ○ Mitotic activity and necrosis are not seen
  ○ May show presence of lipid droplets, similar to that in nonneoplastic RMIC, and this finding may be confirmed on oil red O stain
- Tumors with mixed patterns are common
- Occasional tumors may have amyloid deposition in stroma
- Entrapped normal tubules are frequently seen, particularly at periphery of tumor
  ○ Rarely, some entrapped tubules may show cystic dilatation

ANCILLARY TESTS

Immunohistochemistry
- Stromal cells in RMICT show some immunohistochemical features resembling myofibroblasts
  ○ Stain positive for smooth muscle actin
  ○ Cells are also positive for COX-2 and PGE2
  ○ Tumors have not been investigated for ER and PR
  ○ CD34 and S100 proteins are negative
  ○ Immunohistochemistry is rarely required in diagnostic practice

Electron Microscopy
- Ultrastructural features similar to nonneoplastic RMIC

  ■ Electron dense osmiophilic droplets (lipid), cisternae, and cytoplasmic processes are most consistent features

DIFFERENTIAL DIAGNOSIS

Mixed Epithelial and Stromal Tumor (MEST)
- MEST is usually larger mass lesion and primary reason for nephrectomy; RMICT is almost invariably incidental finding
- Epithelial component in MEST is distributed randomly and throughout tumor; RMICT usually have entrapped renal tubules only in periphery
- Stroma in MEST is usually ER and PR positive
  ○ No reports of ER and PR positivity in RMIC tumors, although nontumorous RMICs have been reported to be ER &/or PR positive

DIAGNOSTIC CHECKLIST

Pathologic Interpretation Pearls
- Benign stromal tumor of kidney that is incidentally detected and which is composed of bland stellate cells

SELECTED REFERENCES

1. Faris G et al: Urosepsis as a presenting symptom of renomedullary interstitial cell tumor causing renal obstruction. Isr Med Assoc J. 11(8):509-10, 2009
2. Gatalica Z et al: COX-2 gene polymorphisms and protein expression in renomedullary interstitial cell tumors. Hum Pathol. 39(10):1495-504, 2008
3. Tickoo SK et al: Estrogen and progesterone-receptor-positive stroma as a non-tumorous proliferation in kidneys: a possible metaplastic response to obstruction. Mod Pathol. 21(1):60-5, 2008
4. Agras K et al: Adolescent renomedullary interstitial cell tumor: a case report. Tumori. 91(6):555-7, 2005
5. Horita Y et al: Incidental detection of renomedullary interstitial cell tumour in a renal biopsy specimen. Nephrol Dial Transplant. 19(4):1007-8, 2004

RENOMEDULLARY INTERSTITIAL CELL TUMOR

Gross and Microscopic Features

(Left) Very rarely, renomedullary interstitial cell tumors may be quite large and detected radiologically. An occasional case may compress the pelvicalyceal system and result in hydronephrosis. *(Right)* Although renomedullary interstitial tumor is almost always well circumscribed, it does not show any encapsulation. This hematoxylin and eosin image shows a well-circumscribed renomedullary interstitial tumor imperceptibly invading the surrounding renal medullary tissue.

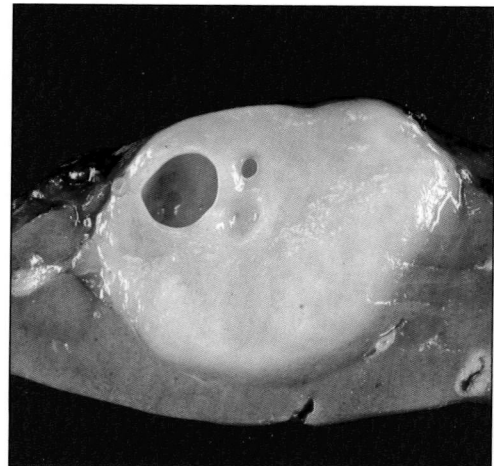
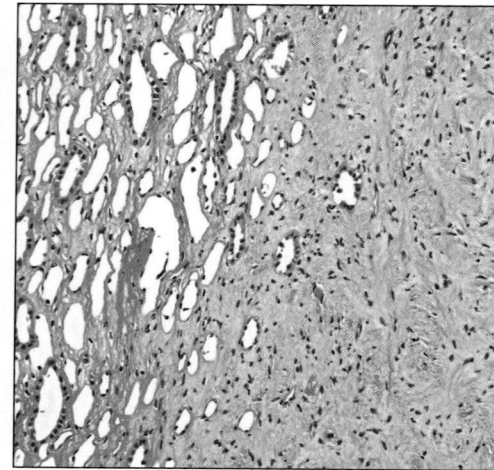

(Left) Some renomedullary interstitial cell tumors show sclerotic stroma and relatively scant spindle or stellate cells. However, the stroma is more loose ➡ and faintly basophilic, at least focally, in most cases. *(Right)* In some renomedullary interstitial tumors, the stroma may be entirely myxoid or basophilic ➡. In many tumors, however, both the sclerotic and basophilic type stroma are present in combination, in variable proportions.

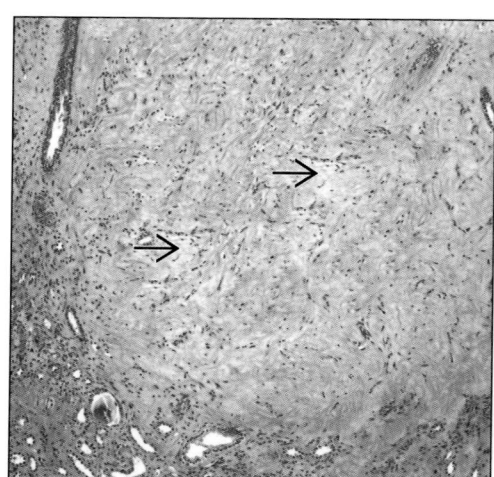
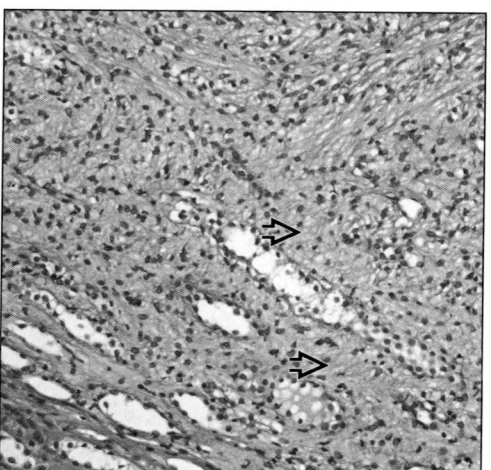

(Left) In some cases of renomedullary interstitial cell tumor, in addition to the loose myxoid and fibrotic-like stroma in variable proportions, keloid-like ➡ hyalinized bands of collagen may also be present. Rare cases with stromal amyloid deposition are also reported. *(Right)* Most renomedullary interstitial cell tumors are paucicellular, with dispersed spindle or stellate cells dispersed within the stroma. This image shows loose myxoid stroma in a tumor with low cellularity.

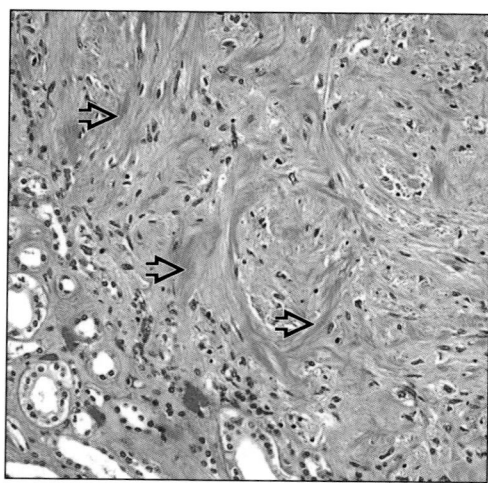
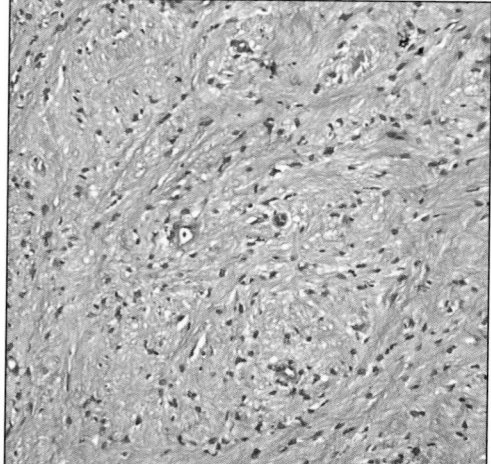

1

Microscopic Features and Differential Diagnosis

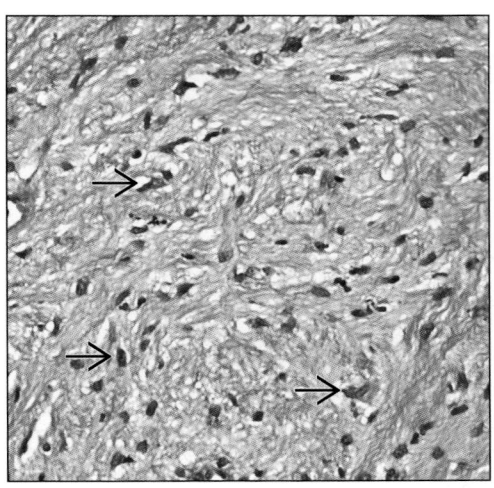

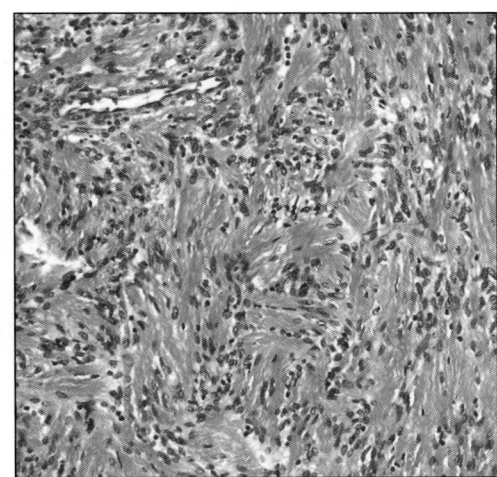

(Left) The spindled or stellate cells ⇨ in renomedullary interstitial cell tumors show open chromatin, minimal atypia, and usually absence of any mitotic activity. Oil red O histochemical stain often reveals lipid droplets in these cells, similar to that found in nonneoplastic RMICs. (Right) Some RMIC tumors are quite cellular. This cellular tumor has a fibrotic/sclerotic stroma. These tumors are negative for CD34 and S100 (unlike solitary fibrous tumor or schwannoma).

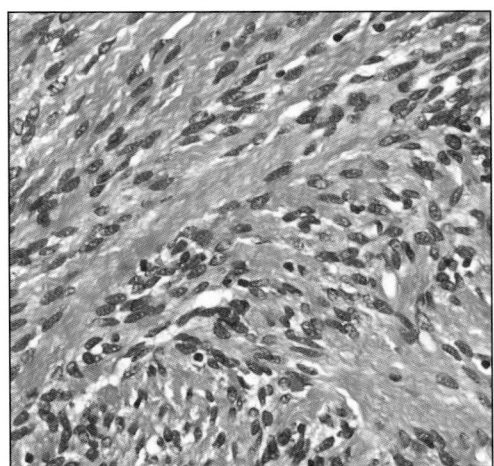

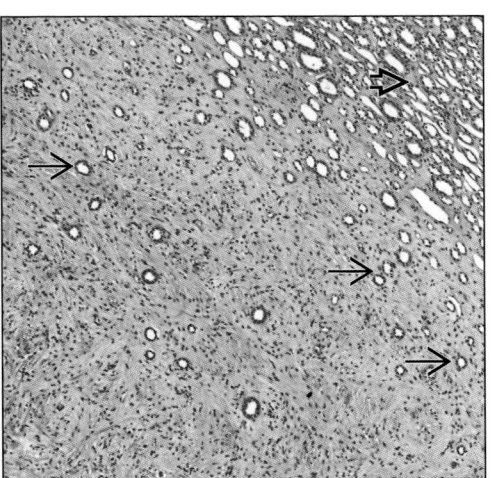

(Left) Cellular renomedullary interstitial cell tumor shows the bland nuclear features characteristic of the tumor. The nuclei depict minimal variation in shape and size, and open chromatin. Mitotic activity is almost always nonexistent. (Right) A consistent feature in renomedullary interstitial cell tumors is the presence of entrapped tubules ⇨, particularly in the periphery of the tumor. Notice the adjacent renal medulla ⇨, in which all of these tumors are located.

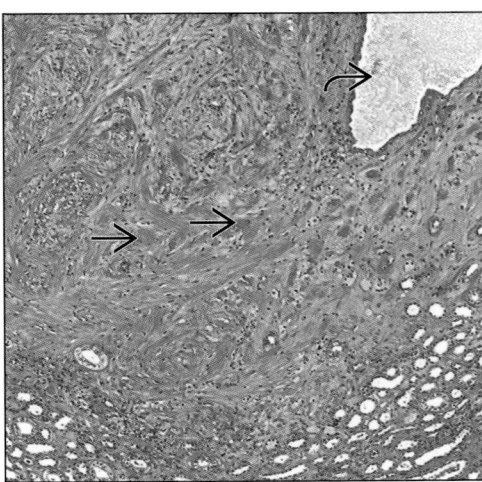

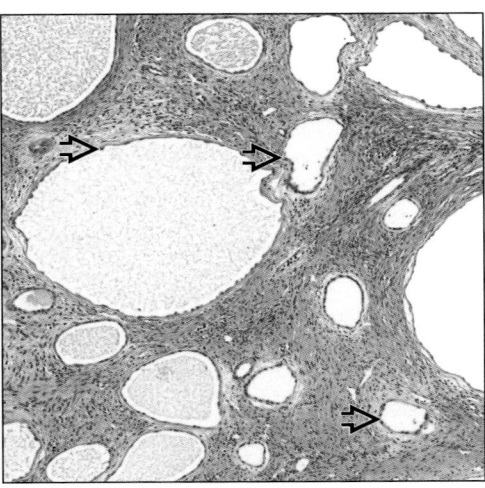

(Left) Rarely, renomedullary interstitial cell tumors may show cystic dilatation ⇨ of the entrapped tubules. Notice the stromal sclerosis and keloid-like collagen ⇨ in this tumor. (Right) Renal mixed epithelial and stromal tumors (MEST) may sometimes be difficult to distinguish from renomedullary interstitial cell tumor. Unlike RMICT, MEST is a large, radiologically identifiable tumor. The epithelial component ⇨ is widely dispersed throughout the tumor, unlike RMICT.

OTHER RARE TUMORS

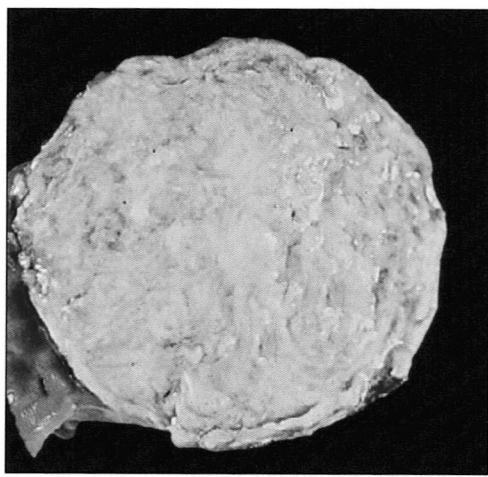

Other than angiomyolipoma, benign mesenchymal tumors are very rare in kidney. Leiomyoma, as depicted here, may arise within the renal parenchyma, or from the renal capsule or walls of hilar vessels.

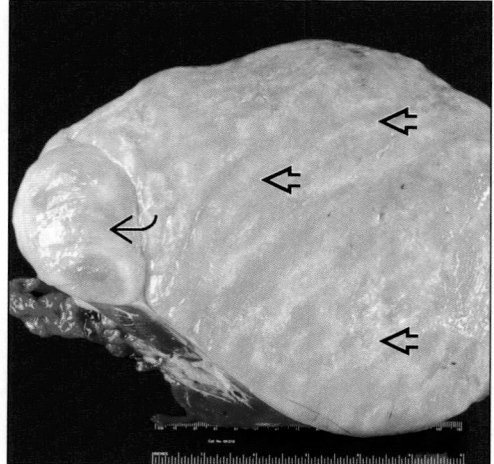

This liposarcoma shows a predominant fleshy cut surface ⬒, suggesting dedifferentiation, and smaller yellow-tan well-differentiated component ➨. Most sarcomas involving the kidney originate in perirenal soft tissue.

TERMINOLOGY

Definitions
- Uncommon tumors that include
  - Benign and malignant mesenchymal neoplasms, neuroendocrine tumors other than carcinoid tumor, and other rare tumors

EPIDEMIOLOGY

Incidence
- Primary mesenchymal tumors of kidney constitute ≤1% of all renal tumors
- Among the sarcomas, largest reported series of 26 cases represents 25 years of experience at Memorial Sloan-Kettering Cancer Center, New York
- After angiomyolipoma, leiomyoma is 2nd most common benign mesenchymal tumor of kidney
  - Based on older autopsy series, reported incidence is > 5%
    - However, we are now aware that most renal leiomyomatous tumors in fact represent leiomyomatous angiomyolipomas
    - Therefore, actual incidence of renal leiomyomas is likely much lower than reported in literature
- Other rarer benign mesenchymal tumors described in kidneys include
  - Hemangioma, lipoma, solitary fibrous tumor, schwannoma, neurofibroma, myxoma, and lymphangioma
- < 20 primary high-grade neuroendocrine carcinomas (mostly small cell carcinoma) and < 10 renal glomus tumors are described in the literature
- Very few cases of renal-adrenal fusion are reported
  - However, ectopic adrenal tissue is more common
  - Very occasional adrenal cortical tumor arising from renal-adrenal fusion or ectopic adrenal tissue has been also described

CLINICAL IMPLICATIONS

Clinical Presentation
- Most benign or low-grade tumors are detected incidentally on evaluation of unrelated symptoms
  - Others may present with palpable mass or hematuria
- Sarcomas and other high-grade tumors often present with flank or abdominal pain and palpable mass, or occasionally with hematuria
  - Rare cases may present with symptoms related to metastases

Clinical Risk Factors
- Prognostic factors and risk
  - Sarcomas of kidney are usually aggressive tumors with reported 5-year survival rates of < 30%
    - Tumor size and metastasis at presentation are most significant predictors of disease specific survival in genitourinary, including renal, sarcomas
  - Renal high-grade neuroendocrine carcinomas are highly aggressive neoplasms, like their counterparts in other sites
    - Metastasis from another site should be ruled out before tumor is reported as primary
    - Distant metastases to brain, bone, adrenal gland, and liver are frequent
    - Prognosis is highly dependent on stage and complete resectability of tumor
    - Approximately 75% of patients are reported to be dead of disease within 1 year of diagnosis
    - However, with current therapies available for small cell carcinoma, the prognosis may not be so dismal
  - Visceral location, size > 2 cm, nuclear atypia, significant mitotic activity, or atypical mitoses reported to predict aggressive behavior in glomus tumors

- However, most reported renal glomus tumors have been > 2 cm, and all have had benign clinical course on relatively short follow-ups
- Degenerative-type nuclear atypia also reported in renal glomus tumors, with no adverse influence on biologic behavior

MACROSCOPIC FINDINGS

General Features

- Leiomyomas and lipomas: Well circumscribed, usually small; rare large tumors, including a 37 kg lipoma, also described
  - Gross appearance similar to that in soft tissue counterparts
- Hemangiomas are usually small (1-2 cm), mostly localized but not well circumscribed
  - Rare tumors as large as 8 cm in size and filling the pelvicalyceal system have been also described
  - Usually hemorrhagic-appearing cut surface; rarely solid-tan appearance
- Glomus tumors are well circumscribed and encapsulated
  - Cut surface may be uniform and tan or with variegated mucoid/myxoid appearance
- Sarcomas are usually large tumors
  - Mean size: 10.5 cm (range: 2.5-30 cm); tumor size closely related to biologic behavior
- Most patients with renal high-grade neuroendocrine carcinoma present with locally advanced disease and regional lymph node metastases
  - Majority of tumors located close to pelvicalyceal system
  - Size ranges from 2.5-23 cm (median: 8 cm)
    - Invasion into renal sinus adipose tissue very frequent
  - Cut surface usually soft, whitish, gritty, and necrotic

MICROSCOPIC FINDINGS

General Features

- Leiomyomas, lipomas, and hemangiomas: Morphologic features similar to those in soft tissue
  - Possibility of angiomyolipoma needs to be excluded in all smooth muscle and lipomatous tumors of kidney
  - As in soft tissue, mitotic activity, nuclear atypia, necrosis, and large size in leiomyomatous tumor favor leiomyosarcoma
  - Hemangiomas are usually of cavernous type; capillary hemangiomas are unusual
  - Recently described rare hemangioma variant, anastomosing hemangioma, appears unique to kidney vascular tumors
    - Shows anastomosing sinusoidal capillary-sized vessels with scattered "hobnail" endothelial cells
    - Morphology displays overlapping features of both sinusoidal hemangioma and "hobnail" hemangioma of soft tissue and skin
    - May mimic angiosarcoma

- Glomus tumor: Represents a group of tumors composed of glomus cells, blood vessels, and smooth muscle cells in various proportions
  - Glomus cells are typically small, round to oval uniform cells with distinct cell borders
  - These have moderate amount of eosinophilic to amphophilic cytoplasm, and smooth nuclear contours with open and speckled chromatin
  - Areas with marked nuclear pleomorphism, likely representing symplastic/degenerative changes, may be present
  - Based on histologic features, 3 subtypes described
    - Solid glomus tumors, with sheets of glomus cells usually within background of compressed capillary framework
    - Glomangiomas that are highly vascular, with dilated vascular channels and dispersed glomus cells in stroma between vessels
    - Glomangiomyomas showing large branching and gaping vessels with spindled cells in stroma resembling smooth muscle cells
- Sarcomas: Most sarcomas involving the kidney originate in retroperitoneum with invasion of kidney
  - Primary sarcomas of kidney extremely rare
    - Leiomyosarcoma most common renal sarcoma, followed by liposarcoma
    - Leiomyosarcoma involving kidney frequently arises from renal vein or its major branches
    - Some apparent leiomyosarcomas in kidney may actually be dedifferentiated liposarcomas with smooth muscle differentiation
    - Other subtypes of sarcoma exceedingly rare
    - Morphologic features are similar to those in soft tissues
- High-grade neuroendocrine carcinoma: Very uncommon primary renal tumor
  - Before accepting it as a primary renal neoplasm, metastasis from other more common sites needs to be excluded
  - Many of the tumors associated with nonneuroendocrine carcinomas, particularly renal pelvic urothelial carcinoma
  - Most reported cases with features of small cell carcinoma, morphologically similar to those in lung
    - Very rare large cell neuroendocrine carcinoma also described
- Renal-adrenal fusion and ectopic adrenal tissue
  - Adrenal tissue fused to kidney often lacks a capsule, and in areas lacking capsule, adrenal cortical tissue shows infiltrative growth
  - Ectopic adrenal tissue always lacks the medulla and is composed of cortical tissue only
  - Clear cells of adrenal cortical tissue almost always show "bubbly" cytoplasm and not transparent clear cytoplasm

DIFFERENTIAL DIAGNOSIS

Angiomyolipoma

- In all leiomyomatous and lipomatous tumors in kidney, smooth muscle or fat-predominant angiomyolipoma needs to be excluded

- Performing immunostaining for melanocytic markers is prudent in all such cases
- Leiomyomatous angiomyolipoma may show focal adipocytes or dysmorphic vessels
- Dysmorphic vessels &/or leiomyomatous foci in lipomatous angiomyolipomas should be carefully searched for, although they are frequently absent
- Epithelioid cells cuffing small vessels may be present and point toward actual diagnosis in many of these lesions
- At least focal positivity for HMB-45 and Melan-A(MART-1) will resolve differential diagnostic issues in most cases

Extrarenal or Metastatic Tumors

- Tumors arising in retroperitoneum usually impinge on and compress/deform renal parenchyma without invading it
- Extrarenal tumors invading renal parenchyma usually show bulk of tumor in extrarenal location often with focal renal parenchymal invasion
- Clinical history of prior neuroendocrine carcinoma in lung or other organs is useful in separating primary from metastatic neuroendocrine carcinoma

Clear Cell Renal Cell Carcinoma

- Ectopic adrenal tissue and adrenal cortical neoplasms involving kidney may be mistaken for clear cell RCC
- Adrenal cortical cells with clear cell features almost always show bubbly, and not optically clear, cytoplasm
- Adrenal cortical cells are immunoreactive for inhibin, Melan-A(MART-1), and synaptophysin, and usually negative for EMA/MUC1, cytokeratins, and CA9

IMMUNOHISTOCHEMISTRY

Leiomyoma and Lipomatous Tumors

- Stains for HMB-45, Melan-A(MART-1), and other melanocytic markers are completely negative
- Liposarcomas are usually mdm2 and CDK4 positive

Glomus Tumor

- Tumors are actin-sm and common muscle actin positive
- Desmin and CD34 is usually negative, although focal positivity for CD34 may be observed
- Unlike juxtaglomerular tumor, CD117 is negative in glomus tumor

Adrenal Cortical Lesions

- These are EMA/MUC1, cytokeratin, and CA9 negative
- Stains for inhibin, Melan-A(MART-1), and synaptophysin are usually positive

Angiosarcoma

- Immunostains may be required in poorly differentiated or epithelioid variants
  - Tumors are CD31, CD34, and FLI-1 positive
  - Cytokeratins may show variable positivity, especially in tumors with epithelioid features

DIAGNOSTIC CHECKLIST

Diagnostic Interpretation Pearls

- Tumors with unusual morphologic features mainly require exclusion of metastases from other primary sites
- In case of mesenchymal neoplasm involving kidney, direct extension from extrarenal, retroperitoneal neoplasms needs to be excluded
- Primary smooth muscle or lipomatous tumors of kidney are extremely rare
  - In all such cases, exclusion of angiomyolipoma with predominant leiomyomatous or lipomatous differentiation is imperative
    - Immunostains for melanocytic markers in all such tumors is essential

SELECTED REFERENCES

1. Mazzucchelli R et al: Neuroendocrine tumours of the urinary system and male genital organs: clinical significance. BJU Int. 103(11):1464-70, 2009
2. Ye H et al: Intrarenal ectopic adrenal tissue and renal-adrenal fusion: a report of nine cases. Mod Pathol. 22(2):175-81, 2009
3. Magro G et al: Solitary fibrous tumour of the kidney with sarcomatous overgrowth. Case report and review of the literature. APMIS. 116(11):1020-5, 2008
4. Al-Ahmadie HA et al: Glomus tumor of the kidney: a report of 3 cases involving renal parenchyma and review of the literature. Am J Surg Pathol. 31(4):585-91, 2007
5. Kuroda N et al: Renal leiomyoma: an immunohistochemical, ultrastructural and comparative genomic hybridization study. Histol Histopathol. 22(8):883-8, 2007
6. Lee TY et al: Renal angiosarcoma: a case report and literature review. Can J Urol. 14(1):3471-6, 2007
7. Dotan ZA et al: Adult genitourinary sarcoma: the 25-year Memorial Sloan-Kettering experience. J Urol. 176(5):2033-8; discussion 2038-9, 2006
8. Leggio L et al: Primary renal angiosarcoma: a rare malignancy. A case report and review of the literature. Urol Oncol. 24(4):307-12, 2006
9. Shum CF et al: Symptomatic renal leiomyoma: report of two cases. Pathology. 38(5):454-6, 2006
10. Moazzam M et al: Leiomyosarcoma presenting as a spontaneously ruptured renal tumor-case report. BMC Urol. 2:13, 2002
11. Tamboli P et al: Benign tumors and tumor-like lesions of the adult kidney. Part II: Benign mesenchymal and mixed neoplasms, and tumor-like lesions. Adv Anat Pathol. 7(1):47-66, 2000
12. Berkmen F et al: Adult genitourinary sarcomas: a report of seventeen cases and review of the literature. J Exp Clin Cancer Res. 16(1):45-8, 1997
13. Melamed J et al: Renal myxoma. A report of two cases and review of the literature. Am J Surg Pathol. 18(2):187-94, 1994
14. Steiner M et al: Leiomyoma of the kidney: presentation of 4 new cases and the role of computerized tomography. J Urol. 143(5):994-8, 1990
15. Dineen MK et al: Pure intrarenal lipoma--report of a case and review of the literature. J Urol. 132(1):104-7, 1984
16. Xipell JM: The incidence of benign renal nodules (a clinicopathologic study). J Urol. 106(4):503-6, 1971

Gross, Microscopic, and Ancillary Features

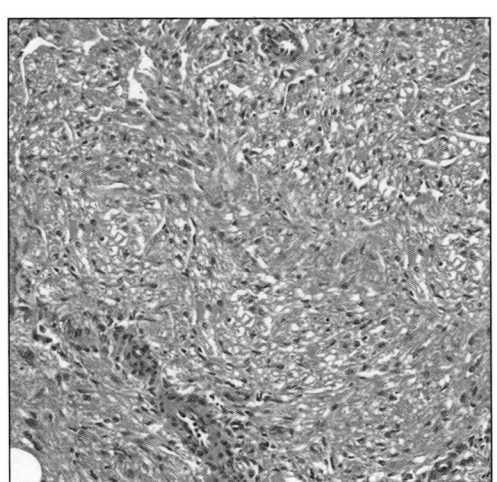

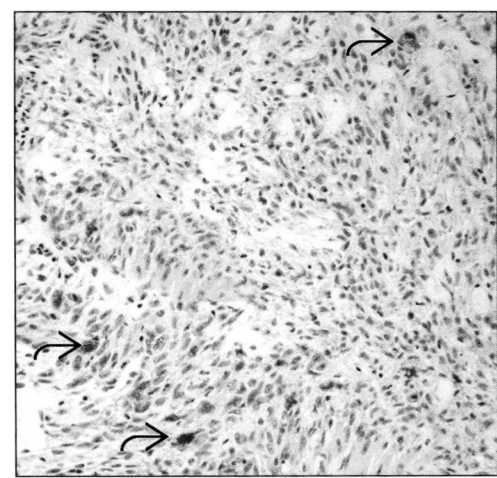

(Left) Leiomyoma is the 2nd most common benign mesenchymal tumor of the kidney. In some old autopsy series, the incidence of renal leiomyomas has been reported to be as high as > 5%. *(Right)* A large proportion of the leiomyomatous tumors of the kidney are now known to be smooth-muscle predominant angiomyolipomas. This image depicts HMB-45 immunoreactivity ⊿ in a renal smooth muscle tumor, confirming it to be an angiomyolipoma, rather than a leiomyoma.

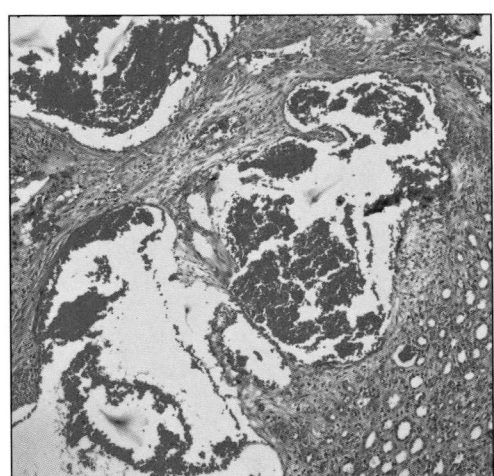

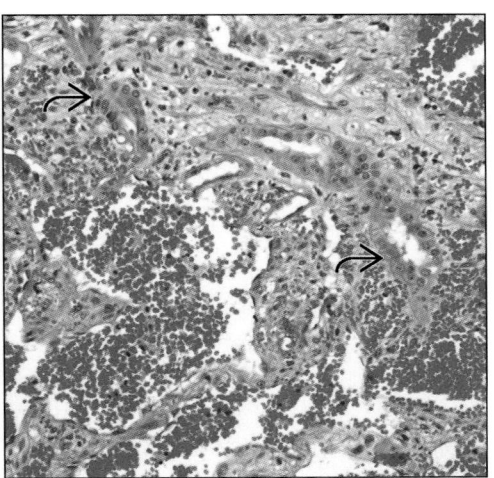

(Left) After angiomyolipoma and leiomyoma, hemangioma and lipoma are the other most frequent benign mesenchymal renal tumors, although both are extremely uncommon. This image shows a primary renal hemangioma. *(Right)* Renal hemangiomas usually have irregular, infiltrative-appearing borders ⊿. Both capillary and cavernous hemangiomas are described, and most described cases have been of the cavernous type. This image depicts a cavernous hemangioma of the kidney.

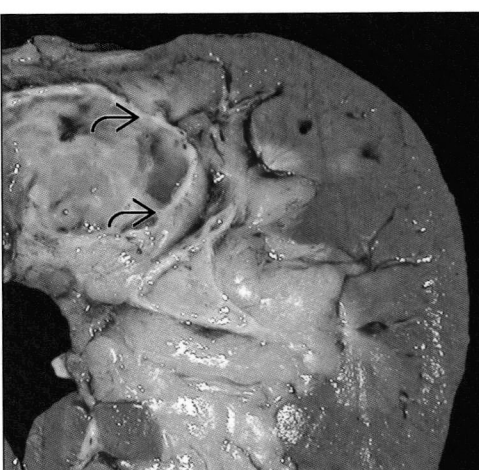

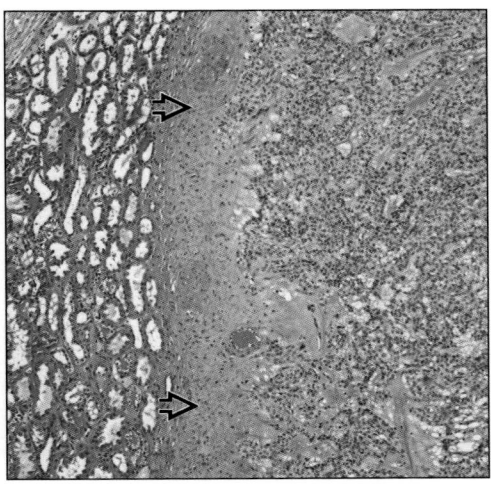

(Left) This well-circumscribed and encapsulated ⊿ tumor represents a glomus tumor. It shows a prominent myxoid cut surface. Glomus tumors of the kidney are quite rare, and at both the gross and microscopic levels need distinction from juxtaglomerular cell tumor. *(Right)* Renal glomus tumors are well circumscribed and mostly encapsulated ⊵. Unlike juxtaglomerular cell tumors, which often contain glomus-like areas, glomus tumors are not associated with hypertension.

OTHER RARE TUMORS

Gross, Microscopic, and Ancillary Features

(Left) Microscopically, glomus tumors show relatively uniform cells, with smooth nuclear contours, open and speckled chromatin, moderate amount of eosinophilic to amphophilic cytoplasm, and distinct cell borders. *(Right)* Glomus tumors are composed of a mixture of glomus cells, blood vessels, and smooth muscle cells in various proportions. This example shows sheets of glomus cells within a background of compressed capillary framework. Such tumors are designated as solid glomus tumors.

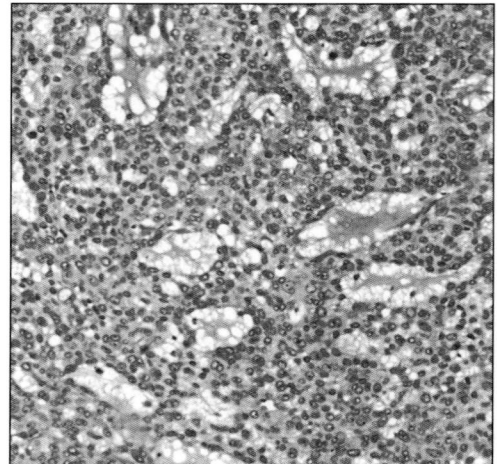
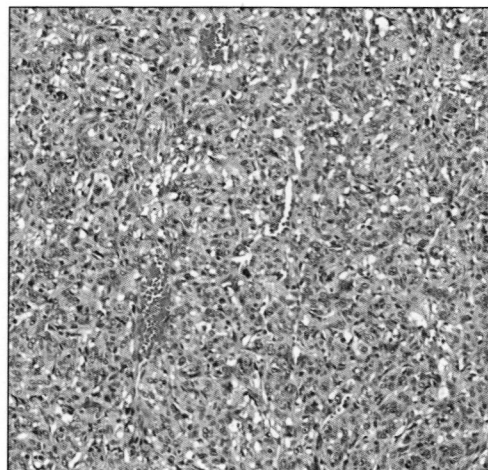

(Left) Some glomus tumors are highly vascular, with dilated vascular channels and round to oval glomus cells dispersed in the stroma between the vessels ➡. Such tumors have been designated as glomangiomas. *(Right)* Some other glomus tumors may show large branching and gaping vessels with spindled cells ➡ in the stroma resembling smooth muscle cells. Such tumors have been called glomangiomyomas. All 3 architectural patterns may sometimes be noted within the same tumor.

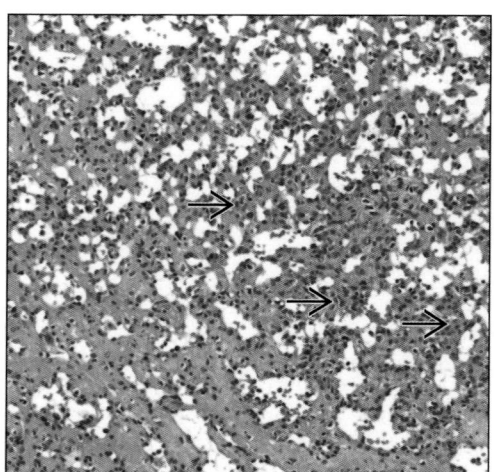
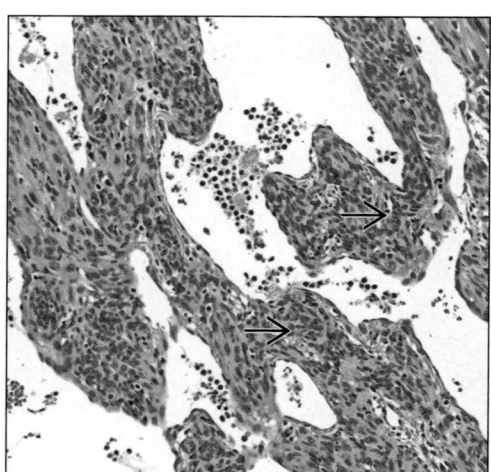

(Left) Glomus tumors show diffuse immunoreactivity for actin-sm and common muscle actin. However, staining for desmin is negative, even in tumors with glomangiomyoma features. *(Right)* This photomicrograph shows diffuse pericellular staining for laminin in a renal glomus tumor, a consistent and characteristic finding in the tumor. Unlike the peripheral glomus tumors, renal and other visceral glomus tumors are usually negative for CD34. However, focal reactivity has been reported in some renal tumors.

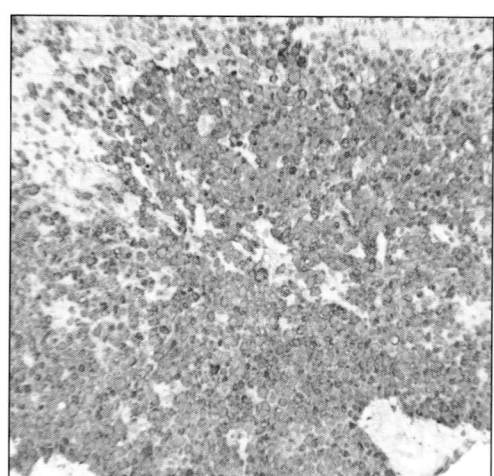
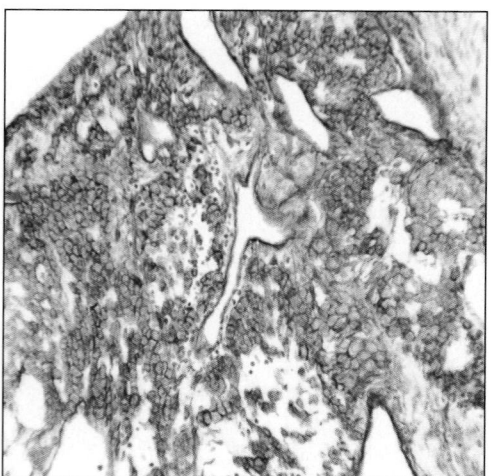

OTHER RARE TUMORS

Gross and Microscopic Features

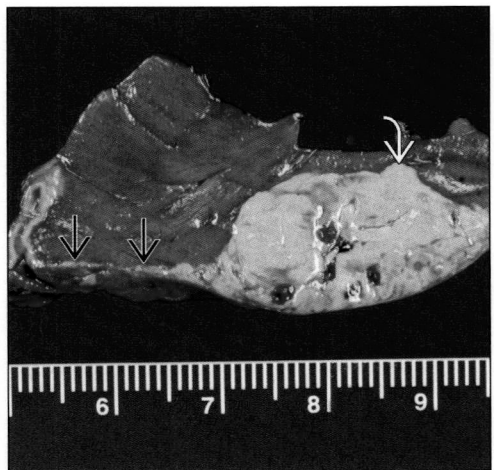

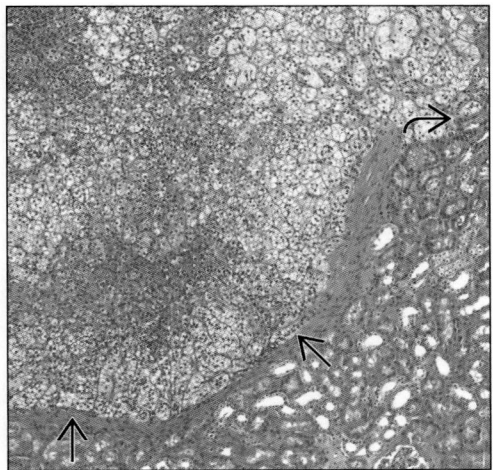

(Left) Renal-adrenal fusion and adrenal cortical neoplasms arising therefrom are not uncommon in spite of few reported cases. Adrenal tissue fused to kidney often lacks a capsule ⟹, and cortical nodules arising from fused adrenal may have infiltrative edges ⟹. (Right) This instance of renal-adrenal fusion shows partial encapsulation ⟹ delimiting renal from adrenal tissue. In the area lacking the capsule, adrenal cortical tissue shows an infiltrative pattern of growth ⟹.

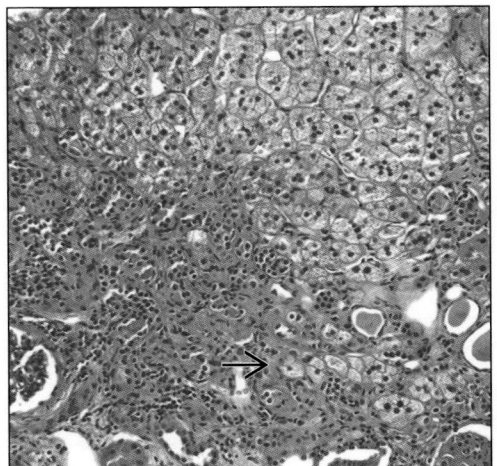

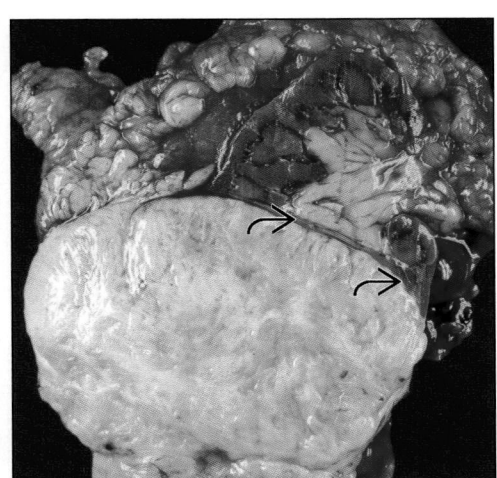

(Left) Ectopic intrarenal adrenal tissues usually show gross circumscription, but on microscopy often depict infiltrative ⟹ growth pattern. Such nodules are mostly noted in superior pole but may be seen elsewhere in kidney. (Right) Leiomyosarcoma (LMS) is the most common sarcoma of the kidney. Most LMS involving the kidney arise in the retroperitoneal soft tissue or renal vein, and due to marked compression ⟹ and distortion of the kidney, are clinically thought to arise from it.

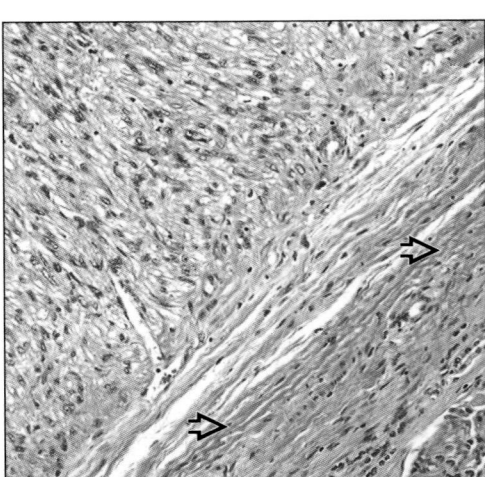

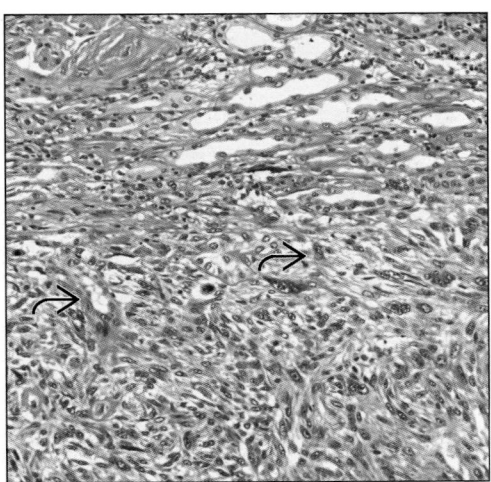

(Left) This H&E image shows a retroperitoneal leiomyosarcoma compressing the kidney, separated from it by a pseudocapsule ⟹. (Right) Rare LMSs do arise in the kidney, and usually show infiltrative borders ⟹. LMS is the most common renal sarcoma, but leiomyomatous angiomyolipoma (AML) is more common. Immunostaining for melanocytic markers in all renal smooth muscle tumors is imperative to exclude AML.

OTHER RARE TUMORS

Gross, Microscopic, and Ancillary Features

(Left) Like leiomyomatous tumors anywhere else, smooth muscle tumors in the kidney, whether representing an angioleiomyoma or a true leiomyoma, show diffuse immunoreactivity for desmin. (Right) This gross image shows an extrarenal angiosarcoma (ANGS) with the typical hemorrhagic cut surface, compressing ⬌ and markedly deforming adjacent renal parenchyma. While primary ANGSs of the kidney do occur, renal involvement by ANGS arising in the retroperitoneum is more common.

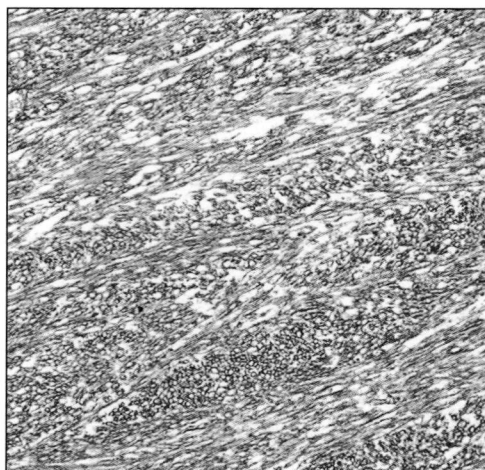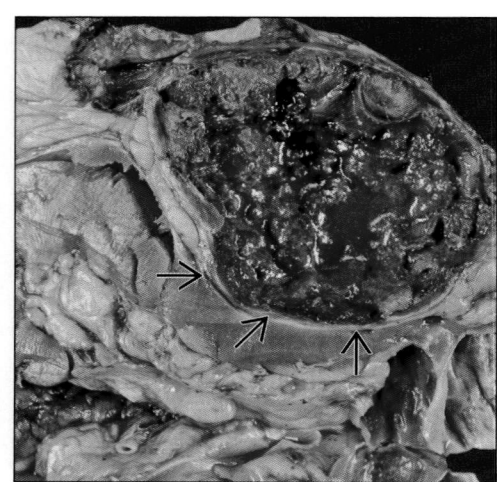

(Left) This primary angiosarcoma of the kidney shows an infiltrative tumor within the renal parenchyma. In this field, the tumor is predominantly composed of nondiagnostic pleomorphic large cells, necessitating immunostaining to confirm the diagnosis. (Right) This light microscopic image from a renal angiosarcoma shows the most characteristic features of the tumor: A vasoformative neoplasm with the vascular spaces lined by high-grade tumor cells.

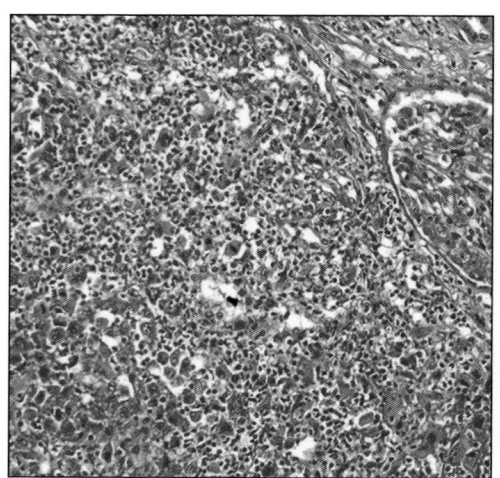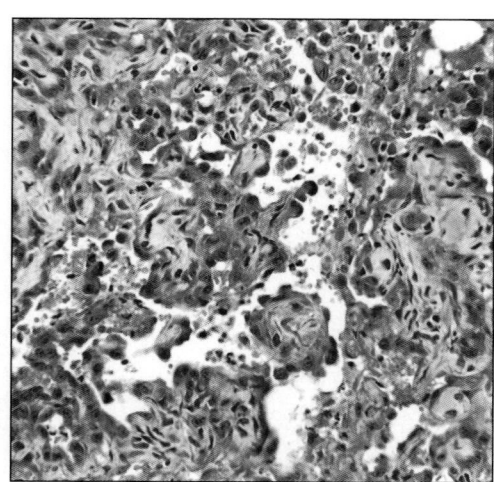

(Left) Immunostaining for CD31 is confirmatory ⬌ in renal angiosarcoma, similar to that in other sites. Immunostains are particularly useful in poorly differentiated tumors. Stains for CD34 and FLI-1 may also help in the diagnosis. (Right) Rare ANGS, particularly those with epithelioid features, may show immunoreactivity for cytokeratins like PAN-CK(AE1/AE3) ⬌. If immunostaining for endothelial markers is not performed, this may lead to misdiagnosis as a carcinoma.

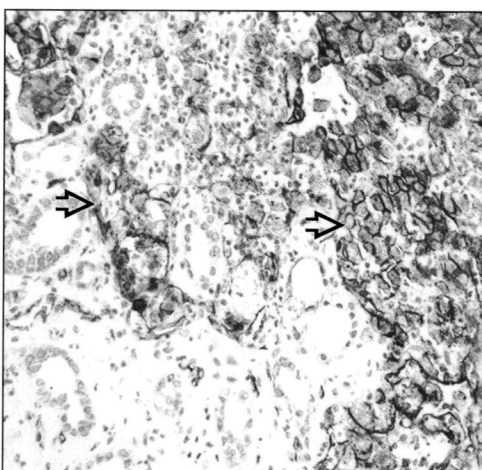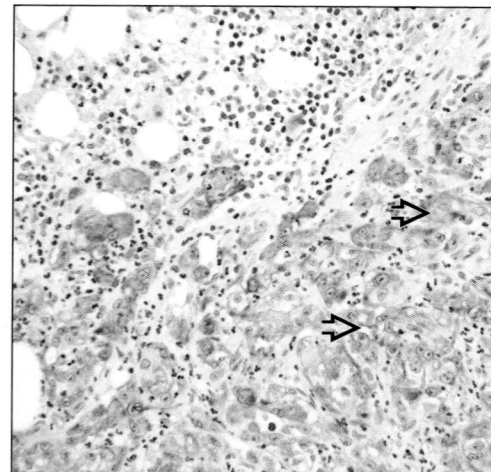

OTHER RARE TUMORS

Microscopic and Ancillary Features

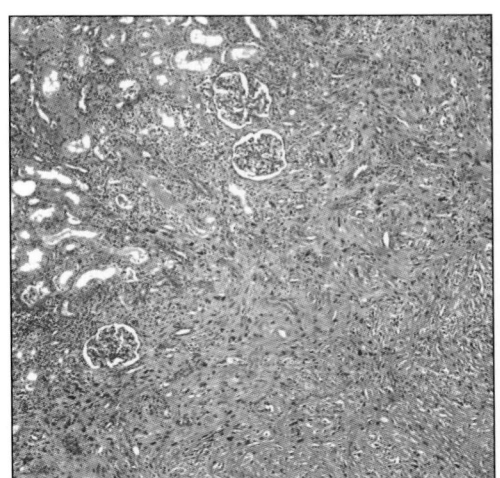
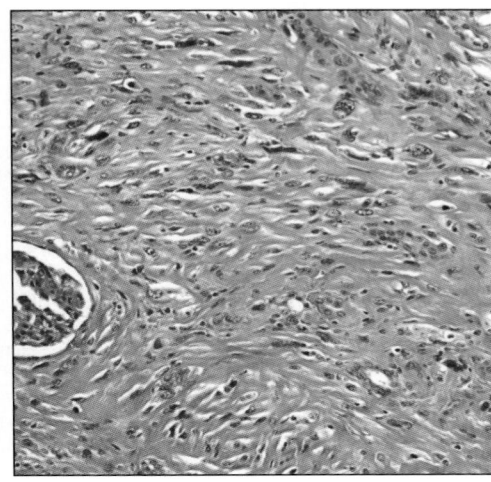

(Left) Adequate sampling and ancillary studies (e.g., immunostaining) are essential for proper classification of malignant spindle cell tumors. Most of these are sarcomatoid carcinomas, although rare cases may represent true sarcoma. *(Right)* This high-grade spindle cell neoplasm invading the kidney was a retroperitoneal liposarcoma with dedifferentiation. The diagnosis was revealed by adequate sampling of perirenal soft tissue that showed its well-differentiated liposarcomatous component.

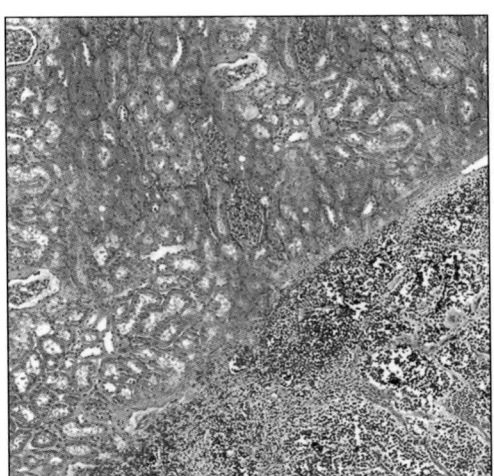
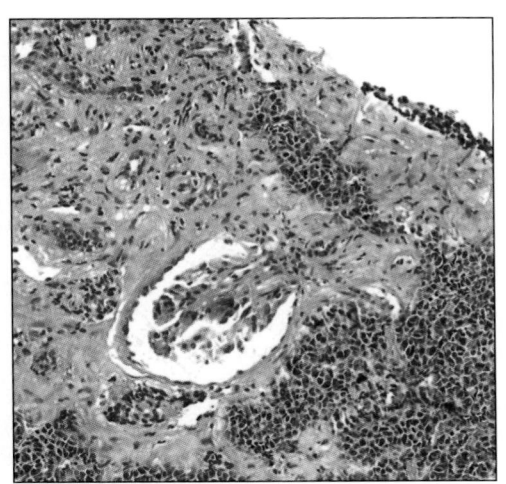

(Left) Small blue round cell tumors in the kidney raise many differential diagnostic possibilities. In children, most of these are Wilms tumor. However, rare primary renal neuroblastomas do exist. This image depicts a primary renal neuroblastoma, undifferentiated type. *(Right)* This tumor represents a small cell carcinoma involving the kidney. Most such tumors are metastases from other sites. However, very occasional primary small cell carcinomas of kidney are described.

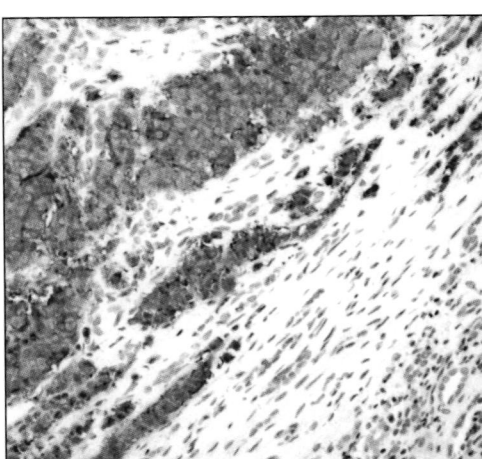
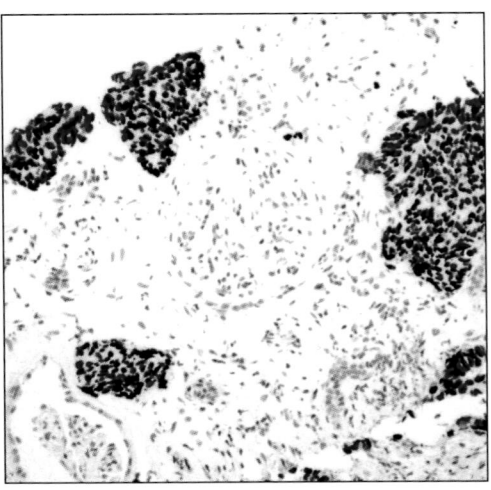

(Left) Most small blue round cell tumors in the kidney need ancillary studies, including immunostaining and molecular analysis, for proper diagnosis. This image depicts a small cell carcinoma showing diffuse immunoreactivity for synaptophysin. *(Right)* Immunostaining for TTF-1 shows diffuse and strong nuclear staining in this small blue round cell tumor of the kidney, supporting the diagnosis of a small cell carcinoma. Stains for CD99, WT1, and muscle markers were negative in this tumor.

METASTATIC TUMORS

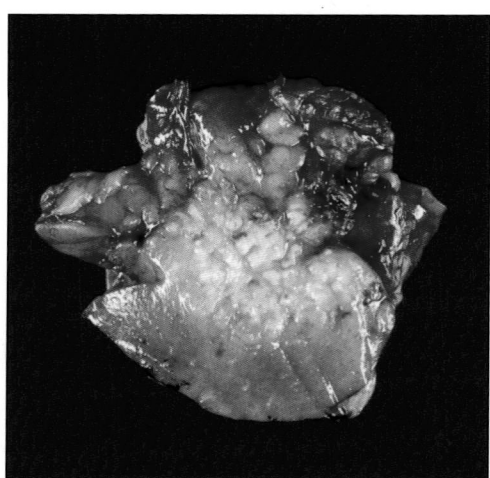

This gross image shows a colonic adenocarcinoma metastatic to the kidney. Most metastatic tumors are multifocal and often bilateral. Solitary metastasis makes such a presumption clinically difficult.

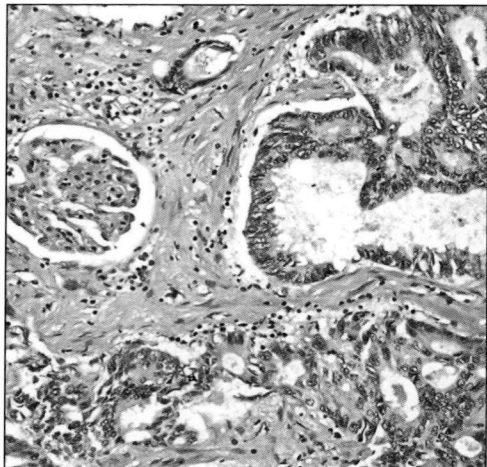

This photomicrograph depicts a metastatic adenocarcinoma from a colorectal primary. In cases with atypical morphologic features for a renal primary, the clinical history is often crucial for proper diagnosis.

TERMINOLOGY

Definitions
- Involvement of kidney by tumors originating in other organs
  - Word "metastasis" is derived from Greek, meaning next placement or displacement
  - Almost always result of vascular or lymphatic spread from primary tumor
    - Direct extension from adjacent organs does not qualify as metastasis
    - Metastasis from contralateral kidney vs. bilateral primary tumors is extremely difficult to prove even when morphologically similar
    - Some hematopoietic malignancies involving kidney may also be considered metastatic but are not discussed here

CLINICAL ISSUES

Epidemiology
- Incidence
  - Reported to constitute up to approximately 3% of all malignant renal tumors in surgical specimens
  - Kidney and ureter most common sites with metastatic tumors in urinary and male genital tract, followed closely by bladder
  - Metastases to kidney are reported to be higher in autopsy series, ranging from 9-20% in patients dying of tumors
- Gender
  - Reported male to female ratio: 2.2:1 in older series
    - Higher incidence in males believed to be due to difference in lung cancer incidences over that time period

Presentation
- Often occurs as part of widespread tumor dissemination

- Renal involvement is frequently bilateral and multinodular in such situations
- In some cases, tumor may be solitary and mimic primary renal tumor
  - Metastatic tumors to kidney presenting in surgical specimens these days are more likely to be mimickers of primary tumor
  - History of extrarenal primary in remote past may be obtained in most such cases on careful scrutiny
- Very rarely, metastasis in kidney may be initial manifestation of primary tumor elsewhere
- Most common reported sources of metastasis to kidney include
  - Lung (most common), colon-rectum, stomach, pancreas, uterus, and skin (malignant melanoma)
  - Other, much rarer sources include breast, salivary gland, and thyroid, among others

MACROSCOPIC FEATURES

General Features
- Metastatic carcinomas are often multifocal and bilateral, particularly at autopsy
  - Concurrent metastatic involvement of other organ systems is very frequent in such a scenario
- Occasionally, tumor may be unicentric, with no other clinically detectable metastatic tumors
  - In such cases, nephrectomy is usually performed with clinical impression of primary renal tumor

MICROSCOPIC PATHOLOGY

Histologic Features
- Based on a large study of 443 cases of tumors metastatic to kidney, and published as an abstract, histologic features are commonly that of
  - Adenocarcinoma (30%), squamous cell carcinoma (28%), small cell carcinoma (8%), and malignant melanoma (6%)

METASTATIC TUMORS

Key Facts

Terminology
- Involvement of kidney by tumors originating in other organs
- Direct extension from adjacent organs does not qualify as metastasis

Clinical Issues
- Reported to constitute up to approximately 3% of all malignant renal tumors in surgical specimens
- Kidney and ureter most common sites with metastatic tumors in urinary and male genital tract, followed closely by bladder
- Often occurs as part of widespread tumor dissemination
- In some cases, tumor may be solitary and mimic primary renal tumor

- Most common reported sources of metastasis to kidney include lung (most common), colon-rectum, stomach, pancreas, uterus, and skin (melanoma)

Microscopic Pathology
- Histologic features in metastatic carcinoma are commonly that of
  - Adenocarcinoma (30%), squamous cell carcinoma (28%), small cell carcinoma (8%), and malignant melanoma (6%)
- Often show multinodular growth pattern, even when apparently well circumscribed on gross evaluation
- Tumor emboli in vessels frequently present

Top Differential Diagnoses
- Collecting duct carcinoma
- Urothelial carcinoma

- Other rare histologic patterns, depending on primary tumor, are also seen and some of these include
  - Salivary gland-type, including adenoid cystic, myoepithelial, and epithelial-myoepithelial carcinoma
  - Thyroid type, including follicular, papillary, undifferentiated, anaplastic, and medullary carcinoma
  - Carcinoid tumor
  - Lobular or signet ring cell type, from breast or gastrointestinal tract
- Often show multinodular growth pattern, even when apparently well circumscribed on gross evaluation
- Tumor emboli in vessels frequently present
- Sometimes tumors centered on pelvicalyceal system and ureter
  - Rarely, tumor cells may replace lining urothelium, giving impression of in situ carcinoma of urothelium
- Occasionally, particularly when metastasis is clinically suspected, needle core biopsies or fine needle aspirations may be performed
  - Morphologic features unusual for renal cell tumor, even on biopsies, should always raise suspicion of metastasis and be investigated for it

DIFFERENTIAL DIAGNOSIS

Collecting Duct Carcinoma
- Stromal desmoplasia, multinodular growth pattern, usual glandular phenotype common to both metastases and collecting duct carcinoma
- Clinical history of primary tumor elsewhere and immunoprofile typical of primary tumor site is often crucial in distinction

Urothelial Carcinoma
- Variety of morphologic phenotypes, and stromal desmoplasia may be similar to that in metastatic carcinoma

- Presence of noninvasive papillary or in situ components supports urothelial carcinoma
- Urothelial carcinomas usually CK7, CK20, HMCK(34βE12), and p63 positive; this immunophenotype is uncommon in other tumors

DIAGNOSTIC CHECKLIST

Pathologic Interpretation Pearls
- Morphologic features unusual for distinctive subtypes of RCC or urothelial carcinoma should always alert one to possibility of metastatic carcinoma
- Clinical history of primary carcinoma elsewhere is often crucial in arriving at definitive diagnosis
- Immunohistochemical profile may also be useful in differential diagnosis

SELECTED REFERENCES

1. Hadley DA et al: A Solitary Seminoma Renal Metastasis Presenting as an Incidental Renal Mass. Urology. Epub ahead of print, 2009
2. Morichetti D et al: Secondary neoplasms of the urinary system and male genital organs. BJU Int. 104(6):770-6, 2009
3. Sterlacci W et al: Primary thyroid-like renal tumor or renal metastasis from the thyroid? Virchows Arch. 455(1):97-8, 2009
4. Bates AW et al: The significance of secondary neoplasms of the urinary and male genital tract. Virchows Arch. 440(6):640-7, 2002
5. Chin-Aleong J et al: Secondary neoplasms of the kidney: a clinico-pathological review of 443 cases. J Pathol. 190[Suppl]:42A, 2000
6. Gattuso P et al: Utilization of fine-needle aspiration in the diagnosis of metastatic tumors to the kidney. Diagn Cytopathol. 21(1):35-8, 1999
7. Wagle DG et al: Secondary carcinomas of the kidney. J Urol. 114(1):30-2, 1975

METASTATIC TUMORS

Gross, Microscopic, and Immunohistochemical Features

(Left) Core biopsy shows an adenocarcinoma that raises the differential of a collecting duct carcinoma. There was a history of lung adenocarcinoma, diagnosed 2 years earlier, that initiated comparison with prior material and rendering of the appropriate diagnosis of metastatic lung carcinoma. *(Right)* Immunohistochemical stain for TTF-1 showed diffuse nuclear positivity ➡ in this tumor. In addition to the comparison with the patient's lung primary, this confirmed a metastasis from the lung.

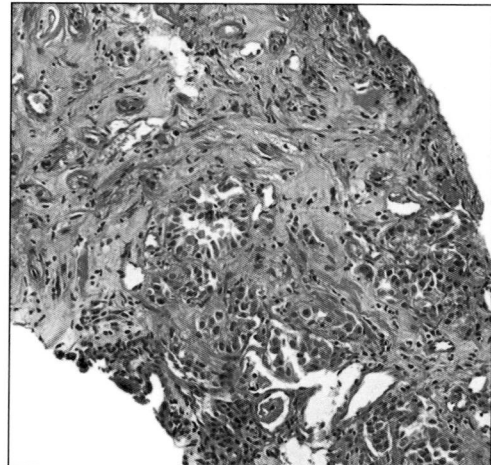
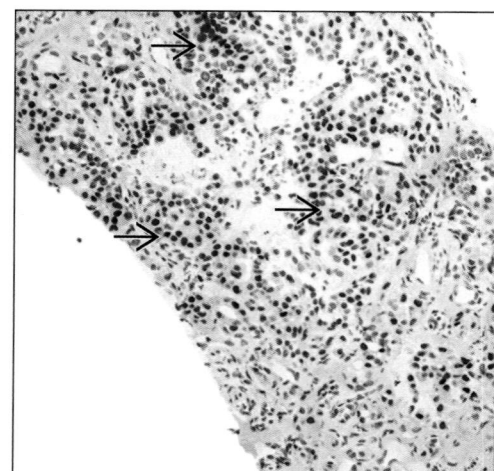

(Left) This image depicts a metastatic squamous cell carcinoma (SCC) from the lung. While a primary urothelial SCC may have similar morphologic features, this patient had bilateral cortical-based tumors with no in situ or papillary urothelial components. *(Right)* This metastatic colorectal adenocarcinoma, centered in the renal pelvis, completely replaces ➡ the surface urothelial lining ➡ in some areas. Such events are rare but raise the possibility of in situ component of a primary tumor.

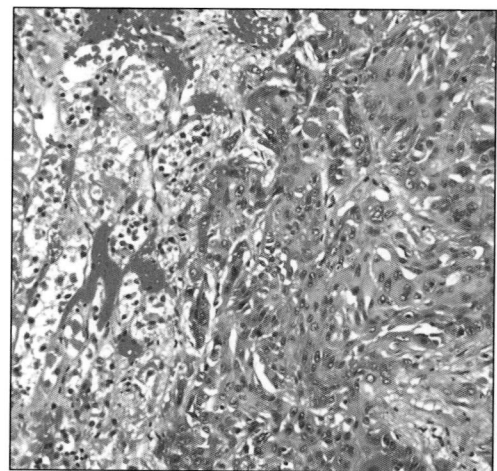
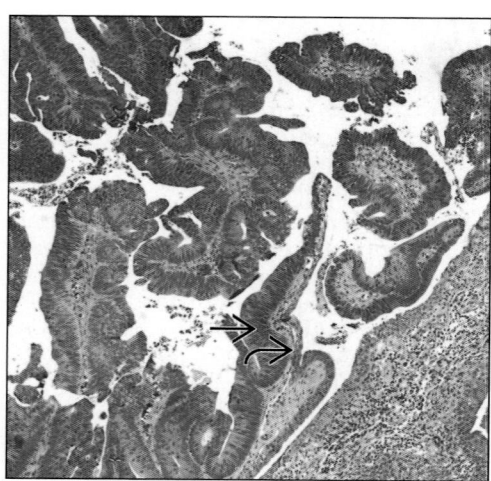

(Left) This solitary tumor in the kidney was resected with the clinical diagnosis of a primary renal tumor. History of a parotid tumor, 15 years earlier, was present. Considering the solitary tumor and very remote history, a new renal primary was clinically favored. *(Right)* Microscopic evaluation revealed a metastatic adenoid cystic carcinoma ➡. Review of the slides obtained from the prior salivary gland resection showed a primary salivary gland adenoid cystic carcinoma.

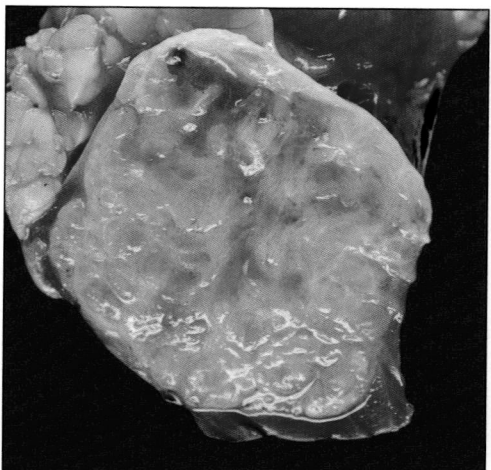
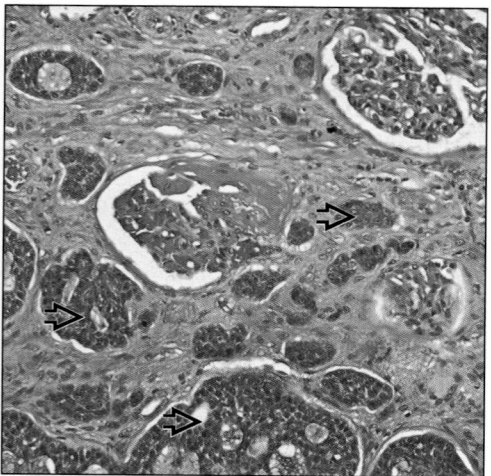

METASTATIC TUMORS

Immunohistochemical Features and Differential Diagnosis

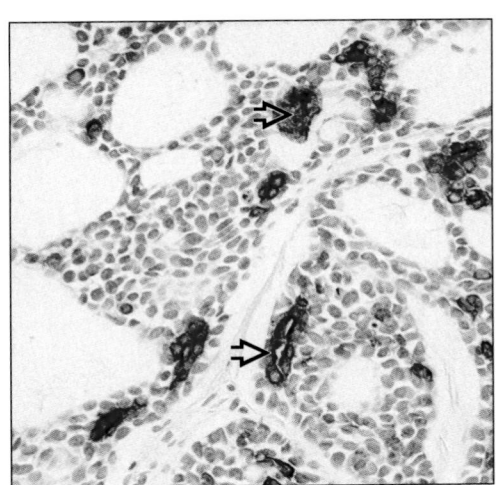

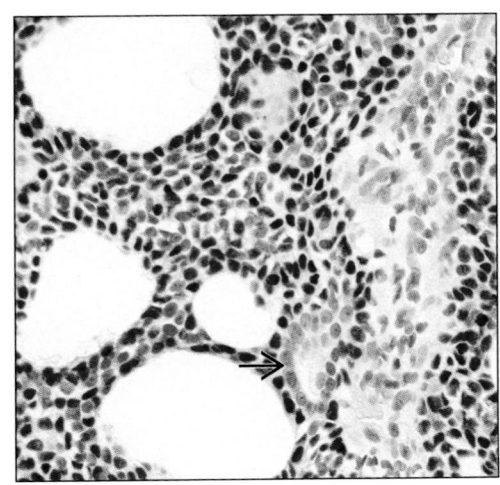

(Left) Immunostain for PAN-CK(AE1/AE3) reveals focal positivity only in the epithelial cells ⊅ of this adenoid cystic carcinoma. (Right) p63 highlights the myoepithelial cells in the tumor, without staining the epithelial component ➡. Unusual morphology in a biopsy or resection specimen requires obtaining clinical history. Metastatic tumors often mimic the morphology of primary renal tumors, leading to misdiagnoses in the absence of available clinical history.

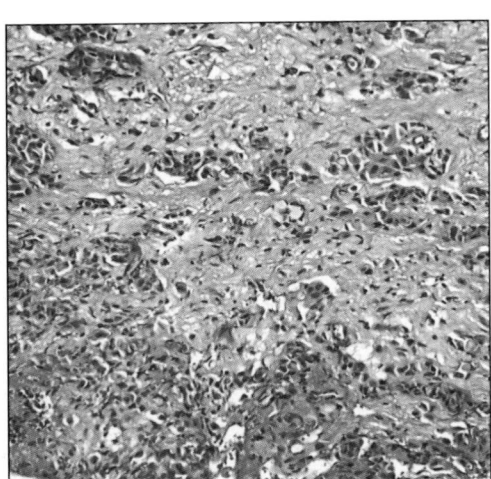

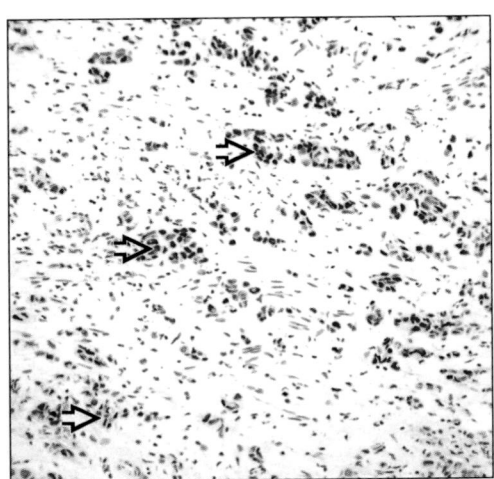

(Left) Needle core biopsy of a renal mass shows a high-grade carcinoma with differential diagnostic possibilities of a urothelial, collecting duct, or metastatic carcinoma. The known history of invasive ductal carcinoma with focal micropapillary features in this case helped in taking the proper approach, including comparison with the prior material from the breast. (Right) Like the breast primary, this renal tumor also was ER positive ⊅ and PR and Her2 negative.

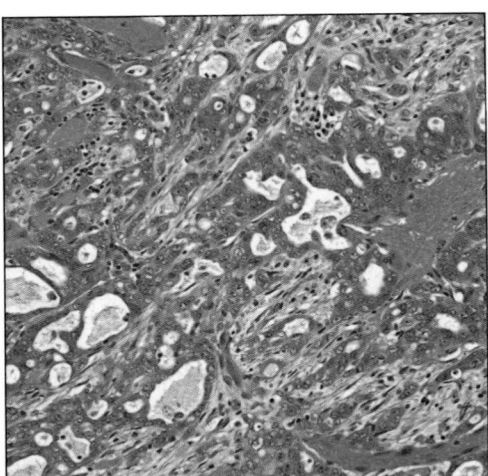

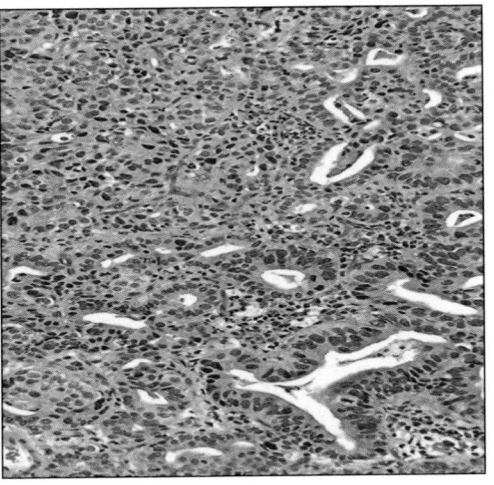

(Left) In the differentiation of adenocarcinomas in the kidney, collecting duct carcinoma is always a consideration. Clinical history and immunostains for HMCK(34βE12), ULEX-1, pax-2, and pax-8 may help in the distinction, but the staining patterns, especially for the 1st 2 antibodies, are not consistent. (Right) Invasive urothelial carcinoma may also mimic metastatic carcinoma. Careful evaluation for urothelial in situ change is a must. Stains for CK7, CK20, HMCK, and p63 may also help.

PROTOCOL FOR RENAL TUBULAR CANCER SPECIMENS

Kidney: Biopsy

Surgical Pathology Cancer Case Summary (Checklist)

*Procedure

*____ Biopsy, needle core

*____ Incisional biopsy, wedge

*____ Other (specify): _____

*____ Not specified

*Specimen Laterality

*____ Right

*____ Left

*____ Not specified

*Histologic Type

*____ Clear cell renal cell carcinoma

*____ Multilocular cystic renal cell carcinoma

*____ Papillary renal cell carcinoma

*____ Chromophobe renal cell carcinoma

*____ Carcinoma of the collecting ducts of Bellini

*____ Renal medullary carcinoma

*____ MiTF/TFE family translocation-associated renal cell carcinoma

*____ Carcinoma associated with neuroblastoma

*____ Mucinous tubular and spindle cell carcinoma

*____ Tubulocystic renal cell carcinoma

*____ Renal cell carcinoma, unclassified

*____ Clear cell papillary renal cell carcinoma

*____ Acquired cystic disease-assoicated renal cell carcinoma

*____ Other (specify): _____

*Sarcomatoid Features

*____ Not identified

*____ Present

*Specify percent sarcomatoid element: _____ %

*Histologic Grade (Fuhrman Nuclear Grade)

*____ Not applicable

*____ GX: Cannot be assessed

*____ G1: Nuclei round, uniform, approximately 10 µm; nucleoli inconspicuous or absent

*____ G2: Nuclei slightly irregular, approximately 15 µm; nucleoli evident

*____ G3: Nuclei very irregular, approximately 20 µm; nuclei large and prominent

*____ G4: Nuclei bizarre and multilobulated, 20 µm or greater; nucleoli prominent; chromatin clumped

*Additional Pathologic Findings

*____ None identified

*____ Other pathology present (specify): _____

*Data elements with asterisks are not required. However, these elements may be clinically important but are not yet validated or regularly used in patient management. Adapted with permission from College of American Pathologists, "Protocol for the Examination of Specimens from Patients with Invasive Carcinoma of Renal Tubular Origin." Web posting date October 2009, www.cap.org.

Kidney: Nephrectomy, Partial or Radical

Surgical Pathology Cancer Case Summary (Checklist)

Procedure

____ Partial nephrectomy

____ Radical nephrectomy

____ Other (specify): _____

____ Not specified

PROTOCOL FOR RENAL TUBULAR CANCER SPECIMENS

Specimen Laterality

____ Right

____ Left

____ Not specified

*Tumor Site (select all that apply)

*____ Upper pole

*____ Middle

*____ Lower pole

*____ Other (specify): _____

*____ Not specified

Tumor Size (largest tumor if multiple)

Greatest dimension: _____ cm

*Additional dimensions: _____ x _____ cm

____ Cannot be determined (see "Comment")

Tumor Focality

____ Unifocal

____ Multifocal

Macroscopic Extent of Tumor (select all that apply)

____ Tumor limited to kidney

____ Tumor extension into perinephric tissues/renal sinus

____ Tumor extension beyond Gerota fascia

____ Tumor extension into major veins (renal vein or its segmental [muscle-containing] branches, inferior vena cava)

____ Tumor extension into pelvicalyceal system

____ Tumor extension into adrenal gland

    ____ Direct invasion (T4)

    ____ Noncontiguous (M1)

____ Tumor extension into other organ(s)/structure(s) (specify): _____

Histologic Type

____ Clear cell renal cell carcinoma

____ Multilocular cystic renal cell carcinoma

____ Papillary renal cell carcinoma

____ Chromophobe renal cell carcinoma

____ Carcinoma of collecting ducts of Bellini

____ Renal medullary carcinoma

____ MiTF/TFE family translocation-associated renal cell carcinoma

____ Carcinoma associated with neuroblastoma

____ Mucinous tubular and spindle cell carcinoma

____ Tubulocystic renal cell carcinoma

____ Renal cell carcinoma, unclassified

____ Clear cell papillary renal cell carcinoma

____ Acquired cystic disease-associated renal cell carcinoma

____ Other (specify): _____

Sarcomatoid Features

____ Not identified

____ Present

    Specify percentage of sarcomatoid element: ____ %

*Tumor Necrosis (any amount)

*____ Not identified

*____ Present

Histologic Grade (Fuhrman Nuclear Grade)

____ Not applicable

PROTOCOL FOR RENAL TUBULAR CANCER SPECIMENS

____ GX: Cannot be assessed

____ G1: Nuclei round, uniform, approximately 10 μm; nucleoli inconspicuous or absent

____ G2: Nuclei slightly irregular, approximately 15 μm; nucleoli evident

____ G3: Nuclei very irregular, approximately 20 μm; nucleoli large and prominent

____ G4: Nuclei bizarre and multilobulated; 20 μm or greater; nucleoli prominent; chromatin clumped

____ Other (specify): _____

Microscopic Tumor Extension (select all that apply)

____ Tumor limited to kidney

____ Tumor extension into perinephric tissue (beyond renal capsule)

____ Tumor extension into renal sinus

____ Tumor extension beyond Gerota fascia

____ Tumor extension into major vein (renal vein or its segmental [muscle-containing] branches, inferior vena cava)

____ Tumor extension into pelvicalyceal system

____ Tumor extension into adrenal gland

    ____ Direct invasion (T4)

    ____ Noncontiguous (M1)

____ Tumor extension into other organ(s)/structure(s) (specify): _____

Margins (select all that apply)

____ Cannot be assessed

____ Margins uninvolved by invasive carcinoma

____ Margin(s) involved by invasive carcinoma

    ____ Renal parenchymal margin (partial nephrectomy only)

    ____ Renal capsular margin (partial nephrectomy only)

    ____ Perinephric fat margin (partial nephrectomy only)

    ____ Gerota fascial margin

    ____ Renal vein margin

    ____ Ureteral margin

    ____ Other (specify): _____

*Lymph-Vascular Invasion (excluding renal vein and its muscle containing segmental branches and inferior vena cava)

*____ Not identified

*____ Present

*____ Indeterminate

Pathologic Staging (pTNM)

TNM descriptors (required only if applicable) (select all that apply)

____ m (multiple primary tumors)

____ r (recurrent)

____ y (posttreatment)

Primary tumor (pT)

____ pTX: Primary tumor cannot be assessed

____ pT0: No evidence of primary tumor

____ pT1: Tumor ≤7 cm in greatest dimension, limited to the kidney

    ____ pT1a: Tumor ≤4 cm in greatest dimension, limited to the kidney

    ____ PT1b: Tumor > 4 cm but ≤7 cm in greatest dimension, limited to the kidney

____ pT2: Tumor > 7 cm in greatest dimension, limited to the kidney

    ____ pT2a: Tumor > 7 cm but ≤ to 10 cm in greatest dimension, limited to the kidney

____ pT3: Tumor grossly extends into major veins or perinephric tissues but not into the ipsilateral adrenal gland and not beyond Gerota fascia

    ____ pT3a: Tumor grossly extends into the renal vein or its segmental (muscle-containing) branches, or tumor invades perirenal &/or renal sinus fat but not beyond Gerota fascia

    ____ PT3b: Tumor grossly extends into the vena cava below the diaphragm

    ____ PT3c: Tumor grossly extends into vena cava above diaphragm or invades the wall of the vena cava

____ pT4: Tumor invades beyond Gerota fascia (including contiguous extension into the ipsilateral adrenal gland)

Regional lymph nodes (pN)

PROTOCOL FOR RENAL TUBULAR CANCER SPECIMENS

____ pNX: Regional lymph nodes cannot be assessed

____ pN0: No regional lymph node metastasis

____ pN1: Metastasis in regional lymph node(s)

Specify: Number examined: _____

Number positive: _____

Distant metastasis (pM)

____ Not applicable

____ pM1: Distant metastasis

Pathologic Findings in Nonneoplastic Kidney (select all that apply)

____ Insufficient tissue (partial nephrectomy specimen with < 5 mm of adjacent nonneoplastic kidney)

____ Significant pathologic alterations

____ None identified

____ Glomerular disease (specify type): _____

____ Tubulointerstitial disease (specify type): _____

____ Vascular disease (specify type): _____

____ Other (specify): _____

*Other Tumors &/or Tumor-like Lesions (select all that apply)

*____ Cyst(s) (specify type): _____

*____ Tubular (papillary) adenoma(s)

*____ Other (specify): _____

*Data elements with asterisks are not required. However, these elements may be clinically important but are not yet validated or regularly used in patient management.

Stage Groupings

Stage	Tumor	Node	Metastasis
I	T1	N0	M0†
II	T2	N0	M0
III	T1 or T2	N1	M0
	T3	N0 or N1	M0
IV	T4	Any N	M0
	Any T	Any N	M1

†M0 is defined as no distant metastasis. Used with the permission of the American Joint Committee on Cancer (AJCC), Chicago, Illinois. The original source for this material is the AJCC Cancer Staging Manual, Seventh Edition (2010) published by Springer Science and Business Media LLC, www.springerlink.com.

PROTOCOL FOR URETER AND RENAL PELVIS CANCER SPECIMENS

Ureter, Renal Pelvis: Biopsy

Surgical Pathology Cancer Case Summary (Checklist)

*Specimen

*____ Renal pelvis

*____ Ureter

*____ Other (specify): _____

*____ Not specified

*Specimen Laterality

*____ Left

*____ Right

*____ Not specified

*Histologic Type

*____ Urothelial (transitional cell) carcinoma

*____ Urothelial (transitional cell) carcinoma with squamous differentiation

*____ Urothelial (transitional cell) carcinoma with glandular differentiation

*____ Urothelial (transitional cell) carcinoma with other variant histology (specify): _____

*____ Squamous cell carcinoma, typical

*____ Squamous cell carcinoma, variant histology (specify): _____

*____ Adenocarcinoma, typical

*____ Adenocarcinoma, variant histology (specify): _____

*____ Small cell carcinoma

*____ Undifferentiated carcinoma (specify): _____

*____ Mixed cell type (specify): _____

*____ Other (specify): _____

*____ Carcinoma, type cannot be determined

*Associated Epithelial Lesions (select all that apply)

*____ None identified

*____ Urothelial (transitional cell) papilloma (World Health Organization [WHO]/International Society of Urologic Pathology [ISUP], 1998; WHO 2004)

*____ Urothelial (transitional cell) papilloma, inverted type

*____ Papillary urothelial (transitional cell) neoplasm, low malignant potential (WHO/ISUP 1998; WHO 2004)

*____ Cannot be determined

*Histologic Grade

*____ Not applicable

*____ Cannot be determined

*Urothelial carcinoma (WHO/ISUP 1998; WHO 2004)

*____ Low grade

*____ High grade

*____ Other (specify): _____

*Adenocarcinoma and squamous cell carcinoma

*____ GX: Cannot be assessed

*____ G1: Well differentiated

*____ G2: Moderately differentiated

*____ G3: Poorly differentiated

*____ Other (specify): _____

*Tumor Configuration (select all that apply)

*____ Papillary

*____ Solid/nodule

*____ Flat

*____ Ulcerated

*____ Indeterminate

*____ Other (specify): _____

1

PROTOCOL FOR RENAL TUBULAR CANCER SPECIMENS

____ pNX: Regional lymph nodes cannot be assessed

____ pN0: No regional lymph node metastasis

____ pN1: Metastasis in regional lymph node(s)

Specify: Number examined: _____

Number positive: _____

Distant metastasis (pM)

____ Not applicable

____ pM1: Distant metastasis

Pathologic Findings in Nonneoplastic Kidney (select all that apply)

____ Insufficient tissue (partial nephrectomy specimen with < 5 mm of adjacent nonneoplastic kidney)

____ Significant pathologic alterations

___ None identified

____ Glomerular disease (specify type): _____

____ Tubulointerstitial disease (specify type): _____

____ Vascular disease (specify type): _____

____ Other (specify): _____

*Other Tumors &/or Tumor-like Lesions (select all that apply)

*____ Cyst(s) (specify type): _____

*____ Tubular (papillary) adenoma(s)

*____ Other (specify): _____

*Data elements with asterisks are not required. However, these elements may be clinically important but are not yet validated or regularly used in patient management.

Stage Groupings

Stage	Tumor	Node	Metastasis
I	T1	N0	M0†
II	T2	N0	M0
III	T1 or T2	N1	M0
	T3	N0 or N1	M0
IV	T4	Any N	M0
	Any T	Any N	M1

†M0 is defined as no distant metastasis. Used with the permission of the American Joint Committee on Cancer (AJCC), Chicago, Illinois. The original source for this material is the AJCC Cancer Staging Manual, Seventh Edition (2010) published by Springer Science and Business Media LLC, www.springerlink.com.

Ureter, Renal Pelvis: Biopsy

Surgical Pathology Cancer Case Summary (Checklist)

*Specimen

* ____ Renal pelvis

* ____ Ureter

* ____ Other (specify): _____

* ____ Not specified

*Specimen Laterality

* ____ Left

* ____ Right

* ____ Not specified

*Histologic Type

* ____ Urothelial (transitional cell) carcinoma

* ____ Urothelial (transitional cell) carcinoma with squamous differentiation

* ____ Urothelial (transitional cell) carcinoma with glandular differentiation

* ____ Urothelial (transitional cell) carcinoma with other variant histology (specify): _____

* ____ Squamous cell carcinoma, typical

* ____ Squamous cell carcinoma, variant histology (specify): _____

* ____ Adenocarcinoma, typical

* ____ Adenocarcinoma, variant histology (specify): _____

* ____ Small cell carcinoma

* ____ Undifferentiated carcinoma (specify): _____

* ____ Mixed cell type (specify): _____

* ____ Other (specify): _____

* ____ Carcinoma, type cannot be determined

*Associated Epithelial Lesions (select all that apply)

* ____ None identified

* ____ Urothelial (transitional cell) papilloma (World Health Organization [WHO]/International Society of Urologic Pathology [ISUP], 1998; WHO 2004)

* ____ Urothelial (transitional cell) papilloma, inverted type

* ____ Papillary urothelial (transitional cell) neoplasm, low malignant potential (WHO/ISUP 1998; WHO 2004)

* ____ Cannot be determined

*Histologic Grade

* ____ Not applicable

* ____ Cannot be determined

*Urothelial carcinoma (WHO/ISUP 1998; WHO 2004)

* ____ Low grade

* ____ High grade

* ____ Other (specify): _____

*Adenocarcinoma and squamous cell carcinoma

* ____ GX: Cannot be assessed

* ____ G1: Well differentiated

* ____ G2: Moderately differentiated

* ____ G3: Poorly differentiated

* ____ Other (specify): _____

*Tumor Configuration (select all that apply)

* ____ Papillary

* ____ Solid/nodule

* ____ Flat

* ____ Ulcerated

* ____ Indeterminate

* ____ Other (specify): _____

PROTOCOL FOR URETER AND RENAL PELVIS CANCER SPECIMENS

*Adequacy of Material for Determining T Category

*____ Muscularis propria not identified

*____ Muscularis propria present

*____ Indeterminate

Pathologic Staging (pTNM)

*TNM descriptors (select all that apply)

*____ None

*____ m (multiple primary tumors)

*____ r (recurrent)

*____ y (post-treatment)

*Primary tumor (pT)

*____ pTX: Cannot be assessed

*____ PT0: No evidence of primary tumor

*____ pTa: Noninvasive papillary carcinoma

*____ pTis: Flat carcinoma in situ

*____ pT1: Tumor invades subepithelial connective tissue (lamina propria)

*____ pT2: Tumor invades muscularis propria

*Additional Pathologic Findings (select all that apply)

*____ Urothelial carcinoma in situ

*____ Urothelial dysplasia (low-grade intraurothelial neoplasia)

*____ Inflammation/regenerative changes

*____ Therapy-related changes

*____ Cautery artifact

*____ Ureteritis or pyelitis cystica &/or glandularis

*____ Keratinizing squamous metaplasia

*____ Intestinal metaplasia

*____ Other (specify): _____

*Data elements with asterisks are not required. However, these elements may be clinically important but are not yet validated or regularly used in patient management. Adapted with permission from College of American Pathologists, "Protocol for the Examination of Specimens from Patients with Carcinoma of the Ureter and Renal Pelvis." Web posting date October 2009, www.cap.org.

Renal Pelvis: Resection/Nephroureterectomy, Partial or Complete

Surgical Pathology Cancer Case Summary (Checklist)

Procedure

____ Nephroureterectomy, partial

____ Nephroureterectomy, complete

____ Other (specify): _____

____ Not specified

Specimen Laterality

____ Right

____ Left

____ Not specified

Tumor Size

Greatest dimension: _____ cm

*Additional dimensions: _____ x _____ cm

____ Cannot be determined

Histologic Type

____ Urothelial (transitional cell) carcinoma

____ Urothelial (transitional cell) carcinoma with squamous differentiation

____ Urothelial (transitional cell) carcinoma with glandular differentiation

____ Urothelial (transitional cell) carcinoma with other variant histology (specify): _____

____ Squamous cell carcinoma, typical

____ Squamous cell carcinoma, variant histology (specify): _____

PROTOCOL FOR URETER AND RENAL PELVIS CANCER SPECIMENS

____ Adenocarcinoma, typical

____ Adenocarcinoma, variant histology (specify): _____

____ Small cell carcinoma

____ Undifferentiated carcinoma (specify): _____

____ Mixed cell type (specify): _____

____ Other (specify): _____

____ Carcinoma, type cannot be determined

Associated Epithelial Lesions (select all that apply)

____ None identified

____ Urothelial (transitional cell) papilloma (World Health Organization [WHO]/International Society of Urologic Pathology [ISUP], 1998; WHO 2004

____ Urothelial (transitional cell) papilloma, inverted type

____ Papillary urothelial (transitional cell) neoplasm, low malignant potential (WHO/ISUP 1998; WHO 2004)

____ Cannot be determined

Histologic Grade

____ Not applicable

____ Cannot be determined

Urothelial carcinoma (WHO/ISUP 1998; WHO 2004)

____ Low grade

____ High grade

____ Other (specify): _____

Adenocarcinoma and squamous cell carcinoma

____ GX: Cannot be assessed

____ G1: Well differentiated

____ G2: Moderately differentiated

____ G3: Poorly differentiated

____ Other (specify): _____

*Tumor Configuration (select all that apply)

*____ Papillary

*____ Solid/nodule

*____ Flat

*____ Ulcerated

*____ Indeterminate

*____ Other (specify): _____

Margins (select all that apply)

____ Cannot be assessed

____ Margins uninvolved by invasive carcinoma

    *Distance of invasive carcinoma from closest margin: _____ mm

    *Specify margin: _____

____ Margin(s) uninvolved by carcinoma in situ

____ Margin(s) involved by carcinoma in situ

    Specify margin(s): _____

    ____ Other(s) (specify): _____

*Lymph-Vascular Invasion

*____ Not identified

*____ Present

*____ Indeterminate

Pathologic Staging (pTNM)

TNM descriptors (required only if applicable) (select all that apply)

____ m (multiple)

____ r (recurrent)

____ y (post-treatment)

Primary tumor (pT)

PROTOCOL FOR URETER AND RENAL PELVIS CANCER SPECIMENS

____ pTX: Cannot be assessed

____ pT0: No evidence of primary tumor

____ pTa: Papillary noninvasive carcinoma

____ pTis: Flat carcinoma in situ

____ pT1: Tumor invades subepithelial connective tissue (lamina propria)

____ pT2: Tumor invades muscularis propria

____ pT3: Tumor invades beyond muscularis into peripelvic fat or the renal parenchyma

____ pT4: Tumor invades adjacent organs, or through the kidney into the perinephric fat

Regional lymph nodes (pN)

____ pNX: Cannot be assessed

____ pN0: No regional lymph node metastasis

____ pN1: Metastasis in a single regional lymph node, ≤2 cm in greatest dimension

____ PN2: Metastasis in a single regional lymph node, > 2 cm but not > 5 cm in greatest dimension, or multiple lymph nodes, none > 5 cm in greatest dimension

____ PN3: Metastasis in a regional lymph node > 5 cm in greatest dimension

Specify: Number examined: _____

Number involved (any size): _____

Distant metastasis (pM)

____ Not applicable

____ pM1: Distant metastasis

*Specify site(s), if known: _____

*Additional Pathologic Findings (select all that apply)

*____ Urothelial carcinoma in situ

*____ Urothelial dysplasia (low-grade intraurothelial neoplasia)

*____ Inflammation/regenerative changes

*____ Therapy-related changes

*____ Pyelitis cystica &/or glandularis

*____ Keratinizing squamous metaplasia

*____ Intestinal metaplasia

*____ Lithiasis

*____ Other (specify): _____

*Data elements with asterisks are not required. However, these elements may be clinically important but are not yet validated or regularly used in patient management.

Ureter: Resection

Surgical Pathology Cancer Case Summary (Checklist)

Procedure

____ Ureterectomy

____ Nephroureterectomy

____ Other (specify): _____

____ Not specified

Specimen Laterality

____ Right

____ Left

____ Not specified

Tumor Size

Greatest dimension: _____

*Additional dimensions: _____ x _____

____ Cannot be determined

Histologic Type

____ Urothelial (transitional cell) carcinoma

____ Urothelial (transitional cell) carcinoma with squamous differentiation

____ Urothelial (transitional cell) carcinoma with glandular differentiation

____ Urothelial (transitional cell) carcinoma with other variant histology (specify): _____

PROTOCOL FOR URETER AND RENAL PELVIS CANCER SPECIMENS

____ Squamous cell carcinoma, typical

____ Squamous cell carcinoma, variant histology (specify): _____

____ Adenocarcinoma, typical

____ Adenocarcinoma, variant histology (specify): _____

____ Small cell carcinoma

____ Undifferentiated carcinoma (specify): _____

____ Mixed cell type (specify): _____

____ Other (specify): _____

____ Carcinoma, type cannot be determined

Associated Epithelial Lesions (select all that apply)

____ None identified

____ Urothelial (transitional cell) papilloma (World Health Organization [WHO]/International Society of Urologic Pathology [ISUP] 1998; WHO 2004)

____ Urothelial (transitional cell) papilloma, inverted type

____ Papillary urothelial (transitional cell) neoplasm, low malignant potential (WHO/ISUP 1998; WHO 2004)

____ Cannot be determined

Histologic Grade

____ Not applicable

____ Cannot be determined

Urothelial Carcinoma (WHO/ISUP 1998; WHO 2004)

____ Low grade

____ High grade

____ Other (specify): _____

Adenocarcinoma and squamous cell carcinoma

____ GX: Cannot be assessed

____ G1: Well differentiated

____ G2: Moderately differentiated

____ G3: Poorly differentiated

____ Other (specify): _____

*Tumor Configuration (select all that apply)

*____ Papillary

*____ Solid/nodule

*____ Ulcerated

*____ Flat

*____ Indeterminate

*____ Other (specify): _____

Margins (select all that apply)

____ Cannot be assessed

____ Margins uninvolved by invasive carcinoma

   *Distance of invasive carcinoma from closest margin: _____ mm

   *Specify margin(s): _____

____ Margin(s) involved by invasive carcinoma

   Specify margin(s): _____

____ Margin(s) involved by carcinoma in situ

____ Margin(s) uninvolved by carcinoma in situ

____ Other(s) (specify): _____

*Lymph-Vascular Invasion

*____ Not identified

*____ Present

*____ Indeterminate

Pathologic Staging (pTNM)

TNM descriptors (required only if applicable) (select all that apply)

____ m (multiple)

PROTOCOL FOR URETER AND RENAL PELVIS CANCER SPECIMENS

____ r (recurrent)

____ y (post-treatment)

Primary tumor (pT)

____ pTX: Cannot be assessed

____ pT0: No evidence of primary tumor

____ pTa: Papillary noninvasive carcinoma

____ pTis: Carcinoma in situ

____ pT1: Tumor invades subepithelial connective tissue (lamina propria)

____ pT2: Tumor invades the muscularis propria

____ PT3: Tumor invades beyond muscularis propria into periureteric fat

____ pT4: Tumor invades adjacent organs

Regional lymph nodes (pN)

____ pNX: Cannot be assessed

____ pN0: No regional lymph node metastasis

____ pN1: Metastasis in a single regional lymph node, ≤ 2 cm in greatest dimension

____ PN2: Metastasis in a single regional lymph node, > 2 cm but not > 5 cm in greatest dimension, or multiple lymph nodes, none > 5 cm in greatest dimension

____ pN3: Metastasis in a regional lymph node > 5 cm in greatest dimension

    Specify: Number examined: _____

    Number involved (any size): _____

Distant metastasis (pM)

____ Not applicable

____ pM1: Distant metastasis

    *Specify site(s), if known: _____

*Additional Pathologic Findings (select all that apply)

*____ Urothelial carcinoma in situ

*____ Urothelial dysplasia (low-grade intraurothelial neoplasia)

*____ Inflammation/regenerative changes

*____ Therapy-related changes

*____ Ureteritis cystica &/or glandularis

*____ Keratinizing squamous metaplasia

*____ Intestinal metaplasia

*____ Other (specify): _____

Pathologic Findings in Nonneoplastic Kidney (select all that apply)

____ Insufficient tissue (partial nephrectomy specimen with < 5 mm of adjacent nonneoplastic kidney)

____ Significant pathologic alterations

____ None identified

____ Glomerular disease (type): _____

____ Tubulointerstitial disease (type): _____

____ Vascular disease (type): _____

____ Inflammation (type): _____

____ Other (specify): _____

*Data elements with asterisks are not required. However, these elements may be clinically important but are not yet validated or regularly used in patient management.

Anatomic Stage/Prognostic Groups

Stage	Tumor	Node	Metastasis
0a	Ta	N0	M0
0is	Tis	N0	M0
I	T1	N0	M0
II	T2	N0	M0
III	T3	N0	M0
IV	T4	N0	M0
	Any T	N1, N2, N3	M0
	Any T	Any N	M1

IMMUNOHISTOCHEMISTRY, KIDNEY

Renal Tumors with Clear/Light-Staining Cytoplasm

Antibody	Clear Cell RCC	Chromophobe RCC	MITF/TFE Family Translocation-associated Carcinoma	Clear Cell Papillary RCC	Epithelioid Angiomyolipoma
CK7	-	+ (diffuse, occasionally patchy)	-	+ (diffuse, almost 100% tumor cells)	-
CD10	+ (membranous)	-/(rarely +)	+ (but often - in TFEB carcinoma)	-	-
Vimentin	+	- (rarely +)	-/+	+	-
Ksp-cadherin	-	+	-	ND	-
CD117	-	+ (diffuse, often peripheral membranous accentuation)	-	ND	-
AMACR	- (rarely focal +)	-	+ (usually)	-	-
EMA/MUC1	+	+	- (rarely focal +)	+	-
PAN-CK(AE1/AE3)	+	+	- (rarely focal +)	+	-
CAIX	+ (diffuse membranous)	- (+ perinecrotic areas)	- (+ in some cases)	+ (diffuse membranous)	-
TFE3/TFEB	-	-	+	-	-
Parvalbumin	-	+	-	-	-
Melan-A(MART-1)	-	-	+ in TFEB carcinoma, rarely + in TFE3	-	+
HMB-45	-	-	+ in TFEB carcinoma, rarely + in TFE3	-	+
MiTF	-	-	+ in TFEB carcinoma, rarely + in TFE3	-	+
Actin-sm	-	-	-	-	+/-

Renal Tumors with Papillary or Tubulopapillary Architecture

Antibody	Papillary RCC	Collecting Duct Carcinoma	Metanephric Adenoma	Mucinous Tubular and Spindle Cell Carcinoma	Clear Cell Papillary RCC
CK7	+	+	- (may be + in branching tubules or papillary structures)	+	+
CD10	+ (often luminal pattern)	-	-	-/+ (focal)	-
RCC	+	-	-	V	-/+
AMACR	+	-	-/+	+	-
EMA/MUC1	+	+	- (may be + in branching tubules or papillary structures)	+	+
WT1	-	-	+	-	-
HMCK(34βE12)	-	+/-	-	-/+	+
CD57	-	ND	+	-	ND
INI1	+	+ (lost in renal medullary carcinoma)	+	+	+
Ulex-1	-	+	-	-	ND
CAIX	- (+ perinecrotic areas and papillary tips)	-/+(perinecrotic area)	ND	ND	+

(V = Variable, ND = No Data)

Kidney Tumors and Tumor-like Conditions

1

242

IMMUNOHISTOCHEMISTRY, KIDNEY

Renal Tumors with Granular/Eosinophilic Cytoplasm

Antibody	Clear Cell RCC, Eosinophilic	Chromophobe RCC, Eosinophilic	Oncocytoma	MiTF/TFE Family Translocation-associated Carcinoma	Epithelioid Angiomyolipoma
Vimentin	+/-	- (rarely +)	-	-/+	+
CD117	-	+	+	-	-
Pax-2	+	- (rarely +)	+	V	-
RCC	+	-/+	-/+	+	-
CK7	-	+/-	-	-	-
CD10	+	-/+	+	+ in TFE3 carcinoma, often (-) in TFEB	-
Ksp-cadherin	-	+	+	V	-
Parvalbumin	-	+	+	ND	-
EpCAM/BER-EP4	V	+	- (occasionally focal or patchy +)	V	--
TFE3/TFEB	-	-	-	+	-
Melan-A(MART-1)	-	-	-	+ in TFEB carcinoma, rarely + in TFE3	+
HMB-45	-	-	-	+ in TFEB carcinoma, rarely + in TFE3	+
MiTF	-	-	-	+ in TFEB carcinoma, rarely + in TFE3	+
Actin-sm	-	-	-	-	+/-
HMCK(34βE12)	-	- (rarely focal +)	-	- (occasionally focal +)	-
EMA/MUC1	+	+ (occasionally only focal +)	+ (occasionally only focal +)	- (occasionally focal +)	-
CAIX	+	-	-	- (+ in some cases)	-

Tumors with Spindle Cell Morphology

Antibody	Spindle Cells in Sarcomatoid RCC	Mucinous Tubular and Spindle Cell Carcinoma	Sarcoma	Angiomyolipoma
PAN-CK(AE1/AE3)	+ (may be focal/rare cells)	+	- (may be focal + in leiomyosarcoma)	-
Cam5.2	+ (may be focal/rare cells)	+	- (may be focal + in leiomyosarcoma)	-
EMA/MUC1	+ (may be focal/rare cells)	+	- (may be focal + in leiomyosarcoma)	-
Desmin	- (may occasionally be +)	-	+ in myosarcomas, occasionally in others	+
Actin-sm	- (may occasionally be +)	-	+ in myosarcomas, occasionally in others	+
CD99	-	-	+ in synovial sarcoma	V
S100	-	-	V	V
Melan-A(MART-1)	-	-	-	+
HMB-45	-	-	-	+
MiTF	-	-	-	+
HMCK(34βE12)	- /(rarely focal +)	-/+	-	-
CK7	- /(rarely focal +)	+	-	-
CAIX	+ (usually)	-	- (+ in perinecrotic areas)	-

(V = Variable, ND = No Data)

IMMUNOHISTOCHEMISTRY, KIDNEY

Poorly Differentiated Carcinomas

Antibody	RCC, Unclassified	Collecting Duct Carcinoma	Urothelial Carcinoma
CK7	-/+	+	+
CK20	-	- (rarely focal +)	+/-
p63	-	-	+
HMCK(34βE12)	-/+	+/ -	+
Thrombomodulin	-	-	+/-
RCC	+/-	-	-
Uroplakin-3	-	-	+/-
Vimentin	+/-	+	-/+
CD10	+/-	-	-/+
CK5/6	-	-	+/-
CK17	-	-	+/-
INI1	+	+ (loss in medullary)	+
Ulex-1	-	+	-/+

Small Blue Round Cell Tumors of Kidney

Antibody	Wilms Tumor	Ewing Sarcoma/ PNET	Small Cell Carcinoma	Lymphoma	Desmoplastic Small Round Cell Tumor	Synovial Sarcoma, Poorly Differentiated
Vimentin	+	+	-	-	+	+
WT1	+	-	-	-	+	-
S100	-	-	-	-	V	-/+
FLI-1	-	+	-	-	-	-
CD99	+/-	+	-	+/-	-/+	-/+
NSE	-	-	-/+	-	+	ND
HMCK(34βE12)	-	-/+	+ (often dot-like)	-	-	-/+
EMA/MUC1	-/+	-	-/+	-	-	-/+
CD45(LCA)	-	-	-	+	-	-
Chromogranin	-	-	+	-	-	-
Desmin	-	-	-	-	+	-
Pax-2	+	ND	ND	ND	ND	ND
PAN-CK(AE1/AE3)	+ (in tubules)	+/- (focal)	+ (often dot-like)	-	+	-/+

(V = Variable, ND = No Data)

Renal Cell Tumors with Clear Cell Cytology

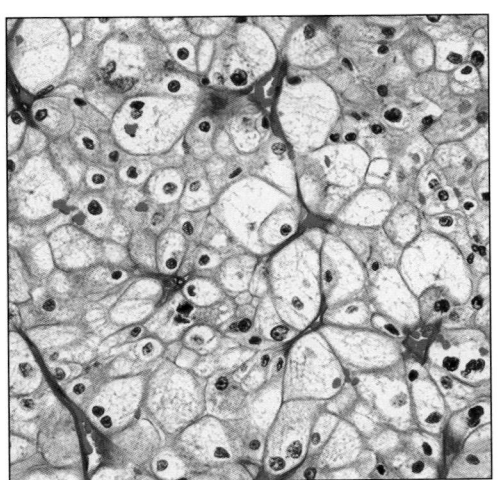

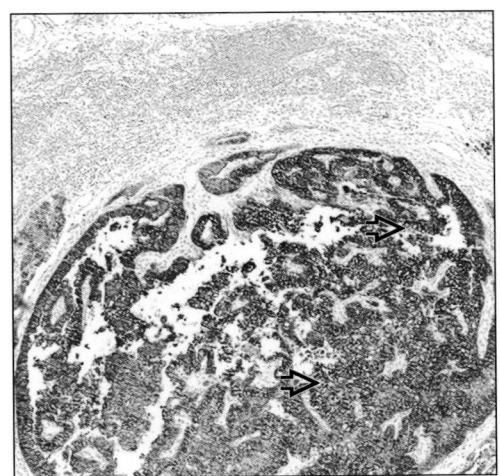

(Left) Differentiation of renal tumors with clear cytoplasm is primarily based on histomorphology. However, immunohistochemistry may be helpful, or needed in rare instances, such as in metastatic settings and on limited material (i.e., biopsy specimens). (Right) Currently, CA9 is the among the most valuable antibody in the differentiation of renal cell tumors, showing diffuse, membranous positivity in > 90% of clear cell RCCs, even at metastatic sites ⊵. Other tumors are negative or only focally positive.

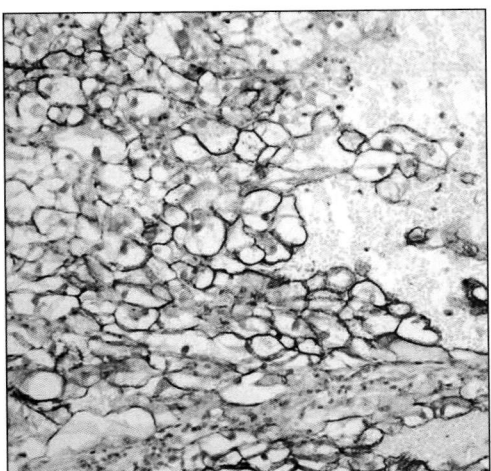

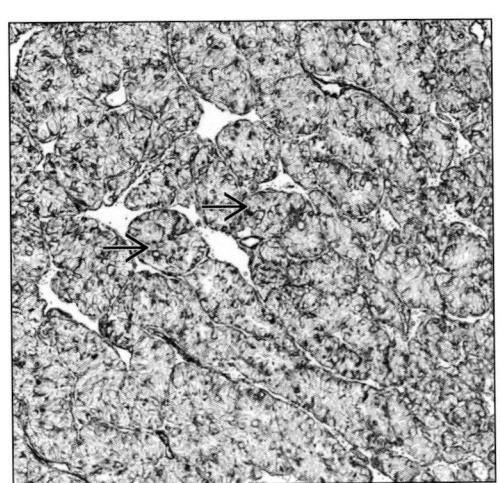

(Left) CD10 shows diffuse membranous reactivity in clear cell RCC but may be negative in high-grade tumors. Translocation-associated carcinomas also show frequent diffuse positivity. Nonspecific cytoplasmic positivity for CD10 is often present in a number of renal and nonrenal tumors. (Right) Vimentin positivity may help in distinguishing clear cell ⊡ from chromophobe RCC. But rare chromophobes, and many high-grade renal and extrarenal tumors, may also be positive for vimentin.

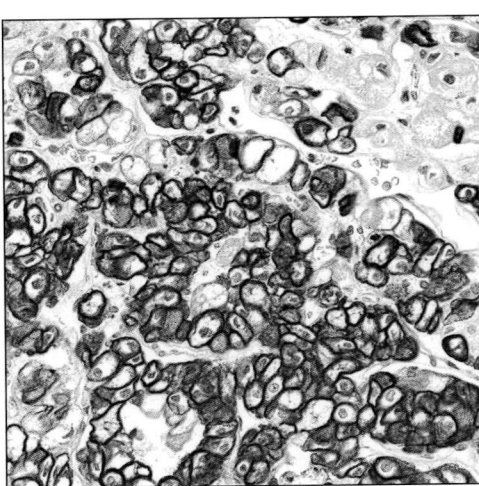

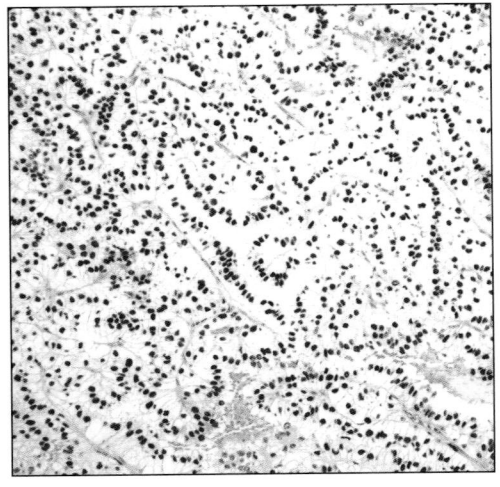

(Left) CK7 usually shows patchy to diffuse membrane-predominant immunoreactivity in chromophobe RCC. In most clear cell RCCs, CK7 is negative, or focally positive in cystic or fibrotic areas. Papillary RCCs with clear cytoplasm show diffuse immunoreactivity, but translocation-associated carcinomas are negative. (Right) In clear cell tumors lacking reactivity for CK and EMA/MUC1, stains for TFE3 and TFEB are essential to exclude the possibility of MiTF/TFE family tumors.

Renal Cell Tumors with Papillary Architecture

(Left) Histomorphologic features are the main defining criteria in diagnosing papillary RCC. However, papillary architecture may be a prominent or predominant feature in a variety of other renal cell carcinomas. *(Right)* CK7 is positive in > 80% of papillary RCCs, but the positivity may be less prominent in type 2 tumors. Diffuse CK7 immunoreactivity is not limited to papillary RCC and may be seen in other renal tumors that enter into differential diagnoses for papillary RCC.

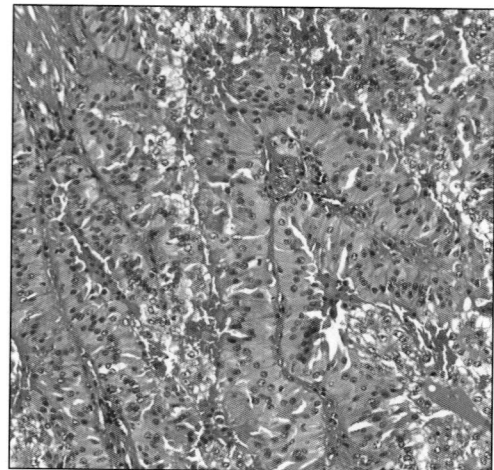
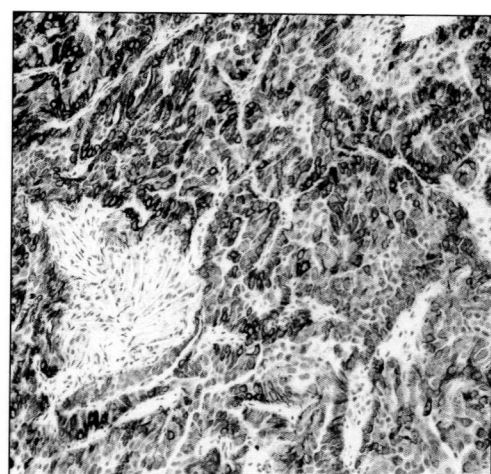

(Left) Diffuse CK7 positivity is often observed in mucinous tubular and spindle cell, collecting duct, renal medullary, and clear cell papillary RCCs. *(Right)* AMACR immunostain shows diffuse, granular cytoplasmic reactivity ➡ in a vast majority of papillary RCCs, but similar diffuse staining may also be seen in many other renal tumors with or without papillary architecture. In the absence of reactivity for CK7 and AMACR, alternative diagnostic possibilities should be considered.

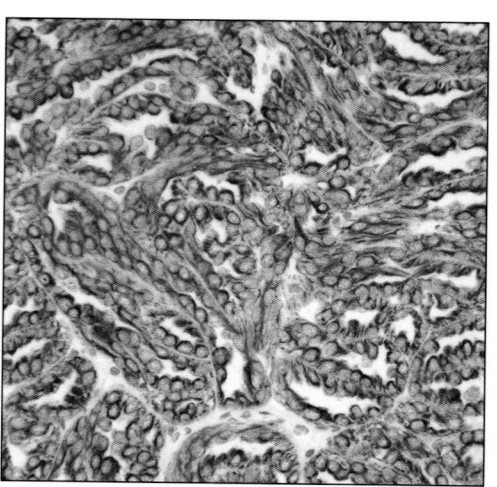
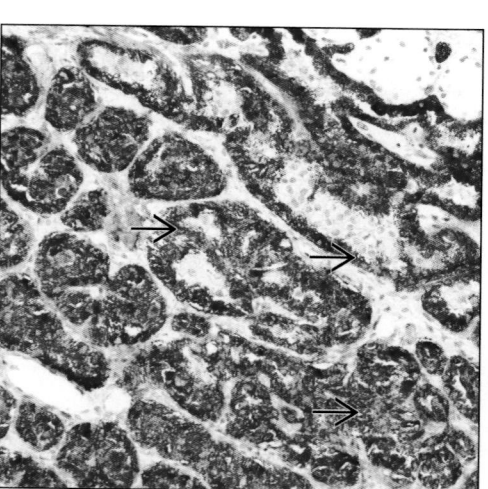

(Left) This renal tumor with papillary architecture is completely (-) for CK7, with (+) staining in the surrounding renal tubules ➡. Negative staining for CK7 is frequent in TFE family translocation-associated, HLRCC syndrome-associated, and some unclassified RCCs with papillary architecture. *(Right)* Metanephric adenoma is sometimes difficult to differentiated from solid, type 1 papillary RCC. In addition to morphologic features, CD57 ➡ and WT1 positivity may help in the distinction.

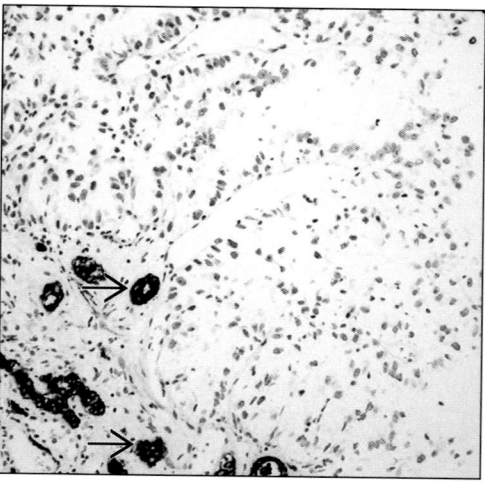
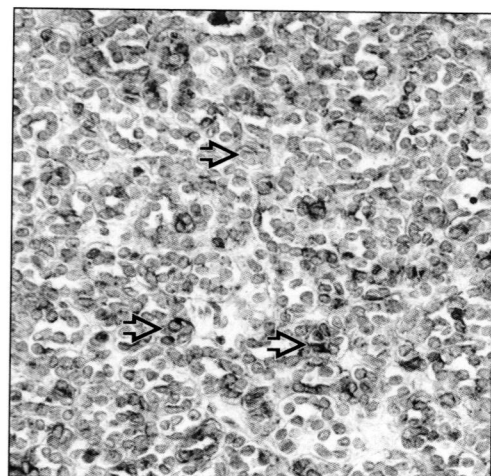

Other Useful Immunohistochemical Stains

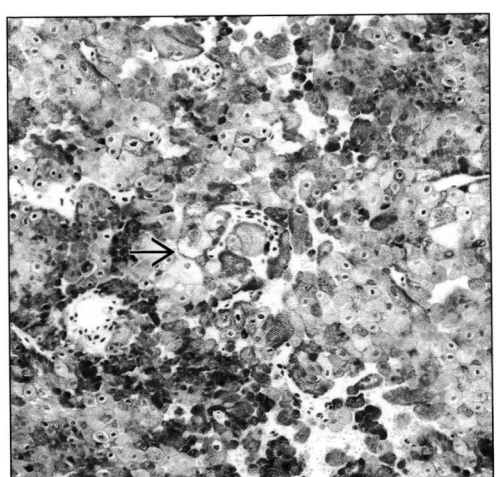 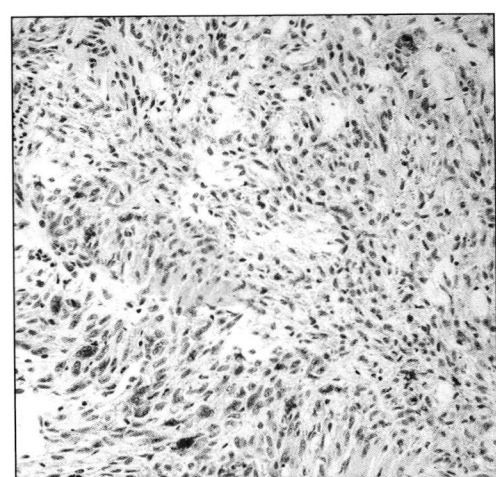

(Left) CD117 immunostaining is useful in the distinction of chromophobe RCC and oncocytoma from eosinophilic, clear cell RCC. Reactivity is diffuse in chromophobe (often, but not always, with peripheral accentuation ⮕), focal to diffuse cytoplasmic in oncocytoma, and (-) in clear cell RCC. *(Right)* Staining for HMB-45 is usually necessary to make the diagnosis in angiomyolipoma showing variant histologic features or in epithelioid AML. Positivity is frequently focal.

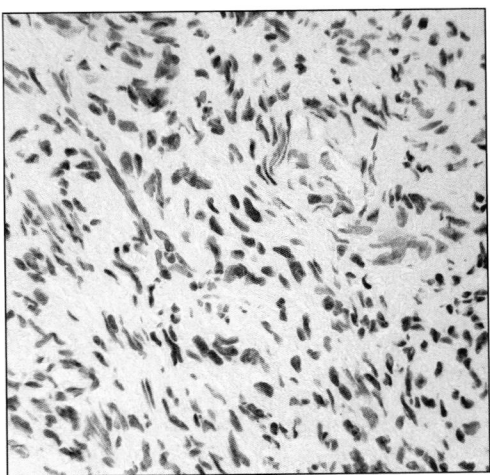 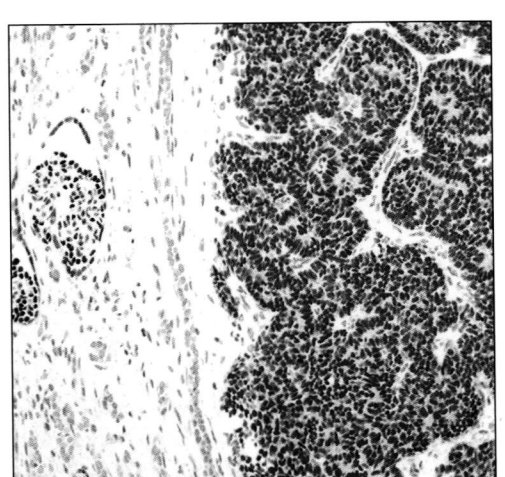

(Left) MITF positivity (nuclear) is seen in about 50% of the cases of AML. SMA, HMB-45, Melan-A(MART-1), and tyrosinase are other positive markers in these tumors. *(Right)* Immunostaining for WT1 may be needed in the distinction of small, blue round cell tumors. WT1 usually shows diffuse nuclear immunoreactivity in the blastemal and epithelial components of Wilms tumor. Positivity may also be observed in desmoplastic small round cell tumor and some metanephric adenomas.

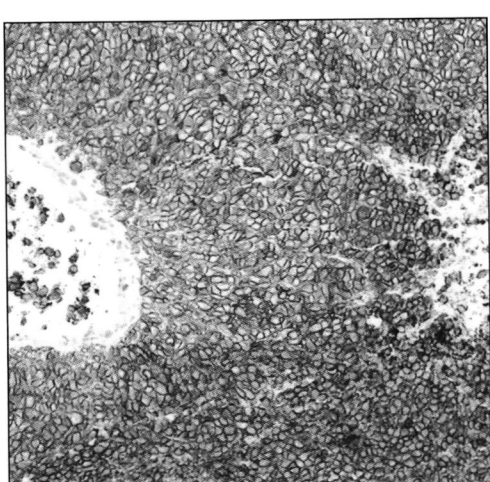 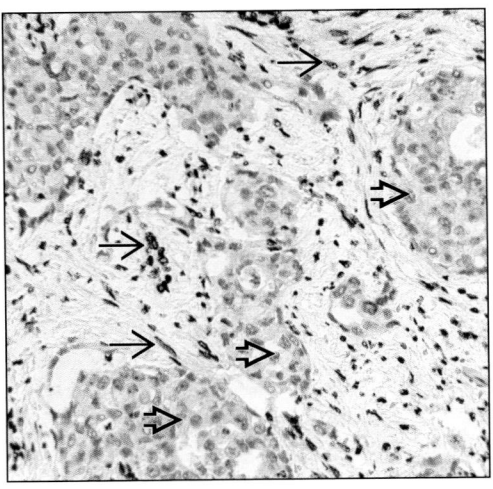

(Left) Diffuse, strong membranous positivity for CD99 is characteristic in PNET. However, focal positivity may occasionally also be seen in synovial sarcoma, Wilms tumor, and other small round cell tumors. Genetic confirmation of the diagnosis is imperative. *(Right)* SNF5 immunostain shows complete loss of the nuclear expression in rhabdoid tumor of the kidney, as well as renal medullary carcinoma ⮕. The background stromal cells and lymphocytes retain positivity ⮕.

Urinary Bladder

CLASSIFICATION OF BLADDER TUMORS & TUMOR-LIKE LESIONS

NONNEOPLASTIC LESIONS

Tumor-like Lesions
- Amyloidosis
- Cystitis
  - Emphysematous
  - Encrusted
  - Eosinophilic
  - Follicular
  - Gangrenous
  - Giant cell
  - Granulomatous
  - Hemorrhagic
  - Infectious
  - Interstitial
  - Radiation
- Cystitis cystica and glandularis
  - ± intestinal metaplasia
  - ± mucin extravasation
- Fibroepithelial polyp
- Malakoplakia
- Müllerian lesions
- Nephrogenic adenoma
- Papillary-polypoid cystitis
- Postoperative lesions
  - Granulomas
  - Spindle cell nodule
- Prostatic-type polyps
- Pseudocarcinomatous hyperplasia
- Schistosomiasis
- Squamous lesions
  - Squamous metaplasia (keratinizing and nonkeratinizing)
  - Squamous hyperplasia, papillary and flat
- von Brunn nests

NEOPLASMS

Flat Urothelial Lesions
- Flat urothelial lesions other than carcinoma in situ
  - Flat urothelial hyperplasia
  - Reactive urothelial atypia
  - Urothelial atypia of unknown significance
  - Dysplasia

Noninvasive Urothelial Neoplasms
- Benign
  - Urothelial papilloma
  - Inverted papilloma
  - Papillary urothelial neoplasm of low malignant potential
- Malignant
  - Papillary (typical)
    - Low-grade papillary urothelial carcinoma
    - High-grade papillary urothelial carcinoma
    - Variant (squamous or glandular differentiation)
  - Micropapillary
  - Nonpapillary
    - Urothelial carcinoma in situ

Invasive Neoplasms
- Microinvasive urothelial carcinoma
- Invasive urothelial carcinoma
  - Typical
  - Urothelial carcinoma with divergent differentiation
    - Squamous differentiation
    - Glandular differentiation
    - Trophoblastic differentiation
  - Deceptively benign features
    - Nested
    - Small tubular
    - Microcystic
    - Inverted
  - Unusual cytoplasmic features
    - Clear cell (glycogen rich)
    - Plasmacytoid
    - Rhabdoid
    - Lipoid (lipid cell) features
  - Unusual stromal reactions
    - Pseudosarcomatous stroma
    - Stromal osseous or cartilaginous metaplasia
    - Osteoclast-type giant cells
    - With prominent lymphoid infiltrate
    - With myxoid stroma
  - Micropapillary
  - Lymphoepithelioma-like
  - Small cell carcinoma
  - Sarcomatoid carcinoma
  - Large cell undifferentiated carcinoma

Glandular Lesions
- Villous adenoma
- Adenocarcinoma in situ
- Invasive adenocarcinoma
  - Adenocarcinoma NOS
  - Signet ring
  - Enteric
  - Mucinous/colloid
  - Hepatoid
  - Mixed
- Clear cell adenocarcinoma
- Urachal adenocarcinoma

Squamous Lesions
- Squamous papilloma
- Condyloma
- Squamous dysplasia
- Squamous cell carcinoma

Smooth Muscle Tumors
- Leiomyoma
- Leiomyosarcoma
- Epithelioid angiomyolipoma/PEComa

Skeletal Muscle Tumors
- Rhabdomyosarcoma (embryonal, alveolar)

Other Mesenchymal Neoplasms
- Pleomorphic undifferentiated sarcoma (malignant fibrous histiocytoma)
- Myofibroblastic proliferations
  - Inflammatory myofibroblastic tumor/ pseudosarcomatous myofibroblastic proliferation
- Neurofibroma
- Solitary fibrous tumor
- Granular cell tumor

CLASSIFICATION OF BLADDER TUMORS & TUMOR-LIKE LESIONS

- Hemangioma/vascular malformation
- Angiosarcoma
- Postradiation sarcoma

Other Tumors, Including Hematopoietic Tumors

- Carcinoid
- Paraganglioma
- Lymphoma
- Plasmacytoma
- Melanoma

Metastatic Tumors

- Prostatic carcinoma
- Colonic adenocarcinoma
- Other (rectum, cervix, endometrium, breast, ovary)

OVERVIEW OF CYSTITIS

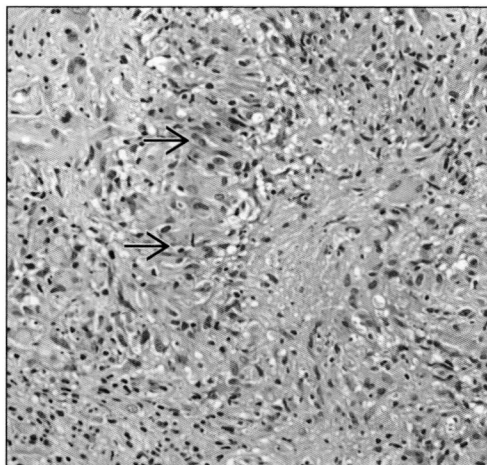

The palisading histiocytes ➡ forming this granuloma are secondary to intravesical bacillus Calmette-Guerin therapy that was administered for urothelial carcinoma.

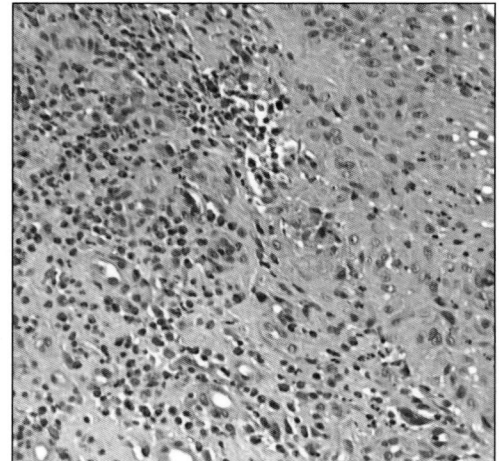

This infiltrate in the bladder, which is rich in eosinophils, has been described as eosinophilic cystitis. The etiology may be allergic, infectious, local injury (e.g., neoplasm), or idiopathic.

TERMINOLOGY

Abbreviations
- Bacillus Calmette-Guérin (BCG)

Definitions
- Spectrum of nonneoplastic inflammatory conditions may involve urinary bladder

CYSTITIS SUBTYPES

Granulomatous Cystitis
- BCG effect following intravesical therapy for bladder carcinoma
  - Caseating or noncaseating granulomatous inflammation
  - Overlying urothelium may show reactive atypia or ulceration
  - Ziehl Neelsen stain may reveal acid-fast bacilli
    - Not generally performed
- Postsurgical granuloma (postsurgical necrobiotic granuloma)
  - Develops after transurethral resection of bladder
  - Traumatic granulomatous process
    - Linear or serpiginous contours with central fibrinoid necrosis
    - Rimmed by palisading histiocytes, some multinucleated
    - May resemble rheumatoid nodule
    - Surrounding inflammation comprised of lymphocytes and plasma cells
    - Eosinophils prominent following post excision to biopsy interval of less than 1 month
    - Necrotic outlines of surrounding vessels may be seen
  - Tuberculous cystitis
    - Usually caseating granulomas with central necrosis surrounded by histiocytes and multinucleated giant cells

- Early lesions generally in region of ureteral orifice
- Systemic or localized tuberculosis infection
- Most commonly caused by *Mycobacterium tuberculosis*
- *Mycobacterium bovus* may rarely be causative agent
- Acid-fast bacilli may be seen on Ziehl Neelsen stain
- Typically no history of prior transurethral procedure or intravesical therapy
- Urine or tissue cultures may be needed for diagnosis
  - Other rare noninfectious causes
    - Sarcoidosis
    - Crohn disease
    - Rheumatoid arthritis (rheumatoid nodule)

Follicular Cystitis
- Nonspecific pattern of inflammation
  - Lymphoid follicles with germinal center formation in lamina propria
  - Associated with bladder cancer or urinary tract infection
  - More prevalent in children but spans all ages
- Differential diagnosis
  - Low-grade lymphoma, such as follicular
  - Readily distinguished by immunohistochemistry as in other sites

Eosinophilic Cystitis
- Descriptive term applied to mixed inflammatory infiltrates of lamina propria rich in eosinophils
  - Not a single diagnostic entity
- Often has polypoid appearance
  - May mimic polypoid cystitis or urothelial carcinoma in adults or rhabdomyosarcoma in children
- 3 clinical settings
  - Nonspecific localized process
    - Pattern of injury associated with a variety of etiologies

- Prostatic hyperplasia, bladder carcinoma, or prior transurethral biopsy
  ○ Allergy associated
    - In children, seen in association with allergic gastroenteritis, asthma, or other allergic disorders
    - May rarely be drug induced
    - Peripheral blood eosinophilia may seen
  ○ Rarely, may be secondary to parasitic infection

Emphysematous Cystitis
- Presence of gas-filled vesicles in bladder that are visible by cystoscopy or gross examination
- More common in women
- Clinical associations
  ○ Adults
    - Most commonly associated with diabetes mellitus/hyperglycemia
  ○ Children
    - Most commonly seen as complication of necrotizing enterocolitis
- By histology, multiple blebs (empty cavities) within lamina propria
  ○ Histiocytes, often multinucleate, or thin fibrous tissue surround clear spaces
- Caused by gas-forming bacteria
  ○ *Aerobacter aerogenes*
  ○ *E. coli*
  ○ *Clostridium perfringens*

Interstitial Cystitis
- Chronic inflammatory process of unknown etiology
- Occurs almost exclusively in middle-aged and older women
- Some research has suggested possibility of autoimmune disorder
- Clinical symptoms
  ○ Urinary frequency, urgency, suprapubic pressure, and pain with either bladder distention or voiding
- Cystoscopy
  ○ Early nonulcer type
    - Small submucosal hemorrhagic foci (glomerulations) and linear cracks under hydrodistention
  ○ Classic ulcer type (Hunner ulcer)
    - Multiple reddened foci with small vessels radiating toward central scar or ulcer with fibrin accumulation
    - Increasing hydrodistention causes mucosal rupture at ulcer with oozing of blood
    - Bullous edema also common after distension
- Clinical diagnosis of exclusion
  ○ Urodynamic studies typically reveal decreased bladder-filling capacity
  ○ Urine cultures are negative, by definition
  ○ Prior therapies with known bladder irritants, concomitant urothelial neoplasia, and infections exclude interstitial cystitis
- Histologic features
  ○ No pathognomonic features
    - Important role for pathologists is exclusion of urothelial carcinoma in situ or specific form of cystitis
  ○ Common findings

- Ulceration with variably admixed fibrin, erythrocytes, and inflammatory cells, especially neutrophils
    - Associated granulation tissue and perineural lymphocytic infiltrates are common
    - Urothelial denudation is frequent
    - Ulcers typically extend deep into lamina propria with surrounding edema and congestion
    - Without ulcers, morphologic changes may be subtle: Suburothelial hemorrhage, edema, and mucosal tears
    - Fibrosis of muscularis propria in longstanding disease
  ○ Considerable debate regarding utility of mast cell counts in distinction from other inflammatory processes
    - Specificity in distinction from other inflammatory processes is questionable
    - Reports of increased intravesical mast cell infiltrates in patients with interstitial cystitis are cited
- Final diagnosis of interstitial cystitis requires close clinical (i.e., history, cystoscopy, and voiding studies) and pathologic correlation

Infectious Cystitis
- Not typically histologic diagnosis
  ○ Culture and serum tests are usually used for diagnosis
- Bacterial
  ○ Sexually active women (20-40 years old)
  ○ Dysuria, frequency, urgency, voiding small quantity
  ○ Common etiologies
    - *E. coli*, *Staphylococcus*, *Klebsiella*, *Proteus*, *Enterococci*
  ○ Tissue biopsy plays little role in diagnosis
    - Diagnosis by urine culture, urinalysis, and clinical symptoms
- Viral
  ○ Human papilloma virus
    - Associated with condyloma
  ○ Adenovirus
    - Important cause of hemorrhagic cystitis in children, particularly types 11 and 21
    - May occur after bone marrow or solid organ transplantation in any age group or in otherwise healthy children
  ○ Polyoma (BK) virus
    - Infection of immunocompromised (such as renal transplant patients)
    - Results in large nuclear inclusions in urothelial cells, so-called "decoy cells," which may mimic carcinoma in situ
  ○ Other viral causes of hemorrhagic cystitis
    - Polyomavirus and herpes simplex type 2
  ○ Herpes zoster may be associated with reversible voiding dysfunction
  ○ Cytomegalovirus may rarely involve bladder in immunocompromised patients
- Fungal
  ○ Fungal cystitis is uncommon
  ○ Debilitated patients on antibiotics or diabetics
  ○ *Candida albicans* most common; rarely *Aspergillus*

- Secondary to ascending urethral infection or hematogenous spread
  - Cystoscopically
    - Small white mucosal plaques, but large fungal balls may rarely be seen
  - Histology
    - Ulceration and inflammation in lamina propria
    - Fungal hyphae may be visible on routine stains
    - Pseudohyphae and yeast forms in tissue section with PAS and silver stain

Giant Cell Cystitis
- Similar cells may be seen in patients treated with chemotherapeutic agents and radiation
- Not a clinical entity
  - Normal histologic finding
    - Commonly seen in bladder biopsy specimen without apparent pathology
  - Presence of atypical stromal cells in lamina propria of bladder
    - Enlarged, hyperchromatic, multilobated nuclei
    - Degenerative atypia
    - Mitoses absent or rare
- Differential diagnosis
  - Radiation atypia
    - More pronounced atypia with nucleoli
  - Sarcoma
    - Bladder sarcomas are almost always more cellular

Hemorrhagic Cystitis
- Severe hematuria shortly after exposure to inciting agent
  - Chemotherapeutic agents
    - Cyclophosphamide
    - Busulfan and thiotepa
  - Industrial exposure
    - Aniline and toluidine derivatives used in dyes and insecticides
  - Viral etiologies also well described
    - Adenovirus, types 11 and 21
    - Polyomavirus
    - Herpes simplex type 2
- Morphology
  - Extensive hemorrhage into lamina propria with vascular congestion and edema
  - Overlying epithelium with ulceration, necrosis, and nuclear atypia
    - Similar to radiation or intravesical chemotherapy-associated changes

Encrusted Cystitis
- Deposition of inorganic salts in bladder mucosa
- Caused by urea-splitting bacteria that alkalinize urine
- Most common in women
- Presenting symptoms are similar to other urinary tract infections
- Cystoscopically
  - Diffuse gritty appearance
- Morphologically
  - Fibrinous exudate with admixed calcified, necrotic debris, and inflammatory infiltrates
- Differential diagnosis
  - Carcinoma may have overlying calcification

- Correlation with cystoscopic impression is important

Radiation Cystitis
- Urothelium may show striking cytologic atypia
  - Cytoplasmic and nuclear vacuolation with normal nuclear/cytoplasmic ratio
  - Karyorrhexis
- Stromal changes also seen
  - Atypical mesenchymal cells similar to those seen in giant cell cystitis in lamina propria
    - Usually have more pronounced atypia with nucleoli
  - Marked stromal edema or fibrosis
  - Prominent telangiectatic vessels with hyalinization and thrombosis
- Pseudocarcinomatous hyperplasia of epithelium may be seen
  - Close mimic of invasive carcinoma
  - Epithelium closely associated with vessels and fibrin
- Differential diagnosis
  - Urothelial carcinoma in situ
    - Lack cytoplasmic vacuolization
    - More uniform nucleomegaly and hyperchromasia
    - Diffuse cytoplasmic cytokeratin 20 immunoreactivity throughout urothelium

Gangrenous Cystitis
- Necrosis generally begins in mucosa and may progress to involve entire wall to serosa
- Most commonly complication of infection
- Other causes
  - Systemic disorders
    - Severe diabetes mellitus
    - Sepsis
    - Vascular disease
  - Corrosive chemical injury

SELECTED REFERENCES

1. Meria P et al: Encrusted cystitis and pyelitis. J Urol. 160(1):3-9, 1998
2. White MD et al: Gangrenous cystitis in the elderly: pathogenesis and management options. Br J Urol. 82(2):297-9, 1998
3. Eble JN et al: Post-surgical necrobiotic granulomas of urinary bladder. Urology. 35(5):454-7, 1990
4. Hansson S et al: Follicular cystitis in girls with untreated asymptomatic or covert bacteriuria. J Urol. 143(2):330-2, 1990
5. Gillenwater JY et al: Summary of the National Institute of Arthritis, Diabetes, Digestive and Kidney Diseases Workshop on Interstitial Cystitis, National Institutes of Health, Bethesda, Maryland, August 28-29, 1987. J Urol. 140(1):203-6, 1988
6. Hellstrom HR et al: Eosinophilic cystitis. A study of 16 cases. Am J Clin Pathol. 72(5):777-84, 1979
7. Rubin JS et al: Cyclophosphamide hemorrhagic cystitis. J Urol. 96(3):313-6, 1966

OVERVIEW OF CYSTITIS

Microscopic Features

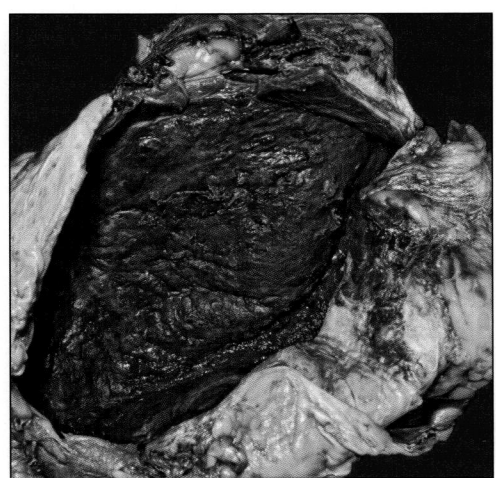

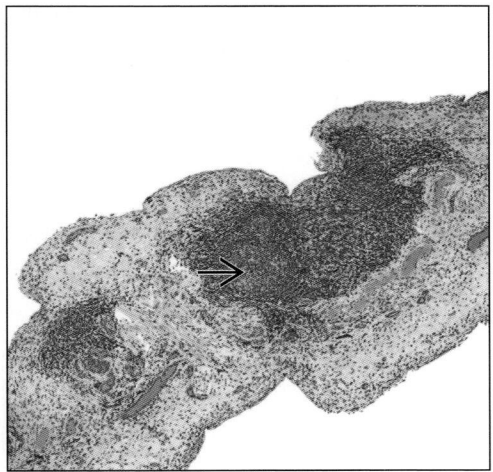

(Left) This urinary bladder specimen from a patient with hemorrhagic cystitis shows diffuse mucosal hemorrhage. Tissue biopsies are rarely performed in such patients. (Courtesy D. Regula, MD.) *(Right)* Follicular cystitis shows a dense lymphocytic inflammatory infiltrate in the lamina propria with central germinal center formation ➡. This pattern of inflammation is nonspecific but is most commonly associated with urinary tract infection.

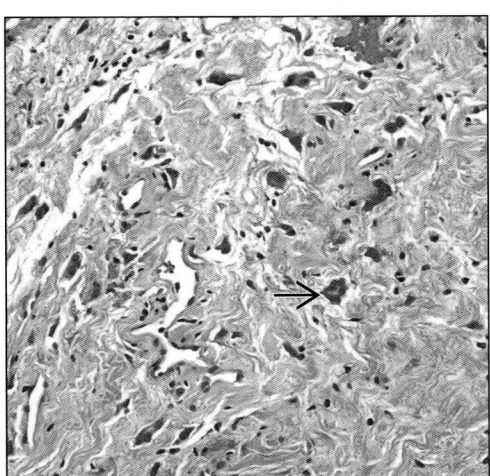

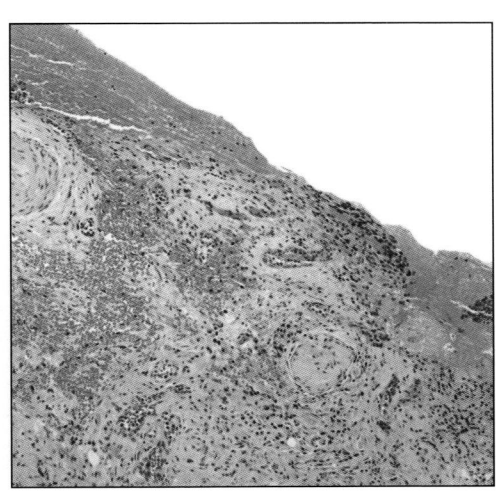

(Left) Atypical stromal cells, often with multilobated smudgy nuclei ➡, are commonly seen in the lamina propria of the urinary bladder and represent a variation of normal histology. When prominent, the term "giant cell cystitis" has been applied. *(Right)* Many of the histologic changes seen in interstitial cystitis are nonspecific, such as ulceration, hemorrhage, and a mixed inflammatory infiltrate. Biopsy is important to exclude other causes, such as urothelial carcinoma in situ.

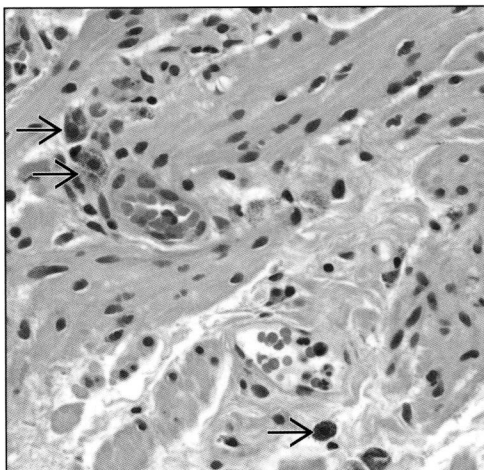

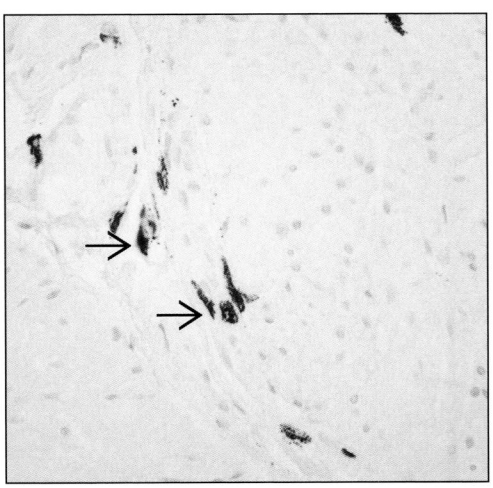

(Left) Increased numbers of mast cells ➡ may be seen within the muscularis propria in interstitial cystitis. *(Right)* A pinacyanol erythrosinate stain highlights mast cells ➡ within the muscularis propria in interstitial cystitis. CD117 immunohistochemistry may also be used. The specificity of this finding for interstitial cystitis is controversial. Ultimately, the diagnosis of interstitial cystitis requires close correlation with voiding studies and cystoscopic findings.

Microscopic Features

(Left) Radiation may induce a variety of histologic changes, such as stromal hemorrhage, as seen in this example. Radiation therapy for prostate and gynecologic tract cancers is the most common association. *(Right)* Neovascularity, telangiectasia, and stromal fibrin deposition in the lamina propria are other histologic findings that may be seen in radiation cystitis. Ischemia secondary to any etiology may induce similar changes.

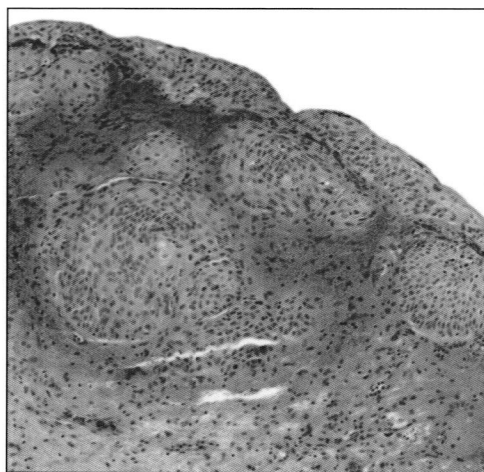
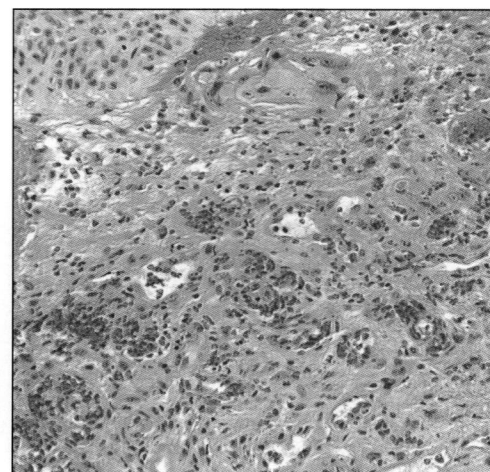

(Left) Eosinophilic cystitis is a nonspecific inflammatory infiltrate that is rich in eosinophils, which may form a mass lesion that clinically mimics malignancy in some cases. *(Right)* In this example of eosinophilic cystitis, the eosinophilic infiltrate is striking. This may rarely be seen with allergic conditions in children. In adults, parasitic infection or association with an adjacent carcinoma or prior biopsy may be seen.

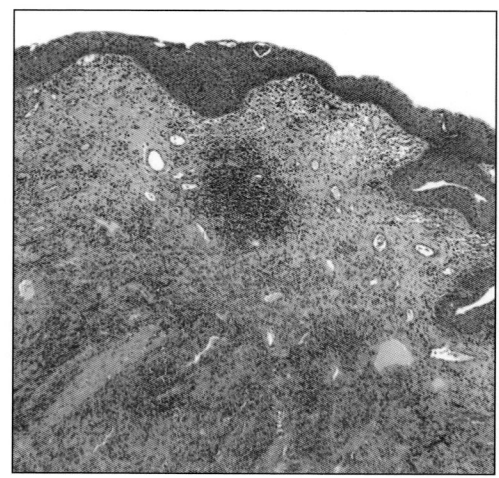
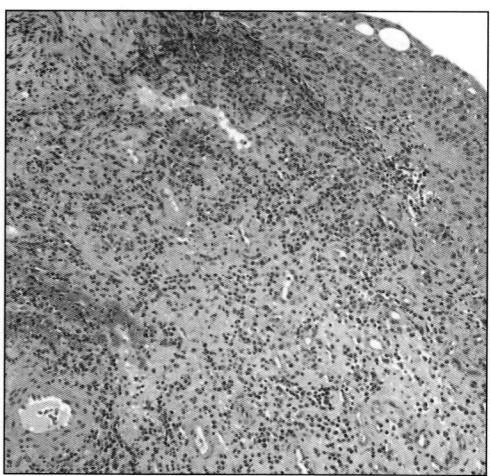

(Left) This bladder biopsy specimen shows evidence of ulceration ⇉ and a mixed inflammatory infiltrate filling the lamina propria with rare lymphoid follicles ➔. This pattern is nonspecific and in some cases an etiology is not known. Such cases are best diagnosed descriptively. *(Right)* Occasionally, reactive lymphoid infiltrates of the bladder, as in this case of unknown etiology, may mimic lymphoma. B- and T-cell immunohistochemical markers show a mixed population in reactive lesions.

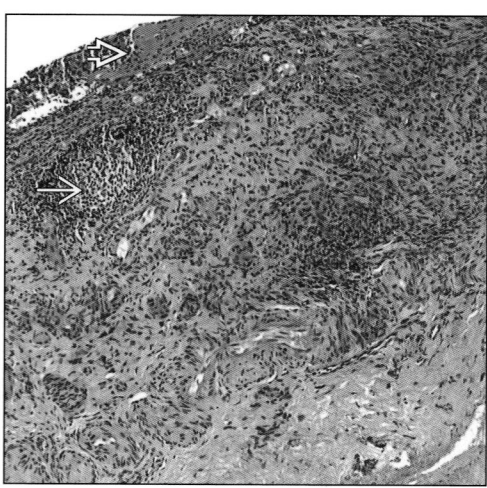
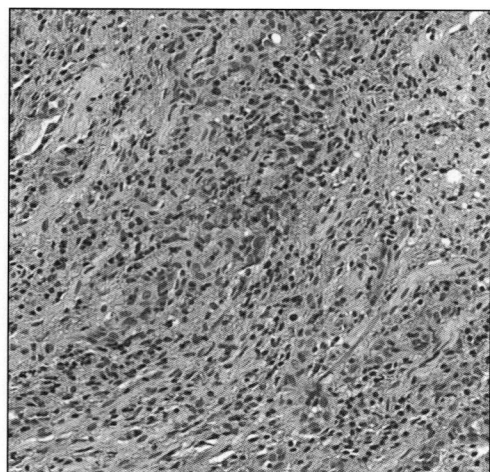

OVERVIEW OF CYSTITIS

Microscopic Features

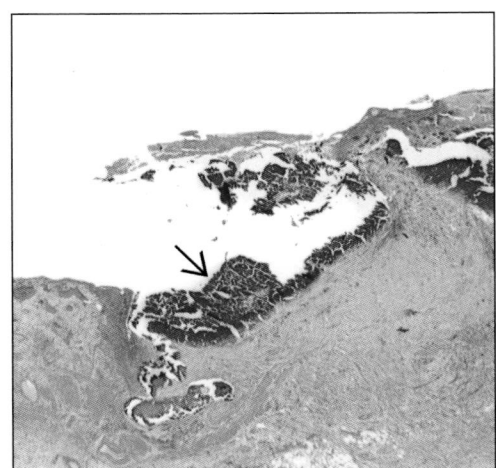 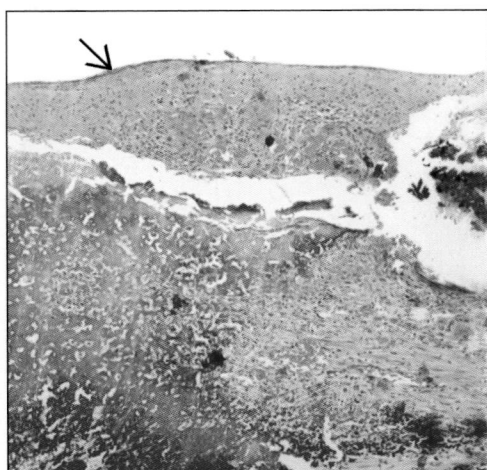

(Left) Occasionally, urea-splitting bacteria may alkalinize the urine and cause precipitation of inorganic salts. Morphologically, this results in calcified debris ➡ in the bladder mucosa, often with associated inflammatory infiltrates. *(Right)* Calcified debris is associated with fibrin deposition ➡ in this encrusted cystitis. This may also be seen in other conditions that cause necrosis. Calcification overlying a necrotic carcinoma is the major differential consideration.

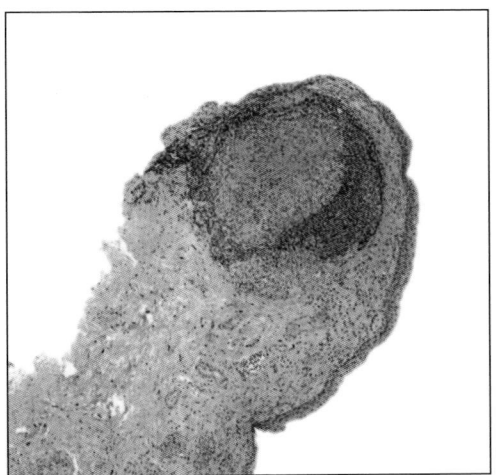 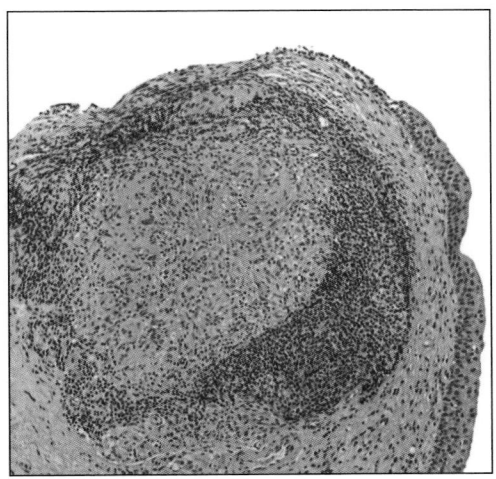

(Left) Intravesical bacillus Calmette-Guerin therapy often causes scattered granulomas within the bladder that may be caseating or noncaseating. These have a similar appearance to tuberculosis-associated granulomas. *(Right)* This tightly formed, noncaseating granuloma with a cuff of lymphocytes was associated with prior bacillus Calmette-Guerin therapy. In the appropriate clinical context, stains for infectious organisms are not required.

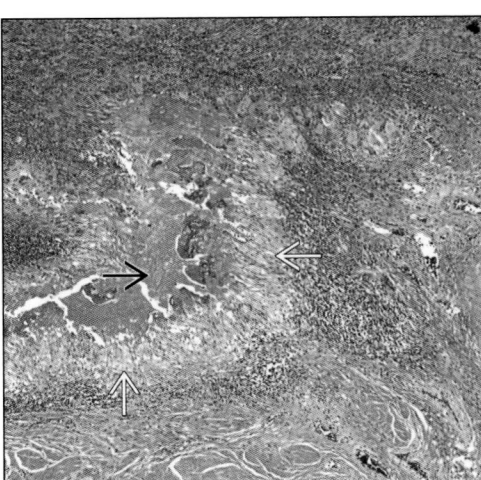 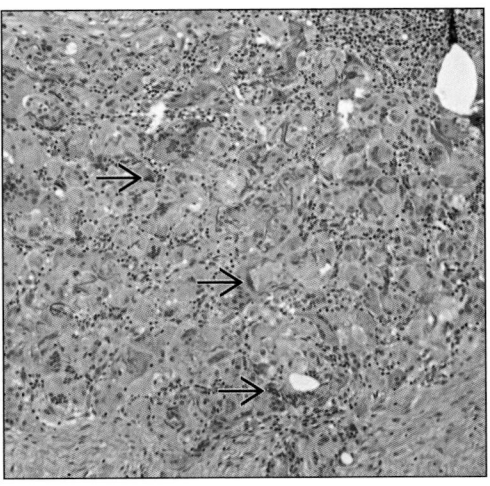

(Left) This granuloma is associated with a prior transurethral resection for a noninvasive papillary urothelial carcinoma. These granulomas commonly have linear or serpiginous contours with central fibrinoid necrosis ➡ and a rim of palisading histiocytes ➡, some multinucleated. *(Right)* Post-biopsy granulomas may also be associated with pigment deposition ➡ from hemorrhage and subsequent red cell breakdown products.

PAPILLARY-POLYPOID CYSTITIS

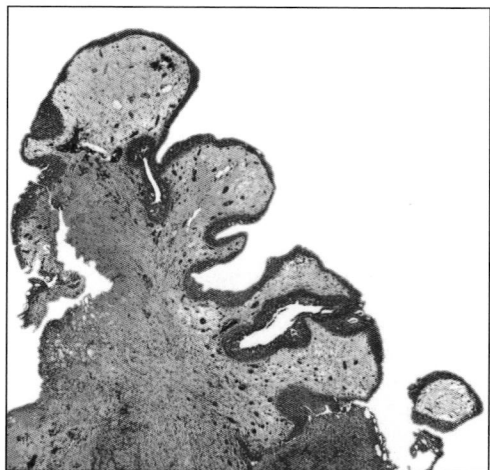

Papillary-polypoid cystitis is characterized by exophytic processes with broad-based connections of the flat bladder mucosa. The cores are edematous without significant branching.

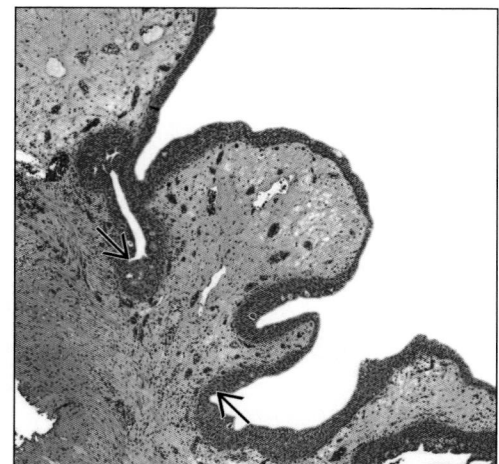

This example of papillary-polypoid cystitis shows a typical bulbous excrescence with a broad base ➡. The absence of complex branching aids in the distinction from a papillary urothelial neoplasm.

TERMINOLOGY

Synonyms
- Papillary cystitis
- Polypoid cystitis
- Bullous cystitis

Definitions
- Nonneoplastic inflammatory lesion of urinary bladder
  - Characterized by edema of lamina propria
  - Exophytic polypoid or papillary projections

ETIOLOGY/PATHOGENESIS

Instrumentation
- Many cases are related to indwelling catheter and vesical fistula

Radiation Therapy
- May follow regional radiation therapy
  - Gynecologic, prostatic, or bladder cancer most common

Tumor Association
- May be seen in association with urothelial carcinoma

CLINICAL ISSUES

Epidemiology
- Age
  - May affect any age group
- Gender
  - Equal gender distribution

Presentation
- Hematuria
- Irritative bladder symptoms from underlying cause

Endoscopic Findings
- Multifocal

- Appears as friable mucosal irregularity or edematous broad papillae adjacent to inflamed area
- Generalized edema common

Treatment
- No excision needed
- Removal of inciting inflammatory factors required

Prognosis
- Benign lesion with no risk of evolving into carcinoma

MACROSCOPIC FEATURES

Size
- Usually small lesions (up to 5 mm)

MICROSCOPIC PATHOLOGY

Histologic Features
- Variable exophytic projections of urothelium secondary to lamina propria edema
- Papillae lack complex secondary or tertiary branching typical of papillary urothelial neoplasia
- Stromal cores are composed of edema and fibrosis
  - Characteristically broader at base and taper to point toward lumen
  - Not typical fibrovascular cores of papillary urothelial neoplasia
- Acute and chronic inflammation may be seen in underlying lamina propria
- Hyperplastic urothelium may be seen
- Reactive urothelial atypia may be prominent
  - May add to morphologic overlap with papillary urothelial carcinoma

Cytologic Features
- Reactive

Predominant Pattern/Injury Type
- Papillary

PAPILLARY-POLYPOID CYSTITIS

Key Facts

Terminology
- Papillary cystitis is nonneoplastic inflammatory lesion of urinary bladder
- Characterized by edema of lamina propria and exophytic polypoid or papillary projections

Etiology/Pathogenesis
- Many cases are related to indwelling catheter or vesical fistula

Clinical Issues
- May affect any age group
- Hematuria
- Irritative bladder symptoms from underlying cause
- No excision required

Microscopic Pathology
- Characterized by variable exophytic projections of urothelium secondary to lamina propria edema
- Papillae lack complex branching typical of papillary urothelial neoplasia
- Stromal cores are comprised of edema and fibrosis, not typical fibrovascular cores of papillary urothelial neoplasia
- Stromal cores are characteristically broader at base and taper to point distally
- Reactive urothelial atypia may be prominent

Top Differential Diagnoses
- Papillary urothelial neoplasia
- Papillary nephrogenic adenoma

- Interstitial edema

Predominant Cell/Compartment Type
- Epithelial, urothelial

Bullous Cystitis
- Elevations are broad; width greater than height
- Extensive edema

Polypoid Cystitis
- Broad-based thick papillae

Papillary Cystitis
- Well-developed slender finger-like papillae with associated lamina propria fibrosis

DIFFERENTIAL DIAGNOSIS

Papillary Urothelial Neoplasia
- Urothelial papilloma and papillary urothelial neoplasm of low malignant potential are closest mimics
- Papillary cores are typically thin and delicate in lower grade papillary urothelial neoplasms
  - Compared to broad and edematous in papillary-polypoid cystitis
  - Detached distal papillary fronds of papillary cystitis without underlying lamina propria may closely mimic papillary urothelial neoplasia
- Papillary urothelial neoplasms generally branch into smaller papillae
  - Complex anastomosis or secondary/tertiary branching favors carcinoma
- Low-grade and high-grade papillary urothelial carcinomas have greater degree of cytologic atypia
  - Must be distinguished from reactive atypia common to papillary-polypoid cystitis

Papillary Nephrogenic Adenoma
- May have admixed architectural patterns
  - Papillary
  - Tubular/tubulocystic
  - Solid/diffuse

- Recognition of solid or tubular patterns excludes papillary/polypoid cystitis
- Lined by single layer of cytologically bland cuboidal epithelium
  - In contrast to stratified layer of urothelial cells in papillary urothelial lesions

DIAGNOSTIC CHECKLIST

Clinically Relevant Pathologic Features
- Gross appearance
  - May be cystoscopically similar to papillary neoplasm
  - Edema and inflammatory changes are common

Pathologic Interpretation Pearls
- Papillary-polypoid cystitis must be considered in differential of papillary urothelial neoplasms
- Urothelial neoplasms should be diagnosed with caution in patients with indwelling catheters or vesical fistulas

SELECTED REFERENCES

1. Lane Z et al: Polypoid/papillary cystitis: a series of 41 cases misdiagnosed as papillary urothelial neoplasia. Am J Surg Pathol. 32(5):758-64, 2008
2. Young RH: Papillary and polypoid cystitis. A report of eight cases. Am J Surg Pathol. 12(7):542-6, 1988
3. Buck EG: Polypoid cystitis mimicking transitional cell carcinoma. J Urol. 131(5):963, 1984
4. Ekelund P et al: The reversibility of catheter-associated polypoid cystitis. J Urol. 130(3):456-9, 1983
5. Milles G: Catheter-induced hemorrhagic pseudopolyps of the urinary bladder. JAMA. 193:968-9, 1965

PAPILLARY-POLYPOID CYSTITIS

Microscopic Features

(Left) This low-power appearance, characterized by broad bulbous excrescences of the urothelium, is typical of papillary-polypoid cystitis. Occasional slender papillary excrescences are also seen in this example ➡. *(Right)* Marked stromal edema is striking within the exophytic polypoid excrescences in this example of papillary-polypoid cystitis. There are associated urothelial changes, including extensive denudation. Where present, the mucosa is unremarkable or shows reactive atypia.

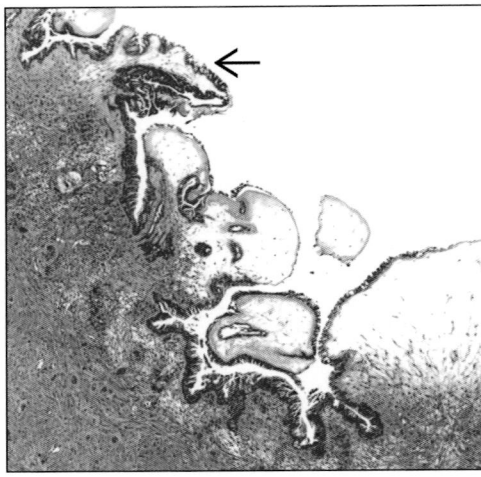 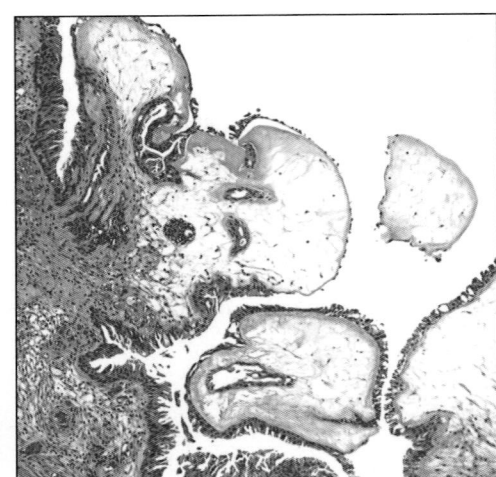

(Left) The bulbous tips ➡ of these simple papillae are characteristic of papillary-polypoid cystitis. This expansion is secondary to edema within the stalk and lamina propria. *(Right)* A more polypoid example of papillary-polypoid cystitis highlights the prototypical broad base ➡. The focus with a thinner papillary-like process ➡ is simple without complex secondary branching. More complexity would be expected in papillary urothelial neoplasms.

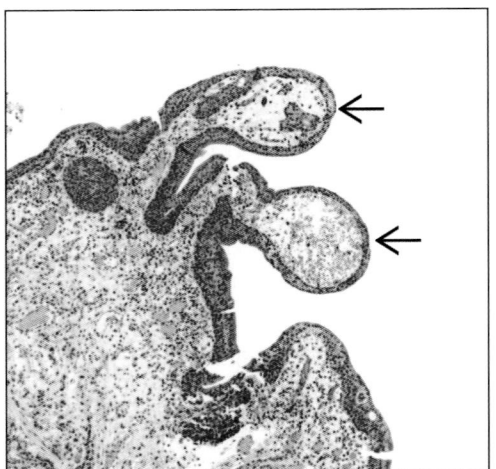 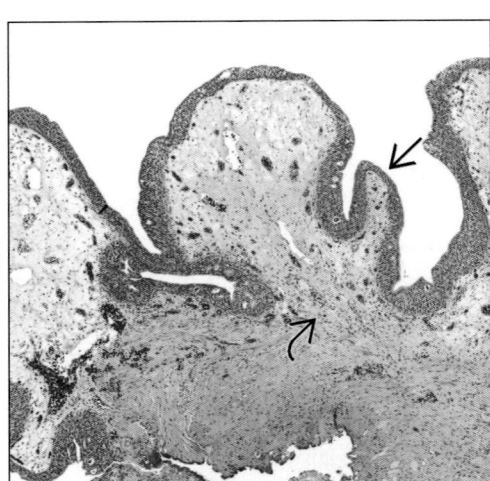

(Left) Admixed large edematous papillae ➡ are characteristic of papillary-polypoid cystitis. *(Right)* When the distal tips of papillary-polypoid cystitis are biopsied, there may be significant overlap with a papillary urothelial neoplasm because of the smaller, tapered ends. Recognition of the more broad papillae toward the base, scattered edematous cores ➡, and the absence of complex anastomosing or hierarchical branching aids in recognition as a reactive papillary proliferation.

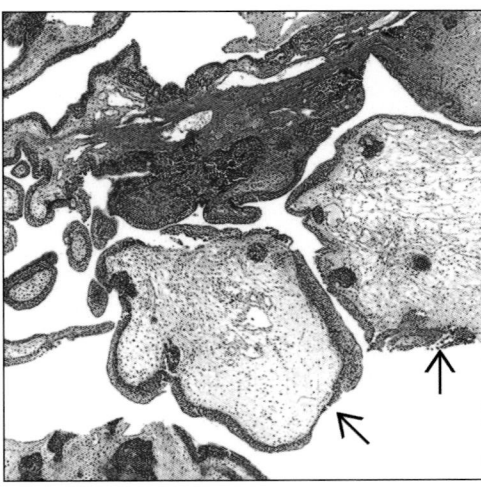 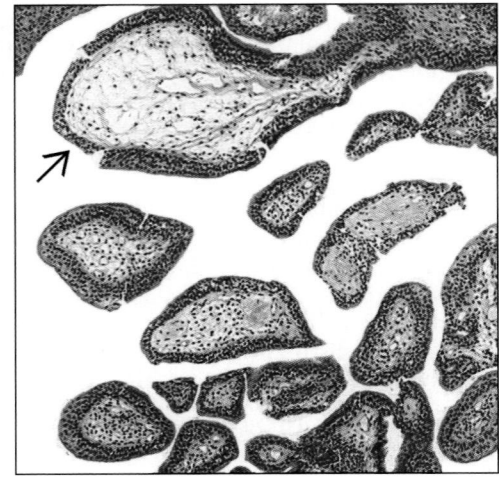

PAPILLARY-POLYPOID CYSTITIS

Differential Diagnosis

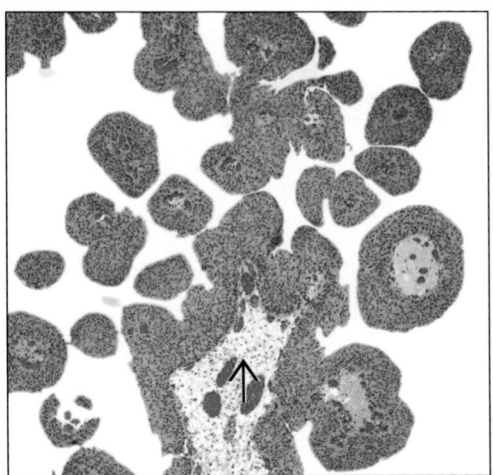 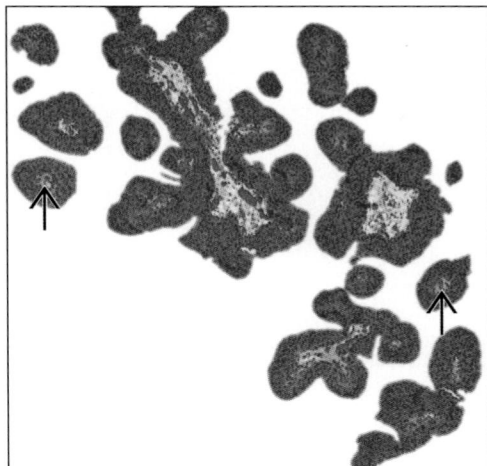

(Left) This urothelial papilloma has prominent secondary branching from a central fibrovascular core ➡, a feature typical of papillary urothelial neoplasms. (Right) Very thin fibrovascular cores ➡, as seen in this example of urothelial papilloma, are typical of papillary urothelial neoplasms. The papillae of papillary-polypoid cystitis generally have a greater amount of stroma with prominent edema.

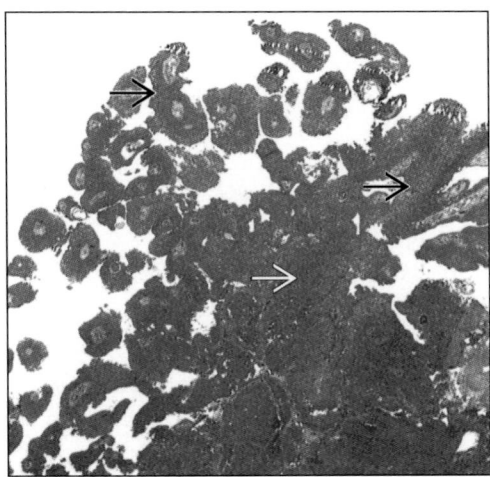 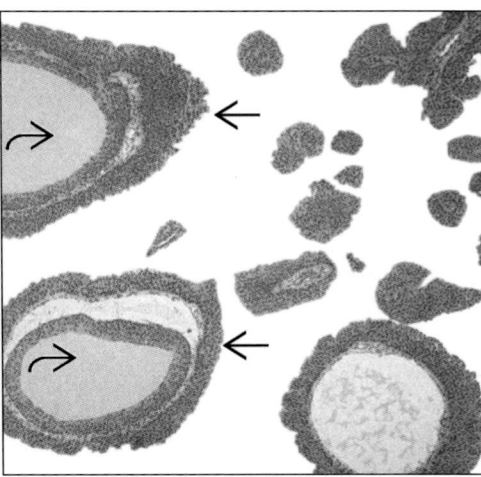

(Left) This degree of epithelial confluence ➡ and the areas of solid growth ➡ are diagnostic of a papillary urothelial neoplasm and would preclude a reactive diagnosis, such as papillary cystitis. (Right) Urothelial papilloma may have some unique architectural patterns within the cores. This example highlights an unusual gland-in-gland pattern ➡ and dilated lymphatics with prominent fluid within the core ➡, features not typical of papillary-polypoid cystitis.

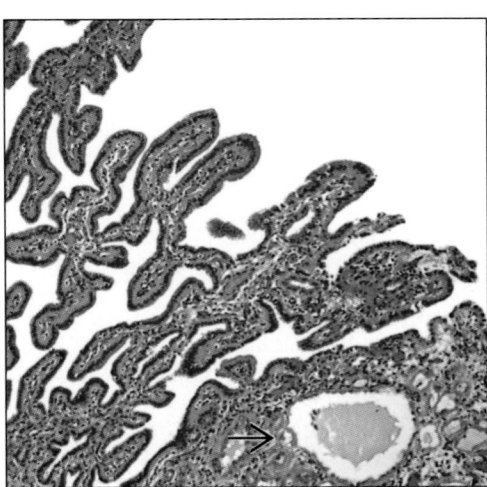 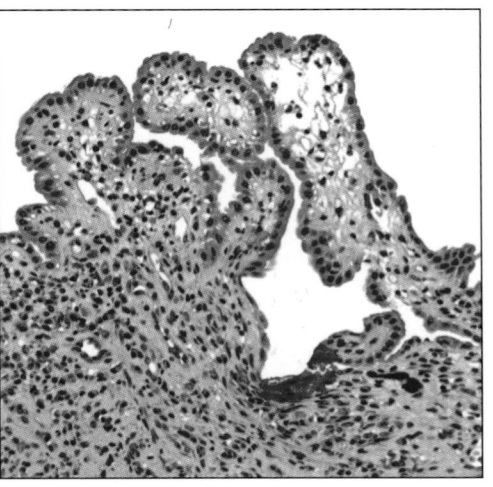

(Left) Papillary nephrogenic adenoma may have variably sized papillae, but they are lined by a single cuboidal epithelial layer. Associated edema is not prominent. Admixed glandular/tubular patterns may also be seen ➡, aiding in the diagnosis. (Right) Papillary nephrogenic adenoma is characteristically lined by a single cuboidal layer of epithelium with bland cytologic figures. In contrast, papillary cystitis has larger and thicker papillae with a stratified urothelial layer.

MALAKOPLAKIA

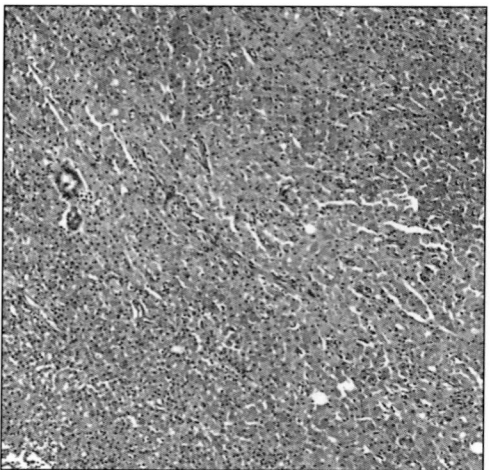

Malakoplakia is characterized by sheets of histiocytes with abundant eosinophilic cytoplasm. This sheet-like growth may mimic a variety of malignant neoplasms.

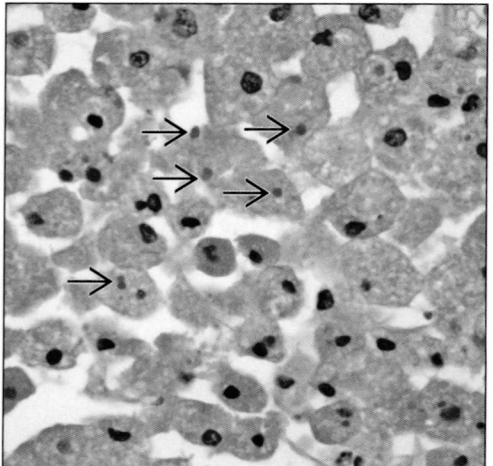

The histiocytes of malakoplakia have abundant eosinophilic cytoplasm and intracytoplasmic inclusions (Michaelis-Guttman bodies) ➔. Inclusions aid in the distinction from other histiocytic lesions.

TERMINOLOGY

Synonyms
- Malacoplakia

Definitions
- Mass-forming histiocytic infiltrate with characteristic cytoplasmic inclusions

ETIOLOGY/PATHOGENESIS

Infectious Agents
- *E. coli* and other gram-negative coliform bacilli
  - Defective phagocytosis of bacterial products by macrophages or monocytes
    - Secondary to defective phagolysosomal activity

CLINICAL ISSUES

Epidemiology
- Age
  - Wide age range from children to adults
    - Peak in 5th to 7th decades
- Gender
  - More common in females

Site
- Most common in bladder
  - Trigone region
- May also be seen in variety of other genitourinary and nonurinary sites

Presentation
- Bladder irritability and hematuria

Endoscopic Findings
- Polypoid mass covered by intact mucosa
- When large, may be confused with neoplastic process

Treatment
- Control of urinary tract infection
  - Antibiotics that concentrate in macrophages (e.g., quinolone, trimethoprim-sulfamethoxazole)
- Cholinergic agents may be beneficial

MACROSCOPIC FEATURES

General Features
- Single or multiple, soft yellow or yellow-brown plaques on mucosal surface
  - Vary greatly in size and number
- May appear nodular or polypoid
- Central umbilication or ulceration on larger nodules

MICROSCOPIC PATHOLOGY

Histologic Features
- Collection of histiocytes with granular eosinophilic cytoplasm (von Hansemann cells)
  - Scattered histiocytes contain Michaelis-Guttman bodies
    - Rounded concentric basophilic intracytoplasmic inclusions
    - In early lesions, may be small dot with surrounding halo
    - Accentuated by special stains
- Overlying urothelium may be ulcerated, hyperplastic, or metaplastic
- Associated inflammatory infiltrate composed of lymphocytes, plasma cells, and eosinophils
  - Abscess formation or granulation tissue may obscure typical findings
- Stromal reaction may be variable with fibroblastic proliferation or fibrosis

Predominant Pattern/Injury Type
- Diffuse

MALAKOPLAKIA

Key Facts

Terminology
- Mass-forming histiocytic infiltrate with characteristic cytoplasmic inclusions

Etiology/Pathogenesis
- *E. coli* and other gram-negative coliform bacilli
- Secondary to defective phagolysosomal activity

Clinical Issues
- Typically polypoid bladder mass covered with intact mucosa
- Treated by eradicating infection

Microscopic Pathology
- Sheets of round histiocytes with abundant eosinophilic granular cytoplasm (von Hansemann cells)
  - Round nuclei
  - Nucleoli variable
  - Rounded concentric basophilic intracytoplasmic inclusions (Michaelis-Guttman bodies)
  - Admixed acute and chronic inflammation common

Ancillary Tests
- Periodic acid-Schiff, von Kossa, and iron stains highlight intracytoplasmic inclusions
- Histiocytic markers (CD68 and CD163) show diffuse cytoplasmic immunoreactivity
- Cytokeratins are nonreactive in lesional cells

Top Differential Diagnoses
- Granulomatous inflammation
- Urothelial carcinoma
- Prostatic adenocarcinoma

Predominant Cell/Compartment Type
- Histiocyte/macrophage

ANCILLARY TESTS

Histochemistry
- von Kossa, iron stain, and periodic acid-Schiff
  - Highlight intracytoplasmic inclusions
  - PAS may be only positive stain in early lesions
    - Mineralization occurs later in disease process, so calcium and iron stains are negative

Immunohistochemistry
- Cytokeratins are nonreactive in lesional cells
- CD68 and CD163 show diffuse cytoplasmic reactivity

DIFFERENTIAL DIAGNOSIS

Urothelial Carcinoma
- Sheets of cells may suggest urothelial carcinoma
  - Poorly differentiated morphology
  - Lymphoma-like variant
- Cytokeratin stains should resolve difficult cases
  - Negative in malakoplakia; positive in carcinoma
- Urothelial carcinoma usually more pleomorphic with sheet-like growth pattern

Prostatic Adenocarcinoma
- Usually monomorphic, even if poorly differentiated
- May have areas with luminal formation
- Express cytokeratin, PSA, and PAP

Tuberculosis-associated Granulomatous Inflammation
- Acid-fast bacilli present by special stains
- Intracytoplasmic inclusions typical of malakoplakia not seen

Xanthogranulomatous Inflammation
- Morphologically and pathogenetically similar to malakoplakia
- Lack Michaelis-Guttman bodies

Histiocytic Sarcoma
- Generally have larger cells with more prominent cytoplasm
- More severe cytologic atypia may be present
- Michaelis-Guttman bodies absent

Myeloid Leukemia with Monocytic or Megakaryocytic Differentiation
- Myelomonocytic and megakaryocytic leukemias commonly have mass-forming disease outside bone marrow
- Usually show larger nuclei with greater cytologic atypia compared to reactive histiocytes
- May express blast markers by immunohistochemistry or flow cytometry

Extranodal Rosai-Dorfman Disease
- Histiocytes with emperipolesis

DIAGNOSTIC CHECKLIST

Pathologic Interpretation Pearls
- Michaelis-Guttman bodies may be difficult to visualize on H&E in early disease process
  - von Kossa (calcium), Perls stain (iron), and periodic acid-Schiff highlight inclusions

SELECTED REFERENCES

1. Long JP Jr et al: Malacoplakia: a 25-year experience with a review of the literature. J Urol. 141(6):1328-31, 1989
2. Curran FT: Malakoplakia of the bladder. Br J Urol. 59(6):559-63, 1987
3. McClure J: Malakoplakia. J Pathol. 140(4):275-330, 1983
4. Lou TY et al: Malakoplakia: pathogenesis and ultrastructural morphogenesis. A problem of altered macrophage (phagolysosomal) response. Hum Pathol. 5(2):191-207, 1974
5. Smith BH: Malacoplakia of the Urinary Tract: a study of twenty-four cases. Am J Clin Pathol. 43:409-17, 1965

MALAKOPLAKIA

Microscopic Features

(Left) Sheets of histiocytes with abundant eosinophilic cytoplasm are characteristic of malakoplakia. This pattern may suggest a carcinoma, but the cells stain with histiocytic markers, not keratin. *(Right)* Numerous intracytoplasmic inclusions (Michaelis-Guttman bodies) ⇨ are present within the eosinophilic histiocytes of malakoplakia. Identification of these characteristic inclusions are diagnostic of malakoplakia and help to exclude the possibility of other histiocytic infiltrates.

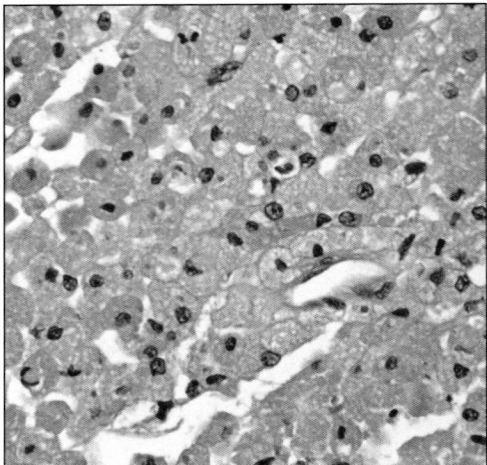
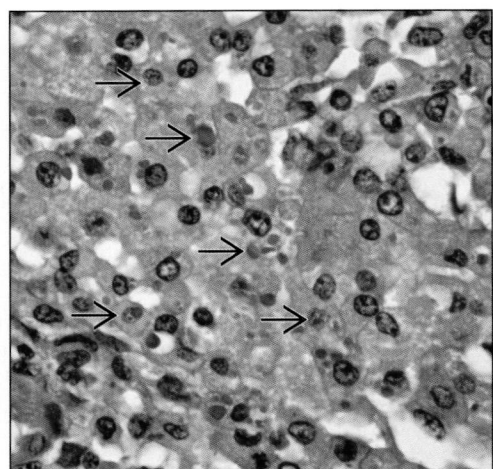

(Left) The eosinophilic histiocytes of malakoplakia ⇨ are often admixed with acute inflammation ⇨ as seen in this case. This may cause consideration of tuberculosis or fungal-associated granulomas. The nature of the inflammatory reaction varies between lesions. *(Right)* Under high-power examination with oil immersion, the lamellated nature of the intracytoplasmic Michaelis-Guttman bodies is evident ⇨. These inclusions are sufficient for a diagnosis of malakoplakia.

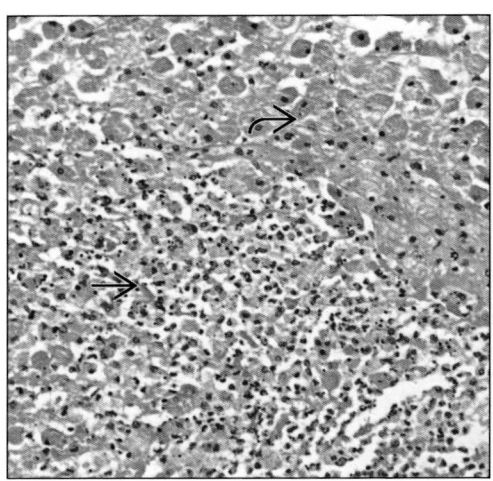
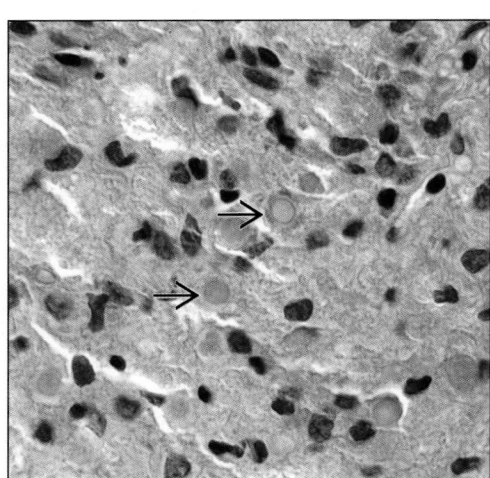

(Left) A von Kossa stain highlights innumerable intracytoplasmic inclusions (black dots) in this example of malakoplakia. In early lesions, prior to mineralization, von Kossa stains may be negative. PAS stains may be more useful in that setting. *(Right)* On high-power evaluation of this malakoplakia with of a von Kossa stain, there is a large Michaelis-Guttman body ⇨. Histiocytic markers may be useful if carcinoma is in the differential diagnosis.

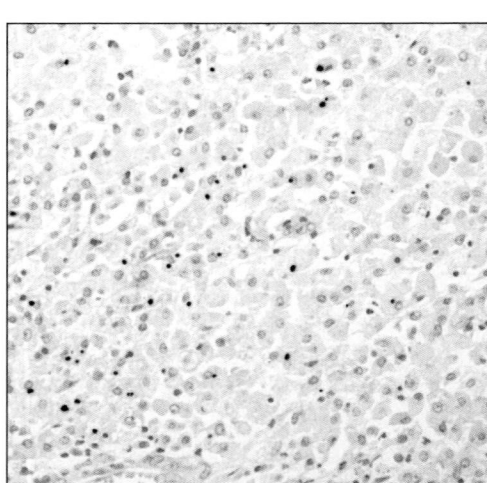
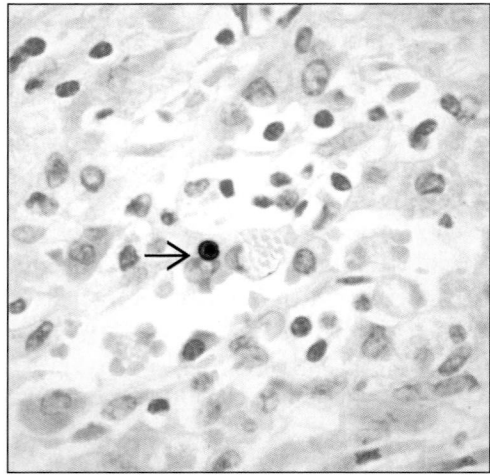

MALAKOPLAKIA

Differential Diagnosis with Carcinoma

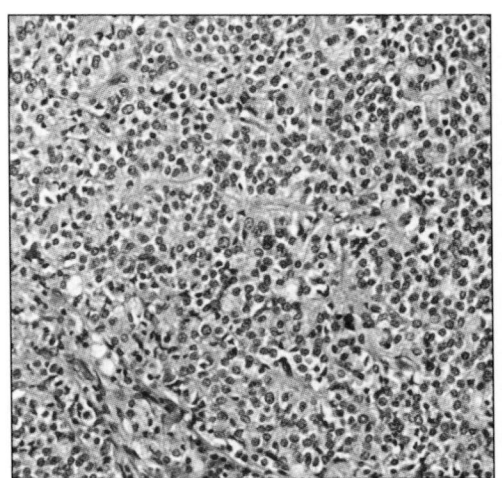
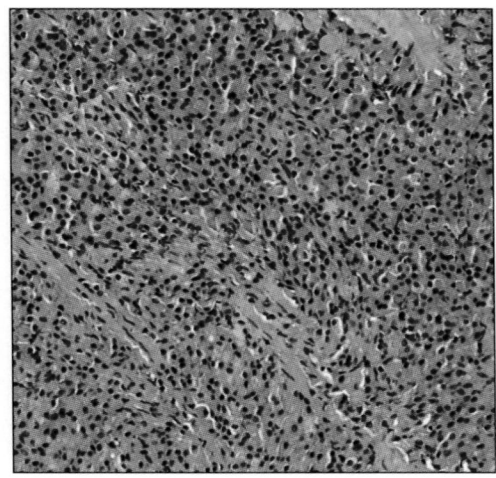

(Left) Gleason pattern 5 prostatic adenocarcinoma involving the urinary bladder may occasionally have a histiocyte-like appearance because of the round nuclei and sheet-like growth. (Right) This example of Gleason pattern 5 prostatic adenocarcinoma involving the bladder has eosinophilic cytoplasm that may prompt consideration of malakoplakia. Immunohistochemistry is helpful in difficult cases. Prostatic adenocarcinoma should express cytokeratin and PSA/PAP.

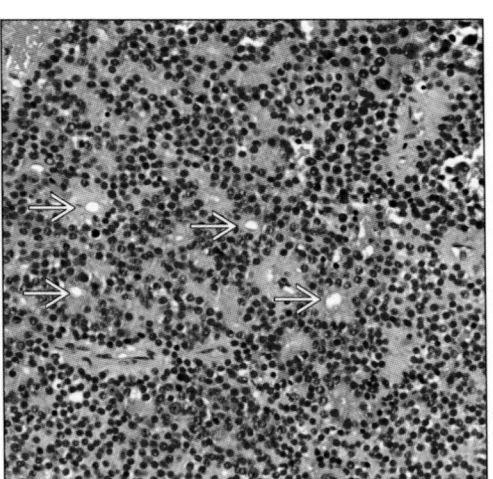
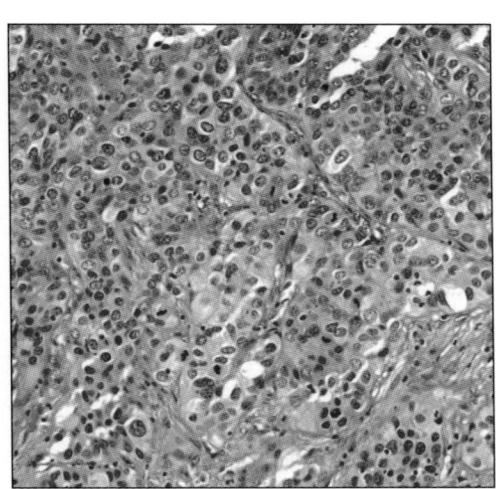

(Left) The identification of foci with luminal differentiation in this neoplasm greatly aids in recognizing prostatic adenocarcinoma ➡. (Right) Occasionally, invasive urothelial carcinoma of the usual type may have a sheet-like growth that may potentially raise the differential diagnostic consideration of a histiocytic infiltrate or inflammatory process. Plasmacytoid urothelial carcinoma is another pattern of urothelial carcinoma, which may mimic malakoplakia.

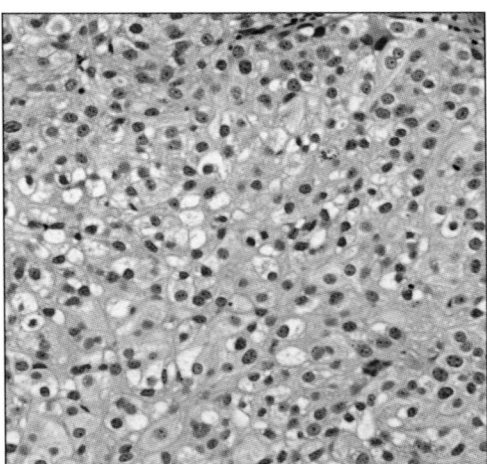
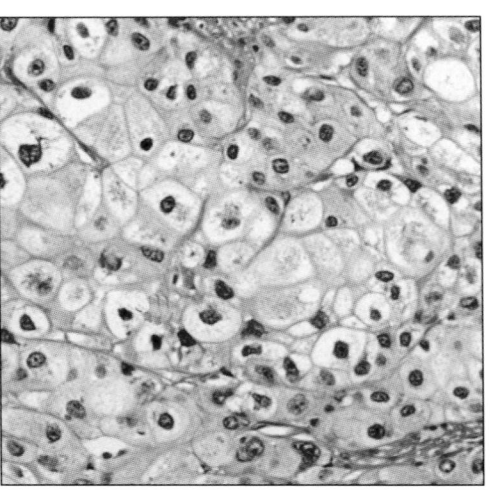

(Left) In this example of invasive urothelial carcinoma, the sheet-like growth is associated with more abundant frothy and lightly eosinophilic cytoplasm. These cells are more uniformly cohesive than typically expected in a histiocytic infiltrate, such as malakoplakia. (Right) At high-power evaluation of this invasive urothelial carcinoma, the abundant lightly eosinophilic cytoplasm with a frothy appearance and the relatively round nuclei may suggest histiocytes.

MALAKOPLAKIA

Differential Diagnosis with Carcinoma

(Left) This example of invasive urothelial carcinoma with an associated mixed inflammatory infiltrate has a morphology with striking resemblance to histiocytes ➡. *(Right)* On high-power evaluation, the neoplastic cells ➡ of this invasive urothelial carcinoma have abundant "frothy" cytoplasm that has marked overlap with histiocytes. Demonstration of cytokeratin reactivity with a broad spectrum keratin is important in difficult cases.

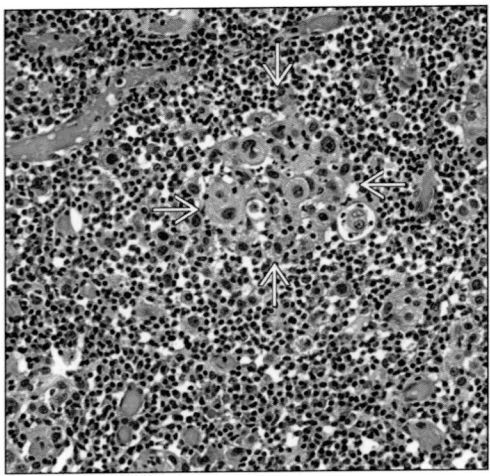 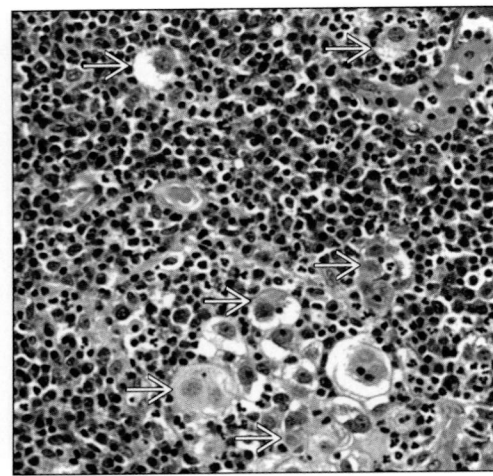

(Left) In this primary vesical signet ring cell adenocarcinoma, the cells infiltrate separately, which may suggest inflammatory cells, but the peripheral nuclei are more atypical ➡ than seen in histiocytes. *(Right)* Primary signet ring cell adenocarcinoma of the urinary bladder, as in other anatomic sites, may have morphologic overlap with histiocytes. The peripheral nuclei and intracytoplasmic mucin are distinctive features. The nuclei are often indented by the cytoplasmic contents.

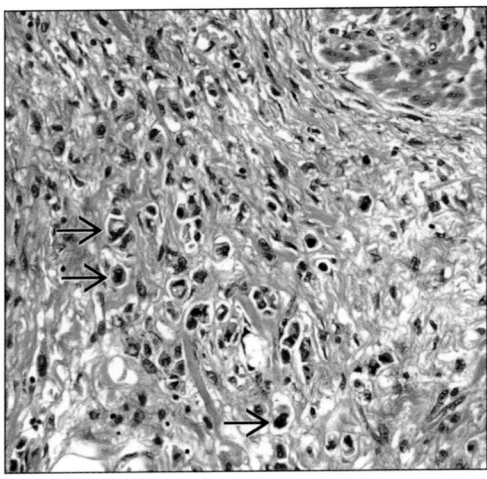 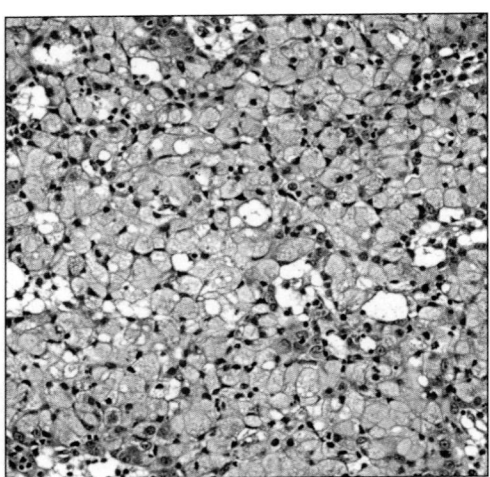

(Left) Invasive urothelial carcinoma may occasionally have a plasmacytoid or lymphoma-like morphology that may mimic a histiocytic infiltrate because of the round nuclei, discohesion, and sheet-like growth. *(Right)* On high-power evaluation, this invasive urothelial carcinoma has round nuclei and lightly eosinophilic cytoplasm that may potentially mimic a histiocytic infiltrate. Cytokeratin immunohistochemistry is very useful to confirm epithelial lineage.

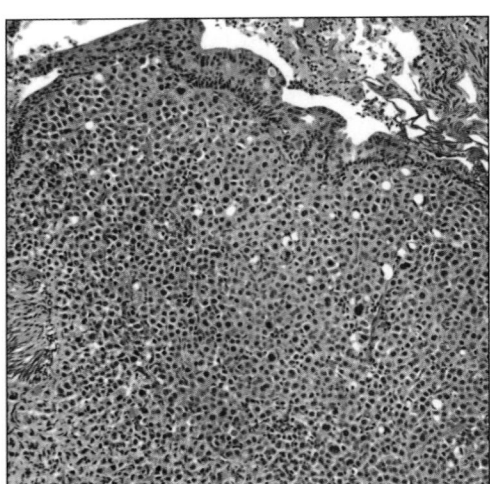 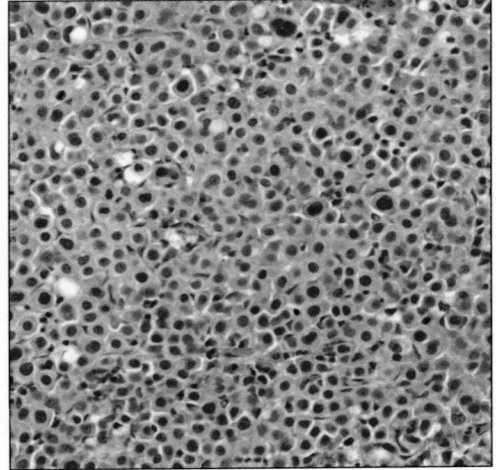

MALAKOPLAKIA

Differential Diagnosis

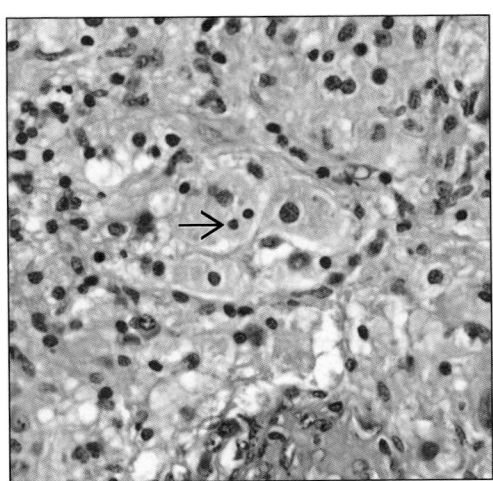
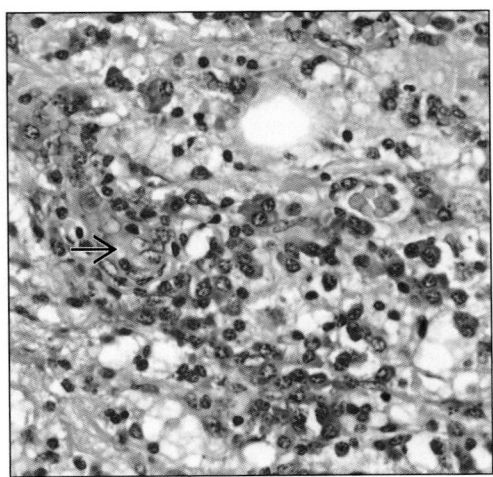

(Left) Extranodal Rosai-Dorfman disease is well documented in the genitourinary tract and may closely resemble other histiocytic infiltrates, such as malakoplakia. The histiocytes of Rosai-Dorfman disease often contain more voluminous cytoplasm and emperipolesis may be present ⇨. Emperipolesis may potentially mimic inclusions. (Right) Perivascular plasma cells (endothelial cells highlighted ⇨) are also characteristic of Rosai-Dorfman disease.

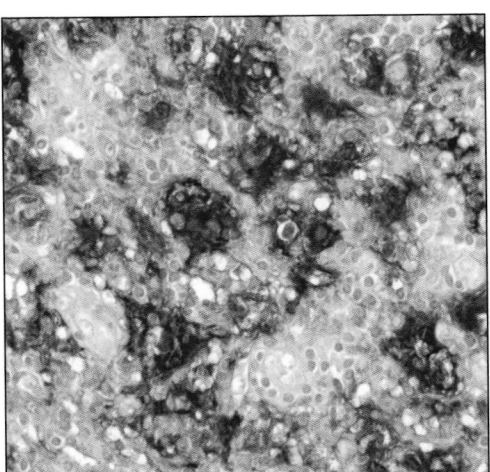
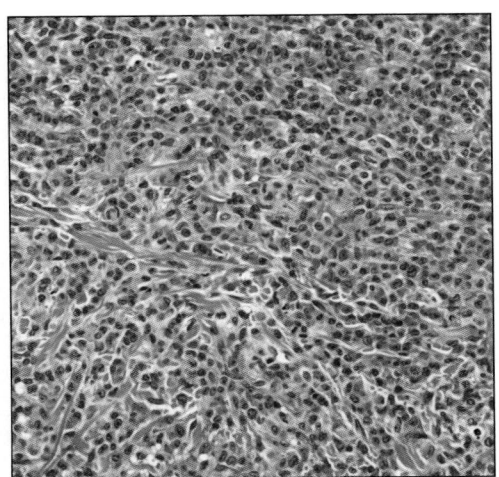

(Left) The histiocytes of Rosai-Dorfman disease, unlike malakoplakia, show diffuse cytoplasmic and nuclear reactivity for S100. (Right) Myeloid sarcoma, especially those with histiocytic or megakaryocytic differentiation, may present in parenchymal organs. The sheets of cells with amphophilic cytoplasm may provoke a differential that includes malakoplakia, especially since histiocytic markers may be positive.

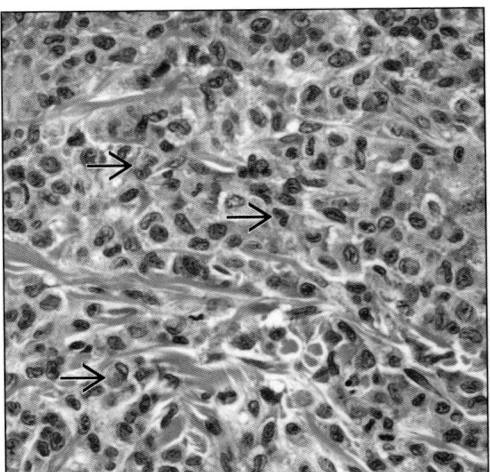
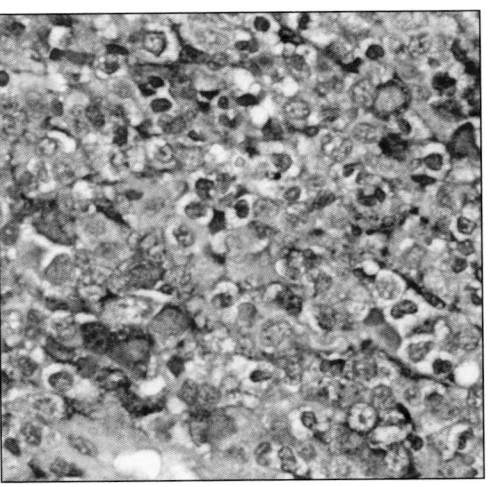

(Left) At high-power magnification of this myeloid sarcoma (myelomonocytic), the nuclear membranes are more irregular ⇨ than typically seen in reactive histiocytic lesions, and the nuclear to cytoplasmic ratio is higher. Flow cytometry and immunohistochemistry are important diagnostic adjuncts in this setting. (Right) Documentation of intracytoplasmic myeloperoxidase by immunohistochemistry establishes the diagnosis of acute myeloid leukemia in this case.

SCHISTOSOMIASIS

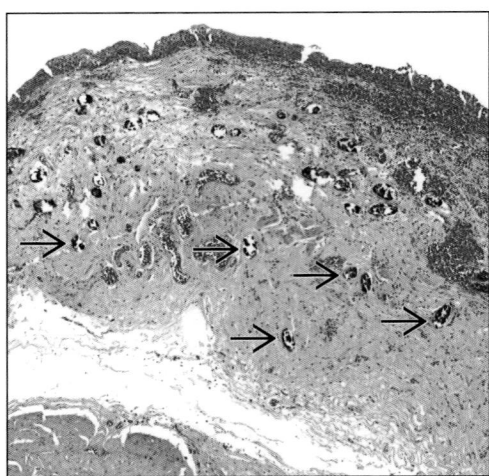

In this section of the urinary bladder, calcified Schistosoma haematobium eggs → fill the lamina propria and are associated with fibrosis and chronic inflammation.

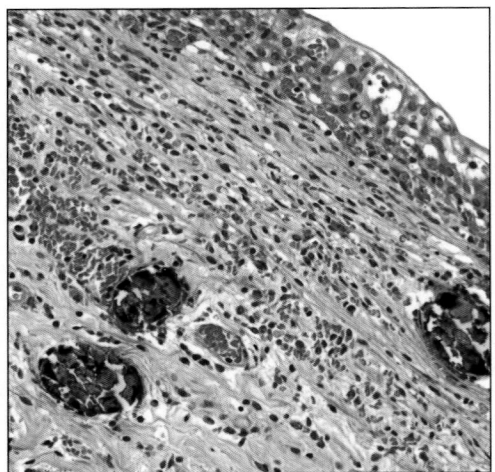

This high-power photomicrograph shows typical oval calcified Schistosoma haematobium eggs in the lamina propria of the urinary bladder.

TERMINOLOGY

Definitions
- Urinary bladder infection by *Schistosoma*

ETIOLOGY/PATHOGENESIS

Infectious Agents
- Water-borne trematode infection
  - *Schistosoma haematobium* infects bladder
  - *Schistosoma mansoni* and *Schistosoma japonicum* are typically intestinal infections
- Acquired by exposure to infected water
  - Eggs enter fresh water through urine or feces contamination
  - Larval stages develop in water
    - Freshwater snails are intermediate host
  - Infection of humans by penetration through skin within water source

CLINICAL ISSUES

Epidemiology
- Incidence
  - Endemic areas
    - Mediterranean and sub-Saharan Africa

Presentation
- Hematuria most common

Laboratory Tests
- Diagnosed by identifying eggs in urine
- Newer serologic tests
  - ELISA specific for *Schistosoma* antigens
    - Circulating cathodic antigen

Natural History
- Ova are deposited in veins of muscularis propria of bladder where they become permeable

  - Infiltrates bladder tissues and incites inflammatory reaction

Treatment
- Drugs
  - Medications with antischistosomal effect

Prognosis
- Morbidity and mortality is determined by parasitic burden, risk of reinfection, and chronicity
  - Untreated chronic infection has serious morbidity
    - Hydronephrosis
    - Pyelonephritis
    - Renal failure
- Predisposing factor for bladder carcinoma
  - Primary squamous cell carcinoma
    - Arises through squamous metaplasia-dysplasia-carcinoma sequence
  - Urothelial carcinoma or adenocarcinoma (less common)

MACROSCOPIC FEATURES

General Features
- Rough granular mucosal surface
  - "Sandy patches"
- Sharp ulcerations and transverse fissures
- Polyps less common

MICROSCOPIC PATHOLOGY

Histologic Features
- Numerous ova are present with surrounding inflammatory response
  - Granulomas
  - Chronic inflammation
  - Hemorrhage
  - Ulceration

SCHISTOSOMIASIS

Key Facts

Terminology
- Urinary bladder infection by *Schistosoma*

Etiology/Pathogenesis
- Water-borne trematode infection
  - *Schistosoma haematobium* infects bladder

Clinical Issues
- Endemic in eastern Mediterranean and sub-Saharan Africa

- Hematuria most common presentation
- Morbidity and mortality is determined by parasitic burden, risk of re-infection, and chronicity
  - Untreated chronic infection has serious morbidity
- Predisposing factor for squamous cell carcinoma

Top Differential Diagnoses
- Encrusted cystitis
- Selective internal radiation therapy (SIRT) microspheres

- In chronic infection, bladder wall may show extensive fibrosis
- Eggs calcify over time
- Associated keratinizing squamous metaplasia and dysplasia may be seen
- *Schistosoma haematobium* vs. *Schistosoma mansoni/Schistosoma japonicum*
  - Terminal spines seen in *S. haematobium*
    - *S. mansoni* has lateral spine
    - *S. japonicum* has no spine or small inconspicuous subterminal spine
  - *S. mansoni* and *S. japonicum* infection typically based in intestines

DIFFERENTIAL DIAGNOSIS

Encrusted Cystitis
- Irregular calcified aggregates distinct from rounded/oval calcified eggs
- May be seen in urinary bladder infections or overlying carcinoma
  - Usually in areas of necrosis

Selective Internal Radiation Therapy (SIRT) Microspheres
- Round microspheres may resemble *Schistosoma* ova
  - Greater awareness of this potential therapy effect reduces possibility of misidentification
    - More spherical than *Schistosoma* eggs

- Seen mostly in stomach and duodenum following intrahepatic treatment of metastatic colorectal adenocarcinoma
  - Other clinical uses may be emerging

DIAGNOSTIC CHECKLIST

Pathologic Interpretation Pearls
- Occasionally, infection is 1st diagnosed on bladder biopsy

SELECTED REFERENCES

1. Obeng BB et al: Application of a circulating-cathodic-antigen (CCA) strip test and real-time PCR, in comparison with microscopy, for the detection of Schistosoma haematobium in urine samples from Ghana. Ann Trop Med Parasitol. 102(7):625-33, 2008
2. Ghoneim MA: Bilharziasis of the genitourinary tract. BJU Int. 89 Suppl 1:22-30, 2002
3. Paul JF et al: Urinary schistosomiasis. Emerg Med J. 19(5):483-4, 2002
4. Elem B et al: Carcinoma of the urinary bladder in Zambia. A quantitative estimation of Schistosoma haematobium infection. Br J Urol. 55(3):275-8, 1983
5. El-Bolkainy MN et al: The impact of schistosomiasis on the pathology of bladder carcinoma. Cancer. 48(12):2643-8, 1981
6. Zahran MM et al: Bilharziasis of urinary bladder and ureter: comparative histopathologic study. Urology. 8(1):73-9, 1976

IMAGE GALLERY

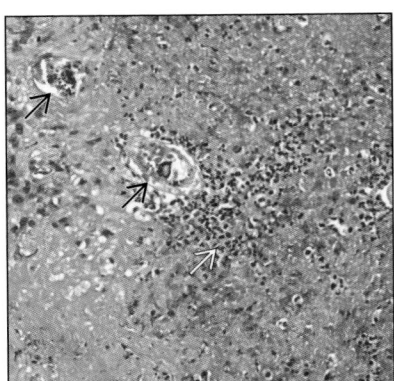 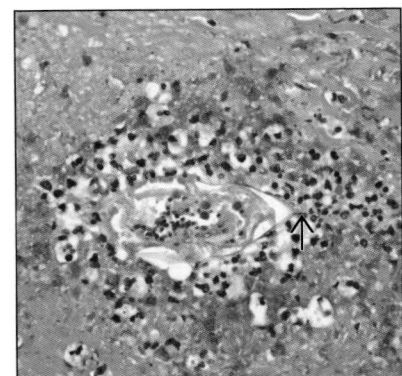 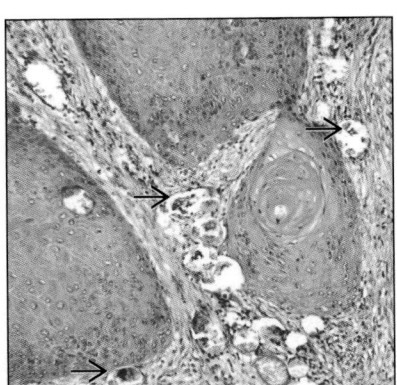

(Left) These noncalcified Schistosoma eggs ⊞ are associated with a marked acute inflammatory infiltrate ⊞, as typically seen. *(Center)* On high-power examination, the terminal spine ⊞ of this noncalcified Schistosoma haematobium egg is evident. *(Right)* This invasive keratinizing squamous cell carcinoma is associated with Schistosoma eggs ⊞.

VON BRUNN NESTS

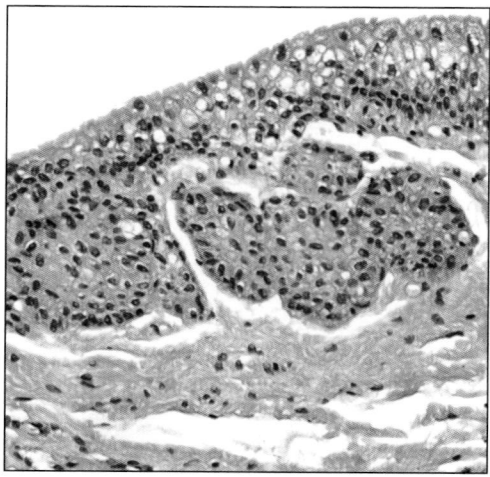

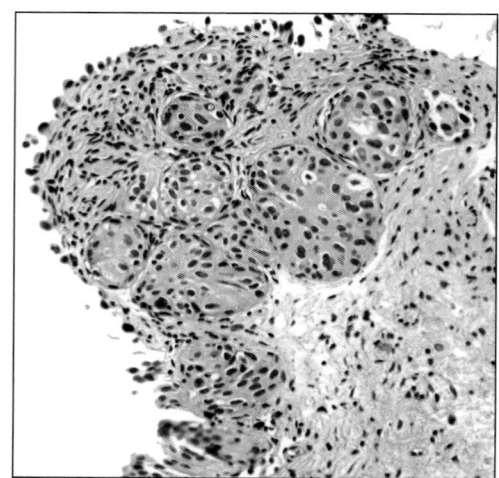

von Brunn nests are cytologically benign invaginations of urothelium into the lamina propria. These nests are very common and represent a variant of normal histology.

von Brunn nests are characterized by aggregated individual urothelial nests with a lobular arrangement. There is typically a sharp linear border at the junction with the lamina propria.

TERMINOLOGY

Synonyms
- Proliferative cystitis

Definitions
- Reactive proliferative change of urothelium
- Invaginated nests of cytologically benign urothelial cells in lamina propria
  - May or may not have continuity with surface epithelium

ETIOLOGY/PATHOGENESIS

Etiology
- Variant of normal urothelial histology
- May occur as a result of local inflammation

CLINICAL ISSUES

Epidemiology
- Incidence
  - Common finding in 85-95% of bladders
- Age
  - Frequency increases with age

Site
- Bladder trigone, renal pelvis, and ureter, in decreasing order of frequency

Presentation
- Usually incidental microscopic finding

Prognosis
- Entirely benign
  - Not a neoplastic precursor lesion
  - Does not require therapy

MACROSCOPIC FEATURES

General Features
- Typically < 5 mm in diameter
- Most are not grossly visible
  - May occasionally be cystoscopically visible when prominent
  - May appear as mucosal blebs

MICROSCOPIC PATHOLOGY

Histologic Features
- Solid nests of urothelial cells in superficial lamina propria; variable continuity with surface urothelium
  - Nests typically have smooth, round contours
    - Some examples have minor branching of nests and some minimal confluence
  - Clustered individual nests have orderly arrangement
    - Evenly spaced with lobular configuration
  - Sharp epithelial-stromal interface with linear border at deep aspect
  - Urothelial cells within nests do not have dysplastic features
    - Normal cytology similar to overlying surface urothelium
- May be associated with other florid conditions, including cystitis cystica and cystitis glandularis
- Inflammation is typically minimal
- Stromal reaction is absent

Cytologic Features
- Identical to normal urothelium

Predominant Pattern/Injury Type
- Nests

VON BRUNN NESTS

Key Facts

Terminology
- Reactive proliferative change of urothelium
- Invaginated nests of cytologically benign urothelial cells in lamina propria

Etiology/Pathogenesis
- Variant of normal urothelial histology
- May occur as a result of local inflammation

Clinical Issues
- Common finding in 85-95% of bladders
- Usually incidental microscopic finding
- Entirely benign

Microscopic Pathology
- Solid nests of urothelial cells in superficial lamina propria
- Nests have smooth, round contours
- Some examples have minimal branching of nests
- Evenly spaced nests with lobular configuration
- Sharp linear border at deep junction with lamina propria
- Urothelial cells do not have dysplastic features
- Variable continuity with surface urothelium

Top Differential Diagnoses
- Nested variant of urothelial carcinoma
- Inverted papilloma
- Carcinoid tumor
- Paraganglioma and normal paraganglionic cells

Diagnostic Checklist
- In superficial biopsies, may have significant morphologic overlap with nested urothelial carcinoma

DIFFERENTIAL DIAGNOSIS

Nested Variant of Urothelial Carcinoma
- Typically larger lesion
- In very superficial biopsies, may be histologically indistinguishable from von Brunn nests
- In contrast to von Brunn nests, has disorganized arrangement of nests
  - Nonlobular configuration with random distribution often into deep lamina propria
  - Irregular invasion of muscularis propria is diagnostic of carcinoma
  - Nests often have greater confluence at least focally
  - Subtle stromal retraction may also be seen around invasive nests
  - May be associated with more typical urothelial carcinoma

Inverted Papilloma
- More numerous and crowded urothelial nests
- Peripheral basal palisading of neoplastic cells is common
- Trabecular architecture are also common
- Spindling of cells, particularly in the center, within nests may be seen
- Distinction of florid von Brunn nests from inverted papilloma may be arbitrary in some cases
  - Size of lesion and presence of cystoscopic lesion are helpful in diagnosis of lesion
  - Greater epithelial to stromal presence in lesion favors neoplasia

Carcinoid Tumor
- Rare tumor in urinary bladder
- Mixed nested and trabecular architecture common
  - May create significant morphologic overlap with von Brunn nests in superficial biopsies
- Typically larger tumor
- More crowded and numerous epithelial nests
- Neoplastic cells with stippled chromatin
- Coexpresses cytokeratin and neuroendocrine markers by immunohistochemistry

Paraganglioma and Normal Paraganglionic Cells
- Nests usually more numerous and crowded
- Vascular septae may be prominent
- Not confined to superficial location
- Scattered "neuroendocrine type" nuclear atypia
- Express synaptophysin and chromogranin
- Do not express cytokeratin, as would be expected in urothelial cells
- Rarely, paraganglionic cells are present as small nests with amphophilic cytoplasm

DIAGNOSTIC CHECKLIST

Pathologic Interpretation Pearls
- In superficial biopsies, may have significant morphologic overlap with nested urothelial carcinoma
- Florid proliferations and those associated with inflammation (greater cytologic atypia and distortion of contours of nests) result in diagnostic difficulty
- Clinical presentation should be carefully reviewed in superficial biopsies thought to represent a mass lesion
  - Nested urothelial carcinoma should be considered in cases with any aggressive clinical findings, such as large mass lesion or ureteral obstruction

SELECTED REFERENCES

1. Volmar KE et al: Florid von Brunn nests mimicking urothelial carcinoma: a morphologic and immunohistochemical comparison to the nested variant of urothelial carcinoma. Am J Surg Pathol. 27(9):1243-52, 2003
2. Wiener DP et al: The prevalence and significance of Brunn's nests, cystitis cystica and squamous metaplasia in normal bladders. J Urol. 122(3):317-21, 1979
3. Goldstein AM et al: New concepts on formation of Brunn's nests and cysts in urinary tract mucosa. Urology. 11(5):513-7, 1978
4. Mostofi FK: Potentialities of bladder epithelium. J Urol. 71(6):705-14, 1954

Microscopic Features

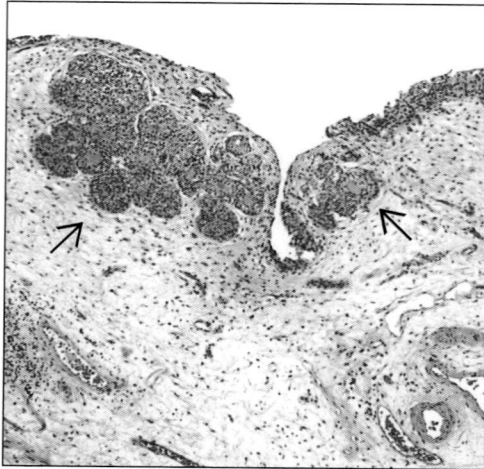
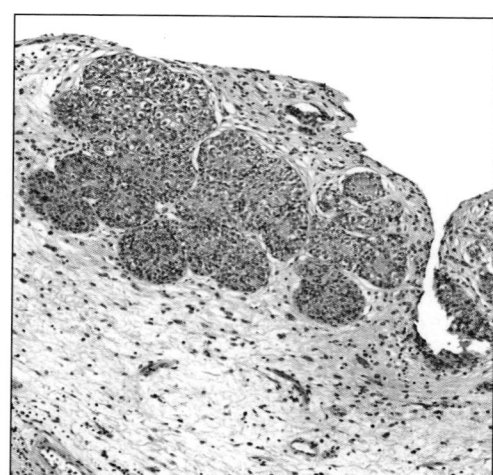

(Left) This low-power image shows the characteristic superficial location of von Brunn nests ➡. There is a sharp linear border at the base of the urothelial nests, a feature that is key to the distinction from urothelial carcinoma. *(Right)* These von Brunn nests have the typical rounded contours and are aggregated into tight superficial clusters. Carcinomas typically have a more random distribution and deeper extension into the lamina propria (or muscularis propria).

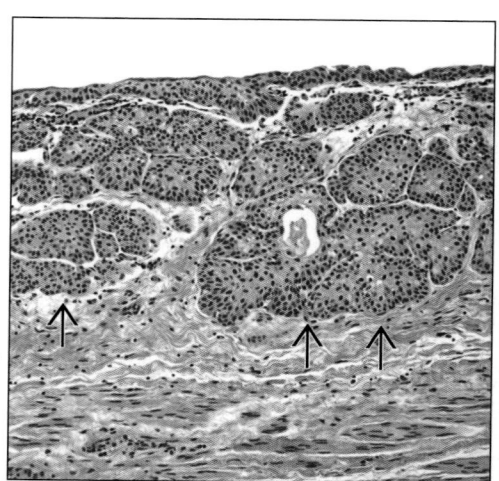
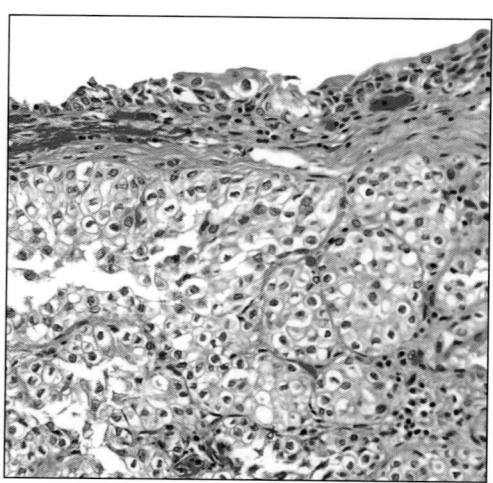

(Left) This example of von Brunn nests is characterized by multiple groups of clustered urothelial nests with a superficial location and sharp border ➡ at the lower junction with the lamina propria. *(Right)* Some examples of von Brunn nests have clear cytoplasm, which may occasionally suggest the possibility of renal cell carcinoma. The superficial location of the nests and well-delineated/lobular architecture, as well as the clinical history, should help in this distinction.

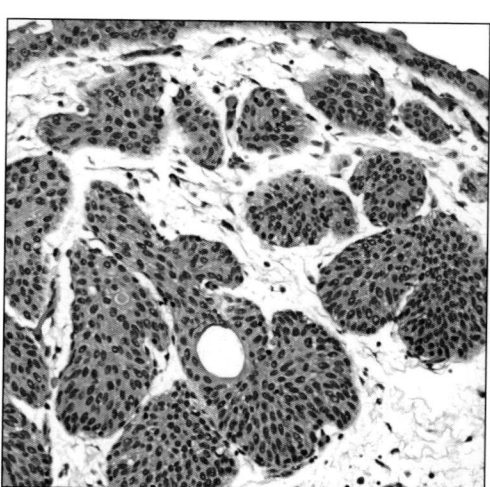
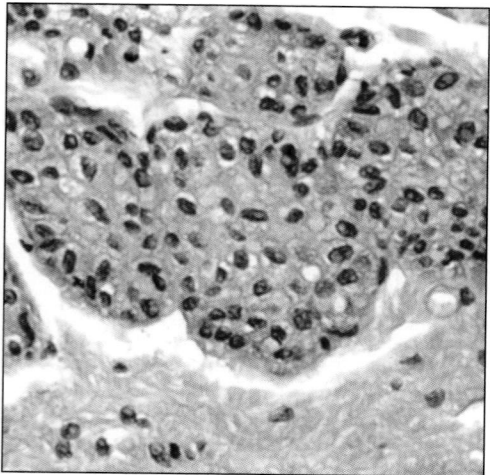

(Left) The individual urothelial aggregates of von Brunn nests may have some degree of branching, as in this example. There is often no demonstrable connection with the overlying urothelium. The overall organized architecture argues for a benign designation. *(Right)* von Brunn nests have small nuclei and bland cytologic features. Some nested carcinomas share similar features; hence, appreciation of the architecture is important to distinguish von Brunn nests from subtle patterns of carcinoma.

VON BRUNN NESTS

Differential Diagnosis

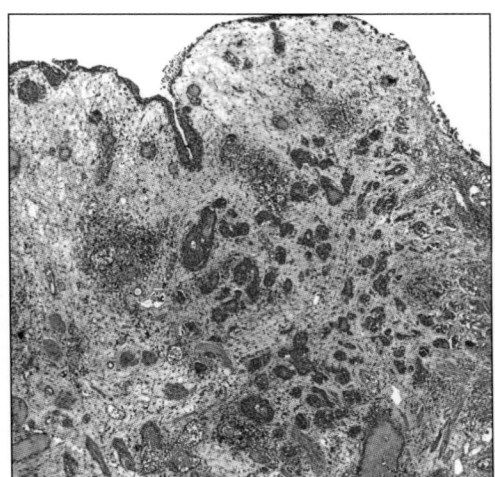
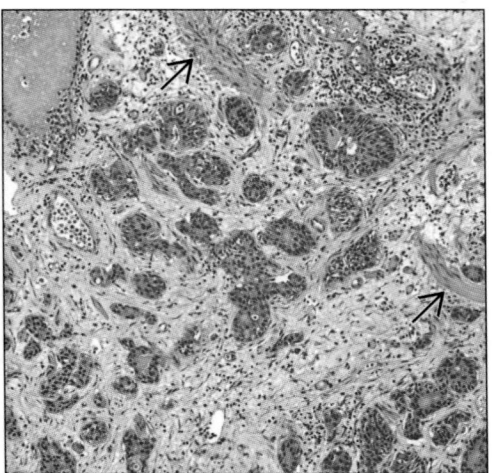

(Left) This photomicrograph highlights the deep, irregular invasion of the lamina propria by nested urothelial carcinoma. The nests lack the aggregated, lobular arrangement typical of von Brunn nests, which are more superficial with a sharp linear border at the base. *(Right)* Nested urothelial carcinomas show deeper invasion into the lamina propria with involvement of the muscularis mucosae ➡. Deep involvement is not seen with von Brunn nests and is diagnostic of neoplasia.

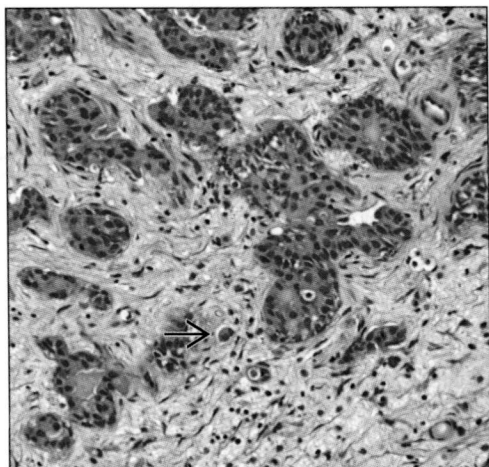
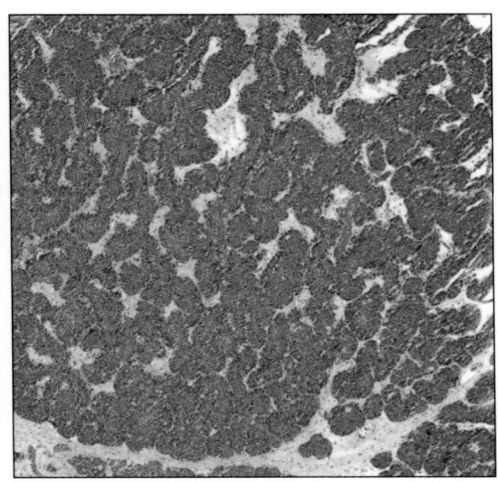

(Left) Clues to the diagnosis of nested carcinoma include more variation in size and shape of urothelial nests and small clusters with retraction ➡. The cytology of the malignant cells is extremely bland, which adds to the degree of histologic overlap with von Brunn nests. *(Right)* Inverted papillomas also have an endophytic growth into the lamina propria, but they typically show a more trabecular, anastomosing growth pattern.

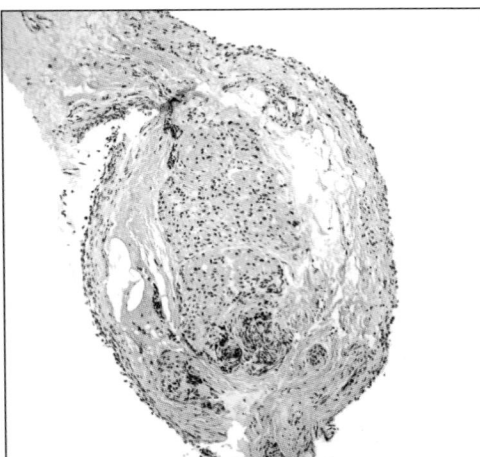
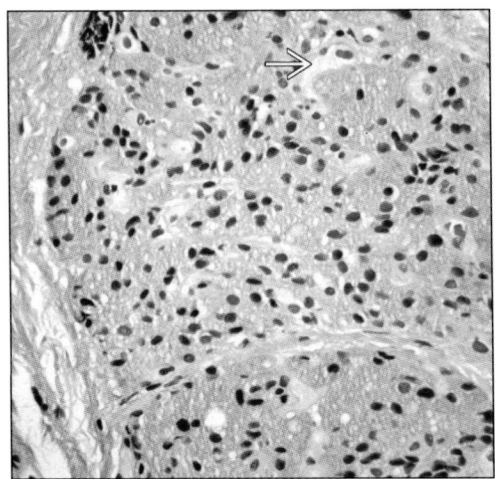

(Left) Paraganglionic tissue in a biopsy specimen shows the lesion is well demarcated & unrelated to urothelium. Paraganglia are present in the lamina propria, rarely in muscularis propria or deeper. Distinction from von Brunn nests is not that critical. *(Right)* In this paraganglionic tissue, note nested architecture with abundant amphophilic cytoplasm & fine blood vessels (sinusoidal pattern) ➡ between nests. In small biopsy specimens, distinction from a paraganglioma may not be tenable.

NEPHROGENIC ADENOMA

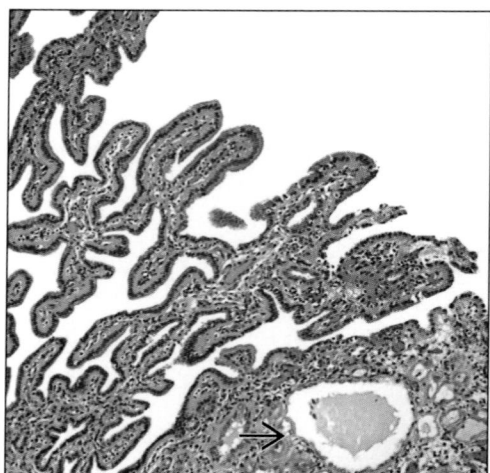

Mixed exophytic papillary, cystic, and tubular patterns ⊅ of nephrogenic adenoma are common. The papillary cores are characteristically lined by a single layer of cuboidal epithelial cells.

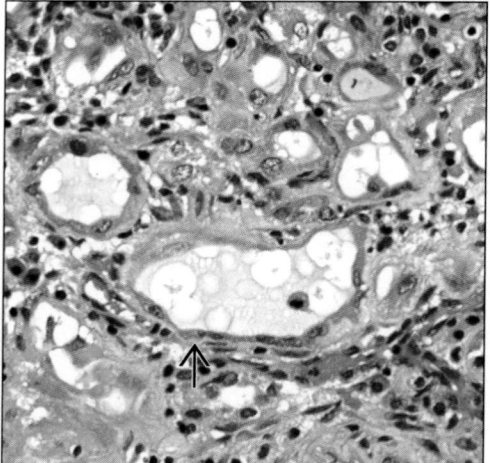

Nephrogenic adenoma commonly shows a tubular pattern in the lamina propria with variably sized lumina lined by flattened atrophic epithelium ⊅. Intraluminal mucinous material is also common.

TERMINOLOGY

Abbreviations
- Nephrogenic adenoma (NA)

Synonyms
- Nephrogenic metaplasia

Definitions
- Benign epithelial lesion of urinary tract characterized by tubular, glandular, &/or papillary growth pattern that commonly occurs secondary to injury of urothelium or renal transplant

ETIOLOGY/PATHOGENESIS

Injury of Urothelium
- Many are secondary to urothelial injury
  - Infections, calculi, instrumentation, intravesical bacillus Calmette-Guérin (BCG) therapy, and surgery

Renal Transplant
- Frequent in these patients; supports proposed renal tubular origin

CLINICAL ISSUES

Presentation
- Usually incidental microscopic finding
  - Difficult to attribute irritative voiding symptoms to NA given other associated inflammatory findings

Treatment
- Simple curetting for larger lesions

Prognosis
- Completely benign, but recurrence is described

MACROSCOPIC FEATURES

General Features
- May appear as papillary-polypoid mass or irregular, flat, velvety lesion

MICROSCOPIC PATHOLOGY

Histologic Features
- Broad architectural spectrum
  - Tubular/glandular pattern most common
    - Low-power architecture may appear pseudoinfiltrative
  - Exophytic papillary cores lined by single cuboidal epithelial layer
  - Lining cells may have "hobnail" appearance
  - Cystic pattern with dilated tubules lined by variably atrophic epithelium
  - Single cells with minute lumen may closely mimic blood vessels or signet ring cells
  - Rare cases have myxoid stroma and cording or spindling of cells (fibromyxoid pattern)
  - Rare cases have diffuse sheet-like growth
- Thick basement membrane/hyalinized sheath may underlie epithelium
- Cytoplasm varies from eosinophilic to clear
- Nucleoli may be present
- Degenerative-type atypia may be present

Predominant Pattern/Injury Type
- Glandular

Predominant Cell/Compartment Type
- Epithelial

ANCILLARY TESTS

Immunohistochemistry
- Express cytokeratins, pax-2, and pax-8

NEPHROGENIC ADENOMA

Key Facts

Etiology/Pathogenesis
- Many are secondary to urothelial injury

Clinical Issues
- Usually incidental microscopic findings
  - May have irritative symptoms from underlying inflammatory process

Macroscopic Features
- May appear as papillary-polypoid mass or irregular flat velvety lesion

Microscopic Pathology
- Papillary cores lined by single cuboidal epithelial layer
- Tubular pattern with "hobnail" arrangement of epithelial cells

- Rare cases have myxoid stroma and cording or spindling of cells (fibromyxoid pattern)
- Rare cases have diffuse sheet-like growth
- Thick basement membrane/hyalinized sheath may underlie epithelium
- Degenerative-type atypia may be present

Ancillary Tests
- Express cytokeratins, pax-2, and pax-8
- May express PSA, PAP, and AMACR

Top Differential Diagnoses
- Clear cell adenocarcinoma of bladder
- Prostatic adenocarcinoma
- Urothelial carcinoma with glandular differentiation
- Nested or tubular variant of urothelial carcinoma
- Papillary urothelial neoplasia

- May express PSA, PAP (rare), and AMACR (common)
  - Potential confusion with prostate cancer

DIFFERENTIAL DIAGNOSIS

Clear Cell Adenocarcinoma of Urinary Bladder
- Often mixed papillary and cystic tubular patterns
  - Histologic overlap with NA may be striking
- Prominent nuclear pleomorphism
- Mitotically active
- May show high proliferation rate by Ki-67
- May express p53 and CA125

Prostatic Adenocarcinoma
- Typically more homogeneous glands
  - Cystic and atrophic patterns uncommon
  - Thick hyalinized sheaths not typical of prostate cancer
- Prostatic adenocarcinoma involving urinary bladder is typically high Gleason grade
  - Solid or cribriform architecture common
- Does not express pax-2 and pax-8
- Often has elevated serum PSA

Urothelial Carcinoma with Glandular Differentiation
- Admixed typical urothelial carcinoma may be present
  - Papillary, in situ, or invasive
- Subset express uroplakin and GATA3
- Typically deeply invasive

Nested or Tubular Variant of Urothelial Carcinoma
- Admixed typical urothelial carcinoma may be present
  - Papillary, in situ, or invasive
- More irregular nests of urothelium
- Deep, irregular infiltration of lamina propria or muscularis propria
- Stromal clefting around invasive foci is common
- Usually express p63

Papillary Urothelial Carcinoma
- Lined by stratified layer of urothelium
- Admixed tubular/glandular pattern uncommon
- Frequently express urothelial markers
  - Uroplakin, GATA3, p63, and CK20

DIAGNOSTIC CHECKLIST

Clinically Relevant Pathologic Features
- Frequently misinterpreted as adenocarcinoma

Pathologic Interpretation Pearls
- Knowledge of wide spectrum of morphologic patterns is essential
- NA may express immunohistochemical markers expected in prostate cancer

SELECTED REFERENCES

1. Rahemtullah A et al: Nephrogenic adenoma: an update on an innocuous but troublesome entity. Adv Anat Pathol. 13(5):247-55, 2006
2. Tong GX et al: PAX2: a reliable marker for nephrogenic adenoma. Mod Pathol. 19(3):356-63, 2006
3. Skinnider BF et al: Expression of alpha-methylacyl-CoA racemase (P504S) in nephrogenic adenoma: a significant immunohistochemical pitfall compounding the differential diagnosis with prostatic adenocarcinoma. Am J Surg Pathol. 28(6):701-5, 2004
4. Allan CH et al: Nephrogenic adenoma of the prostatic urethra: a mimicker of prostate adenocarcinoma. Am J Surg Pathol. 25(6):802-8, 2001
5. Oliva E et al: Nephrogenic adenoma of the urinary tract: a review of the microscopic appearance of 80 cases with emphasis on unusual features. Mod Pathol. 8(7):722-30, 1995
6. Young RH et al: Nephrogenic adenoma. A report of 15 cases, review of the literature, and comparison with clear cell adenocarcinoma of the urinary tract. Am J Surg Pathol. 10(4):268-75, 1986

NEPHROGENIC ADENOMA

Microscopic Features

(Left) Mixed papillary ➡ and tubular patterns (visible in lower half of slide) are common in nephrogenic adenoma. This example of nephrogenic adenoma also shows variation from eosinophilic to clear cytoplasm. *(Right)* Other mixed patterns of nephrogenic adenoma are also common and include predominant tubular pattern, more atrophic-appearing tubular structures ➡, and cystically dilated tubules lined by "hobnail" cells ➡.

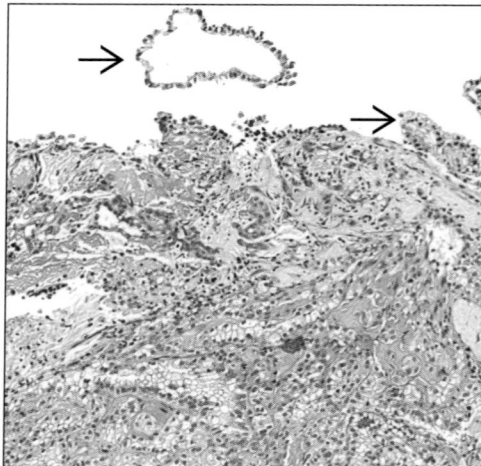
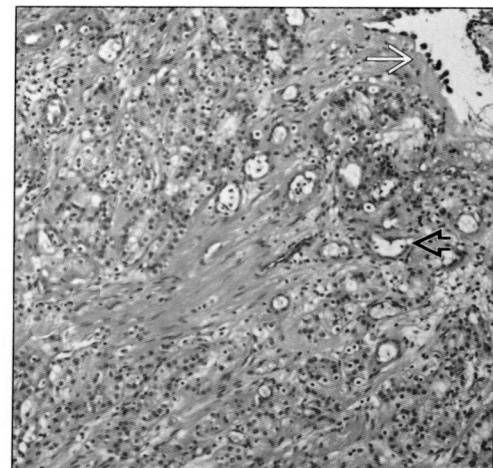

(Left) Nephrogenic adenoma commonly has cystically dilated glands ➡ and signet ring-like cells with intraluminal mucin ➡. Plump single epithelial cells, as seen in the upper right ➡, are also common. *(Right)* Tightly packed tubules of nephrogenic adenoma may create a solid appearance simulating a carcinoma or paraganglioma. This architectural pattern may be difficult to recognize, but multiple patterns are often intermixed to aid in the differential diagnosis.

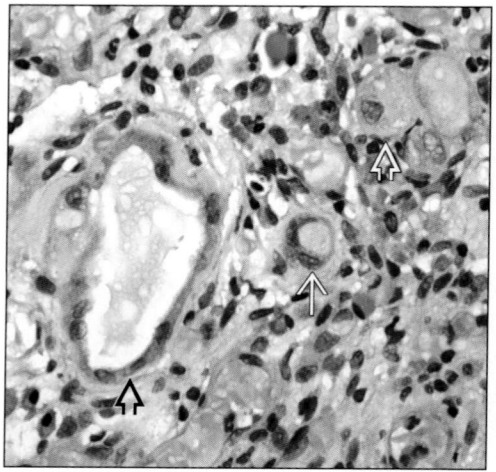
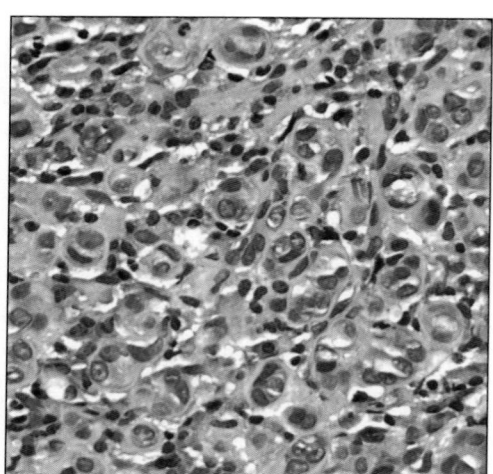

(Left) This example of nephrogenic adenoma has a pure tubular pattern. The monotonous round nuclear contours, as seen in this case, may closely mimic invasive prostatic adenocarcinoma. *(Right)* The tubular pattern of nephrogenic adenoma may appear pseudoinfiltrative, another feature that may be confused with prostatic carcinoma. It is important to carefully consider nephrogenic adenoma in bladder and urethral biopsies. The immunohistochemical overlap further compounds the problem.

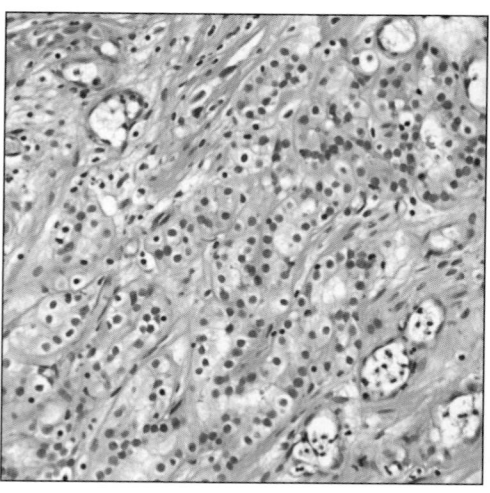
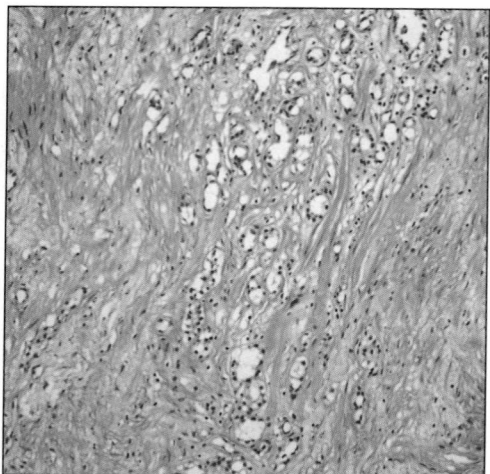

NEPHROGENIC ADENOMA

Variant Microscopic Features and Immunohistochemistry

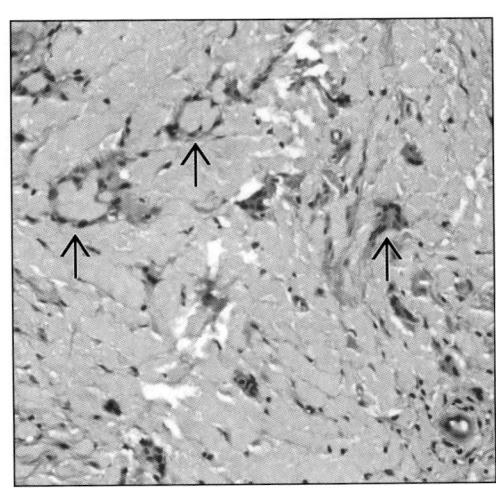
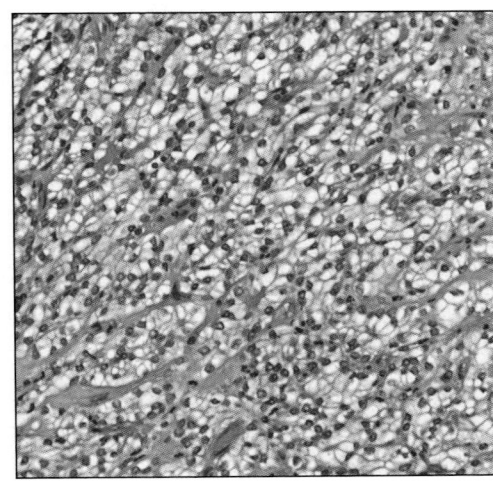

(Left) The fibromyxoid pattern of nephrogenic adenoma is characterized by prominent myxoid stroma and scattered irregular cords of epithelium ➡️. Awareness of this rare pattern is important since it may possibly mimic myxoid mesenchymal neoplasms. *(Right)* Solid growth in nephrogenic adenoma has been described as having a diffuse pattern, which is usually admixed with more typical patterns of nephrogenic adenoma but may be confused with renal cell carcinoma.

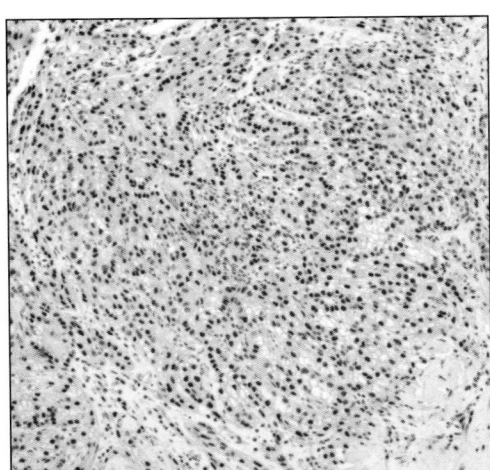
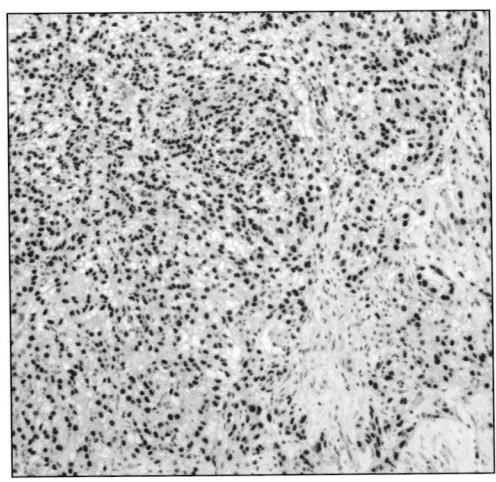

(Left) Diffuse nuclear pax-2 expression is characteristic of nephrogenic adenoma; however, it is also seen in other lesions, such as clear cell renal cell carcinoma and clear cell adenocarcinoma. *(Right)* Diffuse nuclear pax-8 expression is also seen in nephrogenic adenoma but is not entirely specific. Pax-8 stains a spectrum of other benign and malignant neoplasms similar to pax-2 but has not been shown to stain prostate carcinoma.

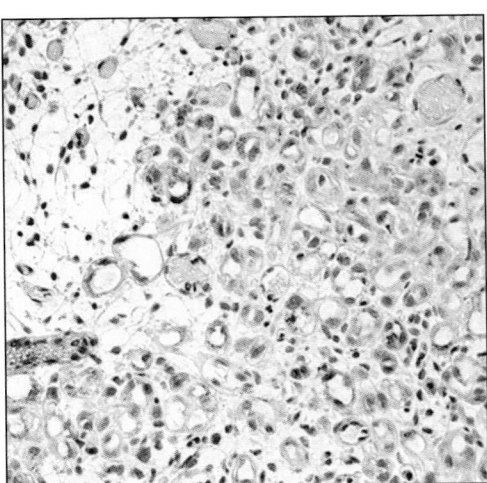
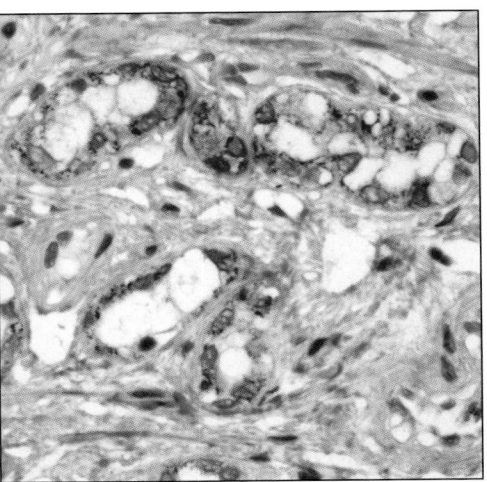

(Left) AMACR reactivity in nephrogenic adenoma is well documented and may cause added diagnostic confusion with prostatic adenocarcinoma. It is important to realize that AMACR is not a lineage-specific marker and may stain a spectrum of carcinomas. *(Right)* Strong cytoplasmic immunoreactivity for PSA may be seen in nephrogenic adenoma. This finding represents a major diagnostic pitfall in the distinction from prostatic adenocarcinoma.

Differential Diagnosis

(Left) Invasive prostatic adenocarcinoma may closely mimic nephrogenic adenoma given the tubular pattern and monomorphic nuclei. Prostatic adenocarcinoma involving the urinary bladder is typically of higher Gleason grade. *(Right)* This prostatic carcinoma shows the potential morphologic overlap with nephrogenic adenoma. In difficult cases, pax-2/pax-8 immunohistochemistry may be useful as it is positive in nephrogenic adenoma. Strong PSA/PAP argues for a diagnosis of prostate cancer.

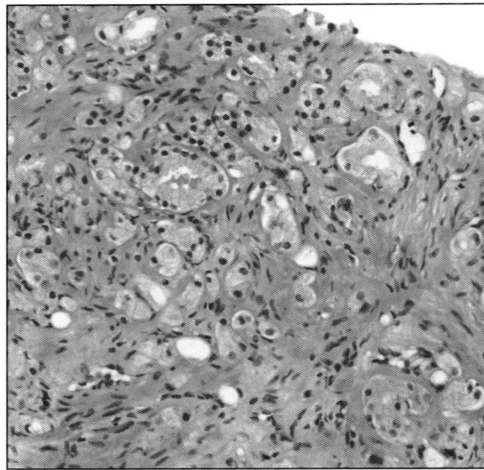
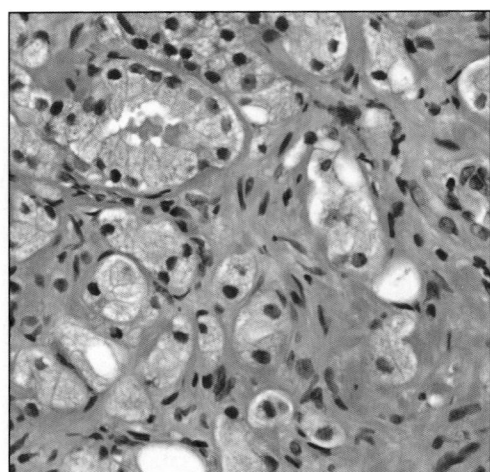

(Left) Papillary urothelial carcinoma is distinct from the papillary component of nephrogenic adenoma because of the stratified layer of epithelium. *(Right)* In contrast to papillary NA that is characterized by a single cuboidal layer of epithelium lining the papillary cores, papillary urothelial neoplasms have a stratified layer of epithelium. An accompanying endophytic component is rare in urothelial neoplasms, whereas it is typical in NA.

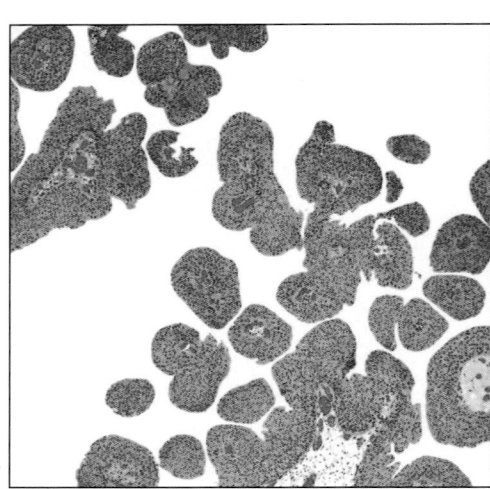
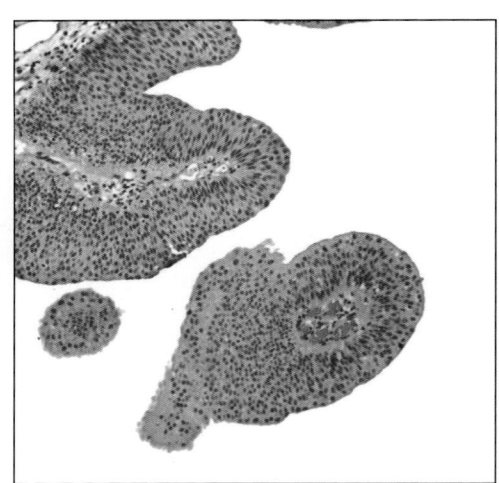

(Left) Clear cell adenocarcinoma of the urinary bladder, as seen in this example, may also have a papillary growth pattern with a single cuboidal lining. In contrast to papillary nephrogenic adenoma, clear cell adenocarcinoma has a greater degree of nuclear atypia and may have areas of epithelial stratification and tufting. *(Right)* Papillary areas of clear cell adenocarcinoma may closely mimic nephrogenic adenoma but have a greater degree of cytologic atypia.

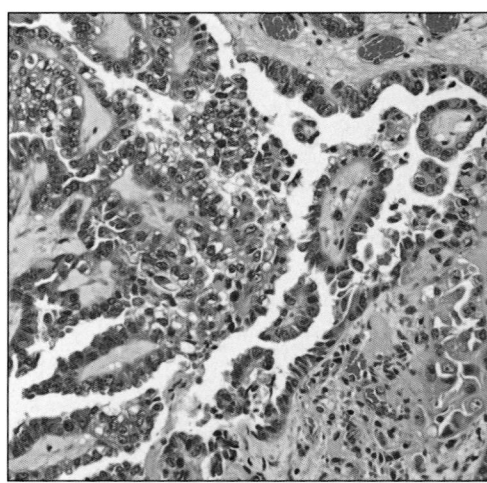
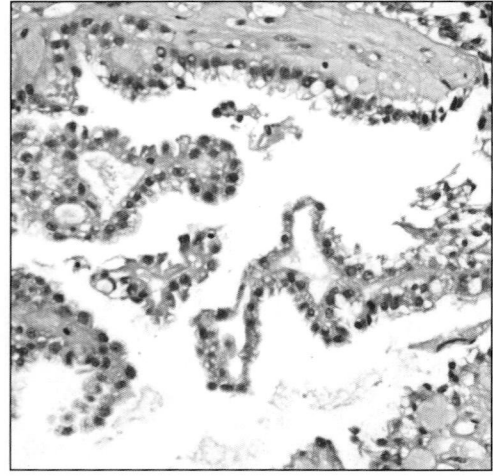

NEPHROGENIC ADENOMA

Differential Diagnosis

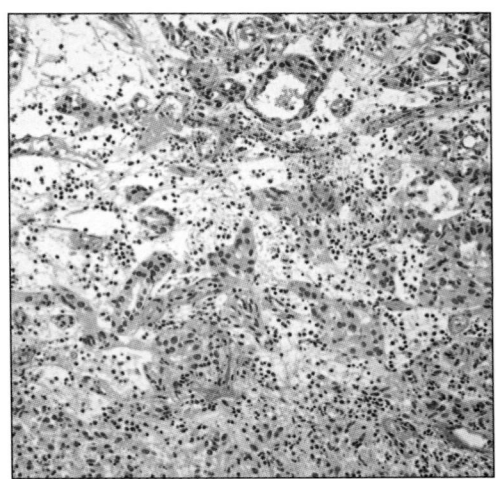

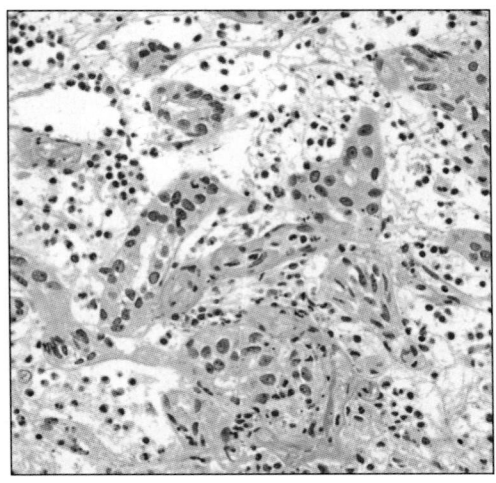

(Left) Clear cell adenocarcinoma of the urinary bladder with a tubular/glandular pattern may mimic nephrogenic adenoma, especially on low-power evaluation. (Right) This tubular/glandular pattern of clear cell adenocarcinoma has significant morphologic overlap with nephrogenic adenoma, but subtle degree of variation in nuclear size and shape warrant careful consideration of malignancy. Overt destructive invasion is not seen in nephrogenic adenoma.

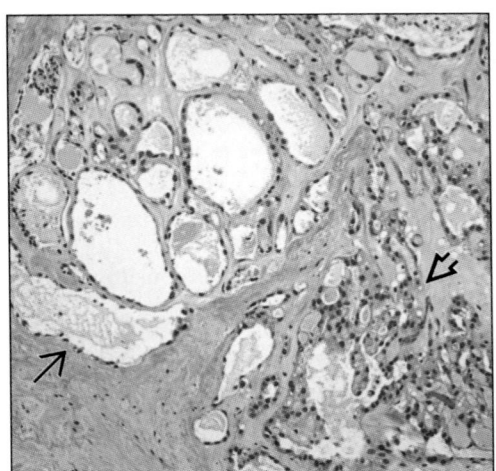

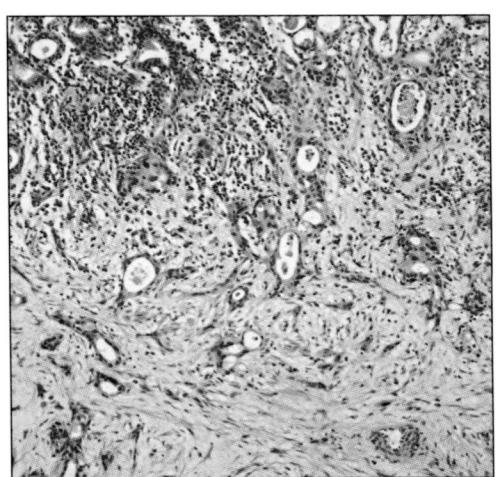

(Left) Histologically bland tubulocystic areas in clear cell adenocarcinoma ⇥ may closely mimic nephrogenic adenoma. Foci with more epithelial confluence and cytologic atypia are usually present ⊃. (Right) This example of invasive urothelial carcinoma with small tubules may also mimic nephrogenic adenoma. The stromal reaction and typically deep irregular invasion help in the distinction from nephrogenic adenoma.

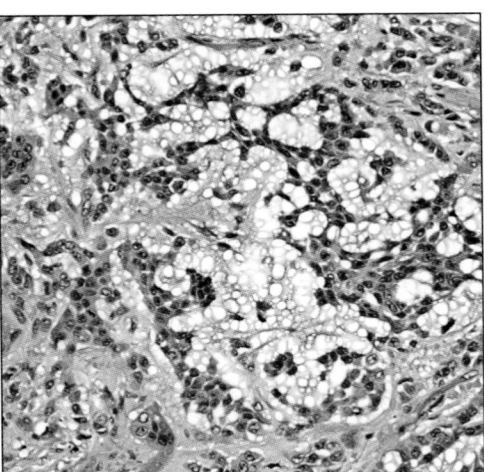

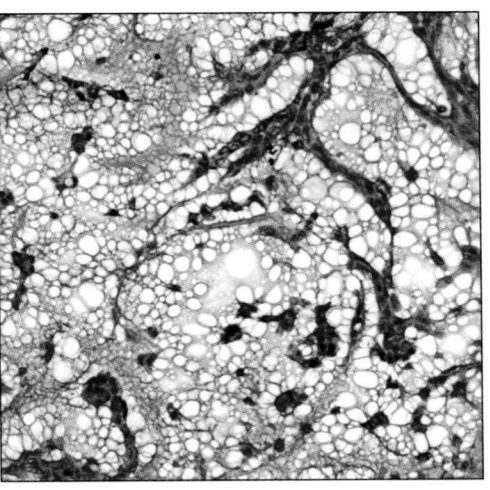

(Left) Invasive urothelial carcinoma with myxoid stroma may mimic fibromyxoid nephrogenic adenoma, especially in small biopsy specimens. Carcinomas have more prominent epithelium, and other typical patterns of urothelial carcinoma are commonly present. (Right) Prominent myxoid stroma and epithelial cording in invasive urothelial carcinoma (so-called chordoid features) closely mimics fibromyxoid nephrogenic adenoma.

FIBROEPITHELIAL POLYP

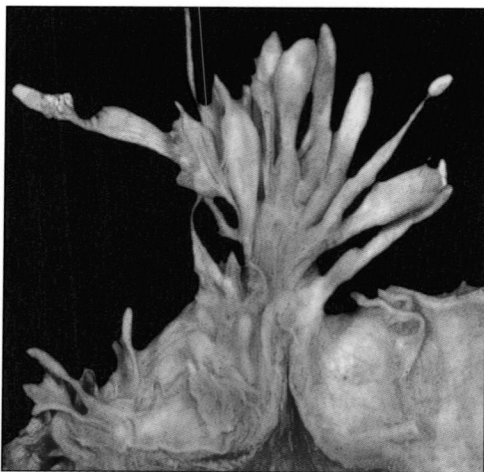

Fibroepithelial polyp with cloverleaf-like projections is shown. In contrast to papillary tumors, each papillary structure is more distinct due to a more prominent fibrous component.

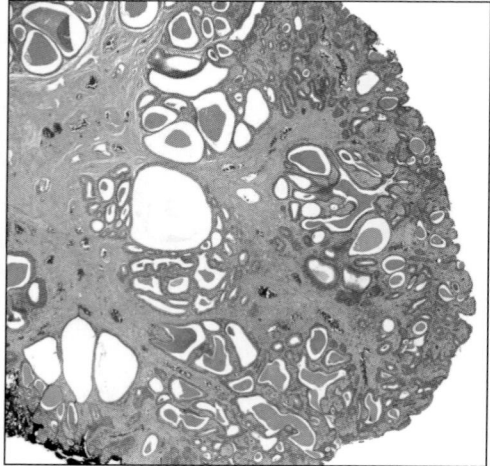

Low-power view of a FEP shows a polypoidal growth with an admixture of epithelial structures and fibrous stroma. The epithelial proliferation is more haphazard than with inverted papillary tumors.

TERMINOLOGY

Abbreviations
- Fibroepithelial polyp (FEP)

Synonyms
- Congenital posterior urethral polyp
- Botryoid fibroepithelial polyp

Definitions
- Nonneoplastic polyp of bladder
  - May be hamartomatous process

CLINICAL ISSUES

Epidemiology
- Incidence
  - Rare lesion
    - Approximately 180 reported
- Age
  - Usually reported in children and adolescents
  - In adults, median age is 44 years old
- Gender
  - Almost exclusively in males

Site
- Usually near verumontanum or bladder neck
- More commonly occurs in urethra and ureter

Presentation
- Acute urinary retention
- Bladder outlet obstruction
- Hematuria

Treatment
- Conservative transurethral resection

Prognosis
- Benign
  - Nonrecurring

MACROSCOPIC FEATURES

General Features
- Papillary or polypoid lesion
  - Usually 1-2 cm

MICROSCOPIC PATHOLOGY

Histologic Features
- Polypoid excrescence with variably bulbous to elongated papillae
  - Cloverleaf-like projections
    - Architecture reminiscent of adenofibromas of gynecologic tract
  - Florid cystitis glandularis of nonintestinal type in stalk
  - Urothelial lining typical
  - Secondary papillae with elongated, finger-like projections may be seen
  - Typically fibrous stroma
    - Rarely, scattered atypical stromal cells may be present
    - Myofibroblastic proliferation has also been described

DIFFERENTIAL DIAGNOSIS

Embryonal Rhabdomyosarcoma
- Polypoid "botryoid" growth pattern of fibroepithelial polyp may closely resemble embryonal rhabdomyosarcoma
- Usually more cellular stroma
  - Cambium layer is typically present
  - May have obvious rhabdomyoblasts
- Coexpression of cytoplasmic desmin with nuclear myogenin &/or MYOD1 is diagnostic of rhabdomyosarcoma

FIBROEPITHELIAL POLYP

Key Facts

Terminology
- Nonneoplastic polyp of bladder

Clinical Issues
- Usually reported in children and adolescents
- Almost exclusively in males
- More commonly occurs in urethra and ureter
- Conservative transurethral resection
- Nonrecurring

Microscopic Pathology
- Polypoid excrescence with variably bulbous to elongated papillae
- Cloverleaf-like projections
- Florid cystitis glandularis of nonintestinal type in stalk
- Urothelial lining typical
- Typically fibrous stroma
- Rarely, scattered atypical stromal cells may be present

Florid Cystitis Cystica/Glandularis
- Endophytic nests in fibroepithelial polyp are identical to cystitis cystica/glandularis
- No exophytic papillary component

Papillary-Polypoid Cystitis
- More edematous stroma with admixed chronic inflammation
- More simple papillary architecture
- Cystitis cystica/glandularis component not prominent feature
- Some reported "fibroepithelial polyps" may represent papillary-polypoid cystitis
  - Fibroepithelial polyp may be end stage of papillary-polypoid cystitis

Urothelial Papilloma
- More slender papillae with secondary branching
  - Less bulbous appearance
- Prominent umbrella cells are common
  - May have extensive vacuolization

Inverted Papilloma
- Endophytic growth with thin anastomosing cords
- More epithelial predominant lesion

Bladder Hamartoma
- Extremely rare lesion
- More extensive epithelial nests distributed haphazardly within stalk
- Squamous metaplasia may be present

Prostatic-Type Polyp
- Contains admixed prostatic secretory cells and urothelium
  - Express PSA and PAP by immunohistochemistry

DIAGNOSTIC CHECKLIST

Pathologic Interpretation Pearls
- In children, botryoid rhabdomyosarcoma must be excluded
  - Some embryonal rhabdomyosarcomas are deceptively bland
  - Immunohistochemistry with myogenin may be useful

SELECTED REFERENCES

1. Natsheh A et al: Fibroepithelial polyp of the bladder neck in children. Pediatr Surg Int. 24(5):613-5, 2008
2. Tsuzuki T et al: Fibroepithelial polyp of the lower urinary tract in adults. Am J Surg Pathol. 29(4):460-6, 2005
3. Al-Ahmadie H et al: Giant botryoid fibroepithelial polyp of bladder with myofibroblastic stroma and cystitis cystica et glandularis. Pediatr Dev Pathol. 6(2):179-81, 2003
4. Musselman P et al: The spectrum of urinary tract fibroepithelial polyps in children. J Urol. 136(2):476-7, 1986
5. Young RH: Fibroepithelial polyp of the bladder with atypical stromal cells. Arch Pathol Lab Med. 110(3):241-2, 1986

IMAGE GALLERY

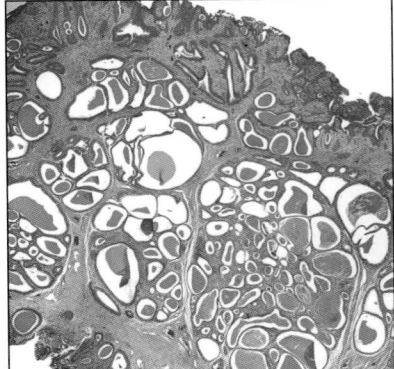
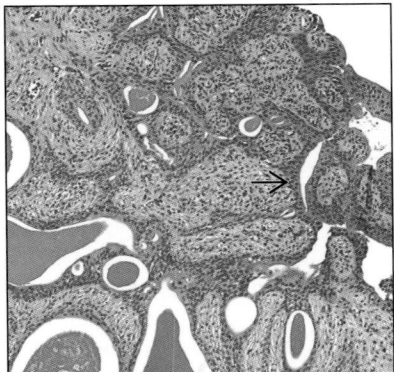
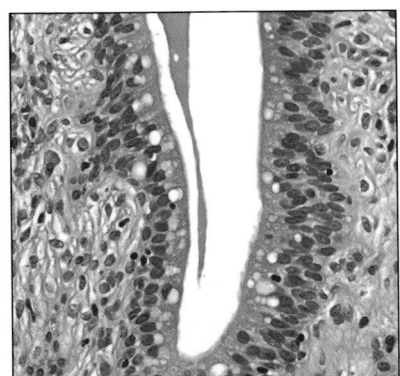

(Left) FEP shows a prominent epithelial proliferation within the stalk of the lesion. Some areas resemble cystitis cystica. *(Center)* The lining of a FEP is typically urothelial ➡. The rest of the epithelial component varies from resembling florid von Brunn nests to cystitis cystica. *(Right)* High power of FEP shows stromal proliferation and bland cytology of the epithelium.

PROSTATIC-TYPE POLYP (ECTOPIC PROSTATE)

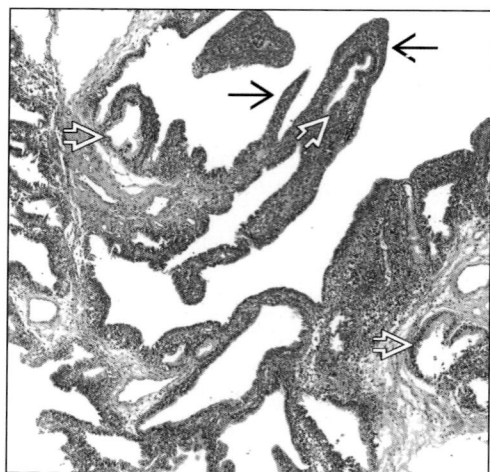

Prostatic-type polyps range from polypoid to villiform ➡, as seen in this example. The key diagnostic feature is the presence of prostatic secretory glands within the stroma ➡.

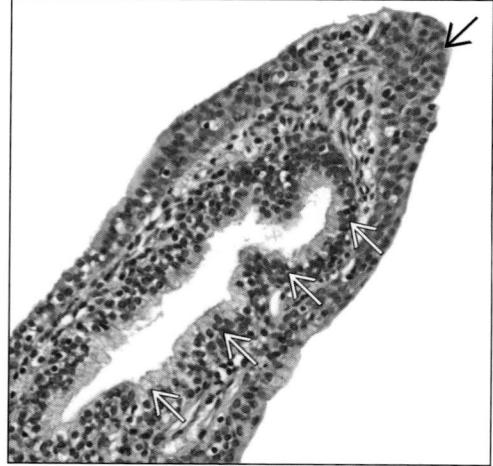

On high-power examination of this prostatic-type polyp, the contrast between the lining urothelial cells ➡ and the prostatic secretory epithelium ➡ is highlighted.

TERMINOLOGY

Synonyms
- Ectopic prostate
- Benign prostatic epithelial polyp

Definitions
- Urothelial tract polyp comprised of benign prostatic glands and stroma

ETIOLOGY/PATHOGENESIS

Controversial, Unproven Etiology
- Multiple theories proposed
  - Metaplastic process
  - Prostate gland ectopia
  - Developmental anomaly
  - Prolapse

CLINICAL ISSUES

Epidemiology
- Age
  - Broad range: 19-89 years

Site
- Most common in prostatic urethra
- Trigone most common in bladder
  - 2/3 of bladder cases

Presentation
- Hematuria
  - Gross or microscopic
- Hematospermia

Endoscopic Findings
- Polypoid mass with variable exophytic fronds
  - Typically bladder neck/trigone or around ureteral orifices

Treatment
- Simple excision
  - Biopsy may be curative

Prognosis
- Benign

MACROSCOPIC FEATURES

General Features
- Papillary or polypoid
- May have multiple lesions

MICROSCOPIC PATHOLOGY

Histologic Features
- Polypoid or papillary/filiform exophytic process
  - Stroma contains benign prostatic-type secretory glandular epithelium
    - Light, faintly eosinophilic cytoplasm
    - Round nuclei
    - Prostatic glands vary greatly in number and may contain crystalloids
    - Prominent nucleoli not seen
  - Admixed urothelium, often with cystitis glandularis
  - Excrescences lined by cytologically benign prostatic secretory cells &/or urothelium
  - Long, finger-like projections are rarely seen

Predominant Cell/Compartment Type
- Epithelial, glandular

ANCILLARY TESTS

Immunohistochemistry
- Immunoreactivity for PSA and PAP in prostatic secretory cells

PROSTATIC-TYPE POLYP (ECTOPIC PROSTATE)

Key Facts

Etiology/Pathogenesis
- Multiple theories proposed

Clinical Issues
- Broad range: 19-89 years
- Trigone is most common site in bladder
- Most common in prostatic urethra
- Hematuria, hematospermia
- Polypoid mass with variable exophytic fronds

Microscopic Pathology
- Polypoid or papillary/filiform exophytic process
- Stroma contains benign prostatic-type secretory glandular epithelium and admixed urothelium
- Excrescences lined by cytologically benign prostatic secretory cells &/or urothelium
- Long, finger-like projections are rarely seen

Ancillary Tests
- Immunoreactivity for PSA and PAP in prostatic secretory cells

Top Differential Diagnoses
- Prostatic ductal adenocarcinoma
- Papillary urothelial neoplasm
- Benign prostatic hyperplasia
- Nephrogenic adenoma
- Papillary-polypoid cystitis
- Cystitis cystica/glandularis

Diagnostic Checklist
- Prostatic ductal carcinoma must be carefully considered and excluded by morphology

DIFFERENTIAL DIAGNOSIS

Prostatic Ductal Adenocarcinoma
- Most important differential consideration
  - Aggressive malignancy that occurs in prostatic urethra
    - May extend superiorly to involve bladder
  - Potential morphologic overlap with prostatic-type polyp on small superficial biopsies
- Typical cellular features
  - Columnar cells lining glands
  - Nucleoli prominent
- More complex architectural growth patterns than prostatic-type polyp
  - Cribriform
  - Anastomosing cords
- Immunohistochemical overlap
  - Shares PSA and PAP reactivity with prostatic-type polyp

Papillary Urothelial Neoplasm
- Absence of prostatic secretory cells is distinctive
- More complex papillary architecture with secondary or tertiary branching

Benign Prostatic Hyperplasia
- May protrude into bladder lumen, forming polypoid mass lesion
  - Commonly called "median lobe hypertrophy"
  - May cause obstruction
- Admixture of prostatic glands and spindled cells in prostatic stroma

Nephrogenic Adenoma
- Mixed papillary and tubular pattern is common
  - Tubules may closely resemble prostate glands
- Express nuclear pax-2 and pax-8 by immunohistochemistry
- May occasionally show weak immunoreactivity for PSA &/or PAP
  - Leads to confusion with prostate secretory epithelium
- Papillae lined by single cuboidal layer of epithelial cells without admixed urothelium

Papillary-Polypoid Cystitis
- No admixed prostatic secretory cells

Cystitis Cystica/Glandularis
- Glands are of varying size and shape without basal cell layer
- Corpora amylacea are absent
- PSA is negative

DIAGNOSTIC CHECKLIST

Pathologic Interpretation Pearls
- Prostatic ductal carcinoma must be considered and excluded by morphology
- Recognition of lightly eosinophilic, frothy cytoplasm in prostatic secretory cells with corpora amylacea is key feature in distinction from papillary urothelial neoplasia

SELECTED REFERENCES

1. Anjum MI et al: Benign polyps with prostatic-type epithelium of the urethra and the urinary bladder. Int Urol Nephrol. 29(3):313-7, 1997
2. Chan JK et al: Prostatic-type polyps of the lower urinary tract: three histogenetic types? Histopathology. 11(8):789-801, 1987
3. Klein HZ et al: Ectopic prostatic tissue in bladder trigone. Distinctive cause of hematuria. Urology. 23(1):81-2, 1984
4. Remick DG Jr et al: Benign polyps with prostatic-type epithelium of the urethra and the urinary bladder. A suggestion of histogenesis based on histologic and immunohistochemical studies. Am J Surg Pathol. 8(11):833-9, 1984
5. Butterick JD et al: Ectopic prostatic tissue in urethra: a clinocopathological entity and a significant cause of hematuria. J Urol. 105(1):97-104, 1971
6. Gutierrez J et al: Ectopic prostatic tissue in bladder. J Urol. 98(4):474-8, 1967

PROSTATIC-TYPE POLYP (ECTOPIC PROSTATE)

Microscopic Features

(Left) Prostatic-type polyps may have a polypoid growth pattern. Prostatic glands ➡ are present in the stroma underlying the urothelium ➡. The presence of corpora amylacea ➡ is helpful. *(Right)* The lightly eosinophilic frothy cytoplasm of the prostatic glands ➡ is distinct from the stratified urothelium that lines the surface of the polyp ➡. This admixture of cell types is characteristic of a prostatic-type polyp (ectopic prostate).

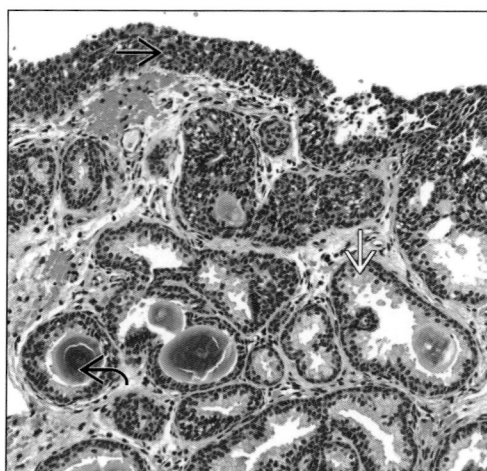
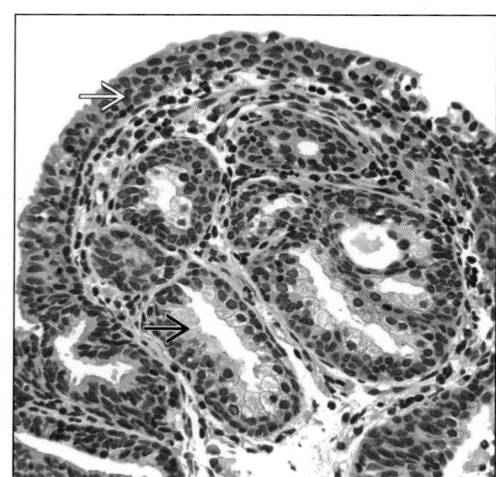

(Left) In some prostatic-type polyps, the prostate glands may predominate. The characteristic bland cytologic features and the presence of 2 cell types (secretory ➡ and basal cells ➡) points to a benign diagnosis. *(Right)* This prostatic-type polyp has urothelial-lined papillae ➡ mimicking a papillary urothelial neoplasm, but prostatic glands are present throughout the underlying stroma ➡. Corpora amylacea may occasionally be seen in the prostate glands ➡.

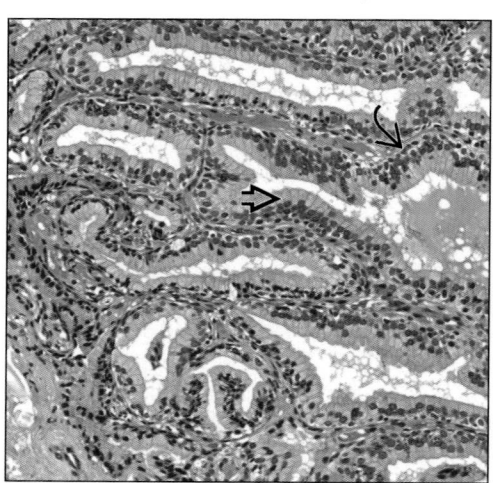
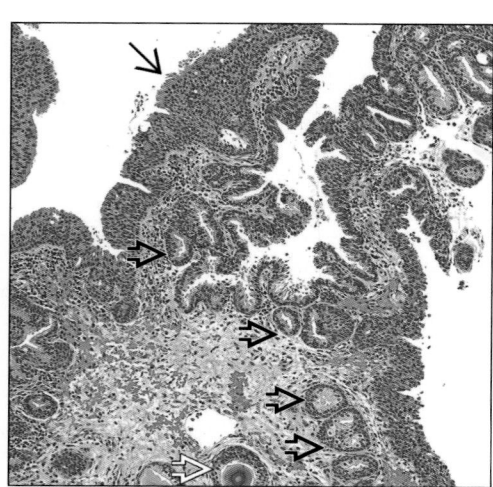

(Left) Villiform prostatic-type polyps may mimic papillary urothelial neoplasms because the tips of the papillae may be morphologically indistinguishable ➡. The benign prostate glands ➡ are diagnostic of a prostatic-type polyp. *(Right)* Strong PSA positivity helps confirm the diagnosis. Cystis cystica/glandularis may be in the differential diagnosis. Although PSA positivity confirms prostatic origin, the difference between benign and malignant is identified with light microscopy.

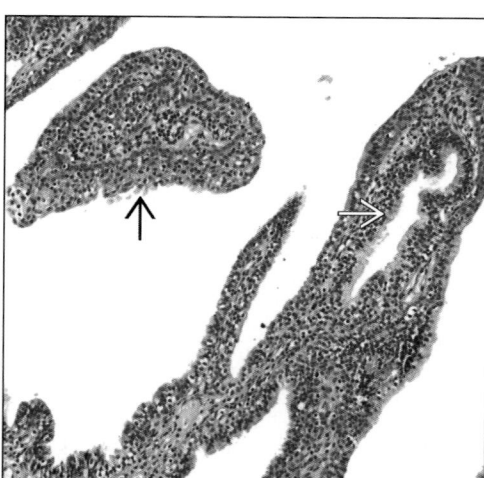
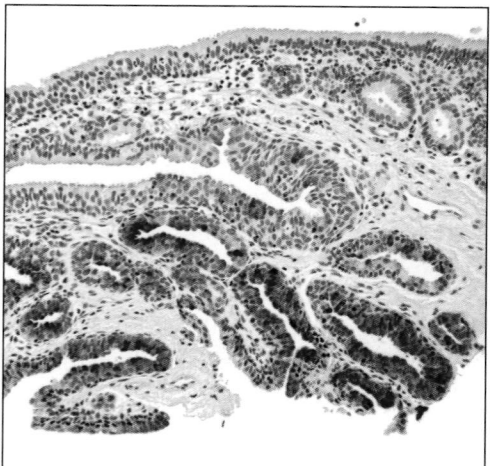

PROSTATIC-TYPE POLYP (ECTOPIC PROSTATE)

Differential Diagnosis

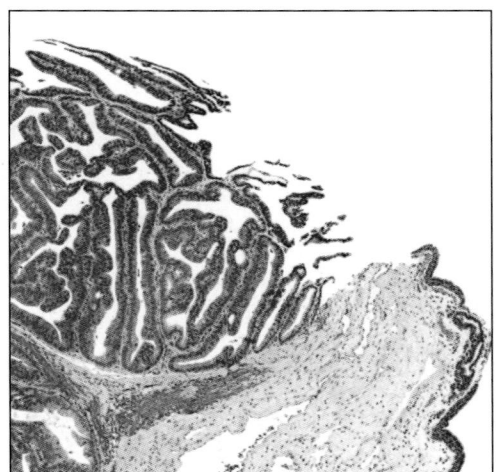

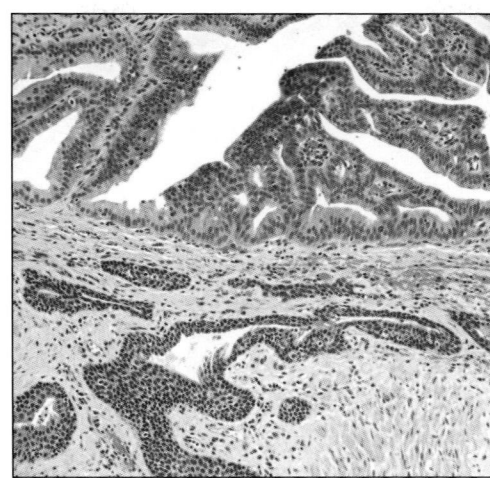

(Left) Prostatic ductal carcinoma may extend intraluminally within the prostatic urethra to involve the urinary bladder. In small biopsies, these carcinomas may potentially have morphologic overlap with a prostatic-type polyp due to the low-grade nuclear features. (Right) The admixture of prostatic epithelium and urothelium may suggest a prostatic-type polyp (ectopic prostate), but the degree of architectural complexity would strongly suggest a carcinoma in this example.

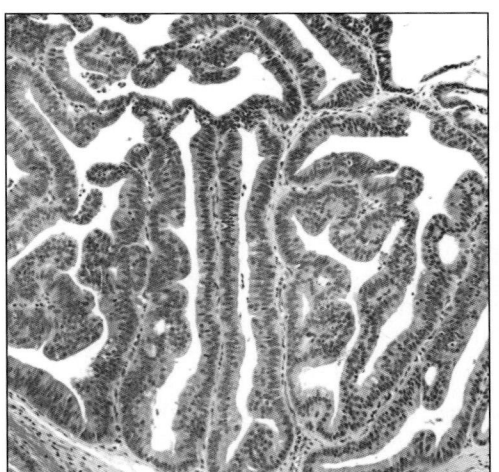

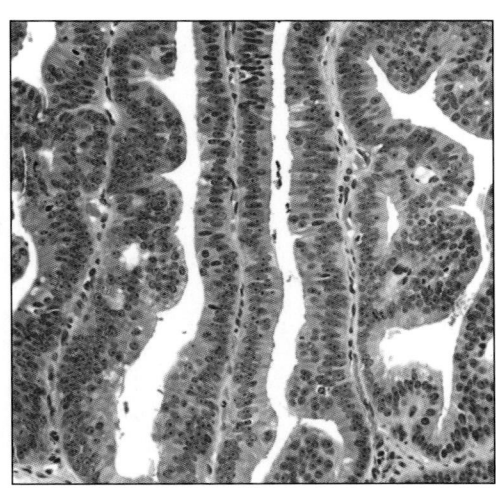

(Left) The degree of nucleomegaly with prominent nucleoli and anastomosing glandular growth are diagnostic of carcinoma in this example of prostatic adenocarcinoma involving the bladder. (Right) The columnar alignment of the lesional cells and prominent nucleoli are both typical of prostatic ductal adenocarcinoma. The nuclear features of prostatic-type polyp are bland and the lining is of 2 cell types, including a basal cell layer.

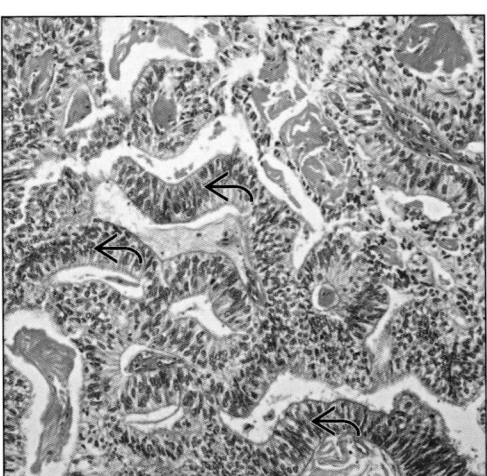

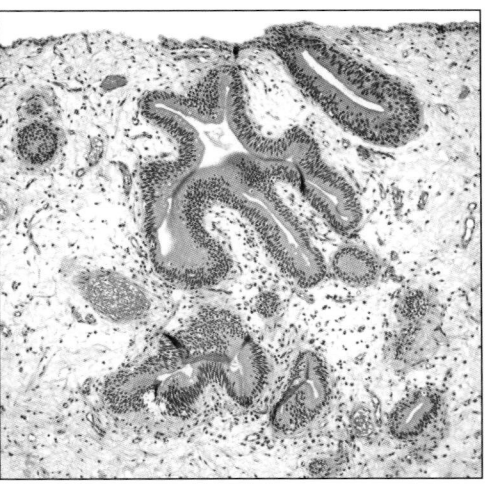

(Left) The lining cells ➡ are characteristic of prostatic ductal adenocarcinoma. The degree of glandular complexity is beyond what would be seen in a prostatic-type polyp. (Right) Cystis glandularis of the bladder has greater variation of glandular size and shape without corpora amylacea. The PSA stain is negative. Cystis glandularis and prostatic-type polyp are both benign lesions and hence, distinction between them is not as critical as with prostatic ductal carcinoma.

AMYLOIDOSIS

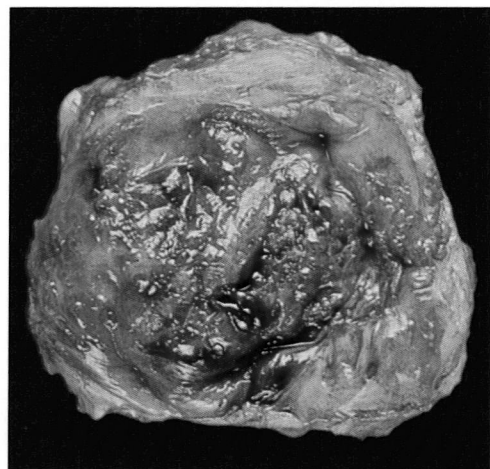

Partial cystectomy shows "tumor" forming amyloidosis (amyloidoma). Large lesions may ulcerate the overlying mucosa due to a large submucosal and mural mass.

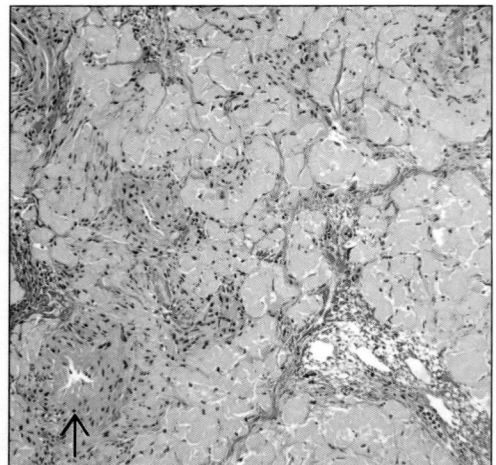

Dense homogeneous eosinophilic material is characteristic of amyloid. In the localized form, the amyloid entraps blood vessels ⇒ but is not typically confined to the vascular walls.

TERMINOLOGY

Synonyms
- Amyloid tumor (if localized)

Definitions
- Deposition of amyloid protein in urinary bladder
  - 2 types
    - Primary localized process
    - Systemic amyloidosis

ETIOLOGY/PATHOGENESIS

Systemic
- Primary
  - AL-type amyloid
- Secondary
  - Associated with chronic inflammatory conditions
    - Autoimmune causes, such as rheumatoid arthritis and ankylosing spondylitis
    - Infectious causes, such as tuberculosis and osteomyelitis
  - AA-type amyloid
- Familial
  - Transthyretin mutations most common
    - Transthyretin deposits
  - Other proteins are extremely rare

Localized Type
- Unknown etiology
- Most commonly AL type
- Rarely transthyretin

CLINICAL ISSUES

Epidemiology
- Incidence
  - Rarely bladder is primary site of disease
- Age
  - After 5th decade

Site
- Posterior and posterolateral walls most common

Presentation
- Hematuria
  - Rarely, frank hemorrhage

Treatment
- Surgical approaches
  - Local excision or laser ablation for localized amyloid
  - Partial cystectomy occasionally required for larger mass-forming lesions

Prognosis
- Primary, localized amyloid has high local recurrence rate (> 50%)
- Secondary amyloid depends on primary cause

MACROSCOPIC FEATURES

General Features
- Diffuse amyloidosis
  - Mucosal erythema, sometimes petechial hemorrhage and necrosis
- Localized amyloidosis
  - On cystoscopy, may be polypoid mass ± ulceration
    - May closely mimic neoplastic process

MICROSCOPIC PATHOLOGY

Histologic Features
- Deposition of eosinophilic amorphous material in lamina propria and superficial muscularis propria
  - Deposition in vessel wall is less common and usually seen in systemic form
- Florid histiocytic and foreign body type giant cell reaction may be seen
- Rarely associated with urothelial carcinoma

AMYLOIDOSIS

Key Facts

Terminology
- Deposition of amyloid protein in urinary bladder
- 2 types
  - Primary localized process
  - Systemic amyloidosis

Microscopic Pathology
- Deposition of eosinophilic amorphous material in lamina propria and superficial muscularis propria

Ancillary Tests
- "Apple green" birefringence on Congo red under polarized light
- Thioflavin T fluorescence is seen
- Randomly arranged, rigid, nonbranching, 8-10 nm fibrils by electron microscopy

Top Differential Diagnoses
- Fibrosis

ANCILLARY TESTS

Histochemistry
- Congo red
  - Amorphous material has dense orange "congophilia" under light microscopy
  - "Apple green" birefringence under polarized light

Immunohistochemistry
- Amyloid panel of κ light chain, λ light chain, prealbumin, β-2 microglobulin, and SAA1 may help

Immunofluorescence
- Fluorescence with Thioflavin T stain is seen

Electron Microscopy
- Randomly arranged, rigid, nonbranching, 8-10 nm fibrils

DIFFERENTIAL DIAGNOSIS

Fibrosis
- Collagen deposition may appear similar to amyloid
  - Highlighted by trichrome stain
  - No green birefringence on Congo red stain
  - No thioflavin T fluorescence

Follicular Lymphoma
- Occasionally associated with dense fibrosis that may closely mimic amyloid

DIAGNOSTIC CHECKLIST

Clinically Relevant Pathologic Features
- May be interpreted as neoplasm on cystoscopy
- Determination of amyloid type may aid clinical work-up of patient

Pathologic Interpretation Pearls
- Because of rarity, may be overlooked as organizing fibrosis
- Does not necessarily indicate systemic process
  - Diagnosis of localized amyloid requires clinicopathologic correlation

SELECTED REFERENCES

1. Tirzaman O et al: Primary localized amyloidosis of the urinary bladder: a case series of 31 patients. Mayo Clin Proc. 75(12):1264-8, 2000
2. Farah RN et al: Primary localized amyloidosis of bladder. Urology. 13(2):200-2, 1979
3. Akhtar M et al: Solitary primary amyloidosis of urinary bladder. Light and electron microscopic study. Urology. 12(6):721-4, 1978
4. Strong GH et al: Primary amyloid disease of the bladder. J Urol. 112(4):463-6, 1974

IMAGE GALLERY

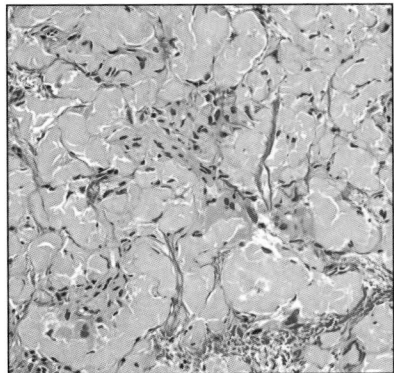
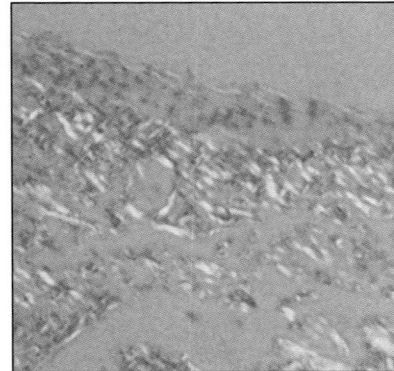
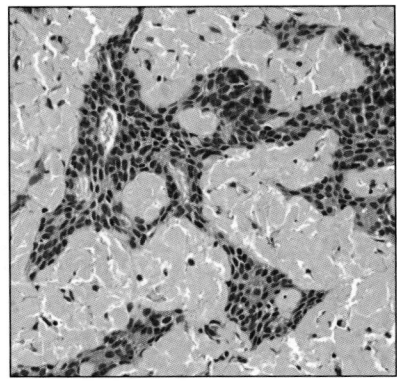

(Left) Amorphous eosinophilic material is characteristic of amyloid, as in other anatomic sites. Congo red is useful in the distinction from collagen. *(Center)* With Congo red stain, amyloid deposits produce characteristic "apple green" birefringence under polarized light. *(Right)* This is a rare example of localized amyloid deposition in the urinary bladder, which was found in association with an invasive urothelial carcinoma.

MULLERIAN LESIONS

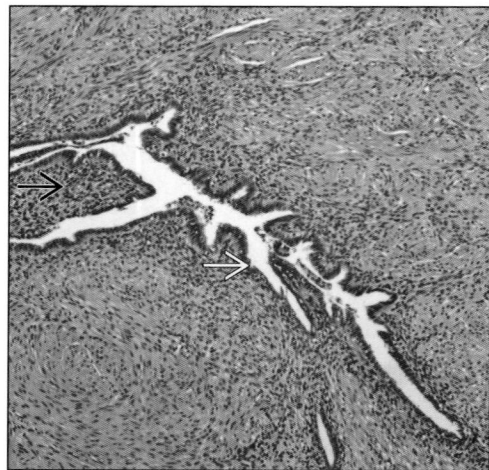

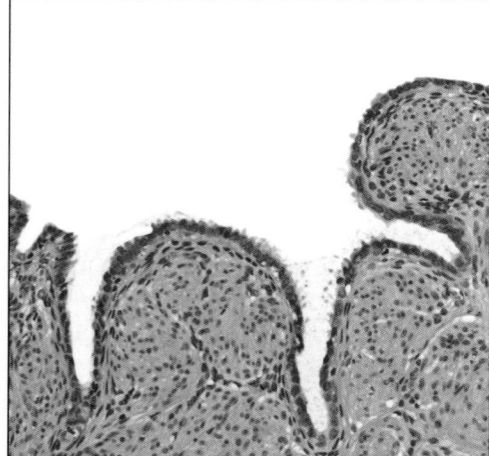

Endometriosis within the muscularis propria of the bladder wall shows the characteristic admixture of endometrial glands ➡ *and stroma* ➡. *The stroma may contain hemosiderin-laden macrophages.*

Endosalpingiotic gland with tubal-type epithelium, but without endometrial stroma, is shown. Some of the glands may have a combination of endometriotic, endocervical-type, or endosalpingiotic stroma.

TERMINOLOGY

Definitions
- Ectopic müllerian tissue within wall of urinary bladder
  - Endometriosis
    - Endometrial glands and stroma
  - Endocervicosis
    - Endocervical-type glands
  - Endosalpingosis
    - Tubal-type glands
  - Müllerianosis
    - Admixture of different types of müllerian epithelium

ETIOLOGY/PATHOGENESIS

Predisposing Factors
- 50% of cases have history of previous pelvic surgery

CLINICAL ISSUES

Epidemiology
- Incidence
  - Endometriosis: Involvement of urinary tract in 1% of cases
    - Bladder most common genitourinary site
  - Endocervicosis/müllerianosis: Less common than endometriosis
- Age
  - Typically reproductive age
  - Rarely postmenopausal if receiving hormones
- Gender
  - Female
  - Rare cases reported in males receiving estrogen therapy

Presentation
- Dysuria

  - Urinary urgency, frequency, suprapubic pain
- Hematuria
- > 50% of patients have no vesical symptoms
- Endometriosis may produce pain with menstrual cycle

Treatment
- Surgical approaches
  - Conservative surgery and hormonal therapy in women who desire fertility
  - Definitive surgery for women beyond reproductive age

Prognosis
- Benign
- Malignant transformation of endometriosis in bladder has been reported

IMAGE FINDINGS

General Features
- Location
  - Cystoscopy
    - Submucosal nodule
    - Appear as congested, edematous mucosal elevations overlying cysts

MACROSCOPIC FEATURES

General Features
- Palpable suprapubic mass in almost 50% of cases
- Hemorrhagic ill-defined mass may project into bladder lumen

MICROSCOPIC PATHOLOGY

Histologic Features
- Cytologically benign glands of müllerian type within bladder wall
  - Endometriosis

MULLERIAN LESIONS

Key Facts

Terminology
- Ectopic benign müllerian tissue within wall of urinary bladder

Clinical Issues
- Typically reproductive age women

Microscopic Pathology
- Cytologically benign glands of müllerian type within bladder wall

- o Endometriosis
- o Endocervicosis
- o Endosalpingiosis
- o Müllerianosis

Top Differential Diagnoses
- Invasive adenocarcinoma
- Urothelial carcinoma with glandular differentiation
- Microcystic urothelial carcinoma

- ▪ Resemble endometriosis at other sites
- ▪ Admixed endometrial-type glands with admixed endometrial stroma
- o Endocervicosis
  - ▪ Epithelium lining the glands consists of single layer of columnar cells with abundant pale cytoplasm
  - ▪ Ciliated cells are often interspersed among mucinous cells
  - ▪ When glands are dilated, epithelium is cuboidal or flattened
- o Endosalpingiosis
  - ▪ Tubal-type glands lined by ciliated cells
- o Müllerianosis
  - ▪ Admixture of tubal, endocervical, &/or endometrial-type glands
- Most involve muscularis propria, but mucosa and adventitia also may be involved
- Fibrosis and hyperplastic muscle around lesional glands may thicken bladder wall

DIFFERENTIAL DIAGNOSIS

Invasive Carcinoma
- Includes adenocarcinoma and urothelial carcinoma with glandular differentiation
- Obvious cytologic atypia with complex glands
- Stromal reaction common

Microcystic Urothelial Carcinoma
- May have bland cytologic features compared to conventional urothelial carcinoma
- May have admixed urothelial carcinoma
- More glandular structures with destructive invasion

DIAGNOSTIC CHECKLIST

Pathologic Interpretation Pearls
- Bland-appearing, well-formed glandular structures deep in bladder wall should raise possibility of müllerianosis over invasive carcinoma

SELECTED REFERENCES

1. Young RH et al: Müllerianosis of the urinary bladder. Mod Pathol. 9(7):731-7, 1996
2. Clement PB et al: Endocervicosis of the urinary bladder. A report of six cases of a benign müllerian lesion that may mimic adenocarcinoma. Am J Surg Pathol. 16(6):533-42, 1992

IMAGE GALLERY

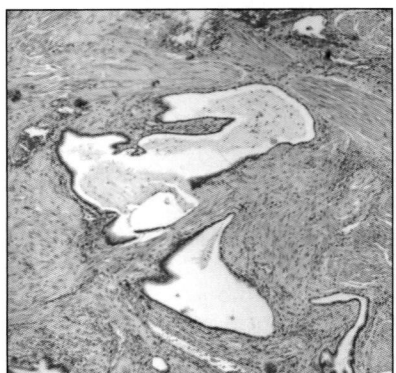 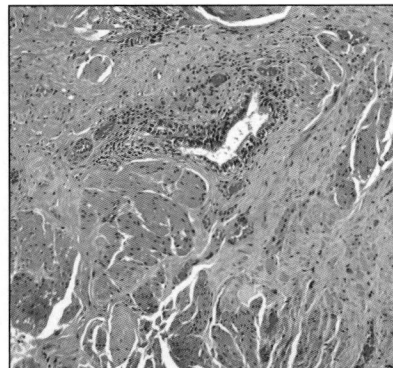 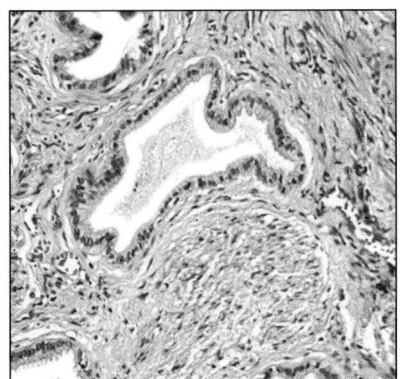

(Left) Endocervicosis is seen with deep presence of glands within the muscularis propria. The well-formed nature of the glands with adequate stromal separation argues against adenocarcinoma. (Center) In this example of endocervicosis, the benign glandular structure is admixed with thick smooth muscle bundles of the muscularis propria. (Right) The bland cytologic features and mucinous appearance of these glands within the muscularis propria are characteristic of endocervicosis.

PSEUDOCARCINOMATOUS HYPERPLASIA

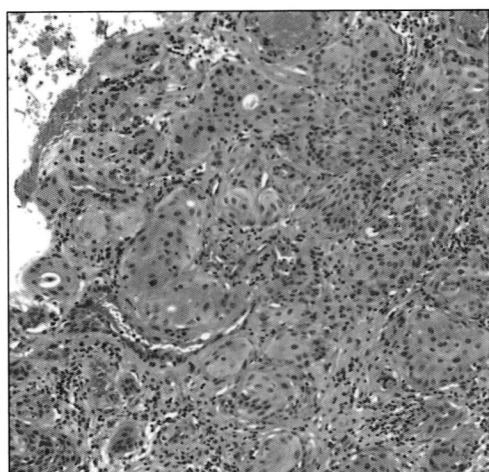

This florid reactive urothelial proliferation is from a patient who underwent radiation therapy for prostate cancer. Despite the back to back nests, the cytology of the urothelial cells is bland.

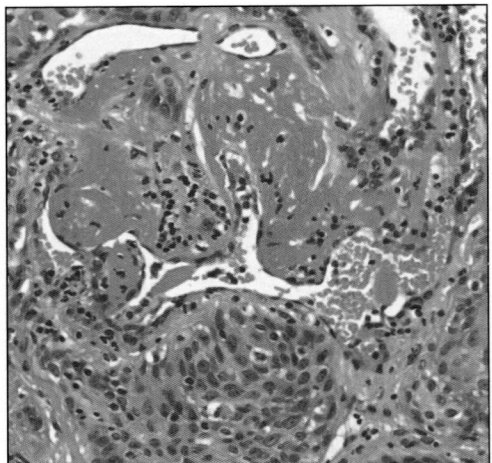

The association between the urothelial nests and intravascular and stromal fibrin is characteristic of this florid reactive process known as pseudocarcinomatous hyperplasia.

TERMINOLOGY

Synonyms
- Radiation/chemotherapy cystitis
- Radiation-induced pseudocarcinomatous hyperplasia
- Post-chemotherapy pseudocarcinomatous hyperplasia

Definitions
- Florid benign urothelial proliferation with pseudoinfiltrative growth pattern
  - Usually in patients with prior radiation &/or chemotherapy

ETIOLOGY/PATHOGENESIS

Environmental Exposure
- Described in association with chemotherapy (thiotepa, mitomycin, cyclophosphamide, BCG therapy) &/or radiation therapy
  - Radiation therapy most commonly for prostatic or gynecologic malignancy (e.g., cervical squamous cell carcinoma)
- Subset of cases with no prior therapy
  - Nontherapy associations suggest underlying ischemic etiology
    - Atrial fibrillation
    - Diabetes
    - Indwelling catheter
    - Prior local surgery

CLINICAL ISSUES

Epidemiology
- Incidence
  - Rare
- Age
  - Range: 40-85 years; mean: 69 years
- Gender
  - Most commonly reported in males

Site
- Urinary bladder

Presentation
- Symptoms of radiation/chemotherapy cystitis
  - Hematuria

Endoscopic Findings
- Most appear polypoid

Natural History
- Morphologic features of radiation cystitis may persist for years

Treatment
- Options, risks, complications
  - Symptomatic care and follow-up
  - Remove inciting factors if possible
- Surgical approaches
  - None required

Prognosis
- Benign condition

MACROSCOPIC FEATURES

General Features
- Small polypoid lesion

MICROSCOPIC PATHOLOGY

Histologic Features
- Urothelial proliferation
  - Small to intermediate-sized urothelial nests with rounded or irregular, jagged borders
  - Prominent cytoplasmic eosinophilia imparting "squamoid" appearance
  - Some have frankly squamous differentiation

PSEUDOCARCINOMATOUS HYPERPLASIA

Key Facts

Etiology/Pathogenesis
- Described in association with chemotherapy &/or radiation therapy
- Subset of cases with no prior therapy

Clinical Issues
- Symptoms of radiation/chemotherapy cystitis
- Most appear polypoid

Microscopic Pathology
- Small urothelial nests with rounded or irregular, jagged borders
- Prominent cytoplasmic eosinophilia imparting "squamoid" appearance
- Some have frankly squamous differentiation
- Epithelium characteristically encircles vessels and fibrin aggregates

- Mitotic figures usually absent
- Stromal hemorrhage and hemosiderin deposition
- Vascular ectasia
- Stromal &/or intravascular fibrin deposition
- Associated ulceration common
- Stromal fibrosis
- Typical radiation-induced epithelial changes
- Atypical fibroblasts

Top Differential Diagnoses
- Invasive urothelial carcinoma
- Nested variant of urothelial carcinoma
- Florid von Brunn nests

Diagnostic Checklist
- Attention to associated background ischemic/radiation changes is crucial to avoid misdiagnosis

---

- o Epithelium characteristically encircles or wraps around vessels and fibrin aggregates
- o Extent of lamina propria involvement varies (> 50% in some cases)
- o Variation in nuclear size and shape
- o Mitotic figures usually absent
- More typical radiation-induced epithelial changes may be present in adjacent urothelium
  - o Cytoplasmic ballooning
  - o Smudged chromatin
  - o Nuclear and cytoplasmic vacuoles
  - o Karyorrhectic cellular debris
- Other associated stromal changes
  - o Vascular ectasia and edema
  - o Stromal hemorrhage and hemosiderin deposition
  - o Stromal &/or intravascular fibrin deposition
  - o Atypical fibroblasts
  - o Stromal fibrosis
  - o Variable acute and chronic inflammation
- Associated ulceration is common

Predominant Pattern/Injury Type
- Hyperplasia

Predominant Cell/Compartment Type
- Urothelial

DIFFERENTIAL DIAGNOSIS

Invasive Urothelial Carcinoma
- Lacks epithelial cells encircling blood vessels with fibrin deposition
- Background radiation cystitis typically less pronounced in post-radiation setting
- More pronounced cytologic atypia
- Invasion of muscularis propria diagnostic

Nested Variant of Urothelial Carcinoma
- Nests and cords of cytologically bland urothelial cells within lamina propria
- More irregular anastomosing growth pattern

- Lacks epithelial cells encircling blood vessels with fibrin deposition
- Invasion of muscularis propria is most definitive feature
- Background radiation cystitis typically less pronounced (if post-radiation setting)

Florid von Brunn Nests
- Background hemorrhage and vascular changes absent
- More uniformly rounded nests
- Lobular configuration of nests
- Sharp line of demarcation with underlying lamina propria

DIAGNOSTIC CHECKLIST

Clinically Relevant Pathologic Features
- Benign mimic of carcinoma
  - o Cystoscopic impression may suggest radiation injury

Pathologic Interpretation Pearls
- Attention to associated background ischemic/radiation changes is crucial to avoid misdiagnosis
- Epithelial nests wrapping around abnormal blood vessels
  - o Specific diagnostic feature of this hyperplastic process

SELECTED REFERENCES

1. Lane Z et al: Pseudocarcinomatous epithelial hyperplasia in the bladder unassociated with prior irradiation or chemotherapy. Am J Surg Pathol. 32(1):92-7, 2008
2. Chan TY et al: Radiation or chemotherapy cystitis with "pseudocarcinomatous" features. Am J Surg Pathol. 28(7):909-13, 2004
3. Baker PM et al: Radiation-induced pseudocarcinomatous proliferations of the urinary bladder: a report of 4 cases. Hum Pathol. 31(6):678-83, 2000
4. Fajardo LF et al: Radiation injury in surgical pathology. Part I. Am J Surg Pathol. 2(2):159-99, 1978

PSEUDOCARCINOMATOUS HYPERPLASIA

Microscopic Features

(Left) This biopsy specimen, which represents pseudocarcinomatous hyperplasia secondary to radiation therapy for cervical cancer, shows nests of urothelium with associated blood vessels ➡ and collagen. *(Right)* The blood vessels with extravasated red blood cells ➡ and collagenized stroma ➡ should suggest the possibility of pseudocarcinomatous hyperplasia.

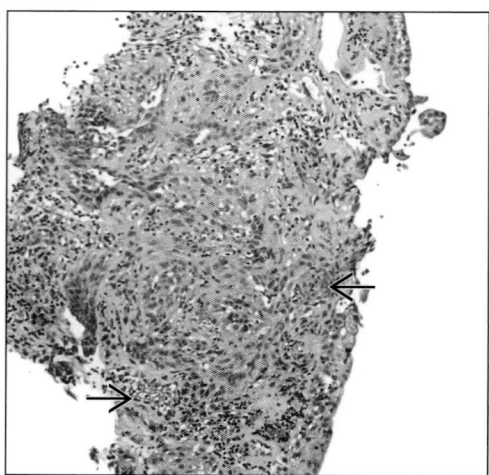

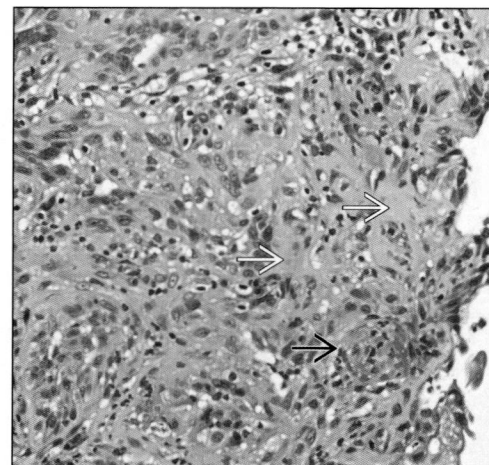

(Left) The epithelial nests in pseudocarcinomatous hyperplasia often have a "squamoid" appearance. The nuclear features remain bland, in contrast to urothelial carcinoma with squamous differentiation. *(Right)* These nests of urothelium can be seen encircling dense collagen ➡ or fibrin in this hyperplastic lesion. This is one of the most important histologic features for distinguishing pseudocarcinomatous hyperplasia from carcinoma.

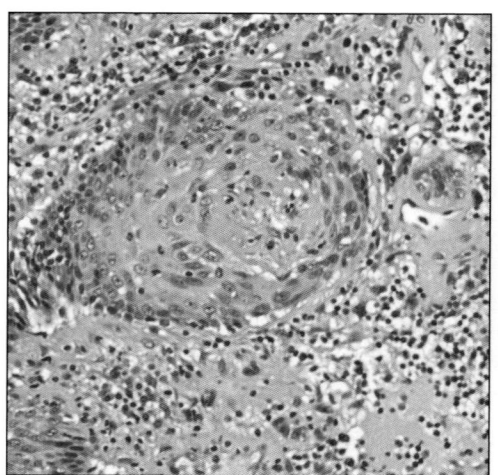

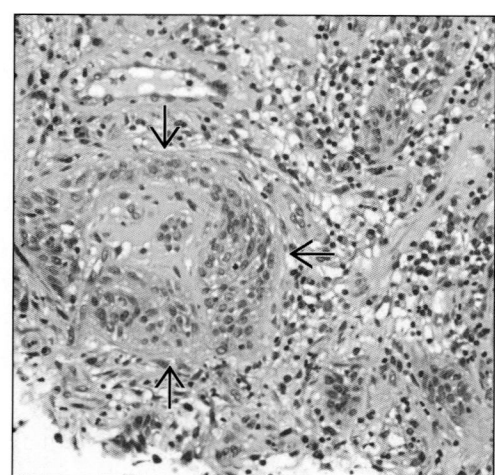

(Left) The overlying surface urothelium in pseudocarcinomatous hyperplasia shows reactive urothelial changes characterized by mild nucleomegaly, fine nuclear chromatin, and pinpoint nucleoli. The absence of associated urothelial carcinoma in situ or papillary urothelial neoplasia is important. *(Right)* Extensive hemorrhage and fibrin deposition is typically associated with the invaginated urothelium in pseudocarcinomatous hyperplasia.

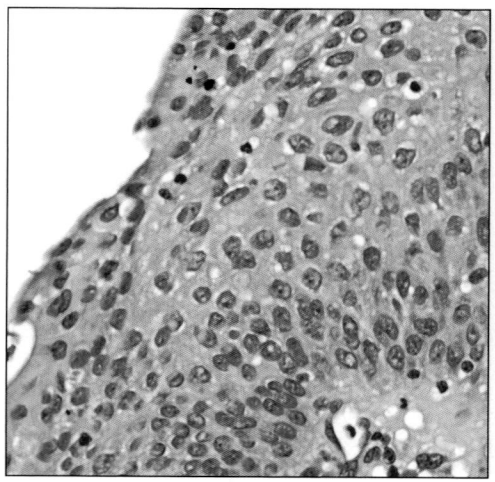

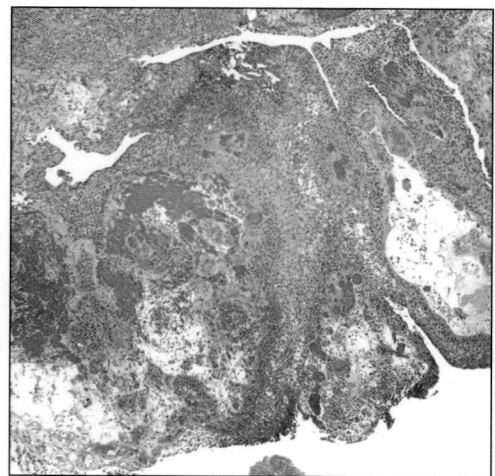

PSEUDOCARCINOMATOUS HYPERPLASIA

Associated Microscopic Features

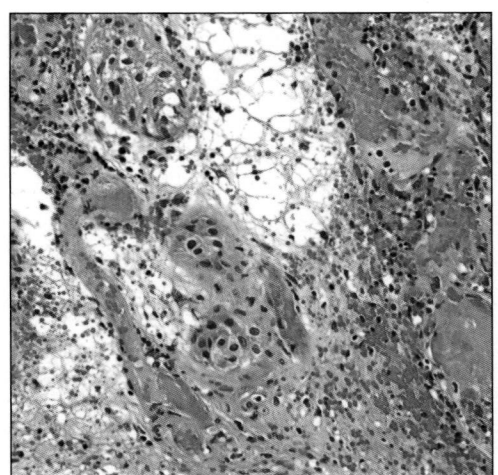

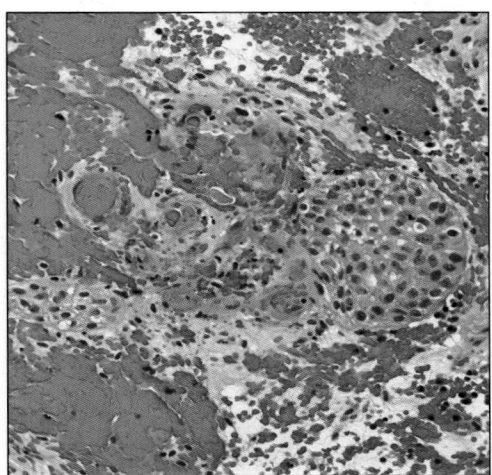

(Left) The nests of urothelium are present deep in the lamina propria with associated stromal hemorrhage and intravascular fibrin accumulation. The urothelial nests have bland cytologic features. (Right) The extensive hemorrhage is a strong clue to the diagnosis of a pseudocarcinomatous hyperplasia, especially when associated with fibrin. The epithelial nests may be more dispersed in some examples, which makes the diagnosis somewhat easier.

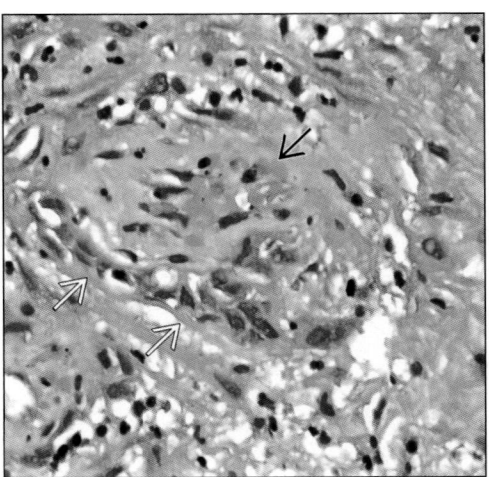

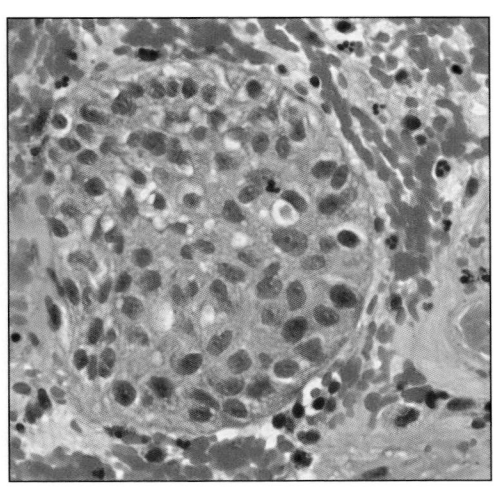

(Left) This demonstrates the typical epithelial-stromal relationship of pseudocarcinomatous hyperplasia, which is characterized by epithelial nests encircling an abnormal blood vessel with dense hyalinization ➡. The urothelial nest in this example is irregular and jagged, a feature that closely mimics invasive carcinoma ➡. (Right) This high-power photomicrograph shows minimal variation in the size of the nuclei and variably prominent pinpoint nucleoli in the urothelial nests.

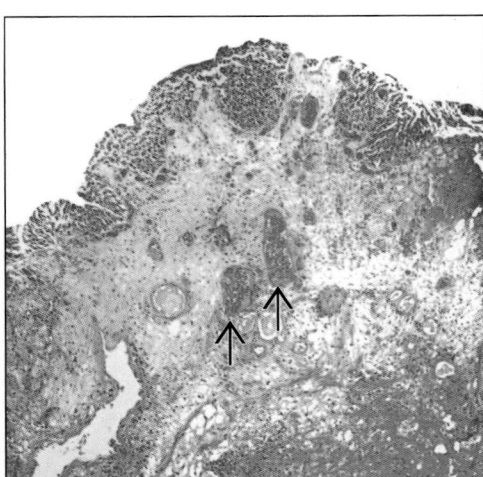

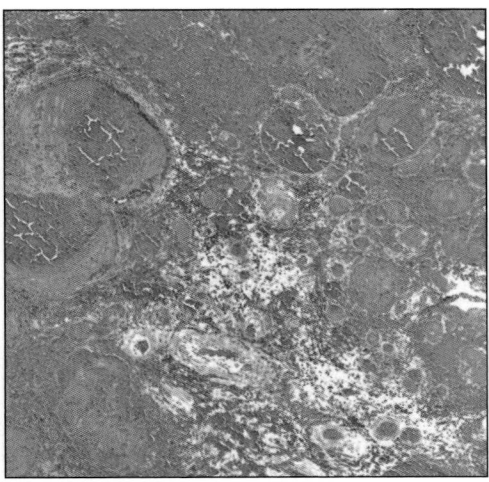

(Left) Lamina propria edema is commonly found in the background/adjacent tissues. This example also shows subtle vascular changes with mild ectasia and intravascular fibrin ➡. (Right) This is a florid example of vascular ectasia with both extensive intravascular and stromal fibrin. This feature in the tissue surrounding an epithelial proliferation should prompt strong consideration of a nonneoplastic process, possibly related to prior therapy.

PSEUDOCARCINOMATOUS HYPERPLASIA

Microscopic Features

(Left) This example of pseudocarcinomatous hyperplasia shows the characteristic "wrapping" of urothelium around abnormal blood vessels ➡ with hyalinization &/or intravascular fibrin. *(Right)* This blood vessel has fibrin within the wall ➡, is encircled by cytologically bland urothelium, and has associated extravasated red blood cells and acute inflammation. These features are typical of pseudocarcinomatous hyperplasia.

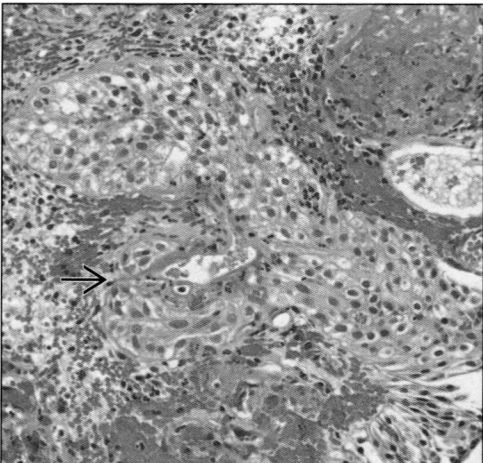
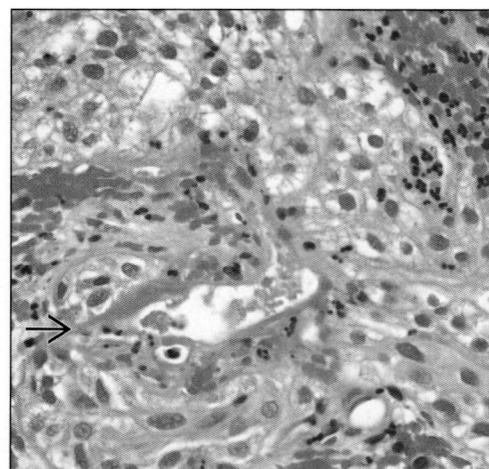

(Left) Admixed acute and chronic inflammation is a common finding because of tissue ischemia and may obscure the fibrin deposition. *(Right)* More subtle vascular changes in tissue surrounding a hyperplastic proliferation show mild dilatation, minimal mural hyalinization, and rare associated atypical stromal cells ➡. These are features that are highly suggestive of prior radiation therapy.

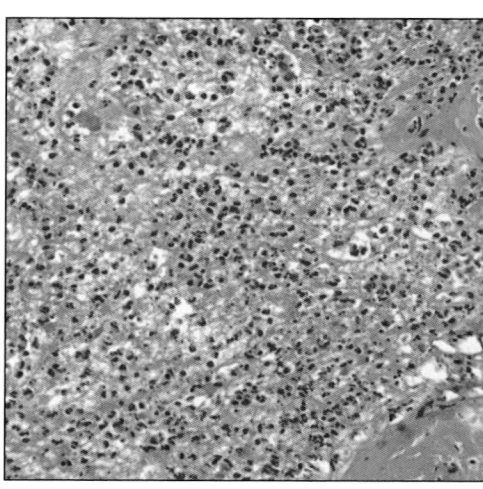
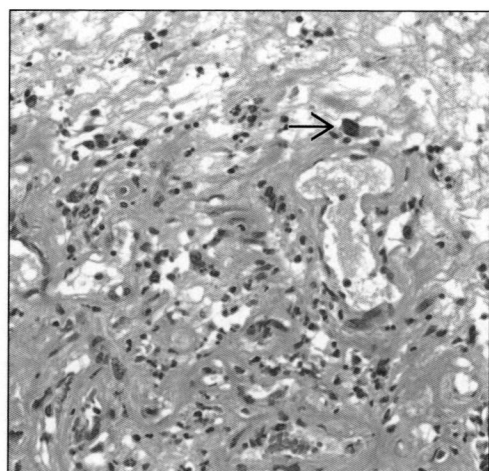

(Left) Prominent vascular ectasia with intravascular fibrin ➡ is present in this example with an associated history of radiation therapy. Scattered atypical fibroblasts are present in the background stroma ➡ as well. *(Right)* This high-power photomicrograph of atypical stromal cells is from a patient with a history of radiation therapy for prostate cancer. The admixed inflammatory cells are also common with prior radiation.

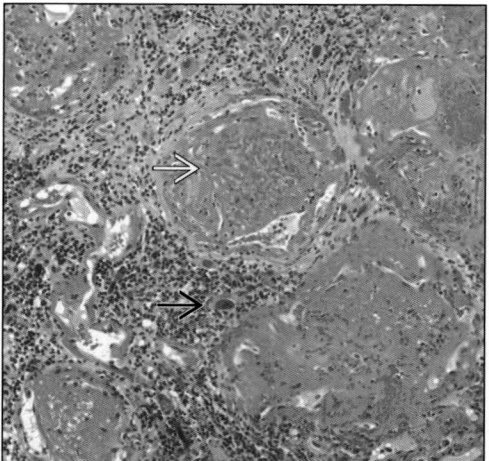
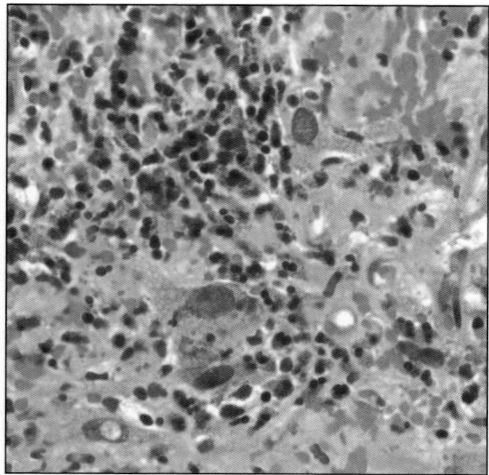

PSEUDOCARCINOMATOUS HYPERPLASIA

Differential Diagnosis

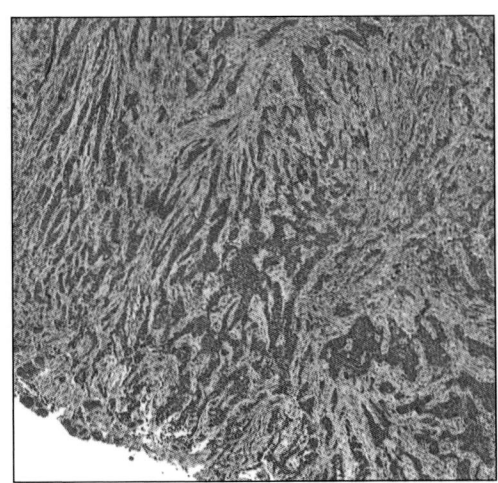
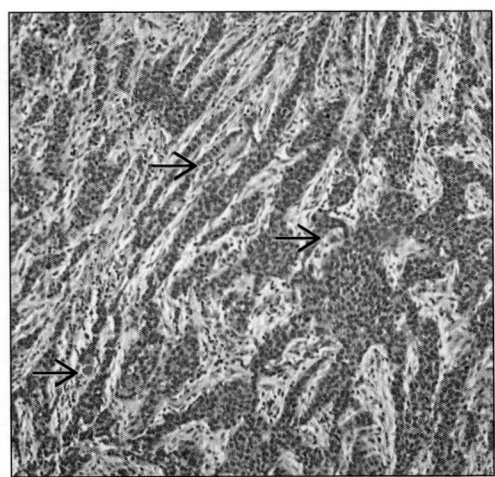

(Left) This is an example of invasive urothelial carcinoma in a patient with a history of radiation therapy. The nests of urothelium are more complex and interanastomosing than typically seen in pseudocarcinomatous hyperplasia. *(Right)* This degree of epithelial confluence should suggest the diagnosis of carcinoma in this case. The associated blood vessels are not associated with fibrin and are not hyalinized ➡.

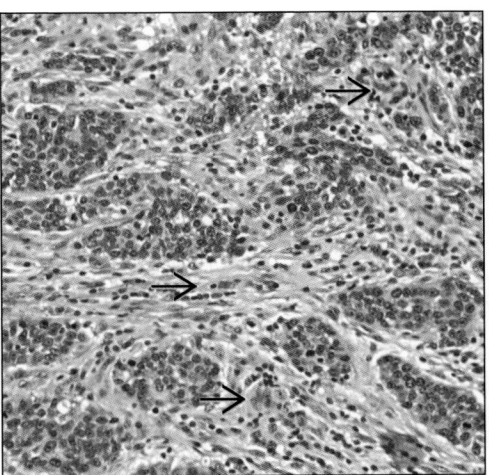
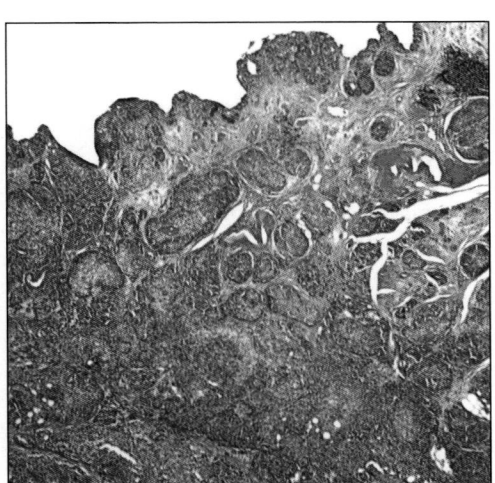

(Left) This invasive urothelial carcinoma, although monomorphic, has a higher nuclear to cytoplasmic ratio and larger nucleoli compared to pseudocarcinomatous hyperplasia. In addition, the blood vessels appear normal ➡. *(Right)* In nested urothelial carcinoma, the low-power architecture shows a greater degree of epithelial confluence and crowding than is typical of a benign process. The absence of blood and fibrin is important in the distinction from hyperplasia.

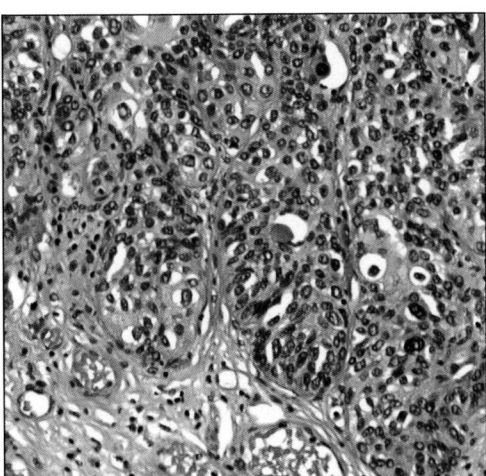
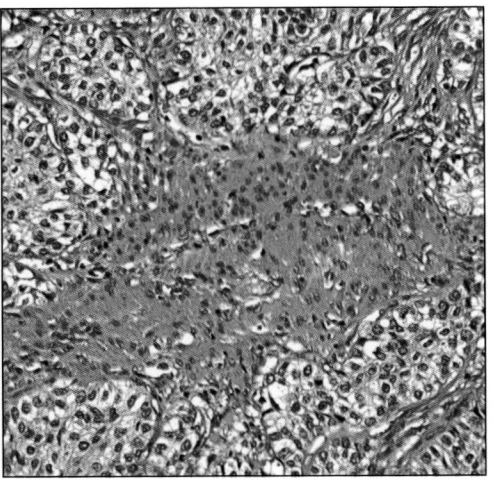

(Left) A high-power examination of nested urothelial carcinoma may be misleading given the bland cytologic features as seen in this example. A low-power architectural examination is important to assess the overall growth pattern. *(Right)* The presence of definitive muscularis propria invasion, as in this example, is the most specific morphologic feature of carcinoma in the differential diagnosis of a hyperplastic lesion.

OVERVIEW OF URINARY BLADDER NEOPLASMS

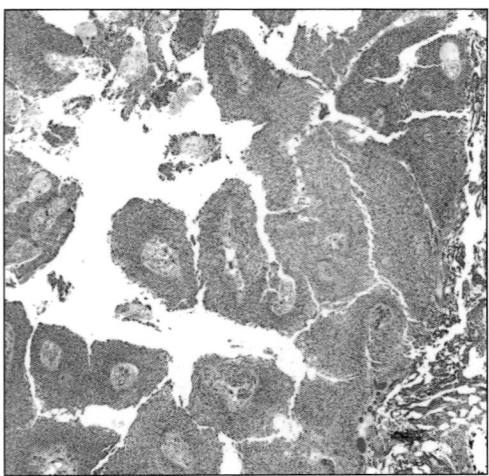

The spectrum of neoplasia in the bladder includes noninvasive papillary urothelial carcinomas. These may progress to invasive urothelial carcinoma; the risk of progression is related to grade.

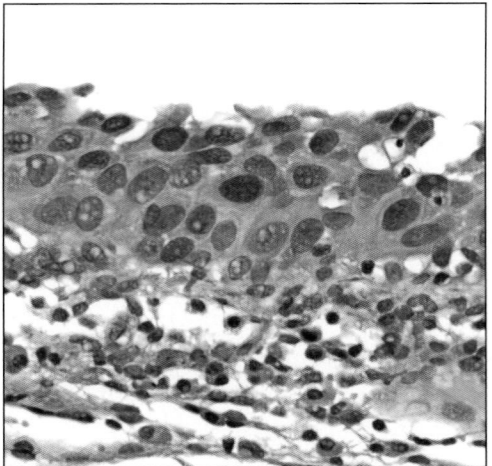

Nonpapillary forms of urothelial carcinoma also occur, as demonstrated by this urothelial carcinoma in situ. Progression to invasion may also arise in these flat urothelial carcinomas.

EPIDEMIOLOGY

Incidence
- 7th most common cancer worldwide
  - 260,000 new cases each year in men
  - 76,000 new cases each year in women
- In USA, over 90% are urothelial in origin
  - Pure squamous cell carcinoma and adenocarcinoma represent < 5%
- In regions of endemic schistosomiasis, squamous cell carcinoma is most common

Ethnicity Relationship
- Highest incidence in Western Europe, North America, and Australia
- Incidence in developed countries is 6x higher than nondeveloped countries
- 2x more common in American white men than African-American men

Gender
- Approximately 3x more common in men than women

Natural History
- For noninvasive tumors, recurrence and progression rates depend on grade
  - Urothelial papilloma
    - Recurrence: 0-8%
    - Grade or stage progression: 0%
  - Papillary urothelial neoplasm of low malignant potential
    - Recurrence: 25-47%
    - Grade or stage progression: 8%
  - Low-grade carcinoma
    - Recurrence: 48-71%
    - Progression and death due to disease: < 5%
  - High-grade carcinoma
    - Almost all disease-related deaths are secondary to high-grade tumors

- 40-45% of newly diagnosed bladder cancer is high grade
- Stage progression: 20% progress to invasion and 12% die of disease
- For invasive tumors, outcome depends on stage
  - Superficial (pT1)
    - For some patients, conservative management is sufficient
    - Subset will progress to pT2 disease and require cystectomy
  - Invasion of muscularis propria and beyond (greater than pT2)
    - 50% of patients with pT2 or greater disease have occult metastases at diagnosis
    - Most of these develop overt signs of metastasis within 1 year
  - Distant metastasis
    - Very poor prognosis
    - Poor response to adjuvant therapy

Age Range
- Typically seen in adults
  - More common after 60 years of age
- In children and adolescents, urothelial papilloma and papillary urothelial neoplasm of low malignant potential may be seen
  - Urothelial carcinoma is extraordinarily rare in young patients

Environmental Factors
- Tobacco smoking
  - Major established risk factor for bladder cancer
    - 2.6x increased risk in smokers
    - Risk increases with duration and intensity (pack years)
- Occupational exposure
  - Aniline dye
  - Aromatic amines
    - Benzidine
    - 2-naphthylamine

- Chronic inflammation
  - Chronic urinary tract infection and calculi proposed as risk factor
- Other drugs
  - Chronic abuse of analgesics that include phenacetin
  - Cyclophosphamide for cancer therapy
  - Chlornaphazine

Infectious Etiology
- Schistosomiasis
  - Squamous cell carcinoma
  - Urothelial carcinoma
- Human papilloma virus
  - Condyloma
  - Squamous dysplasia
  - Squamous cell carcinoma

CLINICAL IMPLICATIONS

Anatomic Considerations
- Microscopic anatomy of bladder is key to proper staging
  - Lamina propria
    - Connective tissues present between urothelium and detrusor muscle (muscularis propria)
    - Contains loose stroma and variably sized blood vessels
    - Includes thin muscle bands of muscularis mucosae
  - Muscularis propria
    - Thick aggregated muscle bundles of detrusor muscle
  - Perivesical soft tissue
    - Adipose tissue deep to muscularis propria
    - Adipose tissue does not define extravesical location as it is also present in lamina propria and muscularis propria

Intraoperative (Frozen Section) Evaluation
- Usually urothelial margin evaluation
  - Ureters
    - Generally sectioned en face
    - En face sections should include entire wall (urothelium, muscularis, and adventitia)
    - Examination usually for carcinoma in situ
    - Invasion may rarely be seen in soft tissues around ureter
    - von Brunn nests are common and should be distinguished from tumor
  - Urethra
    - Not as frequently examined intraoperatively
    - Generally sectioned en face
    - Examination usually for carcinoma in situ
    - Invasion may rarely be seen in soft tissues around urethra
  - General intraoperative issues
    - Frozen section artifact may induce "atypical" features in urothelium
    - Using stromal lymphocytes as a gauge of nuclear size is useful
    - Establishing minimal threshold for carcinoma in situ is key on frozen section analysis of flat lesions

- Variant invasive patterns, as plasmacytoid, mimic inflammatory cells, but more commonly have subtle soft tissue spread along ureter

Staging Issues
- Transurethral biopsy
  - WHO/ISUP 2004 grade should be given for noninvasive tumors
  - Depth of invasion should be clearly documented
    - Invasion into lamina propria (including muscularis mucosae) should be clearly distinguished from invasion into muscularis propria in report
- Cystectomy
  - Depth of invasion is key feature
    - Into lamina propria
    - Into superficial (inner half) or deep (outer half) muscularis propria
    - Into perivesical soft tissue (macroscopic or not)
    - Into adjacent organs (if present)
    - Into pelvic or abdominal wall
- Staging with invasion of prostatic stroma
  - Invasion of prostate stroma directly from bladder carcinoma is pT4a disease
  - Invasion from a tumor involving/colonizing prostatic urethra is staged for urethral origin

Specimen Handling Issues
- Initial evaluation of transurethral biopsy may be based on representative sections if specimen size precludes initial complete submission
  - If high grade and noninvasive
    - Complete submission to rule out invasion
  - If invasive but does not involve muscularis propria
    - Complete submission to rule out involvement of muscularis propria
- Evaluation of cystectomy specimen based on representative sections
  - Tumor with deepest invasion
  - Random sampling of bladder wall regions: Trigone, anterior, left lateral, right lateral, posterior, dome
  - Other focal lesions, including potential lesions, in bilateral opened ureters
- Fixation of cystectomy specimen (2 acceptable methods)
  - Formalin inflation of bladder through urethra
  - Specimen opened anteriorly and pinned out for fixation
- Gross inspection of cystectomy specimen
  - Since multifocality is common, important to document number and location of lesions
  - Ureters should be fully opened and inspected
  - Substaging of pT3 disease is based on presence of gross extension into surrounding soft tissues
    - Must be documented in gross description as positive or negative finding
- Surgical margin evaluation
  - Distal margin (urothelial)
    - Urethra in women: Usually taken en face
    - Prostatic urethra at apex in men: May be taken en face or as apical cone (perpendicular)
    - Apical margin in men more frequently involved by incidental prostate cancer

OVERVIEW OF URINARY BLADDER NEOPLASMS

- ○ Ureter margins
  - ▪ Often examined intraoperatively by frozen section
- ○ Soft tissue
  - ▪ Careful gross examination will identify deepest point of invasion to sample
  - ▪ Usually taken perpendicular to inked outer surface
- Lymph node identification
  - ○ Cystectomy
    - ▪ Not commonly identified in cystectomy specimens
  - ○ Separate dissection specimen
    - ▪ Grossly identified nodes are completely submitted (if not obviously positive)
    - ▪ For each specimen, all tissue can usually be submitted in 5 or fewer cassettes
    - ▪ For very large specimens, adequate sampling of grossly normal fat may yield small subcentimeter lymph nodes
    - ▪ Identification of 12 or more total lymph nodes is recommended
    - ▪ Anatomic node groups sampled &/or involved should be clearly reported (e.g., paraaortic)

Grading Issues

- Multiple grading schemes have been used, but WHO/ISUP 2004 is now widely accepted
  - ○ Adopted by American Joint Committee on Cancer (7th ed.) and American Urologic Association
  - ○ High-grade carcinoma under WHO/ISUP 2004 definition is commonly underdiagnosed
    - ▪ Subset of WHO 1973 grade 2 carcinomas are now classified as high grade
    - ▪ WHO 2004 and 1973 grade categories cannot be directly translated
- WHO/ISUP 2004 classification of papillary neoplasia
  - ○ Urothelial papilloma
  - ○ Papillary urothelial neoplasm of low malignant potential
  - ○ Papillary urothelial carcinoma, low grade
  - ○ Papillary urothelial carcinoma, high grade
- WHO/ISUP 2004 classification of flat lesions with atypia
  - ○ Reactive urothelial atypia
  - ○ Urothelial atypia of uncertain significance
  - ○ Urothelial dysplasia
  - ○ Urothelial carcinoma in situ
- Endophytic neoplasia
  - ○ Inverted papilloma
  - ○ Endophytic urothelial neoplasm of low malignant potential
  - ○ Endophytic urothelial carcinoma, low grade
  - ○ Endophytic urothelial carcinoma, high grade
- Invasive carcinoma
  - ○ No consensus grading scheme
  - ○ Evidence suggests grade of invasive component is not prognostic
    - ▪ We consider all invasive carcinomas as high grade despite lower grade cytology in rare cases, such as nested variant
    - ▪ Prognosis is dependent on depth of invasion rather than grade

Management

- "Superficial" bladder cancer (pTcis, pTa, pT1 disease)
  - ○ Urothelial carcinoma in situ, high-grade papillary, and invasive urothelial carcinoma involving lamina propria
    - ▪ Usually treated with intravesical therapy, such as bacillus Calmette-Guérin
    - ▪ Cystectomy for tumors refractory to conservative management
  - ○ Low-grade carcinoma and papillary urothelial neoplasm of low malignant potential
    - ▪ Usually treated by surveillance
    - ▪ Urine cytology screening
    - ▪ Adjunctive molecular screening
- Urothelial carcinoma invasive into muscularis propria
  - ○ Generally warrants radical cystectomy
  - ○ Use of neoadjuvant/adjuvant therapy is common, but its use varies between institutions

Prognostic Factors

- Depth of invasion in bladder wall determines stage and prognosis
- Some variants may portend worse prognosis
  - ○ Small cell carcinoma
  - ○ Micropapillary carcinoma
  - ○ Sarcomatoid carcinoma
  - ○ Undifferentiated carcinoma
  - ○ Carcinoma with rhabdoid features
  - ○ Plasmacytoid carcinoma
- Lymphovascular invasion
  - ○ Controversial prognostic factor
  - ○ Utilized for management decisions in some centers
  - ○ Because of frequent retraction artifact in invasive carcinoma, reproducibility of lymphovascular invasion diagnosis is problematic
  - ○ When recognized, strict morphologic criteria should be used
  - ○ Immunohistochemistry with endothelial markers may rarely be required
- Lymph node and distant metastasis portend poor prognosis
- Associated urothelial carcinoma in situ &/or tumor multifocality portend higher risk of separate new occurrence

SELECTED REFERENCES

1. American Joint Committee on Cancer: AJCC Cancer Staging Manual. 7th ed. New York: Springer. 2009
2. Eble et al: Tumors of the urinary system. In: World Health Organization Classification of Tumors. Pathology & Genetics. Tumors of the Urinary System and Male Genital Organs. Lyon: IARC Press. 89-149; 2004
3. Epstein JI et al: The World Health Organization/International Society of Urological Pathology consensus classification of urothelial (transitional cell) neoplasms of the urinary bladder. Bladder Consensus Conference Committee. Am J Surg Pathol. 22(12):1435-48, 1998

Microscopic Features

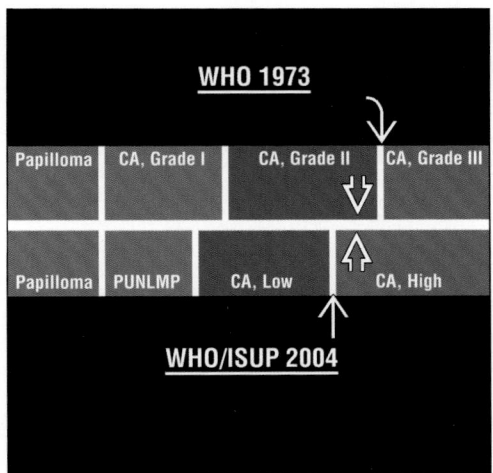

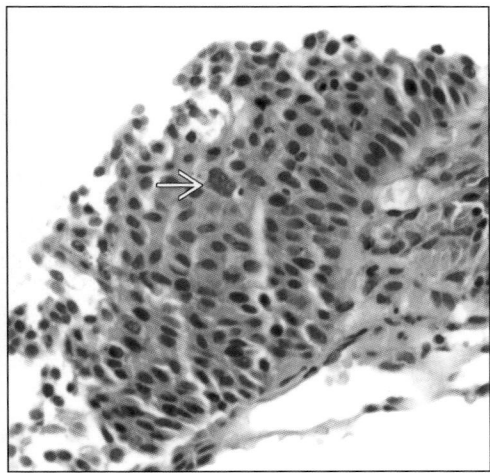

(Left) The WHO/ISUP 2004 threshold for high grade ➡️ was lowered relative to the 1973 system ➡️. A subset of cases classified as "grade II" ➡️ would now be classified as high grade ➡️. This is important for treatment because some "grade II" tumors would now receive therapy. Urologists should understand that "grade II" does not equal low grade in all cases. *(Right)* Scattered large hyperchromatic cells ➡️ are sufficient for a high-grade diagnosis in the WHO/ISUP 2004 system.

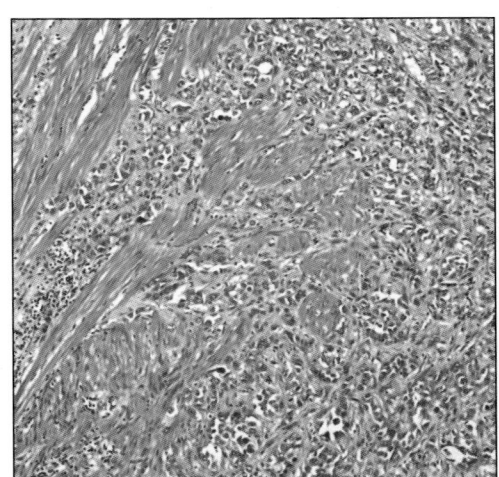

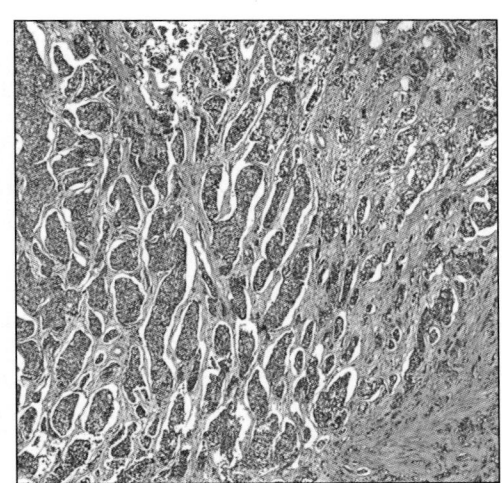

(Left) Invasion of urothelial carcinoma into the muscularis propria of the urinary bladder, as seen here, is the key histologic parameter for determining subsequent therapy (i.e., cystectomy). *(Right)* In a partially submitted bladder biopsy specimen, the initial findings should guide the necessity of processing additional tissue. This case with extensive invasion of fibrous tissue (lamina propria) would require complete tissue submission in search of muscularis propria involvement.

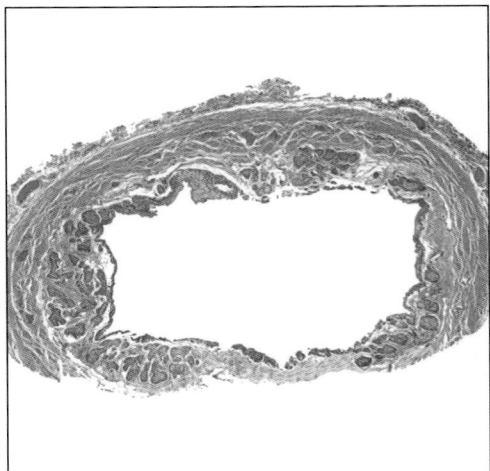

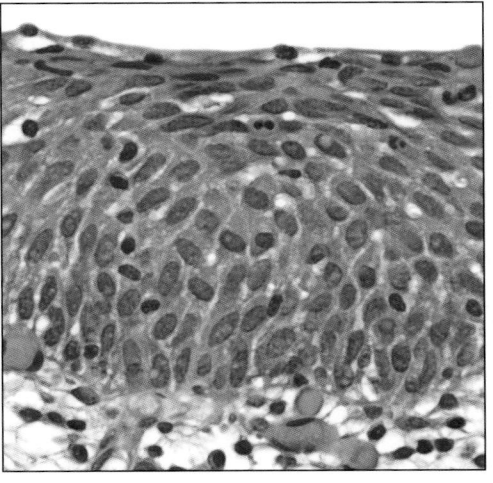

(Left) Ureter margins are evaluated intraoperatively by frozen section analysis. The lumen should be evaluated en face, as seen here, to ensure that the rim of lining urothelium is fully examined for carcinoma in situ. The surrounding fibrous tissue and muscle should also be examined as some invasive urothelial carcinomas may "track down" these tissue planes. *(Right)* Mild disorganization is within the spectrum of normal urothelium and should not be interpreted as neoplasia.

UROTHELIAL CARCINOMA IN SITU

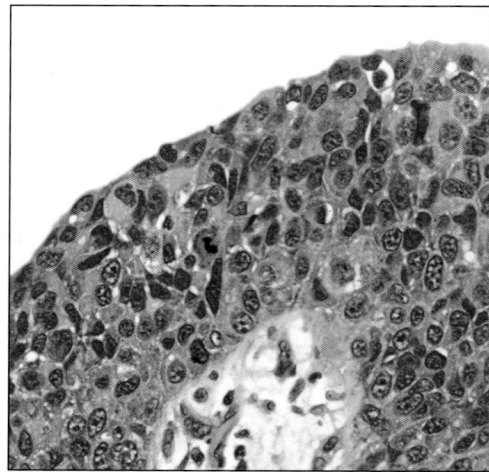

CIS shows a range of histologic diversity, with unequivocal high-grade nuclear atypia, which may include pleomorphism, prominent nucleoli, and atypical mitoses toward the surface.

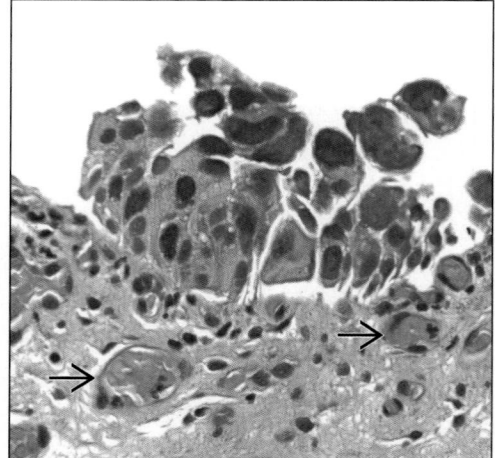

This CIS has marked nuclear pleomorphism. Cellular discohesion, as seen in this example, is common. Frequently, there is neovascularization in the superficial lamina propria ➔.

TERMINOLOGY

Abbreviations
- Urothelial carcinoma in situ (CIS)
- Bacillus Calmette-Guérin (BCG)

Synonyms
- Urothelial carcinoma in situ = only appropriate term for this lesion under the WHO 2004/ISUP classification system

Definitions
- Flat urothelial lesion comprised of cytologically malignant cells, which may involve either full or partial thickness of urothelium
  - 3 clinical forms of CIS
    - 1 = primary (de novo) CIS: Isolated CIS with no prior or concurrent papillary tumors
    - 2 = secondary CIS: Detected on follow-up of patients with papillary tumors
    - 3 = concurrent CIS: Accompanied by papillary tumors at time of diagnosis

ETIOLOGY/PATHOGENESIS

Environmental Exposure
- Tobacco smoking, analgesic abuse, and arylamine compounds are known predisposing factors

Molecular Pathogenesis
- Molecular data have identified several genetic changes that are associated with CIS
  - Amplification/mutation of *p53* gene
  - Aneuploidy common

CLINICAL ISSUES

Epidemiology
- Incidence
  - Primary (de novo) CIS is rare (< 3% of all urothelial neoplasms)
  - CIS is commonly detected with high-grade papillary and invasive urothelial carcinoma
- Age
  - Most typically seen in men in 6th or 7th decade

Presentation
- Asymptomatic, or may present with dysuria, nocturia, urgency, or frequency of micturition
- Hematuria, if present, is typically microscopic

Treatment
- Different forms of intravesical therapy
  - BCG is most common treatment
- Cystectomy is common treatment for patients refractory to intravesical therapy

Prognosis
- Behavior of CIS is somewhat unpredictable
  - ~ 50% of patients develop invasive carcinoma within 5 years
  - Primary (de novo) CIS seems to have lower progression rate than secondary or concomitant CIS

MACROSCOPIC FEATURES

General Features
- Cystoscopic appearance of CIS may range from normal to erythematous, edematous, or erosive
- Multifocality of CIS is common

MICROSCOPIC PATHOLOGY

Histologic Features
- Unequivocal high-grade cytologic atypia may involve either full or partial thickness of urothelium
  - Nuclear anaplasia may be obvious
  - Spectrum of cytologic atypia exists

UROTHELIAL CARCINOMA IN SITU

Key Facts

Terminology
- Malignant flat lesion comprised of cytologically high-grade cells

Etiology/Pathogenesis
- Multiple predisposing environmental factors are known

Clinical Issues
- Most common in men, 6th-7th decade

Microscopic Pathology
- Unequivocal high-grade cytologic atypia may involve either full or partial thickness of urothelium
- Marked nucleomegaly is typical
- Nuclear hyperchromasia with coarse condensed chromatin is typical
- Spectrum of atypia and growth patterns exist

- Loss of polarity to basement membrane is common

Ancillary Tests
- CK20, CD44, and p53 immunohistochemistry may be useful in distinction from nonneoplastic reactive atypia

Top Differential Diagnoses
- Urothelial dysplasia and flat atypia of uncertain significance
- Reactive atypia (including therapy effect)

Diagnostic Checklist
- Key to interpreting flat lesions is developing appropriate minimal threshold for CIS
- Definite nucleomegaly with nuclear hyperchromasia/irregular chromatin is required

---

- Marked nucleomegaly is typical (3-6x size of a normal lymphocyte nucleus)
- Coarse, condensed nuclear chromatin is typical
- Mitoses are variable, but atypical forms may be present, even toward surface
- Cellular discohesion may be prominent
- Loss of polarity and crowding is common
- Urothelial thickness varies greatly in CIS
  o May be denuded, normal, or hyperplastic
- Different morphologic patterns are described

ANCILLARY TESTS

Immunohistochemistry
- CK20, CD44, and p53 may be useful in distinction of reactive atypia from CIS
- Normal urothelium and reactive atypia
  o CK20 expressed in superficial umbrella cells only
  o CD44 stains only basal and parabasal cell layer with increased staining in reactive atypia
  o Nuclear staining for p53 is absent or weak & patchy
- In contrast, CIS has distinct immunophenotype
  o Full thickness cytoplasmic staining for CK20
  o CD44 is absent or confined to residual basal cells
  o Diffuse, strong, nuclear staining for p53 may be seen; full-thickness positivity is diagnostic

DIFFERENTIAL DIAGNOSIS

Urothelial Dysplasia and Flat Atypia of Uncertain Significance
- Unequivocal nuclear atypia (beyond reactive changes) that falls short of threshold for CIS

Reactive Atypia
- Intraepithelial inflammation is usually prominent
- Although there is nuclear enlargement, it is usually uniform
  o Usually < 3x size of a normal lymphocyte nucleus
- Nucleoli are common
- Chromatin remains relatively evenly dispersed

- Mitotic figures may be increased and may extend into upper levels of urothelium but are not atypical

Radiation/Chemotherapy Effect
- May induce full-thickness nuclear atypia
- Cells often have intracytoplasmic & nuclear vacuolization
- Often bizarre nuclear shapes with multinucleation
- Associated radiation-induced atypical fibroblasts &/or vascular changes

DIAGNOSTIC CHECKLIST

Clinically Relevant Pathologic Features
- Multifocality and microinvasion

Pathologic Interpretation Pearls
- Key to interpreting flat lesions is developing appropriate minimal threshold for CIS
  o Definite nucleomegaly with nuclear hyperchromasia/irregular chromatin is required
  o Elevated mitotic rates are not sufficient as they may be seen in reactive lesions

SELECTED REFERENCES

1. Sesterhenn IA: Urothelial carcinoma in situ. In Eble JN et al: World Health Organization Classification of Tumours. Pathology & Genetics. Tumours of the Urinary System and Male Genital Organs. Lyon: IARC Press, 2004
2. McKenney JK et al: Discriminatory immunohistochemical staining of urothelial carcinoma in situ and non-neoplastic urothelium: an analysis of cytokeratin 20, p53, and CD44 antigens. Am J Surg Pathol. 25(8):1074-8, 2001
3. McKenney JK et al: Morphologic expressions of urothelial carcinoma in situ: a detailed evaluation of its histologic patterns with emphasis on carcinoma in situ with microinvasion. Am J Surg Pathol. 25(3):356-62, 2001
4. Epstein JI et al: The World Health Organization/International Society of Urological Pathology consensus classification of urothelial (transitional cell) neoplasms of the urinary bladder. Bladder Consensus Conference Committee. Am J Surg Pathol. 22(12):1435-48, 1998

Microscopic Features

(Left) Marked nucleomegaly is a very useful diagnostic feature of CIS and involves the full thickness in this example. The neoplastic nuclei are approximately 5-6x the size of the underlying lymphocytes ➡ in this case, a useful gauge of nucleomegaly. *(Right)* CIS is characterized by cellular disorder, pronounced nucleomegaly, and variable pleomorphism. There may be cellular discohesion, as seen toward the surface. The thickness of the mucosa involved by CIS varies considerably.

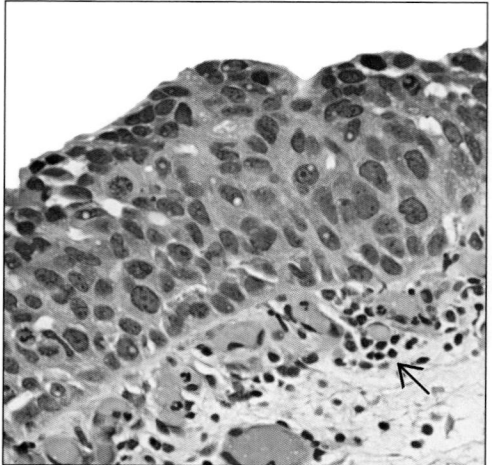
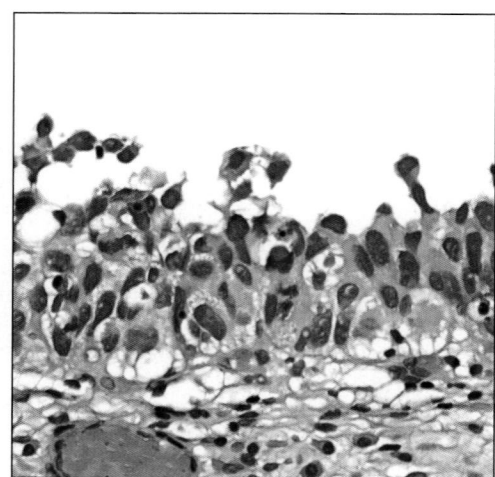

(Left) The degree of nucleomegaly of the CIS ➡ is obvious when compared to the normal urothelium below ➡. The diagnosis of CIS is made on the basis of the overall constellation of nuclear abnormalities. *(Right)* CIS ➡ in this example is characterized by marked nucleomegaly, nuclear hyperchromasia, and some degree of pleomorphism. The nuclei of the normal urothelium ➡ are only 1-2x the size of a stromal lymphocyte ➡, in contrast to at least 4x in this CIS.

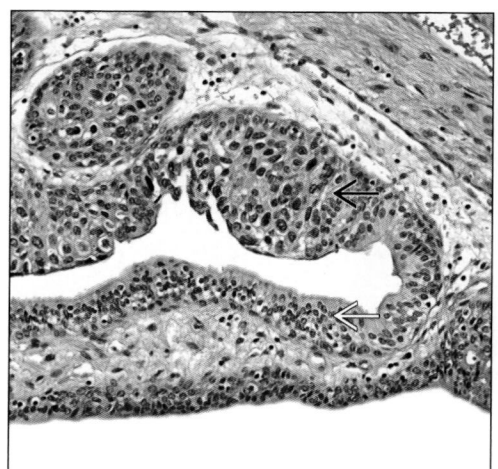
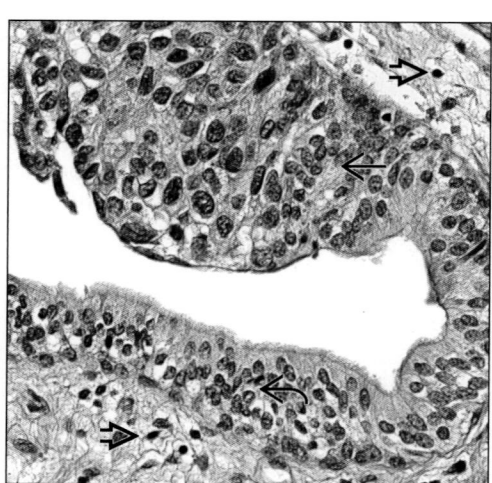

(Left) CIS may show the presence of maturation on the surface (there is a subtle thin layer of residual superficial umbrella cells ➡). Although the cells are large and atypical, pleomorphism is absent. This is referred to as "nonpleomorphic large cell" CIS. *(Right)* CIS may occasionally consist of a very thin urothelium. The urothelial cells are markedly enlarged with irregular coarse chromatin and obvious mitotic figures ➡, features useful in the diagnosis of CIS.

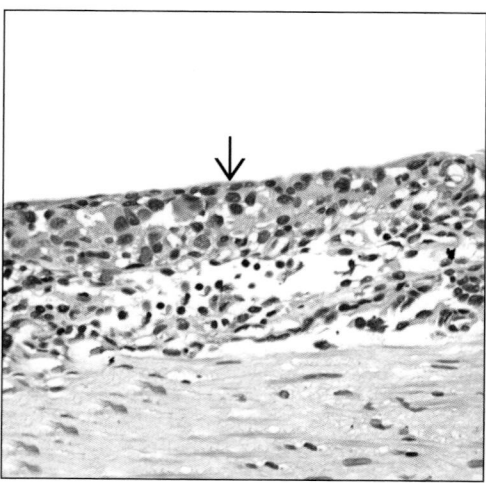
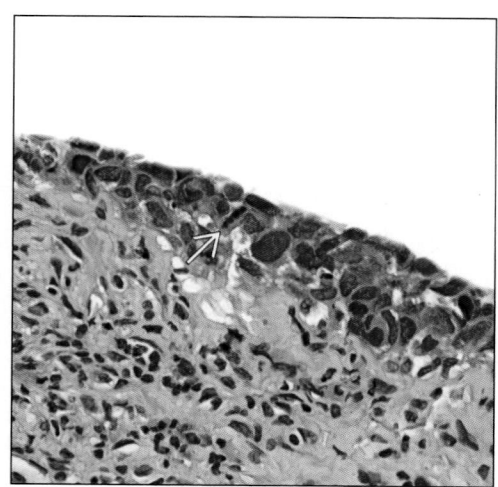

Microscopic Features

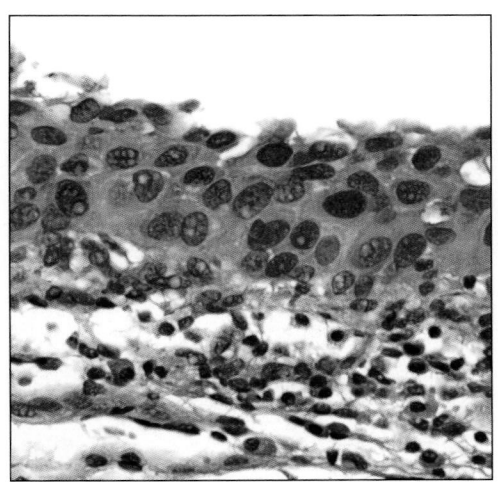

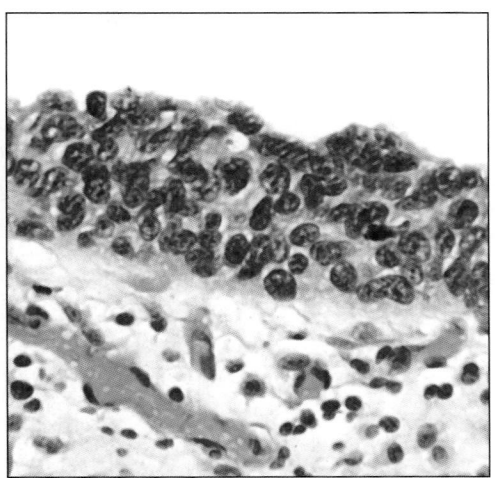

(Left) Some examples of CIS referred to as "non-pleomorphic large cell CIS" have less significant pleomorphism and may have more abundant eosinophilic cytoplasm. The degree of nucleomegaly and coarse nuclear chromatin, however, are diagnostic of CIS. *(Right)* So-called small cell CIS has a high nuclear to cytoplasmic ratio. This term does not imply neuroendocrine differentiation or relation to small cell carcinoma.

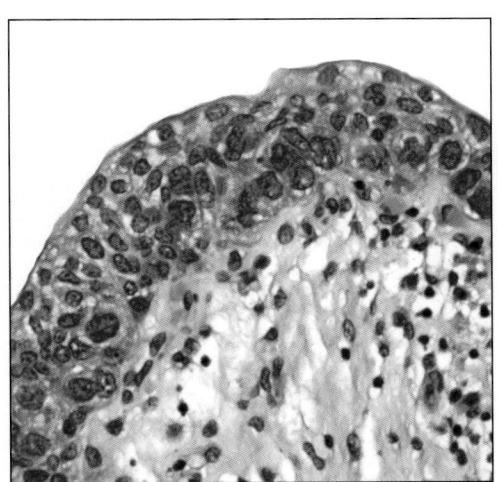

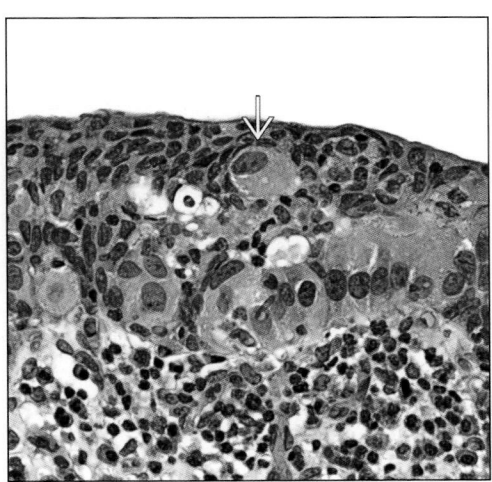

(Left) In CIS, the neoplastic cells may not show full-thickness involvement. In this example, they are confined to the lower 2/3 of the urothelium. In contrast to precursor lesions in other anatomic sites, the presence of markedly atypical cells at any level is sufficient for the diagnosis as CIS. *(Right)* Pagetoid urothelial CIS is characterized by clusters or individual carcinoma cells ➡ that colonize normal urothelium in a pattern similar to mammary Paget disease.

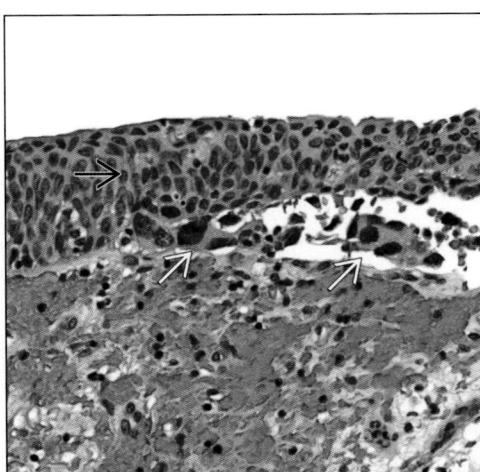

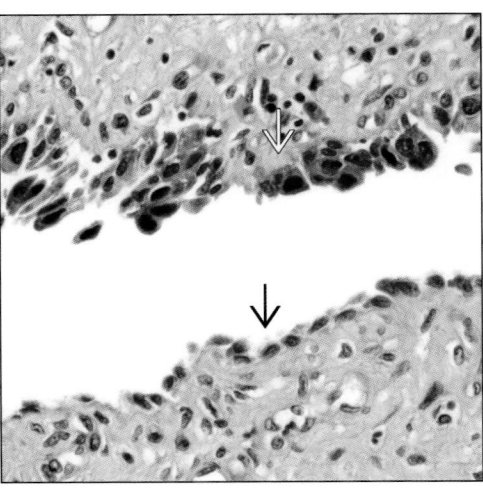

(Left) Undermining urothelial CIS is characterized by extension of carcinoma cells ➡ underneath adjacent normal urothelium ➡. The difference in nuclear size between the 2 populations is striking. *(Right)* Clinging urothelial CIS is characterized by individual residual carcinoma cells ➡ attached to the basement membrane. The nucleomegaly and nuclear hyperchromasia of this clinging CIS are contrasted to the normal residual basal cells below ➡.

UROTHELIAL CARCINOMA IN SITU

Colonization and Immunohistochemistry

(Left) These von Brunn nests are colonized by urothelial CIS. The sharp linear border at the underlying junction with the lamina propria and the rounded borders of the nests help in the distinction from invasive carcinoma. *(Right)* Cells of urothelial CIS colonizing a von Brunn nest on the left ➡ show obvious marked nucleomegaly and coarse chromatin compared to the von Brunn nest with normal urothelial cells on the right ➡.

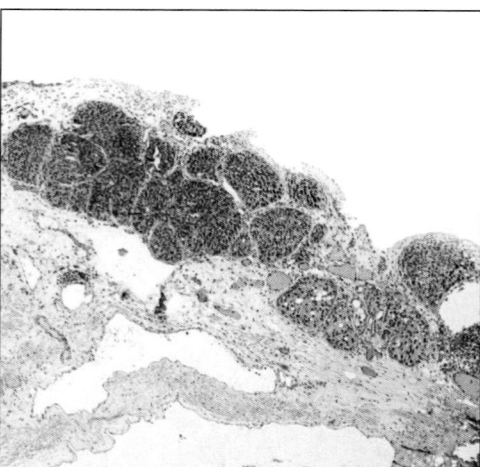
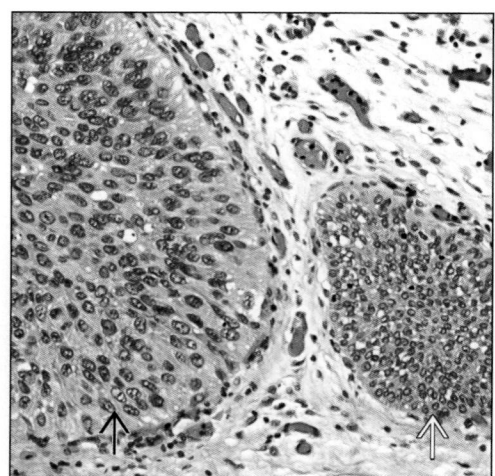

(Left) Diffuse cytoplasmic reactivity for CK20 is commonly seen in urothelial CIS. In normal and reactive urothelium, CK20 staining is confined to the superficial umbrella cell layer; staining may be completely negative if these cells are not present. *(Right)* Denuding urothelial CIS commonly shows diffuse strong cytoplasmic reactivity for CK20. Normal basal and parabasal cells do not express CK20, even in cases with significant reactive atypia.

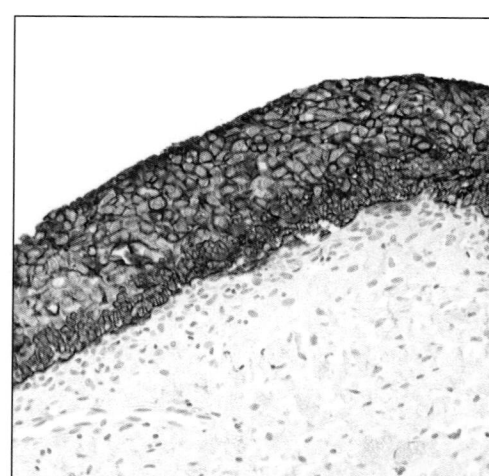
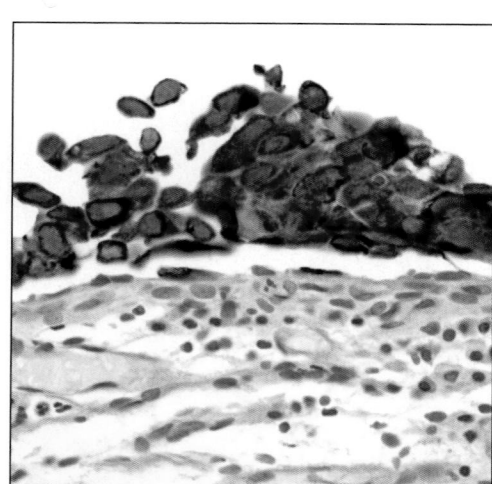

(Left) In this cystectomy specimen with pagetoid urothelial CIS, immunohistochemistry for CD44 isoform shows strong membranous reactivity in the normal reactive urothelial cell population, as expected. The scattered negative cells represent CIS ➡. *(Right)* Scattered neoplastic cells of pagetoid CIS ➡ are highlighted by nuclear immunoreactivity for p53, which is less sensitive than CK20. A combination of 3 markers constitutes an appropriate panel.

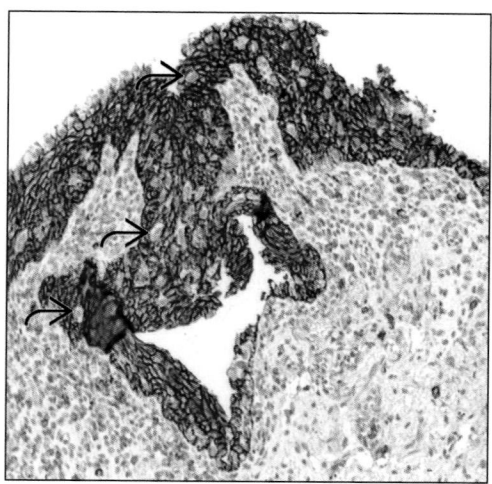
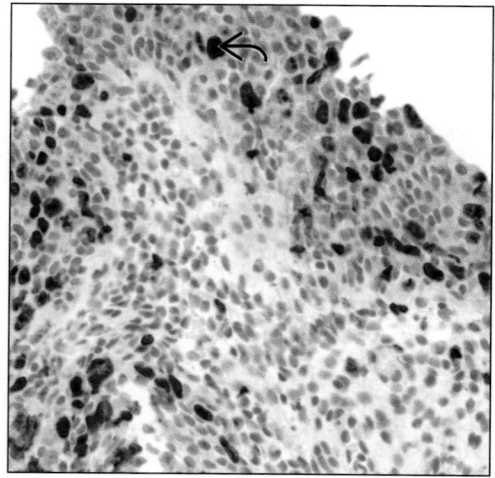

Differential Diagnosis

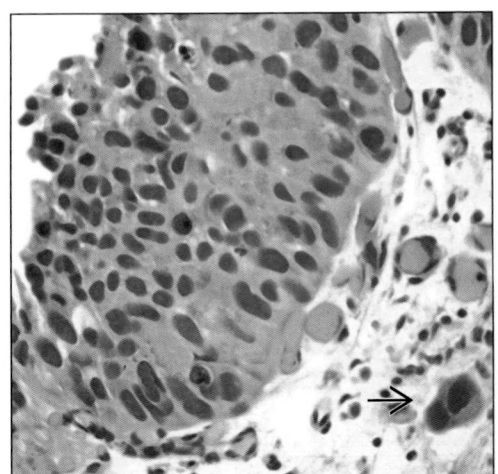

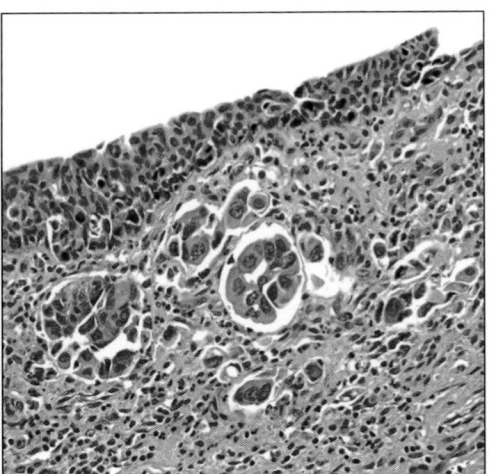

(Left) The small cluster of neoplastic cells ⤐ indicates focal invasion into lamina propria (pT1). Invasion to a depth of < 2 mm is referred to as CIS with microinvasion. *(Right)* These neoplastic cells in the superficial lamina propria, which are characterized by individual cells and clusters with surrounding retraction spaces, represent lamina propria invasion. Stromal clefts are characteristic of invasion and exclude the possibility of von Brunn nests colonized by CIS.

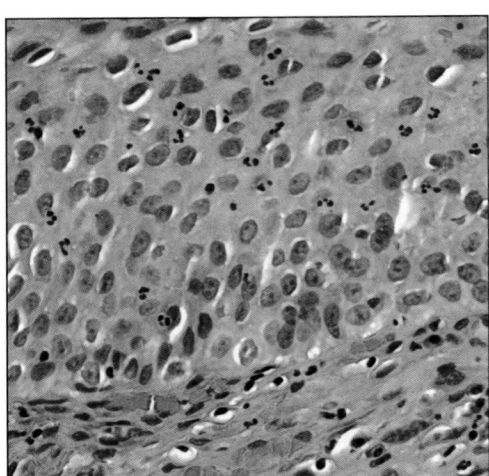

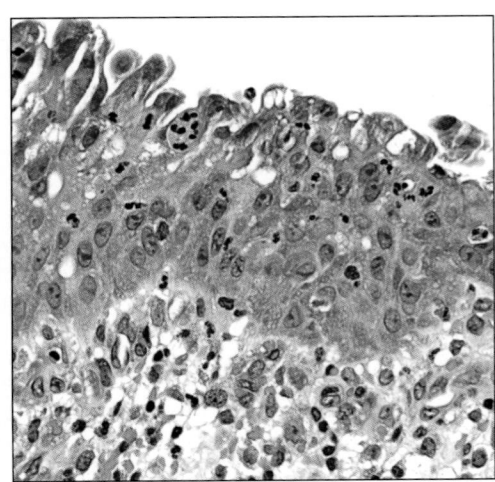

(Left) In this example of reactive atypia, the nuclei are more rounded, but maintain fine nuclear chromatin and show small nucleoli. The homogeneously even chromatin and associated intraurothelial neutrophils support a designation as a reactive lesion. *(Right)* This florid example of reactive atypia in a young patient is associated with an indwelling catheter. Despite the enlarged nucleoli, the relatively fine chromatin and intraurothelial neutrophils support a reactive diagnosis.

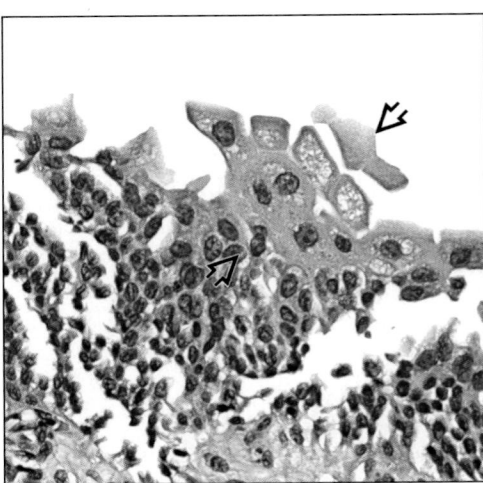

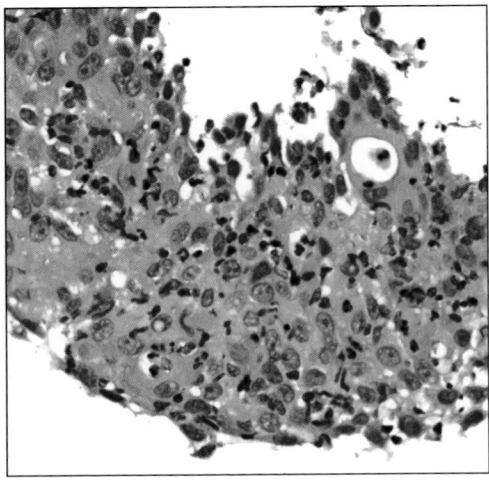

(Left) Normal superficial umbrella cells ⇨ may show some level of cytologic atypia with nucleomegaly and multinucleation that may potentially mimic urothelial CIS, especially if sectioned somewhat tangentially. *(Right)* In this bladder biopsy, the urothelial cells show macronucleoli, some variation in size and shape, and cellular disorder. Given the amount of associated inflammation, this example would be designated as urothelial atypia of uncertain significance.

FLAT UROTHELIAL LESIONS OTHER THAN CARCINOMA IN SITU

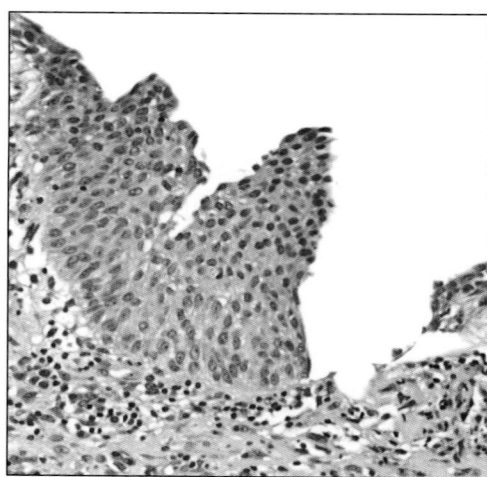

In this example of reactive urothelial atypia, the nuclei of the urothelial cells are only slightly enlarged with small and rarely prominent nucleoli. There is nuclear monotony.

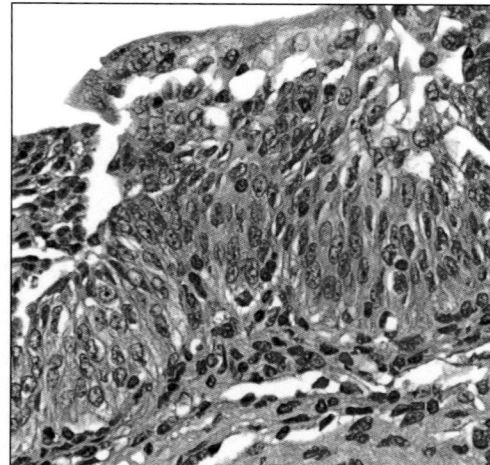

The nuclei in this reactive urothelial atypia are characterized by fine, evenly dispersed nuclear chromatin and prominent nucleoli, typical features of a reactive process.

TERMINOLOGY

Abbreviations
- Carcinoma in situ (CIS)

Definitions
- Urothelial hyperplasia
  - Markedly thickened flat urothelium without cytologic atypia
- Reactive urothelial atypia
  - Benign reactive or regenerative epithelial changes
  - Most often associated with inflammatory infiltrate
- Urothelial atypia of uncertain significance
  - Flat lesions with subtle but definite alterations that are not categorically either reactive or neoplastic
  - Not a diagnostic entity
    - Descriptive diagnosis to ensure clinical follow-up in difficult to classify cases
- Urothelial dysplasia
  - Lesions with unequivocal cytologic and architectural changes felt to be preneoplastic, but that fall below threshold for diagnosis of urothelial CIS
    - Controversial category with poor reproducibility

CLINICAL ISSUES

Presentation
- Irritative bladder symptoms

Treatment
- Urothelial hyperplasia
  - None
- Reactive urothelial atypia
  - Treatment should be based on alleviating underlying cause
    - Infection
    - Radiation
    - Intravesical catheter
    - Prior intravesical therapy

- Urothelial atypia of uncertain significance
  - Requires clinical follow-up
    - Urine cytology and cystoscopy
- Urothelial dysplasia
  - Requires clinical follow-up
    - Urine cytology and cystoscopy

Prognosis
- Urothelial hyperplasia
  - When seen without concomitant papillary neoplasia, no evidence to suggest preneoplastic state
- Reactive atypia
  - Benign
- Urothelial atypia of uncertain significance
  - Not fully known
- Urothelial dysplasia
  - In rare series diagnosed as dysplasia, progression to bladder neoplasia, including CIS, seen in 5-19% of cases

MACROSCOPIC FEATURES

General Features
- May have hyperemic mucosa at cystoscopy

MICROSCOPIC PATHOLOGY

Urothelial Hyperplasia
- Markedly thickened flat urothelium
  - Normal cytology and cellular order
- May be seen in flat mucosa adjacent to low-grade papillary neoplasms

Reactive Urothelial Atypia
- Nucleomegaly with prominent nucleoli
  - Usually 2-3x the size of lymphocyte nucleus
    - Nucleoli usually pin-point but may be larger
- Nuclear chromatin fine and evenly dispersed
- Cells often fusiform but may become rounded

FLAT UROTHELIAL LESIONS OTHER THAN CARCINOMA IN SITU

Key Facts

Terminology
- Urothelial hyperplasia
  - Markedly thickened flat urothelium without cytologic atypia
  - No evidence of potential for progression
  - May be seen adjacent to low-grade papillary lesions
- Reactive urothelial atypia
  - Benign reactive or regenerative epithelial changes, secondary to infection, prior therapy, or intravesical catheter
  - Typically associated with intraurothelial inflammatory infiltrate
  - Mild nucleomegaly, fine chromatin, and prominent nucleoli
  - No pleomorphism
- Urothelial atypia of uncertain significance
  - Subtle but definite alterations that are not categorically either reactive or dysplastic
  - Descriptive diagnosis to ensure clinical follow-up in difficult to classify cases
- Urothelial dysplasia
  - Controversial category with poor reproducibility and poorly understood significance
  - Unequivocal cytologic and architectural changes felt to be preneoplastic but below threshold for urothelial carcinoma in situ
  - Mild nucleomegaly
  - Subtle loss of polarity
  - Minimal irregularity of nuclear contours
  - Increased cytoplasmic eosinophilia

- Cells maintain polarity perpendicular to basement membrane
- Intraurothelial acute or chronic inflammation
- Increased mitotic activity may be present, even in upper layers; not atypical forms
- Radiation therapy may induce additional changes
  - Vacuolated cytoplasm and enlarged cells with dark, smudgy chromatin

Urothelial Atypia of Uncertain Significance
- Used as diagnostic category in cases with inflammation in which severity of atypia appears to be out of proportion to extent of inflammation
  - Preneoplastic lesion cannot be confidently excluded

Urothelial Dysplasia
- Some genitourinary pathologists diagnose such lesions as urothelial atypia of uncertain significance
  - Controversial category with poor reproducibility
  - Poorly understood clinical significance
  - No known treatment implication
- Clear-cut nuclear atypia is evident but is not severe enough to merit diagnosis of CIS
  - Mild nucleomegaly with subtle loss of polarity
    - Nuclear crowding and rounded to polygonal cells
  - Minimal irregularity of nuclear contours and chromatin distribution
  - Increased cytoplasmic eosinophilia

DIFFERENTIAL DIAGNOSIS

Urothelial Carcinoma In Situ
- Marked nucleomegaly (often 4x or more the size of lymphocyte nucleus)
- Nuclear pleomorphism and hyperchromasia
- Loss of normal polarity and presence of nuclear crowding common
- Immunohistochemistry may have utility in distinction from reactive atypia
  - CIS commonly has full-thickness cytoplasmic expression of CK20 and may have diffuse reactivity for p53

- Normal or reactive urothelium shows reactivity for CK20 only in superficial umbrella cell layer
- Reactive atypia may have increased CD44 membranous reactivity, and p53 is usually patchy and weak

Polyoma Virus Inclusions
- Intranuclear inclusions in superficial cells may mimic neoplastic process
- Immunohistochemistry for polyoma virus is diagnostic

Normal Urothelium
- Flat lesions with benign cytology and minimal disorder should be considered within spectrum of "normal"

DIAGNOSTIC CHECKLIST

Pathologic Interpretation Pearls
- Developing appropriate threshold for urothelial CIS is critical in diagnosing flat lesions
  - Nuclear size and chromatin character are critical morphologic features
- Great caution should be exercised before lesion is diagnosed as de novo dysplasia (i.e., with no prior history of urothelial neoplasia)
  - Designating these cases as "atypia of unknown significance" is recommended

SELECTED REFERENCES

1. Eble JN et al: World Health Organization Classification of Tumour. Pathology & Genetics. Tumour of the Urinary System and Male Genital Organs. Lyon: IARC Press. 111-12; 2004
2. Epstein JI et al: The World Health Organization/ International Society of Urological Pathology consensus classification of urothelial (transitional cell) neoplasms of the urinary bladder. Bladder Consensus Conference Committee. Am J Surg Pathol. 22(12):1435-48, 1998

FLAT UROTHELIAL LESIONS OTHER THAN CARCINOMA IN SITU

Microscopic Features

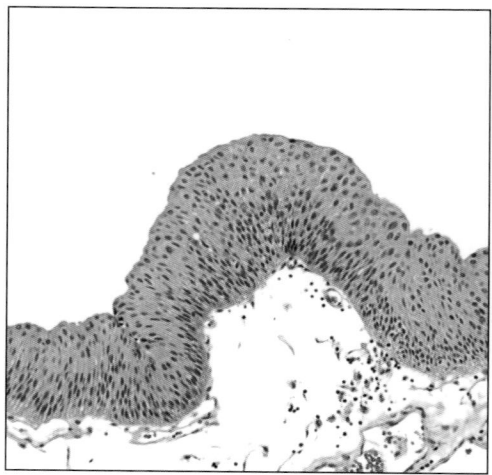
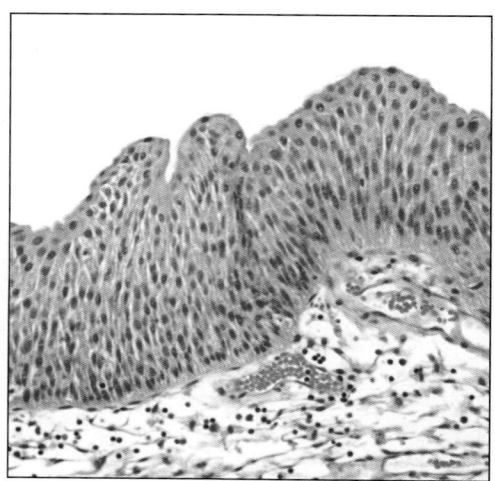

(Left) This example shows flat urothelium with increased thickness, characteristic of urothelial hyperplasia. This lesion is common adjacent to low-grade papillary urothelial neoplasms but may also be seen in isolation. *(Right)* High-power evaluation of urothelial hyperplasia shows preservation of polarity with the urothelial cells streaming upward perpendicular to the basement membrane. In addition, the cytology of the cells appears normal.

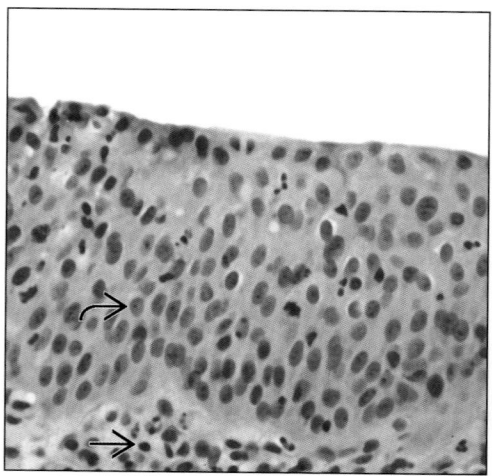
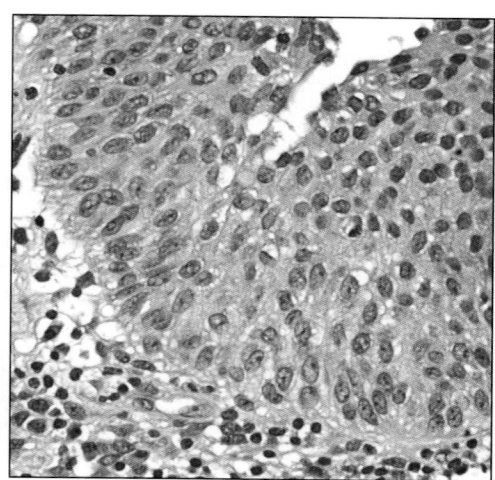

(Left) In this example of reactive urothelial atypia, numerous intraurothelial neutrophils are present. The nuclei of the urothelial cells ⇗ are only 2-3x the size of a stromal lymphocyte ⇥, as expected, and the chromatin remains evenly dispersed with small nucleoli. *(Right)* In reactive atypia, prominent nucleoli are obvious, but the nuclear chromatin is evenly dispersed. There is overall maintained polarity and monotony of nuclei. Inflammation is variable in reactive atypia.

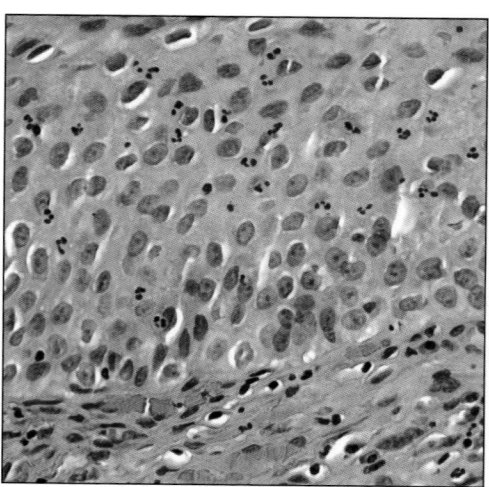
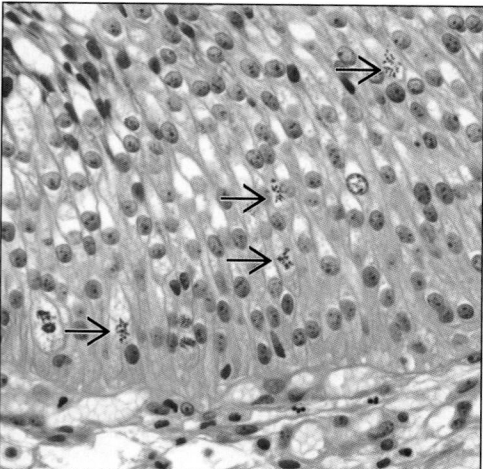

(Left) In this reactive urothelial atypia, there is marked intraurothelial acute inflammation. As typical, the chromatin is fine and nucleoli are prominent. *(Right)* Florid reactive urothelial atypia may have brisk mitotic activity ⇥ that extends into the upper urothelial layers as seen in this case. The fine nuclear chromatin, small pin-point nucleoli, and normal polarity (upward streaming of the urothelial cells) all support a reactive diagnosis.

FLAT UROTHELIAL LESIONS OTHER THAN CARCINOMA IN SITU

Ancillary Techniques

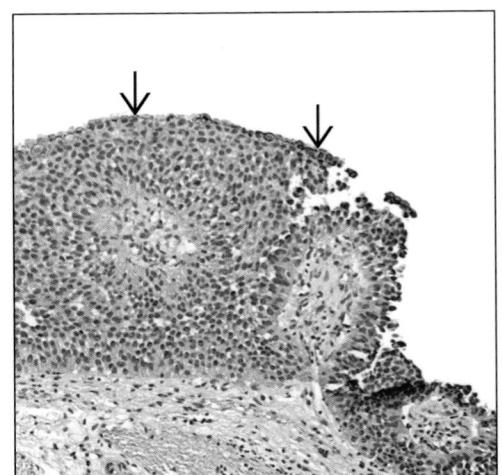

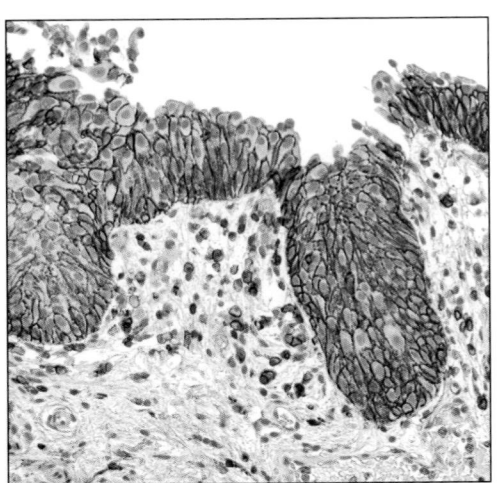

(Left) Immunohistochemistry is useful in the distinction of carcinoma in situ from reactive atypia. CK20 stains only umbrella cells in normal or reactive urothelium ➡. Diffuse full-thickness staining is common in carcinoma in situ. *(Right)* Membranous immunoreactivity with CD44 extending into the intermediate/upper levels of the urothelium is characteristic of reactive atypia. Carcinoma in situ has absent CD44 expression or staining only in residual basal cells.

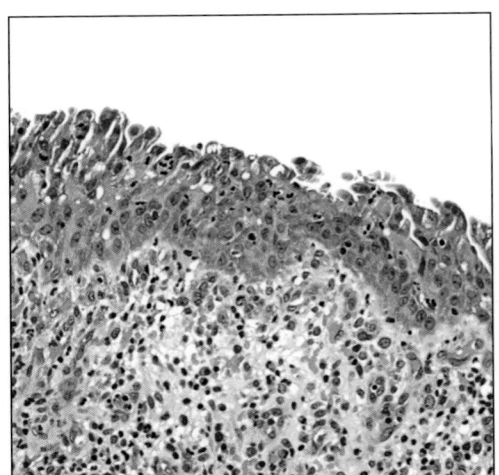

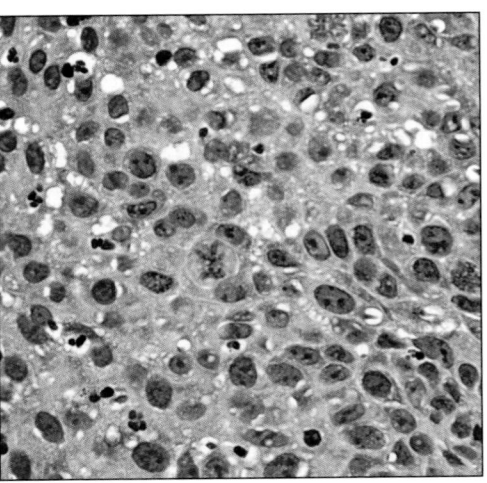

(Left) In this example of florid reactive urothelial atypia associated with intravesical catheterization, intraurothelial inflammation may be present with associated nuclear enlargement and one or more prominent nucleoli. *(Right)* Despite the subtle variation in nuclear size and the mitotic activity, the fine, evenly dispersed nuclear chromatin, prominent nucleoli, and intraurothelial inflammation all support a reactive atypia diagnosis. The nuclei do not show crowding and overlapping.

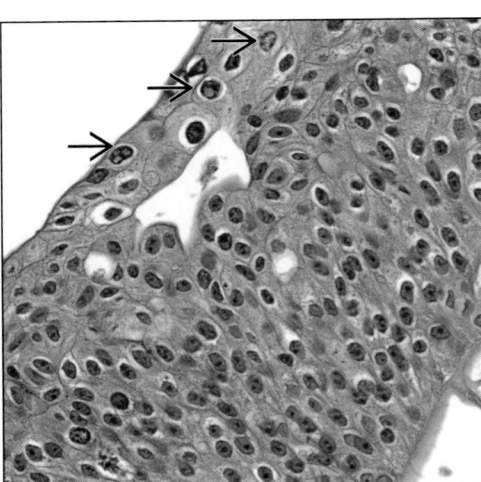

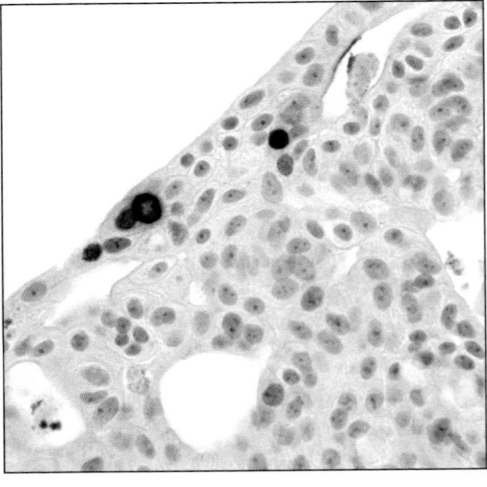

(Left) Specific forms of reactive nonneoplastic urothelial changes, such as this example of polyoma virus infection, may also mimic urothelial neoplasia. In this example, there is "smudgy" nuclear chromatin and intranuclear inclusions ➡ in scattered superficial urothelial cells. The urothelium in the lower levels has a typical reactive appearance. *(Right)* Strong nuclear reactivity for polyoma virus, which is typically superficial, is diagnostic of infection.

FLAT UROTHELIAL LESIONS OTHER THAN CARCINOMA IN SITU

Reactive Atypia

(Left) Multinucleation ⇨ and fibrin aggregates ⇨ are commonly seen in radiation-associated atypia. Other features associated with radiation injury, such as stromal hemorrhage and vascular changes, may be seen in the lamina propria. *(Right)* This example of reactive urothelial atypia secondary to radiation therapy shows characteristic radiation changes that include large nuclei with "smudgy" chromatin and cytoplasmic vacuolization ⇨.

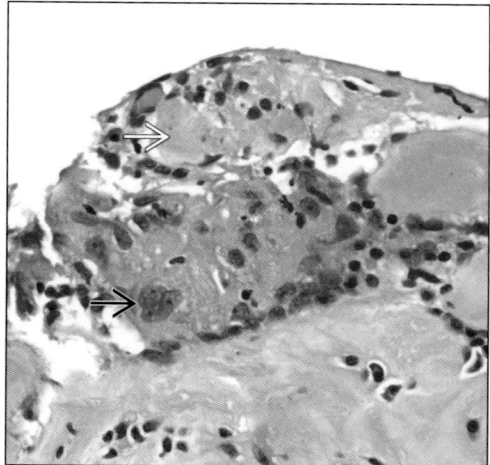
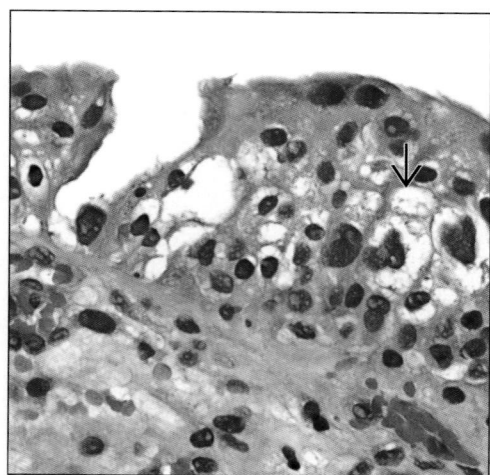

(Left) In this flat urothelial lesion, the nuclei are rounded with some overlapping; however, the fine nuclear chromatin and small pin-point nucleoli are typical of reactive urothelial atypia. *(Right)* Nuclear rounding, mild variation in nuclear size and shape, and macronuclei are present. With this degree of intraurothelial inflammation, the suggested diagnosis would be "atypia of uncertain significance," as the possibility of an underlying neoplasia cannot be entirely ruled out.

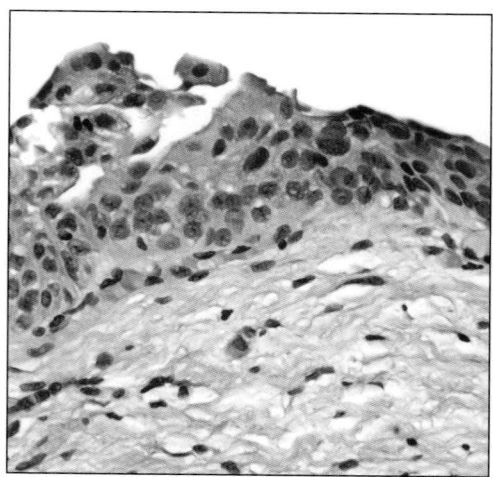
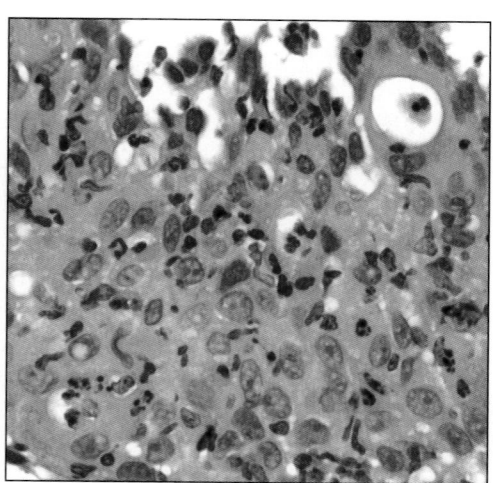

(Left) This lesion has round nuclei with mild enlargement, some polarity loss, and no significant chromatin abnormality. We would classify this lesion as "atypia of uncertain significance," but some might regard such lesions as urothelial dysplasia. *(Right)* Occasional cells are enlarged with mild chromatin alteration ⇨, and there is some crowding and nuclear rounding. This atypia falls short of CIS. Some experts might regard this lesion as "urothelial dysplasia."

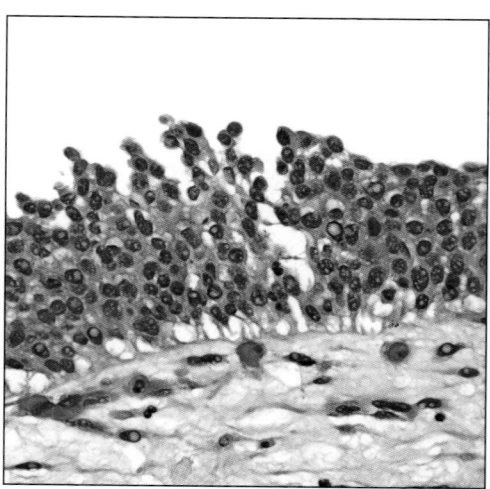
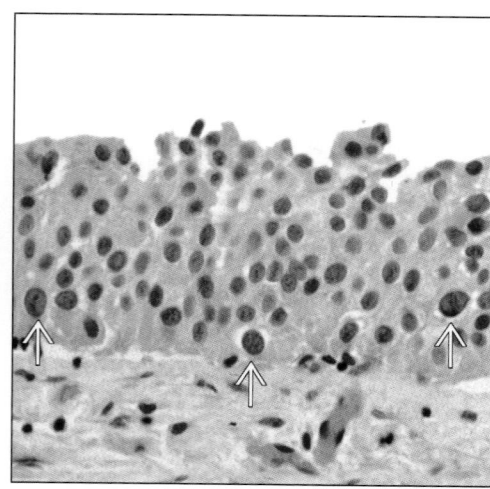

FLAT UROTHELIAL LESIONS OTHER THAN CARCINOMA IN SITU

Differential Diagnosis of Carcinoma in Situ

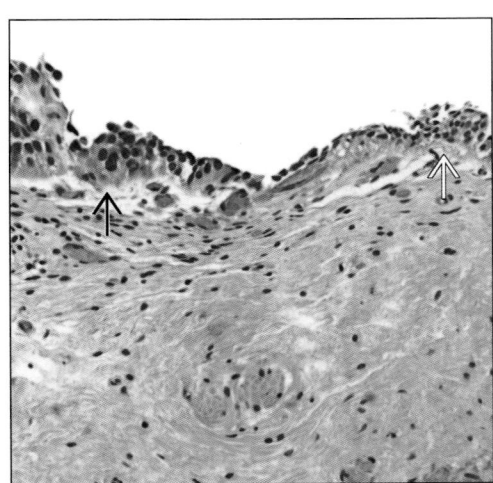
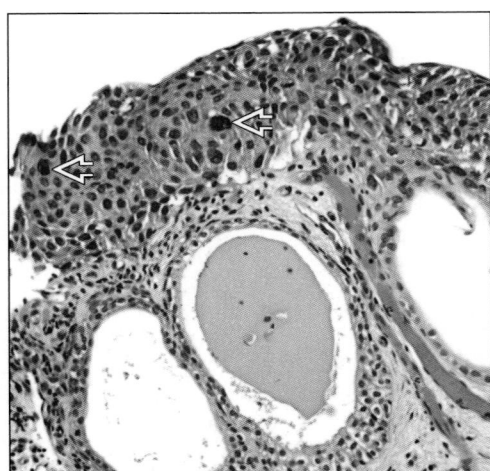

(Left) When present, comparison of the region of flat urothelial atypia to nonatypical foci may be very helpful. In this example, the marked nucleomegaly of urothelial carcinoma in situ on the left ➡ is obvious when contrasted with adjacent normal urothelium ➡. (Right) This degree of nuclear pleomorphism and hyperchromasia ➡ precludes a reactive diagnosis and is sufficient for classification as urothelial carcinoma in situ. Underlying von Brunn nests are not involved.

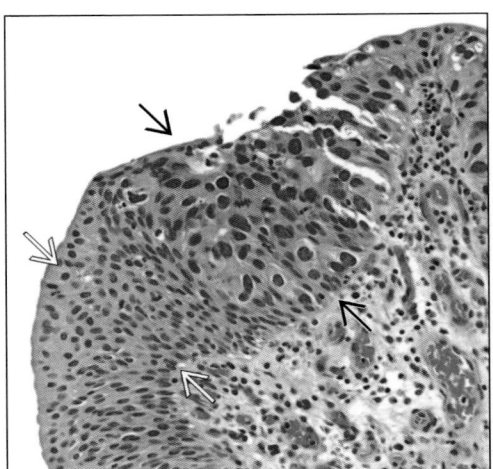
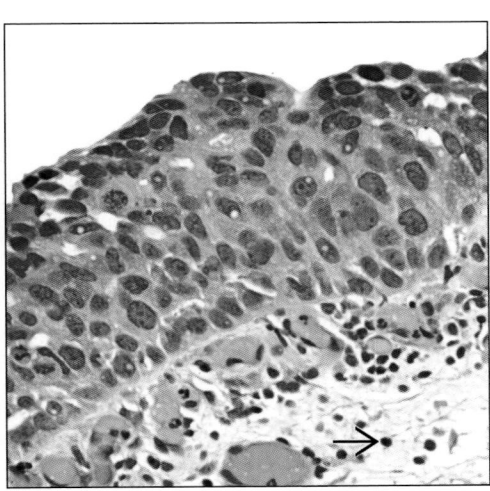

(Left) The marked nucleomegaly and loss of polarity of the urothelial CIS cells ➡ is obvious when compared to the adjacent normal urothelium ➡. CIS may be abrupt or subtle. (Right) Although nucleoli are prominent, the degree of nucleomegaly (more than 5x the size of lymphocyte nuclei ➡ in some cells), marked variation in nuclear size and shape, loss of polarity, and nuclear membrane irregularity all support a diagnosis of urothelial carcinoma in situ in this case.

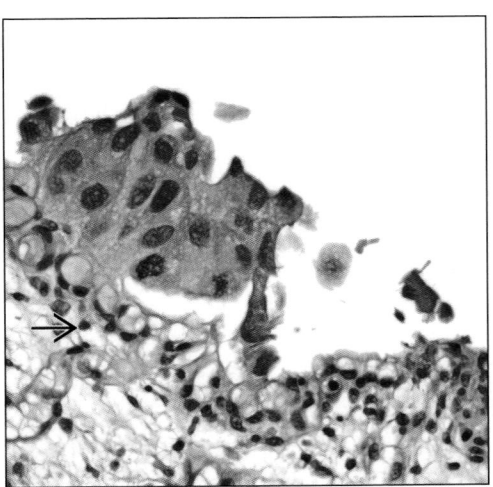
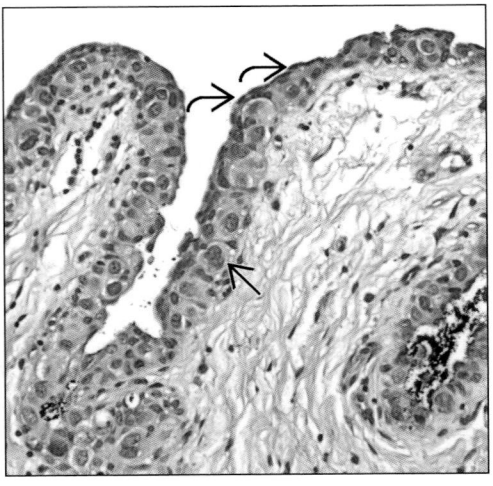

(Left) Using the stromal lymphocytes as a gauge of nuclear size is a useful in the evaluation of flat urothelial atypia. In this example of urothelial carcinoma in situ, the neoplastic nuclei are more than 4-5x the size of the lymphocyte nucleus ➡. (Right) An intact umbrella cell layer ➡ does not preclude a diagnosis of carcinoma in situ, as seen in this example of pagetoid carcinoma in situ. The enlarged pleomorphic cells ➡ are beyond what is allowed in reactive atypia.

UROTHELIAL PAPILLOMA

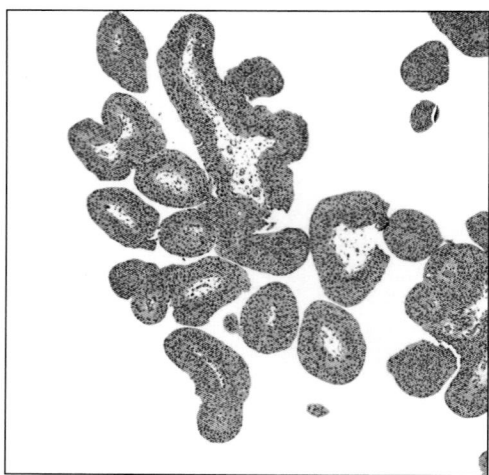

Urothelial papilloma typically has a simple, minimally branching papillary architecture without confluent epithelial aggregates and has a urothelial lining of normal thickness.

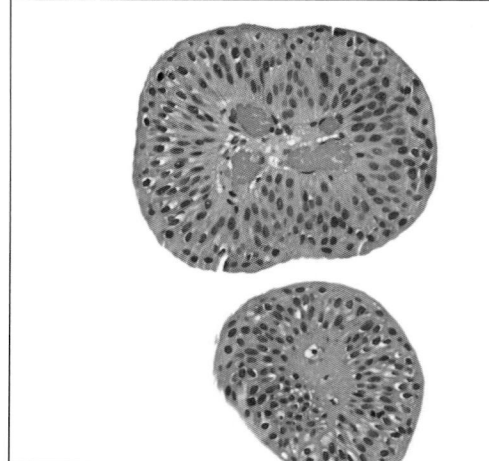

The lining epithelium of urothelial papilloma has normal thickness, normal polarity (perpendicular to the basement membrane), and often a distinct umbrella cell layer.

TERMINOLOGY

Synonyms
- Transitional cell papilloma

Definitions
- Exophytic papillary urothelial neoplasm
  - Fibrovascular cores lined by histologically normal urothelium
    - No significant atypia or mitotic activity

CLINICAL ISSUES

Epidemiology
- Incidence
  - Very uncommon urothelial lesion (~ 1% of papillary urothelial neoplasms)
- Age
  - Tends to occur in younger adult patients
  - May be seen in children
- Gender
  - M:F = 1.9:1

Site
- Posterior or lateral walls of bladder
  - Close to ureteral orifices
- Urethra is another common site of occurrence

Presentation
- Gross or microscopic hematuria
- Frequently present *de novo* in patients without history of bladder neoplasia
  - Particularly in children
- May occur in patients with prior or simultaneous papillary bladder neoplasms
  - Including higher grade lesions

Endoscopic Findings
- Cystoscopic features are identical to other low-grade papillary urothelial neoplasms

Treatment
- Surgical approaches
  - Complete transurethral resection

Prognosis
- Clinical course is benign
- Recurrence is rare (from 0-8%)

MACROSCOPIC FEATURES

General Features
- Most are solitary
- May extensively involve bladder mucosa (rare)

MICROSCOPIC PATHOLOGY

Histologic Features
- Exophytic papillary neoplasm lined by normal-appearing urothelium
  - No significant cytologic atypia
  - Slender, minimally branching papillary architecture
  - Cores may contain prominent dilated lymphatics
  - Cores occasionally show gland-in-gland pattern
- Superficial umbrella cells often prominent
  - Varying from inconspicuous to complete layer
  - Prominent vacuolization of umbrella cells common
  - May be enlarged and multinucleated
- Stroma may show edema &/or scattered inflammatory cells
- Mitoses are typically absent
- Concomitant inverted pattern may be seen

Predominant Pattern/Injury Type
- Papillary

Predominant Cell/Compartment Type
- Epithelial

UROTHELIAL PAPILLOMA

Key Facts

Clinical Issues
- Very uncommon urothelial lesion (~ 1% of papillary urothelial neoplasms)
- Typically occur in younger adult patients and are seen in children
- Gross or microscopic hematuria
- Recurrence is rare (0-8%)
- Posterior or lateral walls of bladder, close to ureteral orifices
- Urethra is another common site of occurrence

Microscopic Pathology
- Exophytic papillary neoplasm lined by normal-appearing urothelium
- No significant cytologic atypia
- Slender, minimally branching papillary architecture
- Superficial umbrella cells often prominent
- Prominent vacuolization of umbrella cells is common
- Umbrella cells may be enlarged and multinucleated

Ancillary Tests
- CK20 expression typically confined to umbrella cells, as in normal urothelium
- Alteration of p53 expression is not seen

Top Differential Diagnoses
- Papillary urothelial neoplasm of low malignant potential
- Papillary-polypoid cystitis

Diagnostic Checklist
- More common in younger patients
- Important not to interpret umbrella cells in assessment of atypia

ANCILLARY TESTS

Immunohistochemistry
- Papillomas are low proliferative lesions by Ki-67 index
- Alteration of p53 is not seen
- CK20 expression typically confined to umbrella cells, as in normal urothelium

DIFFERENTIAL DIAGNOSIS

Papillary Urothelial Neoplasm of Low Malignant Potential
- Lined by multilayered urothelium that is thicker than papilloma
- Cell density appears to be increased compared to normal
  - Nuclear polarity maintained as in papilloma

Papillary Urothelial Carcinoma, Low Grade
- Urothelium with some atypical features
  - Subtle variation in nuclear size, shape, outlines, or chromatin distribution
  - Nuclear polarity shows mild disarray
- More complex papillae
  - Greater degree of branching
  - Anastomosis of papillae may be seen

Papillary Urothelial Carcinoma, High Grade
- Nuclear hyperchromasia and pleomorphism seen
  - Nuclear polarity is often lost
- Cellular discohesion common
- More complex papillae
  - Anastomosis of papillae common
- May be associated with invasive component

Papillary-Polypoid Cystitis
- Broader papillary bases that taper toward tips
- Underlying lamina propria often edematous with admixed chronic inflammatory cells
  - May have bullous polypoid component
- May have history of indwelling catheter or fistula

Nephrogenic Adenoma
- Pure papillary forms may mimic papilloma
- Single layer of cuboidal epithelial cells
  - In contrast to multilayered urothelium of papilloma
- Underlying tubular or cystic glandular component is diagnostic
- Express pax-2 and pax-8 by immunohistochemistry

Papillary Clear Cell Adenocarcinoma
- Focal areas may be histologically bland
  - More atypical areas are almost always present
- Lined by single layer of cuboidal epithelium

DIAGNOSTIC CHECKLIST

Clinically Relevant Pathologic Features
- More common in younger patients
  - Urothelial carcinoma would be rare in children, adolescents, and young adults

Pathologic Interpretation Pearls
- Important not to interpret umbrella cells in assessment of atypia
- Papilloma should be considered in children

SELECTED REFERENCES

1. Fine SW et al: Urothelial neoplasms in patients 20 years or younger: a clinicopathological analysis using the world health organization 2004 bladder consensus classification. J Urol. 174(5):1976-80, 2005
2. Magi-Galluzzi C et al: Urothelial papilloma of the bladder: a review of 34 de novo cases. Am J Surg Pathol. 28(12):1615-20, 2004
3. McKenney JK et al: Urothelial (transitional cell) papilloma of the urinary bladder: a clinicopathologic study of 26 cases. Mod Pathol. 16(7):623-9, 2003
4. Cheng L et al: Urothelial papilloma of the bladder. Clinical and biologic implications. Cancer. 86(10):2098-101, 1999

UROTHELIAL PAPILLOMA

Microscopic Features

(Left) At low magnification, this urothelial papilloma has the typical slender papillae with minimal branching. Significant anastomosing or confluent sheet-like epithelial growth, which is more common in higher grade lesions, is not seen. (Right) The characteristic elongated slender papillae are seen in this urothelial papilloma. The normal thickness of the urothelium distinguishes papilloma from papillary urothelial neoplasm of low malignant potential.

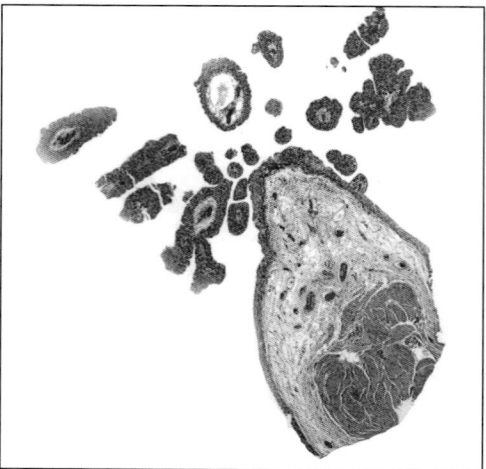
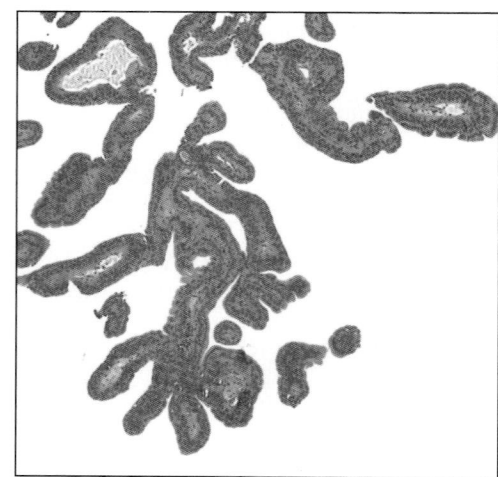

(Left) This typical urothelial papilloma is characterized by a simple branching architecture and an urothelium of normal thickness. The homogeneous thin papillae help distinguish papilloma from papillary cystitis, which would have more broad bulbous papillae toward the base. (Right) This urothelial papilloma shows slender papillae branching from a larger central core ➡. There is normal cytology and nuclear polarity, features that allow classification as papilloma.

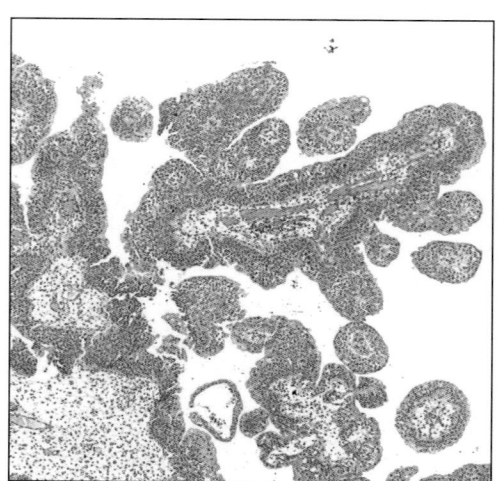
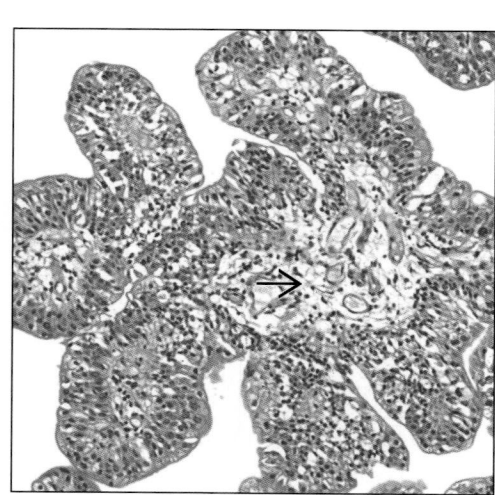

(Left) In urothelial papilloma, the simple papillary architecture may be very similar to papillary urothelial neoplasm of low malignant potential. The urothelium in this example is of normal thickness, consistent with papilloma. (Right) This high-power photomicrograph of the surface lining demonstrates the characteristic normal urothelium of urothelial papilloma. The nuclei are small with fine chromatin and stream upward from the basement membrane.

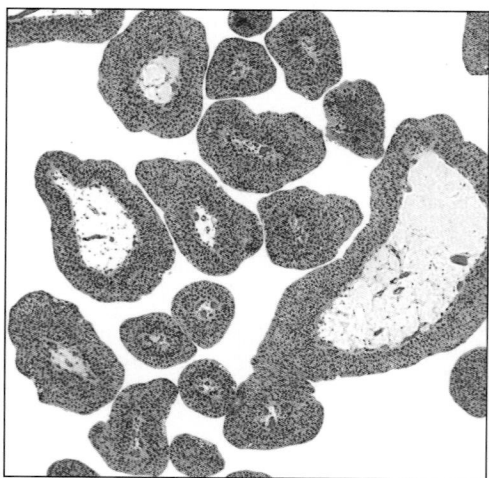
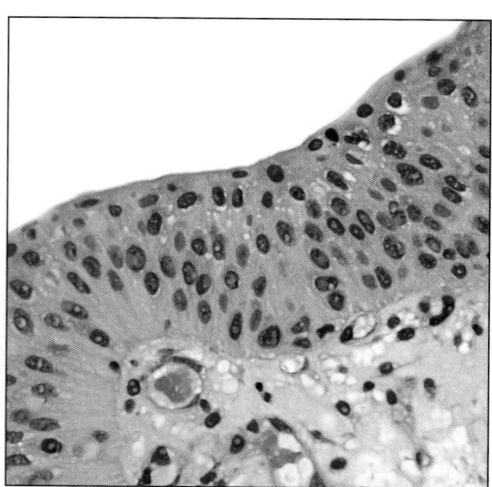

UROTHELIAL PAPILLOMA

Microscopic Features

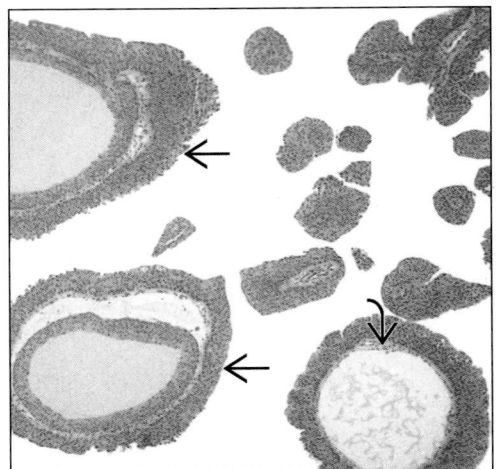

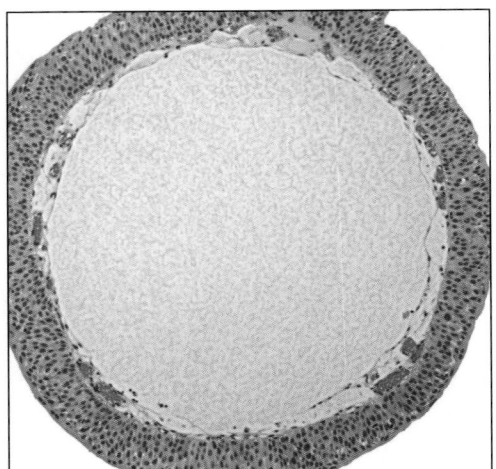

(Left) Urothelial papillomas may show dilated lymphatics in the papillary cores ➔ and occasionally a unique gland-in-gland pattern ➔. The urothelium is of normal thickness, as required for a diagnosis of papilloma. (Right) Dilated lymphatics within the papillary cores are sometimes prominent in urothelial papilloma. This feature is not commonly seen in other reactive or neoplastic papillary urothelial lesions.

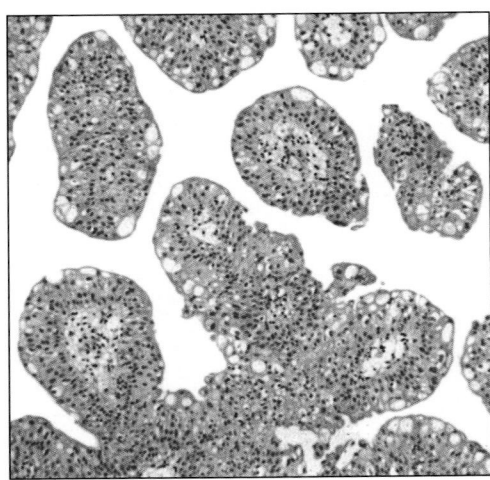

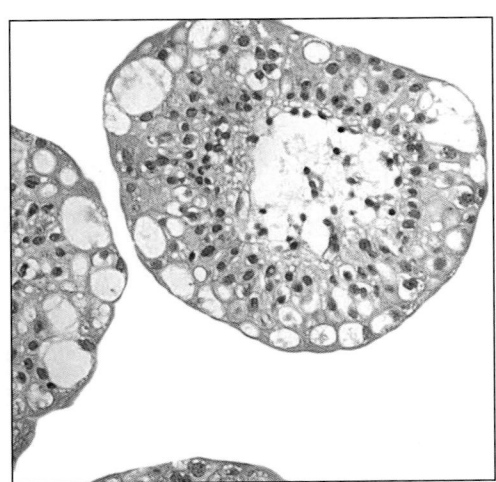

(Left) Urothelial papillomas often have a prominent umbrella cell layer, which may show extensive cytoplasmic vacuolization. (Right) Prominent umbrella cells with cytoplasmic vacuolization are commonly seen in urothelial papillomas. Because normal umbrella cells may have marked nucleomegaly and multilobation, atypia within the umbrella cell layer should not be assessed in grading papillary urothelial lesions.

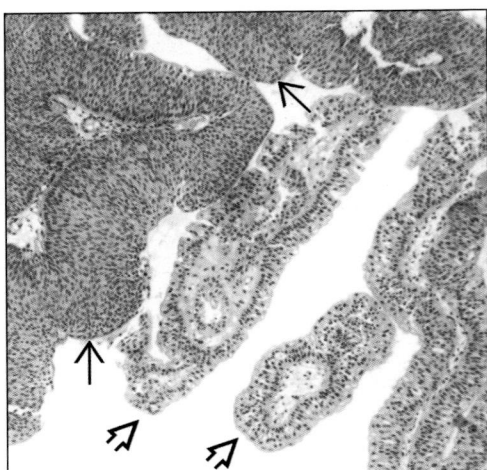

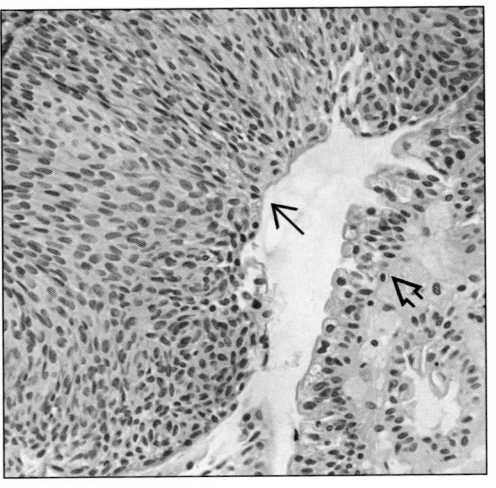

(Left) Papillary urothelial neoplasm with mixed features contrasts foci with a morphology of urothelial papilloma on the right ➘ and papillary urothelial neoplasm of low malignant potential (PUNLMP) on the left ➘. (Right) Increased thickness of the urothelium in PUNLMP ➔ is compared to the papilloma-like component ➘. It would be classified by its highest grade focus as a PUNLMP, but this example contrasts the difference in thickness.

UROTHELIAL PAPILLOMA

Differential Diagnosis

(Left) On low-power examination, this papillary urothelial carcinoma has more epithelial confluence than urothelial papilloma, which would maintain simple discrete papillae. *(Right)* This example of papillary urothelial carcinoma shows complex epithelial growth that encases multiple different papillary cores ➡. This degree of epithelial confluence would preclude classification as urothelial papilloma.

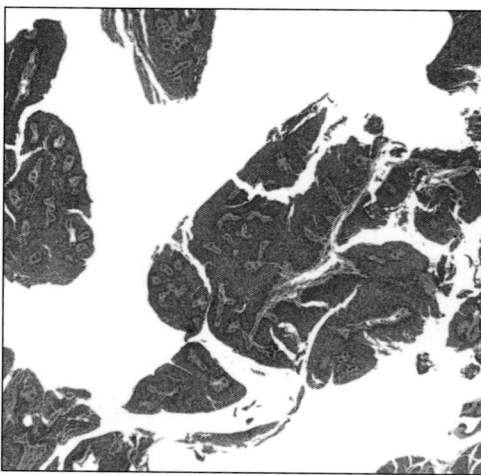
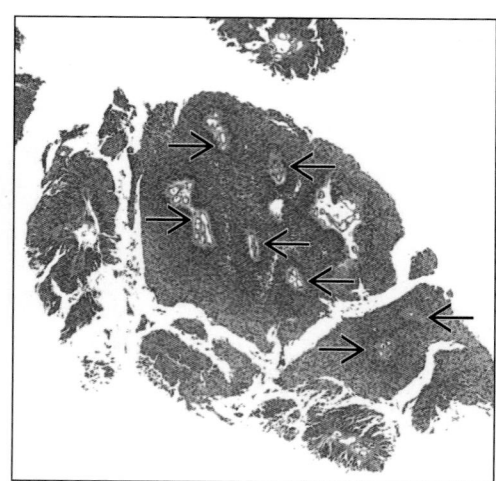

(Left) Papillary urothelial neoplasm of low malignant potential (PUNLMP) has a hyperplastic urothelial lining, in contrast to the urothelium of normal thickness seen in papilloma. *(Right)* On high-power examination of this papillary neoplasm, this urothelium has bland cytology and normal perpendicular orientation to the basement membrane. Despite this normal cytology, the hyperplastic urothelium warrants designation as PUNLMP over papilloma.

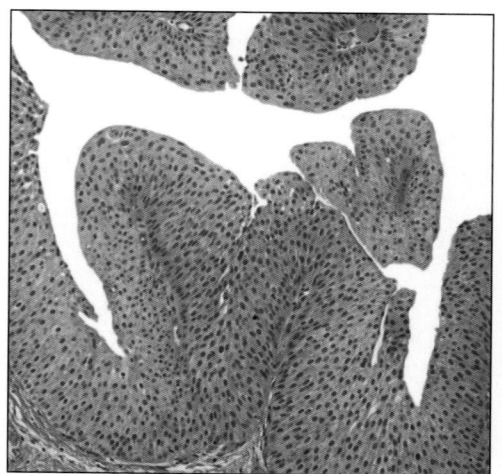
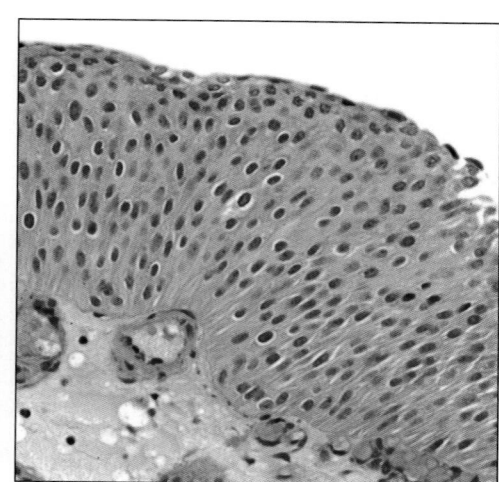

(Left) This papillary urothelial carcinoma has foci with obviously thickened urothelium (hyperplasia) ➡ and more epithelial confluence ➡ than seen in urothelial papilloma. *(Right)* On high-power examination, the disordered urothelium (loss of polarity) with increased thickness warrants classification as low-grade carcinoma. The adjacent normal urothelium ➡ allows comparison with normal thickness.

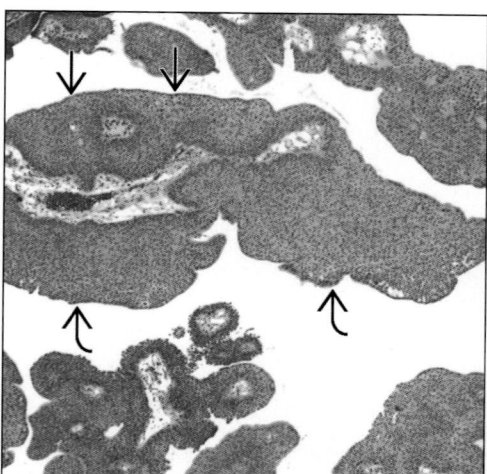
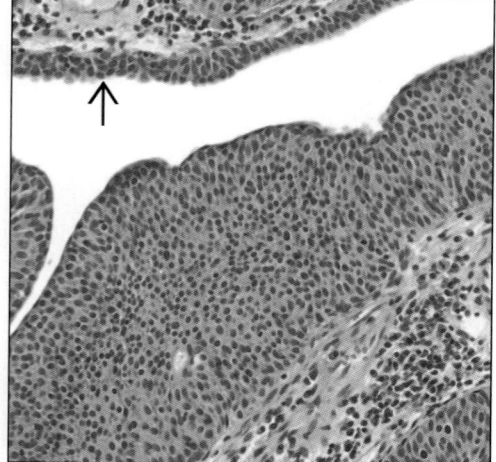

UROTHELIAL PAPILLOMA

Differential Diagnosis

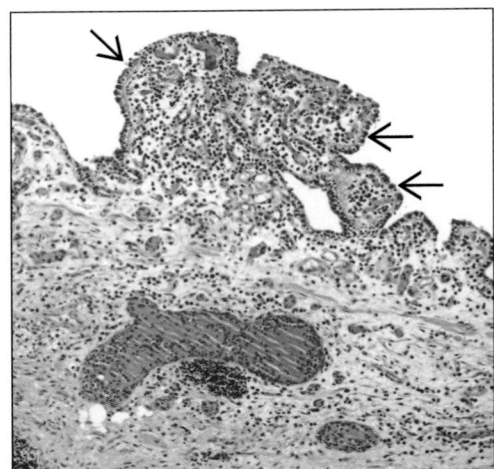
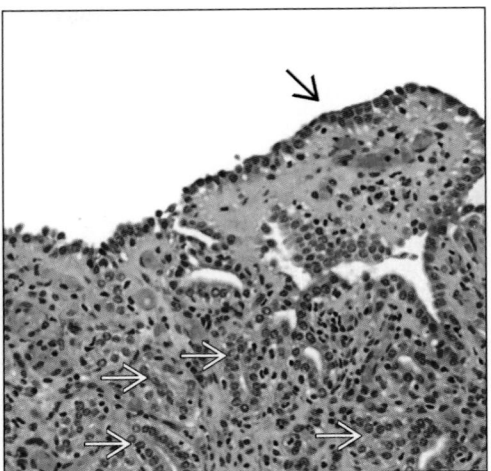

(Left) Papillary nephrogenic adenoma is distinguished from urothelial papilloma by the single cuboidal layer of lining epithelium ⇥. (Right) The admixed tubular component in the lamina propria ⇨ is a distinctive feature of nephrogenic adenoma. In addition, the papillae are lined by a single cuboidal layer of epithelium ⇥. In contrast, urothelial papilloma is lined by multilayered urothelium.

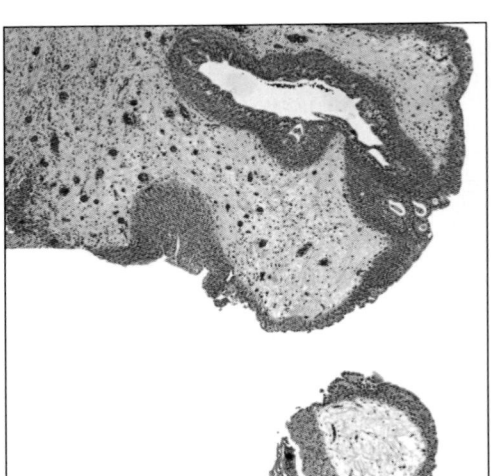
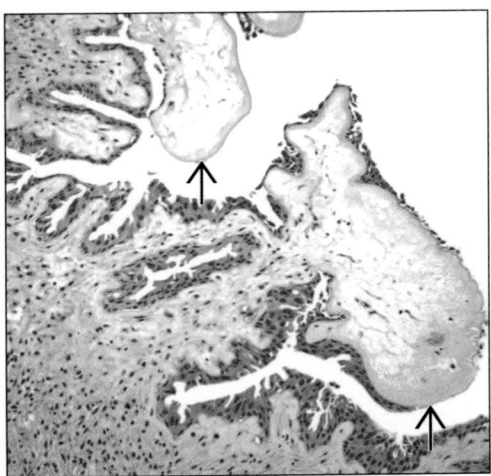

(Left) Papillary-polypoid cystitis is a reactive lesion that may closely mimic urothelial papilloma. In contrast to the thin papillae of urothelial papilloma, papillary-polypoid cystitis is characterized by broad bulbous excrescences with stromal edema. (Right) This example of papillary-polypoid cystitis shows the typical bulbous tips ⇥ of the papillary excrescences.

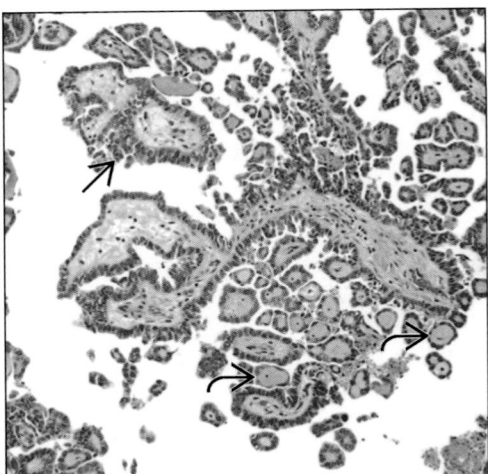
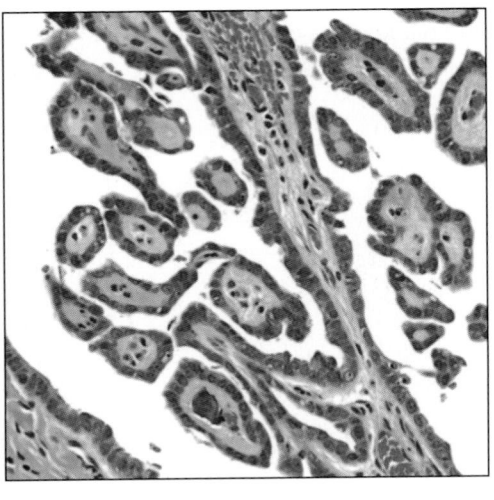

(Left) Papillary foci of clear cell adenocarcinoma may also potentially mimic a benign lesion, such as papilloma. Although there is some stratification ⇥, most of the papillae are lined by a single epithelial lining. The papillae are smaller than typically seen in papilloma, and some have a hyalinized core ⇥. (Right) As seen here, papillary clear cell adenocarcinomas may have deceptively bland foci, but other areas with typical levels of cytologic atypia are usually present.

INVERTED PAPILLOMA

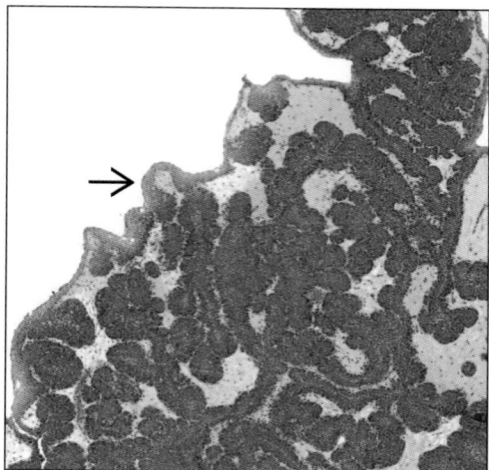

Inverted urothelial papilloma is characterized by endophytic growth into the lamina propria with anastomosing thin trabecular architecture. The overlying urothelium is normal ⇒.

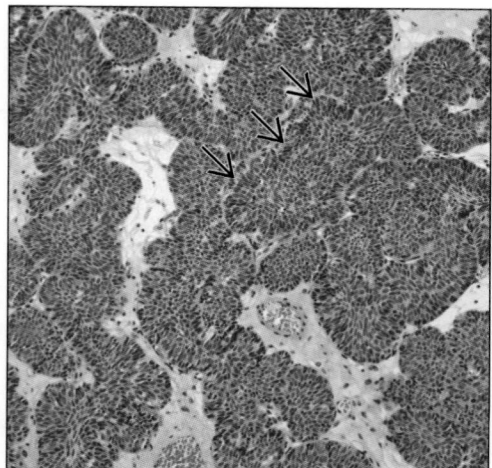

This typical inverted urothelial papilloma shows the usual endophytic growth into the lamina propria, a distinct trabecular architecture, and nuclear palisading ⇒ at the periphery.

TERMINOLOGY

Definitions
- Benign urothelial neoplasm with predominantly endophytic growth pattern
  - Involves lamina propria

CLINICAL ISSUES

Epidemiology
- Incidence
  - Very uncommon urothelial lesion (1% of urothelial neoplasms)
- Age
  - 1st to 8th decade
- Gender
  - Male predominance

Site
- Occurs anywhere along urothelial tract
  - Most common in trigone and bladder neck region

Presentation
- Gross or microscopic hematuria

Endoscopic Findings
- Smooth or nodular polypoid structures
  - May be sessile or contain short stalk

Treatment
- Surgical approaches
  - Complete transurethral resection

Prognosis
- Recurrence rate: < 1%

MACROSCOPIC FEATURES

General Features
- Polypoid with smooth mucosal surface

Size
- Most are < 3 cm
- Rare tumors may be up to 8 cm or more
  - Larger tumors require extensive or complete sampling

MICROSCOPIC PATHOLOGY

Histologic Features
- Urothelium invaginates into lamina propria
  - Forms thin interconnecting cords/trabeculae
- Surface epithelium is normal
  - Presence of more than occasional exophytic papillae argues for mixed inverted and exophytic patterns of urothelial papilloma
- Periphery of cords typically show palisading of basal cell nuclei
  - Mitotic figures are rarely seen at basal layer
- Central areas of cords may show cellular spindling
- Lesion has smooth pushing contours
  - Distinct from irregular nests of invasive carcinoma
  - No stromal reaction
- Epithelial nests may become centrally cystic with cuboidal epithelial lining
  - Cystitis cystica or cystitis glandularis-like patterns
- Bland cytologic features
  - Scattered cells with "degenerative" atypia may be seen
- Rare cases may contain foamy or vacuolated cytoplasm
- Nonkeratinizing squamous metaplasia may be present

Predominant Pattern/Injury Type
- Inverted trabeculae/cord

Predominant Cell/Compartment Type
- Epithelial, urothelial

INVERTED PAPILLOMA

Key Facts

Terminology
- Benign urothelial neoplasm with predominantly endophytic growth pattern

Clinical Issues
- Very uncommon urothelial lesion (1% of urothelial neoplasms)
- Most common in trigone and bladder neck region
- Recurrence rate: < 1%

Microscopic Pathology
- Surface urothelium is normal
- Urothelium invaginates into lamina propria
- Forms thin interconnecting cords/trabeculae
- Periphery of cords typically show palisading of basal cells
- Central areas of cords may be spindled

- Lesion has smooth pushing contour
- Epithelial nests may become centrally cystic with cuboidal epithelial lining
- Rare tumors have mixed inverted and exophytic patterns of urothelial papilloma
- Scattered cells with "degenerative" atypia may be seen
- Rare cases may contain foamy or vacuolated cytoplasm

Top Differential Diagnoses
- Urothelial carcinoma with endophytic growth pattern
- Nested urothelial carcinoma
- Paraganglioma
- Florid von Brunn nests/cystitis cystica
- Carcinoid tumor

DIFFERENTIAL DIAGNOSIS

Other Urothelial Neoplasms with Endophytic Growth Pattern
- Same spectrum of tumors as papillary urothelial neoplasia
  - Papillary urothelial neoplasm of low malignant potential, low- to high-grade carcinoma
  - Subtype based on thickness and cytology of neoplastic cells
  - Distinction has therapeutic significance
- Endophytic component has expansion of trabeculae
  - Most useful feature on low-power examination
- Surface lining shows true papillae in some cases
- Lamina propria invasion may also be present in high-grade lesions

Nested Urothelial Carcinoma
- More irregular distribution of urothelial nests
- Trabecular growth pattern not predominant
- More expansile nests may be present
- Irregular invasion of lamina propria/muscularis propria is common
- Surrounding retraction spaces may be seen

Paraganglioma
- Nested (zellballen) pattern
- Often show marked variation in nuclear size (endocrine anaplasia)
- Immunoreactivity for synaptophysin and chromogranin
  - S100 positive sustentacular cells
  - Cytokeratin negative

Florid von Brunn Nests/Cystitis Cystica
- Rounded nests of urothelium
  - Often lobular distribution
  - Lacks trabecular pattern
- Distinction from cystitis cystica-like pattern of inverted papilloma may be arbitrary in some cases

Carcinoid Tumor
- May have similar trabecular/nested architecture
- Neuroendocrine type nuclear features
  - Stippled chromatin
- Immunoreactivity for synaptophysin &/or chromogranin

DIAGNOSTIC CHECKLIST

Clinically Relevant Pathologic Features
- May be cystoscopically similar to other bladder neoplasms
- Clinically benign despite unusual morphologic patterns (e.g., spindling)

Pathologic Interpretation Pearls
- Urothelial carcinoma with endophytic growth pattern must be considered
  - Contain more expansile trabeculae or solid areas
  - Greater degree of cytologic atypia often present
- Inverted papilloma-like areas may be present in other endophytic lesions of higher grade/stage

SELECTED REFERENCES

1. Fine SW et al: Inverted urothelial papillomas with foamy or vacuolated cytoplasm. Hum Pathol. 37(12):1577-82, 2006
2. Sung MT et al: Natural history of urothelial inverted papilloma. Cancer. 107(11):2622-7, 2006
3. Broussard JN et al: Atypia in inverted urothelial papillomas: pathology and prognostic significance. Hum Pathol. 35(12):1499-504, 2004
4. Amin MB et al: Urothelial transitional cell carcinoma with endophytic growth patterns: a discussion of patterns of invasion and problems associated with assessment of invasion in 18 cases. Am J Surg Pathol. 21(9):1057-68, 1997
5. Kunze E et al: Histology and histogenesis of two different types of inverted urothelial papillomas. Cancer. 51(2):348-58, 1983

Microscopic Features

(Left) On scanning power, the endophytic growth of anastomosing thin urothelial cords/trabeculae can be observed, findings characteristic of inverted papilloma. **(Right)** Inverted urothelial papilloma commonly displays well-formed invaginated epithelial trabeculae/cords that create an anastomosing network. The relatively thin cords aid in the distinction from endophytic urothelial neoplasm of low malignant potential or carcinoma.

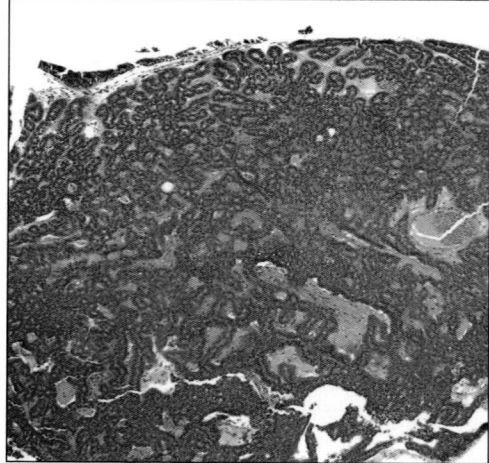
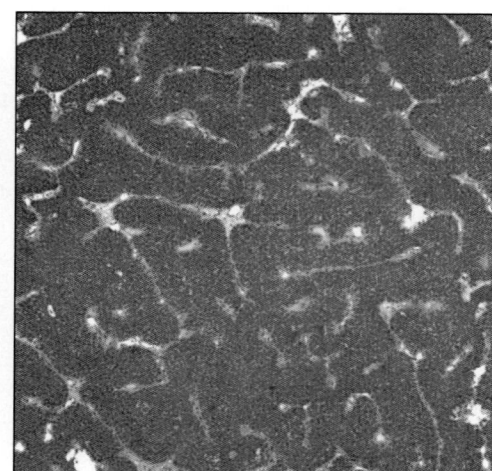

(Left) This example of inverted urothelial papilloma has a striking trabecular architecture with prominent basal palisading ➡. In addition, there is an admixture of more rounded nests ➡, a feature typical of inverted papilloma. **(Right)** On high-power examination of this inverted urothelial papilloma, the bland cytologic features of the urothelial cells within the thin trabeculae are evident.

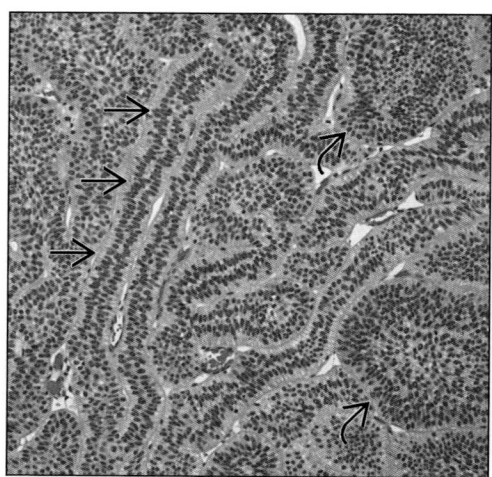
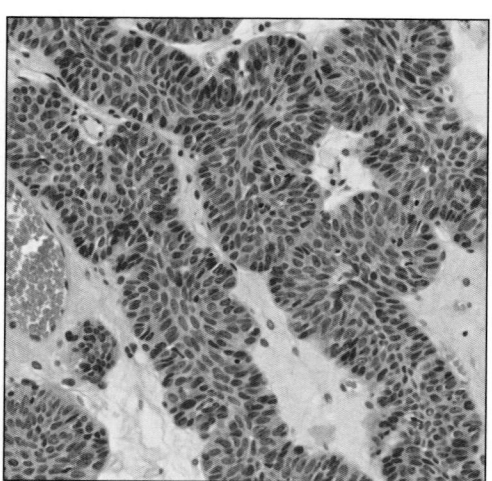

(Left) In this high-power field showing inverted urothelial papilloma, there is striking basal palisading that is accentuated by a reverse polarity ➡ reminiscent of ameloblastoma. **(Right)** This inverted urothelial papilloma demonstrates the characteristic bland monomorphic nuclear features at high-power examination. Mitotic figures and apoptotic debris are typically absent, in contrast to urothelial carcinoma.

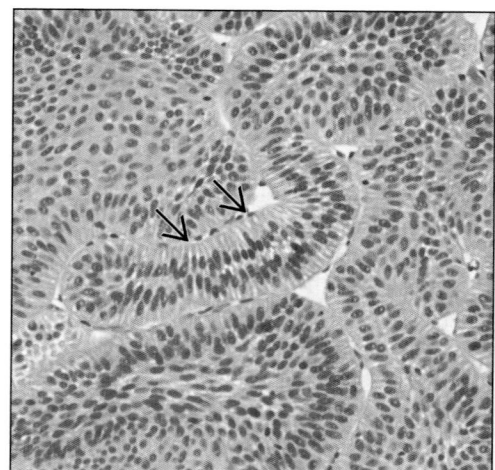
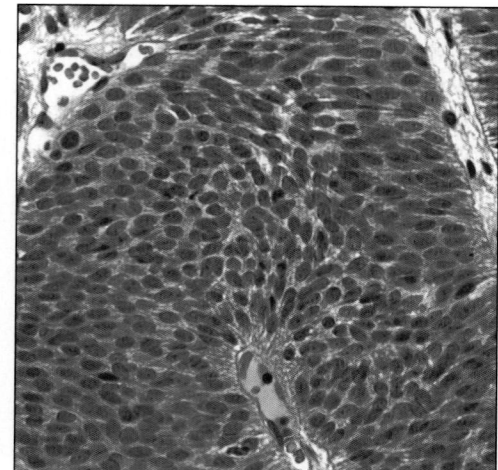

INVERTED PAPILLOMA

Microscopic Features

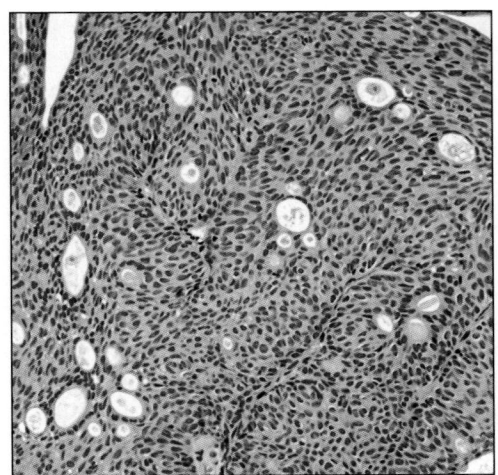

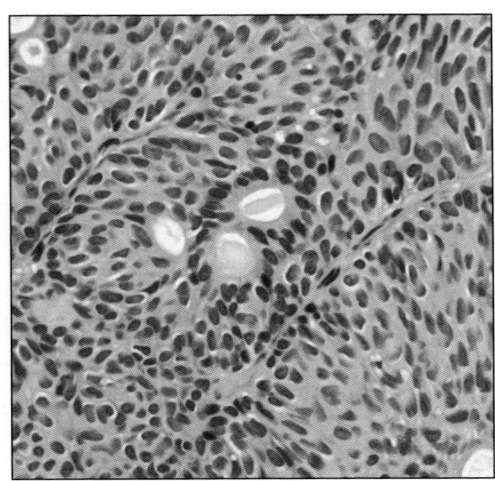

(Left) Inverted urothelial papillomas may have areas with luminal formation that are reminiscent of cystitis glandularis or cystitis cystica. *(Right)* This high-power photomicrograph of an inverted urothelial papilloma highlights scattered lumen with surrounding neoplastic cells containing apical cytoplasm. This cystitis glandularis-like pattern is well described in a subset of inverted papillomas.

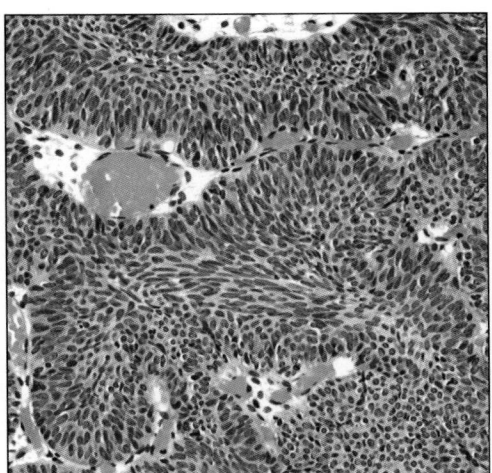

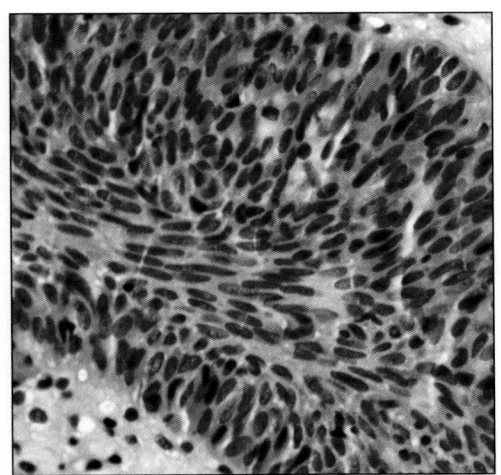

(Left) This inverted urothelial papilloma has the characteristic trabecular growth and also demonstrates prominent basal palisading and central spindling of the neoplastic cells, features that are commonly seen. *(Right)* This high-power photomicrograph highlights the basal palisading and central streaming/spindling of the neoplastic urothelial cells, features that are characteristic of inverted urothelial papilloma.

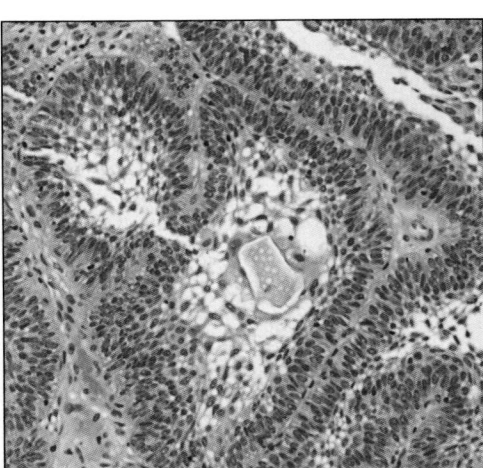

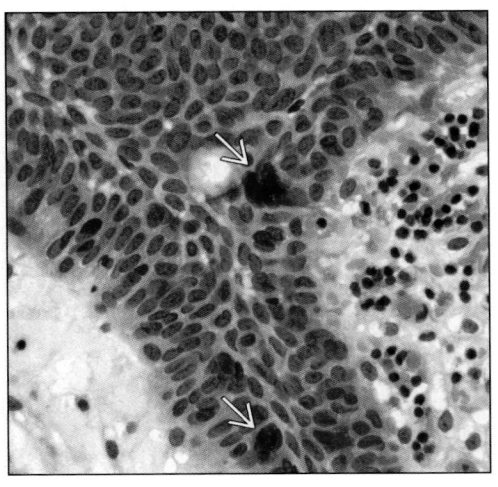

(Left) Rare examples of inverted urothelial papilloma, as seen in this H&E, have endophytic nests with central edema creating a stellate reticulum-like appearance. In this example, the basal palisading is also prominent. *(Right)* Inverted urothelial papillomas occasionally have scattered, enlarged multilobated cells with a degenerative appearance ➡. This feature should not be regarded as high-grade cytologic atypia; therefore, it should not warrant a diagnosis of carcinoma.

Differential Diagnosis: Endophytic Carcinoma

(Left) In this inverted PUNLMP, tissue fragments appear polypoid, but the endophytic and corded growth is distinct from a papillary tumor. Expansile areas ➡️ with loss of thin cord-like growth ➡️ are distinct from inverted papilloma. *(Right)* This endophytic urothelial carcinoma displays prominent trabecular growth that has significant morphologic overlap with inverted papilloma; however, it shows a greater expansion (width) of the cords ➡️ than typically seen in inverted papilloma.

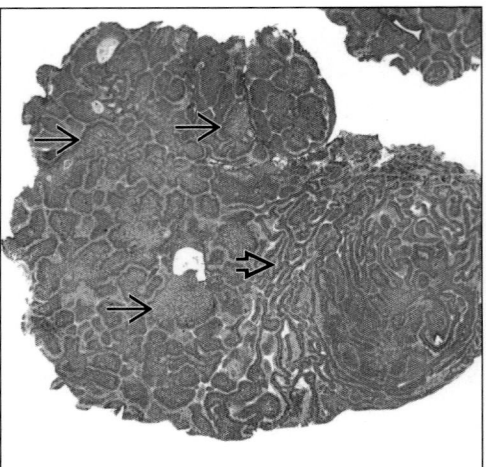
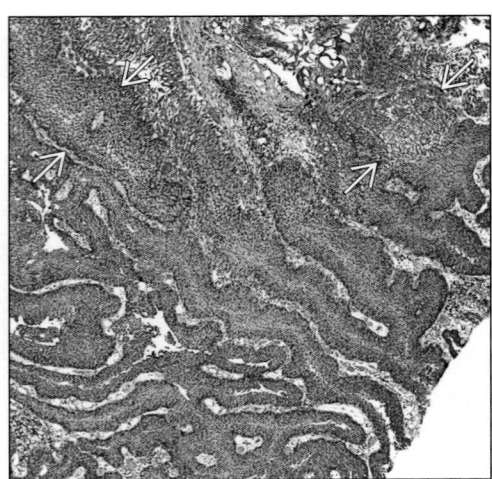

(Left) Despite the endophytic architecture of this neoplasm, the degree of expansile and solid growth ➡️ is diagnostic of endophytic urothelial carcinoma. *(Right)* On low-power examination, this endophytic urothelial carcinoma has a growth pattern that is superficially similar to inverted urothelial papilloma. There is some expansile, solid growth ➡️, which should prompt consideration of a carcinoma. Cytologic features of malignancy were present at higher power.

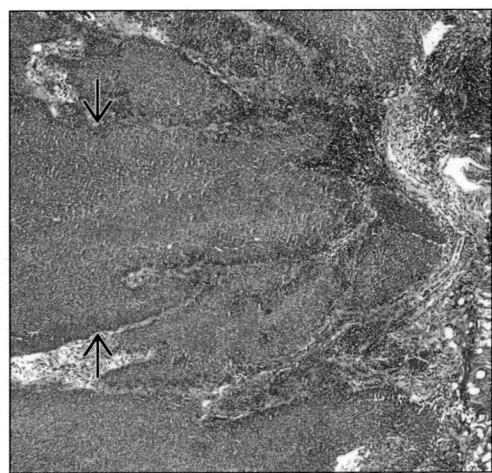
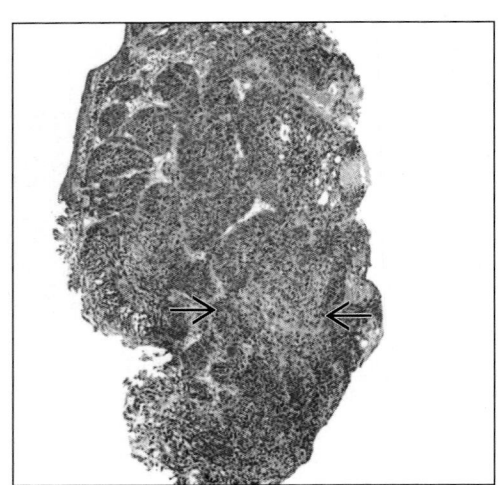

(Left) Even at low-power examination, scattered nuclear pleomorphism ➡️ may be appreciable in high-grade endophytic urothelial carcinomas. The nests and cords are more expansile than typical of inverted urothelial papilloma. *(Right)* On higher power examination, significant nuclear pleomorphism is evident in this high-grade endophytic urothelial carcinoma. In addition, there is loss of polarity with disorganization of the neoplastic cells within the nests and mitotic activity ➡️.

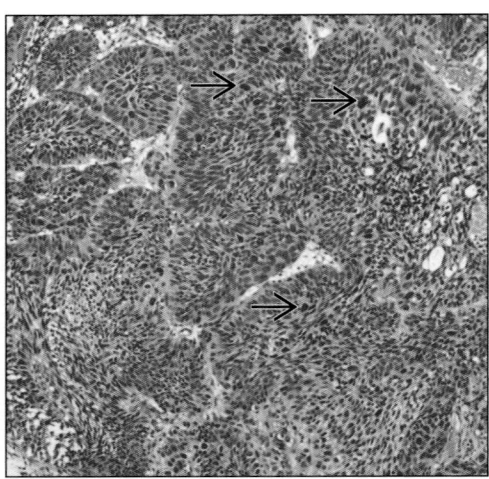
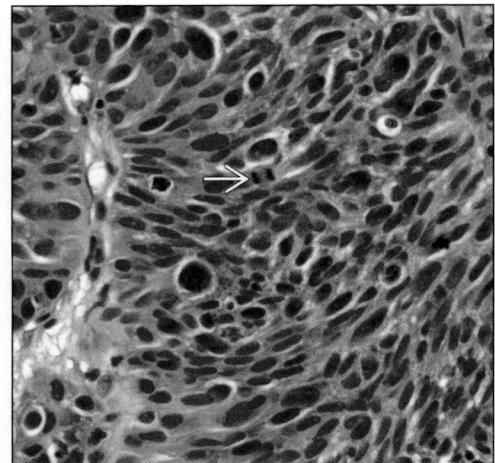

INVERTED PAPILLOMA

Differential Diagnosis

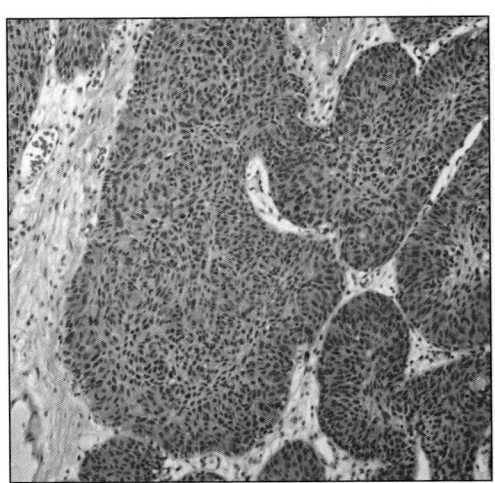
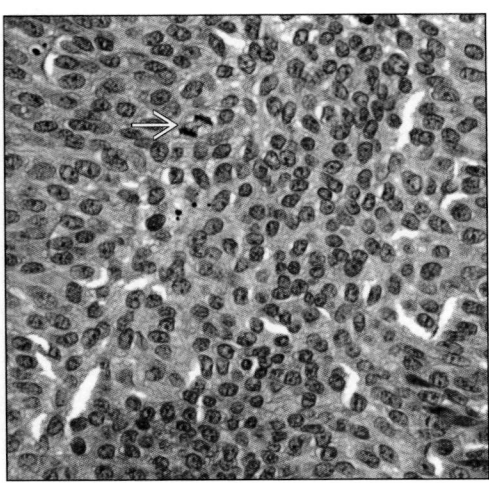

(Left) This endophytic low-grade urothelial carcinoma shows expansion of trabeculae and has a very disordered urothelium with loss of polarization to the surrounding basement membrane. The overall smooth contours of the urothelial proliferation argue for endophytic growth rather than destructive invasion. *(Right)* This endophytic low-grade carcinoma shows nuclear rounding with small nucleoli and scattered mitotic figures ➔, which should not be present in an inverted papilloma.

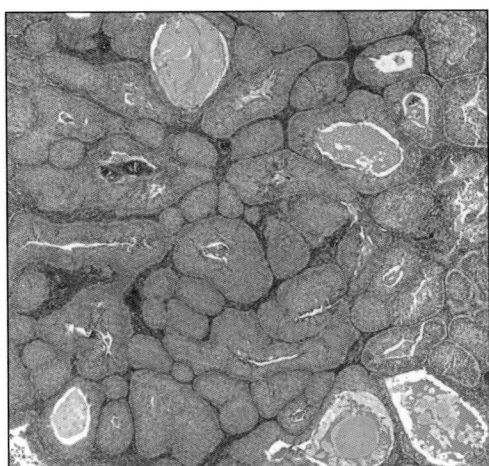
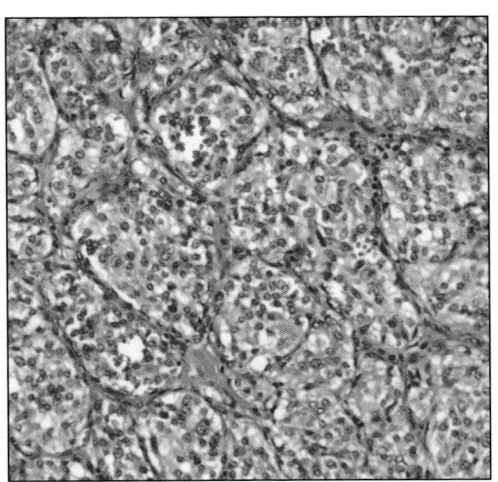

(Left) Inverted papilloma with a cystitis cystica-like pattern is shown. The differential diagnosis is with florid von Brunn nests. In occasional cases where the urothelial proliferation is not pronounced, this diagnostic distinction may be arbitrary. *(Right)* Paraganglioma is characterized by neoplastic cells randomly distributed within nests; inverted papilloma would be expected to show a distinctly palisaded basal layer. A sinusoidal architecture and synaptophysin reactivity is confirmatory.

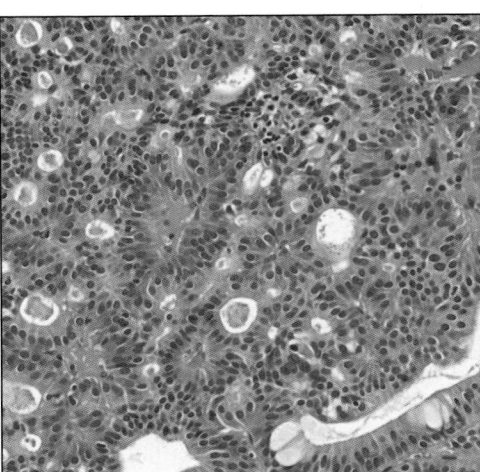
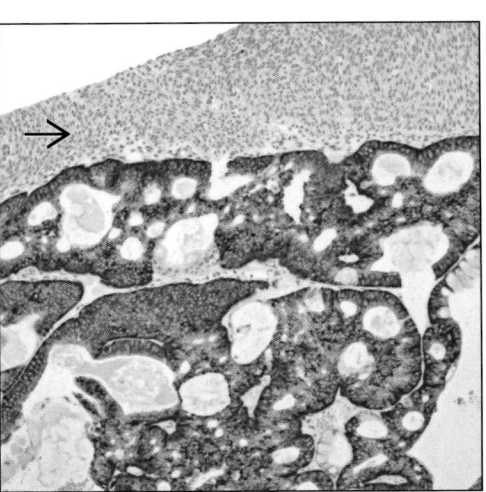

(Left) This trabecular and cystitis cystica-like growth pattern in a rare carcinoid tumor of the urinary bladder may suggest the diagnostic possibility of inverted papilloma with cystitis cystica-like pattern. *(Right)* Strong, diffuse synaptophysin reactivity is seen in this carcinoid tumor, but negative in the overlying urothelium ➔. Neuroendocrine immunohistochemical markers may be very useful in diagnostically challenging superficial biopsies.

PAPILLARY UROTHELIAL NEOPLASM OF LOW MALIGNANT POTENTIAL

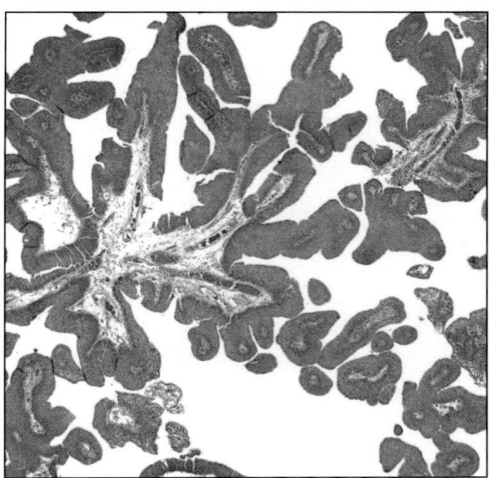

The simple papillary architecture of this PUNLMP with minimal branching may be also be seen in urothelial papilloma, but the hyperplastic urothelial lining is diagnostic of PUNLMP.

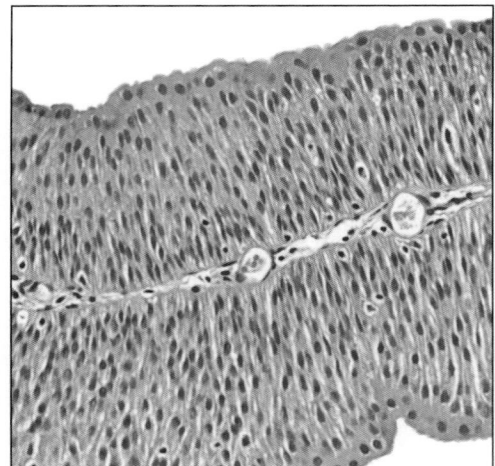

PUNLMP is characterized by papillae lined by a thickened urothelium with normal cytology and preserved cellular order (i.e., streaming of the neoplastic cells perpendicular to the basement membrane).

TERMINOLOGY

Abbreviations
- Papillary urothelial neoplasm of low malignant potential (PUNLMP)

Synonyms
- Represents subset of tumors previously classified as transitional cell carcinoma, grade 1 (WHO 1973)
- Includes tumors classified as "papilloma" by 3rd series AFIP fascicle classification

Definitions
- Papillary urothelial tumor, which resembles exophytic urothelial papilloma, but with increased thickness &/ or cell density of lining urothelium
  - Cytologic features of normal urothelium

CLINICAL ISSUES

Epidemiology
- Incidence
  - Rare bladder lesion: Incidence is approximately 3/100,000 individuals per year
- Age
  - Wide age range
    - May occur in children and adolescents
- Gender
  - Male predominance (M:F = 3-5:1)

Presentation
- Gross or microscopic hematuria
- Urine cytology is usually negative
  - Papillary fragments may be identified

Treatment
- Surgical approaches
  - Complete transurethral resection

Prognosis
- Recurrence rate: 25-47%
- Progression rate to higher grade is approximately 8%
- Stage progression seems very rare

MACROSCOPIC FEATURES

General Features
- Typically 1-2 cm exophytic papillary tumor

MICROSCOPIC PATHOLOGY

Histologic Features
- Papillae of PUNLMP are typically discrete and slender
  - Lined by hyperplastic urothelium (increased cell layers or increased cell density)
  - Minimal to absent cytologic atypia and normal architecture (should be evaluated in well-oriented section)
    - Cells are monotonous with normal size, shape, and chromatin distribution
    - Cells stream upward, perpendicular to basement membrane (polarity is preserved)
    - Umbrella cell layer is often preserved
    - Mitoses are extremely rare and, if present, have basal location
    - Basal layer may show palisading
  - Loss of polarity is minimal to absent and distinct nuclear atypia is not allowed
- Endophytic pattern may also be seen, but rare

Predominant Pattern/Injury Type
- Papillary

DIFFERENTIAL DIAGNOSIS

Urothelial Papilloma
- Papillae are lined by urothelium of normal thickness

PAPILLARY UROTHELIAL NEOPLASM OF LOW MALIGNANT POTENTIAL

Key Facts

Terminology
- Papillary urothelial hyperplasia now considered PUNLMP

Clinical Issues
- Incidence is 3/100,000 individuals per year
- Wide age range that includes children and adolescents
- Male preponderance (M:F = 3-5:1)
- Gross or microscopic hematuria
- Recurrence rate: 25-47%
- Progression rate to higher grade: 8%

Macroscopic Features
- Typically 1-2 cm exophytic papillary tumor

Microscopic Pathology
- Papillae of PUNLMP are typically discrete and slender

- Lined by hyperplastic urothelium
- Minimal to absent cytologic atypia and normal architecture
- Cells are monotonous with normal size, shape, and chromatin distribution
- Cells stream upward, perpendicular to basement membrane (polarity is preserved)
- Mitoses are extremely rare and, if present, have basal location
- Endophytic pattern may also be seen but rare

Top Differential Diagnoses
- Urothelial papilloma
- Low-grade papillary urothelial carcinoma
- Papillary-polypoid cystitis
- High-grade papillary urothelial carcinoma
- Nephrogenic adenoma

- o Key distinction from PUNLMP, which is hyperplastic
- Cytology may be identical to PUNLMP
- Prominent umbrella cells often with vacuolization

Low-Grade Papillary Urothelial Carcinoma
- Papillary architecture is similar to PUNLMP but may have more confluence/complexity
- Lining urothelial cells show obvious loss of orientation to basement membrane (i.e., disorder/loss of polarity)
- Mild but distinct cytologic atypia
  - o Subtle variation in nuclear size and shape
  - o Distinct nuclear border and chromatin abnormalities; usually infrequent nucleoli
- Mitoses may be present but usually rare

High-Grade Papillary Urothelial Carcinoma
- At least focal marked atypia
  - o Marked nucleomegaly with pleomorphism and nuclear hyperchromasia
    - Spectrum of atypia ranging from relatively monomorphic to anaplastic
- Mitotic rate may be brisk
- Cellular discohesion common
  - o May be denuded
- Loss of cellular polarity

Papillary-Polypoid Cystitis
- Exophytic papillary-polypoid structures on low power
  - o Edematous or fibrotic papillary cores
    - No significant branching architecture
    - No anastomosing epithelial growth
    - Broad base of excrescences may taper to slender papillae toward lumen
- Lining urothelium may be normal, hyperplastic, or show reactive urothelial atypia

Nephrogenic Adenoma
- Papillae lined by single layer of cuboidal epithelium
- May have other associated growth patterns, including glandular and tubulocystic
- Typically express nuclear pax-2 and pax-8 by immunohistochemistry

DIAGNOSTIC CHECKLIST

Clinically Relevant Pathologic Features
- Clinical follow-up for PUNLMP similar to low-grade carcinoma

Pathologic Interpretation Pearls
- Strict criteria for PUNLMP must be applied
  - o Little morphologic heterogeneity allowed under WHO 2004/ISUP criteria
    - Relatively uncommon but preserves prognostic distinction from low-grade papillary urothelial carcinoma

SELECTED REFERENCES

1. Fine SW et al: Urothelial neoplasms in patients 20 years or younger: a clinicopathological analysis using the world health organization 2004 bladder consensus classification. J Urol. 174(5):1976-80, 2005
2. Campbell PA et al: Papillary urothelial neoplasm of low malignant potential: reliability of diagnosis and outcome. BJU Int. 93(9):1228-31, 2004
3. Johansson SL et al: Papillary urothelial neoplasm of low malignant potential. In Eble JN et al: World Health Organization Classification of Tumours. Pathology & Genetics. Tumours of the Urinary System and Male Genital Organs. Lyon: IARC Press, 2004
4. Yin H et al: Histologic grading of noninvasive papillary urothelial tumors: validation of the 1998 WHO/ISUP system by immunophenotyping and follow-up. Am J Clin Pathol. 121(5):679-87, 2004
5. Fujii Y et al: Long-term outcome of bladder papillary urothelial neoplasms of low malignant potential. BJU Int. 92(6):559-62, 2003
6. Epstein JI et al: The World Health Organization/ International Society of Urological Pathology consensus classification of urothelial (transitional cell) neoplasms of the urinary bladder. Bladder Consensus Conference Committee. Am J Surg Pathol. 22(12):1435-48, 1998

PAPILLARY UROTHELIAL NEOPLASM OF LOW MALIGNANT POTENTIAL

Microscopic Features

(Left) This papillary urothelial neoplasm is lined by a markedly thickened urothelium, a feature that would raise a differential of PUNLMP vs. low-grade carcinoma. High-power examination of the cytology and cellular orientation are needed for distinction. **(Right)** The cells of the hyperplastic urothelium lining the papillae of PUNLMP have uniform cytology, usually with an elongated fusiform shape and stream perpendicular between the basement membrane and bladder lumen.

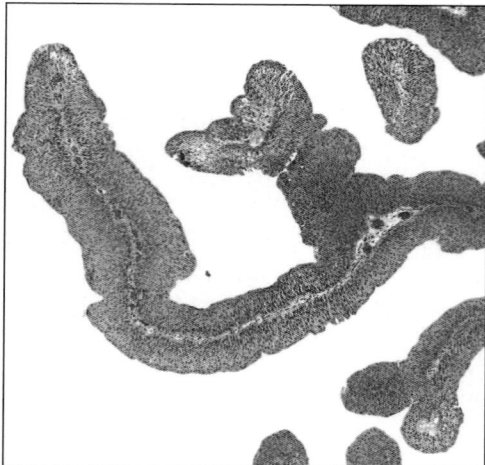
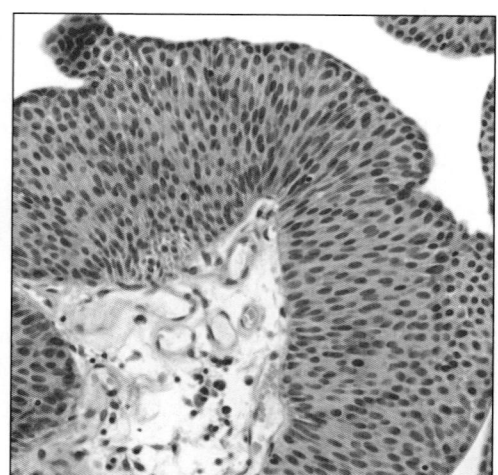

(Left) The normal polarity of the lining neoplastic urothelium in this papillary urothelial neoplasm is characteristic of PUNLMP. **(Right)** Tangentially sectioned superficial (umbrella) cells ➡ may occasionally be seen in a PUNLMP. The normal degree of nucleomegaly and the occasional multilobation of umbrella cells should be discounted and not prompt designation as a higher grade lesion. It is also important to evaluate well-oriented sections in the evaluation of polarity.

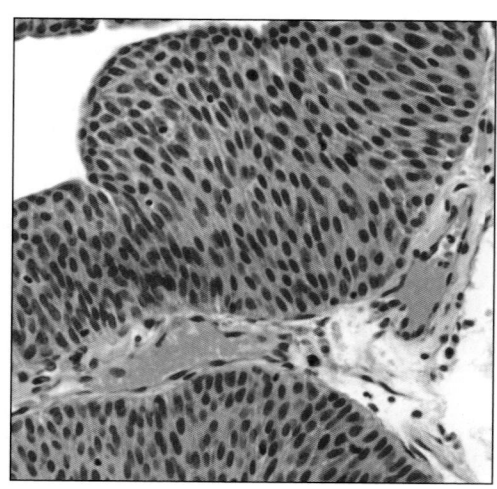
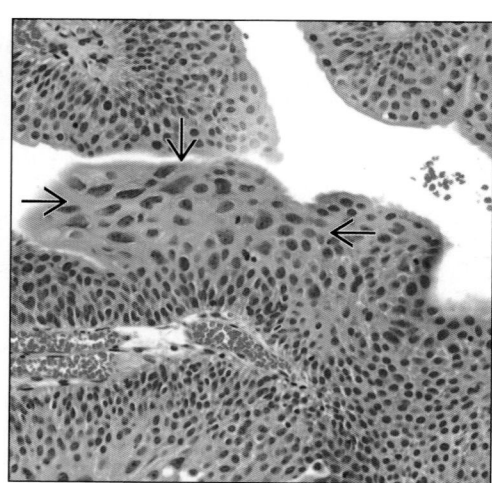

(Left) PUNLMPs may have an endophytic (inverted) growth pattern mimicking inverted papilloma. Broad expansion of multiple nests ➡ contrasts with thin, cord-like/trabecular growth of inverted papilloma. Other areas showed more typical exophytic component. **(Right)** At high-power evaluation of this endophytic urothelial neoplasm, the expanded nests have bland nuclear cytology and maintain an orderly arrangement, features warranting classification as noninvasive endophytic PUNLMP.

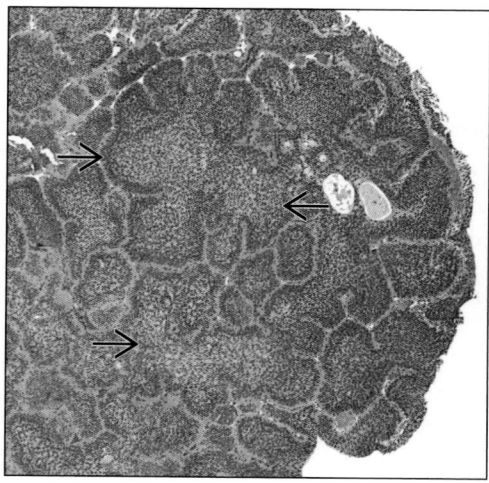
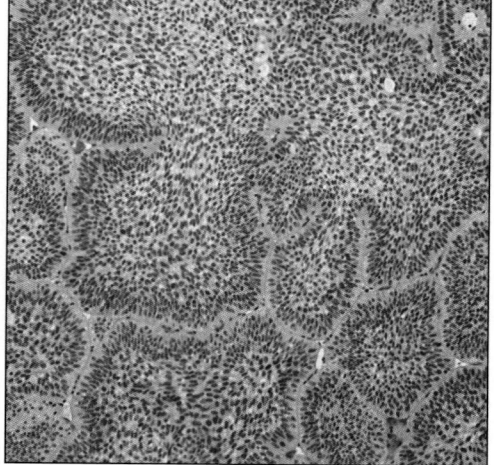

Differential Diagnosis

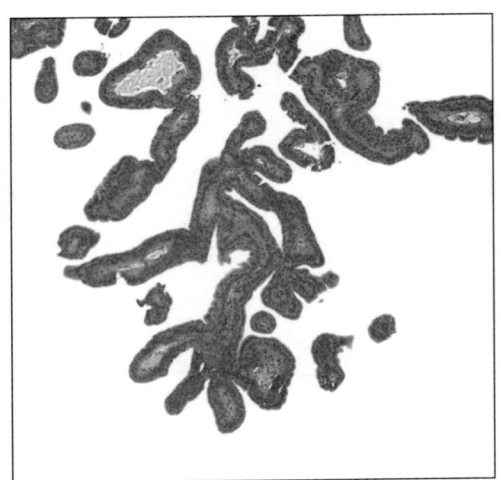

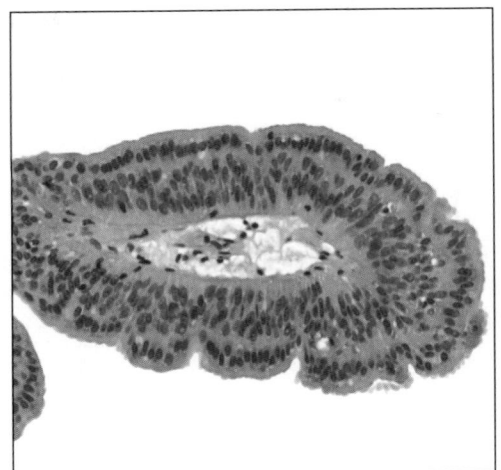

(Left) The thin, simple branching in this urothelial papilloma is similar to that seen in PUNLMP. In contrast to PUNLMP, the lining urothelium is of normal thickness. (Right) The prominent umbrella cell layer and the normal cytology and polarity are all features that may be seen in urothelial papilloma and PUNLMP. The thin (normal) lining urothelium warrants classification of this tumor as urothelial papilloma.

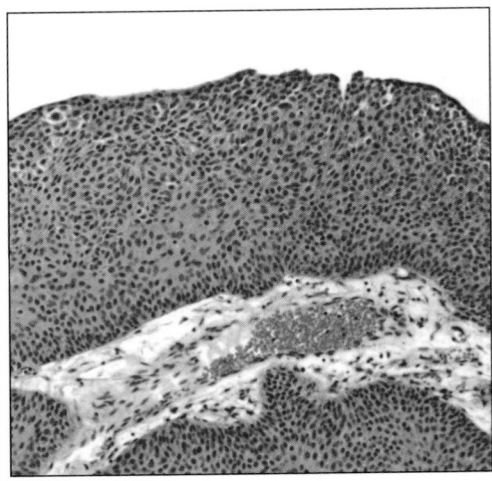

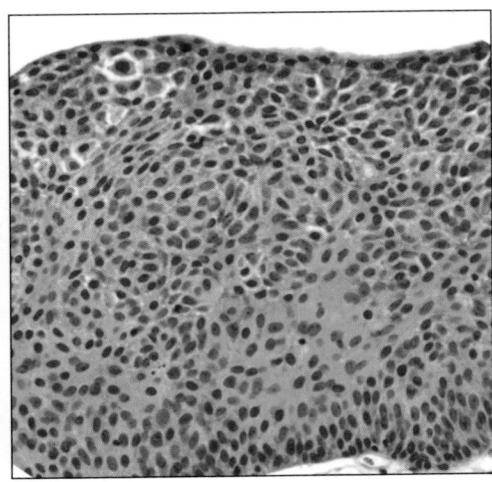

(Left) Although the lining urothelium of this papillary tumor is thickened, the cells do not have the orderly arrangement of PUNLMP. This architectural disorder is sufficient for classification as low-grade papillary urothelial carcinoma. (Right) In this low-grade papillary urothelial carcinoma, the nuclei are small and the chromatin is evenly dispersed; however, there is loss of orientation to the basement membrane, which precludes a diagnosis of PUNLMP.

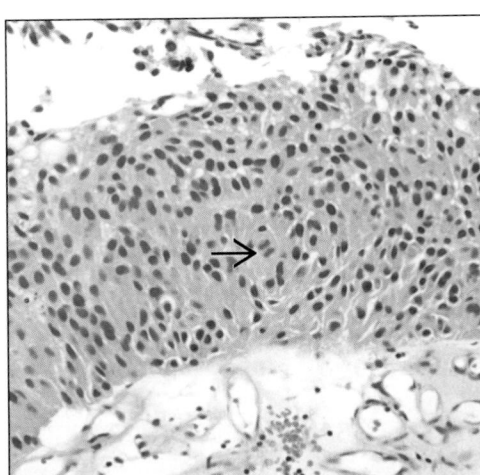

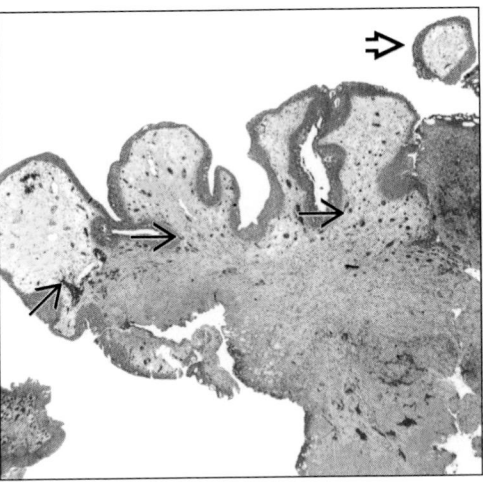

(Left) This low-grade carcinoma has marked architectural disorder to qualify as PUNLMP. In addition, rare mitotic figures are seen ⇨, a feature that should prompt careful consideration of low-grade carcinoma over PUNLMP. (Right) The edematous polypoid stalks with a broad base ⇨ are characteristic of papillary-polypoid cystitis. The sectioned ends of the papillae ⇨ may mimic a PUNLMP, which typically has more slender papillae with at least some degree of simple branching.

LOW-GRADE PAPILLARY UROTHELIAL CARCINOMA

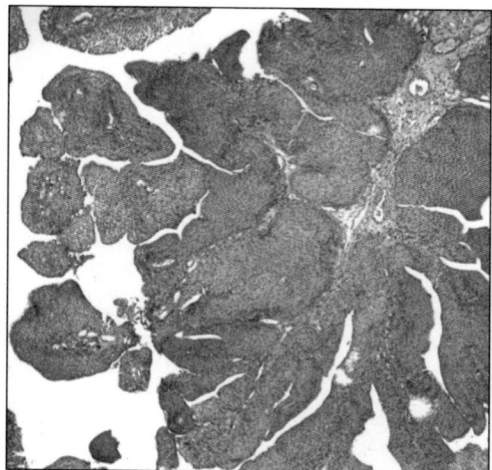

This low-grade papillary urothelial carcinoma has well-formed papillae with minimal urothelial confluence between adjacent papillae. Grading is based on the cytologic features at high magnification.

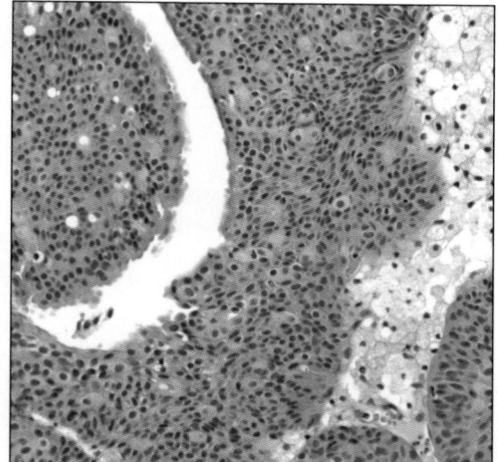

The neoplastic cells show loss of polarity, distinct nuclear atypia, but no significant pleomorphism. These are cytoarchitectural features of a low-grade papillary urothelial carcinoma.

TERMINOLOGY

Synonyms
- None
  - Categories do not translate between nomenclature systems
  - Low-grade papillary urothelial carcinoma is not synonymous with WHO 1973 grade 1

Definitions
- Papillary urothelial neoplasm with some degree of cytoarchitectural disorder and distinct but low-grade cytologic abnormality
  - No high-grade cytologic features (pleomorphism, mitoses toward surface and nucleoli throughout)

CLINICAL ISSUES

Epidemiology
- Incidence
  - 5 per 100,000 individuals per year
- Age
  - Mean: 70 years
- Gender
  - Male predilection (M:F = 3:1)

Site
- Commonly on posterior bladder wall
- Lateral wall close to ureteral orifices also common

Presentation
- Gross or microscopic hematuria common
- Cytology of urine may show cellular clusters/papillae suspicious for carcinoma

Treatment
- Surgical approaches
  - Complete transurethral resection
- Adjuvant therapy
  - Intravesical therapies not generally used for low-grade carcinomas

Prognosis
- Progression and death from disease occurs in < 5% of patients
- Recurrence/new occurrence is common (48-71%)

MACROSCOPIC FEATURES

General Features
- Cystoscopy shows exophytic fronds of tumor
  - Solitary or multiple lesions

Size
- Wide variation

MICROSCOPIC PATHOLOGY

Histologic Features
- Cells are relatively uniform in size without significant nuclear pleomorphism or nucleomegaly
  - Subtle variation in nuclear size may be present
- Loss of cellular polarity, random distribution of cells in urothelium
  - Loss of linear perpendicular orientation to basement membrane
- Nuclei are often rounded with occasional irregularities of nuclear contour
- Relatively fine to slightly abnormal chromatin distribution
- Mitotic figures are rare and distributed randomly
- Nucleoli may be present, but inconspicuous

ANCILLARY TESTS

Immunohistochemistry
- Not routinely used for classifying papillary urothelial neoplasms

LOW-GRADE PAPILLARY UROTHELIAL CARCINOMA

Key Facts

Terminology

- Papillary urothelial neoplasm with some degree of cytoarchitectural disorder and distinct but low-grade cytologic abnormality
- No high-grade cytologic features (pleomorphism, mitoses toward surface and nucleoli throughout)

Clinical Issues

- Mean age is 70 years
- Male predilection (M:F = 3:1)
- Gross or microscopic hematuria common
- Complete transurethral resection
- Intravesical therapies not generally used for low-grade carcinomas
- Progression and death from disease occurs in < 5% of patients
- Recurrence/new occurrence is common (48-71%)

Microscopic Pathology

- Cells are relatively uniform in size without significant nuclear pleomorphism or nucleomegaly
- Subtle variation in nuclear size may be present
- Relatively fine nuclear chromatin
- Loss of cellular polarity
- Random distribution of cells in urothelium
- Loss of linear perpendicular orientation to basement membrane
- Mitotic figures are rare and distributed randomly

Top Differential Diagnoses

- Papillary urothelial neoplasm of low malignant potential (PUNLMP)
- High-grade papillary urothelial carcinoma
- Papillary-polypoid cystitis
- Papillary nephrogenic adenoma

DIFFERENTIAL DIAGNOSIS

Papillary Urothelial Neoplasm of Low Malignant Potential (PUNLMP)

- Similar to low-grade papillary urothelial carcinoma at low and intermediate magnification
- Lacks distinct nuclear abnormalities
  - No variation in nuclear shape or size
  - Maintains normal perpendicular polarity to basement membrane (order)
  - Lack of nucleoli and mitotic figures

High-Grade Papillary Urothelial Carcinoma

- Wide morphologic spectrum
  - High-grade features may be diffuse, focal, or patchy
  - Even focal high-grade features warrant a high-grade designation
- Marked nucleomegaly common
  - Also marked variation in size and shape of nuclei
- Irregular clumped nuclear chromatin
- Irregular nuclear membranes
- Mitotic figures may be easily identified
- May be associated with invasive carcinoma

Papillary-Polypoid Cystitis

- Exophytic papillary excrescences on low power
  - Edematous or fibrotic papillary cores
    - No significant branching architecture
    - No anastomosing epithelial growth
  - Broad base of excrescences may taper to slender papillae toward lumen
- May have associated reactive atypia

Papillary Nephrogenic Adenoma

- Papillae lined by single cuboidal epithelial layer
- Underlying tubular, cystic, or diffuse pattern may be present

DIAGNOSTIC CHECKLIST

Pathologic Interpretation Pearls

- Distinction between low-grade and high-grade noninvasive papillary urothelial carcinoma is often therapeutic threshold for intravesical therapy
  - Establishing morphologic threshold for high-grade carcinoma is important
    - Evenly scattered cells (apparent order) with high-grade cytologic features warrant high-grade diagnosis under WHO 2004/ISUP
    - Well-oriented longitudinal sections of papillae should be chosen for evaluation to avoid artifactual crowding from tangential sectioning
    - Atypia in superficial umbrella cells should be discounted while grading, as these may have inherent atypia

SELECTED REFERENCES

1. Montironi R et al: The 2004 WHO classification of bladder tumors: a summary and commentary. Int J Surg Pathol. 13(2):143-53, 2005
2. Johansson SL et al: Non-invasive Papillary Urothelial Carcinoma, Low Grade. In Eble JN et al: World Health Organization Classification of Tumours. Pathology & Genetics. Tumours of the Urinary System and Male Genital Organs. Lyon: IARC Press, 2004
3. Yin H et al: Histologic grading of noninvasive papillary urothelial tumors: validation of the 1998 WHO/ISUP system by immunophenotyping and follow-up. Am J Clin Pathol. 121(5):679-87, 2004
4. Epstein JI et al: The World Health Organization/International Society of Urological Pathology consensus classification of urothelial (transitional cell) neoplasms of the urinary bladder. Bladder Consensus Conference Committee. Am J Surg Pathol. 22(12):1435-48, 1998

LOW-GRADE PAPILLARY UROTHELIAL CARCINOMA

Microscopic Features

(Left) High- and low-grade papillary urothelial carcinomas may show complex anastomosing epithelial growth that entraps cores of adjacent papillae ➡. Final grading, however, should be based on cytoarchitectural features of the neoplastic urothelium as evaluated at high power. *(Right)* Although there is minimal epithelial fusion and loss of order at low power in this low-grade papillary urothelial carcinoma, no obvious nuclear pleomorphism or hyperchromasia is seen.

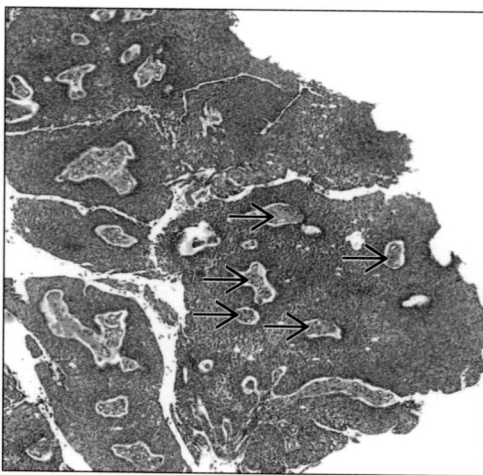 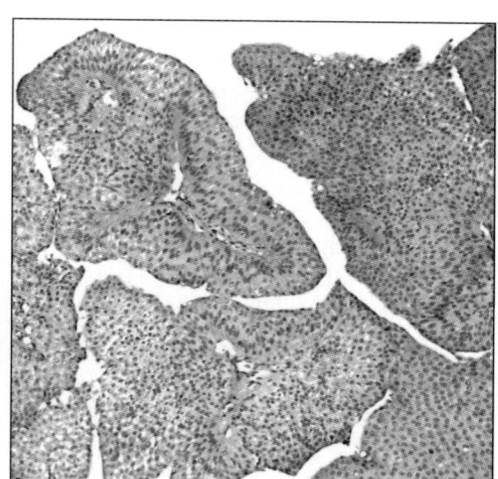

(Left) There is thickened urothelium, marked nuclear rounding, and disorder in this low-grade papillary urothelial carcinoma. *(Right)* The urothelium in this papillary tumor shows neoplastic cells with nuclear rounding, loss of polarity, and subtle variation in nuclear size and shape. This cellular and architectural disorder supports the diagnosis of low-grade carcinoma over PUNLMP. The degree of nuclear pleomorphism and hyperchromasia of a high-grade carcinoma is not seen.

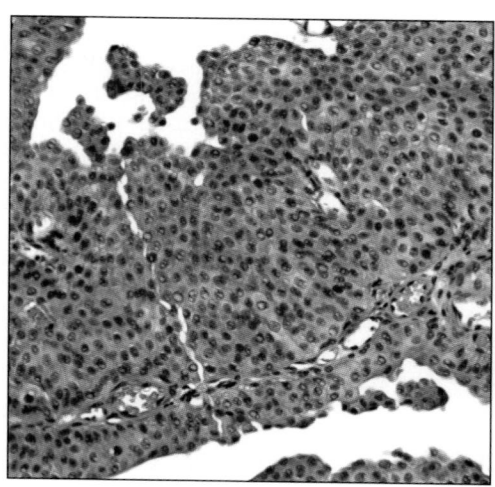 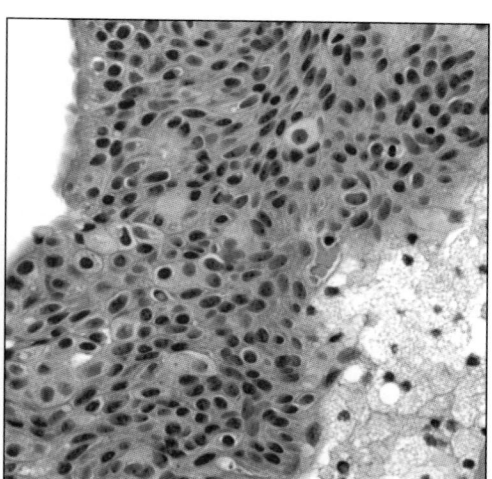

(Left) Papillary urothelial neoplasms frequently show heterogeneity with an admixture of foci showing varying grades and architectural patterns. In this example of low-grade papillary carcinoma, both complex markedly thickened urothelium ➡ and simple papillae with a thin urothelial lining ⬧ are present. *(Right)* This low-grade papillary urothelial carcinoma shows the prototypical loss of polarity with randomly distributed nuclei oriented in varying directions.

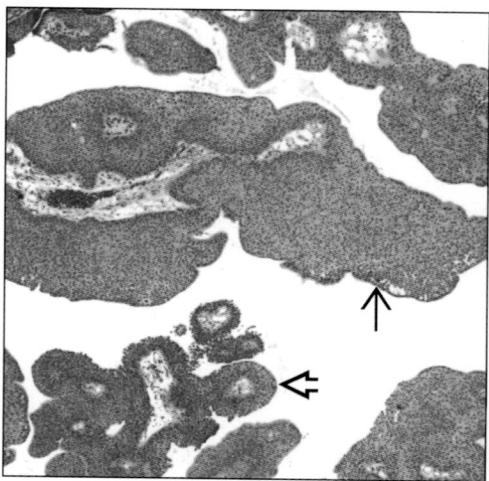 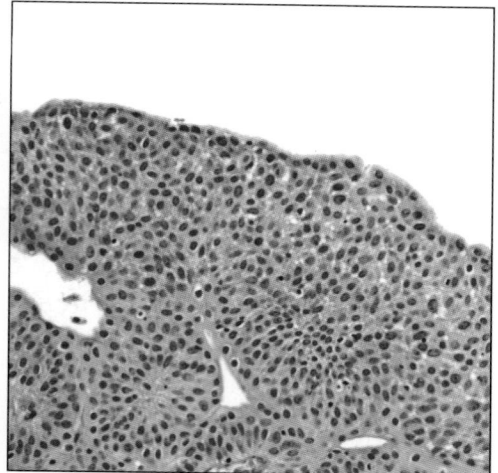

LOW-GRADE PAPILLARY UROTHELIAL CARCINOMA

Microscopic Features

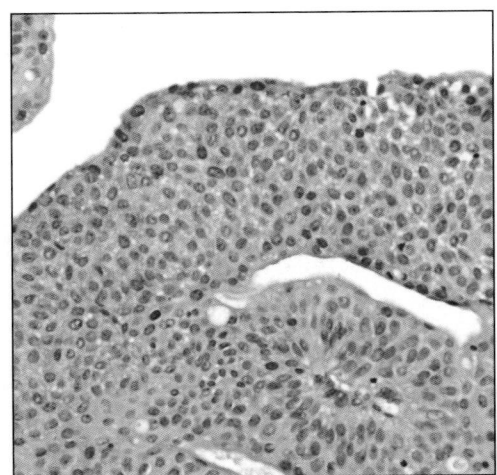
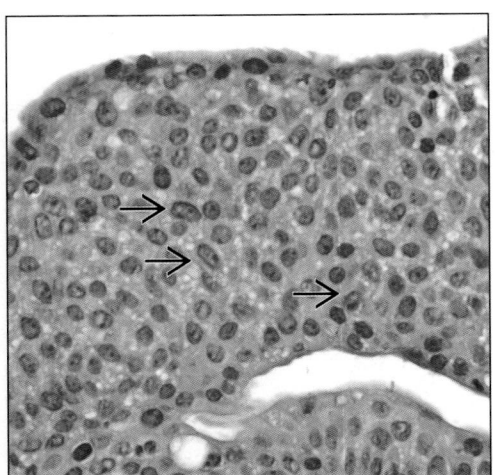

(Left) The degree of nuclear crowding and random distribution of nuclei warrant classification as low-grade papillary urothelial carcinoma over papillary urothelial neoplasm of low malignant potential. *(Right)* At high-power examination, the nuclei of this neoplasm have only subtle variation in size and fine nuclear chromatin. The nuclei occasionally have irregular nuclear contours ➡. These features support classification as low-grade over high-grade papillary urothelial carcinoma.

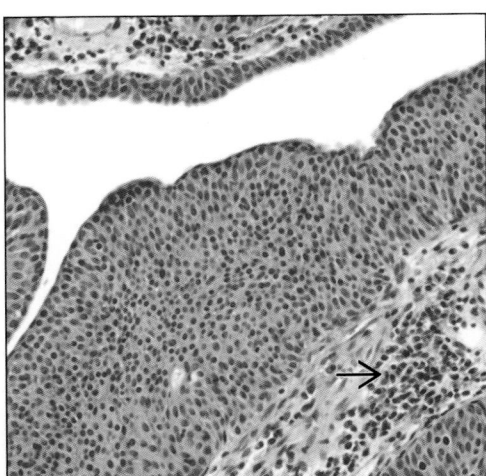
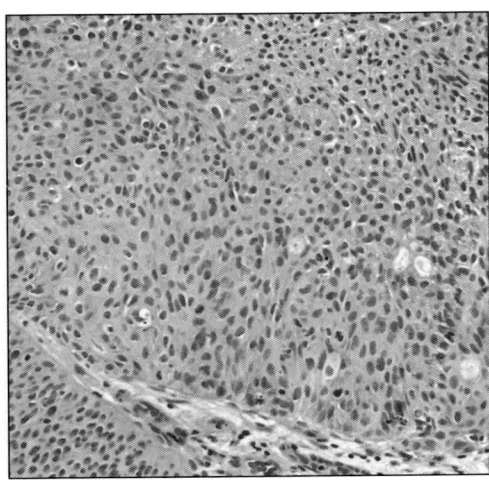

(Left) Low-grade papillary urothelial carcinoma shows cellular disorder, but no pleomorphism. The small size of the neoplastic cells are seen by comparison to the stromal inflammatory cells ➡. *(Right)* Low-grade papillary urothelial carcinoma shows cellular disorder that is distinct from papillary urothelial neoplasm of uncertain malignant potential. In addition, significant nucleomegaly, pleomorphism, or hyperchromasia are not present, excluding a high-grade carcinoma.

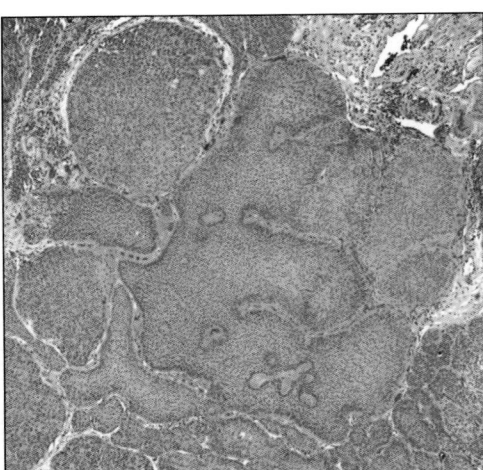
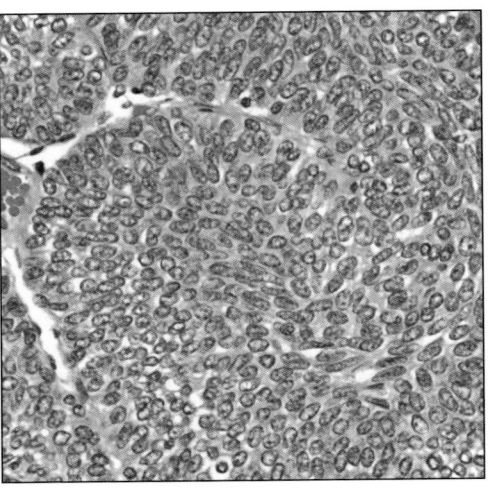

(Left) Low-grade carcinomas may have an endophytic growth pattern that may potentially mimic an inverted papilloma. *(Right)* On high-power examination of this endophytic urothelial neoplasm, the cells have only mild variation in nuclear size and shape with mild disorder. Some areas have slightly enlarged nuclei with small nucleoli. These minimal features warrant classification as low-grade urothelial carcinoma over papillary urothelial neoplasm of uncertain malignant potential.

LOW-GRADE PAPILLARY UROTHELIAL CARCINOMA

Differential Diagnosis

(Left) This papillary urothelial neoplasm of uncertain malignant potential (PUNLMP) has a thickened urothelial lining, but simple papillary architecture, maintained polarity, and no significant atypia. *(Right)* The urothelial lining shows upward linear streaming from the basement membrane ⇨ without significant nuclear atypia. These features support classification as PUNLMP over low-grade carcinoma. The umbrella cell layer is more commonly preserved in lower grade lesions.

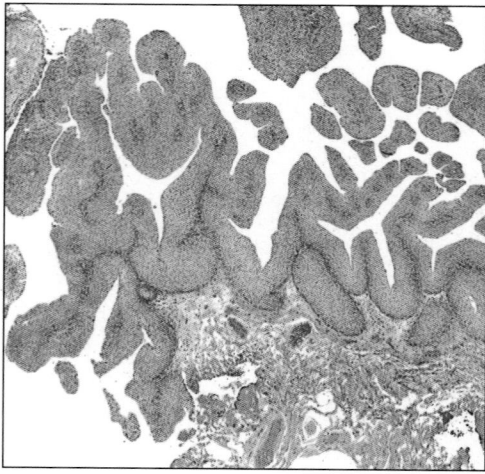
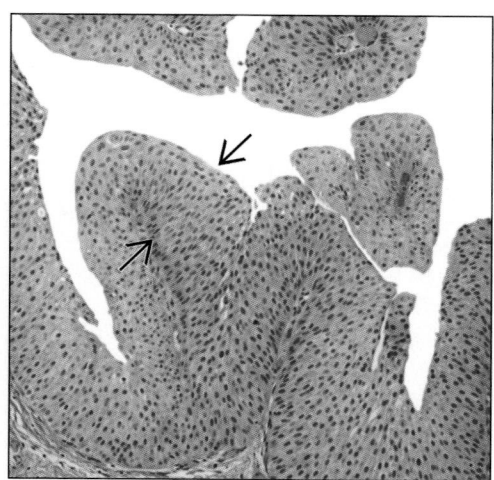

(Left) This papillary urothelial neoplasm has a thickened urothelial lining that maintains perpendicular orientation to the basement membrane and is consistent with PUNLMP. *(Right)* The absence of cytoarchitectural disorder with the perpendicular orientation of neoplastic cells streaming upward from the basement membrane (i.e., normal polarity), combined with the absence of pleomorphism or hyperchromasia, supports interpretation as PUNLMP over low-grade carcinoma.

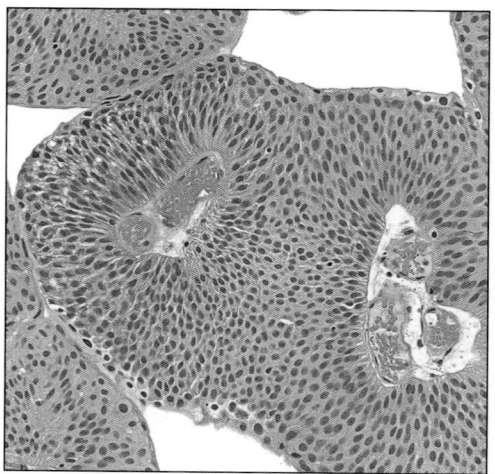
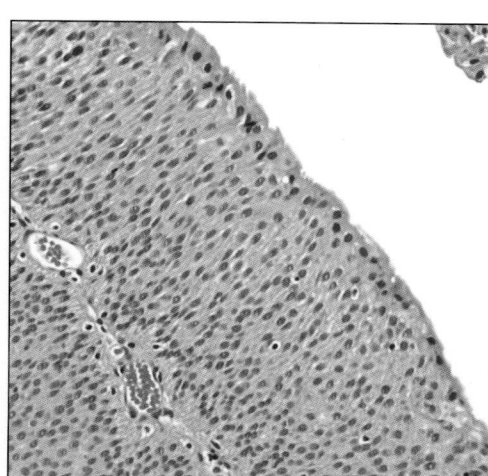

(Left) The simple papillae of this urothelial papilloma have a thin urothelial lining. Architecturally simple papillary patterns without epithelial overgrowth are more common in lower grade tumors. The final grade would require evaluation of the nuclear cytology at high-power examination. *(Right)* The perfectly oriented, cytologically bland urothelial cells of thickness compared to normal urothelium and prominent umbrella cells are diagnostic of urothelial papilloma.

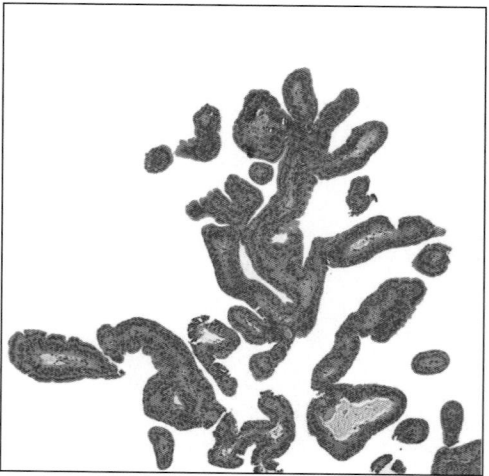
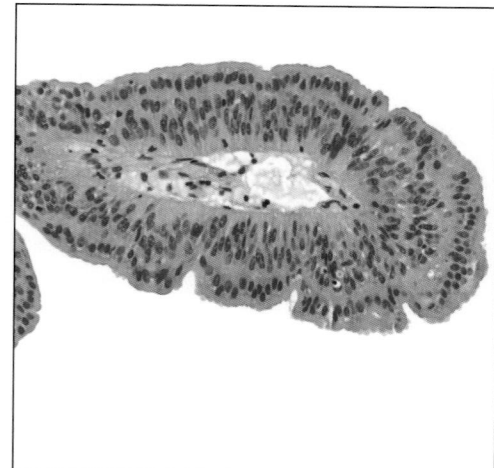

LOW-GRADE PAPILLARY UROTHELIAL CARCINOMA

Differential Diagnosis

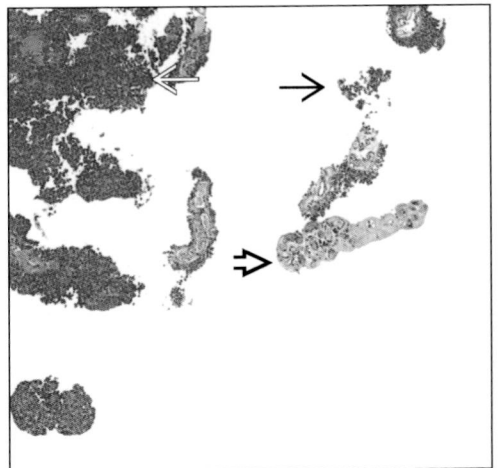

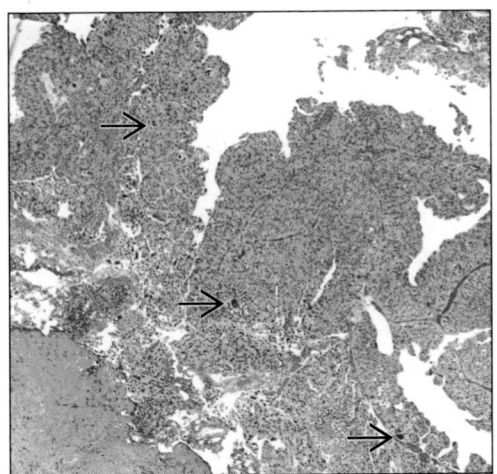

(Left) The presence of nuclear discohesion ➡ or completely denuded papillae ⊡ suggest a high-grade urothelial carcinoma, especially if a cold cup biopsy was performed. The diagnosis, however, is based on the cytologic features of the cells lining the papillae. Some of the papillae are fused and more solid in appearance ➡. *(Right)* The presence of nuclear pleomorphism visible at low-power magnification ➡ warrants a diagnosis of high-grade papillary urothelial carcinoma.

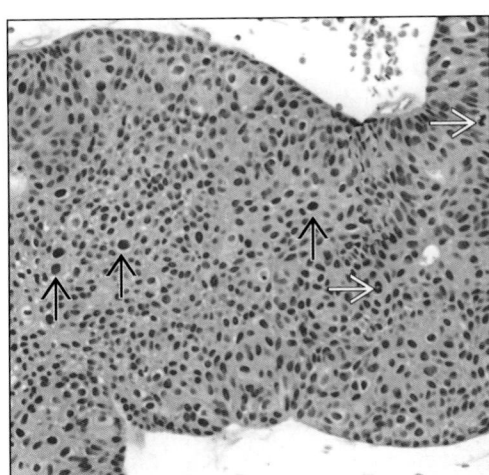

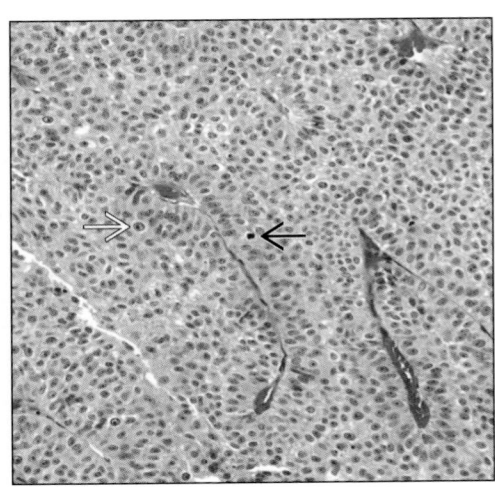

(Left) In this example, the diagnosis of high-grade papillary urothelial carcinoma is based on scattered pleomorphic/ hyperchromatic cells ➡. There are also easily identified mitotic figures ➡. Such lesions would have been classified as grade 2 in the WHO 1973 system but should now be classified as high grade. *(Right)* This high-grade papillary urothelial carcinoma has cellular disorder, scattered mitotic activity ➡, distinct nuclear atypia, and only rare prominent nucleoli ➡.

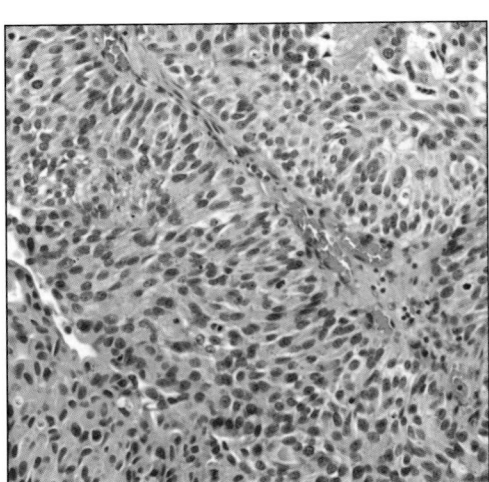

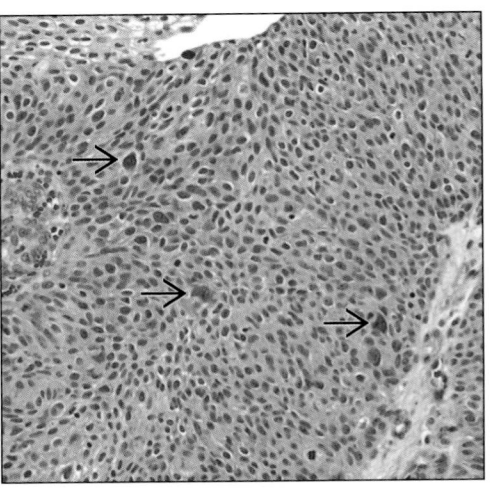

(Left) This high-grade papillary urothelial carcinoma does not show marked pleomorphism, but the hyperchromatic nuclei with irregular, clumped chromatin warrant a high-grade designation. *(Right)* The urothelium lining this papillary neoplasm shows cellular disorder as well as scattered pleomorphic cells ➡; the later feature is sufficient for a high-grade carcinoma diagnosis. Under the WHO 2004/ ISUP system, diffuse nuclear anaplasia is not required for a high-grade diagnosis.

HIGH-GRADE PAPILLARY UROTHELIAL CARCINOMA

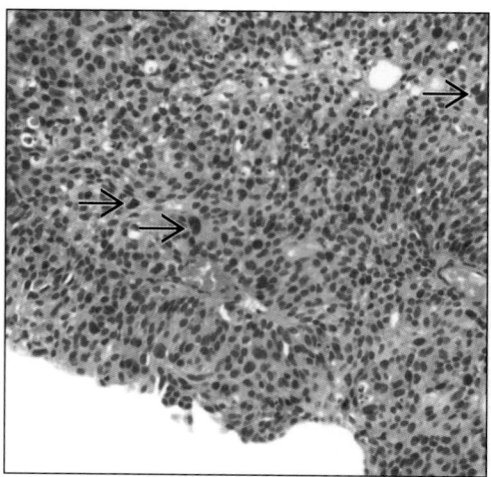

This noninvasive urothelial carcinoma shows typical architectural and cytologic features of high-grade carcinoma, including loss of cellular polarity and scattered nuclear pleomorphism ⇨.

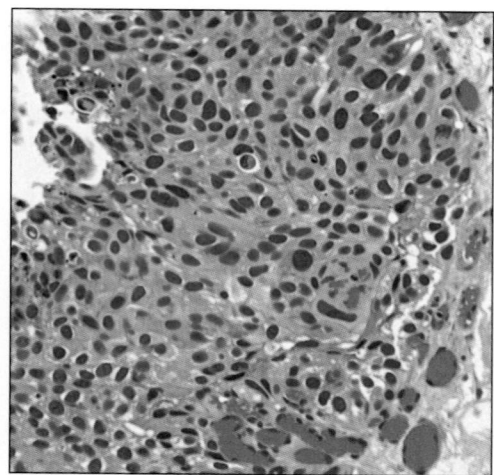

High-grade urothelial carcinoma commonly has rounded nuclear contours, obvious pleomorphism, mitotic activity/apoptotic debris, and loss of normal perpendicular alignment to the basement membrane.

TERMINOLOGY

Definitions
- Papillary urothelial carcinoma with distinct nuclear abnormalities, including presence of moderate to marked nuclear atypia, nucleoli, and pleomorphism

CLINICAL ISSUES

Epidemiology
- Age
  - Most occur in 6th decade or later
- Gender
  - Strong male predominance (M:F = 6-8:1)

Presentation
- Gross or microscopic hematuria is common
- Urine cytology often shows carcinoma

Treatment
- Surgical approaches
  - Transurethral resection and fulguration of visible tumor
- Adjuvant therapy
  - Intravesical immunotherapy with bacillus Calmette-Guérin (BCG)
  - Intravesical chemotherapy with thiotepa or mitomycin-C

Prognosis
- High rate of progression to invasive disease

MACROSCOPIC FEATURES

General Features
- Exophytic papillary growth

MICROSCOPIC PATHOLOGY

Histologic Features
- Often have complex papillary architecture on low-power examination
  - Anastomosis of papillae and confluence is common
  - Cellular discohesion and denudation are common
- Range of nuclear atypia is included in this category
  - Some have obvious nuclear pleomorphism
    - Subset shows marked nuclear anaplasia
  - Other tumors have more monomorphic nuclei
    - Nucleomegaly with irregular clumped nuclear chromatin typical
    - Nuclear rounding is common
- Neoplastic cells are often crowded and overlapping
  - Cells typically lose linear orientation perpendicular to basement membrane (urothelial disorder)
- Nuclear contours typically irregular
- Mitotic activity may be brisk, including on surface
- Nucleoli may be prominent and often in a majority of cells
- May be admixed with lower grade foci of carcinoma

ANCILLARY TESTS

Immunohistochemistry
- Not required for diagnosis
- Expression of CK20 and p53 is more frequent in high-grade carcinomas
  - Compared to lower grade papillary urothelial neoplasms

DIFFERENTIAL DIAGNOSIS

Low-Grade Urothelial Carcinoma
- Nuclear features are less atypical than in high-grade carcinoma

HIGH-GRADE PAPILLARY UROTHELIAL CARCINOMA

Key Facts

Terminology
- Papillary urothelial neoplasm with moderate to marked nuclear atypia

Clinical Issues
- Most occur in 6th decade or later
- Strong male predominance (M:F = 6-8:1)
- Gross or microscopic hematuria is common
- High rate of progression to invasive disease

Microscopic Pathology
- Often have complex papillary architecture on low-power examination
- Range of nuclear atypia is included in this category
- Some have obvious nuclear pleomorphism
- Other tumors have more monomorphic nuclei
- Some degree of nucleomegaly is present
- Irregular clumped nuclear chromatin typical
- Neoplastic cells are often crowded and overlapping
- Cells lose linear orientation perpendicular to basement membrane
- Mitotic activity may be brisk
- Cellular discohesion is common

Ancillary Tests
- Not required for diagnosis

Top Differential Diagnoses
- Low-grade urothelial carcinoma
- Papillary-polypoid cystitis
- Papillary nephrogenic adenoma
- Prostatic-type polyp
- Inverted papilloma
- Prostatic ductal carcinoma

- Cells are more uniform in size and evenly distributed at low-power magnification
- Nuclei may be rounded
- More evenly distributed chromatin
- Large nucleoli may occupy some nuclei but are not prominent feature of low-grade carcinoma
- Mitoses are variable but not on surface
- Cellular discohesion less common
- Prominent umbrella cells are occasionally seen

Papillary-Polypoid Cystitis
- Broad papillae with stromal edema
  - Papillae may taper to thin point distally, but base remains broad
- Do not have complex secondary or tertiary branching typical of papillary urothelial neoplasia
- May have reactive urothelial atypia
  - Nucleoli and mild nucleomegaly but maintains fine nuclear chromatin
  - Mitotic activity is common
- Clinical impression is usually reactive

Papillary Nephrogenic Adenoma
- Papillae are lined by single cuboidal layer
- May have other admixed morphologic patterns
  - Tubular/tubulocystic
    - May mimic invasion
  - Diffuse/solid
    - May mimic poorly differentiated component
    - Does not have nuclear pleomorphism
- Immunoreactivity for pax-2 and pax-8 is characteristic

Prostatic-Type Polyp
- Papillae lined by admixed prostatic secretory and urothelial cells
- Express PSA and PAP in secretory cell component

Inverted Papilloma
- May mimic endophytic growth in high-grade urothelial carcinoma
- Thin trabecular architecture without solid expansile growth

- Usually maintain prominent basal palisading in nests and trabeculae
- Cytologically bland
  - Scattered cells with smudged multilobated nuclei (characteristic of "degenerative" atypia) may be seen
- Nonkeratinizing squamous metaplasia may rarely be present

Prostatic Ductal Carcinoma
- Papillary neoplasm that may extend into bladder from prostatic urethra
- Papillae typically lined by monomorphic columnar cells
- PSA and PAP positive by immunohistochemistry

DIAGNOSTIC CHECKLIST

Clinically Relevant Pathologic Features
- High-grade designation is clinical threshold for adjuvant intravesical therapy
- Nonpapillary urothelium may show carcinoma in situ
- Invasion must be meticulously excluded

Pathologic Interpretation Pearls
- The WHO 2004/ISUP has lowered threshold for diagnosis as high grade
  - High-grade category includes subset of tumors previously considered grade 2 by WHO 1973
    - Therefore, grades cannot be simply translated

SELECTED REFERENCES

1. Reuter VE. Non-invasive Papillary Urothelial Carcinoma, High Grade. In Eble JN et al: World Health Organization Classification of Tumours. Pathology & Genetics. Tumours of the Urinary System and Male Genital Organs. Lyon: IARC Press, 2004
2. Epstein JI et al: The World Health Organization/ International Society of Urological Pathology consensus classification of urothelial (transitional cell) neoplasms of the urinary bladder. Bladder Consensus Conference Committee. Am J Surg Pathol. 22(12):1435-48, 1998

HIGH-GRADE PAPILLARY UROTHELIAL CARCINOMA

Microscopic Features

(Left) This low-power H&E highlights the complex exophytic papillary architecture common in high-grade papillary urothelial carcinoma. There is fusion between the lining urothelium of adjacent papillary cores & some almost solid areas ➡. *(Right)* H&E shows high-grade papillary urothelial carcinoma with confluent urothelial growth entrapping multiple fibrovascular cores ➡. This degree of architectural complexity and fusion between papillae is more common with higher grade lesions.

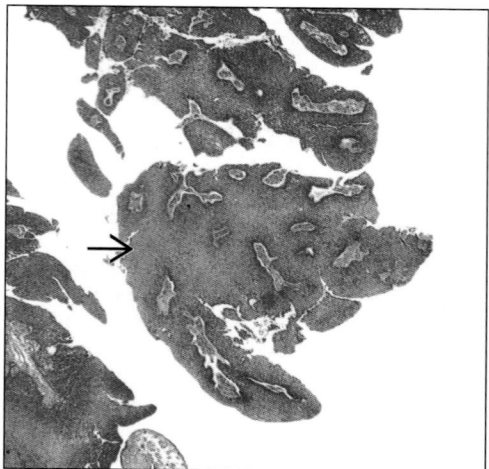 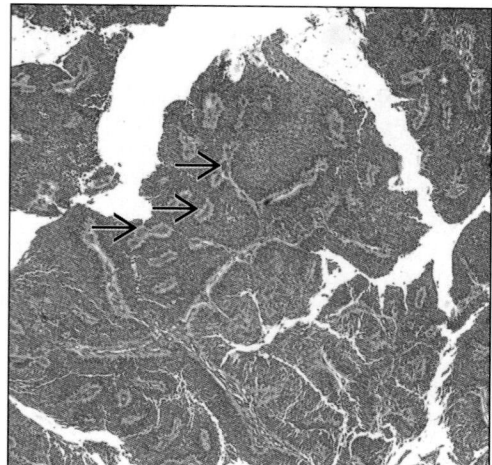

(Left) H&E at high power shows features of high-grade urothelial carcinoma, including nuclear rounding (in contrast to normal fusiform to spindled shape), nuclear pleomorphism, nuclear hyperchromasia, & cellular disorganization. In this example, the orientation of the cells in relation to the basement is not appreciable secondary to loss of polarity. *(Right)* In high-grade urothelial carcinoma, marked nucleomegaly with associated mitotic activity ➡ and apoptotic debris ➡ is common.

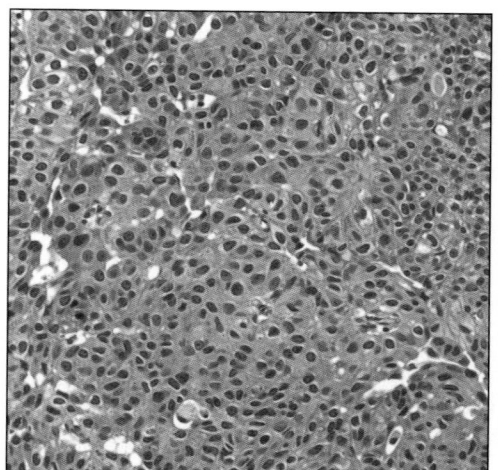 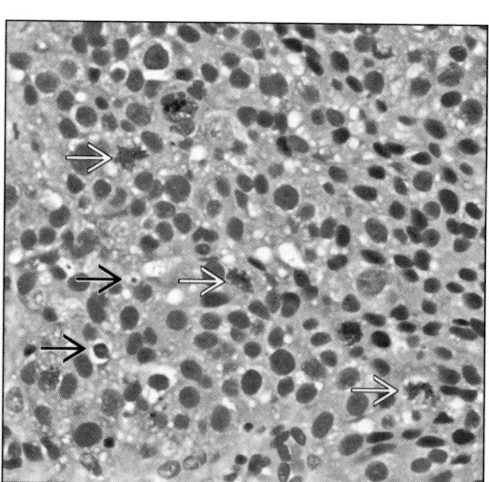

(Left) In the most atypical examples of high-grade papillary urothelial carcinoma, nuclear anaplasia is present ➡. These changes represent the extreme end of the atypia spectrum and are not required for this diagnosis. *(Right)* Obvious cytologic atypia and marked nuclear anaplasia with 5-10x variation in nuclear size ➡ are evident in this high-grade papillary urothelial carcinoma. Anaplasia is not graded separately but may be noted in the report.

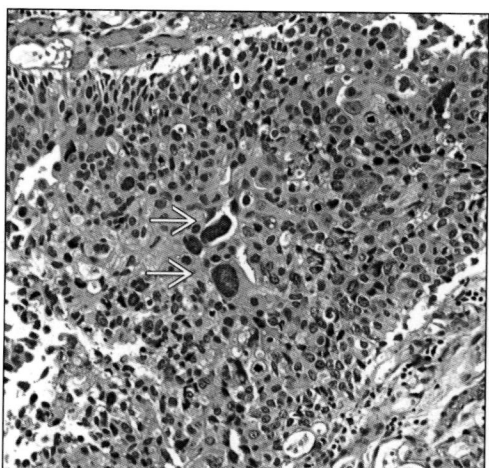 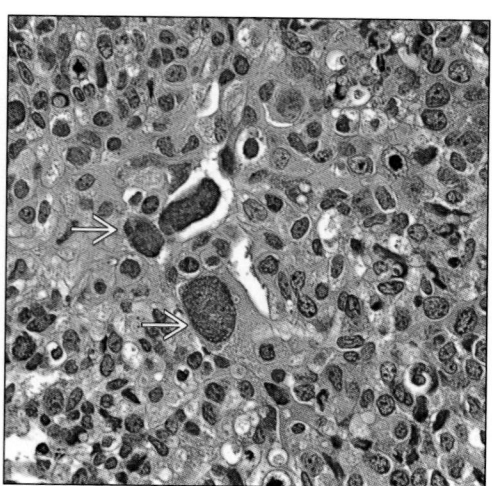

HIGH-GRADE PAPILLARY UROTHELIAL CARCINOMA

Microscopic Features

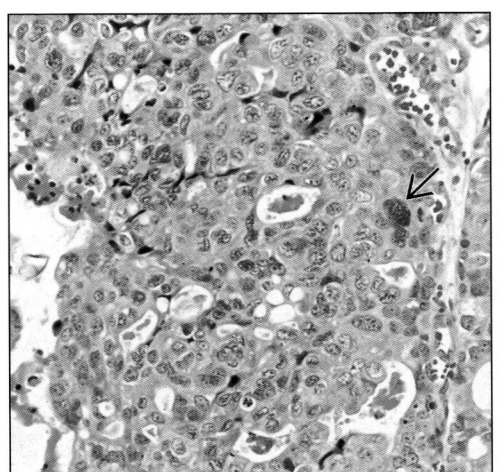
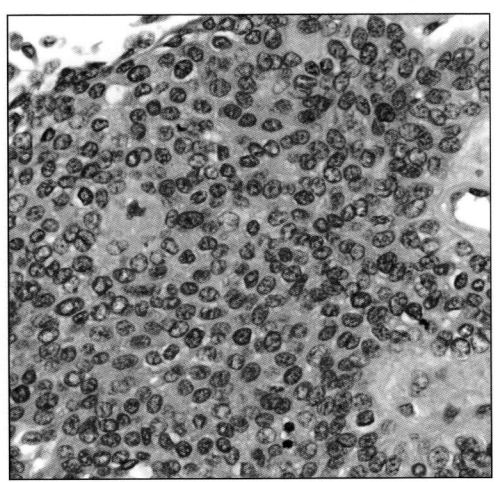

(Left) The features of carcinoma in this case include rounded nuclei, nucleomegaly, variation in nuclear size and shape, loss of polarity, and nuclear membrane irregularity. Hyperchromasia ➡ and marked nuclear pleomorphism, even if focal, are diagnostic of high-grade carcinoma. (Right) This high-grade carcinoma does not have marked pleomorphism. The degree of nucleomegaly, cellular disorder, and nuclear chromatin irregularity are sufficient for high-grade designation.

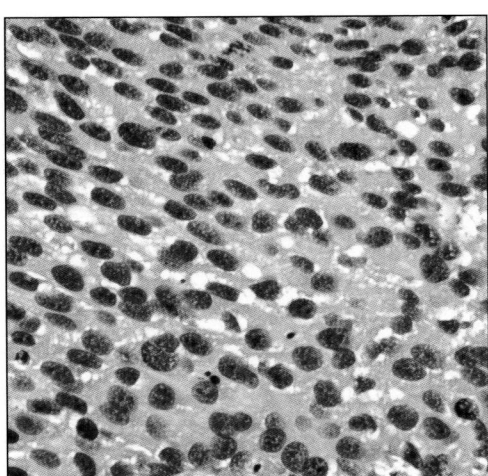
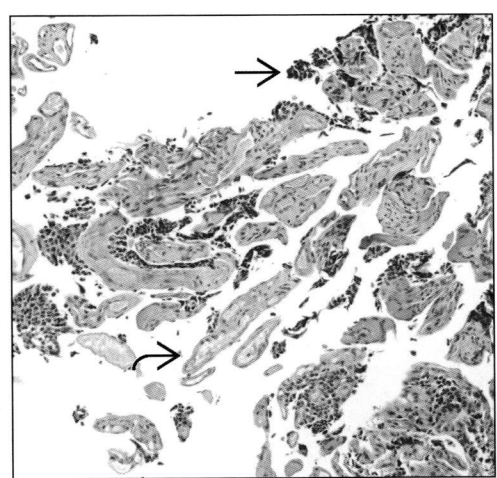

(Left) This high-grade carcinoma is more monomorphic with apparent "order." The nuclear chromatin is very irregular and clumped in all cells, creating marked hyperchromasia. This would have been classified as grade 2 in the WHO 1973 classification system. (Right) The papillae in high-grade papillary urothelial carcinoma may show extensive denudation ➢ and discohesion ➥. Denudation is uncommon in low-grade tumors unless cautery is utilized.

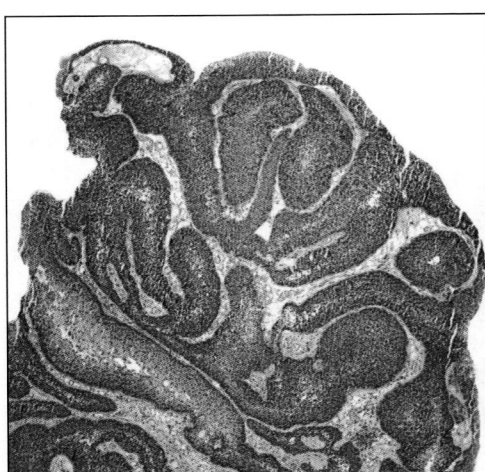
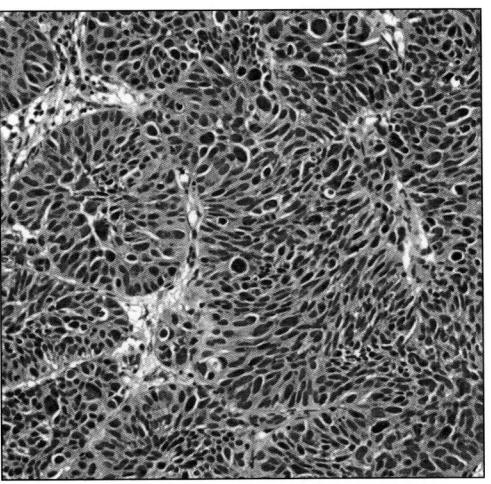

(Left) This represents an uncommon noninvasive endophytic pattern of high-grade urothelial carcinoma. The trabecular growth is reminiscent of inverted papilloma, but the individual cords are broader and more expansile in carcinomas. (Right) The urothelial nests and trabeculae have obvious nuclear pleomorphism, a feature diagnostic of high-grade urothelial carcinoma. Assessment of invasion is better performed on low power and grading of the tumor is best assessed on a higher power.

HIGH-GRADE PAPILLARY UROTHELIAL CARCINOMA

Differential Diagnosis

(Left) Tangentially cut umbrella cells with the expected degree of nucleomegaly and superficial cell atypia ➡ may suggest the possibility of focal high-grade cytology in low-grade urothelial neoplasms. (Right) On high-power examination, the tangentially cut umbrella cells show the expected degree of nucleomegaly and atypia ➡ compared to the underlying low-grade cells ➡. These superficial cells should not be assessed in grading papillary urothelial neoplasia.

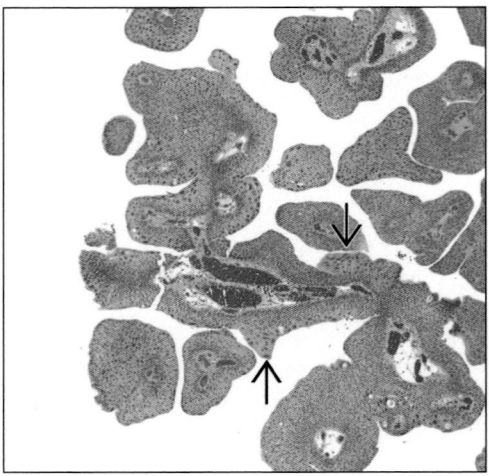 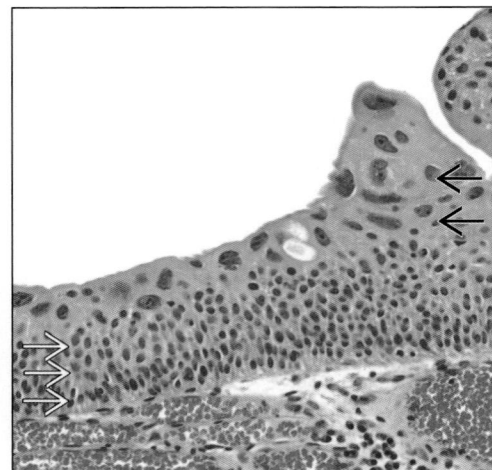

(Left) Papillary nephrogenic adenoma has a single layer of low cuboidal lining cells. The possibility of denudation in a high-grade carcinoma might be considered in such cases. (Right) In this papillary nephrogenic adenoma, the lining epithelial cells from adjacent papillae abut each other, creating a stratified appearance. They may also show some unusual nuclear features, such as nucleoli. There are usually foci with more classic nephrogenic adenoma present to aid in the diagnosis.

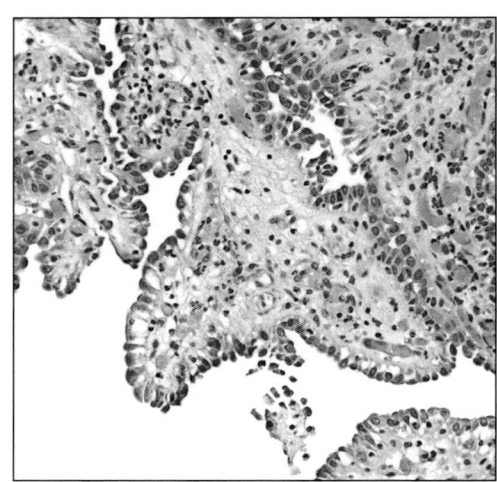 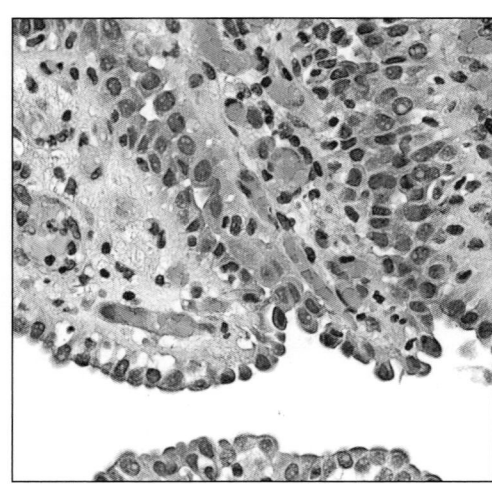

(Left) In papillary-polypoid cystitis, the exophytic processes are broad with more prominent stroma. The tips of some papillary structures may be thin ➡, but they lack the complex branching architecture typical of urothelial neoplasia. (Right) The urothelium in papillary-polypoid cystitis may show reactive changes as in this example with nucleomegaly, some nuclear rounding, and nucleoli. In contrast to high-grade carcinoma, the nuclear membranes are sharp and the chromatin is fine.

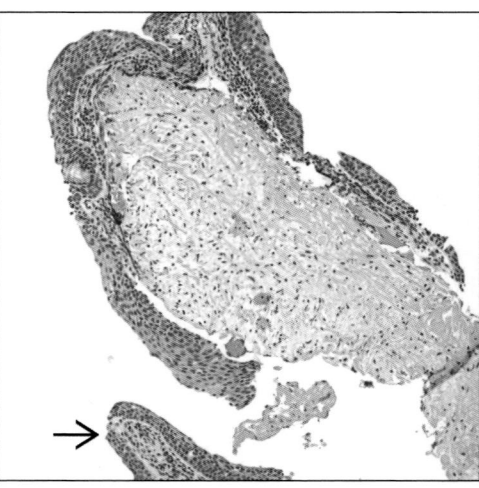 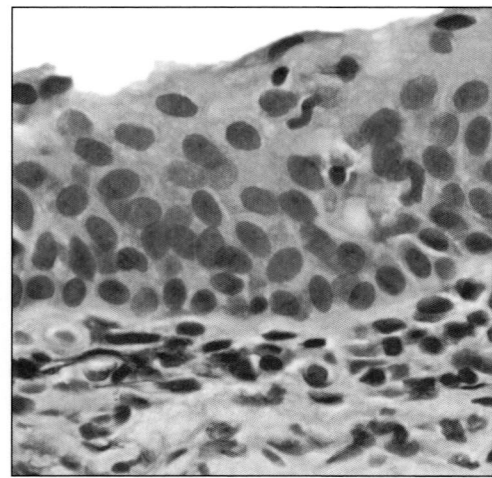

HIGH-GRADE PAPILLARY UROTHELIAL CARCINOMA

Differential Diagnosis

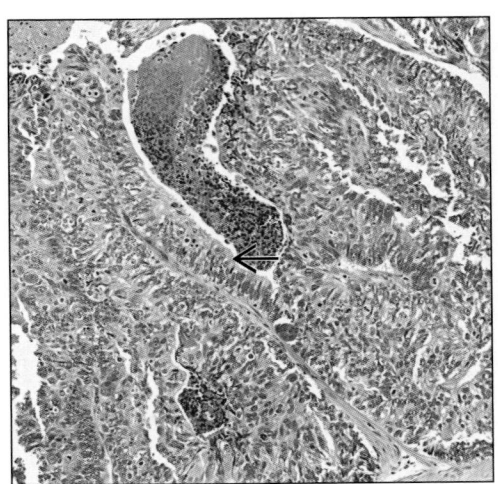

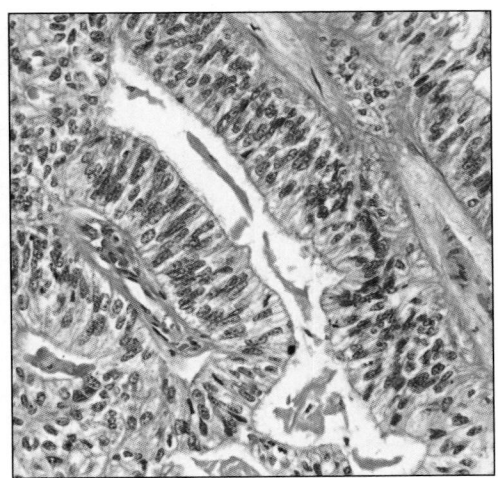

(Left) Prostatic ductal carcinomas with a prominent papillary pattern commonly involve the prostatic urethra and may extend into the bladder, mimicking a papillary urothelial neoplasm. Columnar cells ➡ are not typical of urothelial neoplasia. *(Right)* The rather monomorphic columnar cells with fine chromatin and nucleoli suggest prostatic origin. Immunoreactivity for PSA and PAP (prostate markers) may be helpful in difficult cases.

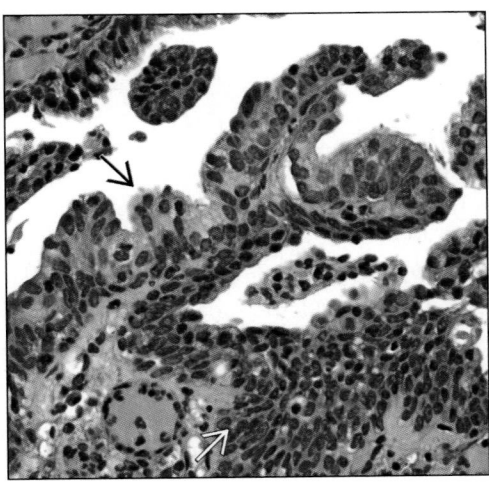

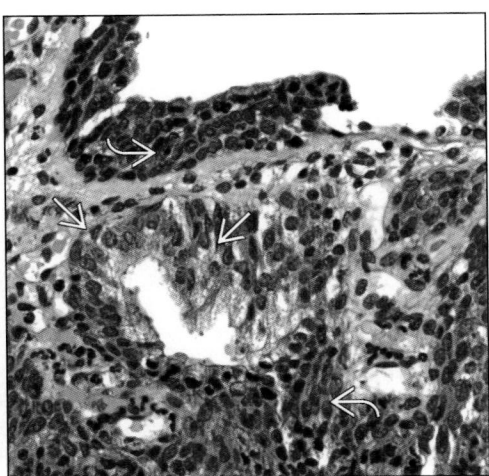

(Left) Prostatic-type polyps are comprised of both prostatic secretory ➡ and urothelial ➡ cells. The urothelial cells are cytologically bland and have normal perpendicular streaming from the basement membrane. *(Right)* Prostatic secretory cells have a more "frothy" cytoplasm ➡ and can be highlighted by PSA immunostains in difficult cases. Admixed urothelial cells are also present in this case ➡. The underlying lamina propria often shows benign-appearing prostatic acini.

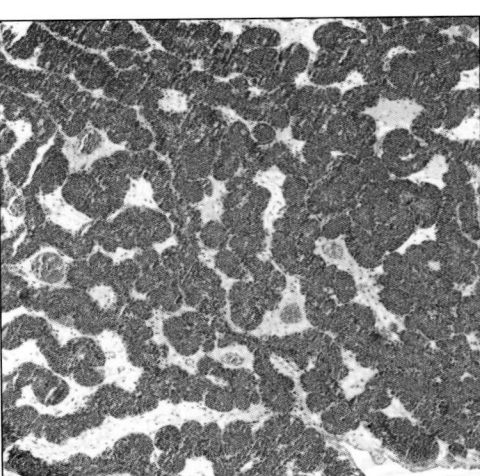

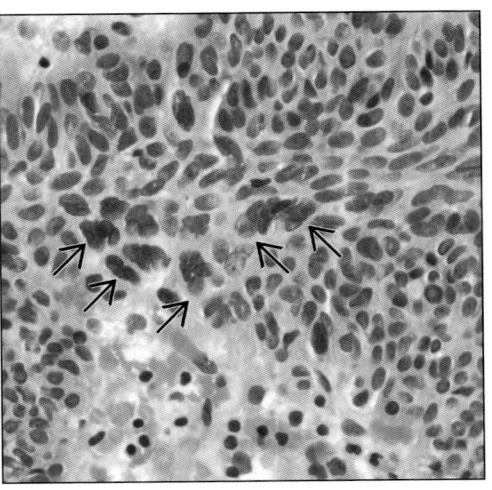

(Left) The thin anastomosing trabeculae in this endophytic urothelial neoplasm are typical of inverted urothelial papilloma. Endophytic carcinomas typically show greater expansion of the invaginated nests and cords. *(Right)* Inverted urothelial papilloma may occasionally contain scattered multinucleated cells with "degenerative" type atypia ➡. This finding should not be regarded as evidence of high-grade carcinoma. The overall features of the cells in the background are benign.

INVASIVE UROTHELIAL CARCINOMA

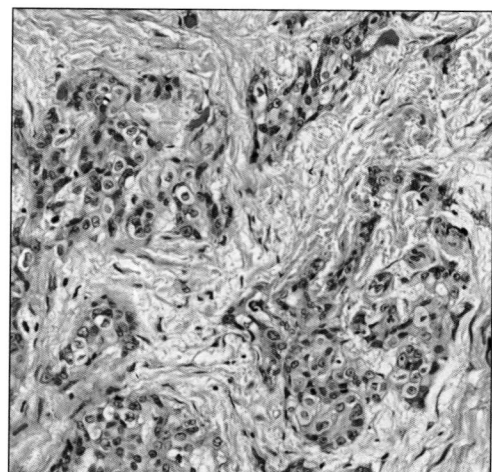

The irregular, jagged nests of urothelium present in this example of urothelial carcinoma are diagnostic of stromal invasion into the lamina propria. No muscularis propria is seen.

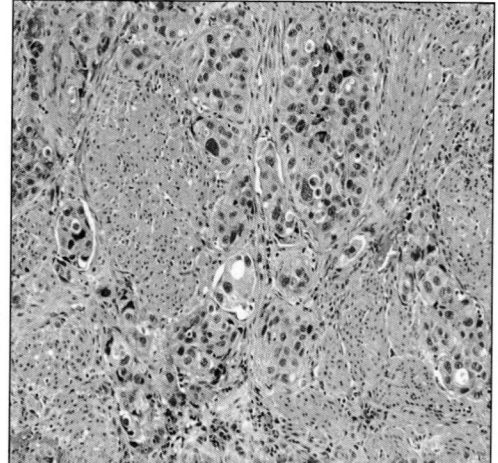

This invasive urothelial carcinoma invades muscularis propria, which is characterized by thick bundles of smooth muscle. This feature classifies the tumor as at least pathologic stage pT2.

TERMINOLOGY

Synonyms
- Invasive transitional cell carcinoma

Definitions
- Urothelial carcinoma that invades beyond basement membrane

CLINICAL ISSUES

Treatment
- Surgical approaches
  - Transurethral resection of visible tumor to base
    - Required for accurate assessment of invasion
  - Invasion into lamina propria usually managed conservatively with intravesical therapy
    - Bacillus Calmette-Guérin
    - Mitomycin and other intravesical therapies
    - Radical cystectomy rarely performed, institution dependent
  - Invasion into muscularis propria usually managed by radical cystectomy
    - ± neoadjuvant therapy
    - Radiation therapy is primary treatment modality in some cases

Prognosis
- Stage dependent
  - Deeply invasive tumors (pT2 or greater/muscularis propria and beyond)
    - Poor prognosis
  - Superficially invasive tumors (pT1/lamina propria)
    - May have excellent prognosis

MACROSCOPIC FEATURES

General Features
- May be papillary, polypoid, nodular, solid, or ulcerated

- Background urothelium may be normal or erythematous
- Frequently multifocal

MICROSCOPIC PATHOLOGY

Key Descriptors
- Predominant Cell/Compartment Type
  - Epithelial, urothelial

Normal Histologic Anatomy of Bladder Wall
- Detailed knowledge of bladder microanatomy is required for proper pathologic staging
- Lamina propria
  - Hypocellular collagenized or edematous stroma
    - Stromal cells may be hyperchromatic and multilobated
  - Associated small to medium caliber blood vessels
  - Muscularis mucosae
    - Classically has thin, wispy fascicles of smooth muscle
    - When hyperplastic, fascicles may be thicker and disorganized with dispersion in multiple directions
    - Occasionally, individual small rounded thick muscle bundles separated by stroma are present in lamina propria
  - May contain adipose tissue
- Muscularis propria (detrusor muscle)
  - Large aggregates of confluent dense smooth muscle
  - Often contains adipose tissue
  - May be very superficially located in some regions

Patterns of Invasion
- Small nests or clusters/single cells within lamina propria
  - Surrounding retraction artifact is common
  - Other stromal reactions include desmoplasia, sclerosis, and myxoid change

INVASIVE UROTHELIAL CARCINOMA

Key Facts

Terminology
- Urothelial carcinoma that invades beyond basement membrane

Clinical Issues
- Invasion into lamina propria usually managed with intravesical therapy
- Invasion into muscularis propria usually managed by radical cystectomy

Microscopic Pathology
- Small nests, clusters, &/or single cells within lamina propria
- Surrounding retraction artifact is common
- Other stromal reactions include desmoplasia, sclerosis, and myxoid change
- May have irregular, jagged tongues of epithelium in continuity with overlying noninvasive component

Top Differential Diagnoses
- Prostatic adenocarcinoma involving bladder
- Gynecologic carcinomas involving bladder
- Paraganglioma
- Inverted patterns of noninvasive urothelial neoplasia
- Nephrogenic adenoma
- Pseudocarcinomatous hyperplasia

Diagnostic Checklist
- Important to state depth of invasion by clearly reporting invasion of "lamina propria" or "muscularis propria"
- Recognizing heterogeneity of urinary bladder microanatomy is important to avoid overstaging

---

- o Microinvasion: Focal invasion of single cells or small clusters, < 2 mm in depth
- May have more abundant eosinophilic cytoplasm than adjacent noninvasive component
  - o "Paradoxical maturation"
- May have irregular, jagged tongues of epithelium in continuity with overlying noninvasive component
- Most invasive urothelial carcinomas are high grade
  - o Exceptions are nested and tubular variants
  - o Grade of invasive component does not affect prognosis as all have recurring and metastatic potential

ANCILLARY TESTS

Immunohistochemistry
- Usually immunoreactive for p63, CK20, and HMCK(34βE12)
  - o Low specificity
- Uroplakin, thrombomodulin, GATA3, and S100p are more specific markers of urothelial lineage
  - o Relatively low sensitivity
- Smoothelin immunostains may be helpful in distinguishing muscularis mucosae from muscularis propria
  - o Weak, patchy staining in muscularis mucosae
  - o Strong, diffuse reactivity in muscularis propria
    - ■ May be useful when tumor obliterates muscularis propria and only scant residual muscle is seen
- Cytokeratin stains may be useful in identifying subtle foci of invasive carcinoma
  - o Should not be confused with cytokeratin positive myofibroblasts
    - ■ Spindled cells with tapered cytoplasmic processes
    - ■ Also coexpress actin-sm

DIFFERENTIAL DIAGNOSIS

Other Nonurothelial Neoplasms
- Prostatic adenocarcinoma involving bladder
  - o Monomorphic round cells with prominent nucleoli

- o May have gland/acinar formation
- o Immunoreactive for PSA &/or PAP
- o Usually negative for p63 and HMCK(34βE12)
- o CK7/CK20 immunophenotype is highly variable in high-grade prostatic adenocarcinomas
- Gynecologic carcinomas involving bladder
  - o Cervical squamous cell carcinomas may mimic urothelial carcinoma with squamous differentiation
  - o High-grade uterine carcinomas may mimic poorly differentiated urothelial carcinoma or urothelial carcinoma with glandular differentiation
    - ■ Often express ER &/or WT1
  - o Clinical/radiographic correlation is critical
- Paraganglioma
  - o Nested aggregates of epithelioid cells
    - ■ Often have closely associated surrounding vascular network
  - o Sclerotic/hyalinized examples may be pseudoinfiltrative
    - ■ Closely mimics invasive carcinoma
  - o May have scattered pleomorphic cells
    - ■ "Endocrine anaplasia"
  - o Immunophenotype is distinctive
    - ■ Positive for synaptophysin but not cytokeratins
    - ■ S100(+) sustentacular cells may be seen
- Inverted patterns of noninvasive urothelial neoplasia
  - o Crowded endophytic nests or trabeculae of urothelium with sharp rounded contours
    - ■ Range from inverted papilloma to inverted high-grade carcinoma, based on cytologic features
  - o No surrounding retraction or other stromal changes
  - o No jagged nests

Benign Mimics
- Nephrogenic adenoma
  - o Small papillae lined by single cuboidal epithelial layer
  - o Small tubules in lamina propria
    - ■ Tubules often possess thick basement membrane
    - ■ Lined by flattened or "hobnail" cells
    - ■ Small lumina may resemble blood vessels

INVASIVE UROTHELIAL CARCINOMA

- Rare "diffuse" or solid pattern may closely mimic malignancy
  - Diffuse nuclear pax-2/pax-8 immunoreactivity
  - May also stain with AMACR (P504s)
- Pseudocarcinomatous hyperplasia
  - Often associated with prior radiation or chemotherapy
  - Rare cases have no prior therapy
    - Often have factors predisposing to ischemia
  - "Squamoid" epithelial nests in lamina propria may be jagged but are associated with fibrin and blood vessels
    - Epithelial aggregates characteristically envelop blood vessels that are obliterated by fibrin
  - Lamina propria is often hemorrhagic with extravasated fibrin
  - Other radiation-associated changes may be seen
- Cystitis cystica/glandularis
  - Invaginated urothelial nests with superficial location in lamina propria
    - Rounded contours of nests
    - May have lobular architecture
  - Sharp border with lamina propria at base
  - No stromal reaction
  - Intestinal type may have associated mucin extravasation
    - May closely mimic malignancy clinically

DIAGNOSTIC CHECKLIST

Clinically Relevant Pathologic Features

- "Hypertrophied" patterns of muscularis mucosa are not restricted to men with prostatic hyperplasia

Pathologic Interpretation Pearls

- Recognizing heterogeneity of urinary bladder microanatomy is important to avoid overstating
  - Morphology of muscularis mucosae is more variable than originally reported
- Stromal retraction should not be overinterpreted as vascular invasion
  - In some centers, presence of vascular invasion may affect clinical management (controversial)

STAGING

Difficult Staging Distinctions

- Noninvasive urothelial carcinoma involving prostatic glands
  - Usually in biopsies of "bladder neck"
  - Rounded contours of epithelial nests
    - May be expansile
    - No irregular jagged nests or small nests with surrounding retraction
    - No stromal response
  - May have residual basal cells
  - Adjacent normal prostatic glands are strong clue to this possibility
  - Because of thick fibromuscular stroma in this location, may mimic muscularis propria invasion
- Muscularis mucosae invasion vs. muscularis propria

- Nonclassic patterns of muscularis mucosa may be difficult
  - Individual small rounded aggregates of thick smooth muscle separated by stroma
  - In contrast, muscularis propria has large confluent aggregates of thick muscle
  - In some bladders, junction of muscularis propria and lamina propria is not well defined
    - Dispersed thick muscle extending luminally toward lamina propria particularly in trigone
- Invasion of perivesical tissue (pT3 disease)
  - Cannot be diagnosed on biopsy
    - Adipose tissue is present throughout normal bladder wall, including lamina propria and muscularis propria
    - Should not be used as gauge of location within bladder wall

REPORTING CRITERIA

Staging on Transurethral Biopsy

- Important to state depth of invasion by clearly reporting invasion of "lamina propria" or "muscularis propria"
  - Reporting "muscle invasion" without further specification is inappropriate
    - Does not distinguish between muscularis mucosae (pT1) and propria (at least pT2)
- Diagnosis of "invasive urothelial carcinoma, involving muscle of indeterminant type" is warranted in some cases
  - Carcinoma involving smooth muscle (difficulty in determining mucosae vs. propria)
    - Requires restaging biopsies

SELECTED REFERENCES

1. Paner GP et al: Diagnostic utility of antibody to smoothelin in the distinction of muscularis propria from muscularis mucosae of the urinary bladder: a potential ancillary tool in the pathologic staging of invasive urothelial carcinoma. Am J Surg Pathol. 33(1):91-8, 2009
2. Paner GP et al: Further characterization of the muscle layers and lamina propria of the urinary bladder by systematic histologic mapping: implications for pathologic staging of invasive urothelial carcinoma. Am J Surg Pathol. 31(9):1420-9, 2007
3. Vakar-Lopez F et al: Muscularis mucosae of the urinary bladder revisited with emphasis on its hyperplastic patterns: a study of a large series of cystectomy specimens. Ann Diagn Pathol. 11(6):395-401, 2007
4. Jimenez RE et al: pT1 urothelial carcinoma of the bladder: criteria for diagnosis, pitfalls, and clinical implications. Adv Anat Pathol. 7(1):13-25, 2000
5. Philip AT et al: Intravesical adipose tissue: a quantitative study of its presence and location with implications for therapy and prognosis. Am J Surg Pathol. 24(9):1286-90, 2000
6. Ro JY et al: Muscularis mucosa of urinary bladder. Importance for staging and treatment. Am J Surg Pathol. 11(9):668-73, 1987

INVASIVE UROTHELIAL CARCINOMA

Gross and Microscopic Features of Lamina Propia

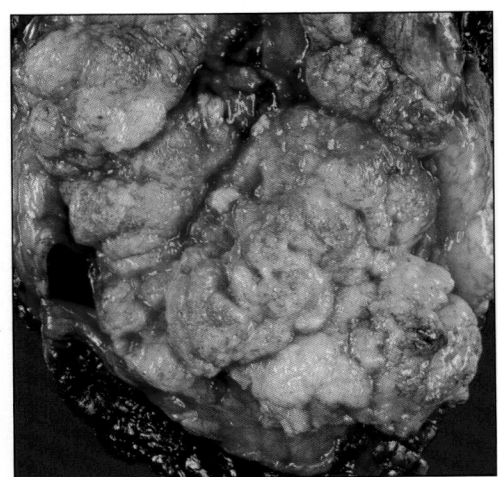

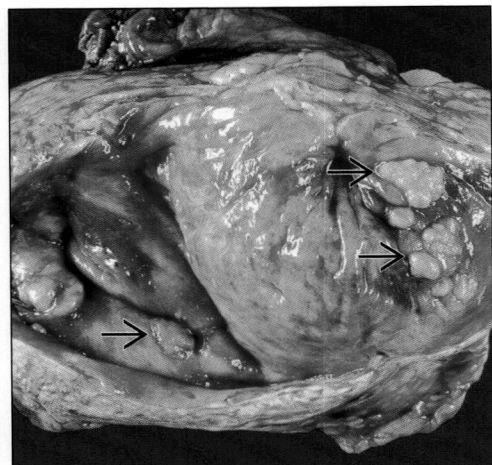

(Left) This radical cystectomy specimen with urothelial carcinoma contains a fungating, ulcerative mass involving the entire mucosal surface of the bladder. There are areas of hemorrhage and necrosis. *(Right)* This radical cystectomy specimen contains multiple urothelial carcinomas ➡. Multifocality of urothelial carcinoma is common and includes disease in the upper tract and prostatic and penile urethra. Tumors vary from being papillary to polypoid to sessile and nodular.

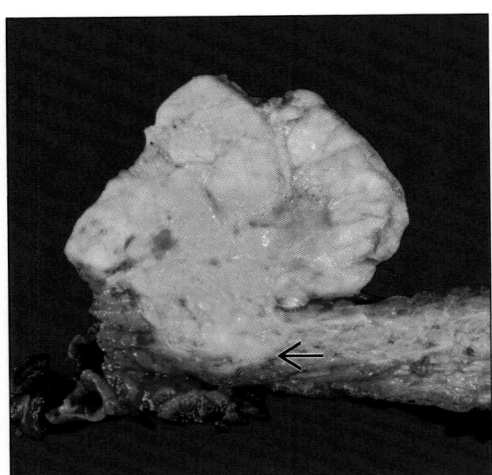

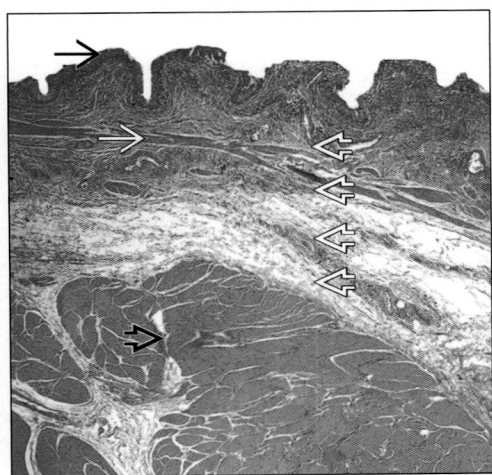

(Left) This cut section of the bladder wall in a pelvic exenteration specimen shows a yellow-tan fleshy cut surface, which infiltrates the outer half of the bladder wall ➡. *(Right)* The normal urinary bladder wall consists of the lining urothelium ➡, the lamina propria that extends from the basement membrane to the muscularis propria ➡ (and contains the muscularis mucosae ➡), the muscularis propria ➡, and the surrounding perivesical soft tissue (not shown).

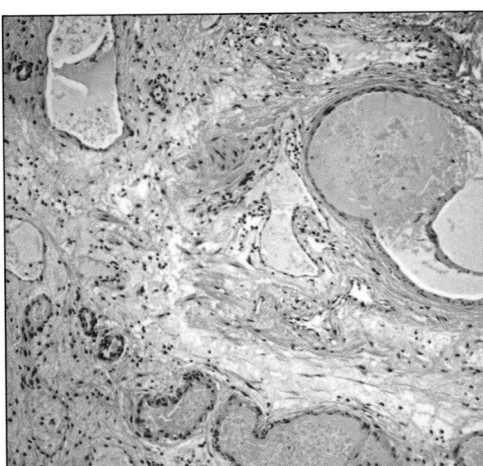

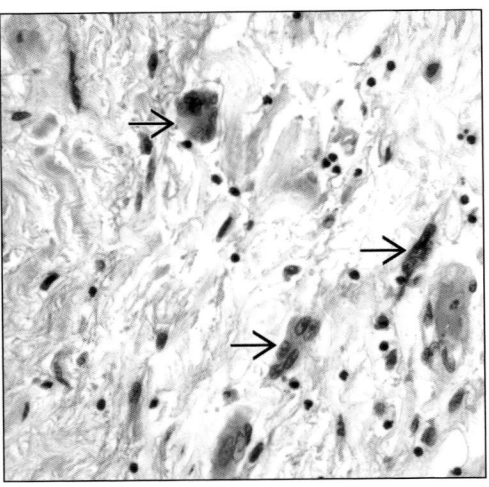

(Left) The lamina propria of the urinary bladder, seen here, typically consists of loose hypocellular stroma and variably small to medium-sized blood vessels. Muscularis mucosae muscle bundles are frequently associated with this vascular plexus. *(Right)* The stromal cells of the lamina propria are often multilobated with dark smudgy chromatin ➡. This normal variation in stromal cells should not be confused with a malignant spindle cell neoplasm and does not indicate prior radiation.

Types of Muscle

(Left) Disorganized, thin wispy bundles of smooth muscle are characteristic of muscularis mucosae. Their location varies from being superficial to deep in the lamina propria. The term "muscle invasion" should not be used in reports as it does not distinguish muscularis mucosae from muscularis propria. (Right) Large aggregates of smooth muscle ➡, separate from the underlying muscularis propria ➡, are unusual but may be present in the lamina propria.

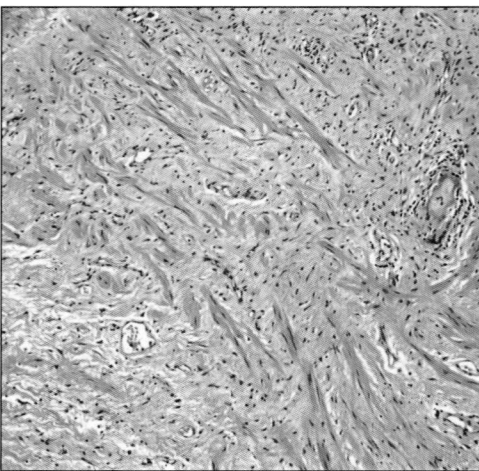 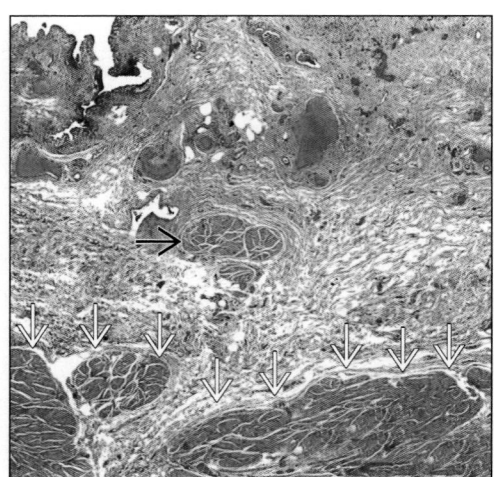

(Left) The muscularis propria may be extremely superficial in some regions of the bladder, as seen in this example. The confluent mass of tightly aggregated smooth muscle bundles is characteristic of muscularis propria. (Right) Even in biopsies with cautery artifact, confluent compact bundles of smooth muscle characteristic of muscularis propria are recognizable. The presence or absence of muscularis propria should be reported in all biopsies with urothelial carcinoma.

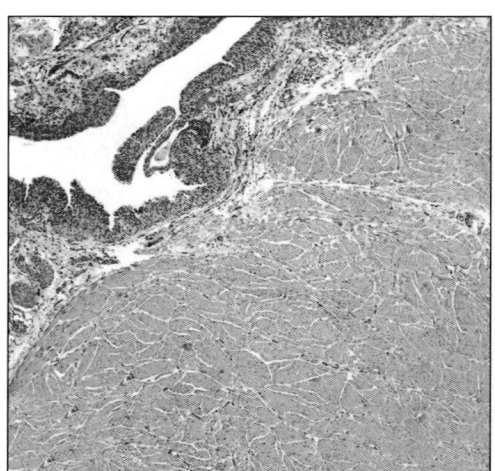 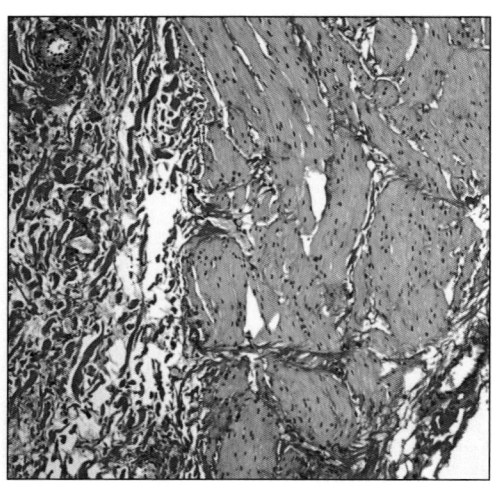

(Left) The large size of this smooth muscle bundle, which is arranged in a fascicular pattern, is diagnostic of muscularis propria. (Right) Confluent compact bundles of smooth muscle of the muscularis propria are cut on end and are distinct from the thin, wispy, disorganized fascicles or separate individual bundles of smooth muscle that characterize muscularis mucosae. Invasion of muscularis propria often constitutes the crossroads between conservative and aggressive management.

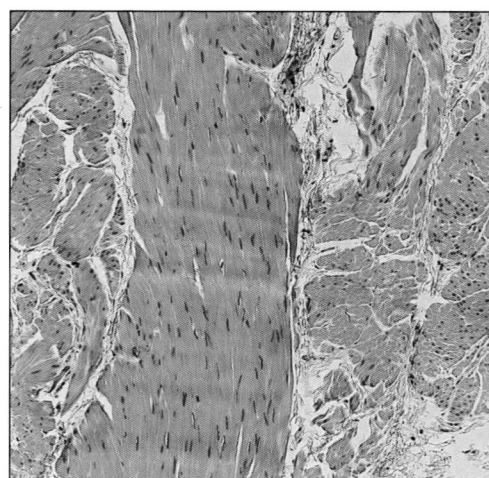 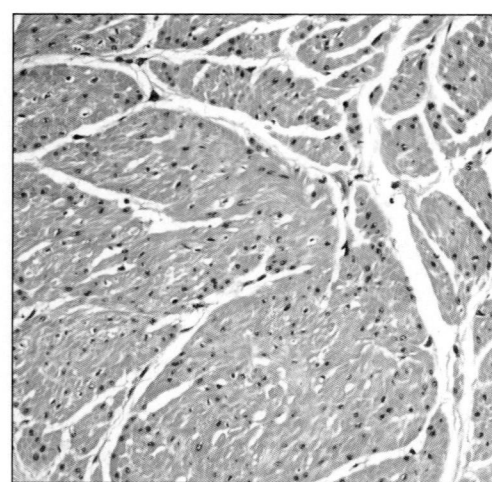

INVASIVE UROTHELIAL CARCINOMA

Lamina Propria Invasion

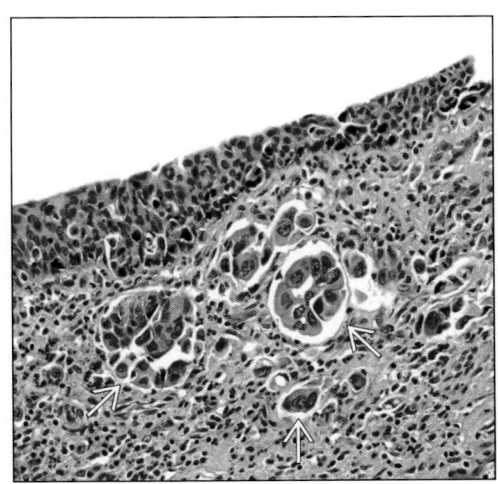

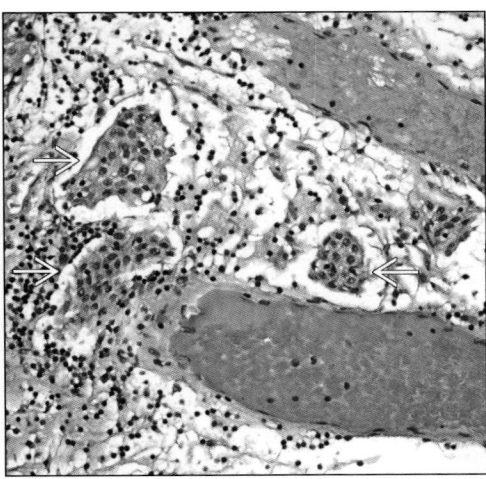

(Left) Small aggregates and individual cells with surrounding retraction spaces ➡ are diagnostic of invasion in urothelial carcinoma. This is a common pattern of invasion and should be distinguished from true vascular invasion. (Right) These rounded aggregates of invasive urothelial carcinoma with surrounding retraction ➡ were present in the deep lamina propria. The edematous stroma, chronic inflammation, and blood vessels are characteristic of lamina propria.

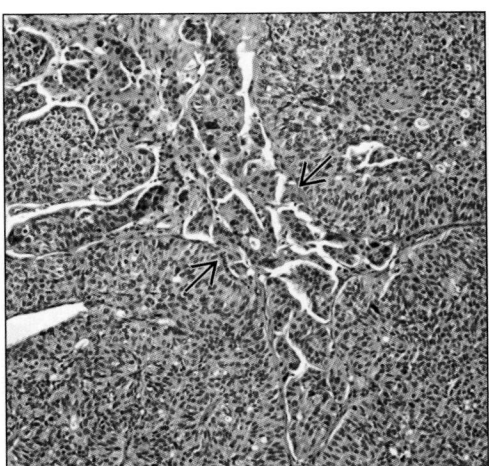

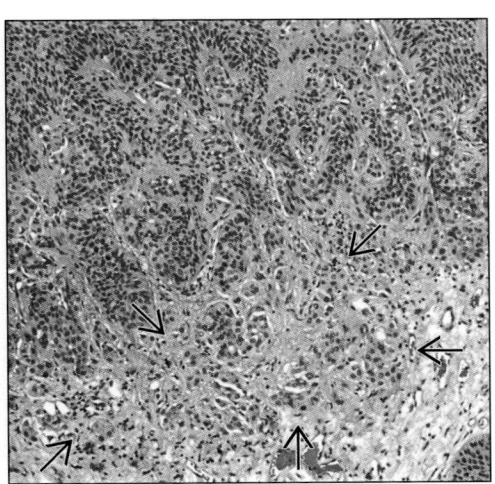

(Left) Invasion into the stalk of a papillary urothelial carcinoma is often characterized by small aggregates and nests of urothelium with surrounding retraction artifact ➡. This would be designated as lamina propria invasion and staged as pT1. (Right) The base of this high-grade papillary urothelial carcinoma, the most frequent site of invasion in papillary carcinoma, shows irregular nests ➡ associated with stromal response that are diagnostic of lamina propria invasion.

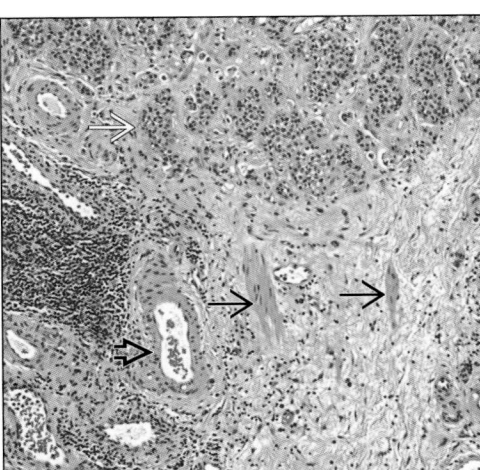

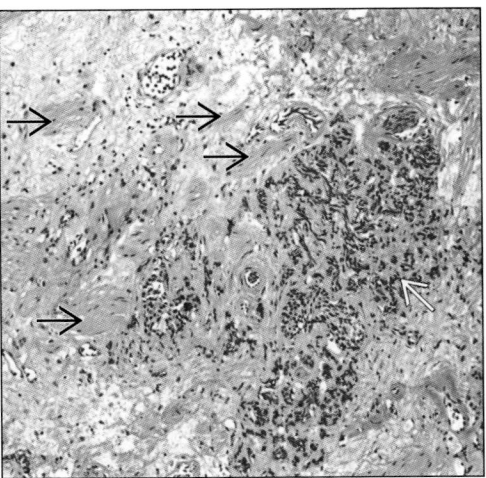

(Left) The irregular nests of this invasive urothelial carcinoma ➡ invade the lamina propria. Typical features of lamina propria, variably sized blood vessels ➡ and wispy fascicles of the muscularis mucosae ➡, are seen. (Right) This invasive urothelial carcinoma ➡ also involves the lamina propria. The separate, individual smooth muscle bundles represent muscularis mucosae ➡. In contrast, muscularis propria is comprised of confluent aggregates of smooth muscle.

INVASIVE UROTHELIAL CARCINOMA

Muscularis Propria Invasion

(Left) At low-power evaluation of this cystectomy specimen, invasive urothelial carcinoma extends deep into the muscularis propria ➡. In biopsy and transurethral resection specimens, this helpful low-power evaluation is often not possible, given the small tissue fragments. *(Right)* This invasive urothelial carcinoma invades muscularis propria. When there is destructive invasion, the residual smooth muscle bundles may appear thin, mimicking the wispy bundles of muscularis mucosae.

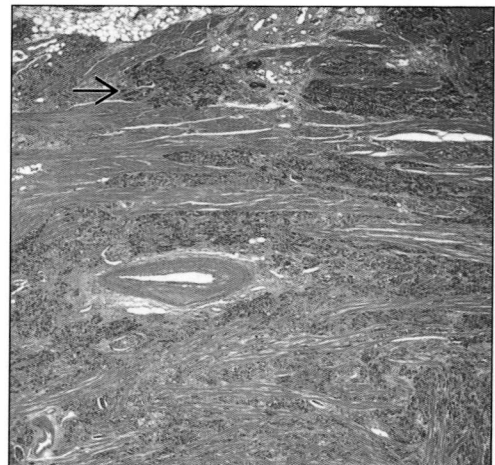 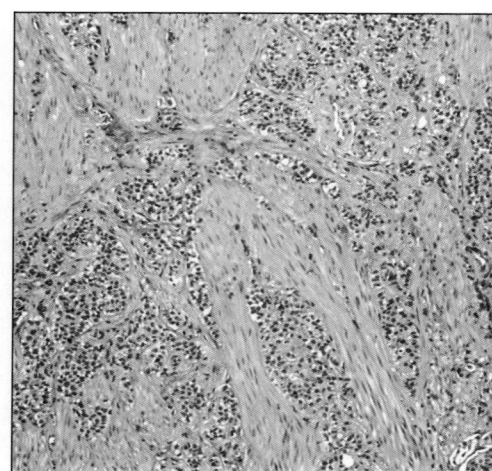

(Left) This example of invasive urothelial carcinoma shows prototypical invasion of the muscularis propria, which is characterized by carcinoma that surrounds large confluent aggregates of compact smooth muscle. *(Right)* Invasive urothelial carcinoma dissects between confluent bundles of smooth muscle, a finding diagnostic of muscularis propria invasion (at least pT2 disease in transurethral resections). There is cautery artifact that, if severe, may preclude recognition of carcinoma.

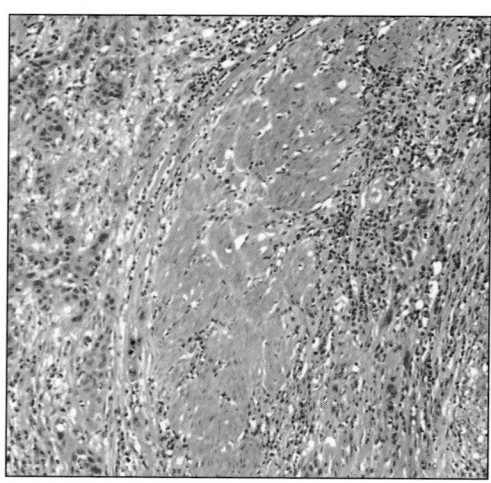 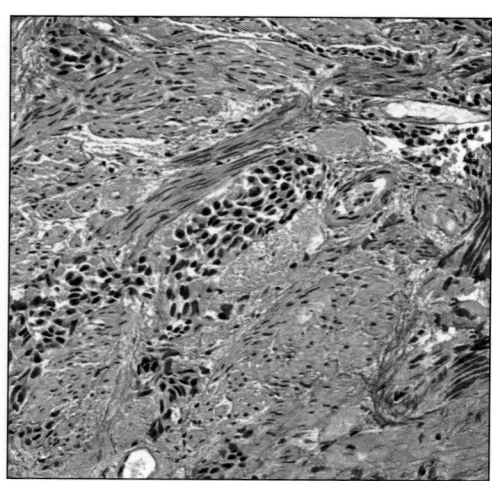

(Left) This invasive urothelial carcinoma involves scattered thin smooth muscle aggregates. The differential diagnosis includes muscularis mucosae invasion or destructive permeation of muscularis propria. The presence of such muscle throughout an entire tissue fragment is strongly suggestive of muscularis propria. *(Right)* Strong and diffuse immunoreactivity for smoothelin in the entrapped smooth muscle cells supports the diagnosis of muscularis propria invasion.

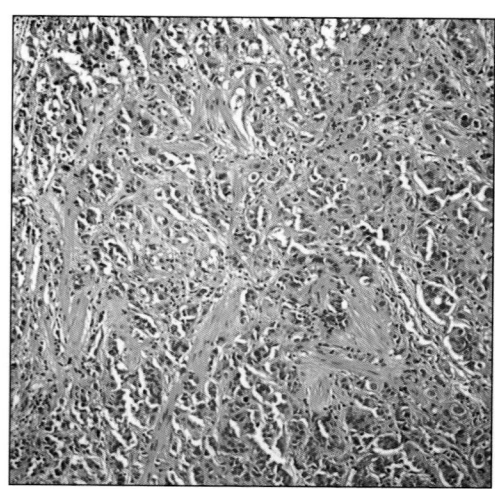 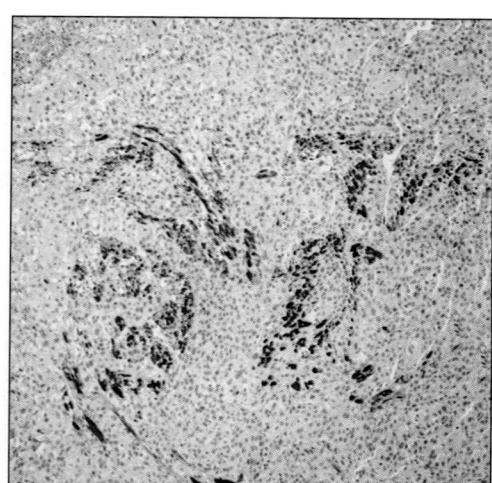

INVASIVE UROTHELIAL CARCINOMA

Differential Diagnosis

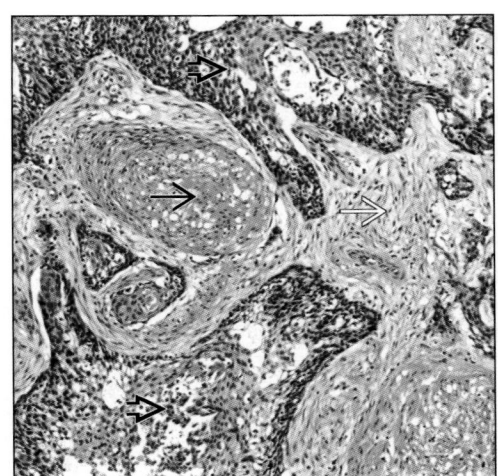

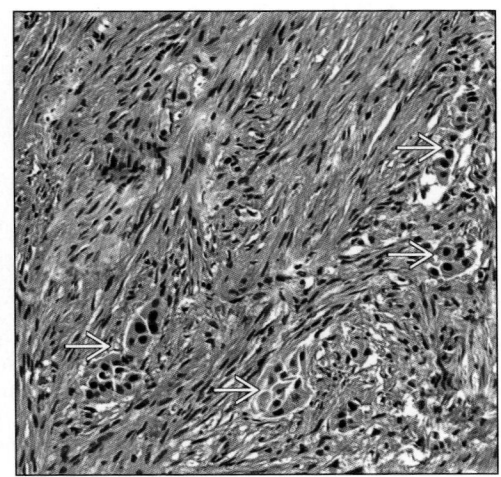

(Left) This invasive urothelial carcinoma ⊵ contrasts the eosinophilic muscle bundles of the muscularis propria ➡ with the more myxoid and spindled reactive myofibroblastic proliferation ➡. *(Right)* This pseudosarcomatous myofibroblastic proliferation is associated with invasive urothelial carcinoma ➡. The cytologically bland tapered spindled cells with a blue hue are typical of myofibroblasts. This may potentially be confused with muscle invasion or sarcomatoid carcinoma.

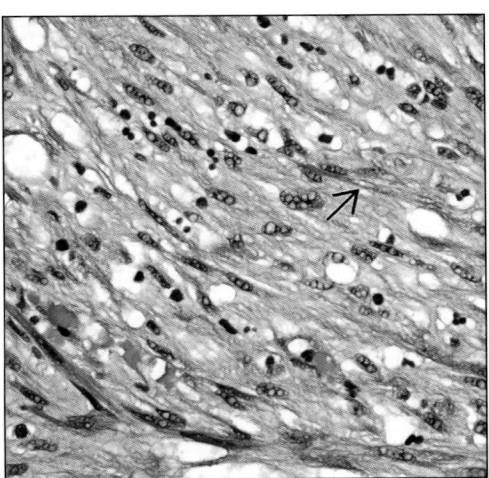

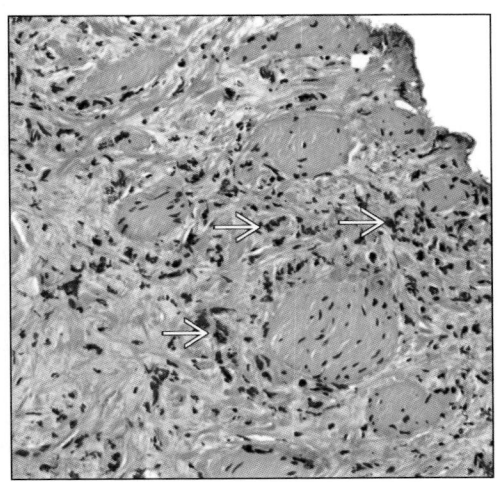

(Left) Elongated cytoplasmic processes ➡ and fine nuclear chromatin are typical of myofibroblasts. Such reactive lesions often lack the eosinophilia of smooth muscle. *(Right)* Invasive urothelial carcinomas ➡ may be masked by biopsy artifact. This case also shows a challenging pattern of muscle involvement with separate individual rounded bundles, a rare pattern of muscularis mucosae. Cytokeratin may be required to highlight infiltrating tumor cells in cases of severe artifact.

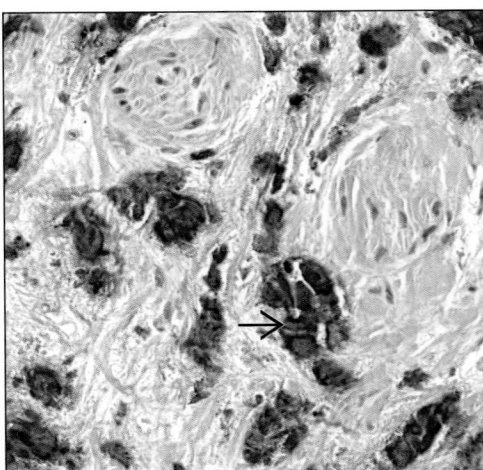

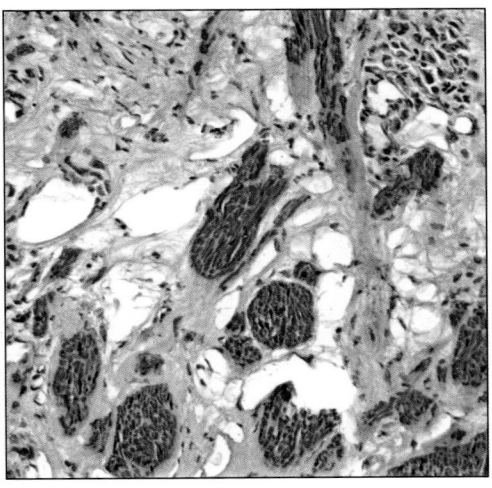

(Left) This PAN-CK(AE1/AE3) immunostain highlights the invasive carcinoma cells ➡ that are masked by crush artifact. Cytokeratin may also stain reactive myofibroblasts; therefore, careful correlation with the morphology is essential. *(Right)* Actin-sm stain in a case with severe artifact highlights individual, round, compact aggregates of smooth muscle. This pattern may be seen rarely in muscularis mucosae. Muscularis propria has more confluent aggregated bundles.

OVERVIEW OF INVASIVE CARCINOMA SUBTYPES

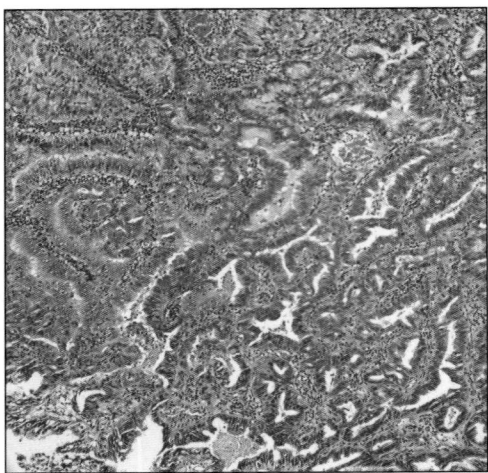

Invasive urothelial carcinoma may show glandular differentiation that is morphologically identical to adenocarcinoma. The presence of a component of conventional urothelial carcinoma is distinctive.

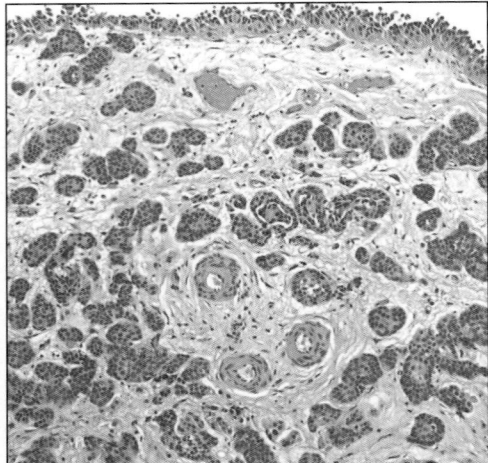

The nested variant of urothelial carcinoma is cytologically bland, but the presence of irregularly distributed nests throughout the lamina propria and the complex epithelial growth is diagnostic.

TERMINOLOGY

Definitions
- Invasive urothelial carcinoma (UC) with morphology distinct from usual or typical pattern

CLINICAL IMPLICATIONS

Gender
- Variants are most common in older men
  - Similar to urothelial carcinoma in general

Clinical Presentation
- Hematuria most common

Treatment
- Urothelial carcinoma variants are treated similarly to conventional urothelial carcinoma with some exceptions
  - Small cell carcinoma treated by separate chemotherapy regimen
  - Pure lymphoepithelioma-like carcinoma may be more responsive to chemotherapy
  - Micropapillary carcinoma may be treated surgically at low stage (pT1) in some centers
  - Urothelial carcinoma with squamous differentiation is less responsive to adjuvant therapy

Prognosis
- Variant invasive urothelial carcinomas have poor prognosis
  - Generally present at high stage
  - Uncertain whether prognosis is worse than urothelial carcinoma of similar stage in some variants

MACROSCOPIC FINDINGS

General Features
- Typically large infiltrative mass lesion

UC WITH ALTERNATIVE/ABERRANT DIFFERENTIATION

Microscopic Features
- By definition, contains component of typical papillary, in situ, or invasive urothelial carcinoma at least focally
  - Squamous differentiation
    - Keratinization and intracellular bridges
    - May be focal or extensive
  - Glandular differentiation
    - Glandular component identical to adenocarcinoma
  - Trophoblastic differentiation
    - Scattered syncytiotrophoblasts within high-grade urothelial carcinoma
    - Rarely choriocarcinomatous differentiation

NESTED CARCINOMA

Microscopic Features
- Nests of infiltrative tumor cells with relatively bland cytologic appearance
  - Irregular infiltrating border with lamina propria is characteristic
  - Muscularis propria is commonly involved
  - Tumor nests often have some degree of complex anastomosis at least focally
  - Invasion with surrounding retraction may be present focally
  - Generally show increasing levels of atypia toward deeper portions of tumor

○ May be admixed with urothelial carcinoma with small tubules

Differential Diagnosis

- von Brunn nests
  ○ More rounded urothelial nests
  ○ Lobular configuration
  ○ Superficial location with sharp border at deep interface with lamina propria
- Cystitis cystica/glandularis
  ○ More superficially located
  ○ Also has sharp border at interface with lamina propria
- Nephrogenic adenoma
  ○ More tubular appearance
  ○ Prominent basement membranes may surround tubules
  ○ Lining epithelium may have "hobnail" appearance
  ○ Other admixed patterns may be present: Papillary, solid/diffuse, cystic

UC WITH SMALL TUBULES

Microscopic Features

- Invasive carcinoma with small gland-like spaces lined by urothelial cells
  ○ No intracellular mucin
  ○ No columnar lining
- May be admixed with nested variant
  ○ Same differential considerations as nested variant

MICROCYSTIC CARCINOMA

Microscopic Features

- Dilated microcysts in invasive component
  ○ Microcysts may reach 1-2 mm in diameter
  ○ Urothelial lining
- May be associated with nested variant

Differential Diagnosis

- Urothelial carcinoma with glandular differentiation
  ○ Glandular component lined by columnar cells or has abundant intracytoplasmic mucin
- Nephrogenic adenoma
  ○ More superficial location
  ○ No destructive invasion
- Cystitis cystica/glandularis
  ○ Sharp linear base at junction with lamina propria
- Müllerianosis
  ○ Endocervical, tubal, or endometrial-type glands
  ○ Bland cytologic features

PLASMACYTOID CARCINOMA

Microscopic Features

- Malignant cells closely resemble plasma cells set in myxoid or loose edematous stroma
  ○ Eccentric nuclei
  ○ Abundant glassy eosinophilic cytoplasm
- Clusters of neoplastic cells may be surrounded by retraction spaces

- Concomitant conventional urothelial carcinoma may be admixed
- Often have more extensive spread in abdominal cavity than other variants of urothelial carcinoma

Differential Diagnosis

- Plasmacytoma and lymphoma
  ○ Plasmacytoid carcinoma may express CD138
  ○ Strong cytokeratin reactivity supports carcinoma
  ○ Evaluation of κ and λ ratio may be helpful

MICROPAPILLARY CARCINOMA

Microscopic Features

- Small nests and papillae with surrounding retraction spaces
  ○ Resembles ovarian serous carcinoma
  ○ Confluent retraction spaces are characteristic
  ○ Multiple nests in same retraction space is common
- Although nuclear grade is typically high, may also have relatively low-grade appearance
- Most are muscle invasive with vascular invasion
  ○ CD31, CD34, and Podoplanin(D2-40) may help to distinguish true lymphatic invasion from retraction artifact
- Immunohistochemically, tumor is reactive for EMA/MUC1, CK7, CK20
  ○ Immunoreactivity for HER2 and CA125 may also be seen

Differential Diagnosis

- Ovarian serous carcinoma
  ○ Clinical/radiographic correlation is needed
  ○ Immunohistochemical expression of ER and WT1 is common in ovarian primary
- Typical invasive urothelial carcinoma with stromal retraction
  ○ Larger nests
  ○ Does not typically show multiple small nests in same retraction space
  ○ Significant immunophenotypic overlap with micropapillary carcinoma: May also express EMA/MUC1, CA125, and HER2
  ○ In some cases, distinction may be very difficult

LYMPHOEPITHELIOMA-LIKE CARCINOMA

Microscopic Features

- Resembles undifferentiated carcinomas of nasopharynx
  ○ Individual neoplastic cells arranged in syncytia with obscuring chronic inflammation
    ■ Cytoplasmic borders are most often indistinct
    ■ Inflammation consists of a mixture of polyclonal B and T lymphocytes, histiocytes, eosinophils, and plasma cells
- Pure forms are reportedly more responsive to chemotherapy
  ○ Percentage of lymphoepithelioma-like areas should be reported

OVERVIEW OF INVASIVE CARCINOMA SUBTYPES

Differential Diagnosis

- Lymphoma or chronic inflammation
  - CD45(LCA) reactivity in neoplastic cells
  - No cytokeratin-positive population
- Small cell carcinoma
  - Neuroendocrine chromatin features
  - Cellular molding
  - High mitotic and apoptotic index
  - Coexpress cytokeratin and synaptophysin
  - May also express TTF-1

SMALL CELL CARCINOMA

Microscopic Features

- Sheets and occasionally nests of cells with scant cytoplasm and high nuclear/cytoplasmic ratio
  - Chromatin is finely stippled, and nucleoli are inconspicuous
  - Geographic areas of necrosis, high mitotic rate, and areas of crush artifact are also frequent
- Other subtypes of primary bladder carcinoma may be admixed
  - Urothelial carcinoma in situ, invasive urothelial carcinoma, squamous cell carcinoma, adenocarcinoma, or sarcomatoid carcinoma
  - Identical pattern of allelic loss in small cell carcinoma and adjacent conventional urothelial carcinoma suggest shared lineage
- Highly aggressive clinical behavior
- Even focal small cell component should be reported

Differential Diagnosis

- Metastatic small cell carcinoma
  - Histologically and immunophenotypically indistinguishable unless conventional urothelial carcinoma is present
  - CK7(+)/CK20(-) phenotype common
  - Both metastases and primary tumors may express TTF-1
- Lymphoma
  - Express hematopoietic markers
  - Cytokeratin negative
- Poorly differentiated urothelial carcinoma
  - Does not express synaptophysin or chromogranin
- Rhabdomyosarcoma
  - May express synaptophysin
  - Nuclear myogenin reactivity diagnostic of skeletal muscle differentiation

SARCOMATOID UC

Microscopic Features

- Neoplasms containing both epithelial and mesenchymal differentiation by morphology or immunohistochemistry
  - Epithelial component may be any subtype of bladder carcinoma
    - Urothelial carcinoma in situ, invasive urothelial carcinoma, squamous cell carcinoma, or adenocarcinoma
  - Mesenchymal component usually has high-grade spindle cell morphology
  - Heterologous elements may be present
    - Osteosarcoma, chondrosarcoma, and rhabdomyosarcoma
- Immunohistochemical expression of HMCK(34βE12) and p63 in both epithelial and spindled component

Differential Diagnosis

- Pseudosarcomatous myofibroblastic proliferation
  - Fine nuclear chromatin
  - Actin expression common
  - In contrast to carcinoma, cytokeratin expression limited to low molecular weight forms
  - Does not express p63
  - Subset expresses ALK1 by immunohistochemistry
- Primary leiomyosarcoma
  - Expresses desmin and actin
  - In contrast to carcinoma, cytokeratin expression limited to low molecular weight forms
  - Up to 23% express p63
- Other primary vesical sarcoma
  - No carcinomatous component or recent history of urothelial carcinoma
  - Nonepithelial immunophenotype

UNDIFFERENTIATED UC WITH OSTEOCLAST-LIKE GIANT CELLS

Microscopic Features

- Prominent osteoclast-type giant cells are seen in rare undifferentiated carcinomas
  - Giant cells are histiocytic in origin
- Background spindled and mononuclear cells are cytokeratin positive

UC WITH RHABDOID FEATURES

Microscopic Features

- Very rare morphologic subtype
- Neoplastic cells with large vesicular nuclei, prominent nucleoli, and eosinophilic cytoplasmic inclusions
  - Resembles malignant extrarenal rhabdoid tumor
  - Does not have deletion of INI1 at 22q11
  - Usually adult tumor, unlike malignant extrarenal rhabdoid tumor
- Very aggressive clinical course

UC WITH MYXOID STROMA

Microscopic Features

- Typical urothelial carcinoma almost always present
- Prominent myxoid stroma
  - Proportion of tumor highly variable
- Neoplastic cells may "float" in myxoid matrix in aggregates or chains
  - Small round cells with eosinophilic cytoplasm are common

Differential Diagnosis

- Myxoid sarcoma

○ Urothelial carcinomas with myxoid stroma maintain epithelial immunophenotype

UC WITH CLEAR CYTOPLASM (GLYCOGEN RICH)

Microscopic Features
- Abundant clear cytoplasm secondary to glycogen accumulation
- Typically focal pattern in otherwise typical urothelial carcinoma

Differential Diagnosis
- Renal cell carcinoma
  ○ Obvious renal mass present
  ○ Expression of pax-2 may be seen
- Clear cell adenocarcinoma, primary or gynecologic
  ○ Distinct mixed tubulocystic and papillary pattern with "hobnail" cells typical

UC WITH LIPOID FEATURES (LIPID-RICH/LIPID CELL)

Microscopic Features
- Rare urothelial carcinomas have foci with intracellular lipid
  ○ Closely resemble lipoblasts
- Most admixed with typical urothelial carcinoma
- Maintain cytokeratin immunoreactivity, even in lipid-rich cells

Differential Diagnosis
- Primary liposarcoma
  ○ Lack component of typical urothelial carcinoma
  ○ Epithelioid variant of pleomorphic liposarcoma is close mimic that may express keratin
- Sarcomatoid urothelial carcinoma with heterologous liposarcoma
  ○ Usually has pleomorphic spindled component
  ○ Lipoblasts do not express cytokeratin
  ○ Other heterologous components may be admixed
- Signet ring cell adenocarcinoma
  ○ Smaller cells with single intracytoplasmic vacuoles
  ○ Often infiltrate as individual cells

LARGE CELL UNDIFFERENTIATED CARCINOMA

Microscopic Features
- Poorly differentiated pleomorphic carcinoma without histologic features typical of urothelial carcinoma

Differential Diagnosis
- Lymphoma
  ○ Expresses hematopoietic markers
- Secondary carcinoma from another anatomic site
  ○ Requires clinical correlation
- Melanoma
  ○ Expresses S100

DIFFERENTIAL DIAGNOSIS

Secondary Carcinomas from Nonbladder Sites
- Variant morphologic patterns of urothelial carcinoma may suggest nonbladder primary
- Most urothelial carcinoma variants maintain urothelial immunophenotype
  ○ CK7 and CK20 coexpression common
  ○ Express HMCK(34βE12)
  ○ Nuclear p63 reactivity

DIAGNOSTIC CHECKLIST

Pathologic Interpretation Pearls
- Variant morphology carcinoma: Primary carcinoma involving bladder and not conforming to morphology of typical urothelial carcinoma
- Variant histology must be documented, including percentage, if not pure in histology
  ○ Variant histology may present at metastatic site; facilitates association with bladder primary
- Variant histology may have diagnostic, prognostic, or therapeutic significance
- Metastatic carcinoma or carcinoma secondarily involving bladder must be ruled out in all cases

SELECTED REFERENCES

1. Amin MB: Histological variants of urothelial carcinoma: diagnostic, therapeutic and prognostic implications. Mod Pathol. 22 Suppl 2:S96-S118, 2009
2. Nigwekar P et al: Plasmacytoid urothelial carcinoma: detailed analysis of morphology with clinicopathologic correlation in 17 cases. Am J Surg Pathol. 33(3):417-24, 2009
3. Drew PA et al: The nested variant of transitional cell carcinoma: an aggressive neoplasm with innocuous histology. Mod Pathol. 9(10):989-94, 1996
4. Amin MB et al: Micropapillary variant of transitional cell carcinoma of the urinary bladder. Histologic pattern resembling ovarian papillary serous carcinoma. Am J Surg Pathol. 18(12):1224-32, 1994
5. Young RH et al: Unusual forms of carcinoma of the urinary bladder. Hum Pathol. 22(10):948-65, 1991

Carcinoma with Squamous and Glandular Differentiation

(Left) Invasive urothelial carcinomas may show squamous differentiation. The cytoplasm is more eosinophilic than typical urothelial carcinoma, and keratin formation ⮕ is seen. These carcinomas are frequently associated with a florid stromal myofibroblastic proliferation ⮕. The presence of typical urothelial carcinoma precludes a diagnosis of primary squamous cell carcinoma. (Right) Squamous differentiation with keratin formation ⮕ may also be seen in the noninvasive component.

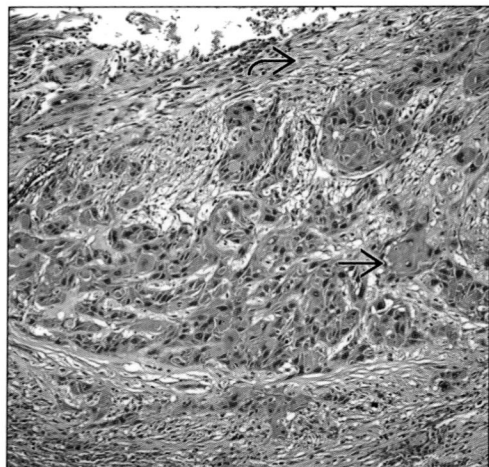
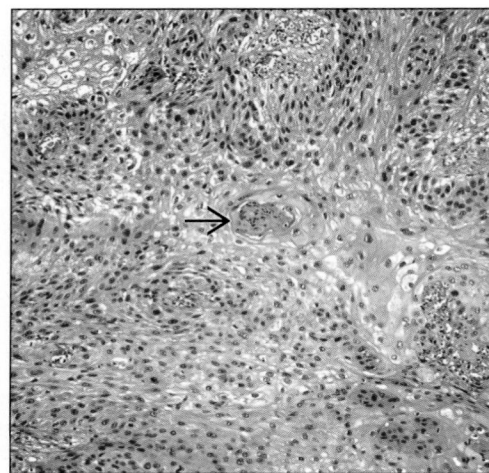

(Left) Focal keratin formation ⮕ is seen in this example of urothelial carcinoma with squamous differentiation. (Right) Keratin pearl formation ⮕ is the prototypical feature of squamous differentiation. In contrast to primary squamous cell carcinoma, urothelial carcinoma with squamous differentiation has areas of conventional papillary, invasive, or in situ urothelial carcinoma. In addition, primary squamous cell carcinoma arises in a background of squamous metaplasia/dysplasia.

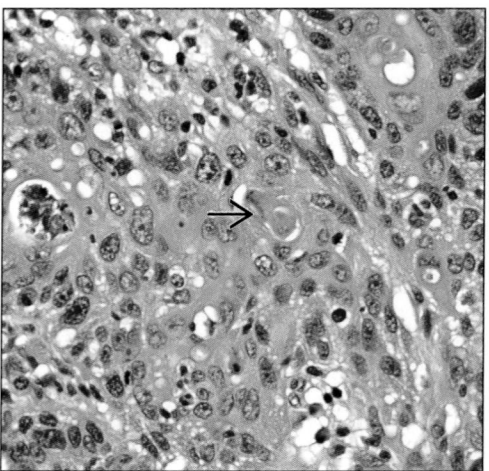
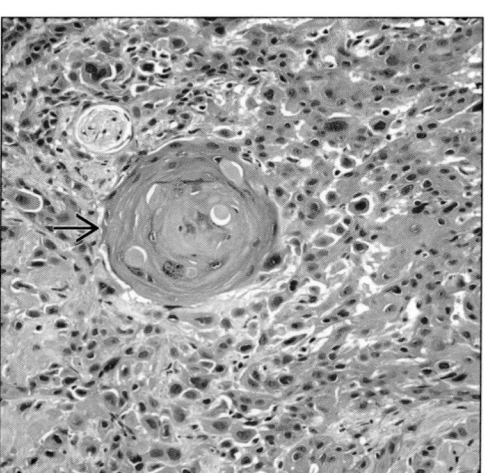

(Left) This invasive urothelial carcinoma with glandular differentiation is indistinguishable from primary bladder adenocarcinoma in this field. By definition, conventional papillary, invasive, or in situ urothelial carcinoma is also present. (Right) The presence of associated urothelial carcinoma in situ, as seen here, is diagnostic of urothelial carcinoma when alternative differentiation is present. Typical noninvasive papillary or invasive urothelial carcinoma is also sufficient.

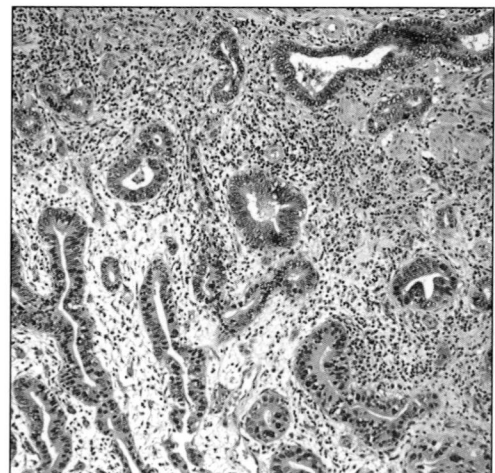
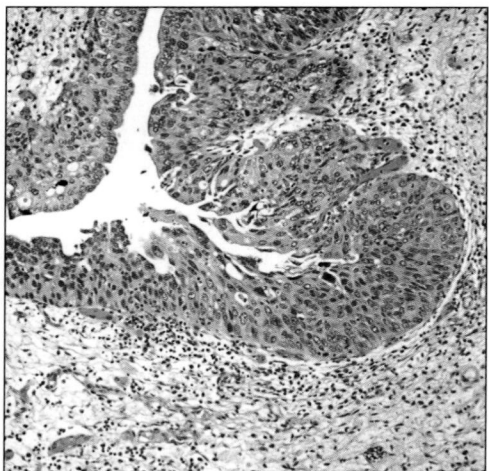

Carcinoma with Trophoblastic Differentiation

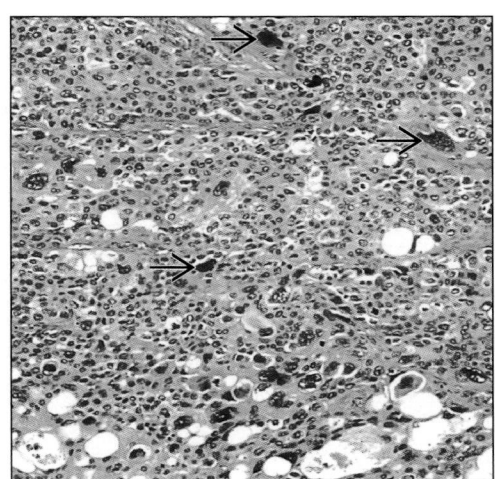

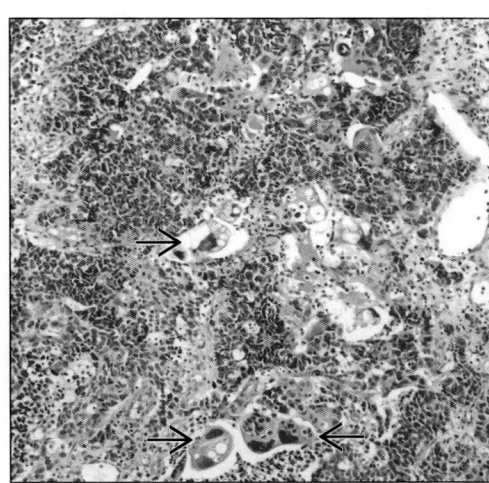

(Left) Multinucleated cells with dense nuclear chromatin ⇨, characteristic of syncytiotrophoblasts, are present amidst this high-grade invasive urothelial carcinoma. This is distinct from choriocarcinoma, which would also contain central nests of cytotrophoblasts. (Right) This example of poorly differentiated urothelial carcinoma of the urinary bladder had both small cell differentiation and numerous scattered syncytiotrophoblasts ⇨.

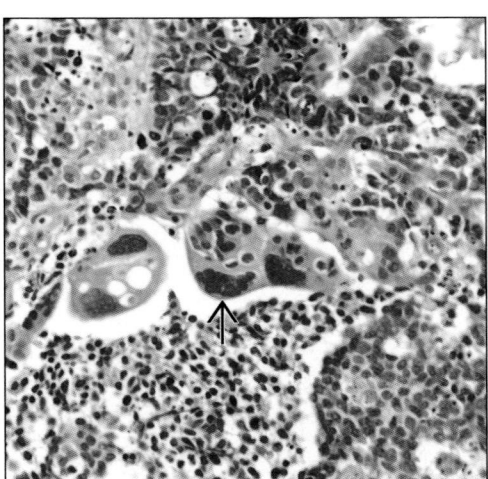

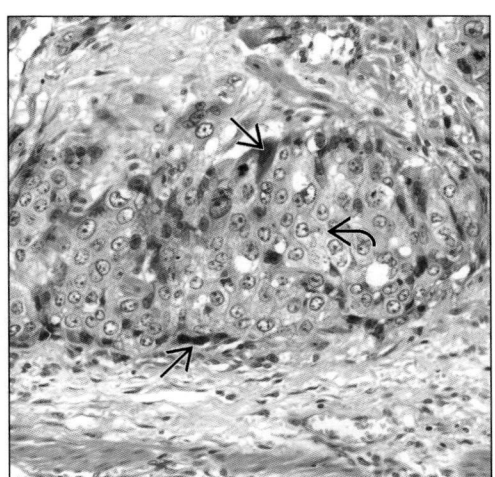

(Left) This photomicrograph shows the characteristic multinucleation of syncytiotrophoblasts ⇨. (Right) To diagnose urothelial carcinoma with choriocarcinomatous differentiation, the classic architecture of choriocarcinoma must be seen: Nests of mononuclear cytotrophoblasts ⇨ enveloped by syncytiotrophoblasts ⇨. Scattered syncytiotrophoblasts are not sufficient for a diagnosis of choriocarcinoma.

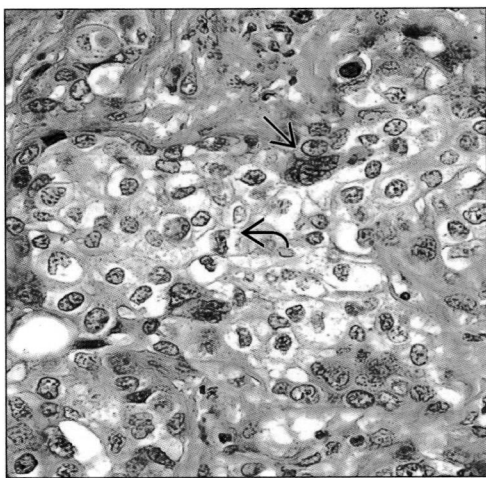

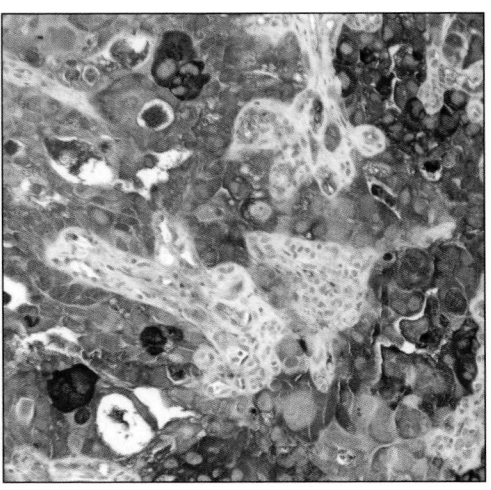

(Left) In this case of urothelial carcinoma with choriocarcinomatous differentiation, multinucleated syncytiotrophoblasts ⇨ are seen wrapping around mononuclear cytotrophoblasts ⇨. (Right) As in this example with choriocarcinomatous differentiation, β-HCG reactivity is typically strong; however, β-HCG reactivity may also be seen in poorly differentiated urothelial carcinoma without trophoblasts. Morphologic context is critical.

Nested Urothelial Carcinoma

(Left) On low-power examination, nested urothelial carcinoma has more epithelial nests present deeper in the lamina propria and areas with more complex architecture than seen in benign mimics, such as florid von Brunn nests and cystitis cystica. (Right) Nested variant is a histologically subtle form of malignancy that has relatively bland cytologic features. The haphazard distribution of the nests, seen here at low power, is helpful in recognizing this variant of bladder cancer.

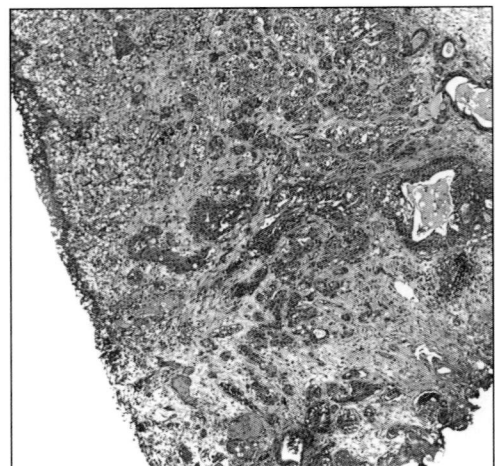
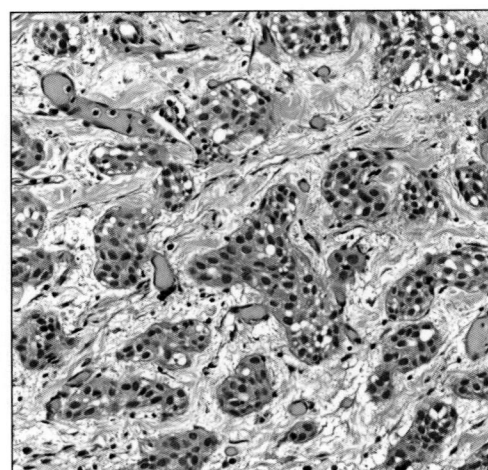

(Left) This nested urothelial carcinoma highlights the bland cytologic features of the neoplastic cells ➔ compared to the normal overlying urothelium ➔. (Right) The neoplastic cells of nested urothelial carcinoma have a subtle increase in the nuclear/cytoplasmic ratio. A mitotic figure ➔ is also seen in this nest. It is difficult to recognize this form of carcinoma only by cytology. In small superficial bladder biopsy specimens, a definitive diagnosis may sometimes be impossible.

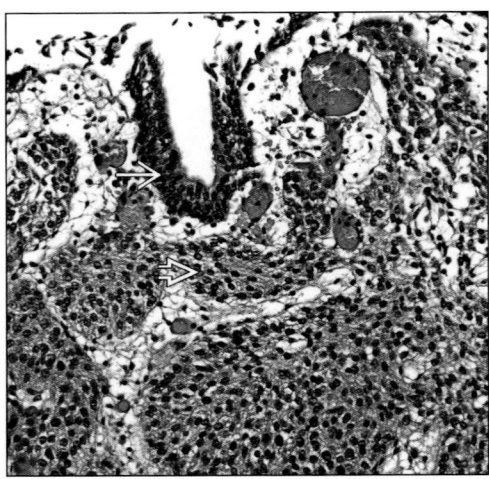
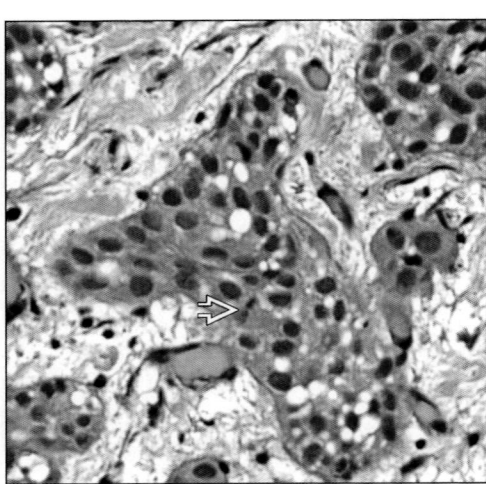

(Left) Invasion of the muscularis propria is diagnostic of carcinoma. In some cases, re-biopsy may be necessary to document invasion. Even in the deeply invasive areas, the bland cytology may be retained, as in this example. (Right) Lymph node metastases ➔ are not uncommon in nested carcinoma, as seen in this photomicrograph. The nested architecture and bland cytology are retained. These tumors should be treated similar to conventional high-grade invasive urothelial carcinoma.

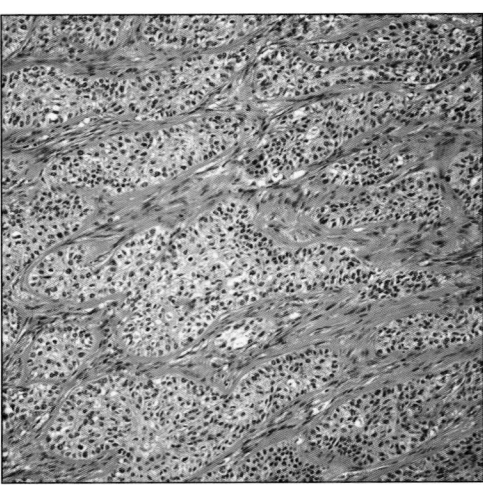
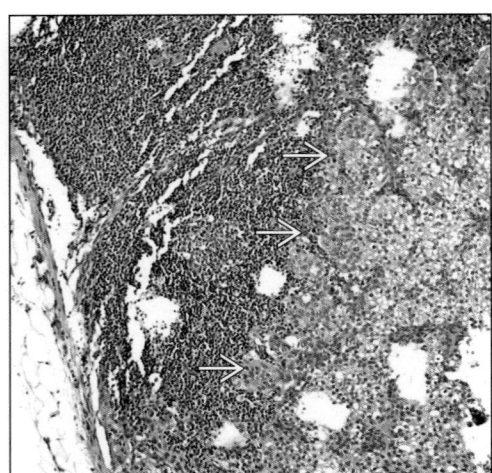

OVERVIEW OF INVASIVE CARCINOMA SUBTYPES

Tubular and Microcystic Carcinoma

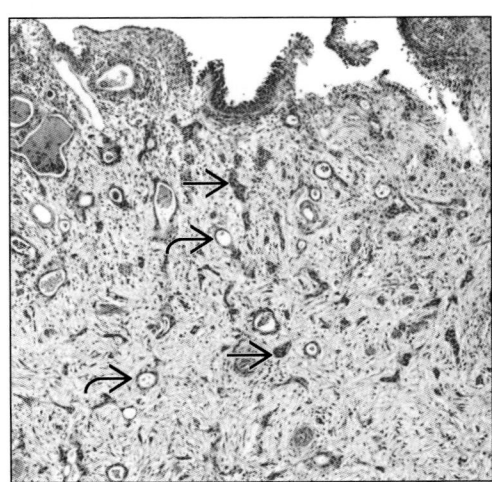

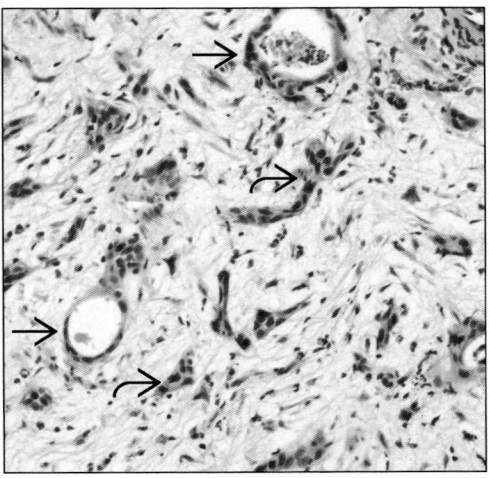

(Left) This invasive urothelial carcinoma has an admixture of nests ⊡ and tubules ⊡. The distribution in the lamina propria is more irregularly dispersed than in benign mimics. *(Right)* On high-power examination, this invasive urothelial carcinoma is comprised of elongated nests ⊡ with occasional tubule formation ⊡. The reactive stromal changes and the irregular, randomly distributed nests are features that should suggest a diagnosis of carcinoma.

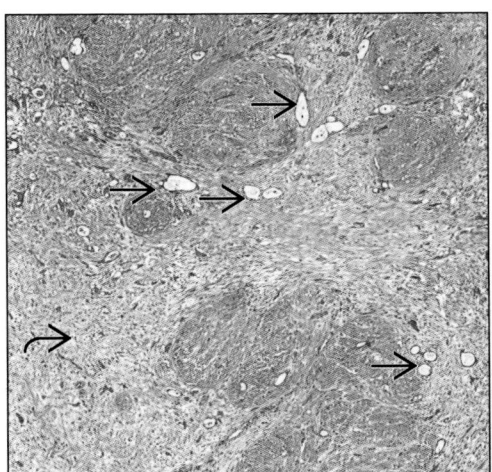

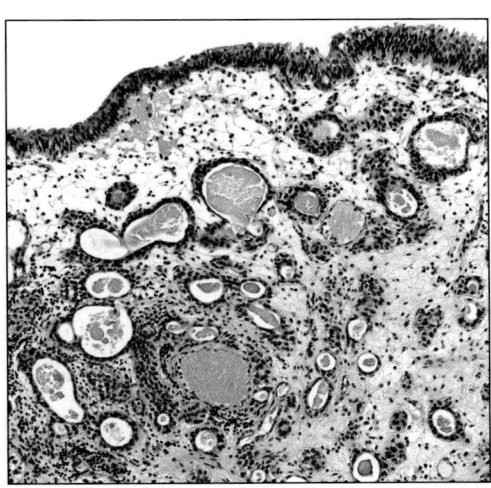

(Left) This deeply invasive carcinoma has a deceptively bland appearance with small luminal structures that mimic blood vessels on low-power evaluation ⊡. The associated stromal reaction ⊡ should suggest a neoplastic process. *(Right)* Microcystic urothelial carcinoma shows deceptively bland features mimicking cystitis glandularis. The irregular and haphazard nature of the proliferation, as well as widespread involvement of lamina propria, aid in recognition as carcinoma.

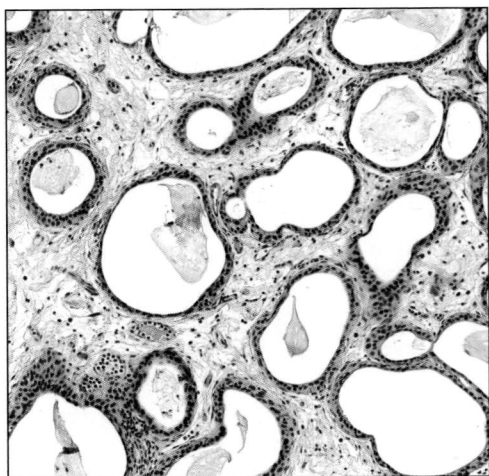

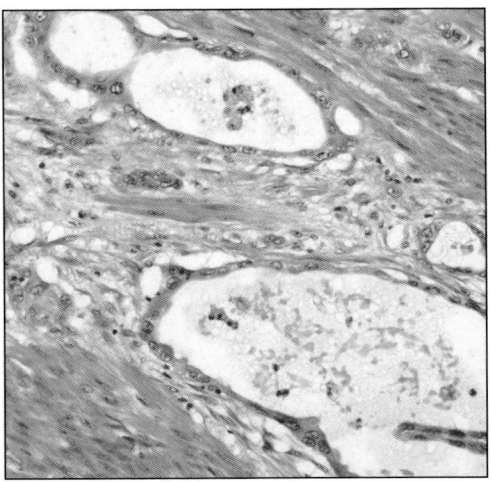

(Left) Microcystic urothelial carcinoma is shown with innocuous nuclear features. The variably sized and shaped cysts are lined by flattened to columnar epithelium or multilayered urothelium. *(Right)* On high-power examination, the extremely bland cytology of the neoplastic cells in this microcystic carcinoma may be appreciated. In contrast to the typical pseudostratified columnar lining cells of adenocarcinoma, these neoplastic cells are flattened.

OVERVIEW OF INVASIVE CARCINOMA SUBTYPES

Plasmacytoid Urothelial Carcinoma

*(Left) Plasmacytoid urothelial carcinoma is characterized by individual round neoplastic cells with eccentric nuclei and deep eosinophilic cytoplasm. They often infiltrate in a pattern similar to signet ring adenocarcinoma. **(Right)** This low-power image shows the subtle morphology of plasmacytoid urothelial carcinoma ➡ adjacent to an inflammatory infiltrate ➡. The neoplastic cells are easily confused with plasma cells or histiocytes at this magnification.*

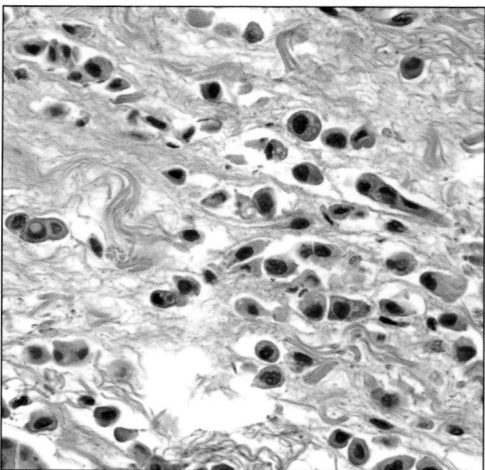
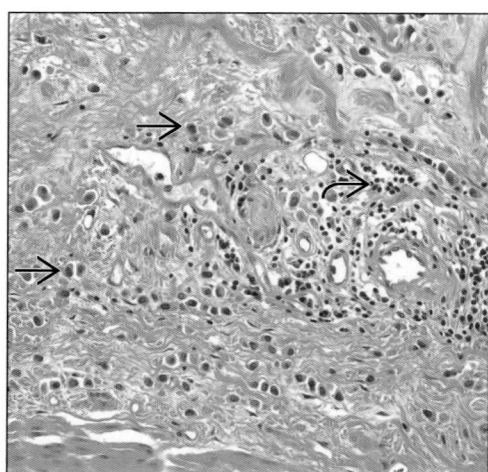

*(Left) The large size of the neoplastic plasmacytoid urothelial carcinoma cells ➡ can be compared to the smaller adjacent normal plasma cells ➡. This pattern may be very difficult to recognize on intraoperative frozen section evaluation of margins. A typical urothelial carcinoma component may be present in some cases. **(Right)** The presence of multiple discohesive neoplastic cells within retraction spaces is typical of the plasmacytoid variant of urothelial carcinoma.*

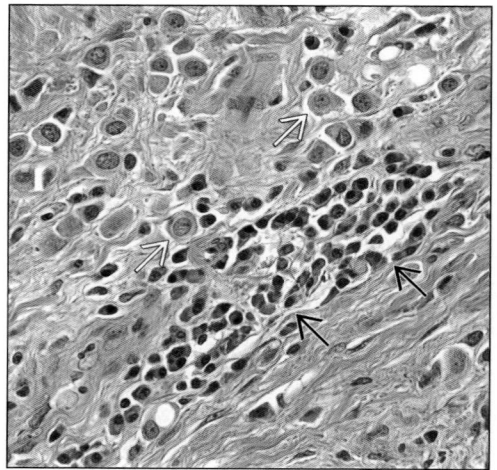
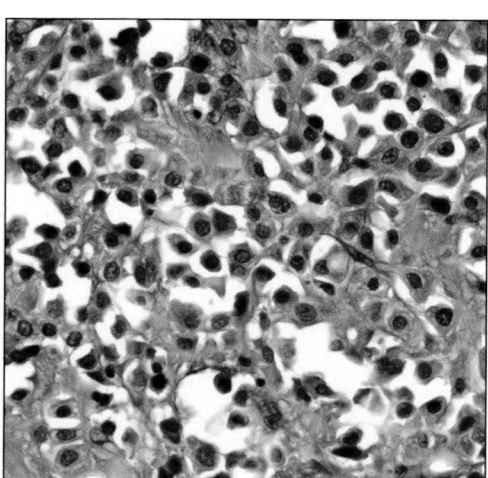

*(Left) The round eccentric nuclei and the eosinophilic cytoplasm are characteristic of plasmacytoid urothelial carcinoma. In difficult cases, immunohistochemistry may aid in the distinction from inflammatory cells. **(Right)** Diffuse cytoplasmic immunoreactivity for broad spectrum cytokeratin is very helpful in establishing the diagnosis of carcinoma in difficult cases. It is important to realize that these carcinomas may also express CD138, further mimicking a plasma cell infiltrate.*

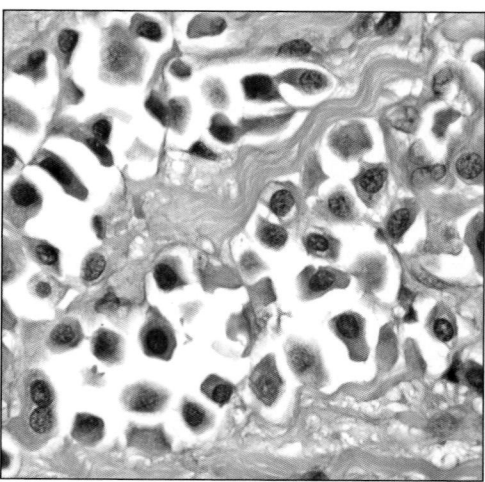
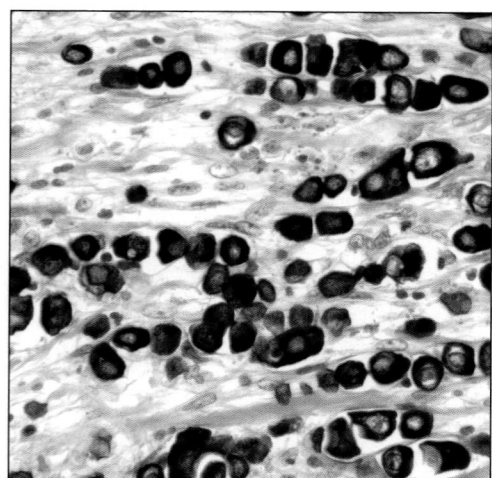

Micropapillary Carcinoma

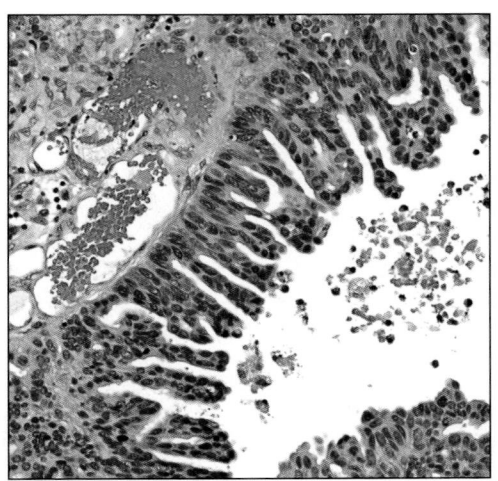

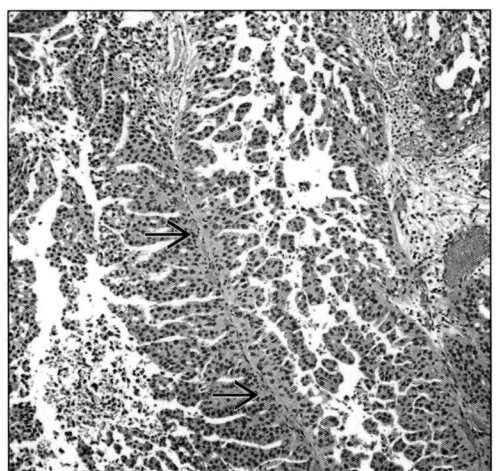

(Left) Noninvasive papillary urothelial carcinomas may also have a micropapillary architecture characterized by thin elongated micropapillae that have a greater length than width. *(Right)* This example of noninvasive urothelial carcinoma also has extensive micropapillary architecture characterized by elongated filiform papillae arising from the main papillary core ➡. The significance of this morphologic pattern in the absence of invasion is not fully known.

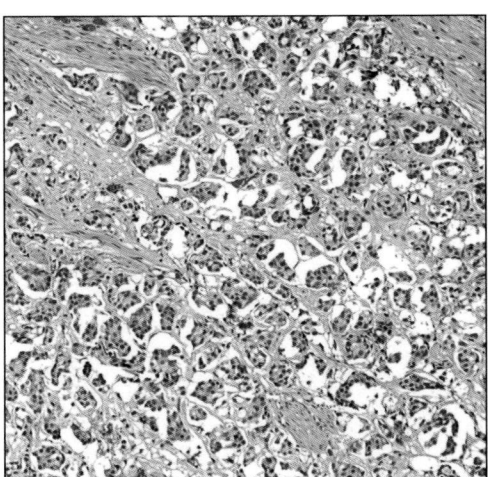

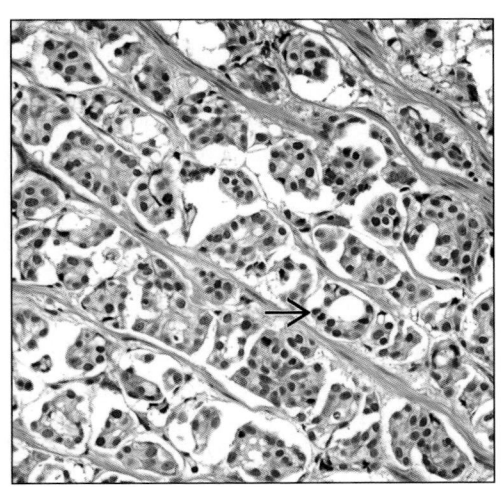

(Left) Invasive micropapillary carcinoma is characterized by back-to-back lacunar spaces containing small nests of carcinoma, as seen in this example. *(Right)* Nests and ring forms ➡ within back-to-back lacunar spaces are characteristic of invasive micropapillary carcinoma. The cytology of the neoplastic cells may be rather bland, despite the deeply invasive growth and the common presentation with metastases. Vascular invasion is typically present in this variant.

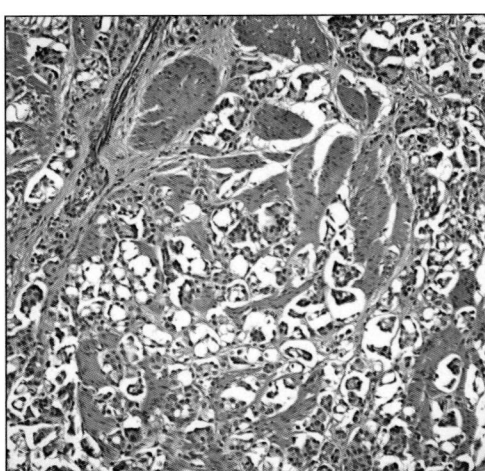

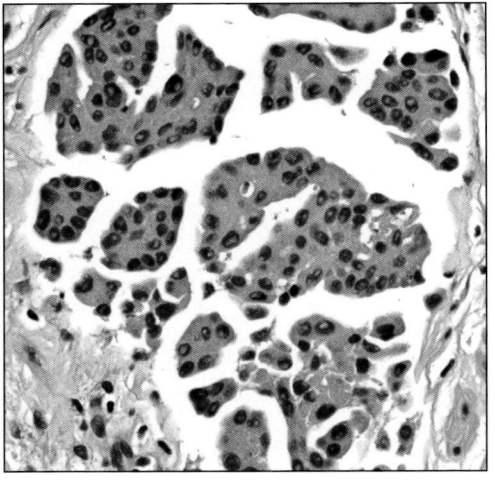

(Left) This invasive micropapillary carcinoma shows permeation of the muscularis propria. Given the frequency of high-stage disease, re-staging biopsies should be performed for apparent pT1 micropapillary carcinomas. *(Right)* Micropapillary carcinoma may have a striking resemblance to ovarian serous carcinoma. Micropapillary carcinoma of the urinary bladder maintains a urothelial phenotype and typically lacks a true fibrovascular core.

OVERVIEW OF INVASIVE CARCINOMA SUBTYPES

Micropapillary Carcinoma

(Left) Although not present in all cases, the peripheral orientation of the nuclei in these nests ⇨ is another feature that may be seen in micropapillary carcinoma. The back-to-back lacunar spaces and the presence of multiple nests in a single lacunar space are other characteristic features. *(Right)* There is a broad spectrum of cytologic atypia in micropapillary carcinoma. This example shows more nuclear pleomorphism ⇨ than typically seen in micropapillary carcinoma.

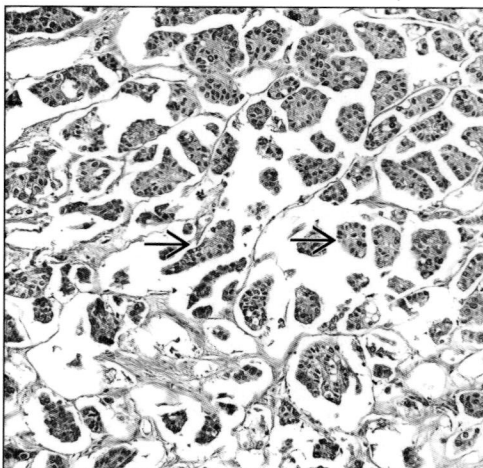 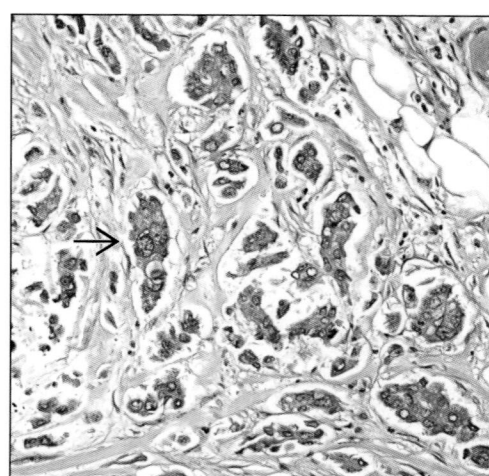

(Left) In this example of urothelial carcinoma with admixed components, sheets of conventional urothelial carcinoma ⇨ are adjacent to the small epithelial nests in lacunar spaces ⇨, characteristic of micropapillary carcinoma. *(Right)* Lymph node metastases maintain the micropapillary architecture, which may cause diagnostic confusion with metastasis from an ovarian or breast primary. Immunohistochemistry may be useful if a primary site is not clinically apparent.

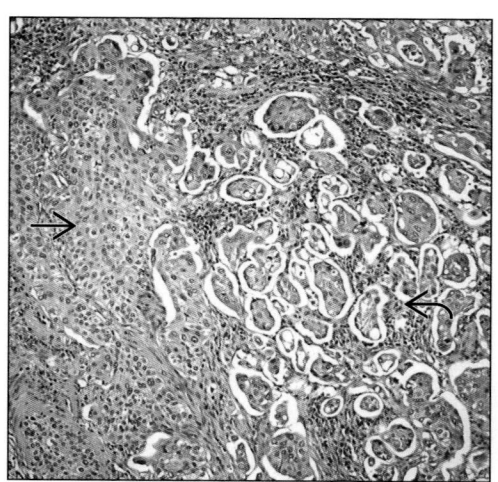 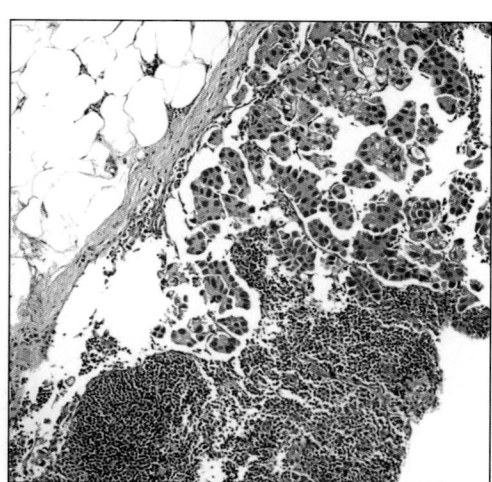

(Left) Despite the prominent retraction spaces, this should be regarded as typical invasive urothelial carcinoma. The epithelial nests are much larger than those seen in micropapillary carcinoma. *(Right)* On higher power evaluation, this typical invasive urothelial carcinoma has larger nests and more confluent, branching epithelium than micropapillary carcinoma. These urothelial carcinomas with extensive retraction may have an identical immunophenotype to micropapillary carcinoma.

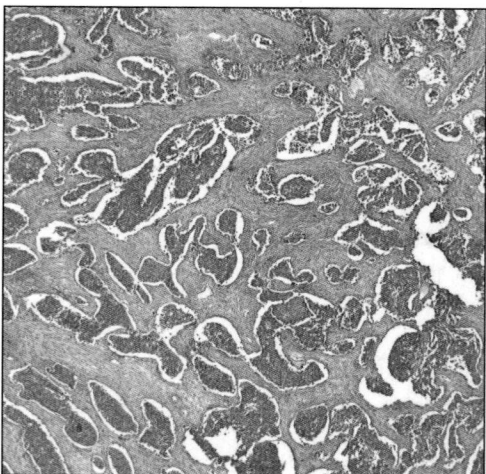 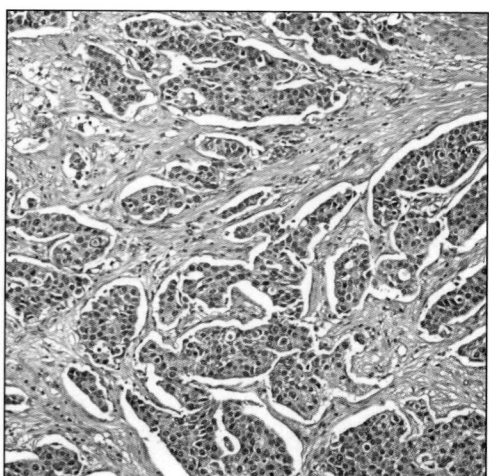

Lymphoepithelioma-like Carcinoma

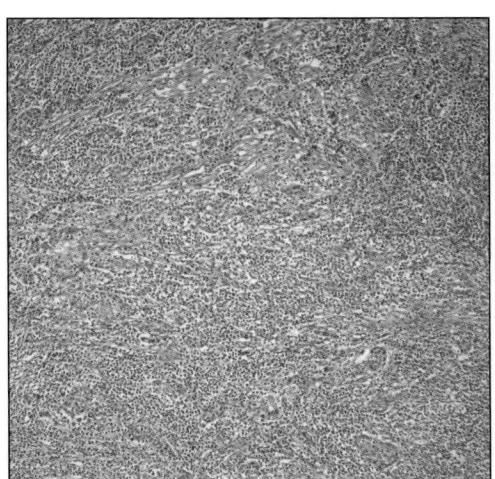

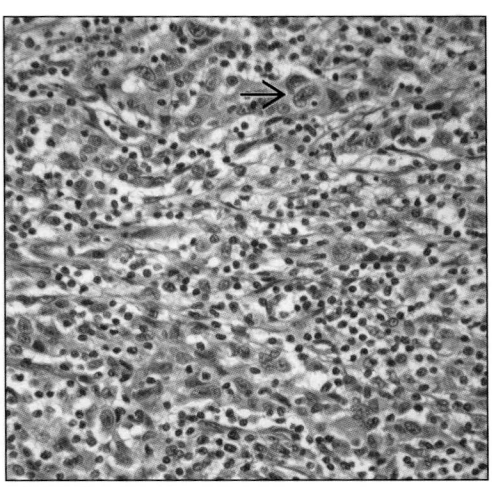

(Left) At low-power evaluation, lymphoepithelioma-like carcinoma closely mimics an inflammatory infiltrate or lymphoma. Recognition as carcinoma depends on identification of the carcinomatous component at high magnification. *(Right)* At high-power evaluation, there is a dense inflammatory infiltrate, but a 2nd subtle population of cells is also seen ➡. This 2nd population is the carcinomatous component and may be highlighted by cytokeratin immunostains.

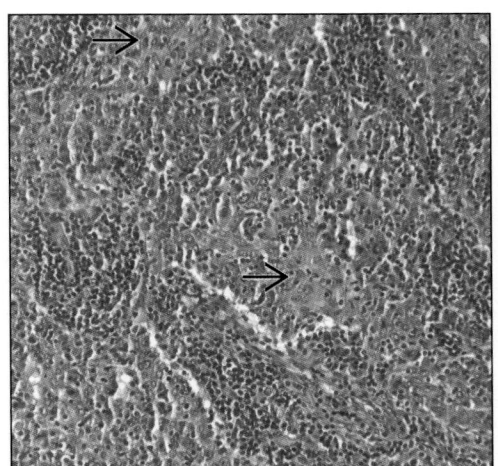

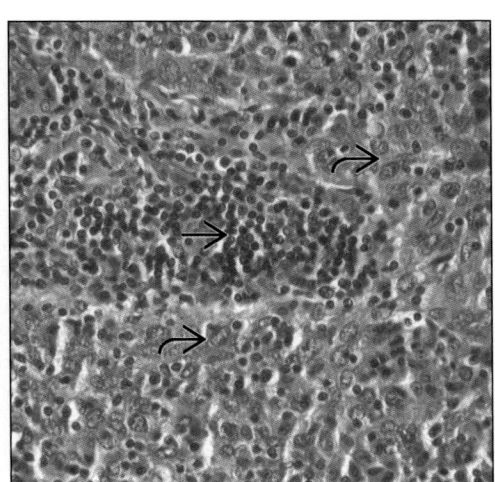

(Left) This example of lymphoepithelioma-like carcinoma in the urinary bladder has a more pronounced epithelial component ➡, even at low-power magnification. *(Right)* On high power, the larger size of the cells in the carcinomatous component ➡ are contrasted with the lymphocytes ➡. Bladder lymphoepithelioma-like carcinoma is not associated with EBV infection. Lymphoepithelioma-like carcinomas may be pure, predominant, or a focal finding.

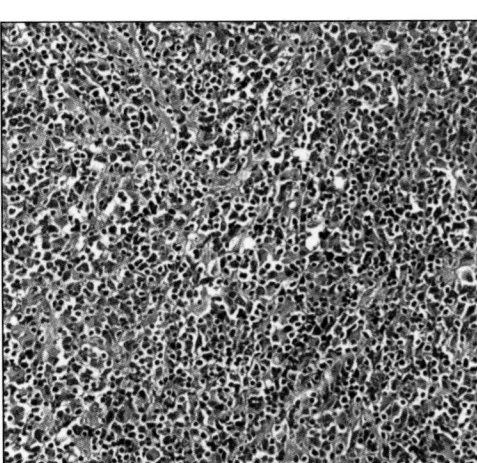

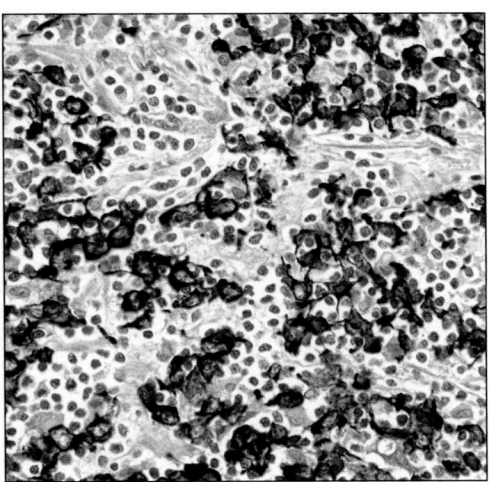

(Left) This lymphoepithelioma-like carcinoma has an absence of epithelial aggregates and closely mimics a lymphomatous process. Immunohistochemical evaluation is important is such cases. *(Right)* This lymphoepithelioma-like carcinoma is highlighted by PAN-CK(AE1/AE3) immunostains. A broad spectrum cytokeratin stain is helpful in excluding other diagnoses, such as lymphoma, that would not show an admixed population of epithelial cells.

Small Cell and Glycogen-Rich Carcinoma

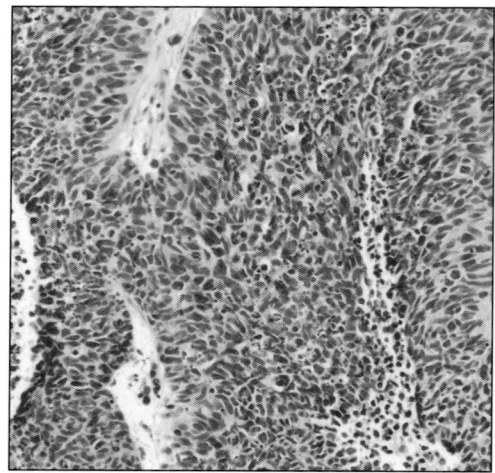 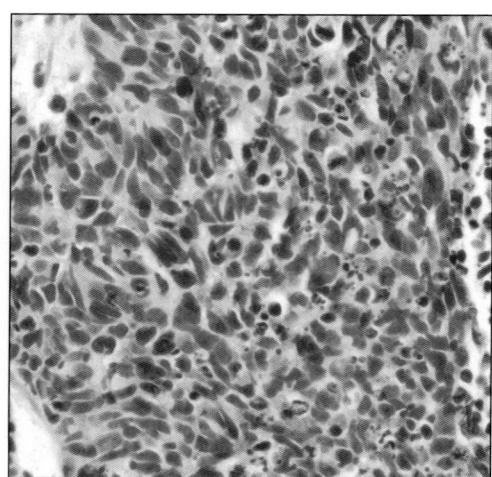

(Left) Small cell carcinoma of the urinary bladder is morphologically similar to pulmonary primaries with high nuclear/cytoplasmic ratio, nuclear molding, and high mitotic rate. In the urinary bladder, this pattern is often interpreted as undifferentiated urothelial carcinoma, but recognition as small cell carcinoma is important because it requires a different chemotherapeutic regimen. *(Right)* At high power, the abundant apoptotic bodies typical of small cell carcinoma are seen.

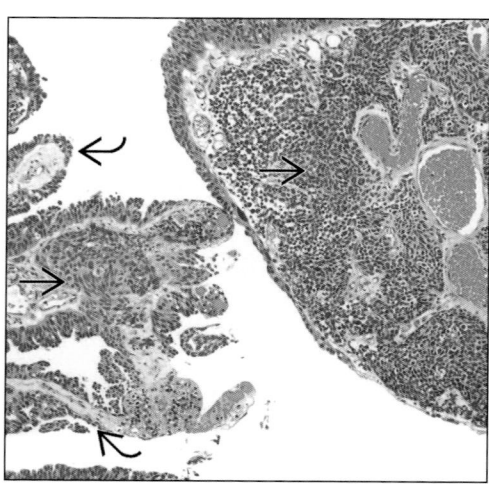 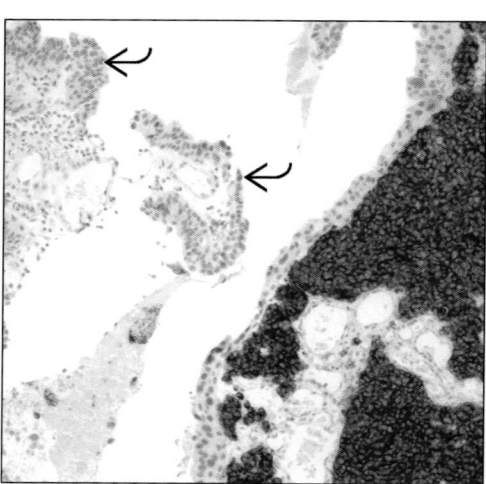

(Left) The small cell carcinoma component ➡ is adjacent to a conventional papillary urothelial carcinoma ➡. *(Right)* Strong diffuse synaptophysin immunoreactivity is seen in this small cell carcinoma component, but not in the adjacent conventional papillary urothelial carcinoma ➡. Synaptophysin stains must be carefully interpreted in the context of the morphology, as prostatic adenocarcinomas secondarily involving the bladder often express synaptophysin.

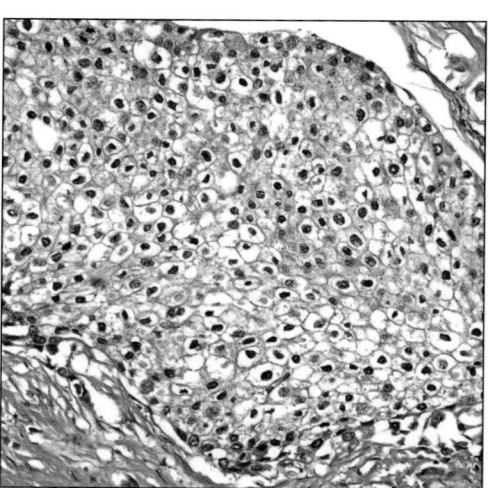 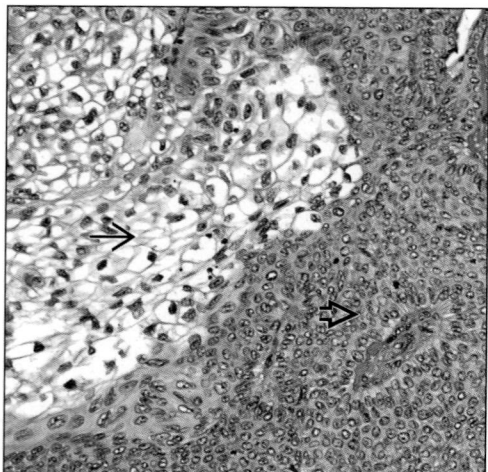

(Left) Rare urothelial carcinomas have abundant clear cytoplasm secondary to intracytoplasmic glycogen accumulation. This feature is typically present only focally in an otherwise typical urothelial carcinoma, which allows distinction from other clear tumors, such as renal cell carcinoma. *(Right)* This urothelial carcinoma of the urinary bladder has a component with intracytoplasmic glycogen ➡ adjacent to a more typical urothelial carcinoma ➡.

Undifferentiated Carcinoma, Including Osteoclast Rich

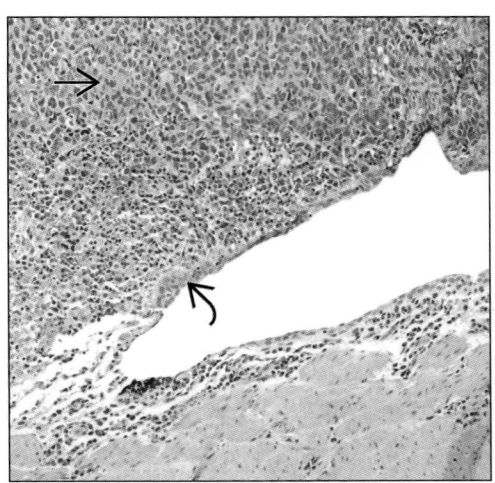 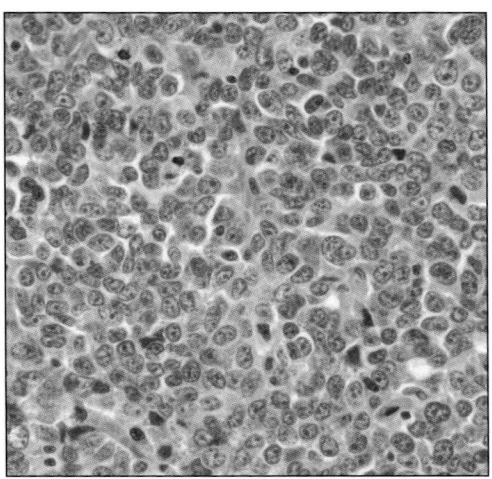

(Left) In this section of the urinary bladder, an undifferentiated round cell malignancy ⮕ is identified underlying the urothelium ⮕. (Right) On high-power examination of a bladder resection specimen, this undifferentiated urothelial carcinoma has a morphology that overlaps with lymphoma, rhabdomyosarcoma, small cell carcinoma, and other round cell malignancies. A broad panel of immunohistochemical stains is critical in evaluating such cases.

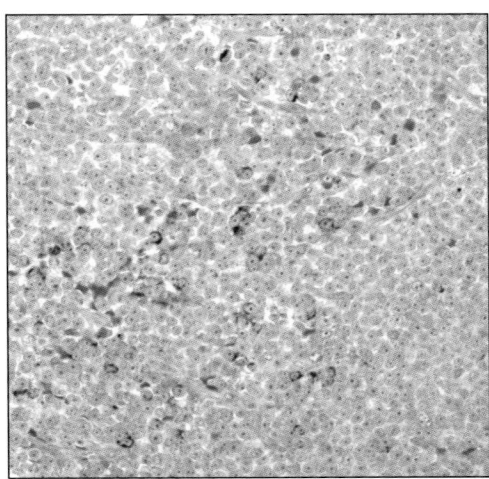 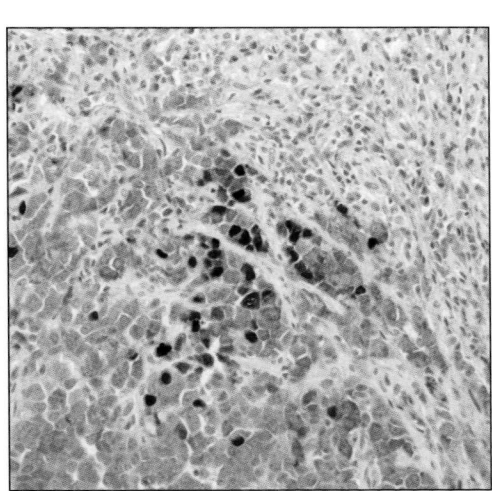

(Left) Patchy cytoplasmic immunoreactivity for HMCK(34βE12) is seen in this undifferentiated urothelial carcinoma. Hematopoietic (CD45[LCA] and CD43), skeletal muscle (desmin and myogenin), and neuroendocrine markers (synaptophysin) were all negative. (Right) Patchy nuclear p63 immunoreactivity is also seen in this undifferentiated neoplasm, supporting classification as undifferentiated urothelial carcinoma.

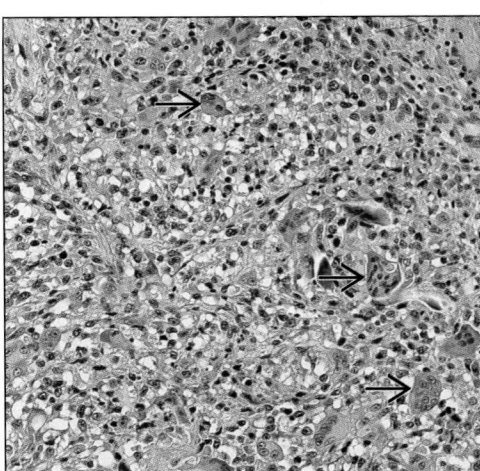 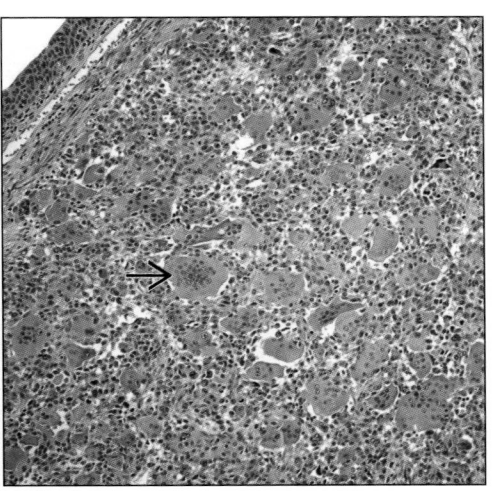

(Left) Undifferentiated urothelial carcinomas may have admixed osteoclast-like giant cells ⮕. This population of multinucleated giant cells stains with histiocytic markers but not cytokeratin. (Right) Rare undifferentiated carcinomas have abundant osteoclast-like giant cells ⮕ that create a morphologic appearance similar to giant cell tumor of bone or soft tissue. The background mononuclear cells express cytokeratin, confirming an epithelial lineage.

Sarcomatoid Urothelial Carcinoma

(Left) The presence of infiltrating urothelial carcinoma ➡ adjacent to a malignant spindle cell neoplasm ➡ is diagnostic of sarcomatoid urothelial carcinoma. When a carcinomatous component is not present, immunohistochemistry may be essential in arriving at the appropriate diagnosis. **(Right)** This sarcomatoid carcinoma has a degree of nuclear chromatin irregularity diagnostic of malignancy. Cytology is the most useful feature in the distinction from a myofibroblastic proliferation.

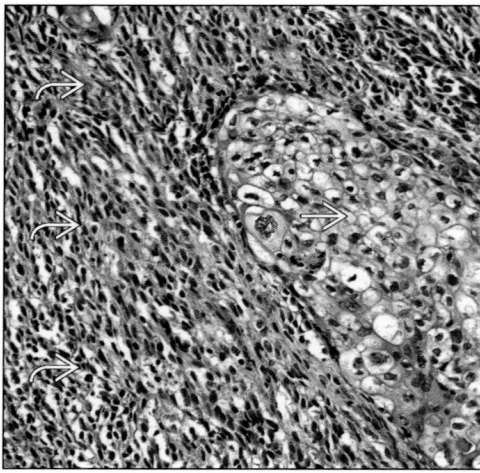
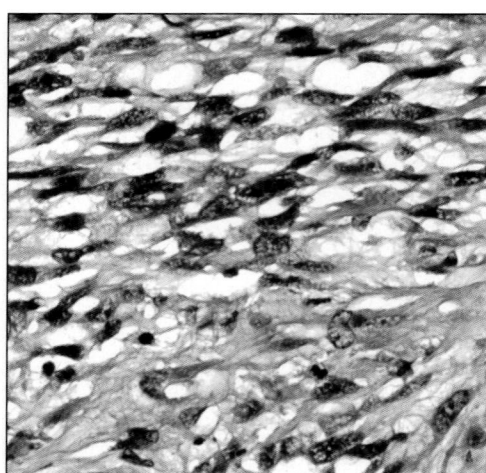

(Left) Spindled sarcomatoid carcinoma may be indistinguishable from a variety of soft tissue sarcomas. Expression of epithelial markers, such as HMCK(34βE12) and p63, are helpful; myofibroblastic and smooth muscle tumors only express low molecular weight keratin. **(Right)** Pure spindled sarcomatoid carcinomas may be deceptively bland with only subtle nuclear chromatin changes. Evaluation of the entire tumor usually reveals areas with more pronounced atypia.

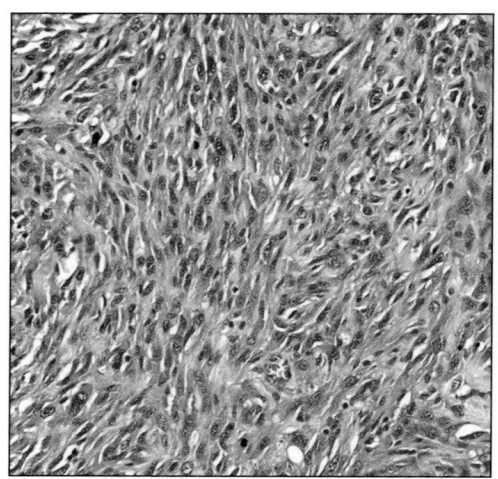
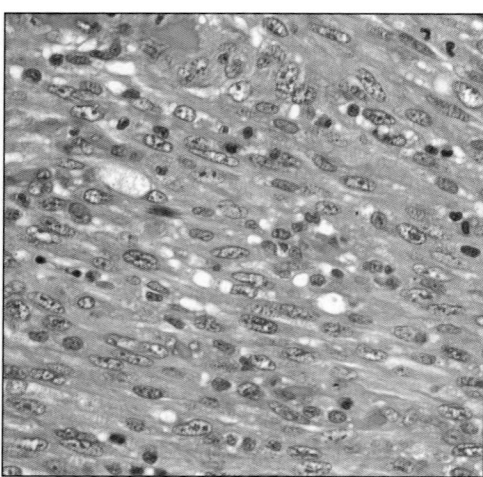

(Left) This example of sarcomatoid urothelial carcinoma shows areas with obvious nuclear pleomorphism and nuclear chromatin abnormalities that are beyond that seen in myofibroblastic lesions. If a carcinomatous component is not seen, leiomyosarcoma should still be excluded immunohistochemically. **(Right)** The presence of foci with a more epithelioid morphology should prompt careful consideration of a carcinoma and appropriate immunohistochemical evaluation.

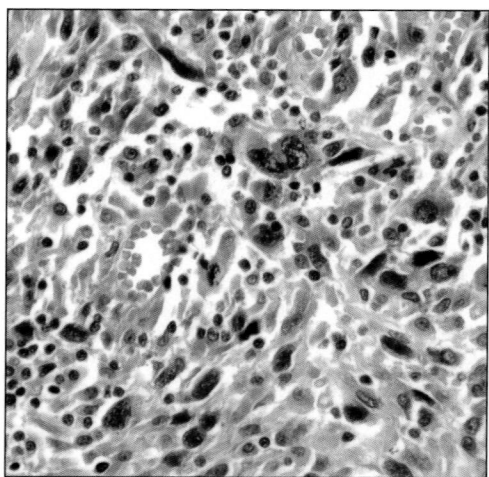
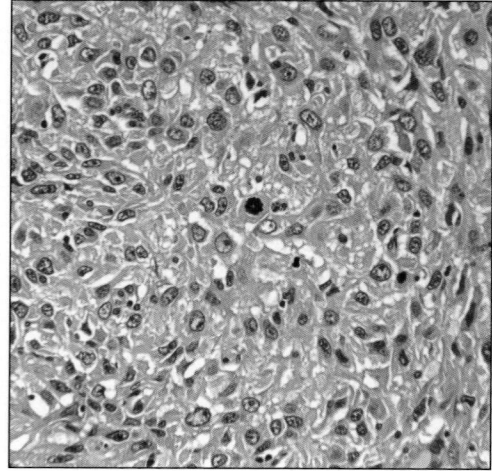

Sarcomatoid Urothelial Carcinoma

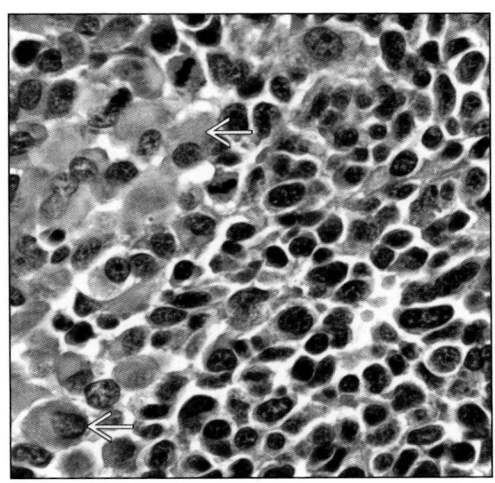
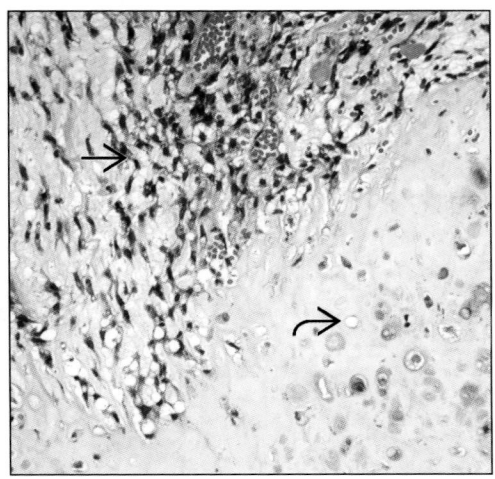

(Left) This sarcomatoid urothelial carcinoma shows a focus of heterologous rhabdomyosarcoma. Numerous rhabdomyoblasts are seen ➡, which showed nuclear immunoreactivity of myogenin, confirming skeletal muscle differentiation. *(Right)* The malignant spindle cell component ➡ merges with a focus of heterologous chondrosarcoma ➡. Osteosarcoma and chondrosarcoma are rare and, when present, should prompt search for a carcinomatous component.

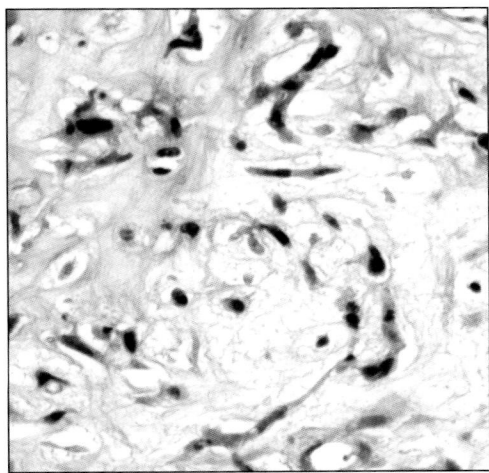
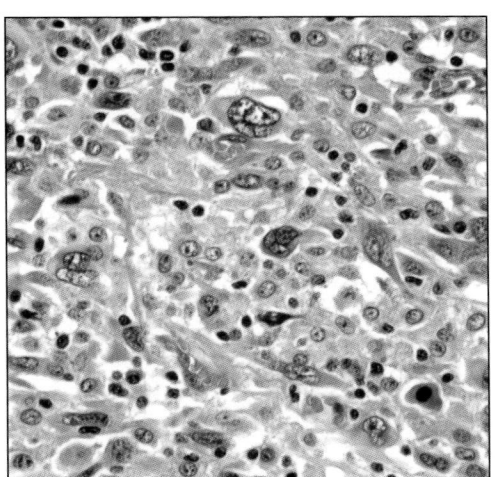

(Left) A subset of sarcomatoid carcinomas have prominent myxoid stroma. Although this may cause confusion with myofibroblastic lesions, the degree of nuclear chromatin changes is more than that seen in myofibroblastic lesions. In this case, conventional urothelial carcinoma was present elsewhere. *(Right)* Some sarcomatoid carcinomas have pleomorphic undifferentiated foci. This neoplasm also had both typical urothelial carcinoma and spindled areas.

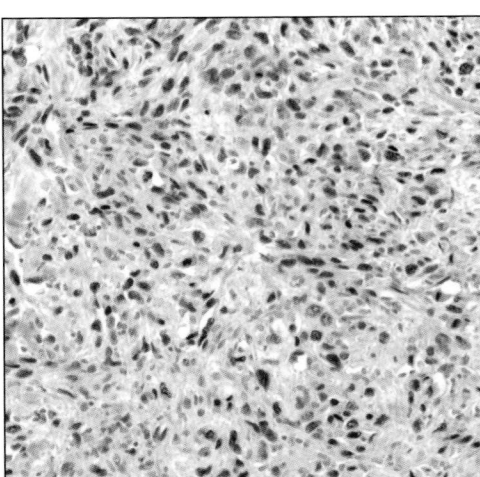
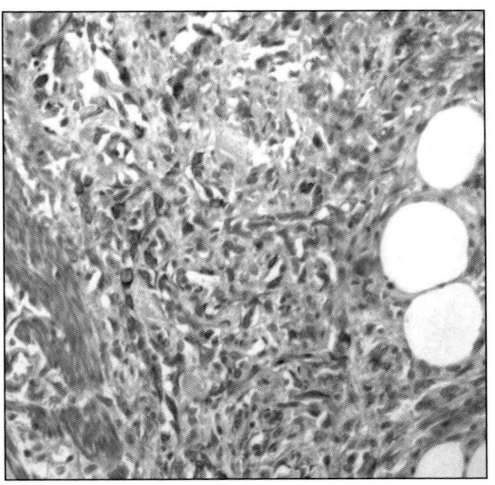

(Left) Nuclear p63 immunoreactivity is characteristic of sarcomatoid urothelial carcinoma. Other spindle cell mimics, such as florid myofibroblastic proliferations, do not show p63 expression. *(Right)* Sarcomatoid urothelial carcinoma typically expresses HMCK(34βE12). In contrast, when keratin expression is present, myofibroblastic proliferations and leiomyosarcomas only show immunoreactivity with low molecular weight cytokeratin.

Urothelial Carcinoma with Myxoid Stroma

(Left) Rare examples of invasive urothelial carcinoma are associated with abundant myxoid stroma that may mimic an adenocarcinoma or a spectrum of mesenchymal neoplasms, raising the possibility of sarcomatoid urothelial carcinoma. *(Right)* In the early phases, the neoplastic cells within the epithelial aggregates of these urothelial carcinomas become separated by gradual accumulation of myxoid matrix. More developed neoplasms are hypocellular with a predominance of myxoid stroma.

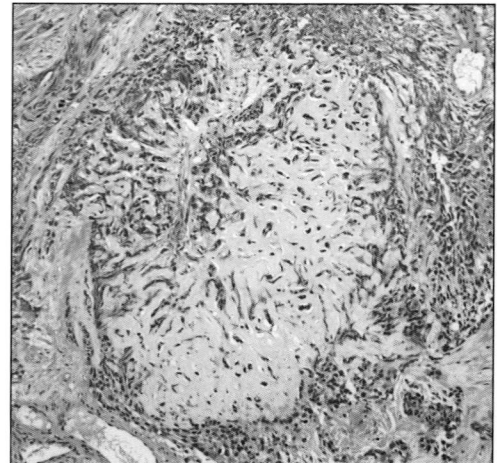
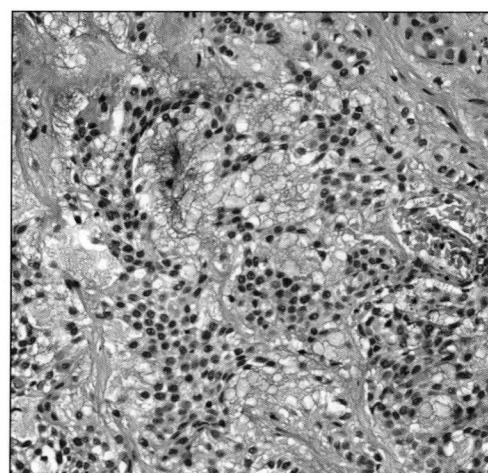

(Left) In urothelial carcinomas with myxoid stroma, the cord-like growth, absence of columnar epithelium or intracytoplasmic mucin, and the histochemical characterization as stromal mucin all help exclude a mucinous adenocarcinoma. *(Right)* Invasive urothelial carcinomas with myxoid stroma may have a complex cord-like epithelial architecture. This pattern of carcinoma may mimic a variety of myxoid mesenchymal neoplasms, especially if seen in metastatic lesions.

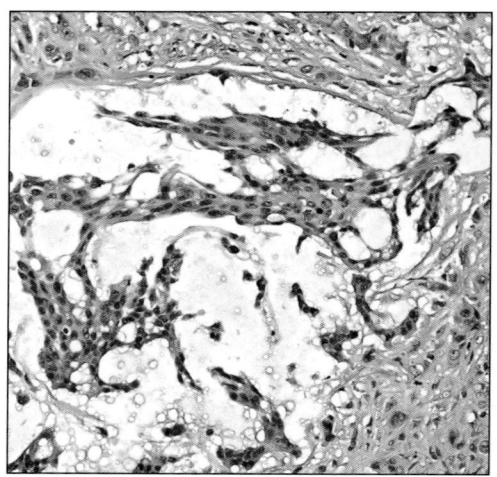
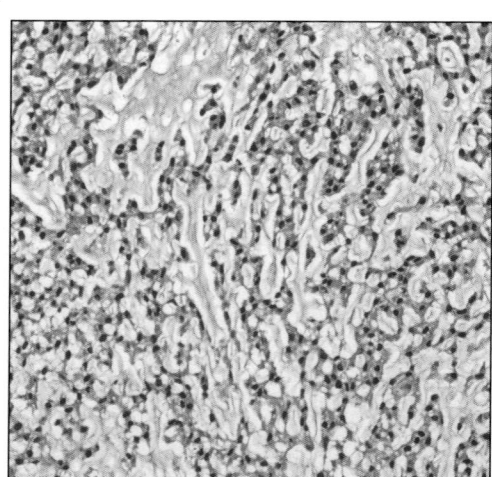

(Left) Diffuse cytoplasmic HMCK(34βE12) immunoreactivity is generally retained in these urothelial carcinomas despite the unusual morphologic features. *(Right)* p63 is maintained in urothelial carcinomas with myxoid stroma, a finding that supports epithelial lineage. The expression of any or all of HMCK(34βE12), p63, CK20, CK5/6, and thrombomodulin help confirm urothelial differentiation in the appropriate clinical context. Uroplakin is specific but not sensitive.

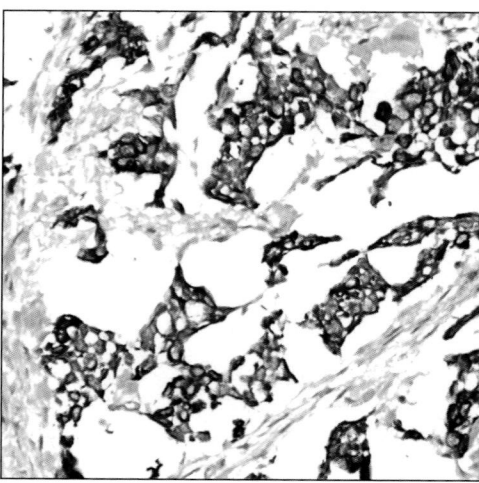
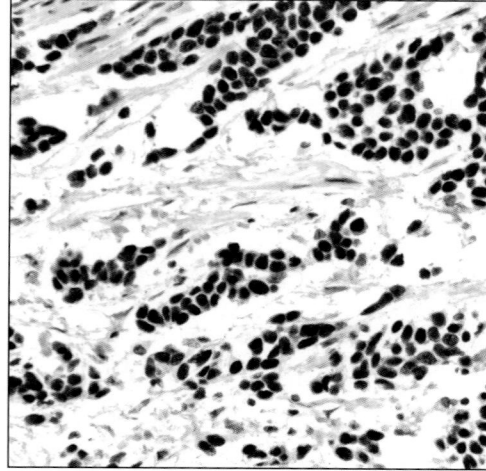

Urothelial Carcinoma with Rhabdoid and Lipoid Features

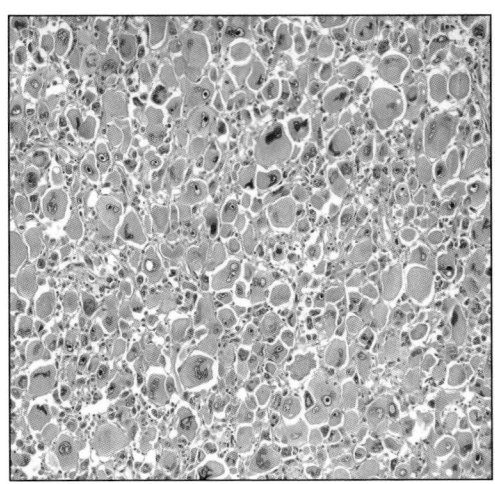 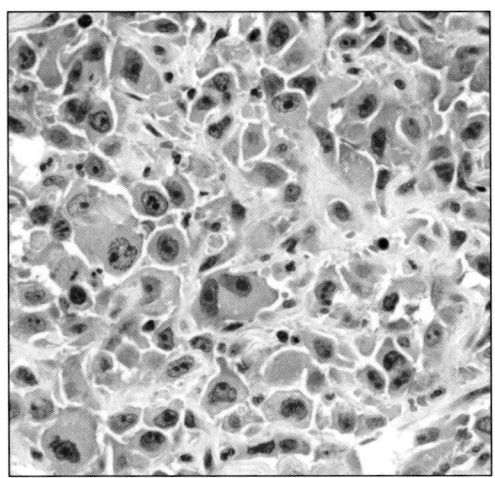

(Left) Invasive urothelial carcinoma with rhabdoid features is characterized by sheets of neoplastic cells showing abundant eosinophilic cytoplasm and eccentric nuclei with vesicular chromatin. These tumors resemble malignant extrarenal rhabdoid tumors but do not have chromosome 22 deletion or INI1 mutation. (Right) Urothelial carcinoma with rhabdoid features has obvious features of malignancy, with marked nucleomegaly and prominent macronucleoli.

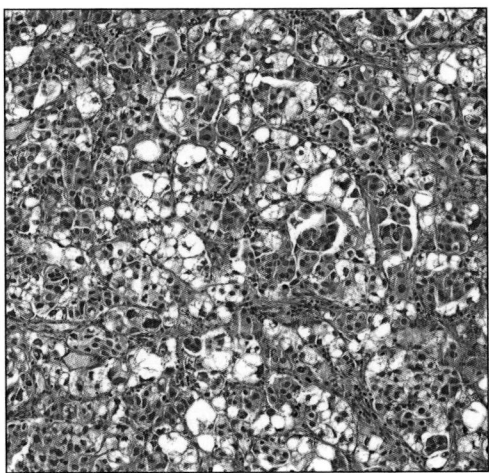 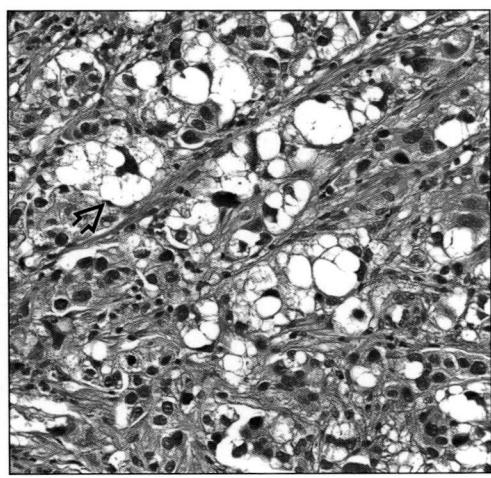

(Left) On low-power examination of this invasive lipid cell urothelial carcinoma, there are scattered neoplastic cells with clear multivacuolated cytoplasm admixed with more conventional urothelial carcinoma. (Right) These rare high-grade carcinomas contain scattered neoplastic cells with intracytoplasmic lipid ⊅ that resemble pleomorphic lipoblasts. This may closely mimic pleomorphic liposarcoma, but obvious typical urothelial carcinoma is usually admixed.

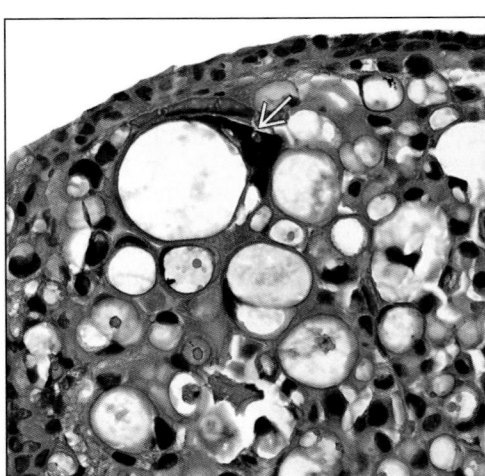 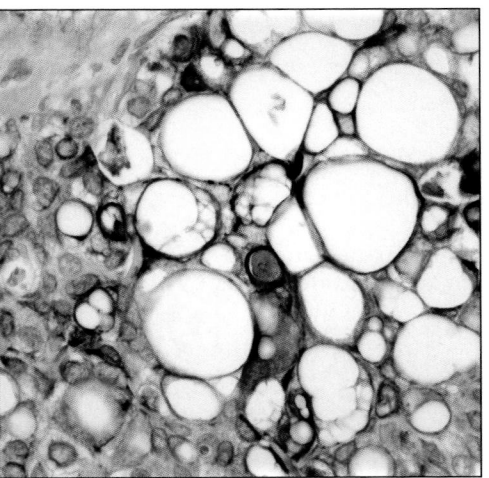

(Left) This invasive urothelial carcinoma with lipid cell features has foci with intracytoplasmic lipid that indent the nuclei ⇥, creating an appearance similar to lipoblasts. (Right) PAN-CK(AE1/AE3) immunohistochemistry shows strong cytoplasmic staining in the neoplastic cells, even in the scant peripheral cytoplasm of the population with intracytoplasmic lipid. S100 stain is negative. These findings should aid in the distinction from primary or heterologous liposarcoma.

CYSTITIS CYSTICA AND GLANDULARIS

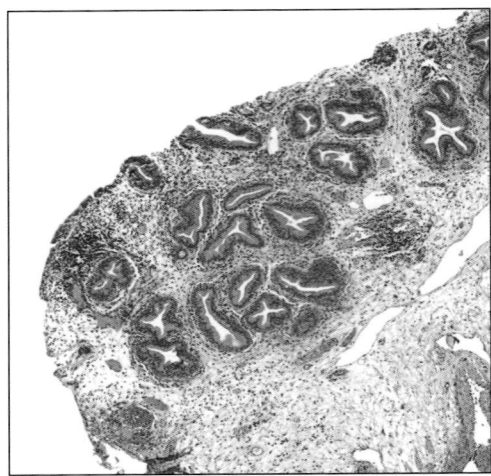

This collection of glandular structures within the superficial lamina propria has overall lobularity and a sharp linear border at the base, features typical of cystitis glandularis.

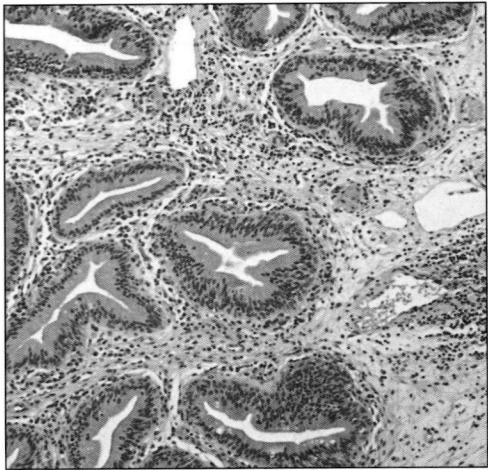

On high-power examination, the glandular epithelium within the lamina propria has abundant luminally oriented cytoplasm, a feature that distinguishes cystitis glandularis from cystitis cystica.

TERMINOLOGY

Definitions
- Cystitis cystica
  - Invaginated urothelial nests in superficial lamina propria with cystic dilatation forming luminal space
  - No cuboidal or columnar luminal cells are present
- Cystitis glandularis
  - Cystitis cystica with luminal cuboidal or columnar lining cells
- Cystitis glandularis with intestinal metaplasia (intestinal type)
  - Cystitis glandularis with at least focal intestinal-type goblet cells

ETIOLOGY/PATHOGENESIS

Environmental Exposure
- May be secondary to localized inflammatory response
- May be a variation in normal bladder microanatomy

CLINICAL ISSUES

Presentation
- Usually incidental finding
- When florid, small raised lesion with intact urothelium may be seen
- Rare cases with intestinal metaplasia and extensive mucin extravasation may form large mass lesion that can mimic malignancy

Treatment
- None

Prognosis
- No convincing evidence that cystitis cystica or glandularis represents neoplastic precursor lesion

MACROSCOPIC FEATURES

General Features
- May form polypoid mass in some florid examples
  - Intact overlying mucosa with variable translucent appearance
- Usually < 1 cm

MICROSCOPIC PATHOLOGY

Histologic Features
- Cystitis cystica
  - Superficial nests of invaginated urothelium in lamina propria
    - Connection to surface urothelium is variable
    - May be organized into lobules
    - In contrast to von Brunn nests, have cystically dilated lumen
    - No glandular-lining cells are present
    - Often admixed with von Brunn nests
- Cystitis glandularis
  - Identical to cystitis cystica, except glandular cells line central lumen
    - Cuboidal or columnar cells with luminally oriented cytoplasm
- Cystitis glandularis with intestinal metaplasia
  - Identical to cystitis glandularis with at least scattered intestinal-type goblet cells
  - Rare cases may have extensive mucin extravasation
    - No significant cytologic atypia
    - No irregular epithelial aggregates
    - No destructive invasion of muscularis propria

DIFFERENTIAL DIAGNOSIS

Invasive Adenocarcinoma
- Usually high stage with destructive invasion into muscularis propria

CYSTITIS CYSTICA AND GLANDULARIS

Key Facts

Terminology

- Invaginated urothelial nests in superficial lamina propria with cystic dilatation forming luminal space
- Cystitis glandularis has luminal cuboidal or columnar lining cells
- Cystitis glandularis of intestinal type contains goblet cells

Etiology/Pathogenesis

- May be normal variant or secondary to localized inflammatory response

Clinical Issues

- Usually incidental finding
- When florid, may have polypoid appearance clinically

- No convincing evidence of neoplastic precursor lesion

Microscopic Pathology

- Cystitis cystica has superficial nests of urothelium with central cysts
- Glandular cells line central lumen in cystitis glandularis
- Cystitis glandularis with intestinal metaplasia contains goblet cells
- Rare cases have extensive mucin extravasation

Top Differential Diagnoses

- Invasive adenocarcinoma
- Noninvasive urothelial carcinoma with glandular differentiation (adenocarcinoma in situ)
- Nested urothelial carcinoma with associated tubules

- Greater degree of nuclear atypia
- In mucinous (colloid) variant, epithelium forms irregular aggregates within stromal mucin
  - Distinctive feature from cystitis glandularis with mucin extravasation

Noninvasive Urothelial Carcinoma with Glandular Differentiation (Adenocarcinoma In Situ)

- Exophytic papillary urothelial carcinoma component may be present
- Glandular component has more atypia than cystitis cystica
  - Columnar cells with nucleomegaly, hyperchromasia, and mitotic activity
- May also have complex exophytic papillary glandular pattern

Nested Urothelial Carcinoma with Associated Tubules

- Individual nests may have significant overlap with cystitis cystica on superficial biopsy
  - Have subtle nucleomegaly
- Typically extends deeply into lamina propria or muscularis propria
  - Invasive clusters may have surrounding retraction

Prostatic-Type Polyp

- Glands within stroma have prostatic secretory phenotype
  - Lightly eosinophilic, frothy cytoplasm
  - Round nuclei
  - PSA and PAP positive

Inverted Urothelial Papilloma

- May have cystitis cystica-like pattern
- Endophytic thin anastomosing cords are typical
  - More complex architecture compared to separate individual nests/glands of cystitis glandularis
- Basal nuclear palisading around nests is typical
- In some cases, distinction from cystitis cystica may be arbitrary

Carcinoid Tumor

- Glandular pattern may closely mimic cystitis glandularis in superficial biopsy
- Immunoreactivity for synaptophysin and chromogranin
- Usually has more complex cribriform or cord-like growth pattern

Clear Cell Adenocarcinoma

- May have cytologically bland foci with cystically dilated tubules
  - Foci with more characteristic nuclear features &/or papillary architecture are typically seen
  - Usually large invasive mass lesion

DIAGNOSTIC CHECKLIST

Clinically Relevant Pathologic Features

- Extensive cystitis glandularis with intestinal metaplasia and mucin extravasation may closely mimic bladder cancer by cystoscopy

Pathologic Interpretation Pearls

- Low-power architectural evaluation is very helpful in distinction from carcinomas
  - Superficial location with sharp base at junction with lamina propria

SELECTED REFERENCES

1. Corica FA et al: Intestinal metaplasia is not a strong risk factor for bladder cancer: study of 53 cases with long-term follow-up. Urology. 50(3):427-31, 1997
2. Young RH et al: Florid cystitis glandularis of intestinal type with mucin extravasation: a mimic of adenocarcinoma. Am J Surg Pathol. 20(12):1462-8, 1996
3. Davies G et al: Cystitis glandularis. Urology. 10(2):128-9, 1977
4. Mostofi FK: Potentialities of bladder epithelium. J Urol. 71(6):705-14, 1954

Microscopic Features

(Left) Hematoxylin & eosin of von Brunn nest ➡️ and cystitis cystica ➡️ shows the lumen with a flattened urothelial lining but without luminally oriented cytoplasm. Columnar cells/glandular epithelia argue for a cystitis glandularis designation. *(Right)* The superficial location of the invaginated nests/glands is an important clue to the diagnosis of cystitis cystica or glandularis. Deceptively bland patterns of invasive urothelial carcinoma typically show irregular infiltration deeper into the lamina propria.

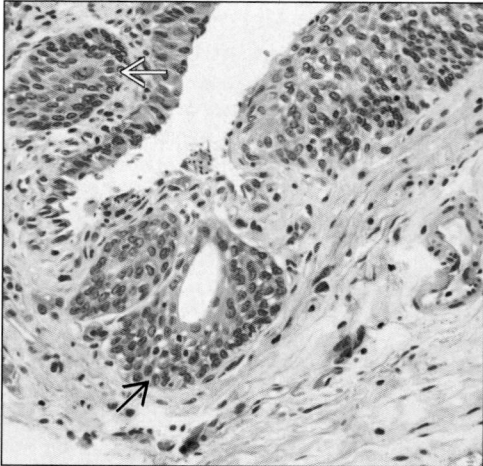
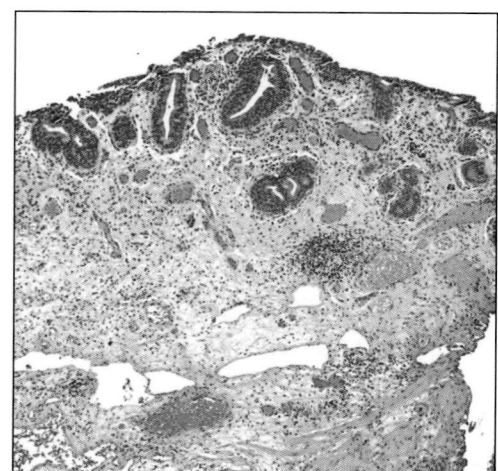

(Left) This photomicrograph shows von Brunn nests ➡️ interspersed with cystitis glandularis ➡️, a common combination. The superficial location and sharp linear border at the base help in the distinction from invasive mimics, such as nested urothelial carcinoma. *(Right)* The luminally oriented cytoplasm of cystitis glandularis ➡️ contrasts with the flattened urothelial lining in cystitis cystica ➡️. These 2 patterns may occur together along with florid von Brunn nests.

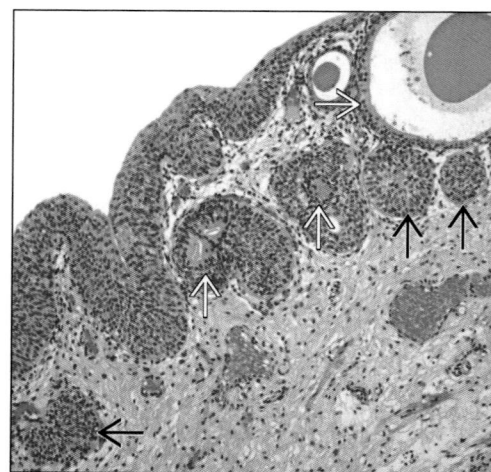
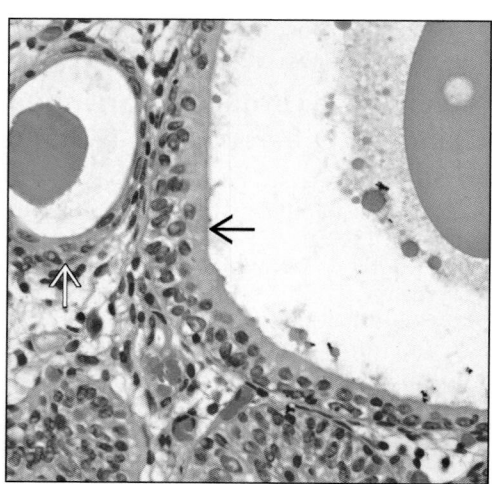

(Left) This superficial collection of tightly aggregated urothelial nests with central lumina is characteristic of florid cystitis glandularis. These florid examples may form a cystoscopic lesion. *(Right)* Florid cystitis glandularis has the characteristic well-developed luminally oriented cytoplasm ➡️. The lesional cells lack the degree of cytologic atypia expected in adenocarcinoma in situ. Overall low-power features of organization are key to recognize the lesion as benign.

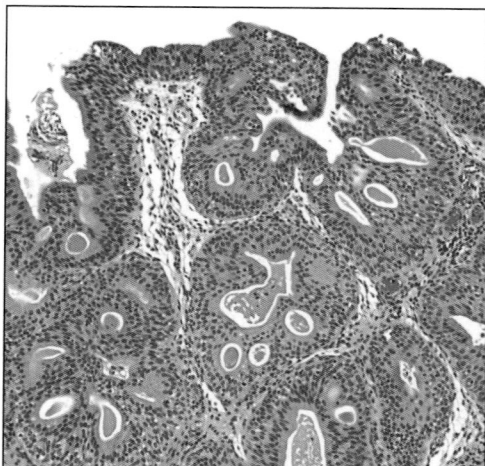
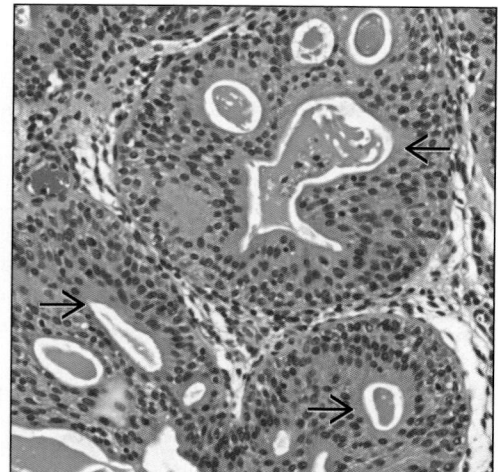

CYSTITIS CYSTICA AND GLANDULARIS

Microscopic Features

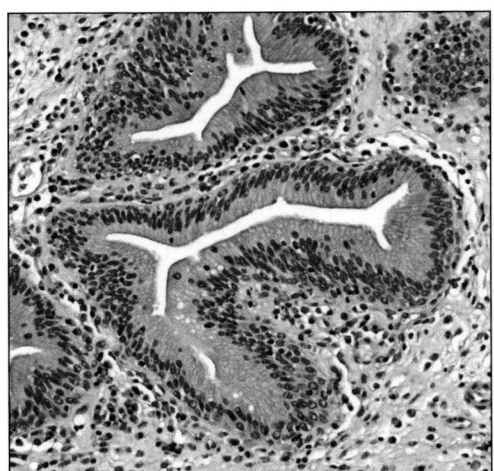
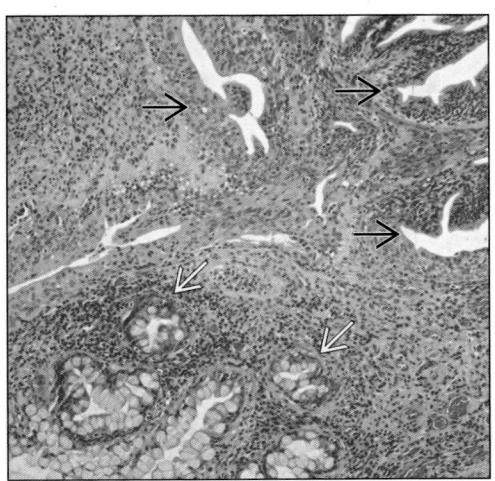

(Left) On high-power examination, this example of cystitis glandularis (nonintestinal type) shows the prototypical lining columnar cells with abundant luminal cytoplasm. The nuclei are cytologically bland and no intestinal metaplasia is present. *(Right)* This example shows an admixture of typical cystitis glandularis without intestinal metaplasia ⇨ and areas with almost complete intestinal metaplasia ➡. Inflammation may vary between cases and may not be conspicuous.

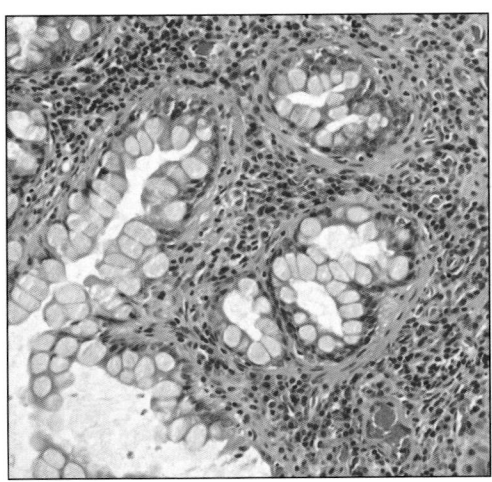
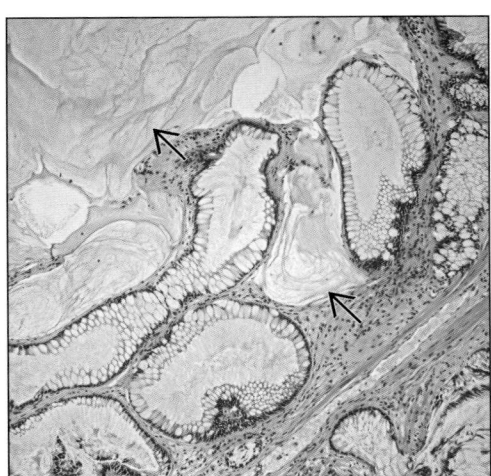

(Left) Cystitis glandularis with intestinal metaplasia is characterized by abundant intracytoplasmic intestinal-type mucin (goblet cells). *(Right)* Some cases of cystitis glandularis with intestinal metaplasia show extensive mucin extravasation ➡. The intact glands and absence of epithelial aggregates in the mucin distinguish this lesion from mucinous adenocarcinoma. Such lesions may mimic a bladder carcinoma on cystoscopic examination and on microscopy.

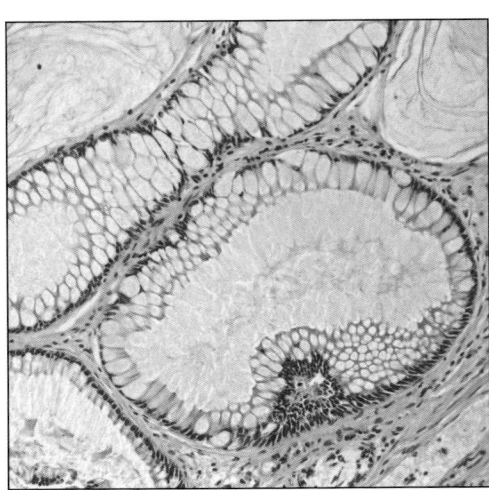
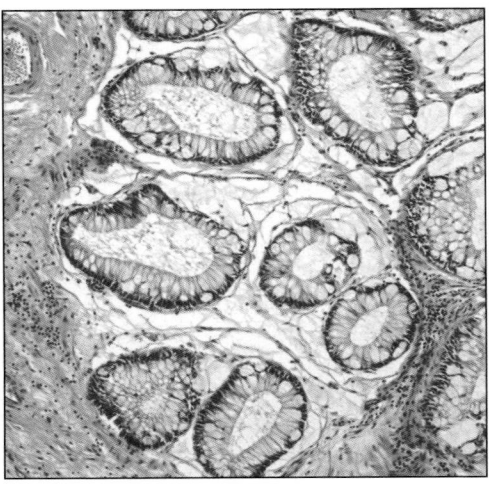

(Left) This cystitis glandularis with intestinal metaplasia is distinguished from adenocarcinoma in situ by small bland nuclei and abundant intracytoplasmic mucin. *(Right)* In rare cases with extensive mucin extravasation, the round contours of the normal benign-appearing intestinal-type glands in cystitis glandularis with intestinal metaplasia allows distinction from invasive mucinous adenocarcinoma, which is comprised of irregular aggregates of epithelium with greater cytologic atypia.

CYSTITIS CYSTICA AND GLANDULARIS

Differential Diagnosis

(Left) *This degree of atypia, characterized by loss of mucin, nucleomegaly, and nuclear hyperchromasia, excludes the diagnosis of cystitis glandularis. This lesion was superficial without evidence of invasion and, therefore, represents adenocarcinoma in situ of the urinary bladder.* *(Right)* *The irregularly shaped clustered aggregates of epithelium floating in pools of mucin would not be seen in cystitis glandularis with mucin extravasation but are typical of mucinous adenocarcinoma.*

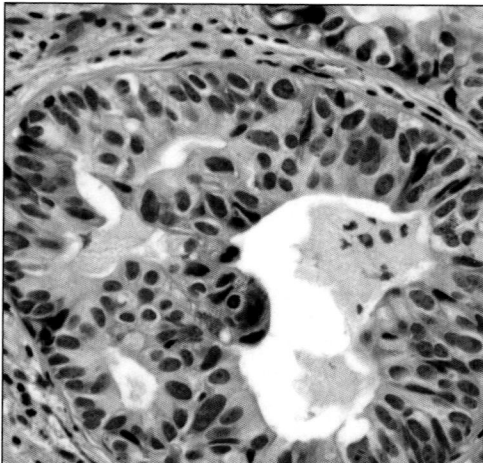
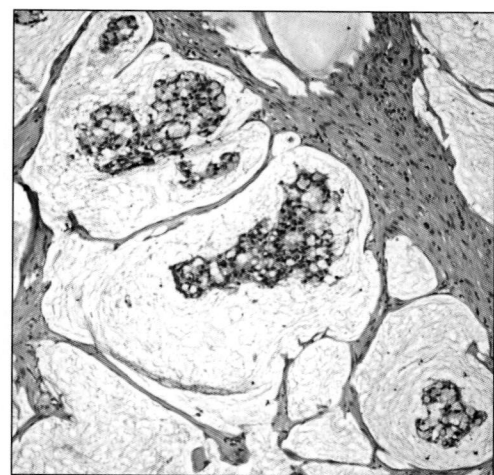

(Left) *Microcystic urothelial carcinoma is shown. On low power, there is remarkable overlap with cystitis cystica/ glandularis. The degree of proliferation and the variation in glandular size and shape are marked.* *(Right)* *In this microcystic carcinoma, higher power shows solid urothelial nests with variably sized cystic spaces in a haphazard growth pattern. There is subtle but distinct nuclear atypia. Appreciation of other features, including invasion into muscularis propria, may be necessary in some cases.*

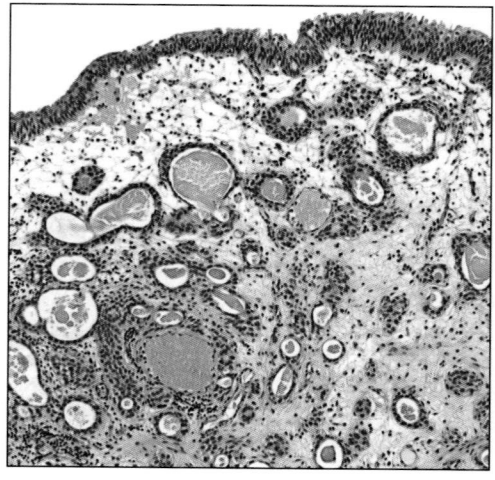
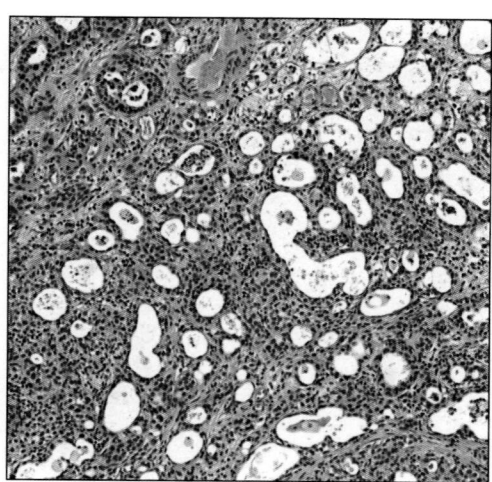

(Left) *As seen here, invasive urothelial carcinomas may show some tubular differentiation or microcystic changes. The low-power architecture shows irregular infiltration of the lamina propria with stromal response, helpful features in the distinction of invasive carcinoma from cystitis cystica or glandularis.* *(Right)* *In this invasive urothelial carcinoma with tubules, the cytology is bland, but there is an irregular distribution and stromal response that warrants a carcinoma diagnosis.*

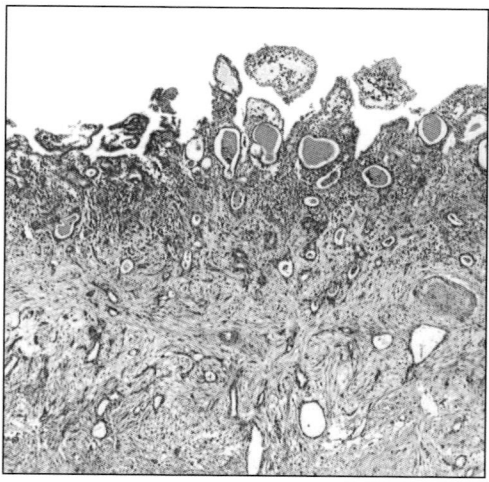
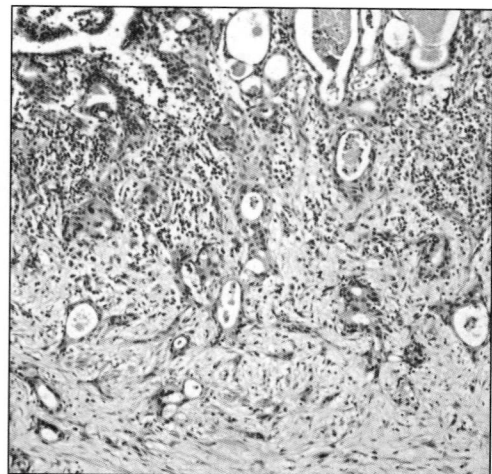

CYSTITIS CYSTICA AND GLANDULARIS

Differential Diagnosis

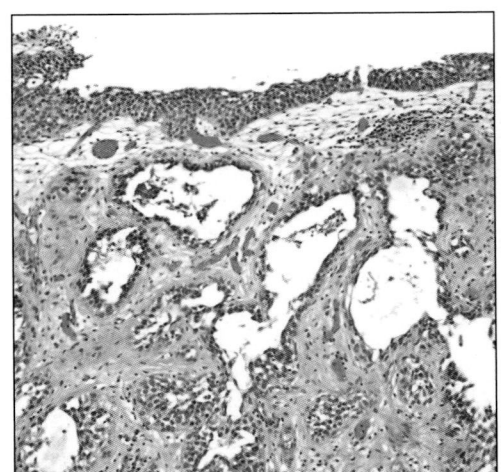

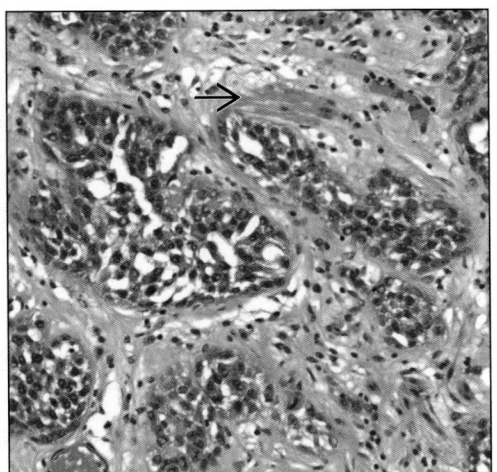

(Left) The nested variant of invasive urothelial carcinoma may have central cystic dilatation in the nests of some foci, a feature that may cause diagnostic confusion with cystitis cystica on small superficial biopsies. *(Right)* Nested urothelial carcinomas are cytologically bland compared to typical urothelial carcinomas but have a subtle degree of nucleomegaly with high nuclear to cytoplasmic ratio. Invasion into the deep lamina propria, including muscularis mucosae ➡, is present.

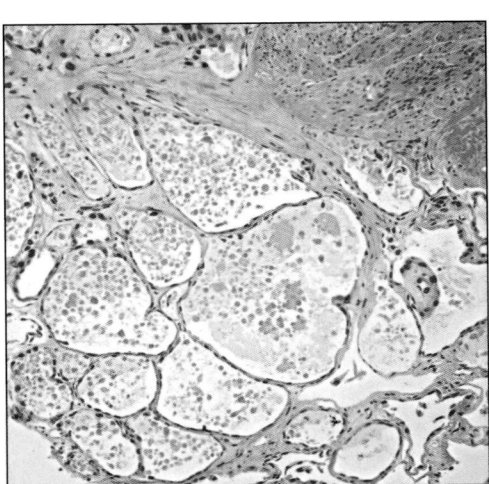

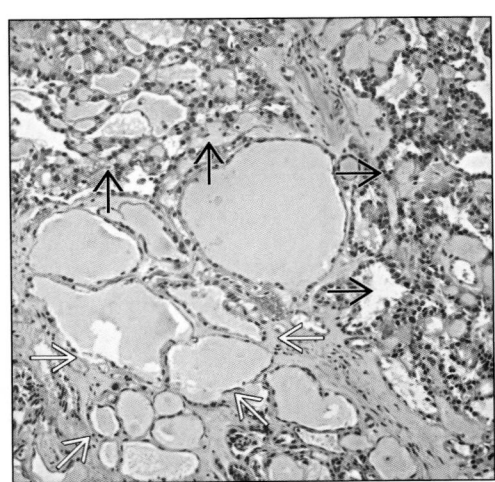

(Left) The tubulocystic pattern of clear cell adenocarcinoma may be deceptively bland in some foci, mimicking a spectrum of benign glandular lesions, including nephrogenic adenoma. Other more typical patterns of clear cell adenocarcinoma should be sought in such cases. *(Right)* Clear cell adenocarcinoma with deceptively bland tubulocystic areas ➡ border foci with more typical glandular & papillary growth ➡. Most tumors show a spectrum of morphologic patterns in the same case.

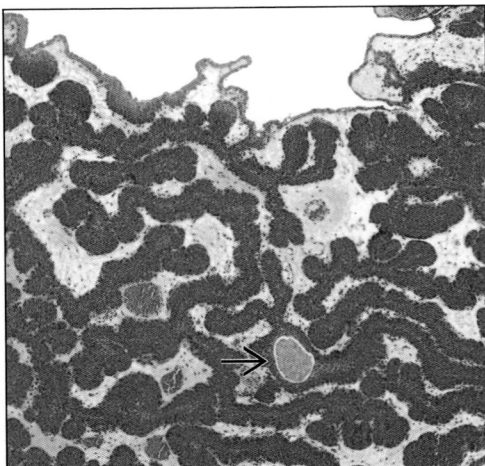

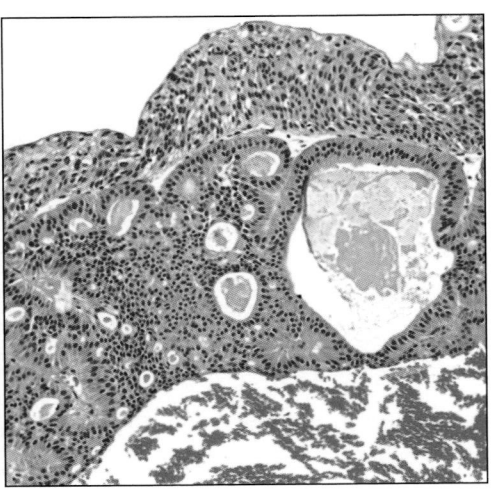

(Left) Despite the focal cystitis cystica pattern ➡, the prominent anastomosing cord-like growth and peripheral nuclear palisading are characteristic of inverted urothelial papilloma. *(Right)* The glandular pattern of a carcinoid tumor may closely mimic cystitis glandularis. The complex cribriform growth pattern is distinct from the individual round urothelial nests expected in cystitis glandularis. Immunohistochemistry may be necessary to confirm the diagnosis.

VILLOUS ADENOMA

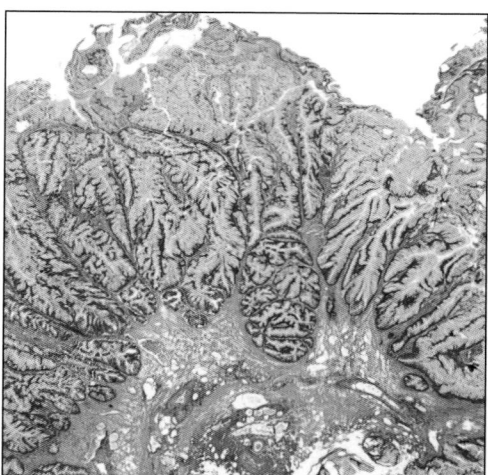

Villous adenoma of the urinary bladder has an identical morphology to its more common colorectal counterpart with variable papillary architecture and obvious intracellular mucin.

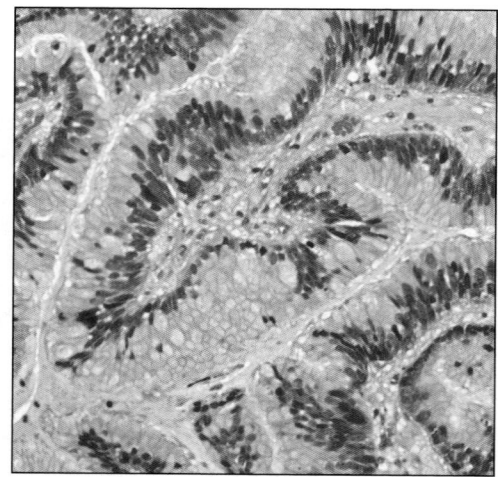

On high-power examination, villous adenoma is characterized by pseudostratified columnar epithelium showing nuclear crowding and hyperchromasia.

TERMINOLOGY

Definitions
- Benign glandular neoplasm of urinary bladder
  - Histologically identical to colorectal adenomas

CLINICAL ISSUES

Epidemiology
- Incidence
  - Rare primary bladder neoplasm
- Age
  - Wide age range
    - Mean: 65 years
- Gender
  - Male predominance

Site
- Common sites include bladder dome and trigone
- May also occur in urachus

Presentation
- Hematuria
- Irritative bladder symptoms
- Rarely, mucosuria can be seen

Natural History
- Rare cases may progress to invasive adenocarcinoma

Treatment
- Complete transurethral resection

Prognosis
- Excellent for villous adenoma with no invasive component and complete resection
- Prognosis for invasive lesions depends on stage of disease

MACROSCOPIC FEATURES

General Features
- Exophytic papillary/villiform tumor
  - May be identical to papillary urothelial neoplasm on cystoscopy

MICROSCOPIC PATHOLOGY

Histologic Features
- Papillary architecture
  - Central fibrovascular cores lined by pseudostratified columnar epithelium
    - Stratification
    - Crowding
    - Nuclear hyperchromasia
- May have high-grade dysplasia/adenocarcinoma in situ
- Invasive adenocarcinoma of enteric type may arise from villous adenoma

Predominant Pattern/Injury Type
- Papillary

Predominant Cell/Compartment Type
- Epithelial, glandular

ANCILLARY TESTS

Immunohistochemistry
- Enteric immunophenotype
  - Immunoreactivity for CK20, CK7, and CEA

DIFFERENTIAL DIAGNOSIS

Invasive Adenocarcinoma of Urinary Bladder
- Irregular gland contours with stromal reaction

VILLOUS ADENOMA

Key Facts

Terminology
- Benign glandular neoplasm arising from urothelium

Clinical Issues
- Presenting symptoms
  - Hematuria and irritative bladder symptoms
  - Rarely, mucosuria can be seen
- Therapy: Complete transurethral resection
- Excellent prognosis for villous adenoma with no invasive component and complete resection

Microscopic Pathology
- Villoglandular architecture
  - Fibrovascular cores lined by pseudostratified columnar epithelium
- Invasive adenocarcinoma of enteric type may arise from villous adenoma

Diagnostic Checklist
- All tissue should be submitted for histologic evaluation to exclude invasive component

---

- May have complex gland formation, such as cribriforming
- Typically deeply invasive into muscularis propria

Papillary Urothelial Carcinoma with Glandular Differentiation
- Obvious urothelial component typically seen
  - Invasive, papillary, or in situ
- More heterogeneous glandular component
  - Intracytoplasmic mucin is rare pattern

Secondary Involvement by Adenocarcinoma
- Colonic adenocarcinoma
  - Superficial biopsies may appear deceptively bland
  - Invasion should be obvious on adequate biopsies
    - Deep involvement of bladder wall
  - Continuity with adjacent bowel on imaging
- Endometrial adenocarcinoma
  - Endometrioid type may appear enteric
  - Typically express PR &/or ER by immunohistochemistry

Cystitis Cystica/Glandularis with Intestinal Metaplasia
- May form conspicuous mass lesion
- Associated with pools of mucin containing intact glands with enteric-type epithelium
  - In large lesions, mucin extravasation may be extensive
- Lining epithelium may be bland or occasionally reactive

DIAGNOSTIC CHECKLIST

Pathologic Interpretation Pearls
- All tissue should be submitted for histologic evaluation
  - Invasive component must be excluded
- Secondary involvement by adenocarcinoma may have surface villous component mimicking primary

SELECTED REFERENCES

1. Lane Z et al: Immunohistochemical expression of prostatic antigens in adenocarcinoma and villous adenoma of the urinary bladder. Am J Surg Pathol. 32(9):1322-6, 2008
2. Sung W et al: Villous adenoma of the urinary bladder. Int J Urol. 15(6):551-3, 2008
3. Tamboli P et al: Villous adenoma of urinary tract: a common tumor in an uncommon location. Adv Anat Pathol. 7(2):79-84, 2000
4. Cheng L et al: Villous adenoma of the urinary tract: a report of 23 cases, including 8 with coexistent adenocarcinoma. Am J Surg Pathol. 23(7):764-71, 1999
5. Trotter SE et al: Villous adenoma of the bladder. Histopathology. 24(5):491-3, 1994
6. Channer JL et al: Villous adenoma of the bladder. J Clin Pathol. 46(5):450-2, 1993
7. Miller DC et al: Villous adenoma of the urinary bladder: a morphologic or biologic entity? Am J Clin Pathol. 79(6):728-31, 1983

IMAGE GALLERY

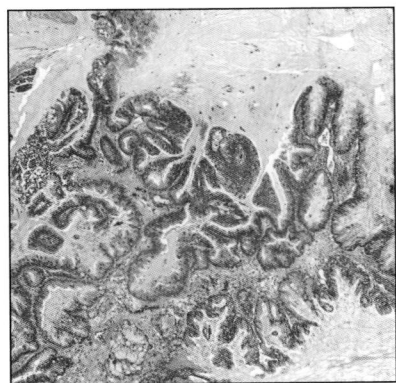 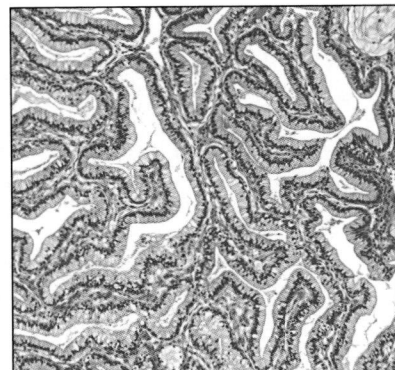 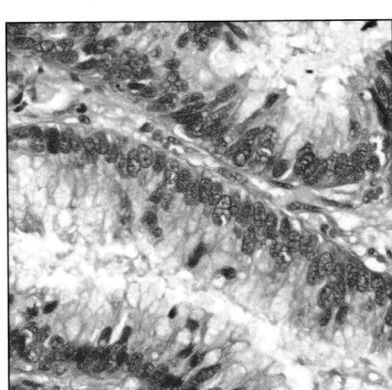

(Left) Hematoxylin & eosin shows typical exophytic, papillary appearance of villous adenoma. *(Center)* The main differential diagnostic considerations for villous adenoma include primary and secondary adenocarcinoma, which are distinguished by the absence of destructive invasion. *(Right)* The cytologic features of villous adenoma are identical to colorectal adenomas with nuclear stratification, hyperchromasia, and variable nucleoli.

ADENOCARCINOMA IN SITU

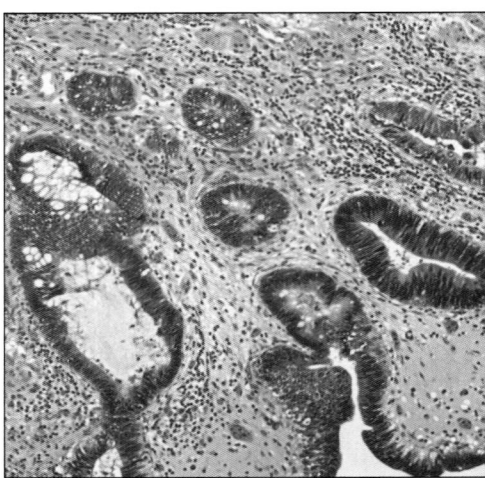

The bladder surface epithelium and underlying invaginations are lined by hyperchromatic columnar epithelial cells, features typical of adenocarcinoma in situ (noninvasive carcinoma with glandular differentiation).

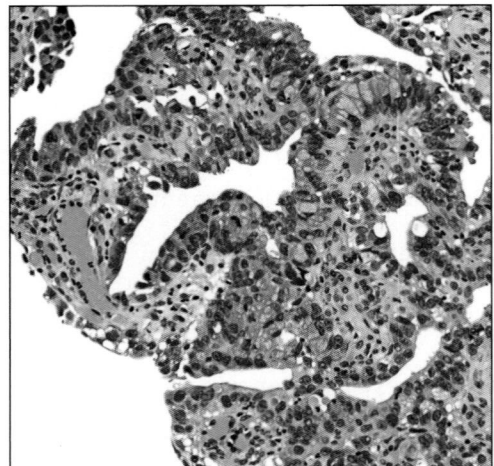

Adenocarcinoma in situ of the urinary bladder typically has a single lining cell layer and may have intracytoplasmic mucin as seen in this example.

TERMINOLOGY

Synonyms
- Noninvasive urothelial carcinoma with glandular differentiation
- Urothelial carcinoma with villoglandular differentiation
- Papillary adenocarcinoma in situ

Definitions
- Noninvasive glandular neoplasm of urinary bladder
  - Characterized by atypical columnar epithelium
  - Often admixed with urothelial carcinoma
  - Recent proposal to rename this lesion noninvasive urothelial carcinoma with glandular differentiation
    - To distinguish from glandular carcinoma in situ arising in cystitis glandularis, which may be precursor of adenocarcinoma

CLINICAL ISSUES

Presentation
- Hematuria
  - Gross or microscopic

Treatment
- Surgical approaches
  - Transurethral excision
    - Similar to high-grade papillary urothelial carcinoma
- Adjuvant therapy
  - Intravesical chemotherapy
  - Intravesical BCG therapy

Prognosis
- Many progress to invasive urothelial carcinoma (50%)
  - Subsequent invasion may have aggressive variant morphology
    - Not typically associated with invasive adenocarcinoma

MACROSCOPIC FEATURES

General Features
- Varies from exophytic papillary lesions to flat lesions

MICROSCOPIC PATHOLOGY

Histologic Features
- May have multiple growth patterns
  - Flat
  - Papillary
  - Cribriform
- Lining neoplastic cells are columnar with luminal cytoplasm
  - Intracytoplasmic mucin occasionally present
- Apoptotic debris and mitotic activity common
- Necrosis is rare
- Frequently associated with other morphologic patterns of urothelial neoplasia
  - Noninvasive papillary urothelial carcinoma
  - Urothelial carcinoma in situ
  - Invasive urothelial carcinoma
    - Frequent association with aggressive variants: Small cell and micropapillary carcinoma
    - Not commonly associated with invasive adenocarcinoma

DIFFERENTIAL DIAGNOSIS

Urothelial Carcinoma In Situ
- Comprised of rounded to polygonal neoplastic cells
- Stratified urothelial cells without luminal cytoplasm
  - Stratified neoplastic urothelial cells are very disorganized
    - Loss of polarity to basement membrane
- Broad range of nuclear pleomorphism

ADENOCARCINOMA IN SITU

Key Facts

Terminology
- Noninvasive glandular lesion characterized by atypical columnar epithelium
- Also called "noninvasive urothelial carcinoma with glandular differentiation" and "urothelial carcinoma with villoglandular differentiation"

Clinical Issues
- Hematuria
- Similar to high-grade papillary urothelial carcinoma
- Many progress to invasive urothelial carcinoma (50%)
- Subsequent invasion may have variant morphology (small cell and micropapillary)

Macroscopic Features
- Varies from exophytic papillary lesions to flat lesions

Microscopic Pathology
- Lining neoplastic cells are columnar with luminal cytoplasm
- Frequently associated with other urothelial neoplasia
- Intracytoplasmic mucin occasionally present
- May have multiple growth patterns (flat, papillary, and cribriform)

Top Differential Diagnoses
- Urothelial carcinoma in situ
- Urothelial carcinoma with gland-like spaces
- Cystitis glandularis ± intestinal metaplasia
- Villous adenoma
- Noninvasive micropapillary carcinoma
- Clear cell adenocarcinoma

Urothelial Carcinoma with Gland-like Spaces
- Typical urothelial carcinoma with admixed small cystic spaces
  - Intraluminal mucin is variable
    - Mucin is not intracytoplasmic
- Not lined by columnar epithelium
- No luminal cytoplasm

Cystitis Glandularis ± Intestinal Metaplasia
- Invaginations from surface urothelium with central luminal space
- Lining epithelial cells may be columnar
- Luminal cytoplasm is characteristic
- Nuclear features are benign
- When intestinal metaplasia is present, nuclei are eccentric with abundant intracytoplasmic mucin
  - Nuclear cytology remains bland
- Mucin extravasation may be present

Villous Adenoma
- Distinct large sessile mass lesion
- Characteristic long finger-like projections
- Not associated with urothelial carcinoma
  - May be associated with invasive adenocarcinoma
- Morphologically identical to colorectal villous adenoma

Noninvasive Micropapillary Carcinoma
- Delicate filiform processes, arising from papillary cores or from flat urothelium
- Glomeruloid structures seen on cross section
- May have admixed adenocarcinoma in situ
  - Creates difficulty in definitive diagnosis of noninvasive micropapillary component in some cases

Clear Cell Adenocarcinoma
- Greater degree of nuclear pleomorphism typical
- "Hobnail" arrangement of lining epithelium common
- Dense hyalinization or myxoid change in papillary cores is also common
- Cytoplasmic features vary
  - Abundant clear cytoplasm typically present at least focally
- Other more classic patterns may be admixed
  - Solid
  - Tubulocystic
    - Focal tubulocystic areas may be deceptively bland

DIAGNOSTIC CHECKLIST

Pathologic Interpretation Pearls
- Adenocarcinoma in situ is frequently associated with invasive urothelial carcinoma
  - Aggressive variant patterns are frequently seen
    - Compared to more typical patterns of noninvasive urothelial carcinoma
    - Small cell and micropapillary carcinoma should be carefully considered
    - These variant patterns may have therapeutic implications (e.g., small cell carcinoma requires different chemotherapy regimen)
- Distinction from villous adenoma is important
  - No risk of urothelial carcinoma with villous adenoma
    - Complete excision is typically curative
  - Villous adenoma must be entirely evaluated to exclude associated invasive adenocarcinoma

SELECTED REFERENCES

1. Lim M et al: Urothelial carcinoma with villoglandular differentiation: a study of 14 cases. Mod Pathol. 22(10):1280-6, 2009
2. Miller JS et al: Noninvasive urothelial carcinoma of the bladder with glandular differentiation: report of 24 cases. Am J Surg Pathol. 33(8):1241-8, 2009
3. Chan TY et al: In situ adenocarcinoma of the bladder. Am J Surg Pathol. 25(7):892-9, 2001
4. O'Brien AM et al: Papillary adenocarcinoma in situ of bladder. J Urol. 134(3):544-6, 1985

ADENOCARCINOMA IN SITU

Microscopic Features

(Left) The columnar cells are characterized by nuclear hyperchromasia and a very thin rim of luminal cytoplasm. This pattern is morphologically similar to the more common endocervical adenocarcinoma in situ. *(Right)* Adenocarcinoma in situ ⇉ is frequently admixed with typical papillary urothelial carcinoma ⇗. The papillary urothelial carcinoma has obvious stratification with multiple layers of urothelial cells and more rounded nuclear contours.

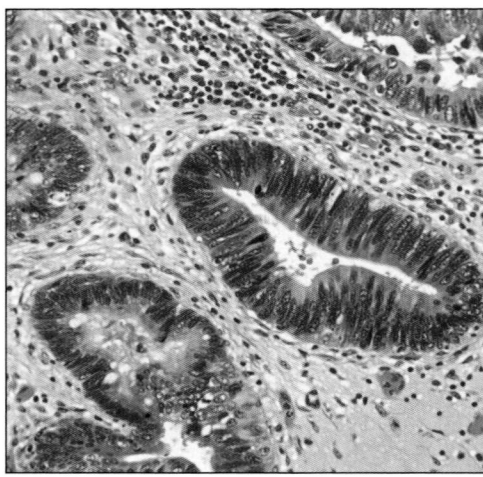
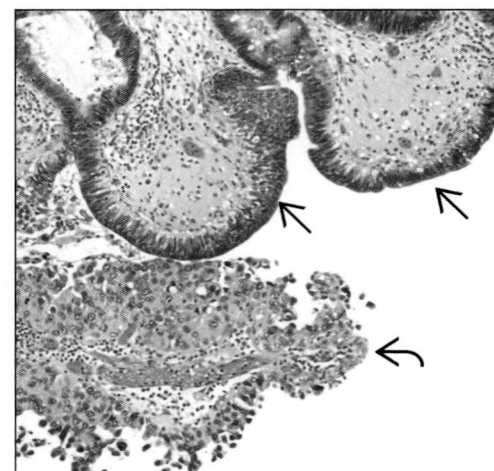

(Left) The characteristic columnar epithelium of adenocarcinoma in situ ⇉ is contrasted with rounded nuclei in the adjacent high-grade urothelial carcinoma below ⇗. *(Right)* Exophytic papillary patterns of adenocarcinoma in situ are also reported, similar to this example. Recent publications have referred to this pattern of bladder carcinoma as "noninvasive urothelial carcinoma of the bladder with glandular differentiation" and "villoglandular."

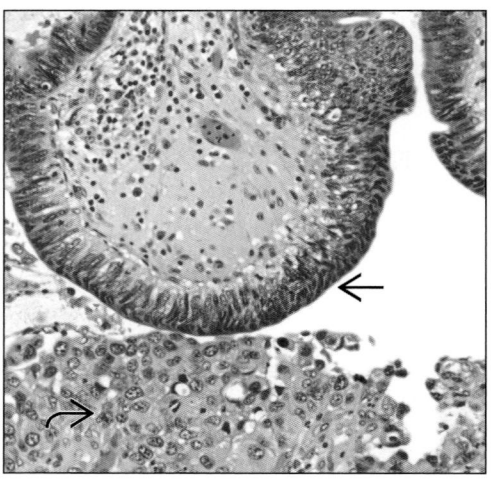
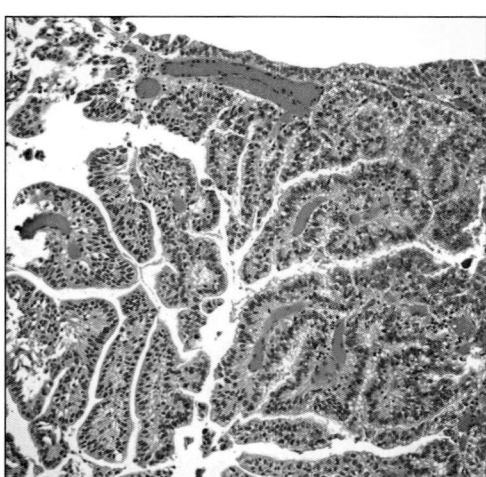

(Left) The columnar lining epithelium in this papillary pattern of adenocarcinoma in situ is striking. In our experience, this pattern is frequently seen in association with micropapillary carcinoma. *(Right)* Some examples of adenocarcinoma in situ have a cribriforming architectural pattern. The columnar arrangement of the cells oriented toward the lumen ⇉ distinguishes cribriform adenocarcinoma in situ from urothelial carcinoma with gland-like spaces.

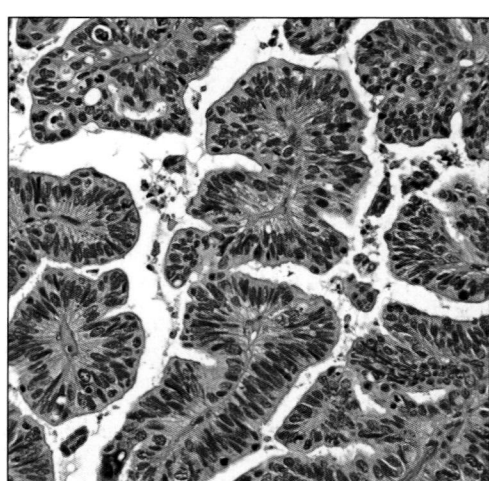
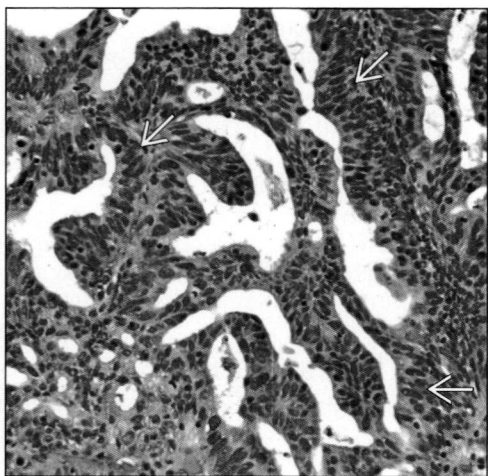

ADENOCARCINOMA IN SITU

Differential Diagnosis

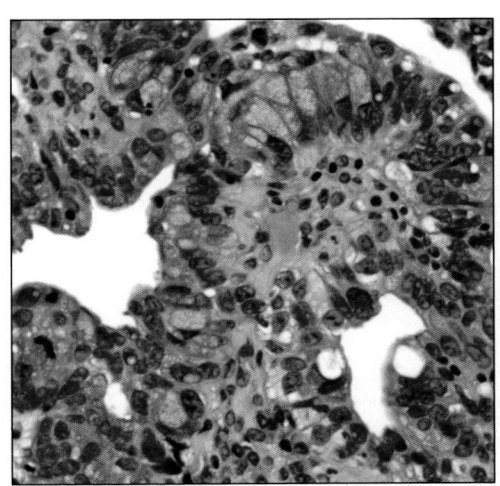

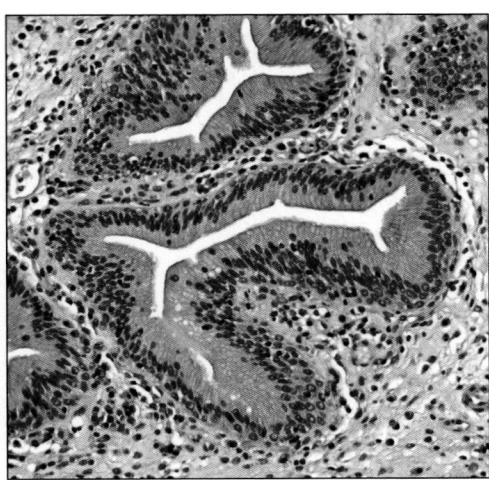

(Left) This example of adenocarcinoma in situ has abundant intracytoplasmic mucin. The degree of nuclear atypia, however, is beyond what is seen in typical cystitis glandularis. **(Right)** Cystitis glandularis is characterized by columnar epithelium with luminal cytoplasm, but the nuclei remain small with bland nuclear chromatin. There is also generally more appreciable cytoplasm, compared to adenocarcinoma in situ, because of the absence of significant nucleomegaly.

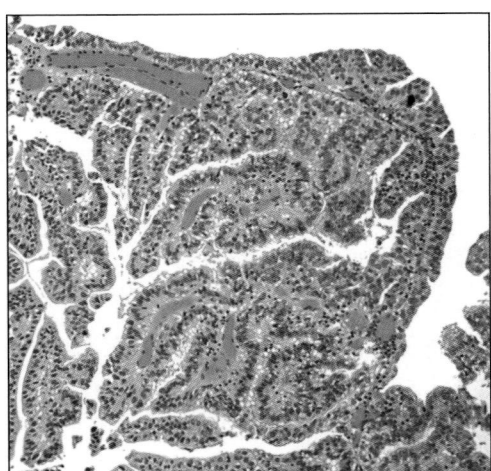

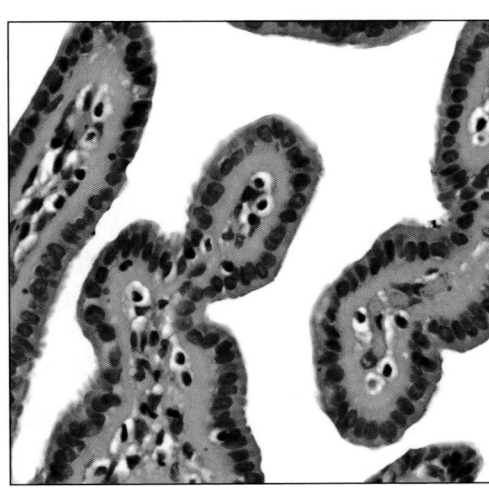

(Left) The exophytic papillary pattern of adenocarcinoma in situ may suggest the possibility of papillary nephrogenic adenoma, but the neoplastic cells of this carcinoma appear more proliferative and typically have a more columnar morphology. **(Right)** Nephrogenic adenoma may also have an exophytic papillary component, but the lining epithelium is comprised of very small columnar cells, typically with very bland cytology.

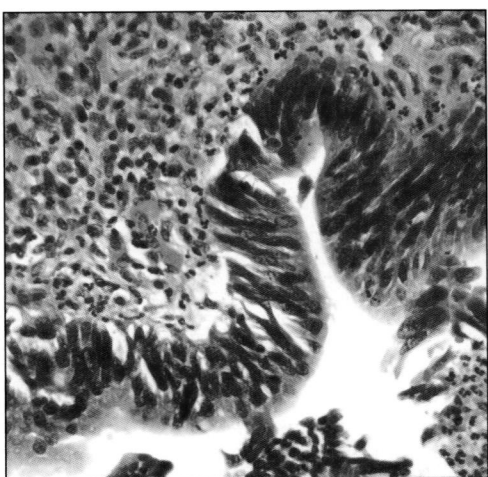

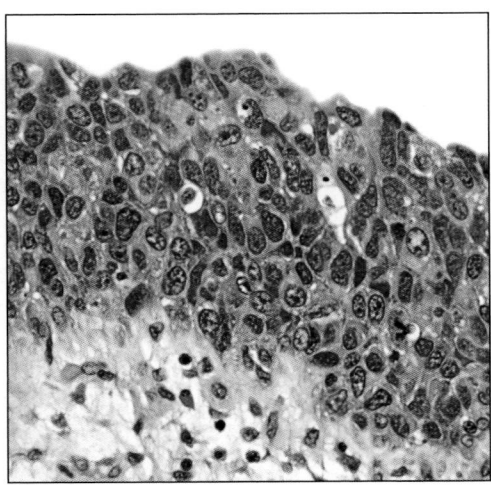

(Left) This high-power photomicrograph of adenocarcinoma in situ highlights columnar-type epithelium with scant luminally oriented cytoplasm, features that are distinct from the rounded nuclei and stratification typical of urothelial carcinoma in situ. **(Right)** In contrast to adenocarcinoma in situ, this urothelial carcinoma in situ is comprised of cells with more rounded nuclei and obvious cellular stratification.

INVASIVE ADENOCARCINOMA

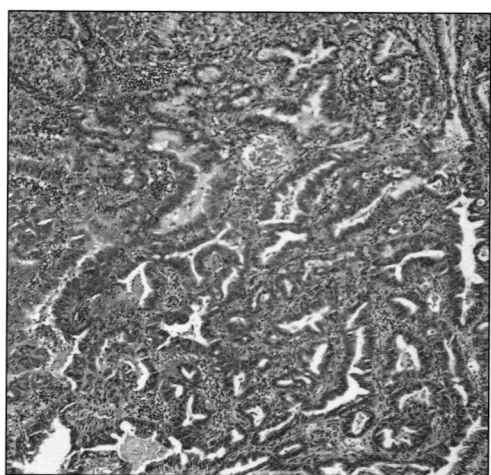

Primary adenocarcinoma is a gland-forming carcinoma with no associated component of urothelial carcinoma. Metastatic carcinoma is always a consideration when dealing with these tumors.

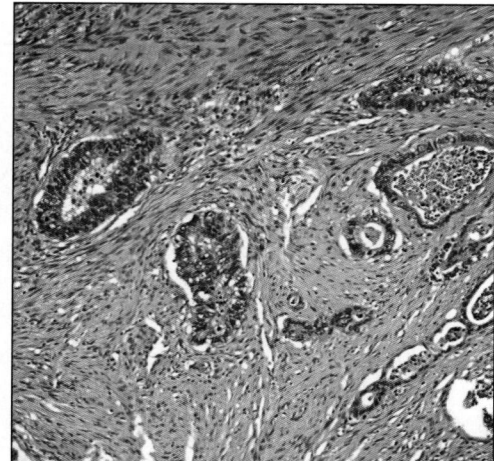

Primary adenocarcinoma with invasion into muscularis propria may be morphologically indistinguishable from colorectal adenocarcinoma. Clinical history is of paramount importance.

TERMINOLOGY

Definitions
- Primary gland-forming carcinoma of urinary bladder not associated with urothelial or squamous carcinoma component

ETIOLOGY/PATHOGENESIS

Developmental Anomaly
- Associated with bladder exstrophy (~ 4-7% risk)

Chronic Irritation
- Nonfunctioning bladder
- May occur within urachal remnant or cyst
- Obstruction
- Schistosomiasis

CLINICAL ISSUES

Epidemiology
- Incidence
  - Rare primary bladder neoplasm (< 2% of bladder malignancies)
- Age
  - Peak incidence in 6th decade
- Gender
  - M:F = 2.6:1

Site
- Bladder base is most common

Presentation
- Hematuria most common
- Dysuria
- Rarely mucusuria

Treatment
- Radical cystectomy

- Adjuvant radiation &/or chemotherapy may be employed

Prognosis
- Poor prognosis (5-year survival rate varies from 18-47%) secondary to high stage at presentation

MACROSCOPIC FEATURES

General Features
- Exophytic, papillary, sessile, or infiltrating mass

MICROSCOPIC PATHOLOGY

Histologic Features
- Pure glandular differentiation
- Varying patterns are described
  - Enteric
  - Adenocarcinoma, not otherwise specified
  - Mucinous/colloid
  - Signet ring cell
  - Hepatoid
  - Mixed
- Not uncommonly associated with intestinal metaplasia
- Associated adenocarcinoma in situ may be seen

ANCILLARY TESTS

Immunohistochemistry
- Enteric adenocarcinoma may have significant overlap with colonic adenocarcinoma
  - CK20 typically positive
  - CK7 phenotype is variable, usually negative
  - May express villin and CDX-2
  - Does not express nuclear β-catenin
- PAP reactivity is reported, but PSA is typically negative
- Uroplakin-3 negative

INVASIVE ADENOCARCINOMA

Key Facts

Etiology/Pathogenesis
- Predisposing factors
  - Associated with bladder exstrophy
  - Nonfunctioning bladder

Clinical Issues
- Rare primary bladder neoplasm (< 2% of bladder malignancies)
- Peak incidence in 6th decade
- Most common presentation is hematuria
- Poor prognosis (5-year survival rate varies from 18-47%) secondary to high stage at presentation

Microscopic Pathology
- Pure glandular differentiation
- Associated adenocarcinoma in situ may be seen

Ancillary Tests
- CK20 positive, CK7 negative
- May express villin and CDX-2
- Does not express nuclear β-catenin
- PAP reactivity is reported, but PSA is typically negative

Top Differential Diagnoses
- Direct invasion by prostatic adenocarcinoma
- Direct invasion or metastatic colorectal adenocarcinoma
- Metastatic adenocarcinoma
- Cystitis glandularis
- Invasive urothelial carcinoma with glandular differentiation or small tubules
- Müllerianosis
- Urachal adenocarcinoma

DIFFERENTIAL DIAGNOSIS

Direct Invasion by Prostatic Adenocarcinoma
- More common than primary adenocarcinoma
- Monomorphic round nuclei with prominent nucleoli suggest prostate origin
- Ductal adenocarcinoma of prostate has significant morphologic overlap
- Often expresses PSA and PAP
  - Primary bladder adenocarcinoma may express PAP
  - PSMA and P501S may also be expressed by bladder adenocarcinoma
- Serum PSA may be elevated

Direct Invasion or Metastatic Colorectal Adenocarcinoma
- Morphologically indistinguishable from bladder primary
- Frequently (80%) expresses nuclear β-catenin
- Colonoscopy is often required for more definitive distinction

Other Metastatic Adenocarcinoma
- Gastric signet ring cell and ovarian serous and clear cell carcinomas may be indistinguishable morphologically

Extensive Cystitis Glandularis
- Superficial location and bland nuclear cytology
- Sharp linear border with underlying lamina propria
- Rare cases have mucin extravasation, which may more closely mimic mucinous adenocarcinoma
  - Irregular epithelial aggregates are not present in mucin

Invasive Urothelial Carcinoma with Glandular Differentiation or Small Tubules
- Identifiable component of papillary, in situ, or invasive urothelial carcinoma

Müllerianosis
- Endocervical, tubal, or endometrial-type glands

- May be present deeply in muscularis propria or adventitia
- Bland nuclear cytology and lack of stromal response aids in distinction from adenocarcinoma

Urachal Adenocarcinoma
- Must be distinguished by its anatomic location in urachus (bladder dome)

DIAGNOSTIC CHECKLIST

Pathologic Interpretation Pearls
- Primary adenocarcinoma of bladder is extremely rare
  - Possibility of origin from distant or contiguous anatomic site should be carefully considered before diagnosis is rendered

SELECTED REFERENCES

1. Zaghloul MS et al: Long-term results of primary adenocarcinoma of the urinary bladder: a report on 192 patients. Urol Oncol. 24(1):13-20, 2006
2. Suh N et al: Value of CDX2, villin, and alpha-methylacyl coenzyme A racemase immunostains in the distinction between primary adenocarcinoma of the bladder and secondary colorectal adenocarcinoma. Mod Pathol. 18(9):1217-22, 2005
3. Wang HL et al: Immunohistochemical distinction between primary adenocarcinoma of the bladder and secondary colorectal adenocarcinoma. Am J Surg Pathol. 25(11):1380-7, 2001
4. Grignon DJ et al: Primary adenocarcinoma of the urinary bladder. A clinicopathologic analysis of 72 cases. Cancer. 67(8):2165-72, 1991
5. Grignon DJ et al: Primary signet-ring cell carcinoma of the urinary bladder. Am J Clin Pathol. 95(1):13-20, 1991

INVASIVE ADENOCARCINOMA

Microscopic Features

(Left) Primary bladder adenocarcinoma with exophytic and invasive components is shown. The exophytic areas also have a glandular phenotype. In contrast, urothelial carcinoma with glandular differentiation has a urothelial morphology in some areas. *(Right)* This invasive bladder adenocarcinoma has a well-formed glandular pattern and a desmoplastic stromal response. This degree of low-power complexity helps in the distinction from benign mimics, such as florid cystitis glandularis.

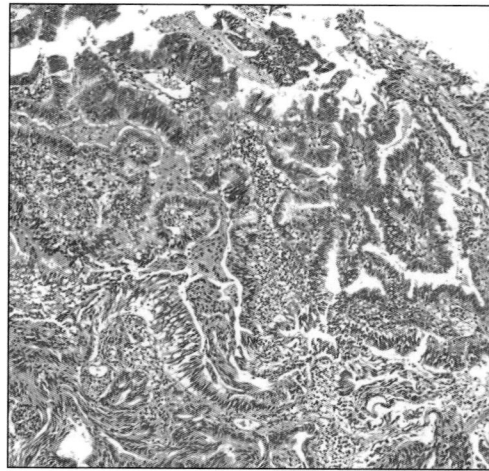 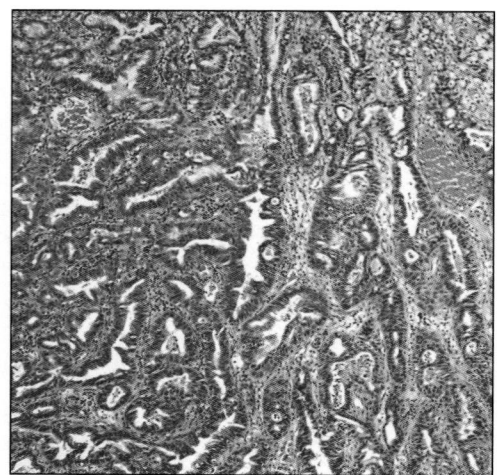

(Left) On high power, this primary vesical adenocarcinoma, enteric morphology, has high nuclear to cytoplasmic ratio, elongated nuclei, and nuclear membrane irregularities. *(Right)* Complex cribriform architecture with dirty necrosis is present in this primary bladder adenocarcinoma that closely resembles colorectal carcinoma. Since colorectal carcinoma may directly invade into the bladder, this diagnostic possibility must be carefully considered prior to diagnosing a bladder primary.

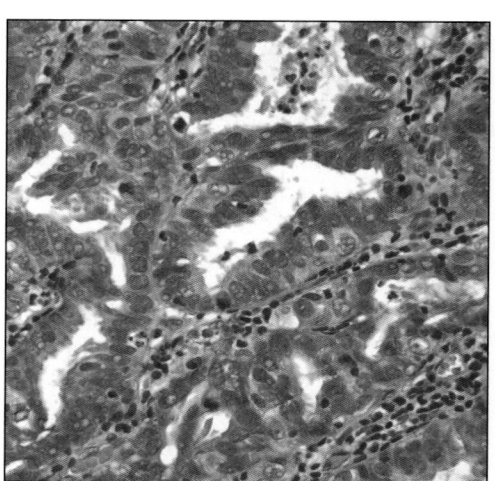 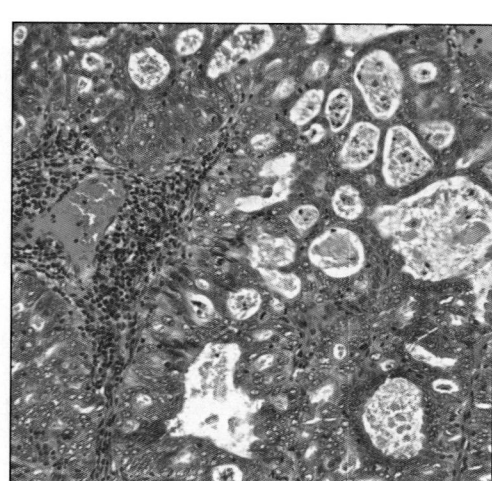

(Left) Enteric-type adenocarcinoma with comedonecrosis may be morphologically indistinguishable from colon cancer. Clinical correlation is essential in this setting, and colonoscopy is often useful if there is no prior diagnosis. *(Right)* Primary vesical adenocarcinoma (enteric and colloid type) is typically high stage and shows obvious destructive invasion of the muscularis propria. This feature is very useful in the distinction from cystitis glandularis with mucin extravasation.

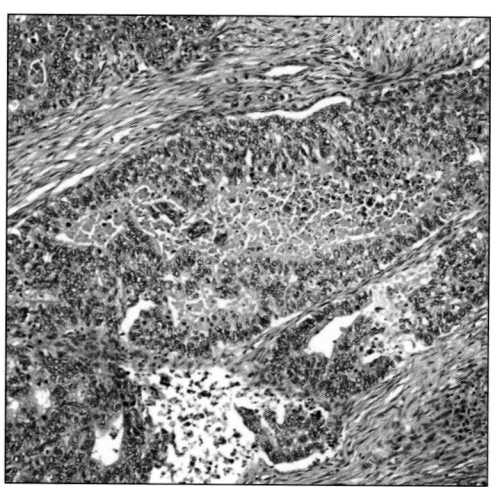 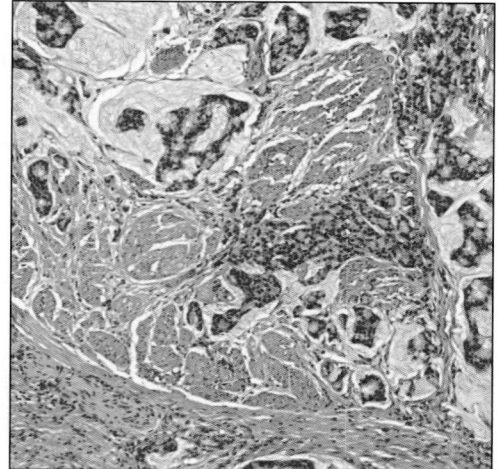

INVASIVE ADENOCARCINOMA

Microscopic Features

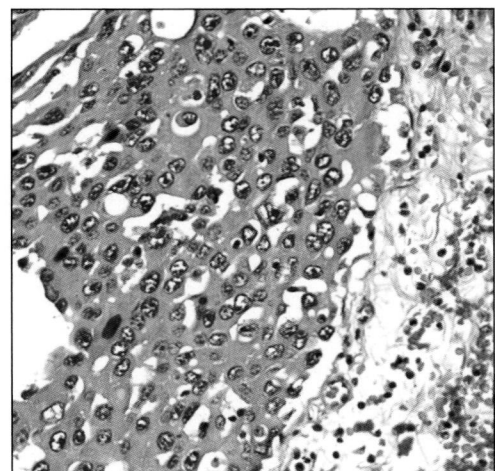

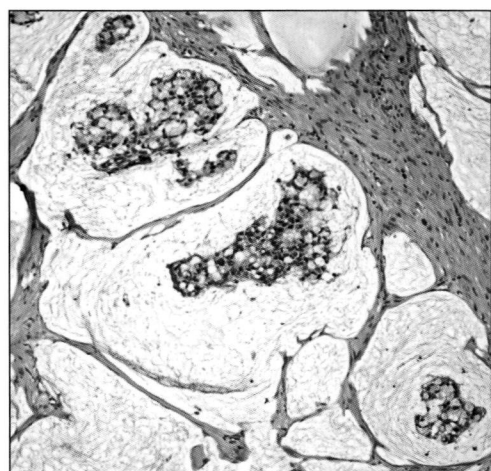

(Left) The "hepatoid" pattern of adenocarcinoma is characterized by trabeculae with a distinct sinusoidal framework and dense cytoplasmic eosinophilia. *(Right)* In this primary mucinous adenocarcinoma of the urinary bladder, irregularly contoured epithelial nests are seen floating in the mucin. This is in contrast to cystitis glandularis with intestinal metaplasia and mucin extravasation, which has, at most, intact glands and simple strips of epithelium within the mucin.

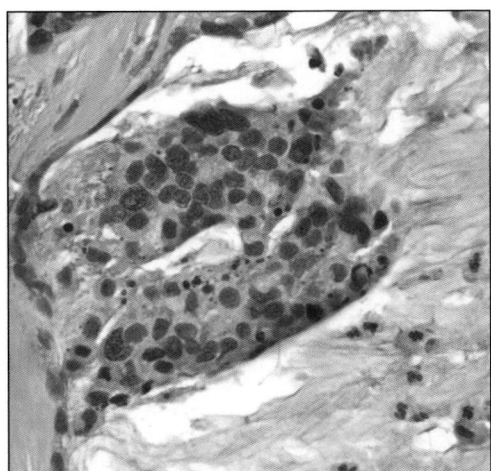

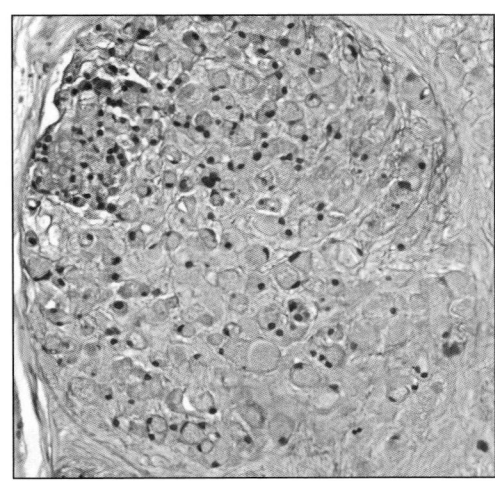

(Left) At higher magnification, the degree of nucleomegaly, nuclear membrane irregularity, and nuclear hyperchromasia is more obvious. Many of the benign mimics of adenocarcinoma may be distinguished by an absence of this degree of atypia. *(Right)* Signet ring cell adenocarcinoma of the urinary bladder is rare but is morphologically indistinguishable from metastatic gastric signet ring cell adenocarcinoma. Mixed patterns of adenocarcinoma are common in the bladder.

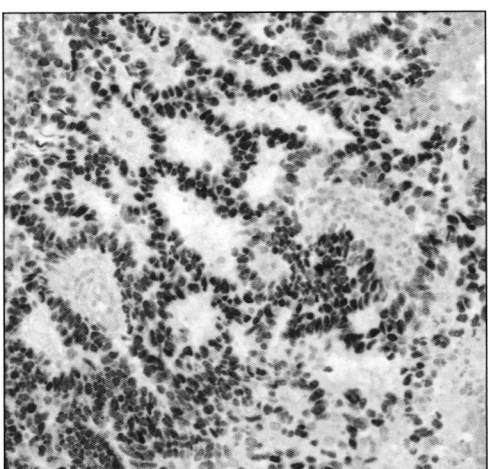

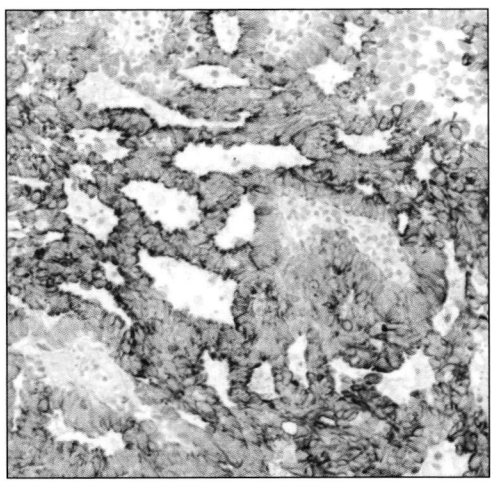

(Left) Nuclear immunoreactivity for CDX-2 may be seen in primary bladder adenocarcinoma but is not present as frequently as in colorectal adenocarcinoma. There may be complete immunophenotypic overlap between these 2 lesions. *(Right)* Primary adenocarcinoma of the urinary bladder may have a complete enteric immunophenotype with strong and diffuse CK20 expression. CK7 reactivity is more variable.

INVASIVE ADENOCARCINOMA

Differential Diagnosis

(Left) Prostatic adenocarcinoma with secondary involvement of the bladder may have a gland-forming pattern that mimics a primary adenocarcinoma. In comparison to vesical adenocarcinomas, prostatic carcinoma has more rounded monomorphic nuclei. *(Right)* Prostatic ductal adenocarcinomas typically involve the lumen of the prostatic urethra and may extend superiorly to involve the bladder. The columnar cells of ductal carcinoma more closely mimic enteric-type vesical adenocarcinoma.

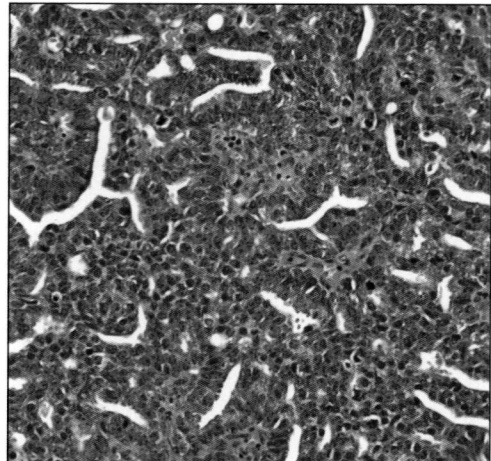
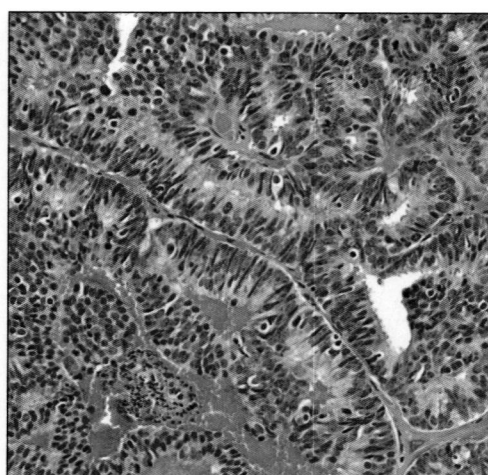

(Left) Immunoreactivity for PSA is useful in the distinction of prostatic adenocarcinoma with secondary involvement of the bladder from a primary vesical adenocarcinoma. For primary vesical adenocarcinomas, there is no specific marker that indicates origin from the bladder. *(Right)* Urachal adenocarcinomas are indistinguishable from primary vesical adenocarcinoma. The presence of a muscularis propria based tumor in the dome and absence of surface lesions favors a urachal primary.

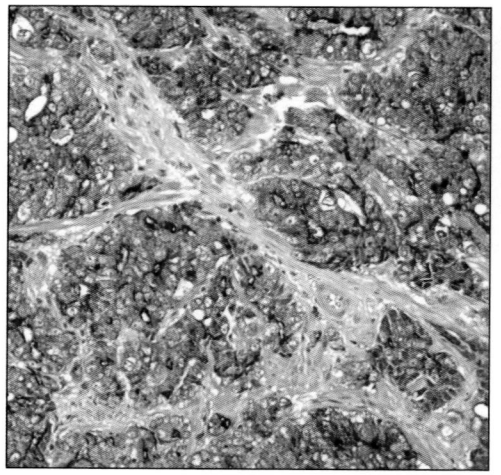
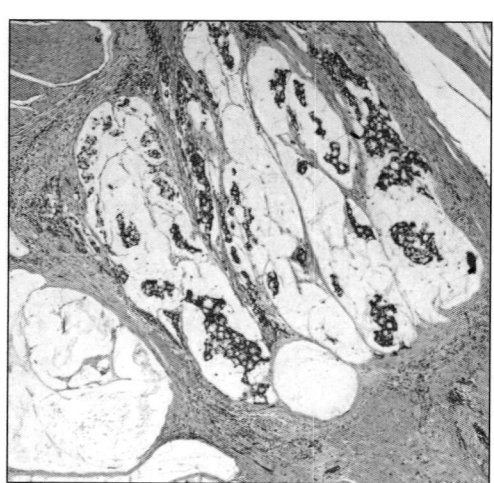

(Left) Urachal adenocarcinomas, such as this mucinous adenocarcinoma, must be distinguished from vesical adenocarcinoma by the location in the dome. Close clinical and radiographic correlation is essential to confirm the tumor's exact anatomic location. *(Right)* Urachal adenocarcinoma is seen with enteric morphologic appearance. The entire range of primary mucosal-based vesical adenocarcinoma histology may also be seen in urachal adenocarcinomas.

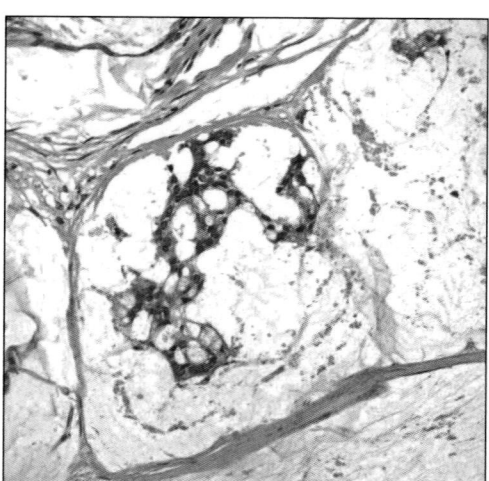
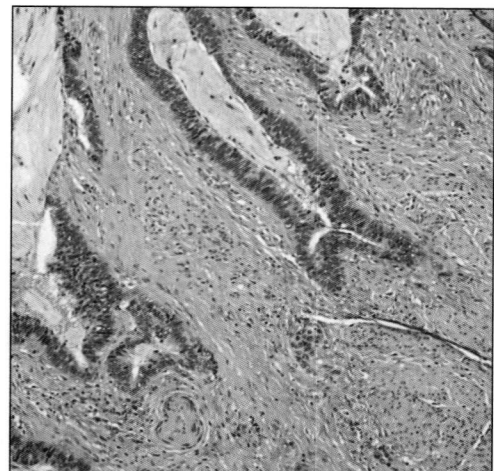

INVASIVE ADENOCARCINOMA

Differential Diagnosis

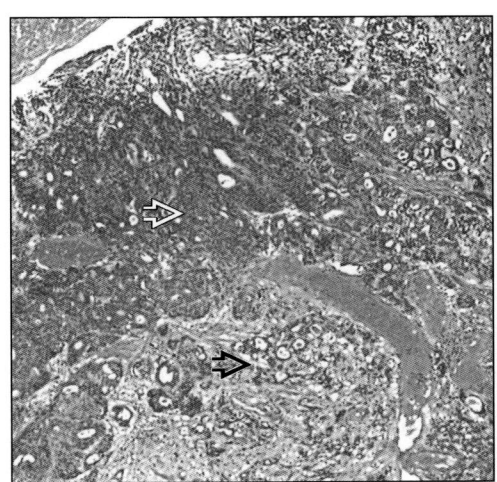

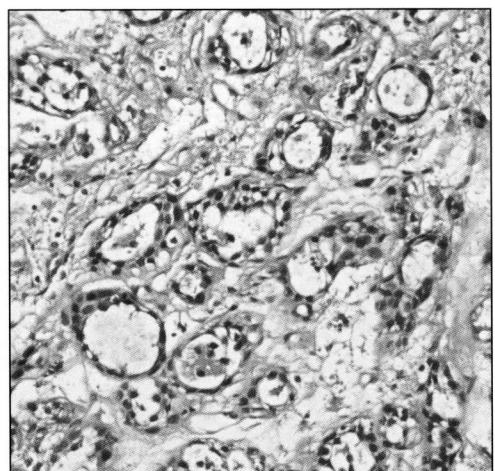

(Left) This example of invasive urothelial carcinoma with small tubular differentiation highlights the dimorphic appearance with an admixture of both typical urothelial carcinoma ⇒ and distinct tubules ⇉. (Right) The bland cytologic features of the tubular pattern in invasive urothelial carcinoma may closely mimic a benign lesion, but obvious invasion into the lamina propria or deeper is characteristic.

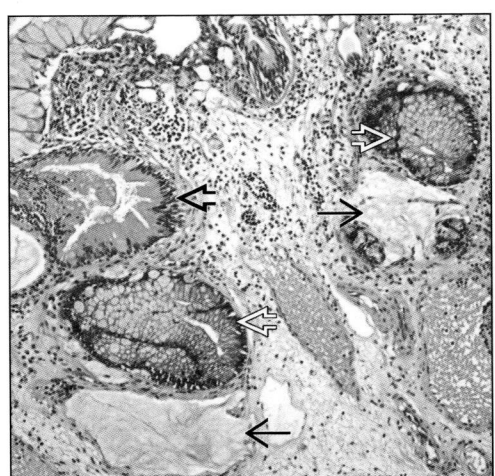

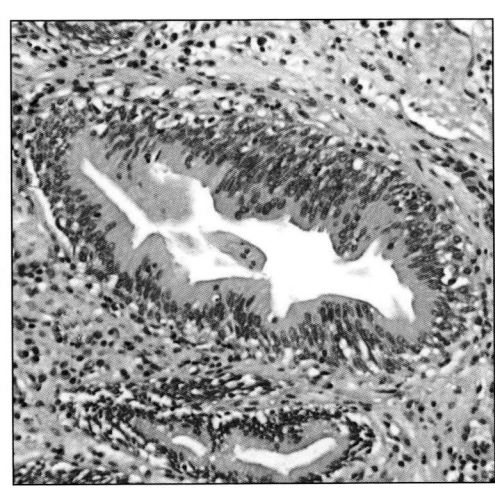

(Left) Cystitis glandularis with intestinal metaplasia may mimic adenocarcinoma in some cases. Some glands have prominent luminal cytoplasm ⇉ and others show extensive goblet cell metaplasia ⇒. Mucin extravasation may be present and is occasionally extensive ⇒. (Right) The cells of cystitis glandularis are cytologically benign. Cystitis glandularis is also confined to the superficial lamina propria, another distinctive feature. Adenocarcinomas usually have significant atypia.

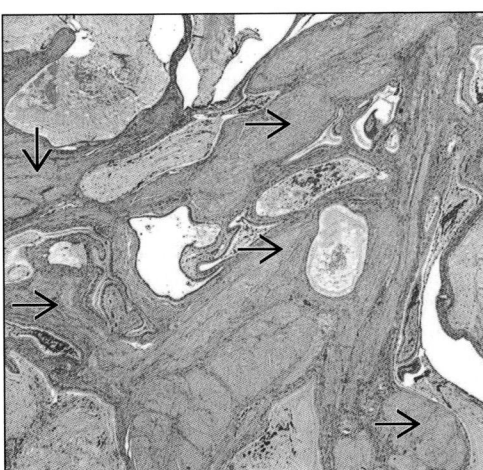

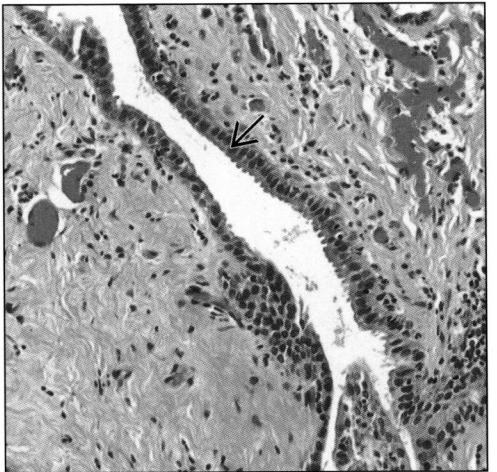

(Left) Lesions in the spectrum of müllerianosis may also enter the differential diagnosis of adenocarcinoma because of the presence of glands deep within the bladder wall, including the muscularis propria ⇒. (Right) Endocervicosis containing glands are comprised of cytologically bland cuboidal cells ⇒. Invasive adenocarcinomas have a greater degree of cytologic atypia with nucleomegaly and irregular nuclear chromatin, and they are typically associated with a stromal reaction.

CLEAR CELL ADENOCARCINOMA

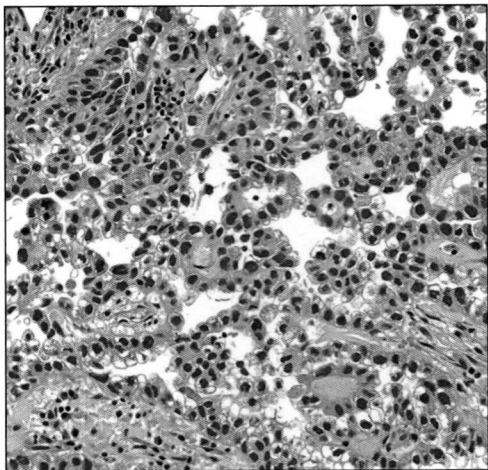

Clear cell adenocarcinoma of the bladder is characterized by papillary architecture with cuboidal lining cells showing clear to eosinophilic cytoplasm and multiple areas with a "hobnail" arrangement.

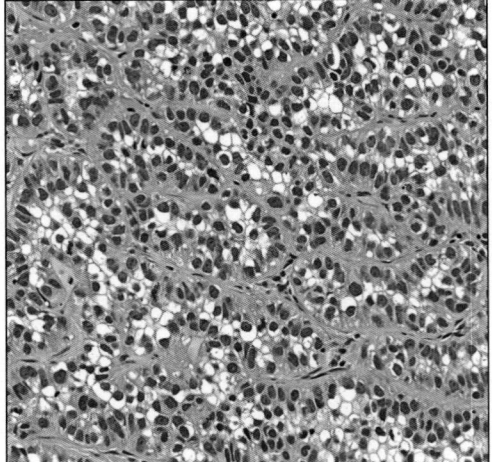

This classic clear cell adenocarcinoma has interconnecting glandular spaces with marked nuclear atypia, prominent clear cytoplasm, and hyalinized fibrovascular septae.

TERMINOLOGY

Abbreviations
- Clear cell adenocarcinoma (CCC)

Synonyms
- Mesonephric adenocarcinoma

Definitions
- Distinct morphologic variant of bladder adenocarcinoma
  - Identical to Müllerian-type clear cell adenocarcinoma of female genital tract

ETIOLOGY/PATHOGENESIS

Urothelial Origin
- Some cases arise in background of typical urothelial carcinoma
  - Represents alternative differentiation

Müllerian Origin
- Subset of CCC in females arise in association with endometriosis or ectopic Müllerian glands

Unknown
- In many cases, origin cannot be determined
  - No immunohistochemical stains aid in this determination

CLINICAL ISSUES

Epidemiology
- Incidence
  - Extremely rare
- Age
  - Wide age range (22-83 years)
- Gender
  - Female predominance

Presentation
- Hematuria and dysuria

Prognosis
- Stage dependent
  - Deeply invasive CCC is highly aggressive
  - Noninvasive exophytic tumors may have long-term survival

MACROSCOPIC FEATURES

General Features
- Papillary &/or polypoid mass
- Rarely ulcerative

MICROSCOPIC PATHOLOGY

Histologic Features
- Mixed tubulocystic, papillary, and solid/diffuse patterns
- Tumor cells typically range from flat to cuboidal
- Neoplastic cells may have clear to eosinophilic cytoplasm
- Papillae may have densely hyalinized cores
- "Hobnail" arrangement of cells may be seen
- Cytologic atypia is usually moderate to severe
- Mitotic figures are frequent
- Level of cytologic atypia may be heterogeneous
  - Foci may closely resemble nephrogenic adenoma
- Typically have obvious invasion
- Associated myxoid stroma is also common

Predominant Pattern/Injury Type
- Neoplastic

Predominant Cell/Compartment Type
- Glandular

CLEAR CELL ADENOCARCINOMA

Key Facts

Etiology/Pathogenesis
- Some cases arise in background of typical urothelial carcinoma
- Subset of CCC in females arise in association with endometriosis or ectopic Müllerian glands

Clinical Issues
- Extremely rare
- Female predominance
- Hematuria and dysuria
- Deeply invasive CCC is highly aggressive

Microscopic Pathology
- Mixed tubulocystic, papillary, and solid/diffuse patterns
- Tumor cells typically range from flat to cuboidal
- Mixed clear and eosinophilic cytoplasm

- "Hobnail" arrangement of cells can be seen
- Papillae may have densely hyalinized cores
- Cytologic atypia usually moderate to severe
- Mitotic figures are frequent

Ancillary Tests
- Positive for CK7, CEA, and CA125; occasionally for CK20
- Also express pax-8 and AMACR

Top Differential Diagnoses
- Nephrogenic adenoma
- Secondary involvement (direct extension) from gynecologic tract CCC
- Urothelial carcinoma with clear cytoplasm
- Urothelial carcinoma with glandular differentiation
- Renal cell carcinoma

ANCILLARY TESTS

Immunohistochemistry
- Usually positive for CK7, CEA, and CA125
  - Occasionally positive for CK20
- No immunoreactivity for PSA, ER, or PR
- Also expresses pax-2, pax-8, and AMACR
- Frequently shows nuclear p53 expression

DIFFERENTIAL DIAGNOSIS

Nephrogenic Adenoma
- Low-power architecture may be identical to CCC
  - Mixed tubulocystic and papillary
  - Solid, diffuse pattern rare but well described
- Nucleoli may be present
  - Lacks significant nuclear pleomorphism
- Noninvasive
- Mitotic figures very rare or absent
- Also expresses pax-2 and pax-8

Secondary Involvement (Direct Extension) from Gynecologic Tract CCC
- Morphologically identical to bladder CCC
- In females, gynecologic origin must be excluded clinically
  - Imaging studies
  - Clinical examination

Urothelial Carcinoma with Clear Cytoplasm
- Cytoplasmic clearing is typically focal
  - Adjacent typical invasive urothelial carcinoma is usually present
- Does not show mixed papillary, tubular, and cystic patterns typical of CCC
- Contains cytoplasmic glycogen

Papillary Adenocarcinoma In Situ (Urothelial Carcinoma with Glandular Differentiation)
- Papillary architecture may mimic CCC
- Neoplastic cells are columnar

Renal Cell Carcinoma
- Associated renal mass
  - Metastatic renal cell carcinoma almost invariably has obvious mass radiographically
- Typically lack mixed clear cell and papillary pattern
- "Hobnail" architecture not seen
- Expression of pax-8/pax-2 in both renal cell carcinoma and CCC may be pitfall

DIAGNOSTIC CHECKLIST

Clinically Relevant Pathologic Features
- Extent of invasion is key prognostic feature

Pathologic Interpretation Pearls
- CCC should be considered when considering large nephrogenic adenoma
  - Significant morphologic overlap

SELECTED REFERENCES

1. Tong GX et al: Expression of PAX8 in nephrogenic adenoma and clear cell adenocarcinoma of the lower urinary tract: evidence of related histogenesis?. Am J Surg Pathol. 32(9):1380-7, 2008
2. Oliva E et al: Clear cell carcinoma of the urinary bladder: a report and comparison of four tumors of mullerian origin and nine of probable urothelial origin with discussion of histogenesis and diagnostic problems. Am J Surg Pathol. 26(2):190-7, 2002
3. Gilcrease MZ et al: Clear cell adenocarcinoma and nephrogenic adenoma of the urethra and urinary bladder: a histopathologic and immunohistochemical comparison. Hum Pathol. 29(12):1451-6, 1998
4. Young RH et al: Clear cell adenocarcinoma of the bladder and urethra. A report of three cases and review of the literature. Am J Surg Pathol. 9(11):816-26, 1985

Microscopic Features

(Left) The dense stromal hyalinization present between nests of tumor cells and the abundant clear cytoplasm are typical features of clear cell adenocarcinoma. *(Right)* This clear cell adenocarcinoma has interconnecting tubules lined by neoplastic cells with a "hobnail" appearance. This example shows subtle, yet distinct variation in nuclear size, a feature that greatly aids in the distinction from nephrogenic adenoma.

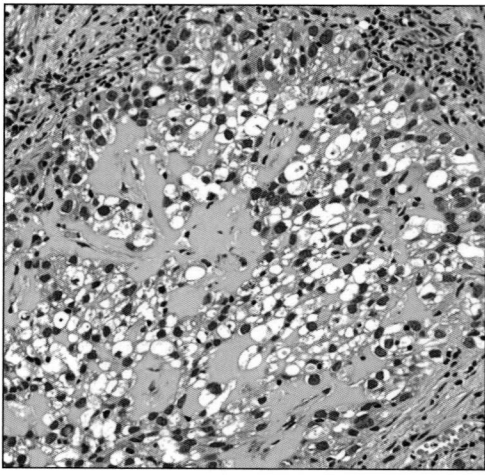
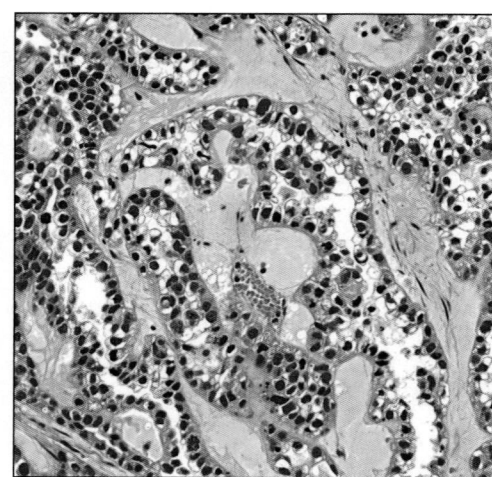

(Left) Mitotic figures ⇨ are variable in clear cell adenocarcinoma but should be easily identifiable. This feature is also helpful in the distinction from nephrogenic adenoma. *(Right)* Some examples of clear cell adenocarcinoma have a predominant exophytic papillary appearance that may mimic nephrogenic adenoma. The papillae are lined by a single layer of cuboidal cells, a feature distinct from typical papillary urothelial carcinoma.

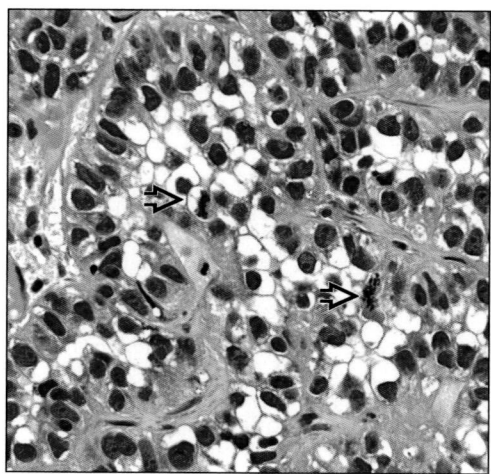
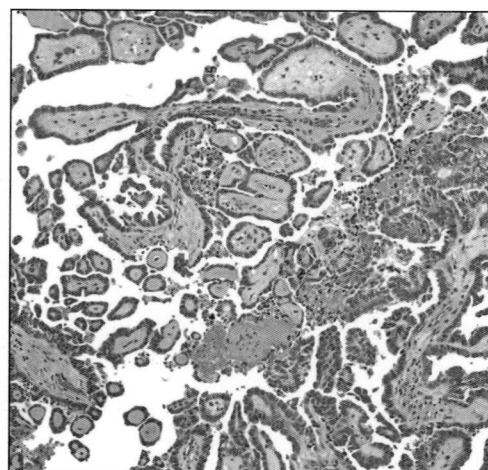

(Left) This example of clear cell adenocarcinoma with a papillary growth pattern shows prominent epithelial tufting. There is subtle stalk invasion ⇨ that, when present, is diagnostic of adenocarcinoma. *(Right)* The degree of cytologic atypia may be very heterogeneous within a given clear cell adenocarcinoma. This papillary focus is relatively bland, which may lead to confusion with nephrogenic adenoma. Areas with more typical cytologic features of carcinoma should be sought.

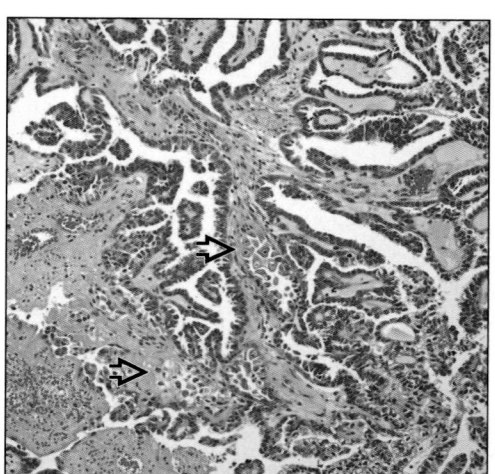
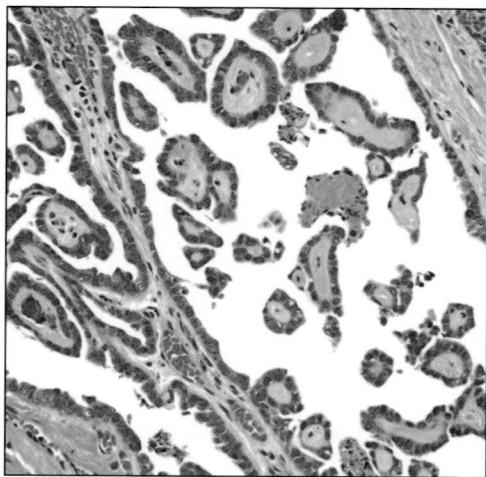

CLEAR CELL ADENOCARCINOMA

Microscopic Features

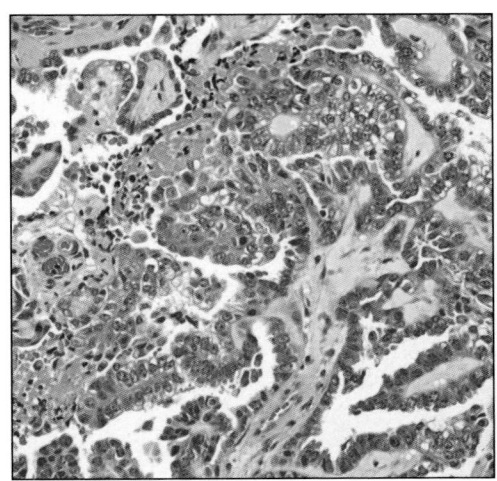

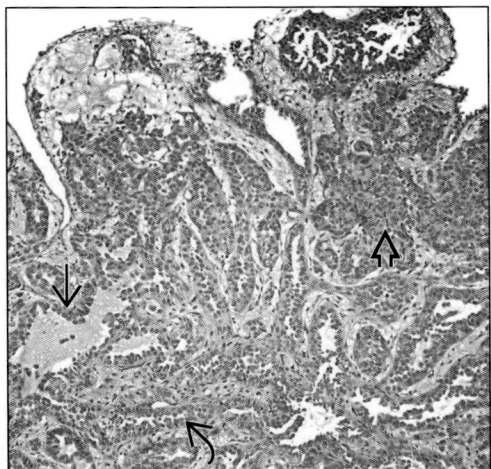

(Left) High-power examination of this clear cell adenocarcinoma shows the typical degree marked nuclear atypia with nucleomegaly, some degree of nuclear pleomorphism, and prominent macronucleoli. *(Right)* Multiple admixed architectural growth patterns are common in clear cell adenocarcinoma of the bladder. On this low-power field, there are cystic ➡, tubular ➡, and solid ▶ components.

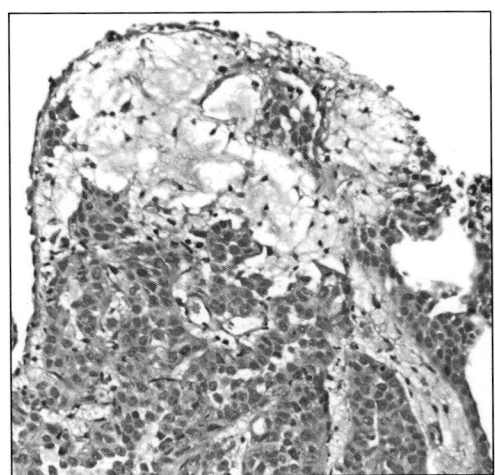

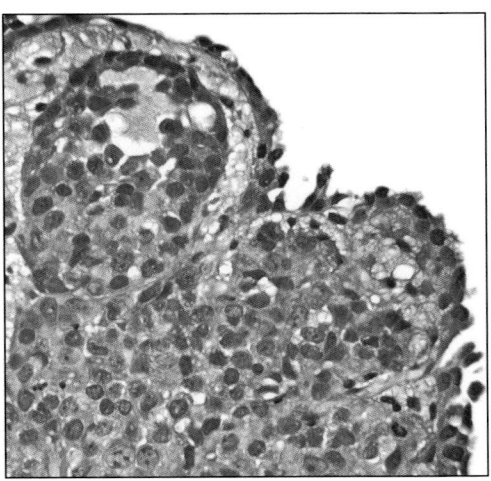

(Left) Clear cell adenocarcinoma may show a tubular pattern with solid intraluminal growth, and occasionally, the neoplastic cells have a more eosinophilic cytoplasm. *(Right)* The foci of solid intratubular growth may mimic a poorly differentiated urothelial carcinoma, especially if the cytoplasm is more eosinophilic as in this example. Identification of more characteristic patterns of clear cell adenocarcinoma is helpful.

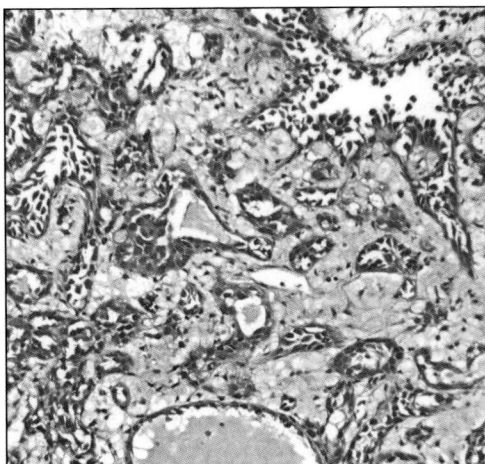

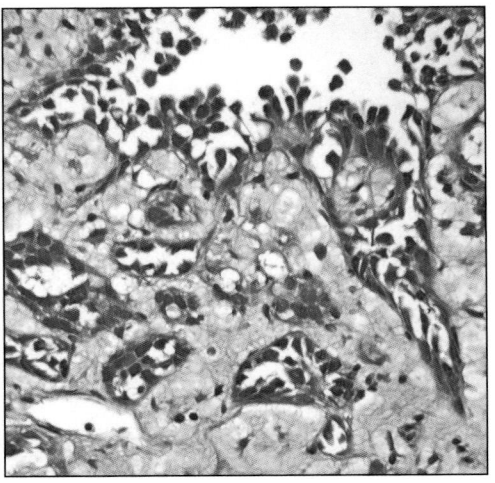

(Left) A low-power photomicrograph shows clear cell adenocarcinoma with a classic tubulocystic pattern. The lining neoplastic cells have a striking "hobnail" appearance in this example. There is also associated myxoid stroma, which is a common finding. *(Right)* This high-power photomicrograph of the tubulocystic growth pattern highlights this typical "hobnail" arrangement of the neoplastic cells in clear cell adenocarcinoma.

CLEAR CELL ADENOCARCINOMA

Microscopic Features

(Left) This example of clear cell adenocarcinoma has dilated tubulocystic foci with very bland cytologic features. This pattern could cause diagnostic confusion with a cystic nephrogenic adenoma or other benign glandular lesion. *(Right)* In this clear cell adenocarcinoma, a morphologically subtle tubulocystic pattern in the lower right ⊡ merges into a more obviously malignant pattern in the upper left ⊡. This degree of intratumoral heterogeneity is not uncommon.

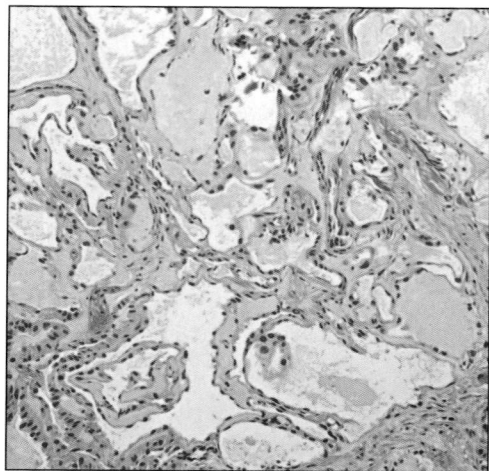 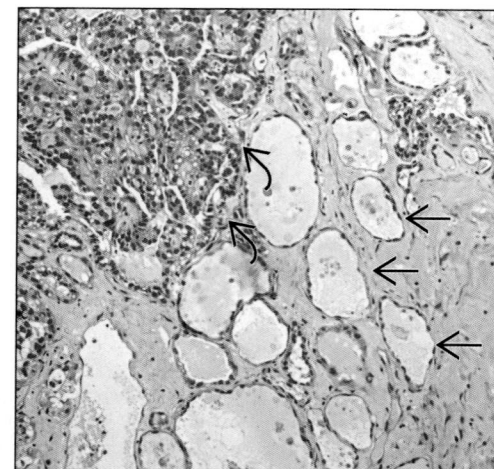

(Left) Tubulocystic patterns of clear cell adenocarcinoma may mimic direct extension from other anatomically adjacent adenocarcinomas. This example does not have a striking "hobnail" arrangement of the neoplastic cells, and cytoplasmic clearing is not a prominent feature in this example. *(Right)* The round nuclear contours are typical of clear cell adenocarcinoma and contrast with the columnar cells present in many other adenocarcinomas.

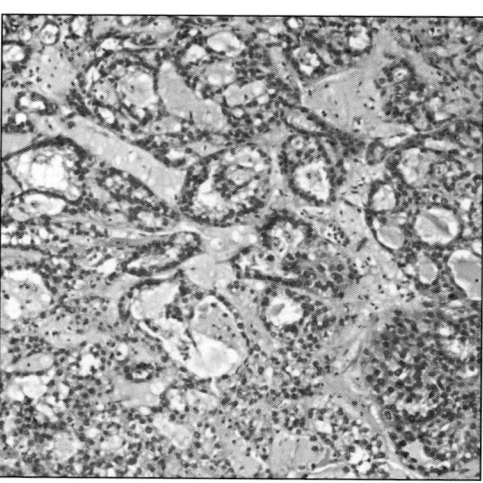 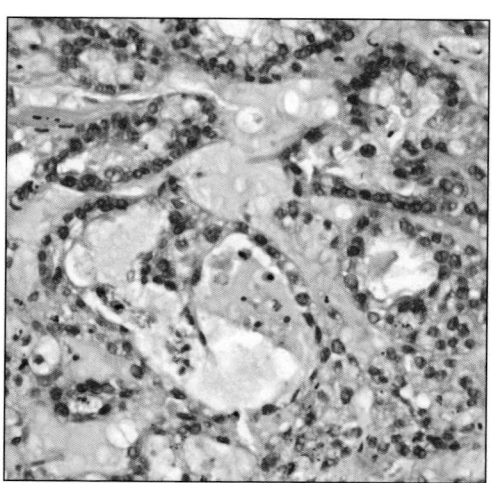

(Left) Solid growth may also be seen in clear cell adenocarcinoma of the urinary bladder, which may mimic other poorly differentiated carcinomas, including renal cell carcinoma. *(Right)* This high-power photomicrograph shows areas of solid growth in clear cell adenocarcinoma of the urinary bladder. The small rim of clear cytoplasm, the rounded nuclei, and the prominent nucleoli are typical of this tumor.

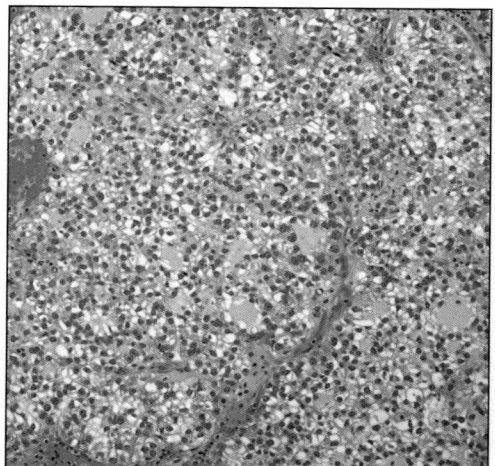 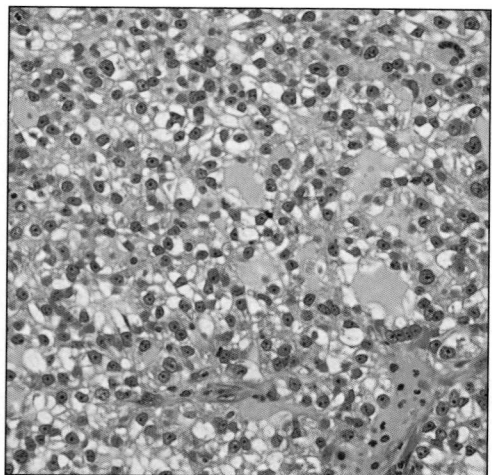

CLEAR CELL ADENOCARCINOMA

Differential Diagnosis

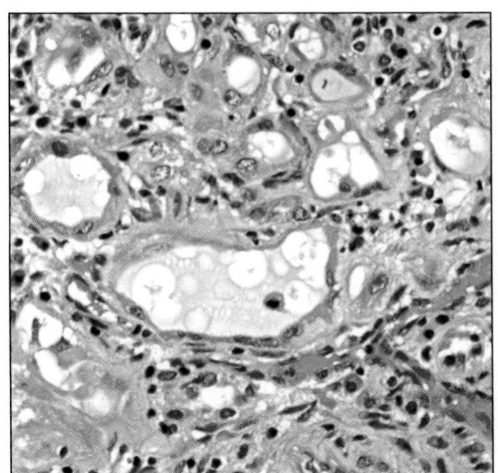

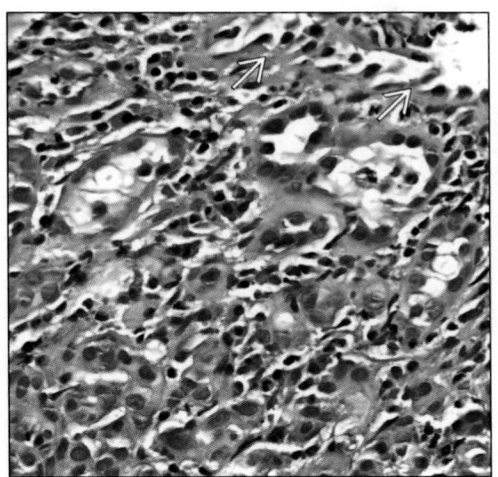

(Left) *Nephrogenic adenoma, shown here, may cause diagnostic confusion with clear cell carcinoma. The lack of significant cytologic atypia and the flattened lining epithelium are characteristic of nephrogenic adenoma.* *(Right)* *Rare examples of nephrogenic adenoma may have "hobnail" architecture* ⮕*, as this example shows. Other patterns of more typical nephrogenic adenoma are usually present, and mitotic figures are usually absent.*

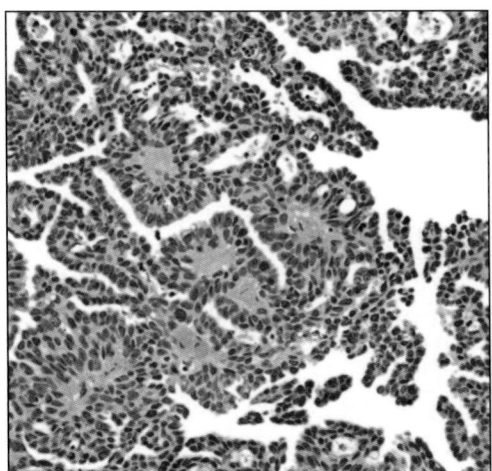

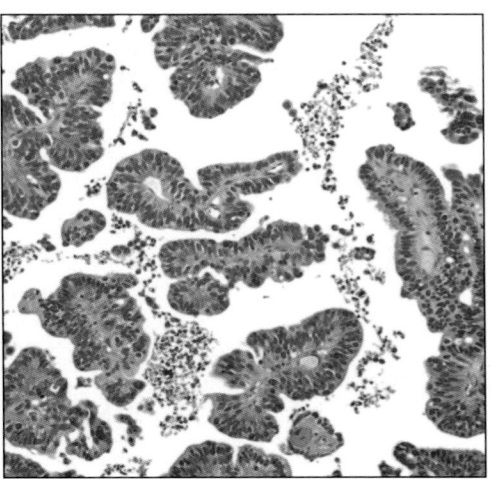

(Left) *This papillary lesion has been described as papillary adenocarcinoma in situ and urothelial carcinoma with glandular/villoglandular differentiation. The thin papillae may suggest clear cell adenocarcinoma.* *(Right)* *Papillary adenocarcinoma in situ (urothelial carcinoma with glandular differentiation) has a columnar lining epithelium that is distinct from clear cell carcinoma. In addition, the papillary cores are not typically hyalinized.*

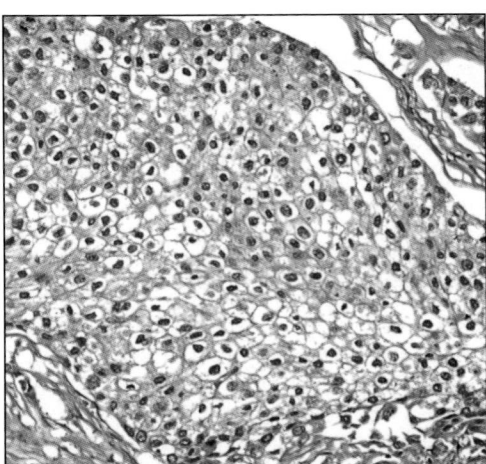

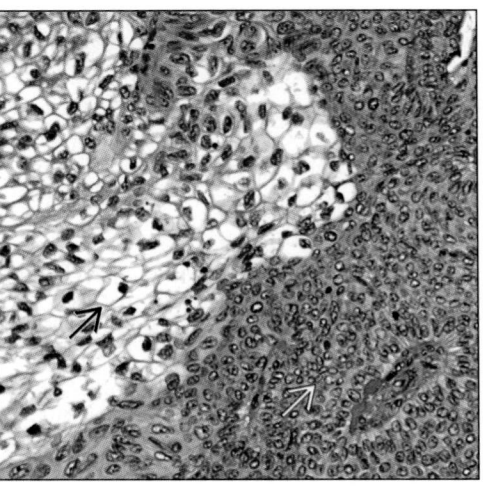

(Left) *Rare urothelial carcinomas contain abundant intracytoplasmic glycogen that imparts a clear appearance. This is typically focal and should be distinguished from clear cell carcinoma.* *(Right)* *This urothelial carcinoma shows an abrupt transition from typical morphology* ⮕ *to areas with prominent clear glycogenated cytoplasm* ⮕*. The focality of this glycogen-rich appearance is typical and is distinct from clear cell carcinoma.*

URACHAL ADENOCARCINOMA

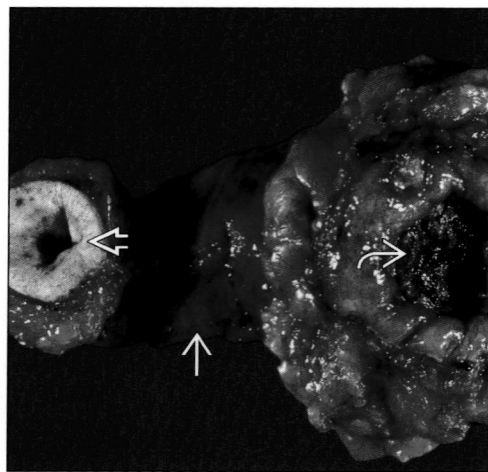

This specimen includes a partial cystectomy with ulcerative tumor ⇗, the urachal tract ➡, and umbilectomy ⬌. This is the typical surgery required for urachal carcinomas.

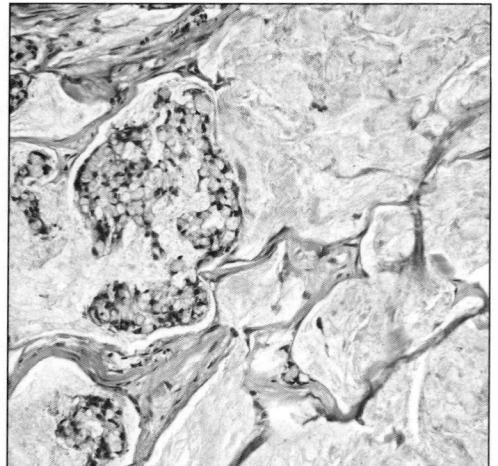

Mucinous adenocarcinoma may arise within urachal remnants at the dome of the bladder. Correlation with clinical/imaging evaluation is critical to establish a urachal origin.

TERMINOLOGY

Definitions
- Primary carcinoma of any morphologic subtype originating from urachus and fulfilling following criteria
  - Tumor primarily located in dome of bladder
  - Epicenter of mass is in wall (muscularis propria) of bladder
  - Absence of surface intestinal metaplasia or precursor lesions
  - Absence of adenocarcinoma elsewhere

ETIOLOGY/PATHOGENESIS

Developmental Anomaly
- Urachal remnants
  - May undergo malignant transformation

CLINICAL ISSUES

Epidemiology
- Incidence
  - Rare
- Age
  - 5th and 6th decades
- Gender
  - More common in men (M:F = 2:1)

Site
- Dome of bladder
  - Anatomic location of urachus
    - Refining feature of urachal origin
- Intramural bladder

Presentation
- Hematuria is most common symptom
- Irritative bladder symptoms, such as voiding difficulties

- Mass lesion
- Mucusuria seen rarely

Treatment
- Partial or radical cystectomy, usually with umbilectomy, is treatment of choice
- Adjuvant therapy depends on stage
  - Chemotherapy
  - Radiotherapy

Prognosis
- Poor prognosis
  - Usually diagnosed at advanced stage
  - 5-year survival rate reported from 25-61%

IMAGE FINDINGS

CT Findings
- Thickened bladder dome
  - May extend along urachus to umbilicus

MACROSCOPIC FEATURES

General Features
- Mucosa is intact in early stages
  - Becomes ulcerated as tumor grows endophytically
- Mass localized to dome of bladder

MICROSCOPIC PATHOLOGY

Histologic Features
- Malignant epithelial neoplasm of diverse morphology
  - Adenocarcinoma or urothelial, squamous, and other rarer carcinomas
    - Enteric, mucinous, signet ring, or mixed histology adenocarcinoma
  - Low-grade mucinous neoplasm
    - Identical to appendiceal primaries
    - May be associated with pseudomyxoma peritonei

URACHAL ADENOCARCINOMA

Key Facts

Terminology
- Primary carcinoma of any morphologic subtype originating from urachus

Clinical Issues
- Very rare
- Hematuria is most common symptom
- Mucusuria rarely seen
- Partial or radical cystectomy, usually with umbilectomy, is treatment of choice
- Prognosis is variable

Macroscopic Features
- Mucosa is intact in early stages

Microscopic Pathology
- Malignant epithelial neoplasm of diverse morphology
  - Enteric
  - Mucinous
  - Signet ring cell
  - Low-grade mucinous neoplasm
- Presence of urachal remnants offer important clue of urachal origin

Top Differential Diagnoses
- Primary adenocarcinoma of urinary bladder
- Colonic adenocarcinoma (or other secondary adenocarcinoma)
- Invasive urothelial carcinoma with glandular differentiation

Diagnostic Checklist
- Urachal carcinoma is clinicopathologic diagnosis
- Recognition of urachal carcinoma is important
  - Different surgical approach than bladder primary

- Presence of urachal remnants offer important clue to urachal origin

ANCILLARY TESTS

Immunohistochemistry
- Urachal carcinomas may have some differences in immunophenotype compared to colonic primary carcinomas
  - CK7 and CK20 are positive in urachal carcinomas
    - CK7 expression is more frequent than colorectal carcinomas
  - Do not express nuclear β-catenin (in contrast to colon)
    - Most specific marker in distinction from colorectal primaries
  - CDX-2 may be expressed by enteric and nonenteric urachal carcinomas
  - Reg4 is more commonly expressed in urachal primaries, compared to enteric-type colon primaries

DIFFERENTIAL DIAGNOSIS

Primary Adenocarcinoma of Urinary Bladder
- May have associated adenocarcinoma in situ in surrounding urothelial mucosa
- Usually based in posterior wall or trigone
- Requires close clinical and imaging correlation

Colonic Adenocarcinoma (or Other Secondary Adenocarcinoma)
- Radiographic location is critical
  - Not typically based in dome
  - Adherent bowel may be seen
- Colonoscopy may be necessary in difficult cases
- Other primary carcinomas may also directly invade bladder
  - Gynecologic tract
    - Endometrial, ovarian, or cervical carcinomas most common
  - Prostatic
    - More monomorphic nuclei with prominent nucleoli
    - Expresses PSA &/or PAP by immunohistochemistry

Invasive Urothelial Carcinoma with Glandular Differentiation
- Usually located in trigone or posterior wall
- Typical urothelial carcinoma may be seen
  - Adjacent urothelial carcinoma in situ
  - Papillary urothelial neoplasm in bladder

DIAGNOSTIC CHECKLIST

Clinically Relevant Pathologic Features
- Positive surgical margin is important negative prognostic factor
- Determining urachal origin at initial diagnosis is often important
  - Different surgical approach
    - Partial cystectomy with umbilectomy

Pathologic Interpretation Pearls
- Urachal carcinoma is clinicopathologic diagnosis
  - Must be located in bladder dome
  - Adenocarcinoma elsewhere must be ruled out

SELECTED REFERENCES

1. Gopalan A et al: Urachal carcinoma: a clinicopathologic analysis of 24 cases with outcome correlation. Am J Surg Pathol. 33(5):659-68, 2009
2. Herr HW et al: Urachal carcinoma: contemporary surgical outcomes. J Urol. 178(1):74-8; discussion 78, 2007
3. Molina JR et al: Predictors of survival from urachal cancer: a Mayo Clinic study of 49 cases. Cancer. 110(11):2434-40, 2007
4. Ashley RA et al: Urachal carcinoma: clinicopathologic features and long-term outcomes of an aggressive malignancy. Cancer. 107(4):712-20, 2006

URACHAL ADENOCARCINOMA

Microscopic Features

(Left) *Mucinous adenocarcinoma, characterized by aggregates of neoplastic cells with malignant cytology floating in pools of extracellular mucin, is a common morphologic subtype of primary urachal adenocarcinoma.* *(Right)* *Some urachal adenocarcinomas have an enteric phenotype that is morphologically indistinguishable from primary vesical adenocarcinoma and secondary involvement from a colorectal adenocarcinoma. In males, prostatic ductal adenocarcinoma is also in the differential.*

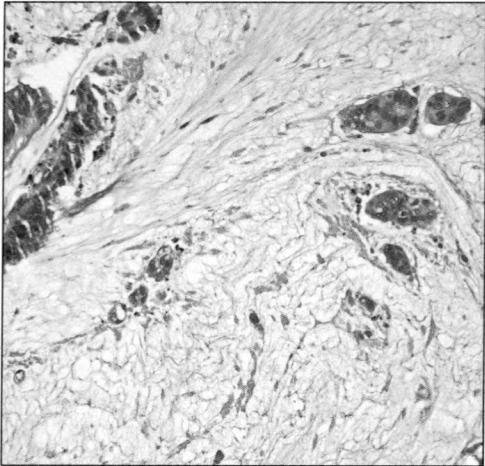
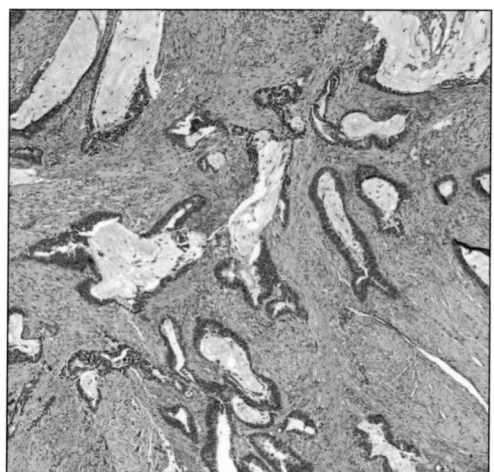

(Left) *Urachal enteric-type adenocarcinoma may have central "dirty" necrosis similar to metastatic colorectal carcinoma. A primary muscularis propria-based tumor with minimal or secondary involvement of lamina propria or mucosa should raise the possibility of a urachal primary.* *(Right)* *Cribriforming architectural growth patterns may mimic endometrioid-type endometrial or colorectal adenocarcinoma. Clinical/radiographic correlation is essential to rule out colorectal or uterine origin.*

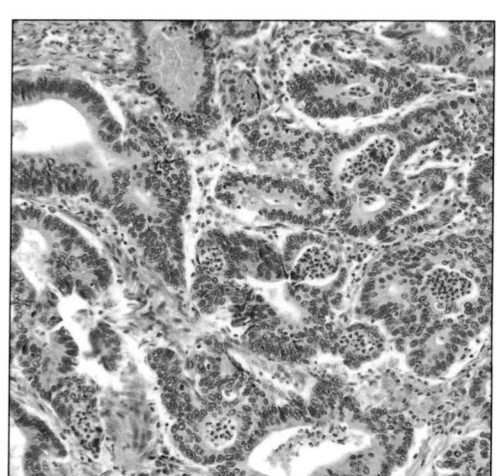
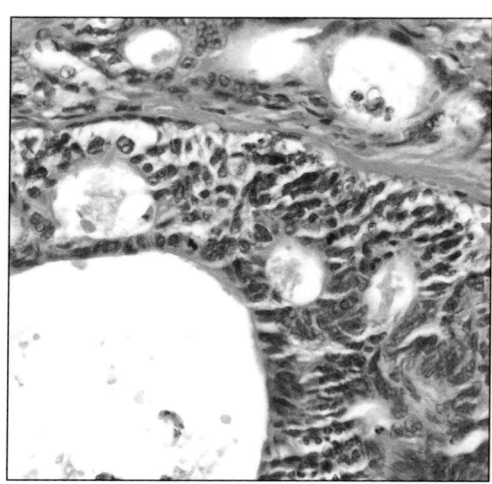

(Left) *Rare primary urachal carcinomas may have adenosquamous differentiation. This example shows squamous morular differentiation* ⇨ *admixed with an enteric-type gland forming adenocarcinoma.* *(Right)* *The morphologic spectrum of primary urachal carcinomas also includes invasive adenocarcinomas of no special type (not otherwise specified), as seen in this example. Such cases could morphologically mimic metastases from a variety of anatomic locations.*

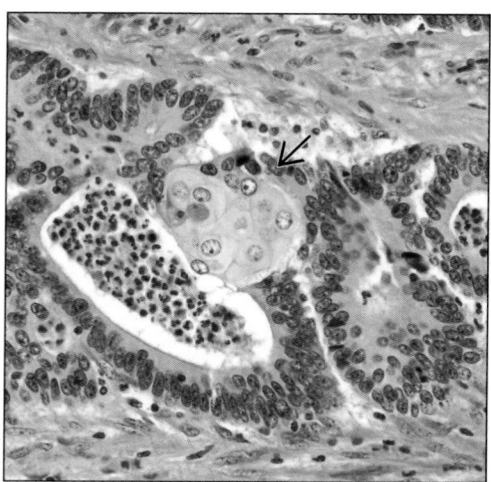
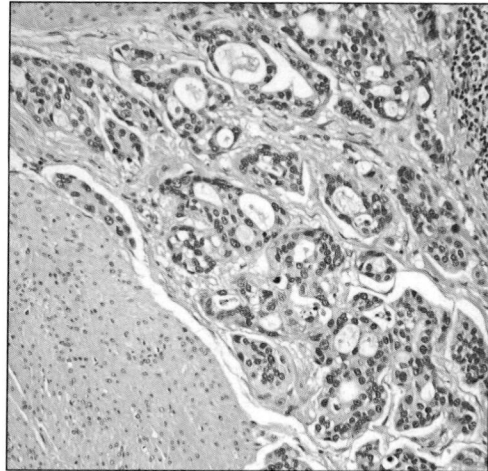

Microscopic Features

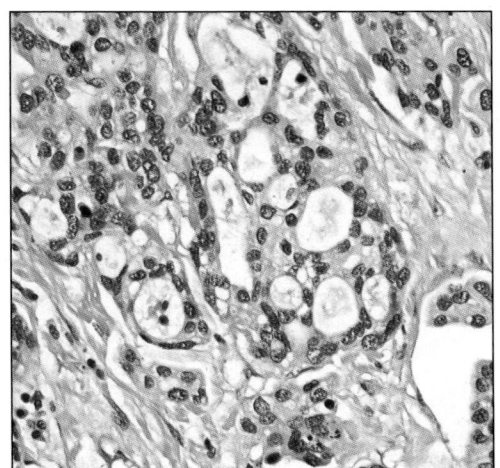

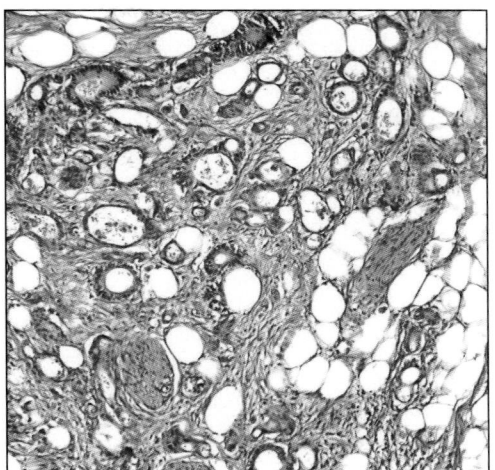

(Left) This primary urachal adenocarcinoma, not otherwise specified, may mimic a wide spectrum of adenocarcinomas from various other primary anatomic sites. Recognition of the anatomic location in the dome of the bladder is critical to determining the site of origin for appropriate surgical intervention. (Right) This urachal adenocarcinoma presented at a high stage with extensive permeation of surrounding adipose tissue. Urachal carcinomas are invariably high stage at presentation.

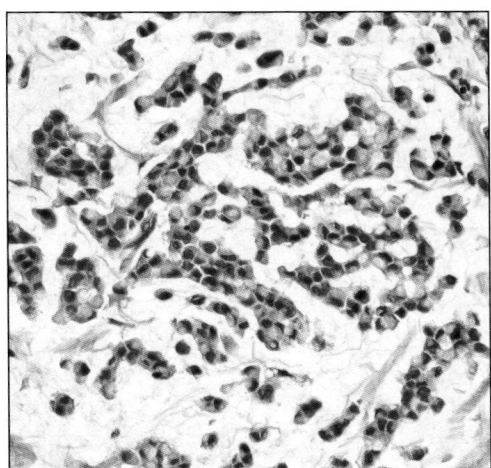

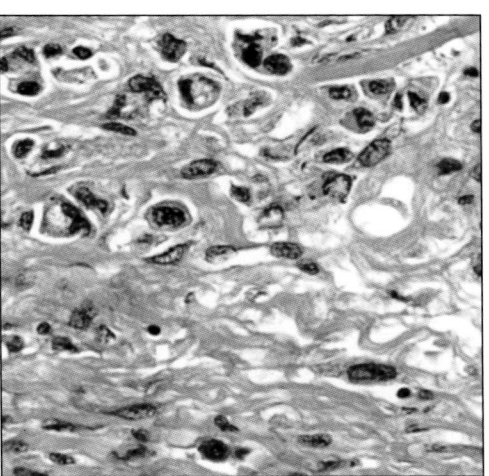

(Left) The morphologic spectrum of primary urachal adenocarcinoma includes signet ring cell adenocarcinoma. This urachal adenocarcinoma is comprised of extensive extracellular mucin and has a signet ring cell phenotype. (Right) This example of signet ring adenocarcinoma is more pleomorphic than is typically seen. Both primary vesical adenocarcinoma and metastatic adenocarcinoma, such as gastric, must be excluded clinically/ radiographically.

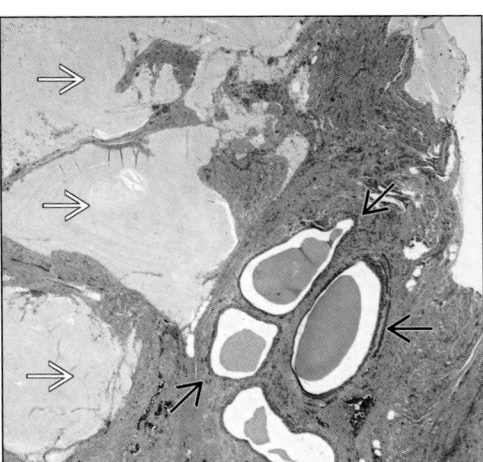

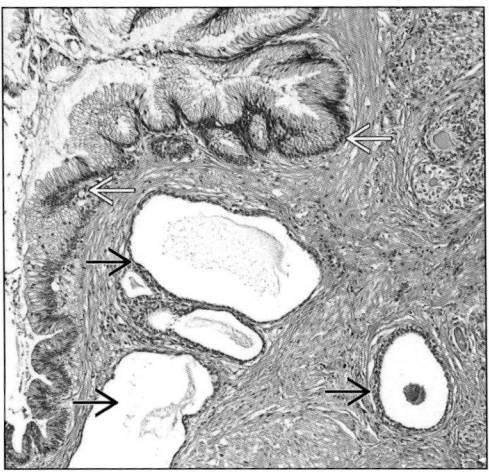

(Left) This low-grade epithelial mucinous neoplasm (mucinous epithelial neoplasm of low malignant potential) has extensive mucin extravasation ⇒ and adjacent urachal remnants ⇨, a clue to urachal origin. (Right) This low-grade mucinous epithelial neoplasm (mucinous epithelial neoplasm of low malignant potential) of the urachus ⇒ directly abuts a focus of urachal remnants ⇨. Extensive sampling is necessary to exclude an invasive component.

URACHAL ADENOCARCINOMA

Microscopic Features

(Left) Low-grade urachal mucinous epithelial neoplasms (mucinous tumors of low malignant potential), like those of the appendix, have relatively bland mucinous epithelium with loss of mucin and nuclear stratification. *(Right)* This example of a low-grade mucinous epithelial neoplasm (mucinous tumor of low malignant potential) of the urachus has abundant epithelium floating in extracellular mucin. Typical mucinous adenocarcinoma has a greater degree of cytologic atypia.

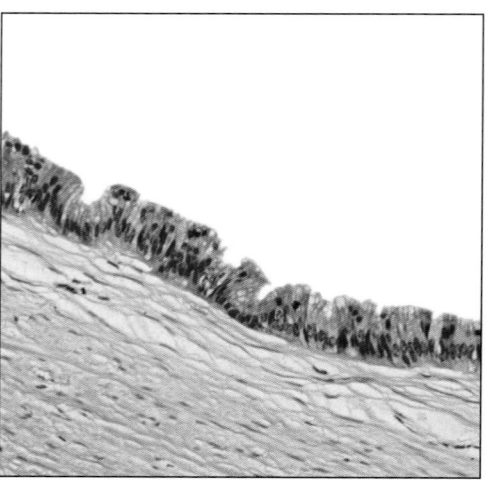 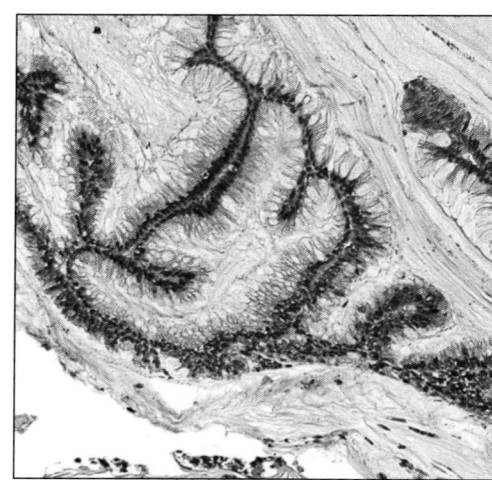

(Left) Primary urachal carcinomas may also have purely urothelial differentiation. This example of a carcinoma arising in the urachus is a noninvasive high-grade papillary urothelial carcinoma. The distinction from a urinary bladder primary is based entirely on the anatomic location of the tumor. *(Right)* This noninvasive urothelial carcinoma arose in the urachus. Colonization of urachal remnants ➡ similar to involvement of von Brunn nests is seen in this example.

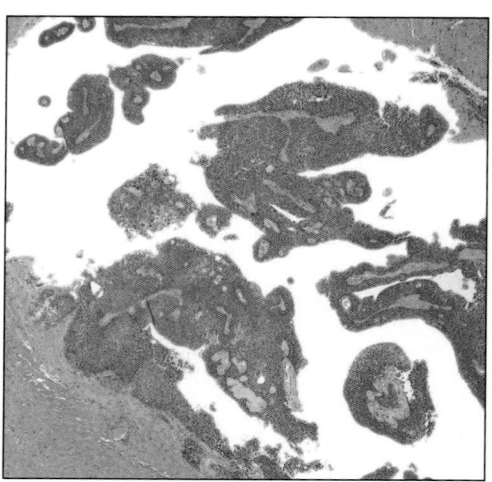 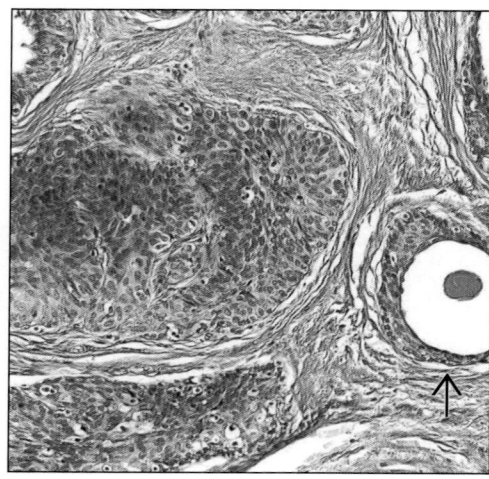

(Left) This primary urachal carcinoma with pure urothelial differentiation has high-grade cytology and lacks gland formation or intracytoplasmic mucin. *(Right)* Immunohistochemistry is usually not helpful in the distinction between urachal and bladder carcinoma. This urachal urothelial carcinoma shows nuclear p63 positivity, as would be expected in urothelial carcinoma arising in any location. Clinicopathologic correlation and absence of surface precursor lesion is necessary.

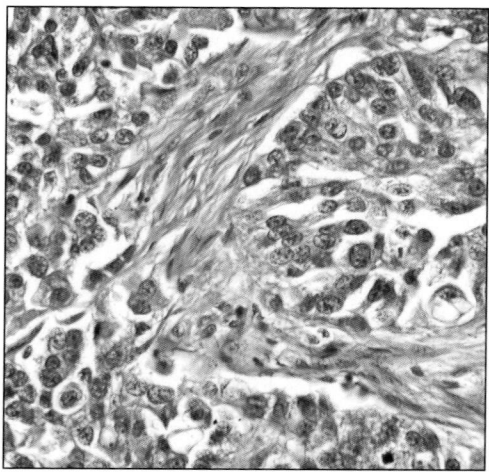 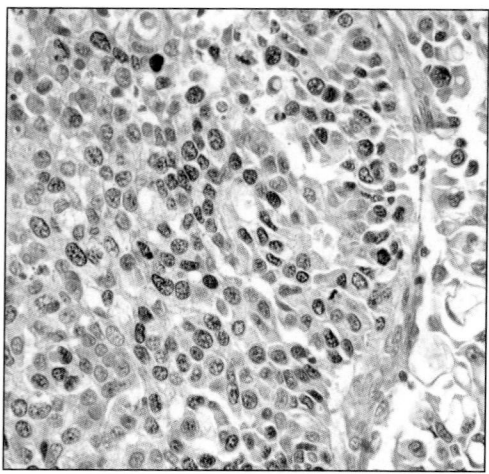

URACHAL ADENOCARCINOMA

Ancillary Techniques

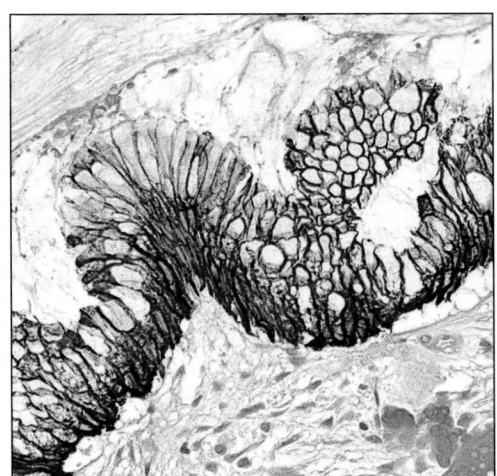

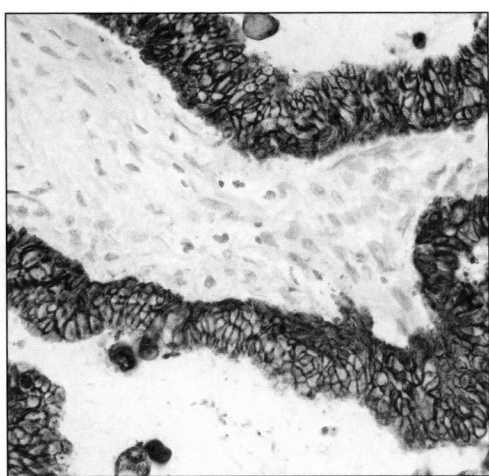

(Left) This mucinous adenocarcinoma of urachal origin shows strong cytoplasmic immunoreactivity for CK20. This finding is not helpful as it is also typically seen in colorectal adenocarcinomas. *(Right)* Urachal adenocarcinoma shows strong cytoplasmic reactivity for CK7. This degree of staining is more common in urachal adenocarcinomas compared to colorectal carcinoma. Immunohistochemistry has a limited role, but β-catenin staining may have value.

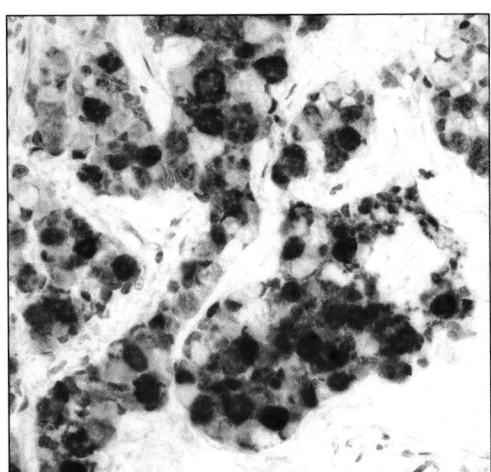

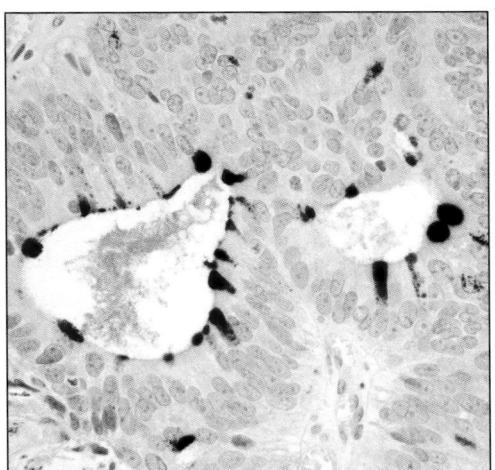

(Left) This urachal carcinoma with a signet ring morphology shows strong immunoreactivity for Reg4, similar to that seen in colorectal signet ring adenocarcinomas. *(Right)* Reg4 immunoreactivity is also seen in this example of an enteric-type adenocarcinoma primary to the urachus. In contrast to signet ring adenocarcinoma of the colon, Reg4 expression is uncommon in enteric-type colorectal carcinomas.

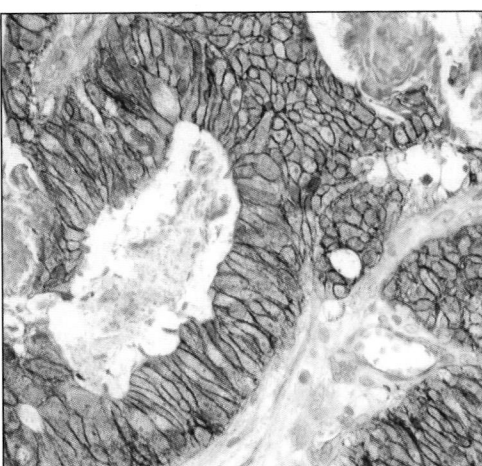

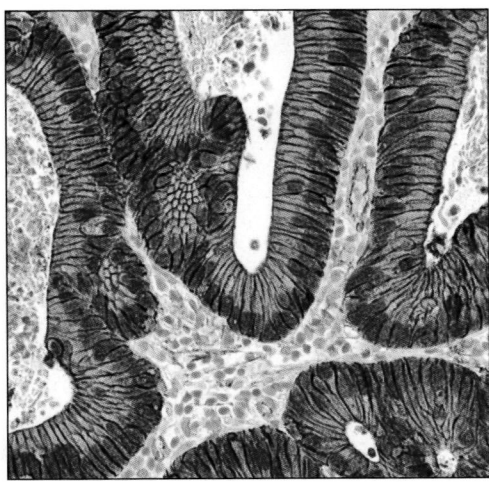

(Left) This primary urachal adenocarcinoma shows membranous immunoreactivity to β-catenin but no nuclear reactivity. Nuclear reactivity appears to be specific to colorectal adenocarcinomas. *(Right)* This example of colonic adenocarcinoma invading the bladder shows strong nuclear immunoreactivity for β-catenin. Nuclear reactivity to β-catenin is specific for colonic primary carcinomas and is not reported in urachal adenocarcinomas.

SQUAMOUS PROLIFERATIONS OTHER THAN CARCINOMA

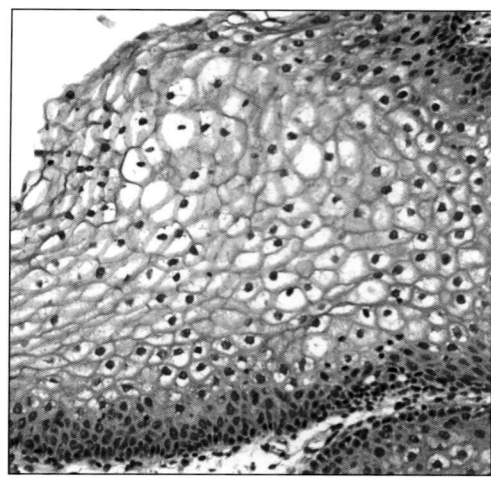

Glycogenated nonkeratinizing squamous mucosa commonly occurs in the trigone and bladder neck of women. This is a normal finding and does not have any pathologic risk for progression to neoplasia.

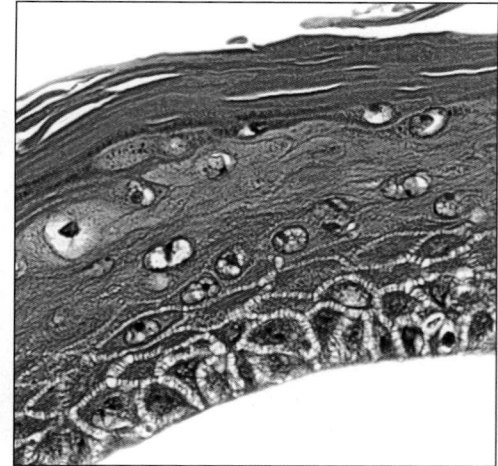

Keratinizing squamous metaplasia may be seen in longstanding inflammatory conditions. This finding should be reported, as it may be associated with risk of obstruction or progression to neoplasia.

TERMINOLOGY

Definitions
- Squamous metaplasia
  - Replacement of urothelium by stratified squamous epithelium
    - Nonkeratinized (except trigone) and keratinized subtypes
- Squamous papilloma
  - Rare benign exophytic papillary squamous neoplasm
    - Unrelated to human papilloma virus (HPV) infection
- Condyloma
  - Exophytic squamous proliferation with HPV viral cytopathic effect
- Squamous hyperplasia, papillary and flat
  - Multiple layers of cytologically bland metaplastic squamous epithelium with flat or papillary architecture

ETIOLOGY/PATHOGENESIS

Environmental Exposure
- Keratinizing squamous metaplasia
  - May be associated with chronic irritation
    - Catheters, stones, parasitic infection

Infectious Agents
- Condyloma of bladder
  - Contains HPV DNA

CLINICAL ISSUES

Epidemiology
- Incidence
  - Isolated urinary tract involvement by condyloma is rare

- Associated urethral, vulvar, vaginal, anal, or perineal condyloma is common
- Age
  - Squamous papilloma
    - Elderly women
  - Condyloma
    - Young sexually active population

Endoscopic Findings
- Squamous metaplasia
  - Pale gray-white with irregular borders, often with surrounding zone of erythema
- Condyloma and squamous papilloma
  - Appear as exophytic polypoid lesions

Prognosis
- Keratinizing squamous metaplasia
  - Risk of malignant transformation to squamous dysplasia/carcinoma
- Condyloma
  - Risk of malignant transformation to squamous dysplasia/carcinoma
- Squamous papilloma
  - Benign clinical course

MICROSCOPIC PATHOLOGY

Squamous Metaplasia
- Nonkeratinizing glycogenated squamous metaplasia, nontrigonal location
  - When it occurs in trigone, it is normal variation and not metaplasia
- Keratinizing squamous metaplasia
  - Hyperkeratotic squamous epithelium lining bladder lumen

Condyloma Acuminatum
- Rarely involves bladder, usually by direct extension from genital lesions
- Resembles condyloma at other sites

SQUAMOUS PROLIFERATIONS OTHER THAN CARCINOMA

Key Facts

Etiology/Pathogenesis
- Keratinizing squamous metaplasia
  - May be associated with chronic irritation
  - Catheters, stones, or parasitic infection
  - Neurogenic bladder
- Condyloma of bladder
  - Contains HPV DNA

Clinical Issues
- Squamous papilloma
  - Elderly women
- Condyloma
  - Young sexually active population

Microscopic Pathology
- Nonkeratinizing glycogenated squamous mucosa
  - Very common in trigone of women
- Normal variation in histology
- Keratinizing squamous metaplasia
  - Hyperkeratotic squamous epithelium lining bladder lumen
- Condyloma
  - Resembles condyloma at other sites
  - Koilocytotic cytologic features
- Squamous papilloma
  - Papillary cores lined by cytologically benign squamous epithelium
  - No viral cytopathic effect is seen

Top Differential Diagnoses
- Squamous dysplasia
- Urothelial carcinoma in situ
- Noninvasive papillary urothelial carcinoma
- Verrucous carcinoma

- Papillary fronds lined by hyperplastic squamous epithelium with koilocytosis
  - Perinuclear halos and hyperchromatic wrinkled nuclei
  - Parakeratosis, hyperkeratosis, and granular layer may be seen

Squamous Papilloma
- Papillary cores lined by cytologically benign squamous epithelium
  - No viral cytopathic effect is seen

Squamous Hyperplasia
- Metaplastic squamous mucosa with increased cell thickness and normal cytology; reactive changes may be present

ANCILLARY TESTS

In Situ Hybridization
- Condyloma is positive for HPV

DIFFERENTIAL DIAGNOSIS

Squamous Dysplasia
- Condyloma may progress to moderate or severe squamous dysplasia
  - Characterized by lack of maturation from basal layer
  - Epithelium becomes colonized by cells with high nuclear to cytoplasmic ratio
  - Mitotic activity may extend to upper levels of epithelium

Urothelial Carcinoma In Situ
- Lacks features of squamous epithelium
  - No keratinization and no intercellular bridges
  - Flat surface with no papillomatous architecture
  - Nuclear membranes are not as irregular as condyloma

Noninvasive Papillary Urothelial Carcinoma
- Papillary urothelial carcinoma has distinct papillary architecture from condyloma
  - Fine papillary cores
  - Longer branching papillae
  - Occasional cases have squamous metaplasia
    - Absence of koilocytes
    - No identifiable HPV by adjunctive studies

Verrucous Carcinoma
- Bland cytology without koilocytic changes
- More striking verrucoid architecture
- Generally larger mass lesion

Radiation Atypia
- Squamoid appearance with multinucleation and cytoplasmic vacuolization may mimic koilocytes
- No history of HPV-related lesions elsewhere
  - Most bladder condylomas have other lesions
- Clinical history of prior radiation therapy

Polyoma Virus
- May have nuclear inclusions in superficial urothelium
- Maintain smooth nuclear membranes
- Immunoreactivity with polyoma virus antibodies

DIAGNOSTIC CHECKLIST

Pathologic Interpretation Pearls
- Presence and extent of keratinizing squamous metaplasia should be reported
- Nonkeratinizing glycogenated squamous epithelium is normal in trigone and bladder neck in women
  - Should not be diagnosed as "squamous metaplasia"

SELECTED REFERENCES
1. Guo CC et al: Noninvasive squamous lesions in the urinary bladder: a clinicopathologic analysis of 29 cases. Am J Surg Pathol. 30(7):883-91, 2006

SQUAMOUS PROLIFERATIONS OTHER THAN CARCINOMA

Condyloma

(Left) At low-power evaluation, condyloma of the urinary bladder, as in other anatomic sites, is characterized by hyperplastic squamous epithelium with a papillomatous architecture ⇒. *(Right)* Even at low-power magnification, enlarged koilocytes may be seen ⇒. Condyloma of the urinary bladder is typically associated with other human papilloma virus-associated lesions, such as perineal squamous dysplasia or urethral condylomas.

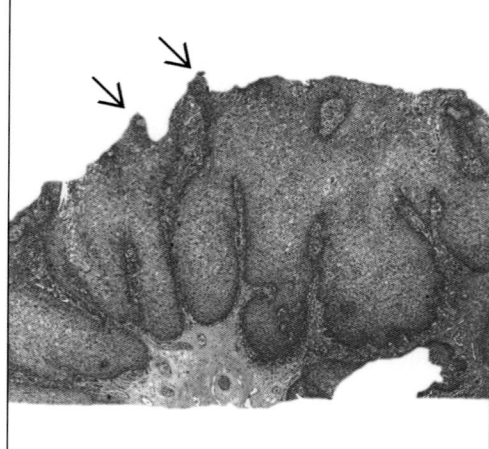
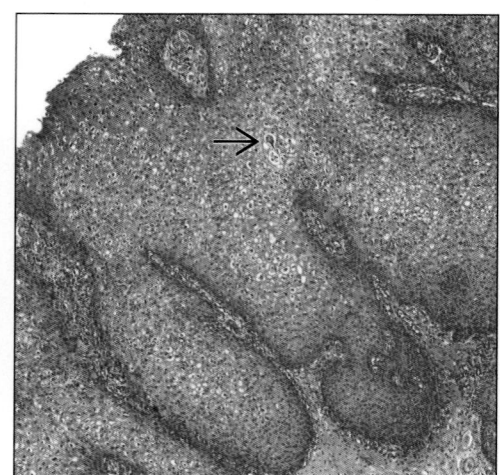

(Left) The degree of viral cytopathic effect in condyloma may vary greatly. In some foci, the perinuclear clearing and nuclear hyperchromasia/membrane irregularity are striking ⇒. Other foci in the same lesion do not show these nuclear changes ⇒. *(Right)* In situ hybridization studies for HPV show diffuse nuclear positivity. This is not usually needed to render a diagnosis of condyloma but demonstrates the viral etiology. This study is negative in a squamous papilloma.

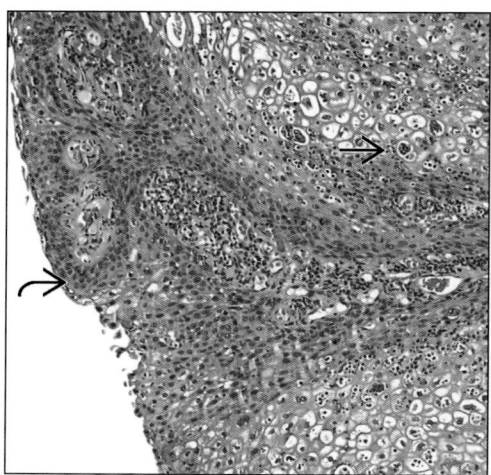
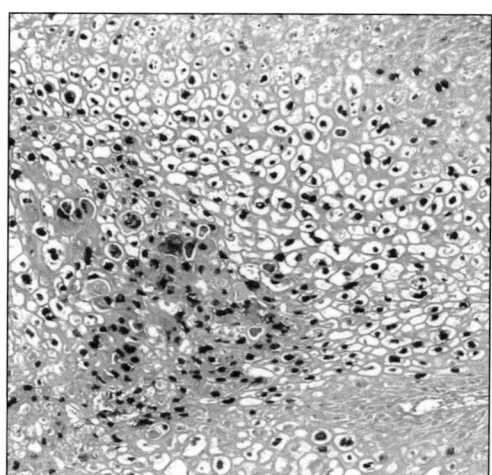

(Left) In squamous papilloma of the bladder, hyperplastic, well-differentiated squamous mucosa shows distinct papillomatosis. The low-power differential diagnoses include condyloma acuminatum and squamous papilloma. *(Right)* High-power evaluation of squamous papilloma shows absence of nuclear atypia and koilocytic change. There is a distinct central vascular core ⇒ surrounded by hyperplastic squamous mucosa. Associated inflammation is usually minimal.

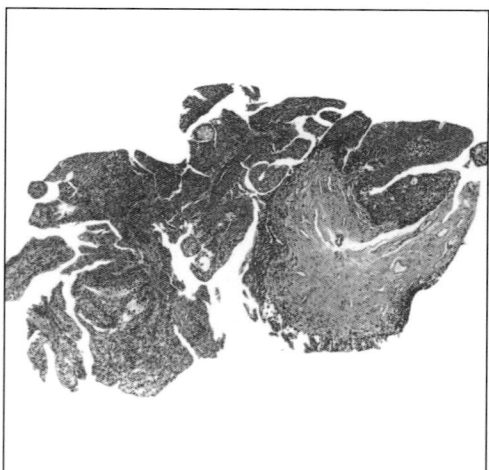
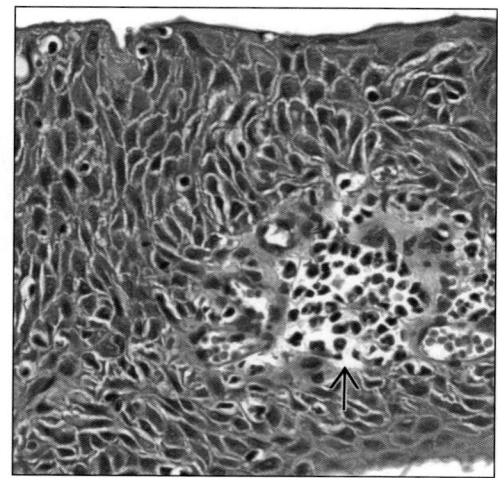

Other Squamous Proliferations

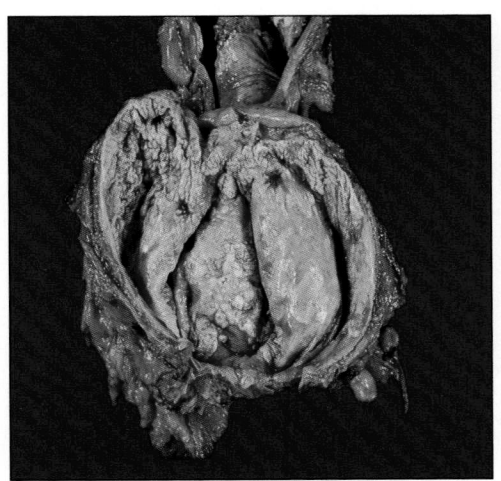

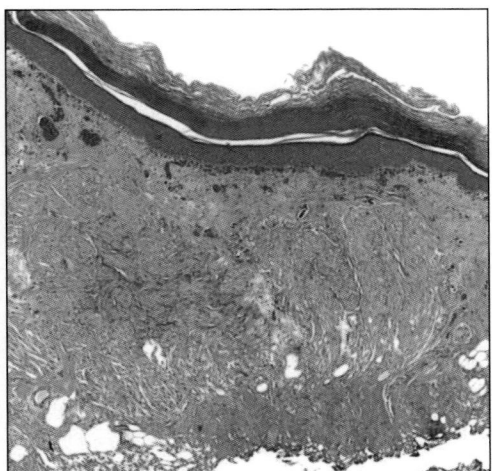

(Left) This radical cystectomy was performed for intractable symptoms secondary to multifocal, widespread keratinizing squamous metaplasia. Different regions showed a spectrum from metaplasia to keratinizing dysplasia. (Right) Keratinizing squamous metaplasia is characterized by hyperkeratosis and parakeratosis without dysplasia. When this is extensive, sampling of multiple areas is key to evaluate for the possibility of in situ neoplasia.

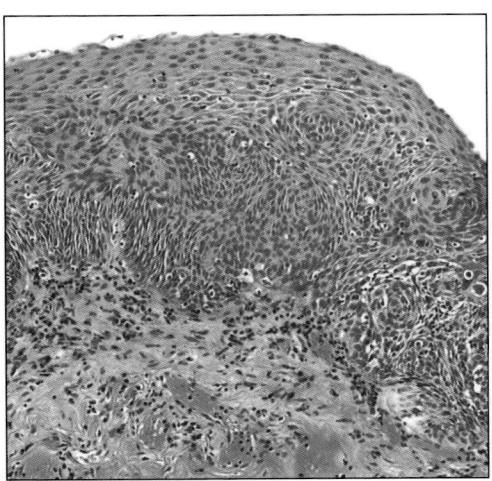

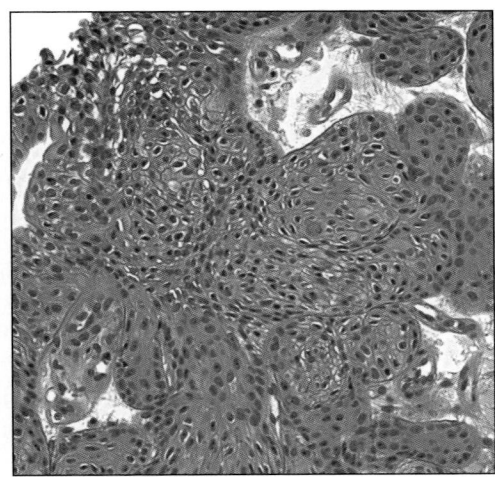

(Left) This hyperplastic squamous mucosa shows reactive squamous changes with accompanying inflammation. Higher power evaluation of cytologic features is necessary to rule out in situ neoplasia. (Right) This focus shows metaplastic squamous changes involving von Brunn nests with focal aberrant keratinization but bland cytology. When florid and associated with inflammation, the superimposed reactive changes may raise concern for neoplasia.

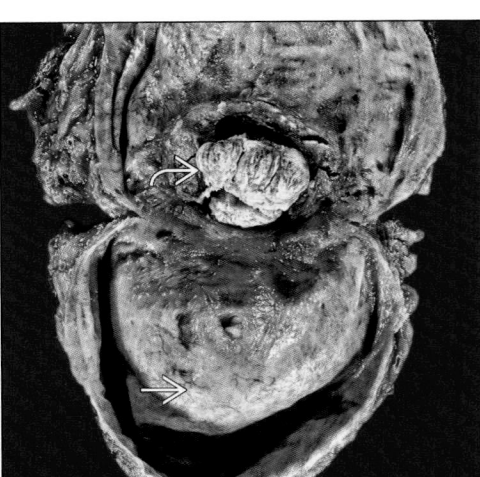

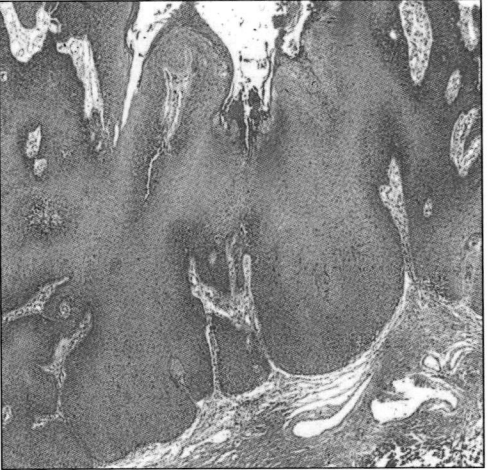

(Left) This cystectomy specimen shows a white, exophytic squamous cell carcinoma ➤ arising in the background of widespread plaque-like keratinizing squamous metaplasia ➤ and keratinizing dysplasia. (Right) Verrucous carcinoma involving the bladder may be confused with squamous papilloma or squamous hyperplasia. The typical large size and the rounded contours at the base of the proliferation, which extend/push into the lamina propria, aid in this distinction.

INVASIVE SQUAMOUS CELL CARCINOMA

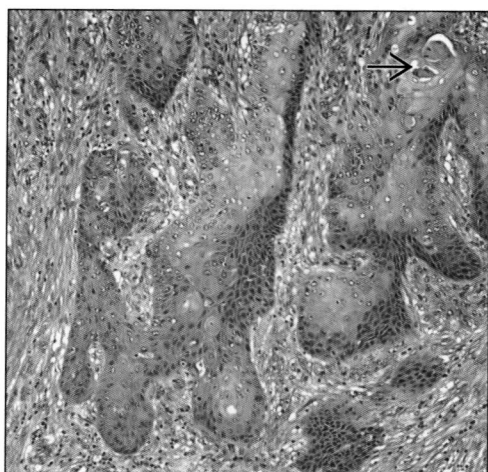

Irregular jagged nests of epithelium with eosinophilic cytoplasm and keratinization ➡ are features of typical/classic invasive squamous cell carcinoma of the urinary bladder.

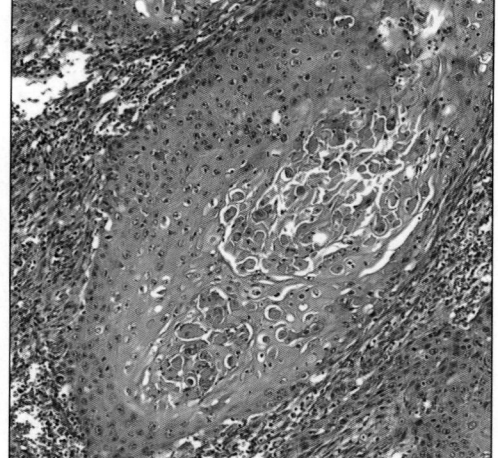

Keratinization is usually obvious in invasive squamous cell carcinoma. By definition, no component of papillary, invasive, or in situ urothelial carcinoma or glandular component is present.

TERMINOLOGY

Abbreviations
- Squamous cell carcinoma (SCC)

Definitions
- Malignant epithelial neoplasm of bladder with pure squamous cell phenotype

ETIOLOGY/PATHOGENESIS

Developmental Anomaly
- Bladder exstrophy

Environmental Exposure
- Associated with tobacco smoking
  - 5x increased risk over nonsmokers

Infectious Agents
- Chronic inflammatory conditions with squamous metaplasia are risk factors
  - Bladder stones
  - Chronic indwelling catheters
  - Neurogenic bladder
  - Prolonged cyclophosphamide treatment
- Strongly associated with schistosomal infection
  - Includes *Schistosoma haematobium* and *Schistosoma mansoni*
  - Common in Egypt and Sudan
  - Verrucous carcinoma is more specifically associated with *Schistosoma* infection
- HPV association is probably very rare
  - May be seen in cases associated with condyloma

CLINICAL ISSUES

Epidemiology
- Incidence

  - Varies by geographic region (incidence higher in areas with endemic schistosomiasis)
    - 5% of bladder tumors in USA
    - 75% in Egypt/Sudan (bladder cancer represents 1/3 of all cancers in Egypt)
  - Verrucous carcinoma of urinary bladder is very rare in USA
    - 3% of bladder cancers in regions of endemic schistosomiasis
- Age
  - Most common in 6th decade
- Gender
  - Male predominance, but lower than in urothelial carcinoma

Presentation
- Hematuria
- Dysuria

Endoscopic Findings
- Large white exophytic mass
- Surface of bladder may show white, plaque-like thickening

Treatment
- Surgical approaches
  - Radical cystectomy is standard therapy
- Adjuvant therapy
  - Often have neoadjuvant or adjuvant radiation
  - Adjuvant chemotherapy is less standardized

Prognosis
- Poor prognosis (nonverrucous SCC)
  - High-stage disease at presentation is common
  - Reported 5-year survival = 7-50%
    - Survival in pT3 disease = 13%
- Pure verrucous carcinoma has favorable prognosis with no metastatic risk

INVASIVE SQUAMOUS CELL CARCINOMA

Key Facts

Terminology
- Malignant epithelial neoplasm of bladder with pure squamous cell phenotype

Etiology/Pathogenesis
- Chronic inflammatory conditions with squamous metaplasia are risk factors
- Strongly associated with *Schistosoma* infection

Clinical Issues
- Varies with geographic region (incidence higher in areas of endemic schistosomiasis)
- Hematuria
- Dysuria
- Radical cystectomy is standard therapy

Microscopic Pathology
- Typical/classic squamous cell carcinoma

- Irregular jagged invasive aggregates distributed randomly in lamina propria
- By definition, no component of urothelial carcinoma is present
- Verrucous carcinoma
  - Verrucous fronds of well-differentiated, acanthotic squamous epithelium with hyperkeratosis
  - Sharp rounded "pushing" base at junction with lamina propria
  - Minimal cytologic atypia
  - Almost exclusively associated with *Schistosoma* infection

Top Differential Diagnoses
- Invasive urothelial carcinoma with squamous differentiation
- Metastatic or secondary squamous cell carcinoma

MACROSCOPIC FEATURES

General Features
- Fungating, tan-white mass
  - Often ulcerated and necrotic
  - Typically large and deeply invasive

MICROSCOPIC PATHOLOGY

Invasive Squamous Cell Carcinoma, Typical/Classic Type
- Irregular jagged invasive aggregates of malignant squamous cells distributed randomly in lamina propria
  - Associated stromal myofibroblastic proliferation common
- Displays range of differentiation
  - Well differentiated: Keratinization, prominent intercellular bridges, and minimal nuclear pleomorphism
  - Poorly differentiated: Marked nuclear pleomorphism and only focal evidence of squamous differentiation
- By definition, no component of urothelial carcinoma or adenocarcinoma is present
  - Includes urothelial carcinoma in situ, papillary urothelial carcinoma, &/or invasive urothelial carcinoma
- Often associated with keratinizing metaplasia and squamous dysplasia

Pure Verrucous Squamous Cell Carcinoma
- Verrucous fronds of well-differentiated, acanthotic squamous epithelium with hyperkeratosis
- Sharp rounded "pushing" base at junction with lamina propria
  - Admixed lymphocytic infiltrate common at base
  - No jagged, irregularly invasive nests (no typical invasive SCC)
- Minimal cytologic atypia

DIFFERENTIAL DIAGNOSIS

Invasive Urothelial Carcinoma with Squamous Differentiation
- Associated component of urothelial carcinoma
  - At least focally

Keratinizing Squamous Metaplasia
- May mimic verrucous carcinoma
  - No deep extension into lamina propria

Condyloma Acuminatum
- Koilocytic atypia is present
- No deep extension into lamina propria

Metastatic or Secondary Squamous Cell Carcinoma
- May be morphologically identical to primary vesical SCC
- Requires close clinical and radiographic correlation
- Background squamous dysplasia argues for primary process

DIAGNOSTIC CHECKLIST

Pathologic Interpretation Pearls
- Carcinoma must be of pure squamous histology to classify as primary SCC

SELECTED REFERENCES

1. Lagwinski N et al: Squamous cell carcinoma of the bladder: a clinicopathologic analysis of 45 cases. Am J Surg Pathol. 31(12):1777-87, 2007
2. Rundle JS et al: Squamous cell carcinoma of bladder. A review of 114 patients. Br J Urol. 54(5):522-6, 1982
3. Faysal MH: Squamous cell carcinoma of the bladder. J Urol. 126(5):598-9, 1981
4. Bessette PL et al: A clinicopathologic study of squamous cell carcinoma of the bladder. J Urol. 112(1):66-7, 1974

INVASIVE SQUAMOUS CELL CARCINOMA

Microscopic Features

(Left) Irregularly formed, jagged tongues of neoplastic squamous epithelium extend into the deep lamina propria with associated stromal inflammatory changes in this biopsy specimen of primary squamous cell carcinoma. *(Right)* Obvious keratinization, often with dyskeratosis ⇨, is commonly seen in primary invasive squamous cell carcinoma. These carcinomas are indistinguishable from squamous carcinomas arising in other anatomic sites.

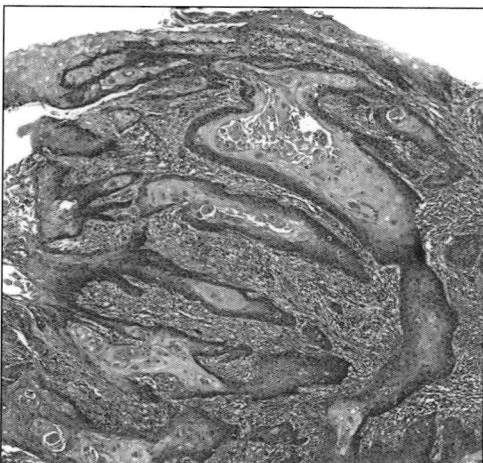
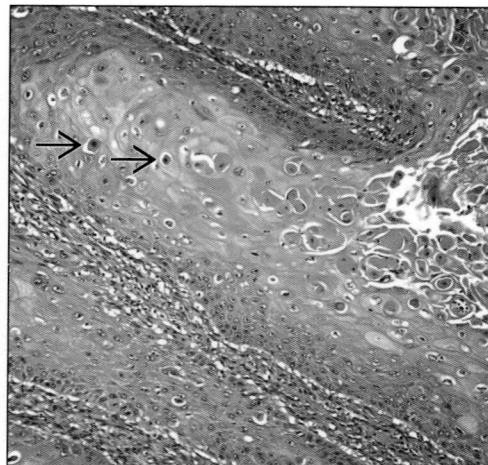

(Left) On low-power evaluation, the jagged outlines of epithelial tongues and associated stromal reaction are diagnostic of invasion in this primary squamous cell carcinoma of the urinary bladder. *(Right)* This primary vesical invasive squamous cell carcinoma has typical features, including irregular nests, stromal reaction, keratin pearl formation ⇨, and dyskeratosis. These features distinguish typical/classic squamous cell carcinoma from verrucous carcinoma.

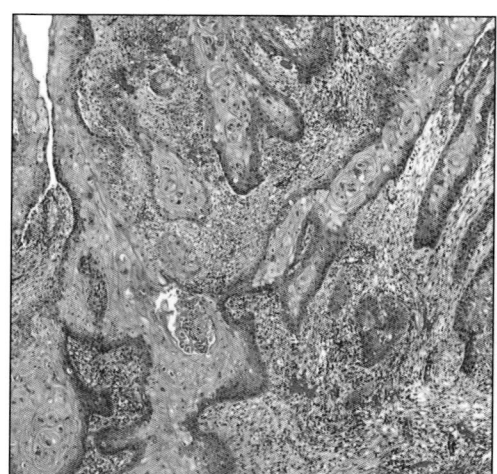
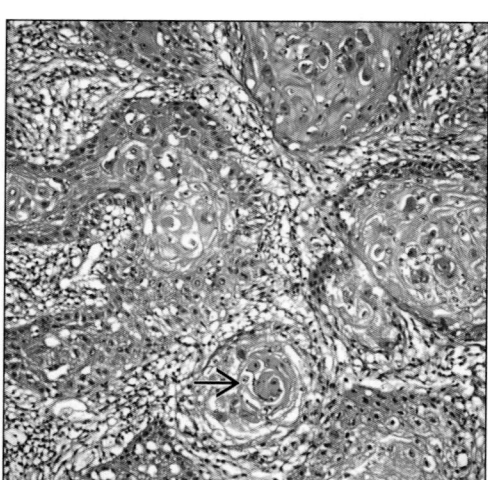

(Left) The jagged irregular nests of invasive SCC are commonly associated with a myofibroblastic proliferation, which, if prominent, may raise the diagnostic possibility of sarcomatoid carcinoma. *(Right)* The spindle cells associated with this SCC are cytologically bland with elongated cytoplasmic processes, features typical of myofibroblasts. In contrast, the spindle cell component of sarcomatoid carcinoma usually has marked nuclear hyperchromasia and obvious pleomorphism.

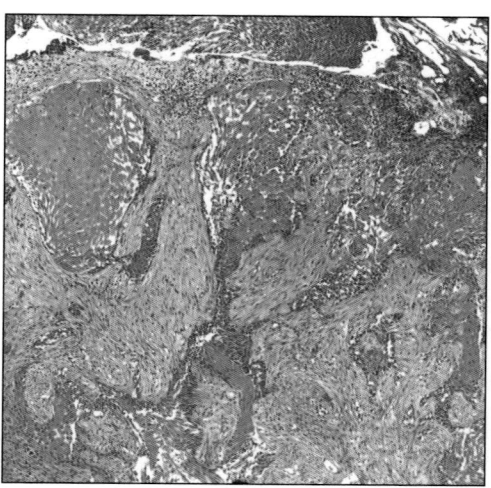
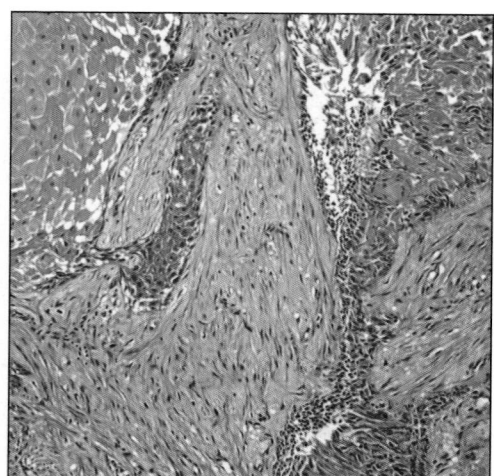

INVASIVE SQUAMOUS CELL CARCINOMA

Microscopic Features

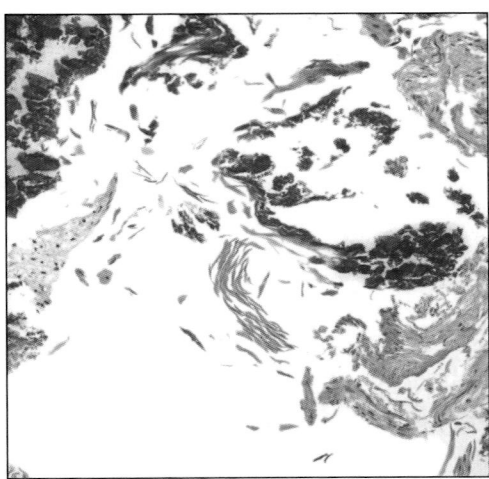
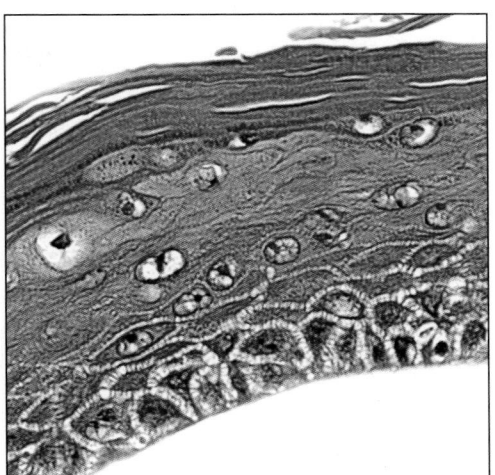

(Left) The presence of calcification and keratin debris should suggest the possibility of an unsampled SCC. Since secondary infection, ulceration, and necrosis are not uncommon with SCC, "encrusted" features may be seen in superficial biopsy specimens. *(Right)* Keratinizing squamous metaplasia is commonly seen in the mucosa surrounding SCC. This is a useful feature in distinguishing primary SCC from urothelial carcinoma with squamous differentiation.

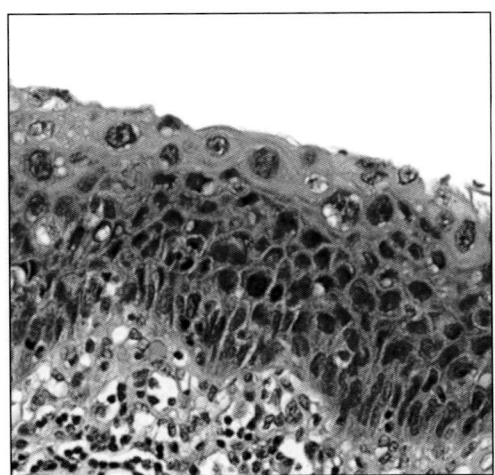
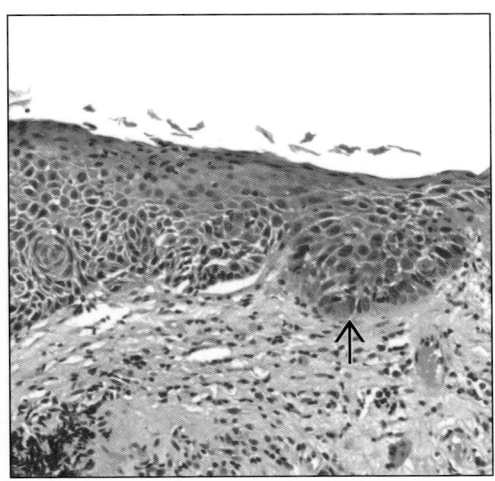

(Left) The background mucosa in SCC may show a spectrum from low-grade dysplasia to squamous carcinoma in situ. Dysplastic changes, including nucleomegaly and hyperchromasia, are seen here. *(Right)* Associated squamous dysplasia may show more subtle "differentiated" type without full-thickness involvement by basaloid cells with high nuclear to cytoplasmic ratio. Note nucleomegaly, hyperchromasia, and mitoses at the base ➡, features of dysplasia.

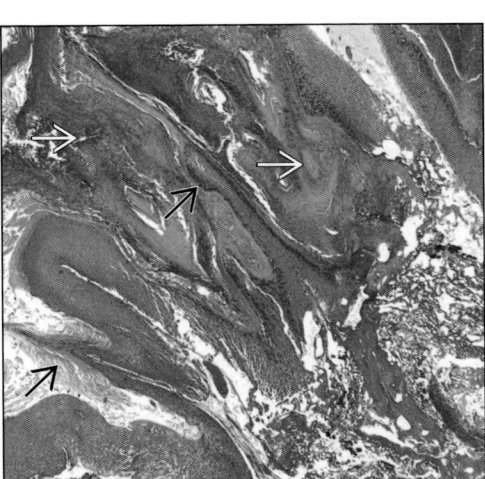
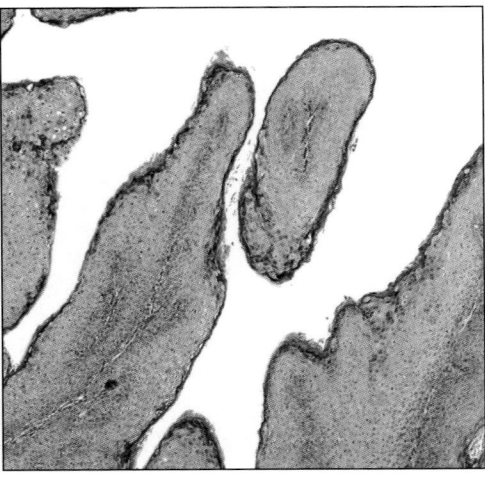

(Left) Long exophytic papillary processes ➡ are typical of verrucous carcinoma and may produce a "warty" appearance. Marked hyperkeratosis may also be seen ➡. *(Right)* The tips of the papillae in this verrucous carcinoma show keratinizing squamous epithelium with bland cytologic features. Hybrid tumors with areas of conventional squamous cell carcinoma may be seen, such that extensive sampling of the gross specimen is essential.

INVASIVE SQUAMOUS CELL CARCINOMA

Microscopic Features

(Left) The round "pushing" base at the deep aspect ⇨ is characteristic of the invasion pattern of verrucous carcinoma. Typical invasive squamous cell carcinoma has more irregular nests at the base of the tumor. *(Right)* In contrast to typical invasive SCC, verrucous carcinoma lacks significant nuclear pleomorphism with bland cytologic features. If the entire lesion is not sampled, diagnostic terminology, such as "well-differentiated SCC with verrucous carcinoma histology," may used.

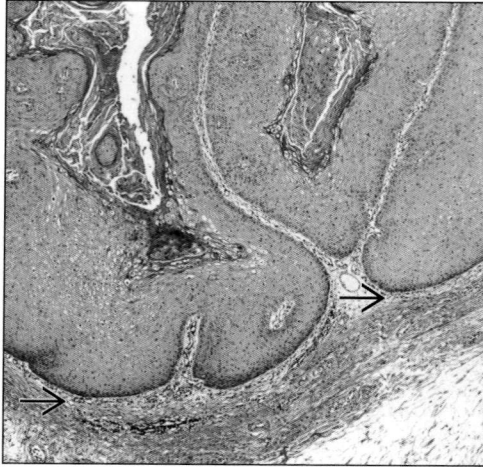
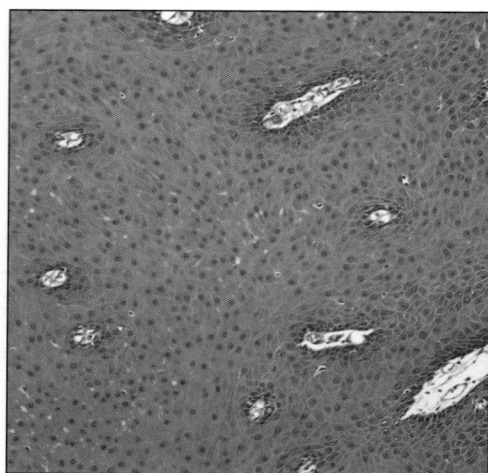

(Left) This SCC ⇨ arose in association with schistosomiasis infection. Numerous calcified eggs ⇨ are present in the adjacent tissue. A spectrum of bladder tumors, including urothelial carcinoma, occurs with schistosomiasis. *(Right)* At high-power evaluation of this transurethral biopsy specimen, oval calcified Schistosoma eggs are present in the lamina propria ⇨. The presence of eggs may help in establishing the bladder as the primary site of a carcinoma.

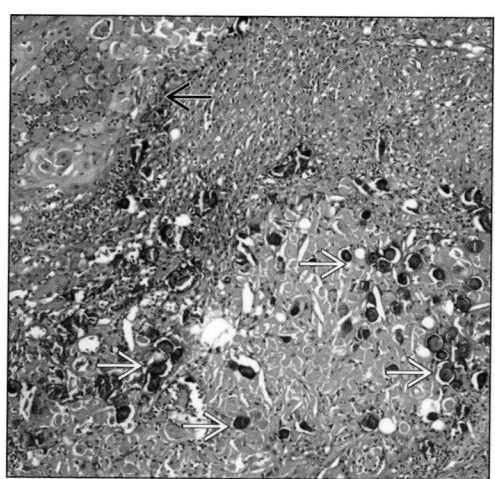
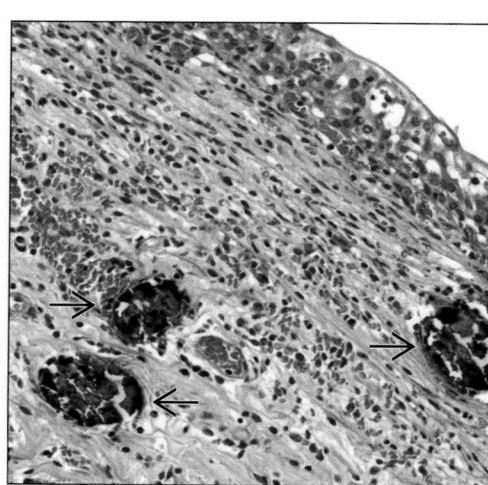

(Left) Noncalcified Schistosoma haematobium eggs with characteristic terminal spines ⇨ may be identified in the urinary bladder of infected patients. *(Right)* The terminal spine of Schistosoma haematobium eggs ⇨ may also be identified in completely calcified forms. Identification of associated Schistosoma eggs provides strong evidence of a primary bladder squamous cell carcinoma over secondary spread.

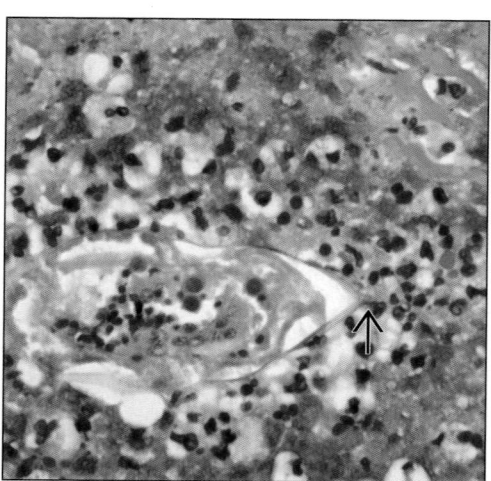
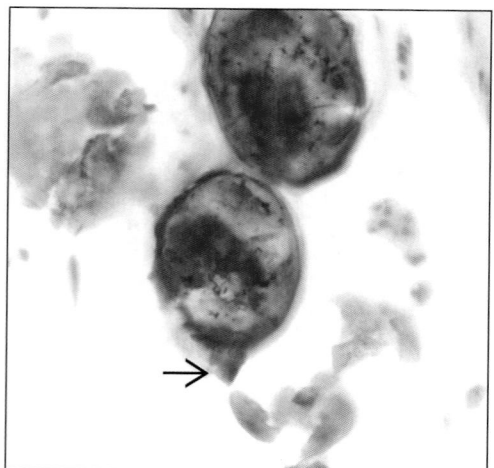

INVASIVE SQUAMOUS CELL CARCINOMA

Differential Diagnosis

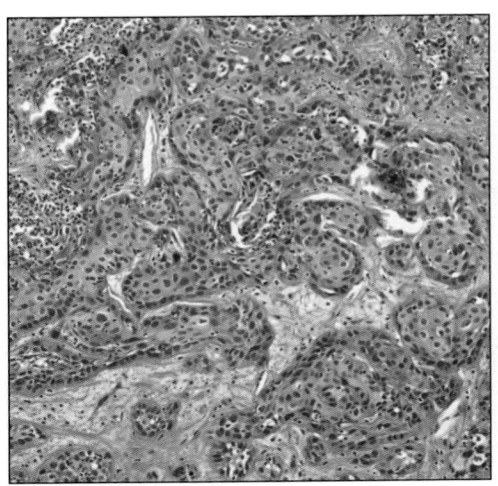

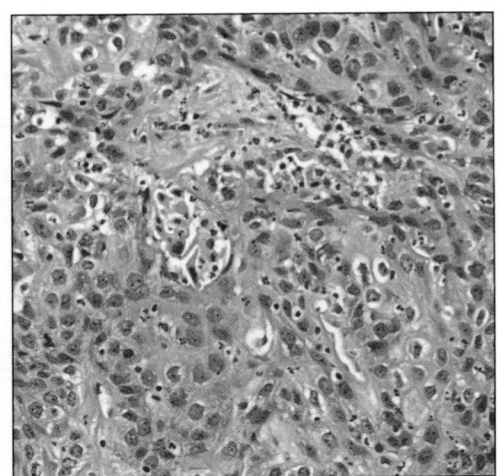

(Left) Invasive squamous cell carcinoma from adjacent anatomic regions may involve the urinary bladder by direct extension, as seen in this example of cervical squamous cell carcinoma in a transurethral biopsy specimen of the bladder. *(Right)* This cervical squamous cell carcinoma in a bladder biopsy specimen is indistinguishable from a primary bladder squamous carcinoma. Very close clinical and imaging correlation is essential in this differential diagnostic setting.

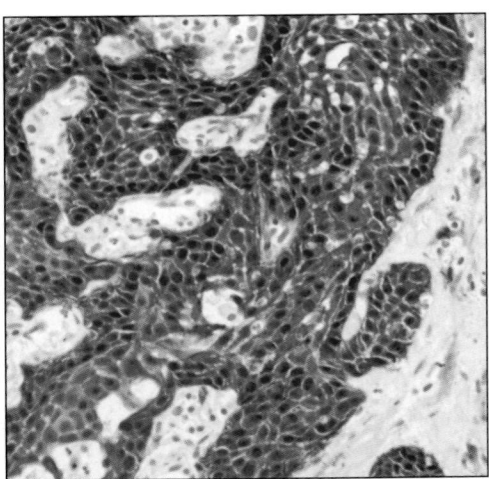

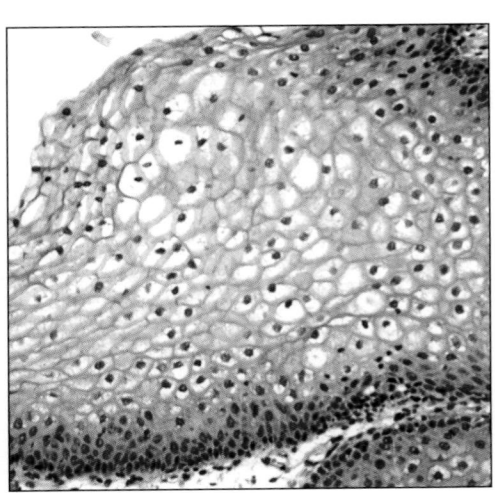

(Left) Diffuse cytoplasmic and nuclear p16 immunoreactivity is seen in this cervical squamous cell carcinoma that involved the urinary bladder by direct extension. p16 is a surrogate marker for HPV that is not specific, as it may occasionally be seen in bladder cancers that are not HPV related. *(Right)* Glycogenated squamous metaplasia is a common finding in the trigone of women and should not be used as evidence in support of diagnosis of primary urinary bladder SCC.

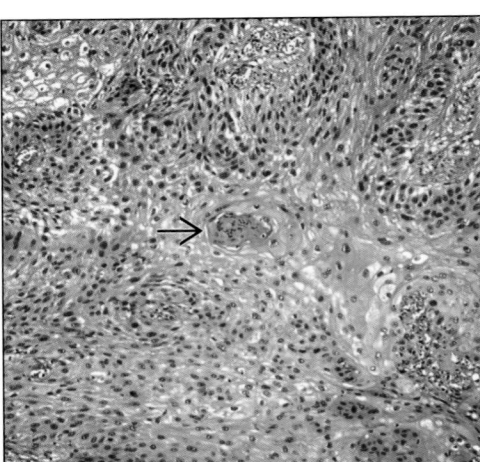

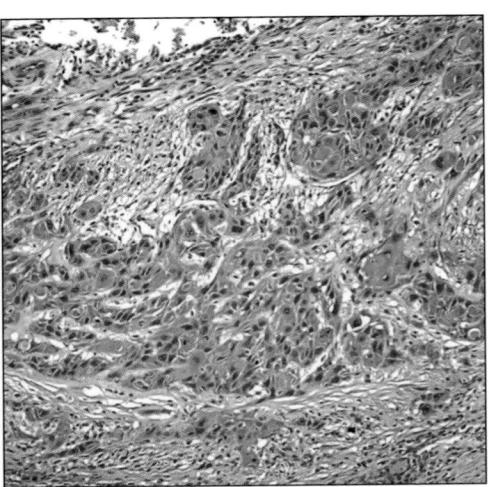

(Left) Squamous differentiation ⇥ may be seen in urothelial carcinoma. Components of both papillary urothelial carcinoma and urothelial carcinoma in situ were present in other areas. *(Right)* Urothelial carcinoma with squamous differentiation may be indistinguishable from primary SCC. The presence of any urothelial component warrants classification as urothelial carcinoma. The relative percentage of both components should be specified.

MYOFIBROBLASTIC PROLIFERATIONS

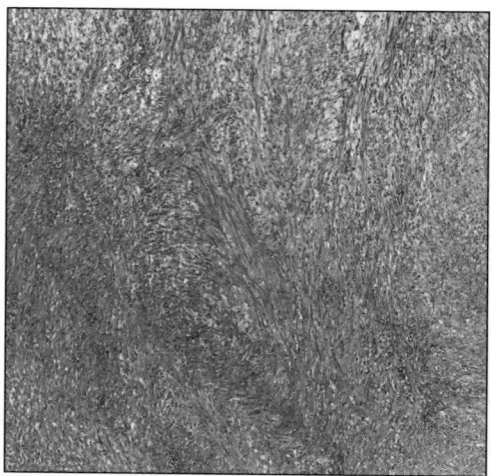

Urinary bladder pseudosarcomatous myofibroblastic proliferations are typically characterized by spindle cells with a loose fascicular architecture and variable myxoid stroma.

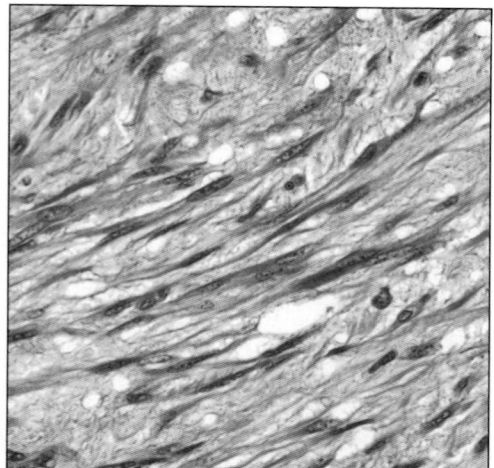

These cells are typical myofibroblasts with elongated tapered cytoplasmic processes, fine nuclear chromatin, and pinpoint nucleoli. Individual cells are commonly separated by myxoid stroma.

TERMINOLOGY

Synonyms
- Pseudosarcomatous myofibroblastic proliferation
- Pseudosarcomatous fibromyxoid tumor
- Inflammatory myofibroblastic tumor (IMT)
- Postoperative spindle cell nodule
- Inflammatory pseudotumor

Definitions
- Cytologically benign myofibroblastic proliferation of urinary bladder
- Different names have been used for identical lesions

ETIOLOGY/PATHOGENESIS

Infectious Agents
- No known inflammatory or infectious etiology

Associations
- May have history of trauma/prior instrumentation (postoperative spindle cell nodule)
- Some invasive urothelial carcinomas have florid myofibroblastic proliferation

CLINICAL ISSUES

Epidemiology
- Incidence
  - Rare
- Age
  - Typically occurs in 2nd to 4th decade; may occur in children

Site
- Urinary bladder
  - Most common site in urogenital system

Presentation
- Gross hematuria (most common), abdominal pain, irritative or obstructive voiding symptoms

Treatment
- Transurethral resection or partial cystectomy for larger lesions

Prognosis
- 10% local recurrence rate
- No metastases reported

MACROSCOPIC FEATURES

General Features
- Polypoid or submucosal nodule
- Cut surface is often pale, firm, and gelatinous

Size
- 1.5-13 cm

MICROSCOPIC PATHOLOGY

Histologic Features
- Proliferation of spindle cells
  - Loose fascicular architecture
  - Elongated cytoplasmic processes
  - Chromatin fine and evenly distributed
  - Scattered nuclei enlarged with macronucleoli
  - Cellularity variable with loose and edematous, or myxoid stroma
  - Mitotic activity may be brisk, but not atypical mitoses
- Hypocellularity common superficially with higher cellularity deeper (zonation)
- Granulation tissue-type vascularity
- Invasion of muscularis propria does not denote malignancy
- Necrosis may be seen

MYOFIBROBLASTIC PROLIFERATIONS

Key Facts

Terminology
- Different names have been used for identical, cytologically benign myofibroblastic proliferations

Clinical Issues
- Rare
- 10% local recurrence rate
- No metastases reported

Microscopic Pathology
- Loose fascicular architecture
- Individual cells tapered with elongated cytoplasmic processes
- Chromatin fine and evenly distributed
- Scattered nuclei enlarged with macronucleoli
- Invasion of muscularis propria does not denote malignancy

- Cellularity variable with loose and edematous, or myxoid stroma
- Mitotic activity may be brisk
- Admixed inflammatory cells present, including eosinophils and plasma cells

Ancillary Tests
- Commonly coexpress actin-sm and cytokeratin (low molecular weight forms)
- *ALK1* expression by immunohistochemistry varies widely (8-89%)

Top Differential Diagnoses
- Rhabdomyosarcoma
- Sarcomatoid carcinoma
- Leiomyosarcoma
- Fibromyxoid nephrogenic adenoma

- Admixed inflammatory cells present including eosinophils and plasma cells

Predominant Cell/Compartment Type
- Myofibroblast

ANCILLARY TESTS

Immunohistochemistry
- Commonly coexpress actin-sm and cytokeratin (low molecular weight forms)
- Typically nonreactive for HMCK(34βE12), such as CK5/6
- ALK1 expression by immunohistochemistry varies widely (8-89%)
  - Subset of cases show *ALK* rearrangements by FISH
- Desmin reactivity is variable

DIFFERENTIAL DIAGNOSIS

Rhabdomyosarcoma
- Cambium layer
- More cellular foci with nuclear hyperchromasia
- Rhabdomyoblasts
- Must be carefully considered in children
- Express desmin and nuclear myogenin &/or MYOD1

Sarcomatoid Urothelial Carcinoma
- Admixed papillary or in situ urothelial carcinoma
- Heterologous elements may be seen
- Myxoid and sclerosing pattern may mimic myofibroblastic process
- Nuclear pleomorphism and hyperchromasia present
- Expression of p63 and HMCK(34βE12)

Leiomyosarcoma
- Morphologically heterogeneous
  - Cellular form with tight intersecting fascicles
  - Myxoid pattern may mimic myofibroblastic process
- Nuclear pleomorphism and hyperchromasia
- Commonly express desmin and actin-sm

- Aberrant low molecular weight keratin expression

Fibromyxoid Nephrogenic Adenoma
- Prominent myxoid background
- Scattered corded or spindled epithelial cells
- Other concurrent patterns of nephrogenic adenoma
- Express cytokeratin, pax-2, and pax-8

Urothelial Carcinoma with Myxoid Stroma
- Rarely have prominent myxoid stroma and cording of epithelial cells
- Immunoprofile typical of urothelial carcinoma

DIAGNOSTIC CHECKLIST

Clinically Relevant Pathologic Features
- Nuclear features are key to distinguish from malignant process

Pathologic Interpretation Pearls
- Nuclear chromatin distinguishes myofibroblastic proliferations from malignancy
  - Chromatin is fine and evenly dispersed with marked variation in nuclear size and scattered macronucleoli

SELECTED REFERENCES

1. Westfall DE et al: Utility of a comprehensive immunohistochemical panel in the differential diagnosis of spindle cell lesions of the urinary bladder. Am J Surg Pathol. 33(1):99-105, 2009
2. Sukov WR et al: Utility of ALK-1 protein expression and ALK rearrangements in distinguishing inflammatory myofibroblastic tumor from malignant spindle cell lesions of the urinary bladder. Mod Pathol. 20(5):592-603, 2007
3. Harik LR et al: Pseudosarcomatous myofibroblastic proliferations of the bladder: a clinicopathologic study of 42 cases. Am J Surg Pathol. 30(7):787-94, 2006
4. Montgomery EA et al: Inflammatory myofibroblastic tumors of the urinary tract: a clinicopathologic study of 46 cases, including a malignant example inflammatory fibrosarcoma and a subset associated with high-grade urothelial carcinoma. Am J Surg Pathol. 30(12):1502-12, 2006

MYOFIBROBLASTIC PROLIFERATIONS

Microscopic Features

(Left) Spindled myofibroblasts, as seen in pseudosarcomatous myofibroblastic proliferation, are typically arranged into loose, poorly formed fascicles and are commonly associated with myxoid stroma. *(Right)* These typical myofibroblasts highlight the characteristic tapered nuclei and thin elongated cytoplasmic processes ➡. The fine nuclear chromatin distinguishes myofibroblasts from malignant lesions, such as leiomyosarcoma and sarcomatoid carcinoma.

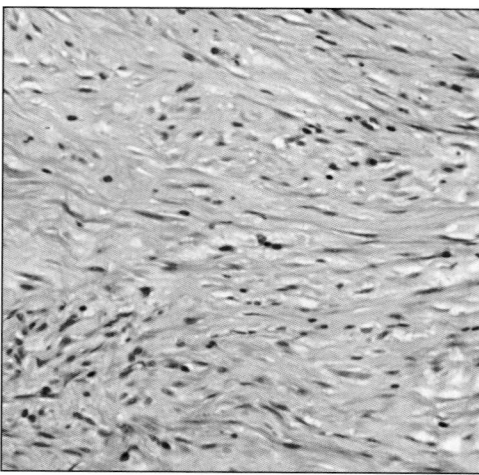 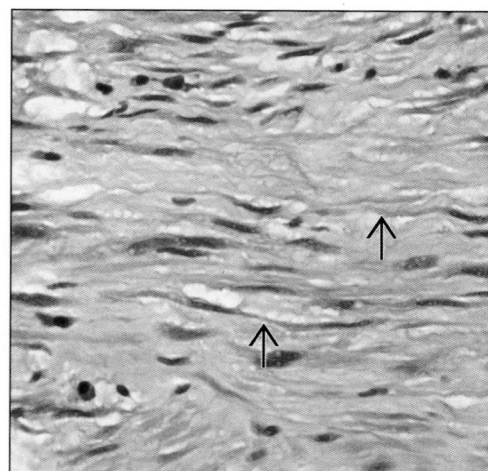

(Left) This cellular myofibroblastic proliferation is arranged into a distinct fascicular architecture and has admixed inflammatory cells, a feature that is common. More cellular lesions may closely mimic a true smooth muscle tumor. *(Right)* Involvement of the muscularis propria by these florid myofibroblastic proliferations is common and may be extensive. This infiltrative growth does not denote malignancy.

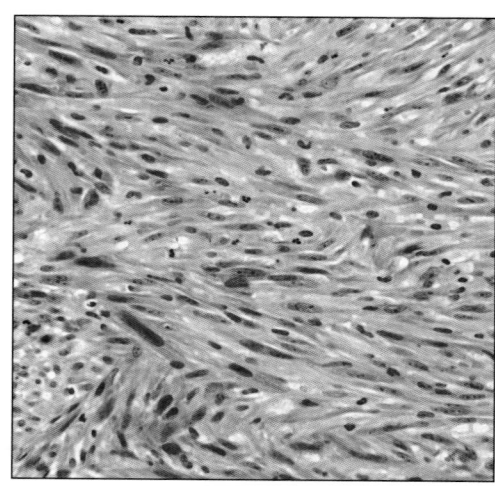 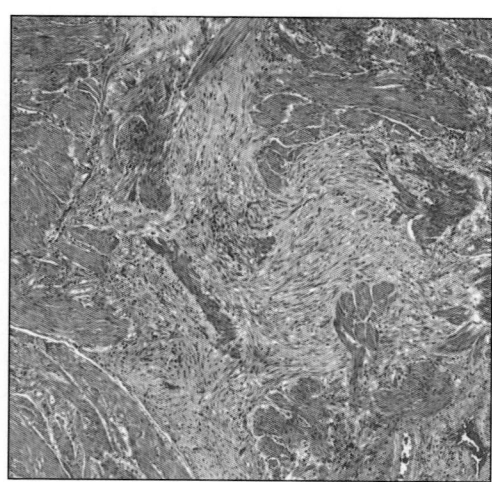

(Left) Myofibroblasts may show variation in nuclear size and may have prominent nucleoli ➡. Despite these features, the chromatin is fine and evenly dispersed. Malignant spindle cell lesions typically show coarse nuclear chromatin. *(Right)* This myofibroblastic proliferation shows the spectrum of nuclear size and shape that may be seen. This variation in cell size and the presence of prominent nucleoli ➡ are common and should not prompt a diagnosis of malignancy.

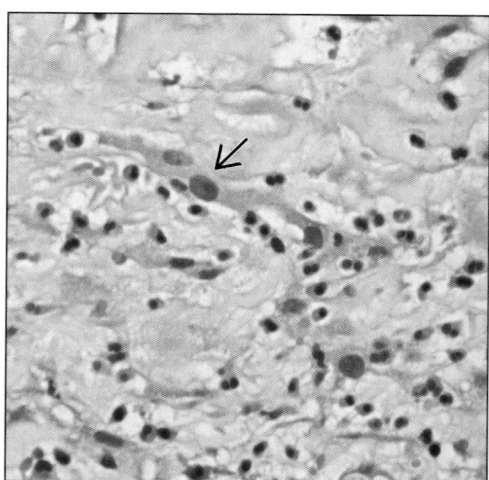 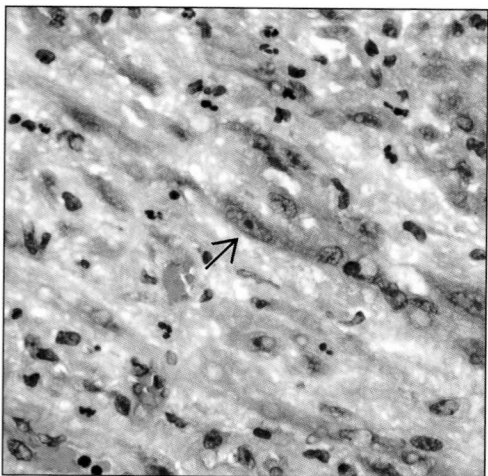

MYOFIBROBLASTIC PROLIFERATIONS

Ancillary Techniques

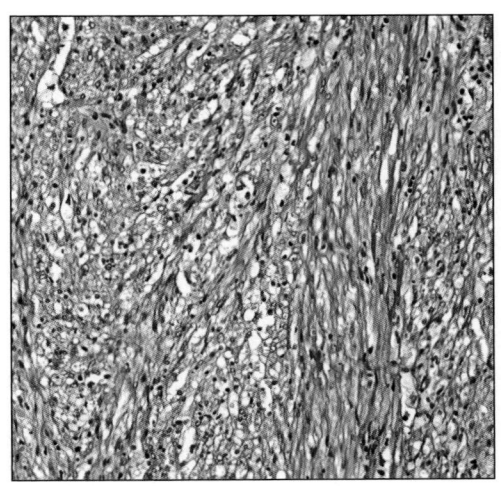
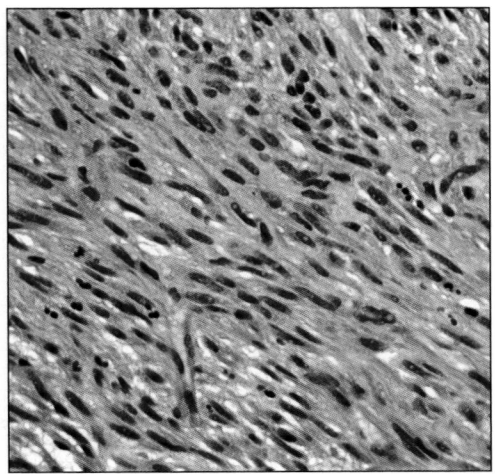

(Left) Some myofibroblastic proliferations are more cellular and eosinophilic, closely mimicking a smooth muscle neoplasm. This example arose 1 month following a transurethral biopsy (postoperative spindle cell nodule). (Right) On high-power examination, the lesional cells are monomorphic with fine nuclear chromatin. Immunostains may be needed in these cellular examples to distinguish from a true smooth muscle neoplasm.

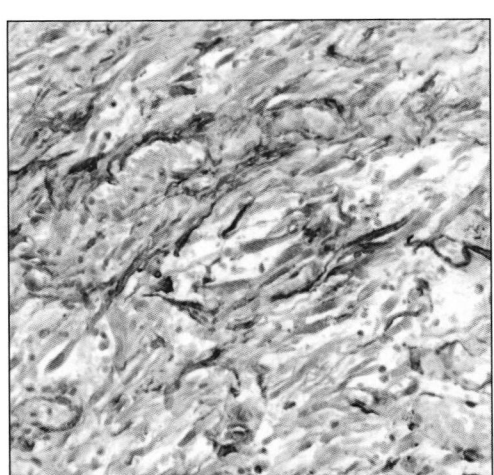
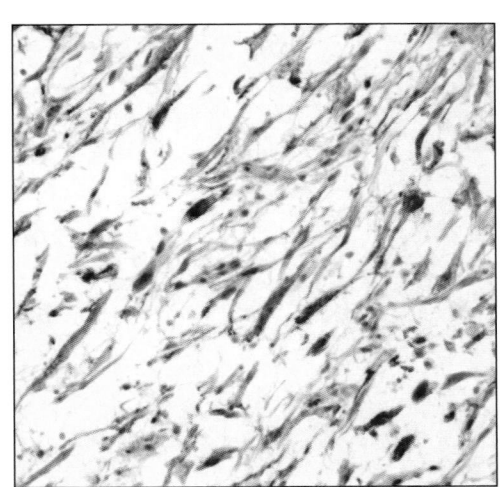

(Left) Diffuse actin-sm immunoreactivity is typical of myofibroblasts. Myofibroblasts do not commonly coexpress desmin, a distinguishing feature from smooth muscle. (Right) Strong cytoplasmic immunohistochemical staining with ALK1 may be seen in these myofibroblastic proliferations, but this finding varies widely in the literature. This feature has suggested a relationship to inflammatory myofibroblastic tumor.

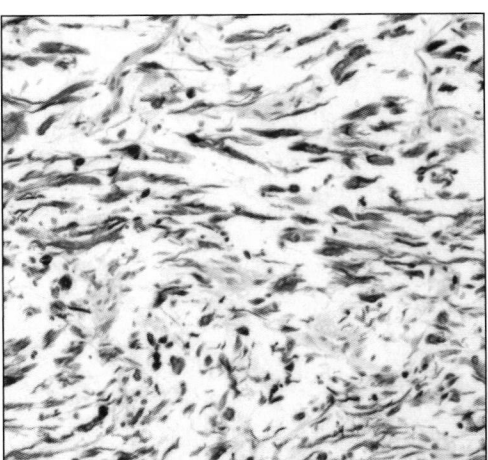
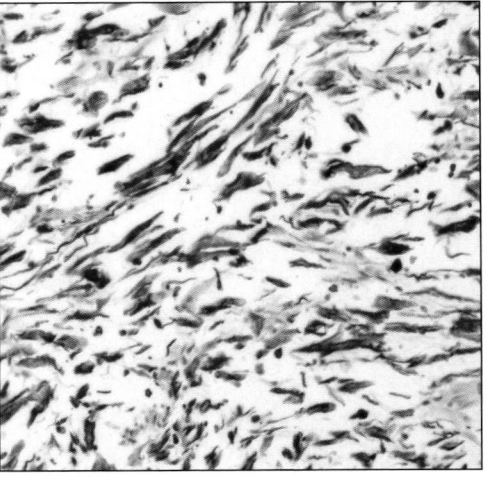

(Left) Cytoplasmic immunoreactivity to cytokeratin AE1/3 may cause diagnostic confusion with sarcomatoid urothelial carcinoma, but low molecular weight keratin staining is fairly common in these bladder myofibroblastic proliferations. (Right) Keratin subtyping reveals that the myofibroblastic cells express only low molecular weight cytokeratin. In contrast, sarcomatoid urothelial carcinoma expresses HMCK(34βE12) as well as nuclear p63.

Carcinoma-associated Myofibroblastic Proliferation

(Left) Invasive urothelial carcinoma ➡ may be associated with a florid myofibroblastic proliferation that may mimic a primary myofibroblastic process. *(Right)* This example has a florid myofibroblastic proliferation that is associated with scant, subtle aggregates of invasive carcinoma ➡. The individual myofibroblasts are identical to those seen in other myofibroblastic lesions. It is important to exclude the possibility of a morphologically subtle carcinoma in this setting.

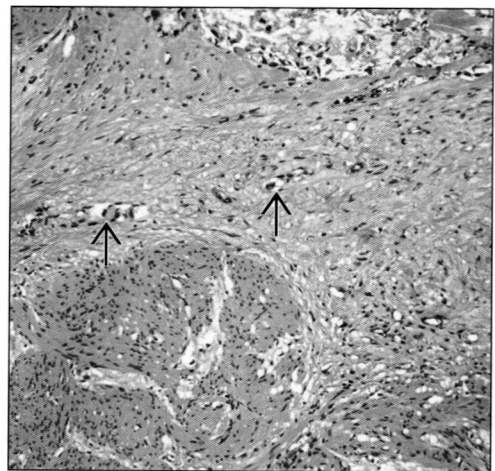
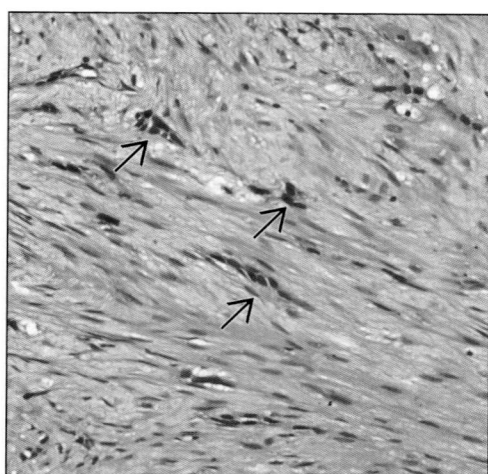

(Left) This invasive urothelial carcinoma involves the muscularis propria ➡ and is also associated with a myofibroblastic proliferation ➡. *(Right)* The myofibroblastic proliferation ➡ that is associated with carcinoma has less eosinophilic cytoplasm than the adjacent smooth muscle of the muscularis propria ➡. The myofibroblasts are cytologically bland, which aids in distinction from sarcomatoid carcinoma.

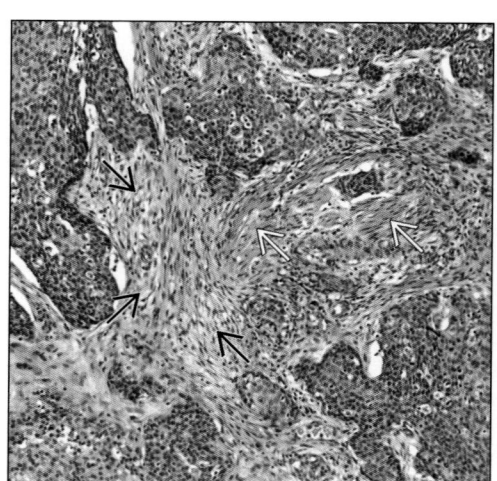
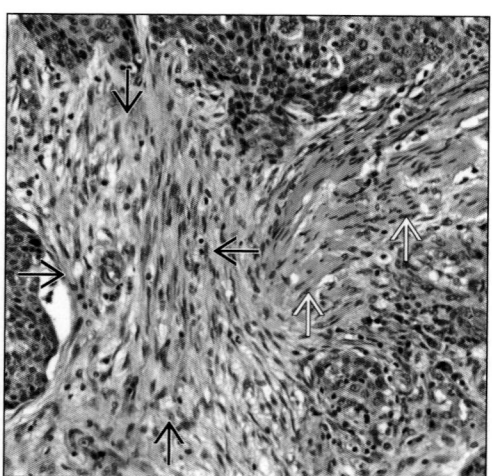

(Left) Invasive urothelial carcinoma with associated "pseudosarcomatous" stroma may suggest sarcomatoid carcinoma when the carcinomatous component ➡ is prominent. These myofibroblasts are associated with an inflammatory infiltrate similar to primary myofibroblastic proliferations. *(Right)* On high-power examination, these spindle cells that were associated with carcinoma in other fields show the long cytoplasmic processes ➡ and fine nuclear chromatin, typical of myofibroblasts.

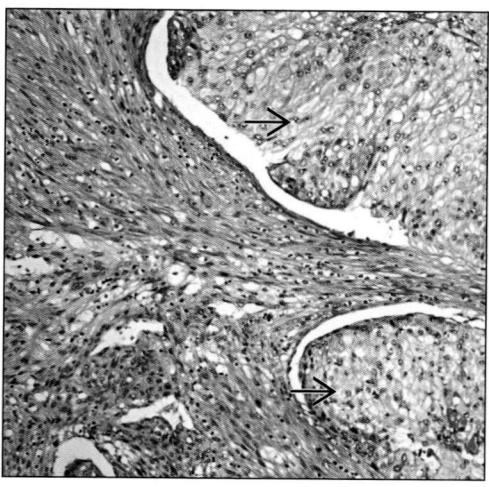
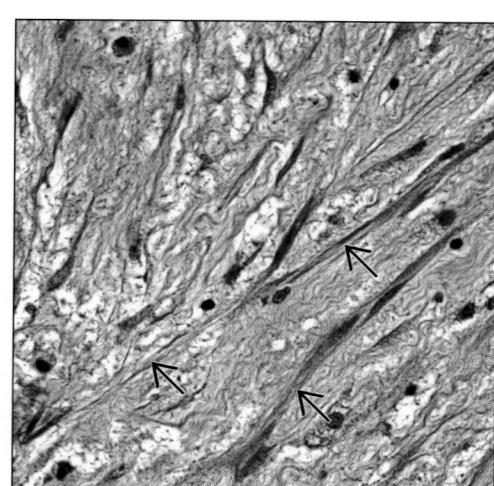

Differential Diagnosis

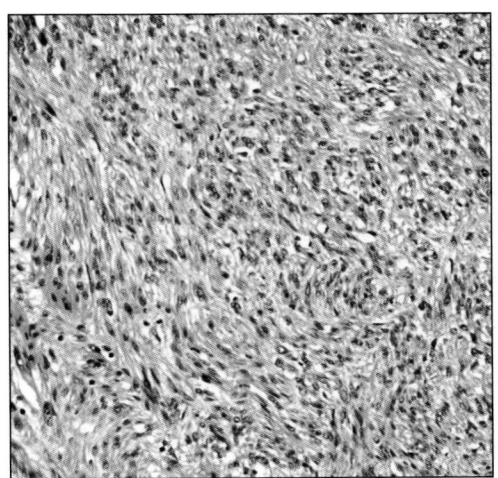
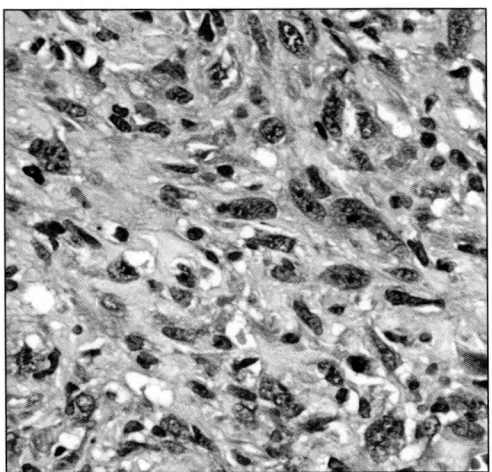

(Left) True smooth muscle tumors of the urinary bladder, as in this example of leiomyosarcoma, typically have more eosinophilic cytoplasm compared to myofibroblasts and have more cellular and better developed fascicular growth. (Right) The degree of cytologic atypia in this smooth muscle tumor, which was desmin and actin-sm positive, is diagnostic of malignancy (i.e., leiomyosarcoma).

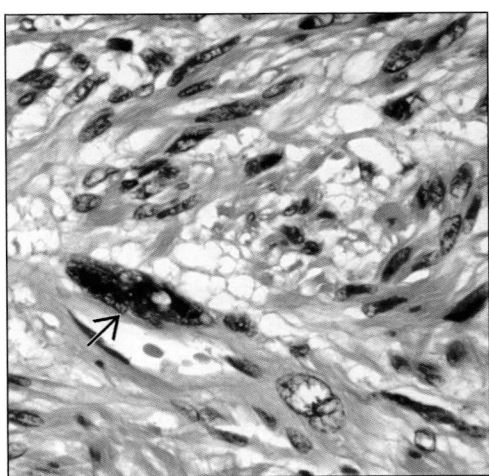
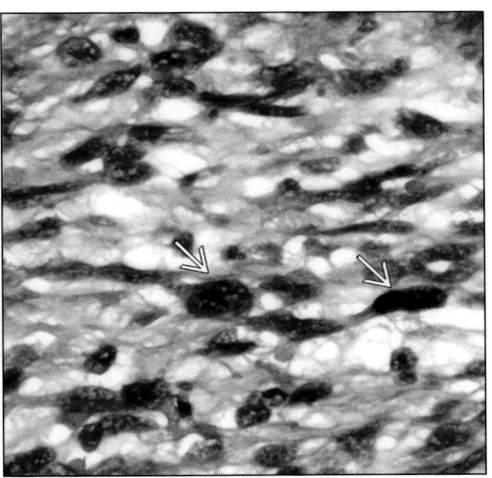

(Left) This example of leiomyosarcoma shows individual neoplastic cells with marked nuclear pleomorphism and nuclear hyperchromasia ➔, features that are most useful in the distinction from myofibroblasts. (Right) The degree of nuclear hyperchromasia/irregular clumped chromatin ➔ in this sarcomatoid urothelial carcinoma is diagnostic of malignancy and should exclude the diagnosis of a benign myofibroblastic process.

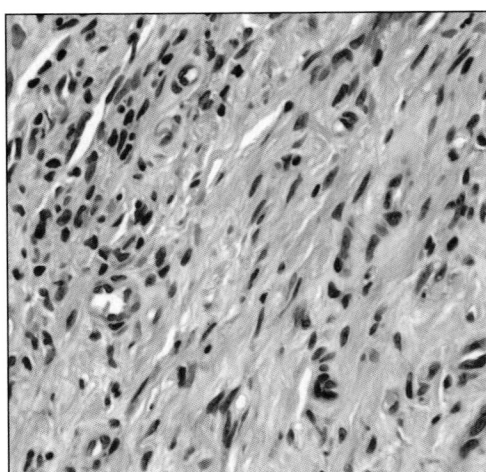
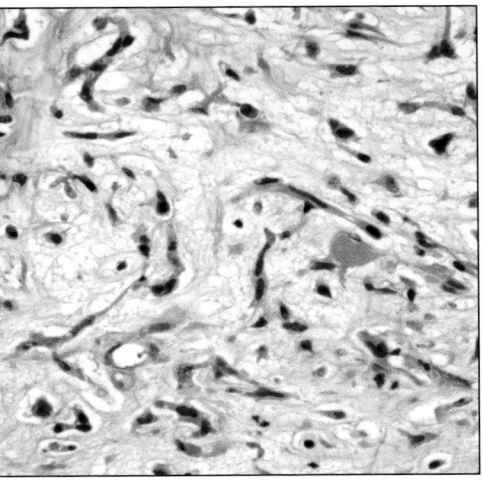

(Left) Focal areas in malignant tumors may have significant overlap with pseudosarcomatous myofibroblastic proliferation. This example of sarcomatoid urothelial carcinoma had more striking nuclear atypia in other areas of the tumor. (Right) Sarcomatoid urothelial carcinoma may also be associated with myxoid stroma. This morphologic pattern may very closely mimic a myofibroblastic proliferation. More conventional areas with definitive malignant cytology should be sought.

SMOOTH MUSCLE TUMORS

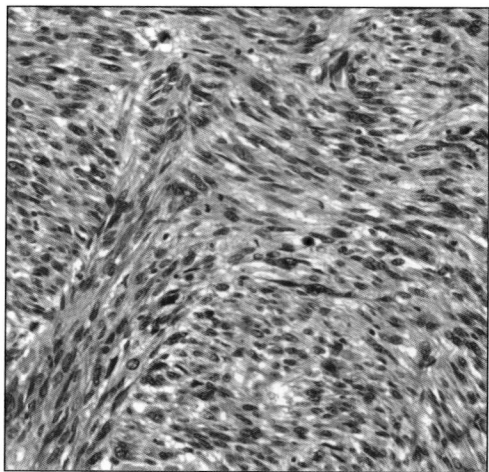

Intersecting fascicular growth and variable eosinophilic cytoplasm are characteristic of smooth muscle tumors. Tumors with this cellularity should be carefully examined for features of leiomyosarcoma.

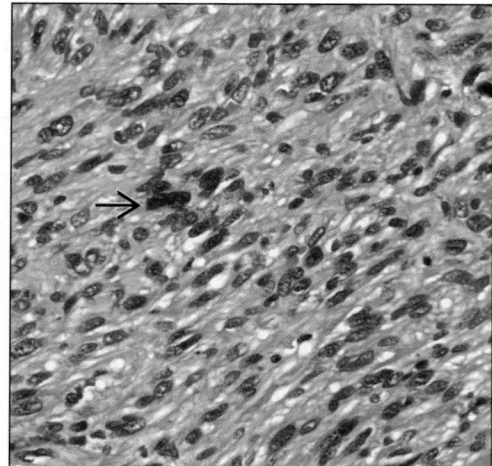

This degree of nuclear pleomorphism ⇨ and hyperchromasia is diagnostic of malignancy and supports a diagnosis of leiomyosarcoma if sarcomatoid urothelial carcinoma is excluded.

TERMINOLOGY

Definitions
- Leiomyoma
  - Benign mesenchymal neoplasm showing smooth muscle differentiation
- Leiomyosarcoma
  - Morphologically and clinically malignant mesenchymal neoplasm with smooth muscle differentiation

ETIOLOGY/PATHOGENESIS

Iatrogenic
- History of chemotherapy reported in some cases of leiomyosarcoma

CLINICAL ISSUES

Epidemiology
- Incidence
  - Leiomyoma is most common benign mesenchymal neoplasm of bladder
  - Leiomyosarcoma is rare, but most common primary vesical sarcoma in adults
    - < 1% of all bladder malignancies
- Age
  - Wide range for both leiomyoma and leiomyosarcoma
- Gender
  - Female predilection for leiomyoma
  - Male predominance in leiomyosarcoma (M:F = 2:1)

Presentation
- Urinary symptoms
  - Obstruction, irritative symptoms, and hematuria

Treatment
- Leiomyoma

- Transurethral resection or open resection
- Leiomyosarcoma
  - Radical surgical resection

Prognosis
- Leiomyoma
  - Complete excision is curative
- Leiomyosarcoma
  - High recurrence/metastatic rate (approximately 70%)

MACROSCOPIC FEATURES

Leiomyoma
- Typically small circumscribed mass lesion within bladder wall
- Mean size is < 2 cm
- Rare leiomyomas up to 25 cm are reported
- Usually lack necrosis; infarction may be present in large tumors

Leiomyosarcoma
- Typically large, solid, infiltrating intramural mass
- Mean size is 7 cm
- Foci of geographic necrosis are common

MICROSCOPIC PATHOLOGY

Histologic Features
- Leiomyoma
  - Interlacing fascicles of spindle cells with prominent eosinophilic cytoplasm
  - Low cellularity and circumscription is typical
  - No nuclear pleomorphism and fine nuclear chromatin
  - Mitotic figures are rare or absent
  - No areas of coagulative necrosis
- Leiomyosarcoma

SMOOTH MUSCLE TUMORS

Key Facts

Clinical Issues
- Leiomyosarcoma is rare, but most common primary vesical sarcoma
- Complete excision is curative for leiomyoma
- Leiomyosarcoma has high recurrent and metastatic rate

Microscopic Pathology
- Leiomyoma
  ○ Interlacing fascicles of spindle cells with prominent eosinophilic cytoplasm
  ○ Low cellularity is typical
  ○ No nuclear pleomorphism and fine nuclear chromatin
- Leiomyosarcoma
  ○ Fascicles of spindle cells with variable eosinophilic cytoplasm

○ Scattered pleomorphic, hyperchromatic cells are common
○ Rarely, marked nuclear anaplasia is seen
○ Mitotic figures are usually easily identified

Ancillary Tests
- Express actin-sm and desmin
- Focal expression of cytokeratin may be seen

Top Differential Diagnoses
- Sarcomatoid urothelial carcinoma
- Pseudosarcomatous myofibroblastic proliferation (inflammatory myofibroblastic tumor)

Diagnostic Checklist
- Nuclear cytology is key feature in distinguishing leiomyosarcoma from benign mimics

---

○ Interlacing fascicles of spindle cells with prominent eosinophilic cytoplasm
○ Wide range of cytologic atypia, infiltrative growth pattern
  ▪ Scattered pleomorphic, hyperchromatic cells are common
  ▪ Rarely, marked nuclear anaplasia is seen
○ Coagulative necrosis may be present
○ Mitotic figures are usually easily identified

Leiomyosarcoma Grading Scheme
- Low grade
  ○ Mitoses < 5 per 10 high-power fields
  ○ Usually mild to moderate cytologic atypia
- High grade
  ○ Mitoses > 5 per 10 high-power fields
  ○ Marked nuclear pleomorphism and hyperchromasia
  ○ Necrosis common

ANCILLARY TESTS

Immunohistochemistry
- Diffuse cytoplasmic smooth muscle actin and desmin
  ○ Stronger staining more common in leiomyoma
- Focal expression of cytokeratin may be seen
  ○ Typically found with low molecular weight subtypes
- No immunoreactivity for ALK1, p63, or HMCK(34βE12)

DIFFERENTIAL DIAGNOSIS

Sarcomatoid Urothelial Carcinoma
- Spindled component may be histologically indistinguishable from leiomyosarcoma
- Previous history, associated papillary, in situ, or invasive urothelial carcinoma is diagnostic of carcinoma
- Positivity for p63 and HMCK(34βE12)
- May have heterologous differentiation
  ○ Skeletal muscle and cartilage most common

Pseudosarcomatous Myofibroblastic Proliferation (Inflammatory Myofibroblastic Tumor)
- Distinguished from leiomyosarcoma by cytologic features
  ○ Enlarged nuclei with nucleoli and fine chromatin
- Myxoid stroma and granulation tissue type vascularity are common
- Commonly express smooth muscle actin, but desmin staining is variable
- ALK1 immunoreactivity is identified in subset of cases

Benign Nerve Sheath Tumor
- May have degenerative atypia (ancient change) that mimics malignancy
- Diffuse cytoplasmic and nuclear immunoreactivity for S100 protein is diagnostic

DIAGNOSTIC CHECKLIST

Pathologic Interpretation Pearls
- Nuclear cytology is key feature in distinguishing leiomyosarcoma from benign mimics
- Immunohistochemistry is commonly required to exclude sarcomatoid urothelial carcinoma

SELECTED REFERENCES

1. Westfall DE et al: Utility of a comprehensive immunohistochemical panel in the differential diagnosis of spindle cell lesions of the urinary bladder. Am J Surg Pathol. 33(1):99-105, 2009
2. Martin SA et al: Smooth muscle neoplasms of the urinary bladder: a clinicopathologic comparison of leiomyoma and leiomyosarcoma. Am J Surg Pathol. 26(3):292-300, 2002
3. Goluboff ET et al: Leiomyoma of bladder: report of case and review of literature. Urology. 43(2):238-41, 1994
4. Mills SE et al: Leiomyosarcoma of the urinary bladder. A clinicopathologic and immunohistochemical study of 15 cases. Am J Surg Pathol. 13(6):480-9, 1989

SMOOTH MUSCLE TUMORS

Microscopic Features

(Left) This leiomyoma is characterized by a relatively hypocellular proliferation of spindled cells with a fascicular growth and prominent eosinophilic cytoplasm. No obvious nuclear pleomorphism is appreciable at this magnification. *(Right)* On high-power examination of this bladder leiomyoma, the neoplastic cells are evenly spaced, and the nuclei are cytologically bland with fine chromatin and no pleomorphism.

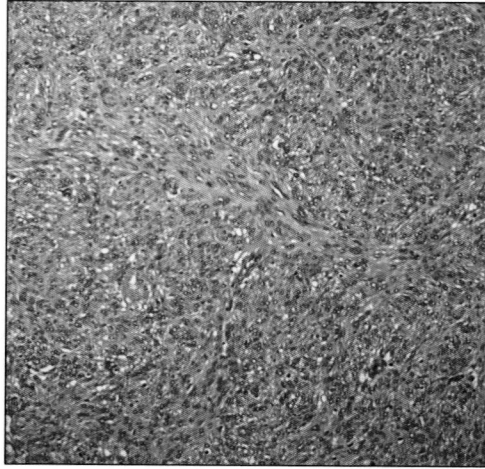
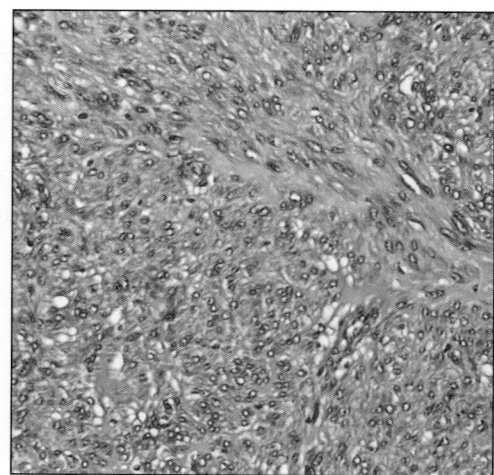

(Left) The small, monotonous smooth muscle cells in this leiomyoma have a very bland cytology with fine nuclear chromatin. The tumor is very hypocellular, a feature typical of benign leiomyomas. The cytologic features in smooth muscle tumors are the key in distinguishing benign from malignant tumors. *(Right)* In contrast to leiomyoma, this leiomyosarcoma has scattered hyperchromatic cells ➡ visible at low-power magnification. Such findings should prompt careful consideration of malignancy.

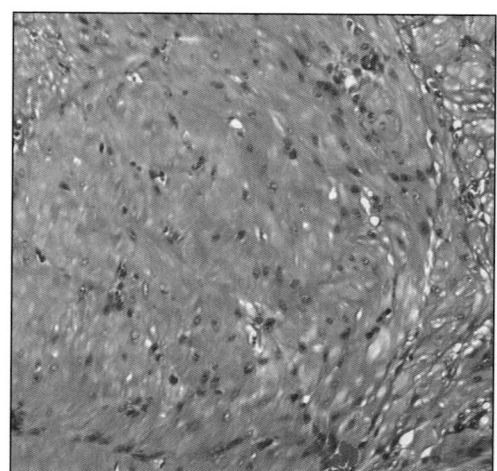
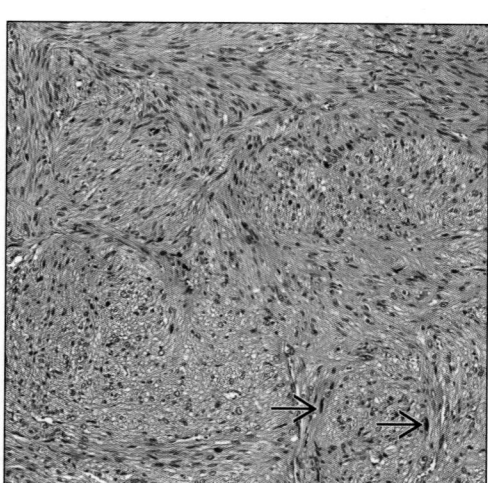

(Left) This spindle cell neoplasm had evidence of smooth muscle differentiation by immunohistochemistry (diffuse desmin reactivity). The variation in nuclear size, nuclear hyperchromasia ➡, and mitotic activity ➡ all support a diagnosis of leiomyosarcoma. *(Right)* Leiomyosarcomas have a wide spectrum of atypia. This example does not show significant nuclear pleomorphism, but there is nuclear membrane irregularity and clumped chromatin imparting a hyperchromatic appearance.

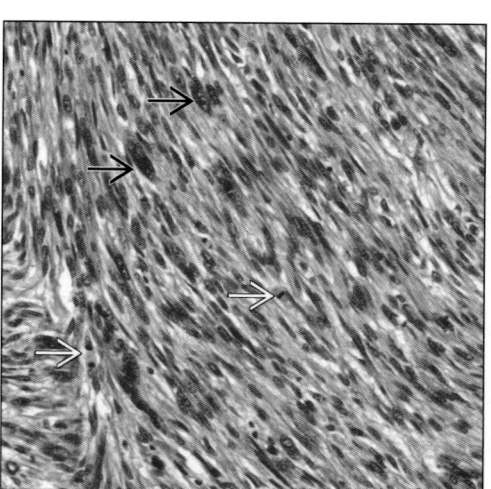
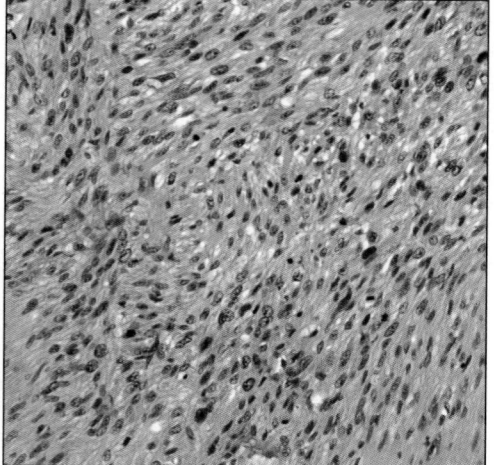

SMOOTH MUSCLE TUMORS

Microscopic Features

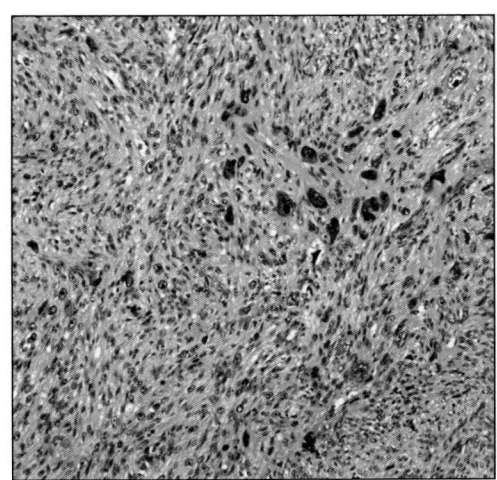

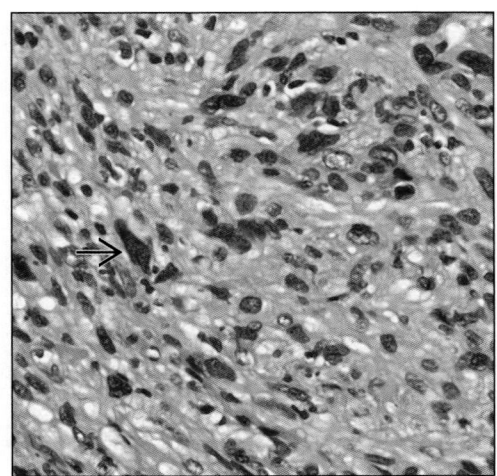

(Left) This leiomyosarcoma contains scattered cells with obvious nuclear pleomorphism. Most of these tumors have easily identifiable mitotic figures at higher power examination. (Right) Scattered neoplastic cells with nucleomegaly and nuclear hyperchromasia are typically found in leiomyosarcoma ➡. This degree of atypia would not be seen in leiomyoma or pseudosarcomatous myofibroblastic proliferation (inflammatory myofibroblastic tumor).

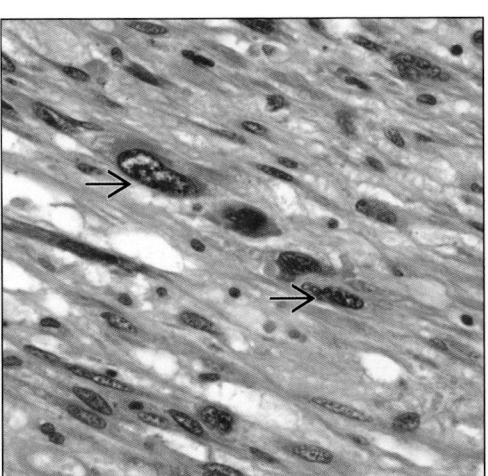

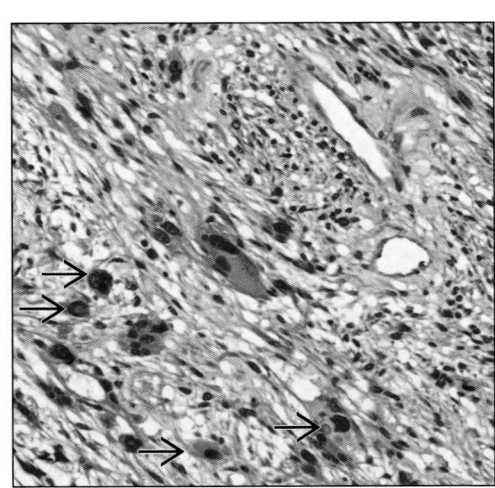

(Left) The clumped irregular nuclear chromatin of leiomyosarcoma ➡ is a key feature in the morphologic distinction of leiomyosarcomas from pseudosarcomatous myofibroblastic proliferations (inflammatory myofibroblastic tumors). (Right) Marked nuclear pleomorphism, focal or diffuse, may be seen in high-grade leiomyosarcomas. Epithelioid histology ➡ may mimic a carcinomatous component.

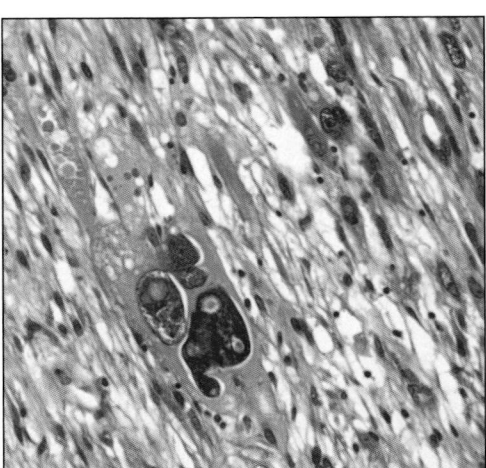

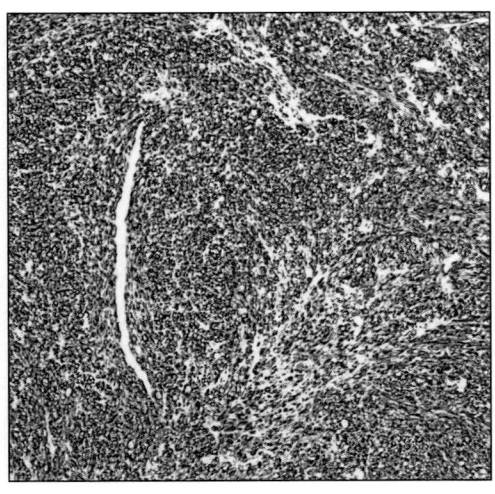

(Left) This example of leiomyosarcoma shows extreme nuclear anaplasia. (Right) Immunohistochemistry is very useful in establishing the lineage of spindle cell neoplasms in the urinary bladder. Diffuse cytoplasmic desmin reactivity, as seen here, is strong evidence for a smooth muscle phenotype. It should be remembered that smooth muscle tumors may have aberrant cytokeratin expression, but this is typically seen only with low molecular weight keratins.

Differential Diagnosis: Sarcomatoid Carcinoma

(Left) This biphasic sarcomatoid carcinoma has an adenocarcinoma component ⊳ adjacent to the malignant spindle cell component ⊳. This biphasic morphology is diagnostic of sarcomatoid carcinoma. *(Right)* This myxoid and sclerosing sarcomatoid carcinoma mimics a leiomyosarcoma or pseudosarcomatous myofibroblastic proliferation. The cellularity and nuclear hyperchromasia are diagnostic of malignancy, but a smooth muscle lineage should be excluded by immunohistochemistry.

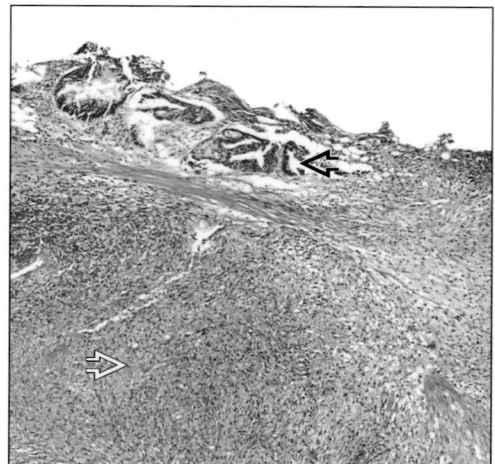
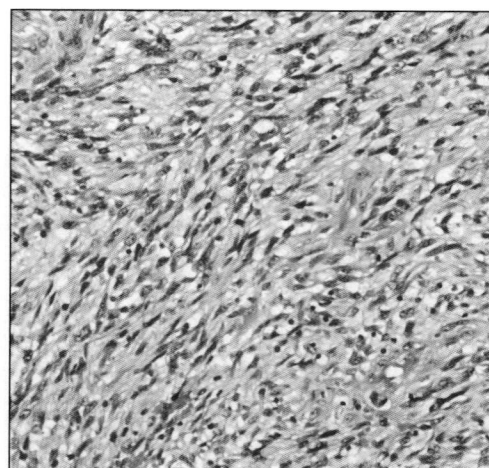

(Left) Pure spindled sarcomatoid carcinomas may closely mimic a primary vesical sarcoma, such as leiomyosarcoma. *(Right)* A mixed spindled and epithelioid appearance should suggest the possibility of a sarcomatoid urothelial carcinoma. If a typical component of in situ, papillary, or invasive urothelial carcinoma is not present, then immunohistochemistry is typically required. History of prior urothelial carcinoma in the bladder is usually sufficient evidence for a carcinoma diagnosis.

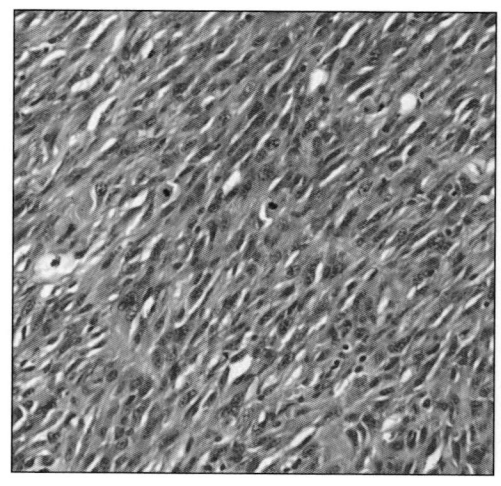
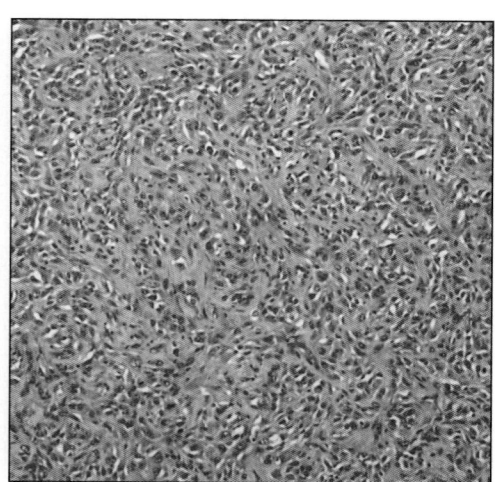

(Left) Nuclear p63 immunoreactivity provides strong evidence of an epithelial origin and is maintained in the spindle cell components. *(Right)* Cytoplasmic positivity for HMCK(34βE12) is a feature of epithelial lineage. Keratin expression in smooth muscle cells and myofibroblasts is typically only found with low molecular weight cytokeratins. Due to the marked overlap in morphology and immunohistochemistry, a broad panel of markers is necessary.

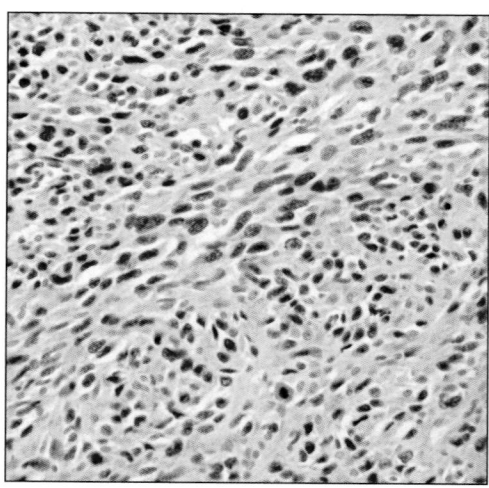
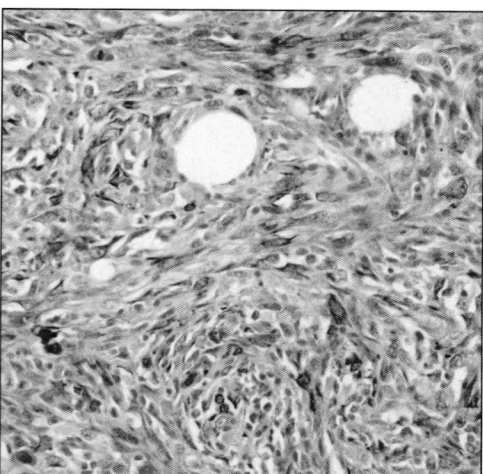

SMOOTH MUSCLE TUMORS

Differential Diagnosis: Myofibroblastic Proliferation

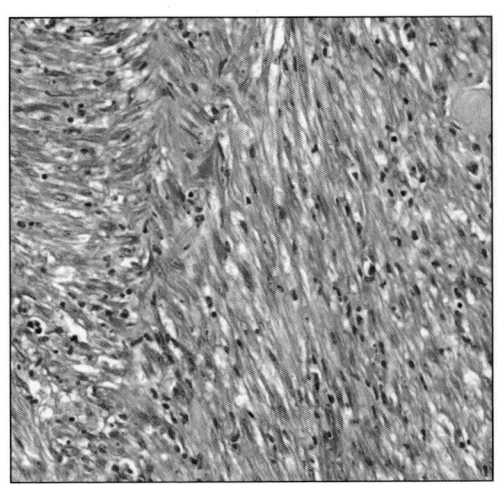

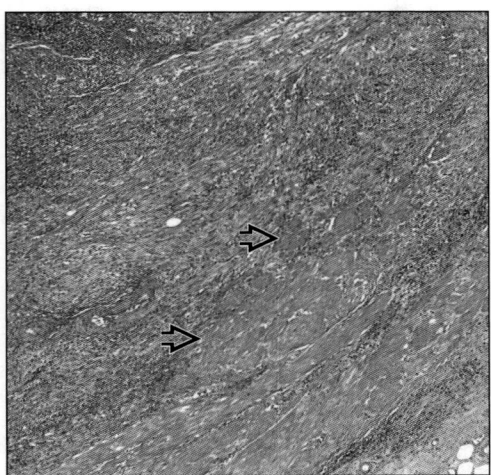

(Left) This pseudosarcomatous myofibroblastic proliferation (inflammatory myofibroblastic tumor) has a fascicular growth pattern that closely resembles a smooth muscle tumor. Cytologic features are most important in the distinction from a malignant tumor. *(Right)* Invasion of muscularis propria ⇛ is common in pseudosarcomatous myofibroblastic proliferations. This finding should not be regarded as a feature of malignancy.

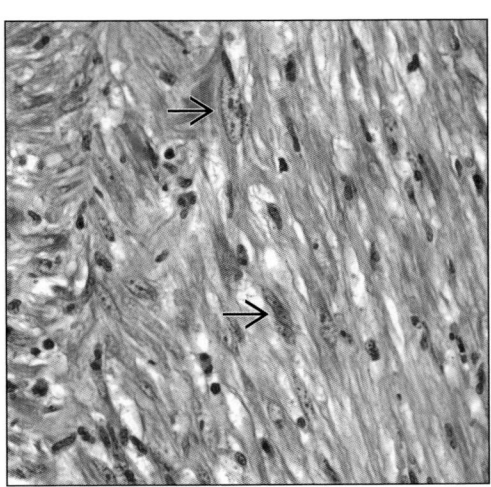

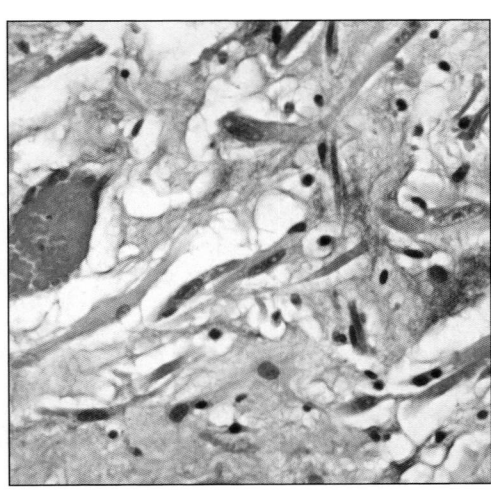

(Left) Pseudosarcomatous myofibroblastic proliferations may have obvious variation in nuclear size and prominent nucleoli, but the nuclear chromatin is evenly dispersed ⇨. This is the most important morphologic feature in the distinction from leiomyosarcoma. *(Right)* Some examples of pseudosarcomatous myofibroblastic proliferation (inflammatory myofibroblastic tumor) are relatively hypocellular with prominent myxoid stroma. Neoplastic cells have a tissue culture-like appearance.

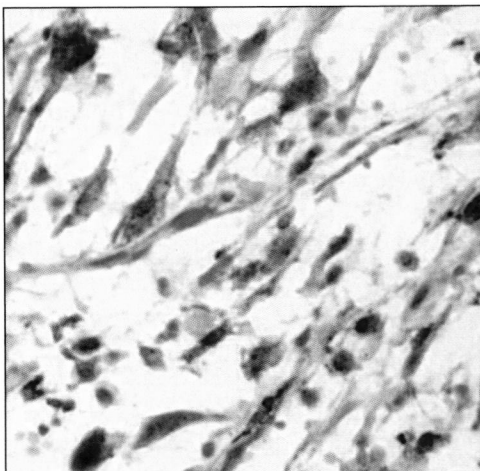

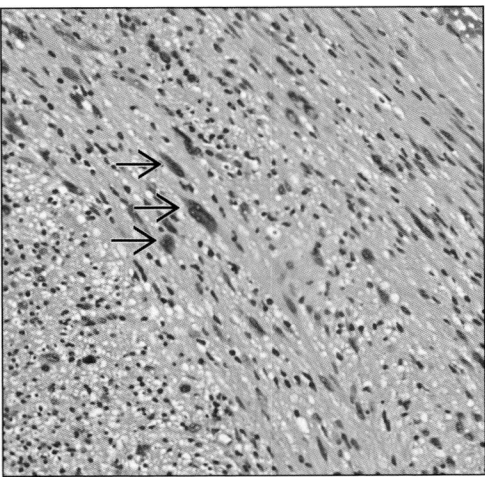

(Left) Cytoplasmic ALK1 reactivity is seen in a subset of pseudosarcomatous myofibroblastic proliferations, but it is not typically seen in sarcomatoid carcinoma or leiomyosarcoma. *(Right)* This benign nerve sheath tumor (schwannoma) shows scattered cells with degenerative-type atypia ⇨ that may mimic malignancy. Demonstration of diffuse immunoreactivity for S100 is an important diagnostic feature in this distinction.

SKELETAL MUSCLE TUMORS

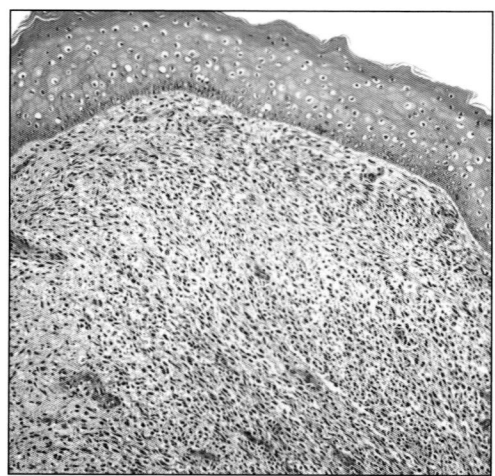

A subepithelial proliferation of spindle cells is characteristic of the botryoid variant of embryonal rhabdomyosarcoma, the most common rhabdomyosarcoma of the urinary bladder.

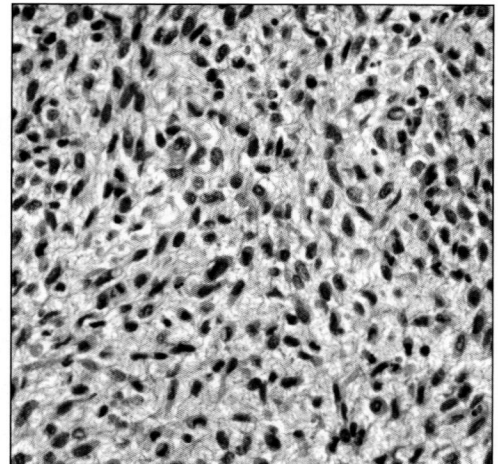

Spindled to round or fusiform neoplastic cells with a variable rim of eosinophilic cytoplasm is typical of embryonal rhabdomyosarcoma. The associated myxoid stroma is also common.

TERMINOLOGY

Abbreviations
- Rhabdomyosarcoma (RMS)

Definitions
- Malignant neoplasm recapitulating morphologic and molecular features of skeletal muscle

CLINICAL ISSUES

Epidemiology
- Incidence
  - Most common urinary bladder tumor in childhood and adolescence
  - Extraordinarily rare in adults
- Age
  - Mean at diagnosis is 4 years
- Gender
  - Male predominance (M:F = 3:2)

Presentation
- Gross hematuria is most common initial symptom

Treatment
- Combined surgery and chemotherapy have greatly improved survival in pediatric group

Prognosis
- Excellent in children with newer chemotherapy regimens
- Extremely poor in adults

MACROSCOPIC FEATURES

General Features
- Typically polypoid (botryoid)

MICROSCOPIC PATHOLOGY

Histologic Features
- Embryonal RMS is composed of proliferation of spindled tumor cells with variable cellularity
  - Botryoid subtype has condensation of tumor cells (cambium layer) beneath covering surface epithelium
  - Marked variability with fusiform, spindled, and rounded neoplastic cells may be seen
  - May have scattered rhabdomyoblasts ("strap cells")
  - Foci may be markedly hypocellular with bland cytology
  - Myxoid stroma is common
- Classic alveolar RMS
  - Characterized by back-to-back "round cells" with high nuclear-to-cytoplasmic ratio
  - Neoplastic cells have nuclear morphology reminiscent of lymphoma
  - May have alveolar septae or may grow in solid pattern
  - May have scattered wreath-like cells
- Vesical RMS in adults
  - Often have alveolar or unclassifiable RMS histology
  - Areas of nuclear anaplasia are common

Predominant Pattern/Injury Type
- Spindled

Predominant Cell/Compartment Type
- Skeletal muscle

ANCILLARY TESTS

Immunohistochemistry
- Desmin and actin-sm are typically strongly positive
- Nuclear myogenin and MYOD1 expression define skeletal muscle phenotype

SKELETAL MUSCLE TUMORS

Key Facts

Clinical Issues
- Most common bladder tumor of childhood
- Extraordinarily rare in adults
- Current therapies have greatly improved survival in pediatric group

Microscopic Pathology
- Embryonal RMS is composed of proliferation spindled tumor cells with variable cellularity
- Classic alveolar RMS has back-to-back "round cells" with high nuclear to cytoplasmic ratio
- Vesical RMS in adults often have alveolar or unclassifiable RMS histology with anaplasia

Ancillary Tests
- Desmin and smooth muscle actin are typically strongly positive

- Nuclear myogenin and MYOD1 expression characteristic
- Alveolar RMS may have *FKHR (FOX01a)* rearrangements

Top Differential Diagnoses
- Inflammatory myofibroblastic tumor
- Fibroepithelial polyp
- Small cell carcinoma in adults
- Sarcomatoid urothelial carcinoma/carcinosarcoma in adults
- Lymphoma

Diagnostic Checklist
- Embryonal RMS should be ruled out when considering vesical inflammatory myofibroblastic tumor in a child

---

   o MYOD1 commonly has nonspecific cytoplasmic staining, which is nondiagnostic
   o Myosin and myoglobin have been largely replaced by myogenin

In Situ Hybridization
- Alveolar RMS may have rearrangements involving *FKHR (FOX01a)* and either *PAX3* or *PAX7*

DIFFERENTIAL DIAGNOSIS

Inflammatory Myofibroblastic Tumor
- Important differential diagnosis in children
- Hypocellular proliferation of spindle cells with elongated, eosinophilic cytoplasmic processes
- Myxoid stromal matrix is common
- Admixed inflammatory cells, including eosinophils and plasma cells
- Tumor cells typically coexpress actin-sm and cytokeratin
- Subset are positive for anaplastic lymphoma kinase (ALK) immunostain
- Do not express nuclear myogenin or MYOD1
- Do not have cambium layer

Small Cell Carcinoma in Adults
- May be morphologically indistinguishable from alveolar RMS
- Typical urothelial carcinoma may also be present
- Immunohistochemistry for synaptophysin and chromogranin are positive
   o Synaptophysin may also be positive in RMS
- Typically express cytokeratin
- Tumor cells are negative for myogenin and MYOD1 by immunohistochemistry

Fibroepithelial Polyp
- Polypoid exophytic growth may clinically simulate botryoid RMS
- Does not have cambium layer
- Does not express myogenin or MYOD1

Sarcomatoid Urothelial Carcinoma/ Carcinosarcoma in Adults
- Component of urothelial carcinoma (carcinosarcoma) should be excluded
- RMS is common heterologous element in carcinosarcoma

Lymphoma
- Lymphomas may have identical cytology to alveolar RMS
- CD45(LCA), CD20, and CD3 immunohistochemistry help exclude hematopoietic lineage

DIAGNOSTIC CHECKLIST

Pathologic Interpretation Pearls
- Embryonal RMS should be ruled out when considering diagnosis of vesical inflammatory myofibroblastic tumor in child
- RMS and small cell carcinoma may be morphologically indistinguishable in adults

SELECTED REFERENCES

1. Paner GP et al: Rhabdomyosarcoma of the urinary bladder in adults: predilection for alveolar morphology with anaplasia and significant morphologic overlap with small cell carcinoma. Am J Surg Pathol. 32(7):1022-8, 2008
2. Parham DM et al: Correlation between histology and PAX/ FKHR fusion status in alveolar rhabdomyosarcoma: a report from the Children's Oncology Group. Am J Surg Pathol. 31(6):895-901, 2007
3. Leuschner I et al: Rhabdomyosarcoma of the urinary bladder and vagina: a clinicopathologic study with emphasis on recurrent disease: a report from the Kiel Pediatric Tumor Registry and the German CWS Study. Am J Surg Pathol. 25(7):856-64, 2001
4. Kumar S et al: Myogenin is a specific marker for rhabdomyosarcoma: an immunohistochemical study in paraffin-embedded tissues. Mod Pathol. 13(9):988-93, 2000
5. Scholtmeijer RJ et al: Embryonal rhabdomyosarcoma of the urogenital tract in childhood. Eur Urol. 9(2):69-74, 1983

2

SKELETAL MUSCLE TUMORS

Microscopic Features

(Left) The cambium layer (subepithelial condensation of the neoplastic cells) is typical of the botryoid variant of embryonal RMS. In children, the clinical presentation of an exophytic bladder mass should strongly suggest the diagnosis of RMS. *(Right)* There is a broad morphologic spectrum for RMS. This example of embryonal RMS has a more cellular fascicular pattern of growth with scant myxoid stroma. The patient's age is important in arriving at the appropriate diagnosis.

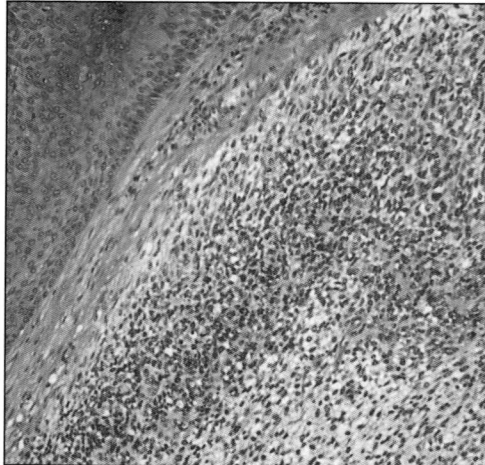 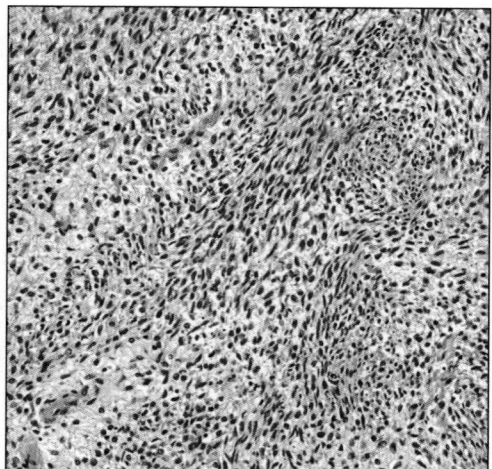

(Left) Myxoid stroma is common in embryonal RMS. In the urinary bladder, this may cause diagnostic consideration of an inflammatory myofibroblastic tumor/pseudosarcomatous myofibroblastic proliferation, which may also occur in children. *(Right)* Some foci in embryonal RMS may have very bland nuclear cytology that may closely mimic a benign process. In children, the index of suspicion for RMS should be high and prompt an immunohistochemical work-up to exclude RMS.

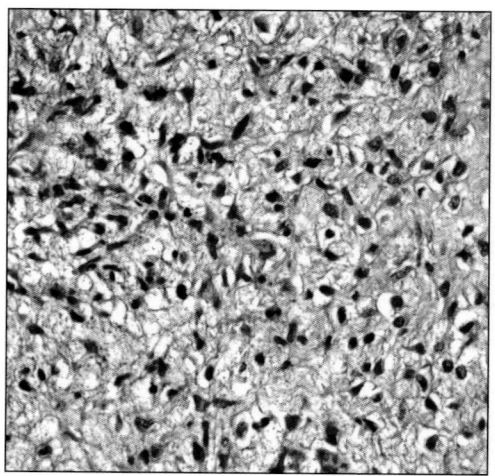 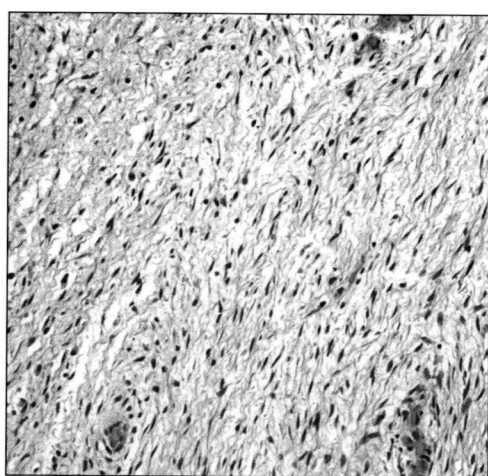

(Left) Classic rhabdomyoblasts or "strap cells" with cross striations may be identified. These are diagnostic of rhabdomyoblastic differentiation. *(Right)* Focal cartilaginous differentiation is well described in RMS of the gynecologic and genitourinary tracts. This may cause diagnostic confusion with a carcinosarcoma. The presence of cartilage does not alter the favorable prognosis for a patient with a childhood bladder RMS.

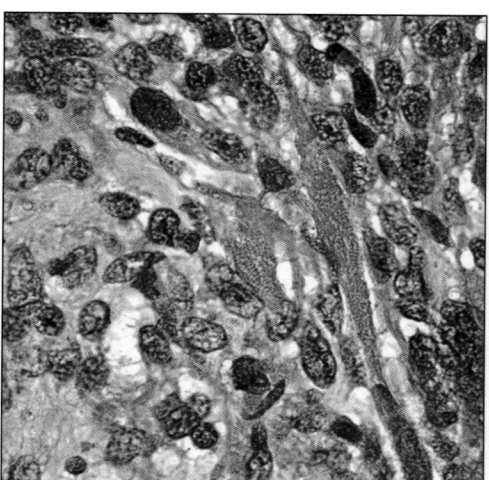 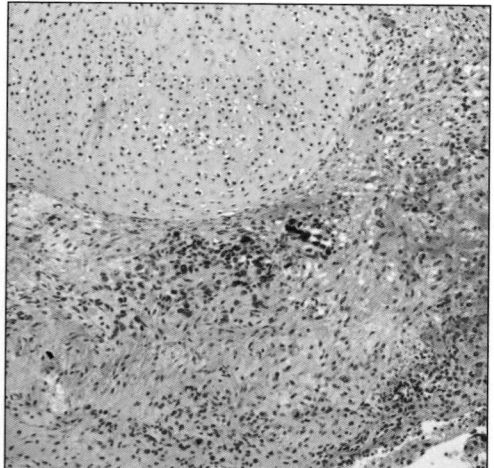

SKELETAL MUSCLE TUMORS

Microscopic Features

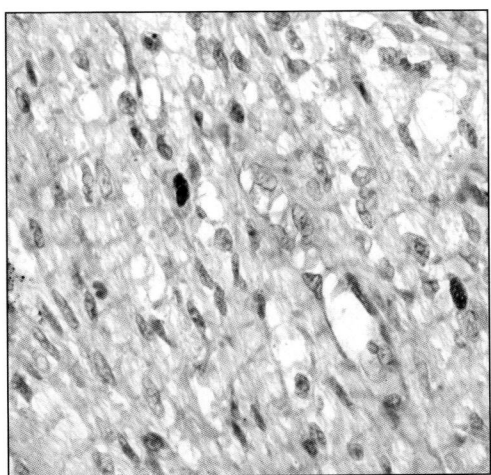

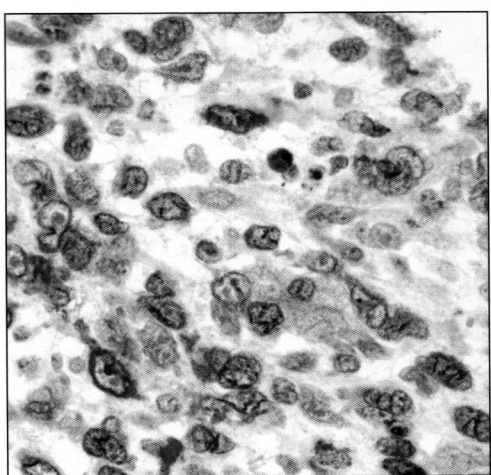

(Left) As in this example of embryonal RMS, nuclear myogenin immunoreactivity may be patchy. In contrast, diffuse immunoreactivity (greater than 80%) is typical of alveolar RMS. (Right) Careful attention to the pattern of staining is important in the interpretation of skeletal muscle markers. As in this example, nonspecific cytoplasmic staining for MYOD1 (a nuclear marker) is common but does not indicate skeletal muscle differentiation.

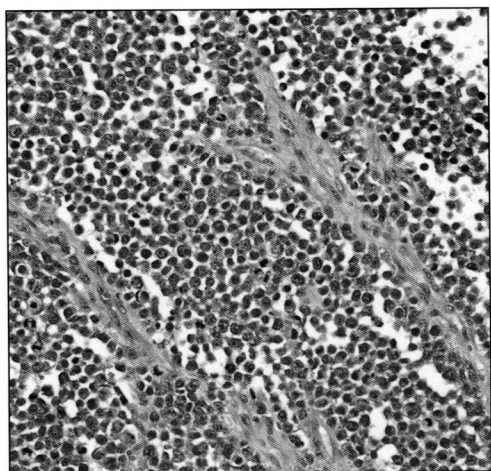

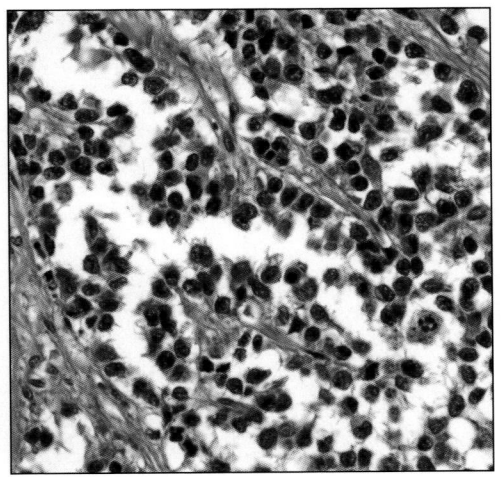

(Left) This is a classic example of alveolar RMS with fibrovascular septae creating the prototypical alveolar architecture. The neoplastic cells typically appear discohesive and have a "malignant small round blue cell" morphology. (Right) The neoplastic small round cells of alveolar RMS often cling to the fibrous septae in a "hobnail" pattern. The alveolar pattern of RMS is extremely rare in the urinary bladder. It may occur in adults where it may mimic small cell carcinoma.

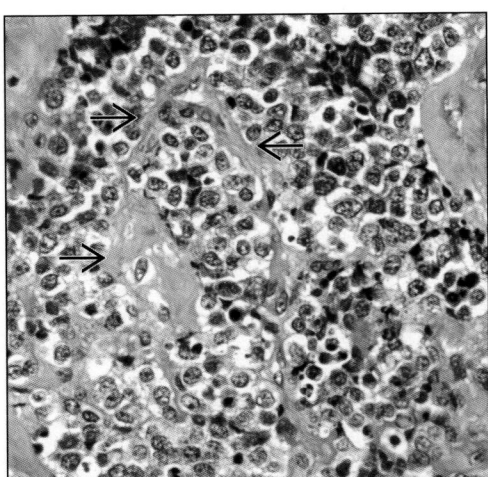

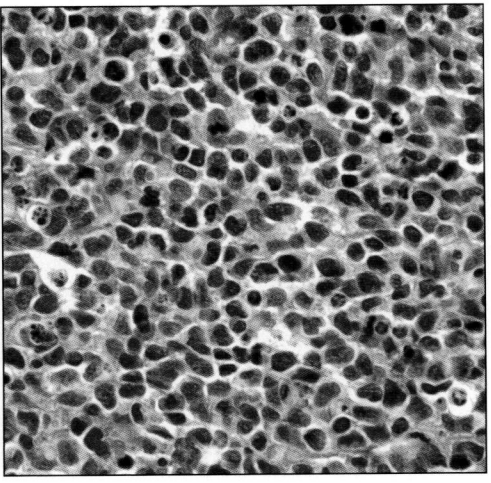

(Left) In some cases of alveolar RMS, the septae are more subtle ⮕, and the tumor has a more solid pattern. The individual neoplastic cells, however, have a round cell lymphoma-like morphology that is distinct from the embryonal subtype of RMS. (Right) This alveolar RMS has a solid pattern that lacks fibrous septae. The alveolar classification is based on the cytologic features that are reminiscent of lymphoma, as in this example.

SKELETAL MUSCLE TUMORS

Rhabdomyosarcoma in Adults

(Left) This example of RMS in an adult has a greater degree of pleomorphism than typically seen in childhood RMS. This appearance suggests the possibility of a carcinoma with or without neuroendocrine differentiation or an aggressive high-grade lymphoma. *(Right)* This example of adult RMS has a round cell morphology strongly suggesting lymphoma or small cell carcinoma. Immunohistochemical evaluation to cover a broad range of differentials is essential in adults.

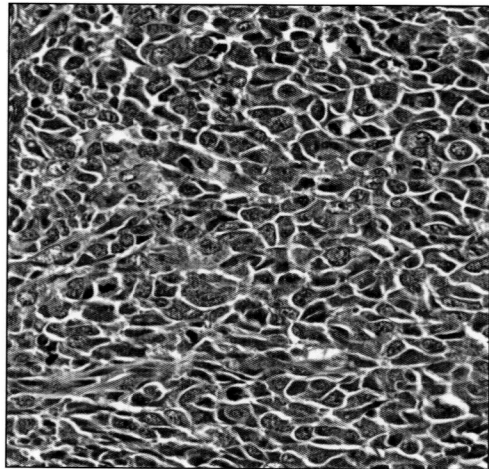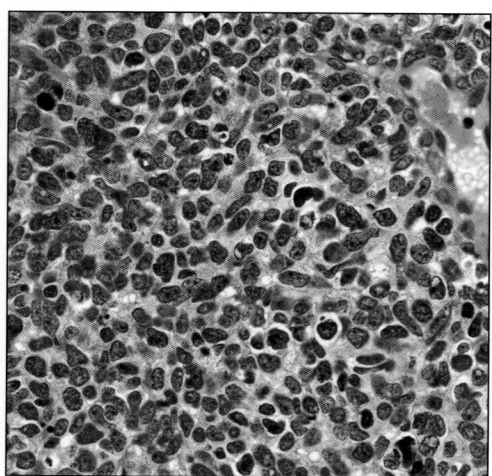

(Left) Adult RMS commonly has an alveolar morphology, as well as scattered neoplastic cells with marked nuclear anaplasia ⊟. Anaplasia is more frequent in adult than pediatric RMS. In adults, pure RMS should be distinguished from carcinosarcoma with rhabdomyoblastic differentiation. *(Right)* Strong cytoplasmic desmin reactivity is typical of RMS. Desmin immunoreactivity is not entirely specific for RMS, so other skeletal muscle markers, such as myogenin and MYOD1, are often utilized.

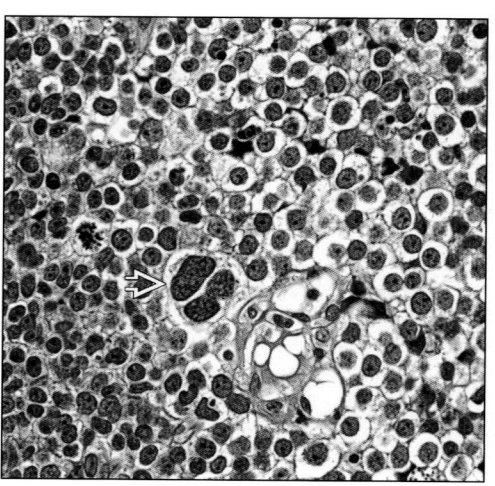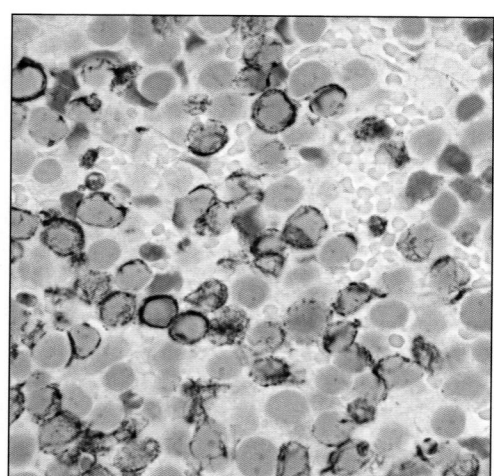

(Left) Strong and diffuse myogenin reactivity is characteristic of alveolar RMS. The percentage of cells expressing myogenin is typically much less in embryonal RMS. *(Right)* This RMS shows "aberrant" synaptophysin reactivity. It is not uncommon for RMS at any site to be positive for synaptophysin. In adults, this finding may result in further diagnostic confusion with small cell carcinoma. Cytokeratin staining is helpful to confirm a small cell carcinoma diagnosis.

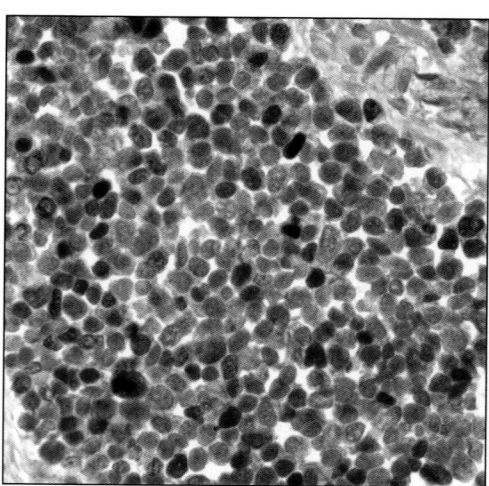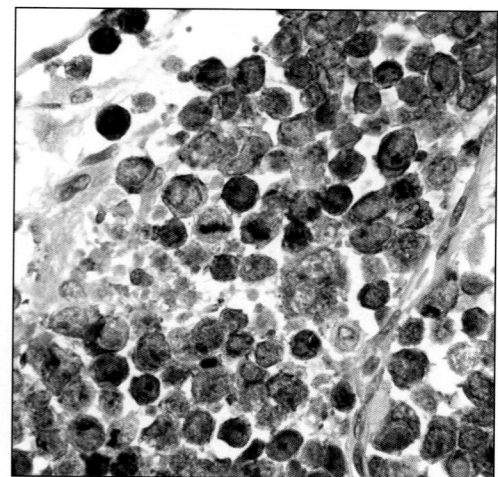

SKELETAL MUSCLE TUMORS

Differential Diagnosis

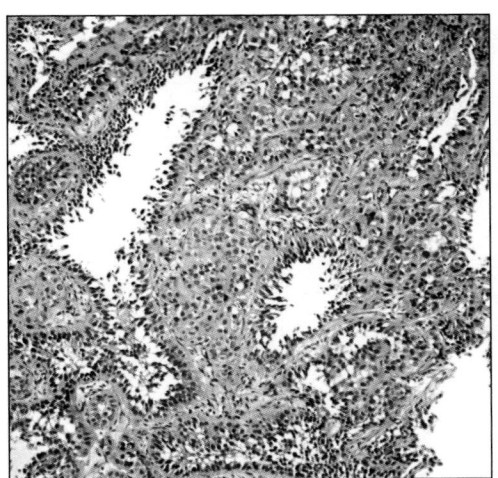
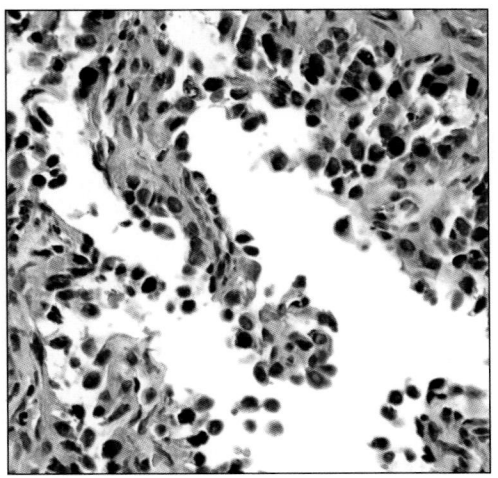

(Left) Morphologically subtle patterns of invasive urothelial carcinoma (e.g., nested or microcystic) may occasionally have cystic change with discohesion that may suggest an alveolar morphology on biopsy. *(Right)* Focal areas of this urothelial carcinoma have cellular discohesion that may suggest an alveolar RMS on a small biopsy specimen. Other foci of more typical urothelial carcinoma are usually present. Immunohistochemistry may be necessary in biopsy specimens.

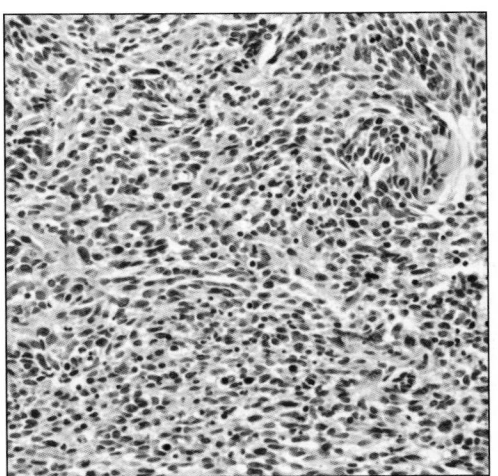
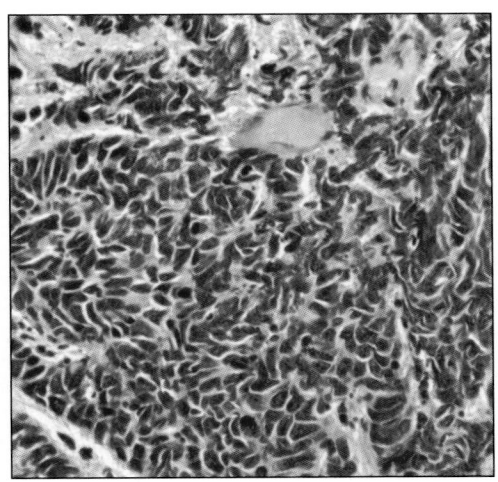

(Left) As seen here, a small cell carcinoma of the urinary bladder in an adult may mimic any small round cell tumor, such as RMS, lymphoma, or malignant melanoma. *(Right)* Small cell carcinoma with high nuclear to cytoplasmic ratio, nuclear molding, apoptotic bodies, and high mitotic index. It is negative for myogenin and MYOD1 but expresses cytokeratin, synaptophysin, and in some cases TTF-1. It is not uncommon for small cell carcinoma to have an associated urothelial carcinoma.

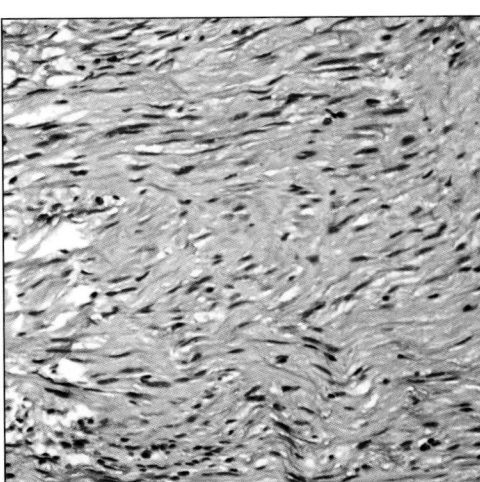
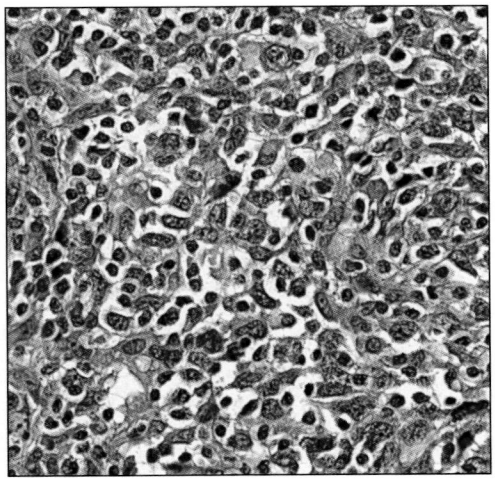

(Left) Myofibroblastic proliferations, as in this example, may closely resemble bland foci of embryonal RMS. In a child, the possibility of RMS should be carefully considered and excluded when a cytologically bland spindle cell proliferation is encountered on a biopsy specimen. *(Right)* A lymphoepithelioma-like carcinoma of the urinary bladder may also closely mimic a round cell tumor. Cytokeratin reactivity is useful in confirming an epithelial lineage.

OTHER MESENCHYMAL TUMORS

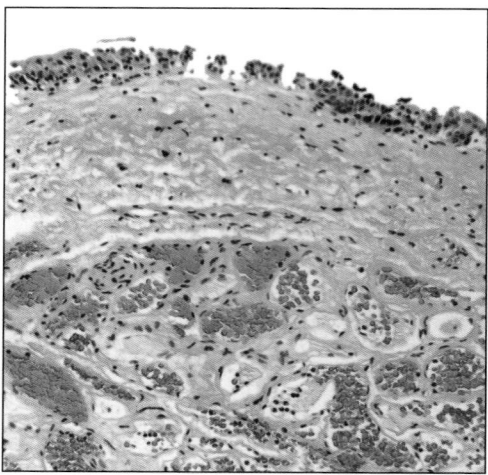

Most vascular lesions in the bladder are vascular malformations or hemangiomas, which are characterized by lobular collections of blood vessels with cytologically benign endothelial cells.

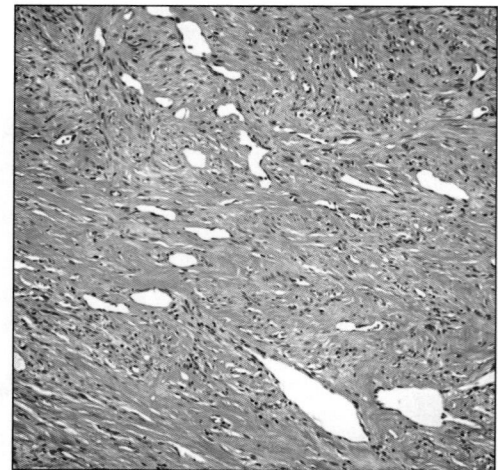

Although not common, solitary fibrous tumors are also well described in the urinary bladder. The angulated (hemangiopericytic) blood vessels and collagenization are both typical features.

TERMINOLOGY

Definitions
- Mesenchymal neoplasms other than muscle and myofibroblastic lineage may occur in urinary bladder

CLINICAL ISSUES

Epidemiology
- Incidence
  - Extraordinarily rare
    - Often present in literature as single case reports

Presentation
- Hematuria
- Obstruction
- Pelvic pain

Treatment
- Surgical approaches
  - Simple transurethral resection for small benign lesions
  - Large benign lesions may need more extensive resection
  - Sarcomas generally require radical cystectomy and consideration of adjuvant therapy

MICROSCOPIC PATHOLOGY

Neurofibroma
- Proliferation of spindled cells with small tapered or wavy nuclei
- Randomly distributed individual bundles of "shredded carrot" collagen are common
- Lack of significant cytologic atypia or mitotic figures
  - Scattered degenerative atypia may be seen
- Neoplastic cells show cytoplasmic and nuclear immunoreactivity with S100

Solitary Fibrous Tumor
- Most behave in benign fashion when completely resected
  - Large size, nuclear pleomorphism, and mitotic activity may predict malignant potential
- Spindle cells arranged in haphazard pattern
- Cellularity varies greatly
- Deposition of intercellular collagen
- Neoplastic cells are positive with CD34

Hemangioma/Vascular Malformation
- Benign lesion composed of blood vessels
  - Cytologically bland endothelial cells
  - Surrounding smooth muscle cells often seen
- Most lesions reported as hemangioma are designated as vascular malformation under recent classification systems

Post-Radiation Sarcoma
- Pleomorphic undifferentiated appearance most common
  - Distinction from sarcomatoid carcinoma may be very difficult
    - Especially if history of genitourinary tract carcinoma
- Commonly arises 8-10 years after radiation therapy
  - Many occur after treatment of prostatic or uterine primaries

Other Sarcoma Subtypes
- Angiosarcoma
  - Wide morphologic spectrum
  - Vasoformative or epithelioid with sheet-like growth
    - Commonly express CD34 and CD31
    - May show aberrant cytokeratin expression, especially if epithelioid
- Osteosarcoma
  - Trabeculae of neoplastic bone associated with malignant cells

OTHER MESENCHYMAL TUMORS

Key Facts

Clinical Issues
- Extraordinarily rare
- Hematuria

Microscopic Pathology
- Neurofibroma
  - Proliferation of spindled cells with small tapered nuclei
  - Randomly distributed collagen bundles common
  - May mimic myofibroblastic proliferation in cellular cases
  - S100 positive
- Solitary fibrous tumor
  - Spindle cells arranged in haphazard pattern
  - Angulated "hemangiopericytic" blood vessels
  - Deposition of intercellular collagen
  - Neoplastic cells are positive with CD34

- Hemangioma/vascular malformation
  - Benign lesion comprised of aggregated blood vessels
  - No destructive invasive growth or significant cytologic atypia
- Post-radiation sarcoma
  - Pleomorphic undifferentiated appearance most common
  - Distinction from sarcomatoid carcinoma may be difficult
- Other tumors
  - Angiosarcoma
  - Osteosarcoma
  - Pleomorphic undifferentiated sarcoma (malignant fibrous histiocytoma)
  - Granular cell tumor

- Pleomorphic undifferentiated sarcoma (malignant fibrous histiocytoma)
  - Pleomorphic spindled malignant neoplasm without evidence of specific line of differentiation
- Granular cell tumor
  - Round cellular infiltrate with abundant granular eosinophilic cytoplasm
  - Express S100

DIFFERENTIAL DIAGNOSIS

Neurofibroma
- Low-grade malignant peripheral nerve sheath tumor
  - Better developed fascicular growth with mitotic activity
- Embryonal rhabdomyosarcoma
  - May have morphologically bland areas with close resemblance to neurofibroma
  - Cytoplasmic desmin and nuclear myogenin &/or MYOD1 immunoreactivity diagnostic
- Leiomyoma
  - Usually more cellular without collagen bundles
  - Express actin-sm but not S100
- Myofibroblastic proliferation
  - Usually have associated mixed inflammatory infiltrate
  - Express actin-sm but not S100

Solitary Fibrous Tumor
- Sarcomatoid carcinoma
  - Usually more cytologic atypia and carcinomatous component may be identified
  - Typically expresses HMCK(34βE12) and p63
- Neurofibroma
  - Diffuse S100 immunoreactivity
- Synovial sarcoma
  - Typically more cellular, tightly organized fascicles
  - Does not express CD34
  - Has characteristic (X;18) translocation

Hemangioma/Vascular Malformation
- Angiosarcoma has infiltrative growth and cytologic atypia
- Kaposi sarcoma typically has cellular fascicles
- Granulation tissue contains tightly aggregated small vessels with associated inflammation

Post-Radiation Sarcoma
- Sarcomatoid urothelial carcinoma
  - Carcinomatous component may be seen
  - Typically expresses high molecular weight cytokeratin and p63

Angiosarcoma
- Kaposi sarcoma
  - Predominantly spindled and expresses HHV8
- Hemangioma
  - Lobulated architecture without infiltration or significant atypia

Pleomorphic Undifferentiated Sarcoma (Malignant Fibrous Histiocytoma)
- Sarcomatoid urothelial carcinoma
  - Component of typical carcinoma or expresses epithelial markers (e.g., p63)

Granular Cell Tumor
- Malakoplakia does not express S100
- Carcinomas express cytokeratin but not S100

SELECTED REFERENCES

1. Tavora F et al: A series of vascular tumors and tumorlike lesions of the bladder. Am J Surg Pathol. 32(8):1213-9, 2008
2. Wang W et al: Benign nerve sheath tumors on urinary bladder biopsy. Am J Surg Pathol. 32(6):907-12, 2008
3. Westra WH et al: Solitary fibrous tumor of the lower urogenital tract: a report of five cases involving the seminal vesicles, urinary bladder, and prostate. Hum Pathol. 31(1):63-8, 2000
4. Cheng L et al: Neurofibroma of the urinary bladder. Cancer. 86(3):505-13, 1999

OTHER MESENCHYMAL TUMORS

Microscopic Features

(Left) *This neurofibroma is seen underlying the surface urothelium of the urinary bladder. On low-power evaluation, neural tumors may mimic a myofibroblastic or other spindle cell process.* *(Right)* *The randomly scattered collagen bundles ("shredded carrot" collagen) are characteristic of neurofibroma at any site. The neoplastic cells are usually cytologically bland, but scattered cells with degenerative atypia may be seen.*

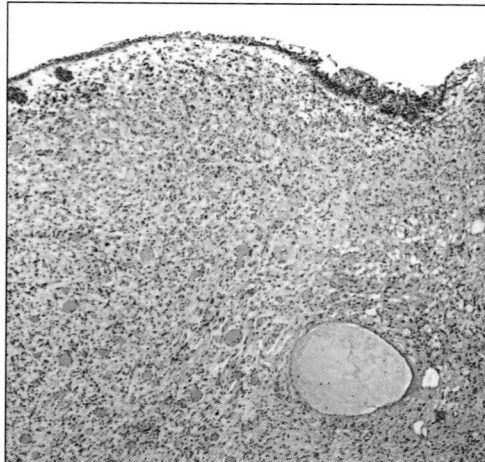
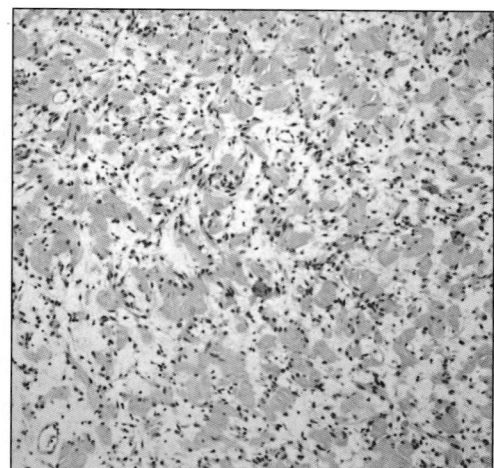

(Left) *More cellular neurofibromas, such as this example, may closely mimic a myofibroblastic proliferation of the urinary bladder. Demonstration of diffuse cytoplasmic and nuclear S100 immunoreactivity is helpful in this diagnostic setting.* *(Right)* *Hemangioma/vascular malformation of the bladder is seen with discrete nonanastomosing capillary-sized structures lined by flattened innocuous endothelial cells. Low-power circumscription is another clue that the lesion is benign.*

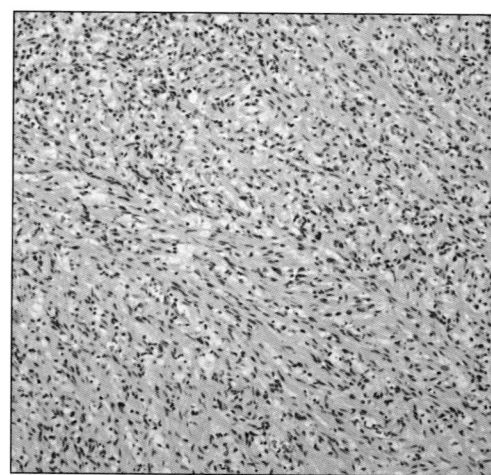
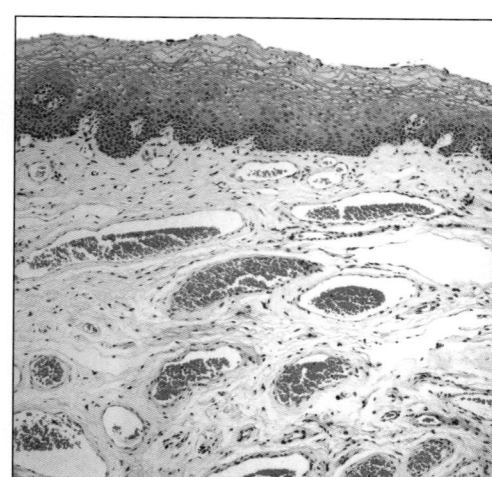

(Left) *In benign vascular lesions, the individual endothelial cells are cytologically bland. Permeation and destructive invasion of normal structures, such as muscularis propria, is not seen.* *(Right)* *Granular cell tumors of the genitourinary tract are similar to those in other sites with a sheet-like growth pattern and abundant granular eosinophilic cytoplasm. The neoplastic cells show diffuse expression of S100.*

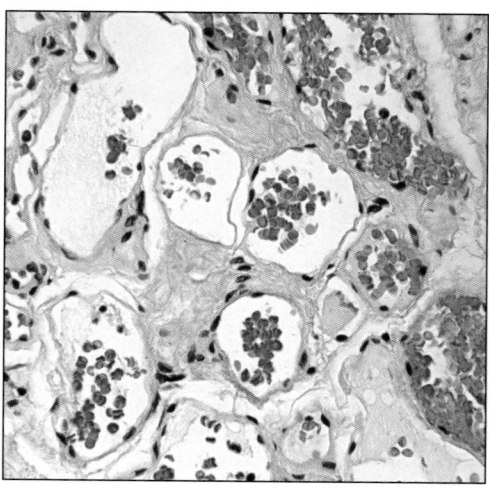
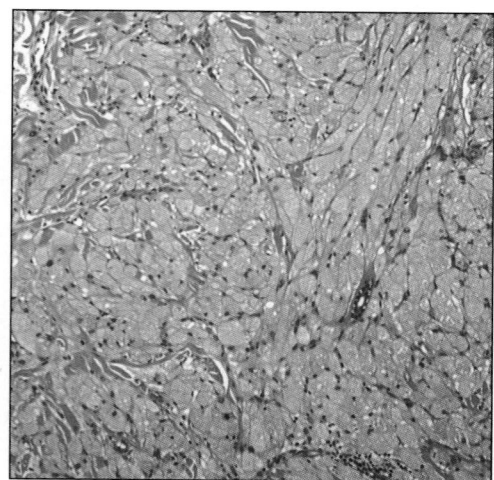

OTHER MESENCHYMAL TUMORS

Microscopic Features

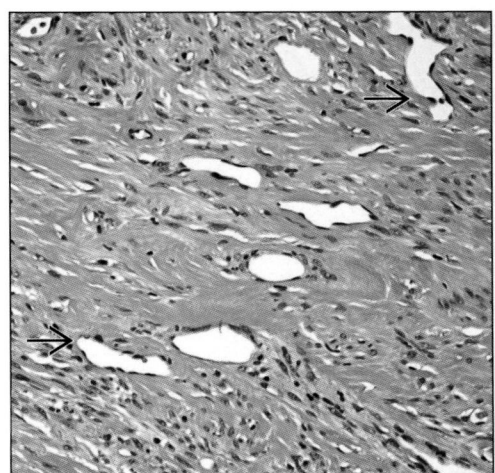
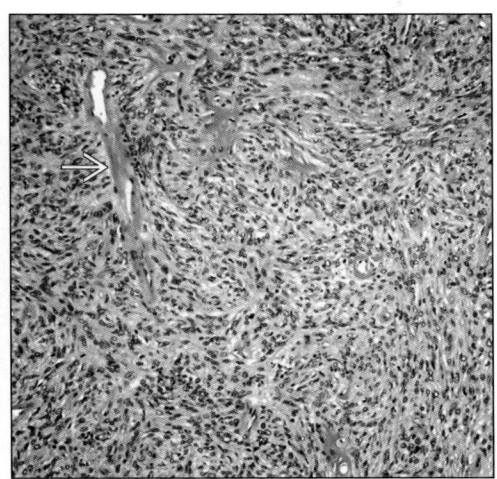

(Left) The hypocellular proliferation of fibroblasts without a distinct architectural growth (so-called "patternless" pattern), the dense collagenization, and the angulated hemangiopericytic blood vessels ⊟ all support a diagnosis of solitary fibrous tumor. (Right) Some examples of solitary fibrous tumor are more cellular and have also been called hemangiopericytoma in the past. The angulated blood vessels with hyalinization ⊟ are typical of solitary fibrous tumor.

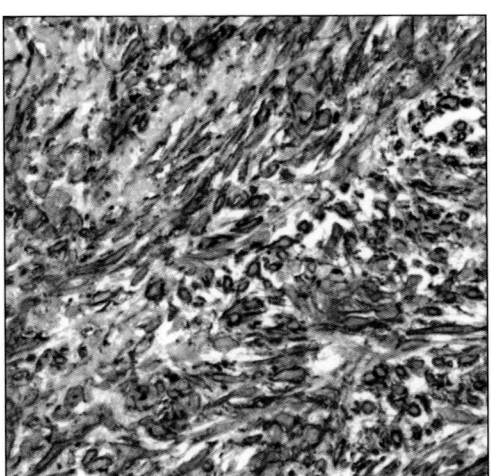
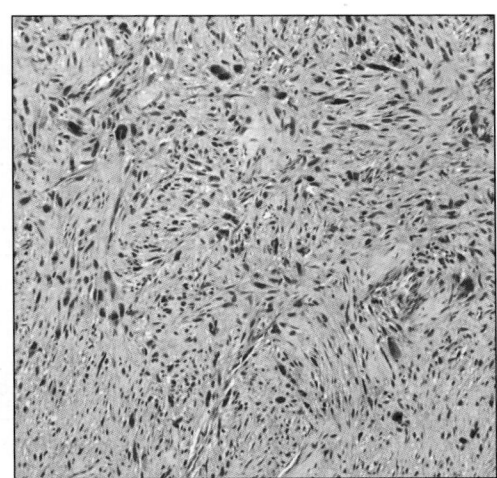

(Left) Diffuse cytoplasmic immunoreactivity with CD34 is characteristic of solitary fibrous tumor, which would typically be negative for cytokeratin staining. Smooth muscle actin may occasionally show immunoreactivity. (Right) Pleomorphic undifferentiated sarcoma may look identical to a high-grade leiomyosarcoma or sarcomatoid carcinoma; however, no immunoreactivity with smooth muscle or epithelial immunohistochemical markers is demonstrable.

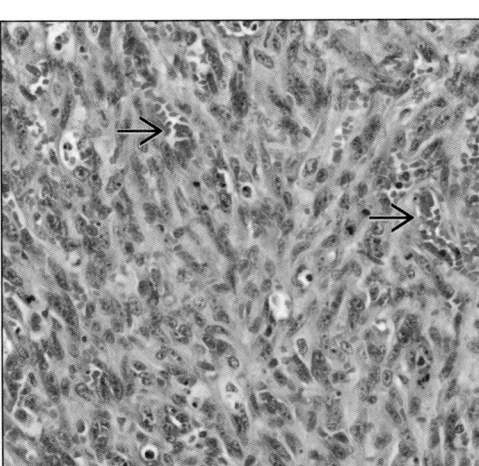
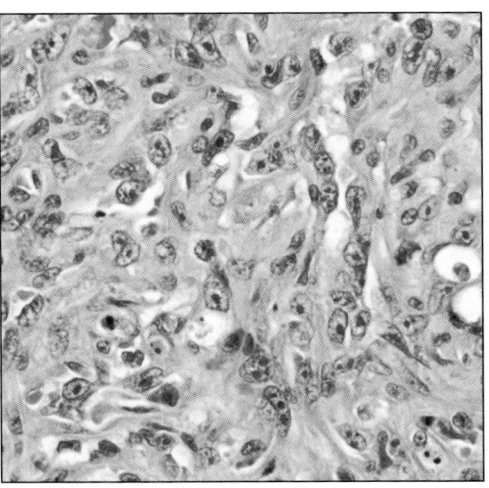

(Left) Vasoformation ⊟ and extravasated red blood cells should suggest angiosarcoma. Spindled areas may mimic leiomyosarcoma or sarcomatoid urothelial carcinoma, which are more common than angiosarcoma. (Right) Epithelioid foci in angiosarcoma may closely mimic poorly differentiated urothelial carcinoma, especially given the frequent immunoreactivity with cytokeratin. CD31, FLI-1, and CD34 immunostains may be helpful.

PARAGANGLIOMA

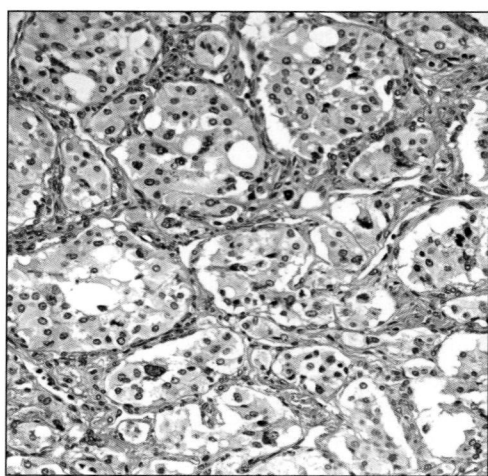

The classic nested or zellballen architecture of paraganglioma may mimic an invasive urothelial carcinoma with a nested growth pattern. An awareness of vesical paraganglioma is important.

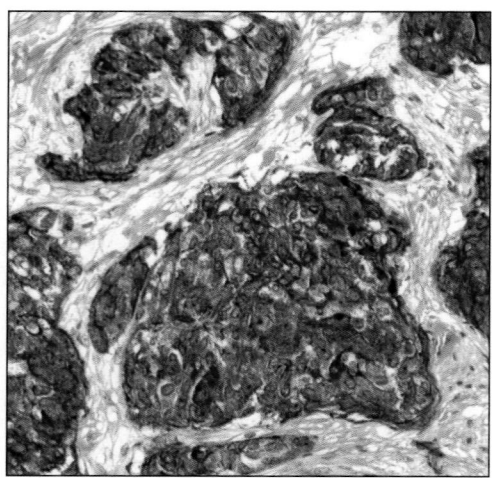

Diffuse cytoplasmic synaptophysin immunoreactivity is a helpful ancillary finding to aid in the differential diagnosis of urothelial carcinoma. The absence of cytokeratin staining is also helpful.

TERMINOLOGY

Synonyms
- Pheochromocytoma of bladder

Definitions
- Neoplasm derived from paraganglia cells in bladder wall in which sole criterion for malignancy is metastasis

CLINICAL ISSUES

Epidemiology
- Incidence
  - Majority described in case reports
  - < 0.05% of bladder tumors
- Age
  - 10-90 years

Site
- Urinary bladder
  - Most frequent extraadrenal site of urinary tract

Presentation
- Hematuria
  - Most common presentation
- Other symptoms (up to 15%)
  - Headache, palpitations, and sweating during micturition
  - Hypertension

Laboratory Tests
- Elevated serum and urine catecholamines are common

Natural History
- Most are clinically benign

Treatment
- Surgical approaches
  - Complete excision

Prognosis
- 10% demonstrate malignant behavior (i.e., metastasis)
- Local recurrence with incomplete excision

MACROSCOPIC FEATURES

General Features
- Intramural nodules
  - Lateral wall common

Size
- Most < 5 cm

MICROSCOPIC PATHOLOGY

Histologic Features
- Typically well-circumscribed
- Classic zellballen or nested arrangement of tumor cells
- Diffuse pattern of growth in subset of cases
- Sclerosing pattern may mimic invasive growth
- Neoplastic cells are round to polygonal
  - Abundant eosinophilic to granular cytoplasm; cytoplasm may be occasionally basophilic
- Central nucleus with vesicular chromatin
- Mitoses can be present
- Scattered pleomorphic cells are often present (i.e., endocrine atypia)
- Surface urothelium is intact and normal

Predominant Pattern/Injury Type
- Neoplastic

Predominant Cell/Compartment Type
- Neuroendocrine

PARAGANGLIOMA

Key Facts

Clinical Issues
- < 0.05% of bladder tumors
- Patients frequently present with hematuria
- Other systemic paraganglioma symptoms in up to 15% of cases
- Elevated levels of catecholamines in serum and urine
- 10% have malignant behavior (i.e., metastasis)

Macroscopic Features
- Commonly intramural nodules on lateral wall

Microscopic Pathology
- Most have classic zellballen pattern
- Rarely, more diffuse &/or sclerosing pattern of growth
- Scattered pleomorphic cells are often present (i.e., endocrine anaplasia)

Ancillary Tests
- Express neuroendocrine markers (e.g., synaptophysin, chromogranin-A, and CD56)
- Sustentacular cells highlighted by S100 protein (not always present)
- Neoplastic cells are typically negative for cytokeratin

Top Differential Diagnoses
- Invasive urothelial carcinoma
- High-grade prostatic adenocarcinoma
- Metastatic renal cell carcinoma
- Malignant melanoma
- Other endocrine neoplasms

ANCILLARY TESTS

Immunohistochemistry
- Express neuroendocrine markers (e.g., synaptophysin, chromogranin-A, and CD56)
- Sustentacular cells highlighted by S100 protein (not always present)
- Neoplastic cells are typically negative for cytokeratin

DIFFERENTIAL DIAGNOSIS

Invasive Urothelial Carcinoma (Nested or Typical Types)
- Associated papillary or in situ urothelial carcinoma
- Varying shapes of infiltrating nests
  - Present diffusely within lamina propria
  - Stromal reaction variable
    - Surrounding retraction spaces common
- Immunoreactive for cytokeratin and p63
- May show reactivity for urothelial specific markers uroplakin-3 or GATA3

Granular Cell Tumor
- Lack fine vascular network
- Abundant eosinophilic granular cytoplasm
- Diffuse S100 protein immunoreactivity

Metastatic Large Cell Neuroendocrine Carcinoma
- Necrosis, abundant mitotic activity, and cellular anaplasia common
- Positive for cytokeratin in addition to neuroendocrine markers
- Negative for S100 protein

Malignant Melanoma
- Anaplasia and prominent nucleoli
- Admixed nested and spindled components are common
- S100 protein is best screening marker
- May be positive for HMB-45, Melan-A, and MITF

Metastatic Renal Cell Carcinoma
- Delicate vascular septae may mimic zellballen pattern
- Clear or eosinophilic cytoplasm
- Variably immunoreactive for renal epithelial markers RCC, pax-2, and pax-8

High-Grade Prostatic Adenocarcinoma
- More prominent nucleoli
- Luminal differentiation typical
- Immunoreactive for PSA and PAP
  - May also express neuroendocrine markers
- Serum PSA often markedly elevated

DIAGNOSTIC CHECKLIST

Clinically Relevant Pathologic Features
- No reliable morphologic features for predicting malignant behavior

Pathologic Interpretation Pearls
- Awareness and consideration of paraganglioma in bladder is key to its distinction from other tumors
- Paraganglioma should be considered in younger females & with nested architecture & endocrine atypia

SELECTED REFERENCES
1. Plaza JA et al: Sclerosing paraganglioma: report of 19 cases of an unusual variant of neuroendocrine tumor that may be mistaken for an aggressive malignant neoplasm. Am J Surg Pathol. 30(1):7-12, 2006
2. Kovacs K et al: Malignant paraganglioma of the urinary bladder: Immunohistochemical study of prognostic indicators. Endocr Pathol. 16(4):363-9, 2005
3. Zhou M et al: Paraganglioma of the urinary bladder: a lesion that may be misdiagnosed as urothelial carcinoma in transurethral resection specimens. Am J Surg Pathol. 28(1):94-100, 2004
4. Cheng L et al: Paraganglioma of the urinary bladder: can biologic potential be predicted? Cancer. 88(4):844-52, 2000
5. Moyana TN et al: Urinary bladder paragangliomas. An immunohistochemical study. Arch Pathol Lab Med. 112(1):70-2, 1988

Microscopic Features

(Left) The interface of paraganglioma with the surrounding bladder soft tissues is usually well delineated ⇨. In carcinomas, a more irregular, infiltrative border is typically seen at scanning magnification. *(Right)* On low-power examination, this paraganglioma has a more vaguely nested growth pattern. Considering the possibility of paraganglioma at this site is important to its recognition. The correct diagnosis has prognostic and therapeutic implications.

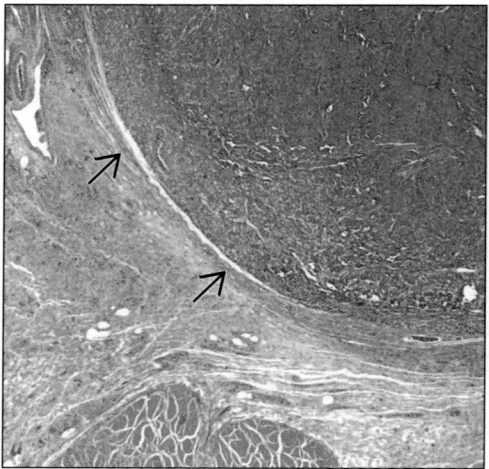
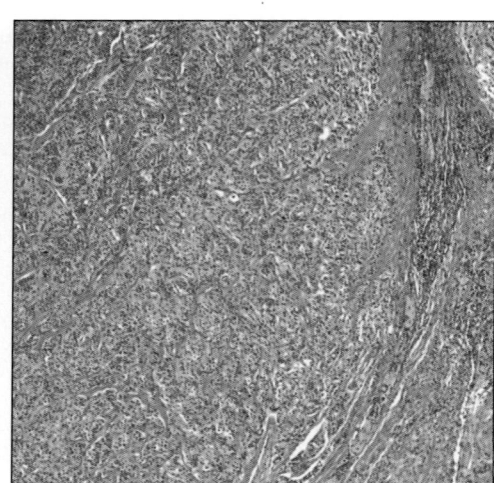

(Left) This example of paraganglioma has a striking nested architecture at low-power examination. This is the prototypical zellballen pattern of paraganglioma. *(Right)* The nests of tumor cells in paraganglioma are encircled by fine vascular septae. The neoplastic cells are round and monomorphic. This pattern may suggest the possibility of an invasive urothelial carcinoma with a nested pattern or possibly a high-grade prostatic adenocarcinoma.

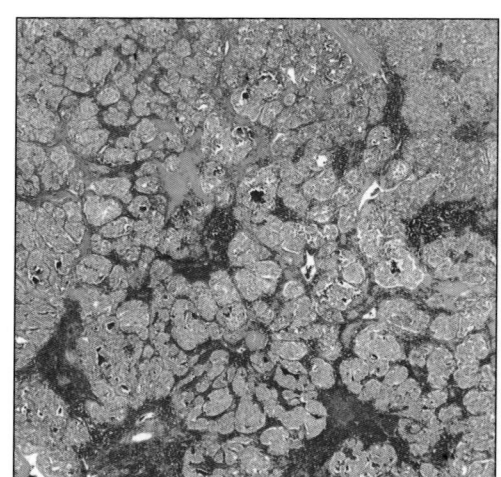
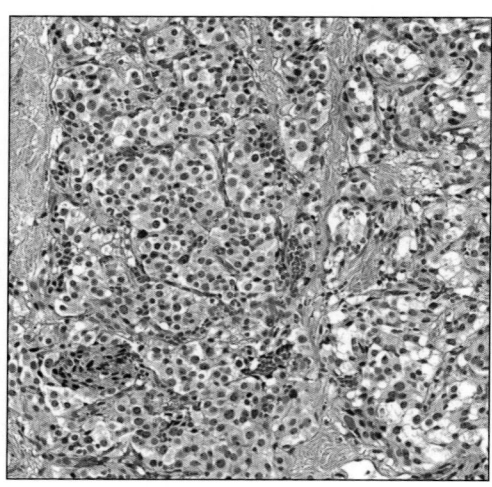

(Left) Surface ulceration due to prior transurethral resection may distort the tissue or impart an artifactual papillary appearance in subsequent excision specimens. These changes may cause additional confusion with urothelial carcinoma. *(Right)* Other morphologic clues may be helpful in recognizing paraganglioma. A normal surface urothelium is typically seen overlying paragangliomas of the urinary bladder.

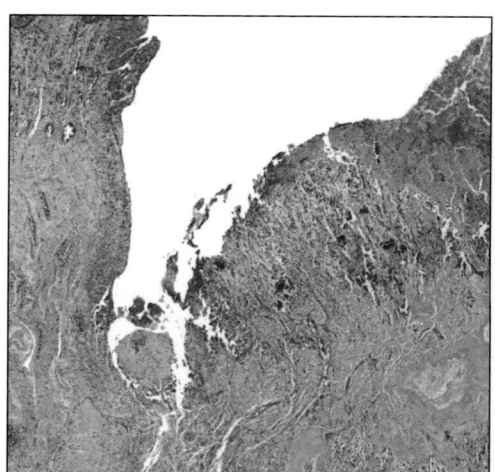
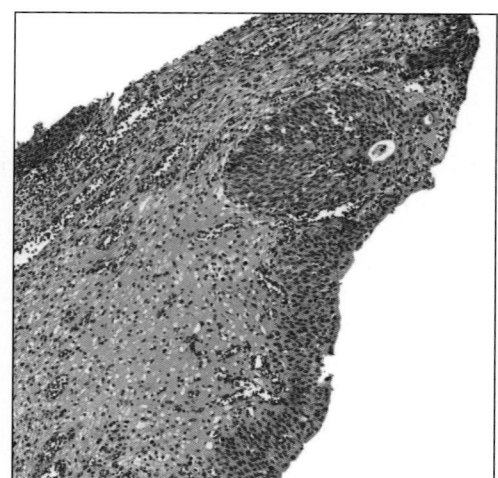

PARAGANGLIOMA

Variant Microscopic Features

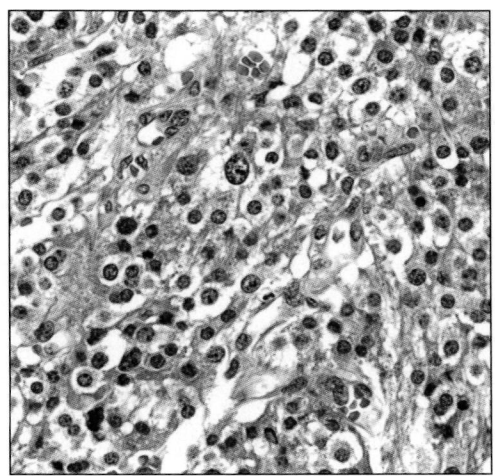

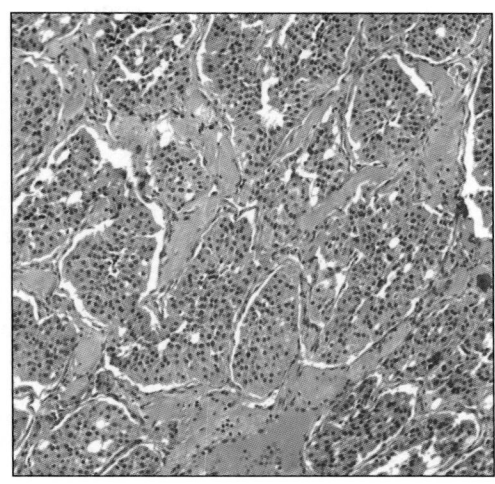

(Left) The nuclear contours of paraganglioma are typically round and sharp, but scattered individual enlarged cells may be present. This monotonous nuclear morphology may suggest prostatic adenocarcinoma, but nucleoli are not typically prominent in paraganglioma. *(Right)* Retraction artifact, as seen in this example of paraganglioma, may closely mimic invasive urothelial carcinoma. An immunohistochemical work-up is useful in such cases.

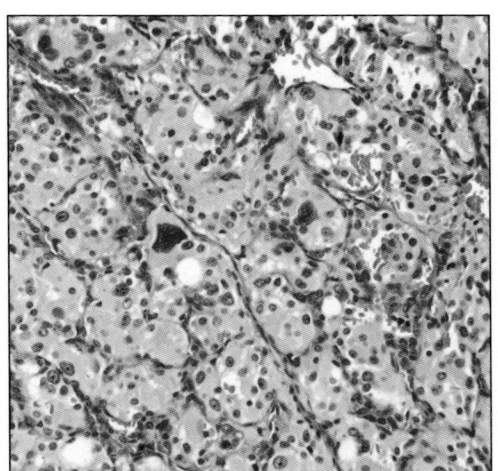

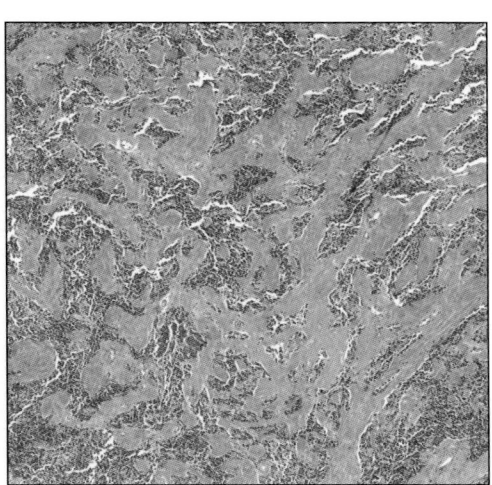

(Left) Scattered neoplastic cells with marked variation in size and shape (i.e., "endocrine anaplasia") are common in paraganglioma and do not denote malignancy. This is a helpful diagnostic feature that should suggest a neuroendocrine tumor. *(Right)* The sclerosing pattern of paraganglioma may mimic invasion, as seen in this example, and cause added diagnostic confusion with urothelial carcinoma.

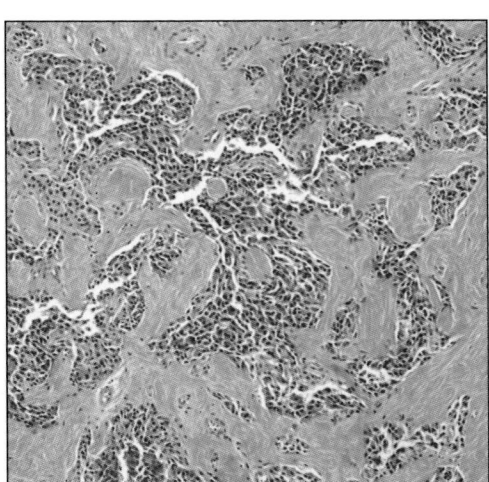

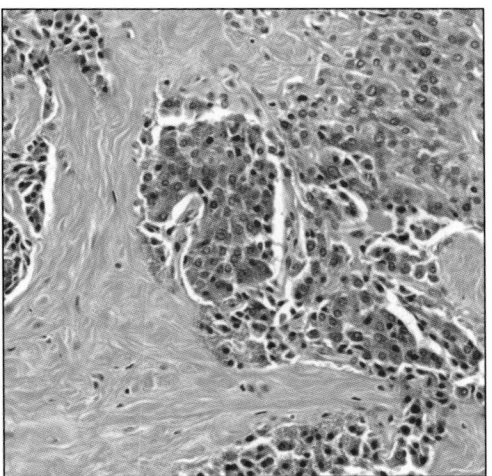

(Left) Because of this significant degree of morphologic overlap with invasive urothelial carcinoma, awareness of this sclerosing pattern of paraganglioma is important. *(Right)* The classic individual cell nests (zellballen pattern) may not be apparent in some examples of paraganglioma, especially those with significant hyalinization.

Variant Microscopic Features

(Left) Despite the pseudo-invasive sclerosing growth pattern, the individual neoplastic cells maintain the typical round nuclear contours. This example of paraganglioma has more amphophilic cytoplasm. *(Right)* In rare examples of sclerosing paraganglioma, the fibrotic tissue may comprise the majority of the lesion. Immunohistochemical confirmation with cytokeratin (negative) and synaptophysin (positive) may be essential in such cases.

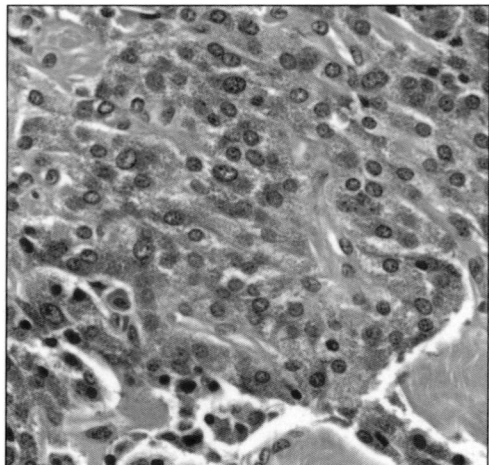
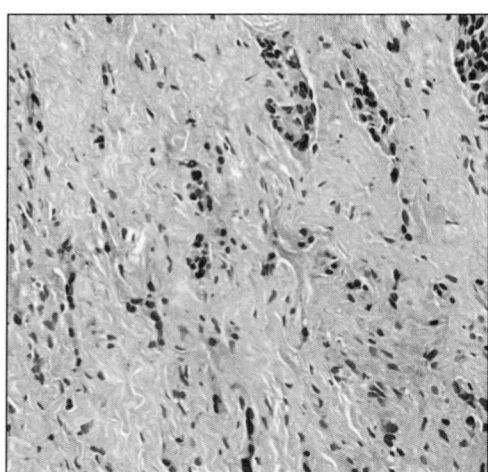

(Left) In this paraganglioma, a poorly differentiated invasive urothelial carcinoma is a strong consideration given the extensive degree of sclerosis and cord-like architectural growth. *(Right)* Recognition of rare scattered nests and high morphologic consideration of paraganglioma in bladder pathology with confirmatory immunostains is critical to properly classifying these morphologically difficult cases.

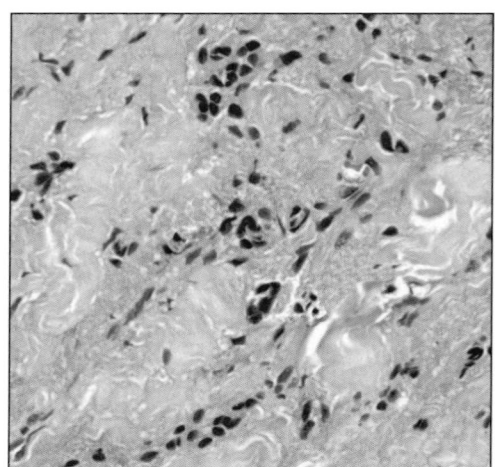
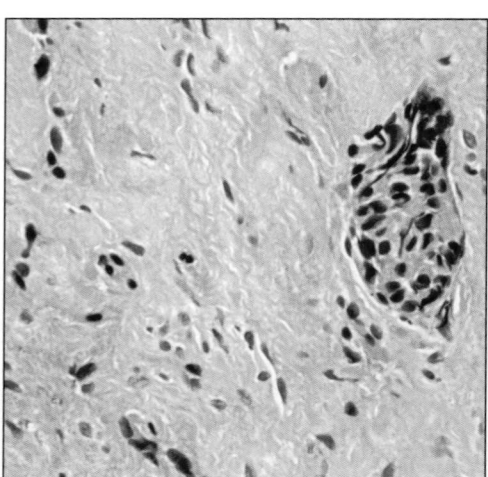

(Left) Definitive lymphovascular invasion was identified in this example of a clinically malignant paraganglioma. Malignant potential may be impossible to predict by morphologic examination. *(Right)* Metastatic paraganglioma may be identified in regional lymph nodes ➡. Histologic features do not adequately predict malignancy in paraganglioma, which is defined by the presence of metastasis.

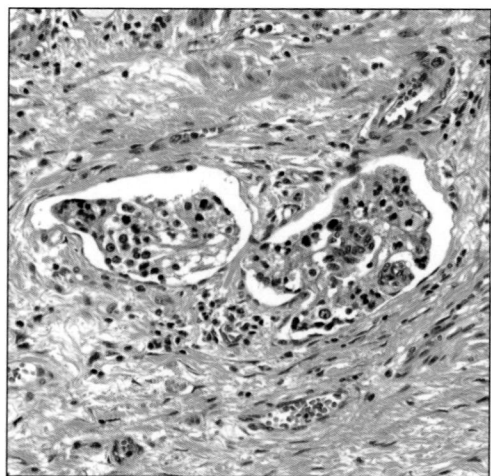
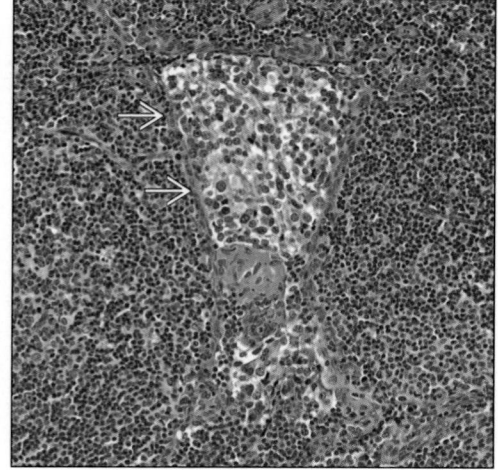

PARAGANGLIOMA

Ancillary Techniques

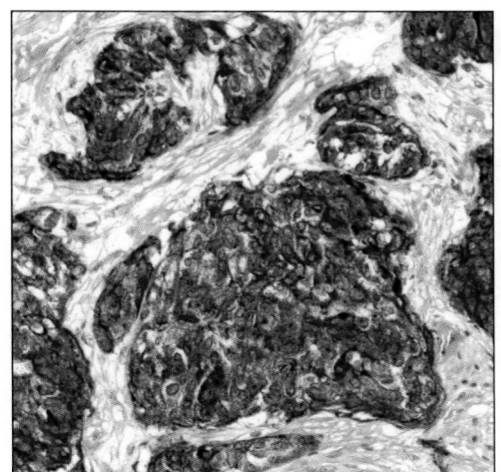

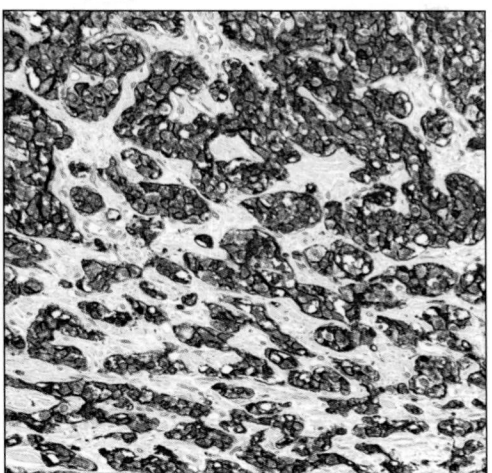

(Left) Strong cytoplasmic immunoreactivity with synaptophysin is seen in this paraganglioma. Demonstration of neuroendocrine markers by immunohistochemistry adds strong support for paraganglioma (if cytokeratin is negative). However, it should be noted that prostatic carcinomas commonly express neuroendocrine markers. *(Right)* Strong cytoplasmic positivity with chromogranin-A is also typical of paraganglioma.

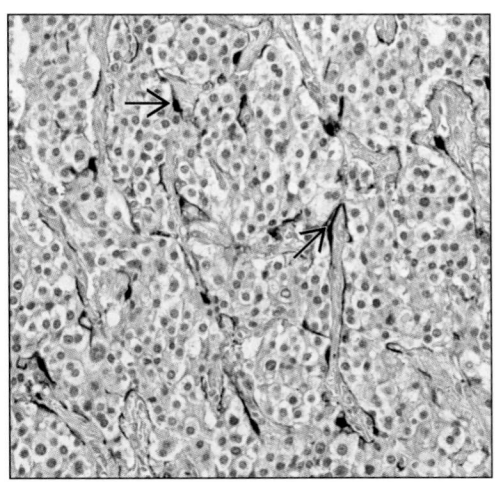

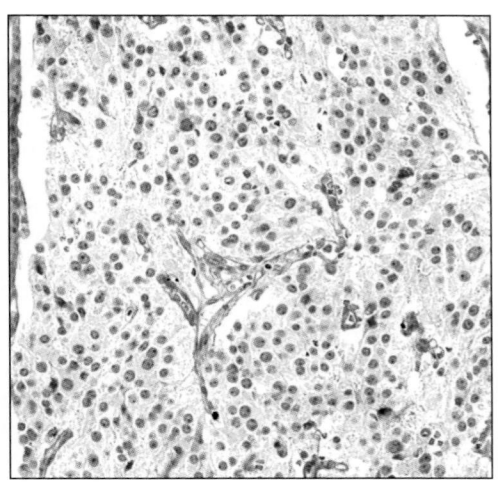

(Left) S100 protein immunohistochemistry highlights obvious sustentacular cells ⇨ in this paraganglioma. These sustentacular cells may not always be readily apparent, even after immunohistochemical evaluation. Synaptophysin is, therefore, the most sensitive marker for paraganglioma. *(Right)* As typical, this paraganglioma does not show immunoreactivity for p63. In contrast, urothelial carcinoma commonly expresses p63.

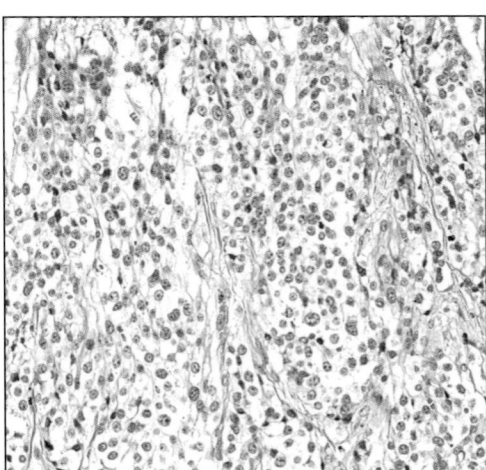

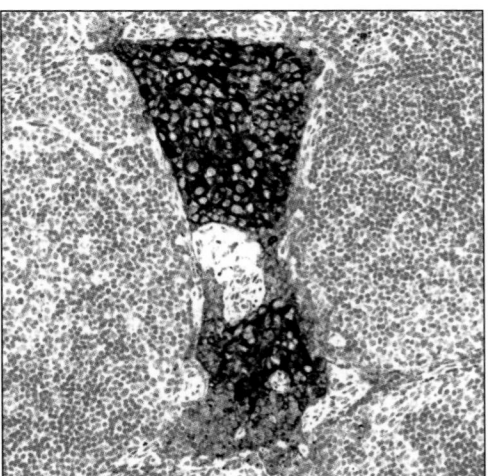

(Left) As expected, no PAN-CK(AE1/AE3) reactivity is found in this paraganglioma. Urothelial or prostatic carcinomas would be expected to diffusely express cytokeratins. *(Right)* Strong cytoplasmic immunoreactivity with chromogranin highlights the metastatic paraganglioma in this lymph node. Expression of endocrine markers, in the absence of keratin expression, is characteristic of paraganglioma.

METASTATIC AND SECONDARY CARCINOMAS

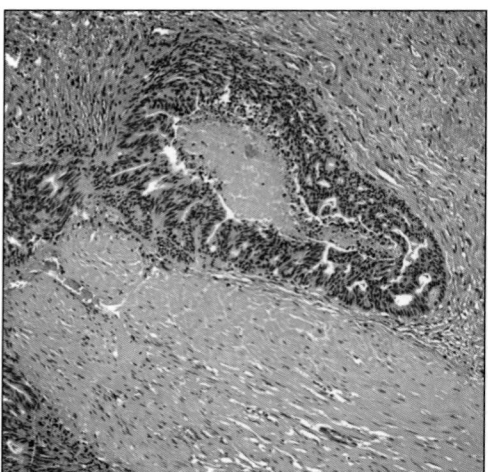

Uterine endometrioid adenocarcinoma may involve the muscularis propria by direct extension. This may be morphologically indistinguishable from primary bladder adenocarcinoma.

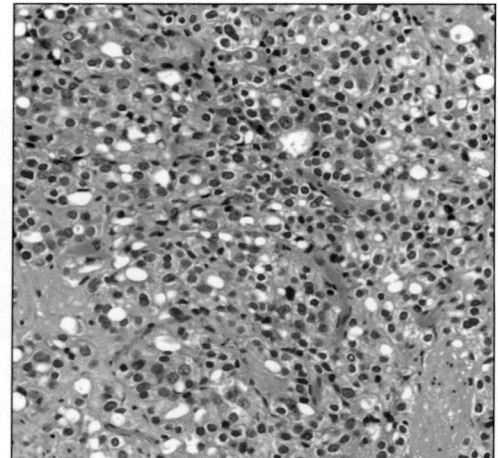

Metastatic lobular carcinoma of the breast may have significant morphologic overlap with some morphologic variants of invasive urothelial carcinoma. ER, mammaglobin, and GCDFP-15 are helpful stains.

TERMINOLOGY

Definitions
- Urinary bladder may be involved secondarily by carcinomas
  - Direct extension from adjacent anatomic sites
  - Metastases from distant anatomic sites

CLINICAL ISSUES

Epidemiology
- Incidence
  - Comprise 2-15% of malignant tumors
  - Possible primary sites include
    - Colon (21%), prostate (19%), rectum (12%), uterine cervix (11%), melanoma and ovary (rare)

Site
- Bladder neck and trigone

Presentation
- Hematuria

Treatment
- Dependent on primary site and tumor subtype
- Resection may be required to stop hemorrhage

Prognosis
- Poor prognosis secondary to high-stage malignancy

MACROSCOPIC FEATURES

General Features
- Polypoid bladder mass
  - May be multiple and often intramural

MICROSCOPIC PATHOLOGY

Histologic Features
- Colorectal adenocarcinoma
  - Enteric-type adenocarcinoma
    - Gland formation with pseudostratified columnar epithelium
    - May be histologically identical to primary bladder adenocarcinoma
    - Surface villous component may be misleading
  - Commonly expresses nuclear β-catenin by immunohistochemistry
  - CK7, CK20, and CDX-2 immunophenotype may be identical to primary bladder adenocarcinoma
- Prostatic adenocarcinoma
  - May have sheet-like growth with occasional lumens
  - Monomorphic nuclei with round nuclear contours
  - Expresses PSA and PAP by immunohistochemistry
- Gynecologic carcinomas
  - Uterine cervical squamous cell carcinoma
    - Identical to primary bladder squamous cell carcinoma or urothelial carcinoma with squamous differentiation
    - Clinical and radiographic correlation is essential
  - Ovarian and endometrial carcinoma
    - Clear cell, serous, and endometrioid carcinomas are potential mimics
- General features of metastatic carcinoma
  - Multiple foci of nodular aggregates of tumors cells
  - Absence of surface mucosal abnormalities
    - No urothelial carcinoma in situ
    - No papillary urothelial carcinoma
  - Tumor may show only muscularis propria involvement
  - Extensive or exclusive angiolymphatic involvement suggests metastasis
  - Unusual morphologies may suggest metastasis

METASTATIC AND SECONDARY CARCINOMAS

Key Facts

Terminology
- Bladder may be involved secondarily by direct extension of tumors from adjacent sites or by metastases from distant site

Clinical Issues
- Comprise 15% of malignant bladder tumors
  - Prostate
  - Colorectal
  - Gynecologic tract
- Bladder neck and trigone are frequent locations for metastasis

Macroscopic Features
- Generally, multiple mass lesions with intramural location

Ancillary Tests
- Immunoreactivity dependent on primary site of origin
  - Colorectal adenocarcinoma and primary bladder adenocarcinoma may have identical phenotype
  - β-catenin may be specific for colonic origin
  - Breast carcinoma may maintain ER, GCDFP-15, and mammaglobin reactivity
- Absence of specific urothelial carcinoma markers

Top Differential Diagnoses
- Primary adenocarcinoma of urinary bladder
- Urothelial carcinoma with glandular differentiation
- Müllerianosis/endometriosis
- Specific variants of urothelial carcinoma

ANCILLARY TESTS

Immunohistochemistry
- Immunoreactivity dependent on primary site of origin
- Absence of specific urothelial carcinoma markers
  - Uroplakin, GATA3, and S100p have low sensitivity in urothelial carcinoma
  - Nonurothelial carcinomas may express HMCK(34βE12) and p63

DIFFERENTIAL DIAGNOSIS

Primary Adenocarcinoma of Urinary Bladder
- May have associated precursor lesion
  - Adenocarcinoma in situ or villous adenoma
- Absence of nuclear β-catenin expression
- May have enteric immunophenotype: CK20 and CDX-2 expression
- Colonoscopy may be needed in difficult cases to exclude colonic primary
- Signet ring adenocarcinoma of bladder may be difficult to distinguish from gastric or breast primary

Urothelial Carcinoma with Glandular Differentiation
- Admixed typical urothelial carcinoma
  - Invasive, papillary, or urothelial carcinoma in situ
- Absence of nuclear β-catenin expression

Müllerianosis/Endometriosis
- Müllerian-type glands present within bladder wall
  - Tubal or endometrial-type epithelium may be seen
    - Cytologically bland with no destructive invasion

Specific Variants of Invasive Urothelial Carcinoma
- Plasmacytoid carcinoma
  - May mimic involvement by plasmacytoma/myeloma
  - Strong cytokeratin reactivity but may express CD138
- Micropapillary carcinoma
  - Closely resembles ovarian serous carcinoma or micropapillary carcinomas in other sites
  - ER, pax-8, mammaglobin, and TTF-1 are negative
- Lymphoma-like carcinoma
  - Close morphology to low-grade lymphoma or lobular breast carcinoma
  - Immunoreactive for cytokeratin
    - Negative for CD45(LCA), ER, GCDFP-15, mammaglobin
- Glycogen-rich carcinoma
  - May mimic renal cell carcinoma
  - Maintains urothelial immunophenotype

DIAGNOSTIC CHECKLIST

Pathologic Interpretation Pearls
- Nonbladder primaries must be considered before accepting diagnosis of primary vesical adenocarcinoma
  - Careful radiographic correlation is often essential
- Multifocality, vascular-lymphatic invasion, and normal surface mucosa should strongly raise possibility of metastasis
- Tumors with only muscularis propria involvement and those with unusual morphologies should strongly raise possibility of nonurothelial origin

SELECTED REFERENCES

1. Bates AW et al: The significance of secondary neoplasms of the urinary and male genital tract. Virchows Arch. 440(6):640-7, 2002
2. Wang HL et al: Immunohistochemical distinction between primary adenocarcinoma of the bladder and secondary colorectal adenocarcinoma. Am J Surg Pathol. 25(11):1380-7, 2001
3. Bates AW et al: Secondary neoplasms of the bladder are histological mimics of nontransitional cell primary tumours: clinicopathological and histological features of 282 cases. Histopathology. 36(1):32-40, 2000

METASTATIC AND SECONDARY CARCINOMAS

Microscopic Features

(Left) Metastatic melanoma in the bladder may resemble any undifferentiated malignancy, such as poorly differentiated urothelial carcinoma. Obvious melanin pigment ➡ may not be present. S100 is the most sensitive screening marker for melanoma. *(Right)* Metastatic papillary serous carcinoma of the ovary may simulate micropapillary urothelial carcinoma. Clinical presentation is helpful as ovarian carcinomas typically have large adnexal masses and peritoneal spread.

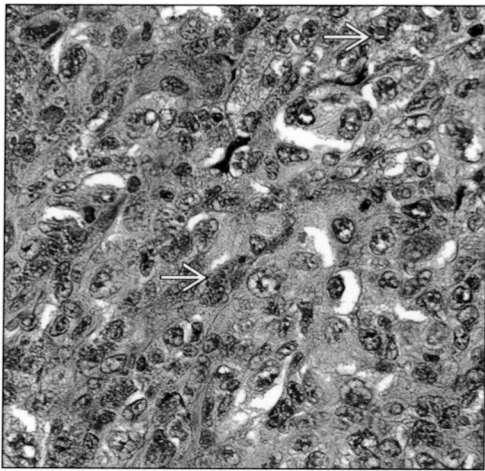
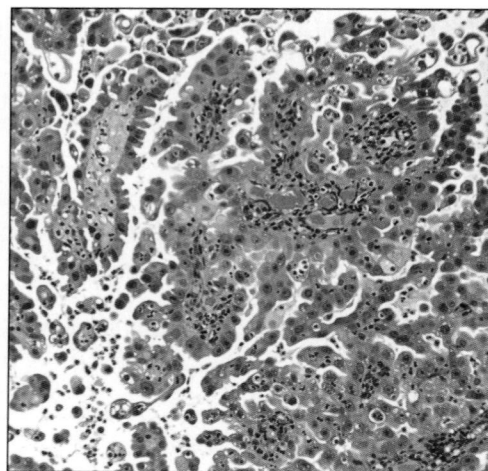

(Left) Prostatic adenocarcinoma may extend to the bladder. The monotonous appearance of cells with relatively round nuclei and prominent nucleoli is characteristic of prostatic primaries. Immunohistochemistry for PSA(+), PAP(+), and high molecular weight keratin(-) often help establish prostatic origin. *(Right)* Direct invasion from gastrointestinal tract adenocarcinomas may be indistinguishable from primary bladder adenocarcinoma.

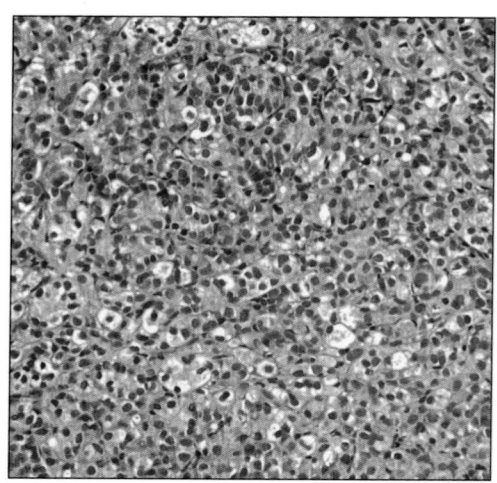
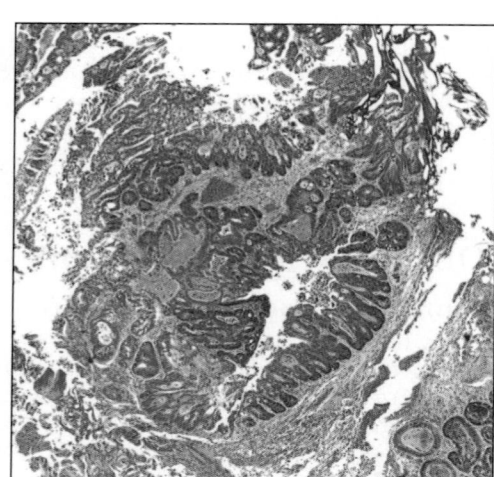

(Left) Metastatic ductal adenocarcinoma from the breast may closely resemble invasive urothelial carcinoma. Preservation of the overlying urothelium ➡ or predominant intravascular growth should suggest the possibility of metastasis. *(Right)* Invasion of the urinary bladder from an adjacent cervical squamous cell carcinoma, as seen here, presents a diagnostic challenge, since squamous differentiation is not uncommon in urothelial carcinomas. Clinical/imaging correlation is essential.

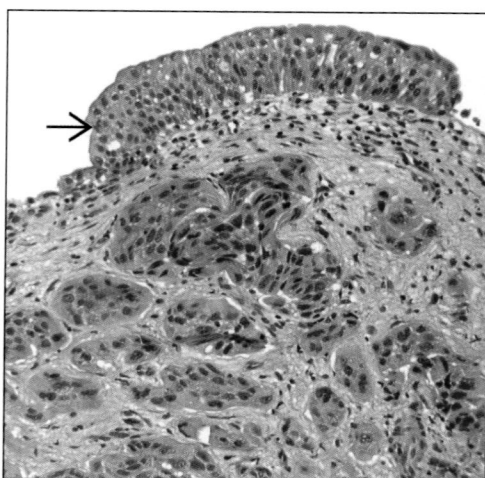
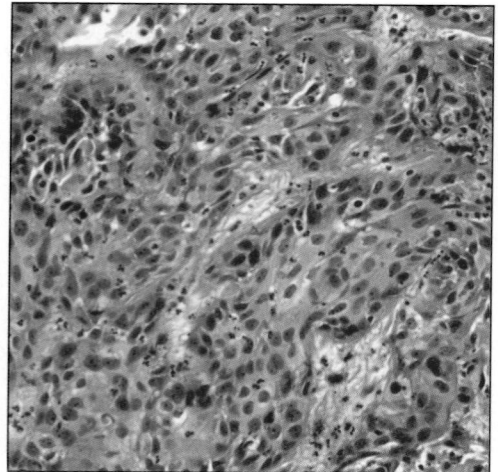

METASTATIC AND SECONDARY CARCINOMAS

Immunohistochemical Features

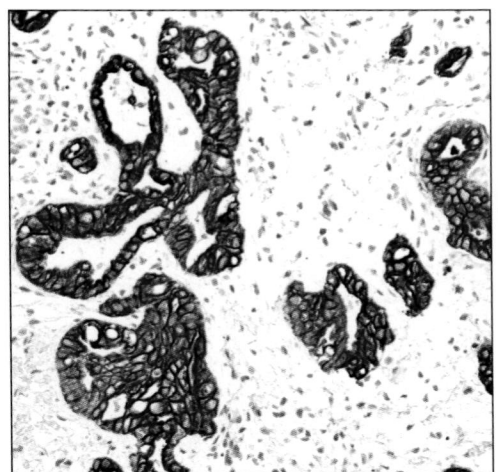

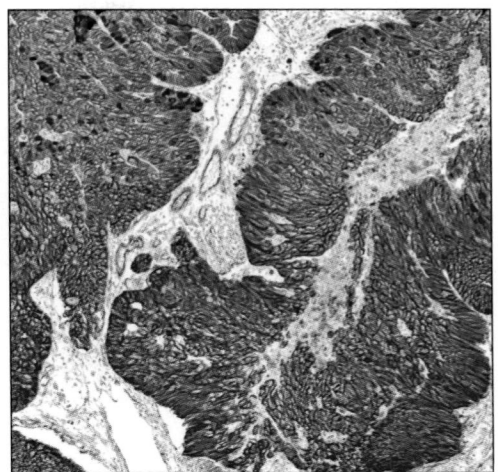

(Left) Colorectal adenocarcinoma involving the bladder shows strong cytoplasmic immunoreactivity for CK20, as in this case. CK20 expression may also be seen in enteric-type adenocarcinomas of urinary bladder origin, which often have an identical enteric immunophenotype. *(Right)* Cytoplasmic and nuclear immunoreactivity for β-catenin is reportedly a specific finding for colorectal primary adenocarcinoma. Close clinical correlation is essential in this distinction.

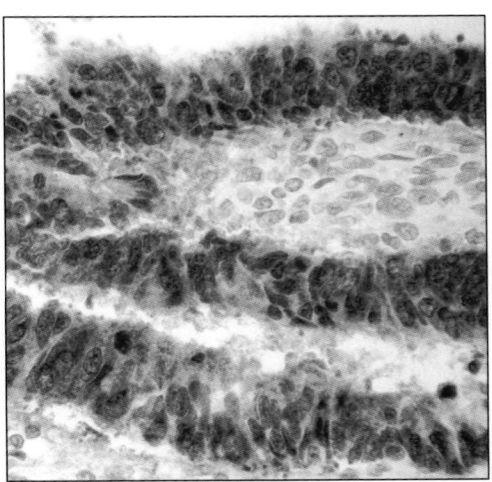

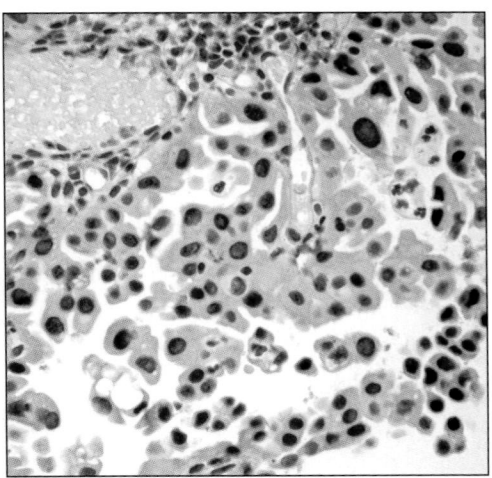

(Left) Nuclear expression of CDX2 in colorectal adenocarcinoma is seen involving the urinary bladder. Clinical history and comparison with the primary are often more useful than immunostains. *(Right)* Nuclear pax-8 expression is common in ovarian surface epithelial tumors, such as this metastatic ovarian papillary serous carcinoma. pax-2 expression may also be seen, but these nuclear transcription factors are not entirely specific, and may occasionally be expressed in urothelial neoplasms.

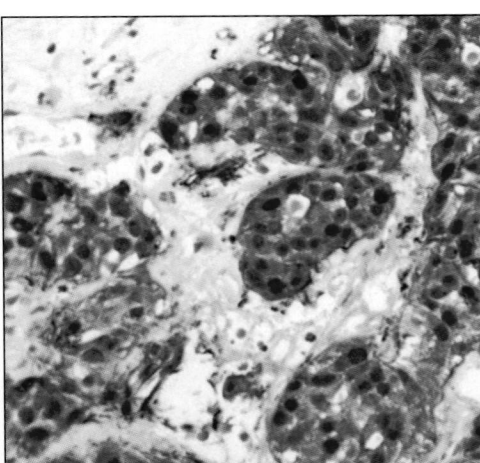

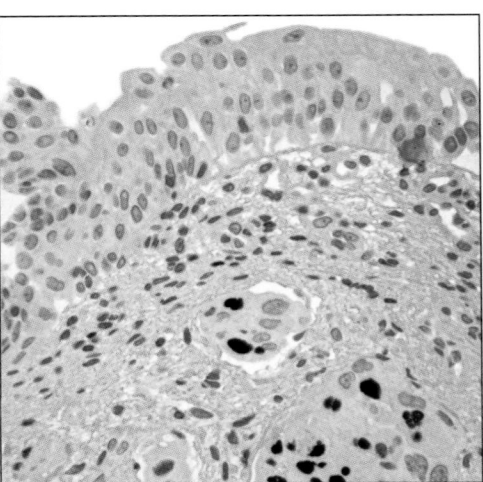

(Left) Strong nuclear and cytoplasmic immunoreactivity for p16 is seen in this cervical squamous cell carcinoma that invaded the bladder. p16 staining is used as an HPV surrogate in cervical squamous lesions but is not specific and may be expressed in urothelial carcinoma. *(Right)* Nuclear immunoreactivity for ER is often maintained by metastatic breast cancer, as in this metastatic ductal carcinoma of breast origin in the superficial lamina propria of the bladder.

Urinary Bladder: Biopsy and Transurethral Resection of Bladder Tumor (TURBT)

Surgical Pathology Cancer Case Summary (Checklist)

Applies primarily to invasive carcinomas &/or associated epithelial lesions, including carcinoma in situ

*Procedure

*____ Biopsy

____ TURBT

*____ Other (specify): _____

Histologic Type

____ Urothelial (transitional cell) carcinoma

____ Urothelial (transitional cell) carcinoma with squamous differentiation

____ Urothelial (transitional cell) carcinoma with glandular differentiation

____ Urothelial (transitional cell) carcinoma with variant histology (specify): _____

____ Squamous cell carcinoma, typical

____ Squamous cell carcinoma, variant histology (specify): _____

____ Adenocarcinoma, typical

____ Adenocarcinoma, variant histology (specify): _____

____ Small cell carcinoma

____ Undifferentiated carcinoma (specify): _____

____ Mixed cell type (specify): _____

____ Other (specify): _____

____ Carcinoma, type cannot be determined

Associated Epithelial Lesions (select all that apply)

____ None identified

____ Urothelial (transitional cell) papilloma (World Health Organization [WHO] 2004/International Society of Urologic Pathology [ISUP])

____ Urothelial (transitional cell) papilloma, inverted type

____ Papillary urothelial (transitional cell) neoplasm, low malignant potential (WHO 2004/ISUP)

____ Cannot be determined

Histologic Grade

____ Not applicable

____ Cannot be determined

Urothelial carcinoma (WHO 2004/ISUP)

____ Low grade

____ High grade

____ Other (specify): _____

Adenocarcinoma and squamous cell carcinoma

____ GX: Cannot be assessed

____ G1: Well differentiated

____ G2: Moderately differentiated

____ G3: Poorly differentiated

____ Other (specify): _____

*Tumor Configuration (select all that apply)

*____ Papillary

*____ Solid/nodule

*____ Flat

*____ Ulcerated

*____ Indeterminate

*____ Other (specify): _____

Adequacy of Material for Determining Muscularis Propria Invasion

____ Muscularis propria (detrusor muscle) not identified

____ Muscularis propria (detrusor muscle) present

____ Presence of muscularis propria indeterminate

PROTOCOL FOR URINARY BLADDER CANCER SPECIMENS

Lymph-Vascular Invasion

____ Not identified

____ Present

____ Indeterminate

Microscopic Extent of Tumor (select all that apply)

____ Cannot be assessed

____ Noninvasive papillary carcinoma

____ Flat carcinoma in situ

____ Tumor invades subepithelial connective tissue (lamina propria)

____ Tumor invades muscularis propria (detrusor muscle)

____ Urothelial carcinoma involving prostatic urethra in prostatic chips sampled by TURBT

____ Urothelial carcinoma in situ involving prostatic ducts and acini in prostatic chips sampled by TURBT

____ Urothelial carcinoma invasive into prostatic stroma in prostatic chips sampled by TURBT

**Additional Pathologic Findings (select all that apply)*

*____ Urothelial dysplasia (low-grade intraurothelial neoplasia)

*____ Inflammation/regenerative changes

*____ Therapy-related changes

*____ Cautery artifact

*____ Cystitis cystica glandularis

*____ Keratinizing squamous metaplasia

*____ Intestinal metaplasia

*____ Other (specify): _____

*Data elements with asterisks are not required. However, these elements may be clinically important but are not yet validated or regularly used in patient management. Adapted with permission from College of American Pathologists, "Protocol for the Examination of Specimens from Patients with Carcinoma of the Urinary Bladder." Web posting date October 2009, www.cap.org.

Urinary Bladder: Cystectomy, Partial, Total, or Radical; Anterior Exenteration

Surgical Pathology Cancer Case Summary Checklist

Specimen

____ Bladder

____ Other (specify): _____

____ Not specified

Procedure

____ Partial cystectomy

____ Total cystectomy

____ Radical cystectomy

____ Radical cystoprostatectomy

____ Anterior exenteration

____ Other (specify): _____

____ Not specified

**Tumor Site (select all that apply)*

*____ Trigone

*____ Right lateral wall

*____ Left lateral wall

*____ Anterior wall

*____ Posterior wall

*____ Dome

*____ Other (specify): _____

*____ Not specified

Tumor Size

Greatest dimension: _____ cm

*Additional dimensions: _____ x _____ cm

____ Cannot be determined

PROTOCOL FOR URINARY BLADDER CANCER SPECIMENS

Histologic Type

____ Urothelial (transitional cell) carcinoma

____ Urothelial (transitional cell) carcinoma with squamous differentiation

____ Urothelial (transitional cell) carcinoma with glandular differentiation

____ Urothelial (transitional cell) carcinoma with variant histology (specify): _____

____ Squamous cell carcinoma, typical

____ Squamous cell carcinoma, variant histology (specify): _____

____ Adenocarcinoma, typical

____ Adenocarcinoma, variant histology (specify): _____

____ Small cell carcinoma

____ Undifferentiated carcinoma (specify): _____

____ Mixed cell type (specify): _____

____ Other (specify): _____

____ Carcinoma, type cannot be determined

Associated Epithelial Lesions (select all that apply)

____ None identified

____ Urothelial (transitional cell) papilloma (World Health Organization [WHO] 2004/International Society of Urologic Pathology [ISUP])

____ Cannot be determined

Histologic Grade

____ Not applicable

____ Cannot be determined

Urothelial carcinoma (WHO 2004/ISUP)

____ Low grade

____ High grade

____ Other (specify): _____

Adenocarcinoma and squamous cell carcinoma

____ GX: Cannot be assessed

____ G1: Well differentiated

____ G2: Moderately differentiated

____ G3: Poorly differentiated

____ Other (specify): _____

*Tumor Configuration (select all that apply)

*____ Papillary

*____ Solid/nodule

*____ Flat

*____ Ulcerated

*____ Indeterminate

*____ Other (specify): _____

Microscopic Tumor Extension (select all that apply)

____ None identified

____ Perivascular fat

____ Rectum

____ Prostatic stroma

____ Seminal vesicle (specify laterality): _____

____ Vagina

____ Uterus and adnexae

____ Pelvic sidewall (specify laterality): _____

____ Ureter (specify laterality): _____

____ Other (specify): _____

Lymph-Vascular Invasion

____ Not identified

____ Present

PROTOCOL FOR URINARY BLADDER CANCER SPECIMENS

____ Indeterminate

Pathologic Staging (pTNM)

TNM descriptors (required only if applicable) (select all that apply)

____ m (multiple primary tumors)

____ r (recurrent)

____ y (post-treatment)

Primary tumor (pT)

____ pTX: Primary tumor cannot be assessed

____ pT0: No evidence of primary tumor

____ pTa: Noninvasive papillary carcinoma

____ pTis: Carcinoma in situ: "Flat tumor"

____ pT1: Tumor invades subepithelial connective tissue (lamina propria)

pT2: Tumor invades muscularis propria (detrusor muscle)

____ pT2a: Tumor invades superficial muscularis propria (inner half)

____ pT2b: Tumor invades deep muscularis propria (outer half)

pT3: Tumor invades perivesical tissue

____ pT3a: Microscopically

____ pT3b: Macroscopically (extravesicular mass)

pT4: Tumor invades any of the following: Prostatic stroma, seminal vesicles, uterus, vagina, pelvic wall, abdominal wall

____ pT4a: Tumor invades prostatic stroma or uterus or vagina

____ pT4b: Tumor invades pelvic wall or abdominal wall

Regional lymph nodes (pN)

____ pNX: Lymph nodes cannot be assessed

____ pN0: No lymph node metastasis

____ PN1: Single regional lymph node metastasis in the true pelvis (hypogastric, obturator, external iliac, or presacral lymph node)

____ PN2: Multiple regional lymph node metastasis in the true pelvis (hypogastric, obturator, external iliac, or presacral lymph node metastasis)

____ pN3: Lymph node metastasis to the common iliac lymph nodes

Specify: Number examined: _____ Number involved (any size): _____

Distant metastasis (pM)

____ Not applicable

____ pM1: Distant metastasis

*Specify site(s), if known: _____

*Additional Pathologic Findings (select all that apply)

____ Adenocarcinoma of prostate (use protocol for carcinoma of prostate)

____ Urothelial (transitional cell) carcinoma involving urethra, prostatic ducts and acini ± stromal invasion (use protocol for carcinoma of urethra)

*____ Urothelial dysplasia (low-grade intraurothelial neoplasia)

*____ Inflammation/regenerative changes

*____ Therapy-related changes

*____ Cystitis cystica glandularis

*____ Keratinizing squamous metaplasia

*____ Intestinal metaplasia

*____ Other (specify): _____

Data elements with asterisks are not required. However, these elements may be clinically important but are not yet validated or regularly used in patient management.

TNM Stage Groupings

Stage	Tumor	Node	Metastasis
0a	Ta	N0	M0†
0is	Tis	N0	M0
I	T1	N0	M0
II	T2a	N0	M0
	T2b	N0	M0
III	T3a	n0	M0
	T3b	N0	M0
	T4a	N0	M0

PROTOCOL FOR URINARY BLADDER CANCER SPECIMENS

IV	T4b	N0	M0
	Any T	N1, 2, 3	M0
	Any T	Any N	M1

†M0 is defined as no distant metastasis. Used with the permission of the American Joint Committee on Cancer (AJCC), Chicago, Illinois. The original source for this material is the AJCC Cancer Staging Manual, Seventh Edition (2010) published by Springer Science and Business Media LLC, www.springerlink.com.

IMMUNOHISTOCHEMISTRY, URINARY BLADDER

High-Grade Undifferentiated Carcinoma

Antibody	Prostate	Urothelial
PSA	68-94%	0%
PAP	78-95%	0%
PSMA	> 95% (best)	0%
HMCK(34βE12)	6-10%	65-100%
Uroplakin-3	0%	57-60%
Thrombomodulin	0%	49-69%
p63	0-18%	70-75%
CD57	94%	17%
S100p	0-1%	78-86%
GATA3	0-3%	67%

Enteric-type Adenocarcinoma

Antibody	Bladder	Colon
CK7(+)/CK20(+)	24%	8%
CK7(+)/CK20(-)	41%	0%
CK7(-)/CK20(+)	29%	82%
CK7(-)/CK20(-)	6%	10%
CDX-2	47-100%	99-100%
β-catenin	0%	81% (best)
Villin	65-100%	82-98%
Thrombomodulin	59%	0%

Spindle Cell Proliferations: Adults

Antibody	Pseudosarcomatous Myofibroblastic Proliferation	Sarcomatoid Carcinoma	Leiomyosarcoma
Actin-sm	63-100%	15-80%	43-100%
Desmin	27-80%	0-40%	0-60%
h-caldesmon	0-66%	ND	100%
PAN-CK(AE1/AE3)	36-89%	67-100%	0-38%
EMA/MUC1	0-50%	50-100%	0-12%
ALK1	75-89%	0%	10%
p63	0%	50%	23%
HMCK(34βE12)	0%	25-27%	0%

Spindle Cell Proliferations: Children

Antibody	Pseudosarcomatous Myofibroblastic Proliferation	Rhabdomyosarcoma
Actin-sm	63-100%	97%
Desmin	27-80%	97%
MyoD1	0%	100%
Myogenin	0%	100%
ALK1	75-89%	20%

Bladder Neoplasms with Nested Morphology

Antibody	Paraganglioma	Carcinoid	Urothelial Carcinoma	Melanoma
PAN-CK(AE1/AE3)	-	+	+	-
Synaptophysin	+	+	-	-
Chromogranin	+	+	-	-
S100	+ (sustentacular cells)	-	-	+

ND = No Data

IMMUNOHISTOCHEMISTRY, URINARY BLADDER

Flat Urothelial Lesions with Atypia (URO3 Cocktail)

Antibody	Normal	Reactive	CIS
CK20 (cytoplasmic, red)	Umbrella layer only	Umbrella layer only	Full thickness urothelium
CD44 (membranous, brown)	Basal layer only	Increased expression in intermediate cells to full thickness urothelium	Basal layer only or loss of expression
p53 (nuclear, brown)	Rare cells; weak reactivity	Rare cells; weak reactivity	Diffuse, strong reactivity

URO3 is a antibody cocktail comprised of three antibodies: CK20, CD44, and p53.

Metastatic Carcinoma

Antibody	Sensitivity for Urothelium	Other Tumors
CK7(+)/CK20(+)	65%	V
CK7(+)/CK20(-)	37%	V
CK7(-)/CK20(+)	3%	V
CK7(-)/CK20(-)	10%	V
Uroplakin-3	57-60%	0%
Thrombomodulin	49-69%	V
HMCK(34βE12)	65-100%	V
p63	60-90%	V
S100p	78-86%	0-1%
GATA3	67%	0-3%

ND = No Data; V = Variable; unknown primary immunostain panel, bladder: CK7, CK20, uroplakin-3, thrombomodulin, S100p, GATA3, p63, HMCK(34βE12)

IMMUNOHISTOCHEMISTRY, URINARY BLADDER

URO3 in Flat Lesions

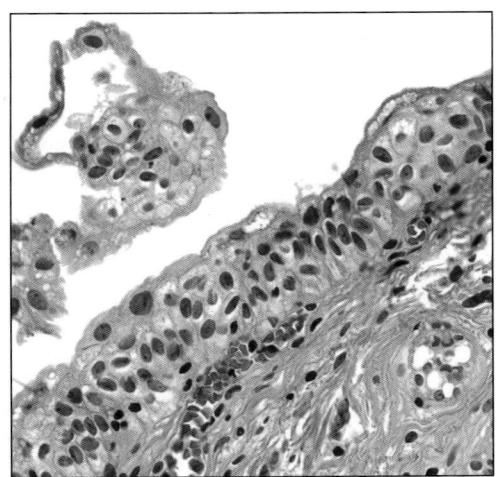

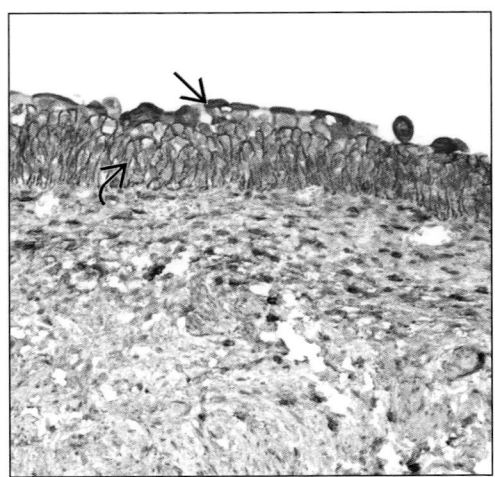

(Left) Reactive urothelial atypia may mimic urothelial carcinoma in situ in some cases. Immunohistochemistry with CK20, CD44, and p53 may be useful for classification in select cases. (Right) URO3, an antibody cocktail containing CK20, p53, and CD44, shows CK20 reactivity (red) ➔ in the umbrella cell layer and strong membranous CD44 immunoreactivity (brown) ➔ in the full thickness of the urothelium, an immunophenotype characteristic of reactive atypia.

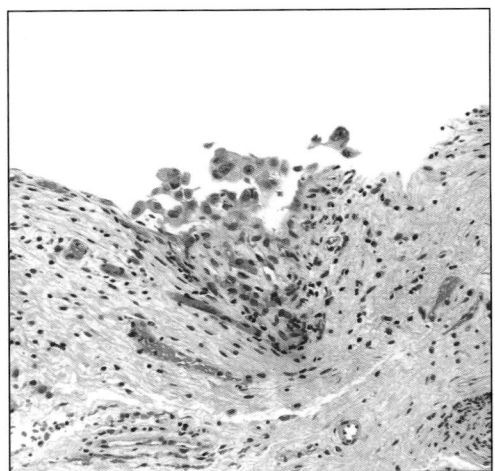

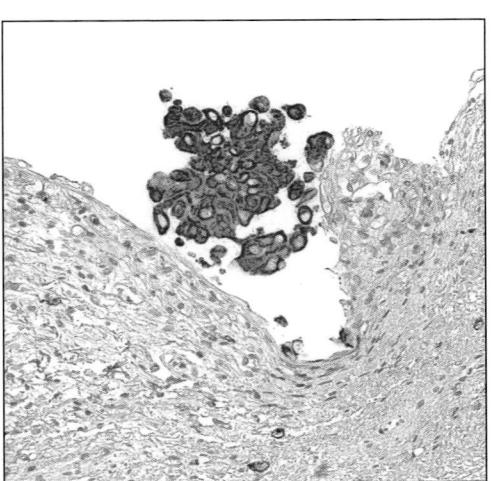

(Left) This photomicrograph shows an example of urothelial carcinoma in situ with a clinging, or denuding, pattern. (Right) The URO3 cocktail (CK20, CD44, and p53) shows diffuse cytoplasmic immunoreactivity for CK20 in the clinging cells of this urothelial carcinoma in situ. Normal or reactive clinging basal urothelial cells would be expected to show strong membranous CD44 staining, but no CK20. There is no nuclear p53 staining, which may be seen in a subset of carcinoma in situ.

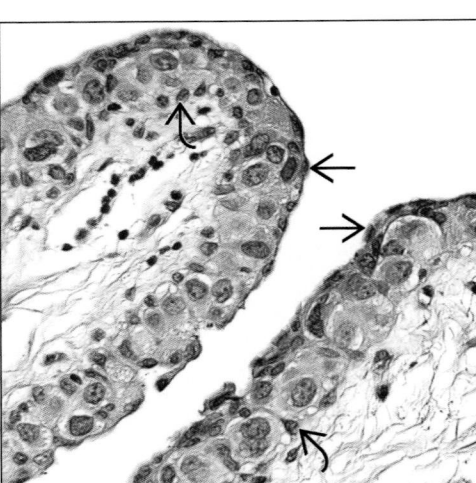

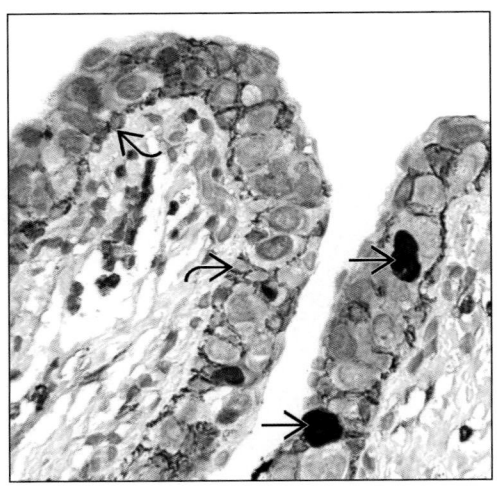

(Left) This example of urothelial carcinoma in situ has a pagetoid pattern with neoplastic cells infiltrating amongst intact umbrella cells ➔ and basal cells ➔. (Right) This URO3 cocktail highlights CIS cells with diffuse staining for CK20 (red). Normal basal cells are CD44 positive (brown) ➔. Scattered cells show nuclear reactivity for p53 ➔; this pattern is nonspecific, as diffuse, strong reactivity with p53 is required to more fully support CIS. The sensitivity of p53 is relatively low.

Urothelial vs. Prostate Carcinoma

(Left) This carcinoma was identified in a biopsy from the prostatic urethra. Because of the relatively monotonous nuclei, the distinction between prostatic and urothelial lineage was difficult by morphologic evaluation alone. Immunohistochemistry for p63, HMCK(34βE12), PSA, and PAP was performed. *(Right)* The neoplastic cells in this carcinoma showed strong and diffuse nuclear immunoreactivity for p63, supporting urothelial carcinoma.

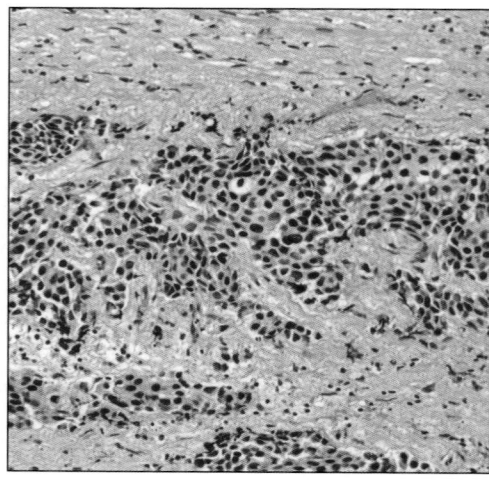 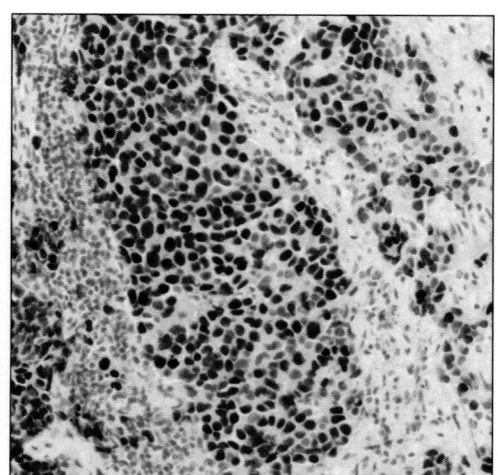

(Left) This carcinoma from the prostatic urethra also expressed strong and diffuse cytoplasmic HMCK(34βE12), but did not express PSA or PAP. This immunophenotype, in conjunction with the positive p63, strongly supports a diagnosis of urothelial carcinoma. *(Right)* This carcinoma with round monotonous nuclei was identified in a biopsy from the urinary bladder. These nuclear features strongly suggested the possibility of prostatic adenocarcinoma.

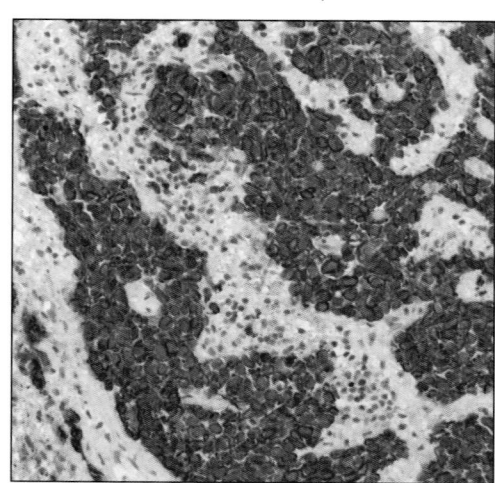 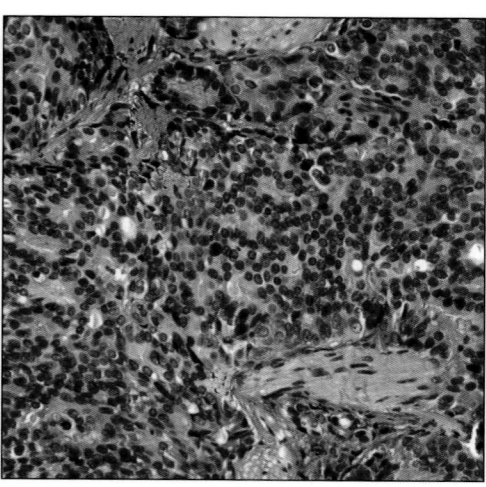

(Left) This carcinoma showed diffuse cytoplasmic immunoreactivity for PSA. *(Right)* Cytoplasmic immunoreactivity for PAP was also identified in this bladder-based carcinoma, supporting the diagnosis of prostatic adenocarcinoma secondarily involving the urinary bladder. Both PSA and PAP immunoreactivity may be patchy in prostatic adenocarcinoma. Performing a full panel of immunostains including p63, HMCK(34βE12), PSA, and PAP is important.

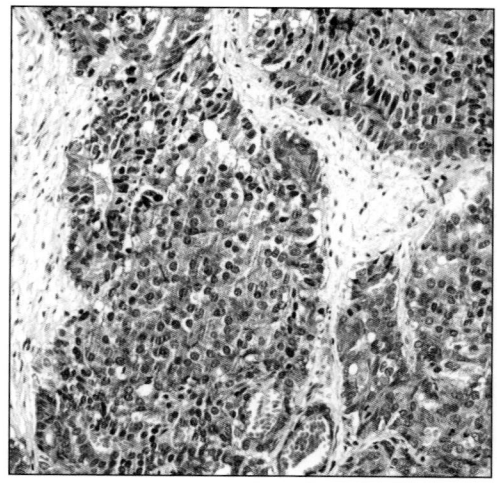 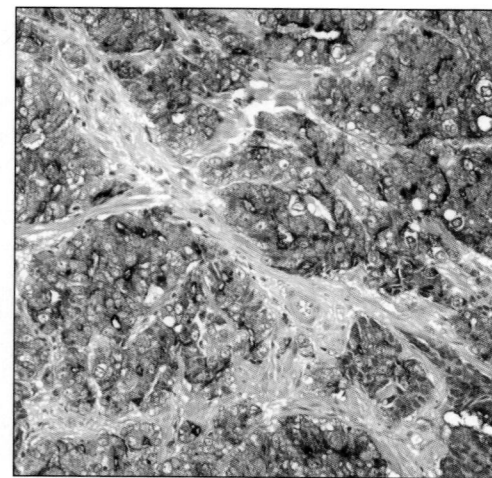

Immunohistochemistry in Spindled Lesions

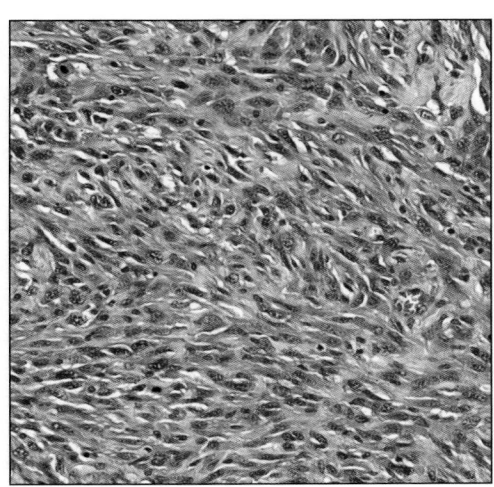
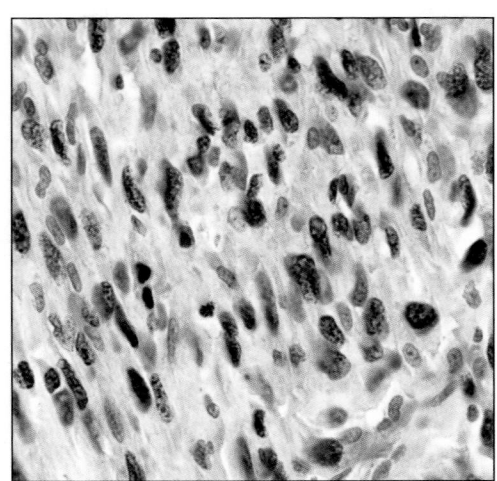

(Left) When the diagnosis of sarcomatoid carcinoma is considered, as in this example, an immunohistochemical panel should include p63 and HMCK(34βE12). (Right) This sarcomatoid urothelial carcinoma shows nuclear immunoreactivity for p63. It also had coexpression of HMCK(34βE12). PAN-CK(AE1/AE3) and low molecular weight cytokeratins should be interpreted with caution, as both smooth muscle and myofibroblastic lesions may show expression.

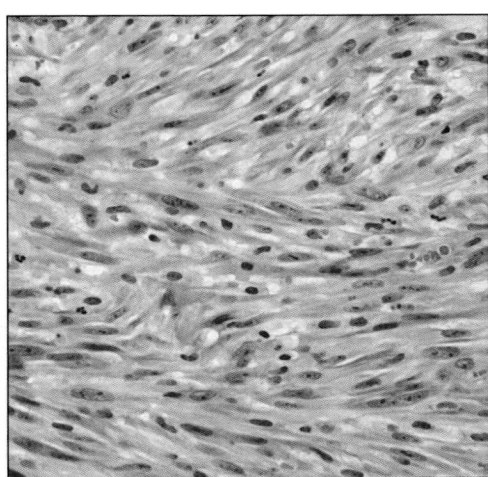
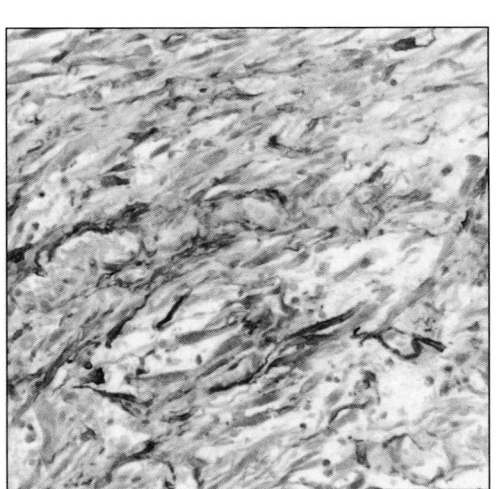

(Left) This pseudosarcomatous myofibroblastic proliferation has a spindle cell pattern that could potentially mimic a sarcoma or spindled carcinoma. If immunohistochemistry is used, a broad panel should be utilized because of immunophenotypic overlap. (Right) Myofibroblasts typically show strong actin-sm reactivity, as seen here. They may also express low molecular weight forms of cytokeratin, which may cause confusion with carcinoma. A subset also expresses ALK1.

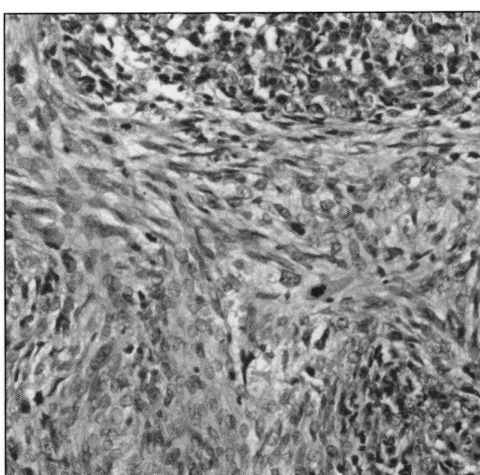
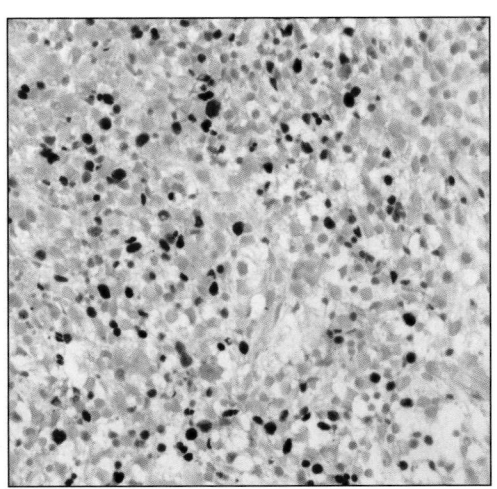

(Left) Rhabdomyosarcoma, as seen here, may have significant morphologic overlap with a myofibroblastic proliferation on biopsy. (Right) Nuclear myogenin immunoreactivity is definitive evidence of skeletal muscle differentiation. Myogenin should be performed if rhabdomyosarcoma is considered because of immunophenotypic overlap with myofibroblasts using other markers. Rhabdomyosarcoma may express ALK1, and myofibroblasts may occasionally express desmin.

Immunohistochemistry in Nested Lesions

(Left) The nested variant of invasive urothelial carcinoma, as seen in this example, may occasionally have histologic overlap with another nested neoplasm, such as carcinoid tumor or paraganglioma. *(Right)* This invasive nested urothelial carcinoma shows the typical strong nuclear expression of p63. Nested urothelial carcinoma also shows immunoreactivity with PAN-CK(AE1/AE3), but are nonreactive for neuroendocrine markers such as synaptophysin and chromogranin.

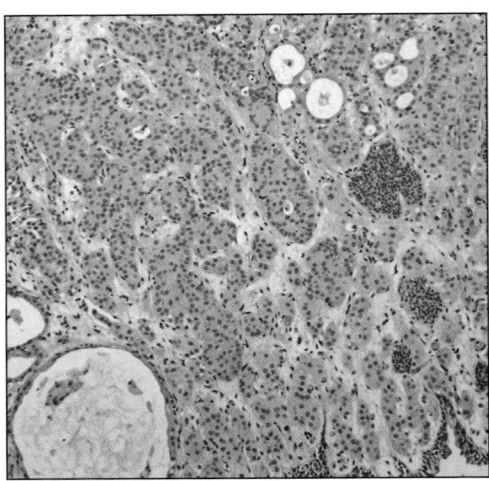 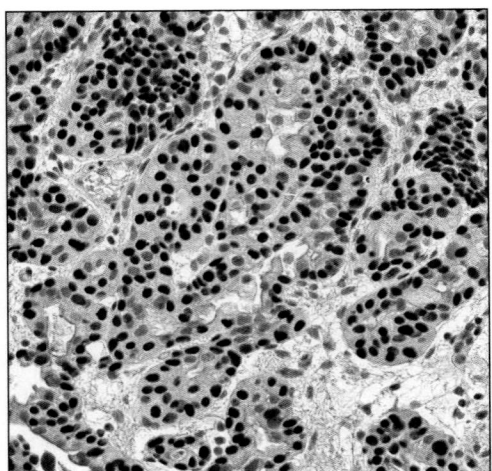

(Left) Paragangliomas may occasionally be identified in the bladder, where they closely mimic urothelial carcinoma. The use of immunohistochemistry is critical to the distinction from carcinoma in this setting. *(Right)* This paraganglioma of the urinary bladder had strong immunoreactivity with synaptophysin, but no staining with cytokeratins. Paragangliomas may also show surrounding sustentacular cells with S100, but these are not always identified.

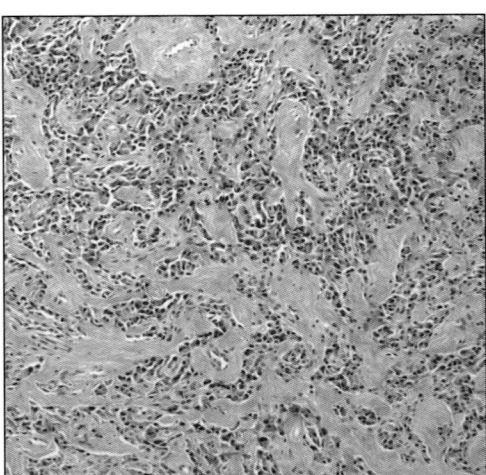 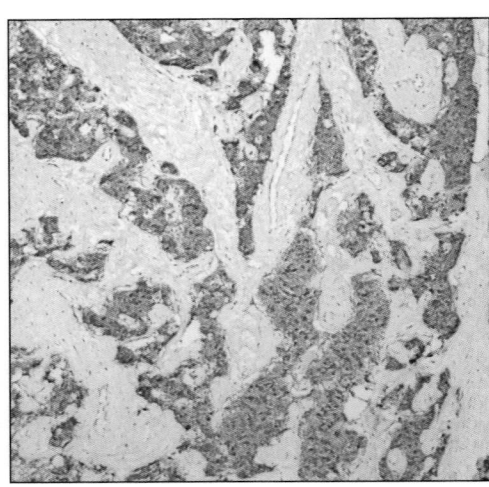

(Left) This carcinoid tumor of the bladder has a pattern that closely mimics a nested urothelial carcinoma with tubule formation. Evaluation of urothelial markers is important because carcinoid tumor, unlike paraganglioma, co-expresses cytokeratin and neuroendocrine markers. *(Right)* This carcinoid tumor is nonreactive for p63, but there is strong nuclear internal control staining in the overlying urothelium. The tumor did coexpress cytokeratin and synaptophysin, as expected.

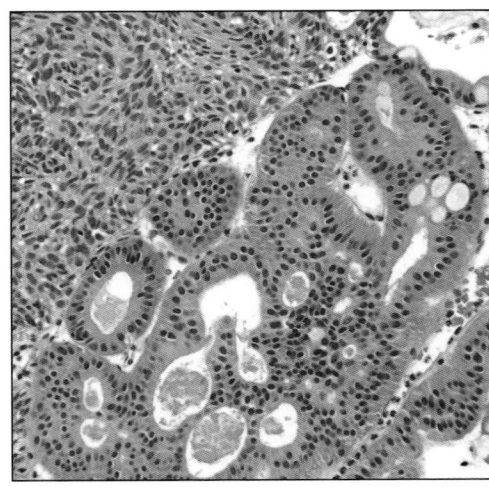 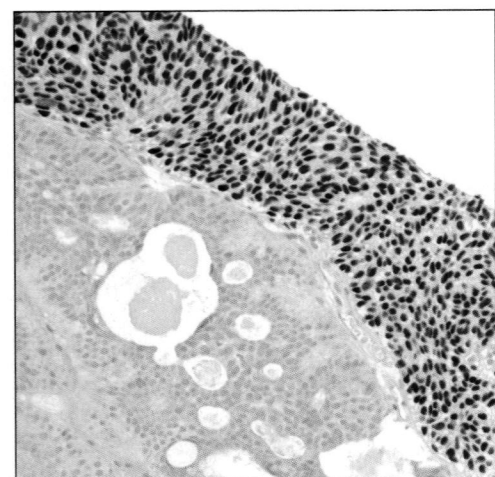

Prostate Gland and Seminal Vesicle

CLASSIFICATION OF PROSTATE TUMORS & TUMOR-LIKE LESIONS

NONNEOPLASTIC LESIONS

Tumor-like Lesions
- Retention cysts
- Prostatitis (acute, chronic, granulomatous, nonspecific granulomatous)
- Atrophy
  - Simple
  - Simple with cyst formation
  - Partial
  - Post atrophic hyperplasia (PAH)
  - Sclerotic
- Sclerosing adenosis
- Inflammatory pseudotumor/pseudosarcomatous myofibroblastic proliferation
- Melanosis
- Amyloid
- Endometriosis
- Post needle biopsy changes

Hyperplasia
- Benign nodular hyperplasia
  - Usual pattern
    - Glandular or epithelial
    - Stromal
    - Mixed
  - Special pattern
    - Epithelial predominant (small glandular, cribriform, basal cell, adenoid cystic-like)
    - Stromal (fibrous, fibromuscular, leiomyomatous)
    - Mixed (fibroadenoma-like, phyllodes-type)
- Basal cell hyperplasia
- Veromontanum mucosal gland hyperplasia
- Mesonephric hyperplasia
- Transitional cell hyperplasia

Metaplasia
- Mucinous metaplasia
- Squamous metaplasia
- Transitional metaplasia

NEOPLASMS

Benign Tumors
- Cystadenoma
- Nephrogenic adenoma of prostatic urethra
- Paraganglia/paraganglioma
- Fibroma
- Hemangioma
- Angioneuroma
- Leiomyoma
- Rhabdomyoma
- Malakoplakia

Putative Premalignant Lesions
- Atypical adenomatous hyperplasia (AAH, adenosis)
- Prostatic intraepitehlial neoplasia (PIN)
  - Low-grade PIN
  - High-grade PIN

Prostate Carcinoma
- Atypical small acinar proliferation (ASAP)

- Acinar adenocarcinoma
  - Atrophic
  - Pseudohypertrophic
  - PIN-like
  - Stratified/double cell layer
  - Foamy gland (xanthomatous)
  - With Paneth cell-like differentiation
  - Oncocytic
- Ductal adenocarcinoma
- Mucinous (colloid) adenocarcinoma
- Signet ring cell adenocarcinoma
- Carcinomas with squamous differentiation
  - Adenosquamous carcinoma
  - Squamous cell carcinoma
- Basal cell carcinoma (adenoid cystic carcinoma)
- Urothelial carcinoma of prostate
- Neuroendocrine tumors of prostate
  - Small cell carcinoma
  - Carcinoid tumor
  - Large cell neuroendocrine carcinoma
- Sarcomatoid carcinoma, prostate (carcinosarcoma)
- Lymphoepithelioma-like carcinoma
- Undifferentiated carcinoma

Tumors of Specialized Prostatic Stroma
- Epithelial-stromal tumor, not otherwise specified (phyllodes tumor)
- Stromal proliferations of uncertain malignant potential (STUMP)
  - Degenerative atypia
  - Hypercellular stroma
  - Myxoid
  - Phyllodes-type growth
- Prostatic stromal sarcoma (PSS)

Mesenchymal Tumors: Malignant
- Leiomyosarcoma
- Rhabdomyosarcoma
- Solitary fibrous tumor
- Malignant fibrous histiocytoma (MFH)
- Synovial sarcoma
- Angiosarcoma

Secondary Tumors of Prostate
- Metastatic tumors
- Direct spread from adjacent organs
  - Urinary bladder cancer
  - Colorectal cancer
  - Gastrointestinal stromal tumors (GIST)

Hematopoietic Tumors
- Lymphoma
- Leukemia
- Plasmacytoma

Tumors of Uncertain Origin
- Angiomyolipoma/PEComa
- Primitive neuroectodermal tumor (PNET)

Tumors of Seminal Vesicles
- Cystadenoma
- Epithelial stromal tumor
- Seminal vesicle adenocarcinoma

PROSTATE, GENERAL CONCEPTS

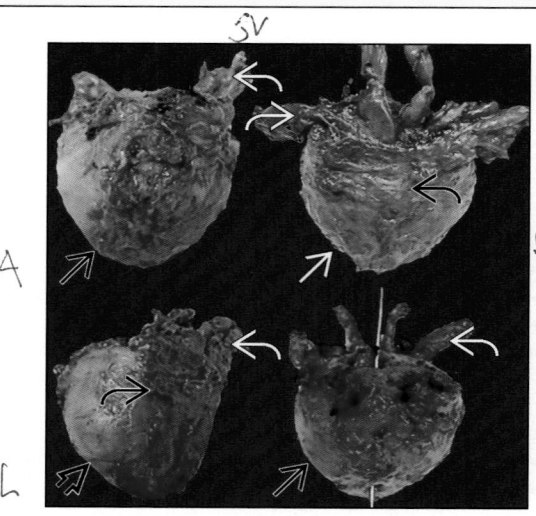

Anterior ➡, posterior ➡, postero-lateral ➡ views show an inverted conical gland with broad base and tapered apex. Seminal vesicles ➡ and flat posterior surface ➡ are orientation landmarks.

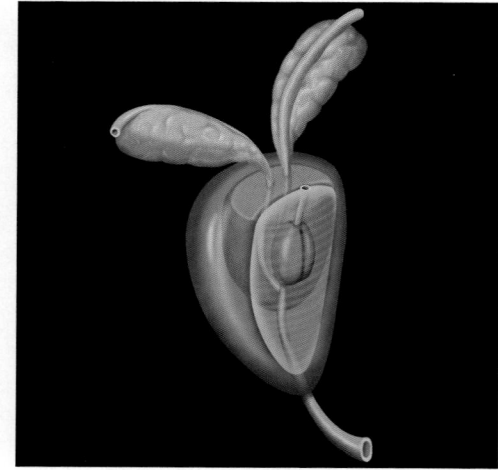

McNeal anatomic model of prostate depicts the internal structural relationship of peripheral (green), central (orange), and transition (blue) zones, and the anterior fibromuscular stroma (yellow).

ANATOMIC FEATURES

Prostate Gland

- Exocrine compound tubulo-alveolar gland
- Located in true pelvis
  - Surrounded by urinary bladder superiorly, transverse urogenital diaphragm inferiorly, inferior aspect of symphysis pubis anteriorly, and rectum posteriorly
- Inverted conical shape: Base is broad superior region, and apex is tapered inferior region
  - Base contiguous with bladder neck superiorly and seminal vesicle attachment posteriorly
  - Apex blends with striated muscle of transverse urogenital diaphragm
- Normal prostate in men (21-30 years old) weighs ~ 20 g (range 14-26 g)
- In adults, usually measures 4 x 3 x 2 cm
  - Widest at transverse dimension of base
- McNeal anatomic model divides prostate into glandular and nonglandular components
  - Glandular component
    - Peripheral zone, central zone, transition zone, periurethral gland region
  - Nonglandular component
    - Anterior fibromuscular stroma, preprostatic sphincter, striated sphincter
- Receives arterial supply from inferior vesical and middle rectal arteries, branches of internal iliac artery
- Prostatic venous plexus lies partly within prostatic fascial sheath and drains into internal iliac vein
- Primary lymphatics drain into regional lymph nodes in true pelvis
  - Hypogastric, obturator, internal and external iliac, and sacral lymph nodes

Prostatic Urethra

- Approximately 3 cm in length and begins at internal urethral orifice at apex of bladder trigone

- Courses through prostate, makes anteriorly concave 35° bend, ends as urethra penetrates fascia of urogenital diaphragm and enters perineum
- Continues distally as membranous urethra
- Posterior wall of prostatic urethra has several unique features related to prostatic secretory function
  - Contains a longitudinal ridge (urethral crest) lined by 2 adjacent grooves (prostatic sinuses)
  - Prostatic ductules enter urethra predominantly in sinuses with fewer entering along lateral aspects of crest
  - Urethral crest also has midline protuberance (verumontanum or colliculus seminalis)

Verumontanum (Colliculus Seminalis)

- Protrusion of prostatic tissue from posterior wall of urethra at angulation, tapers distally as crista urethralis
- Contains epithelium-lined blind sac (utricle) between openings of paired ejaculatory ducts

Ejaculatory Duct

- Passes through central zone entering at cephalad aspect
- Both ducts open into prostatic urethra at verumontanum, lateral to prostatic utricle

Seminal Vesicle

- Attached to superior-posterior aspect of prostate and bladder base
- Paired, highly coiled epithelial-lined tubes with irregular outpouchings
- Small intraprostatic portion is seen
- Excretory duct connects anteriorly with ampullary portion of vas deferens forming ejaculatory duct
- In adults, average 6 x 2 cm and contains up to 5 mL milky fluid, which forms bulk of ejaculatory volume

Periprostatic Structures

- Resected prostate may include adjoining tissues, such as adipose tissue, neurovascular bundle, paraganglia, Denonvilliers fascia, and lateral prostatic fascia
  - Potency-sparing prostatectomy preserves neurovascular bundle, site of cavernous nerves important for erection

SPECIMEN TYPES AND HANDLING

Needle Core Biopsy

- Indication is for histologic diagnosis of prostate cancer and evaluation of mass lesion or hypoechoic region
- Performed for elevated serum PSA level &/or abnormal digital rectal examination (DRE)
- Performed almost universally via transrectal ultrasound (TRUS)-guided using 18-gauge needle as outpatient procedure
- May also be performed perineally or transurethrally
- Different prostate biopsy sampling schemes
  - **Sextant biopsy** (6 cores)
    - Use remains widespread despite becoming the less preferred technique
    - Samples bilateral base, midgland, and apex
  - **Extended biopsy** (10-12 cores)
    - Preferred initial diagnostic procedure
    - Demonstrated increased cancer detection rate without increase in morbidity
    - False-negativity rate of 5% (vs. ~ 25% for sextant biopsy)
    - Optimal extended biopsy includes standard sextant area plus cores that target mid and lateral peripheral zone
    - Transition zone biopsy is not usually recommended at initial biopsy due to low detection rate
  - **Saturation biopsy** (≥ 20 cores)
    - Does not improve cancer detection when performed as initial procedure
    - Considered in men with persistently elevated PSA and several prior negative biopsies
    - Includes biopsy of transition zone
- **Handling of biopsy specimen**
  - If possible, avoid accessioning prostate biopsy specimens in sequence
  - Count and document number of cores per container
    - Ideally core(s) submitted in 1 container per site (> 3 is detrimental for evaluation)
  - Formalin fixative is preferred
    - Bouin solution is not preferred as it may enhance nucleoli in benign glands
  - Hematoxylin or other indelible dye makes tissue cores more visible when cutting paraffin blocks
  - Ideally, submit only 1-2 tissue cores per block to maximize tissue representation
    - More cores per block often leads to undesired tissue loss
  - Prospectively cut intervening unstained slides to ensure presence of atypical focus for adjunctive immunostains
    - Levels 1, 3, and 5 for H&E staining

- Save unstained levels 2, 4, and 6 for potential immunohistochemistry (IHC) or H&E stains
- Attempting immunostains on subsequent deeper levels more frequently results in loss of atypical focus
  - Multiple sections (ideally 3) should be present on each H&E slide to enhance sampling
  - Most of the tissue in the block from superficial to deep should be included in sections

Fine Needle Aspiration Biopsy

- Rarely performed in USA
  - Advocates claim aspiration cytology is cheaper, faster, easier to use, and has less morbidity
  - Major drawback is lack of cancer architecture that precludes Gleason grading and distinction from HGPIN
    - Inability to provide important information for planning therapy and prognostication

Transurethral Resection of Prostate (TURP) or Subtotal Prostatectomy

- TURP is surgical treatment of choice for benign prostatic hyperplasia (BPH)
- Open simple prostatectomy may be performed for bulky BPH
- Incidental prostate cancer encountered in ~ 10%
- TURP specimen consists of elongated rubbery fragments called prostate chips
  - Includes transition zone and areas around proximal prostatic urethra
- **Handling of TURP specimen**
  - Specimens ≤ 12 g: Submit entirely
  - For > 12 g: Submit initial 12 g (6-8 cassettes) and 1 cassette for every additional 5 g
  - Sensitivity for cancer detection may be increased by selectively submitting chips that are firm, yellow, or grossly suspicious for cancer
  - If incidental prostate cancer comprises < 5% of tissues examined, entire remaining tissue should be submitted

Radical Prostatectomy (RP)

- Most common treatment for localized prostate cancer (cT1-T2), when life expectancy is > 10 years
- Retropubic, laparoscopic, or robotic-assisted
  - Increasing popularity of robotic-assisted prostatectomy
  - ~ 40% of radical prostatectomies performed in USA in 2006 were robotic-assisted
  - Data comparing outcomes between surgical methods is starting to emerge
- **Handling of RP specimen**
  - Weigh and measure specimen in 3 dimensions
  - Unless being sampled for research, fix in 10% buffered formalin for 18-24 hours
    - May use microwave-assisted technique to facilitate fixing
  - Ink entire outer surface using 2 colors to identify right and left sides
  - Apex, base, and seminal vesicles should be handled in standardized fashion
  - Apical margin

- Apex amputated (should not be thinly shaved) and subsequently sectioned perpendicular to inked surface
- Perpendicular apex sections may be taken in radial manner (similar to cervical cone) or as series of parallel (parasagittal) sections
- Shaved (en face) margin not recommended as it may lead to a false-positive margin
- Urethra often retracts and urothelium may not be present in apical margin sections
  - Base margin
    - Submit either as perpendicular or shaved (en face) section(s)
    - Perpendicular sections recommended because they avoid possibility of false-positive margin
  - Middle portion serially sectioned coronally at 3-5 mm intervals and sections submitted in quadrants
    - Sections submitted from remainder of gland ranges from systematic partial sampling to entire prostate submission
  - Partial sampling should be systematic to allow for assessment of volume, multifocality, and orientation
    - Random sampling precludes tumor measurements, focality determination, and location of margin and EPE positivity
  - Grossly evident tumor should be sampled with adjacent extraprostatic tissues and margins
  - Seminal vesicle
    - Sections of prostatic tissue at base, including adjacent attached seminal vesicle, are needed to demonstrate direct tumor extension
    - Not necessary to submit entire seminal vesicle
    - Margins of vas deferens optional since cancer spread through this route is highly unusual
  - Few institutions process whole mount prostate sections
    - Advocates report ease in assessing tumor volume and assigning a more precise primary Gleason score in multifocal tumors
    - Location of extraprostatic extension and positive margins easier to determine
    - Expensive, technically cumbersome, and requires special filing and storage

Frozen Section (FS)

- Currently, there is no standard for intraoperative FS in patients undergoing RP
  - Depends on surgeon's preference and preoperative or intraoperative findings
- FS performed mainly for apical margin, bladder neck margin, and posterolateral aspect of prostate for monitoring neurovascular bundle
- Good correlation between FS and permanent section interpretations
  - High positive predictive value
- FS artifacts may compromise interpretation particularly of Gleason 3 pattern carcinoma
- Some studies have reported reduction in margin positivity rate
- Overall, has low sensitivity (42%) in identifying positive margins due to sampling bias
- Utility of FS in improving functional outcomes and biochemical control has not been shown

- Occasionally may be performed to determine whether benign or cancerous glands are present (intraoperative clearance of prostate gland)

IMMUNOHISTOCHEMISTRY

General Principles

- Use of IHC in prostate cancer is primarily for the following scenarios
  - Confirming diagnosis of carcinoma in biopsy materials containing atypical glands
  - Diagnosis of prostatic origin of tumor, whether in prostate or at distant metastatic site
- Principles of IHC used in prostate carcinoma diagnosis
  - Confirm absence of basal cell layer
    - Carcinoma should not contain basal cells
  - Demonstrate overexpression of proteins (i.e., AMACR) upregulated in prostate cancer
  - Diagnosis of carcinoma should always be made in conjunction with H&E morphology

Basal Cell Markers

- Include HMCK(34βE12), CK5/6, CK14, p63, and antibody cocktails
  - HMCK(34βE12) labels intermediate filaments in basal cell cytoplasm
    - Does not stain prostatic secretory cells
  - p63 labels basal cell nuclei
    - Comparable to HMCK(34βE12), although some studies suggested p63 has higher sensitivity
  - Basal cell marker cocktails (HMCK[34βE12] or CK5/6 & p63) provide more intense basal cell staining, combination of nuclear and cytoplasmic
- Interpretation
  - Complete lack of immunoreactivity in suspicious atypical glandular focus is supportive of carcinoma diagnosis
    - All morphologically atypical glands must be identified by H&E, and corresponding glands on IHC slide should be completely negative
    - Consistency of staining reaction should preferably be demonstrated on subsequent section on same slide, if available
- Potential pitfalls
  - Main drawback is staining pattern supportive of carcinoma diagnosis is based on negative staining
    - Absence of basal cell staining is not entirely diagnostic of cancer, as some benign glands may show patchy, discontinuous, or absent staining
    - Weak or nonreactive in 5-23% of benign glands
    - May be absent (up to 24%) in small foci of partial atrophy, post atrophic hyperplasia, and up to 50% of atypical adenomatous hyperplasia (adenosis)
  - Rare aberrant nuclear p63 staining may occur in malignant secretory cells of acinar adenocarcinoma
  - Several preanalytic and analytic factors may interfere with immunoreactivity
    - Should be run with appropriate positive and negative controls

α-methylacyl-CoA-racemase (AMACR, P504S)

- Overexpressed in prostate cancer with marked differential staining between malignant (positive) and benign (negative or weak expression) glands
  - Identified in gene expression array studies
- Highly sensitive, reportedly positive in ~ 75-95% of prostate carcinomas
- Interpretation
  - Positivity in carcinoma is characterized by intense circumferential luminal reactivity with granular quality
  - Staining in malignant glands must be stronger than in adjacent benign glands, if they stain positive
  - Interpretation must always be in conjunction with H&E morphology and in conjunction with basal cell marker(s)
- Potential pitfalls
  - Similar immunoreactivity pattern seen in HGPIN (reported 56-100%)
  - Negative or weakly expressed in some prostatic carcinomas: 5-25% typical, 30% atrophic, 32-38% foamy gland, 23-30% pseudohyperplastic, and up to 29% hormone-treated carcinomas
  - Expressed in benign lesions: 35-58% nephrogenic adenoma, up to 29% luminal staining in partial atrophy and post atrophic hyperplasia, 2-36% benign glands, 18% atypical adenomatous hyperplasia
  - Not specific for prostatic origin in metastatic setting
    - Expressed by variety of other malignancies

Dual Chromogen Antibody Cocktails

- Use gaining widespread popularity
- Combine 1 or 2 basal cell markers with AMACR
- Maximize tissue preservation, which may be critical in small foci of carcinoma
  - May be performed on single unstained or destained section if required
- Utilizes 2 chromogens, usually red for AMACR and brown for basal cell marker
  - Positive marker AMACR complements negative basal cell marker in carcinoma

Epithelial Marker

- PAN-CK(AE1/AE3)
  - Aids distinction of prostate carcinoma cells from nonepithelial process
    - Nonspecific granulomatous prostatitis, crushed or marked inflammation, and xanthoma cells are keratin negative
    - Diagnosis of small cell proliferations involving prostate (small cell carcinoma vs. lymphoma and rhabdomyosarcoma)
  - In post-treatment setting, highlights individual atrophic prostate cancer cells
    - Superior to PSA, which may be suppressed by treatment

Prostate Lineage-Specific Markers

- PSA and PAP

- Newer markers include prostate-specific membrane antigen (PSMA) and proPSA, but experience is limited
- Expressed by both benign and malignant prostatic epithelium
  - Aid in exclusion of nonprostatic lesions that mimic carcinoma
    - Seminal vesicle/ejaculatory duct, mesonephric glands, nephrogenic adenoma, Cowper gland, and paraganglionic tissue
  - Differential diagnosis of unusual variants of prostate carcinoma (e.g., ductal, mucinous, signet ring) vs. secondary tumors involving prostate
- Intensity of expression usually inversely proportional to Gleason grade
  - Gleason pattern 5 tumors may exhibit weak or negative staining (up to 13%)
- In metastatic setting, strong expression of PSA and PAP by adenocarcinoma of unknown origin is strongly suggestive of prostate primary
  - PSA and PAP are not entirely specific for prostate carcinoma

SELECTED REFERENCES

1. Ramirez-Backhaus M et al: Value of frozen section biopsies during radical prostatectomy: significance of the histological results. World J Urol. 27(2):227-34, 2009
2. Srigley JR et al: Protocol for the examination of specimens from patients with carcinoma of the prostate gland. Arch Pathol Lab Med. 133(10):1568-76, 2009
3. Epstein JI et al: Recommendations for the reporting of prostate carcinoma: Association of Directors of Anatomic and Surgical Pathology. Am J Clin Pathol. 129(1):24-30, 2008
4. Paner GP et al: Best practice in diagnostic immunohistochemistry: prostate carcinoma and its mimics in needle core biopsies. Arch Pathol Lab Med. 132(9):1388-96, 2008
5. Scattoni V et al: Extended and saturation prostatic biopsy in the diagnosis and characterisation of prostate cancer: a critical analysis of the literature. Eur Urol. 52(5):1309-22, 2007
6. Eichelberg C et al: Frozen section for the management of intraoperatively detected palpable tumor lesions during nerve-sparing scheduled radical prostatectomy. Eur Urol. 49(6):1011-6; discussion 1016-8, 2006
7. Eichler K et al: Diagnostic value of systematic biopsy methods in the investigation of prostate cancer: a systematic review. J Urol. 175(5):1605-12, 2006
8. Srigley JR: Key issues in handling and reporting radical prostatectomy specimens. Arch Pathol Lab Med. 130(3):303-17, 2006
9. Amin M et al: Prognostic and predictive factors and reporting of prostate carcinoma in prostate needle biopsy specimens. Scand J Urol Nephrol Suppl. (216):20-33, 2005
10. Epstein JI et al: Prognostic factors and reporting of prostate carcinoma in radical prostatectomy and pelvic lymphadenectomy specimens. Scand J Urol Nephrol Suppl. (216):34-63, 2005
11. Tsuboi T et al: Is intraoperative frozen section analysis an efficient way to reduce positive surgical margins? Urology. 66(6):1287-91, 2005
12. McNeal JE: Normal histology of the prostate. Am J Surg Pathol. 12(8):619-33, 1988

Anatomic Features

(Left) Prostate is situated in true pelvis surrounded by urinary bladder superiorly ➘, urogenital diaphragm inferiorly ➘, inferior aspect of symphysis pubis anteriorly ➘, and rectum posteriorly, with intervening Denonvilliers fascia ➘. Seminal vesicles ➘ are attached postero-superiorly. **(Right)** View from robotic prostatectomy shows lateral-posterior prostate ➘ being dissected from neurovascular bundle ➘ along lateral prostatic fascia ➘. (Courtesy M. Woods, MD.)

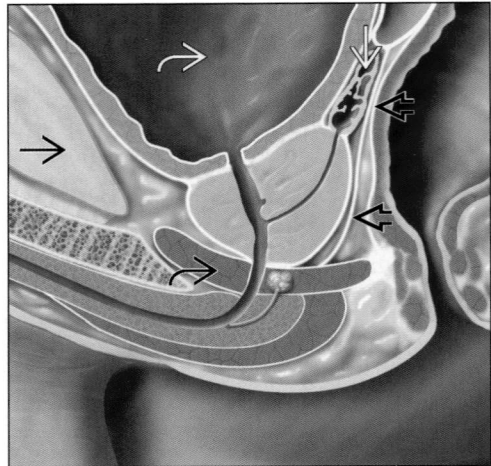
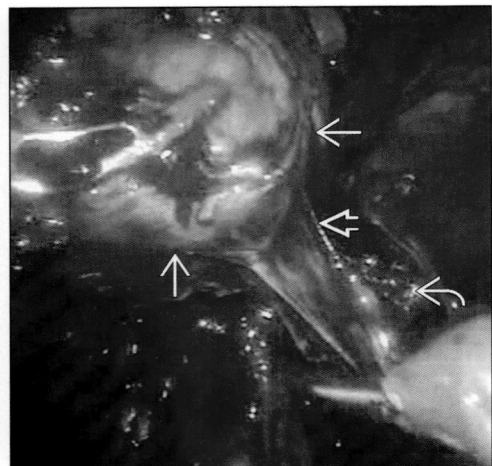

(Left) These different views of the prostate depict the path of the prostatic urethra (tan), which has a 35° anterior angulation ➘ halfway between base and apex that divides urethra into proximal and distal segments. The ejaculatory ducts (blue) are almost continuous with long axis of distal prostatic urethra ➘. **(Right)** The verumontanum forms a protrusion from posterior urethral wall at the urethral angulation and contains openings of paired ejaculatory ducts and utricle ➘.

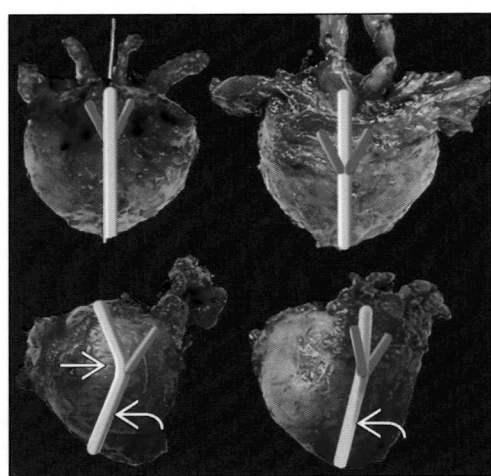
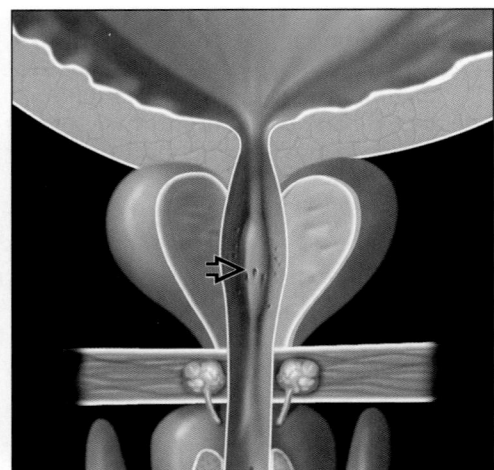

(Left) This coronal section of the prostate at the verumontanum ➘ shows the peripheral zone ➘ extending from posterior aspect ➘, surrounding part of transition zone ➘, and abutting the anterior fibromuscular stroma ➘. The central urethra is enveloped by the transition zone. **(Right)** These anterior ➘ and superior ➘ views of the prostate show paired bilateral seminal vesicles ➘ attached to the posterior aspect of the base ➘, lateral to vas deferens ➘.

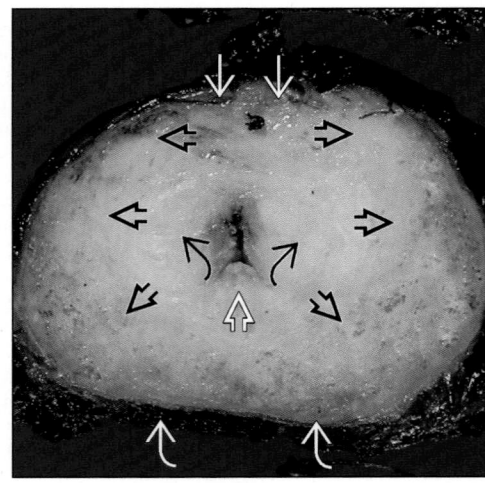
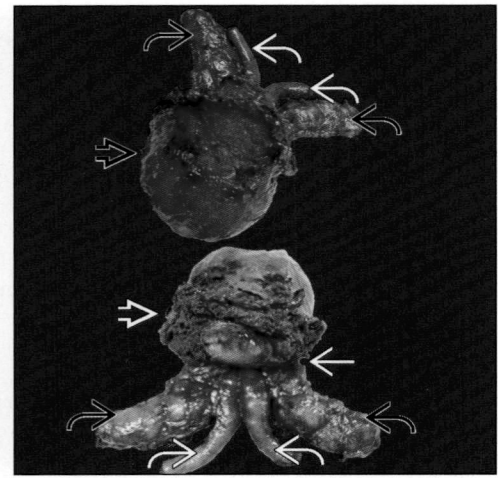

Specimen Handling

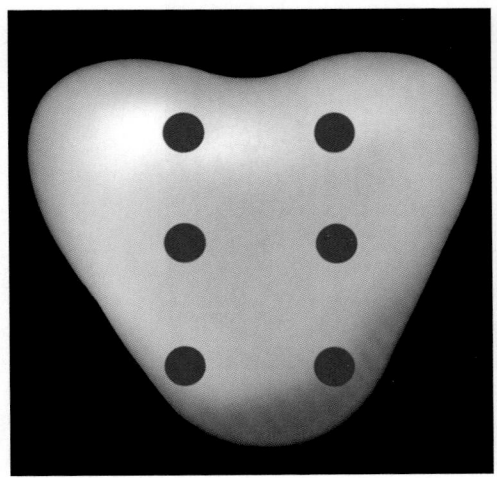 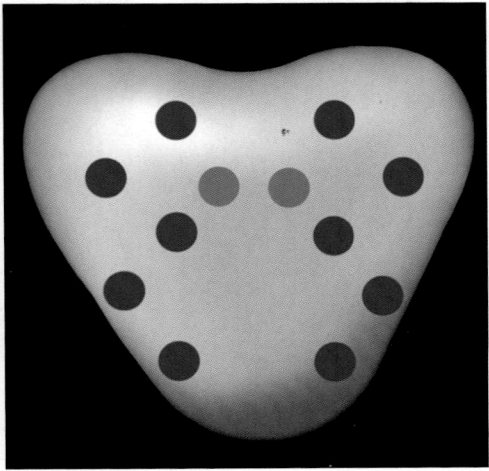

(Left) This anterior view of the prostate shows targets for the classic sextant biopsy scheme, which samples bilateral base, midgland, and apex. *(Right)* The extended biopsy scheme includes standard sextant biopsies with more laterally directed biopsies, and is preferred due to a lower false-negative rate. Biopsy of the transition zone (blue) is not recommended at initial biopsy; the saturation biopsy scheme is reserved for persistent indication and negative prior biopsies.

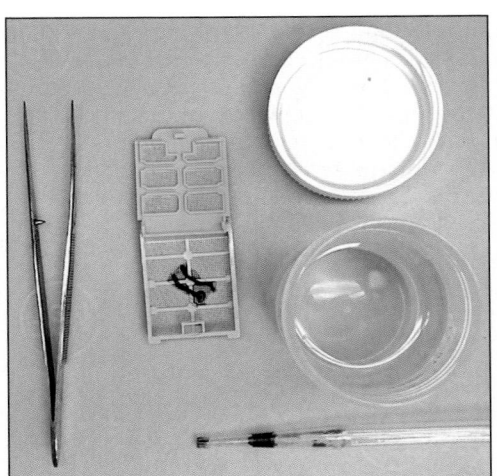 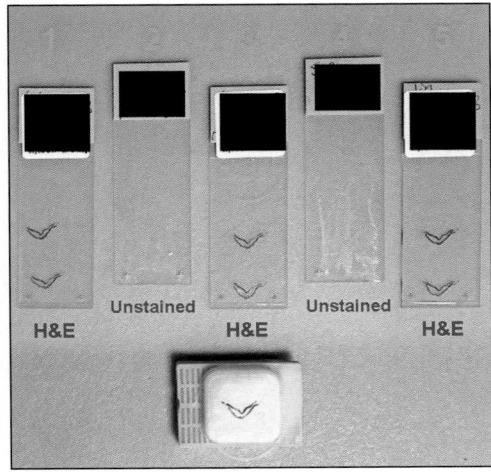

(Left) The prostate cores are ideally submitted with only 1-2 cores per cassette. Too many cores per block may cause tissue loss since cores may be cut at different levels. Inked cores are more visible and aid in the cutting of paraffin blocks. *(Right)* Prospective intervening unstained slides are recommended for possible immunohistochemical studies or additional H&E stains. This approach ensures representation of the focus of interest that may be lost in subsequent deeper levels.

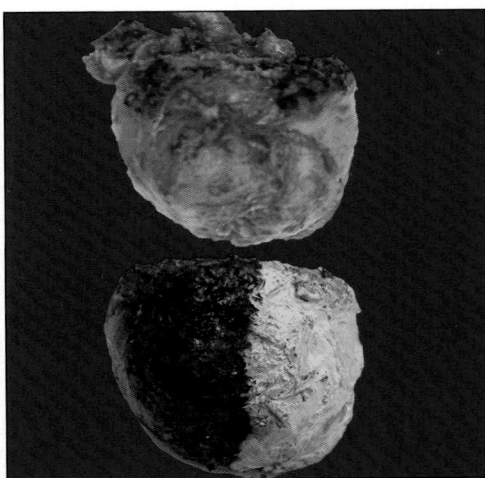 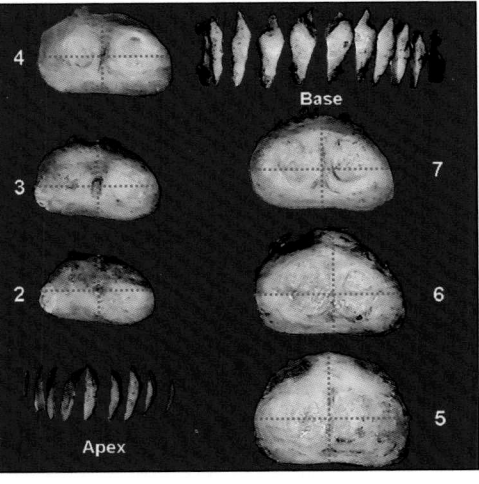

(Left) The entire outer prostate surface must be inked for assessment of margin status. Right and left lobes are designated by different colors. *(Right)* Apical and base margins are transected and submitted as a series of parasagittal (perpendicular) sections. Shaving of the apex (en face margin) is not recommended due to risk of false-positivity. The remaining prostate is coronally sectioned at 3-5 mm intervals and submitted sequentially as quadrants. (Courtesy E. Drinka, MD.)

MICROANATOMY AND ZONAL VARIATIONS

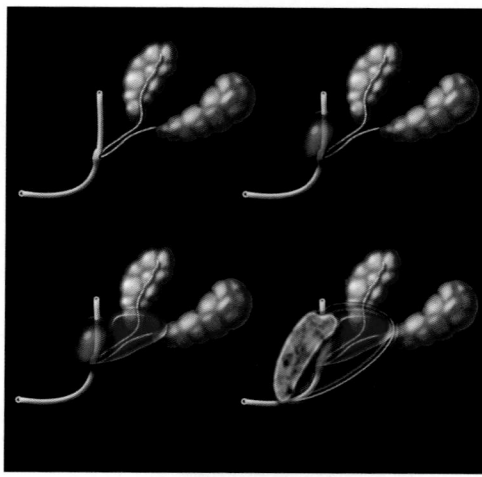

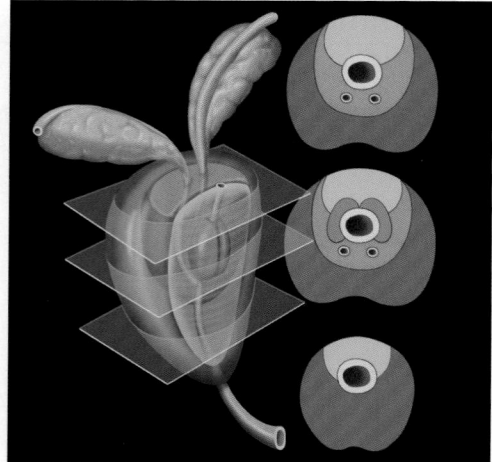

PU is divided into PPU and DPU by a mid angulation. TZ (blue) and CZ (magenta) encase PPU and ED, respectively. PZ (transparent) surrounds CZ and DPU posteriorly. AFS (yellow) is situated anteriorly.

McNeal model uses PU as key anatomic landmark and divides prostate glandular component into PZ (green), CZ (orange), TZ (blue), and PUGR (white). The AFS (yellow) comprises midanterior portion.

TERMINOLOGY

Abbreviations

- Peripheral zone (PZ)
- Central zone (CZ)
- Transition zone (TZ)
- Periurethral gland region (PUGR)
- Anterior fibromuscular stroma (AFS)
- Prostatic urethra (PU)
- Proximal prostatic urethra (PPU)
- Distal prostatic urethra (DPU)
- Ejaculatory duct (ED)
- Seminal vesicle (SV)

DUCTAL-ACINAR UNIT

Ducts and Acini

- Primarily lined by secretory cells, except at proximal ducts close to PU where epithelium is urothelial
- Main cell types: Secretory, basal, and endocrine-paracrine cells
- Cross section of ducts and acini cannot be reliably distinguished histologically, except when longitudinal dimension of duct is appreciated
- All ducts originate from PU and end near the capsule, except main TZ duct, which ends at AFS
- Very rarely, acini may lie within perineural space

Secretory Cells

- Typically cuboidal to columnar with clear to pale cytoplasm and basally located round regular nuclei
- May appear multilayered depending on plane of section
- PSA/PSAP(+)
- HMCK(34βE12), p63, CK5/6, CK14 (-)

Basal Cells

- Believed to be stem cell compartment of acini that divides and matures into secretory cells

- Lack muscle filaments, thus not identical to myoepithelial cells in breast ducts and lobules
- Located between secretory cells and acinar basement membrane and should be internal to acinar outline
- Cuboidal, flattened, attenuated, or triangular cells with long axis parallel to basement membrane
- Contains little or no discernible cytoplasm, dark round to oval nuclei, and occasional small nucleoli
- May not be obvious on H&E or may appear discontinuous or absent, unless highlighted by immunohistochemistry
- PSA/PSAP(-)
- p63, HMCK(34βE12), CK5/6, CK14 (+)

Endocrine-Paracrine Cells

- Typically isolated or irregularly distributed in acini
- May not be readily identifiable on H&E, demonstrable only by immunohistochemistry or special stains
- Contain hormones, such as serotonin, neuron-specific enolase, somatostatin, calcitonin, and bombesin
- Include argentaffin and Paneth-like cells
  - Argentaffin cells contain finer eosinophilic granules situated between secretory cells, rest on basal cells, and usually do not reach lumen
  - Paneth-like cell contains larger intensely eosinophilic granules and extends to luminal aspect of acini
- Exact function not known

Nonglandular &/or Metaplastic Cells

- **Urothelial cells**
  - Lining epithelium of PPU, proximal part of DPU, and proximal portion of prostatic ducts
  - Unlike in bladder, urothelium of PU and ducts have scant cytoplasm and maturation into surface umbrella cells is variable
  - May be seen in deep ducts and acini presumably as metaplastic process
  - Seen in up to 34% of prostate biopsies

- ○ May undergo exuberant hyperplasia that may mimic urothelial carcinoma
- **Mucinous metaplasia**
  - ○ May occur in benign prostate glands
  - ○ Reported in nodular hyperplastic epithelium, transitional cell metaplasia, basal cell hyperplasia, sclerotic atrophy, and postatrophic hyperplasia
  - ○ Postulated to arise from metaplasia of basal cells
  - ○ Mucinous cells contain foamy cytoplasm and basally oriented bland nuclei
  - ○ Contain both neutral and acid mucin (PASD, mucicarmine, Alcian blue [+])
  - ○ Nonreactive to PSA/PSAP
- **Squamous metaplasia**
  - ○ Prostate glands may undergo squamous metaplasia in response to infarction and estrogen
  - ○ Postulated to arise directly from proliferative basal cells
  - ○ Reduces or loses ability to express prostate-associated antigens (PSA/PSAP[-])
  - ○ Differential diagnosis for rare squamous cell carcinoma of prostate, which in contrast has marked atypia and infiltrative growth

PROSTATE ANATOMIC ZONES

Peripheral Zone

- Comprises about 70% of glandular compartment
- Accounts for all glandular tissues surrounding DPU
- Surrounds CZ posteriorly, laterally, and inferiorly
- Ducts exit in double row at posterolateral aspect of DPU extending from verumontanum to apex
- Ducts extend laterally within PZ, major branches curve anteriorly, and minor branches curve posteriorly
- Most common origin for prostate carcinoma (70-75%)
- Most susceptible to inflammation and most common to undergo atrophy

Central Zone

- Comprises about 25% of glandular compartment
- Inverted conical shape with its base comprising entire base of prostate
- Ducts arise around ED opening at verumontanum, follow course of ED, and fan out posteriorly to base
- Relatively resistant to prostate carcinoma and inflammation

Transition Zone

- Comprises about 5% of glandular compartment
- 2 separate small paraurethral lobes at mid prostate
- Ducts of both TZ lobes arise posterolaterally from PPU at lower border of preprostatic sphincter just above urethral angulation
- Main ducts extend laterally around preprostatic sphincter and curve sharply anteriorly
- Most common site for BPH and atypical adenomatous hyperplasia (AAH)/adenosis
- Zone resected in transurethral resection of prostate (TURP) for BPH

Periurethral Gland Region

- Series of tiny ducts and abortive acini embedded within longitudinal smooth muscle of preprostatic sphincter organized around PPU
- Possible origin of uncommon pure primary urothelial carcinoma of prostate

ZONAL VARIATIONS IN HISTOLOGY

Prostatic Ducts and Acini

- PZ and TZ acini are identical, which are small, usually 0.15-0.3 mm, with slight luminal undulations
  - ○ TZ acini are less numerous than in PZ
  - ○ Secretory cells of PZ and TZ are evenly spaced, uniform columnar cells, with pale cytoplasm and small more basally situated nuclei
- CZ acini are larger, up to 0.6 mm, and more complex
  - ○ Luminal borders are uneven, with individual secretory cells protruding into lumen
  - ○ Contain cribriform formations, "Roman bridging," and papillary infolding
  - ○ May be confused with prostatic intraepithelial neoplasia or BPH glands
  - ○ Secretory cells of CZ have more crowded columnar cells, more granular or darker cytoplasm, and relatively larger nuclei at varying levels within cells
- Urothelial cells variably line PUGR glands

Prostatic Stroma

- PZ stroma is loose with random muscle bundles
- TZ stroma relatively more compact than PZ with interlacing, smooth muscles bundles that blend with preprostatic sphincter and AFS
- CZ stroma more compact but less stroma to acini ratio than PZ and TZ
- Contrast of stromal quality is more abrupt between PZ and CZ than with TZ

LUMINAL AND CELLULAR DEPOSITS

Corpora Amylacea

- Common in lumen of benign prostate glands and verumontanum glands
- Present in benign acini of 25% of men ages 20-40 years and frequency increases with age
- Reported in 32% of atypical adenomatous hyperplasia cases, 75% of postatrophic hyperplasia cases, and 20% of needle biopsies with infarcts
- Very rare in prostate carcinoma
- Round pink-purple concretions often with concentric lamination
- Thought to be related to cellular desquamation and degeneration

Intraluminal Crystalloids

- Seen in 5% of benign glands and up to 41% of prostate carcinoma
- Bright, eosinophilic, refractile, with sharp borders and a variety of shapes
- When seen in benign glands, not a significant risk factor for subsequent diagnosis of prostate cancer

MICROANATOMY AND ZONAL VARIATIONS

Intraluminal Secretions
- Occasionally present in gland lumina consisting of light eosinophilic amorphous material on H&E
- Contains neutral mucin (PAS/PASD[+])

Pigments
- **Lipofuscin**
  - Ubiquitously present in SV and ED epithelium
  - May also be seen within benign prostatic secretory cells and rarely in basal and stromal cells
    - Awareness is important and should not be the sole criterion to identify SV and ED epithelium
    - Golden-yellow pigment usually subnuclear or at basal aspect of secretory cells
    - Usually finely granular and sparse although may have coarse clumping where it is abundant
    - Varies from inconspicuous to diffuse and may be found in all prostate zones
    - Exhibits yellow autofluorescence
    - Pigment within basal cells more likely an artifactual overlap of pigment from secretory cells
    - Rare pigment in stroma is scant and appears as isolated clusters
  - May be found in epithelium of benign prostatic hyperplasia, prostatic intraepithelial hyperplasia, and adenocarcinoma
  - SV and ED lipofuscin pigment is more uniform yellow, coarsely granular to globular, more refractile, and found in luminal aspect of cytoplasm
- **Melanin**
  - Seen rarely in prostatic stromal cells (blue nevus)
  - Finely granular brown or black pigment
  - Stromal cells show melanosomes at different stages of differentiation by electron microscopy
  - Pigmented stromal cells are S100(+)
  - Pigment may be seen in adjacent glandular epithelium, which are S100(-) and due to pigment transfer
  - Pigment may also be dispersed extracellularly among cells and collagen fibers

NONGLANDULAR PROSTATE

Anterior Fibromuscular Stroma
- Comprises anterior 1/3 of prostate, at anteromedial aspect extending from bladder neck to apex
- Laterally, covers most anterior aspect of PZ
- Deep aspect always in contact with PU, proximally with preprostatic sphincter and TZ, and distally with striated sphincter
- Composed of large compact smooth muscle bundles similar in bladder neck although more haphazard and some separated by fibrous tissues
- Occasionally may contain benign acini

Preprostatic Sphincter
- Circular smooth muscle fibers surrounding PU, which prevents retrograde ejaculation
- Located "preprostatic" or proximal to openings of ducts from main glandular areas
- More compact at urethra posteriorly, but fibers dispersed more laterally to mingle with TZ ducts and acini
- Not complete anteriorly, where it blends with AFS

Striated Sphincter
- Semicircular cap over anterior and anterolateral surface of gland
- Surrounds distal urethra anteriorly but incomplete posterolaterally where fibers continue to anterior margin of PZ
- Thin, consisting of small compact striated muscle fibers

Prostatic "Capsule"
- Prostate does not have true capsule but outer condensation of fibromuscular tissue that is inseparable component of prostatic stroma
- For convenience, this fibromuscular band is referred to in literature as prostate capsule
- Covers most of posterior and lateral surfaces of prostate
- Blends anteriorly with AFS
- Not well defined or absent at anterolateral aspect of apex and at bladder neck where prostatic stroma blends with bladder musculature
  - Complicates interpretation of extraprostatic tumor extension (EPE) at these sites
- Outer surface of this fibromuscular band gives rise to few fibromuscular bands that blend into periprostatic connective tissue

NONPROSTATIC STRUCTURES

Prostatic Urethra
- PPU lined by urothelium with variable umbrella cells and merges imperceptibly with DPU
- Distal aspect of DPU lined by pseudostratified or stratified columnar cells

Verumontanum (Colliculus Seminalis)
- Elevation from posterior wall at PU angulation
- Contains a mid, blind epithelial-lined sac known as utricle and opening of ED at both sides
- Contains closely apposed small to medium-sized glands, which often contain corpora amylacea or orange-brown luminal secretions
- Glands has 2 layers consisting of glandular cells and readily discernible basal cells
- Glandular cells are cuboidal to low columnar containing clear to eosinophilic cytoplasm and round regular nuclei
- May undergo florid glandular hyperplasia, which may be confused with prostate carcinoma

Ejaculatory Duct
- Paired ducts cross CZ and exit in PU at both sides of prostatic utricle in verumontanum
- Similar to SV, shows complex luminal papillation
- Identical lining epithelium to SV, including presence of lipofuscin pigment and random pleomorphism

Cowper Glands (Bulbourethral Glands)
- Paired tubuloalveolar gland situated in striated muscles of urogenital diaphragm lateral to membranous urethra
- Because of its proximity, may be inadvertently sampled by transurethral resection or rarely by needle biopsy of apex
- May mimic low-grade prostate carcinoma
- Lobular arrangement of numerous mucinous acini with excretory ducts that end in posterior aspect of bulbous urethra
- Acinar structures contain single layer of bland cuboidal to columnar cells with abundant mucin and basally located small nuclei
- Acinar structures contain myoepithelial cells that are not easily discernible on H&E
- PSA/PSAP(-)
- SMA strongly stains myoepithelial cells around acini

PERIPROSTATIC STRUCTURES

Adipose Tissue
- Involvement by prostate cancer constitutes EPE
- Present in periprostatic region in about 1/2 of radical prostatectomy specimens
- Distribution around radical prostatectomy specimen varies: Most frequent in lateral region (57-59%), lowest at posterior surface (36%)
- Nerve sparing radical prostatectomy contains lesser periprostatic adipose tissue
- Very rarely, fat may be seen within prostate

Neurovascular Bundle
- Has short distance anterior to plane of rectal surface
- Consists of nerves and blood vessels in varying amounts of fibroadipose tissue and contains several autonomic ganglia
- "Bundle" formation not always present and may be seen spreading to lateral surface, although larger nerves and vessels tend to be at posterolateral region
- Ganglion cells may be present within prostate in region of neurovascular bundle

Paraganglia
- Present in approximately 8% of radical prostatectomy specimens
- Primarily situated in loose connective and adipose tissue immediately external to prostate
- Mostly located in lateral to slightly posterior extraprostatic tissues, closer to base than apex, and often in association with neurovascular bundle
- Rare in anterior aspect of prostate
- Range from approximately 100 μm to 1.7 mm (median: 0.9 mm)
- Lobular or zellballen pattern of cells with prominent stromal vascular component
- Cells typically have abundant clear to slight granular, basophilic to amphophilic cytoplasm with centrally placed small round to oval nuclei
- Rarely, may have more solid configuration, show single cell "infiltrative" pattern, or contain larger cells

- May mimic prostate carcinoma with hypernephroid features
- Synaptophysin, chromogranin, neuron specific enolase (+)

Denonvilliers Fascia
- Single avascular fascial sheath sometimes referred to as "prostoperitoneal membrane" situated behind prostate, covering posterior surface and SV
- Fused layers of collagenous fibers and occasional muscle
- Often fused with midposterior portion of prostate capsule, separated laterally by investing adipose tissue
- Usually dissected with prostate in radical and nerve sparing radical prostatectomy, being plane of dissection in the latter

Lateral Prostatic Fascia
- Collagenous fascia at variable distance from lateral aspect of prostate
- Either completely separate or fused with prostate capsule with very little adipose tissue in between
- Usually at lateral border of prostate near base; this area overlies boundary of CZ and PZ
- Usually dissected with prostate in radical prostatectomy and spared with preservation of neurovascular bundle

SEMINAL VESICLE

SV Glands
- Adult SV mucosa contains papillary projections and invaginating ducts surrounded by glands in vaguely lobular configuration
- Surrounding glands are small to medium and elongated or slit-like
- Papillae are lined by single layer of cuboidal to columnar secretory cells and underlying basal cells
- Secretory cells
  - Not uniform
  - Randomly contain pseudomalignant pleomorphic cells with nucleomegaly, hyperchromasia, and multinucleation
  - Lipofuscin granules frequent in cytoplasm
  - Nuclei may contain occasional pseudoinclusions
- Secretory cells are PSA/PSAP(-), pax-2(+), and basal cells are basal cell markers(+)
- Localized amyloid deposits seen in subepithelial region and around vessels in 4-12% of SV, usually incidental or identified at autopsy

SV Wall
- Thick inner circular layer and thin outer longitudinal fibromuscular layer
- Thinner at prostate base
- Contain round eosinophilic hyaline bodies thought to be degenerating smooth muscle cells

SELECTED REFERENCES

1. Christian JD et al: Corpora amylacea in adenocarcinoma of the prostate: incidence and histology within needle core biopsies. Mod Pathol. 18(1):36-9, 2005

3

MICROANATOMY AND ZONAL VARIATIONS

Significance of Normal Histoanatomic Structures in Prostate Pathology

Structures	Remarks
PZ	Most common origin for prostate carcinoma (70-75%)
	Most susceptible to inflammation and most common to undergo atrophy
	Uncommon site for benign prostatic hyperplasia (BPH)
TZ	Most common site for BPH and its myriad morphologic patterns
	Common site for atypical adenomatous hyperplasia (AAH)
	Less commonly site of origin of prostate carcinoma (15-20%), which tends to be lower grade
CZ	Relatively resistant to prostate carcinoma and inflammation
	Mimic glands of BPH and prostatic intraepithelial neoplasia
PUGR	Possible origin of uncommon pure primary urothelial carcinoma of prostate
Corpora amylacea	Common in benign prostate glands and rarely seen in carcinoma
Intraluminal crystalloids	Common in prostate carcinoma but may also be seen in benign glands
	Presence in benign glands not a risk factor for subsequent diagnosis of prostate carcinoma
Lipofuscin pigment	Not exclusive for SV and ED epithelium and may also be seen uncommonly in benign and malignant prostate glands
Striated muscles in AFS and apical region	Benign glands may be seen admixed with striated muscles and thus not necessarily an invasive or malignant feature
	Adenocarcinoma involving striated muscles at these sites does not constitute EPE
Prostate capsule	Although not a true capsule, serves as histoanatomic boundary for organ-confined prostate cancer
	Absent in base and not clearly defined in apex complicating interpretation of EPE at these sites
Nerve	Perineural glands not exclusively associated with carcinoma, unless glands completely circles or are present within a nerve
	One of the pathways for EPE by carcinoma
PU	May give rise to urothelial carcinoma (common), squamous carcinoma, adenocarcinoma of prostate and primary of urethra
	Florid nephrogenic adenoma from this site may extend to prostate and mimic prostate carcinoma
	Urothelial carcinoma of PU invading prostate may occur in patients with bladder urothelial carcinoma and should not be staged as pT4 bladder cancer
Verumontanum	May undergo florid glandular hyperplasia, which may be confused with prostate carcinoma
SV	Rare site for primary malignancy
	Secondary involvement by prostate carcinoma relatively more common and denotes higher tumor stage (pT3b)
	Pseudomalignant features of epithelium may be confused with malignancy in limited sample
ED	Involvement by cancer in needle biopsy should not be confused as SV involvement, which denotes higher tumor stage
	Pseudomalignant features of epithelium may be confused with malignancy in limited sample
	Distinction from SV is based on absence of distinct smooth muscle wall
Cowper gland	Resembles minor salivary gland tissue, may mimic low-grade prostate carcinoma
Periprostatic adipose tissue	Involvement by prostate carcinoma constitutes EPE, including in needle biopsy specimens
	May be absent over large areas of prostatic surface in prostatectomy specimen making evaluation of EPE difficult
Paraganglia	May mimic prostate carcinoma with hypernephroid features
	Involvement by carcinoma not always equivalent to EPE since it may be present rarely within prostate

2. Kiyoshima K et al: Anatomical features of periprostatic tissue and its surroundings: a histological analysis of 79 radical retropubic prostatectomy specimens. Jpn J Clin Oncol. 34(8):463-8, 2004
3. Hong H et al: Anatomic distribution of periprostatic adipose tissue: a mapping study of 100 radical prostatectomy specimens. Cancer. 97(7):1639-43, 2003
4. Srodon M et al: Central zone histology of the prostate: a mimicker of high-grade prostatic intraepithelial neoplasia. Hum Pathol. 33(5):518-23, 2002
5. Anton RC et al: The significance of intraluminal prostatic crystalloids in benign needle biopsies. Am J Surg Pathol. 22(4):446-9, 1998
6. Saboorian MH et al: Distinguishing Cowper's glands from neoplastic and pseudoneoplastic lesions of prostate: immunohistochemical and ultrastructural studies. Am J Surg Pathol. 21(9):1069-74, 1997
7. Amin MB et al: Pigment in prostatic epithelium and adenocarcinoma: a potential source of diagnostic confusion with seminal vesicular epithelium. Mod Pathol. 9(7):791-5, 1996
8. Ostrowski ML et al: Paraganglia of the prostate. Location, frequency, and differentiation from prostatic adenocarcinoma. Am J Surg Pathol. 18(4):412-20, 1994
9. Grignon DJ et al: Mucinous metaplasia in the prostate gland. Am J Surg Pathol. 17(3):287-90, 1993
10. Villers A et al: Anatomy of the prostate: review of the different models. Eur Urol. 20(4):261-8, 1991
11. Ayala AG et al: The prostatic capsule: does it exist? Its importance in the staging and treatment of prostatic carcinoma. Am J Surg Pathol. 13(1):21-7, 1989
12. Lager DJ et al: Squamous metaplasia of the prostate. An immunohistochemical study. Am J Clin Pathol. 90(5):597-601, 1988

MICROANATOMY AND ZONAL VARIATIONS

Microscopic Features

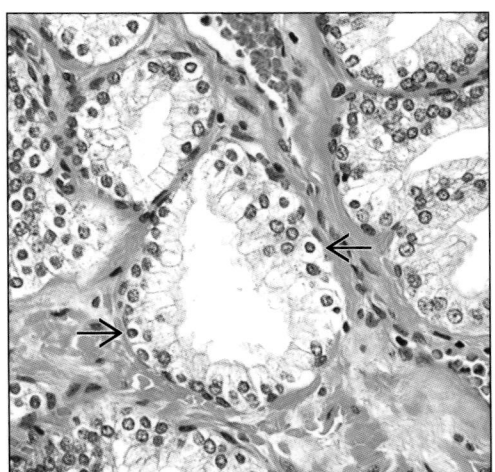
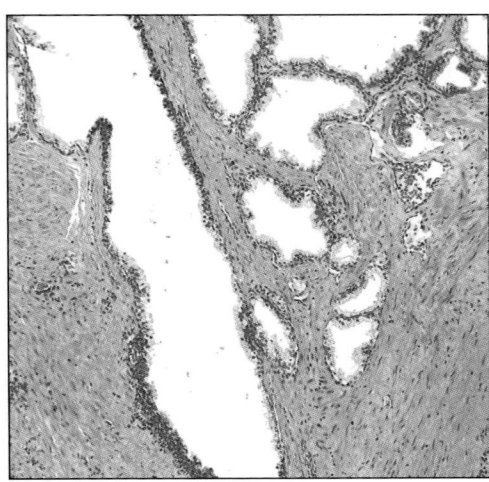

(Left) Typical benign acini show columnar secretory cells with pale cytoplasm and round, regular, basally oriented nuclei, with indistinct nucleoli. Basal cells ⮕ are situated internal to glandular basement membrane outline and contain scant cytoplasm. (Right) The lining of the prostatic duct is similar to the adjacent acini. On cross section, ducts and acini are not reliably distinguished unless the longitudinal dimension of the duct is appreciated.

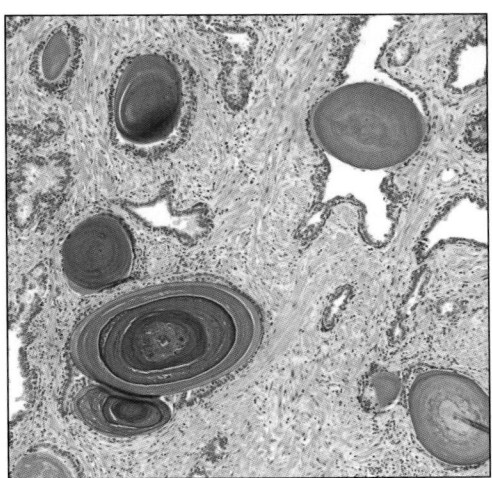
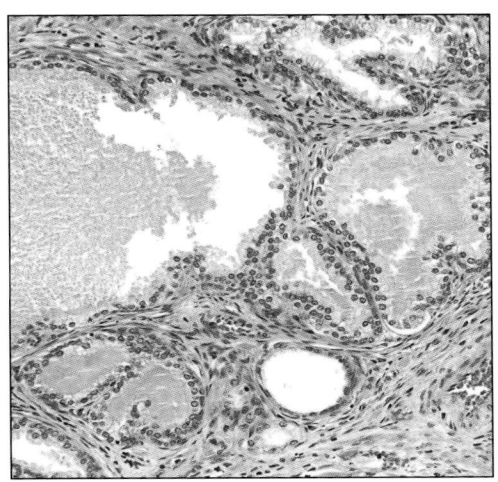

(Left) Benign glands contain corpora amylacea with its distinctive circular lamellation. Corpora amylacea are frequent in benign prostate and verumontanum glands and may only rarely be seen in prostate carcinoma. These concretions are thought to be related to cellular degeneration. (Right) Benign glands show intraluminal pink amorphous secretions. Prostatic secretions are a minor component of ejaculatory volume and contain enzymes, which enhance sperm viability.

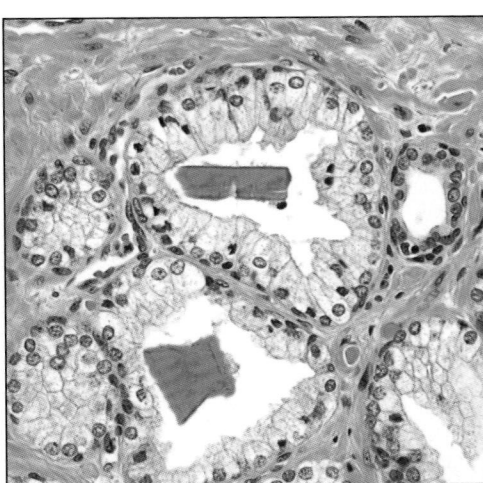
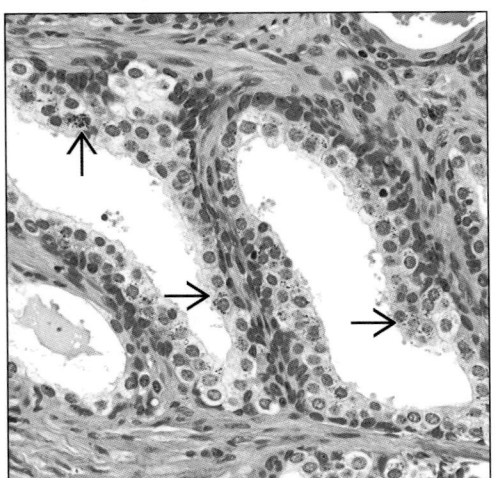

(Left) Benign glands show bright refractile eosinophilic crystals with sharp borders. Intraluminal crystalloids are common in prostate carcinoma and may be seen uncommonly in benign glands. Presence in benign glands is not a risk factor for carcinoma. (Right) Benign glands show intracytoplasmic fine golden-yellow pigment ⮕. The presence of granules should not be used as sole criterion to distinguish SV and ED from prostate epithelium. SV/ED granules are coarser and more abundant.

Microscopic Features

(Left) The periurethral prostatic duct shows urothelium lining its proximal aspect and secretory cells more distally. Urothelial carcinoma that arises primarily within the prostate is believed to originate from these cells. The presence of urothelium in the peripheral prostate indicates metaplasia. **(Right)** Peripheral prostatic gland shows urothelial metaplasia. When inflamed, this may mimic HGPIN. Presence of prostatic intraluminal material indicates the prostatic nature of this acinus.

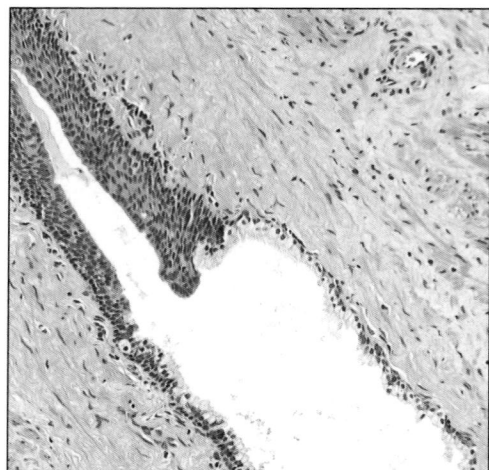
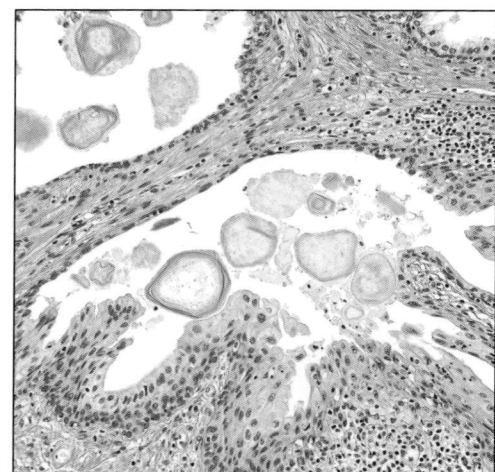

(Left) Biopsy shows florid squamous metaplasia of prostatic glands consisting of nests of squamous cells surrounded peripherally by basal cells. Squamous metaplasia may be seen in infarction or hormonally treated prostate for cancer. Squamous metaplasia should be excluded before the diagnosis of the rare squamous carcinoma of prostate is made. **(Right)** Mucinous metaplasia of prostatic acini shows mucin-containing cells with small basally oriented nuclei. The process may be focal ➡.

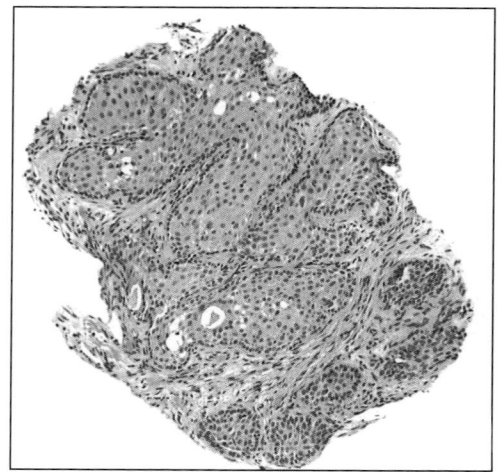
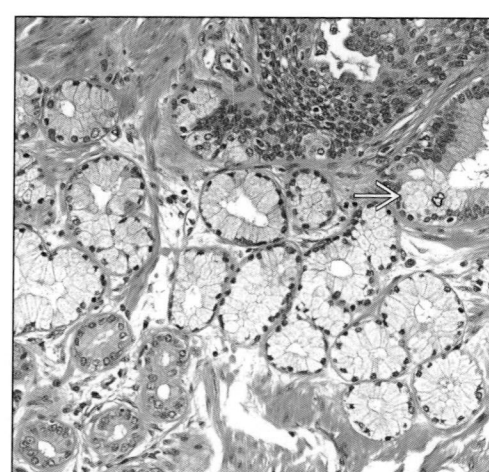

(Left) Coronal section of prostate at level of verumontanum ➡ shows PZ ➤ located posteriorly and extending anteriorly abutting the AFS ➡. The verumontanum is at urethral angulation midway between base and apex, and where both EDs exit into PU. **(Right)** Ducts of PZ (green) exit in DPU and extend laterally within PZ. Ducts of CZ (orange) arise at verumontanum and fan out posteriorly. Ducts of TZ (blue) arise at lower PPU. PUGR is seen as series of ducts and acini in PPU.

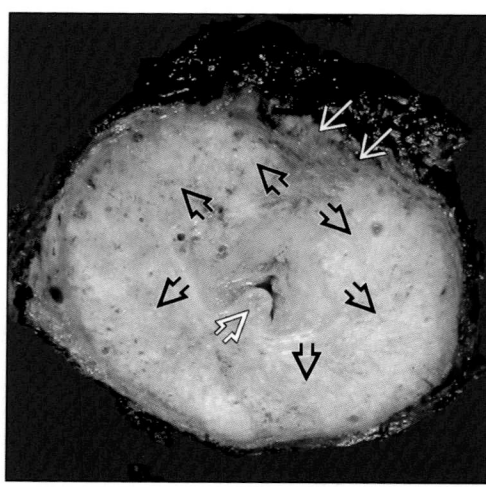
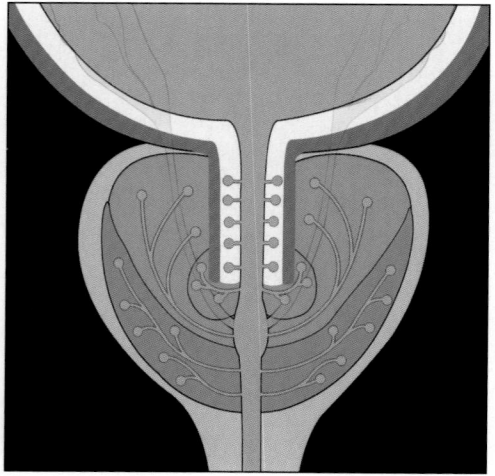

MICROANATOMY AND ZONAL VARIATIONS

Microscopic Features

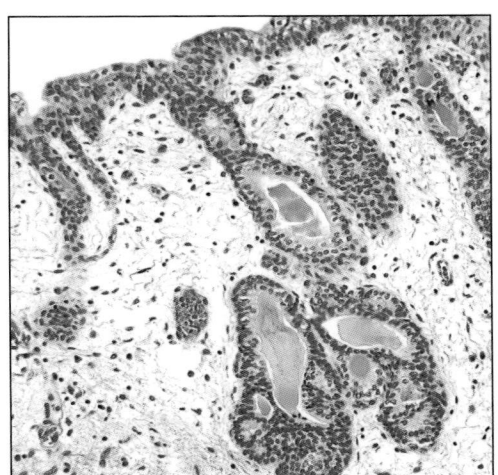

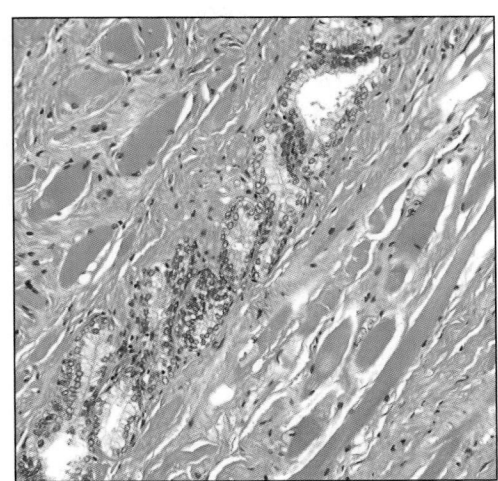

(Left) PU shows surface urothelium and underlying glands forming the PUGR of the prostate in McNeal model. These abortive ducts and acini are lined by urothelium and may give rise to urothelial carcinoma. (Right) This H&E section shows benign glands present in between striated muscle. This may be seen in AFS and apical regions and must not be interpreted as an invasive feature. The presence of glands in striated muscle complicates interpretation of EPE by cancer at these sites.

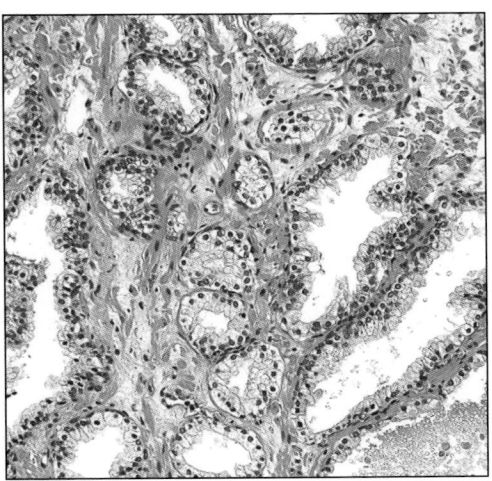

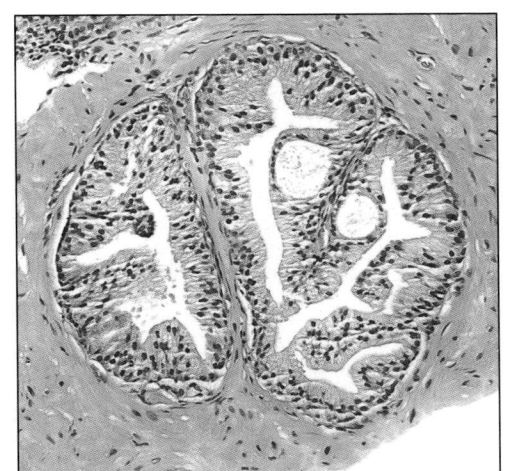

(Left) Normal peripheral zone shows glands that have smaller caliber compared to central zone glands. The stroma is loose and less compact. Most carcinomas of the prostate arise from this zone. (Right) The glands of the central zone are innately larger. There is multilayering, intraluminal ridges, epithelial arches, and papillary infoldings. These features overlap with benign prostatic hyperplasia and high-grade prostatic intraepithelial neoplasia; awareness is important particularly in needle biopsy.

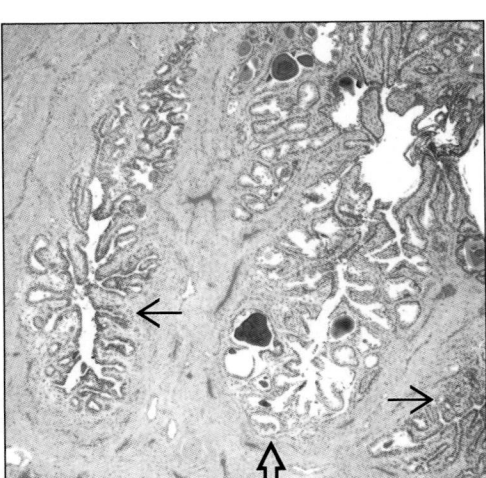

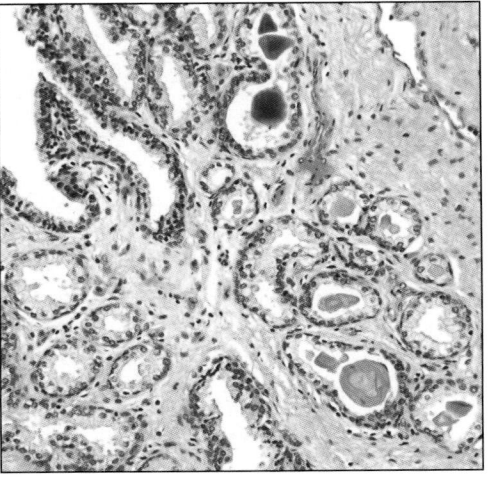

(Left) Low-power view of verumontanum shows the paired EDs ➡ situated lateral to the invagination of the prostatic utricle ⬕. The verumontanum forms an elevation at the PU angulation to the DPU. Verumontanum mucosal glands frequently contain corpora amylacea. (Right) Verumontanum mucosal glands show 2 layers of cells, including distinct basal cells and occasional intraluminal corpora amylacea. Hyperplasia of these glands may mimic prostate carcinoma.

3

MICROANATOMY AND ZONAL VARIATIONS

Microscopic Features

(Left) Perineural glands show intimate association of benign glands to nerve ➡; this feature should not be used as an absolute criterion for malignancy. Circumferential invasion is more diagnostic. *(Right)* The prostate "capsule" is not a true capsule but a condensation of fibromuscular tissue that is an inseparable component of the prostatic stroma. Periprostatic adipose tissues and nerves are present. Involvement of adipose tissue by prostate carcinoma constitutes EPE.

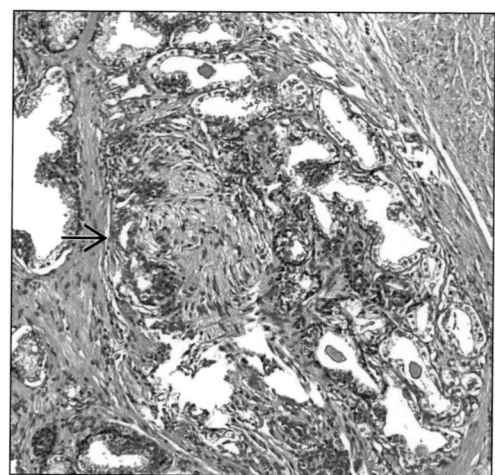
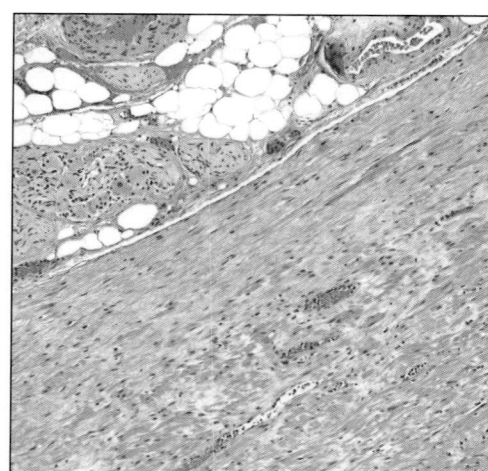

(Left) Cowper glands may occasionally be included in a needle biopsy from the apex. These are tubuloalveolar glands situated within striated muscle. The abundant clear cytoplasm and the crowded lobular architecture of these glands overlap with adenocarcinoma of prostate. *(Right)* Clues to the recognition of Cowper glands include the presence of excretory duct-like structures, as well as glands with abundant, voluminous, and mucinous cytoplasm.

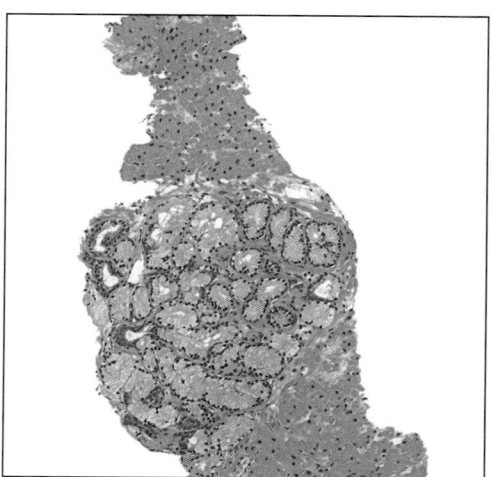
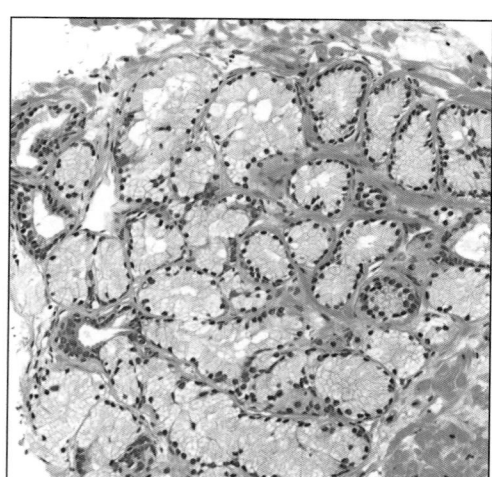

(Left) Low-power view of Cowper glands demonstrates lobular architecture and numerous excretory duct-like structures. The pattern may mimic atrophy and mucinous metaplasia, although this mischaracterization has no clinical relevance. *(Right)* Cowper glands frequently have skeletal muscle at the periphery of the lobular proliferation, which may or may not be sampled. The abundant voluminous cytoplasm may mimic the foamy gland pattern of adenocarcinoma of the prostate.

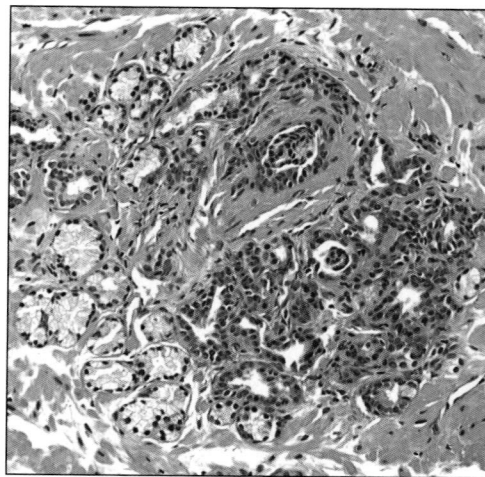
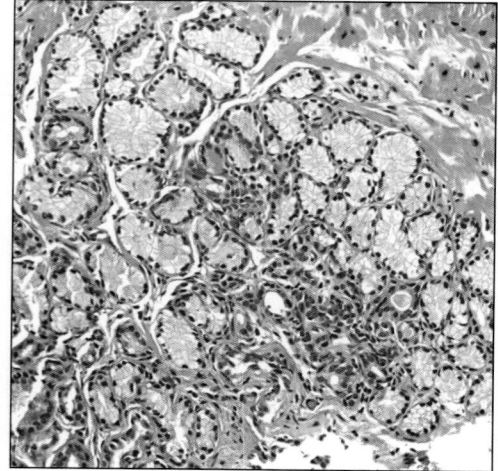

Microscopic Features

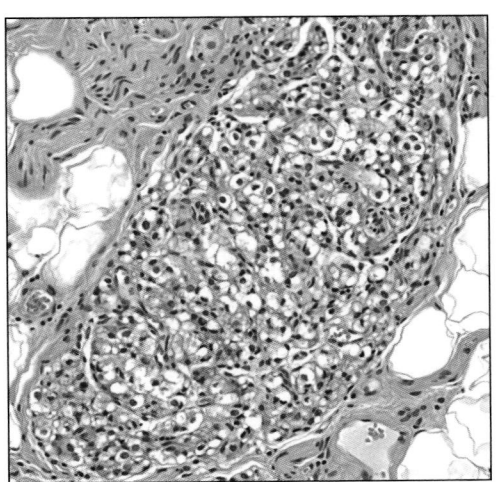
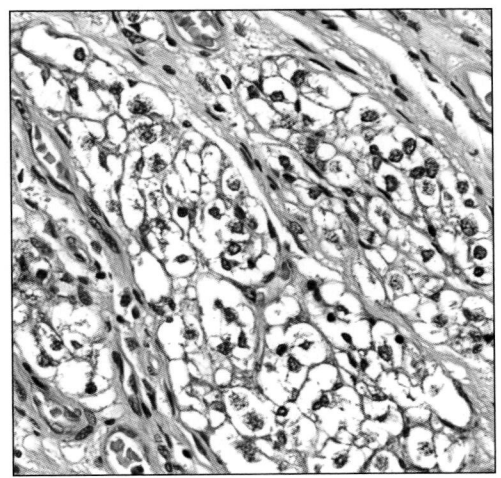

(Left) Paraganglion shows lobular configuration of cells with clear to slightly granular cytoplasm. Location in periprostatic fat, as in this case, and identification of sinusoidal vasculature are useful for accurate recognition. *(Right)* Paraganglia have cells with amphophilic, granular to clear cytoplasm and are associated with a delicate, characteristic vascular pattern. Paraganglia may mimic hypernephroid prostate carcinoma and, if misdiagnosed, may lead to upstaging as EPE.

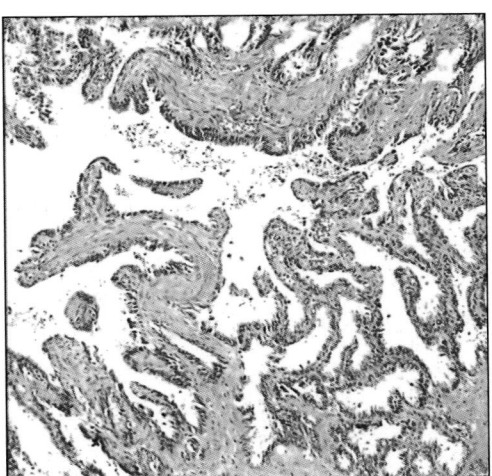
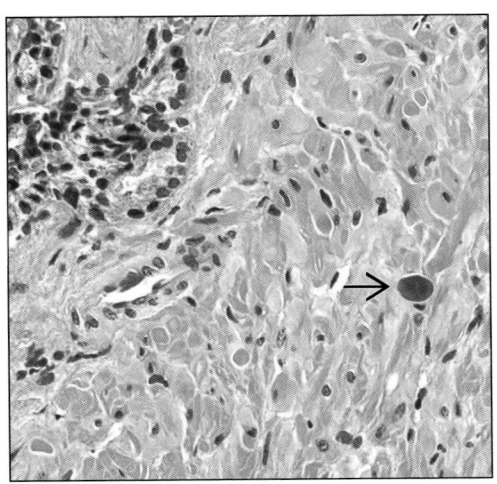

(Left) Seminal vesicles show a central lumen with invaginations and branching of elongated, cleft- and slit-like primary and secondary ducts that extend into a thick muscular coat of 2 cell layers. When the peripheral glands are tangentially sectioned, they may mimic adenocarcinoma of prostate. *(Right)* A hyaline body ➡ within SV wall represents degenerating smooth muscle cell. Involvement of the muscular wall of the SV by carcinoma is required to diagnose SV invasion.

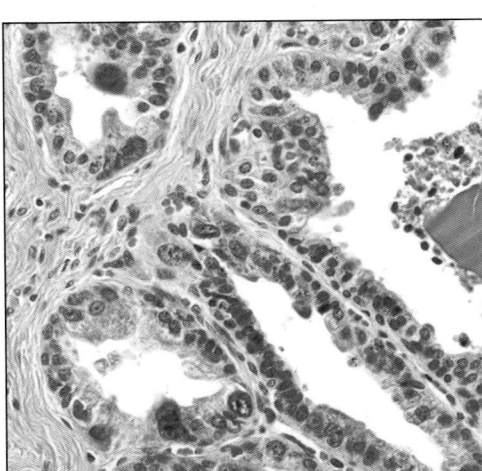
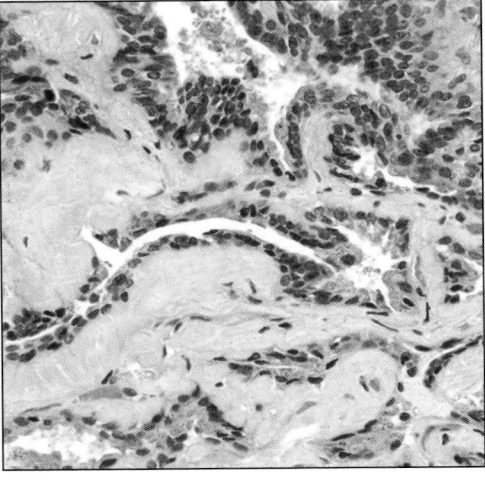

(Left) SV epithelium shows prominent cytoplasmic coarse golden-yellow granules. The epithelium is not uniform and contains random markedly pleomorphic cells containing enlarged hyperchromatic nuclei. Intranuclear inclusions are another hallmark of SV epithelium. *(Right)* Section of SV lumina shows subepithelial amyloid deposits, which may be seen in up to 12% of SV, mostly as an incidental finding. These are localized deposits and not a component of systemic amyloidosis.

PROSTATITIS

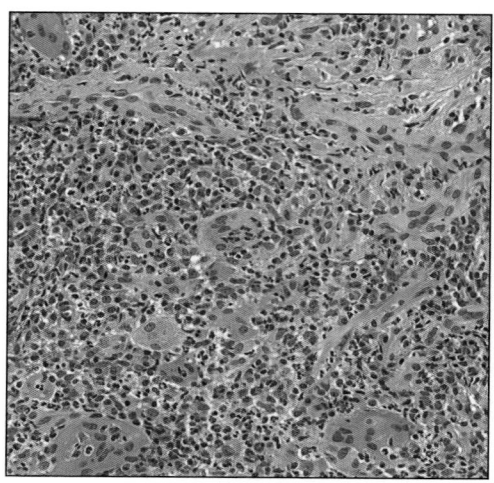

Nonspecific GP shows admixture of multinucleated giant cells, epithelioid histiocytes, lymphocytes, plasma cells, and eosinophils. This is the most common GP.

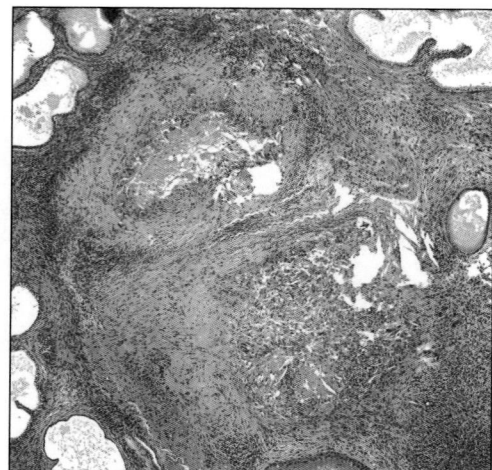

Post-transurethral resection GP shows wedge-shaped granulomas with central fibrinoid necrosis surrounded by palisaded histiocytes. This is the 2nd most common GP.

TERMINOLOGY

Abbreviations
- Granulomatous prostatitis (GP)
- Nonspecific granulomatous prostatitis (NSGP)
- Post-transurethral resection granuloma (PTG)
- Infectious granulomatous prostatitis (IGP)

Definitions
- **GP**
  - Inflammation of prostate containing granulomata
- Types of granulomatous prostatitis
  - Nonspecific granulomatous prostatitis
  - Postprocedural GP
    - Post-transurethral resection GP
    - Post-needle biopsy GP
  - Infectious granulomatous prostatitis
    - Bacillus Calmette-Guérin (BCG)-related granuloma
    - Bacterial, e.g., *Mycobacterium tuberculosis* (most common), *Treponema pallidum*, *Brucella abortus*, *Escherichia coli*
    - Fungal, e.g., *Blastomyces*, *Cryptococcus*
    - Parasitic, e.g., *Schistosoma haematobium*
    - Viral, e.g., herpes zoster
  - Systemic or secondary GP
    - Allergic (eosinophilic) GP
    - Churg-Strauss syndrome
    - Wegener granulomatosis
  - Xanthogranulomatous prostatitis
- **Prostatitis syndrome**
  - Group of inflammatory and noninflammatory conditions of prostate characterized by genitourinary or pelvic pain
    - Defined by International Prostatitis Collaborative Network under the National Institute of Health (NIH)
  - Diagnosis follows clinical, microbiological, and laboratory criteria; histopathologic (i.e., biopsy) diagnosis less crucial or may not be required
  - Histologic changes of prostatic inflammation overlaps among entities of prostatitis syndrome and other causes
- NIH consensus classification of prostatitis syndrome
  - Acute bacterial prostatitis
  - Chronic bacterial prostatitis
  - Chronic prostatitis/chronic pelvic pain syndrome
    - Inflammatory
    - Noninflammatory
  - Asymptomatic inflammatory prostatitis

ETIOLOGY/PATHOGENESIS

Nonspecific Granulomatous Prostatitis
- Inflammatory reaction to altered prostatic acini &/or secretions from duct blockage, bacterial products, or refluxed urine is suggested
- Possibly autoimmune based
  - HLA-DR15-linked T-cell response against proteins in prostatic secretion, principally PSA

Postprocedural Granulomatous Prostatitis
- Inflammatory response to traumatic injury

CLINICAL ISSUES

Epidemiology
- Incidence
  - Granulomatous prostatitis
    - 0.8% of benign prostate specimens
    - 0.36% of prostate needle biopsies
    - Nonspecific GP most common (50-78% of GP)
    - Post-transurethral resection GP (21-24% of GP)
    - Infectious GP (3.5-8% of GP)
    - Systemic GP exceedingly rare
  - BCG-related GP
    - Seen in 1.3% of patients with BCG treatment
    - Intravesical instillation performed 3-55 months (average ~ 1 year) before diagnosis of GP

PROSTATITIS

Key Facts

Terminology
- Granulomatous prostatitis
  - Inflammation of prostate containing granuloma
  - Types: NSGP, postprocedural GP, IGP, systemic GP, xanthogranulomatous prostatitis
- Prostatitis syndrome
  - Group of inflammatory and noninflammatory conditions of prostate characterized by genitourinary or pelvic pain
  - NIH classification: Acute bacterial prostatitis, chronic bacterial prostatitis, chronic prostatitis/chronic pelvic pain syndrome, asymptomatic inflammatory prostatitis

Clinical Issues
- GP seen in 0.8% of benign prostate specimens
  - NSGP most common comprising 50-78% of GP

- Prostatitis syndrome accounts for about 1/4 of male clinic visits with genitourinary complaints

Microscopic Pathology
- NSGP
  - Expansile nodular infiltrates usually involving entire lobules
  - Epithelioid histiocytes, lymphocytes, plasma cells, neutrophils, variable eosinophil infiltrates
- PTG
  - Necrobiotic granulomas or central fibrinoid necrosis surrounded by palisaded histiocytes
- Diagnosis of specific category of prostatitis syndrome requires clinical, microbiologic, and laboratory correlation
  - Acute or chronic inflammation in prostate biopsies should **not** be labeled as "prostatitis"

- Prostatitis syndrome
  - Accounts for about 1/4 of male clinic visits for genitourinary complaints
  - Chronic prostatitis/chronic pelvic pain syndrome most common cause (> 90%)
- Age
  - Granulomatous prostatitis
    - 18-86 years old; mean and median: 62 years
    - 2/3 of patients between 50 and 70 years old

Presentation
- Granulomatous prostatitis
  - Irritative voiding symptoms
    - Urgency, frequency, and dysuria
  - Fever, chills
  - Asymptomatic (11%)
  - Systemic symptoms of allergy in allergic GP
  - Upper and lower respiratory involvement in Wegener granulomatosis
  - May have firm, fixed nodules on digital rectal examination
    - Clinical suspicion of carcinoma in 60% of cases
  - Rare misdiagnosis as prostate cancer in needle biopsy
  - Concomitant prostate carcinoma seen in 10-14% of cases
- Prostatitis syndrome
  - Characterized by genitourinary or pelvic pain
  - Acute bacterial prostatitis presents with symptomatic acute bacterial urinary tract infection
  - Chronic bacterial prostatitis experiences recurrent bacterial urinary tract infection
  - Chronic prostatitis/chronic pelvic pain syndrome clinically identical to chronic bacterial prostatitis but with negative microbiologic study
  - Asymptomatic inflammatory prostatitis diagnosed in patients without genitourinary tract complaints
    - e.g., incidental inflammation encountered in prostate needle biopsy

Laboratory Tests
- Prostate inflammation common cause for serum PSA elevation
- Granulomatous prostatitis
  - Elevated serum PSA level
    - Up to 84% of nonspecific GP
    - Up to 45% of infectious GP
  - Majority of patients have pyuria &/or hematuria
  - May have peripheral blood leukocytosis and eosinophilia
  - Elevated ESR

Treatment
- Granulomatous prostatitis
  - Majority require no treatment
  - Rare prostatectomy to relieve obstructive symptoms in refractory cases
  - Distinction of nonspecific GP from infectious GP and systemic GP important because of different management
    - Antibiotics for infectious GP
    - Chemotherapy and steroids for systemic GP
- Prostatitis syndrome
  - Antimicrobial therapy

Prognosis
- Benign course
- Most symptoms resolve within few months

MACROSCOPIC FEATURES

General Features
- Granulomatous prostatitis
  - Mainly diagnosed in TURP and needle biopsy specimens (94%)
  - May present with firm yellow nodular prostate, with dilated ducts containing inspissated materials

PROSTATITIS

MICROSCOPIC PATHOLOGY

Granulomatous Prostatitis
- Nonspecific GP
  - Expansile nodular infiltrates usually involving entire lobules; discrete granulomas rare
  - Epithelioid histiocytes, lymphocytes, plasma cells, neutrophils, and variable eosinophil infiltrates
  - Well-formed noncaseating granulomas and multinucleated giant cells may rarely be seen
  - Periglandular/periductal pattern of inflammation
  - Dilated and ruptured ducts/acini may be identified
- Post-transurethral resection GP
  - Resembles rheumatoid nodules
  - Necrobiotic granulomas or central fibrinoid necrosis surrounded by palisaded histiocytes
  - Granulomas vary in shape; may be wedge-shaped or long and tortuous
  - Eosinophils may be prominent in early lesions
  - Noncaseating granulomas and multinucleated giant cells frequent in surrounding tissues
  - Multinucleated giant cells may appear to engulf damaged prostatic epithelium
- BCG-related GP
  - Multiple caseating and noncaseating granulomas
  - May be accompanied by extensive necrosis and parenchymal destruction
  - Caseating necrosis more frequent in larger granulomas
  - Acid-fast bacilli demonstrable in up to 38% of cases, seen in areas of caseation
  - Eosinophil infiltrates uncommon
- Allergic GP
  - Necrobiotic granulomas surrounded by palisaded histiocytes containing eosinophil infiltrates
  - Presence of increased eosinophils not specific for allergic GP
- Xanthogranulomatous prostatitis
  - Predominant or pure collections of lipid-laden histiocytes in prostate
  - Histiocytes have abundant xanthomatous cytoplasm and small nuclei with inconspicuous nucleoli
  - Other type of inflammatory cells may be minimal

Prostatitis Syndrome
- When present, inflammation is nongranulomatous
- Acute inflammation of prostate due to acute bacterial prostatitis overlap with those due to noninfectious causes
- Histologic changes of chronic inflammation of prostate similar in
  - Chronic bacterial prostatitis
  - Chronic prostatitis/chronic pelvic pain syndrome inflammatory type
  - Asymptomatic inflammatory prostatitis
- Asymptomatic prostatic inflammation almost universally found in benign prostatic hyperplasia
- Prostate carcinoma and infertility commonly shows prostatic inflammation
- Diagnosis of specific category of prostatitis syndrome requires clinical, microbiological, and laboratory correlation
  - Acute or chronic inflammation encountered in prostate biopsies should **not** be labeled as "acute prostatitis" or "chronic prostatitis"
  - Only descriptive diagnosis should be made for prostate parenchymal inflammation in absence of symptoms related to prostatitis syndrome

DIFFERENTIAL DIAGNOSIS

Prostate Carcinoma
- Prostate carcinoma glands may be mimicked by benign acini with reactive inflammatory atypia
  - Typically lacks background inflammation
  - Contains nucleomegaly, prominent and multiple nucleoli
  - Lacks basal cell layer
- High-grade (Gleason pattern 5 single cell pattern) prostate carcinoma may be mimicked by crushed inflammatory lymphocytic infiltrate
  - PAN-CK(AE1/AE3)(+)
  - CD45(LCA)(-)
- High-grade (Gleason pattern 5 solid pattern) prostate carcinoma may be mimicked by sheets of epithelioid histiocytes
  - PAN-CK(AE1/AE3)(+)
  - CD68(-)
- Hypernephroid prostate carcinoma morphology may be mimicked by xanthogranulomatous prostatitis
  - PAN-CK(AE1/AE3)(+)
  - CD68(-)

Malakoplakia
- Michaelis-Gutman bodies and von Hasseman cells
- Calcium and iron stains may be necessary

DIAGNOSTIC CHECKLIST

Pathologic Interpretation Pearls
- Clinical history important in diagnosis of GP
- Acute or chronic inflammation in prostate biopsies should not be labeled as "prostatitis" since prostatitis syndrome requires clinical diagnostic criteria

SELECTED REFERENCES

1. Uzoh CC et al: Granulomatous prostatitis. BJU Int. 99(3):510-2, 2007
2. Krieger JN et al: NIH consensus definition and classification of prostatitis. JAMA. 282(3):236-7, 1999
3. Matsumoto T et al: Nonspecific granulomatous prostatitis. Urology. 39(5):420-3, 1992
4. Oates RD et al: Granulomatous prostatitis following bacillus Calmette-Guerin immunotherapy of bladder cancer. J Urol. 140(4):751-4, 1988
5. Stillwell TJ et al: The clinical spectrum of granulomatous prostatitis: a report of 200 cases. J Urol. 138(2):320-3, 1987
6. Epstein JI et al: Granulomatous prostatitis: distinction among allergic, nonspecific, and post-transurethral resection lesions. Hum Pathol. 15(9):818-25, 1984

Microscopic Features

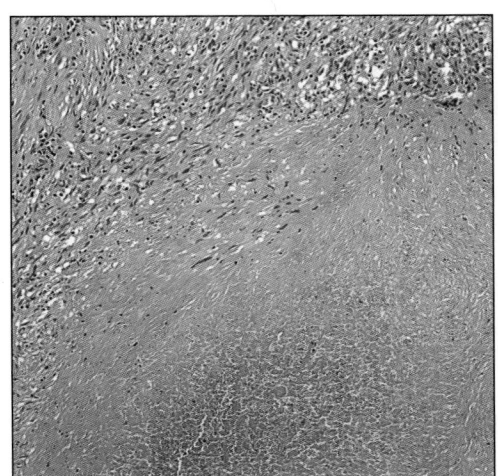
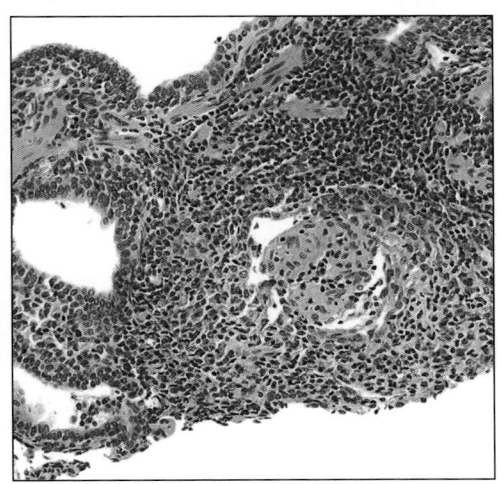

(Left) BCG-related GP shows a large granuloma with central area of caseation. Acid-fast bacilli may be seen in up to 38% of cases. The type of granulomas vary between cases and include epithelioid granulomas without necrosis. *(Right)* Needle biopsy shows GP with a well-formed noncaseating granuloma. Correlation with clinical history is important in the diagnosis and classification of GP. Use of special stains for microorganisms is warranted if infectious GP is suspected.

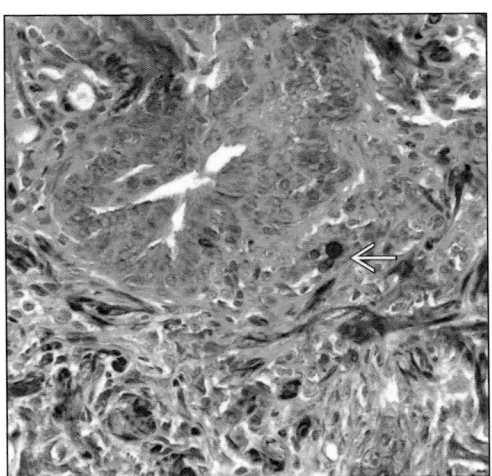
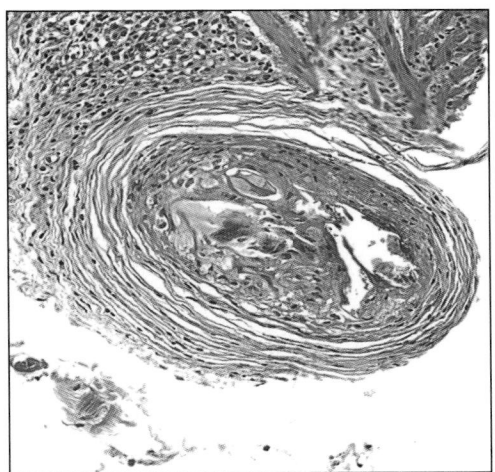

(Left) GMS stain in infectious GP shows budding yeast forms of Blastomyces dermatitidis ➡. IGP may be caused by fungal, bacterial, parasitic, and viral infections. Mycobacterium tuberculosis is the most common etiologic agent for IGP. *(Right)* Prostate needle biopsy shows deposit of Schistosoma ova with associated inflammation. Schistosoma infestation of urinary bladder and association with squamous cell carcinoma is well documented; involvement of prostate is exceedingly rare.

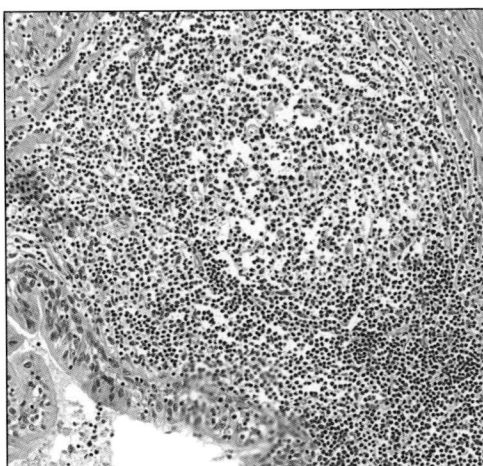
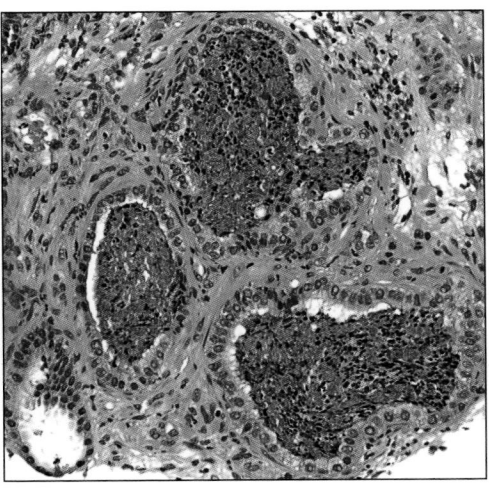

(Left) Periglandular chronic inflammation of the prostate shows reactive germinal center formation. Inflammation in prostate should not be routinely labeled as "prostatitis." Asymptomatic inflammation is common in BPH. *(Right)* Benign acini with acute inflammation shows reactive cytologic atypia, mimicking prostate carcinoma. In contrast to carcinoma, these acini lack multiple nucleoli. Immunohistochemistry may be required in difficult cases. Prominent inflammation may mask a carcinoma.

PROSTATE HYPERPLASIA

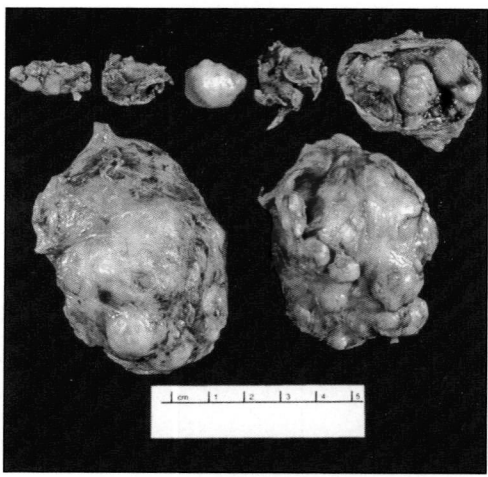

BPH shows marked nodular enlargement and distortion of the prostate. Presence of these hyperplastic nodules is the pathologic hallmark of BPH.

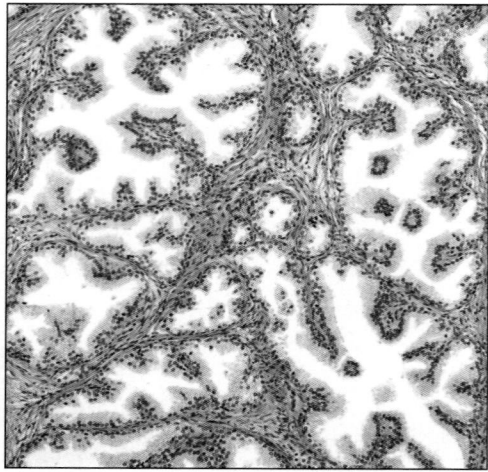

Epithelial predominant hyperplasia is seen composed of tightly clustered medium- to large-sized complex glands.

TERMINOLOGY

Abbreviations
- Benign prostatic hyperplasia (BPH)

Synonyms
- Benign prostatic hypertrophy

Definitions
- Nodular prostate enlargement due to cellular proliferation of prostatic glands and stroma associated with lower urinary tract symptoms (LUTS)

ETIOLOGY/PATHOGENESIS

Origin
- Prostatic glandular hyperplasia
  - Acinar cells and basal cells
- Prostatic stromal hyperplasia
  - Undifferentiated mesenchyme, fibroblasts, and smooth muscle cells
  - Epithelial-mesenchymal transition recently proposed

Etiology
- Pathophysiology remains poorly understood
- Hormonal alteration plays a central role
  - Cellular accumulation of testosterone, particularly active metabolite dihydrotestosterone (DHT)
  - Role of estrogen suggested
- Known risk factors include aging and family history
- No association with tobacco use, weight, sexual libido, diabetes mellitus, hypertension, or cirrhosis

CLINICAL ISSUES

Epidemiology
- Incidence
  - 1 of leading causes of morbidity in elderly men

- Age
  - Increasing incidence with age, particularly in men > 50 years of age
    - Seen in 50% of men in 50s and up to 80-90% of men in 70s and 80s
    - In contrast, seen in only 8% of men in 40s and rarely in younger men

Site
- Mainly in tissues surrounding proximal prostatic urethra
  - Transition zone, submucosal compartment, specialized mesenchyme of preprostatic sphincter
  - Also known as "estrogen sensitive zone"
- Peripheral zone uncommonly involved, reported in 2-15% of prostatectomies

Presentation
- LUTS
  - Obstructive symptoms, such as hesitancy, straining, weak flow, prolonged voiding, retention, and overflow incontinence
  - Irritative symptoms, such as frequency, urgency, nocturia, painful urination, and dribbling
- Digital rectal palpation of enlarged, nodular, often symmetric and rubbery prostate
- No correlation between histology and symptoms
  - Only 50% with histologic disease have clinical prostate enlargement; 50% of these have symptoms
  - Without associated LUTS, features of glandular and stromal proliferation in needle biopsies should **not** be labeled as BPH

Laboratory Tests
- Most common noncancerous cause of serum PSA elevation

Treatment
- Medical therapy is most frequently used approach
  - α-adrenergic blockers or 5-α-reductase inhibitors
- Surgery is more effective in terms of controlling LUTS

PROSTATE HYPERPLASIA

Key Facts

Terminology

- Nodular prostate enlargement due to cellular proliferation of prostatic glands and stroma associated with lower urinary tract symptoms (LUTS)

Clinical Issues

- 1 of leading causes of morbidity in elderly men
- Seen in 50% of men in 50s, up to 80-90% of men in 70s and 80s
- Most common noncancerous cause of serum PSA elevation
- Medical therapy is most frequently used approach
- Surgery is more effective in terms of controlling LUTS
- Without associated LUTS, features of glandular and stromal proliferation in needle biopsies should **not** be labeled as BPH

Macroscopic Features

- Hallmark of BPH is nodular prostatic enlargement
- Hyperplastic nodules are mainly centered on proximal prostatic urethra involving transition zone and submucosal compartment

Microscopic Pathology

- Epithelial predominant hyperplasia shows nodules composed of tightly clustered expanded ductal acinar elements
- Stromal predominant hyperplasia composed of bland spindle cells with little cytoplasm and plump nuclei seen surrounding small blood vessels
- Morphologic variants: Small glandular, cribriform, basal cell, leiomyomatous nodule, and phyllodes-type hyperplasias

---

- o Transurethral resection of prostate (TURP) is standard surgical procedure
- o Open (simple) prostatectomy for very bulky prostate

Prognosis

- Benign course

IMAGE FINDINGS

General Features

- Computed tomography, ultrasound, and magnetic resonance imaging can visualize BPH
- Evidence of urinary retention, dilated bladder, hydroureter, or hydronephrosis in advanced cases

MACROSCOPIC FEATURES

General Features

- Nodular prostatic enlargement is the hallmark of BPH
- Hyperplastic nodules identifiable in prostatic chips or more readily in prostatectomy specimens
  - o Vary from millimeters to large bulging masses; sometimes prostate can be massively enlarged
  - o Typically firm white-tan but can be spongy due to cystically dilated glands
- Hyperplastic nodules are mainly centered on proximal prostatic urethra involving submucosal compartment and transition zone
- Hyperplastic transition zone compresses peripheral zone, which can be markedly attenuated or atrophic
- Uncommon peripheral zone hyperplasia more often presents as solitary hyperplastic nodule

Sections to Be Submitted

- TURP specimen
  - o For 12 g or less, submit entirely (usually 6-8 cassettes)
  - o For > 12 g, submit initial 12 g plus 1 cassette for every additional 5 g

MICROSCOPIC PATHOLOGY

Histologic Features

- **Epithelial predominant hyperplasia**
  - o Proliferative nodules composed of tightly clustered expanded ductal acinar elements
  - o Glands are medium to large or sometimes cystically enlarged
  - o Enlarged glands usually show architectural complexity and papillary infoldings
  - o Distinct acinar and basal cell layers present
  - o Acinar cells are usually columnar or cuboidal to flat when cystic
  - o Cytoplasm is abundant and pale
  - o Nuclei are regular with open chromatin
- **Stromal predominant hyperplasia**
  - o Early stromal nodule seen around urethral submucosal connective tissue
  - o Bland spindle cells with little cytoplasm and plump nuclei containing open chromatin
  - o Contains abundant small capillaries and spindle cells typically condensed around these vessels
  - o Occasionally can be very cellular with dense collagen around small capillaries
  - o Increasing smooth muscle component with increasing nodule size
- **Mixed epithelial and stromal hyperplasia**
  - o Both glandular and stromal proliferations substantially present
- **Special morphologic variants**
  - o Can be seen within the overall spectrum of BPH
- **Small glandular hyperplasia**
  - o Composed of proliferation of relatively small glands in fibromuscular stroma
  - o Acinar cells are more cuboidal, and basal cells are more prominent than in usual hyperplasia
- **Cribriform hyperplasia**
  - o Unique form of nodular hyperplasia wherein glandular component is composed of medium to large glands with cribriform architecture

PROSTATE HYPERPLASIA

- May have clear cytoplasm ("clear cell cribriform hyperplasia")
- **Basal cell hyperplasia**
  - Usually seen, but not exclusively, in cases of BPH
  - Can also be seen associated with glandular atrophy, typically involving peripheral zone, in setting of androgen ablation therapy
  - Proliferation can be "incomplete" preserving acinar cells or "complete" imparting solid nests
  - May have cribriform architecture (adenoid cystic-like hyperplasia)
  - May undergo squamous metaplasia
  - May show nuclear atypia (atypical basal cell hyperplasia)
  - Basal cell markers (p63 or HMCK(34βE12)) helpful in diagnosis of challenging cases
- **Leiomyomatous nodule**
  - Stromal predominant hyperplasia with prominent smooth muscle component
  - Unlike leiomyoma, usually small (< 1 cm), blends into surrounding stroma, contains fibroblastic component, and is sometimes multinodular
- **Fibroadenoma-like hyperplasia**
  - Glandular and stromal proliferations are architecturally arranged to mimic fibroadenoma of breast
- **Phyllodes-type hyperplasia**
  - Stromal predominant proliferation with cleft-like spaces and intramural stromal projections covered peripherally by glandular epithelium
  - In contrast to phyllodes-like tumor of prostate, is focal, lacks significant atypia, and seen in background of BPH

Predominant Pattern/Injury Type
- Hyperplasia

Predominant Cell/Compartment Type
- Epithelial, glandular
- Mesenchymal, spindle

ANCILLARY TESTS

Immunohistochemistry
- Reactivity similar to normal benign glands
- Not routinely needed for diagnosis
- Acinar cells
  - Positive for PSA and PAP
  - Underexpresses AMACR but may be weakly positive
  - Negative for p63 or HMCK(34βE12)
- Basal cells
  - Negative for PSA, PAP, or AMACR
  - Positive for p63 or HMCK(34βE12)

DIFFERENTIAL DIAGNOSIS

Atypical Adenomatous Hyperplasia (AAH)
- Differential diagnosis for small glandular hyperplasia in limited sample, such as needle biopsy
- No associated stromal proliferation

- Contains less uniform glands with presence of "parent duct"

Specialized Stromal Tumors of Prostate
- **Stromal tumors of uncertain malignant potential (STUMP)**
  - Diagnosis may be made when sampling is limited
  - Hypercellular stroma that often shows degenerate-type nuclear atypia
  - Can be admixed with benign glands, with myxoid change, or with phyllodes-type pattern
  - Lacks typical intermixed small blood vessels; may lack multinodularity of BPH
- **Stromal sarcoma**
  - Shows greater degree of cellularity, significant atypia, increased mitosis, and presence of necrosis

Smooth Muscle Tumors
- Differential diagnosis for hyperplastic leiomyomatous nodule
- Leiomyoma is more cellular, lacks stromal vessels, and occurs without background BPH
- Leiomyosarcoma contains significant cytologic atypia that is often high grade with increased mitotic activity, and shows coagulative necrosis

Solitary Fibrous Tumor of Prostate
- Uniform bland spindle cells with haphazard patternless pattern, dense ropey collagen, more variable cellularity, and staghorn vessels
- Borderline and malignant cases with increasing cellularity, mitotic activity, presence of necrosis, and infiltrative growth
- Positive for CD34, bcl-2, and CD99

DIAGNOSTIC CHECKLIST

Pathologic Interpretation Pearls
- Diagnosis of BPH is made when histologic glandular and stromal proliferation is associated with prostatic nodular enlargement accompanied by LUTS

SELECTED REFERENCES

1. Viglione MP et al: Should the diagnosis of benign prostatic hyperplasia be made on prostate needle biopsy?. Hum Pathol. 33(8):796-800, 2002
2. Van de Voorde WM et al: Peripherally localized benign hyperplastic nodules of the prostate. Mod Pathol. 8(1):46-50, 1995
3. Ayala AG et al: Clear cell cribriform hyperplasia of prostate. Report of 10 cases. Am J Surg Pathol. 10(10):665-71, 1986
4. Berry SJ et al: The development of human benign prostatic hyperplasia with age. J Urol. 132(3):474-9, 1984
5. Cleary KR et al: Basal cell hyperplasia of the prostate. Am J Clin Pathol. 80(6):850-4, 1983
6. Kafandaris PM et al: Fibroadenoma-like foci in human prostatic nodular hyperplasia. Prostate. 4(1):33-6, 1983
7. McNeal JE: Origin and evolution of benign prostatic enlargement. Invest Urol. 15(4):340-5, 1978
8. Attah EB et al: Phyllodes type of atypical prostatic hyperplasia. J Urol. 115(6):762-4, 1976
9. Pradhan BK et al: Morphogenesis of nodular hyperplasia--prostate. J Urol. 113(2):210-3, 1975

Gross, Diagrammatic, and Microscopic Features

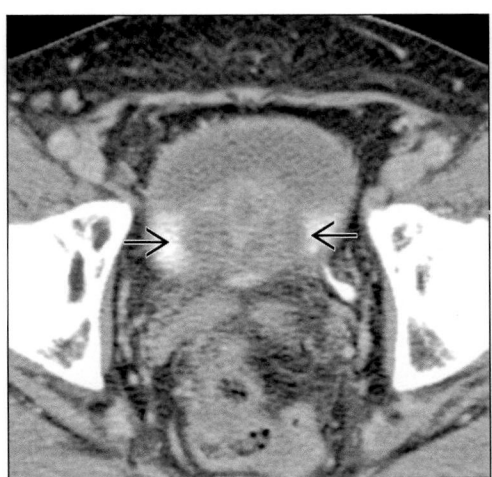

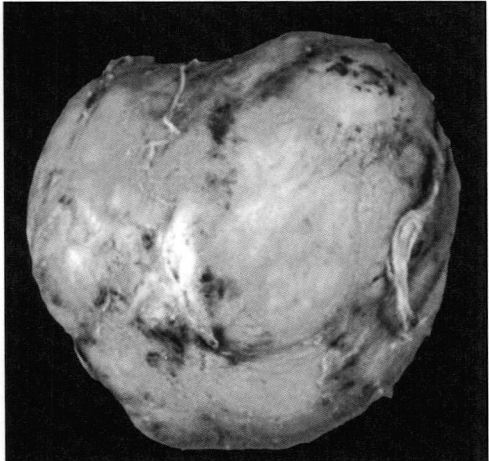

(Left) Axial CECT shows BPH. Note medial lobe hypertrophy of prostate pressing on the base of the bladder ➡. Advanced BPH may show evidence of urinary retention and dilated bladder. Pathologic diagnosis of BPH, particularly in limited samples, requires clinical correlation and must be reserved in absence of LUTS. *(Right)* BPH shows an asymmetrically enlarged prostate due to bulging hyperplastic nodules as seen from external surface. The prostate can be massively enlarged in BPH.

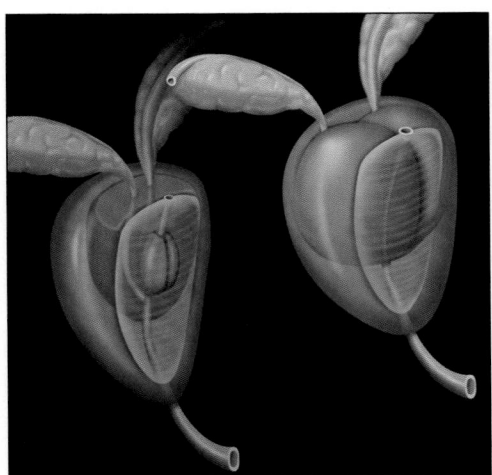

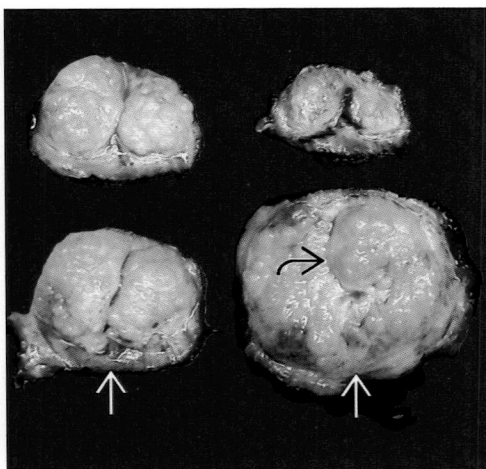

(Left) This drawing compares normal prostate (left) and BPH (right), which shows enlargement of prostatic transition zone (blue). BPH mainly involves transition zone and submucosal compartment around proximal prostatic urethra. *(Right)* Cross section of BPH shows markedly enlarged transition zone compressing the prostatic urethra ➡. Peripheral zone ➡ is compressed and attenuated by the hyperplastic transition zone, causing secondary diffuse atrophy.

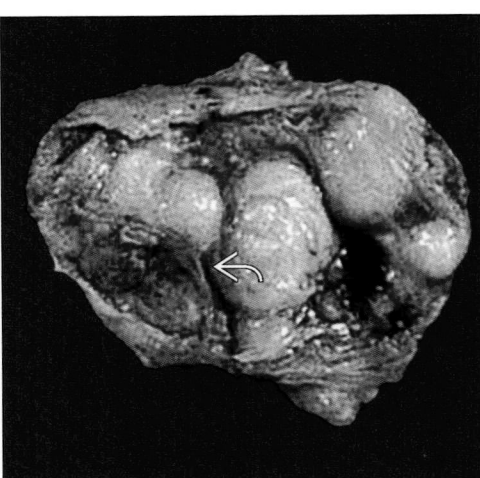

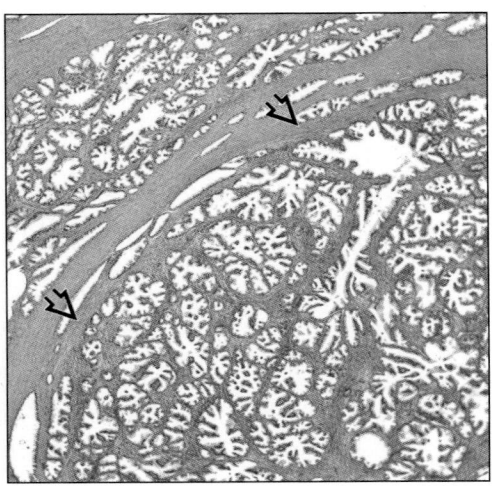

(Left) Cross section of prostate with BPH shows multiple bulging hyperplastic nodules in transition zone compressing prostatic urethra ➡. BPH commonly presents with multiple macro- and microscopic hyperplastic nodules that vary in size. Uncommon peripheral zone hyperplasia more often presents with solitary nodule. *(Right)* Epithelial predominant hyperplastic nodule ➡ shows well-circumscribed expansile cluster of medium to large complex glands.

Microscopic Features

(Left) Hyperplastic gland typically shows papillary infoldings imparting inverted image of luminal branchings. Stroma follows contour of hyperplastic glands. **(Right)** BPH gland shows columnar cells containing abundant pale to clear cytoplasm and round nuclei with open chromatin. Architecture mimics normal central zone glands and high-grade prostatic intraepithelial neoplasia (HGPIN) glands. In contrast, central zone glands are less crowded and HGPIN contains severe nuclear atypia.

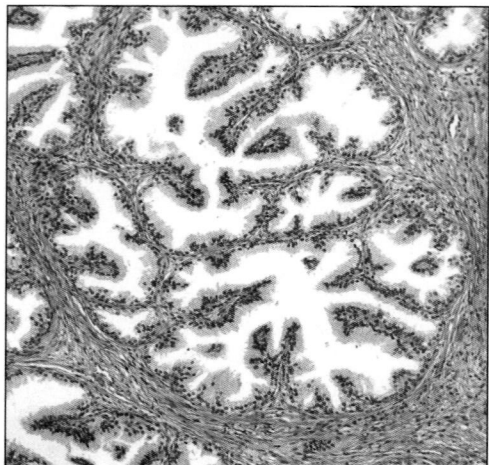 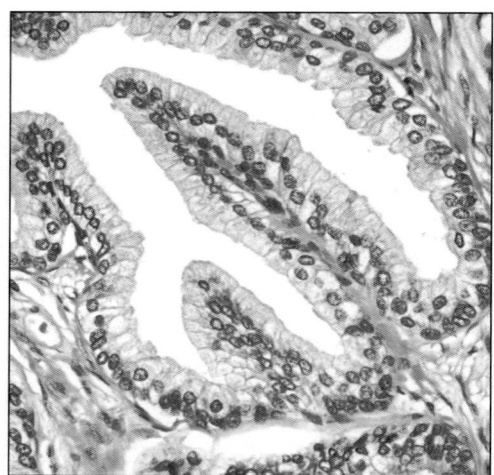

(Left) Stromal predominant hyperplasia shows sheets of spindle cells typically containing abundant capillaries dispersed throughout the stroma. **(Right)** Stromal predominant hyperplasia shows bland spindle cells often condensed around small blood vessels. These small blood vessels are not typically seen in STUMP, a main differential diagnosis. In contrast to BPH, STUMP is often solitary and involves both peripheral and transition zones.

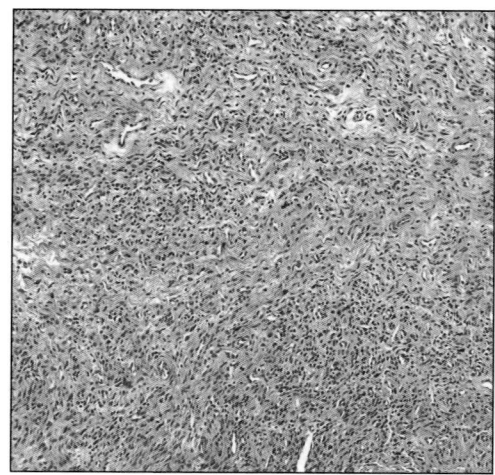 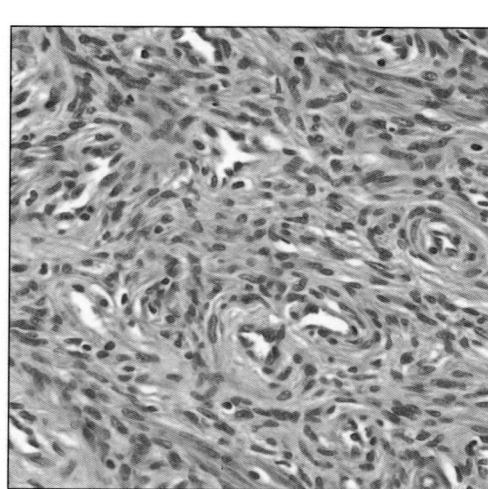

(Left) An "early" stromal nodule ⇨ is seen in submucosal compartment of proximal urethra ⇨ adjoining the transition zone ⇨. This area of the prostate is also known as "estrogen sensitive zone." **(Right)** A large stromal nodule is shown adjacent to prostatic urethra. BPH nodules are believed to begin as pure stromal nodule and later acquire epithelial component with growth. Proximity of proximal prostatic urethra results in obstruction and LUTS with nodule enlargement.

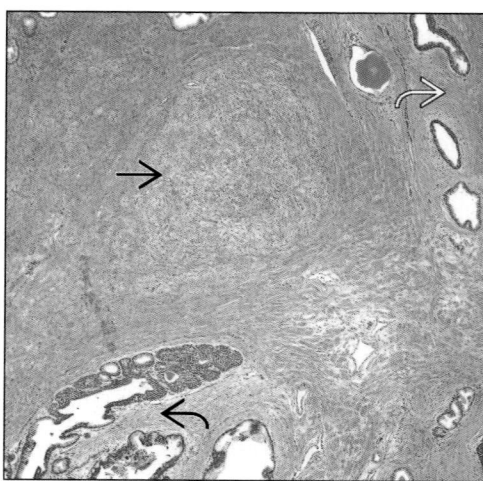 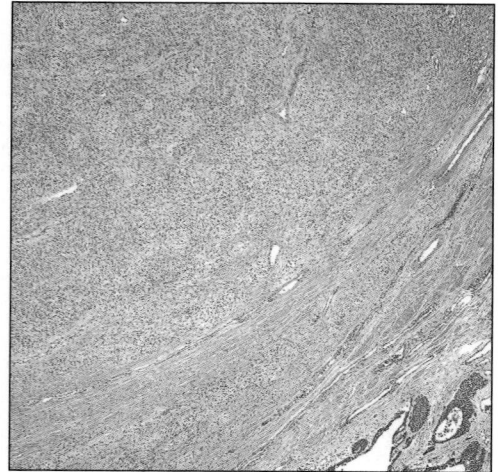

Microscopic Features

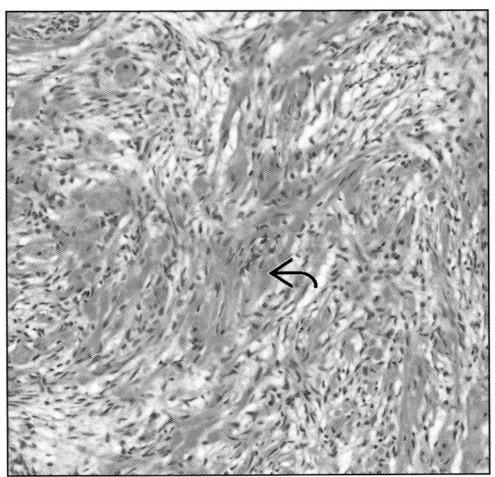

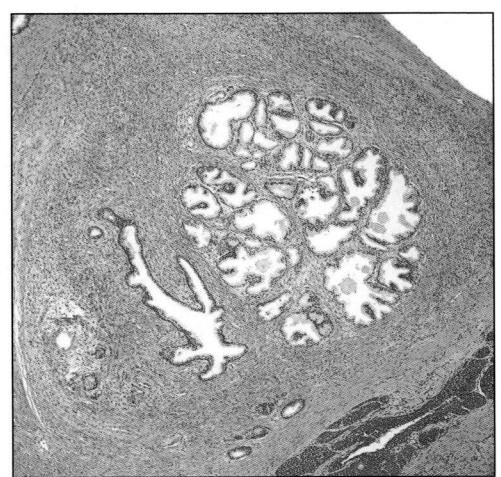

(Left) Stromal predominant hyperplastic nodule shows myoid component ➡ admixed with stromal elements. Myoid component usually becomes much more prominent with increasing size of the hyperplastic nodule. Occasionally, myoid component may become abundant imparting myomatous appearance. *(Right)* Hyperplastic nodule with substantial proliferation of both stromal and glandular elements is seen adjacent to prostatic urethra.

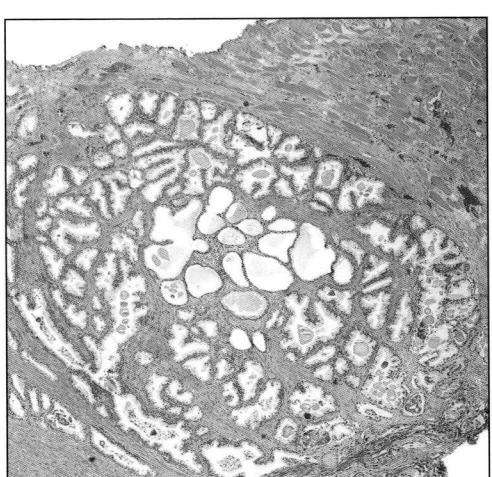

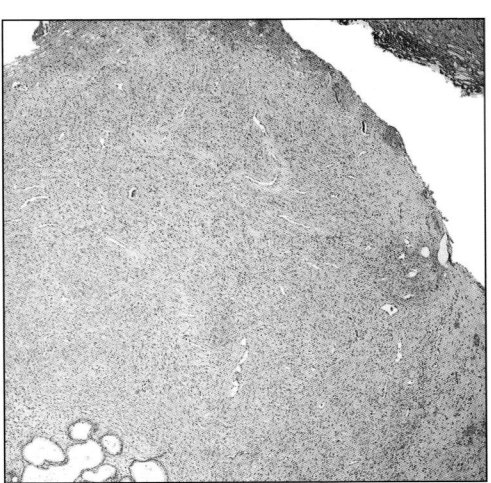

(Left) TURP chip shows an epithelial predominant hyperplastic nodule. *(Right)* TURP chip shows a stomal predominant hyperplastic nodule. In limited samples, pathologic diagnosis of BPH requires clinical evidence of LUTS. Unlike in needle biopsy containing epithelial &/or stromal proliferation, pathologic diagnosis of BPH is readily rendered in TURP specimens since TURP is performed as therapeutic procedure for clinically diagnosed BPH.

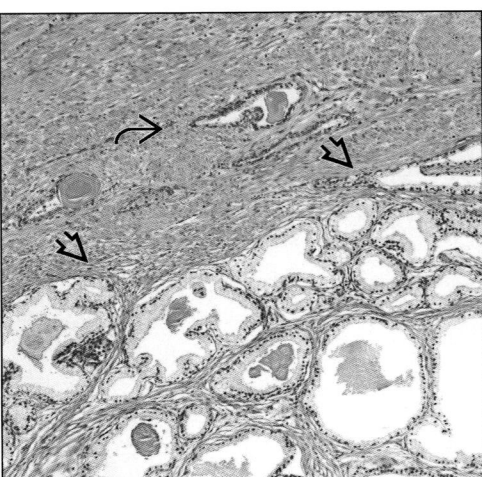

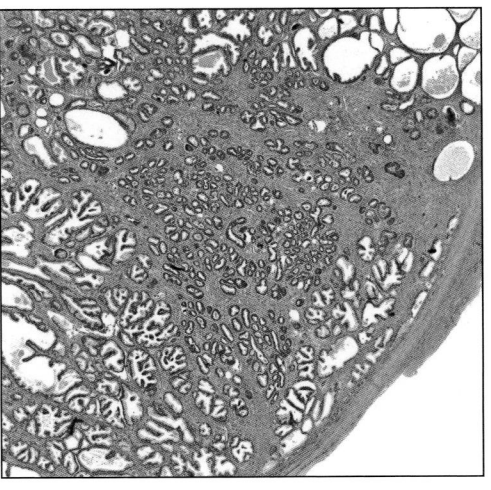

(Left) BPH nodule arising from transition zone ⊡ shows compression with secondary atrophy of surrounding peripheral zone ➡. *(Right)* Small glandular hyperplasia shows well-defined proliferation of relatively small-sized glands adjacent to usual epithelial predominant hyperplasia. Small glandular hyperplasia may mimic AAH. In contrast, AAH has no associated stromal proliferation, contains "parent duct," and occurs without background BPH.

PROSTATE HYPERPLASIA

Microscopic Features

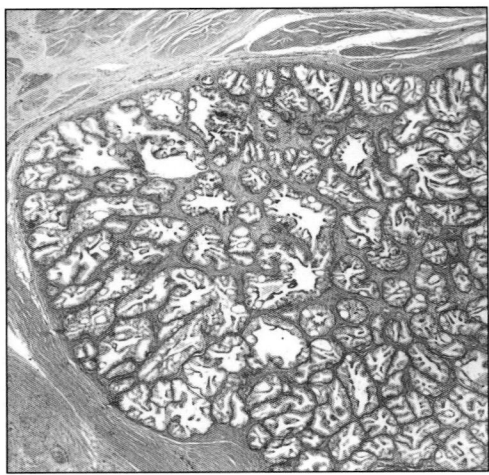 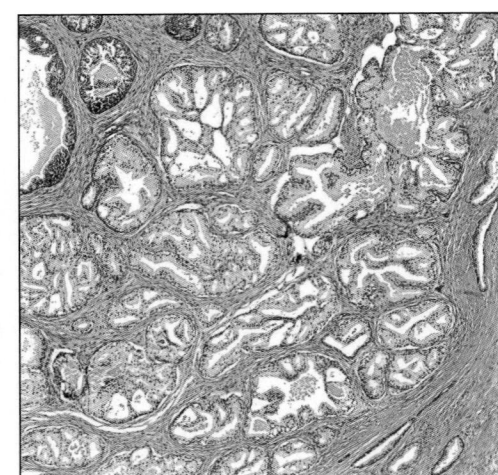

(Left) Cribriform hyperplasia shows a dense nodular cluster of complex glands showing cribriform architecture. *(Right)* Cribriform hyperplasia composed of large glands shows distinctive cribriform or "Roman bridging" architecture. The glandular complexity may mimic cribriform acinar adenocarcinoma, ductal carcinoma, and HGPIN. In contrast, cribriform hyperplasia lacks cytologic atypia or other features associated with malignant glands.

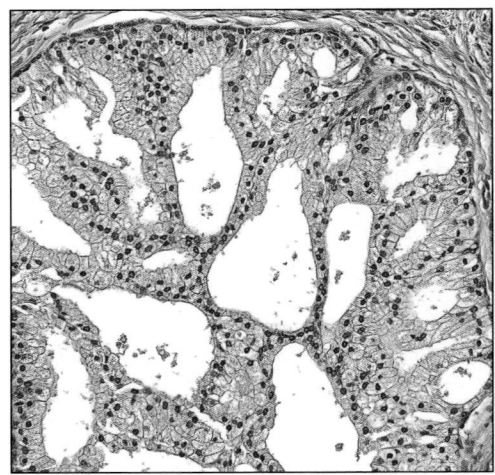 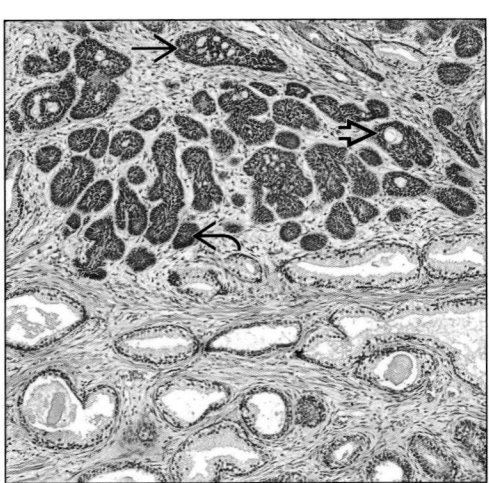

(Left) Cribriform hyperplasia gland shows bland acinar cells with abundant pale to clear cytoplasm and round regular nuclei lacking atypia. Presence of pale cytoplasm is often distinctive ("clear cell cribriform hyperplasia"). *(Right)* Basal cell hyperplasia can be seen uncommonly within spectrum of BPH. Basal cell proliferation is either "complete" ➡, imparting solid nests, or "incomplete" ➡, retaining lumen. Rarely, cribriform pattern ➡ may be seen ("adenoid cystic-like hyperplasia").

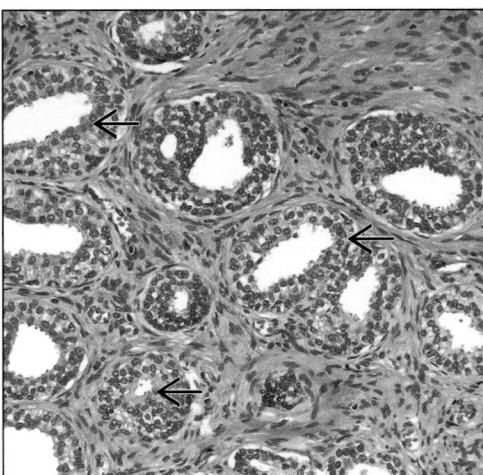 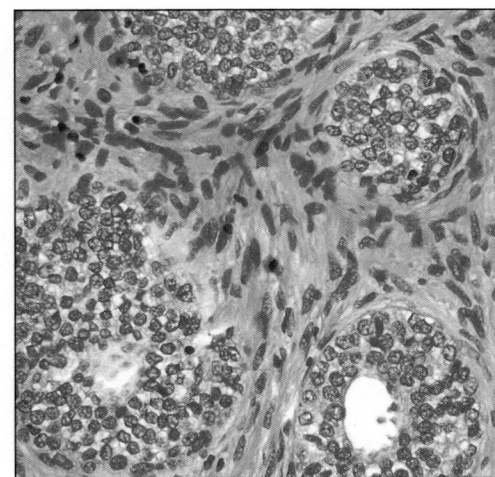

(Left) Incomplete basal cell hyperplasia shows preservation of glandular lumen lined by acinar cells ➡ and surrounded by hyperplastic basal cells. *(Right)* Basal cell hyperplasia shows proliferation of basaloid cells with high nuclear to cytoplasmic ratio. Basal cell hyperplasia when exuberant may mimic basal cell carcinoma (BCC). In contrast to BCC, basal cell hyperplasia exhibits contained growth and lacks invasive features.

3

Microscopic Features

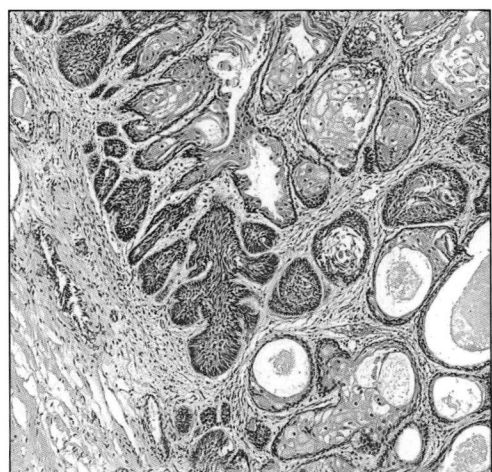

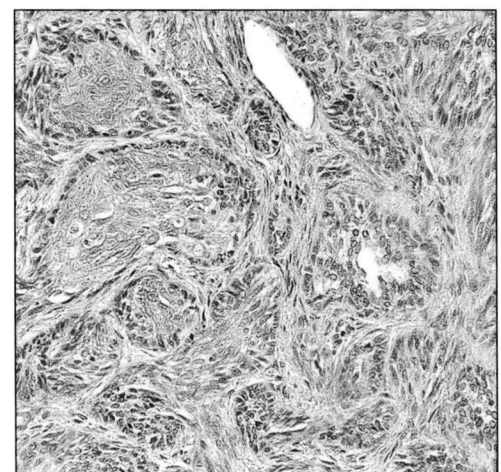

(Left) Basal cell hyperplasia with squamous metaplasia shows some nests containing squamous cells with abundant glassy cytoplasm surrounded peripherally by basal cells. Some cellular nests contain central lumen. (Right) Basal cell hyperplasia with squamous metaplasia shows transition of centrally placed squamous cells and peripherally situated basal cells. Squamous cells lack cytologic atypia or mitosis. Squamous cell metaplasia arises from the proliferative basal cells.

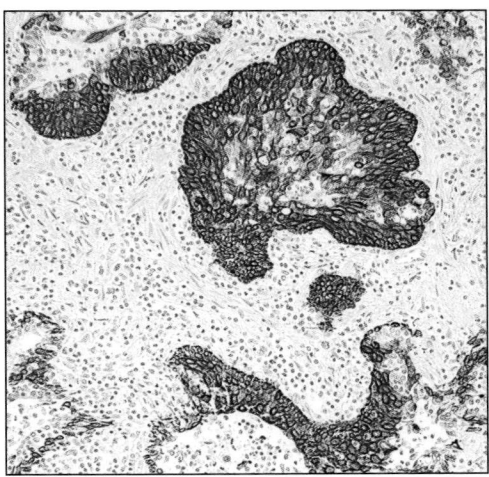

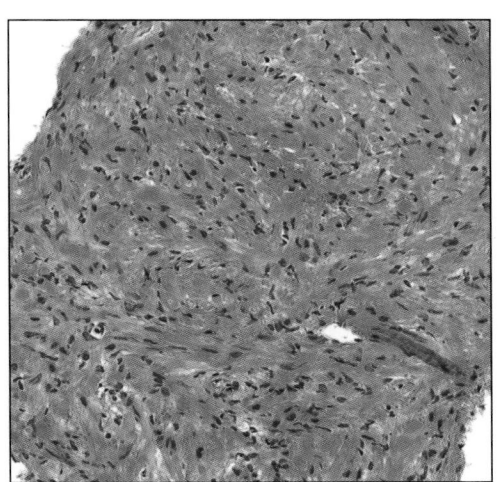

(Left) Basal cell hyperplasia shows basal cells diffusely positive for HMCK(34βE12). Central acinar cells are negative. (Right) Leiomyomatous hyperplasia in prostate biopsy shows prominent myoid elements admixed with stromal cells. Distinction from benign smooth muscle tumor can be difficult. Leiomyomatous hyperplasia is less cellular, may contain abundant small stromal vessels, and may have background typical stromal &/or epithelial hyperplasia.

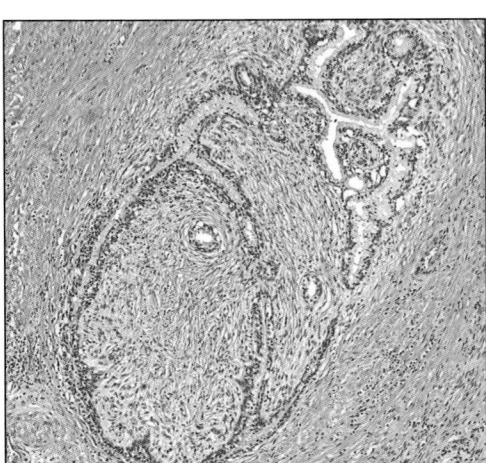

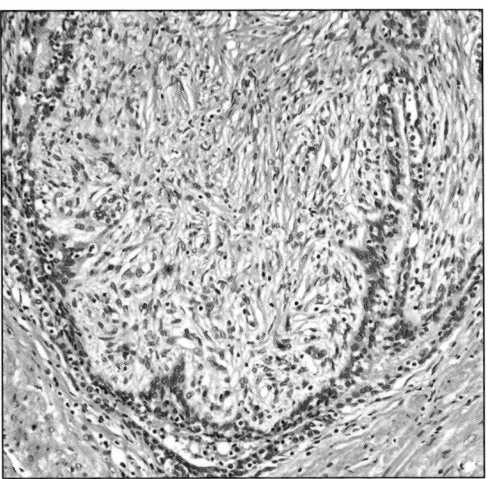

(Left) Fibroadenoma-like hyperplasia shows stromal proliferation surrounding compressed hyperplastic acini, which morphologically mimics mammary fibroadenoma. (Right) Fibroadenoma-like hyperplasia shows proliferation of bland spindle and epithelial cells. This process is typically focal and seen in background of BPH.

3

ATROPHY AND ITS VARIANTS

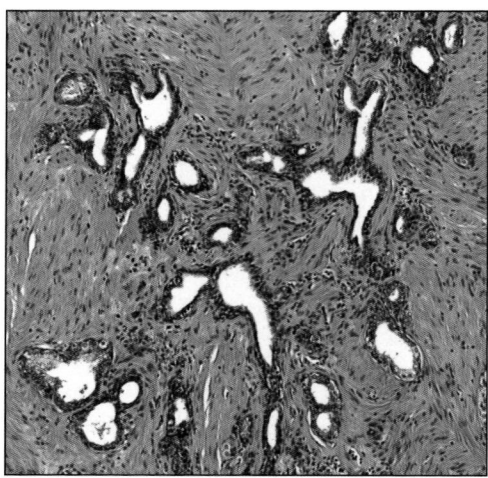

Cluster of atrophic acini composed of attenuated irregular glands is seen with scant amount of cytoplasm, which imparts a more basophilic appearance to the acini.

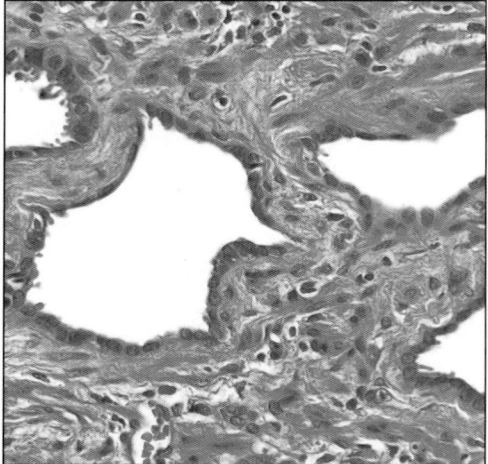

The atrophic glands are typically irregular and are lined by cuboidal to flattened cells with high nuclear to cytoplasmic ratio.

TERMINOLOGY

Abbreviations
- Simple atrophy (SA)
- Postatrophic hyperplasia (PAH)
- Partial atrophy (PA)

Definitions
- Cellular shrinkage with loss of cytoplasmic volume of prostatic ductal acinar unit and surrounding stroma

ETIOLOGY/PATHOGENESIS

Causes
- Diffuse atrophy linked to aging, androgen deprivation, and radiotherapy
- Secondary compression by benign prostate hyperplasia (BPH) nodule, e.g., peripheral zone atrophy in BPH of transition zone
- End result of severe chronic inflammation ("postinflammatory atrophy")
- Chronic local ischemia suggested

CLINICAL ISSUES

Epidemiology
- Incidence
  - Very common
  - Seen in 85% of prostates in autopsies of men > 40 years of age
- Age
  - Frequency increases with age; more common after 6th decade of life

Site
- Commonly involves peripheral zone and, less frequently, central and transition zones

Presentation
- Asymptomatic; incidental histologic finding
- Remarkable in routine practice as morphologic mimicker of adenocarcinoma in prostate biopsy

Treatment
- None

Prognosis
- Benign course
- Possible but very weak current evidence for atrophy as a neoplastic precursor, suggested in post-inflammatory atrophy with high proliferation index ("proliferative inflammatory atrophy")

MICROSCOPIC PATHOLOGY

Histologic Features
- All patterns of atrophy are characterized by acinar cells with scant cytoplasm imparting higher nuclear to cytoplasmic ratio
- Maintains overall lobular configuration with angular or slit-like glands, occasionally with parent duct
- Glands contain crowded and hyperchromatic nuclei, imparting a more basophilic appearance
- Since secretory cells have minimal to no cytoplasm, they resemble basal cells and impart a "single cell type" appearance
- Glands may very rarely contain intraluminal mucin and crystalloids
- Surrounding stroma with a variable amount of fibrosis
- Chronic inflammation may be seen in association with atrophic acini

Predominant Pattern/Injury Type
- Atrophy

Predominant Cell/Compartment Type
- Epithelial, glandular

ATROPHY AND ITS VARIANTS

Key Facts

Terminology
- Cellular shrinkage with loss of cytoplasmic volume of prostatic ductal acinar unit and surrounding stroma

Clinical Issues
- Frequency increases with age; more common after 6th decade of life
- Remarkable in routine practice as morphologic mimicker of adenocarcinoma in prostate biopsy

Microscopic Pathology
- Most commonly involves the peripheral zone
- All patterns of atrophy are characterized by acinar cells with scant cytoplasm producing higher nuclear to cytoplasmic ratio
- Glands contain crowded and hyperchromatic nuclei, imparting a more basophilic appearance

- Atrophy can be diffuse or widespread; linked to aging, androgen deprivation, and radiotherapy
- Main morphologic types of focal atrophy include simple atrophy, simple atrophy with cyst formation, postatrophic hyperplasia, and partial atrophy
- Simple atrophy consists of atrophic acini that are spaced relatively similar to normal glands
- Simple atrophy with cyst formation shows large dilatations of atrophic acini
- Postatrophic hyperplasia consists of proliferative atrophic acini arranged in lobules often surrounding central larger dilated duct
- Unlike other forms of atrophy, partial atrophy contains relatively modest amount of pale or clear cytoplasm and has less crowded nuclei

Diffuse Atrophy
- Widespread atrophy, which shows uniform involvement of all glands
- Basal cells are relatively prominent

Focal Atrophy
- Localized or patchy atrophy of the glands

Morphologic Types of Focal Atrophy
- Proposed by the Working Group Classification of Focal Atrophy of the Prostate in 2006 as SA, SA with cyst formation, PAH, and PA
  - Interobserver reproducibility is less than optimal; no clinical significance of subtyping atrophy at this time
- Admixture of these patterns is commonly seen
- **Simple atrophy (SA)**
  - Atrophic acini are spaced relatively similar to normal glands
  - Glands are about normal in caliber but can be larger and are often irregular in shape
- **SA with cyst formation**
  - SA associated with large dilatations of atrophic acini
  - Dilated glands closely apposed with little amount of intervening stroma and show rounded configuration
- **Postatrophic hyperplasia (PAH)**
  - Atrophic acini arranged in lobules often surrounding central larger dilated duct
  - Acini can be oval, slit-like, or stellate-shaped
  - Nuclei typically bland but can occasionally be enlarged with distinct nucleoli
  - Admixed with variable amount of hyperplastic acini containing clear or pale cytoplasm
- **Partial atrophy (PA)**
  - Unlike other forms of atrophy, has relatively modest amount of pale to clear cytoplasm and less crowded nuclei
  - Acini are small to medium-sized and round or undulating in contour
  - Nucleoli are occasionally moderately enlarged
- **Sclerotic atrophy**
  - Atrophy containing dense fibrotic stroma

  - Atrophic glands are more angulated or irregular

ANCILLARY TESTS

Immunohistochemistry
- Positive for basal cell markers (p63 or HMCK[34βE12])
  - Rare glands within PAH focus may be completely negative (23%)
  - PA shows patchy staining in 73-87% and completely absent staining in 6%
- Underexpress or negative for AMACR
  - 10% of PA show stronger staining than benign glands
  - 24% of PA show combination of AMACR positivity and basal cell marker negativity

DIFFERENTIAL DIAGNOSIS

Acinar Adenocarcinoma
- Malignant acini are relatively smaller, more rigid, or less irregular in contour
- Shows nucleomegaly and presence of prominent &/or multiple nucleoli; most helpful particularly if appreciated in several cells
- Glands may contain blue mucin and crystalloids
- Completely negative for basal cell markers
- Strong circumferential staining with AMACR

Prostate Adenocarcinoma with Atrophic Features
- Carcinoma that is architecturally similar in appearance to atrophic benign glands
- Retains cytologic and other features of adenocarcinoma, and is occasionally admixed with more typical carcinoma histology

SELECTED REFERENCES
1. De Marzo AM et al: A working group classification of focal prostate atrophy lesions. Am J Surg Pathol. 30(10):1281-91, 2006

ATROPHY AND ITS VARIANTS

Microscopic Features

(Left) SA shows normal-spaced atrophic acini lined by cuboidal to flattened cells. Like in most forms of atrophy, the nuclei are bland and appear crowded from the loss of cytoplasmic volume. Nuclear atypia, (seen in adenocarcinoma) such as nucleomegaly, prominent nucleoli, multiple nucleoli, and brisk mitosis, are not seen in atrophic glands. *(Right)* SA shows nuclear crowding from loss of cytoplasmic volume. Unlike adenocarcinoma, these atrophic glands are more irregular and angulated.

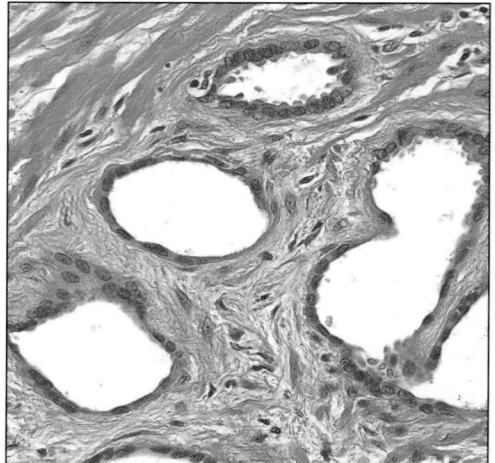 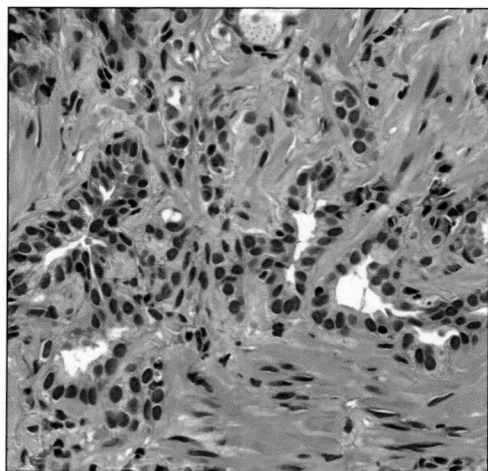

(Left) SA with cyst formation shows cluster of cystically dilated glands, which exhibit nodular configuration. There is relatively less stroma in between the clusters of atrophic acini. In comparison, some relatively normal-sized glands are seen on the right lower side of the image. *(Right)* Higher power magnification of the same SA with cyst formation to the left shows dilated glands that are mostly lined by flattened glandular cells.

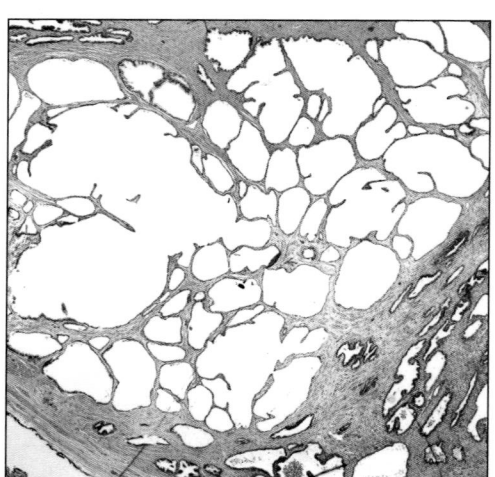 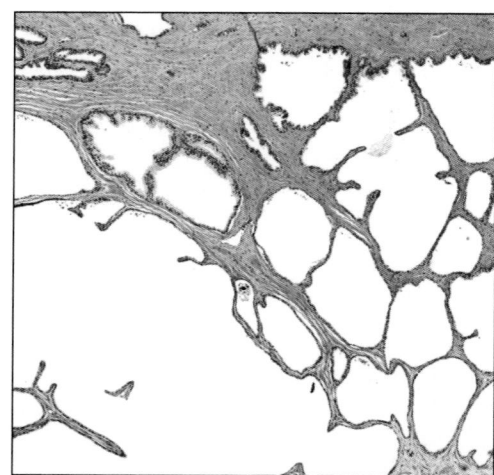

(Left) SA with cyst formation is lined by flattened to cuboidal cells. Like in most forms of atrophy, the nuclei are relatively crowded and do not show atypicality. *(Right)* PAH consists of centrally located dilated atrophic ducts surrounded by benign proliferative atrophic acini ➡. PAH, particularly in limited sample such as biopsy, is one of the many mimics of prostate adenocarcinoma. Contrast the PAH atrophic lobules to the adjacent nonatrophic benign glands ➡.

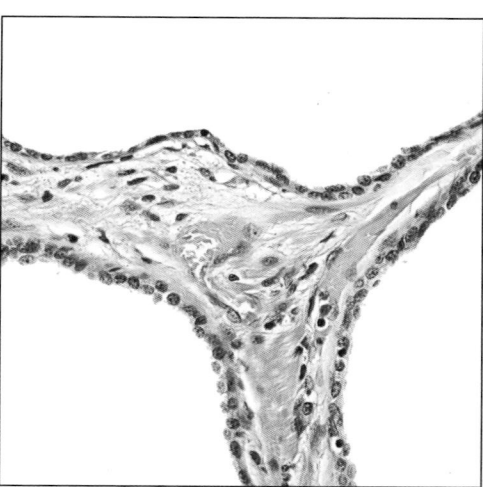 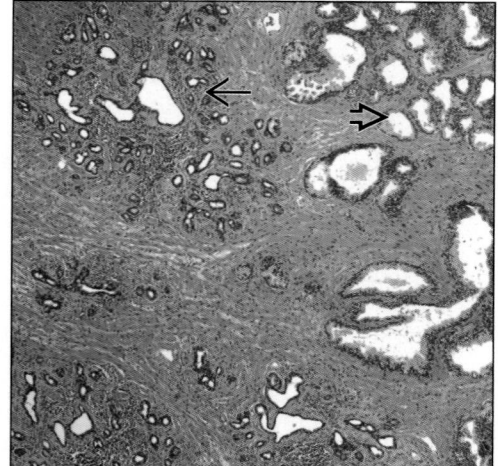

ATROPHY AND ITS VARIANTS

Microscopic Features

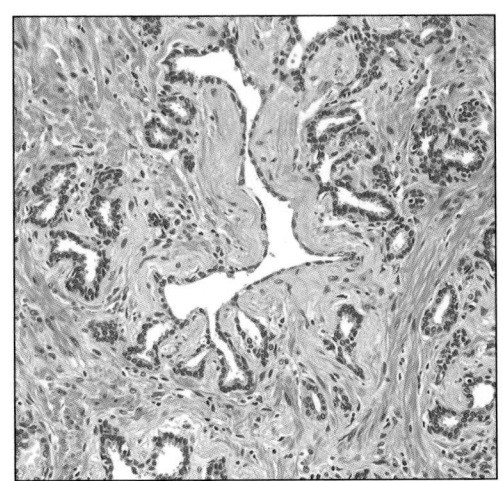

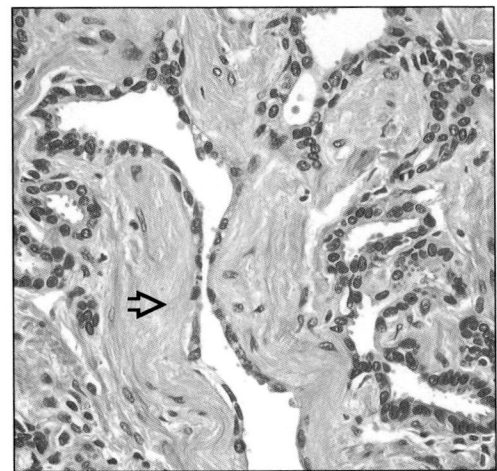

(Left) PAH shows a lobular configuration of atrophic acini surrounding a larger central atrophic duct. These smaller glands, particularly if the lesion is not appreciated in its entirety, may mimic prostate adenocarcinoma. *(Right)* High-power magnification of the same PAH to the left shows the duct and acini are lined by cuboidal to flattened cells with nuclear crowding. Note the presence of sclerotic stroma within the atrophic lobule ➡.

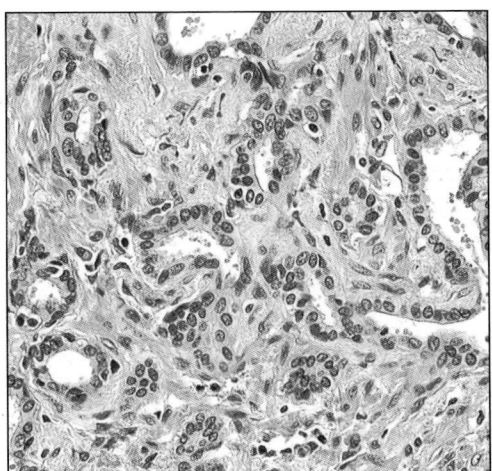

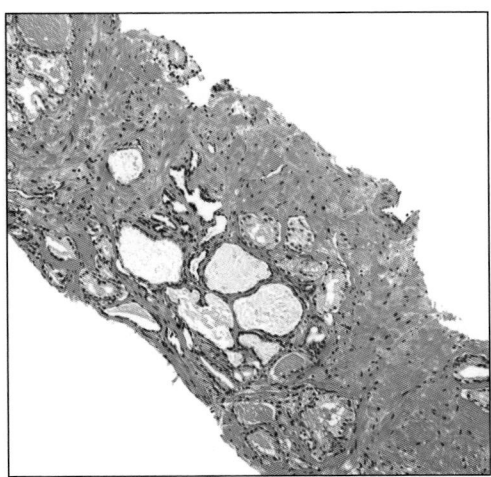

(Left) PAH. In contrast to adenocarcinoma, these atrophic acini are more irregular and lack nuclear atypia, such as nucleomegaly and prominent nucleoli. *(Right)* PAH encountered in needle biopsy is shown. PAH is 1 of the main differential diagnoses for atypical small acinar proliferation (ASAP) in needle biopsy. Diagnosis is relatively less challenging if the entire architecture is appreciated, as in this case.

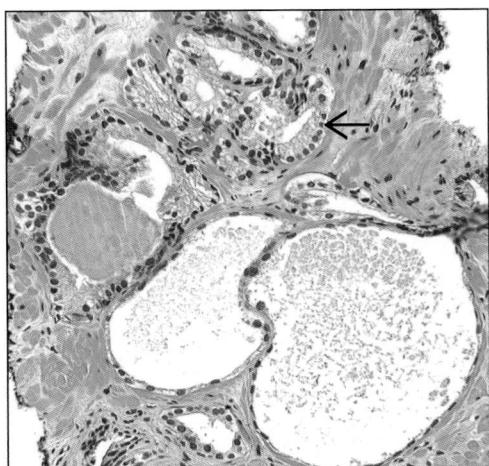

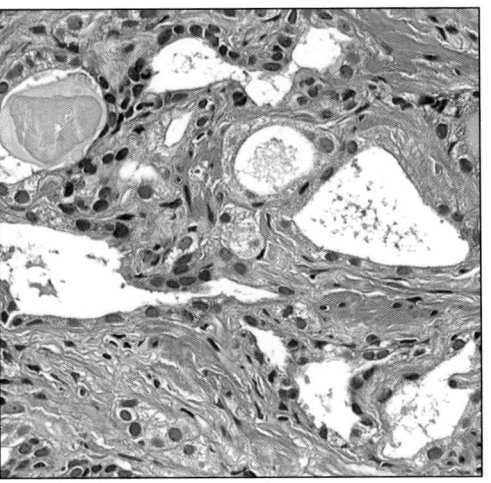

(Left) PAH in needle biopsy is seen. Sometimes admixed with the atrophic acini are hyperplastic acini with relatively abundant pale to clear cytoplasm and less crowded nuclei ➡. *(Right)* The nuclei of PAH typically have inconspicuous nucleoli; however, they may occasionally be prominent. In challenging cases, use of immunohistochemical stains, particularly basal cell markers, can be helpful in establishing definitive diagnosis of PAH.

ATROPHY AND ITS VARIANTS

Microscopic Features

(Left) PA, in contrast to other forms of atrophy, shows a relatively ample amount of pale to clear cytoplasm and less crowded nuclei. *(Right)* PA consists of small to medium-sized glands with pale to clear cytoplasm. In contrast to adenocarcinoma, these glands are more irregular and lack nuclear features of malignancy. However, nucleoli can occasionally be moderately enlarged in PA compounding distinction from carcinoma. Use of immunohistochemical stains is helpful in challenging cases.

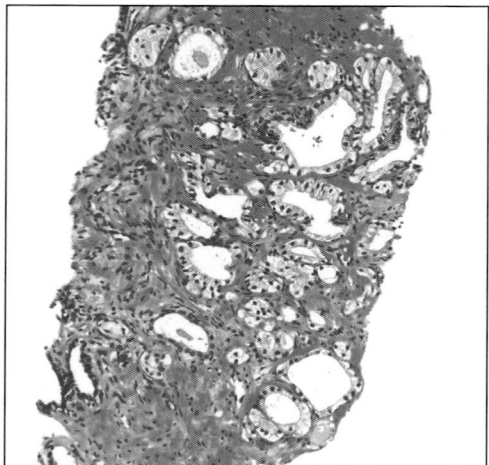
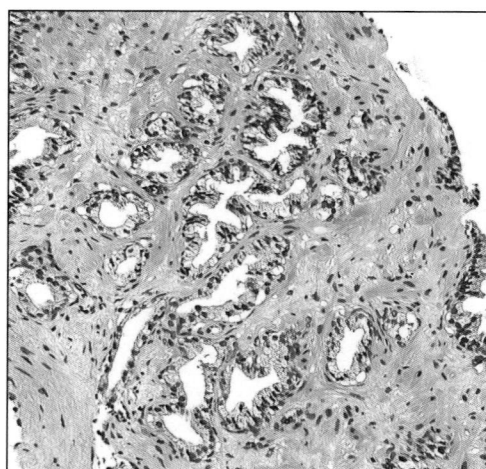

(Left) Sclerotic atrophy shows dense fibrotic stroma surrounding angulated atrophic glands. The atrophic glands show typical features of atrophy, including irregularity in contour or angulation, basophilia, nuclear crowding, and bland nuclei. *(Right)* Diffuse atrophy shows widespread cell shrinkage of all glands. This type of atrophy is linked to aging, androgen deprivation, and radiotherapy, or can be secondary to compression by a BPH nodule.

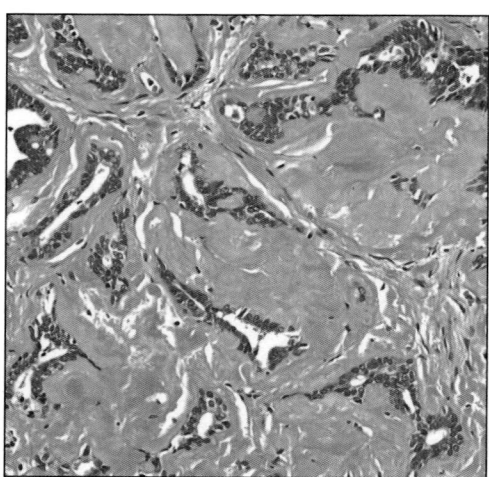
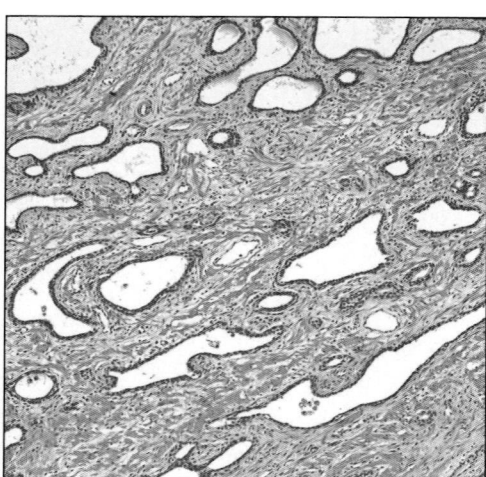

(Left) Diffuse glandular atrophy secondary to androgen ablation therapy for adenocarcinoma is shown. Few residual treated adenocarcinoma glands are present ➡, which are markedly shrunken as a result of hormonal deprivation. Diffuse atrophy should alert for possible prior hormone ablation and careful search for treated cancer. *(Right)* In contrast to focal atrophy, the acini in diffuse atrophy have a relatively distinct basal layer ➡, and 2 cellular layers are often discernible.

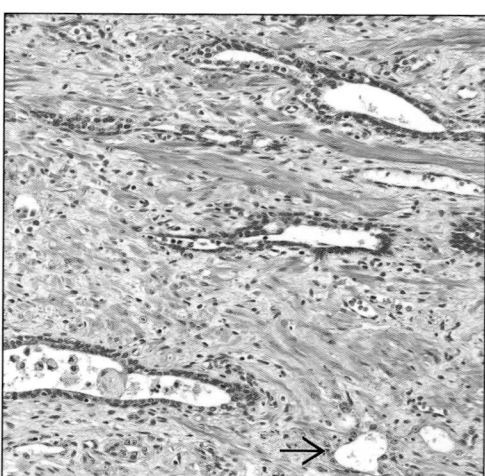
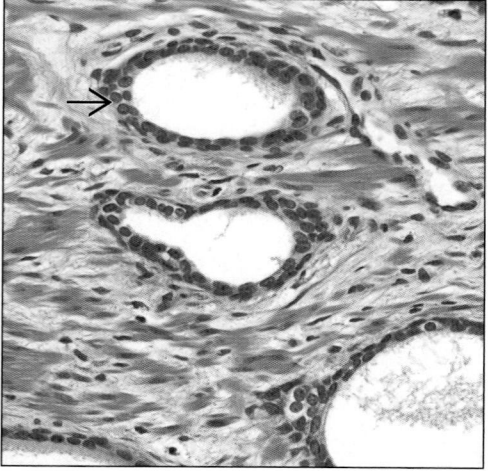

3

ATROPHY AND ITS VARIANTS

Microscopic and Immunohistochemical Features

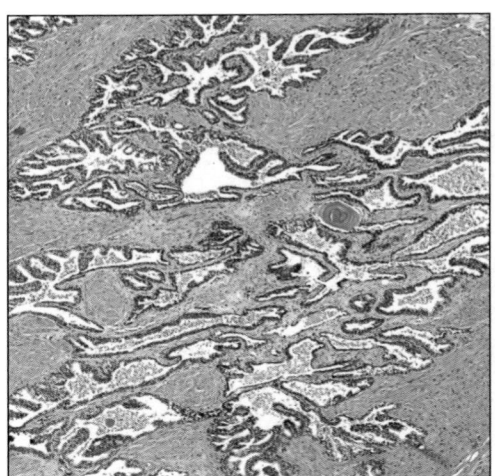
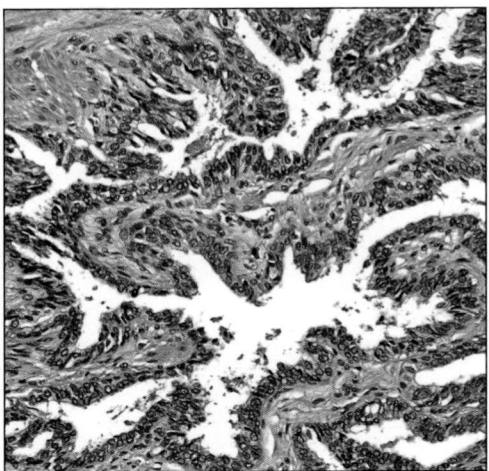

(Left) Diffuse atrophy involving the prostate central zone shows involvement of all central zone glands. *(Right)* High-power view of the same central zone atrophy to the left shows large glands with loss of cytoplasmic volume and nuclear crowding. These atrophic glands maintain their overall architectural complexity typical for glands from this zone.

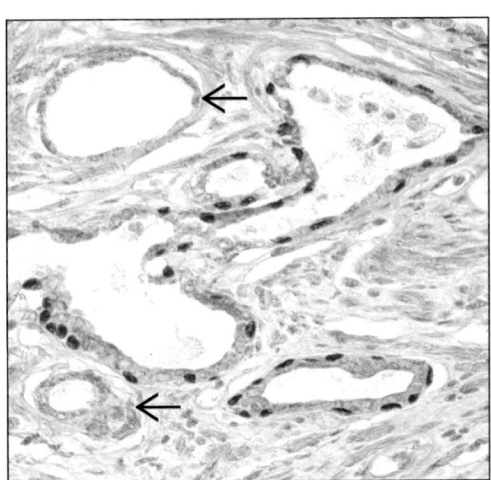
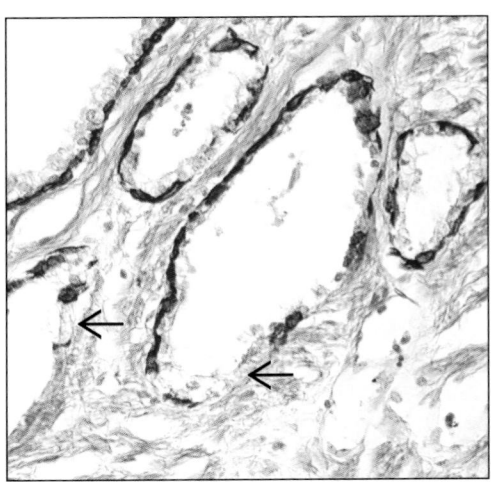

(Left) Basal cells within the atrophic benign acini exhibit nuclear p63 positivity. Note few benign glands within the atrophic focus are completely negative with p63 ⇒. *(Right)* HMCK immunostain highlights the basal cells within these atrophic benign glands. Note the patchy discontinuous (+) staining in portions of the glands ⇒. In contrast, adenocarcinoma (not shown) demonstrates complete lack of basal cell staining in all the atypical acini within a suspicious focus.

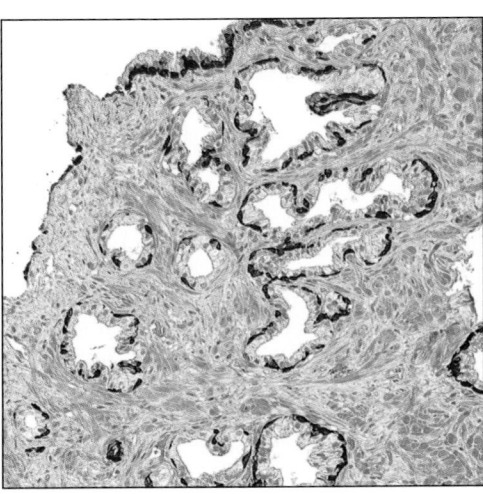
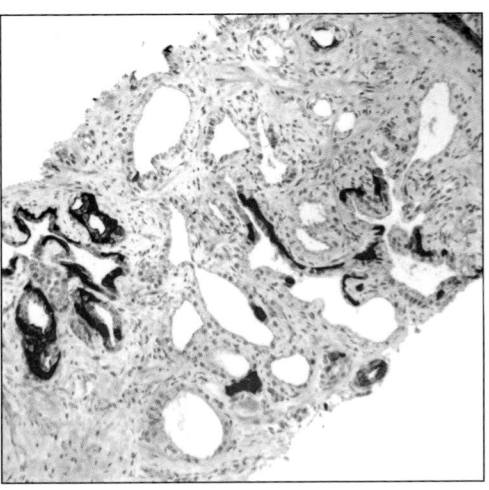

(Left) PA commonly shows patchy (+) staining with basal cell markers (p63 and HMCK[34βE12]). *(Right)* PAH shows patchy to absent basal cell markers (brown) and weak AMACR (red) staining in the benign glands. Unlike PAH or PA, prostate adenocarcinoma (not shown) shows uniformly absent basal cell markers staining in all glands within the suspicious focus and has more intense and circumferential staining for AMACR.

HYPERPLASIA OF MESONEPHRIC REMNANTS

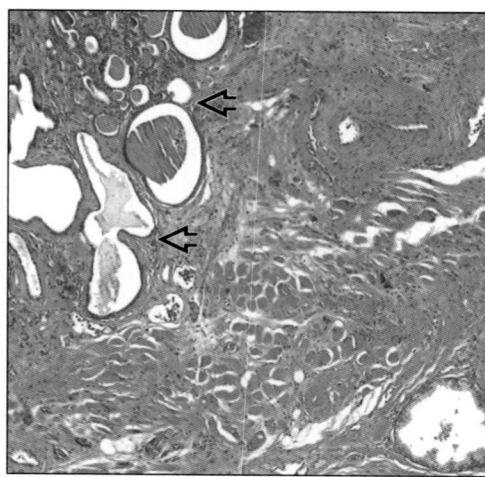

Mesonephric hyperplasia ⊞ involving prostate shows lobular and infiltrative growth of tubules, which characteristically contain intraluminal colloid-like material.

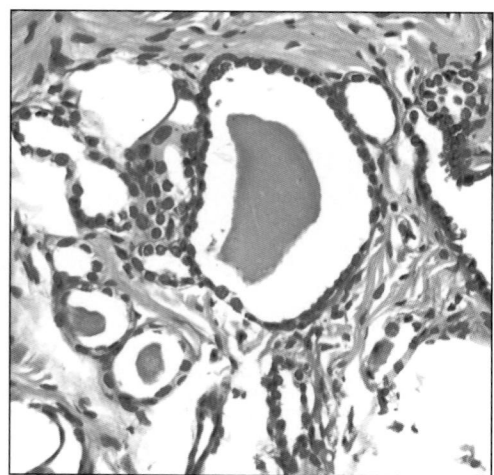

Mesonephric remnant tubules are lined by a single layer of cuboidal cells with scant cytoplasm imparting an "atrophic" appearance. Note the presence of intraluminal eosinophilic material.

TERMINOLOGY

Definitions
- Tubular or acinar proliferation of putative mesonephric duct remnants containing characteristic intraluminal colloid-like material
- Histologically similar to mesonephric remnants that are well recognized in female genital tract

ETIOLOGY/PATHOGENESIS

Origin
- During embryogenesis, mesonephric or wolffian duct gives rise to rete testis, epididymis, vas deferens, and seminal vesicles
- Vestigial mesonephric duct remnants or rests can be seen more commonly in female genital tract and only rarely in male genital tract
- Mesonephric duct remnants may undergo proliferation or hyperplasia, the cause of which is not known

CLINICAL ISSUES

Epidemiology
- Incidence
  - Very rare
  - Seen in only 0.6% of transurethral resection of prostate (TURP) specimens
  - Only 15 cases reported in literature
- Age
  - Mean: 67 years old, range 50-85 years

Site
- Described typically in prostatic base but may extend into bladder neck and periprostatic soft tissues
- Likely involves central region of prostate, since most are seen in TURP specimens

Presentation
- Incidental histologic finding
  - Encountered mainly in patients treated for obstructive urinary symptoms due to benign prostate hyperplasia
  - Few cases encountered in prostatectomy specimens for prostate adenocarcinoma
- Report of misdiagnosis as prostate adenocarcinoma

Treatment
- None required

Prognosis
- Benign course

MACROSCOPIC FEATURES

Size
- Measures 0.1-0.7 cm in TURP specimens

MICROSCOPIC PATHOLOGY

Histologic Features
- Composed of tubules or acini arranged in somewhat lobular clusters
- Tubules may have infiltrative-appearing growth pattern
- Tubules are lined by single layer of bland cuboidal, flattened, or low columnar cells
- Distinctively, tubules often contain dense eosinophilic colloid-like material reminiscent of thyroid follicles
- Cytoplasm is typically scant and pale pink, imparting "atrophic" appearance
- Nuclei are round, regular, and typically with inconspicuous nucleoli, although occasionally they may be prominent
- Occasional intratubular papillary fronds are present
- Infiltrative growth pattern can be seen as clusters of several glands or occasional single glands

HYPERPLASIA OF MESONEPHRIC REMNANTS

Key Facts

Terminology
- Tubular or acinar proliferation of putative mesonephric duct remnants containing characteristic intraluminal colloid-like material

Etiology/Pathogenesis
- During embryogenesis, mesonephric or wolffian duct gives rise to rete testis, epididymis, vas deferens, and seminal vesicles
- Mesonephric remnants may undergo proliferation

Clinical Issues
- Very rare, seen in 0.6% of TURP specimens
- Mean: 67 years old, range: 50-85 years
- Incidental histologic finding
- Typically in prostatic base but can extend into bladder neck and periprostatic soft tissues

Microscopic Pathology
- Lobular or infiltrative growth of tubules that often contains dense eosinophilic colloid-like material
- Lined by single layer of bland cuboidal cells with scant cytoplasm imparting "atrophic" appearance
- Nuclei are regular, round, and typically with inconspicuous nucleolus but can also be prominent
- Hyperplasia may be florid; tubules may appear to infiltrate between bladder neck muscle bundles and into periprostatic connective tissues
- Tubules may be seen intimately associated with nerves or ganglions

Ancillary Tests
- Colloid-like material is PAS(+) and PASD(+)
- PSA/PAP(-)
- Most are HMCK(34βE12)(+)

- Hyperplasia may be florid; tubules may appear to infiltrate between bladder neck muscle bundles and into periprostatic connective tissues
- Tubules may be seen intimately associated with nerves and ganglia
- May contain infiltrative-appearing cords of micro-acini that lack colloid-like material and, along with prominent nucleoli, may mimic prostate adenocarcinoma

Predominant Pattern/Injury Type
- Hyperplasia

Predominant Cell/Compartment Type
- Epithelial

ANCILLARY TESTS

Histochemistry
- Colloid-like material is PAS(+) and PASD(+)

Immunohistochemistry
- PSA/PAP(-)
- Most are HMCK(34βE12)(+)

DIFFERENTIAL DIAGNOSIS

Verumontanum Mucosal Gland Hyperplasia
- Microacinar proliferation along verumontanum and adjacent urethra at openings of utricle and ejaculatory ducts
- Tubules are lined by single layer of cuboidal to columnar cells with underlying basal cell layer
- Tubules are more closely packed and contain abundant intraluminal corpora amylacea
- Unlikely to be seen in TURP, which spares verumontanum

Nephrogenic Adenoma
- May secondarily involve prostate parenchyma
- Cystic tubules may contain colloid-like material
- In contrast, mainly periurethral in location

- Shows thickened peritubular hyaline sheath and characteristic "hobnail" cell lining
- May have exophytic papillary growth overlying tubular parenchyma
- May be PSA/PAP(+)

Benign Small Acinar Proliferations
- Differential diagnosis for atypical small acinar proliferations (ASAP) that includes benign prostate glands, small glandular variant of BPH, atypical adenomatous hyperplasia, atrophy, and sclerosing adenosis
- In contrast, these benign acinar proliferations lack intraluminal colloid-like material
- PSA/PAP(+)
- Contain a basal cell layer that is p63 or HMCK(34βE12)(+)

Acinar Adenocarcinoma
- Mesonephric hyperplasia with infiltrative-appearing architecture that lacks typical intraluminal colloid material; may mimic prostate carcinoma
- Both may be seen around or within nerves
- In contrast, malignant glands are more infiltrative and lacks lobular pattern
- Cytoplasm is slightly more abundant and paler and shows nucleomegaly with prominent nucleoli
- PSA/PAP(+), HMCK(34βE12)(-)

SELECTED REFERENCES

1. Bostwick DG et al: Mesonephric remnants of the prostate: incidence and histologic spectrum. Mod Pathol. 16(7):630-5, 2003
2. Val-Bernal JF et al: Hyperplasia of prostatic mesonephric remnants: a potential pitfall in the evaluation of prostate gland biopsy. J Urol. 154(3):1138-9, 1995
3. Gikas PW et al: Florid hyperplasia of mesonephric remnants involving prostate and periprostatic tissue. Possible confusion with adenocarcinoma. Am J Surg Pathol. 17(5):454-60, 1993

3

HYPERPLASIA OF MESONEPHRIC REMNANTS

Microscopic Features

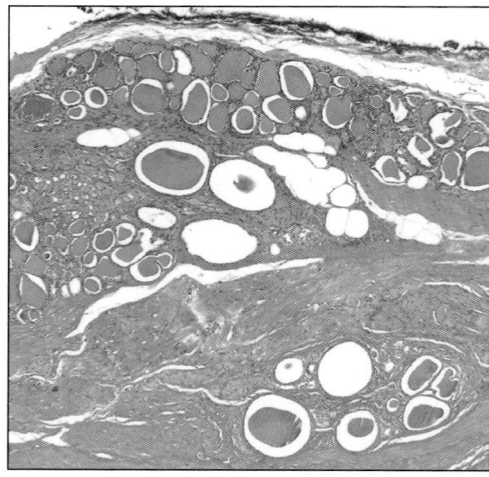
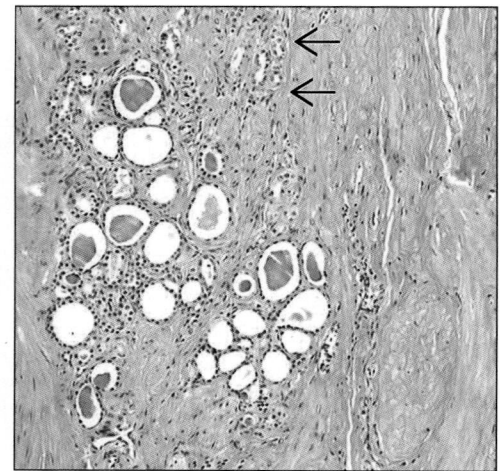

(Left) Mesonephric hyperplasia involving periprostatic neurovascular bundle shows clusters of variably sized tubules arranged in lobular configuration. The intraluminal colloid-like material is distinctive and helpful in making the diagnosis. *(Right)* Mesonephric hyperplasia shows a cluster of tubules in somewhat lobular configuration. Smaller tubules lacking intraluminal eosinophilic material are present at the periphery of the cluster ➡, which may mimic prostate adenocarcinoma.

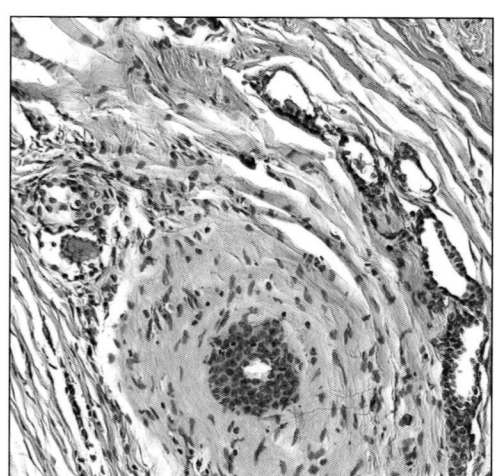
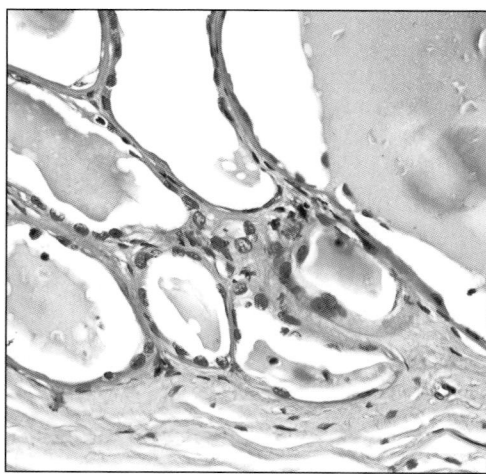

(Left) Small mesonephric remnant tubules show an infiltrative pattern of growth. The infiltrative appearance of these tubules and absence of intraluminal eosinophilic material may cause confusion with prostate adenocarcinoma. *(Right)* High-power view of mesonephric remnants shows tubules lined by a single layer of flattened to cuboidal cells with scant cytoplasm. Nuclei of mesonephric remnant tubules are typically bland and do not contain prominent nucleoli.

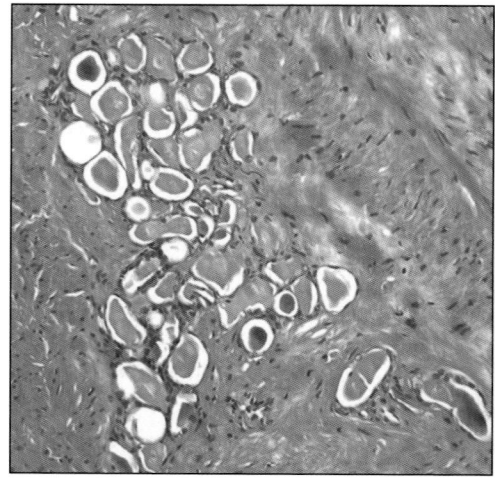
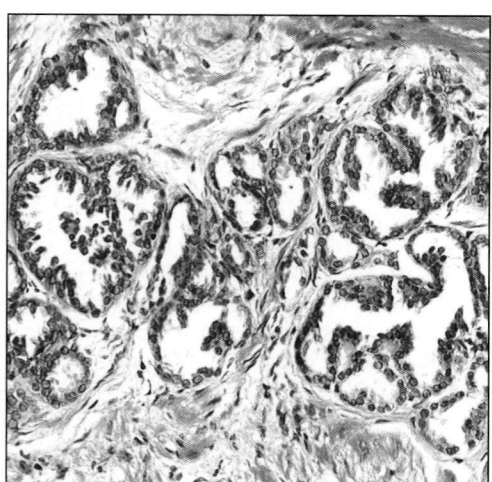

(Left) Lobular cluster of mesonephric hyperplasia shows a group of crowded tubules containing intraluminal eosinophilic material that resemble thyroid follicle colloid. Presence of this material is helpful in the distinction of mesonephric hyperplasia from prostate adenocarcinoma and other benign proliferations. *(Right)* Mesonephric tubules occasionally may contain intratubular papillary fronds, which may be seen admixed with more typical-appearing mesonephric remnant tubules.

HYPERPLASIA OF MESONEPHRIC REMNANTS

Microscopic and Immunohistochemical Features

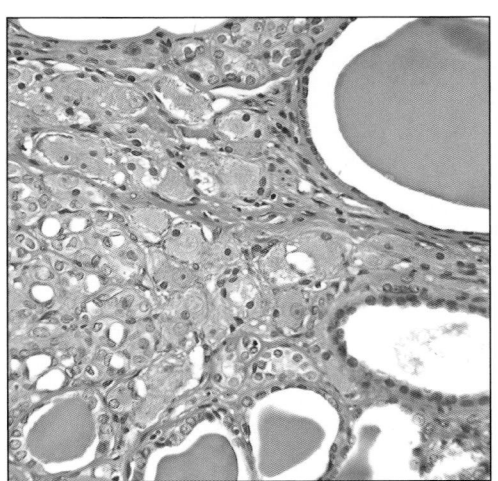

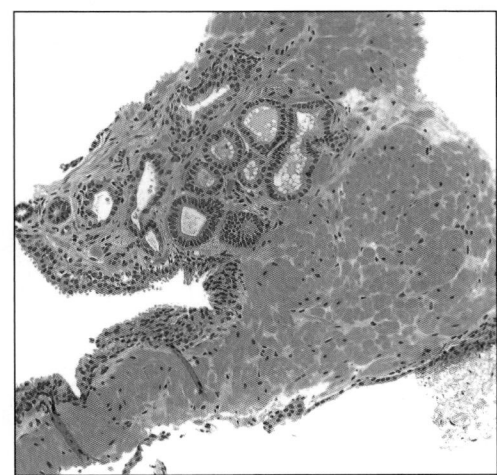

(Left) Mesonephric remnant tubules show intimate association with a paraganglion. Awareness of this feature in mesonephric hyperplasia is important; not to be mistaken as perineural invasion by carcinoma. *(Right)* Prostate needle biopsy shows mesonephric remnant tubules. The tight cluster and rigid appearance of these tubules simulate prostate adenocarcinoma on low-power magnification. Lack of cytologic atypia and presence of luminal secretions in these glands are key in making the diagnosis.

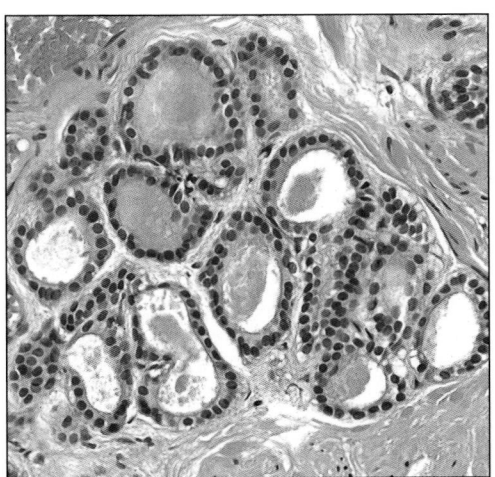

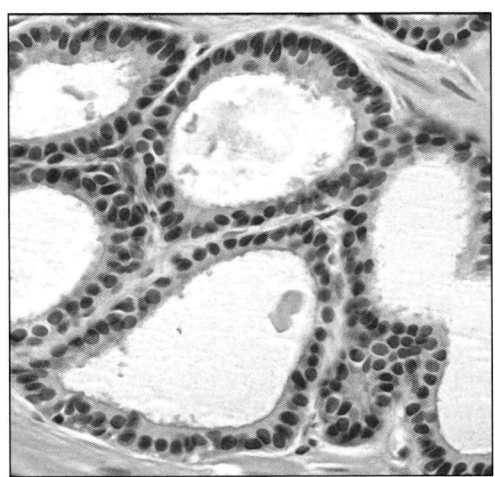

(Left) A cluster of mesonephric remnant tubules mimics prostate adenocarcinoma. These glands are tightly clustered, small, regular, and show monolayer of cells, which are all worrisome features for adenocarcinoma. However, the lack of nuclear atypia and presence of intraluminal eosinophilic material in some of the tubules is helpful in making the diagnosis. *(Right)* Close inspection of the same mesonephric remnant tubules to the left does not reveal the nuclear features of malignancy.

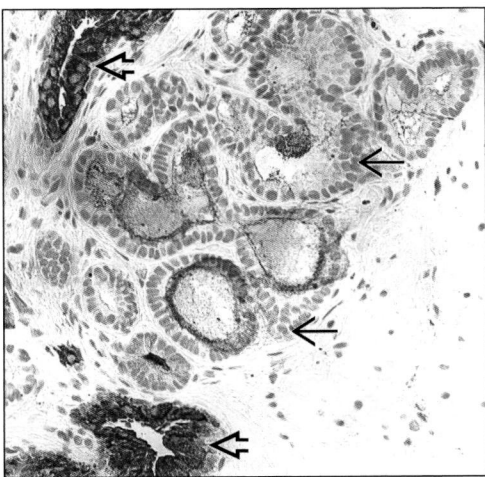

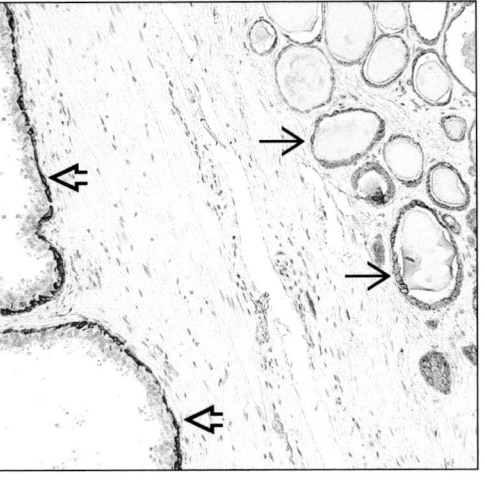

(Left) Mesonephric remnant tubules shows negative staining with PSA ⇥, in contrast to the positive benign prostate glands ⇨. *(Right)* Mesonephric remnant tubules ⇥ show HMCK(34βE12) positivity in the tubular cells, in contrast to basal cell staining pattern in adjacent benign prostate glands ⇨. PSA and HMCK(34βE12) are helpful in differentiating mesonephric hyperplasia (PSA[-], HMCK[34βE12][+]), from acini of prostate adenocarcinoma (PSA[+], HMCK[34βE12][-]).

VERUMONTANUM MUCOSAL GLAND HYPERPLASIA

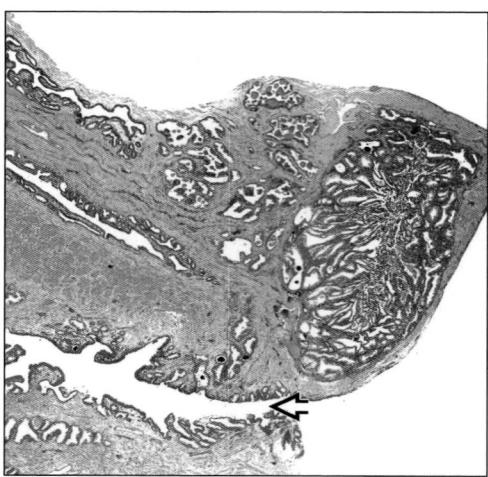

Low-power magnification of VMGH shows well-circumscribed, nodular proliferation of small to medium-sized glands. Adjacent prostatic utricle ⊵ is not involved.

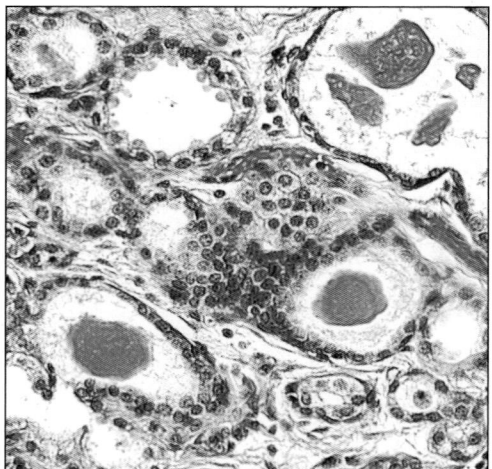

H&E shows small glands lined by cuboidal cells containing amphophilic cytoplasm and regular nuclei lacking atypia. Note presence of intraluminal corpora amylacea, typical for VMGH.

TERMINOLOGY

Abbreviations
- Verumontanum mucosal gland hyperplasia (VMGH)

Definitions
- Benign proliferation of glands indigenously situated along verumontanum of prostatic urethra
- Verumontanum or seminal colliculus is located at posterior prostatic urethral wall where utricle and ejaculatory ducts merge with prostatic urethra

ETIOLOGY/PATHOGENESIS

Origin
- Morphologic evidence suggests origin from urethral mucosal glands, which occupy most distal portion of prostatic ducts, ejaculatory ducts, and utricle
- Another possibility is origin from utricle since this structure developmentally acquires morphological and functional features of prostate
  - However, presence of VMGH exclusively along prostatic urethra argues against this theory

CLINICAL ISSUES

Epidemiology
- Incidence
  - Reported in 14% of prostatectomy specimens
- Age
  - Older patients, range 47-87 years old

Presentation
- Clinically asymptomatic, encountered as incidental histologic lesions more commonly in prostatectomy and less often in needle biopsy specimens
  - Unlikely to be seen in transurethral resection of prostate (TURP) specimens, since verumontanum is spared in this procedure

- Significance in routine practice: Morphologic mimic of adenocarcinoma in prostate biopsy

Treatment
- None

Prognosis
- Benign course

MICROSCOPIC PATHOLOGY

Histologic Features
- Situated along openings of ejaculatory or prostatic ducts (67%), utricle (19%), or adjacent urethral mucosa (14%)
- Seen subjacent to urothelium, demonstrating expansile architectural growth
- Composed of relatively well-circumscribed proliferation of small to medium-sized, closely packed glands
- Glands are often back to back with minimal interglandular stroma
- Glandular cells are cuboidal to low columnar and rarely may be flattened
  - Cytoplasm is clear to eosinophilic
  - Nuclei are round and regular with indistinct nucleoli and absent mitoses
  - Cytoplasmic lipofuscin pigment is often present
- Basal cell layer is readily identifiable in routine H&E stained sections
- Characteristically, lamellated eosinophilic concretions typical of corpora amylacea are seen
- Uncommonly, intraluminal orange-red fragmented concretions may be seen
- True crystalloids or luminal mucin are typically not present

Predominant Pattern/Injury Type
- Hyperplasia

VERUMONTANUM MUCOSAL GLAND HYPERPLASIA

Key Facts

Terminology
- Benign proliferation of glands indigenously situated along verumontanum of prostatic urethra

Clinical Issues
- Encountered as incidental histologic finding
- Significant as morphologic mimic of adenocarcinoma in prostate biopsy specimens

Microscopic Pathology
- Seen along ejaculatory or prostatic ducts (67%), utricle (19%), or adjacent urethral mucosa (14%)
- Composed of relatively well-circumscribed proliferations of closely packed glands
- Frequently contain corpora amylacea
- Glandular cells usually are cuboidal to low columnar, and basal cell layer is readily discernible

Predominant Cell/Compartment Type
- Epithelial, glandular

Immunohistochemistry
- Glandular cells are PSA(+)
- Basal cells are HMCK(34βE12)(+)

DIFFERENTIAL DIAGNOSIS

Nephrogenic Adenoma
- Located in suburethral prostatic stroma
- Tubules lined by cuboidal, flattened, or "hobnailed" cells
- May have thickened or prominent peritubular basement membranes
- May contain intraluminal eosinophilic secretions
- May have exophytic papillary component overlying tubular proliferation
- PSA/PAP(-)

Mesonephric Hyperplasia
- May be situated along urethral aspect of prostate
- Tubules arranged in somewhat lobular and infiltrative-appearing growth pattern
- Characteristically contain dense eosinophilic colloid-like material
- PSA/PAP(-)

Low-Grade Acinar Adenocarcinoma and Its Mimics
- Cytologic features of malignancy, including prominent nucleoli
- Demonstrates infiltrative or expansile growth pattern
- Lacks basal cell layer
  - Basal cell markers useful in challenging cases
- May contain intraluminal crystalloids and mucin
- Corpora amylacea are very rare

DIAGNOSTIC CHECKLIST

Pathologic Interpretation Pearls
- Diagnosis of benign nature is usually straightforward, based on nuclear features and presence of basal cell layer

SELECTED REFERENCES

1. Muezzinoglu B et al: Verumontanum mucosal gland hyperplasia is associated with atypical adenomatous hyperplasia of the prostate. Arch Pathol Lab Med. 125(3):358-60, 2001
2. Gagucas RJ et al: Verumontanum mucosal gland hyperplasia. Am J Surg Pathol. 19(1):30-6, 1995
3. Gaudin PB et al: Verumontanum mucosal gland hyperplasia in prostatic needle biopsy specimens. A mimic of low grade prostatic adenocarcinoma. Am J Clin Pathol. 104(6):620-6, 1995

IMAGE GALLERY

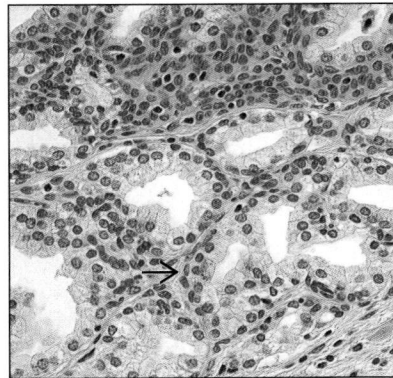
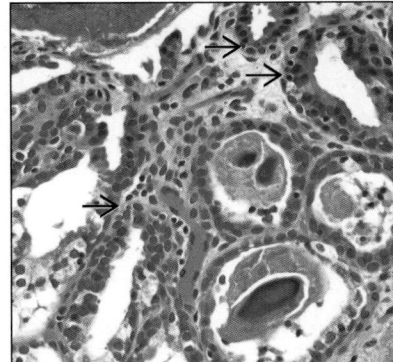
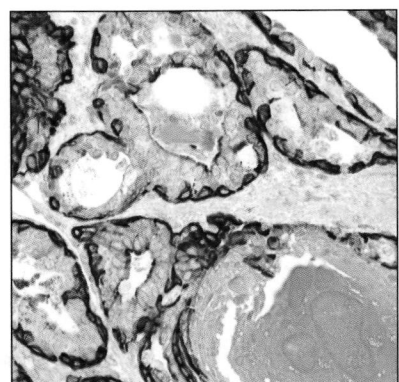

(Left) VMGH glands are often small and back to back; basal cells are readily discernible in some of these glands ➡. *(Center)* VMGH glands may have round rigid contour mimicking adenocarcinoma, in this case, compounded by presence of fragmented concretions simulating crystalloids. VMGH glands, however, do not show nuclear atypia and basal cell layer is readily discernible ➡. *(Right)* Triple PIN cocktail antibody in VMGH glands shows no overexpression of AMACR (red) and basal cells are HMCK(34βE12) (brown) (+).

NEPHROGENIC ADENOMA OF THE PROSTATIC URETHRA

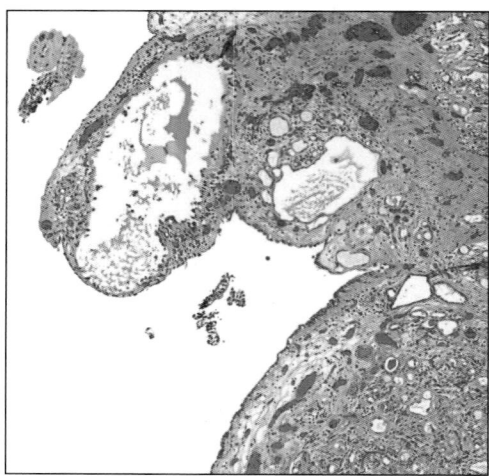

Low-power magnification of NA of the prostatic urethra shows polypoid growth with subjacent tubular and cystic proliferations in the lamina propria.

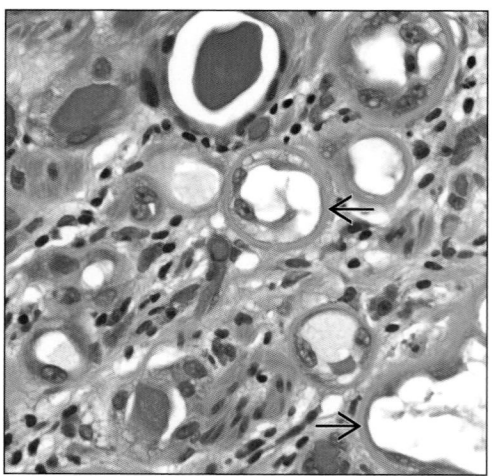

High-power magnification of NA shows variably sized round hollow tubules with characteristic thickened basement membrane ➡. Some of the tubules contain intraluminal eosinophilic secretions.

TERMINOLOGY

Abbreviations
- Nephrogenic adenoma (NA)

Synonyms
- Nephrogenic metaplasia

Definitions
- Benign epithelial lesion of urethra characterized by tubular, glandular, &/or papillary growth pattern that is morphologic and immunohistochemical mimic of prostatic adenocarcinoma

ETIOLOGY/PATHOGENESIS

Renal Tubular Cell Seeding Hypothesis
- In renal transplant patients, NA cells shown to have same sex chromosome status with allografted kidneys and not with surrounding bladder tissue in opposite gender recipients
- May represent seeding implantation and growth of renal tubular cells in injured urothelial mucosa

Nephrogenic Metaplasia Hypothesis
- Metaplastic alteration of urothelium in response to insult or injury

CLINICAL ISSUES

Epidemiology
- Age
  - Mean: 66 years; range: 21-77 years

Site
- Vast majority of NA encountered in urinary bladder
- Prostatic urethra is involved in approximately 15% of cases and may extend into subjacent prostate stroma

Presentation
- Most are incidental findings
  - Mainly seen in transurethral resection of prostate (TURP) specimens for benign prostatic hyperplasia

Natural History
- Majority of cases with preceding genitourinary surgery, instrumentation, urinary tract infection, or calculi

Treatment
- None required

Prognosis
- Benign, but with high "recurrence" rate (37%) if inciting etiology persists

MACROSCOPIC FEATURES

General Features
- Only about 1/3 may assume macroscopic proportions, which may be seen at cystourethroscopically as exophytic papillary or polypoid lesions

Size
- Generally < 1 cm, average 0.3 cm

MICROSCOPIC PATHOLOGY

Histologic Features
- Architectural patterns
  - Most common as small round to oval tubules in laminar fashion
    - Some tubules characteristically have thickened or prominent peritubular basement membrane
    - May contain intraluminal basophilic or eosinophilic secretions, the latter imparting resemblance of tubules to thyroid follicles
    - Tubules may be very small, simulating signet ring cells

NEPHROGENIC ADENOMA OF THE PROSTATIC URETHRA

Key Facts

Terminology
- Tubulo-papillary proliferations along urothelial mucosa that resemble immature renal tubules

Etiology/Pathogenesis
- Renal tubular cell seeding hypothesis
- Nephrogenic metaplasia hypothesis

Microscopic Pathology
- Most common as small round to oval tubules
- Thickened peritubular basement membrane
- May contain intraluminal basophilic or eosinophilic secretions
- Other architectural patterns include cystic, papillary-polypoid, solid growth, and rare fibromyxoid subtype
- Monolayer of cuboidal, flattened, or "hobnailed" cells
- Scanty to modest eosinophilic to clear cytoplasm

- Nuclei with minimal atypia, inconspicuous nucleoli, and absent to rare mitosis
- Tubules may be very small simulating signet ring cells
- Admixture of these different patterns is common
- Polypoid-papillary growth when present is always seen with underlying tubular proliferation
- Extension of tubules into subjacent prostate fibromuscular stroma is common

Ancillary Tests
- Key immunohistochemical panel: PAN-CK(AE1/AE3) (+), pax-2(+), PSA/PAP(-) in majority of cases

Top Differential Diagnoses
- Prostatic acinar adenocarcinoma
- Urethral papillary neoplasms

- ▪ Extension of tubules into subjacent prostate fibromuscular stroma common
- ○ Cystically dilated tubules
- ○ Papillary-polypoid pattern, usually with minimal branching and edematous stroma
- ○ Rare solid or diffuse growth and fibromyxoid appearance with spindled cells
- ○ Admixture of these different patterns is common; polypoid-papillary, when present, is always seen with underlying tubular proliferation
- Cytological features
  - ○ Monolayer of bland cuboidal, flattened, or "hobnailed" cells
  - ○ Scanty to modest amount of eosinophilic to clear cytoplasm
  - ○ Small nuclei with minimal atypia (in range of reactive) and inconspicuous to rarely prominent nucleoli
  - ○ Absent to rare mitotic figures
- Additional findings
  - ○ Stromal edema, inflammatory cell infiltrates, dilated vessels, and occasional microcalcifications

Predominant Pattern/Injury Type
- Metaplastic

Predominant Cell/Compartment Type
- Epithelial, tubular

ANCILLARY TESTS

Immunohistochemistry
- Key panel: PAN-CK(+), pax-2(+), PSA/PAP(-) in majority of cases; rare focal positivity is pitfall
  - ○ Other (+) markers: S100-A1, pax-8, CK7, EMA/MUC1, HMCK(34βE12) (variable and focal); MIB1 (low index)
  - ○ Other (-) markers: p63

Cytogenetics
- Monosomy 9 (24% of cells), trisomy 7 (8% of cells)

DIFFERENTIAL DIAGNOSIS

Prostatic Acinar Adenocarcinoma
- Usually monotonous small acinar pattern (tubular, cystic, papillary components are absent)
- "Hobnail" cells, eosinophilic secretions, stromal edema, and inflammation; rare to absent
- AMACR(+), PSA/PAP(+), pax-2/pax-8(-), and S100-1A(-)

Urethral Papillary Neoplasms
- Papillae lined by multilayered urothelium; presence and extent of atypia determines grade
- Lacks concomitant tubular growth
- p63(+) and pax-2/pax-8(-)

DIAGNOSTIC CHECKLIST

Pathologic Interpretation Pearls
- Proliferation of small round tubules and cysts lined by bland monolayered cuboidal or "hobnail" epithelial cells, often with concomitant papillary or polypoid growth

SELECTED REFERENCES

1. Allan CH et al: Nephrogenic adenoma of the prostatic urethra: a mimicker of prostate adenocarcinoma. Am J Surg Pathol. 25(6):802-8, 2001
2. Malpica A et al: Nephrogenic adenoma of the prostatic urethra involving the prostate gland: a clinicopathologic and immunohistochemical study of eight cases. Hum Pathol. 25(4):390-5, 1994
3. Young RH: Nephrogenic adenomas of the urethra involving the prostate gland: a report of two cases of a lesion that may be confused with prostatic adenocarcinoma. Mod Pathol. 5(6):617-20, 1992
4. Martin SA et al: Adenomatoid metaplasia of prostatic urethra. Am J Clin Pathol. 75(2):185-9, 1981

NEPHROGENIC ADENOMA OF THE PROSTATIC URETHRA

Microscopic Features

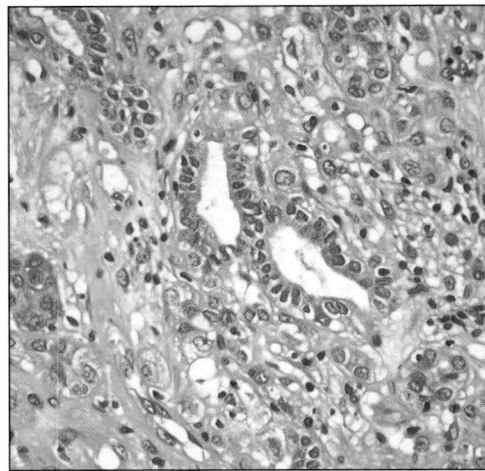
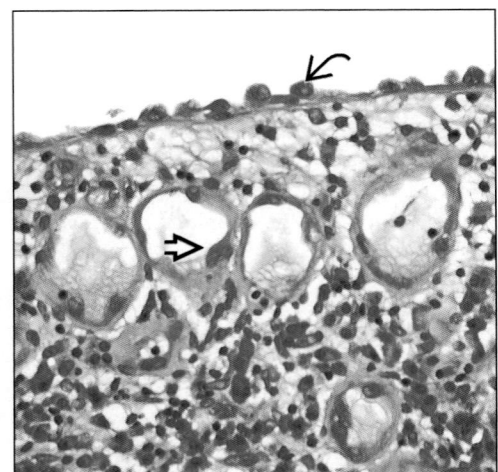

(Left) H&E shows NA tubules lined by cuboidal cells with a modest amount of eosinophilic cytoplasm containing nuclei without significant atypia. (Right) H&E shows NA tubules lined by flattened cells with "hobnail" nuclei protruding in the lumen ➡. Similar cells are seen on the surface lining ➡. Note the presence of chronic inflammation in the background. Identification of the relationship of a small glandular proliferation in the prostate to the urethra is an important clue to diagnose NA.

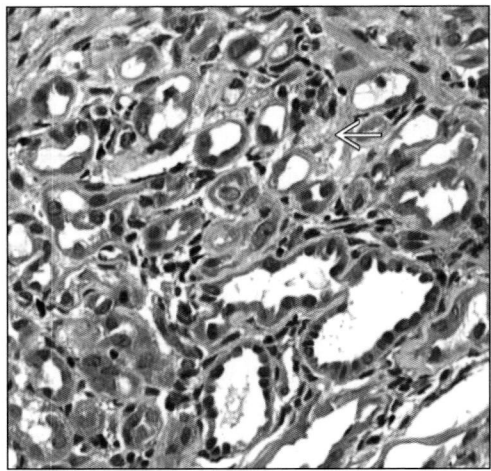
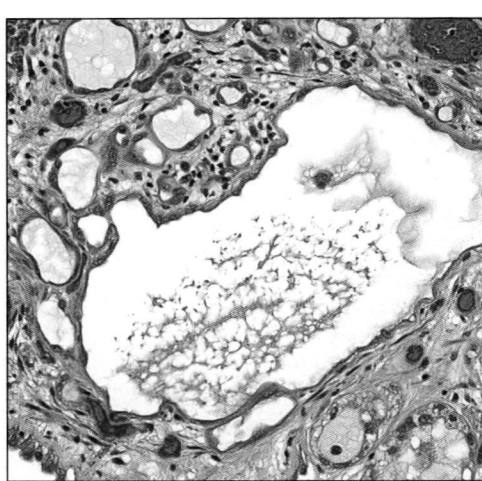

(Left) H&E shows NA tubules lined by "hobnail" cells, some tubules are smaller in caliber and contain intraluminal basophilic secretions. Note the basophilic hue of extracellular mucinous material in the stroma ➡ along with the background inflammation. (Right) H&E shows that there is marked variation in the size and shape of the tubules, a feature that is rare in prostatic carcinoma. The cytoplasm is eosinophilic and the nuclei have a "hobnailed" appearance. There is attendant inflammation.

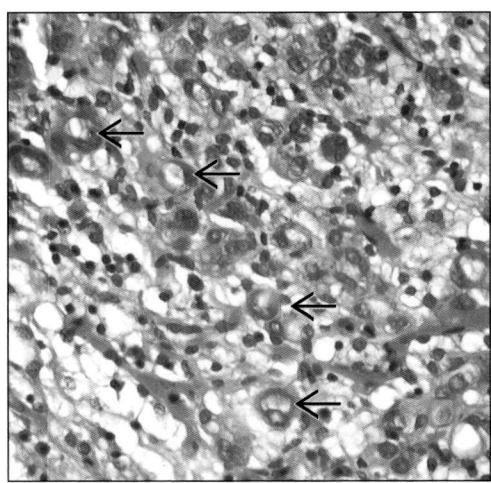
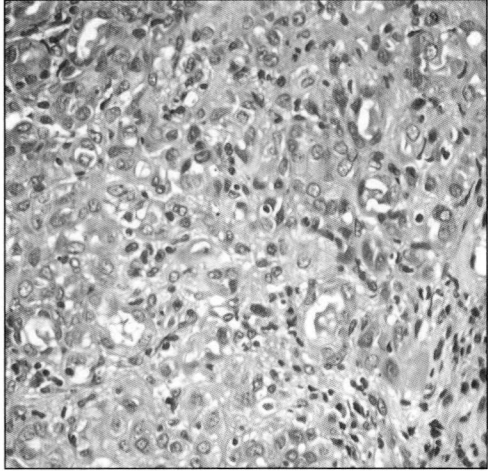

(Left) Occasionally, NA tubules can be very tiny showing small lumina with a single nucleus and may contain basophilic mucin, mimicking the appearance of signet ring cells ➡. This H&E shows the presence of extracellular basophilic mucin in the stroma in. (Right) H&E shows a solid or diffuse pattern of NA. This pattern usually occurs as a minor component and is often admixed with other architectural patterns. Observation of a range of architectural patterns in the same lesion should raise the possibility of NA.

NEPHROGENIC ADENOMA OF THE PROSTATIC URETHRA

Microscopic Features

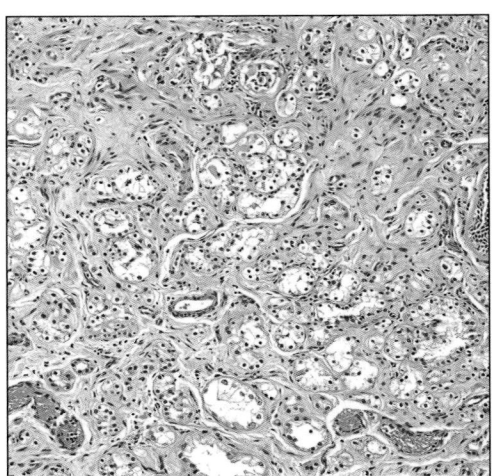

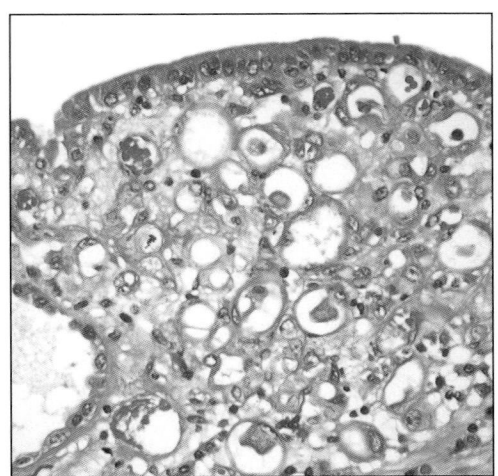

(Left) H&E of NA shows numerous tubules lined by clear cells. Presence of clear cells raises concern for clear cell adenocarcinoma (CCA) or prostatic carcinoma. In contrast to NA, CCA is less common in males and shows obvious cytologic atypia and features of malignancy. *(Right)* H&E of NA shows a tight cluster of hollow tubules mimicking a florid vascular proliferation. Occasional true capillaries (containing RBCs) are seen in this cluster, which may add to the false impression.

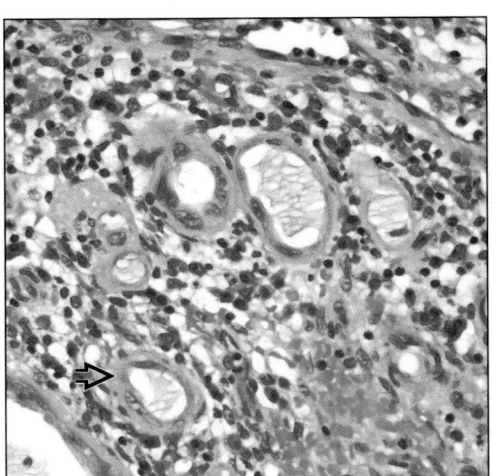

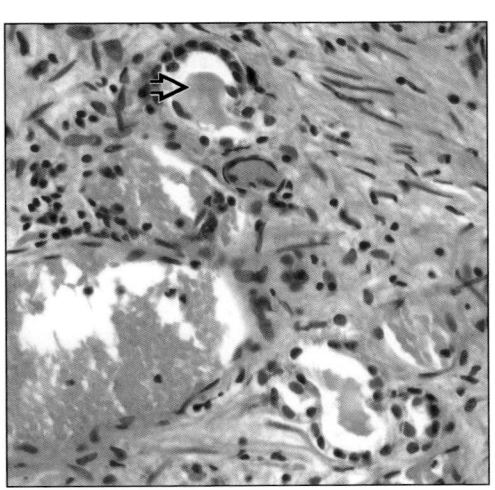

(Left) H&E shows NA tubules with intraluminal basophilic secretions. Note the characteristic thickened basement membrane ⇨ around the tubules, which can be highlighted with PAS stain. *(Right)* H&E shows NA tubules with eosinophilic secretions imparting an appearance that resembles thyroid follicles ⇨. This may also be seen in mesonephric hyperplasia (MH), but distinction is not clinically important. NA, in addition, shows other patterns and does not exhibit the lobularity seen in MH.

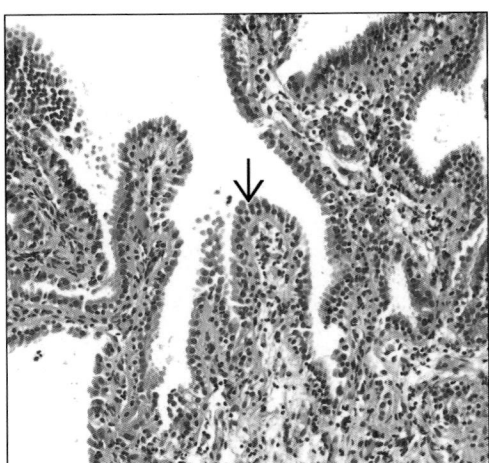

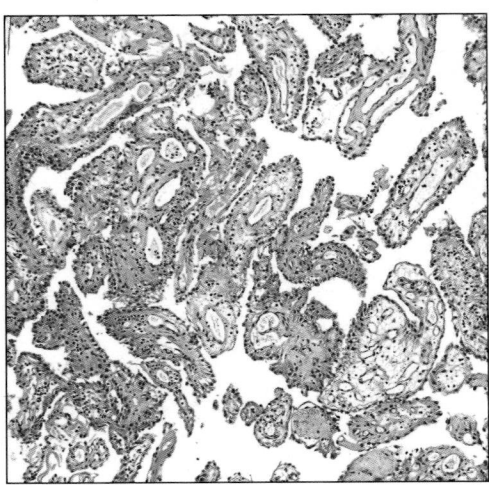

(Left) H&E of exophytic papillary projections of NA shows the papillae are nonbranching or have minimal branching. Papillae, when present, are frequently accompanied by endophytic tubular proliferations. These papillae are lined by a monolayer of cells ⇨ similar to those in tubules. *(Right)* Uncommonly, the papillary growth may be florid & show more complex branching. These papillae may mimic a papillary urothelial neoplasm (PUN). Distinction is tenable, as PUN is typically multilayered.

NEPHROGENIC ADENOMA OF THE PROSTATIC URETHRA

Microscopic Features

(Left) NA may be accompanied by dense chronic inflammation seen here scattered between the tubules in this H&E. Some cases of NA are preceded by history of genitourinary injury or urinary tract infection, which may cause inflammation in the urethral submucosa. *(Right)* Rarely, microcalcifications may be seen in NA. The background stroma is edematous. The variation in the size & shape of the tubules plus stromal edema helps distinguish NA from the atrophic pattern of prostatic adenocarcinoma.

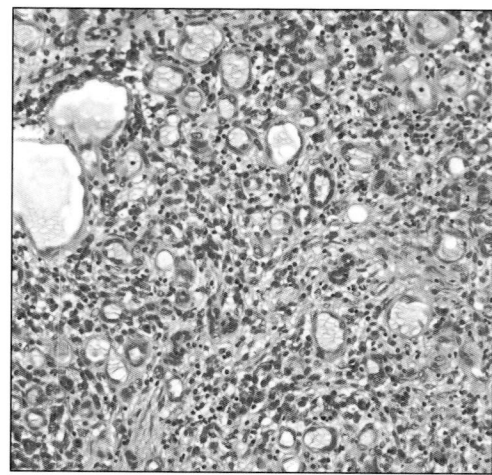
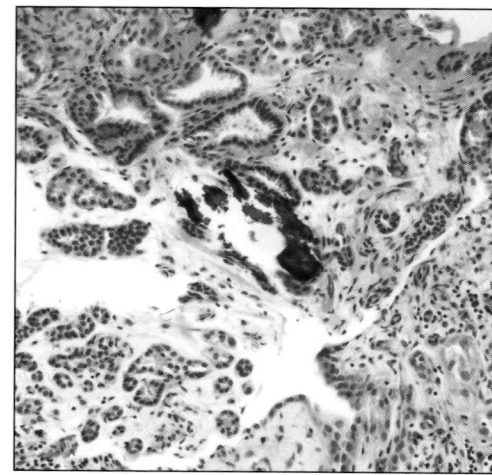

(Left) H&E shows NA tubules in a TURP chip. Extension of urethral NA into the prostate fibromuscular stroma is common and may enter into the differential diagnosis of atypical glandular proliferations of the prostate. *(Right)* Several rigid NA tubules in the prostate stroma are shown. In contrast to prostate adenocarcinoma, these NA tubular cells show frequent "hobnailed" nuclei and do not show nucleomegaly and prominent nucleoli. The differential diagnosis is the atrophic pattern of prostatic cancer.

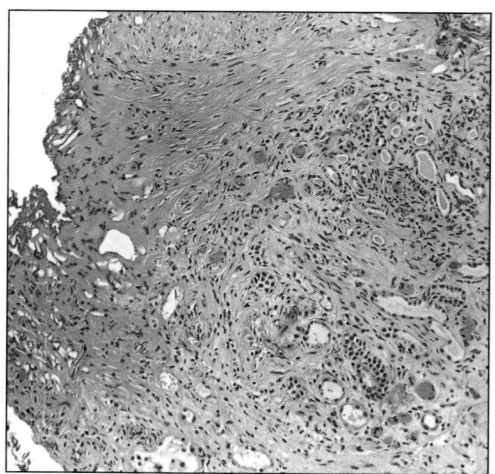
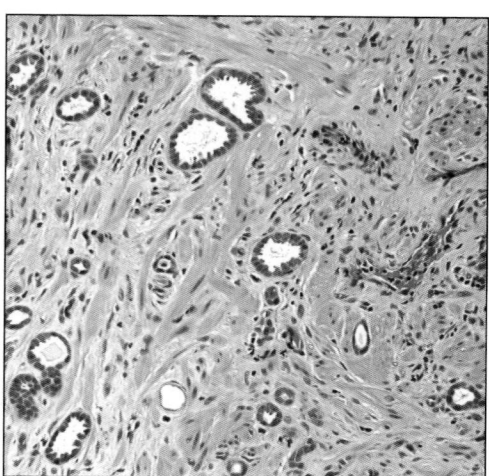

(Left) Cluster of NA tubules and cords with clear to eosinophilic cytoplasm show pseudoinfiltrative growth pattern in the prostate stroma, mimicking microacinar prostate adenocarcinoma. *(Right)* NA showing clusters of small poorly formed tubules and occasional separate single cells, mimicking Gleason pattern 4 and 5 prostate adenocarcinoma, respectively. In challenging cases, appropriate immunohistochemical stains (PSA/PAP[-] and pax-2[+]) may be helpful.

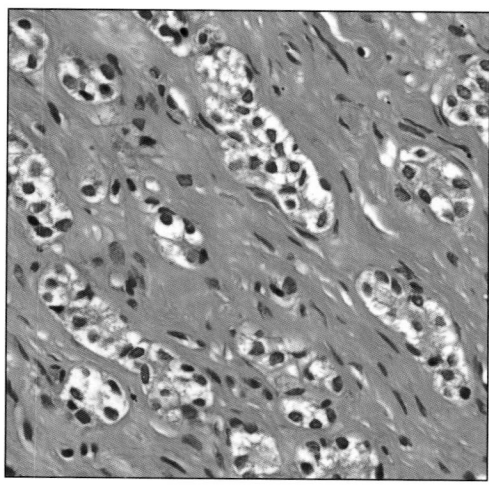
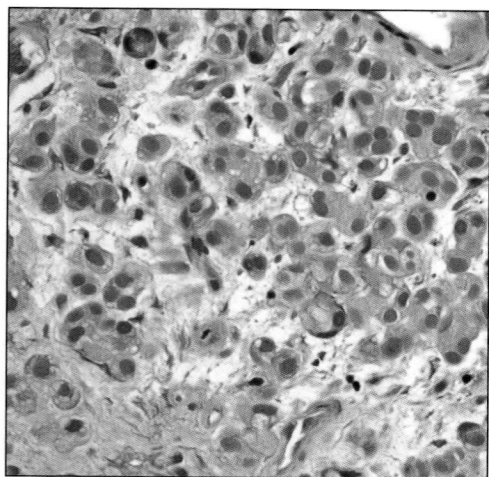

Microscopic and Immunohistochemical Features

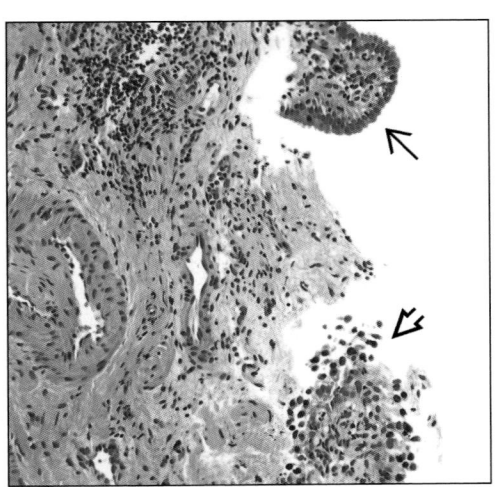

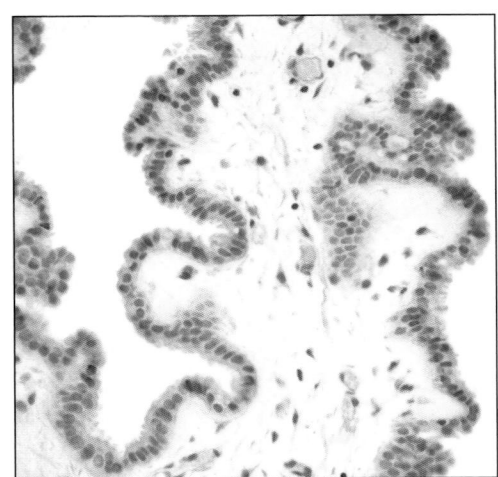

(*Left*) NA papilla ⇥ is adjacent to a focus of urothelial carcinoma in situ ⇥. NA papilla is monolayered and shows only minimal cytologic atypia. In contrast, the focus of urothelial carcinoma shows multiple layers of pleomorphic cells. (*Right*) p63 stain shows negative immunoreactivity in NA papillae. In contrast, papillary urothelial carcinoma is usually diffusely p63 nuclear(+). pax-2 may additionally help in differentiating NA from urothelial carcinoma.

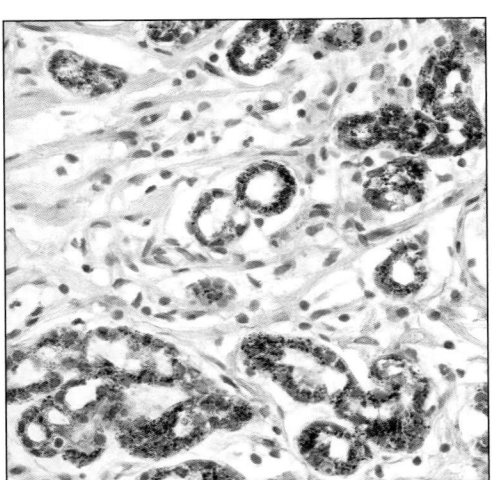

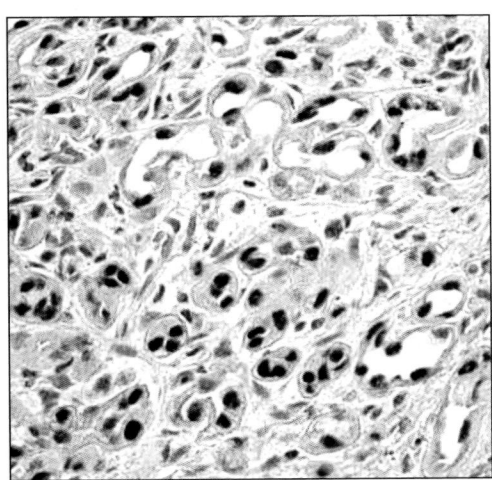

(*Left*) AMACR positivity in NA tubules is shown. Awareness of this pitfall is important in the differential diagnosis of prostate adenocarcinoma. (*Right*) Diffuse pax-2 nuclear expression in NA. pax-2 is normally found in epithelial cells of all tubular segments and of Bowman capsule of fetal kidneys. This marker is not expressed by prostate or urothelial carcinoma and is helpful in the differential diagnosis. pax-8 has a staining range similar to pax-2 and may be used alternatively.

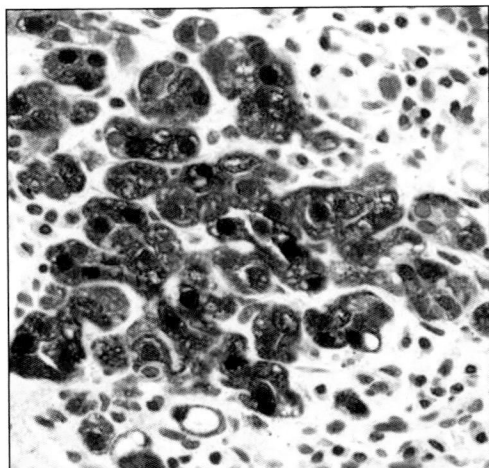

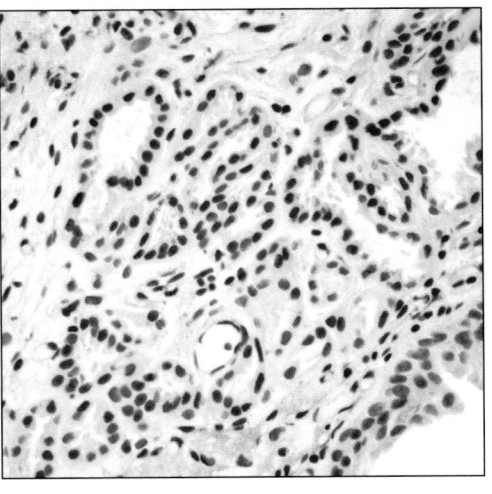

(*Left*) S100-1A nuclear and cytoplasmic expression in NA cells. This marker is not expressed in prostate adenocarcinoma and is helpful in the differential diagnosis. (*Right*) NA shows negative reaction to PSA, which complements positivity to pax-2 and S100-1A in NA (PSA[-] and pax-2/S100-1A[+]) vs. prostate adenocarcinoma (PSA[+] and pax-2/ S100-1A[-]). Rare and focal positivity for PSA and PAP has been reported in NA such that a panel of markers should be employed.

ATYPICAL ADENOMATOUS HYPERPLASIA

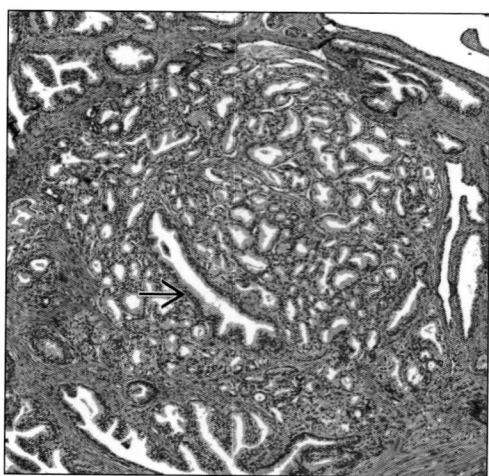

AAH shows relatively well-circumscribed proliferation of variably sized acini. Note the presence of a larger "parent" duct ⇨ in the central aspect of the lesion. The background is that of a BPH.

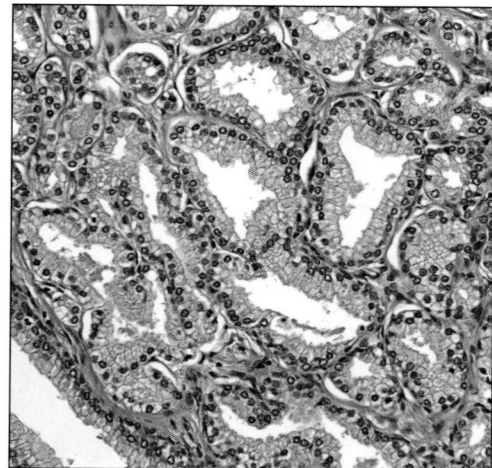

The peripheral small acini show a crowded pattern and bland cytology (nucleomegaly and prominent nucleoli are absent). Distinction may be difficult if the entire lesion is not visualized.

TERMINOLOGY

Abbreviations
- Atypical adenomatous hyperplasia (AAH)

Synonyms
- Adenosis
- Atypical adenosis, small acinar atypical hyperplasia, atypical hyperplasia, atypical primary hyperplasia (outdated terms)
  - 1994 consensus statement by expert GU pathologists recommended use of term AAH, although both AAH and adenosis are used interchangeably

Definitions
- Small to medium-sized acinar proliferation usually forming well-circumscribed nodule in transition zone of prostate, which has basal cell layer and does not fulfill cytologic criteria of carcinoma

CLINICAL ISSUES

Epidemiology
- Incidence
  - Present in 1.5-19.6% of transurethral resections of prostate (TURP) specimens
  - Seen in up to 33% of radical prostatectomies
  - Uncommon in needle core biopsies (< 2%), since transition zone is not often sampled

Presentation
- Asymptomatic, incidental histologic finding
- Comes to attention in routine practice as prostate cancer mimic in needle biopsy or TURP

Treatment
- No treatment is currently warranted

Prognosis
- Weak evidence suggests AAH may represent preneoplastic entity, particularly for low-grade, transition zone adenocarcinoma
- Evidence is circumstantial, mostly based on morphologic findings and little molecular or clinical supporting data

MACROSCOPIC FEATURES

General Features
- No gross abnormality

MICROSCOPIC PATHOLOGY

Histologic Features
- On low power, AHH consists of relatively well-circumscribed proliferation of small to medium-sized glands in transition zone, usually mixed with typical hyperplastic nodules in background
- Some peripheral AAH glands infiltrate surrounding stroma, tending to merge with adjacent benign glands
- More dilated "parent" gland may be centrally located
- Variable size and shape of glands, with similar cytology of surrounding hyperplastic glands
- Acinar cells with clear cytoplasm, round uniform nuclei, and inconspicuous nucleoli
- Fragmented basal cell layer, often requires immunostains for detection
- Occasionally crystalloids, amorphous eosinophilic secretions, corpora amylacea, or mucin may be found intraluminally

Predominant Pattern/Injury Type
- Hyperplasia

Predominant Cell/Compartment Type
- Epithelial, glandular

ATYPICAL ADENOMATOUS HYPERPLASIA

Key Facts

Terminology
- Small to medium-sized acinar proliferation usually forming well-circumscribed nodule in prostate transition zone, which does not fulfill cytologic criteria of carcinoma

Clinical Issues
- Minimal evidence suggests that AAH may represent preneoplastic entity, particularly for low-grade, transition zone adenocarcinoma
- Comes to attention in routine practice as prostate cancer mimic in needle biopsy or TURP

Microscopic Pathology
- Well-circumscribed proliferation of small to medium-sized glands in transition zone, usually mixed with typical hyperplastic nodules in background

- Variable size and shape of glands; similar cytology of surrounding hyperplastic glands
- More dilated "parent" gland may be centrally located
- Some peripheral AAH glands infiltrate surrounding stroma, tending to merge with adjacent benign glands
- Acinar cells with clear cytoplasm, round uniform nuclei with inconspicuous nucleoli
- Fragmented basal cell layer, often requires immunostains for detection

Ancillary Tests
- Basal cell markers frequently show discontinuous basal cell layer
- AMACR is focally positive in 7% and can be diffusely positive in up to 10% of cases

ANCILLARY TESTS

Immunohistochemistry
- Basal cell markers
  - p63, HMCK(34βE12), and CK5/6
  - Frequently show discontinuous basal cell layer, which may be absent in some to many acini within focus
- AMACR is focally positive in 7% and can be diffusely positive in up to 10% of cases

PCR
- 1 study showed allelic imbalances frequently found in adenocarcinoma in 47% of AHH cases

DIFFERENTIAL DIAGNOSIS

Benign Prostatic Hyperplasia (BPH)
- BPH nodules are better circumscribed with no peripheral infiltration by glands
- Glands are larger with papillary infoldings and consistent double cell layer

Sclerosing Adenosis
- Associated with dense fibrotic cellular stroma
- Thickened basement membrane or hyalinized stroma around glands may be present
- Poorly formed budding glands and individual cells
- Basal cell layer usually easy to recognize

Mesonephric Remnants
- Presence of colloid material within lumina
- Less nodular, more haphazardly arranged

Acinar Adenocarcinoma
- Usually demonstrates infiltrative growth
- Difference in cytoplasmic tinctorial qualities and nuclear size between tumor glands and adjacent benign glands
- Cytologic features of macronuclei, multiple nucleoli, and amphophilic cytoplasm
- Absent basal cell layer

  - May be difficult to differentiate from discontinuous basal cell layer of AAH in limited samples
  - Facilitated by use of basal cell immunomarkers

DIAGNOSTIC CHECKLIST

Pathologic Interpretation Pearls
- Well-circumscribed proliferation of glands in transition zone frequently seen in TURP specimens, which on close inspection lack cytologic features for cancer
- Immunohistochemistry shows discontinuous basal cell marker staining, and uncommonly may show focal or diffuse AMACR staining

REPORTING CONSIDERATIONS

Key Elements to Report
- Absence or presence of coexistent adenocarcinoma
- Not required to include AAH in final diagnosis report

SELECTED REFERENCES

1. Yang XJ et al: Expression of alpha-Methylacyl-CoA racemase (P504S) in atypical adenomatous hyperplasia of the prostate. Am J Surg Pathol. 26(7):921-5, 2002
2. Grignon DJ et al: Atypical adenomatous hyperplasia of the prostate: a critical review. Eur Urol. 30(2):206-11, 1996
3. Epstein JI: Adenosis (atypical adenomatous hyperplasia): histopathology and relationship to carcinoma. Pathol Res Pract. 191(9):888-98, 1995
4. Bostwick DG et al: Consensus statement on terminology: recommendation to use atypical adenomatous hyperplasia in place of adenosis of the prostate. Am J Surg Pathol. 18(10):1069-70, 1994
5. Bostwick DG et al: Atypical adenomatous hyperplasia of the prostate: morphologic criteria for its distinction from well-differentiated carcinoma. Hum Pathol. 24(8):819-32, 1993

ATYPICAL ADENOMATOUS HYPERPLASIA

Microscopic Features

(Left) Variable size of acini is a key low-power feature of AAH. The overall circumscribed architecture raises concern for low-grade carcinoma. Some experts argue that some of the original Gleason pattern 1 or 2 tumors may have represented AAH. *(Right)* The peripheral aspect of AAH shows small atypical glands, which may mimic microacinar adenocarcinoma. Lack of cytologic features of malignancy is helpful in the diagnosis, but immunohistochemistry is often necessary.

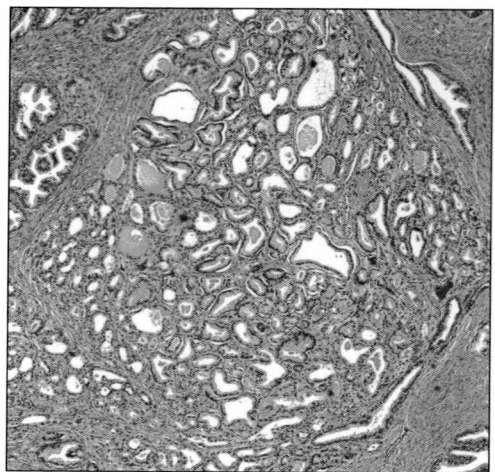
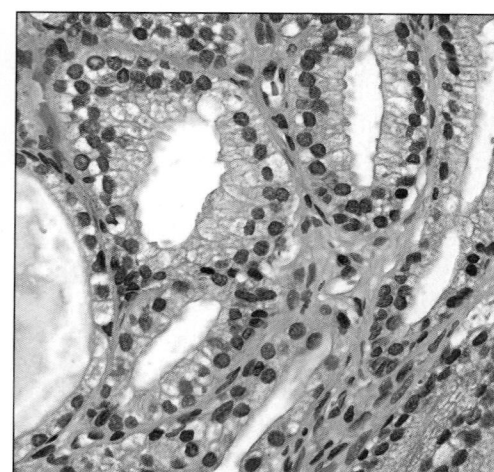

(Left) Some AAH glands may show rigid configuration ➡ and uniformity of caliber closely mimicking cancer. However, other glands in the same focus vary considerably in size and shape. This feature along with overall nodularity would suggest AAH. *(Right)* Crystalloids are not infrequently present in AAH. However, the glandular cells lack the cellular atypia and prominent nucleoli of adenocarcinoma. Basal cells ➡ are discernible on H&E stain in this particular example.

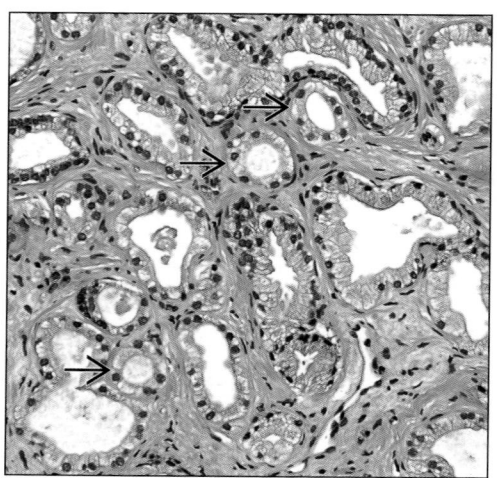
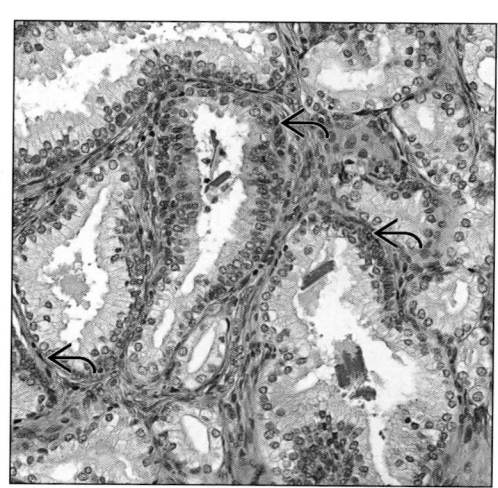

(Left) Intraluminal proteinaceous material and crystalloids may occasionally be seen in AAH. Presence of both these features in atypical glands compounds the diagnostic difficulty (vs. cancer). Use of immunohistochemical stains is often necessary in challenging cases. *(Right)* Staining for basal-associated markers (HMCK(34βE12) and p63) & AMACR shows discontinuous basal cell layer ➡ and positivity for AMACR. Immunostaining must be evaluated in aggregate and not for individual acini.

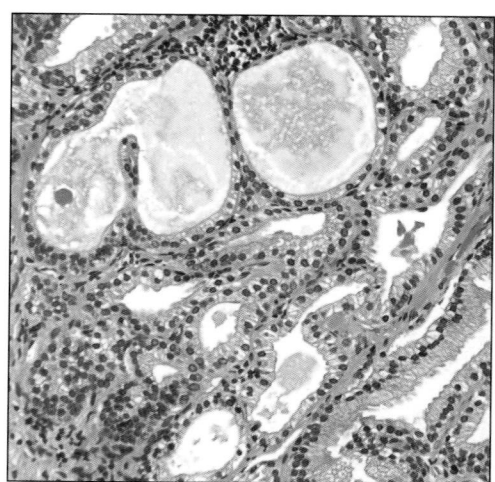
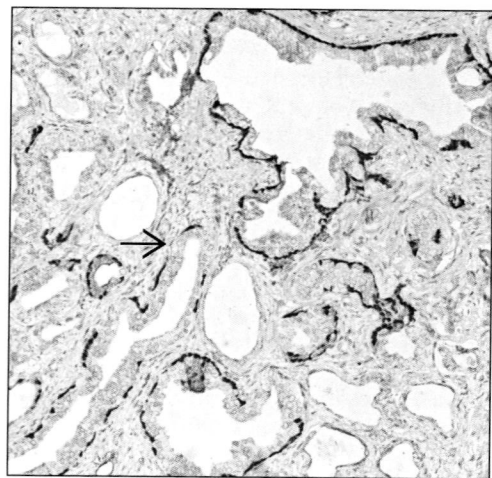

3

Microscopic and Immunohistochemical Features

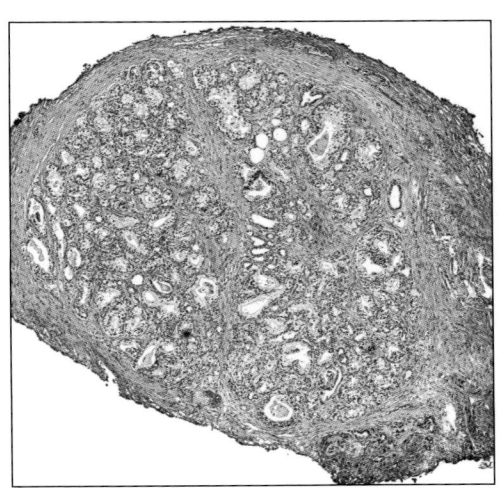
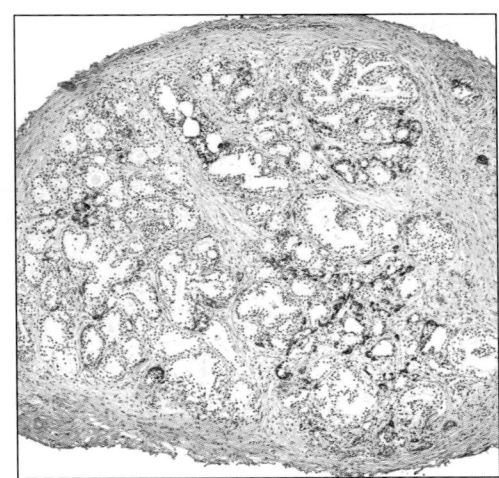

(Left) AAH in TURP chip shows well-circumscribed contour of the small acinar proliferation containing glands of variable size and shape. Most AAH are encountered in TURP specimens since the majority of these lesions arise in the transition zone. A low-grade prostate adenocarcinoma is the main differential diagnosis on low-power magnification. *(Right)* AAH shows patchy positivity with HMCK(34βE12), which is typical for this lesion.

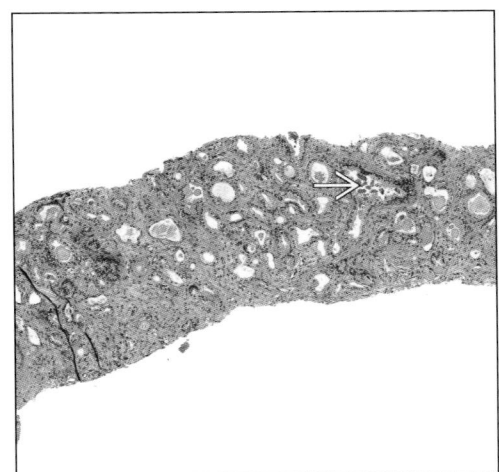
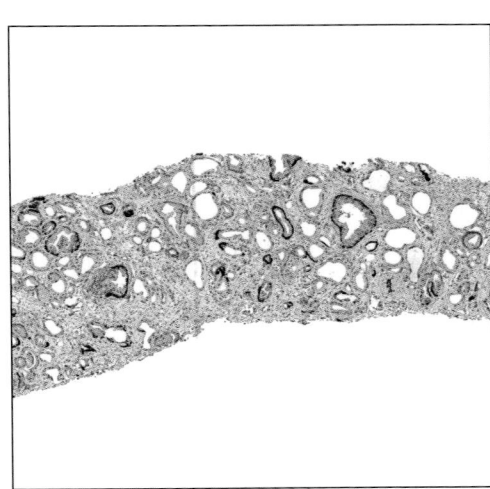

(Left) AAH in needle biopsy may pose a greater challenge in differentiating from cancer since the overall architecture is not appreciated. Small acinar architecture and discernible crystalloids ➡ raise concern for cancer. *(Right)* AAH stained with a triple cocktail shows patchy positivity with basal cell markers (brown) and only weak scattered AMACR (red) positivity. The diagnosis of cancer requires complete absence of basal cell staining in all glands within the suspicious focus.

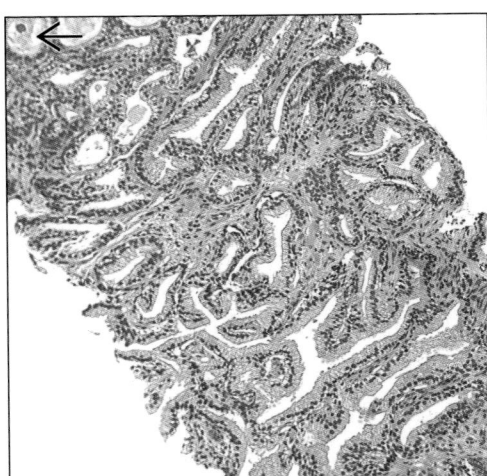
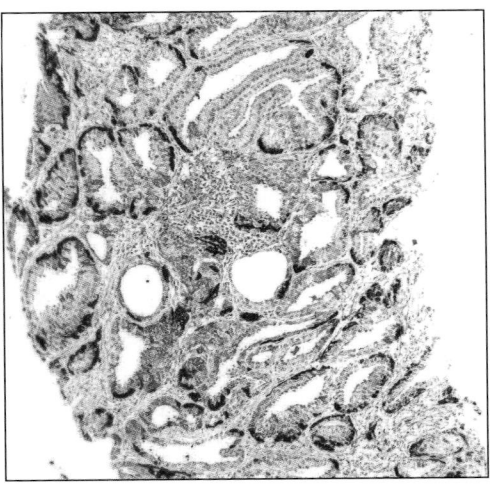

(Left) Crowded glands of AAH are shown, including large and small caliber acini. Note the presence of intraluminal proteinaceous material and a crystalloid ➡. *(Right)* Triple cocktail staining of AAH shows relatively strong AMACR (red) expression in some of the glands. The patchy staining for basal cells (brown) confirms the diagnosis of AAH. Up to 10% of AAH may stain diffusely with AMACR, and awareness of this pitfall is important in the diagnosis of AAH vs. cancer.

PROSTATIC INTRAEPITHELIAL NEOPLASIA

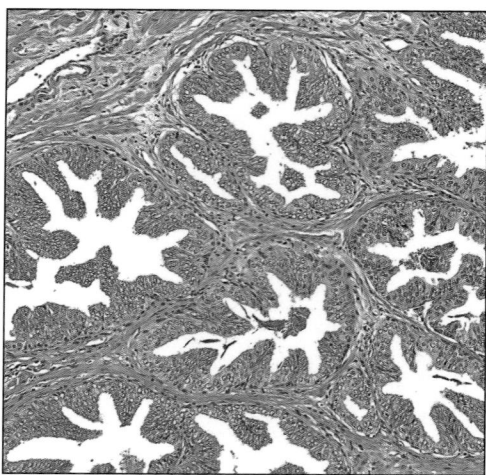

HGPIN shows large and medium-sized glandular structures, which appear expanded and crowded but retain their rounded contours. Basal cell layer in HGPIN is often discernible on H&E stained sections.

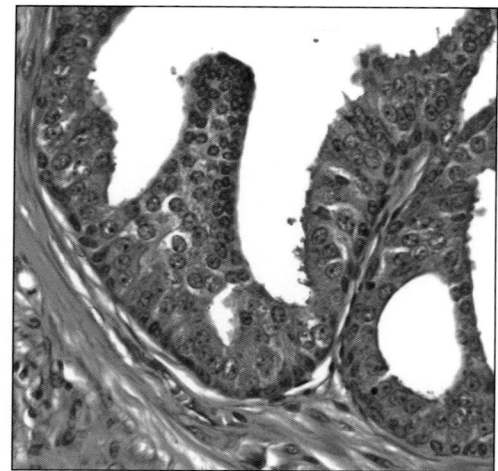

HGPIN lining cells display diagnostic cytologic features of nuclear enlargement, hyperchromasia, and prominent nucleoli. Presence of high-grade nuclei is the diagnostic hallmark of HGPIN.

TERMINOLOGY

Abbreviations
- Prostatic intraepithelial neoplasia (PIN)
  - PIN in routine surgical pathology terms usually refers to high-grade PIN (HGPIN)

Synonyms
- Prostatic duct dysplasia

Definitions
- PIN
  - Noninvasive neoplastic transformation of lining epithelium of preexisting prostatic ducts and acini, categorized into low-grade or high-grade PIN
- HGPIN
  - PIN characterized by severe nuclear atypia (as in carcinoma) and varied, including more complex, architectural patterns

ETIOLOGY/PATHOGENESIS

Genetics
- Provides evidence of association between HGPIN and prostate carcinoma (PCa)
- *TMPRSS-ERG* fusion
  - Seen in 19% of HGPIN intermingling with cancer foci vs. 48.5% for clinically localized PCa
- Aneuploid DNA seen in 32-58% of cases
- Nuclear morphometric studies show characteristics intermediate between cancer and benign glands
- Numeric alterations of chromosomes 7, 8, 10, 12, and Y common in both HGPIN and adenocarcinoma, though mean number higher in adenocarcinoma
- Deletions of chromosome 8p most common allelic loss, detected in both HGPIN and adenocarcinoma
- Increased expression of *p16*, *p53*, *AMACR*, *Bcl-2*, and *MYC* genes
- Hypermethylation of glutathionine S-transferase

CLINICAL ISSUES

Epidemiology
- Incidence
  - HGPIN is present as isolated diagnosis in up to 16% of needle core biopsies (usually 5-6%) and 1-5% in transurethral resection specimens
  - Present in 80-100% of prostate glands harboring adenocarcinoma vs. 43% of age-matched controls
- Age
  - May be seen beginning in 3rd decade of life
  - Incidence increases with age, reaching up to 67% by 8th decade
- Ethnicity
  - Lesion is usually more diffuse and presents earlier in African-Americans compared to Caucasians

Presentation
- Asymptomatic, commonly encountered as incidental histologic finding
- May have abnormal serum PSA level
  - Debatable if it is the cause of increased PSA; difficult to exclude undetected coexistent PCa

Treatment
- Surgical approaches
  - No aggressive treatment (i.e., surgery, radiation) is warranted with diagnosis of HGPIN, unless concomitant adenocarcinoma is documented
- Drugs
  - HGPIN has been studied as potential marker &/or target for chemoprevention of PCa
- Risk of cancer
  - Previously, diagnosis of HGPIN without PCa would prompt rebiopsy, as 50-60% of cases would have PCa in subsequent biopsy
  - Contemporary data, in era of extended sampling biopsy, has shown that median risk of cancer following diagnosis of HGPIN is around 21%

PROSTATIC INTRAEPITHELIAL NEOPLASIA

Key Facts

Terminology
- HGPIN: Noninvasive neoplastic transformation of lining epithelium of existing prostatic ducts and acini characterized by severe nuclear atypia

Etiology/Pathogenesis
- *TMPRSS-ERG* fusion seen in 19% of HGPIN

Clinical Issues
- HGPIN is present as isolated diagnosis in 4-16% of needle core biopsies and < 5% in transurethral resection specimens
- Present in over 80% of prostate glands harboring adenocarcinoma vs. 43% of age-matched controls
- Incidence increases with age, reaching up to 67% in 8th decade

- Median risk of cancer following diagnosis of HGPIN is around 21% in more recent series

Microscopic Pathology
- Preexistent ducts and acini are lined by crowded epithelial cells with abnormal cytologic features
  - Enlarged monomorphic nuclei, prominent nucleoli, hyperchromasia, nuclear overlap, amphophilic cytoplasm
- Preserved or discontinuous basal cell layer may be readily identified on H&E or only with basal cell specific immunostains
- 4 major architectural patterns: Tufted, micropapillary, cribriform, and flat
- Other uncommon types: Signet ring, mucinous, foamy, inverted or "hobnail," and small cell neuroendocrine

---

- This risk is not significantly different from risk following benign diagnosis (around 19%)
  - Thus, recommendations on follow-up of diagnosis of HGPIN are currently controversial
- Patients with multifocal HGPIN (i.e., > 3 cores), bilateral HGPIN, and that associated with ASAP have higher risk of harboring concomitant PCa, and should be more aggressively followed
- Other clinical or pathologic parameters do not appear to identify patients with higher risk of harboring PCa
- Rebiopsy technique
  - PCa is identified with higher frequency in or adjacent to quadrant where HGPIN was detected
  - However, up to 45% of PCas are found in another sextant
  - Incidence of detection of subsequent PCa in patients with isolated HGPIN increases when rebiopsy is performed at 1 and 3 years
  - On rebiopsy, sampling should include all sextants

IMAGE FINDINGS

Ultrasonographic Findings
- May be associated with hypoechoic lesion in peripheral zone

MACROSCOPIC FEATURES

General Features
- Not associated with recognizable gross findings

Sections to Be Submitted
- If only HGPIN (without invasive foci) detected in transurethral resection
  - Submit entire specimen for histologic evaluation or obtain deeper levels of block with HGPIN
  - Biopsy of peripheral zone may be an option, particularly in younger males
- If only HGPIN (without invasive foci) detected in prostate needle biopsy specimen

- May consider deeper levels if extensive or associated with atypical small acinar proliferation (ASAP)

MICROSCOPIC PATHOLOGY

Histologic Features
- Preexisting ducts and acini, usually of medium to large size, lined by crowded epithelial cells with abnormal cytologic features
  - Hyperchromasia
  - Nuclear overlap
  - Enlarged relatively monomorphic nuclei
  - Prominent nucleoli (easily observed at 20x magnification)
  - Amphophilic cytoplasm
  - Diagnostic threshold varies as some individuals require all cells to be atypical and others require at least 10% of cells to have prominent nucleoli
- Preserved or discontinuous basal cell layer may be readily identified on routine slides, or only with basal cell specific immunostains
- 4 major architectural patterns of HGPIN
  - **Tufted** (87%)
    - Stratification of acinar cells imparting luminal undulations or folds
  - **Micropapillary** (85%)
    - Nuclear stratification forming slender filiform projections and cellular budding
  - **Cribriform** (32%)
    - Complex intraluminal proliferation resulting in multiple irregular or round punched-out lumens
    - May show "cellular maturation," wherein peripheral cells show greater nuclear atypia (i.e., nucleomegaly, prominent nucleoli) than cells at luminal aspect
  - **Flat** (25%)
    - Lacks significant cellular stratification, composed of only 1 or 2 cell layers
- Other uncommon types
  - Signet ring
  - Mucinous

PROSTATIC INTRAEPITHELIAL NEOPLASIA

○ Foamy
○ Inverted or "hobnail"
○ Small cell neuroendocrine
- Multiple patterns may be seen concurrently
- Variety of other architectural and cytologic features may be observed in HGPIN
  ○ Luminal cytoplasmic blebs, epithelial arches, cellular trabecular epithelial bars, "Roman bridges," partial gland involvement, and basal cell layer disruption with glandular budding
    ▪ Uncommonly, large cystic gland pattern, involvement in nodular hyperplasia and mucinous metaplasia
- Variety of luminal features may be observed in HGPIN
  ○ Proteinaceous secretions, corpora amylacea, and exfoliated cells of PIN
  ○ Uncommonly, microcalcifications, and crystalloids; comedonecrosis is extremely rare

Predominant Pattern/Injury Type
- Neoplastic

Predominant Cell/Compartment Type
- Epithelial, glandular

Grade
- Low-grade PIN
  ○ Tufted or micropapillary pattern
  ○ Nuclear crowding, stratification, and irregular spacing
  ○ Mild nuclear enlargement, with inconspicuous to rare prominent nucleoli
  ○ Diagnostic reproducibility is very low and has questionable relationship to PCa
  ○ Should not be diagnosed in needle core biopsies, as management and significance is uncertain
- High-grade PIN
  ○ Cellular proliferation within medium to large glands
  ○ Increased basophilia or amphophilia readily detected at low power
  ○ Hyperchromasia, nuclear membrane irregularity, macronucleoli
  ○ Greater reproducibility among pathologists and more established relationship to concomitant or subsequent adenocarcinoma

ANCILLARY TESTS

Immunohistochemistry
- Basal cell markers (p63, HMCK[34βE12]) highlight intact or frequently discontinuous basal cell layer around involved ducts
- Due to discontinuous basal cell layer, these cells may not be apparent in particular plane of section, compounding differential diagnosis with PCa
- AMACR variably stains acinar cells (56-100%)
- PSA/PSAP(+) in acinar cells
- Neuroendocrine HGPIN(+) for synaptophysin &/or chromogranin

DIFFERENTIAL DIAGNOSIS

Prostate Central Zone Glands
- Show architectural complexity, including cribriforming and "Roman bridges," but lack nuclear changes of HGPIN

Seminal Vesicle/Ejaculatory Duct Epithelium
- No prominent nucleoli
- More pleomorphism than HGPIN
- Nuclear pseudoinclusions
- Degenerative nuclear atypia
- Intracellular coarse lipofuscin pigment

Prostate Glands with Reactive Atypia (Inflammation, Infarction, or Radiation)
- Diagnosis of HGPIN should require more stringent criteria or should be questioned in areas of infarction, inflammation, or in previously radiated glands
- Architectural features of HGPIN tend to be absent in mimics

Transitional Cell Metaplasia
- Multilayered cells or solid nests that lack typical patterns of HGPIN
- Uniform, smaller cells with nuclear grooves; secretory cell layer may be focally present

Benign Prostate Hyperplasia Nodule with Prominent Papillary Fronds
- Located in transition zone
- Architectural complexity but lack atypical cytology of HGPIN

Cribriform Hyperplasia
- Located in transition zone
- Frequently clear cytoplasm with no amphophilia
- Lack of nuclear changes of HGPIN

Atypical Basal Cell Hyperplasia
- Atypical nuclei are in basal and not secretory cells; usually patterns of HGPIN absent
- Frequently lumina are obliterated

Low-Grade Acinar Adenocarcinoma
- Small glands adjacent to glands involved by HGPIN may pose particularly difficult differential diagnosis
- May not be possible to determine whether small glands represent adjacent invasive adenocarcinoma or tangentially sectioned outpouching of HGPIN glands
- Immunostains are useful only if basal cells are demonstrated in small glands, indicating outpouching
- If no basal cells present, they still could represent HGPIN, as basal cell layer is frequently discontinuous or markedly attenuated
- Case diagnosed as HGPIN with atypical focus suspicious, but not diagnostic, for carcinoma

High-Grade Acinar Adenocarcinoma with Cribriform Pattern (Gleason Pattern 4 or 5)
- Greater architectural complexity, including consistent cribriforming, back-to-back glands, and solid nests
- Confluence of cribriform structures

3

- Absent basal cell layer with IHC

PIN-like Adenocarcinoma

- Some adenocarcinomas may have stratified epithelium and may form medium-sized glands
- Numerous atypical glands with absence of basal cell layer; may be associated with typical acinar pattern

Ductal Adenocarcinoma

- Commonly involves prostatic urethra and periurethral region; involvement may be diffuse
- Shows expansile large glandular pattern
- Papillae contain true fibrovascular stalks; maturation not present
- Nuclei frequently pseudostratified with elongated appearance; mitoses may be frequent
- Invasive features present, such as crowded back-to-back glands, stromal fibrosis, perineural invasion, extraprostatic extension
- Majority lacks basal cell layer confirmed by use of basal cell markers (p63 and HMCK[34βE12])

Basal Cell/Adenoid Cystic Carcinoma

- Basaloid-appearing cells with smaller nuclei with adenoid cystic pattern
- Basement membrane material may be present
- p63 &/or HMCK(34βE12)(+)
- Typically PSA/PSAP(-)

Urothelial (Transitional Cell) Carcinoma Involving Prostatic Ducts and Acini

- Significant cellular pleomorphism and mitotic activity within large glandular structures
- Cytoplasm is densely eosinophilic and may show squamoid features
- Pagetoid growth by neoplastic cells with elevation and preservation of normal secretory cells
- PSA or PSAP(-); p63, HMCK(34βE12) (+)

Intraductal Carcinoma of the Prostate

- Controversial nomenclature when it is exclusive finding in needle core biopsy
- Suggested to represent either intraductal or intraacinar spread of prostate carcinoma or intraluminal carcinomatous progression of HGPIN
- *TMPRSS-ERG* fusion more common in intraductal carcinoma than HGPIN
- Similar loss of heterozygosity seen with Gleason pattern 4 and 5 adenocarcinoma
- Multivariate analysis confirms independent prognostic value of intraductal carcinoma over Gleason grade, stage, tumor volume, and treatment failure
- Proposed criteria for diagnosing atypical intraductal lesions exceeding HGPIN but lacking features of invasive carcinoma include
  o Major criteria
    ▪ Large glands (> 2x normal), presence of basal cells (confirmed by immunohistochemistry), cytologically malignant cells with frequent mitosis, cells spanning gland lumen, comedonecrosis
  o Minor criteria

      ▪ Right angle gland branching, round smooth gland contour, frequently 2 population of cells
      ▪ Solid or extensive cribriform architecture
- Basal cell layer is present, similar to HGPIN; often continuous
- Without invasive foci, may be impossible to differentiate vs. HGPIN in limited biopsy material
- Limited number of cases with follow-up show that virtually all cases have invasive carcinoma only in rebiopsy
- Closely associated with large volume and high-grade invasive adenocarcinoma (Gleason pattern 4 or 5)

DIAGNOSTIC CHECKLIST

Pathologic Interpretation Pearls

- Screen for HGPIN on low-power magnification and confirm cytologic features on high-power view
- If cytologic threshold for diagnosis is doubtful or borderline, probably not HGPIN

REPORTING CONSIDERATIONS

Key Elements to Report

- Presence or absence of concomitant adenocarcinoma
- Number of biopsy cores involved by HGPIN
- Number of foci of HGPIN (e.g., isolated, focal, multifocal, extensive)

SELECTED REFERENCES

1. Singh PB et al: Risk of prostate cancer after detection of isolated high-grade prostatic intraepithelial neoplasia (HGPIN) on extended core needle biopsy: a UK hospital experience. BMC Urol. 9:3, 2009
2. Cohen RJ et al: A proposal on the identification, histologic reporting, and implications of intraductal prostatic carcinoma. Arch Pathol Lab Med. 131(7):1103-9, 2007
3. Perner S et al: TMPRSS2-ERG fusion prostate cancer: an early molecular event associated with invasion. Am J Surg Pathol. 31(6):882-8, 2007
4. Egevad L et al: Current practice of diagnosis and reporting of prostatic intraepithelial neoplasia and glandular atypia among genitourinary pathologists. Mod Pathol. 19(2):180-5, 2006
5. Epstein JI et al: Prostate needle biopsies containing prostatic intraepithelial neoplasia or atypical foci suspicious for carcinoma: implications for patient care. J Urol. 175(3 Pt 1):820-34, 2006
6. Bishara T et al: High-grade prostatic intraepithelial neoplasia on needle biopsy: risk of cancer on repeat biopsy related to number of involved cores and morphologic pattern. Am J Surg Pathol. 28(5):629-33, 2004
7. Wu CL et al: Analysis of alpha-methylacyl-CoA racemase (P504S) expression in high-grade prostatic intraepithelial neoplasia. Hum Pathol. 35(8):1008-13, 2004
8. Dawkins HJ et al: Distinction between intraductal carcinoma of the prostate (IDC-P), high-grade dysplasia (PIN), and invasive prostatic adenocarcinoma, using molecular markers of cancer progression. Prostate. 44(4):265-70, 2000
9. Bostwick DG et al: Architectural patterns of high-grade prostatic intraepithelial neoplasia. Hum Pathol. 24(3):298-310, 1993

PROSTATIC INTRAEPITHELIAL NEOPLASIA

Microscopic Features

(Left) Common patterns in HGPIN: Tufting (top left), micropapillary (top right), cribriform (bottom left), and flat (bottom right). It is not unusual for HGPIN foci in the same biopsy or rarely within the same gland to show different patterns. *(Right)* HGPIN shows nuclear enlargement, nuclear overlap, hyperchromasia, prominent nucleoli, and amphophilic cytoplasm. Prominent nucleoli in HGPIN can easily be observed at 20x magnification. Discontinuous basal cell layer ➡ is identifiable.

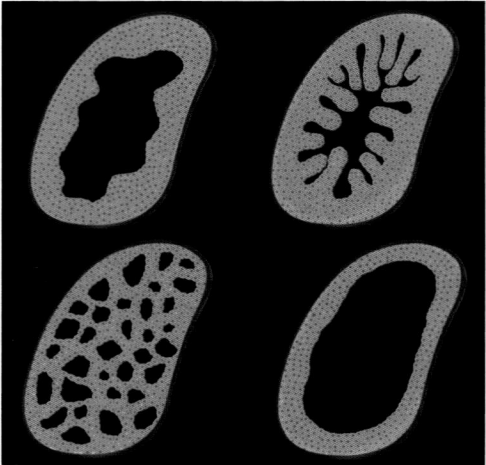
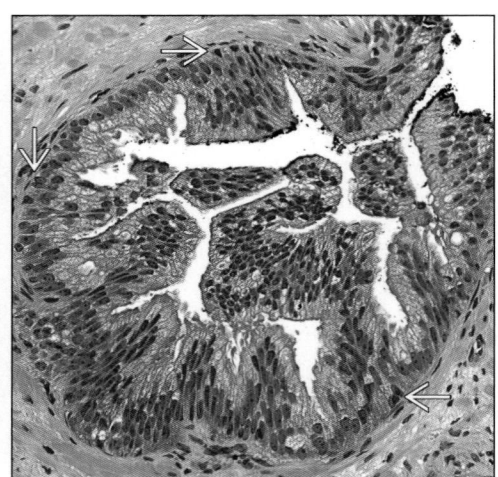

(Left) Tufted pattern of HGPIN shows stratification of acinar cells imparting luminal undulations or folds. These glands retain their rounded contour, and basal cell layer is discernible. *(Right)* High-power view of tufted HGPIN shows cellular stratification of acinar cells with overlapping, enlarged monomorphic and hyperchromatic nuclei. The tufts on the left side ➡ are more cellular and almost form micropapillations. Admixture of different architectural patterns in HGPIN is common.

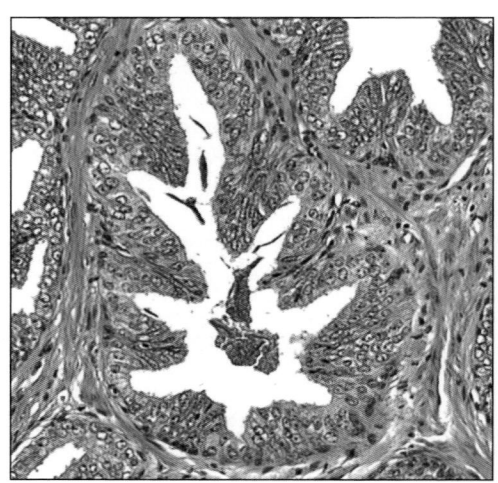
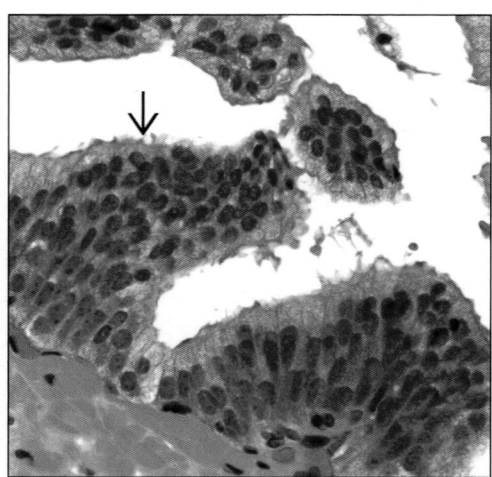

(Left) Micropapillary pattern of HGPIN shows stratification of acinar cells forming slender filiform projections. Detached cellular budding may be seen distally. The micropapillae of HGPIN lack a true fibrovascular core (pseudopapillae). Note prominent centrally placed nucleoli and a basal cell layer ➡ at the periphery. *(Right)* Micropapillary pattern of HGPIN shows slender papillae with cellular stratification of acinar cells containing overlapping nuclei and prominent nucleoli.

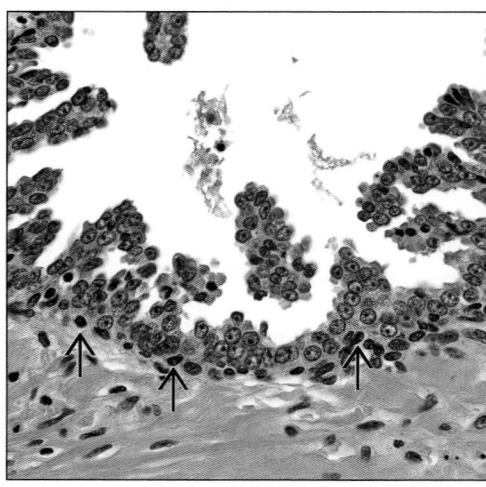
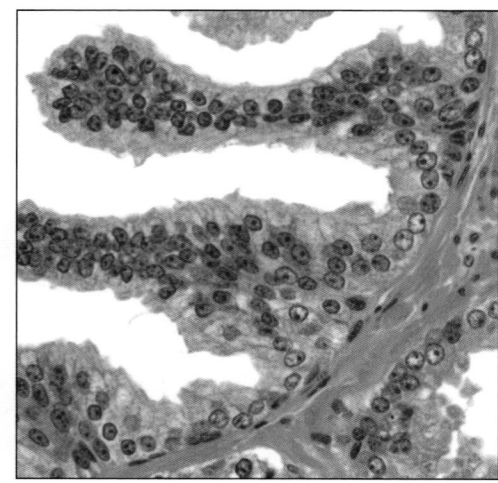

PROSTATIC INTRAEPITHELIAL NEOPLASIA

Microscopic Features

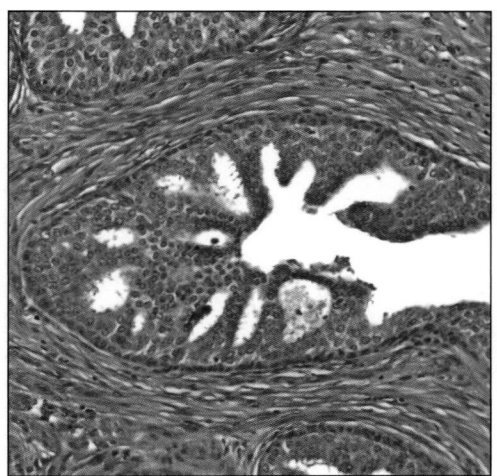

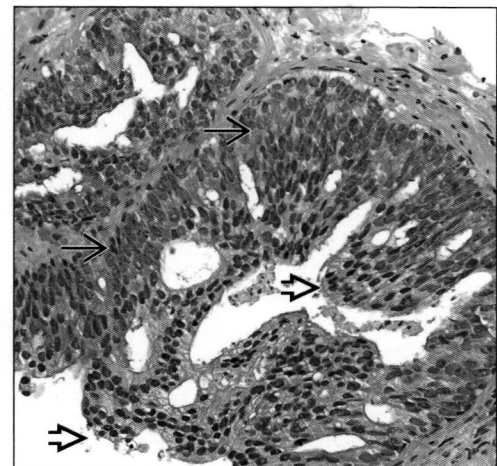

(Left) Cribriform pattern of HGPIN shows luminal cellular proliferation characterized by cribriform or "Roman bridges" resulting in the presence of multiple irregular or rounded lumens. The glands retain their rounded contours, and the basal cell layer is discernible. **(Right)** Cribriform pattern of HGPIN shows "cellular maturation," wherein the peripheral cells ⇒ show greater nuclear atypia (i.e., nucleomegaly, prominent nucleoli) than cells at the luminal aspect ⇒.

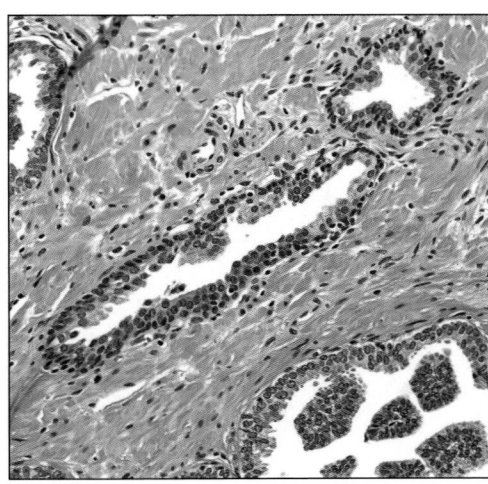

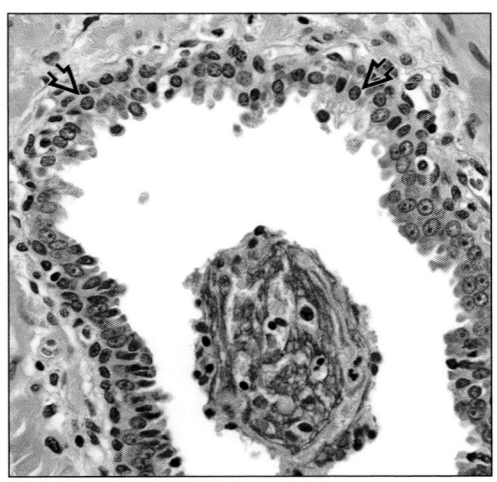

(Left) Admixture of glands show flat and micropapillary patterns of HGPIN. The flat pattern is the least common among the major architectural patterns of HGPIN. **(Right)** Flat pattern of HGPIN shows lack of significant cellular stratification, composed of only 1 or 2 cell layers. This gland is partially involved by HGPIN and shows the presence of normal-appearing acinar cells ⇒. The gland retains its rounded contour, and the basal cell layer is discernible.

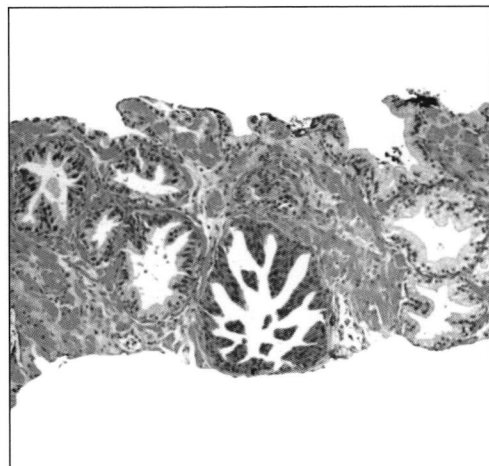

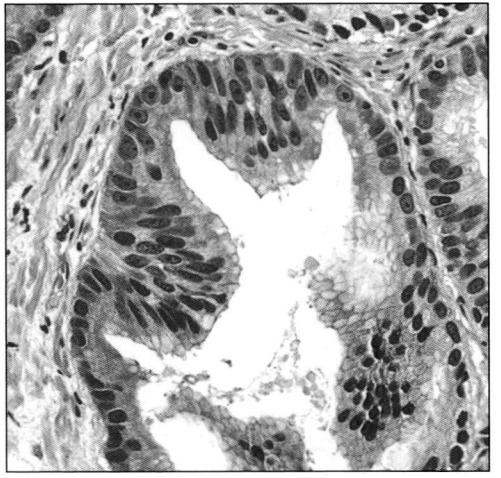

(Left) Needle biopsy with HGPIN. The glands should be screened at low power. HGPIN glands stand out from the surrounding benign glands due to their hyperchromasia. The nuclei reach the surface in stratified epithelium. **(Right)** Needle biopsy with HGPIN. The diagnosis is then confirmed on high-power examination, where nuclear enlargement and prominent nucleoli become evident. Despite the inconspicuous basal cells, the round contour and cellular maturation within the lumen indicate HGPIN.

PROSTATIC INTRAEPITHELIAL NEOPLASIA

Variant Microscopic Features

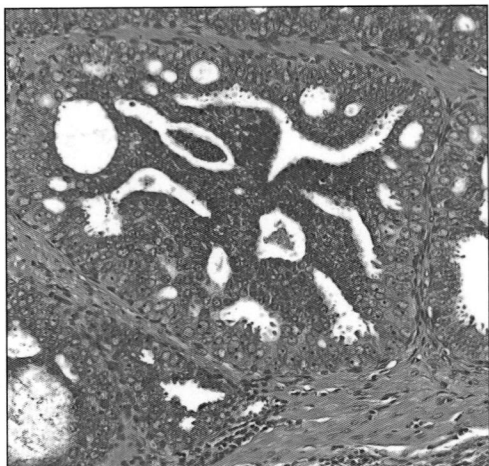
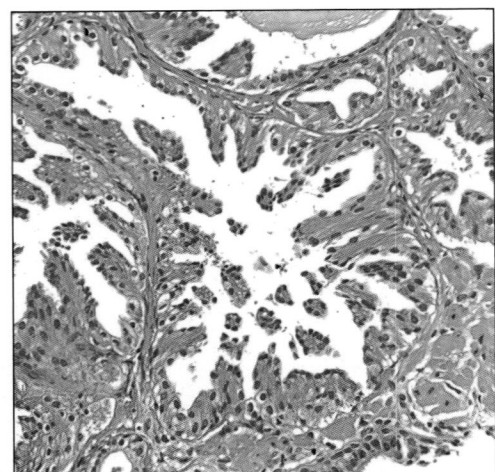

(Left) In this HGPIN with neuroendocrine features, note the population of small cells in the center of the lumen, reminiscent of small cell neuroendocrine carcinoma. This unusual variant expresses neuroendocrine markers, such as synaptophysin or chromogranin. *(Right)* "Hobnail" or inverted pattern of HGPIN is shown. Notice the location of the nuclei, which are toward the apical aspect of the luminal cells. The nuclei should display the classical high-grade cytologic features of HGPIN at higher power.

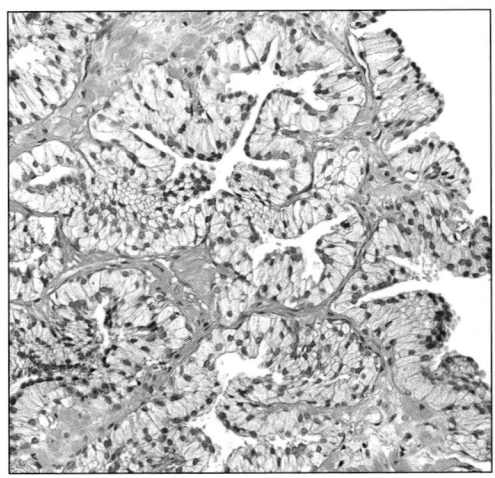
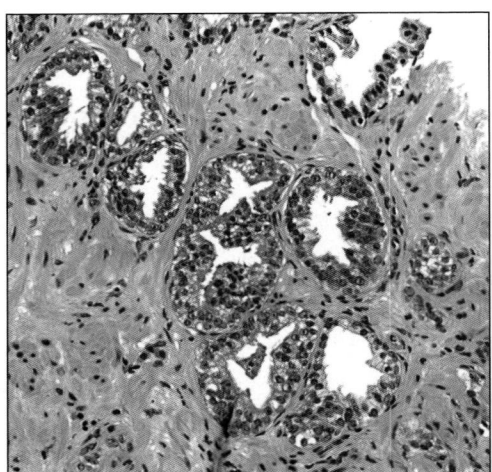

(Left) HGPIN with "hobnail" or inverted pattern with characteristic luminal alignment of nuclei. The glands with HGPIN additionally contain abundant foamy cytoplasm ("foamy gland" HGPIN). *(Right)* HGPIN may extend to involve smaller glands with lobular architecture. The resulting "small glandular" pattern should not be confused with acinar adenocarcinoma, as basal cells are preserved. This pattern of HGPIN may also be designated as flat pattern of HGPIN.

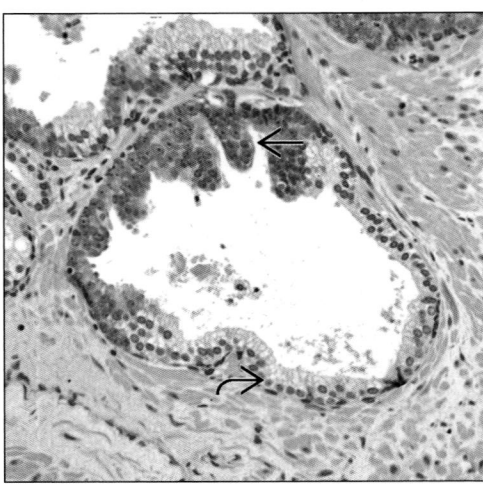
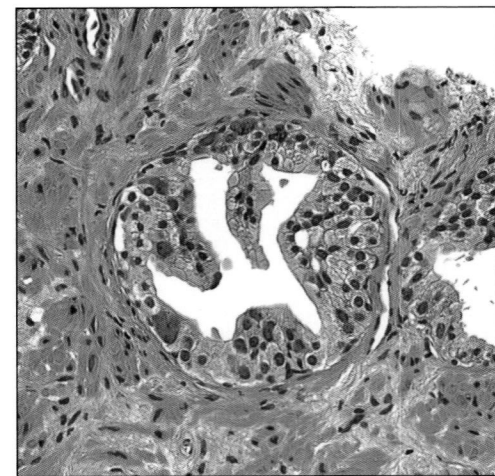

(Left) In partial involvement of a glandular structure by HGPIN, the gland is focally lined by cells displaying hyperchromasia, nuclear enlargement, & prominent nucleoli ⇒ compared to the cytologic features of the benign aspect of the gland ⇗. *(Right)* HGPIN may rarely show prominent nuclear pleomorphism. Isolated presence of pleomorphism may also be seen in seminal vesicle glands, & diffuse atypia should raise concern for intraductal growth of PCa & urothelial carcinoma.

PROSTATIC INTRAEPITHELIAL NEOPLASIA

Microscopic Features

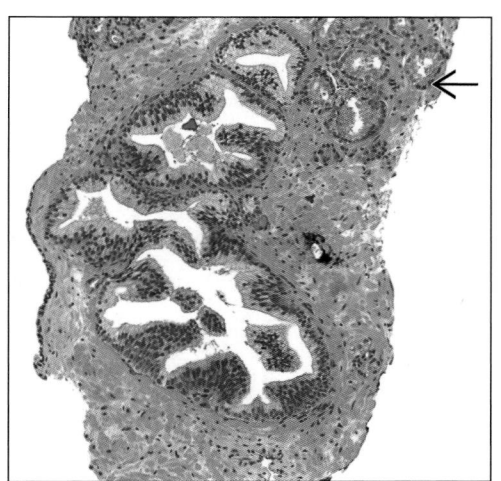

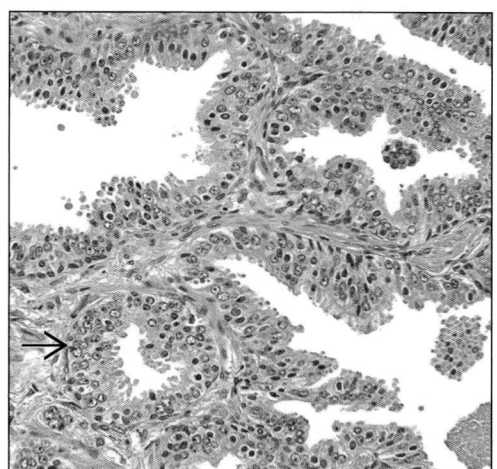

(Left) HGPIN is frequently associated with invasive carcinoma ➡. HGPIN is a large glandular proliferation with nuclear stratification, and carcinoma shows a small glandular proliferation of single cell type. *(Right)* Tangential sectioning of convoluted HGPIN glands may result in smaller glands adjacent to HGPIN ➡. These may be difficult to distinguish from an adjacent adenocarcinoma on H&E sections. Use of IHC may be helpful in this setting.

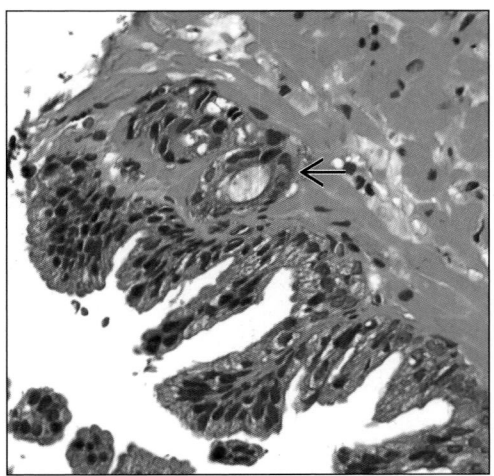

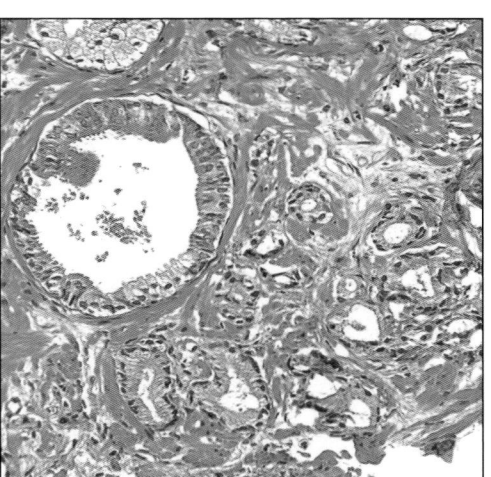

(Left) Occasionally, small glands ➡ adjacent to HGPIN may be too close and too few to ascertain whether they represent a focus of adenocarcinoma, adjacent acini involved by HGPIN, or tangentially sectioned outpouchings of convoluted HGPIN. Intraluminal mucin present in this rigid gland and absent in the HGPIN gland is helpful in supporting the diagnosis of carcinoma. *(Right)* A large gland with flat pattern of high-grade PIN shows admixture with small glands of PCa.

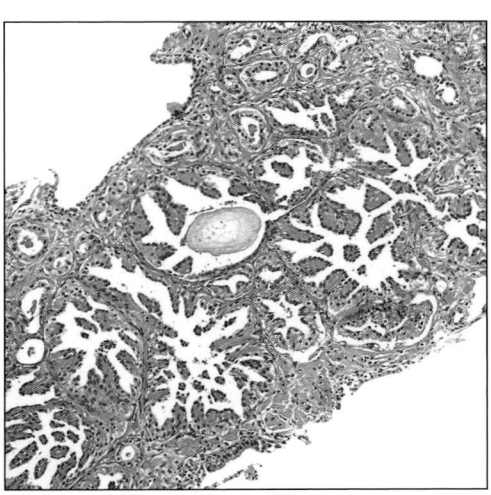

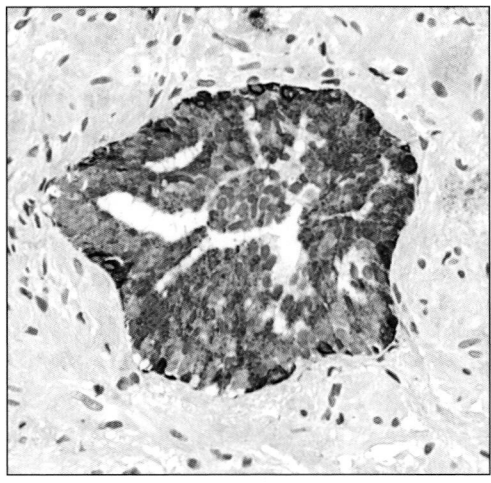

(Left) Inverted gland flat pattern of high-grade PIN is admixed with small glands of prostate carcinoma in needle biopsy. *(Right)* The innovative combination of HMCK(34βE12), p63, and AMACR or triple PIN cocktail has been invaluable in the difficult diagnosis of HGPIN vs. cancer. HGPIN frequently demonstrates a discontinuous but present basal cell layer (brown staining) and strong expression of racemase (red staining).

PROSTATIC INTRAEPITHELIAL NEOPLASIA

Immunohistochemical Features

(Left) HGPIN ⇥ is shown with smaller atypical glands ⇥. Without immunohistochemical support, it may be difficult to distinguish invasive carcinoma from outpouching of glands involved by HGPIN. *(Right)* Triple PIN cocktail confirms the diagnosis of HGPIN with no invasive cancer. The smaller glands ⇥ show strong AMACR expression (red), and the basal cell markers show patchy positivity (brown). Complete lack of basal cell staining in the suspicious focus is required for a cancer diagnosis.

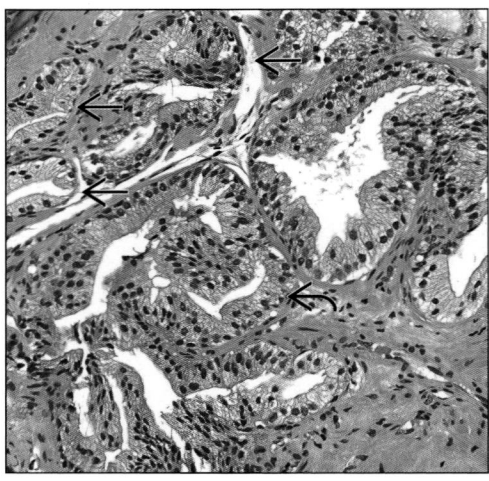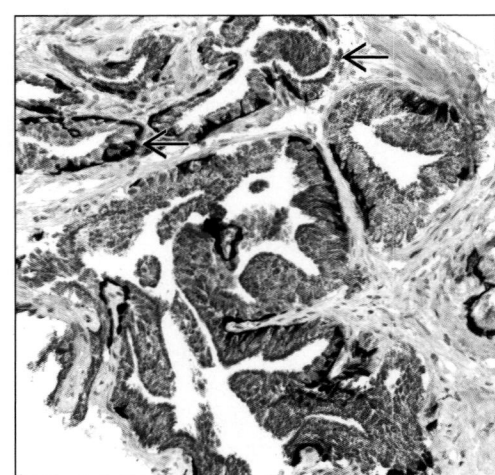

(Left) In this biopsy, the small glands ⇥ raise the possibility of invasive cancer or outpouching of glands involved by adjacent HGPIN. *(Right)* Triple PIN cocktail stain shows absence of a basal cell layer around the smaller glands, supporting a diagnosis of invasive cancer ⇥ adjacent to HGPIN. Other features that should be factored in to rule out outpouching include overall gland configuration and the spatial relationship with HGPIN. Deeper levels may also be helpful.

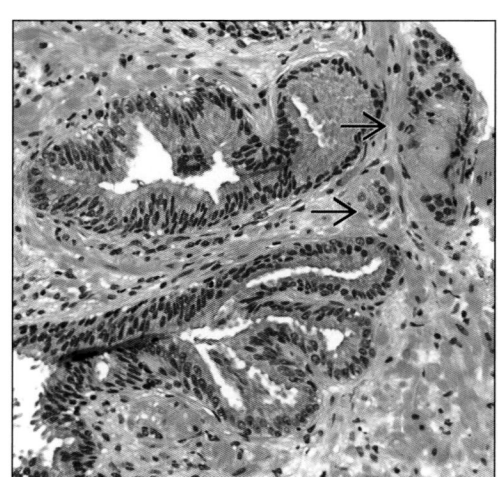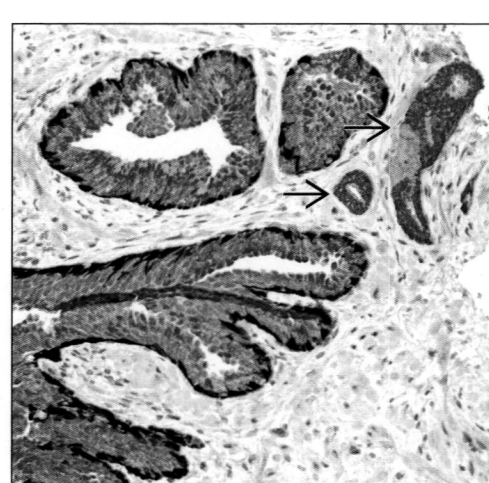

(Left) Needle biopsy shows an isolated focus of atypical large glands. It is difficult to differentiate whether this represents HGPIN or ductal adenocarcinoma. *(Right)* Triple PIN cocktail stain shows strong AMACR expression (red) with scattered basal cells (brown). This pattern may be seen in HGPIN and ductal adenocarcinoma with intraductal growth, hence this focus is not resolved by IHC. A diagnosis of "atypical glandular proliferation" is rendered with a comment.

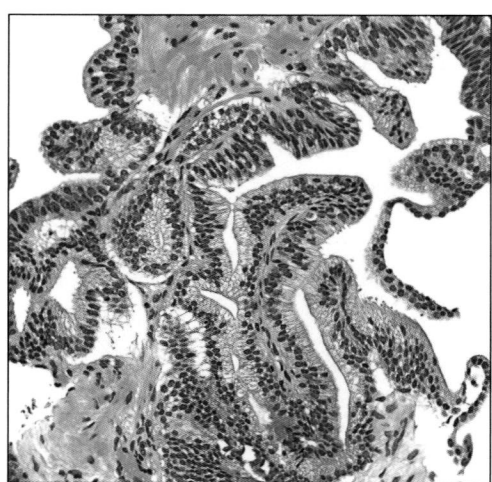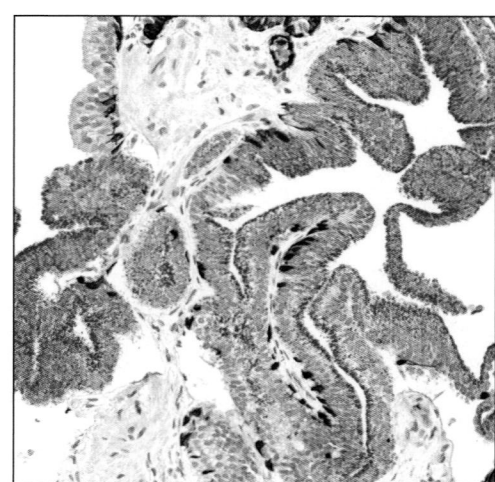

Differential Diagnosis - Intraductal Carcinoma of Prostate

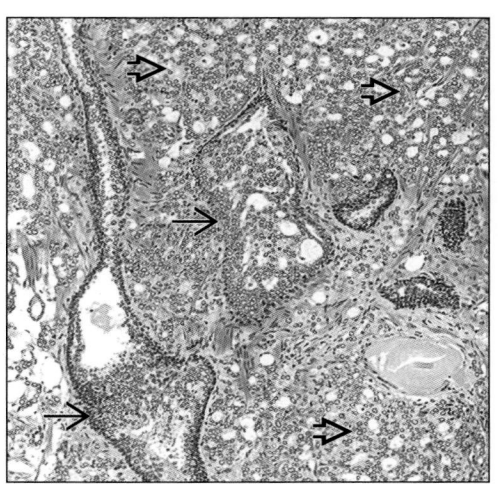

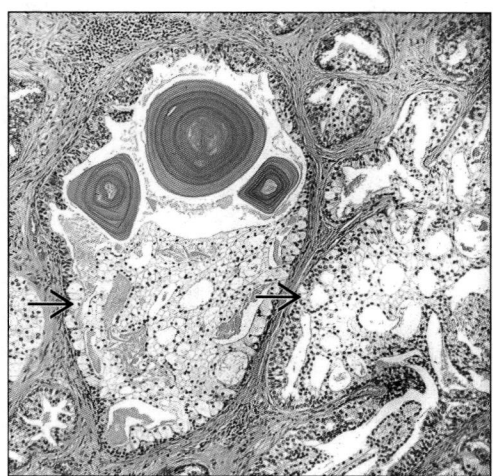

(Left) The terminology of intraductal carcinoma is controversial when seen in a needle biopsy. In this prostatectomy, within an area of invasive carcinoma ⊡, there is an intraglandular proliferation spanning the entire lumen of the ducts ⊡ with easily discernible basal cells indicating intraductal growth or extension of carcinoma. *(Right)* In this intraductal spread ⊡ by foamy gland carcinoma, the growth is usually associated in a prostatectomy with high-grade & high-volume disease.

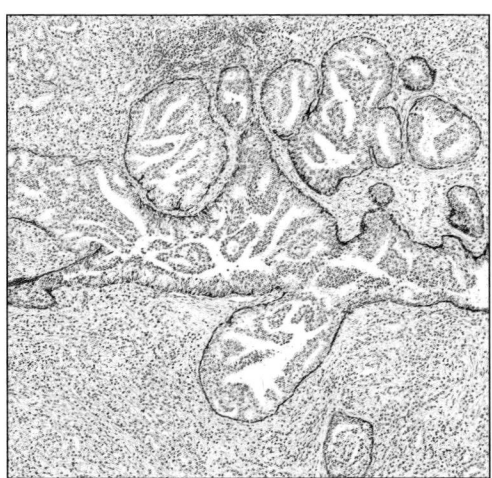

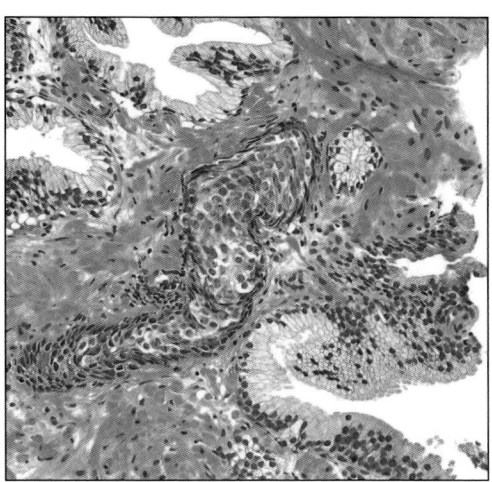

(Left) HMCK(34βE12) highlights the outline of the ducts and confirms the intraluminal proliferation of the high-grade carcinoma cells. The invasive cancer foci surrounding the large duct are negative. *(Right)* A needle biopsy shows a large solid gland completely filled by high-grade cells surrounded by a distinct basal cell layer. This focus likely represents intraductal growth of carcinoma and may be diagnosed as atypical glandular proliferation deserving a comment for rebiopsy.

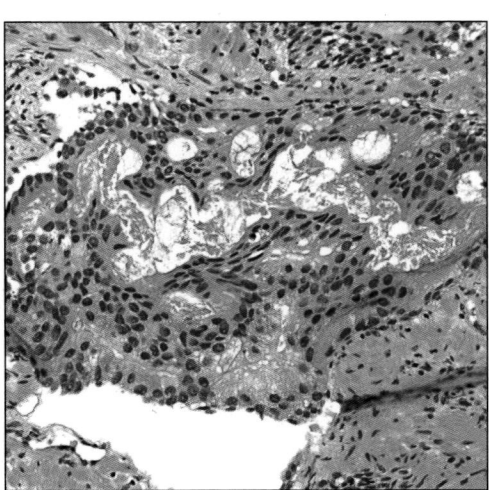

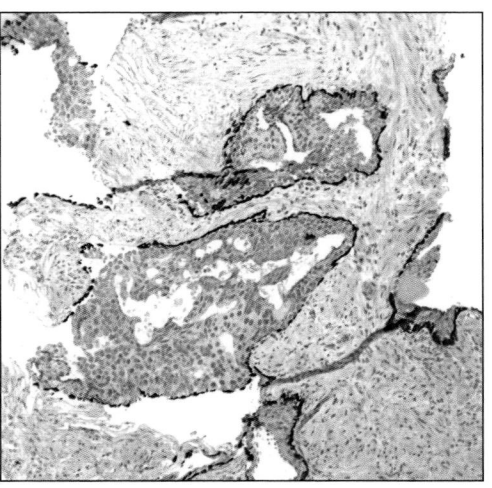

(Left) Needle biopsy shows a single atypical cribriform proliferation with mucin and high-grade cells. The features exceed HGPIN and raise the possibility of invasive carcinoma with cribriform features or intraductal growth. *(Right)* PIN cocktail stain confirms a basal cell layer. In the absence of invasive cancer elsewhere, this intraductal growth may be diagnosed as "atypical glandular proliferation" with a comment that this pattern is highly associated with carcinoma of high volume.

PROSTATE CARCINOMA, GENERAL CONCEPTS

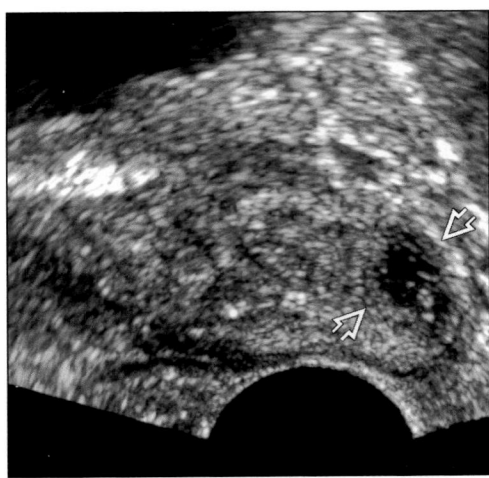

Longitudinal TRUS shows a small, hypoechoic lesion ➡ in the peripheral zone, confirmed as PCa by biopsy. A nodule of benign hyperplasia or infarction may also mimic PCa.

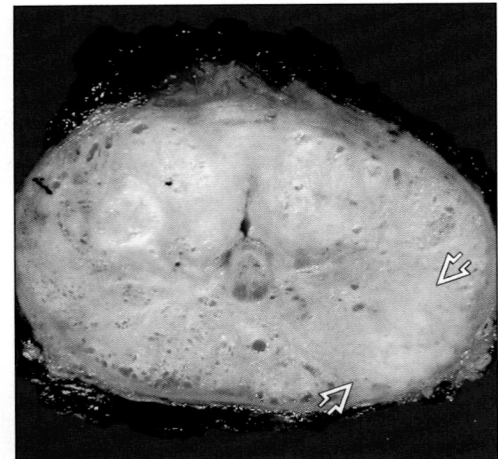

PCa shows a relatively dense, homogeneous solid area ➡ at the postero-lateral aspect of the peripheral zone. PCa most commonly occurs at this site. Most PCas are multifocal.

TERMINOLOGY

Synonyms
- Prostate carcinoma (PCa)

Definitions
- Term "prostate cancer/carcinoma" has been used for varying histologic subtypes
  - Acinar adenocarcinoma and morphologic variants
  - Ductal adenocarcinoma
  - Adenosquamous and squamous cell carcinoma
  - Basaloid and adenoid cystic carcinoma
  - Small cell carcinoma
  - Sarcomatoid (spindle cell) carcinoma
- However, ≥ 95% of PCas are acinar adenocarcinoma
  - Some authors use the term microacinar, acinar, or conventional to describe typical PCa
- Epidemiologic, pathogenetic, and clinical features of PCas mainly based on those of acinar adenocarcinoma

EPIDEMIOLOGY

Age Range
- Common in elderly men; low incidence in < 50 years
- Incidence increases dramatically with age; > 75% occur in patients ≥ 65 years
- Mortality from prostate cancer also increases with age
  - 3rd and 2nd cause of cancer death in ages 60-79 years and ages 80 years or older, respectively
  - Not one of top 5 causes of cancer mortality for ages 40-59 years

Incidence
- 6th most common cancer in the world
- Incidence varies in different parts of the world
  - Attributed to ethnic and environmental factors and detection rates of clinically latent tumors
- High incidence areas include USA, Australia, and Scandinavian countries

- In USA, prostate cancer is most common malignancy in men; 2nd most lethal after lung cancer
  - In 2009: 192,280 new cases of prostate cancer were expected in USA, and 27,360 men expected to die from disease
- Low incidence areas include Asia and North Africa
- Mortality rates
  - High in North America, North and West Europe, Australia, and Caribbean
  - Low in Asia and North Africa
  - Differences in mortality rates less marked than differences in incidence rates in different areas

Ethnicity Relationship
- In USA, African-Americans have highest incidence and mortality rates, up to 70% higher than Caucasians
- Lower rates in Asian-Americans than Caucasians
- Rate differences in ethnic groups also documented in other regions of the world, such as Brazil and Europe

Diet
- Strong positive association with diets rich in animal products, particularly red meat
  - Suggested to be due to heterocyclic amine content
- Weak association with obesity
  - Healthy weight and diet low in total fat associated with lower risk for prostate cancer
  - Fruits and vegetables may have protective effect

ETIOLOGY/PATHOGENESIS

General Concepts
- Migration studies demonstrate that immigrants from low incidence areas acquire intermediate-risk levels after migrating to high-risk areas
  - Suggests role for environmental and genetic factors
- Well-documented familial association
  - 5-11x increased risk among men with 2 or more 1st-degree relatives with prostate cancer
- Proposed higher risk with environmental exposures

PROSTATE CARCINOMA, GENERAL CONCEPTS

- ○ Cadmium, rubber, textile, chemical, drug, fertilizer, and atomic energy industries
- Vitamin D deficiency implicated and may explain geographic differences due to light exposure
- Controversial association with xenotropic murine leukemia virus-related virus (XMRV)

CLINICAL IMPLICATIONS

Clinical Presentation
- Majority of PCa in USA are clinically diagnosed in asymptomatic patients
  - ○ Tumor detected due to early detection programs
- Main indications for prostate biopsy
  - ○ Increased serum PSA level
  - ○ Abnormal digital rectal examination (DRE)
    - ▪ Palpable nodules, firmness, or asymmetry
    - ▪ Majority of prostate cancer (70-75%) arise in posterior zone, which is accessible by palpation
    - ▪ Low sensitivity and positive predictive value
    - ▪ Still considered "gold standard" in clinical staging of prostate cancer
- When symptomatic, prostate cancer presents with signs or symptoms of advanced disease
  - ○ Obstructive bladder symptoms
    - ▪ Transition zone cancers may present earlier
  - ○ Pelvic pain due to local extension
  - ○ Bone pain and tenderness, spinal cord compression, or adenopathy due to metastatic disease
  - ○ Rarely, disseminated intravascular coagulation, nonbacterial thrombotic endocarditis, ascites, or pleural effusion
- Paraneoplastic syndrome more common in certain carcinoma subtypes (i.e., small cell carcinoma)
- ~ 10% of transurethral resection of prostate (TURP) specimens for lower urinary tract obstruction contain incidental prostate cancer

Laboratory Tests
- Prostate specific antigen (PSA)
  - ○ Synthesized by secretory cells of normal, hyperplastic, or malignant prostatic acini and ducts
  - ○ Increased diffusion into serum when basement membrane is breached by invasive PCa
  - ○ Traditional cut off is 4 ng/mL, over which prostate biopsies are recommended
  - ○ PSA serum level above 4 ng/mL has sensitivity of ~ 20% and specificity of 60-70% for PCa
  - ○ Sensitivity in cancer detection increases with lower serum PSA cut-off
  - ○ Modifications of measurement and interpretation used to improve sensitivity and specificity
  - ○ PSA density
    - ▪ Serum PSA level/prostate gland volume
    - ▪ > 0.15 would prompt prostate biopsy
  - ○ Age-specific ranges
    - ▪ Higher PSA levels permissible in older age groups (e.g., 2.5 ng/mL for men 40-49 years vs. 6.5 ng/mL for men 70-79 years)
  - ○ PSA velocity
    - ▪ Relative change in time of PSA value
    - ▪ Increase of > 0.75 ng/mL per year would prompt prostate biopsy
  - ○ Percentage of free PSA
    - ▪ PSA not bound to serum protease inhibitors
    - ▪ Low levels (< 10%) associated with higher risk of cancer
  - ○ PSA levels useful in monitoring patients after therapy for prostate cancer
- National Comprehensive Cancer Network (NCCN) 2009 guidelines
  - ○ Perform biopsy for abnormal DRE regardless of serum PSA level
  - ○ Consider biopsy for PSA 2.6-4 ng/mL or PSA velocity ≥ 0.35 ng/mL/y when PSA ≤ 2.5 ng/mL
    - ▪ Also consider age, comorbidity, percent free PSA, prostate exam/size, family history, African-American race
  - ○ Prefer biopsy when PSA 4-10 ng/mL or do free PSA when risk of biopsy &/or diagnosis and treatment outweighed by comorbid conditions
    - ▪ Perform biopsy if free PSA ≤ 10%
  - ○ Perform biopsy when PSA >10 ng/mL
- American Urological Association (AUA) 2009 Best Practice Policy
  - ○ Baseline serum PSA level at 40 years old
  - ○ No single threshold value for PSA to prompt prostate biopsy is recommended
    - ▪ Decision based primarily on PSA and DRE, but other factors should be considered
    - ▪ Consider multiple factors: Free and total PSA, age, PSA velocity, PSA density, family history, ethnicity, prior biopsy history, and comorbidities
- Prostatic acid phosphatase (PAP)
  - ○ 1st serum marker used for prostate cancer
  - ○ Low sensitivity and specificity limit its role in prostate cancer diagnosis and monitoring
    - ▪ Also elevated in prostatic hyperplasia and inflammation
- Prostate specific membrane antigen (PSMA)
  - ○ Most informative in hormone-resistant states, metastasis, or in tumor recurrence or progression
- Molecular diagnostic tests
  - ○ Currently investigational
    - ▪ Clinical utility in prostate cancer diagnosis and management still to be confirmed
  - ○ May target PCa-associated proteins, mRNA, or DNA
    - ▪ High throughput gene expression profiling and proteinomics have identified genes and proteins specifically overexpressed in prostate cancer
  - ○ Candidate biomarkers include
    - ▪ Human kallikrein 2, urokinase-type plasminogen activator receptor, PSMA, early prostate cancer antigen, prostate carcinoma antigen 3, AMACR, GST-π, *TMPRSS2-ERG* gene fusions
  - ○ Performed in tissues, blood, or urine samples
  - ○ Use varying methods of detection, such as RT-PCR, ELISA, Western blot, or other techniques
  - ○ RT-PCR extremely sensitive assay, capable of detecting 1 prostate cell in 10^8 nonprostate cells
    - ▪ Limits clinical utility of this assay due to possible nonspecific positivity

3

Natural History

- PCa is biologically heterogeneous and some present clinically as "latent" or "quiescent" tumors
  - Latent form PCa extremely common; up to 80% of PCa in 9th decade
  - Unclear whether latent tumors are intrinsically different from clinically significant tumors
- Natural history of nonlatent PCa highly dependent on stage at presentation

Imaging Findings

- Radiographic studies
  - As ancillary tool in diagnosis of primary tumors
  - More useful for staging and detection of metastases
    - Bone scan performed for localized disease with PSA > 20 ng/mL, Gleason score (GS) ≥ 8, or symptomatic T3 or T4 disease
    - Osteoblastic bone metastasis for acinar carcinoma
    - Pelvic CT or MR performed for T3 or T4 disease or in localized cancer with high nomogram probability for lymph node involvement
  - In PSA era of lower stage prostate cancers, false-positivity higher in detecting metastases
    - Staging imaging studies not routinely recommended if GS < 7 or PSA < 20 ng/mL
- Ultrasonography
  - Transrectal ultrasound (TRUS) mainly to guide needle core biopsy sampling
  - Also to measure prostate gland volume and to estimate prostate cancer size
  - Low sensitivity and specificity
    - Most prostate cancers are hypoechoic lesions (40%) but can be hyper- (30%) or isoechoic (30%)
    - Organ-confined prostate cancer isoechoic with prostate parenchyma are difficult to detect
    - Not satisfactory in predicting extraprostatic extension (EPE)

Predictive Tables and Nomograms

- Clinical tool integrating several clinicopathologic variables to predict prostate cancer progression
- Preoperative total serum PSA, GS, and clinical stage predictive of prostate cancer stage at radical prostatectomy (RP)
- Several pre- or post prostatectomy models are proposed
  - Documentation of key prognostic variables from biopsy or RP specimens crucial
    - e.g., GS (primary, secondary, and sum), cancer volume, EPE, margins, seminal vesicle invasion, lymph node involvement

REPORTING CRITERIA

Key Elements to Report

- **Gleason grade**
  - 1 of the most powerful prognostic indicators in PCa; widely used in planning therapy
  - High GS (7-10) associated with worse prognosis than GS 5-6, which has lower progression rates
  - In needle core biopsies
    - Correlates with findings at RP (e.g., stage, Gleason score, tumor volume, and margin status)
    - Correlates with outcome after RP, radiotherapy, and other treatments, such as cryotherapy and neoadjuvant therapy, or no treatment
    - GS 7, 4 + 3 portends poorer prognosis than 3 + 4
    - Predictive value of GS enhanced when combined with PSA level and DRE findings
  - Integral component of predictive nomograms and tables and latest 2009 TNM stage groupings for PCa
- **Tumor quantity**
  - Tumor volume in needle core biopsy
    - Studies show correlation with RP stage, tumor volume, GS, margin status, neurovascular bundle involvement, and post-treatment progression
    - Small amount of tumor in biopsy is not always indicative of small tumor volume in RP
    - Recommended to report as number of positive cores and estimated proportion (percentage) &/or linear extent of tumor in millimeters
    - Optional to report positive core with greatest tumor percentage
  - Tumor volume in TURP
    - Should always be reported, as tumor volume is determinant of substaging T1 in TURP
    - Should report number of involved chips and ratio or percentage of involved to total chips
  - Tumor volume in RP and subtotal prostatectomy
    - Studies show correlation with disease progression; although inconsistently as independent factor
    - Percentage of tumor involvement may be estimated by visual inspection
    - Size of dominant tumor nodule may be provided in 2 measured dimensions &/or by number of blocks involved over total number of blocks
- **Extraprostatic extension (EPE)**
  - Preferred term over "capsular penetration" since prostate does not have true capsule
  - Reported in 36% of prostatectomy specimens
  - Definitions
    - Tumor involvement of fat; intraprostatic fat exceedingly rare
    - In cases with no direct contact to fat, tumor seen in loose connective tissues in plane of fat
    - Peri-/intraneural invasion within or in plane of fat
  - Amount of fat varies with paucity of fat in apex, anterior part of prostate, or base
    - EPE in these 3 regions suggested as tumor outside glandular confines of prostate
    - Rarely, fat may be seen around apex
  - Comment on extent and if positive margin at site of EPE; location is optional
  - EPE descriptors
    - "Focal EPE": Tumor extension < 1 high-power field and not in > 2 sections
    - "Nonfocal or established EPE": More extensive tumor spread
    - Size estimate is optional; greatest linear dimension ± number of blocks involved
  - Comment of EPE may be made in needle biopsy or TURP showing fat involvement by tumor

PROSTATE CARCINOMA, GENERAL CONCEPTS

- ○ Involvement of striated muscles (anterior or apex) &/or ganglion cells alone does not constitute EPE
- **Margin status**
  - ○ "Positive" if tumor cells touch the ink; report extent of positive margin in mm
  - ○ Positive margin reported in 16-41% of RP
  - ○ Should report location of positive margin
    - ▪ Most common in posterolateral aspect of prostate
  - ○ 2 types of positive margins
    - ▪ Iatrogenic or capsular incision (pT2+ or pT2x): Tumor transected within prostate
    - ▪ Noniatrogenic: Tumor transected at EPE
  - ○ Higher progression-free probability with negative (81-83%) than positive (58-64%) RP margin
  - ○ Reporting size, focality (unifocal or multifocal), and presence of benign glands at margin is optional
- **Perineural invasion (PNI)**
  - ○ Defined as presence of prostate cancer juxtaposed intimately along, around, or within a nerve
  - ○ Most studies have shown prognostic significance in univariate analysis only
  - ○ Some studies suggest strong correlation of PNI in biopsy with EPE on RP
  - ○ PNI present in fat is considered as EPE
  - ○ PNI ubiquitously present in RP; reporting not mandated
  - ○ PNI in a needle biopsy has been correlated with recurrence after radiation therapy
    - ▪ Reporting status of PNI in a biopsy is optional; recommend reporting if present
- **Lymphovascular invasion (LVI)**
  - ○ Several studies have shown LVI as independent predictor of disease progression
  - ○ Reporting of LVI in RP is required
- **Seminal vesicle (SV) invasion**
  - ○ Defined as PCa involving muscular wall of SV
  - ○ 3 mechanisms of SV involvement by PCa
    - ▪ Direct spread along ejaculatory duct tissue into SV
    - ▪ Direct extra- or intraprostatic spread into SV
    - ▪ Noncontiguous metastasis to SV
  - ○ Portion of SV may be intraprostatic; only extraprostatic SV involvement should be considered
  - ○ Should note SV involvement in needle biopsy
    - ▪ Caution not to overinterpret ejaculatory duct involvement as SV invasion
    - ▪ SV has thick muscular wall, not present in ejaculatory duct
- **High-grade prostatic intraepithelial neoplasia (HGPIN) and atypical small acinar proliferation (ASAP)**
  - ○ HGPIN or ASAP are predictive of subsequent cancer in 21-31% and 40-50% of patients, respectively; prognostic significance being questioned
  - ○ Extent of HGPIN on biopsy is more predictive of subsequent cancer
  - ○ Reporting of HGPIN optional in biopsy, and RP is optional when PCa is present

STAGING

General Principles
- American Joint Committee on Cancer (AJCC) Tumor-Node-Metastasis (TNM) universally accepted staging for prostate cancer
  - ○ Criteria for pathologic (pT) staging starts at pT2 on RP specimen
  - ○ If biopsied tumor is not resected and highest T,N,M can be confirmed histologically, criteria for pT staging is fulfilled without removal of tumor
  - ○ Latest major change in AJCC anatomic stage/prognostic groups incorporate PSA level and GS in addition to TNM stage
    - ▪ Influenced by increasing application of predictive nomograms that use these variables

T1
- Clinically inapparent tumor; requires combination of clinical, imaging, and histologic evaluation
  - ○ Incidental tumors often encountered in TURP or cystoprostatectomy specimens
  - ○ ~ 10% of TURP contain incidental cancer; divided into pT1a (< 5%) or pT1b (> 5%)
  - ○ May provide pT1 stage if clinical (i.e., asymptomatic) and imaging (i.e., negative) findings known

pT2
- Organ-confined tumor, subdivided by extent of prostate involvement by tumor
  - ○ No evidence of prognostic significance for these subdivisions; to be validated with future data
  - ○ Subdivisions act as surrogate for estimating prostate cancer volume, which correlate with disease relapse

pT3
- EPE
- SV invasion
- Microscopic bladder neck invasion
  - ○ Recently shown to have similar prognosis to EPE by cancer; change in latest TNM staging (7th edition)

pT4
- Extension to adjacent organs other than SV; staging not assessable with RP specimen only

SELECTED REFERENCES

1. Andriole GL et al: Mortality results from a randomized prostate-cancer screening trial. N Engl J Med. 360(13):1310-9, 2009
2. Greene KL et al: Prostate specific antigen best practice statement: 2009 update. J Urol. 182(5):2232-41, 2009
3. Jemal A et al: Cancer statistics, 2009. CA Cancer J Clin. 59(4):225-49, 2009
4. Schröder FH et al: Screening and prostate-cancer mortality in a randomized European study. N Engl J Med. 360(13):1320-8, 2009
5. Srigley JR et al: Protocol for the examination of specimens from patients with carcinoma of the prostate gland. Arch Pathol Lab Med. 133(10):1568-76, 2009
6. Srigley JR: Key issues in handling and reporting radical prostatectomy specimens. Arch Pathol Lab Med. 130(3):303-17, 2006

PROSTATE CARCINOMA, GENERAL CONCEPTS

Prostate Cancer Staging

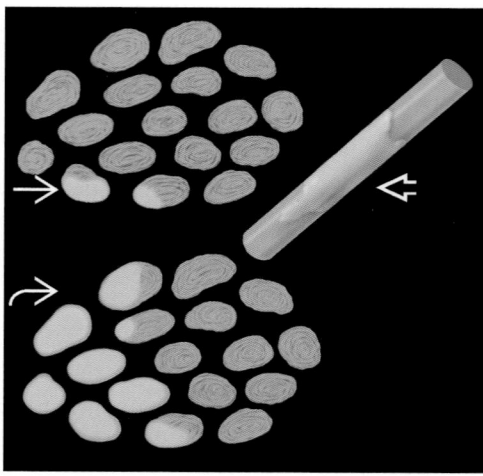
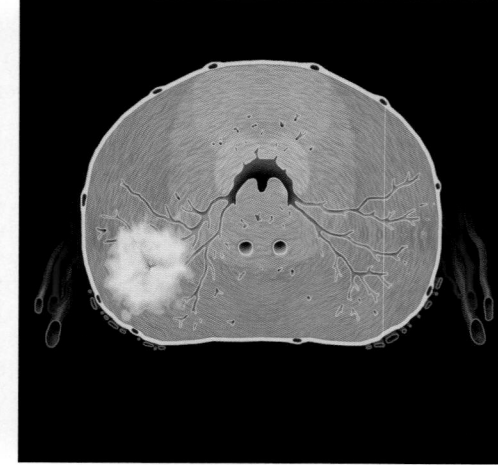

(Left) This graphic shows examples of incidental T1 PCa divided into T1a, < 5% tumor in tissue resected (TURP) ➡; T1b, > 5% tumor in tissue resected (TURP) ➡, and T1c, tumor identified by needle biopsy (e.g., because of elevated PSA) ➡. If unsuspected PCa is identified in tissue submitted and is < 5%, then remainder of tissue should be submitted for histologic evaluation. *(Right)* pT2a shows tumor involving not more than half of 1 lobe of the prostate.

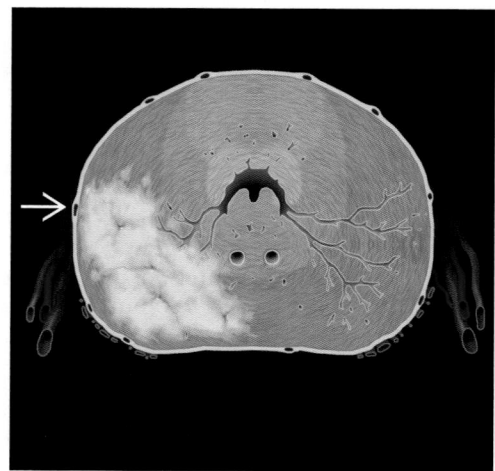
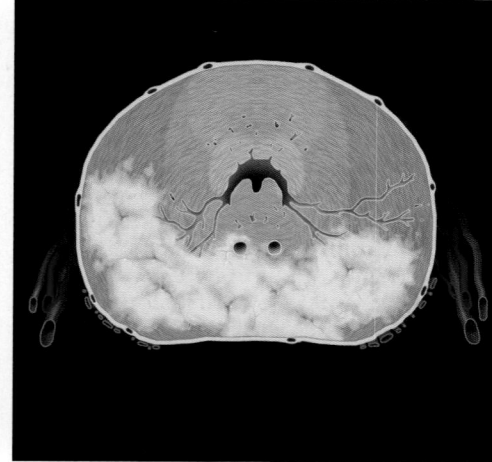

(Left) pT2b shows tumor involving more than half ➡ of 1 lobe of prostate. This pattern of tumor involvement is uncommon, since PCa is usually located at the posterior aspect and larger tumors tend to involve bilateral posterior sides (pT2c), even without anterior involvement. *(Right)* pT2c shows organ-confined tumor involving both lobes of prostate. pT2 subdivisions may act as surrogate for estimating PCa volume, which correlates with disease relapse.

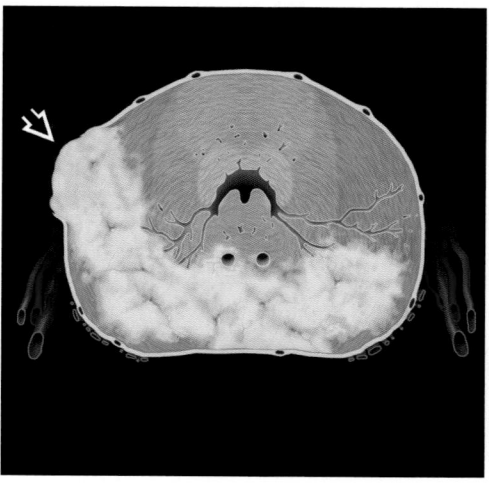
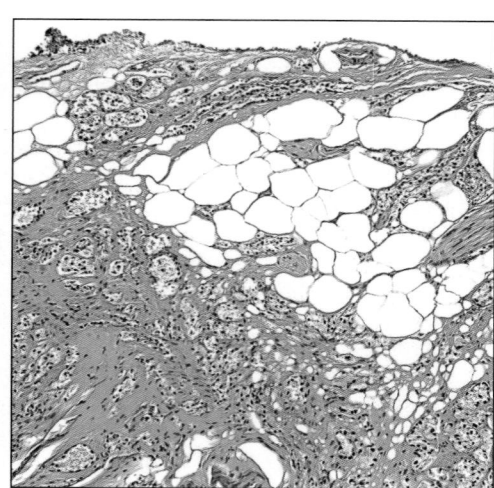

(Left) EPE ➡ by PCa indicates pT3 disease. Detection of EPE is most reliably made by histologic examination. DRE and radiographic studies are not sensitive in detecting EPE. Up to 36% of RP have EPE. *(Right)* EPE with tumor extension into periprostatic fat is shown, which is the most objective evidence for EPE. Intraprostatic fat is vanishingly rare, thus fat involvement by PCa is considered diagnostic for EPE. EPE most commonly occurs at posterior and postero-lateral aspects of prostate.

Prostate Cancer Staging

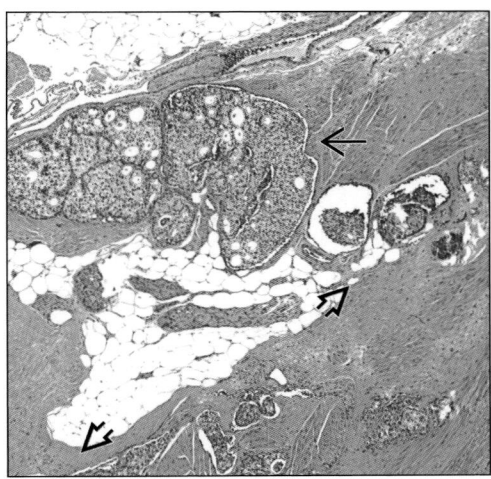

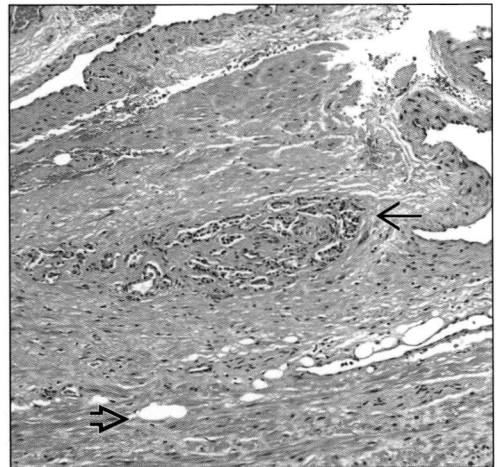

(Left) EPE of PCa ⇥ shows tumor involvement of connective tissues beyond the plane of fat. EPE may not directly involve adipocytes, and diagnosis of EPE is made if tumor involves connective tissues or nerves outside the plane contiguous with internal boundary of adipocyte clusters ⇥. *(Right)* Focal EPE shows focus of PCa ⇥ beyond internal plane of fat ⇥. Focal EPE is defined as tumor extension < 1 high-power field in no more than 2 sections.

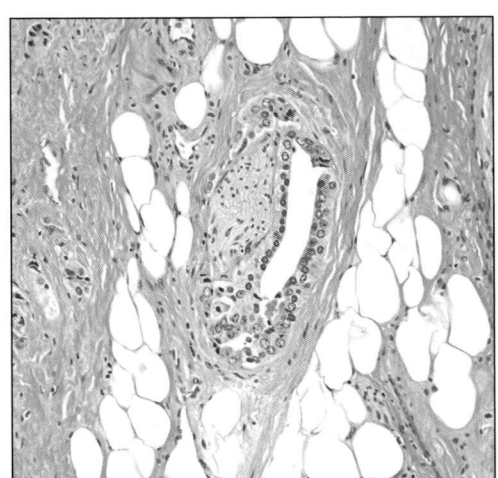

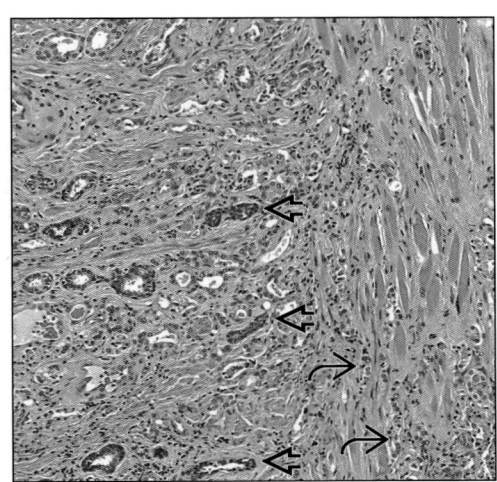

(Left) EPE by PCa shows perineural invasion within plane of fat. Periprostatic fat may not be present in up to ~ 50% of RPs. Without fat, EPE is determined when tumor protrudes and disrupts the normal rounded contour of prostate observed on scanning magnification. *(Right)* PCa glands are seen involving striated muscle at anterior aspect of prostate. There is paucity of fat anteriorly, and EPE may be considered if PCa ⇥ is beyond the normal glandular extent of prostate ⇥.

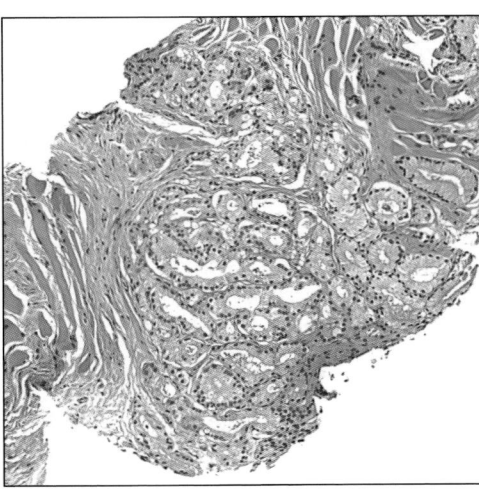

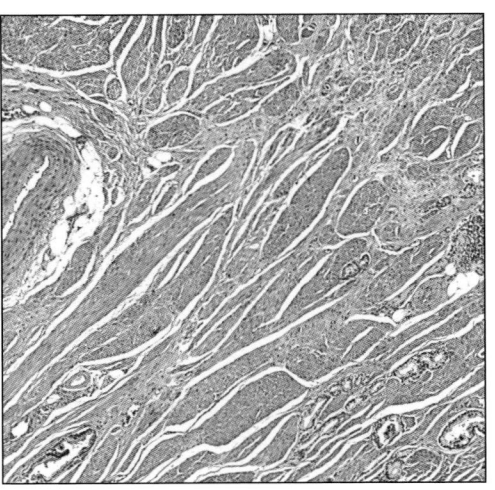

(Left) Apical prostate biopsy shows PCa involving striated muscle. Striated muscle may be seen at the anterior prostate and apex. Benign prostatic glands may extend into striated muscle, thus involvement of striated muscle by PCa does not necessarily constitute EPE. *(Right)* Microscopic involvement of bladder neck shows PCa involving large smooth muscle bundles. Microscopic bladder invasion portends a prognosis similar to SV invasion and is recently recategorized as pT3.

PROSTATE CARCINOMA, GENERAL CONCEPTS

Prostate Cancer Staging

(Left) Positive margin shows PCa transected at EPE ⇨. This suggests lack of complete excision of extraprostatic tissue around EPE. EPE is determined by bulge in desmoplastic tissues beyond fat ⧁. *(Right)* Positive margin shows PCa transected within the prostate parenchyma (pT2+ or pT2x). This type of positive margin most often occurs at the posterolateral aspect of prostate where parenchyma is inadvertently transected during dissection of the neurovascular bundle for potency sparing.

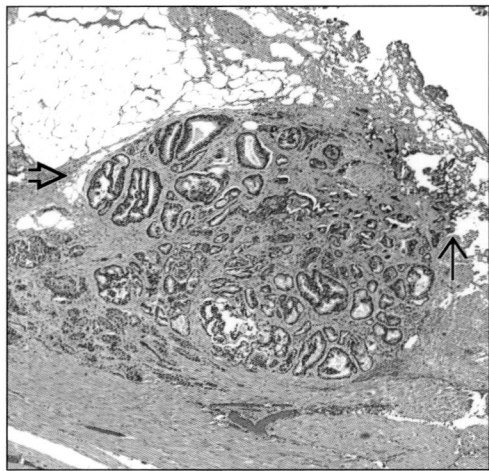
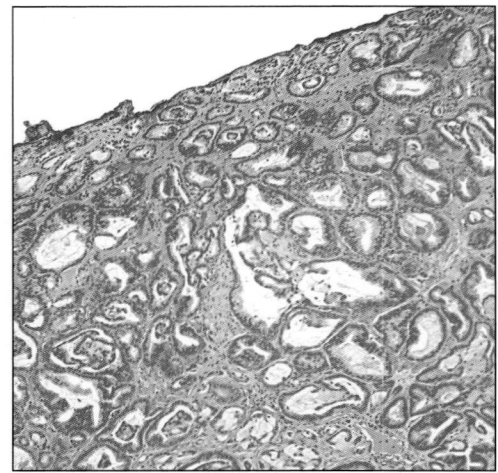

(Left) Mechanisms of SV involvement by PCa includes spread via (a) ejaculatory duct tissue into SV (green), (b) direct extra- (blue) or intraprostatic (red) spread into SV, or (c) noncontiguous metastasis to SV (purple). *(Right)* PCa involving ejaculatory duct (ED) shows tumor adjacent to ED epithelium. PCa may extend to SV via invasion through the wall and not within the lumen of ED. SV invasion is considered only when there is involvement of SV muscular wall.

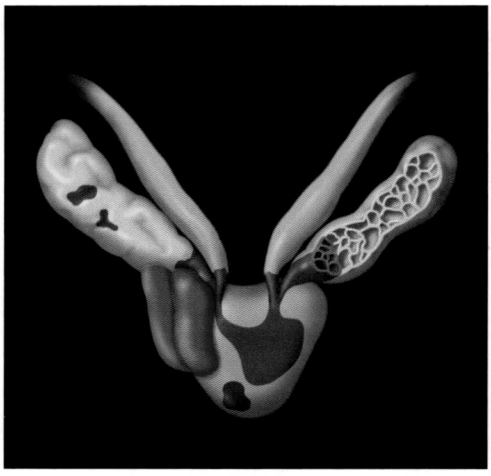
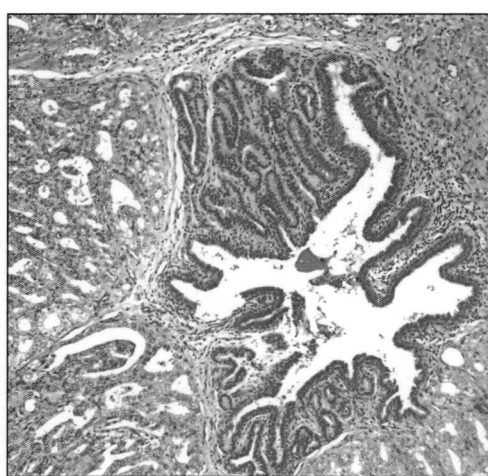

(Left) PCa invasion of SV shows direct extension of PCa from prostate (showing benign glands ⇗) to SV muscular wall ⧁. *(Right)* PCa invasion of SV shows indirect extension of PCa from extraprostatic tissues ⇗ to SV muscular wall ⧁. Direct extension from prostate to SV is the most common mode for SV invasion by PCa. It is suggested that indirect metastasis from prostate to SV has relatively better survival than the other patterns of SV invasion.

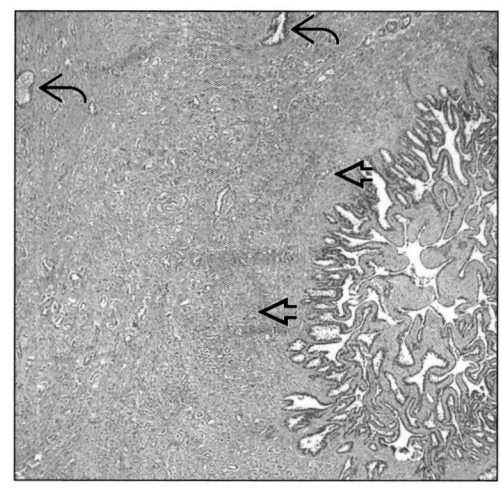
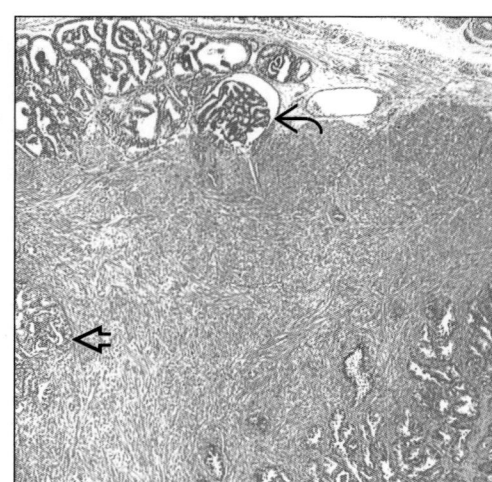

Prostate Cancer Staging

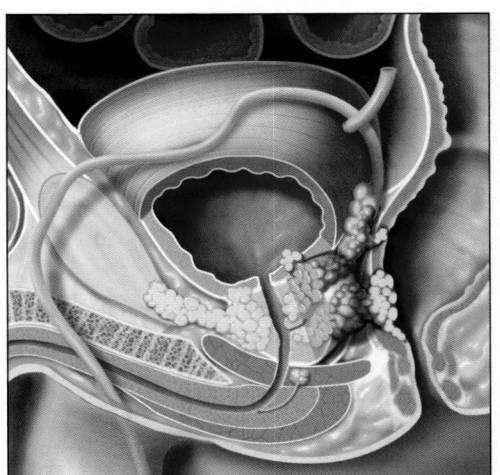

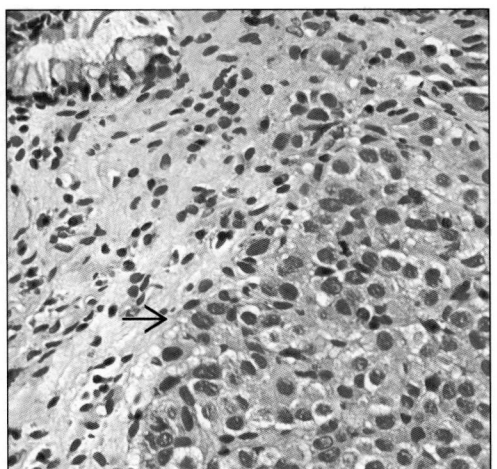

(Left) pT4 PCa shows tumor invading structures other than SV, such as the bladder, rectum, and anterior pelvic wall. This extent of PCa is managed with radiotherapy or hormonal therapy. RP with lymph node dissection may be performed in selected patients (e.g., low volume, no fixation). *(Right)* Rectal biopsy shows poorly differentiated PCa ➡ involving rectal mucosa. Thus, the highest T stage is confirmed histologically and criteria for pT staging is fulfilled without removal of tumor.

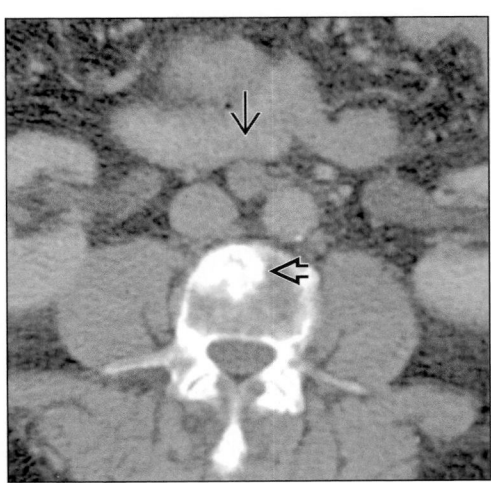

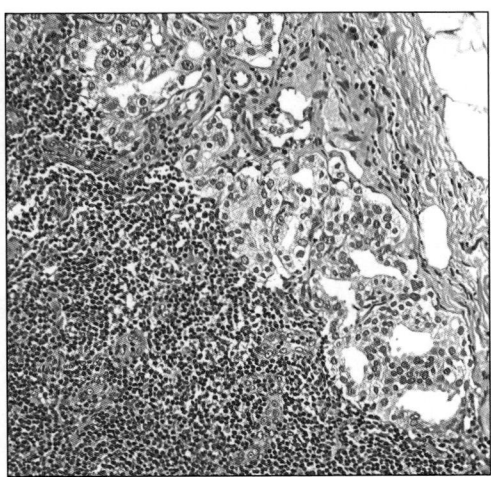

(Left) Axial CT shows retroperitoneal lymphadenopathy ➡ and sclerotic vertebral metastasis by PCa ➡. Staging pelvic CT or MR is performed for T3 or T4 or in localized PCa with high nomogram probability for lymph node involvement. Due to false-positivity, staging MR/CT is usually not performed if GS < 7 or PSA < 20 ng/mL. *(Right)* Lymph node shows subcapsular metastatic PCa. It is important to specify the number of lymph nodes involved and the size of the largest positive lymph node.

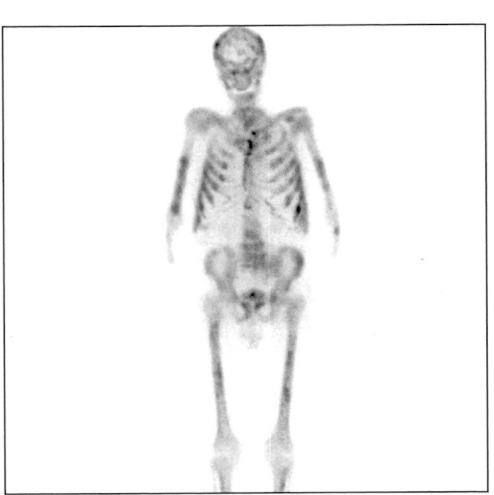

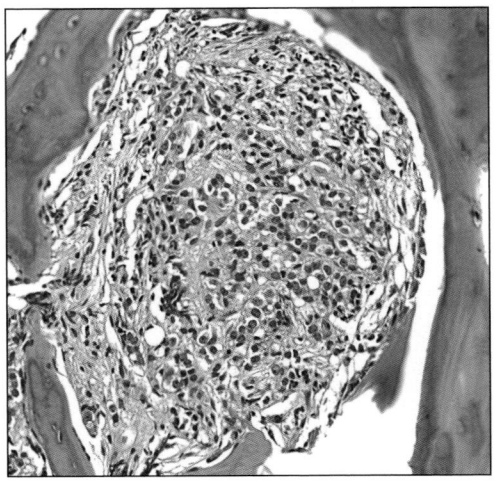

(Left) Anterior bone scan shows multiple osseous metastases by PCa, including to the calvarium, bilateral humeri, multiple ribs, sternum, lumbar spine, pelvis, and both femurs. Bone metastasis by PCa is typically osteoblastic. *(Right)* Bone biopsy shows involvement by metastatic PCa. Adenocarcinoma with low columnar or cuboidal cells and prominent &/or multiple nucleoli are helpful features. PSA or PAP immunostains may be useful for confirmation.

ACINAR ADENOCARCINOMA

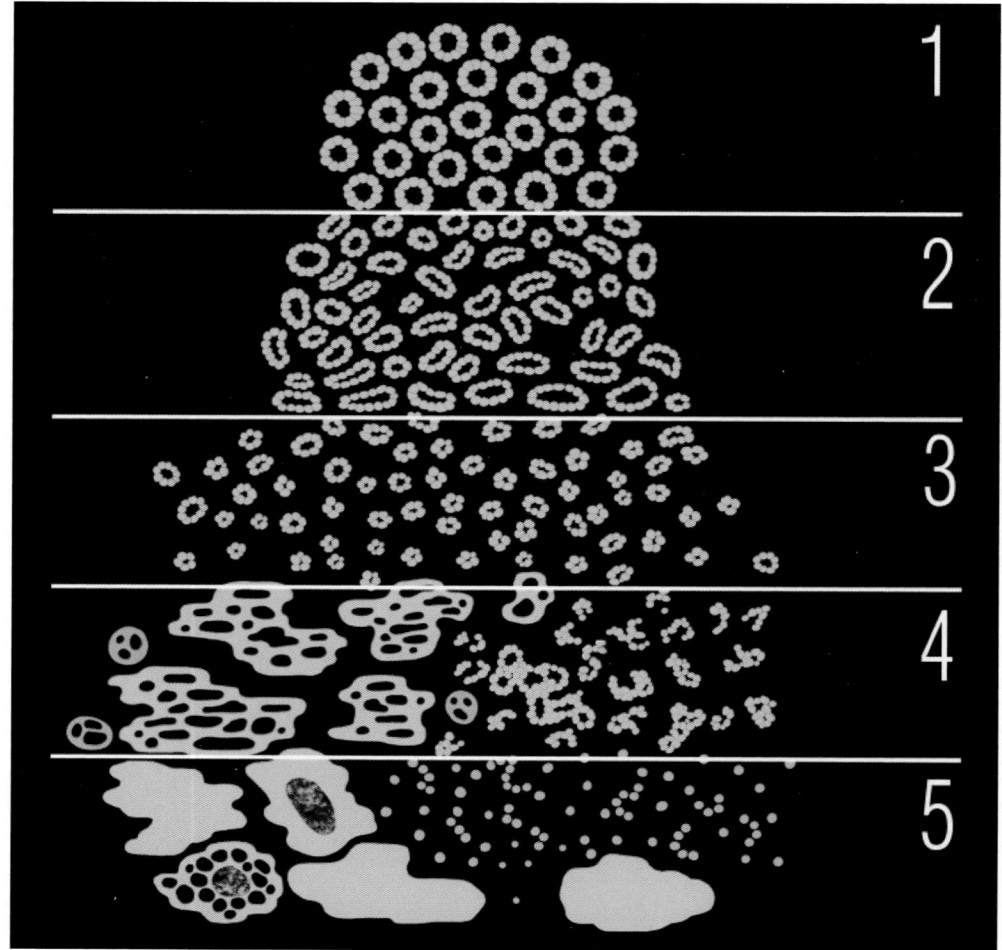

Schematic diagram shows modified Gleason grading system for PCa. The Gleason score is a powerful prognostic variable in predicting PCa behavior. This grading system is based purely on glandular architectural patterns, divided into 5 histologic categories or grades with decreasing differentiation. First developed in 1966 by Dr. Donald F. Gleason, it underwent refinements in 1974 and 1977 and had its latest modification by ISUP in 2005. This grading scheme is now universally accepted and recognized by World Health Organization and by American Joint Committee on Cancer as the grading system of choice for PCa.

TERMINOLOGY

Abbreviations
- Prostate adenocarcinoma (PCa)

Synonyms
- Prostatic adenocarcinoma

Definitions
- Malignant neoplasm arising from secretory cells

ETIOLOGY/PATHOGENESIS

Molecular Genetics
- **TMPRSS2 and ETS gene fusion**
  - Most common recurrent arrangement identified
  - ~ 50% PCa harbor these recurrent gene fusions; individual estimates vary between 15-78%
  - TMPRSS2 encodes for serine protease secreted by prostatic cells in response to androgen exposure
  - ETS family of transcription factors include *ERG*, *ETV1*, *ETV4*, and *ETV5*
  - *TMPRSS2:ERG* gene fusion most common (~ 90%)
    - ERG brought under control of androgen-regulated promoter causing protein overexpression
  - Intra- and interchromosomal genetic rearrangements lead to creation of fusion transcript
    - In ~ 2/3 of cases, fusion results from deletion (intervening 3 Mb between *TMPRSS2* and *ERG*)
    - Fusion may also occur by more complex rearrangement, such as translocation
    - Over 20 *TMPRSS2:ERG* variants now described
  - Morphological features of prostate cancer associated with *TMPRSS2:ERG* gene fusion
    - Blue-tinged mucin, cribriform pattern, intraductal spread, macronucleoli, and signet ring cells
  - Clinical significance of this gene fusion not yet fully understood
    - Conflicting reports in literature
- **Hereditary prostate cancer**

ACINAR ADENOCARCINOMA

Key Facts

Terminology
- Malignant neoplasm arising from secretory cells

Etiology/Pathogenesis
- ~ 50% PCa harbor *TMPRSS2* and *ETS* gene fusion

Macroscopic Features
- 75-80% of PCas arise in PZ; ~ 15-25% arise in TZ

Microscopic Pathology
- Diagnosis based on constellation of architectural, nuclear, cytoplasmic, and intraluminal features
- Crowded uniform glands that infiltrate between preexisting benign glands
  ○ Small caliber, crowded clusters, rigid or "sharp" lumina, tinctorial staining of cytoplasm distinct from adjacent benign glands

- Malignant glands lack basal cells by immunohistochemistry
- Nuclear enlargement and hyperchromasia with prominently enlarged &/or multiple and peripherally located nucleoli
- Pathognomonic features for malignant glands
  ○ Glomerulations or collagenous micronodules
  ○ Circumferential perineural/intraneural invasion or growth within fat
- Less differentiated tumors have poorly formed, fused, or large cribriform glands
- Poorly differentiated tumors may grow as infiltrative single cells or solid sheets
- Treated PCa glands usually poorly formed but retain infiltrative appearance

---

○ Compelling evidence suggests familial predisposition to prostate cancer in some cases
○ High-risk alleles identified with either autosomal dominant or X-linked mode of inheritance
○ 3 candidates genes identified: *HPC2/ELAC2* on 17p, *RNASEL* on 1q25, and *MSR1* on 8p22-23
- **Other genes and molecular alterations**
  ○ Most common chromosomal alterations in prostate cancer are losses at 1p, 6q, 8p, 10q, 13q, 16q, and 18q and gains at 1q, 2p, 7, 8q, 18q, and Xq
  ○ Genes implicated in PCa include *GST-pi*, *NKX3.1*, *PTEN*, *AMACR*, *hepsin*, *KLF-6*, *EZH2*, *p27*, *E-cadherin*
  ○ Mutations in androgen receptor gene may promote cancer growth at lower circulating androgen levels
  ○ Hedgehog pathway has been shown to play a role in growth and metastasis of prostate cancer

MACROSCOPIC FEATURES

General Features
- Unlike most other visceral organ tumors, PCa often has no reliably distinguishable gross mass lesion
  ○ Grossly evident tumors are usually pT3, ≥ Gleason score (GS) 8, or ≥ 1 cm size tumors
    ▪ Indurated yellow to yellow-tan homogeneous areas
    ▪ More dense or firmer than surrounding benign spongy parenchyma
  ○ Typically lack necrosis or hemorrhage
  ○ Tumor border blends imperceptibly with benign parenchyma
  ○ Lesions < 5 mm generally inapparent
  ○ Tumors often larger when examined by microscopy than when measured grossly
  ○ False-positivity rate in gross identification up to 19%
- Tumors usually in posterior or posterolateral aspect (peripheral zone [PZ]) of the gland
- Anterior tumors more difficult to recognize as they are usually admixed with nodular hyperplasia

Site
- 75-80% of PCas arise in PZ, and 15-25% arise in transition zone (TZ)
- Central zone is usually only secondarily involved
- Multifocal tumors present in more than 50% of PCas

MICROSCOPIC PATHOLOGY

Histologic Features
- Diagnosis based on constellation of architectural, nuclear, cytoplasmic, and intraluminal features
  ○ Some individual features may also be seen in benign glands
- **Architectural features**
  ○ Better differentiated tumors consist of compact or loose collections of well-formed glands
    ▪ Small crowded uniform glands infiltrate between preexisting benign glands
  ○ Malignant glands usually differ in appearance from surrounding benign glands
    ▪ Smaller-caliber glands
    ▪ Crowded or compact gland clusters
    ▪ Rigid or "sharp" glandular lumina
    ▪ May have periglandular clefts
  ○ Malignant glands should lack basal cells
  ○ Less differentiated tumors consist of poorly formed, fused, or large cribriform glands
  ○ Poorly differentiated tumors may grow as infiltrative single cells or solid sheets
- **Nuclear features**
  ○ Nuclear enlargement and hyperchromasia
  ○ Prominently enlarged nucleoli
  ○ Multiple and peripherally located nucleoli
  ○ Parachromatin clearing
  ○ Mitoses are rare; highly suggestive of malignancy if present
  ○ Apoptotic bodies (rare)
  ○ Nuclei commonly uniform, nonpleomorphic
- **Cytoplasmic features**
  ○ Typically cuboidal to columnar cells with modest cytoplasm

ACINAR ADENOCARCINOMA

o Amphophilic, clear or pale granular cytoplasm
o Taller cells with clear to pale pink cytoplasm and basally located nuclei more common in TZ
- **Intraluminal features**
  o Blue mucin
    ▪ Usually prominent collection of wispy, blue-tinged intracellular mucin
  o Eosinophilic amorphous secretions
    ▪ Granular eosinophilic luminal material
  o Crystalloids
    ▪ Geometric bright eosinophilic rhomboid to prismatic structures with sharp edges, usually associated with eosinophilic amorphous secretions
    ▪ Present in up to 41% of PCas
    ▪ Seen in atypical adenomatous hyperplasia and uncommonly in benign glands
  o Corpora amylacea are extremely rare in PCa, should strongly suggest benign glands
  o Intraluminal necrosis may be present in high-grade tumors, highly indicative of malignancy
- **Pathognomonic features for malignant glands**
  o Glomerulations
    ▪ Cribriform cellular luminal proliferations in otherwise well-formed glands attached to 1 pole
  o Collagenous micronodules (mucinous fibroplasia)
    ▪ Hyalinized eosinophilic material usually associated with abundant intraluminal blue mucin
    ▪ Often imparts an anastomosing epithelial pattern
  o Circumferential perineural or intraneural invasion
    ▪ Gland should completely surround the nerve or be seen within the nerve
    ▪ Benign glands may focally touch or indent a nerve; very rarely may be intraneural
  o Growth within adipose tissue
    ▪ Intraprostatic fat is exceedingly rare
    ▪ Indicates extraprostatic extension (EPE)

Gleason Grading System
- Universally accepted grading system for PCa
- Assessment of glandular architecture at low/ intermediate magnification: Classified into 5 basic patterns
  o Each pattern may arise de novo without progression from lower grade
- In resection specimens, GS is sum of primary and secondary Gleason patterns
  o Primary pattern is most prevalent pattern and secondary is 2nd most common pattern
- International Society of Urological Pathology (ISUP) 2005 consensus conference proposed several modifications and guidelines
  o In needle biopsies, include tertiary pattern in Gleason score if it is higher than secondary pattern
    ▪ Similar rule applies for transurethral resection and enucleation (simple prostatectomy) specimens
    ▪ In high-grade cancers, ignore lower grade pattern if < 5% (e.g., 4 + 4, if pattern 3 is < 5%)
    ▪ For cancers with more than 1 pattern, include the higher grade even if it is < 5% (e.g., 3 + 4, even if pattern 4 is < 5%)
  o Assign individual GS to all cores as an aggregate if submitted in 1 container; assign GS to each

core separately designated (e.g., ink or separately submitted) by urologist
  o In radical prostatectomy, provide GS (primary and secondary pattern); separately mention tertiary pattern
  o Assign separate GS to dominant tumor(s) for multifocal tumors in radical prostatectomy
  o Individualized Gleason grading approach for some PCa morphologic variants and subtypes
- **Gleason pattern 1**
  o Circumscribed nodule of tightly packed, uniform, round to oval, well-formed glands, with no or minimal infiltration of adjacent parenchyma
  o Using these strict criteria, exceedingly rare and controversial in current practice
    ▪ Most described pre-immunohistochemistry were likely atypical adenomatous hyperplasia
- **Gleason pattern 2**
  o Nodular with minimal peripheral infiltration, less uniform and more loosely arranged glands
  o Also very rare and typically found in TZ
  o Usually incidental with associated higher grades, but occasionally secondary pattern in resection specimens
  o ISUP recommends that GS 3 or 4 should rarely, if ever, be diagnosed in needle biopsy specimens
    ▪ Architecture cannot be assessed in its entirety
    ▪ Poor reproducibility among experts
    ▪ Poor correlation with grade in subsequent prostatectomy (i.e., undergrading)
    ▪ May misguide clinicians and patients with assumption of indolent tumor
- **Gleason pattern 3**
  o Most common pattern
  o Predominantly well-formed, individual glands that infiltrate between benign ducts and acini
  o Includes smaller but well-formed glands (micro-acini)
  o Glands typically smaller than in patterns 1 or 2
  o Inclusion of small cribriform structures is controversial, as most experts include all cribriform patterns in Gleason pattern 4
    ▪ Should have perfectly round contours
    ▪ Size similar to surrounding benign glands
    ▪ Uniform round "punched-out" lumina with bridges not thicker than lumina
    ▪ By this strict definition, cribriform Gleason pattern 3 is extraordinarily rare; we rarely designate cribriform patterns as Gleason 3
- **Gleason pattern 4**
  o Most commonly fused, poorly formed glands
    ▪ Tangentially sectioned pattern 3 glands may mimic fused pattern 4 glands
    ▪ Common cause of overgrading
  o 2nd most common pattern is cribriform structures with either regular or irregular outlines
  o Uncommon "hypernephromatoid" pattern, consists of solid sheets of cells with optically clear cytoplasm
- **Gleason pattern 5**
  o Lacks glandular differentiation: Manifests as solid sheets, cords, or single infiltrative tumor cells

ACINAR ADENOCARCINOMA

o Also includes solid, cribriform, or papillary structures with central comedo-type necrosis

Morphologic Variations and Variants

- **Atrophic variant**
  o PCa with glands lined by cells with scant cytoplasm, resembling atrophy
  o Infiltrative growth, cytology of malignancy
  o Usually admixed with nonatrophic PCa
  o In contrast, benign atrophic glands typically have dense hyperchromatic nuclei and lobular growth
- **Pseudohyperplastic variant**
  o Large-sized or dilated glands, with branching and papillary infolding
  o Tall columnar cells with abundant pale to slight granular luminal cytoplasm
  o Basally located nuclei along basement membrane
  o Commonly with luminal eosinophilic amorphous secretions and may have crystalloids
  o Diagnostic malignant nuclear features retained, in contrast to benign hyperplastic glands
  o ISUP recommends grade of 3 + 3 = 6; if part of a large circumscribed nodule, grade may be 3 + 2 = 5
- **Foamy gland (xanthomatous) variant**
  o PCa with abundant foamy cytoplasm
  o Malignant nuclear features not always present, as nuclei may be small and pyknotic
  o Presence of infiltrative pattern; may require immunostains
  o ISUP recommends discounting foamy cytoplasm and assigning grade based on architecture; most are 3 + 3 = 6 tumors
- **Mucinous (colloid) adenocarcinoma**
  o ≥ 25% of resected tumor shows extracellular mucin
  o Intraluminal mucinous material does not qualify, and extraprostatic origin must be excluded
  o Diagnosis should be made only in resection specimen, as needle biopsy specimen may not show exact proportion of mucinous component
    - In needle biopsy, may be diagnosed as "PCa with mucinous features"
  o With strict diagnostic criteria, suggested to have similar features and behavior with conventional PCa
  o ISUP recommend to grade irregular cribriform glands floating in mucin as 4 + 4 = 8; no consensus if individual discrete glands in mucin
- **Signet ring cell variant**
  o ≥ 25% of resected tumor shows signet ring cell (arbitrary definition)
  o Tumor cells contain optically clear vacuoles displacing nuclei and are widely infiltrative
  o Associated with typical high-grade PCa
  o May be mucin-producing PCa ("mucinous carcinoma with signet ring cells")
    - Not clear if nonmucinous (mucicarmine negative) signet ring PCa is distinct clinically
  o Clinical presentation similar to conventional PCa, with tendency to present at higher stage
- **PCa with Paneth-cell-like differentiation**
  o PCa containing neuroendocrine cells with bright eosinophilic cytoplasmic granules resembling Paneth cells of gastrointestinal tract

o Suggested to have favorable prognosis, including those with nests, cords, or single cell morphology
- **Other rarer variants**
  o **Lymphoepithelioma-like variant**
    - As in other organs, characterized by syncytial growth amid dense lymphocytic background
    - No Epstein-Barr virus association
  o **Oncocytic variant**
    - PCa with abundant granular eosinophilic cytoplasm
    - Like other oncocytic tumors, ultrastructurally contains abundant mitochondria
  o **PCa with stratified epithelium ("PIN-like")**
    - Glands lined by ≥ 2 layers of malignant cells
    - May resemble flat or tufted high-grade PIN but lacks basal cells by immunohistochemistry

Therapy-related Changes

- **Radiation therapy**
  o Treated PCa glands usually poorly formed but retain their infiltrative appearance
    - Foamy vacuolated cytoplasm and pleomorphic nuclei; changes vary from mild to marked
    - Marked radiation effect may artifactually produce architecture resembling GS 9 or 10 cancers
    - Luminal features of malignancy may be retained
  o Cytologic atypia and pleomorphism more pronounced in benign than malignant glands
  o Residual treated PCa with minimal or no radiation effect has higher chance of recurrence
  o PAN-CK(AE1/AE3) useful to highlight treated PCa
- **Hormonal therapy**
  o Treated PCa may be shrunken glands or single cells
  o Glands show xanthomatous cytoplasm, pyknotic and fragmented nuclei, and mucin extravasation
  o Empty spaces representing remnants of shrunken glands may be present
  o Marked atrophy, basal cell hyperplasia, or squamous metaplasia in adjacent benign glands
  o PAN-CK(AE1/AE3) useful to highlight treated PCa

DIFFERENTIAL DIAGNOSIS

General Features

- Given broad morphologic spectrum, differential diagnosis for PCa ranges from innocuous benign normal structures to secondary high-grade cancers
- PCa most often mimicked by benign prostatic glandular lesions; difficulty enhanced in limited samples (e.g., biopsy)
  o Use of ancillary immunohistochemistry helpful in some scenarios
  o Pattern-based approach facilitates work-up and judicious selection of adjuvant stains

Atypical Small Acinar Proliferation (ASAP)

- Focal atypical glands that are suspicious but quantitatively &/or qualitatively insufficient for diagnosis or exclusion of PCa
- Most common differential diagnostic scenario for PCa
- Differential diagnosis includes focal PCa and benign glandular lesions

ACINAR ADENOCARCINOMA

Differential Diagnosis for Prostate Carcinoma

Histologic Pattern	Prostate Carcinoma	Main Differential Diagnoses
Small glandular proliferation	Glandular Gleason pattern 3	Crowded benign glands, not otherwise specified
	Atrophic pattern	Simple atrophy
	Post-treatment cancer	Outpouching of high-grade PIN
		Partial atrophy
		Postatrophic hyperplasia (PAH)
		AAH (adenosis)
		Sclerosing adenosis
		Basal cell hyperplasia
		Seminal vesicle epithelium
		Ejaculatory duct
		Cowper glands
		Mesonephric remnants
		Nephrogenic adenoma
		Verumontanum mucosal gland hyperplasia
		Radiation atypia
Atypical large glandular proliferation	Cribriform Gleason patterns 3, 4, and 5	High-grade PIN
	Ductal adenocarcinoma	Urothelial carcinoma involving prostatic ducts and acini
	Pseudohyperplastic pattern	Colorectal carcinoma involving prostate
		Cribriform hyperplasia
		Squamous metaplasia
		Urothelial metaplasia
Infiltrative single cell pattern	Single cell Gleason 5 pattern	Dense inflammation
	Post-treatment carcinoma	Granulomatous prostatitis
		Lymphoma
		Small cell carcinoma
Clear cell pattern	Hypernephroid Gleason pattern 4	Prostatic xanthoma
	Glandular Gleason pattern 3	
Oncocytic pattern	Gleason pattern 4	Paraganglion/paraganglioma
		Carcinoid tumor
Poorly to undifferentiated carcinoma	Solid Gleason pattern 5	Urothelial carcinoma
Spindle cell pattern	Sarcomatoid carcinoma	Pseudosarcomatous myofibroblastic proliferation
		Stromal sarcoma
		Leiomyosarcoma
Small cell pattern	Small cell carcinoma	Lymphoma
		Rhabdomyosarcoma

- Immunohistochemistry may be helpful
  - PCa lacks basal cell staining and often overexpresses AMACR
    - In some cases, definitive diagnosis of PCa is not possible even with a carcinoma staining pattern

SELECTED REFERENCES

1. Gopalan A et al: TMPRSS2-ERG gene fusion is not associated with outcome in patients treated by prostatectomy. Cancer Res. 69(4):1400-6, 2009
2. Lopez-Beltran A et al: Lymphoepithelioma-like carcinoma of the prostate. Hum Pathol. 40(7):982-7, 2009
3. Epstein JI et al: The 2005 International Society of Urological Pathology (ISUP) Consensus Conference on Gleason Grading of Prostatic Carcinoma. Am J Surg Pathol. 29(9):1228-42, 2005
4. Tomlins SA et al: Recurrent fusion of TMPRSS2 and ETS transcription factor genes in prostate cancer. Science. 310(5748):644-8, 2005
5. Varma M et al: Morphologic criteria for the diagnosis of prostatic adenocarcinoma in needle biopsy specimens. A study of 250 consecutive cases in a routine surgical pathology practice. Arch Pathol Lab Med. 126(5):554-61, 2002
6. Humphrey PA et al: Pseudohyperplastic prostatic adenocarcinoma. Am J Surg Pathol. 22(10):1239-46, 1998
7. Egan AJ et al: Prostatic adenocarcinoma with atrophic features: malignancy mimicking a benign process. Am J Surg Pathol. 21(8):931-5, 1997
8. Nelson RS et al: Prostatic carcinoma with abundant xanthomatous cytoplasm. Foamy gland carcinoma. Am J Surg Pathol. 20(4):419-26, 1996

ACINAR ADENOCARCINOMA

Gross Features

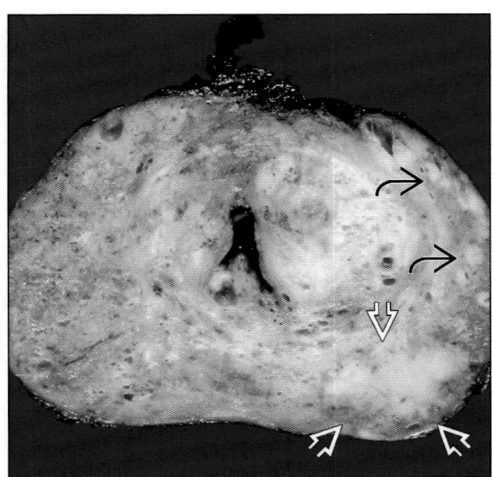
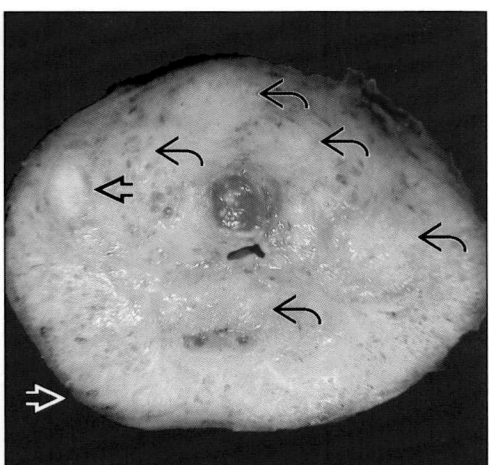

(Left) This coronal section of prostate shows multifocal PCa predominantly involving left lobe with a dominant nodule ⟴ at the posterolateral aspect and additional smaller tumor foci ⟶ at the lateral aspect of the peripheral zone. *(Right)* Coronal section of prostate shows a focus of PCa ⟴ involving the anterior aspect of PZ. Several hyperplastic nodules ⟶ are seen in the adjacent TZ. Note absence of grossly visible tumor in posterior and posterolateral aspect of the PZ ⟴.

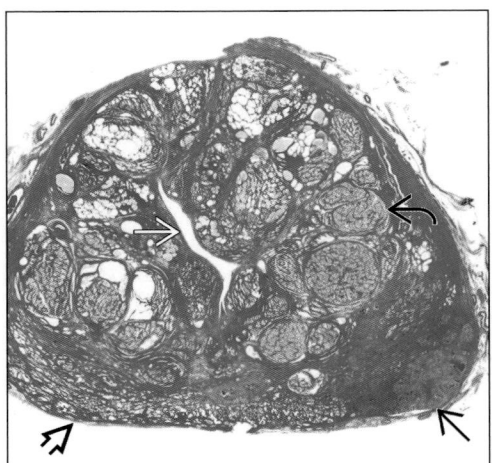
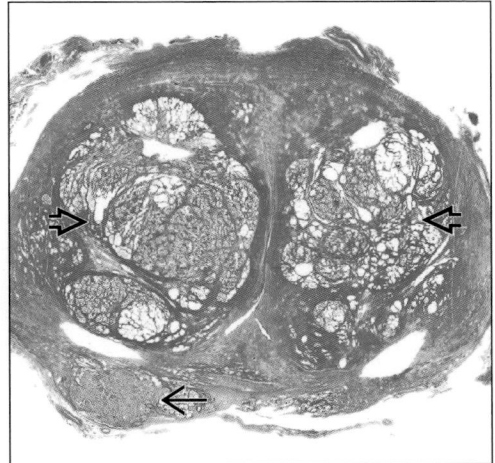

(Left) Coronal section of the prostate shows the urethra ⟶ pushed to the left due to prominent benign fibromuscular and glandular hyperplasia ⟶. The peripheral zone shows evidence of prominent atrophy ⟴ and a carcinoma ⟶ involving the posterolateral aspect. *(Right)* Whole mount coronal section of the prostate shows evidence of prominent fibromuscular hyperplasia ⟴ in the transition zone compressing the urethra and a focus of adenocarcinoma ⟶ in the peripheral zone.

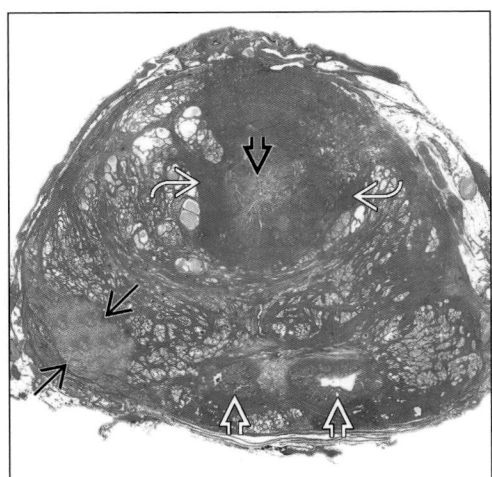
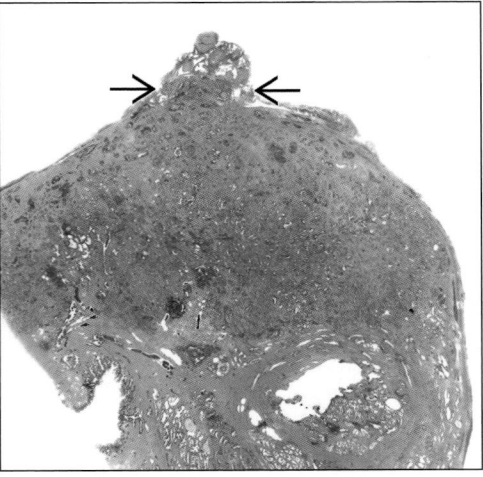

(Left) A nodule of adenocarcinoma ⟶ is present in the right posterolateral aspect of the peripheral zone. There is also prominent stromal hyperplasia ⟴ in the transition zone, which compresses the urethra ⟴. The intraprostatic portion of the seminal vesicles ⟴ is also seen. *(Right)* This macrosection shows extensive adenocarcinoma replacing much of the peripheral zone. Extraprostatic extension ⟶ is present in the neurovascular bundle.

ACINAR ADENOCARCINOMA

Architectural Features

(Left) In contrast to most carcinomas, stromal reaction is rare in PCa; "infiltration" is therefore difficult to define. Most commonly, it is identified as infiltration of small glands between larger, normal, benign glands ➡. *(Right)* This poorly differentiated PCa is characterized by crowded, poorly formed glands infiltrating between normal large-caliber glands ➡. Glandular crowding is another key feature in the recognition of adenocarcinoma.

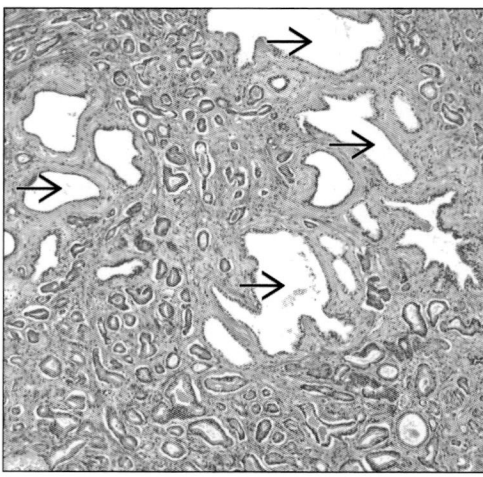
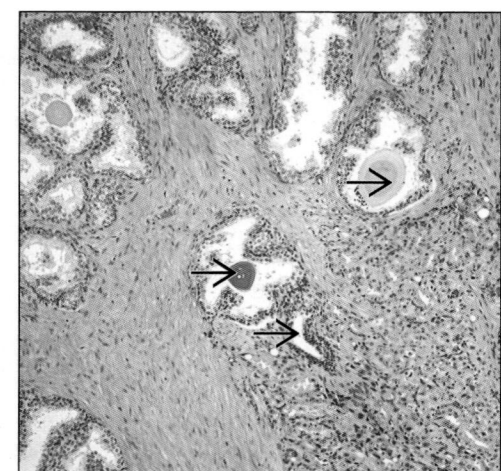

(Left) This low-power magnification of focal PCa shows a collection of tightly clustered, small, crowded glands ➡. Despite the absence of infiltrative growth, these features warrant closer examination to evaluate for adenocarcinoma. *(Right)* This PCa is characterized by crowded medium-caliber glands with extensive retraction spaces surrounding the individual carcinoma glands. This periglandular clearing is not specific but is relatively rare in benign glands.

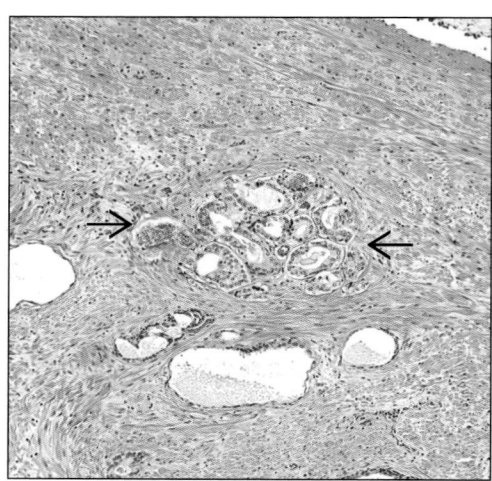
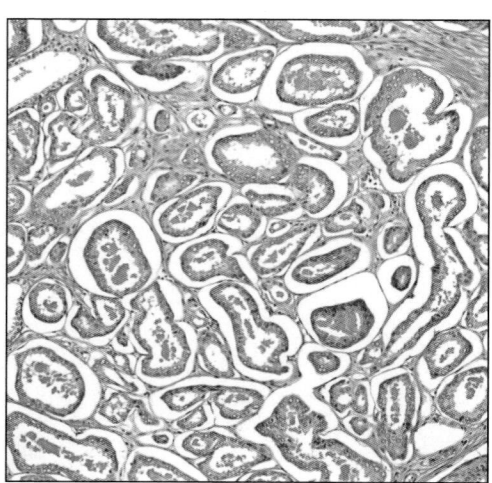

(Left) PCa in needle biopsy may show a linear alignment of glands ➡ that course perpendicular to the long axis of the core. This architectural growth pattern is highly suggestive of adenocarcinoma. *(Right)* PCa glands are tightly clustered and oriented in a linear arrangement. Cytologic features of PCa are not readily apparent. The focus lacked basal cells by immunohistochemistry with p63 and also had strong luminal racemase/AMACR immunoreactivity, features supporting the diagnosis of PCa.

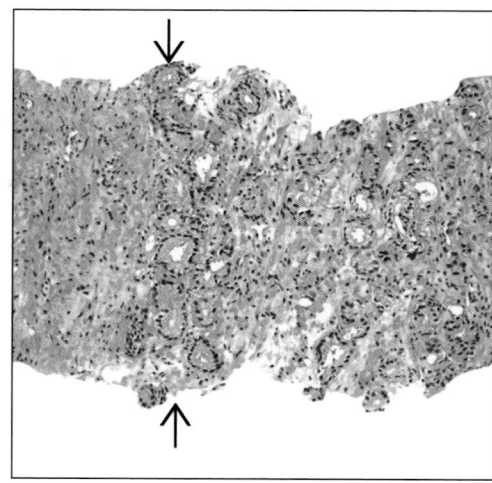
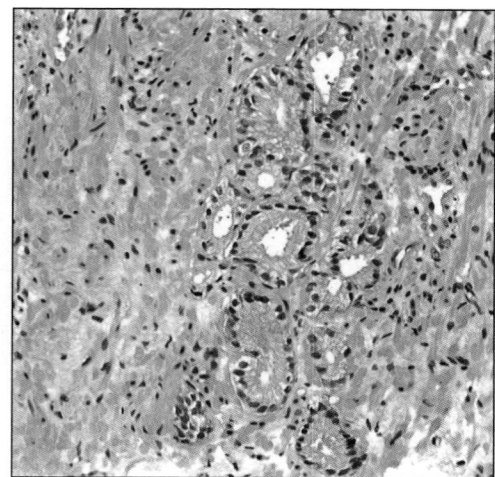

ACINAR ADENOCARCINOMA

Cytologic Features

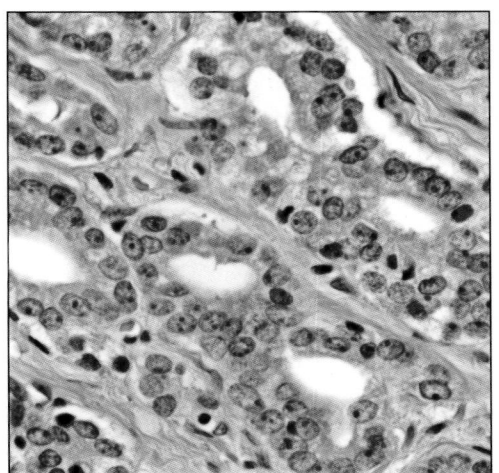

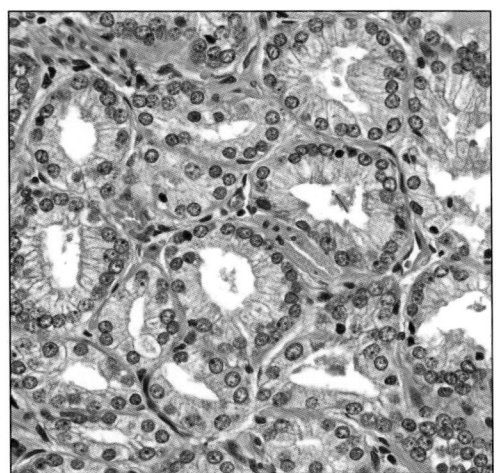

(Left) Prominent nucleoli, as seen here, are characteristic of PCa, but they are not always required for the diagnosis. In addition, nuclei larger than the adjacent nuclei of benign glands and those with double nucleoli and with parachromatin clearing or mitosis are helpful features. *(Right)* PCa shows pale granular cytoplasm and monotonous-appearing round nuclei. PCa nuclei are typically homogeneous. Nuclear pleomorphism should suggest the possibility of a nonprostatic lesion.

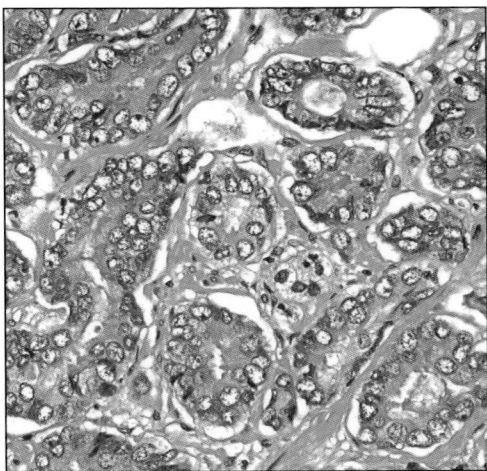

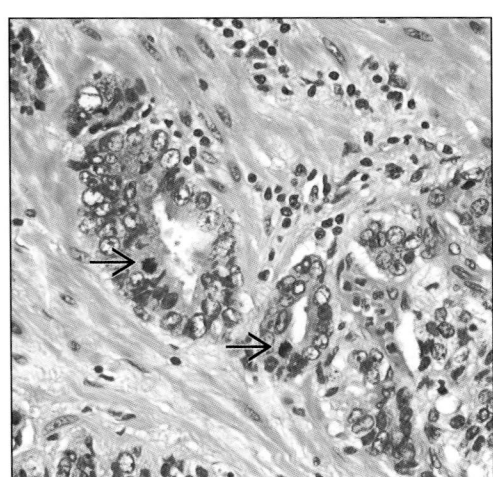

(Left) PCa glands commonly show parachromatin clearing in the malignant nuclei. These nuclei also show a mild degree of nuclear variability and crowding not typically seen in most PCa. PCa nuclei are usually very round and monotonous. Note the absence of any stromal reaction. *(Right)* PCa shows readily identifiable mitotic figures ⊡ within the malignant glands. Mitotic figures are very rare in PCa; however, their presence is highly suggestive of adenocarcinoma.

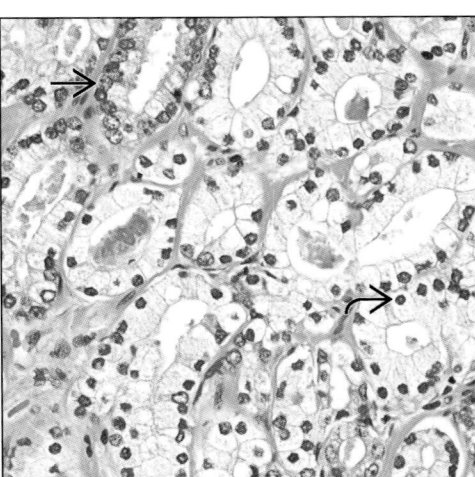

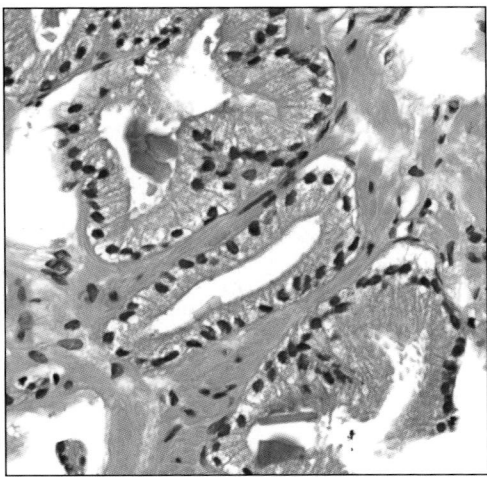

(Left) PCa shows columnar cells with pale cytoplasm and basally situated nuclei. Some nuclei are large with prominent nucleoli ⊡, while others are more condensed ⊡. The size of the nuclei and prominence of nucleoli may vary considerably within the same tumor. *(Right)* Some PCa have relatively bland nuclear features, as seen in this case. The presence of obvious nucleoli is not required for a diagnosis of adenocarcinoma if other sufficient features are present.

Adjunctive Features

(Left) PCa shows abundant intraluminal crystalloids. Luminal crystalloids are relatively more common in PCa than in benign glands; however, abundant crystalloids may be seen in atypical adenomatous hyperplasia (adenosis) and some other small glandular proliferations. *(Right)* Intraluminal blue mucin ⇒ is another feature that, while not entirely specific, is highly suggestive of adenocarcinoma. Glands with luminal mucin should be carefully evaluated for other features of carcinoma.

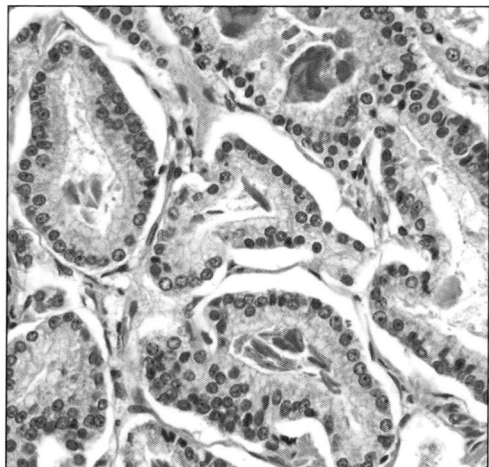
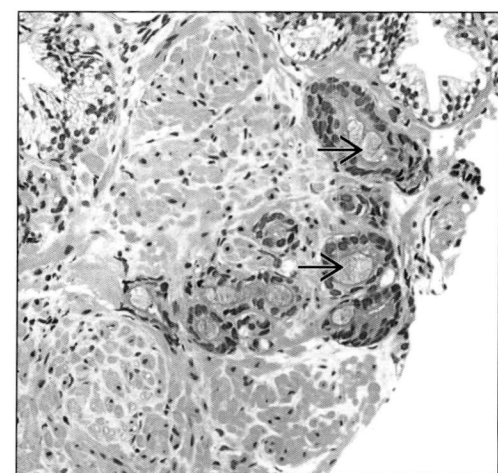

(Left) PCa often has a sharp luminal contour, which is distinct from the undulating or tufted luminal surface typical of benign glands. This PCa also shows basal orientation of the nuclei; in normal glands, nuclei have more variation in their relation to the lumen. *(Right)* This PCa has both corpora amylacea ⇒ and crystalloids ⇒ within the lumina. Despite their presence here, corpora amylacea are very rare in PCa glands and should prompt careful exclusion of a benign process.

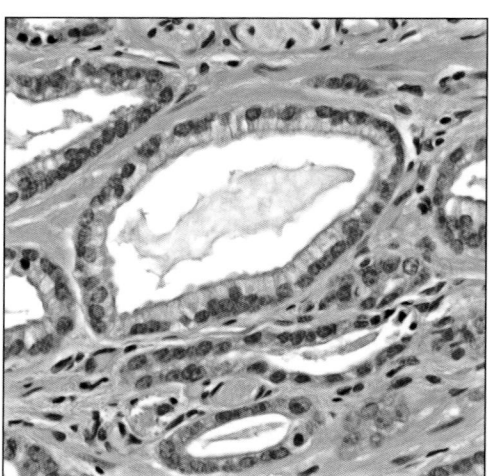
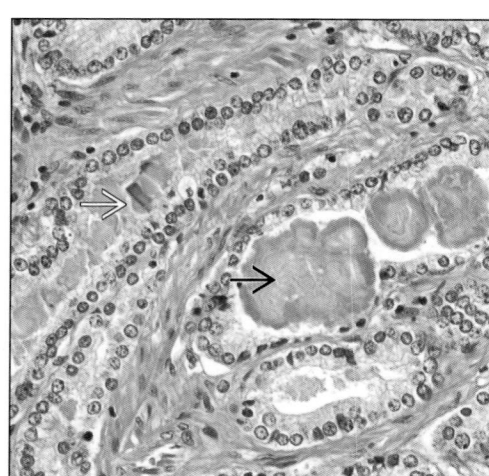

(Left) Intraluminal eosinophilic secretions, while not entirely specific, are commonly seen in PCa. This PCa also shows basally oriented nuclei and prominent luminal cytoplasm, other histologic features that are suggestive of malignancy. *(Right)* This PCa shows multiple foci of lymphovascular invasion ⇒. Retraction artifact may closely mimic lymphovascular invasion, but definite involvement of vascular spaces is diagnostic of malignancy.

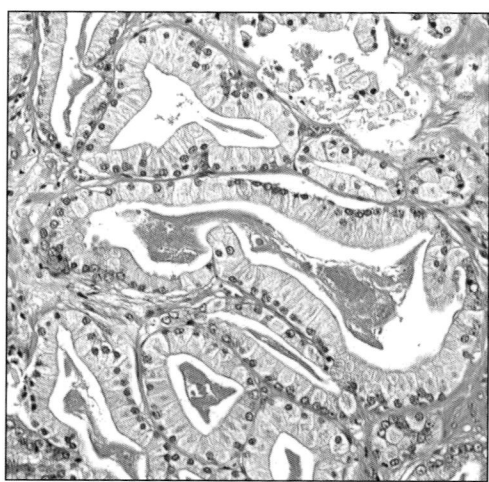
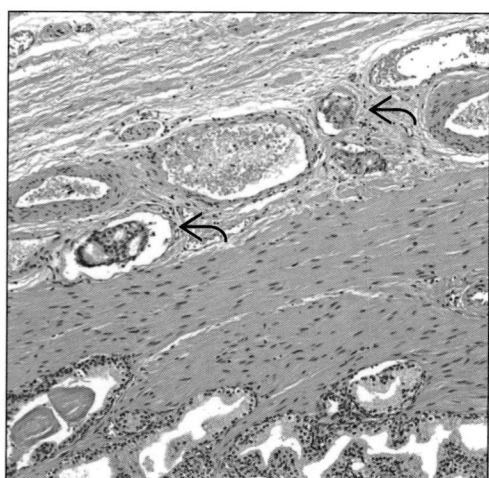

ACINAR ADENOCARCINOMA

Pathognomonic Features

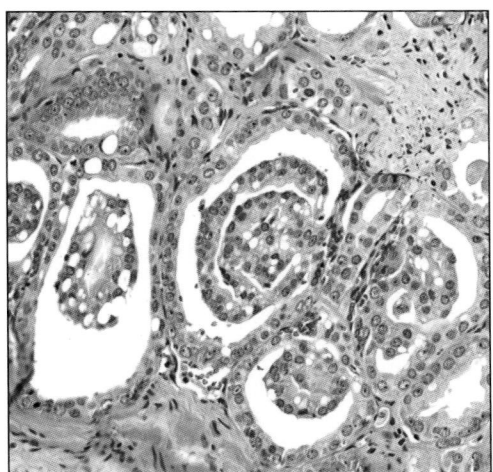

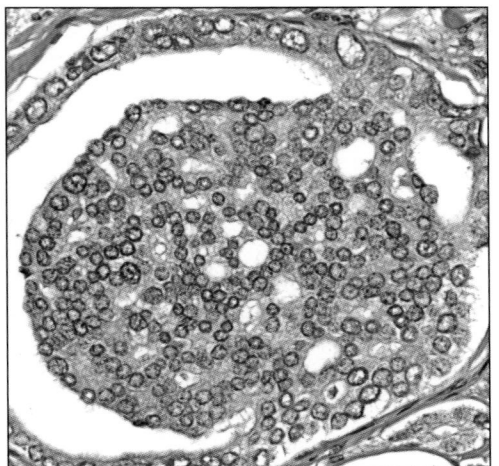

(Left) The presence of glomerulations, defined as a cribriform cellular luminal proliferation attached to 1 pole of the lumen, is diagnostic of adenocarcinoma. *(Right)* High-power view of a PCa gland with a glomerulation shows the cribriform cellular luminal proliferation attached at 1 pole. Although Gleason grading for glomerulations is controversial and no consensus was reached by ISUP, recent data suggest they should be regarded as Gleason pattern 4.

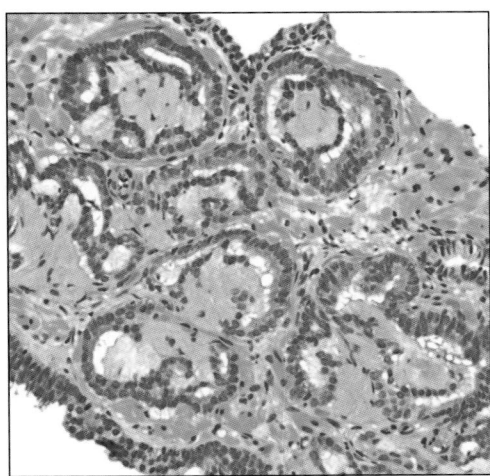

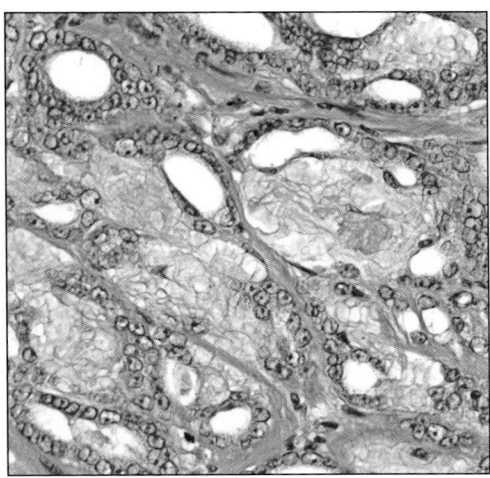

(Left) Collagenous micronodules (mucinous fibroplasia) are a pathognomonic feature of PCa. They are typically associated with mucin and are characterized by dense nodules of fibrous tissue and fibroblasts associated with the epithelium. *(Right)* In early collagenous micronodules, the fibrous tissue is scant and more mucin is seen. Although the epithelium often assumes a complex architecture, mucinous fibroplasia is typically assigned a 3 + 3 = 6 Gleason score.

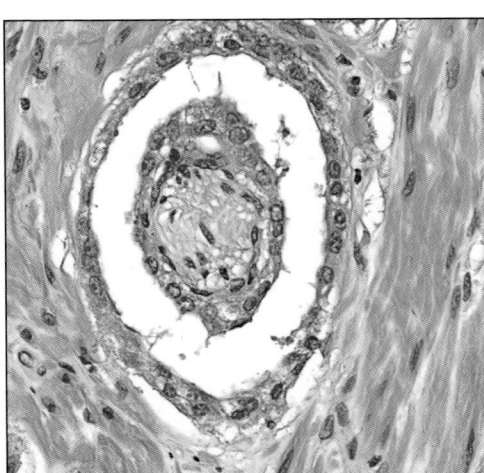

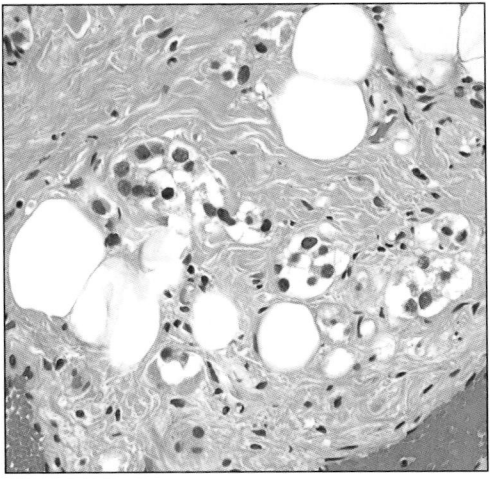

(Left) Circumferential (or intraneural) involvement is required if perineural invasion is used as a diagnostic adjunct. Some benign lesions, such as postatrophic hyperplasia, may contain glands with focal, noncircumferential indentation of a nerve. When present, perineural invasion is supportive of a diagnosis of PCa. *(Right)* This PCa shows invasion into adipose tissue, which is considered by most as a diagnostic feature of adenocarcinoma since intraprostatic fat is exceedingly rare.

ACINAR ADENOCARCINOMA

Gleason Pattern 2-3

(Left) This GS 2 + 2 = 4 PCa is characterized by a circumscribed nodule of mainly medium-sized glands with minimal peripheral infiltration. This pattern is rare and seen almost exclusively in TZ. ISUP recommends that GS 3 or 4 should rarely, if ever, be diagnosed in needle biopsies. *(Right)* This GS 2 + 3 = 5 PCa shows a relatively circumscribed large nodule composed of mostly medium-sized glands (Gleason pattern 2) with focal peripheral infiltration by smaller glands (Gleason pattern 3) ➡.

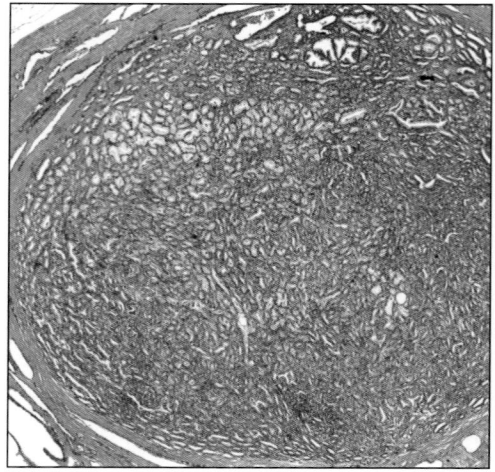 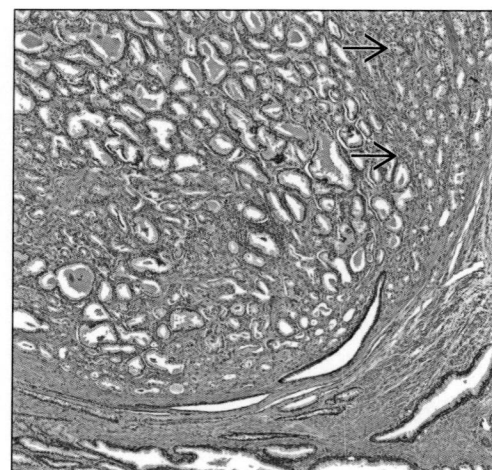

(Left) This GS 3 + 2 = 5 PCa contains more prominent foci of peripheral infiltration by smaller glands (Gleason pattern 3) ➡. This PCa cluster shows overall nodular configuration with relatively larger-sized glands (Gleason pattern 2) ➡. *(Right)* Gleason pattern 3 PCa shows discrete, well-formed glands. These glands are smaller than glands in Gleason patterns 1 or 2 and show an infiltrative pattern of growth. Gleason grade 3 is the most common pattern in the Gleason grading scheme.

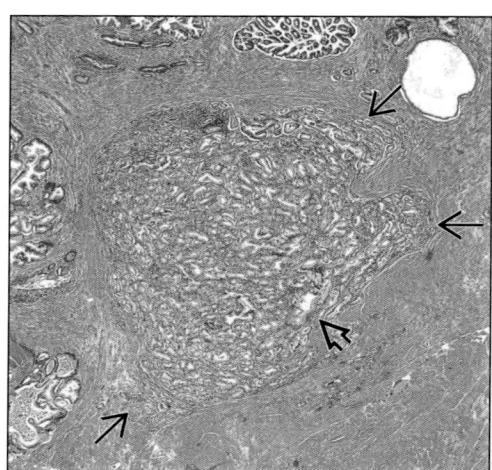 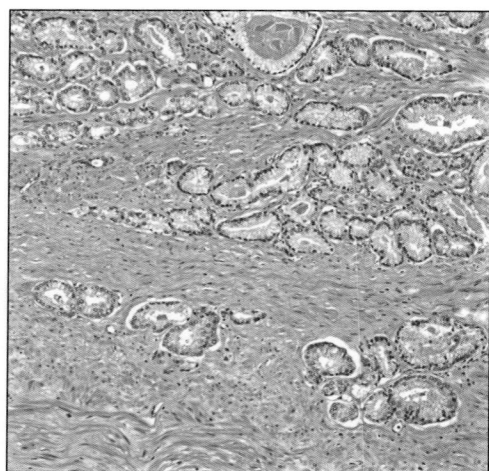

(Left) This Gleason pattern 3 PCa shows well-formed glands with marked variation in gland size and shape, as well as diffuse infiltrative growth without formation of a discrete nodule. *(Right)* High-power view of Gleason pattern 3 PCa shows clusters of small to minute glands (microacinar pattern). These glands have a continuous cell lining around central lumina. Some of these glands display luminal rigidity and contain blue-tinged mucin ➡, typical of PCa.

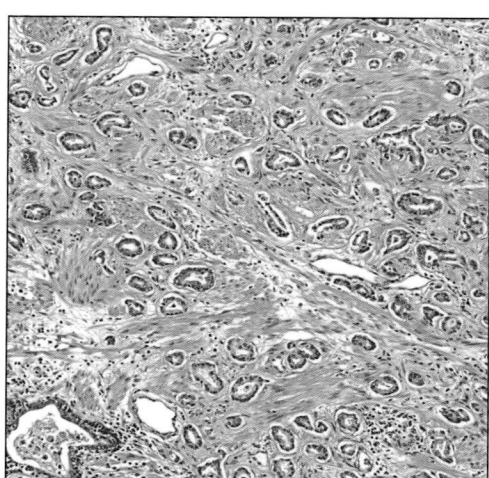 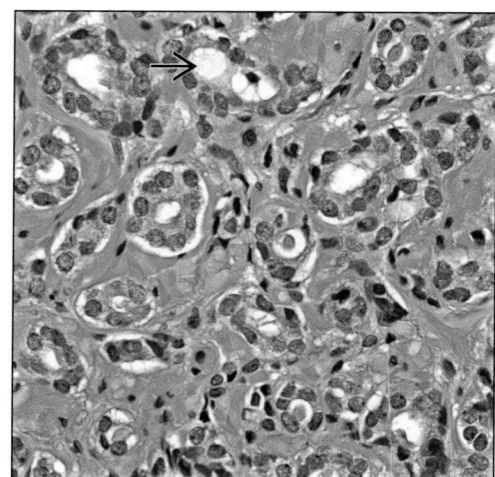

ACINAR ADENOCARCINOMA

Gleason Pattern 4

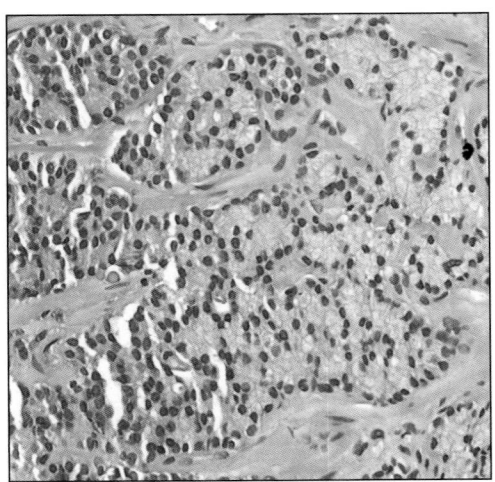

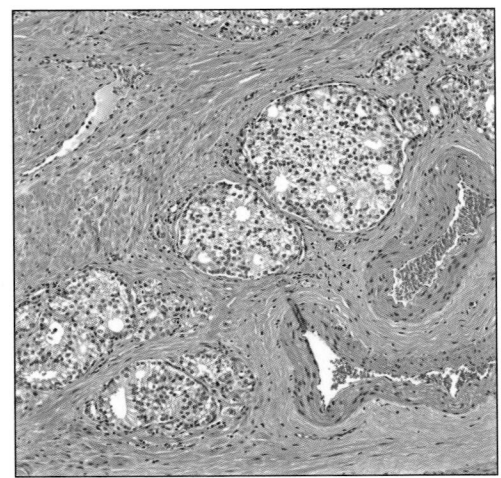

(Left) PCa with extensive confluent anastomosing growth (or fusion) indicates Gleason pattern 4. Fused glands are complex, such that an imaginary line cannot be easily drawn around the individual glands. **(Right)** This Gleason score 4 + 4 = 8 PCa shows large tumor nodules with a well-developed internal cribriform structure. Cribriform patterns should rarely, if ever, be designated as Gleason pattern 3, and cribriform high-grade prostatic intraepithelial neoplasia should also be excluded.

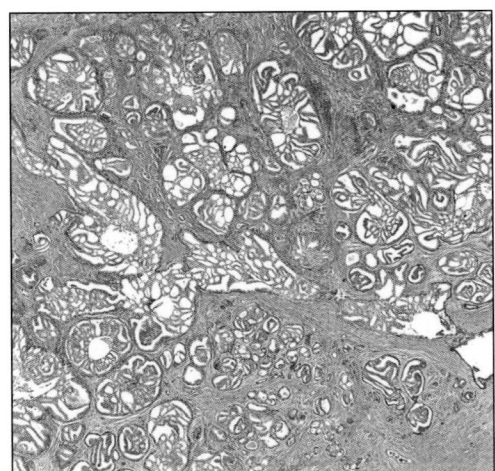

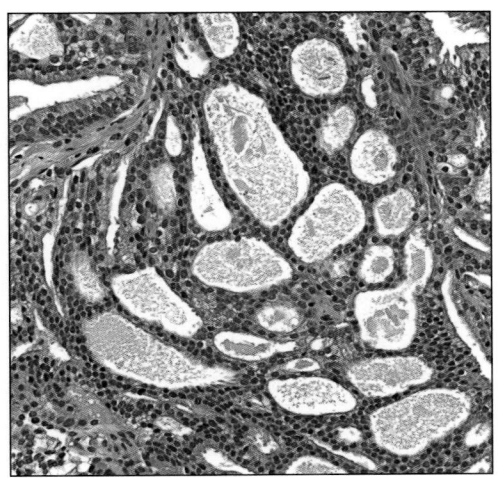

(Left) Most cribriform growth represents Gleason pattern 4, and this may include intraductal growth, especially in high-volume cancer. Central necrosis in any of the glands would indicate pattern 5. **(Right)** This Gleason pattern 4 cribriform pattern shows a large gland with an irregular outline containing multiple lumina separated by cellular bridges. The presence of necrosis or solid growth in a cribriform gland (not seen here) would warrant designation as Gleason pattern 5.

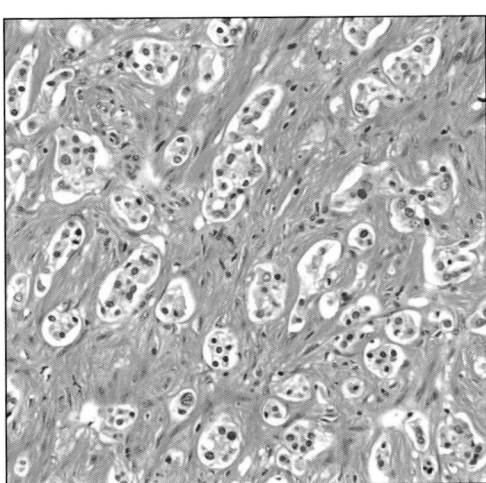

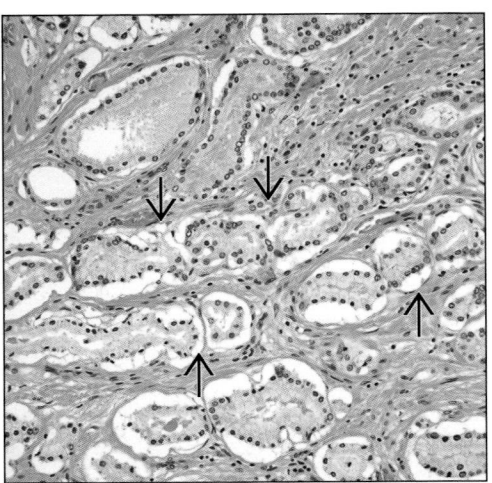

(Left) Irregular clusters of PCa shows no well-formed glands (Gleason 4 pattern). It is important to rule out tangential sectioning and the architecture of accompanying PCa glands. **(Right)** This GS 3 + 3 = 6 PCa has tangentially sectioned, elongated, undulating glands ("tunneling") ⤇ identified by the linear direction of the lumina. The series of luminal compartments represent part of a single continuous lumina (hence not pattern 4), which is not evident in 1 H&E plane.

ACINAR ADENOCARCINOMA

Gleason Pattern 5

(Left) Solid sheet-like growth without luminal formation is considered Gleason pattern 5. *(Right)* This Gleason pattern 5 PCa with comedonecrosis shows a large, partly cribriform gland with a central collection of necrotic tumor "ghost" cells ➡️. The comedonecrosis of Gleason pattern 5 may also be surrounded by solid or papillary growth of cells. Comedonecrosis should be distinguished from amorphous secretions with pyknotic nuclei, which may be seen in Gleason pattern 3 glands.

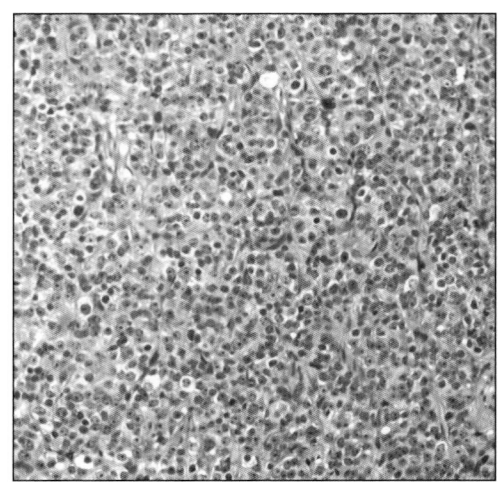 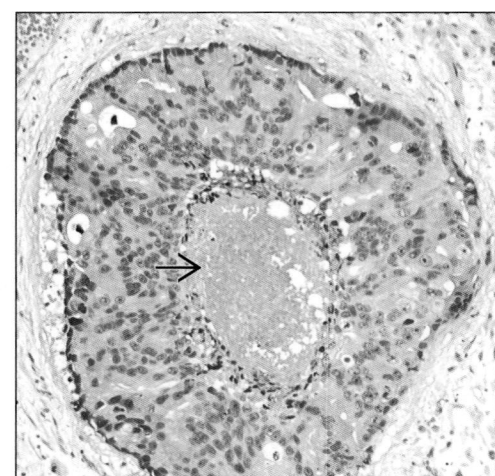

(Left) Gleason pattern 5 PCa solid architecture shows diffuse sheet-like growth without lumina. This pattern may be difficult to distinguish from urothelial carcinoma involving the prostate. Use of p63 &/or HMCK(34βE12) immunostains are helpful in making this distinction. *(Right)* Gleason pattern 5 PCa with central comedonecrosis shows a large, irregular, cribriform gland with central area of necrotic tumor cells ➡️. Stringent criteria should be used in identifying tumor cell necrosis.

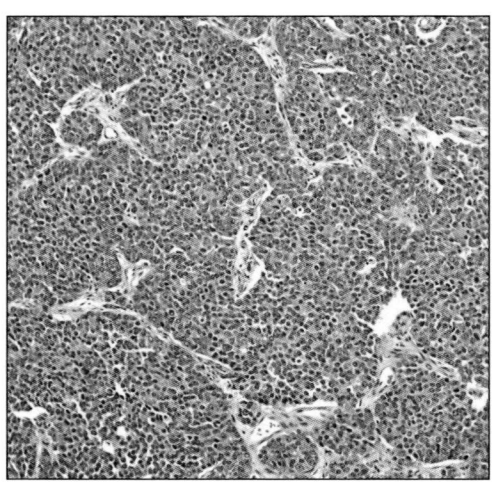 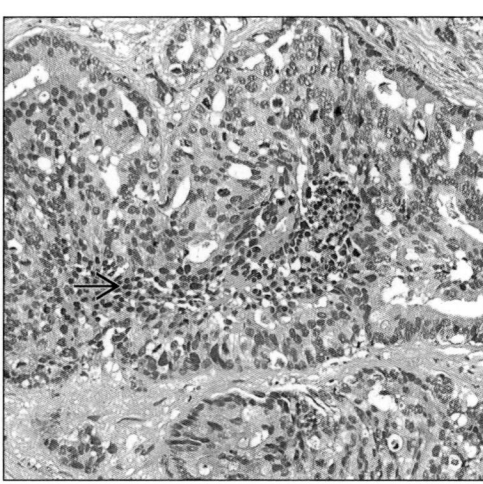

(Left) Infiltration of PCa as linear chains and individual single cells is designated as Gleason pattern 5. *(Right)* This PCa shows prominent cytoplasmic vacuoles, which should not be considered signet ring differentiation (Gleason pattern 5). The ISUP consensus recommends discounting the vacuoles while assigning a grade. In this case, the underlying architecture of the vacuolated cells is that of Gleason pattern 4, poorly formed glands.

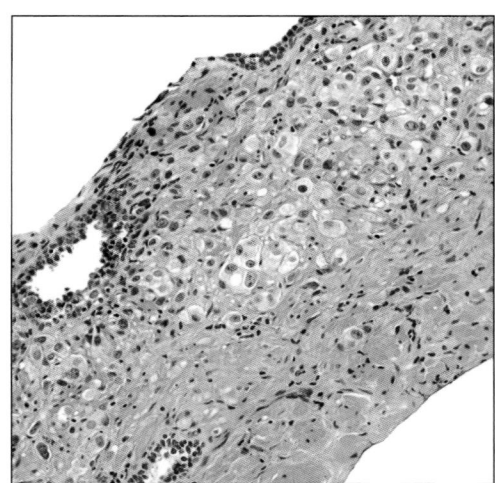 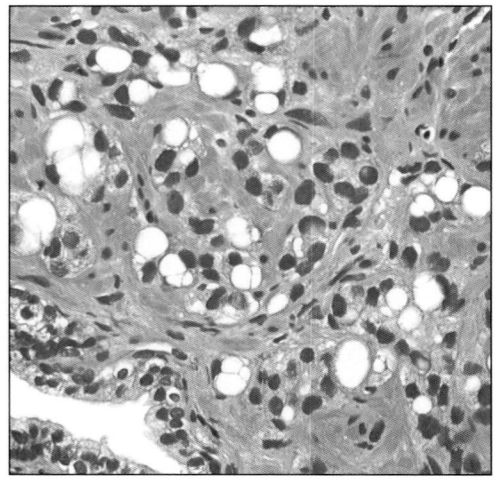

ACINAR ADENOCARCINOMA

Prostatic Adenocarcinoma, Atrophic Variant

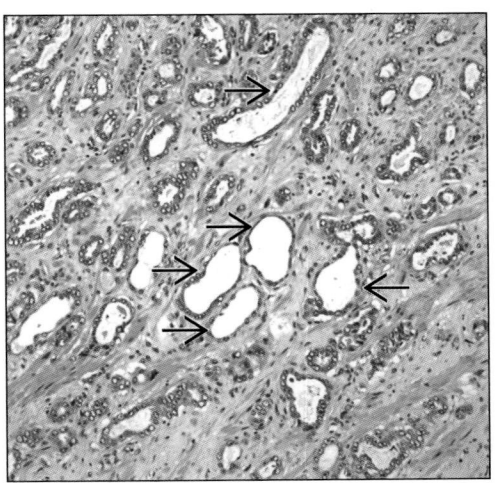
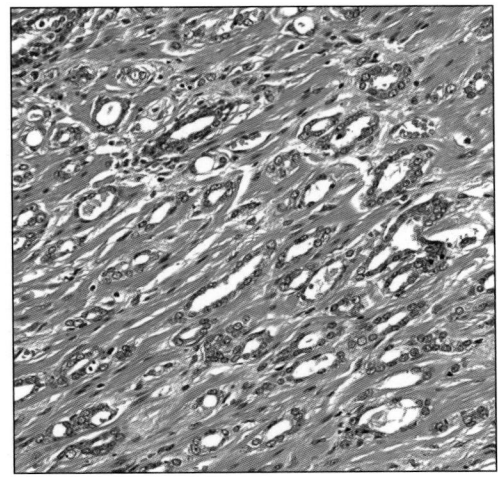

(Left) The atrophic variant of PCa shows infiltration of malignant glands with scant cytoplasm, resembling atrophy. There is often heterogeneity with some markedly atrophic forms ⤐. *(Right)* The atrophic variant of PCa shows acini lined by cells with attenuated cytoplasm. Helpful features indicative of malignancy include malignant nuclear features (e.g., nucleomegaly, prominent nucleoli), nonlobular or infiltrative growth, luminal features of malignancy, and admixed usual PCa morphology.

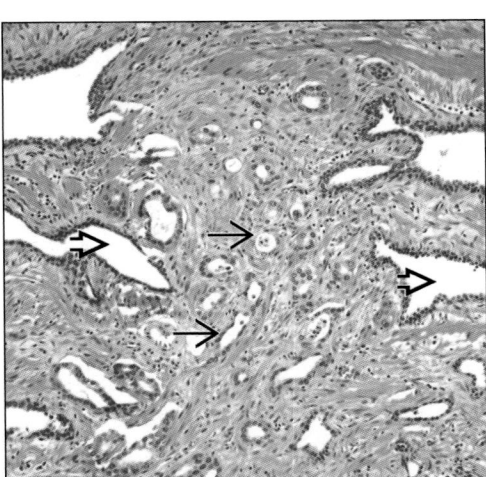
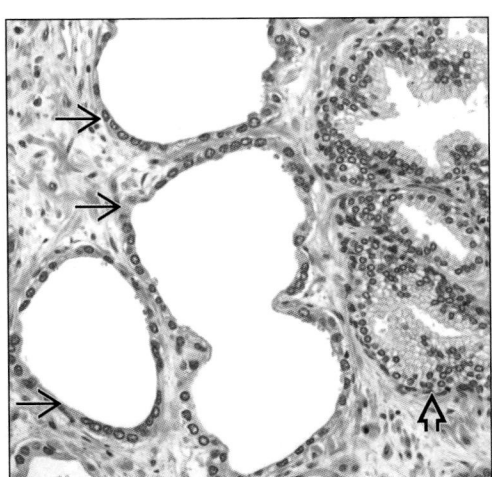

(Left) This PCa with an atrophic morphology allows comparison of the smaller infiltrating carcinoma glands ⤐ with the larger benign atrophic glands ⮚. A nonlobular architecture is key to recognize this subtle variant. *(Right)* At high-power magnification, the nucleomegaly and occasional nucleoli may be appreciated in this atrophic PCa ⤐. In contrast, the adjacent benign glands ⮚ have smaller nuclei and an intact basal cell layer.

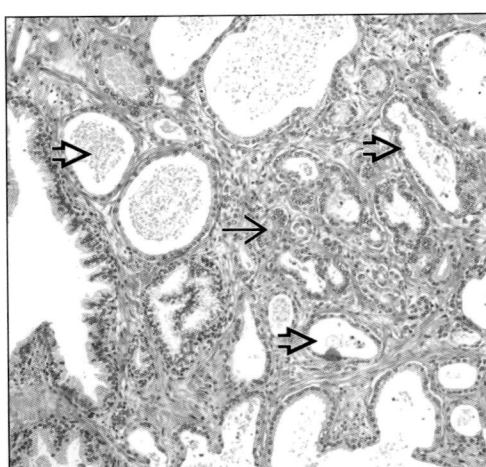
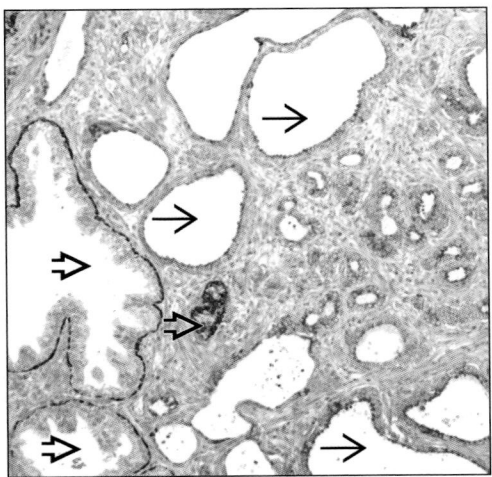

(Left) This example of PCa shows an admixture of both typical ⤐ and markedly atrophic ⮚ carcinoma glands. The nonlobular growth and admixture with more typical areas of PCa are helpful in this case. *(Right)* As expected, the AMACR/p63/HMCK cocktail immunostain shows an absence of basal cells, even in the markedly atrophic-appearing large glands ⤐ (with strong internal control in benign glands ⮚). The carcinoma glands also show strong luminal AMACR immunoreactivity.

ACINAR ADENOCARCINOMA

Prostatic Adenocarcinoma, Foamy Variant

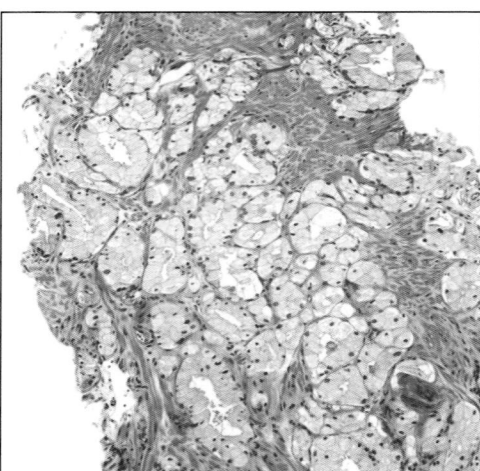 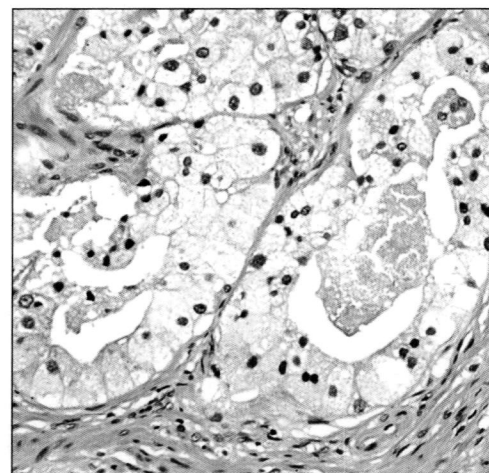

(Left) Invasive foamy carcinoma of the prostate is characterized by abundant xanthomatous cytoplasm. *(Right)* The foamy gland variant of PCa shows cells with abundant xanthomatous cytoplasm, small to pyknotic nuclei, and eosinophilic luminal secretions. The typical malignant nuclear features of PCa may not be present, making recognition as PCa difficult. Infiltrative growth, negativity for basal cell markers, and familiarity with the unique features are helpful in diagnosis.

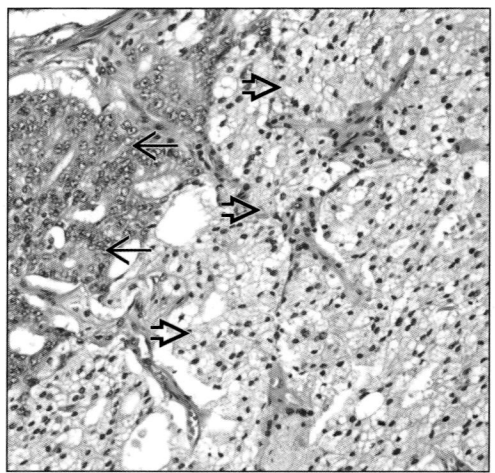 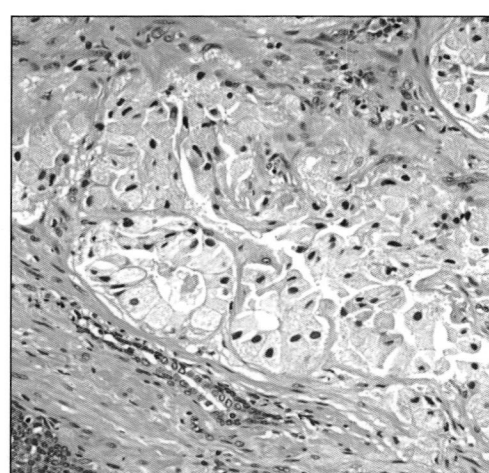

(Left) This photomicrograph contrasts the small, relatively pyknotic nuclei of the foamy gland carcinoma component ⊃ with the large nuclei with prominent nucleoli ➔ in the more conventional acinar PCa. *(Right)* Some studies suggest that foamy gland carcinoma, as seen in this photomicrograph, potentially has a worse prognosis than conventional acinar PCa, although the prognostic significance is debatable. AMACR staining is less frequently positive (32-38%) in foamy gland carcinoma.

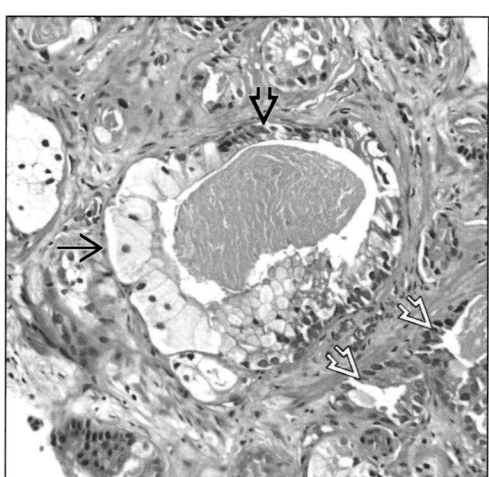 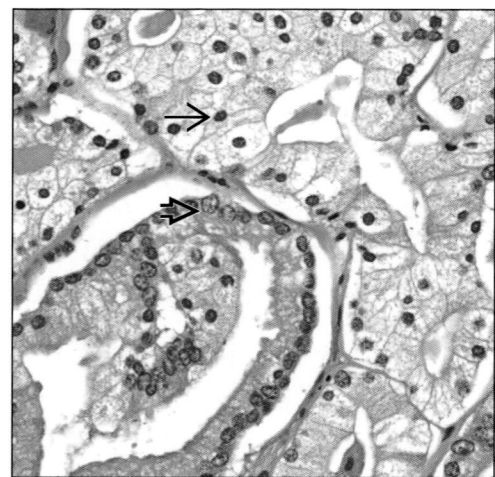

(Left) The central gland in this PCa shows a mixture of foamy features ➔ and conventional morphology ⊃ within the same gland. Adjacent typical PCa is present ⊃. This combination is not infrequent and contributes to difficulty in defining this variant and its prognostic significance. *(Right)* Foamy PCa cells with small pyknotic nuclei ➔ set in a xanthomatous cytoplasm are highlighted and contrasted with the adjacent focus showing more typical nuclear features ⊃.

ACINAR ADENOCARCINOMA

Prostatic Adenocarcinoma, Pseudohyperplastic Variant

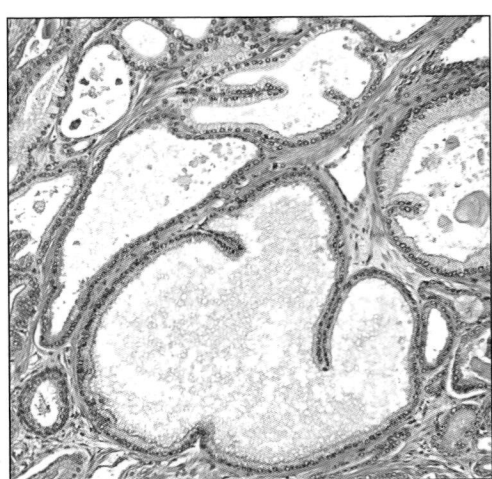

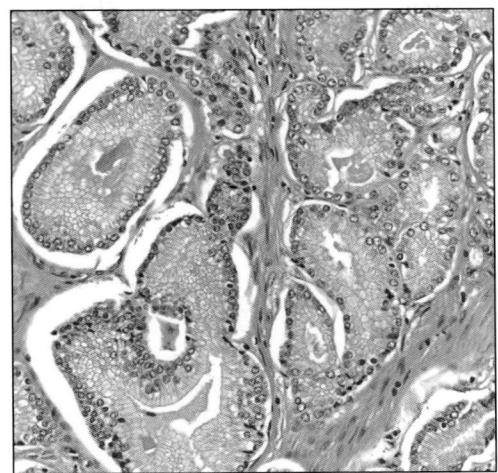

(Left) The pseudohyperplastic variant of PCa shows medium to large dilated glands with papillary infoldings and luminal eosinophilic secretions. These glands are deceptively benign on low-power view and may be mistaken for hyperplastic benign glands. *(Right)* The abundant cytoplasm and larger-caliber glands admixed with smaller glands may impart a deceptively benign appearance. In this case, the intraluminal mucin should raise additional suspicion for carcinoma.

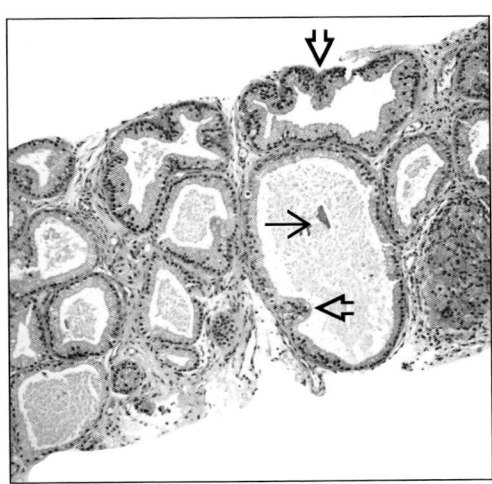

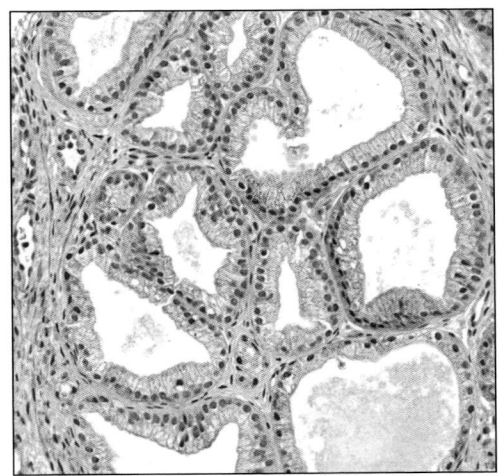

(Left) Prostate biopsy shows a morphologically subtle, pseudohyperplastic PCa characterized by evenly dispersed large-caliber glands with papillary infoldings ⊳ and intraluminal eosinophilic secretions with rare crystalloids ➔. *(Right)* HMCK(34βE12) documents complete absence of basal cells in pseudohyperplastic PCa. Internal positive controls were present in basal cells of benign glands. AMACR staining (not shown here) may be negative in many cases with this pattern.

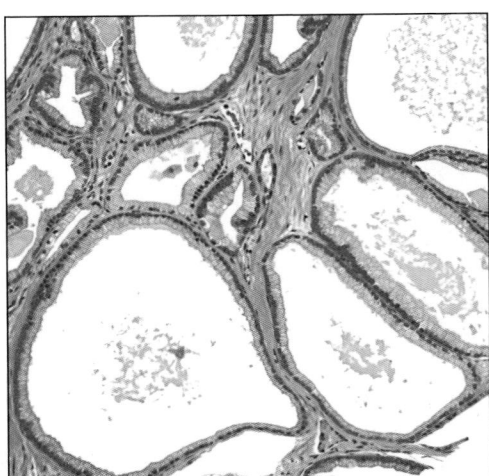

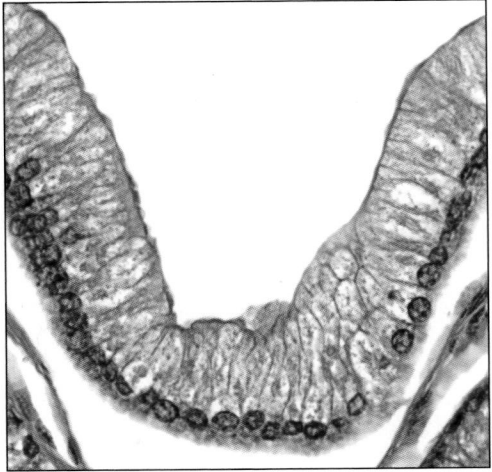

(Left) This pseudohyperplastic PCa also has large-caliber glands, but the abundant luminal cytoplasm and basally oriented nuclei suggest the diagnosis of malignancy at low power. Adjunctive immunohistochemistry (AMACR/p63/HMCK) is often used to confirm histologically subtle patterns of adenocarcinoma. *(Right)* Pseudohyperplastic PCa often has abundant luminal cytoplasm, and nuclei may show alignment at the basal layer, as seen in this example.

Prostatic Adenocarcinoma, PIN-like

(Left) This is an unusual example of the morphologically subtle PIN-like invasive PCa. On low-power evaluation, the architecture suggests normal glands but with some degree of hyperchromasia in the lining cells. *(Right)* The epithelium is pseudostratified columnar, which has led some authors to regard this as a pattern of ductal carcinoma. These "PIN-like invasive PCas" do not seem to be as aggressive as conventional ductal PCa. Immunostaining is necessary to confirm the diagnosis.

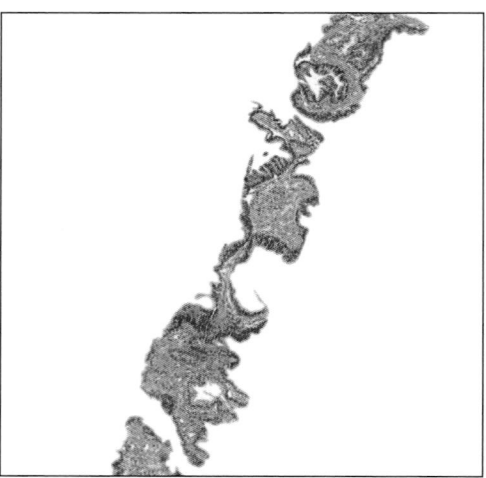
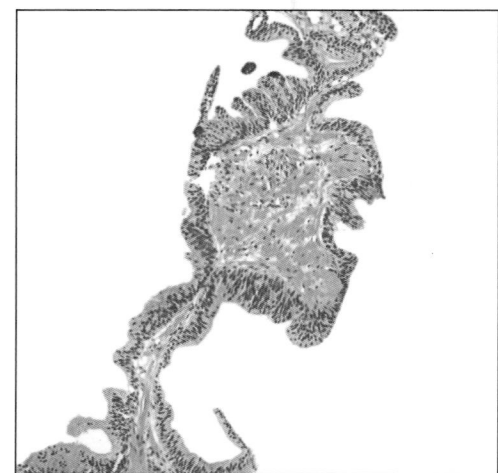

(Left) At high-power magnification, the hyperchromasia and pseudostratified columnar lining of PIN-like invasive PCa ⬒ are distinct from the adjacent benign glands with the usual round nuclei ⬒. Immunohistochemistry confirmed an absence of basal cells. *(Right)* Rare examples of invasive PCa have a multilayered or stratified epithelial layer, as seen here, that closely mimics HGPIN with apparent basal cells. This case mimics the flat pattern of HGPIN.

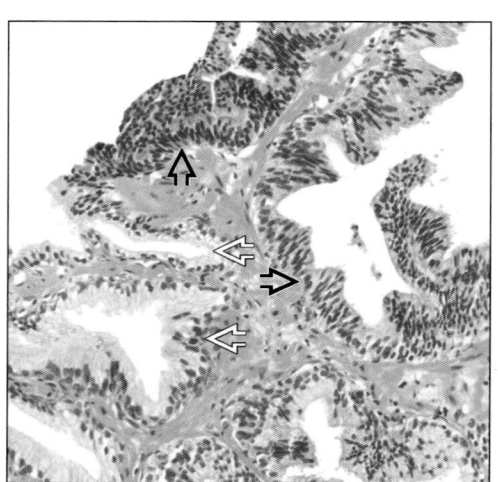
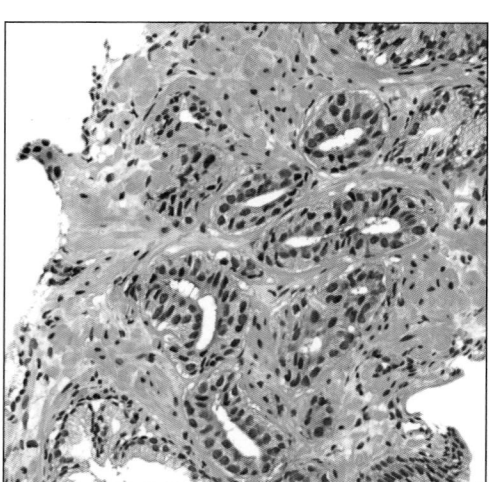

(Left) Unusual PCa pattern with acini shows several layers of secretory cells ➡ with malignant nuclear features similar to that of usual PCa. The architecture and cytology may mimic flat or tufted HGPIN glands, requiring adjunctive confirmatory immunostaining. *(Right)* This p63/HMCK(34βE12) cocktail confirms an absence of basal cells in this PCa ⬒ with an unusual stratified appearance. There is a strong internal control staining in the basal cells of adjacent benign glands ➡.

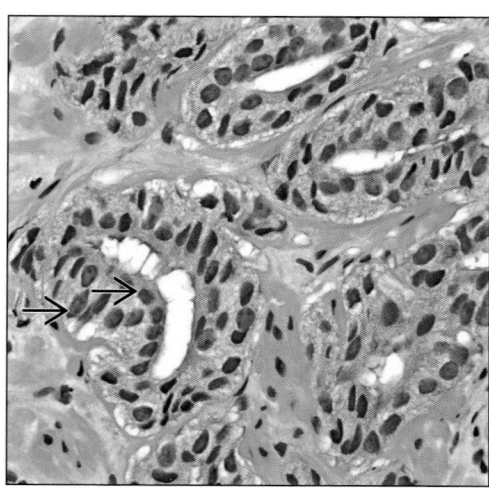
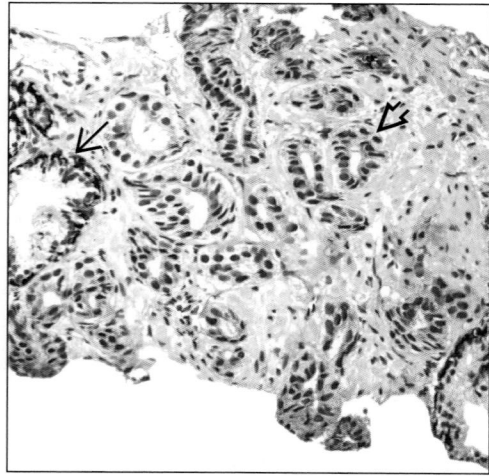

Prostatic Adenocarcinoma, Other Variants

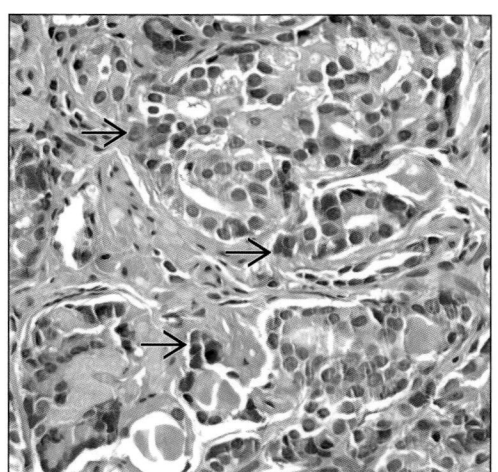

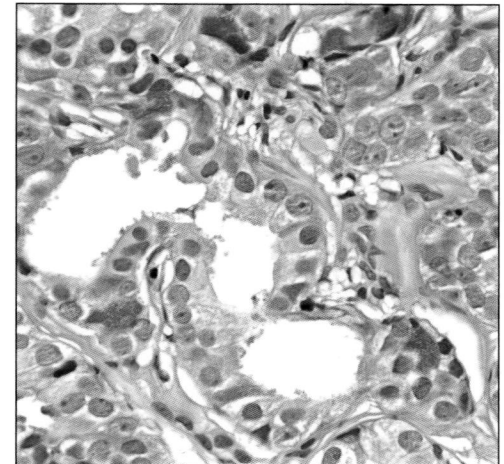

(Left) PCa with Paneth-cell-like differentiation shows occasional neuroendocrine cells ➔ with bright eosinophilic cytoplasmic granules resembling Paneth cells of the gastrointestinal tract. *(Right)* These PCa with Paneth-cell-like differentiation are reportedly indolent even in the presence of more architecturally complex patterns; therefore, it has been suggested that this variant not be graded.

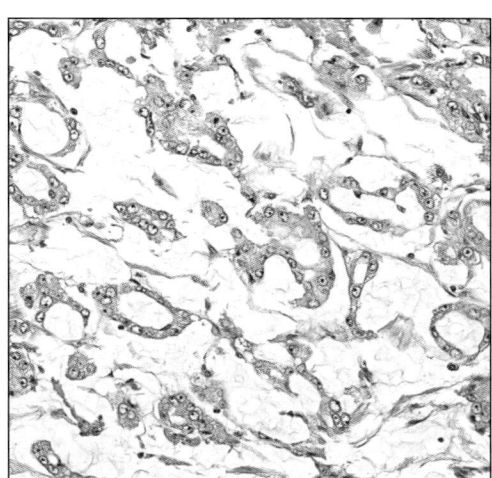

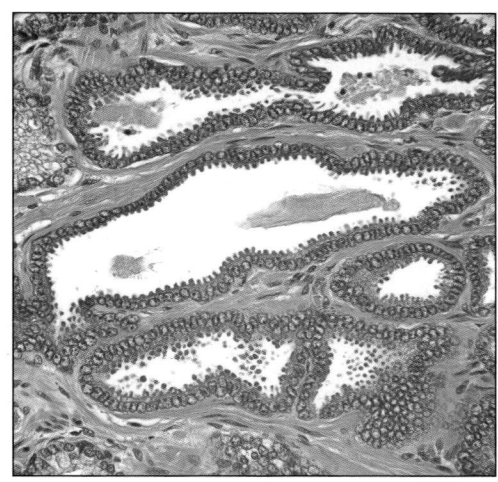

(Left) Mucinous (colloid) carcinoma is characterized by the presence of malignant epithelium "floating" in abundant extracellular mucin. This is distinct from the intraluminal mucin seen in more typical forms of PCa. When this finding is seen exclusively in a biopsy, confirmation of prostatic origin by immunostains is necessary. *(Right)* This highly unusual form of PCa shows luminal cellular apocrine-like snouts. This pattern is usually admixed with typical PCa and may also be seen in HGPIN.

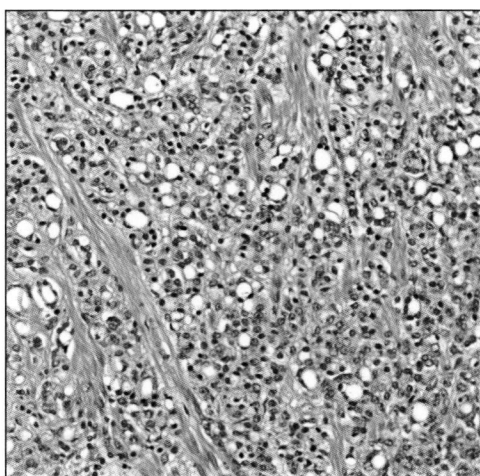

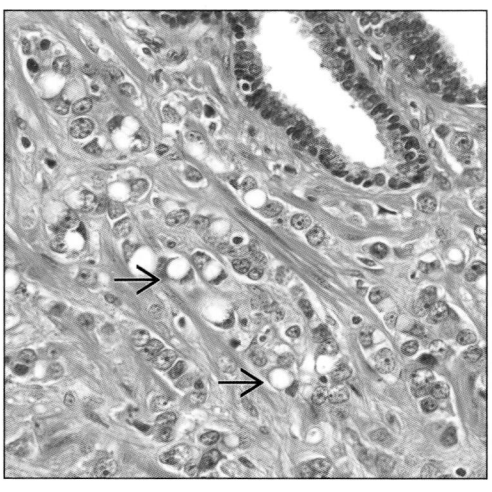

(Left) This signet ring cell PCa is composed of sheets of discohesive round cells with scattered vacuoles displacing the nuclei peripherally. Signet ring cell features may be seen in lymphocytes, rarely in stromal nodular BPH and sarcomas involving the prostate. *(Right)* Signet ring cell variant of PCa shows diffuse infiltrates of individual cells that include some with optically clear vacuoles displacing the nuclei peripherally ➔. This carcinoma is usually Gleason patterns 4 and 5.

ACINAR ADENOCARCINOMA

Therapy-related Changes

(Left) PCa with radiation effect shows poorly formed, atrophic glands with foamy or vacuolated cytoplasm and nucleolomegaly ➡. Gleason grading is not recommended for PCa with treatment effect. Marked radiation effect may artifactually produce an architecture resembling GS 9 or 10 PCa. *(Right)* PCa with radiation effect shows voluminous foamy cells with focal squamous differentiation ➡. Radiation may induce squamous differentiation in both primary and metastatic foci of PCa.

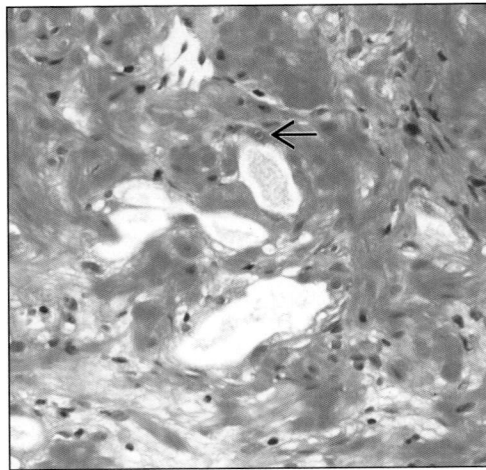
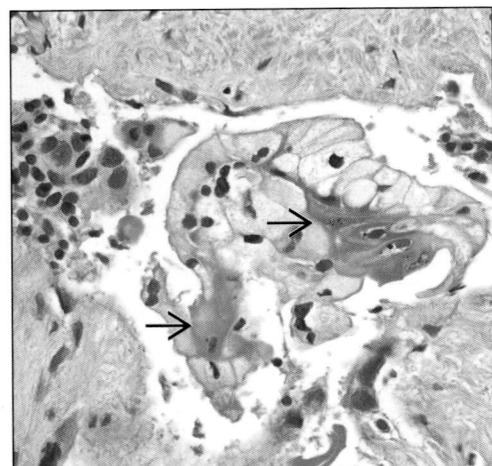

(Left) PCa with radiation effect may show atrophic changes and vacuolated cytoplasm ➡. Adjacent PCa glands ➡ show minimal radiation effect in this case. The effects of radiation in PCa are variable. Minimal or no radiation effect following radiotherapy portends a poorer prognosis. The carcinoma without treatment effect should be graded as usual. *(Right)* PCa with hormonal therapy effect shows shrunken PCa glands. Some PCa cells may resemble inflammatory cells and histiocytes.

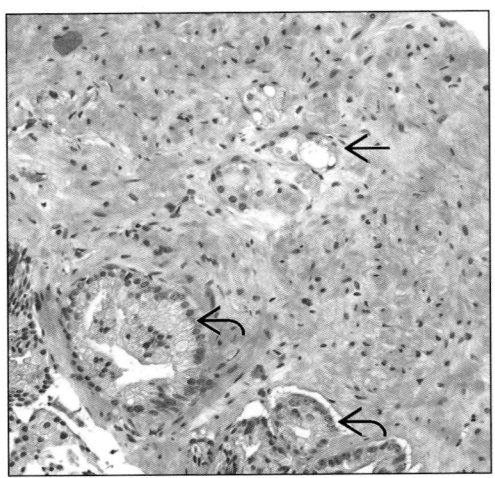
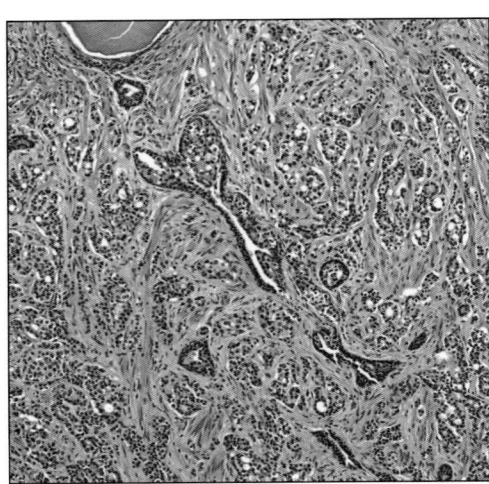

(Left) PCa with hormonal therapy effect shows shrunken cells with vacuolated and xanthomatous cytoplasm. Some cells display pyknotic nuclei. AMACR staining is variable and proportional to the degree of therapy effect. *(Right)* PCa with hormonal therapy effect shows shrunken PCa cells ➡, not readily identifiable on low power, that may mimic inflammatory cells. Use of PAN-CK(AE1/AE3) helps to facilitate detection of residual PCa. Cystic spaces ➡ may also be seen following therapy.

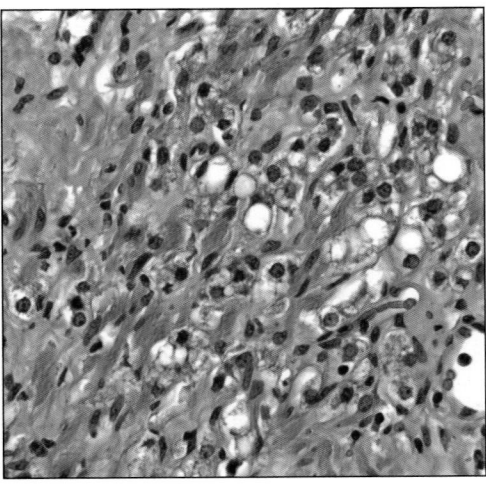
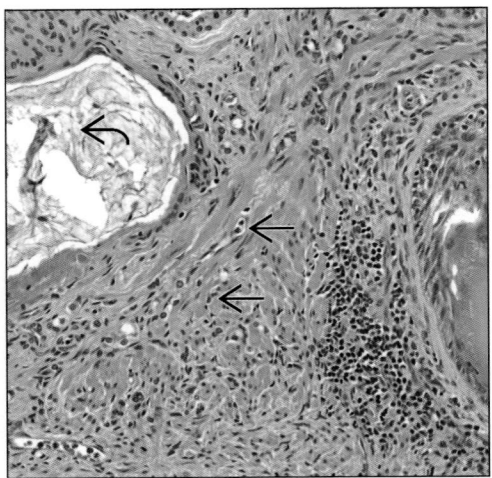

ACINAR ADENOCARCINOMA

Differential Diagnosis

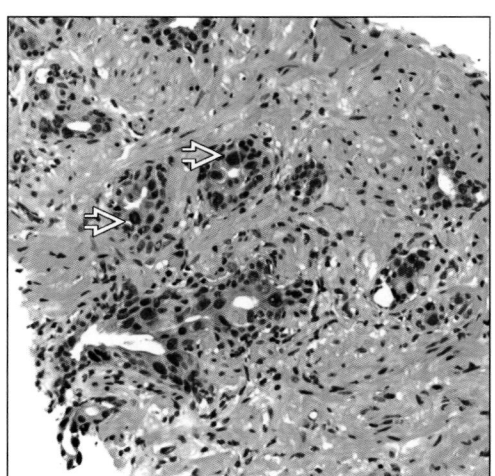

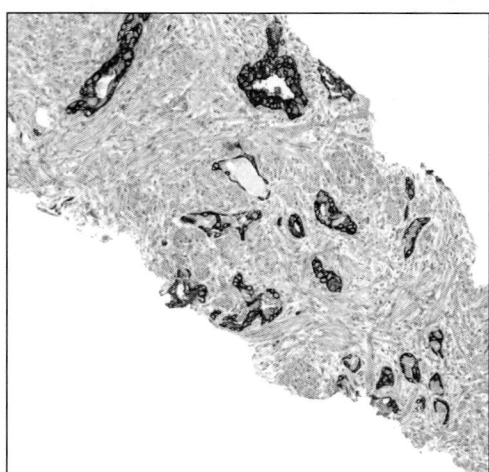

(Left) These benign prostatic glands with radiation therapy effect show marked nuclear pleomorphism ⮚. The pleomorphism is due to variable effect on benign basal cells and secretory cells. Nuclear pleomorphism is extremely uncommon in PCa. *(Right)* Following local radiation therapy, benign glands invariably show strong and diffuse cytoplasmic immunoreactivity for HMCK. This makes the distinction from malignancy relatively straightforward with immunostaining.

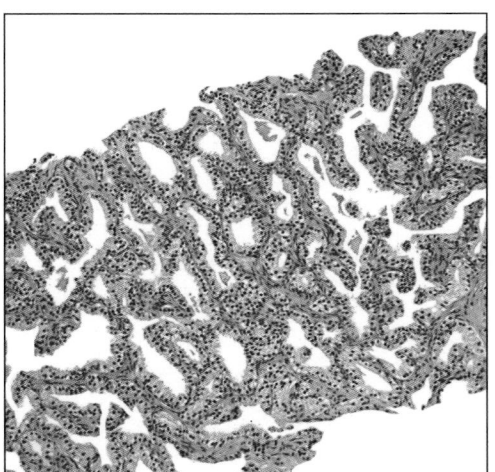

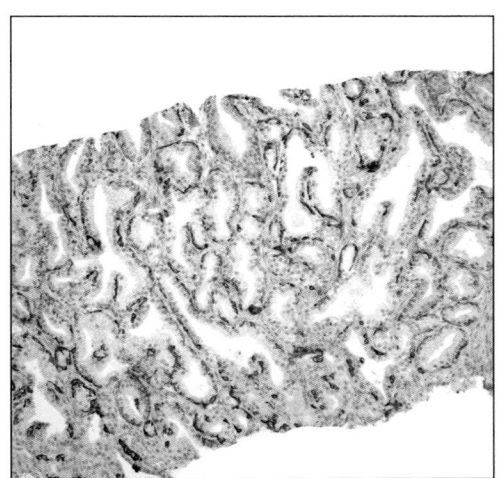

(Left) Atypical adenomatous hyperplasia (adenosis) is characterized by crowded glands, but varying caliber glands with normal cytology and luminal infolding and tufting are common. This lesion occurs mostly within the transition zone, so it is relatively uncommon on needle biopsy. *(Right)* The HMCK(34βE12) staining in this atypical adenomatous hyperplasia (adenosis) demonstrates basal cells. In atypical adenomatous hyperplasia, the basal layer may be patchy or even absent in some acini.

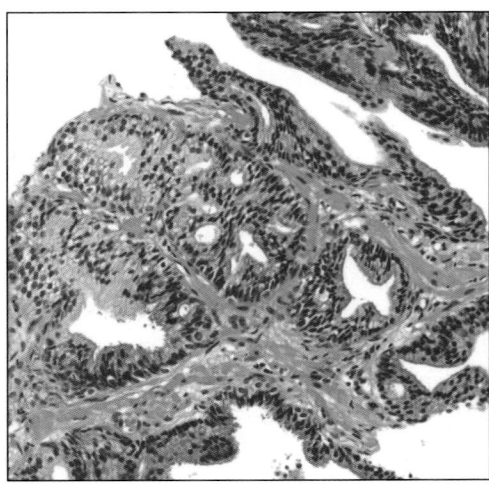

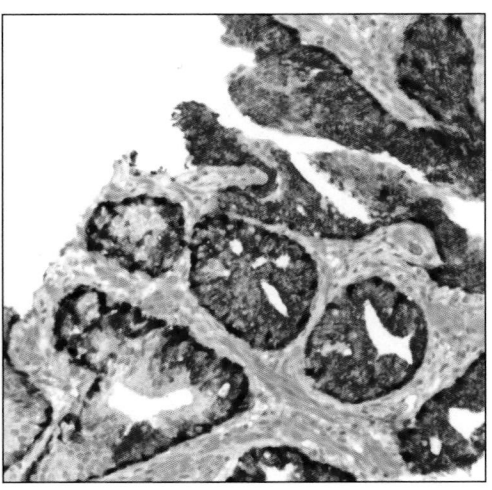

(Left) Cribriform high-grade prostatic intraepithelial neoplasia, as seen in this example, may closely mimic invasive adenocarcinoma with a cribriform pattern (Gleason pattern 4). Central zone glands and clear cell cribriform hyperplasia are also mimics. *(Right)* In this AMACR/p63/HMCK immunostain cocktail, there is strong luminal AMACR reactivity, but the basal layer remains intact, features expected in high-grade prostatic intraepithelial neoplasia.

ACINAR ADENOCARCINOMA

Differential Diagnosis

(Left) *Partial atrophy, atrophy, and postatrophic hyperplasia are the most common mimics of PCa encountered in daily practice. The loss of luminal cytoplasm with preserved lateral cytoplasm is characteristic.* **(Right)** *This HMCK(34βE12) immunostain highlights a patchy discontinuous basal cell layer, a pattern typical for partial atrophy. Some glands in partial atrophy may completely lack basal cells ➡, but the overall staining in the entire focus should be interpreted.*

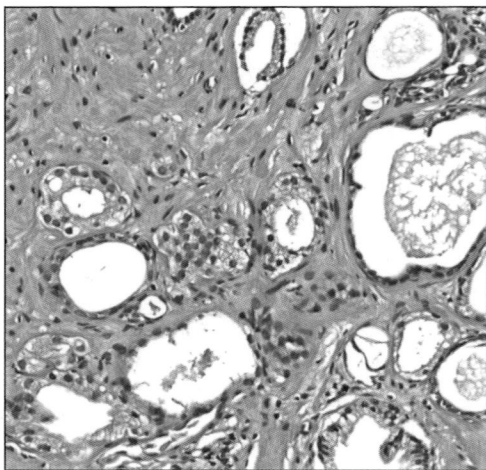
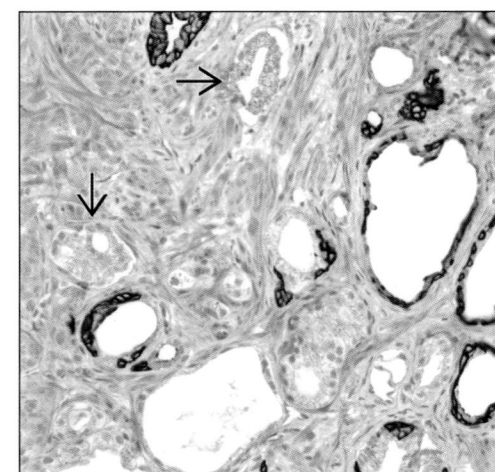

(Left) *Verumontanum gland hyperplasia is typically adjacent to the prostatic urethra epithelium and is characterized by a back-to-back collection of varying sized benign prostate glands. Intraluminal secretions and corpora amylacea are common.* **(Right)** *On high-power examination, this example of verumontanum gland hyperplasia shows varying caliber glands, luminal undulation, and a preserved basal cell layer that may be confirmed by immunohistochemistry.*

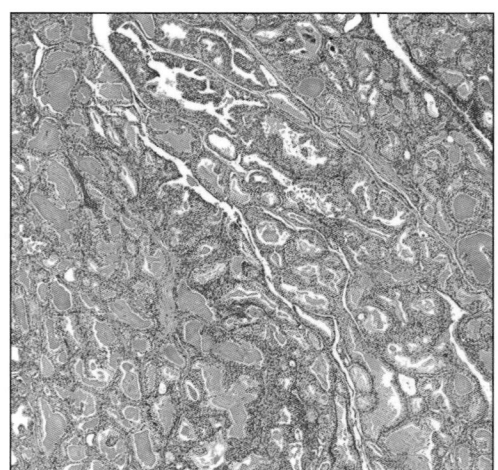
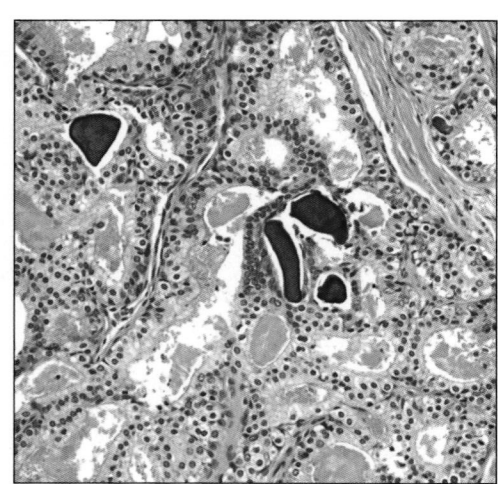

(Left) *Seminal vesicle (SV) epithelium commonly has scattered pleomorphic cells, intranuclear inclusions, and intracytoplasmic coarse yellow pigment, which all aid in the distinction from PCa. It is extraordinarily rare for PCa to show marked nuclear pleomorphism.* **(Right)** *Pax-2 immunostaining shows strong nuclear reactivity in SV epithelium but not in the neoplastic cell population of PCa. This staining pattern is useful, as PSA, PAP, and AMACR may show nonspecific reaction in SV.*

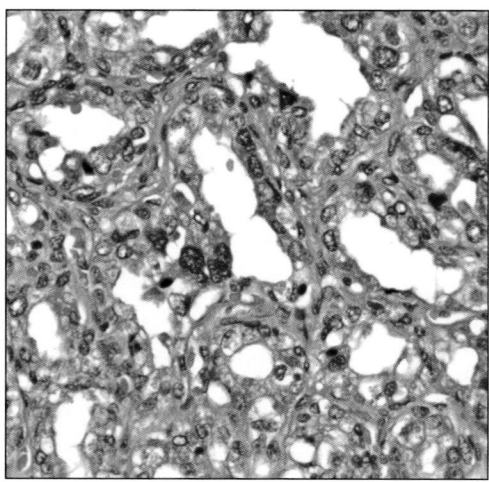
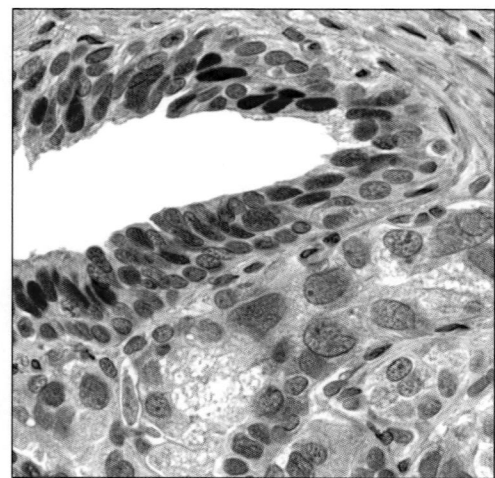

ACINAR ADENOCARCINOMA

Differential Diagnosis

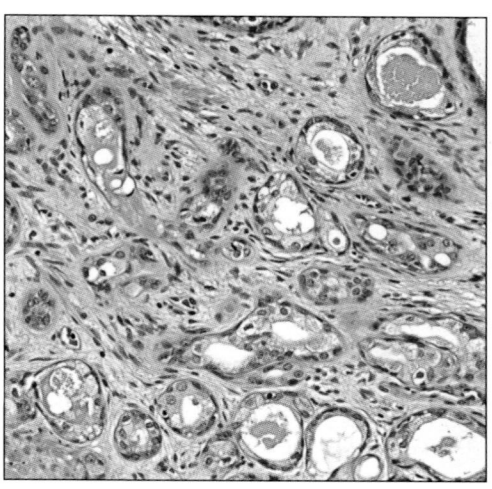

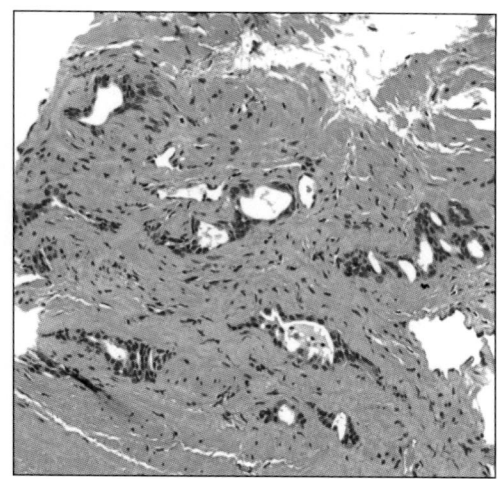

(Left) Sclerosing adenosis is rare and is seen most commonly in the transition zone. It is characterized by crowded benign glands with an associated cytologically benign spindle cell component. The spindle cells commonly have a myoepithelial phenotype not typically found in prostatic basal cells. *(Right)* Sclerotic atrophy may closely mimic the invasive growth of PCa. Nevertheless, the angulated glands with scant cytoplasm and the dense fibrotic stroma are distinctive.

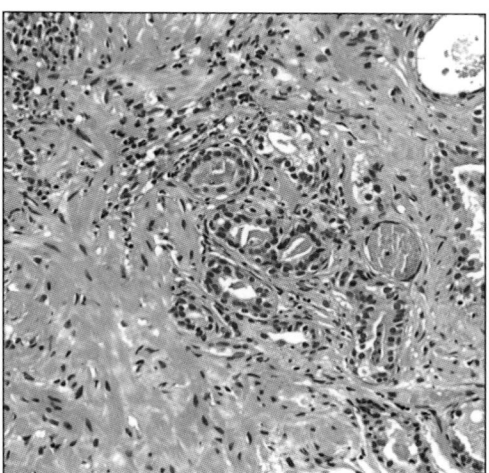

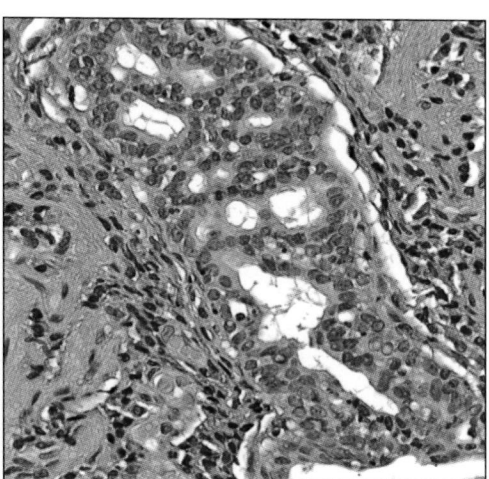

(Left) When associated with inflammatory infiltrates, benign glands may appear crowded and hyperchromatic. In addition, luminal secretions may be present. A diagnosis of malignancy should be rendered with great caution in the setting of inflammatory infiltrates. *(Right)* Benign glands may also show pseudoneoplastic cribriform pattern when associated with significant inflammation. Reactive atypia with nucleoli in the epithelium further compounds the diagnostic dilemma.

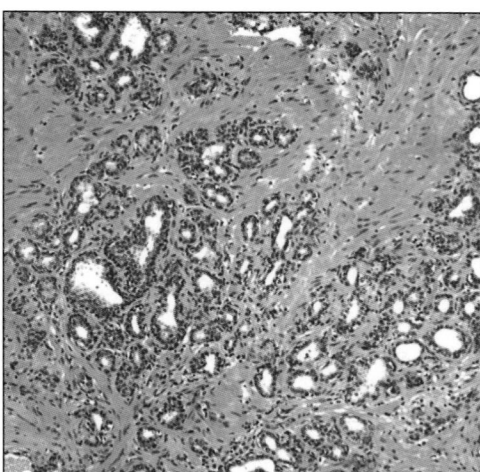

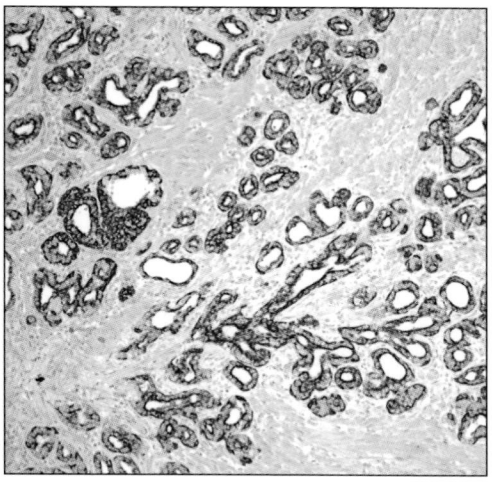

(Left) Postatrophic hyperplasia is characterized by an aggregate of small, crowded benign glands with atrophic features. The glands are usually situated in a lobular arrangement and may have an associated central larger-caliber duct. Lobular architecture and variation in size and shape of the glands are useful diagnostic features. *(Right)* With HMCK(34BE12) immunostaining, postatrophic hyperplasia typically shows strong and diffuse basal cell positivity, as illustrated.

ATYPICAL SMALL ACINAR PROLIFERATIONS

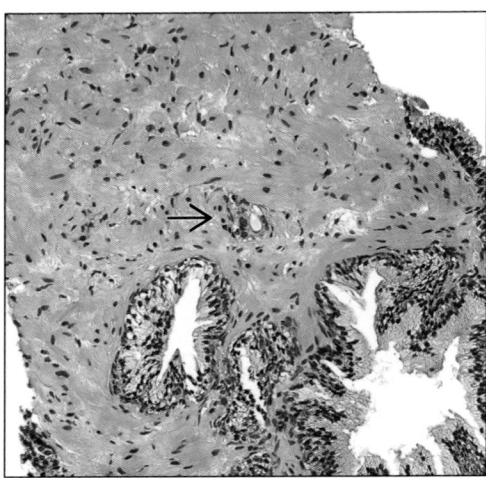

This single atypical gland ➡, with a sharp rigid lumen, nucleomegaly, and subtle intraluminal mucin, is an example of "ASAP suspicious for focal adenocarcinoma."

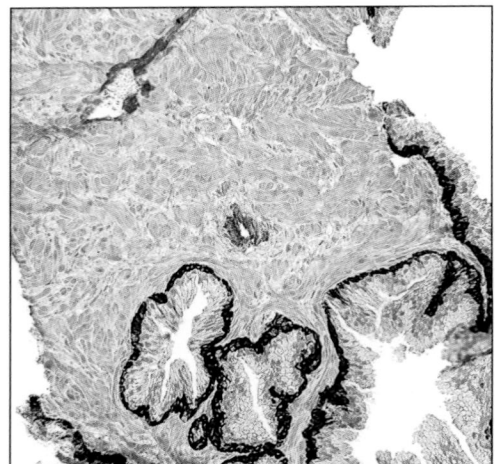

Despite the AMACR overexpression (red) and lack of basal cell markers (brown) typical of carcinoma, this is regarded as "ASAP suspicious for focal adenocarcinoma" given the presence of only 1 gland.

TERMINOLOGY

Abbreviations
- Atypical small acinar proliferation (ASAP)

Synonyms
- Suspicious for cancer
- Focal glandular atypia
- Atypical glands

Definitions
- Focus of atypical glands in needle biopsy quantitatively &/or qualitatively insufficient for definitive diagnosis or exclusion of prostate carcinoma (PCa)
- ASAP is not an entity
  - Represents descriptive diagnosis to guide subsequent clinical management
    - Includes undersampled PCa and various benign mimics of PCa
- ASAP introduced in 1993 and is well-accepted descriptive diagnosis in contemporary practice
  - Term ASAP not entirely accurate as some atypical foci may not be "acinar," "small," or "proliferative"
    - Some atypical glandular lesions suspicious for carcinoma are comprised of large caliber glands (e.g., pseudohyperplastic carcinoma)

CLINICAL ISSUES

Epidemiology
- Incidence
  - Reported in 5% of prostate needle biopsies (individual series vary from 0.7-9%)
    - Threshold for establishing PCa diagnosis has interobserver variability
    - Variation, even amongst experts, dependent on experience and training

Presentation
- Biopsy performed for known indications
  - Elevated serum PSA level
  - Abnormal digital rectal examination
  - Abnormal transrectal ultrasound

Laboratory Tests
- Serum PSA level may be elevated
  - No significant difference in serum PSA level between patients with PCa on initial biopsy and with ASAP diagnosis preceding subsequent PCa on rebiopsy

Treatment
- Patient with ASAP diagnosis should be rebiopsied with extended sampling of prostate gland, including anatomic region where suspicious focus was found

Prognosis
- Carries higher risk of finding PCa in rebiopsy (40-50%; individual series vary between 17-70%)
- Subsequent PCa may also be identified in contralateral side (up to 27%)
- When adjacent to high-grade prostatic intraepithelial neoplasia (HGPIN) (HGPIN and ASAP), higher risk of carcinoma than HGPIN alone
- Most PCa detected on subsequent rebiopsy are Gleason score 6 (up to 80%)
  - May be ≥ Gleason score 8 in some cases (up to 10%)

MICROSCOPIC PATHOLOGY

Histologic Features
- Typically group of small crowded glands that do not meet threshold for definitive carcinoma diagnosis
  - May have too few glands or insufficient qualitative features
- Quantitative factors associated with ASAP diagnosis
  - Inadequate number of glands
    - No absolute cut-off in number of glands is a formal criteria for diagnosis of PCa

ATYPICAL SMALL ACINAR PROLIFERATIONS

Prostate Gland and Seminal Vesicle

Key Facts

Terminology

- Focus of atypical glands in needle biopsy
  - Quantitatively &/or qualitatively insufficient for definitive diagnosis or exclusion of prostatic carcinoma
- Not a diagnostic entity
  - Includes undersampled cancer and various benign mimics
  - Represents descriptive diagnosis to aid in subsequent clinical management

Clinical Issues

- Reported in 5% of prostate needle biopsy (0.7-9%)
- ASAP diagnosis should prompt rebiopsy
  - Particularly in area with previous suspicious focus
- Carries higher risk of finding PCa in rebiopsy
  - Mean: 40%; range: 17-70%

Microscopic Pathology

- Atypical small glands that either are too few or do not show minimum morphologic features for definite diagnosis as PCa
- IHC with AMACR and basal cell markers may be helpful
  - Should be aware of overlap with benign lesions in small foci

Top Differential Diagnoses

- Benign
  - Partial atrophy
  - Atypical adenomatous hyperplasia (adenosis)
  - Crowded benign glands
- Malignant
  - Prostatic acinar adenocarcinoma

- In absence of pathognomonic features, minimum requirement for PCa varies between expert genitourinary pathologists
- Most authors do not recommend diagnosis of PCa on single atypical gland; others favor presence of at least 3 glands
- Threshold largely dependent on extent of other associated qualitative features: Infiltrative growth, cytologic atypia, intraluminal mucin, crystalloids, nucleoli
  - Small size of atypical glandular focus
    - Linear extent usually < 0.8 mm
- Qualitative factors associated with ASAP diagnosis
  - Features may suggest PCa but are insufficient to reach diagnostic threshold for PCa
    - Architecture may not show definite infiltration
    - May lack significant nuclear atypia (i.e., absence of nucleomegaly &/or nucleolomegaly)
    - Glandular lumina may have smooth, sharp contour (no luminal irregularity or infolding) or basal palisading of nuclei without other features
    - Diagnostic threshold for PCa may be more stringent when certain histologic findings are present: Atrophic features, pseudohyperplastic appearance, or foamy cytoplasm
  - ASAP frequently does not have any pathognomonic features of PCa
    - Glomerulations
    - Collagenous micronodules (mucinous fibroplasia)
    - Circumferential perineural or intraneural invasion
    - Invasion of adipose tissue or seminal vesicle
  - Confounding features
    - Presence at edge of biopsy
    - Poor cytologic detail, such as crush artifact
    - Obscuring inflammation
    - Loss of atypical focus on subsequent (and intervening) levels precluding adjunctive immunohistochemistry (IHC)
    - When adjacent to HGPIN, makes distinction from noninvasive outpouchings of HGPIN difficult

Predominant Pattern/Injury Type

- Not applicable

Adjuncts in Work-Up and Diagnosis

- Ancillary IHC helpful in resolving some ASAP cases as PCa or benign glands
  - Prospectively obtaining intervening unstained slides is important and beneficial
- Multiple levels (ideally 3) should be on each H&E slide to enhance representation of atypical focus
- Deeper levels, particularly if atypical focus is present in last level, may produce more diagnostic features
- When atypical glands are present in conjunction with separate cores showing definitive cancer, there may be need for further evaluation if diagnosis of PCa would upstage tumor (e.g., bilateral involvement)
- Internal &/or external expert consultation may help resolve issue of diagnostic uncertainty
  - For some cases, ASAP remains best diagnosis

ANCILLARY TESTS

Immunohistochemistry

- 2 general approaches (philosophies) to interpreting adjunctive IHC in diagnosis of focal PCa
  - Use to establish definitive diagnosis as PCa
    - To confirm very strong impression of carcinoma
    - To confirm carcinoma of morphologically subtle subtype
  - Use to exclude benign process, which would preclude ASAP designation
    - Typically in cases with less diagnostic certainty
    - When partial atrophy and other mimics are considered
    - In this setting, presence of basal cells would determine diagnosis as benign (positive) or ASAP (negative)
  - Decision not to render definitive PCa diagnosis is made on H&E evaluation

3

95

ATYPICAL SMALL ACINAR PROLIFERATIONS

- If qualitative threshold is not met on H&E review, IHC supportive for PCa may not be sufficient to confidently make diagnosis of PCa
- In cases with absence of basal cells, biopsy is diagnosed as ASAP
- Circumferential luminal AMACR overexpression typical of carcinoma
  - Definitive diagnosis of PCa does not require AMACR expression
    - AMACR may be completely negative or show weak noncircumferential staining
  - False-negative AMACR immunoreactivity
    - 5-25% typical PCa (usually < 10%)
    - Morphologic variants more commonly negative
    - 30% atrophic PCa
    - 32-38% foamy gland PCa
    - 23-30% pseudohyperplastic PCa
    - 29% hormonally treated PCa
  - False-positive AMACR immunoreactivity (usually weaker noncircumferential staining)
    - 2-36% benign glands
    - 10% atypical adenomatous hyperplasia (adenosis)
    - Up to 40% partial atrophy and post atrophic hyperplasia
    - 35-58% nephrogenic adenoma
    - 56-100% of HGPIN (usually 50-60%)
- Absence of basal cell markers (p63, HMCK[34βE12], or CK5/6) required in carcinoma
  - Presence of focal or patchy basal cells argues against diagnosis of invasive carcinoma
  - False-negative PCa staining pattern (absence of basal cells by IHC)
    - 5-23% benign glands
    - Approximately 20-25% partial atrophy
    - Up to 50% atypical adenomatous hyperplasia (adenosis)

DIFFERENTIAL DIAGNOSIS

Prostatic Carcinoma (PCa)

- ASAP, in most instances, represents PCa in which diagnostic features are not present
- Minimal volume PCa
  - Quantitatively insufficient glands
- PCa variants
  - Foamy gland variant may have small pyknotic nuclei
  - Atrophic variant may have significant histologic overlap with partial atrophy
- Presence of well-described pathognomonic features of carcinoma in small foci are often diagnostic of cancer regardless of extent
  - Collagenous micronodules (mucinous fibroplasia), circumferential perineural invasion, glomerulations or invasion of adipose tissue
- Clear presence of Gleason pattern 4 or higher warrants definitive diagnosis of carcinoma

Normal Structures

- Benign crowded glands
  - Lack nuclear features of PCa

- If reactivity is present, AMACR typically shows only patchy, granular cytoplasmic staining without luminal accentuation
- Commonly show obvious basal cells by IHC
- Seminal vesicles/ejaculatory duct epithelium
  - Prominent nuclear pleomorphism with scattered hyperchromatic cells
  - Prominent coarse lipofuscin pigmentation
  - Intranuclear inclusions common
  - Express nuclear pax-2
    - Less intense nuclear staining in ejaculatory duct epithelium
- Cowper glands
  - Typically seen in biopsies from apex
  - Lobular architecture
  - Admixture of mucinous acini and ducts
    - Intracytoplasmic mucin but not intraluminal
  - PSAP negative
  - PSA may show focal staining
  - Muscle specific actin may be positive in basal distribution
- Verumontanum mucosal gland hyperplasia
  - Noninfiltrative closely packed glands of variable caliber
  - Usually closely oriented to urothelium
  - Abundant corpora amylacea and intraluminal concretions
  - HMCK(34βE12) typically highlights numerous basal cells
- Paraganglia
  - Found in 8% of radical prostatectomies
  - Usually located in periprostatic soft tissue of posterolateral region
  - Often associated with nerves
  - Prominent vasculature delineates nests of cells
  - Nucleoli usually not prominent
  - Express MAP-2, synaptophysin, and chromogranin by IHC, but cytokeratin negative

Proliferative Lesions

- Outpouching of HGPIN
  - Nuclear features of carcinoma
  - Contains basal cell layer confirmed by IHC
- Atypical adenomatous hyperplasia (adenosis)
  - Crowded glands with lobular configuration
    - Admixed small glands and larger more benign-appearing glands with luminal infolding
  - More common in transition zone
  - Cytologically, glands are similar to adjacent benign glands
    - Small nucleoli occasionally seen
  - May contain abundant crystalloids (up to 39% of cases); intraluminal mucin rare and focal
    - Luminal corpora amylacea are also common
  - Contains patchy basal cell layer by IHC
    - May be present in as few as 10% of total glands
    - Individual glands may have only 1 or 2 basal cells
- Mesonephric remnant hyperplasia
  - Identical to those more commonly seen in gynecologic tract
  - More atrophic glands with dense intraluminal colloid secretions

- o Nonreactive for PSA and PSAP
- o Shows basal cells by IHC
- Sclerosing adenosis
  - o Very rarely seen in needle biopsies
    - ▪ Occurs in transition zone
  - o Glands characteristically associated with intimately admixed spindle cell population
  - o Hyaline membranes around glands
  - o Contain basal cells by IHC
    - ▪ Basal cells have myoepithelial phenotype with actin expression
- Basal cell hyperplasia
  - o Prominent nucleoli common
  - o Strongly reactive for p63, CK5/6, &/or HMCK(34βE12)

Atrophy Variants

- Simple atrophy
  - o Glands retain lobular architecture
  - o Cells with scant cytoplasm imparting basophilic appearance on low-power view
  - o Contains basal cell layer confirmed by IHC
- Post atrophic hyperplasia
  - o More crowded acinar units than simple atrophy
  - o Large "feeder" duct may be identified
  - o Numerous basal cells are typically obvious by IHC
- Partial atrophy
  - o Most common and closest morphologic mimic of PCa
  - o Slightly more disorganized architecturally than other atrophy variants
  - o Comprised of secretory cells with scant pale clear to eosinophilic luminal cytoplasm
    - ▪ Often have abundant cytoplasm lateral to nucleus
  - o Typically have undulating luminal surface
  - o Usually bland nuclear features, but small nucleoli seen in up to 20%
  - o Immunohistochemistry interpretation may be difficult
    - ▪ Presence of any basal cells is diagnostic of benign lesion
    - ▪ Basal cells are typically patchy, but in some small foci they may not be identifiable
    - ▪ In 24% of cases, small foci of partial atrophy may show both AMACR reactivity and absence of basal cells

Inflammatory/Reactive Lesions

- Nephrogenic adenoma
  - o Variably sized tubules with thick basement membrane; "hobnail" cells and inflammation
  - o May have mixed papillary &/or solid growth
  - o AMACR positive
  - o Rarely PSA/PSAP positive
  - o pax-2 and pax-8 positive
  - o S100-1A positive
- Xanthogranulomatous prostatitis
  - o Sheets of foamy histiocytes
  - o Cytokeratin negative
  - o Positive for CD68

DIAGNOSTIC CHECKLIST

Pathologic Interpretation Pearls

- In a small focus not fulfilling diagnostic criteria for PCa, there should be consideration for benign mimics
  - o Benign lesions should be excluded by IHC if at all possible
    - ▪ Avoids overuse of ASAP diagnosis and unnecessary rebiopsy
- ASAP should not be used for lesions with only patchy basal cells
  - o Leads to unnecessary rebiopsy
  - o Should be diagnosed as benign in appropriate morphologic context

REPORTING CRITERIA

Recommendations

- Some authors recommend qualifying ASAP, such as "suspicious" or "highly suspicious for cancer"
  - o No known difference in risk of PCa on follow-up biopsy between ASAP qualifiers
  - o May aid in understanding of ASAP diagnosis
  - o Some clinicians may be unaware of conveyed risk in ASAP diagnosis and need for rebiopsy
    - ▪ Some authors advocate detailed comment relaying risk of subsequent cancer on rebiopsy

SELECTED REFERENCES

1. Van der Kwast TH et al: Variability in Diagnostic Opinion Among Pathologists for Single Small Atypical Foci in Prostate Biopsies. Am J Surg Pathol. Epub ahead of print, 2010
2. Wang W et al: Partial atrophy on prostate needle biopsy cores: a morphologic and immunohistochemical study. Am J Surg Pathol. 32(6):851-7, 2008
3. Bostwick DG et al: Atypical small acinar proliferation in the prostate: clinical significance in 2006. Arch Pathol Lab Med. 130(7):952-7, 2006
4. Egevad L et al: Current practice of diagnosis and reporting of prostatic intraepithelial neoplasia and glandular atypia among genitourinary pathologists. Mod Pathol. 19(2):180-5, 2006
5. Epstein JI et al: Prostate needle biopsies containing prostatic intraepithelial neoplasia or atypical foci suspicious for carcinoma: implications for patient care. J Urol. 175(3 Pt 1):820-34, 2006
6. Girasole CR et al: Significance of atypical and suspicious small acinar proliferations, and high grade prostatic intraepithelial neoplasia on prostate biopsy: implications for cancer detection and biopsy strategy. J Urol. 175(3 Pt 1):929-33; discussion 933, 2006
7. Iczkowski KA: Current prostate biopsy interpretation: criteria for cancer, atypical small acinar proliferation, high-grade prostatic intraepithelial neoplasia, and use of immunostains. Arch Pathol Lab Med. 130(6):835-43, 2006
8. Schlesinger C et al: High-grade prostatic intraepithelial neoplasia and atypical small acinar proliferation: predictive value for cancer in current practice. Am J Surg Pathol. 29(9):1201-7, 2005

Microscopic and Immunohistochemical Features

(Left) This example of ASAP shows a focus with 2 atypical glands ⇨ adjacent to 2 benign glands ⇨. The atypical glands have pale cytoplasm and rigid lumina. *(Right)* On the immunostain level, a few more glands are present with a staining pattern typical of carcinoma (absence of basal cells with circumferential luminal AMACR). However, the very few glands and lack of obvious cytologic atypia are the main reasons for a diagnosis of "ASAP suspicious for adenocarcinoma."

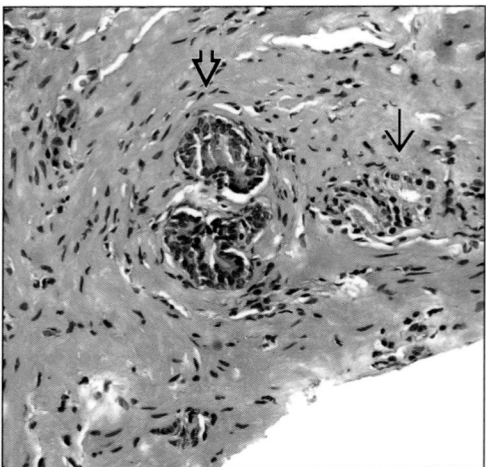
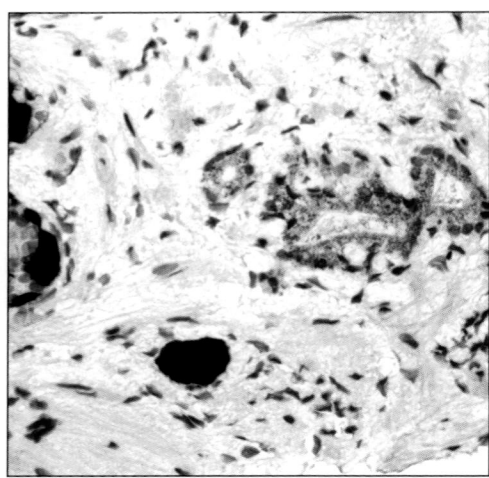

(Left) In this prostate needle biopsy, there is 1 atypical gland identified ⇨ that is characterized by a smaller caliber and more cytoplasmic eosinophilia compared to adjacent glands. *(Right)* This atypical gland ⇨ has cytoplasmic eosinophilia and nuclear atypia with nucleomegaly and prominent nucleoli compared to adjacent benign glands ⇨. Since this is the only atypical focus in a 12 part sampling, many would still consider this as "ASAP suspicious for adenocarcinoma."

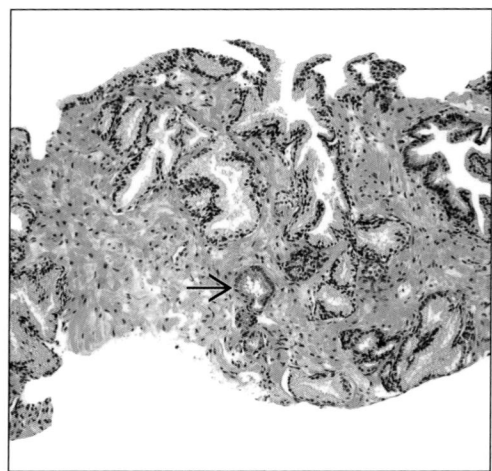
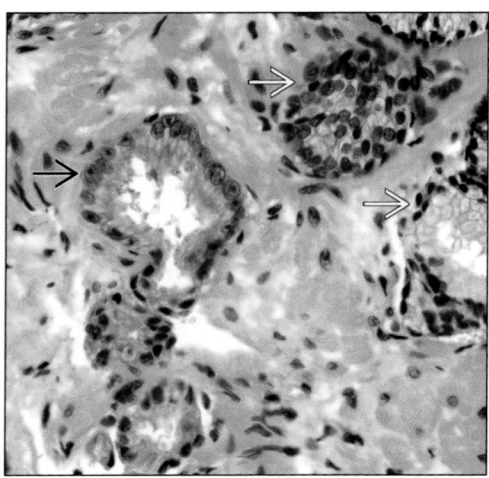

(Left) Some features are pathognomonic of carcinoma. This focus of atypical glands has intraluminal balls of tumor cells attached to 1 pole of the gland ⇨, a feature known as "glomerulations." With the right cytology, this finding warrants a diagnosis of carcinoma regardless of the number of glands present. *(Right)* Another diagnostic feature of carcinoma is the presence of collagenous micronodules, characterized by loose fibrous tissue ⇨ admixed with fibroblasts, mucin, and atypical epithelium.

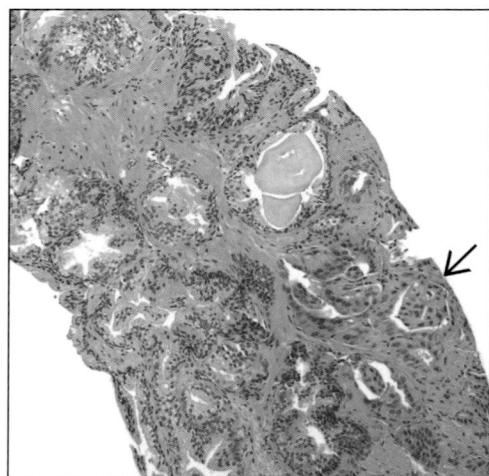
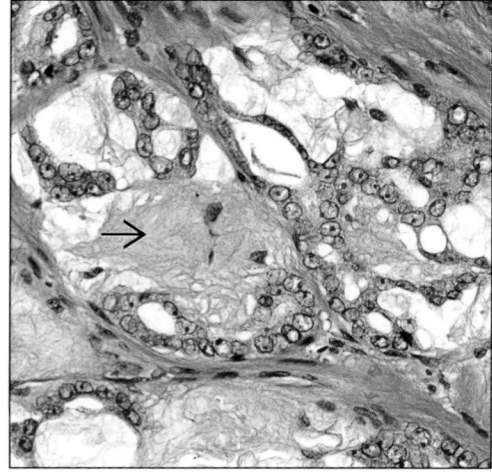

ATYPICAL SMALL ACINAR PROLIFERATIONS

Differential Diagnosis

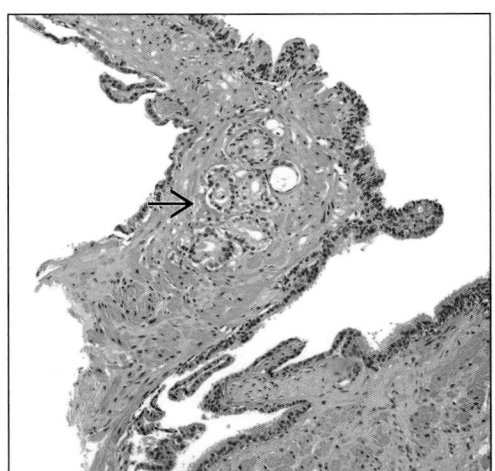

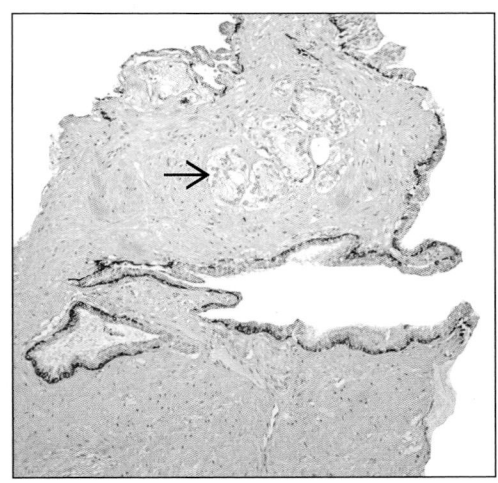

(Left) This area would be regarded as a small focus of prostatic adenocarcinoma ➡, Gleason score 3 + 3 = 6. The small crowded glands have a streaming architecture and are present between larger caliber benign glands. *(Right)* This immunohistochemical cocktail contains both AMACR and basal cell markers. The focal adenocarcinoma ➡ shows an absence of basal cells but no AMACR reactivity. AMACR staining is not required for a definitive diagnosis of carcinoma.

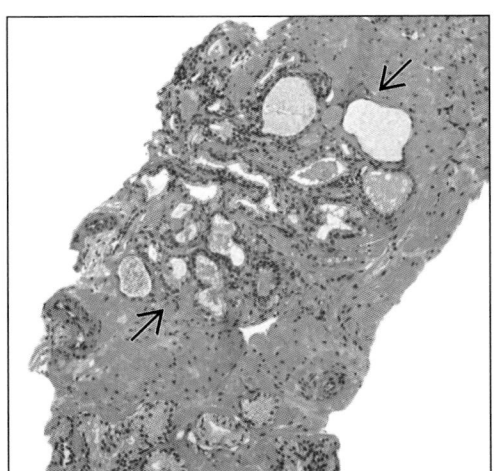

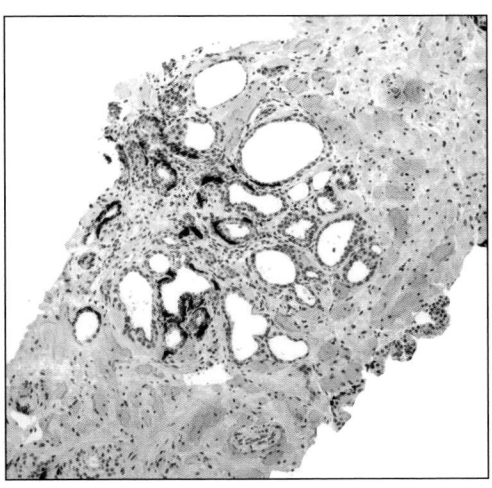

(Left) This aggregate of glands ➡ represents an example of partial atrophy, the most common mimic of adenocarcinoma. *(Right)* In this triple cocktail (AMACR, p63, HMCK[34βE12]), there is patchy basal cell staining within partial atrophy. Some glands show no basal cells and many have immunoreactivity for AMACR. This staining pattern is common in partial atrophy and should not be regarded as ASAP. When evaluating for basal cells, the entire population must be interpreted as a whole.

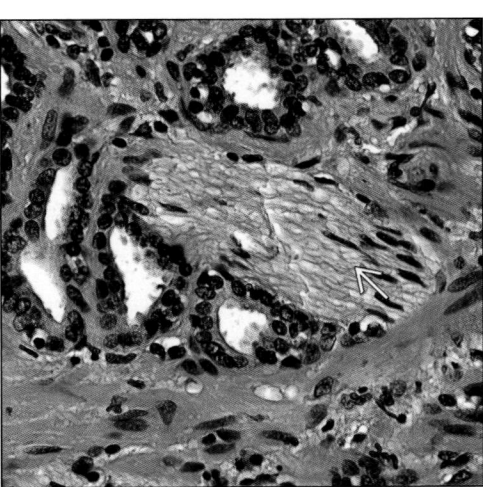

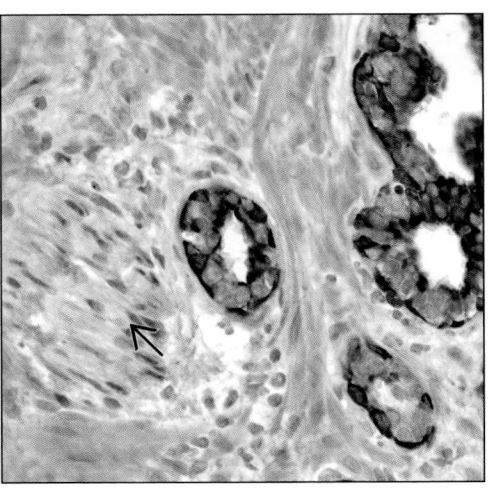

(Left) This is an example of benign atrophic glands showing "indentation" of a nerve ➡. Circumferential envelopment or intraneural invasion (not indentation) of the nerve should be required for a diagnosis of perineural invasion and carcinoma. *(Right)* These benign atrophic glands with "indentation" of a nerve ➡ show strong and diffuse immunoreactivity for HMCK(34βE12), a feature confirming the presence of basal cells and, therefore, a benign process.

DUCTAL ADENOCARCINOMA

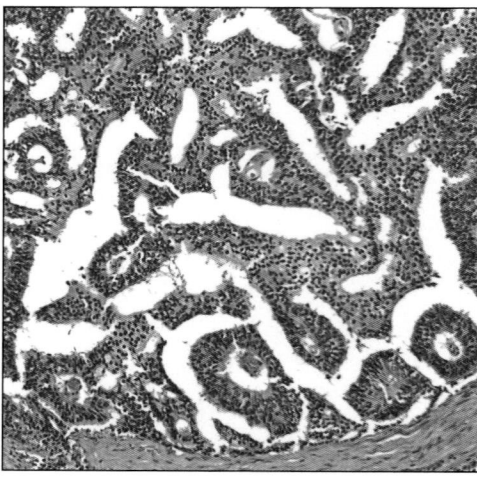

Ductal adenocarcinoma, papillary pattern, shows distinctive papillary architecture with fibrovascular core lined by pseudostratified tall columnar cells.

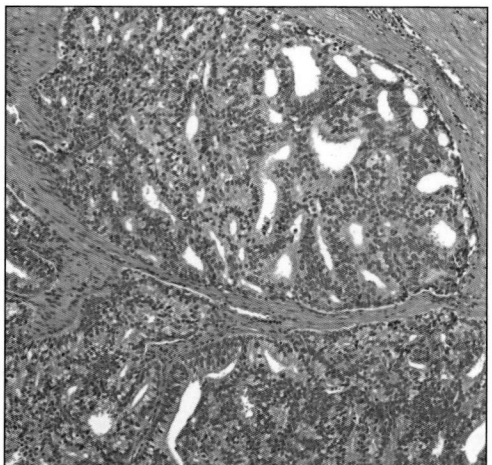

Ductal adenocarcinoma, cribriform pattern, shows large glands with cribriform architecture imparting multiple lumina lined by pseudostratified tall columnar cells.

TERMINOLOGY

Synonyms
- Prostatic duct adenocarcinoma
- Endometrioid carcinoma of the prostate (outdated term)

Definitions
- Adenocarcinoma of prostatic epithelial cell origin with large glandular and papillary architecture lined by tall columnar cells, often with pseudostratified growth
- Features comprising predominant (> 80%) or pure histology of carcinoma in transurethral resection of prostate (TURP) or radical prostatectomy
- Occurs either as pure ductal adenocarcinoma or, more commonly, in combination with acinar adenocarcinoma in microscopy

ETIOLOGY/PATHOGENESIS

Origin
- Prostatic glandular epithelial cell origin
- Previously postulated to arise from the müllerian-derived prostatic utricle due to its morphologic resemblance to adenocarcinoma of endometrium

CLINICAL ISSUES

Epidemiology
- Incidence
  - Rare
  - Pure ductal adenocarcinoma accounts for 0.4-0.8% of all prostate cancers
  - Mixed ductal and acinar adenocarcinoma reported in 5-6.3% of prostate cancers
- Age
  - Mean: 63-72 years, range: 41-89 years

Site
- May be central &/or peripheral in location
- Central tumors occur in periurethral area and involve transition zone and TURP specimens
- Peripheral tumors involve prostate peripheral zone and can extend to transition zone

Presentation
- Central/periurethral tumors
  - Obstructive symptoms
  - Hematuria
- Peripherally located tumors
  - Abnormal digital rectal examination
  - Elevated serum PSA levels
- Bone metastasis are osteoblastic

Laboratory Tests
- Majority of patients have elevated serum PSA level

Treatment
- Reported response to treatment options for prostate acinar adenocarcinoma, including hormonal manipulation

Prognosis
- Data suggest that tumors have a more aggressive clinical behavior than acinar adenocarcinoma
- Overall 5-year survival rate of only 15-24%
- Presence in biopsies indicate more advanced cancer at prostatectomy and shortened progression time than Gleason 7 or less acinar adenocarcinoma
- Extraprostatic extension and seminal vesicle involvement seen in 63% and 10% of prostatectomy specimens, respectively
- Metastasis in 19-44% of cases, mostly to lungs

MACROSCOPIC FEATURES

General Features
- Centrally located tumors

DUCTAL ADENOCARCINOMA

Key Facts

Terminology
- Adenocarcinoma of prostatic epithelial cell origin with large glandular and papillary architecture lined by tall columnar cells, often with pseudostratified growth

Clinical Issues
- Pure ductal adenocarcinoma accounts for 0.4-0.8% of all prostate cancers
- Mixed ductal and acinar adenocarcinoma reported in 5-6.3% of prostate cancers
- Most studies suggest a more aggressive clinical behavior than acinar adenocarcinoma

Macroscopic Features
- Centrally located tumors can have exophytic friable fronds protruding in urethral lumen

- Peripheral tumors are more often posteriorly situated as firm, gray-white parenchymal mass

Microscopic Pathology
- Main architectural patterns: Papillary, cribriform, individual glands, solid
- Tall columnar cells in single or pseudostratified growth pattern
- Cytoplasm usually amphophilic and nucleus oblongated with variably prominent nucleolus
- Can grow intraluminally into preexisting ducts retaining "native" basal cell layer
- Positive for AMACR in 77% of cases
- Majority has no detectable basal cells by p63 or HMCK(34βE12)
- ISUP 2005 consensus recommends grading as Gleason pattern 4; if necrosis is present, pattern 5

- o Can have exophytic friable fronds protruding in urethral lumen around prostatic utricle or verumontanum
  - o Cystoscopic visualization possible
- Peripherally located tumors
  - o More often posteriorly situated
  - o Firm, gray-white parenchymal mass, similar to acinar adenocarcinoma

MICROSCOPIC PATHOLOGY

Histologic Features
- Main architectural patterns
  - o Papillary
  - o Cribriform
  - o Individual glands
  - o Solid
- More than 1 architectural patterns is typical
- Combination of papillary and cribriform patterns most common, seen in 36% of tumors
- Papillary tumors often are centrally located
- Peripheral tumors are often papillary and cribriform
- Neoplastic cells
  - o Tall columnar cells
  - o Single or pseudostratified cell layer
  - o Cytoplasm usually amphophilic but can be pale or clear
  - o Nucleus typically elongated
  - o Variably usually prominent nucleolus
  - o Occasional to frequent mitoses present
  - o Greater degree of chromatin irregularities compared to usual acinar prostate adenocarcinoma
- Can grow intraluminally into preexisting ducts retaining "native" basal cell layer
  - o Invasive component must be present to be diagnosed as ductal adenocarcinoma
  - o Negativity for basal cell marker immunohistochemistry is a must in invasive component
- Glands can be very large, expansile, and crowded back to back

- Background stromal fibrosis often present
- Perineural invasion may be seen
- Almost half admixed with acinar adenocarcinoma
- Concomitant acinar adenocarcinoma usually microacinar Gleason pattern 3, seen in 48% of tumors

Predominant Pattern/Injury Type
- Neoplastic

Predominant Cell/Compartment Type
- Epithelial, glandular

Genetics
- *TMPRSS2-ERG* gene fusion
  - o Less frequent in pure ductal adenocarcinoma (11%) and mixed ductal acinar adenocarcinoma (5%) than pure acinar adenocarcinoma (45%)
  - o When present, mostly through deletion

ANCILLARY TESTS

Immunohistochemistry
- Positive for PSA and PAP
- Positive for AMACR in 77% of cases
- Majority lacks basal cell layer
  - o Negative for p63 or HMCK(34βE12)
  - o 31% have detectable basal cells by p63 or HMCK(34βE12), staining in patchy or discontinuous distribution (intraductal growth)

DIFFERENTIAL DIAGNOSIS

High-Grade Prostatic Intraepithelial Neoplasia (HGPIN)
- Micropapillary, cribriform, and flat HGPIN can mimic ductal adenocarcinomas due to overlap in architecture
- Distinction can be very difficult in limited samples
- Typically lacks predominance of tall columnar cells
- Lacks expansile large glandular growth pattern
- No invasive features, such as crowded back-to-back glands, stromal fibrosis, or perineural invasion

DUCTAL ADENOCARCINOMA

- Micropapillary HGPIN cellular fronds lack a true fibrovascular core
- Occasionally, cells at center of cribriform HGPIN glands tend to have lower grade nuclei (maturation)
- Consistently contains basal cell layer highlighted by basal cell markers, such as p63 or HMCK(34βE12)

Cribriform Hyperplasia

- Unusual form of benign prostatic hyperplasia composed of crowded cribriform glands
- Nodular pattern of growth
- Composed of cells with uniformly bland cytology, often with clear cytoplasm and absent nucleoli
- Contains basal cell layer

Cribriform Gleason Pattern 4 and 5 Acinar Adenocarcinoma

- Overlap and continuum of ductal adenocarcinoma and cribriform acinar carcinoma
- Similarly to ductal adenocarcinoma, shows invasive features, including large expansile growth and glandular crowding
- Morphologic definition limited to invasive large cribriform glands lacking true papillary component and tall columnar cells

Prostatic Urethral Polyp

- Reactive papillary lesions growing along urethra lined by cuboidal to columnar prostatic acinar cells
- More commonly seen in younger patients
- Bland cytology

DIAGNOSTIC CHECKLIST

Pathologic Interpretation Pearls

- Presence of large prostatic glandular proliferations lined by pseudostratified tall columnar cells generally lacking basal cells and showing invasive features
- High-grade tumor morphology compared to acinar adenocarcinoma

REPORTING CONSIDERATIONS

Key Elements to Report

- Biopsy, microscopic evaluation
  - Diagnosis cannot be made in needle biopsy; if present, diagnosis should be "adenocarcinoma of prostate with ductal features" with a comment
    - If prostatectomy is performed, tumor may be diagnosed as ductal adenocarcinoma if 80% or exclusive morphology is of ductal type
  - Gleason score with primary and secondary grades
  - Quantitation of tumor (i.e., percent)
  - Local invasion (i.e., prostatic fat, seminal vesicle)
  - Additional findings, if present
- Prostatectomy, microscopic evaluation
  - Histologic type (ductal adenocarcinoma or mixed)
  - Gleason score with primary and secondary grades
  - Location
  - Extent of local invasion (i.e., extraprostatic extension, seminal vesicle involvement)
  - Margins (location and extent of margins involved with tumor)
  - Regional lymph node status
  - Additional findings, if present

GRADING

Criteria

- International Society of Urological Pathology (ISUP) 2005 consensus conference recommendations
  - Ductal adenocarcinoma must be graded as Gleason score 4 + 4 = 8; if necrosis is present, pattern 5 should be designated
  - Retain diagnostic term when grading, i.e., "ductal adenocarcinoma (Gleason score 4 + 4 = 8)"
  - In mixed ductal and acinar adenocarcinoma, ductal component to be assigned Gleason pattern 4; or pattern 5 if with necrosis

STAGING

Criteria

- American Joint Committee on Cancer (AJCC)/ International Union Against Cancer (UICC) 2009
  - Prostate cancer TNM staging applies for ductal adenocarcinoma

SELECTED REFERENCES

1. Lotan TL et al: TMPRSS2-ERG gene fusions are infrequent in prostatic ductal adenocarcinomas. Mod Pathol. 22(3):359-65, 2009
2. Herawi M et al: Immunohistochemical antibody cocktail staining (p63/HMWCK/AMACR) of ductal adenocarcinoma and Gleason pattern 4 cribriform and noncribriform acinar adenocarcinomas of the prostate. Am J Surg Pathol. 31(6):889-94, 2007
3. Bock BJ et al: Does prostatic ductal adenocarcinoma exist? Am J Surg Pathol. 23(7):781-5, 1999
4. Brinker DA et al: Ductal adenocarcinoma of the prostate diagnosed on needle biopsy: correlation with clinical and radical prostatectomy findings and progression. Am J Surg Pathol. 23(12):1471-9, 1999
5. Samaratunga H et al: Distribution pattern of basal cells detected by cytokeratin 34 beta E12 in primary prostatic duct adenocarcinoma. Am J Surg Pathol. 21(4):435-40, 1997
6. Christensen WN et al: Prostatic duct adenocarcinoma. Findings at radical prostatectomy. Cancer. 67(8):2118-24, 1991
7. Ro JY et al: Prostatic duct adenocarcinoma with endometrioid features: immunohistochemical and electron microscopic study. Semin Diagn Pathol. 5(3):301-11, 1988
8. Epstein JI et al: Adenocarcinoma of the prostate with endometrioid features. A light microscopic and immunohistochemical study of ten cases. Cancer. 57(1):111-9, 1986
9. Bostwick DG et al: Prostatic adenocarcinoma with endometrioid features. Clinical, pathologic, and ultrastructural findings. Am J Surg Pathol. 9(8):595-609, 1985

DUCTAL ADENOCARCINOMA

Microscopic Features

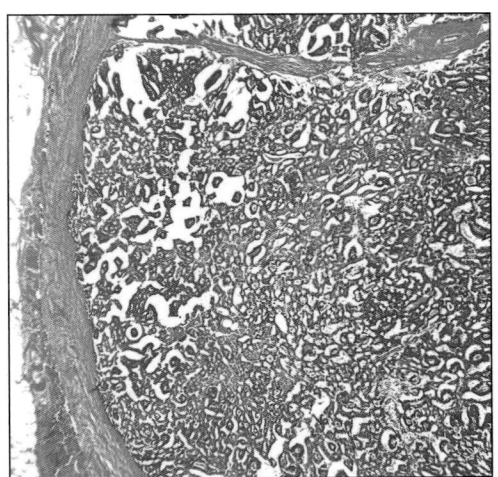
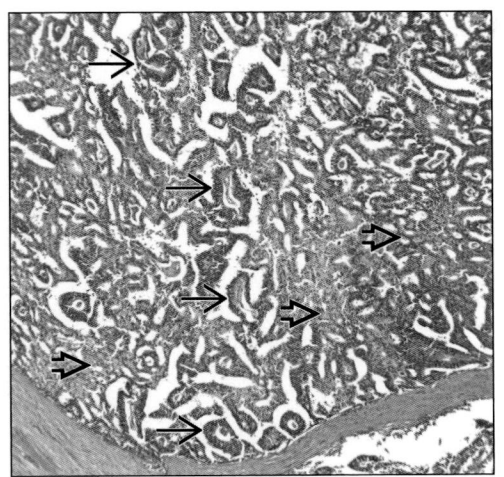

(Left) Large nodule of ductal adenocarcinoma in prostatectomy specimen shows predominance of papillary architectural pattern. This tumor involves the prostate peripheral zone close to the prostate "capsule." (Right) Ductal adenocarcinoma shows numerous papillae containing fibrovascular core ➡ ("true papillae"). Part of this tumor consists of cribriform architecture ▷. Admixture of papillary and cribriform pattens is common in ductal adenocarcinoma.

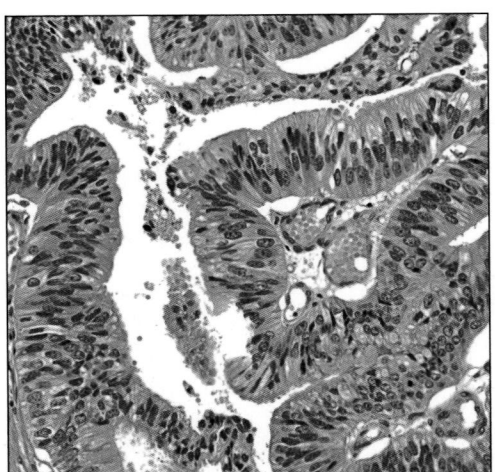
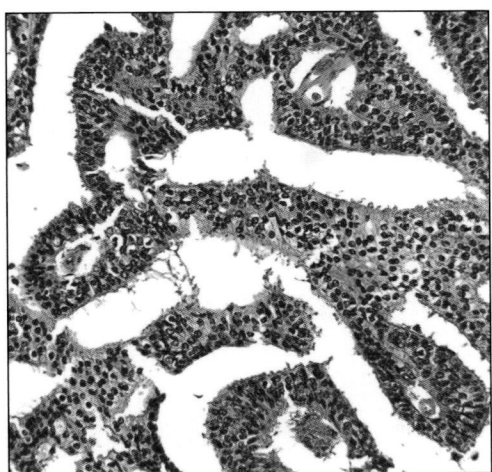

(Left) Ductal adenocarcinoma, papillary pattern, shows cell lining composed of tall columnar cells with pale cytoplasm and elongated nuclei, exhibiting pseudostratification. Presence of tall columnar cell lining is a distinguishing feature of ductal adenocarcinoma. (Right) These papillae of ductal adenocarcinoma shows thin, delicate architecture and contains fibrovascular core. Lining shows cellular pseudostratification with layering of nuclei.

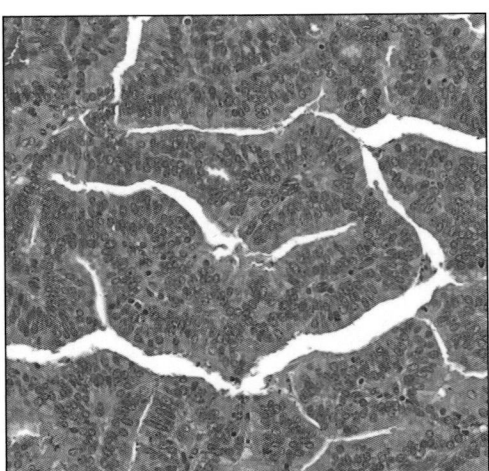
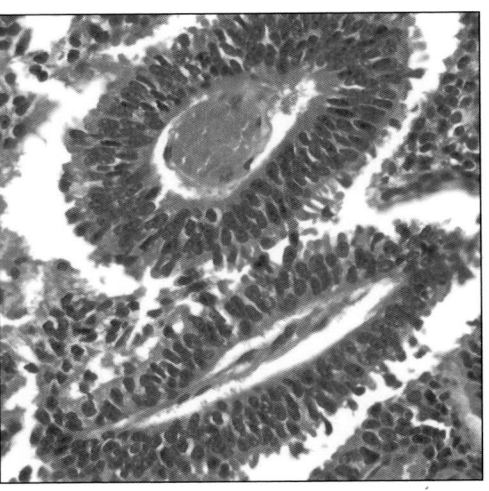

(Left) Ductal adenocarcinoma, papillary pattern, shows tall columnar cells with eosinophilic cytoplasm containing crowded high-grade nuclei. (Right) High-power magnification of ductal adenocarcinoma, papillary pattern, shows nuclei with dense irregular chromatin and occasional prominent nucleoli. Ductal adenocarcinoma nuclei are typically of higher grade compared to conventional prostate adenocarcinoma.

DUCTAL ADENOCARCINOMA

Microscopic Features

(Left) High-power view of ductal adenocarcinoma shows tall columnar cells with pale cytoplasm and oval to elongated nuclei with variably prominent nucleoli. Ductal adenocarcinoma cytoplasm is typically amphophilic but can be pale or clear. *(Right)* Ductal adenocarcinoma, papillary pattern, encountered in TURP specimen, shows multiple papillary fragments lined by tall columnar cells. Papillary architecture is relatively more common in tumors that arise in central region of the prostate.

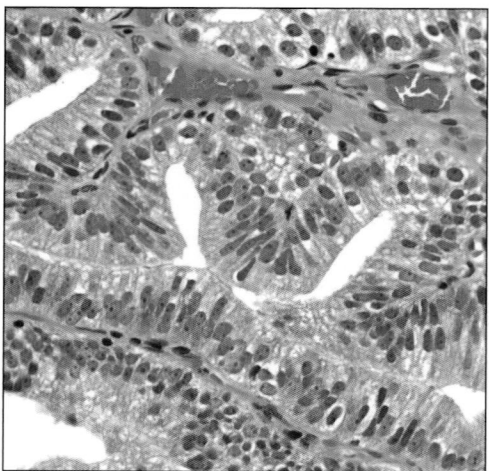
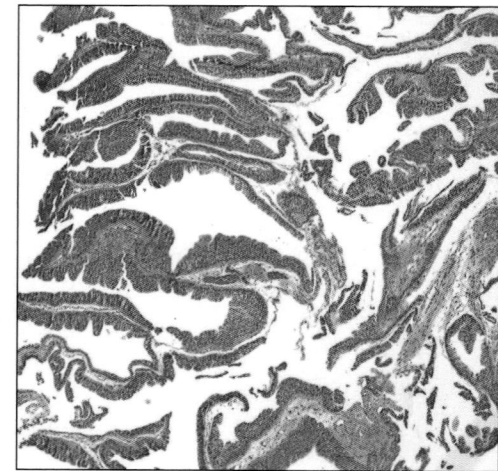

(Left) Low-power magnification of ductal adenocarcinoma, cribriform pattern, in prostatectomy specimen shows large glands containing multiple lumina separated by cell bridges. Note the presence of comedonecrosis ➡, indicating Gleason pattern 5 carcinoma. *(Right)* Ductal adenocarcinoma, cribriform pattern, shows multiple luminal spaces and bridges lined by tall columnar cells. Ductal adenocarcinoma without necrosis are graded as Gleason pattern 4.

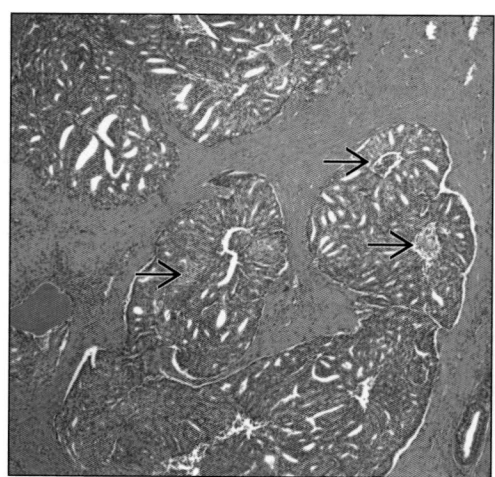
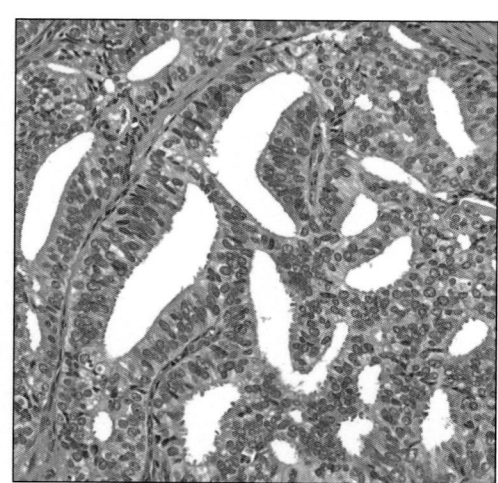

(Left) Ductal adenocarcinoma, cribriform pattern, shows peripheral lumina lined by tale columnar cells with pale eosinophilic cytoplasm. In contrast, cribriform acinar adenocarcinoma are lined by non-tall columnar cells. *(Right)* Ductal adenocarcinoma, cribriform pattern, shows pseudostratified hyperchromatic nuclei. In contrast, cribriform HGPIN lacks large expansile growth, back-to-back glands, and contains basal cell layer that can be confirmed immunohistochemically.

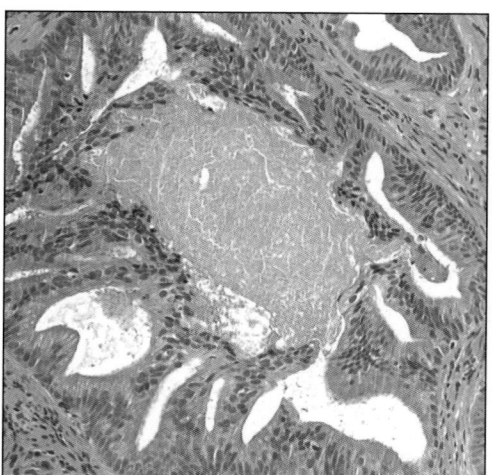
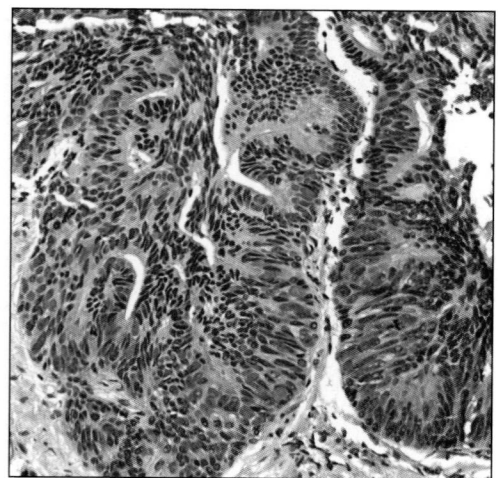

3

DUCTAL ADENOCARCINOMA

Microscopic Features

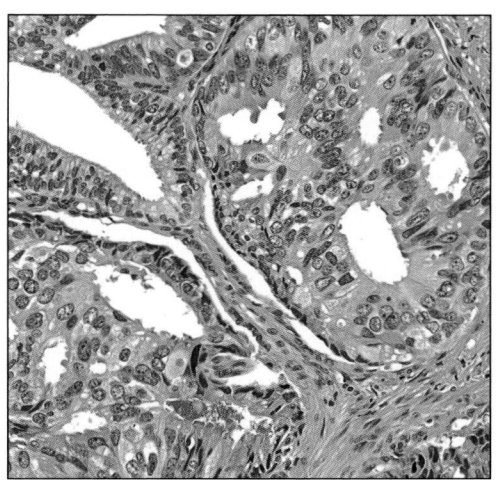

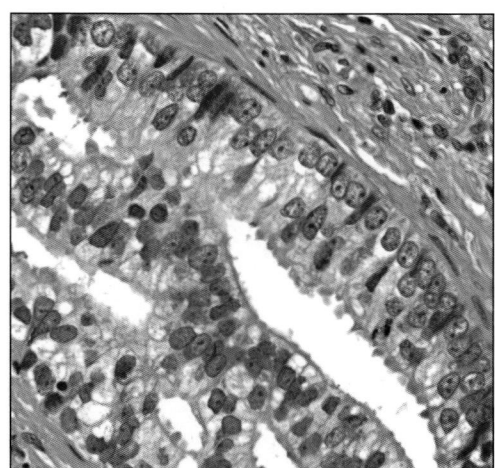

(Left) Ductal adenocarcinoma, cribriform pattern, shows large glands with multiple lumina containing tall columnar cells, some exhibiting atypical nuclear rounding. *(Right)* High-power view of ductal adenocarcinoma, cribriform pattern, shows tall columnar cells with pale cytoplasm and high-grade oval to elongated nuclei. In contrast, cribriform acinar adenocarcinoma is composed of non-tall columnar cells with rounder nuclei of relatively lower grade.

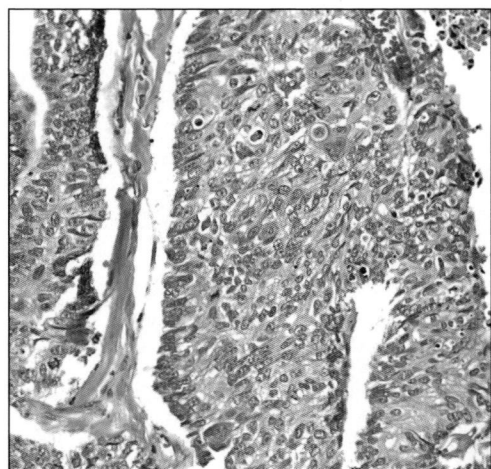

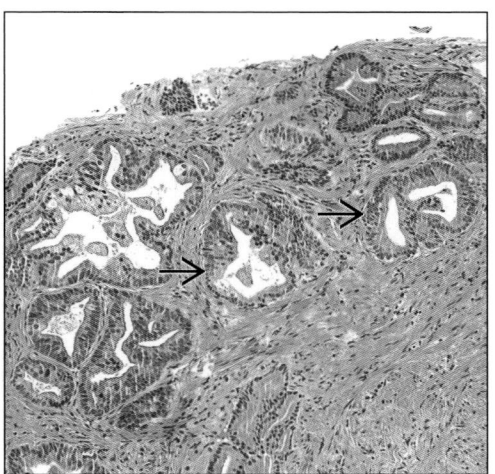

(Left) Ductal adenocarcinoma, solid growth pattern, shows solid nests of columnar cells with crowded elongated nuclei, some with palisaded growth. *(Right)* Ductal adenocarcinoma, individual glands pattern ⇒, shows well-formed glands lined predominantly by single layer of tall columnar cells. The tall columnar cell lining distinguishes these glands from microacinar adenocarcinoma glands and absence of basal cell layer from flat HGPIN, aided by immunohistochemistry.

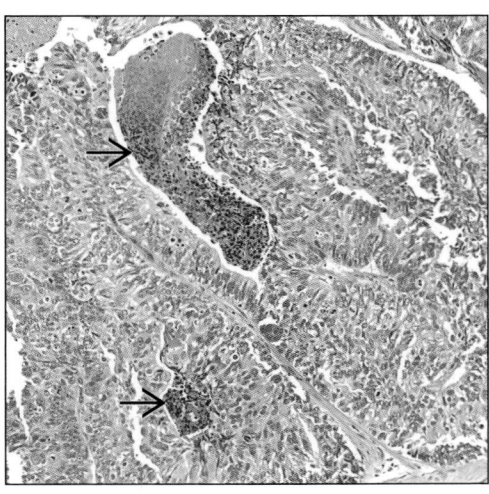

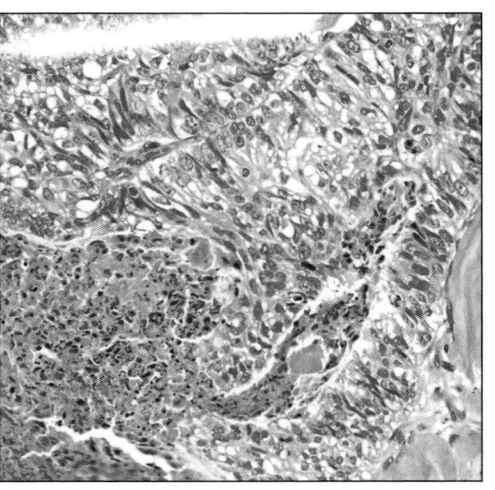

(Left) Ductal adenocarcinoma shows large cribriform and solid glands containing tall columnar cells and contains comedonecrosis ⇒. *(Right)* High-power view of ductal adenocarcinoma with comedonecrosis is characterized by luminal collection of necrotic ghost cells and nuclear debris. Presence of comedonecrosis warrants designation of Gleason pattern 5 for these glands. Without necrosis, ductal adenocarcinoma should be designated as Gleason pattern 4.

DUCTAL ADENOCARCINOMA

Microscopic Features

(Left) Adenocarcinoma with ductal features, papillary pattern, in needle biopsy shows multiple papillae with fibrovascular cores ➡. In contrast to micropapillary HGPIN, these glands are large with expansile growth and papillae contains fibrovascular core. Ductal adenocarcinoma diagnosis is not tenable in needle biopsy. *(Right)* Adenocarcinoma with ductal features in needle biopsy shows large cribriform gland lined by tall columnar cells. Ductal adenocarcinoma diagnosis is not tenable in needle biopsy.

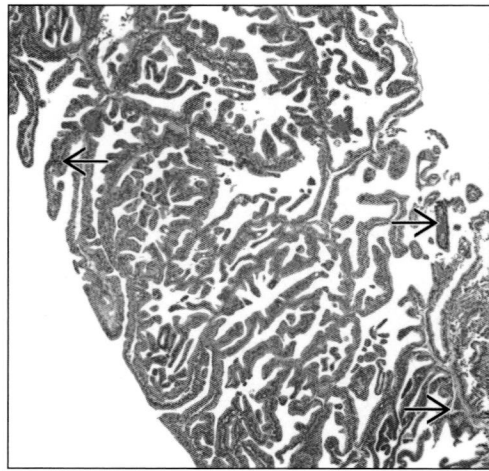 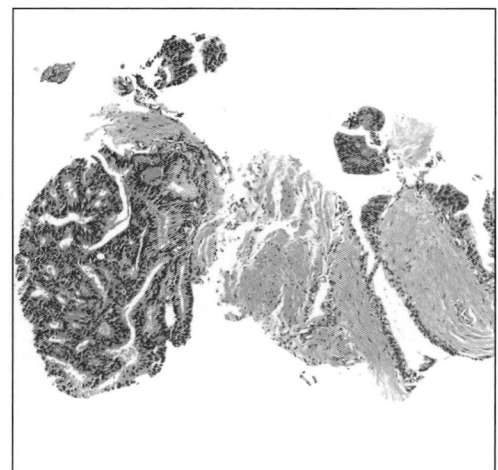

(Left) Mixed ductal and acinar adenocarcinoma shows acinar adenocarcinoma component consisting of individual Gleason 3 pattern glands ➡ interspersed between larger cribriform glands of ductal adenocarcinoma ➡. *(Right)* Mixed acinar (left side) and ductal (right side) adenocarcinoma shows that acinar adenocarcinoma cells are relatively more cuboidal ➡, while ductal adenocarcinoma cells are taller and contain larger and more hyperchromatic nuclei ➡.

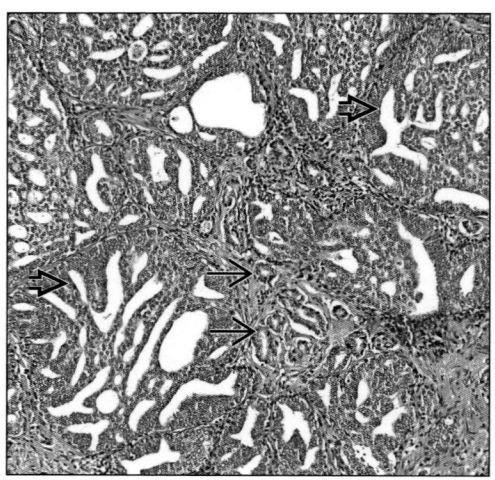 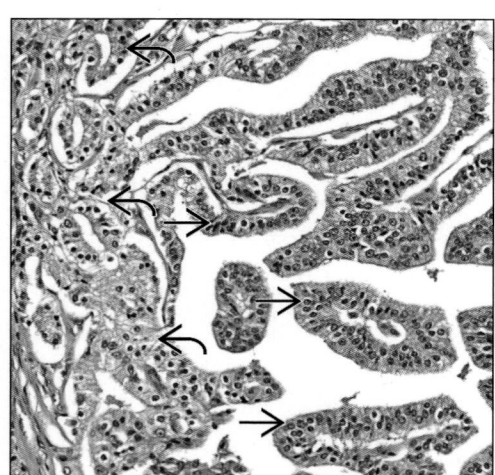

(Left) Adenocarcinoma with mixed acinar ➡ and ductal ➡ features in needle biopsy shows individual glands of acinar adenocarcinoma and ductal adenocarcinoma lined by cuboidal and tall columnar cells, respectively. About half of ductal adenocarcinomas are mixed with acinar adenocarcinoma. In prostatectomy specimens, > 80% ductal features are required for diagnosis of ductal adenocarcinoma. *(Right)* Ductal adenocarcinoma shows cribriform gland of tall columnar cells with perineural invasion.

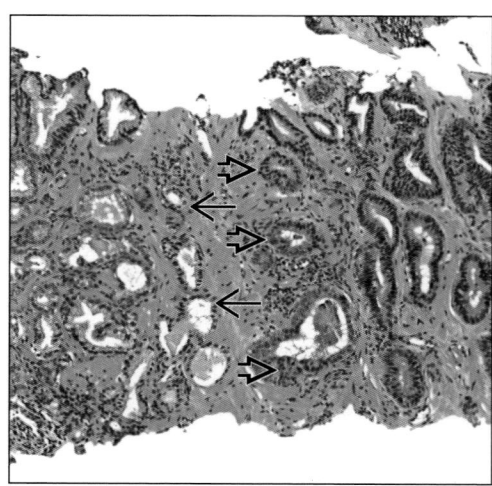 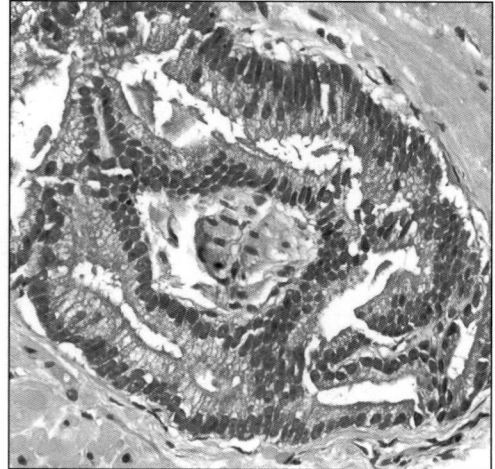

DUCTAL ADENOCARCINOMA

Microscopic and Immunohistochemical Features

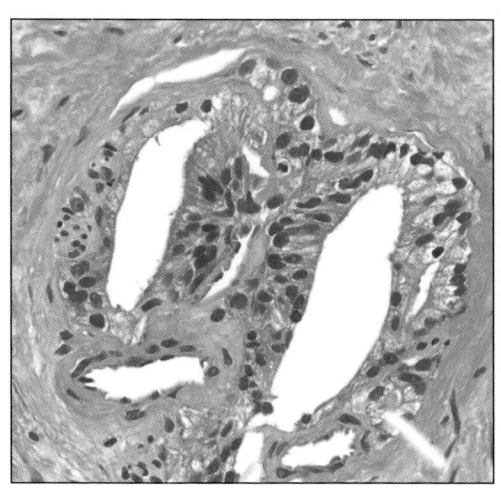

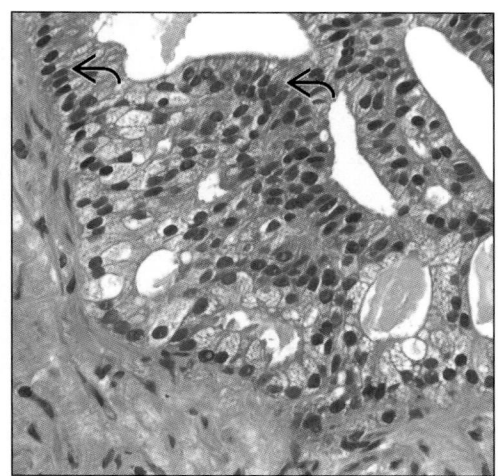

(Left) High-power view of ductal adenocarcinoma individual glands pattern with radiation treatment effect shows relative nuclear pleomorphism and partly foamy cytoplasm. *(Right)* Ductal adenocarcinoma, cribriform pattern with radiation treatment effect, shows foamy appearance of cytoplasm. The tall columnar and palisaded appearance can still be appreciated ⇗. Data suggests that ductal adenocarcinoma has a more aggressive clinical behavior than acinar adenocarcinoma.

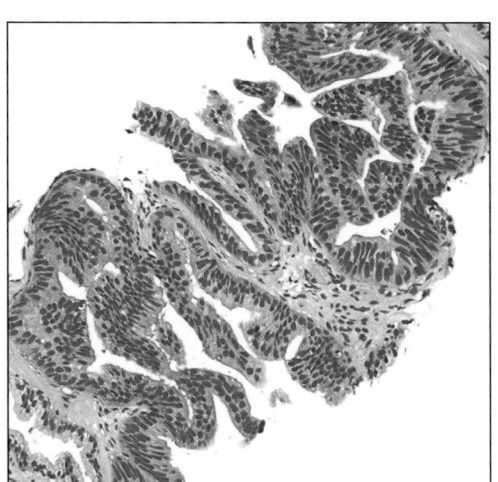

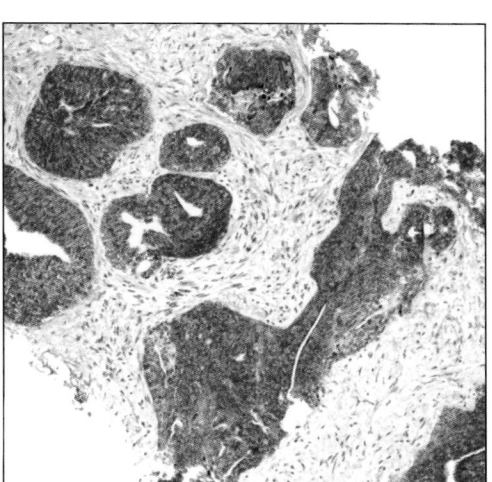

(Left) Adenocarcinoma of prostate with ductal features in needle biopsy shows several large glands with high-grade nuclei. Distinction from high-grade PIN can be difficult and may necessitate use of IHC to confirm absence of basal cells. *(Right)* Triple PIN cocktail immunostain of ductal adenocarcinoma shows strong diffuse cytoplasmic AMACR expression and absence of basal cell markers (p63 and HMCK[34βE12]) staining. In contrast, HGPIN will show basal cell markers staining.

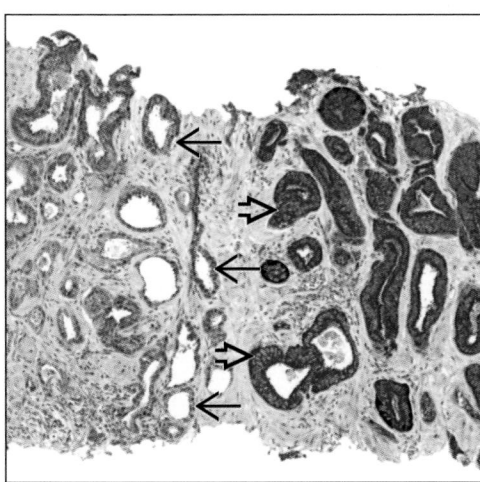

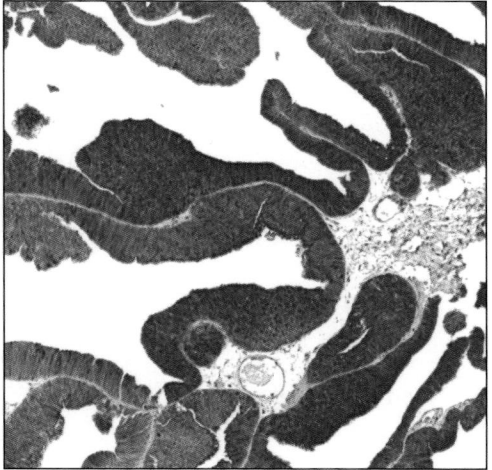

(Left) Triple PIN cocktail immunostain in needle biopsy of adenocarcinoma with mixed acinar → and ductal ⇗ features shows similar AMACR positivity and basal cell markers negativity. *(Right)* Ductal adenocarcinoma, papillary pattern, shows diffuse PSA positivity. PSA is helpful in distinguishing ductal adenocarcinoma from other tumors with similar architecture, such as the rare seminal vesicle papillary adenocarcinoma, which is PSA negative, or in metastatic setting.

UROTHELIAL CARCINOMA OF PROSTATE

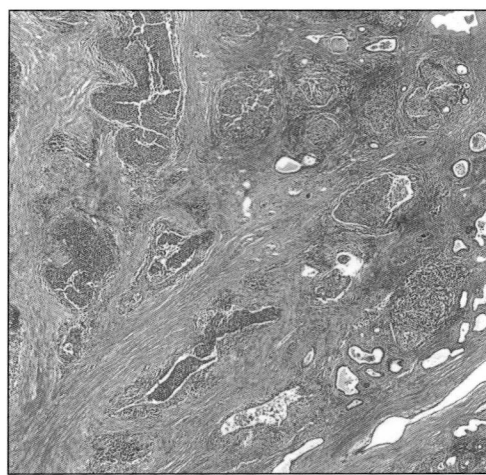

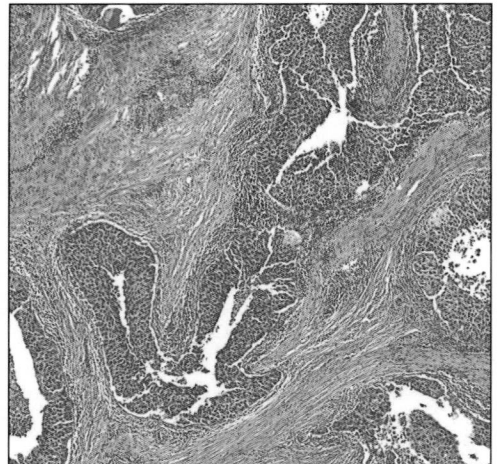

UroCa is shown involving prostatic ducts and acini. Preexisting acini are expanded and completely filled by UroCa. Stromal invasion may arise anywhere along prostatic urethra to the acini.

UroCa is shown involving prostatic ducts without stromal invasion. The outlines of the glands are smooth. Invasion of stroma should be recognized using strict criteria as it is of prognostic importance.

TERMINOLOGY

Abbreviations
- Urothelial carcinoma (UroCa)
- Carcinoma in situ (CIS)

Synonyms
- Intraepithelial carcinoma of periurethral glands and prostatic ducts
- Periurethral prostatic duct carcinoma

Definitions
- UroCa involving prostate arising from prostatic urethra, periurethral glands, and proximal prostatic ducts
- Clinicopathologically distinct from bladder UroCa transmurally invading through bladder wall and extending into prostate (pT4 bladder UroCa)

ETIOLOGY/PATHOGENESIS

Origin
- Urothelium in periurethral mucosal and submucosal glands &/or junction with prostatic ducts
  - In strict terms, UroCa arising from these sites is true primary prostatic UroCa
- Prostatic urethral urothelium
  - Frequently coexists with primary prostatic UroCa

CLINICAL ISSUES

Epidemiology
- Incidence
  - Primary prostate UroCa is uncommon, comprising 1-4% of prostate cancers in adults
    - 64% have concomitant bladder urothelial CIS
    - 24% have no prior or concurrent invasive or in situ bladder UroCa

  - Prostatic involvement in cystoprostatectomy for bladder UroCa is relatively more common, ranging from 12-58%
    - UroCa extending from prostatic urethra and ducts comprises 76-87%
    - UroCa transmurally invading bladder wall into prostate (pT4 bladder UroCa) comprises 13-24%
- Age
  - Similar in age distribution to bladder UroCa
  - Mean: 66 years, range: 52-87 years

Presentation
- More commonly detected in cystoprostatectomies for UroCa of bladder
- Most primary prostatic UroCa present with obstructive urinary symptoms, such as hesitancy, slowed stream, frequency, and dysuria
  - May have rapid progression of obstruction, usually < 6 months
- Other symptoms include hematuria, prostatism, weight loss, and rectal pain
- Prostate may be large on rectal examination, and may be mistaken clinically as benign prostatic hyperplasia, prostatitis, or prostate cancer
- Symptomatic cases more often encountered in transurethral resection of prostate (TURP) specimens performed for obstructive symptoms

Laboratory Tests
- Serum PSA level typically not elevated
  - However, 1 study showed 78% of prostate UroCa detected by needle biopsy had elevated serum PSA levels
    - Although this high percentage is perhaps reflective of specimen type performed for elevated PSA, which may or may not be due to UroCa
- May have elevated serum alkaline phosphatase level, due to bone metastasis

Treatment
- Depends on extent, location, and stage of disease

UROTHELIAL CARCINOMA OF PROSTATE

Key Facts

Terminology
- UroCa involving prostate arising from prostatic urethra, periurethral glands, and proximal prostatic ducts
- Clinicopathologically distinct from bladder UroCa transmurally invading through bladder wall and extending into prostate (pT4 bladder cancer)

Clinical Issues
- Primary prostate UroCa is uncommon, comprising 1-4% of prostate cancers in adults
- Prostate involvement in cystoprostatectomy for invasive bladder UroCa is relatively more common, ranging from 12-58%
- Similar in age distribution to bladder UroCa
- Most primary prostatic UroCa presents with obstructive urinary symptoms

- Disease specific survival higher in CIS of prostatic urethral glands, ducts, and acini vs. urethral submucosal and prostatic stromal invasion
- Prostatic stromal invasion associated with higher incidence of nodal metastasis
- Survival rate poorer for bladder UroCa transmurally invading through bladder wall and extending into prostate (pT4 bladder cancer) vs. with prostatic stromal invasion arising intraurethrally

Microscopic Pathology
- Diagnostic criteria identical to those of bladder UroCa
- CIS can spread from prostatic urethra, involves ducts and acini, or grows along ejaculatory duct to seminal vesicle
- Stromal invasion may arise anywhere along this spread

○ In patients presenting with limited disease in TUR specimens
  ■ Prostatic urethral UroCa with minimal or superficial prostatic acinar involvement without stromal involvement may be treated with bacillus Calmette-Guérin (BCG)
  ■ Cystoscopy should be performed to determine presence of bladder neoplasia
  ■ 1 study reported 87% complete response rate for BCG, but only 17% of these had prostatic acinar involvement and none had stromal invasion
○ For cases involving prostatic stroma and peripheral zone
  ■ Radical cystoprostatectomy is treatment of choice
  ■ Chemotherapy and radiotherapy may have role

Prognosis
- Depends on extent, location, and stage of disease
- **Primary prostatic UroCa with no invasive bladder UroCa**
  ○ Disease-specific survival higher in CIS of prostatic urethra and involvement of prostatic ducts and acini vs. UroCa involving suburethral glands or prostatic stroma
  ○ 5-year disease-specific survival
    ■ Prostatic urethral CIS and CIS involving prostatic ducts and acini without stromal invasion (100%)
    ■ Prostatic stromal invasion (45%)
    ■ Extraprostatic extension (0%)
    ■ Lymph node extension (30%)
    ■ Prostate primary UroCa overall (52%)
  ○ Concurrent prostate adenocarcinoma seen in 8%
  ○ Subsequent UroCa of upper urinary tract seen in 6%
  ○ Metastases most commonly occur in bone, lung, and liver
- **Prostate UroCa in patients with invasive bladder UroCa**
  ○ Bladder UroCa with no prostatic involvement vs. with involvement
    ■ Bladder UroCa patients without prostatic involvement 5-year survival rate: 64%

  ■ Bladder UroCa patients with either prostatic CIS and urethral lamina propria invasion 5-year survival rate: 44%
  ■ Bladder UroCa patients with prostatic stromal/periprostatic/seminal vesical invasion 5-year survival rate: 32%
  ○ Bladder UroCa patients with prostatic urethral UroCa involving prostatic stroma vs. pT4 bladder UroCa
    ■ Prostate involvement by UroCa from urethra 5-year overall survival: 43-64%
    ■ pT4 bladder UroCa 5-year overall survival: 22-25%
  ○ Bladder UroCa patients with prostatic urethral UroCa, noninvasive (involving ducts and acini only) vs. invasive (involving prostatic stroma)
    ■ Survival rates similar for prostatic urethral and noninvasive prostatic urethral UroCa
    ■ Prostatic stromal invasion associated with higher incidence of nodal metastasis and worse survival
    ■ Noninvasive UroCa 5-year overall survival rate: 49%
    ■ Stromal invasive UroCa 5-year overall survival rate: 25%
  ○ Prostate involvement decreases survival of bladder cancer, which varies according to primary stage of bladder cancer
  ○ Age, degree of prostate invasion, and lymph node involvement are independent prognostic variables

Locoregional Involvement in Reported Series
- **Primary prostatic UroCa with no invasive bladder UroCa**
  ○ Prostatic urethra CIS: 8%
  ○ UroCa involving prostatic duct and acini/CIS without stromal invasion: 30%
  ○ Prostatic stromal invasion: 42%
  ○ Extraprostatic extension: 6%
  ○ Lymph node metastasis: 14%
- **Prostatic involvement by bladder UroCa**
  ○ Noninvasive UroCa: 43-47%
    ■ Prostatic urethra CIS: 20%

UROTHELIAL CARCINOMA OF PROSTATE

- UroCa involving prostatic duct and acini/CIS without stromal invasion: 47%
- Combination of prostatic urethral CIS and UroCa involving prostatic duct and acini/CIS without stromal invasion: 33%
  - Invasive UroCa: 53-67%
    - Prostatic urethral lamina propria invasion: 28%
    - Stromal invasion: 33%
    - Periprostatic/seminal vesicle invasion: 13%
    - Direct penetration from bladder UroCa (pT4 bladder UroCa): 26%

IMAGE FINDINGS

Radiographic Findings
- Abnormal excretory urograms in > 1/2 of patients
- Hydronephrosis and enlarged prostatic impression in more advanced disease

Bone Scan
- Bone metastasis is lytic in > 70%

MACROSCOPIC FEATURES

General Features
- Indistinguishable from prostate adenocarcinoma
- Prostate may be enlarged, firm, and fixed with more advanced spread

Cystoscopy
- Majority of prostatic urethral UroCa are flat lesions (86%) and 14% have papillary component

MICROSCOPIC PATHOLOGY

Histologic Features
- Diagnostic criteria identical to those of bladder UroCa
  - **Noninvasive papillary UroCa involving prostatic urethra**
    - Low-grade or high-grade histology
  - **Prostatic urethral CIS**
    - CIS may spread from prostatic urethra, involve ducts and acini, or grow along ejaculatory ducts to seminal vesicle
    - May exhibit different CIS patterns identical to bladder, including large cell pleomorphic, large cell nonpleomorphic, small cell, clinging, pagetoid, and undermining types
    - High-grade dysplastic urothelium confined to urethral basement membrane
    - Invasion of stroma may arise along this spread
  - **Prostatic urethral CIS with invasion of lamina propria**
    - Destructive invasion by nests or single cells through urethral basement membrane often accompanied by desmoplasia or inflammation
  - **UroCa involving prostatic duct and acini/CIS without stromal invasion**
    - High-grade dysplastic urothelium confined within expanded prostatic ducts or acini

- Ducts/acini often completely filled by neoplastic cells
- Ducts/acini have rounded contours and are rimmed by basal cells
- Surrounding basal cells highlighted by more intense and contiguous keratin 34bE12 staining
- May contain central area of necrosis
- Uncommonly, may exhibit pagetoid spread of UroCa within ducts or acini
  - **Prostatic stromal invasion**
    - Destructive invasion by nests or single cells through ductal/acinar basement membranes often accompanied by desmoplasia or inflammation
    - Less commonly may have lymphovascular invasion
    - Invasion may be in absence of duct/acinar involvement
    - Invasive UroCa typically forms small nests with marked nuclear pleomorphism, increased mitosis, and variable nucleoli
    - Invasive UroCa may have squamous differentiation
    - Typically with associated desmoplastic stromal response or inflammation
    - Perineural invasion is not typical finding

Cytologic Features
- High grade

Predominant Pattern/Injury Type
- Neoplastic

Predominant Cell/Compartment Type
- Epithelial, urothelial

ANCILLARY TESTS

Immunohistochemistry
- HMCK, p63(+): Lesional cells(±), native basal cells(+)
- CK7(±) and CK20(±)
- Other positive markers: GATA3, thrombomodulin, CK5/6, uroplakin-3, and S100p
- PSA/PAP(-)
- AMACR(+); not helpful vs. prostate adenocarcinoma

DIFFERENTIAL DIAGNOSIS

Poorly Differentiated Adenocarcinoma of Prostate, ± Intraductal Growth
- Intraductal growth of acinar carcinoma ± comedonecrosis
- Usually associated with invasive Gleason pattern 4 and 5 carcinoma
- Focally may contain glandular formations
- Stromal desmoplasia and inflammatory response to tumor is less common
- Less mitotically active, squamous differentiation is unusual, and perineural invasion is frequent
- Mostly PSA/PAP(+)
- Other new prostate markers include prostate-specific membrane antigen (PSMA), protein (P501s), NKX3, and proPSA (pPSA)

2010 TNM Staging of Urothelial Carcinoma of Prostate

Classification		Description
Primary Tumor (T)		
TX		Primary tumor cannot be assessed
T0		No evidence of primary tumor
Ta		Noninvasive papillary, polypoid, or verrucous carcinoma
Tis	pu	Carcinoma in situ, involvement of prostatic urethra
Tis	pd	Carcinoma in situ, involvement of prostatic ducts
T1		Tumor invades subepithelial connective tissue
T2		Tumor invades any of following: Prostatic stroma, corpus spongiosum, periurethral muscle
T3		Tumor invades any of following: Corpus cavernosum, beyond prostatic capsule, bladder neck (extraprostatic extension)
T4		Tumor invades other adjacent organs (invasion of bladder)
Regional Lymph Nodes (N)		
NX		Regional lymph nodes cannot be assessed
N0		No regional lymph node metastasis
N1		Metastasis in single lymph node 2 cm or less in greatest dimension
N2		Metastasis in single node > 2 cm in greatest dimension, or in multiple nodes
Distant Metastasis (M)		
M0		No distant metastasis (no pathologic M0; use clinical M to complete stage group)
M1		Distant metastasis

Used with the permission of the American Joint Committee on Cancer (AJCC), Chicago, Illinois. The original source for this material is the AJCC Cancer Staging Manual, Seventh Edition (2010) published by Springer Science and Business Media LLC, www.springerlink.com.

High-Grade Prostatic Intraepithelial Neoplasia

- Mimics UroCa involving prostatic ducts and acini
- Atypical cells are prostatic acinar in nature
- Although atypical, including prominent nucleoli, pleomorphism and mitoses are not common

DIAGNOSTIC CHECKLIST

Pathologic Interpretation Pearls

- UroCa involving prostatic ducts and acini raises differential diagnosis with high-grade prostatic intraepithelial neoplasia
- Invasion into stroma should be meticulously ruled out in UroCa involving prostatic ducts and acini
- UroCa involving prostate stroma may occur as result of extension from bladder (pT4 using bladder staging system)
- UroCa involving prostate stroma may occur as result of extension from involvement of prostatic ducts and acini (pT2 using UroCa of prostate staging system)

GRADING

Criteria

- World Health Organization (WHO) 2004/International Society of Urological Pathologists (ISUP) classification for flat and papillary lesions
  - Applicable for prostatic urethral UroCa

STAGING

Criteria

- American Joint Committee on Cancer (AJCC)/ International Union Against Cancer (UICC) 2009
  - UroCa of prostate has separate TNM staging system from prostate or bladder cancer
  - Bladder UroCa transmurally invading through vesical wall and extending into prostate is staged under bladder cancer TNM staging (pT4 bladder ca)

SELECTED REFERENCES

1. Chuang AY et al: Immunohistochemical differentiation of high-grade prostate carcinoma from urothelial carcinoma. Am J Surg Pathol. 31(8):1246-55, 2007
2. Shen SS et al: Prostatic involvement by transitional cell carcinoma in patients with bladder cancer and its prognostic significance. Hum Pathol. 37(6):726-34, 2006
3. Njinou Ngninkeu B et al: Transitional cell carcinoma involving the prostate: a clinicopathological retrospective study of 76 cases. J Urol. 169(1):149-52, 2003
4. Oliai BR et al: A clinicopathologic analysis of urothelial carcinomas diagnosed on prostate needle biopsy. Am J Surg Pathol. 25(6):794-801, 2001
5. Cheville JC et al: Transitional cell carcinoma of the prostate: clinicopathologic study of 50 cases. Cancer. 82(4):703-7, 1998
6. Esrig D et al: Transitional cell carcinoma involving the prostate with a proposed staging classification for stromal invasion. J Urol. 156(3):1071-6, 1996
7. Mahadevia PS et al: Prostatic involvement in bladder cancer. Prostate mapping in 20 cystoprostatectomy specimens. Cancer. 58(9):2096-102, 1986

UROTHELIAL CARCINOMA OF PROSTATE

Microscopic Features

(Left) UroCa growing along prostatic ducts and acini ⇥ shows smooth contours and lack of desmoplasia indicating absence of stromal invasion. Overlying prostatic urethra exhibits features of CIS ⇥; it may be denuded, normal, or show features of a high-grade papillary UroCa. *(Right)* UroCa in situ is shown involving prostatic urethra and periurethral duct. The involvement may be limited to the urethra, submucosal glands, or may more extensively involve prostatic ducts and acini.

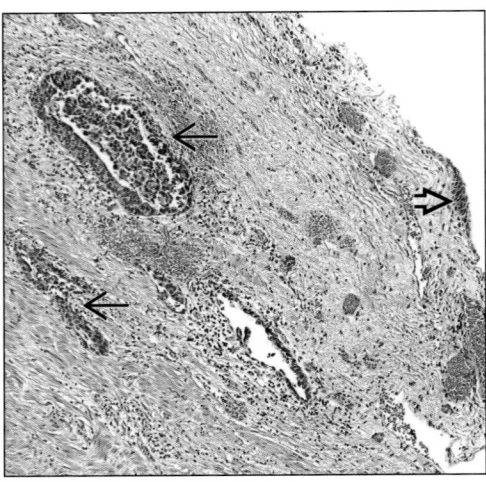
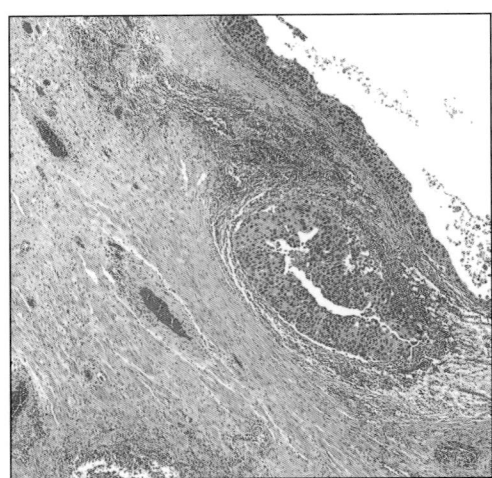

(Left) Noninvasive UroCa involving a prostatic duct shows tumor cells that are pleomorphic, with brisk mitotic activity, and completely fill the duct. Note presence of identifiable basal cells at the periphery ⇥. *(Right)* This duct is expanded by intraductal growth of UroCa with central area of necrosis. Criteria for diagnosis of prostate UroCa is identical to those in the bladder. Ductal involvement by UroCa mimics Gleason pattern 5 prostate adenocarcinoma with comedonecrosis.

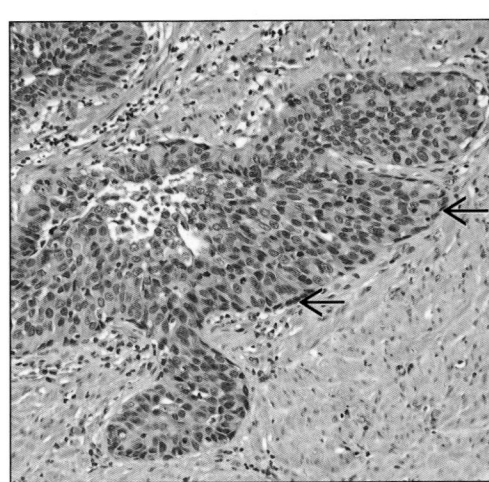
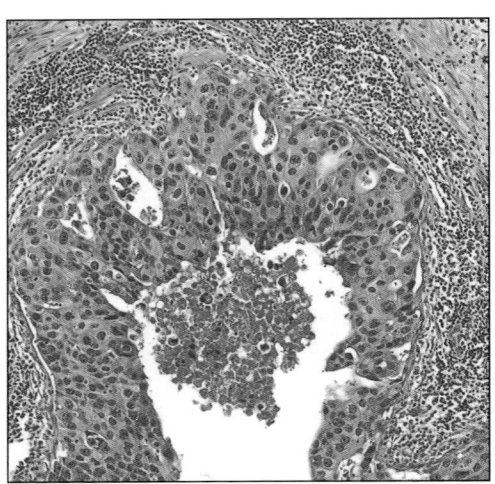

(Left) UroCa involving prostatic ducts and acini with stromal invasion. At low power, there is greater complexity than mere expansion of preexisting ducts and acini; this pattern should raise concern for invasion, which is an adverse prognostic parameter. *(Right)* UroCa involving prostatic ducts and acini associated with stromal invasion shown. There are small irregular nests with desmoplasia and associated inflammatory response. The solid invading nests are unusual for prostatic carcinoma.

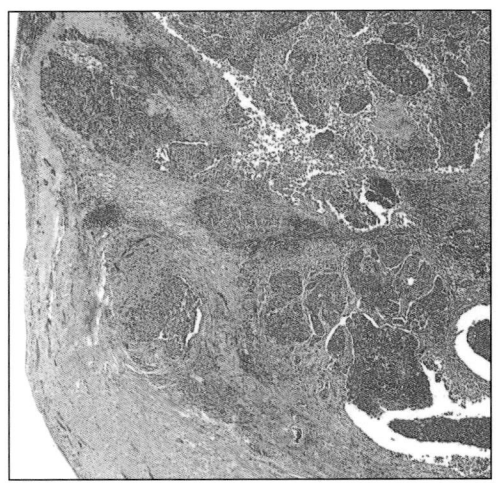
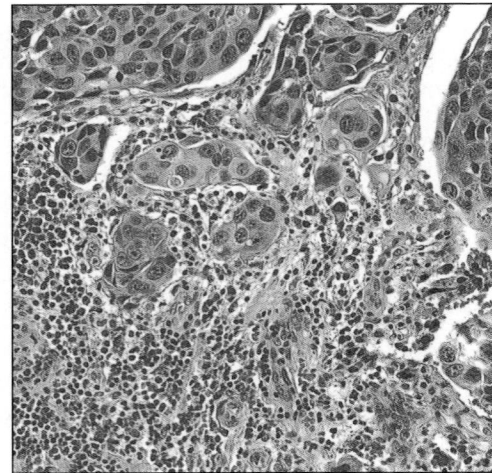

UROTHELIAL CARCINOMA OF PROSTATE

Immunohistochemical Features and Differential Diagnosis

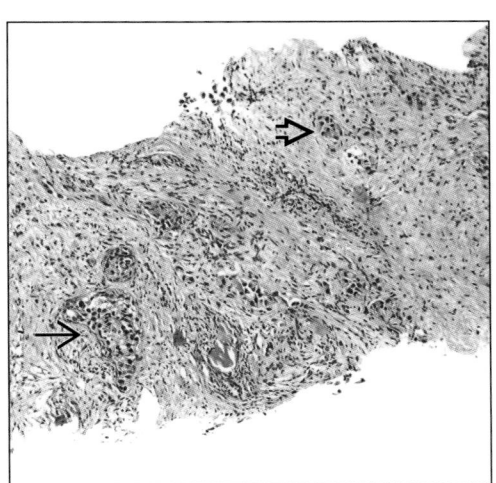

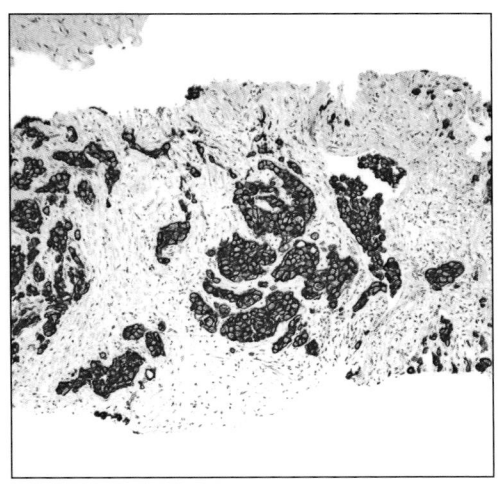

(Left) UroCa involves prostatic ducts and acini ⇨ with associated stromal invasion ⮞. Diagnosis of UroCa in prostate biopsies is uncommon and must be distinguished from poorly differentiated prostate adenocarcinoma. UroCa typically shows marked pleomorphism, increased mitoses, and desmoplasia. The presence of squamous differentiation is more common in UroCa. *(Right)* UroCa involves prostatic ducts with associated stromal invasion showing positivity with CK20.

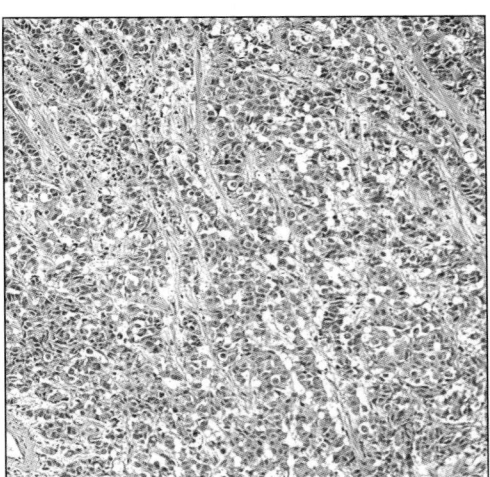

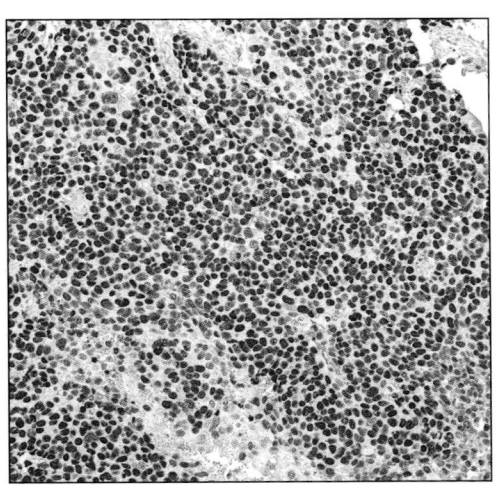

(Left) High-grade UroCa arises from the bladder and diffusely involves the prostate (pT4 bladder UroCa), mimicking poorly differentiated prostate adenocarcinoma. *(Right)* p63 diffusely staining UroCa involves the prostate. p63 is helpful in distinguishing high-grade UroCa vs. prostate adenocarcinoma. Other useful positive markers for UroCa include keratin HMCK(34βE12), CK5/6, and thrombomodulin. AMACR may be positive in UroCa and is not helpful vs. prostate cancer.

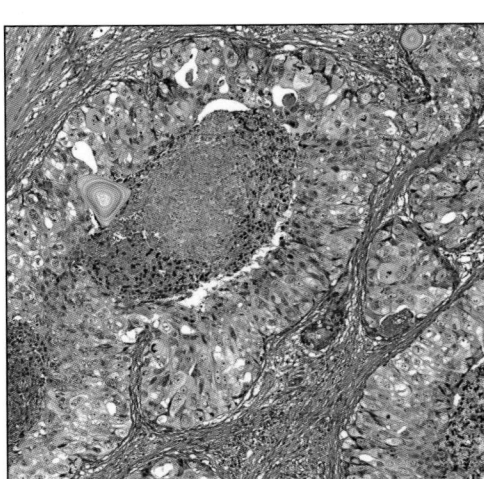

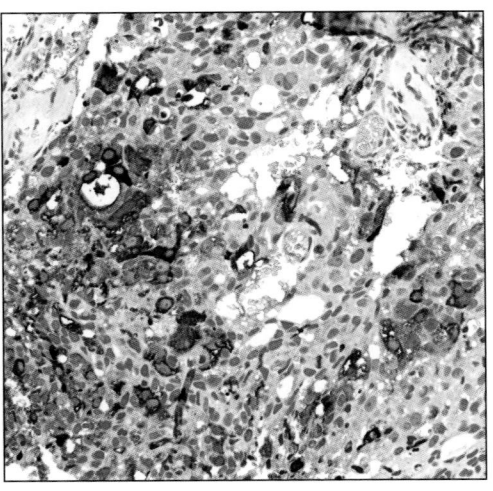

(Left) Large nests of poorly differentiated prostate adenocarcinoma with central necrosis mimic high-grade UroCa. Distinction between these 2 entities is important because of differing treatment options. *(Right)* Poorly differentiated prostate adenocarcinoma is shown marking focally with PSA. Other positive markers that may be used vs. poorly differentiated UroCa include PAP, PSMA, P501s, NKX3, and pPSA. Prostate cancer is typically negative for p63 and HMCK(34βE12).

SMALL CELL CARCINOMA AND OTHER NEUROENDOCRINE TUMORS

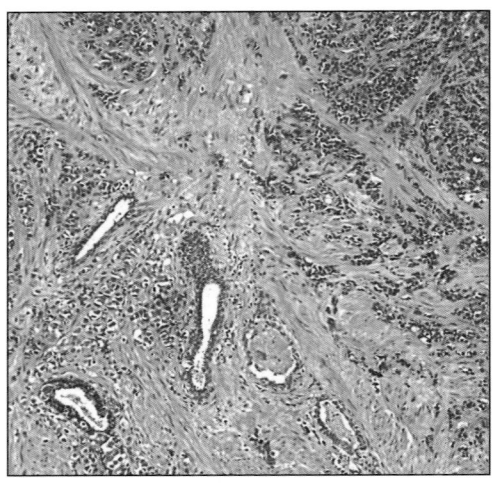

Low-power magnification of SCC involving the prostate shows tumor cells arranged in haphazard nests and trabeculae with infiltration between benign glands.

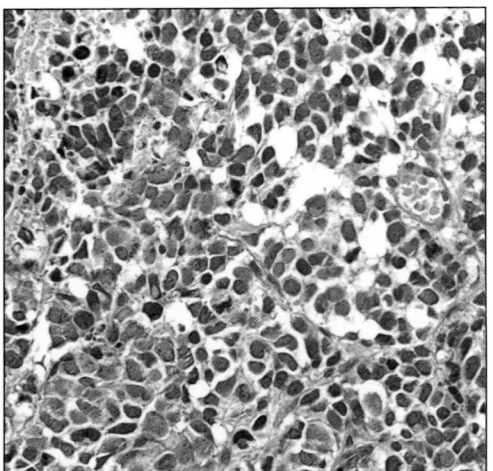

SCC shows tumor cells with scant cytoplasm and nuclei with "salt and pepper" chromatin, indistinct nucleoli, and increased mitosis. Note nuclear molding and abundant apoptosis.

TERMINOLOGY

Abbreviations
- Small cell carcinoma (SCC)

Synonyms
- Small cell neuroendocrine (NE) carcinoma, poorly differentiated NE carcinoma, small cell anaplastic carcinoma, oat cell carcinoma

Definitions
- **NE tumors of prostate**
  - Spectrum of primary prostatic tumors exhibiting NE differentiation which, in pure form, are analogous to NE tumors of other organ sites
  - NE tumors occur either as pure or admixed with acinar adenocarcinoma
  - WHO 2002 classification recognizes 3 forms of prostatic NE tumors
    - SCC, focal NE differentiation in acinar adenocarcinoma, and carcinoid tumor
- **SCC**
  - High-grade NE carcinoma consisting of small to intermediate-sized NE tumor cells
- **Focal NE differentiation in acinar adenocarcinoma**
  - Rare to occasional single or clusters of NE cells present in acinar adenocarcinoma, more often demonstrated by immunohistochemistry
- **Carcinoid tumor**
  - Well-differentiated NE carcinoma
- **Large cell NE carcinoma (LCNEC)**
  - High-grade NE carcinoma consisting of large-sized NE tumor cells, often with prominent nucleoli
  - Recently reported entity
- **Mixed acinar and SCC**
  - Distinct components, ± juxtaposition, of usual acinar carcinoma and SCC

ETIOLOGY/PATHOGENESIS

Origin
- Transdifferentiation or dedifferentiation from non-NE tumor cells
- De novo transformation from prostatic NE cells
  - These are terminally differentiated postmitotic cells that evolved from committed basal cells and share common stem cell origin with acinar and basal cells
  - These NE cells are believed to play role in growth, differentiation, and homeostatic regulation of secretory processes of prostatic glands

Risk Factors
- History of acinar adenocarcinoma, present in about 1/2 of SCC and most carcinoid tumors and LCNEC
- Hormonal treatment or androgen deprivation therapy (ADT) for acinar adenocarcinoma
  - NE cells are devoid of androgen receptors; ADT may lead to clonal propagation
  - Possible clonal progression and evolution of subset of non-NE tumor cells that have been influenced by ADT

CLINICAL ISSUES

Epidemiology
- Incidence
  - SCC accounts for approximately 1% of all prostate cancers, when SCC admixed with adenocarcinoma are included
  - Focal NE differentiation in acinar adenocarcinoma is almost ubiquitous, reported in 10-100% of adenocarcinomas, depending on technique employed
  - Carcinoid tumor and LCNEC are exceedingly rare, described only in isolated case reports and small case series

SMALL CELL CARCINOMA AND OTHER NEUROENDOCRINE TUMORS

Key Facts

Terminology

- NE tumors of prostate include spectrum of primary prostatic tumors exhibiting NE differentiation; in their pure form, they are analogous to NE tumors of other organ sites
- Occur either as pure or admixed with acinar adenocarcinoma
- Includes SCC, focal NE differentiation in acinar adenocarcinoma, carcinoid tumor, and LCNEC

Clinical Issues

- SCC accounts for 1-5% of all prostate cancers, including SCC admixed with adenocarcinoma
- Focal NE differentiation in acinar adenocarcinoma is reported in 10-100% of adenocarcinomas
- Carcinoid tumor and LCNEC are exceedingly rare
- Serum PSA level variable and may be normal

- Prognosis of SCC is poor with mean survival of < 1 year after development of SCC component

Microscopic Pathology

- SCC is histologically similar to SCC of lungs
  - Small blue cell tumor with scant cytoplasm, high nuclear to cytoplasmic ratio, "salt and pepper" chromatin, nuclear molding, single cell necrosis or geographic necrosis, and smearing artifacts
- Focal NE differentiation in acinar adenocarcinoma
  - Characterized by scattered or focal cluster of NE cells blending with adenocarcinoma cellular elements, highlighted by NE markers
  - Paneth cell-like change may occur
- Carcinoid tumor and LCNEC are histologically similar to their pulmonary counterparts
- Up to 90% of NE tumors are NE marker (+)

- Poorly differentiated NE carcinomas arise in approximately 10% of prostate cancer patients with androgen-resistant disease following long-term ADT
- Age
  - Tumors occur predominantly in elderly patients
  - SCC
    - Mean: 69 years; range: 30-92 years

Presentation

- SCC
  - Rapid onset urinary tract obstruction, such as dysuria, nocturia, or urgency, are main presenting symptoms
  - Previous diagnosis of adenocarcinoma in 42-67% cases, some with history of prior hormonal therapy
    - Interval from adenocarcinoma to diagnosis of SCC ranges from 1 to 300 months; mean: 59 months
  - Lack of clinically evident hormone production in most cases
  - Paraneoplastic syndromes: Adrenocorticotrophic hormone (ACTH) or antidiuretic hormone (ADH) production, Eaton-Lambert syndrome, and others
  - Most patients present with extraprostatic extension, large primary tumor masses, advanced stage disease, and distant metastases
- Carcinoid tumor
  - Incidental or may present with hematuria, burning, nocturia, frequency, oliguria, or symptoms of urinary retention
  - May occur following diagnosis of acinar adenocarcinoma
- LCNEC
  - Most patients with initial diagnosis of acinar adenocarcinoma and prior ADT
    - Interval from adenocarcinoma to diagnosis of LCNEC ranges from 2 to 12 years; mean: 4.7 years
  - Advanced stage at time of diagnosis
  - Clinical and therapeutic significance of distinguishing LCNEC from SCC in prostate is not established

Laboratory Tests

- Serum PSA level variable, may be normal
- May show significant drop in serum PSA, as NE component predominates over acinar adenocarcinoma component
- Serum chromogranin-A and pro-gastrin-releasing peptide levels
  - May be diagnostically and prognostically useful in prostate cancers with focal NE differentiation
  - May be useful particularly in androgen-independent cancers

Treatment

- Surgery remains mainstream for therapy of SCC
- Cisplatin-based chemotherapy has been suggested in SCC, but studies showing significant survival impact are lacking

Prognosis

- Prognosis of SCC is poor with mean survival of < 1 year after development of SCC component
  - No difference in prognosis between pure SCC and SCC admixed with adenocarcinoma
  - Response to available treatment modalities is poor
  - Common metastatic sites include bone, liver, lung, and lymph nodes
- Prognostic significance of focal NE differentiation in acinar adenocarcinoma is controversial
  - Some studies show negative effect on prognosis, while some studies show no relationship
  - Paneth cell-like change in adenocarcinoma does not portend poor prognosis
- Prognosis of carcinoid tumor is uncertain because of few cases reported
  - Some tumors with clinically aggressive behavior may represent prostate adenocarcinoma (carcinoid-like adenocarcinoma)
  - True carcinoid is suggested to have indolent behavior, although cases reported are limited
- Prognosis of LCNEC is similar to SCC
  - Most common metastatic site is bone; other sites of metastasis include lung, liver, lymph nodes

SMALL CELL CARCINOMA AND OTHER NEUROENDOCRINE TUMORS

MACROSCOPIC FEATURES

General Features
- Large volume disease frequently, with diffuse involvement of prostatic parenchyma

MICROSCOPIC PATHOLOGY

Histologic Features
- **SCC**
  - Histologically similar to SCC of lung
  - Predominantly diffuse sheet-like growth; may form clusters, trabeculae, cords, and single cell patterns
  - Small blue cell tumor
    - Scant cytoplasm
    - High nuclear to cytoplasmic ratio
    - "Salt and pepper" chromatin
    - Nuclear molding
    - Single cell necrosis or geographic necrosis
    - Smearing artifacts
    - Brisk mitotic activity
    - Frequent apoptosis
  - 2 cell types
    - Oat cell carcinoma consists of small cells (up to 2x size of lymphocytes), pyknotic round to oval nuclei, and indistinct nucleoli
    - "Intermediate cell" histology with overall less uniformity, containing slightly larger nuclei, prominent nucleoli, relatively more cytoplasm, and polygonal or fusiform cells
    - Admixture of these 2 cell types may occur
  - About 50% have recognizable acinar adenocarcinoma component
    - Most adenocarcinoma are high grade: 85% are Gleason score 8 or higher
    - Transition between adenocarcinoma and NE components may be abrupt or tumors may merge imperceptibly
  - Perineural invasion and lymphovascular invasion may be seen
- **Focal NE differentiation in acinar adenocarcinoma**
  - Characterized by scattered or focal clusters of NE cells blending with adenocarcinoma cellular elements and may be highlighted by NE markers
  - Occasionally NE cells contain bright eosinophilic cytoplasmic granules resembling Paneth cells of gastrointestinal tract
- **Carcinoid tumor**
  - Histologically similar to carcinoid tumor at other sites
  - Nested, trabecular, cords, or mixed architectural patterns
  - Uniform round or polygonal cells with round, regular nuclei containing "salt and pepper" chromatin; nucleoli are indistinct
  - Rare to low mitotic activity and absent necrosis
- **LCNEC**
  - Histologically similar to LCNEC of lung
  - Architectural pattern similar to SCC

  - Tumor cells contain large, hyperchromatic nuclei with coarse chromatin and visible nucleoli and pale to amphophilic cytoplasm
  - Brisk mitotic activity

Predominant Pattern/Injury Type
- Neoplastic

Predominant Cell/Compartment Type
- Neuroendocrine

ANCILLARY TESTS

Immunohistochemistry
- Up to 90% of NE tumors are positive for NE
- Reported NE marker immunoreactivity in SCC
  - Synaptophysin 84-89%(+)
  - Chromogranin 61-75%(+)
  - CD56 83-92%(+)
  - NSE 85%(+)
- < 20% are prostate specific markers (PSA, PAP, PSMA) (+)
- Approximately 50% of SCC are TTF-1(+)
- Basal cell markers (p63 and HMCK) typically (-); positivity reported in up to 35% of cases
- About 1/2 of SCC are AMACR(+)
- AR typically (-)
- SCC may show typical paranuclear dot-like immunoreactivity with PAN-CK(AE1/AE3)
- SCC is typically CK7(-)/CK20(-); CK7(+) reported in up to 39%; CK20 rarely positive

DIFFERENTIAL DIAGNOSIS

Secondary SCC Involving Prostate
- Primary and secondary NE tumors of prostate are histologically and immunohistochemically indistinguishable
- Use of lung marker TTF-1 is not helpful, as about 1/2 of prostate or bladder primary SCC are positive
- Distinction from SCC of urinary bladder secondarily involving prostate may be impossible in specimens with limited sampling
- Distinction relies on clinico-pathological correlation, e.g., history of prostate adenocarcinoma, prior hormonal therapy, elevated serum PSA (uncommon)
- Concomitant evidence of prostatic adenocarcinoma or bladder urothelial carcinoma may suggest primary site (for bladder vs. prostate)
  - SCC from these sites often occurs admixed with these primary histologic patterns

Poorly Differentiated Acinar Adenocarcinoma (Gleason Pattern 5)
- High-grade adenocarcinoma with solid sheet and single cell infiltration
- Synaptophysin (in acinar adenocarcinoma component) and PSA (in NE component) positivity compounds diagnostic distinction
  - Strong PSA positivity would favor poorly differentiated acinar adenocarcinoma

SMALL CELL CARCINOMA AND OTHER NEUROENDOCRINE TUMORS

- Does not have typical architectural and cytologic features of SCC
- May lack expression of other NE markers (chromogranin, CD56)
- PAN-CK(AE1/AE3) shows diffuse positivity, in contrast to SCC, which may show dot-like positivity

Poorly Differentiated Urothelial Carcinoma
- Crush artifact in urothelial carcinoma may cause it to mimic SCC on low magnification
- Does not have typical cytologic features of SCC
- Negative for NE markers
- Typically diffusely p63(+), HMCK(34βE12)(+), CK7(+), and CK20(+)

Basal Cell Carcinoma
- Similar to SCC, tumor cells have scant cytoplasm, high nuclear to cytoplasmic ratio, and form nests, cords, or trabeculae
- Does not have typical cytologic features of SCC
- Negative for NE markers
- Typically diffusely (+) for basal cell markers (p63 and HMCK[34βE12])

Malignant Lymphoma
- Does not have typical architectural and cytologic features of SCC
- Simple immunohistochemical panel (CD45 and PAN-CK) should differentiate between both entities

Rhabdomyosarcoma
- Rare in adults; synaptophysin positivity may compound diagnosis

DIAGNOSTIC CHECKLIST

Pathologic Interpretation Pearls
- Diffuse sheets, clusters, cords, or single cell patterns of tumor cells with NE features; spectrum defined by cell or nuclear size, nucleoli, mitotic activity, and amount of necrosis

REPORTING CONSIDERATIONS

Key Elements to Report
- Biopsy, microscopic evaluation
  - Histologic type (SCC, focal NE differentiation in acinar adenocarcinoma, carcinoid tumor, LCNEC, or mixed NE tumors-adenocarcinoma)
  - Grade (Gleason grade for adenocarcinoma if mixed)
  - Local invasion
    - Prostatic fat
    - Seminal vesicle
  - Additional findings, if present
- Prostatectomy, microscopic evaluation
  - Histologic type (SCC, focal NE differentiation in acinar adenocarcinoma, carcinoid tumor, LCNEC, or mixed NE tumors-adenocarcinoma)
  - Grade (Gleason grade for adenocarcinoma if mixed)
  - Specify percentage of any differentiation, if mixed
  - Location
  - Extent of local invasion
    - Extraprostatic extension
    - Seminal vesicle involvement
  - Margins (location and extent of margins involved with tumor)
  - Regional lymph node status
  - Additional findings, if present

GRADING

Criteria
- Gleason grading
  - Not applicable in NE tumors
  - Apply for adenocarcinoma component in mixed NE tumors and adenocarcinoma with focal NE differentiation

STAGING

Criteria
- American Joint Committee on Cancer (AJCC)/ International Union Against Cancer (UICC) 2009
  - Prostate cancer TNM staging applies for SCC of prostate

REPORTING CRITERIA

Diagnostic Criteria for Prostate NE Tumors
- Follows histologic criteria established for pulmonary NE tumors

SELECTED REFERENCES

1. Wang W et al: Small cell carcinoma of the prostate. A morphologic and immunohistochemical study of 95 cases. Am J Surg Pathol. 32(1):65-71, 2008
2. Evans AJ et al: Large cell neuroendocrine carcinoma of prostate: a clinicopathologic summary of 7 cases of a rare manifestation of advanced prostate cancer. Am J Surg Pathol. 30(6):684-93, 2006
3. Tamas EF et al: Prognostic significance of paneth cell-like neuroendocrine differentiation in adenocarcinoma of the prostate. Am J Surg Pathol. 30(8):980-5, 2006
4. Yao JL et al: Small cell carcinoma of the prostate: an immunohistochemical study. Am J Surg Pathol. 30(6):705-12, 2006
5. Reyes A et al: Low-grade neuroendocrine carcinoma (carcinoid tumor) of the prostate. Arch Pathol Lab Med. 128(12):e166-8, 2004
6. Tash JA et al: Metastatic carcinoid tumor of the prostate. J Urol. 167(6):2526-7, 2002
7. Bonkhoff H: Neuroendocrine differentiation in human prostate cancer. Morphogenesis, proliferation and androgen receptor status. Ann Oncol. 12 Suppl 2:S141-4, 2001
8. di Sant'Agnese PA: Neuroendocrine differentiation in carcinoma of the prostate. Diagnostic, prognostic, and therapeutic implications. Cancer. 70(1 Suppl):254-68, 1992
9. Oesterling JE et al: Small cell anaplastic carcinoma of the prostate: a clinical, pathological and immunohistological study of 27 patients. J Urol. 147(3 Pt 2):804-7, 1992

SMALL CELL CARCINOMA AND OTHER NEUROENDOCRINE TUMORS

Small Cell Carcinoma

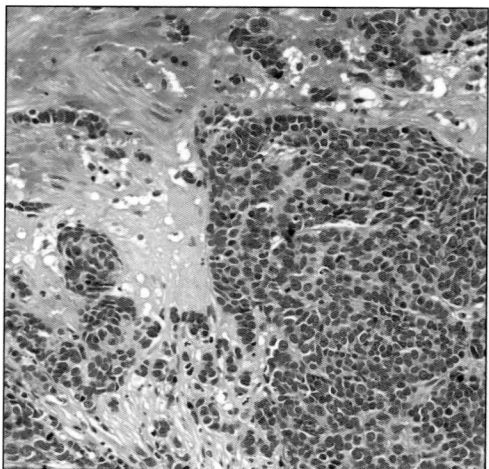
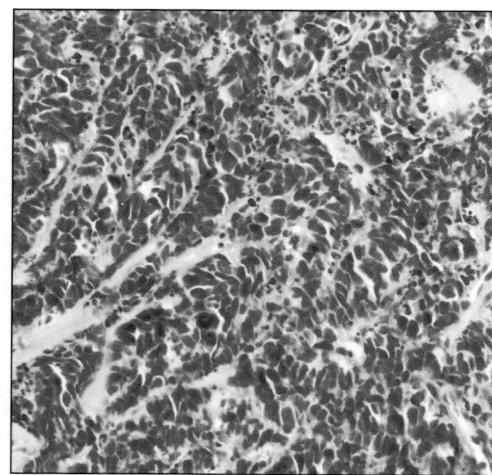

(Left) SCC shows diffuse patternless growth and abundant single cell necrosis. Tumor cells are relatively large or intermediate in size with nuclei containing occasional prominent nucleoli. *(Right)* SCC with small undifferentiated cells shows scant cytoplasm and exhibits nuclear molding, abundant crush artifact, and apoptosis. Sometimes referred to as oat cell carcinoma, SCC of the prostate is morphologically similar to SCC of the lung.

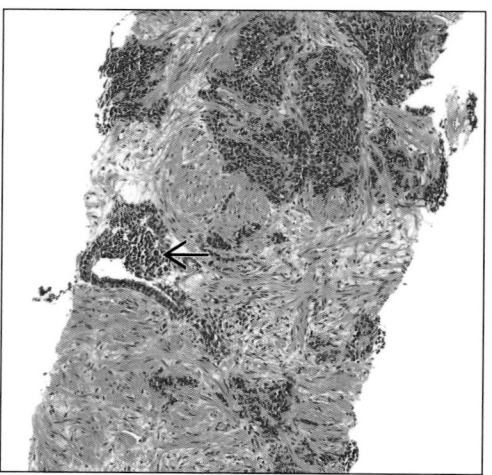
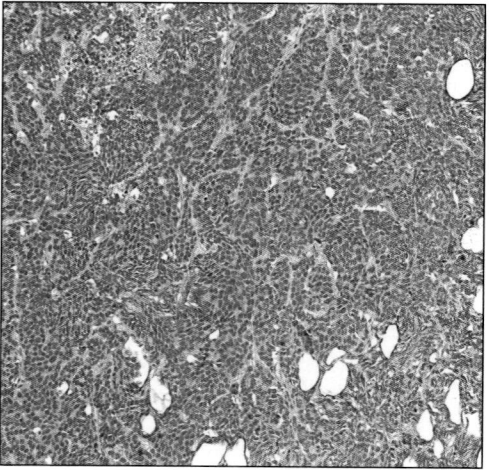

(Left) Needle biopsy of prostate with involvement by SCC shows tumor cells with round blue cell appearance arranged in infiltrative clusters and small nests. Tumor cells are seen invading an adjacent benign gland ➡. *(Right)* SCC shows diffuse infiltration of the prostate by tumor cells exhibiting a variable nested to organoid arrangement. The scant cytoplasm and crowding of tumor cells impart a round blue cell appearance on low magnification.

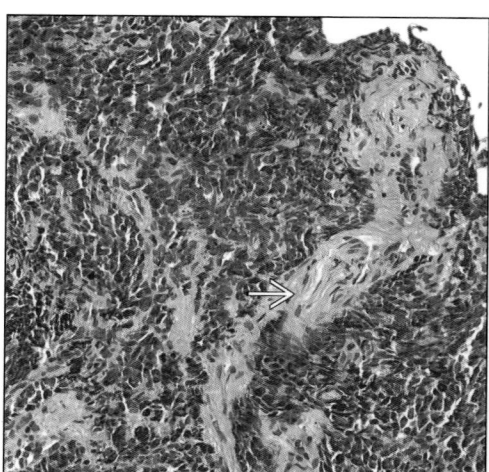
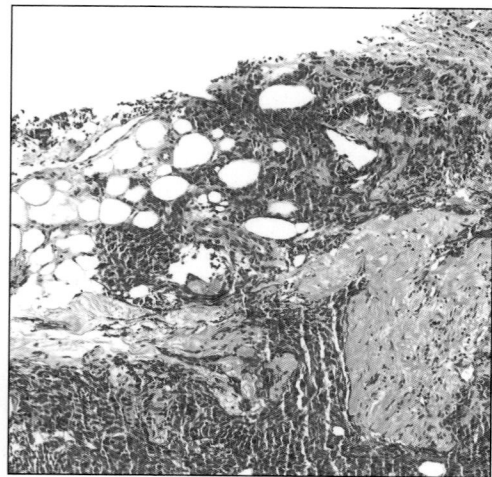

(Left) SCC shows sheets of small cells with extensive crush artifact. This distortion, along with an Azzopardi effect, is a helpful feature in the diagnosis of SCC. Note the presence of perineural invasion ➡. *(Right)* SCC shows extraprostatic extension by tumor cells (pT3 disease) characterized by infiltration of periprostatic adipose tissue. Majority of SCCs present with advanced tumor stage, and the prognosis is poor with an aggressive disease course.

Mixed SCC or NE Differentiation with Adenocarcinoma

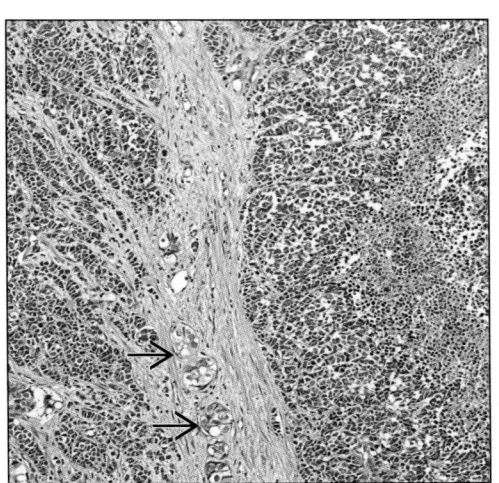

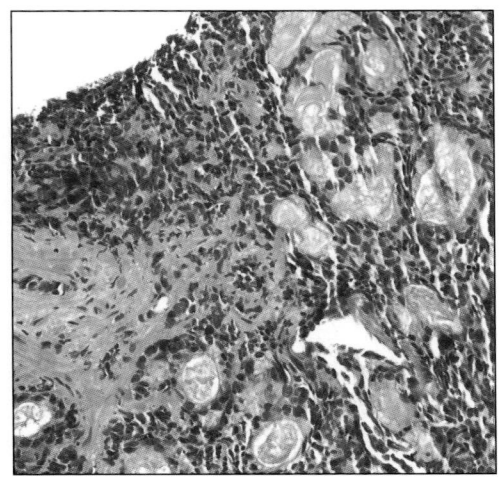

(Left) SCC admixed with acinar adenocarcinoma shows large sheets, nests, and trabeculae of cells with central necrosis. Microacini of usual prostatic adenocarcinoma ➡ are seen infiltrating in fibrous bands between SCC components. About 1/2 of SCC of the prostate occur with acinar adenocarcinoma. *(Right)* SCC admixed with acinar adenocarcinoma shows an intimate admixture of SCC with glands of acinar adenocarcinoma (Gleason pattern 3). Frequently, the Gleason score is higher.

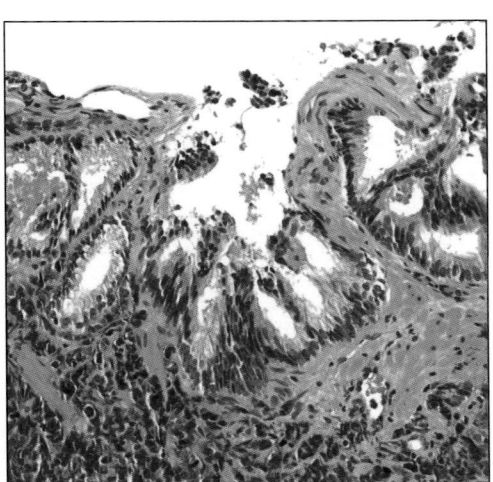

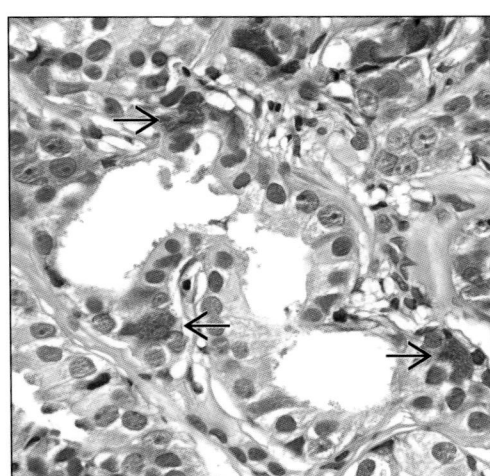

(Left) SCC admixed with acinar adenocarcinoma in needle biopsy shows SCC tumor cells admixed with cribriform pattern of acinar adenocarcinoma. Most adenocarcinomas admixed with SCC are high grade; 85% are Gleason grade 8 or higher. *(Right)* Acinar adenocarcinoma with Paneth cell-like change ➡. Cells with abundant cytoplasm and brightly eosinophilic granules shown to have neuroendocrine differentiation by immunohistochemistry and ultrastructure.

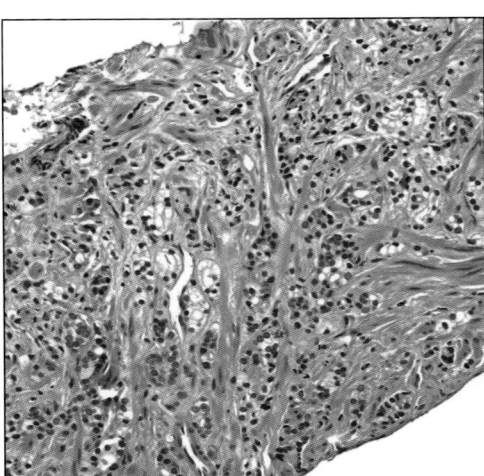

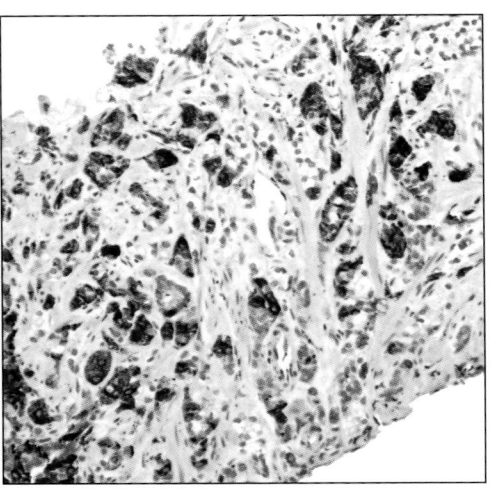

(Left) NE differentiation in conventional adenocarcinoma shows infiltrative and poorly formed glands of adenocarcinoma, some containing cells with relatively less cytoplasm. *(Right)* NE differentiation in this acinar adenocarcinoma is confirmed by immunohistochemical staining with synaptophysin. More often, NE differentiation is confirmed only with use of ancillary techniques, the value of which in clinical practice remains in question.

SMALL CELL CARCINOMA AND OTHER NEUROENDOCRINE TUMORS

Immunohistochemical Features

(Left) SCC shows diffuse and strong expression of synaptophysin. The majority of SCC are positive for multiple NE markers, such as synaptophysin, chromogranin, NSE, and CD56. Strong PSA positivity is unusual in these tumors. *(Right)* Needle biopsy with SCC shows complete negative staining with PSA ⇨. SCC are typically negative for prostate-specific markers, such as PSA, PAP, and PSMA. Note benign prostatic glands in adjacent core are strongly PSA positive.

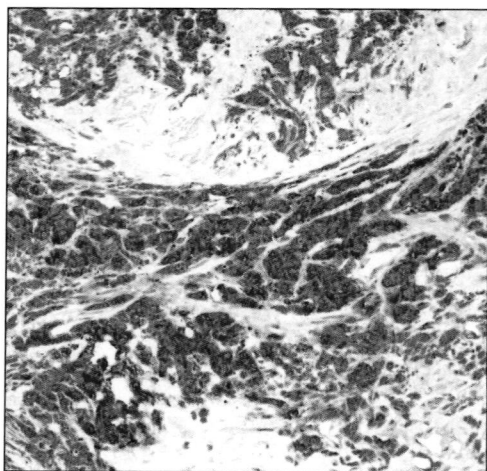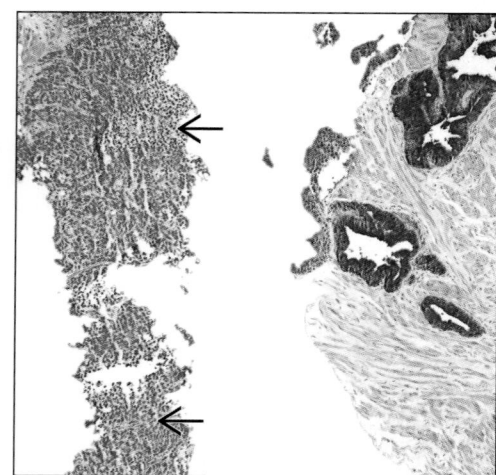

(Left) SCC shows strong and diffuse expression of chromogranin. Studies have shown that synaptophysin and CD56 stains have relatively higher sensitivity than chromogranin. Since some SCC may be negative for any NE markers, use of at least 3 markers is recommended when there is suspicion for NE differentiation. *(Right)* PAN-CK(AE1/AE3) expression in SCC may show dot-like cytoplasmic positivity, which is associated with NE neoplasms.

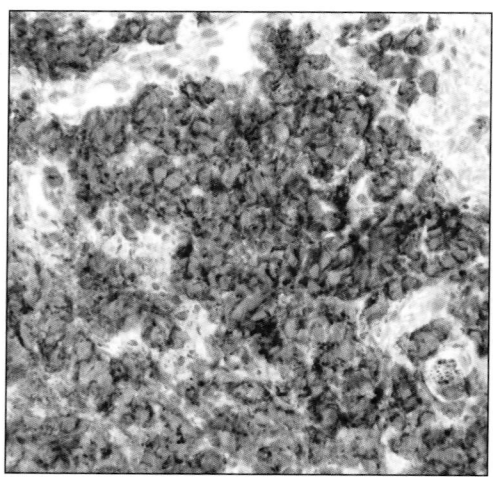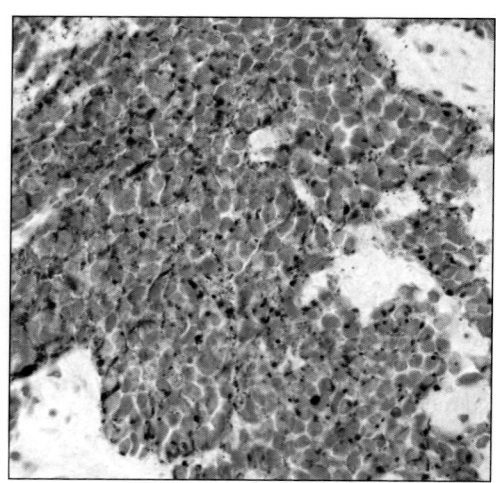

(Left) Triple cocktail (AMACR, p63, and PAN-CK[AE1/AE3]) in prostate needle biopsy with SCC ⇨ shows SCC tumor cells with modest AMACR (red) staining and patchy with basal cell markers (brown) staining. Note adjacent benign glands showing basal cell marker positivity ⇨ and AMACR negativity. *(Right)* SCC shows diffuse reactivity to AMACR (red). Note the focal membranous positivity for PAN-CK(AE1/AE3) (brown) ⇨. Approximately 1/2 of SCC express AMACR.

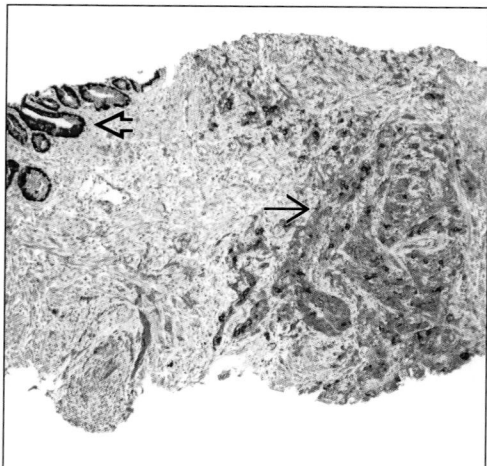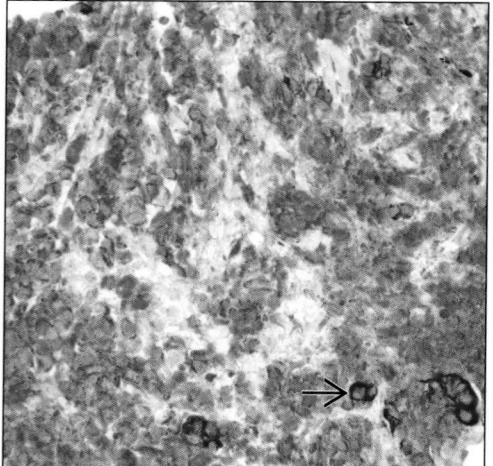

SMALL CELL CARCINOMA AND OTHER NEUROENDOCRINE TUMORS

Carcinoid Tumor and LCNEC

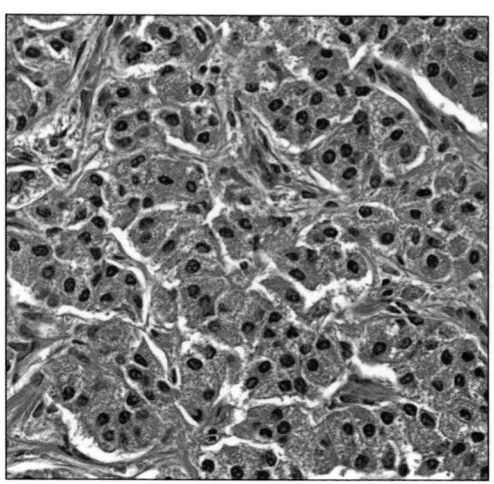

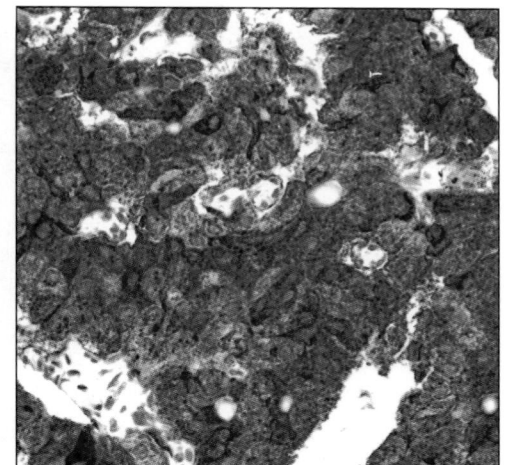

(Left) Well-differentiated neuroendocrine carcinoma (carcinoid tumor) involving the prostate shows classic organoid architecture and low-grade nuclei of carcinoid tumor. Criteria in distinguishing carcinoid tumor from SCC are similar to those applied to NE tumors of the lung. By definition, carcinoid tumors should have absent to rare mitosis and no tumor cell necrosis. *(Right)* Carcinoid tumor of prostate shows strong synaptophysin expression.

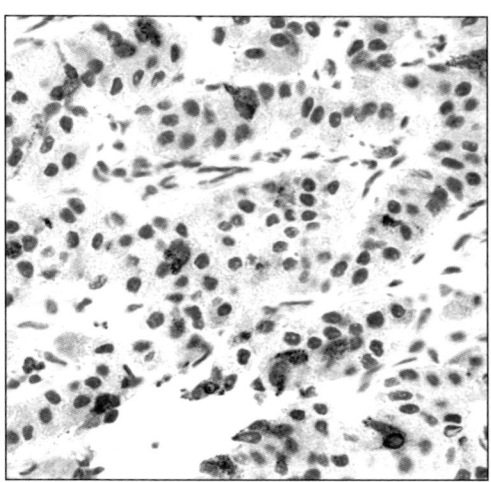

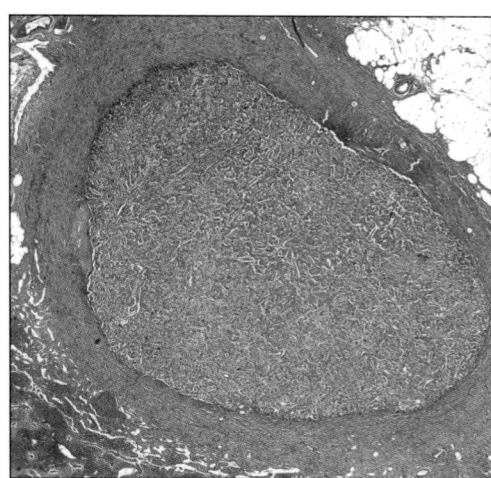

(Left) This carcinoid tumor shows scattered positivity for PSA. Some authors suggest that carcinoid tumors of the prostate should be essentially negative for PSA to distinguish from carcinoid-like prostate carcinoma, which is conventional adenocarcinoma that resembles carcinoid tumor. *(Right)* Carcinoid tumor of the prostate shows metastasis to a pelvic lymph node. Prognosis of carcinoid tumor is uncertain because of few cases reported.

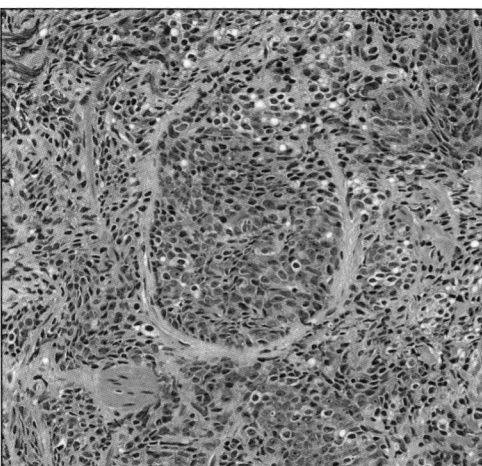

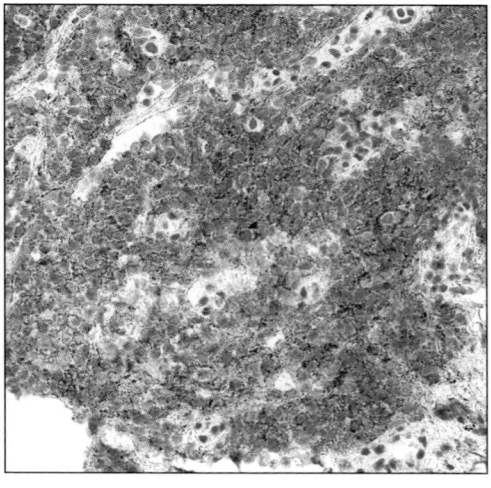

(Left) LCNEC of the prostate shows sheets of NE tumor cells with relatively large nuclei and prominent nucleoli. The tumor cells are less uniform than SCC and some show relatively more cytoplasm. As with SCC, an acinar adenocarcinoma component may be present. The clinical and therapeutic significance of distinguishing SCC from LCNEC of the prostate has not been established. *(Right)* LCNEC shows diffuse expression of chromogranin. Like SCC, LCNEC expresses multiple NE markers.

BASAL CELL AND ADENOID CYSTIC CARCINOMA

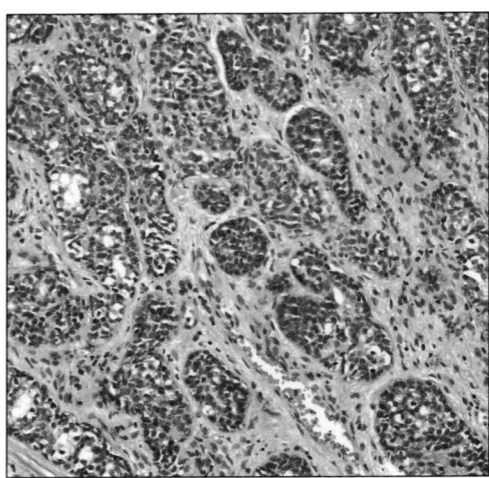

BCC/ACC may present with 2 patterns. The BCC pattern is characterized by infiltrative solid nests of basaloid cells with peripheral cellular palisading, similar in appearance to cutaneous BCC.

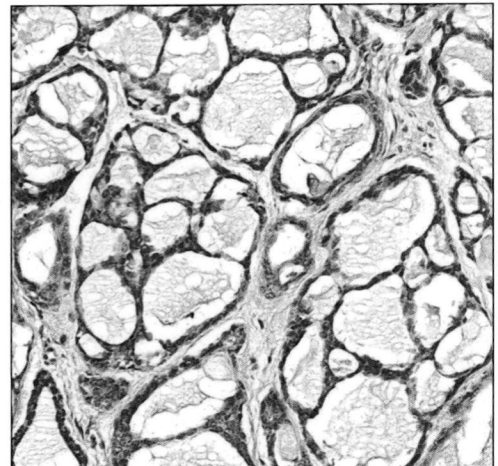

The ACC pattern is characterized by large, invasive nests with cribriform architecture containing multiple lumina resembling ACC at other sites. BCC and ACC patterns may coexist in the same tumor.

TERMINOLOGY

Abbreviations
- Adenoid cystic carcinoma (ACC)
- Basaloid cell carcinoma (BCC)

Synonyms
- Adenoid basal cell tumor, adenoid cystic-like tumor

Definitions
- Malignant neoplasm composed primarily of basaloid cells arising putatively from prostatic basal cells

ETIOLOGY/PATHOGENESIS

Origin
- Considered to arise from basal cells along prostatic ducts and acini

CLINICAL ISSUES

Epidemiology
- Incidence
  ○ Uncommon: Approximately < 75 cases reported in the literature
- Age
  ○ Wide age range (28-89 years), but majority occur in older men

Presentation
- Most commonly presents with obstructive urinary symptoms
  ○ Thus most cases diagnosed on transurethral resection of prostate (TURP) specimens
- Perianal pain
- Few tumors incidentally encountered in needle biopsy during work-up for elevated serum PSA level for other causes

Laboratory Tests
- Serum PSA levels may be normal or elevated

Treatment
- Most reported cases treated with TURP, with a subset undergoing radical prostatectomy
- Advanced stage treated with adjuvant radiotherapy or chemotherapy

Prognosis
- Limited data available on clinical behavior
- Local recurrence, metastasis, and death from disease reported in approximately 30% of cases
- Metastases commonly to lung and liver
- Bone metastasis rare compared to acinar adenocarcinoma
- Presence of large solid nests with central necrosis, high Ki-67 staining, and less immunoreactivity to basal cell markers suggested to be associated with aggressive behavior

MACROSCOPIC FEATURES

General Features
- Grossly apparent tumor that is white and fleshy with ill-defined infiltrative edges
- May have microcystic features

Site of Involvement
- Tumor widely involving prostate, including peripheral zone

MICROSCOPIC PATHOLOGY

Histologic Features
- Basaloid tumor cells have scant cytoplasm, high nuclear to cytoplasmic ratio, and irregular or angulated nuclei with open chromatin

BASAL CELL AND ADENOID CYSTIC CARCINOMA

Key Facts

Terminology
- Malignant neoplasm composed primarily of basaloid cells arising putatively from prostatic basal cells

Clinical Issues
- Wide age range (28-89 years), but majority occur in older men
- Most commonly presents with obstructive urinary symptoms
- Normal serum PSA level
- Local recurrence, metastasis, and death from disease reported in approximately 30% of cases

Macroscopic Features
- White and fleshy tumor with ill-defined infiltrative edges and may have microcystic features

- Tumor primarily centered in transition zone, with variable peripheral zone involvement

Microscopic Pathology
- Basaloid tumor cells have scant cytoplasm, high nuclear to cytoplasmic ratio, and irregular or angulated nuclei with open chromatin
- Infiltration of adjacent parenchyma is hallmark feature for diagnosis of malignancy
- 2 main histologic patterns
  - BCC consisting of variably sized solid nests, cords, or trabeculae with peripheral palisading of cells
  - ACC consisting of infiltrative nests with prominent cribriform architecture

Ancillary Tests
- Basal cell markers(+) and usually PSA/PSAP(-)

- Basaloid cells may exhibit nuclear and cytoplasmic microvacuolation
- Infiltration of adjacent parenchyma is hallmark feature of BCC
- **BCC pattern**
  - Variably sized solid nests, cords, or trabeculae with peripheral palisading of basaloid cells
  - May be associated with extensive central necrosis
- **ACC pattern**
  - Tumor grows in nests with prominent cribriform architecture
  - Eosinophilic, hyaline, basement membrane-like material may be present
  - Basophilic mucinous secretions may be present in lumina
- Additionally, tubuloglandular pattern with collagenous rim and basal cell hyperplasia-like patterns may occur
- Combination of these different architectural patterns is often encountered
- Usually associated with desmoplastic stromal response, which may be fibromyxoid or myxoid
- Rarely acinar, sebaceous, or squamous cell differentiation may be present
- Perineural invasion, angiolymphatic invasion, or necrosis may be present
- Extraprostatic extension is often present, including involvement of bladder neck or seminal vesicle
- Tumor involvement of thick bladder neck muscles detected with relatively high frequency in TURP specimens
- Subset may have synchronous or metachronous prostate cancer, such as acinar adenocarcinoma, sarcomatoid carcinoma, or small cell carcinoma

Predominant Pattern/Injury Type
- Neoplastic

Predominant Cell/Compartment Type
- Epithelial

ANCILLARY TESTS

Immunohistochemistry
- Usually PSA/PSAP(-), or at most focally (+)
- Basal cell markers(+), including p63 or HMCK(34βE12)
  - May stain multiple layers of cells, only peripheral aspect of tumor clusters, or in only few scattered tumor cells
- Typically CK20(-)/CK7(+)
  - CK7 exhibits luminal (+) staining in ACC pattern, inverse to HMCK(34βE12), which stains peripheral aspect
  - CK7(-) in pure solid basal cell nests
- Only minority (27%) of tumors are AMACR(+)
- Synaptophysin(-)
- Bcl-2 staining is strongly and diffusely (+)
- High proliferative rate with Ki-67 nuclear staining, > 20% (+)

DIFFERENTIAL DIAGNOSIS

Adenoid Cystic Pattern of Basal Cell Hyperplasia (AC-BCH)
- Occurs in background of benign prostatic hyperplasia (BPH) and BCH
- When florid may mimic BCC
- Cribriform architecture may be present; glands typically smaller
- Many previously reported "BCC" correspond to exuberant examples of AC-BCH
- Exhibits nodular, well-circumscribed or lobulocentric growth, predominantly in the transition zone
- In contrast to orderly arranged clusters of BCH, BCC shows haphazard widespread or single gland infiltration
- Distinction from BCC based mainly on absence of invasive features
  - Absent desmoplasia, perineural invasion, or necrosis; stroma is cellular, as in BPH

BASAL CELL AND ADENOID CYSTIC CARCINOMA

o Lack of infiltration between normal prostatic glands or extraprostatic extension
- Luminal aspect of AC-BCH is bounded by acinar cells
- Bcl-2 stains more diffusely and strongly in BCC than BCH
- Ki-67 usually labels > 20% of cells in BCC, compared to < 5% in BCH

Cribriform Hyperplasia
- Composed of medium to large glands with cribriform architecture
- Cells have abundant cytoplasm, which may be clear
- Lacks cytologic and invasive features of ACC

Small Cell Carcinoma
- Sheets of small cells with high nuclear to cytoplasmic ratio exhibiting nests, cords, or trabecular growth
- Nuclear molding, "salt and pepper" chromatin, abundant single cell necrosis, and crush artifact
- Neuroendocrine markers(+) and basal cell markers(-)

Poorly Differentiated Acinar Adenocarcinoma (Gleason Pattern 5)
- High-grade adenocarcinoma composed of cribriform and solid nodules may mimic ACC
- Often with markedly elevated serum PSA level
- Basal cell markers(-), PSA/PSAP(+)

Cribriform Pattern Acinar Adenocarcinoma (Gleason Pattern 3 and 4)
- May mimic ACC on low magnification
- Acinar cells have more cytoplasm and exhibit nucleomegaly with prominent nucleoli
- May contain luminal crystalloids
- Basal cell markers(-), PSA/PSAP(+)

Poorly Differentiated Urothelial Carcinoma
- Like BCC/ACC, are p63 &/or HMCK(34βE12)(+)
- Invasive nests with cells containing abundant cytoplasm and higher degree of pleomorphism
- Carcinoma in situ may be present along prostatic urethra, prostatic ducts, or bladder mucosa

Anal Cloacogenic Carcinoma and ACC of Cowper Glands
- Histological and immunohistochemical overlap with BCC; cloacogenic carcinoma indistinguishable from BCC and ACC of Cowper glands similar to ACC of prostate
- Distinction based on epicenter of tumor, with prostate being only secondarily involved

DIAGNOSTIC CHECKLIST

Pathologic Interpretation Pearls
- Infiltrative solid or cribriform nests of basaloid cells showing invasive features

REPORTING CONSIDERATIONS

Key Elements to Report
- Biopsy, microscopic evaluation
  o Histologic type
  o Local invasion
    - Prostatic fat
    - Seminal vesicle
  o Additional findings, if present
- Prostatectomy, microscopic evaluation
  o Histologic type
  o Location
  o Extent of local invasion
    - Extraprostatic extension
    - Seminal vesicle involvement
  o Margins (location and extent of margins involved with tumor)
  o Regional lymph nodes status
  o Additional findings, if present

GRADING

Criteria
- Gleason grading is not applicable for BCC and ACC of prostate

STAGING

American Joint Committee on Cancer (AJCC)/International Union Against Cancer (UICC) 2009
- Prostate cancer TNM staging applies for BCC and ACC of prostate

SELECTED REFERENCES

1. Ali TZ et al: Basal cell carcinoma of the prostate: a clinicopathologic study of 29 cases. Am J Surg Pathol. 31(5):697-705, 2007
2. McKenney JK et al: Basal cell proliferations of the prostate other than usual basal cell hyperplasia: a clinicopathologic study of 23 cases, including four carcinomas, with a proposed classification. Am J Surg Pathol. 28(10):1289-98, 2004
3. Iczkowski KA et al: Adenoid cystic/basal cell carcinoma of the prostate: clinicopathologic findings in 19 cases. Am J Surg Pathol. 27(12):1523-9, 2003
4. Mastropasqua MG et al: Basaloid cell carcinoma of the prostate. Virchows Arch. 443(6):787-91, 2003
5. Hasan N et al: Basal cell carcinoma of the prostate. Histopathology. 28(6):571, 1996
6. Devaraj LT et al: Atypical basal cell hyperplasia of the prostate. Immunophenotypic profile and proposed classification of basal cell proliferations. Am J Surg Pathol. 17(7):645-59, 1993
7. Denholm SW et al: Basaloid carcinoma of the prostate gland: histogenesis and review of the literature. Histopathology. 20(2):151-5, 1992
8. Grignon DJ et al: Basal cell hyperplasia, adenoid basal cell tumor, and adenoid cystic carcinoma of the prostate gland: an immunohistochemical study. Hum Pathol. 19(12):1425-33, 1988

BASAL CELL AND ADENOID CYSTIC CARCINOMA

Basaloid Cell Carcinoma Pattern

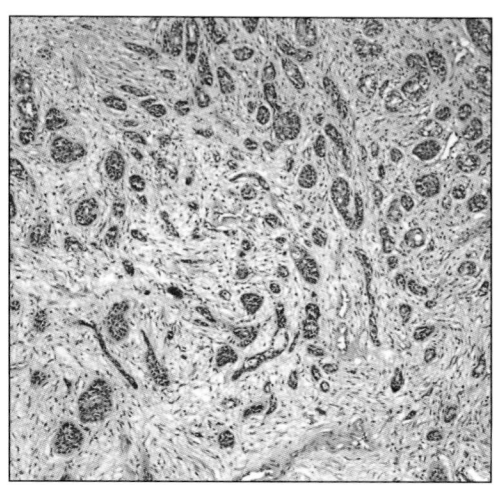
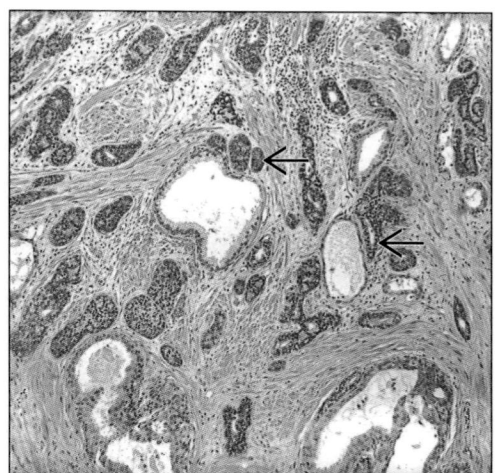

(Left) Haphazardly arranged infiltrative tumor nests and cords of BCC are associated with desmoplastic stromal response. The stroma is fibromyxoid to myxoid in appearance. Stromal desmoplasia is usually present in BCC and is helpful in distinguishing BCC from AC-BCH. *(Right)* Nests of basaloid cells infiltrate between benign acini. Infiltration by tumor cells is the hallmark of BCC vs. florid benign prostatic basal cell proliferations. Note the periglandular pattern of invasion ➡.

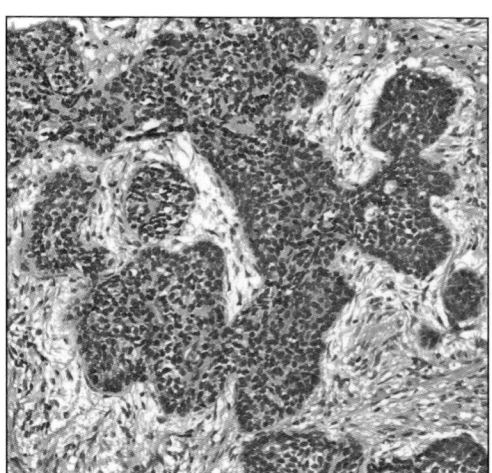
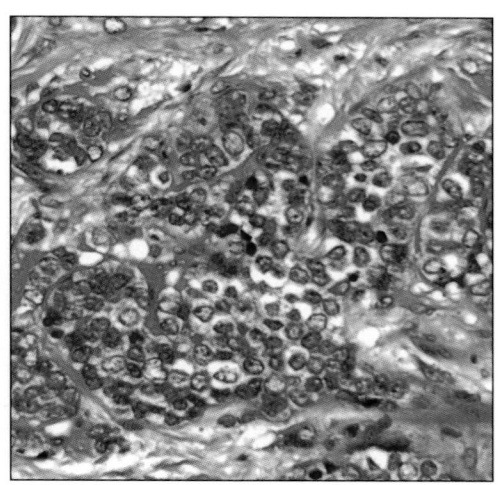

(Left) BCC pattern is shown consisting of basaloid cells arranged in infiltrative large and small solid nests with peripheral palisading. The basaloid tumor cells have scant cytoplasm and are crowded imparting a basophilic appearance. Note the stromal desmoplasia. *(Right)* Higher magnification of BCC shows crowded basaloid cells with high nuclear to cytoplasmic ratio, irregular nuclei, open chromatin, and nuclear overlapping. Mitotic activity is variable in BCC.

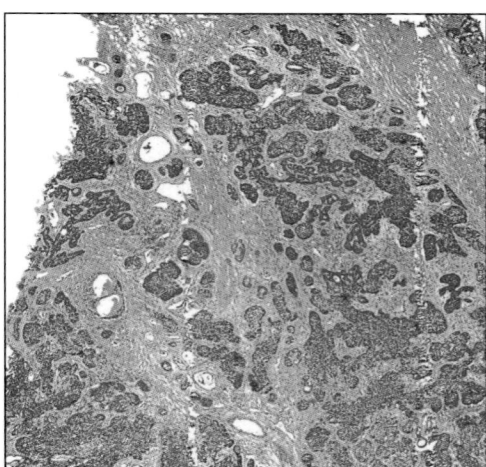
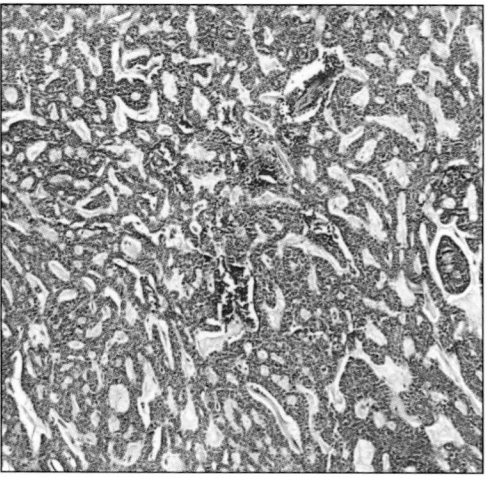

(Left) BCC is shown involving a TURP chip. BCC is commonly centered in the prostatic transition zone and may present with obstructive urinary symptoms and in a TURP specimen. In contrast to BCH, the growth pattern is haphazard. *(Right)* Diffuse growth of BCC forms an expansile trabecular meshwork of tumor cells. The solid and adenoid cystic growth of BCC mimic Gleason pattern 5 (solid) and pattern 4 (cribriform) of adenocarcinoma, respectively. Gleason grading is not applicable to BCC.

BASAL CELL AND ADENOID CYSTIC CARCINOMA

Adenoid Cystic Carcinoma Pattern

(Left) ACC pattern is characterized by infiltrative nests of basaloid tumor cells with prominent cribriform architecture, resembling ACC of the salivary gland. Note the perineural invasion ➡. The growth pattern is haphazard, and the cribriform nests are large and irregular. *(Right)* ACC shows more florid proliferation of variably sized infiltrative cribriform nests with multiple lumina. ACC lumina may contain basophilic material ➡ or collagenous hyaline material ➡.

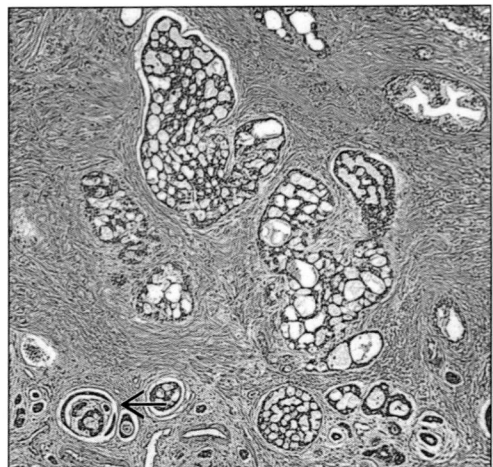
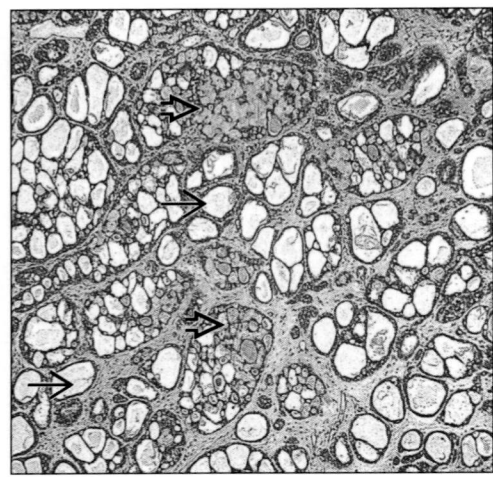

(Left) Combination of BCC and ACC patterns is shown. It is not uncommon for basaloid carcinomas to exhibit both patterns. In contrast to BCH, the nests are irregular, and the stroma is desmoplastic. *(Right)* In this perineural invasion by ACC pattern, the tumor is juxtaposed to a large nerve while maintaining its cribriform architecture, which contains intraluminal eosinophilic hyaline material. Note the separate perineural cluster of basaloid cells rimmed by hyalinized collagen ➡.

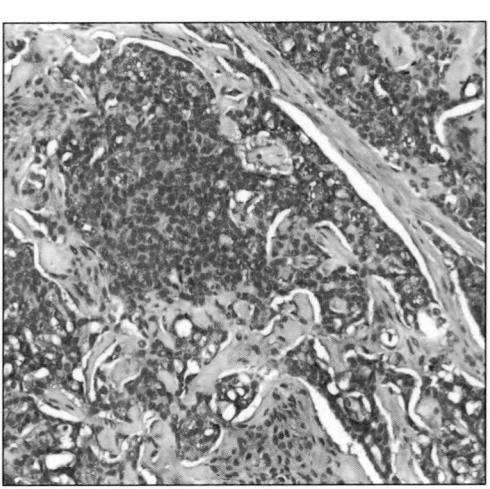
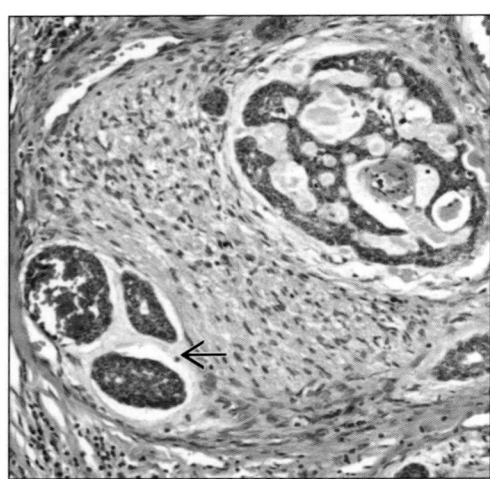

(Left) ACC pattern exhibits extraprostatic extension by the tumor with involvement of periprostatic adipose tissue and nerves. Most cases of BCC show extraprostatic extension in prostatectomy specimens. *(Right)* Cribriform architecture of ACC with several lumina is separated by cellular bridges formed by thin strands of basaloid cells. The lumina contain basophilic mucinous material. The basaloid cells in ACC are similar to those seen in BCC pattern.

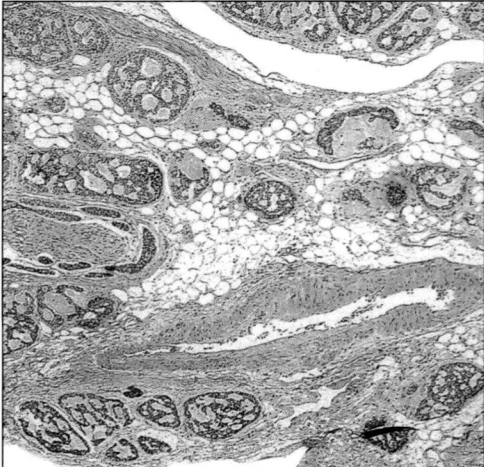
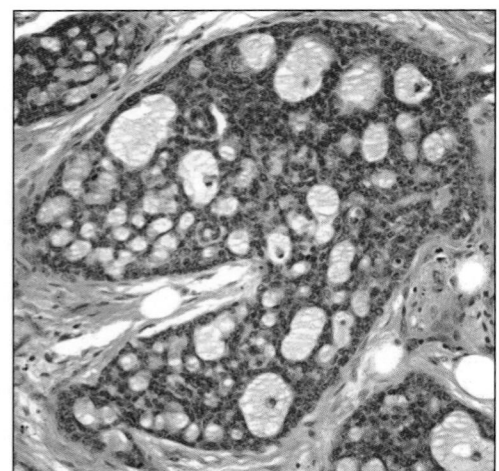

BASAL CELL AND ADENOID CYSTIC CARCINOMA

Differential Diagnosis and Immunohistochemistry

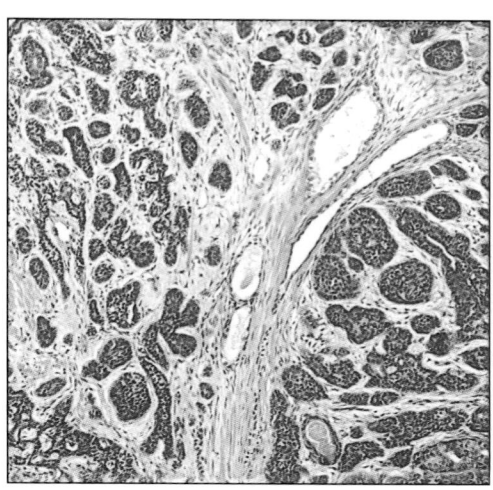

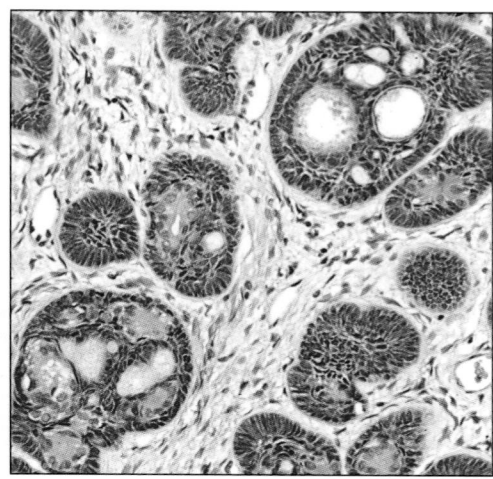

(Left) AC-BCH is shown. Some of these cases were previously designated as BCC. The background is of BPH, and the cribriform nests are small. Appreciation of the nodular architecture, restriction to the transition zone, &/or presence in a transurethral resection are key features to distinguish this lesion as benign. *(Right)* Typical glands in AC-BCH is shown with smaller cribriform nests. The stroma is cellular, resembling that seen in fibromuscular hyperplasia of the prostate.

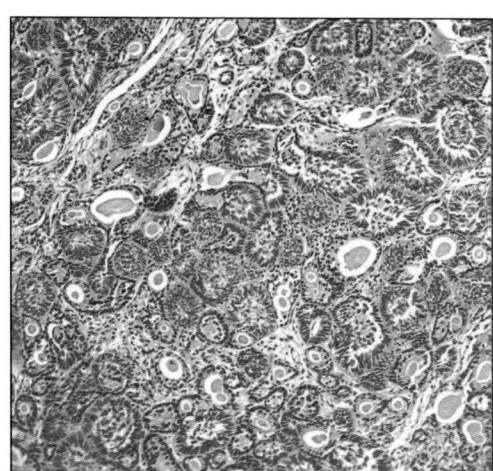

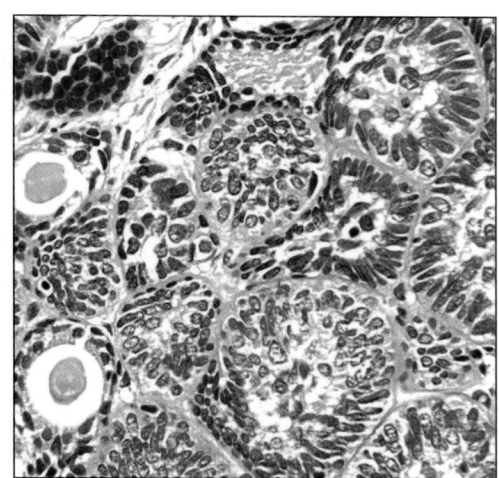

(Left) AC-BCH is the main differential diagnosis for BCC. Note circumscription and background of BPH. Like BCC, the basaloid proliferation shows luminal eosinophilic hyaline material. In contrast, BCC has a haphazard and infiltrative growth (between benign glands), desmoplastic stroma, and may exhibit perineural invasion. *(Right)* The nests of AC-BCH show basaloid cells with peripheral palisading similar to BCC. However, BCH lacks the invasive features seen in BCC.

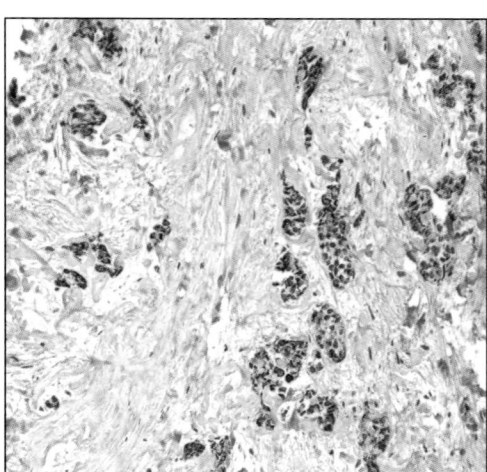

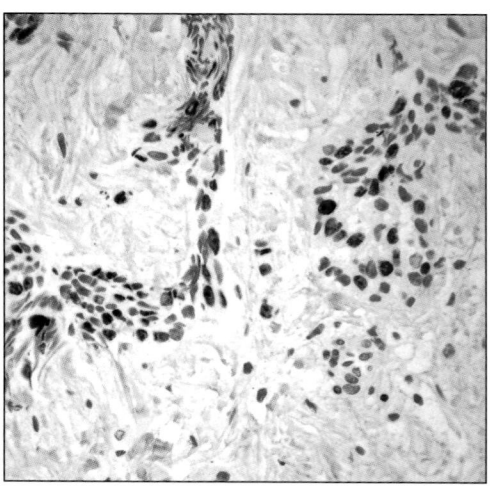

(Left) HMCK(34βE12) is diffusely positivity in BCC. HMCK(34βE12) is typically positive in BCC but may show variable, florid, peripheral, or only scattered staining in some cases. This staining reaction is useful in distinction from acinar PCa, which is HMCK(34βE12) negative. *(Right)* BCC is shown with increased Ki-67 nuclear positivity. BCC usually exhibits higher Ki-67 (> 20%) than AC-BCH (typically < 5%). High Ki-67 staining in BCC is correlated with tumor aggressiveness.

SARCOMATOID CARCINOMA, PROSTATE

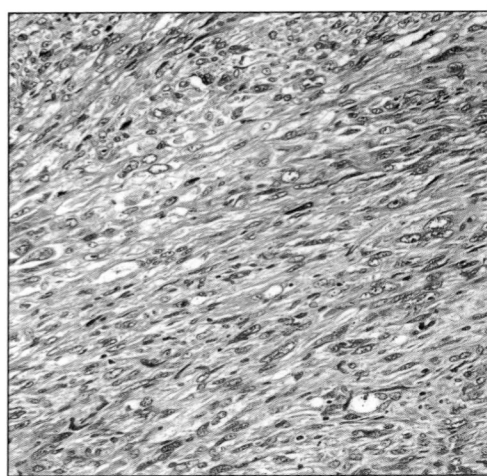

Monophasic malignant spindle cell tumor is shown involving the prostate. Other areas of this neoplasm showed typical high-grade adenocarcinoma of the prostate with acinar histology.

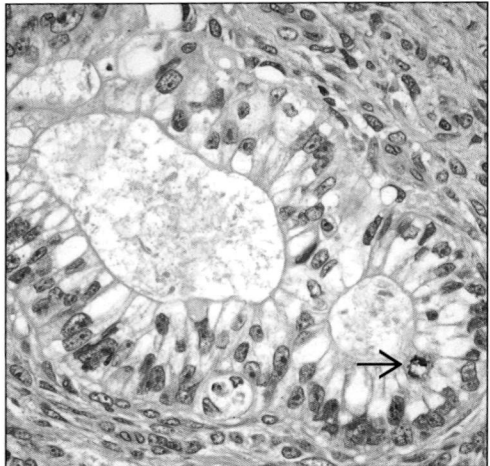

Acinar adenocarcinomatous component of SC shows prominent nucleoli, mitoses ➡, and absence of basal cell layer. Spindle cells surrounding the glands have malignant features.

TERMINOLOGY

Abbreviations
- Sarcomatoid carcinoma (SC)
- Carcinosarcoma (CS)

Definitions
- Malignant biphasic or monophasic neoplasm of prostate, demonstrating epithelial and mesenchymal differentiation by light microscopy or immunohistochemistry
  - CS is employed by some authors for tumors with heterologous sarcomatous elements
  - Rationale for considering SC and CS as single entity is due to similar clinicopathologic features and poor prognosis

ETIOLOGY/PATHOGENESIS

Origin
- Sarcomatoid dedifferentiation in prostatic carcinoma
  - High proportion of SCs have prior diagnosis of prostate adenocarcinoma
  - Focal immunohistochemical expression of PSA &/or PAP is demonstrated in spindle cells
  - Even with heterologous elements present, spindle cells often express keratin or p63 suggesting common origin with carcinomatous component
  - Loss-of-heterozygosity studies show that carcinomatous and sarcomatoid components are clonally related
- Possible collision of epithelial and mesenchymal malignant tumors less accepted

Risk Factors
- Prior diagnosis of prostate adenocarcinoma in almost 1/2 of cases
- Radiotherapy &/or hormonal therapy for prostate carcinoma may play role in SC development

CLINICAL ISSUES

Epidemiology
- Incidence
  - Rare
  - Only ~ 100 cases described in literature
- Age
  - Mean: 70 years, range: 43-91 years

Presentation
- Majority present with obstructive urinary symptoms or metastatic disease
- Uncommonly, tumors are detected in patients with elevated serum PSA level or palpable nodule on digital rectal examination (DRE)

Laboratory Tests
- PSA serum level may be normal or elevated

Natural History
- Prior history of prostate adenocarcinoma seen in 48-66%
  - Time interval from prostate adenocarcinoma to diagnosis of SC range from 6 months to 16 years (mean: 6.8 years)
- About 1/3 of cases arises de novo with no prior history of prostate adenocarcinoma and radiation &/or hormonal therapy

Treatment
- Current therapies, including multimodality approach, are ineffective, as tumor is high grade

Prognosis
- Poor outcome
- Aggressive clinical course characterized by local recurrences and metastasis
- 1 study reports 5-year cancer specific survival of 41% and 7-year survival of 14%
- Another study reports actuarial risk of death at 1 year of 20% after diagnosis of SC

SARCOMATOID CARCINOMA, PROSTATE

Key Facts

Terminology
- Malignant biphasic or monophasic neoplasm of prostate demonstrating epithelial and mesenchymal differentiation by LM/IHC
- Rationale for considering SC and CS as single entity is due to similar clinicopathologic features and poor prognosis

Clinical Issues
- Rare; only about 100 cases described in literature

Microscopic Pathology
- Overall histology falls into 3 categories
  - Carcinoma admixed with sarcomatoid spindle cell component (most common)
  - Carcinoma admixed with sarcomatous component containing heterologous elements

- Monophasic spindle cell tumor with immunohistochemical &/or electron microscopic evidence of epithelial differentiation
- Acinar adenocarcinoma pattern most common
- Sarcomatoid component frequently composed of hypercellular high-grade spindle cells (undifferentiated spindle cell sarcoma)
- Heterologous elements present in 24% of cases, most commonly osteosarcoma
- Carcinoma typically PSA/PAP(+)
- Spindle cells at least focally (+) for at least 1 epithelial marker

Top Differential Diagnoses
- Primary sarcomas of prostate
- Pseudosarcomatous myofibroblastic proliferation of prostate

---

- Systemic metastases in majority of patients are to lungs and bone
  - Other reported sites include brain, lymph node, liver, peritoneum, and skin

MACROSCOPIC FEATURES

General Features
- Most tumors are encountered in transurethral resection of prostate (TURP) specimens for obstructive urinary symptoms
- Large gray-white to yellow-tan with prominent necrosis, hemorrhage, and infiltrative growth
- Tumors extend extraparenchymally into periprostatic soft tissues or adjacent organs, such as seminal vesicles and urinary bladder

MICROSCOPIC PATHOLOGY

Histologic Features
- Carcinomatous and sarcomatoid components are intimately admixed
- Overall histology falls into 3 categories
  - Carcinoma admixed with sarcomatoid spindle cell component (most common)
  - Carcinoma admixed with sarcomatous component containing heterologous elements
  - Monophasic spindle cell tumor with immunohistochemical &/or electron microscopic evidence of epithelial differentiation
- Proportion of components vary, and sarcomatoid elements may range from 5-99% of tumor
  - Florid sarcomatoid overgrowth may be mistaken as pure sarcoma of prostate
- **Carcinomatous component**
  - Variable and may be admixture of the following patterns
  - **Acinar adenocarcinoma**
    - Most frequent epithelial pattern
    - Often are high grade (Gleason score 8-10)

- Typical patterns, such as glandular, cribriform, comedo, and solid, may be seen
  - **Uncommon prostate adenocarcinoma pattern**
    - Foamy gland, ductal, adenosquamous, and signet ring cell carcinoma
  - **Uncommon nonglandular prostate carcinoma pattern**
    - Small cell, basaloid, squamous, and transitional carcinoma
  - **Unusual morphology**
    - Micropapillary pattern and intestinal-type glands
  - **Discrete polygonal cell**
    - Seen intimately admixed with spindle cells, highlighted by epithelial markers
  - **Monophasic spindle cell morphology**
    - Rare, evidence of epithelioid differentiation demonstrated only by immunohistochemistry or electron microscopy
  - Nuclei are often enlarged and can be markedly pleomorphic
- **Sarcomatoid/sarcomatous component**
  - Spindle cell morphology (most frequent)
    - Typically composed of hypercellular fusiform cells lacking specific lineage differentiation (undifferentiated spindle cell sarcoma)
    - Architecture may show storiform, fascicular growth, or patternless appearance
    - Majority are high-grade cells with large hyperchromatic nuclei
    - Mitotic activity is usually brisk
    - May contain bizarre nuclei and tumor giant cells resembling malignant fibrous histiocytoma (MFH)
    - Rarely, spindle cells are less cellular with background myxoid stroma
  - May contain heterologous elements (24%) that resemble
    - Osteosarcoma (most frequent)
    - Leiomyosarcoma
    - Chondrosarcoma
    - Rhabdomyosarcoma
    - Angiosarcoma

SARCOMATOID CARCINOMA, PROSTATE

- - Combination of these sarcomatous elements is common
  - Heterologous elements typically merge with spindle cells
- Necrosis is frequent
- Histology of metastatic tumors is usually carcinomatous, although less commonly both components may be present

Predominant Pattern/Injury Type
- Neoplastic

Predominant Cell/Compartment Type
- Epithelial
- Mesenchymal

ANCILLARY TESTS

Immunohistochemistry
- Carcinomatous component
  - Typically PSA/PAP(+)
  - Epithelial markers (PAN-CK, Cam 5.2, EMA/MUC1) (+)
  - Vimentin(-)
- Sarcomatoid spindle cell component
  - PSA/PAP usually negative; may be focally positive
  - Positive for (PAN-CK), HMCK, CK5/6, p63
  - Vimentin(+)
  - Desmin, SMA (variably +)
- Heterologous sarcomatous elements
  - PSA/PAP(-)
  - Epithelial markers generally (-), although a subset of leiomyosarcomas may express keratin
  - Vimentin(+)
  - SMA(+) in leiomyosarcoma
  - Desmin, myogenin(+) in rhabdomyosarcoma
  - S100(+) in chondrosarcoma

Electron Microscopy
- Structural evidence of epithelial differentiation (e.g., desmosomes, intermediate filaments) may be demonstrated in spindle cell component

DIFFERENTIAL DIAGNOSIS

Primary Sarcomas of Prostate
- Overgrowth of any heterologous sarcomatous component of SC may simulate their pure sarcoma counterpart
- Most common prostate sarcomas are leiomyosarcoma and stromal sarcoma
  - Stromal sarcomas with phyllodes growth: Epithelial component is benign
  - Stromal sarcomas are positive for CD34 and PR; cytokeratin is typically negative
  - Leiomyosarcoma may occasionally show focal positivity for cytokeratin, although diffuse positivity is rare
- Other rare prostate sarcomas include MFH, malignant solitary fibrous tumor, angiosarcoma, osteosarcoma,

chondrosarcoma, malignant peripheral nerve sheath tumor, and synovial sarcoma
  - These entities lack carcinomatous component and have clinicopathological features distinct from SC

Pseudosarcomatous Myofibroblastic Proliferation of Prostate
- Includes inflammatory myofibroblastic tumors and postoperative spindle cell nodule
- Bland spindle cell proliferation with nodular fascitis/tissue culture appearance
- Lack significant cytologic atypia (no nuclear hyperchromasia or pleomorphism)
- Typical granulation tissue-type vascularity with scattered inflammatory cells
- Morphologic features, including necrosis, infiltrative growth, cellularity, and mitotic activity, overlap with sarcomatoid carcinoma
- Tumor cells may demonstrate strong and diffuse positivity for cytokeratin, further compounding the diagnostic difficulty
- ALK1 positive; negative for p63, HMCK, and CK5/6

Gastrointestinal Stromal Tumor
- Tumors of gastrointestinal origin or pelvic soft tissue may secondarily involve prostate, mimicking prostatic primary
- CD117, DOG-1, and CD34 are positive

DIAGNOSTIC CHECKLIST

Pathologic Interpretation Pearls
- Differential diagnosis of malignant spindle cell neoplasm of prostate should always include sarcomatoid carcinoma

SELECTED REFERENCES

1. Huan Y et al: Sarcomatoid carcinoma after radiation treatment of prostatic adenocarcinoma. Ann Diagn Pathol. 12(2):142-5, 2008
2. Hansel DE et al: Sarcomatoid carcinoma of the prostate: a study of 42 cases. Am J Surg Pathol. 30(10):1316-21, 2006
3. Ray ME et al: Clonality of sarcomatous and carcinomatous elements in sarcomatoid carcinoma of the prostate. Urology. 67(2):423, 2006
4. Perez N et al: Carcinosarcoma of the prostate: two cases with distinctive morphologic and immunohistochemical findings. Virchows Arch. 446(5):511-6, 2005
5. Rogers CG et al: Carcinosarcoma of the prostate with urothelial and squamous components. J Urol. 173(2):439-40, 2005
6. Dundore PA et al: Carcinosarcoma of the prostate. Report of 21 cases. Cancer. 76(6):1035-42, 1995
7. Lauwers GY et al: Carcinosarcoma of the prostate. Am J Surg Pathol. 17(4):342-9, 1993
8. Shannon RL et al: Sarcomatoid carcinoma of the prostate. A clinicopathologic study of 12 patients. Cancer. 69(11):2676-82, 1992
9. Wick MR et al: Prostatic carcinosarcomas. Clinical, histologic, and immunohistochemical data on two cases, with a review of the literature. Am J Clin Pathol. 92(2):131-9, 1989

SARCOMATOID CARCINOMA, PROSTATE

Gross and Microscopic Features

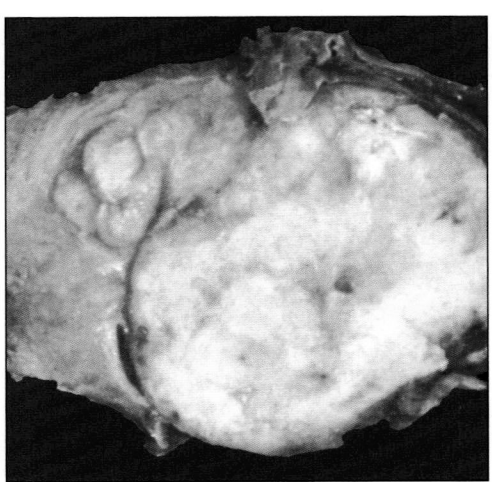

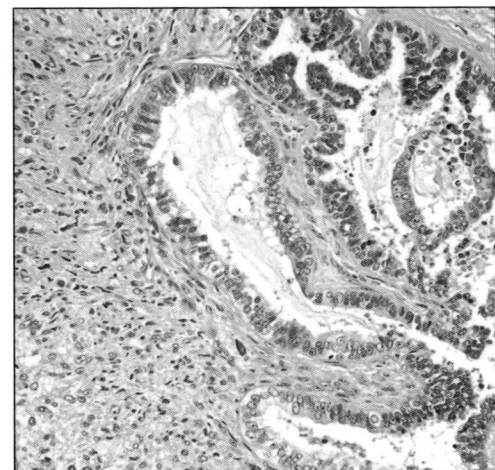

(Left) Gross photograph of SC shows extensive involvement of peripheral and transition zones of prostate. Tumor is tan-white and yellow, fleshy (sarcoma-like) with ill-defined edges. *(Right)* SC shows admixture of adenocarcinoma and high-grade undifferentiated spindle cell sarcoma. Carcinoma and sarcomatoid components are intimately admixed. In contrast to stromal sarcomas with phyllodes pattern, epithelial component in SC is malignant.

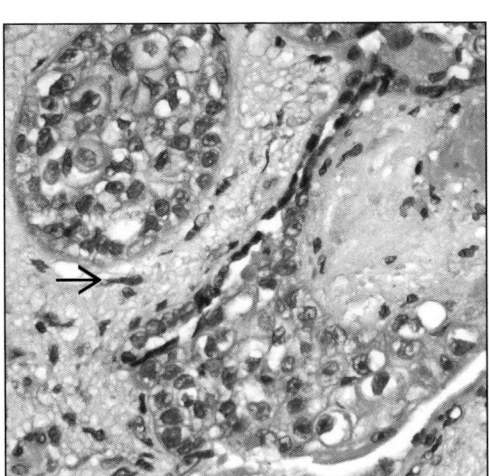

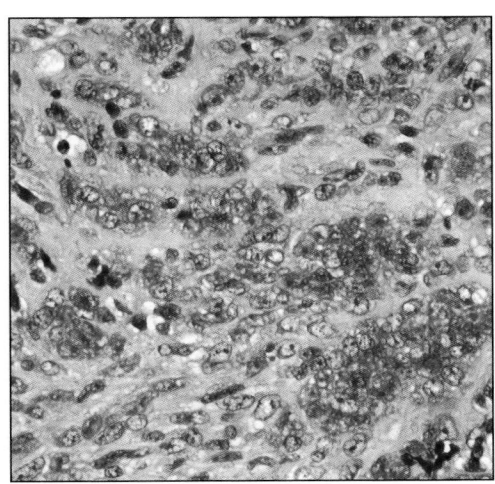

(Left) Adenosquamous carcinoma of prostate with sarcomatoid differentiation shows epithelial nests with squamous features. In other areas, there was more typical acinar and sarcomatoid histology. Few atypical spindle cells ⇒ are seen. *(Right)* Occasionally, carcinomatous component of SC is less obvious and consists of subtle epithelioid cells embedded in sarcomatoid area. Epithelial markers may highlight these carcinomatous foci, facilitating diagnosis of SC.

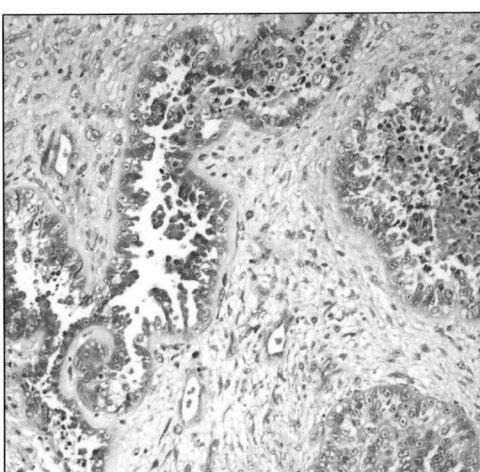

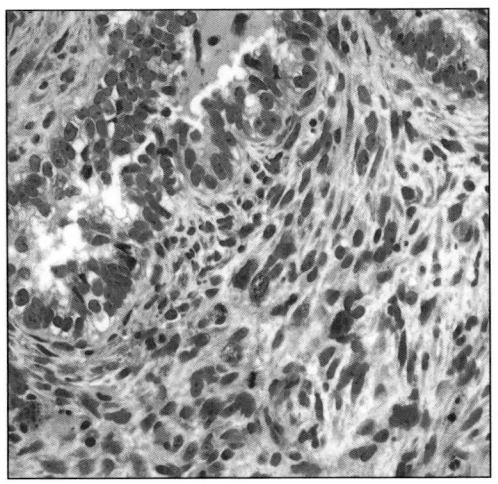

(Left) SC may show unusual carcinomatous morphology, which in this case, the glands show intraluminal papillary & pseudopapillary projections. The DDx should include adenocarcinoma or urothelial carcinoma of the bladder with glandular features secondarily involving the prostate. *(Right)* High-power view of SC shows high-grade pleomorphic glandular and spindle cells. Undifferentiated spindle cell sarcoma is the most frequent sarcomatoid component in SC.

SARCOMATOID CARCINOMA, PROSTATE

Microscopic Features

(Left) Adenosquamous carcinoma with sarcomatoid differentiation shows atrophic appearing Gleason pattern 3 glands ➡ and a focus of neoplastic squamous epithelium ⇨. *(Right)* Sarcomatoid component of SC shows high-grade spindle cells with storiform arrangement simulating MFH. Overgrowth of heterologous sarcomatoid component may simulate its pure sarcoma counterpart involving the prostate. Adequate sampling is important in making accurate diagnosis of SC.

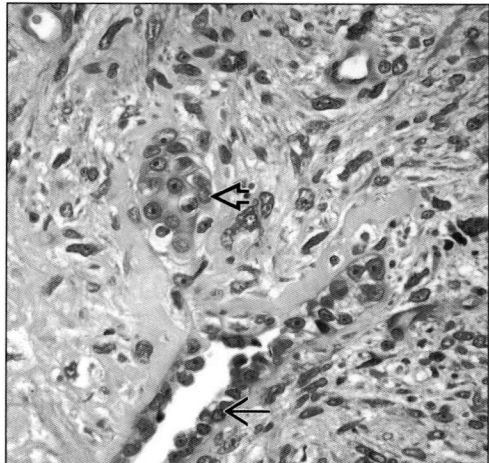 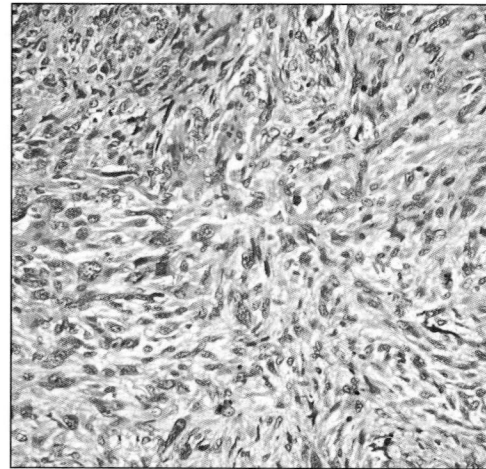

(Left) High-power magnification of sarcomatoid element of SC shows markedly pleomorphic and bizarre cells resembling MFH. *(Right)* Sarcomatoid component of SC shows hypercellular high-grade spindle cells ➡ merging with loose myxoid stroma with malignant cells ⇨. Tumors with heterologous elements (e.g., malignant cartilage, bone, etc.) have similar poor outcome to SC containing only malignant spindle cell component.

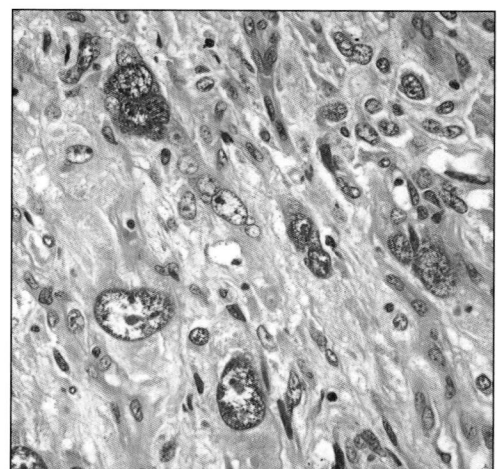 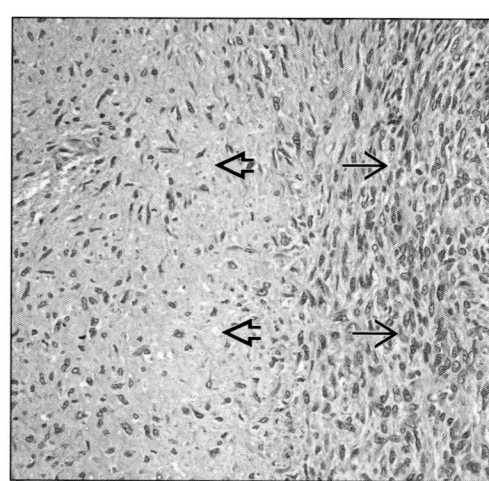

(Left) SC shows malignant epithelial component with ductal histology ➡, whereas malignant stromal component shows association with osteoid ➡ (osteosarcomatous heterologous differentiation). *(Right)* SC is shown containing heterologous osteosarcomatous differentiation. Extensive sampling may be required to detect a malignant epithelial component. Recent history of prostate cancer or elevated serum PSA levels would also support an SC diagnosis.

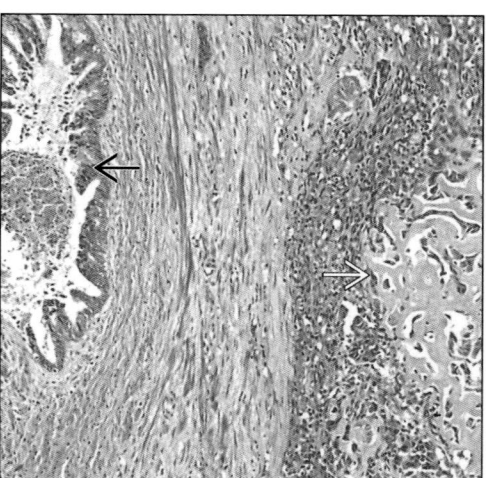 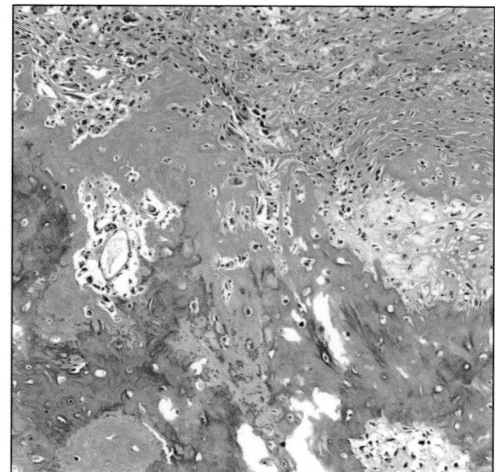

Microscopic and Immunohistochemical Features

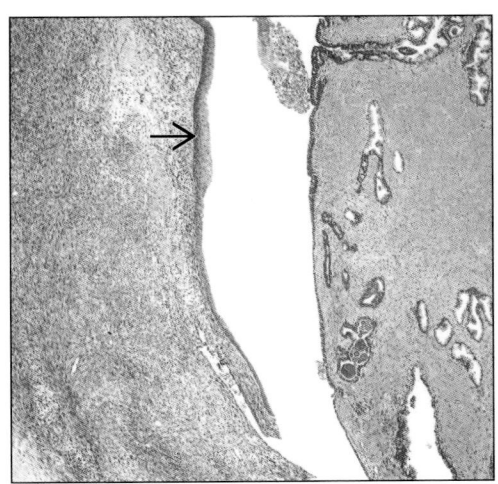
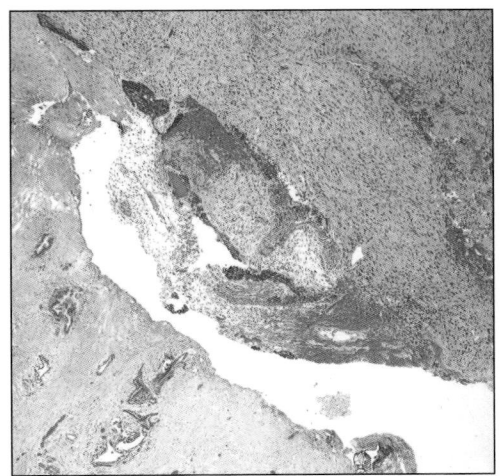

(Left) Sarcomatoid component of SC extends to the prostatic urethra ➡. Due to rapid growth, many SC present with obstructive urinary symptoms and hence may be 1st detected in a TURP specimen. *(Right)* SC in prostatic chip of TURP specimen shows intimate admixture of malignant epithelial and stromal cells. Spindle cell component is hypercellular and markedly atypical.

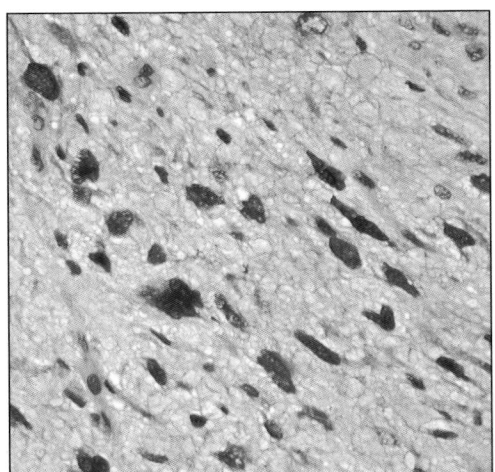
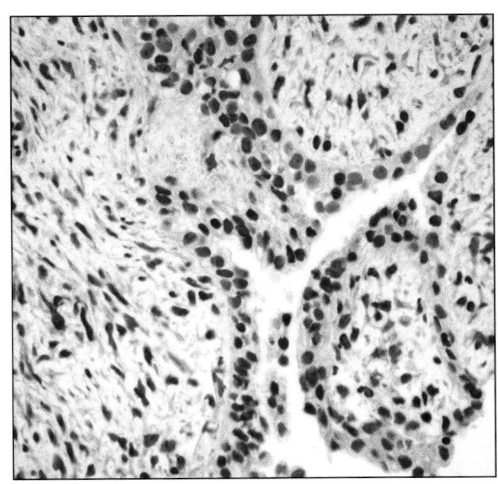

(Left) SC shows myxoid stroma and frankly atypical spindle cells. The DDx is with pseudosarcomatous myofibroblastic proliferations (spindle cells do not appear malignant) and stromal sarcomas (spindle cells are malignant). *(Right)* PSA is positive in adenocarcinomatous component of SC and negative in stromal component. It is important to confirm that epithelial component is malignant and not benign entrapped glands, which may occur in stromal sarcomas.

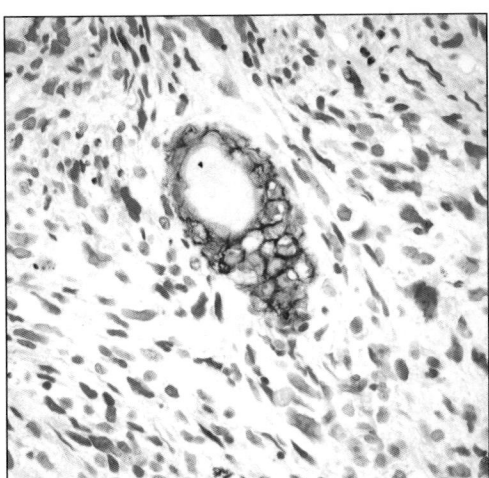
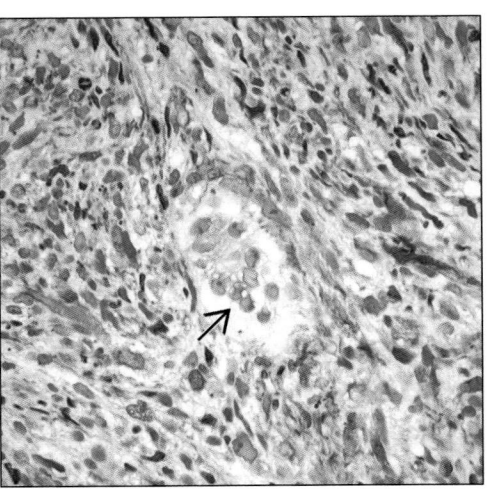

(Left) Focus of adenocarcinoma highlighted by PAN-CK(AE1/AE3). Occasionally, epithelial marker expression may be demonstrated in spindle cell component. Keratin immunohistochemistry is helpful in highlighting discrete carcinoma cells or glands & confirming epithelial differentiation in spindle cells. *(Right)* Vimentin immunoreactivity in SC shows diffuse positivity in malignant spindle cells. In contrast, the malignant gland ➡ shows lack of staining with vimentin.

CARCINOMAS WITH SQUAMOUS DIFFERENTIATION

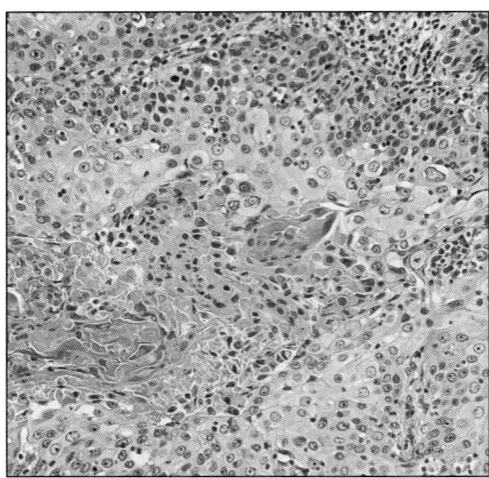

Invasive pure SCC of the prostate shows evidence of squamous differentiation including abundant keratinization.

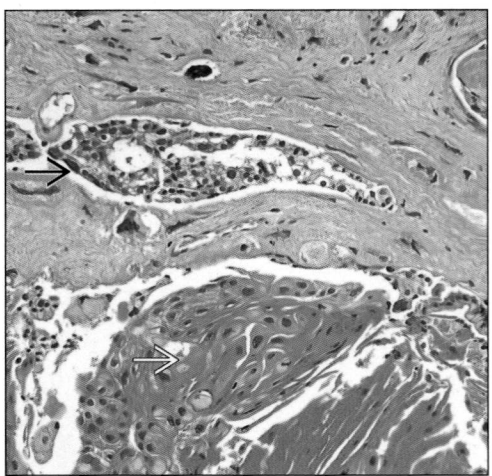

Adenocarcinoma of the prostate treated with radiation therapy shows juxtaposition of acinar adenocarcinoma ➡ and atypical squamous cells with keratinization ➡.

TERMINOLOGY

Abbreviations
- Squamous cell carcinoma (SCC)
- Adenosquamous carcinoma (ASC)

Synonyms
- Mixed adenocarcinoma and SCC, adenocarcinoma with squamous differentiation, adenoacanthoma (outdated term)

Definitions
- Primary prostate carcinoma with squamous cell features, including pure SCC and adenocarcinoma admixed with SCC (ASC)
- Definition requires exclusion of secondary SCC involving prostate from other anatomic sites
- Prostatic urothelial carcinoma with squamous differentiation and sarcoma admixed with SCC not included

ETIOLOGY/PATHOGENESIS

Risk Factors
- Prior history of prostate adenocarcinoma
  - May uncommonly give rise to SCC or ASC 4-10 years after adenocarcinoma diagnosis
- Radiation or hormonal therapy
  - May influence squamous differentiation in primary as well as metastatic adenocarcinoma
- Genitourinary schistosomiasis has been proposed
- May arise de novo without radiation or hormonal therapy or prior prostate adenocarcinoma history

Origin
- Precise cell of origin remains controversial
- Considered to be derived from prostatic glandular cells that show ability to differentiate toward squamous cells

- Both acinar and basal glandular cells proposed as cell of origin
- Other proposed theories of cell derivation
  - Urothelium of prostatic urethra or periurethral ducts
  - Malignant transformation in squamous metaplasia of benign glands
  - Pluripotential stem cells capable of multidirectional differentiation
  - For ASC: Collision-type tumor with de novo origin for SCC and adenocarcinoma

CLINICAL ISSUES

Epidemiology
- Incidence
  - Very rare; < 0.6% of all prostate cancers
    - ~ 55 cases of pure SCC reported
    - ASC even rarer; ~ 30 cases reported
- Age
  - Mean: 64 years; range: 52-79 years

Presentation
- Presenting symptoms resemble advanced prostate adenocarcinoma
- Obstructive urinary symptoms
  - Majority encountered in TURP specimens
- Hematuria
- Bone pain from metastasis
- Most cases with palpable disease on rectal examination at time of presentation

Laboratory Tests
- Serum PSA or acid phosphatase level may be normal, even with advanced disease
  - PSA elevation occurs more often in ASC
- Serum SCC antigen marker elevated; may be useful in monitoring disease

CARCINOMAS WITH SQUAMOUS DIFFERENTIATION

Key Facts

Terminology

- Primary carcinomas of prostate with squamous cell features and include pure SCC and adenocarcinoma admixed with SCC (ASC)
- Requires exclusion of secondary SCC involving prostate from other anatomic sites

Etiology/Pathogenesis

- Both SSC and ASC can arise de novo or preceded by prostate adenocarcinoma ± radiation or hormonal treatment

Clinical Issues

- Incidence: < 0.6% of all prostate cancers
- Serum PSA or acid phosphatase level typically normal, even with advanced disease
- More aggressive than prostate adenocarcinoma

- Generally poor response to surgical, hormonal, chemotherapeutic, or radiation therapies

Microscopic Pathology

- Pure SCC similar to SCC of other anatomic sites
- Well to poorly differentiated with variable cytologic atypia
- Glandular component of ASC similar to acinar adenocarcinoma
- Adenocarcinoma component tends to be higher grade
- Squamous and glandular components intermingled

Ancillary Tests

- SCC negative for PSA and PAP and positive for HMCK(34βE12)
- Glandular component of ASC positive for PSA and PAP and negative for HMCK(34βE12)

Natural History

- Both SCC and ASC may arise de novo or be preceded by prostate adenocarcinoma ± radiation or hormonal treatment
- Relatively greater proportion of ASC (than SCC) encountered in patients with prior adenocarcinoma
- No established relationship with squamous metaplasia of benign prostatic glands

Treatment

- Generally poor response to surgical, hormonal, chemotherapeutic, or radiation therapy
- Some reported success with combination of surgical therapy followed by local radiation and systemic chemotherapy

Prognosis

- More aggressive than prostate adenocarcinoma
- Reported survival ranges from 8 days to 9 years; mean 15 months
- Metastasis occurs in 1/3 of cases, most commonly to bones and lung
- Bone metastasis is osteolytic, in contrast to osteoblastic metastasis in acinar adenocarcinoma

MACROSCOPIC FEATURES

General Features

- Tends to be more localized in transition zone or central region of prostate
- Firm grayish white tumor
- Tumor may be bulky and extend into adjacent organs, such as seminal vesicles and rectum

MICROSCOPIC PATHOLOGY

Histologic Features

- **Pure SCC**
  - Similar to SCC of other anatomic sites
  - By definition does not contain glandular elements

  - Infiltrating nests and sheets of polygonal cells with intercellular bridges
  - Abundant eosinophilic glassy cytoplasm or keratin pearls in better differentiated tumors
- **ASC**
  - Squamous component similar to pure SCC
  - Glandular component demonstrates range seen in morphology of acinar adenocarcinoma
  - Squamous and glandular components intermingled with no distinct transition
  - Amount of adenocarcinoma varies from 5-95% of tumor
  - Adenocarcinoma tends to be higher grade (Gleason score 7 or higher)
- Perineural invasion may be seen
- May have extraprostatic extension

Predominant Pattern/Injury Type

- Neoplastic

Predominant Cell/Compartment Type

- Epithelial, squamous
- Epithelial, biphasic, or mixed

Grade

- SCC
  - Well- to poorly differentiated with variable cytologic atypia (Broder grade)
- Glandular component of ASC
  - Tends to be higher grade (Gleason score 7 or higher)

ANCILLARY TESTS

Immunohistochemistry

- SCC
  - Negative for PSA and PAP
  - Positive for HMCK(34βE12)
- Glandular component of ASC
  - Positive for PSA and PAP
  - Negative for HMCK(34βE12)

CARCINOMAS WITH SQUAMOUS DIFFERENTIATION

Flow Cytometry
- DNA analysis
  - Similarity in DNA peaks observed in both squamous and glandular components of ASC

Electron Microscopy
- SCC demonstrates microvilli lining intercellular spaces and variable desmosomes

DIFFERENTIAL DIAGNOSIS

Squamous Metaplasia of Benign Prostatic Glands ± Inflammation
- Occurs as response to infarction and hormonal or radiation therapy
- Similar to SCC, does not express PSA and PAP
- Lacks cytologic atypia and invasive features of SCC
- Clinical history or recognition of adjacent infarcted prostatic tissue helpful in diagnosis

Secondary SCC Involving the Prostate
- Direct extension from urinary bladder or anal SCC
- Histologic distinction is difficult, if not impossible, especially in limited tissue samples
- Distinction may require clinicopathologic correlation
- SCC metastatic to prostate from distant anatomic sites exceedingly rare, encountered mainly in autopsies

Secondary Urothelial Carcinoma with Squamous Differentiation
- Urinary bladder or prostatic urethral urothelial carcinoma with squamous differentiation may invade into prostate
- Differentiation may be difficult in limited tissue samples
- Admixed invasive urothelial carcinoma ± glandular (nonprostatic type) differentiation
- Presence of urothelial carcinoma in situ or papillary neoplasm in bladder mucosal surface
- Acinar component absent (vs. ASC)
- Distinction may require clinicopathologic correlation

DIAGNOSTIC CHECKLIST

Pathologic Interpretation Pearls
- Neoplastic squamous growth displaying cytologic atypia and invasive features
- Diagnosis requires clinicopathologic exclusion of secondary carcinomas with squamous differentiation from other sites (mainly urinary bladder)

REPORTING CONSIDERATIONS

Key Elements to Report
- Biopsy, microscopic evaluation
  - Histologic type (SCC or ASC)
  - Grade (Gleason grade &/or Broder grade)
  - Local invasion
    - Prostatic fat
    - Seminal vesicle
  - Additional findings, if present
- Prostatectomy, microscopic evaluation
  - Histologic type (SCC or ASC)
  - Grade (Gleason grade &/or Broder grade)
  - Location
  - Extent of local invasion
    - Extraprostatic extension
    - Seminal vesicle involvement
  - Margins (location and extent of margins involved with tumor)
  - Regional lymph node status
  - Additional findings, if present

GRADING

Types
- Gleason grading
  - Applied to glandular component of ASC
  - Not applicable for SCC component
- Broder grading system for SCC of other anatomic sites
  - Applied to prostate SCC
  - Based on degree of squamous differentiation (i.e., keratinization of tumor cells) and nuclear atypicality
  - Well- to undifferentiated tumors (grades I to IV)

STAGING

Criteria
- American Joint Committee on Cancer (AJCC)/ International Union Against Cancer (UICC) 2009
  - Prostate cancer TNM staging applies for prostate carcinomas with squamous differentiation

SELECTED REFERENCES

1. Kanthan R et al: Squamous cell carcinoma of the prostate. A report of 6 cases. Urol Int. 72(1):28-31, 2004
2. Parwani AV et al: Prostate carcinoma with squamous differentiation: an analysis of 33 cases. Am J Surg Pathol. 28(5):651-7, 2004
3. Majeed F et al: Primary squamous cell carcinoma of the prostate: a novel chemotherapy regimen. J Urol. 168(2):640, 2002
4. Helal M et al: Postradiation therapy adenosquamous cell carcinoma of the prostate. Prostate Cancer Prostatic Dis. 3(1):53-56, 2000
5. Orhan D et al: Adenosquamous carcinoma of the prostate. Br J Urol. 78(4):646-7, 1996
6. Miller VA et al: Primary squamous cell carcinoma of the prostate after radiation seed implantation for adenocarcinoma. Urology. 46(1):111-3, 1995
7. Little NA et al: Squamous cell carcinoma of the prostate: 2 cases of a rare malignancy and review of the literature. J Urol. 149(1):137-9, 1993
8. Wernert N et al: Squamous cell carcinoma of the prostate. Histopathology. 17(4):339-44, 1990
9. Lager DJ et al: Squamous metaplasia of the prostate. An immunohistochemical study. Am J Clin Pathol. 90(5):597-601, 1988
10. Moyana TN: Adenosquamous carcinoma of the prostate. Am J Surg Pathol. 11(5):403-7, 1987

CARCINOMAS WITH SQUAMOUS DIFFERENTIATION

Microscopic Features

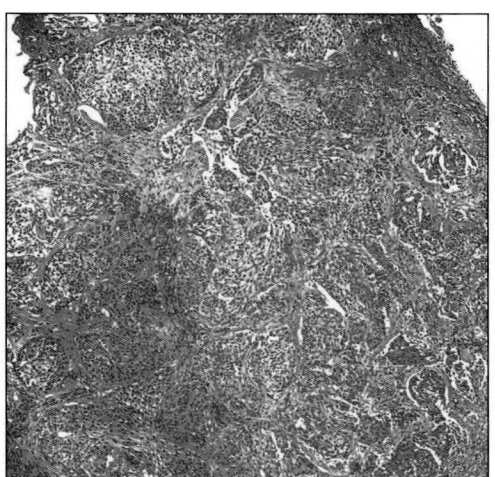

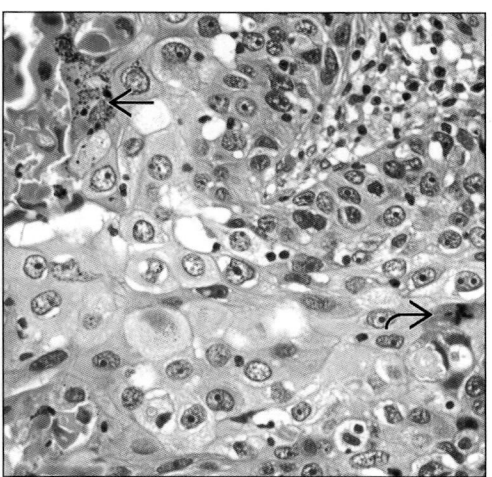

(Left) Pure SCC of the prostate in TURP consists of infiltrating nests of malignant squamous cells amidst a desmoplastic stroma. Before diagnosis of pure SCC is rendered, extensive sampling is required to rule out acinar component. *(Right)* Pure SCC of the prostate shows cells containing abundant glassy eosinophilic cytoplasm with well-defined borders. There are frequent mitoses ➡. Note keratohyaline granules ➡ next to the keratinized cells.

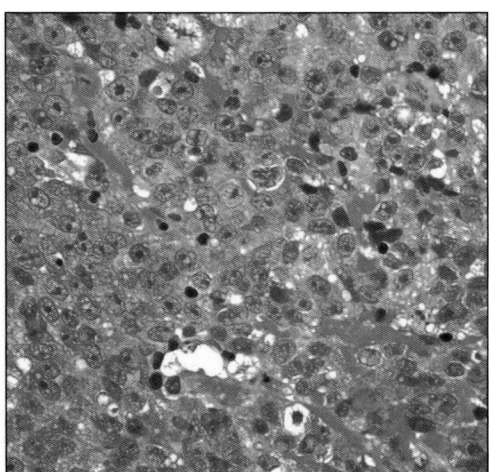

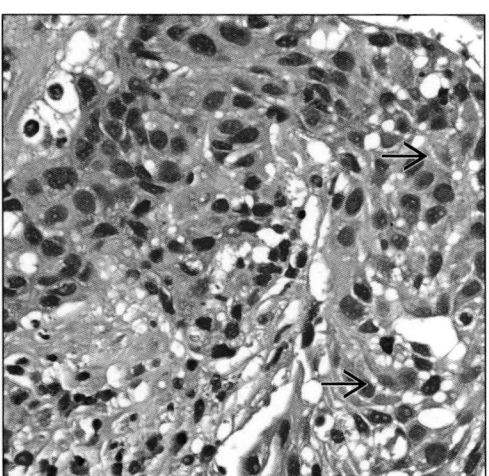

(Left) ASC of the prostate with poorly differentiated adenocarcinoma component shows high-grade cells lacking glandular lumina (Gleason pattern 5). This component was positive for PSA. *(Right)* ASC of the prostate in the same case shows malignant squamous cells with intercellular bridges ➡. In ASC, the glandular component is typically of higher grade (Gleason score 7 or higher).

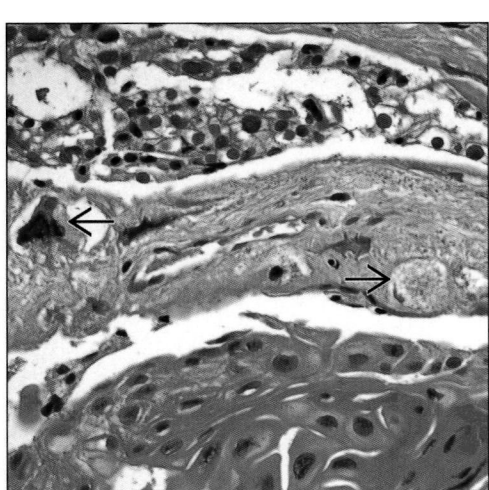

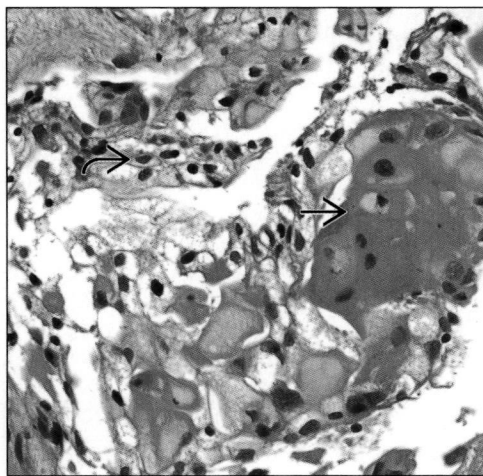

(Left) Radiation-treated prostate ASC shows both prostatic adenocarcinoma and squamous cell differentiation. There are occasional single carcinoma cells with marked treatment effect ➡, including enlarged irregular nuclei and foamy cytoplasm. *(Right)* Radiation-treated prostrate ASC shows squamous differentiation ➡ intimately admixed with the adenocarcinoma cells with treatment effect ➡.

CARCINOMAS WITH SQUAMOUS DIFFERENTIATION

Differential Diagnosis

(Left) Urothelial carcinoma in situ along the prostatic urethra shows focal squamous differentiation. Presence of this feature is a helpful clue in distinguishing invasive urethral urothelial carcinoma with squamous differentiation from primary pure SCC of the prostate. *(Right)* The invasive component from the same case maintains squamous differentiation, including presence of occasional intracytoplasmic keratin ➡.

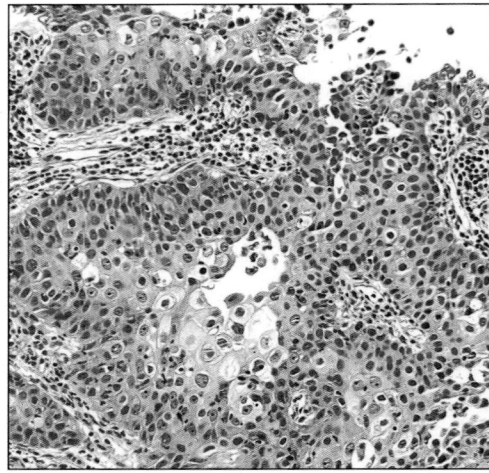
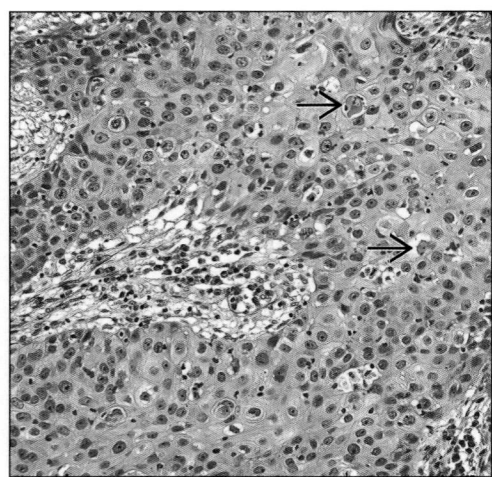

(Left) Bladder urothelial carcinoma with squamous differentiation invading the prostatic stroma. Invasive squamous component is seen adjacent to benign prostatic glands ➡. Urinary bladder carcinoma directly invading the prostatic stroma denotes high-stage bladder cancer (pT4). *(Right)* Primary anal SCC secondarily involving the prostate is indistinguishable from primary prostatic SCC in limited samples. Precise categorization requires clinicopathologic correlation.

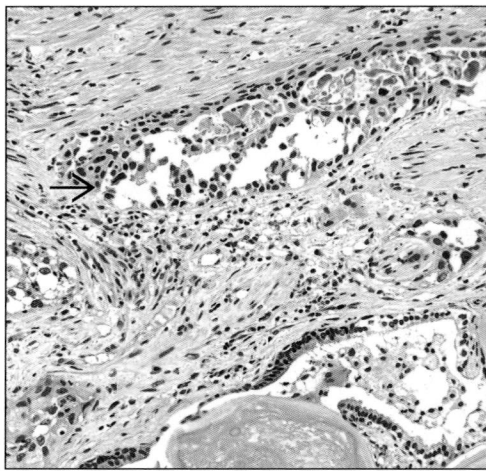
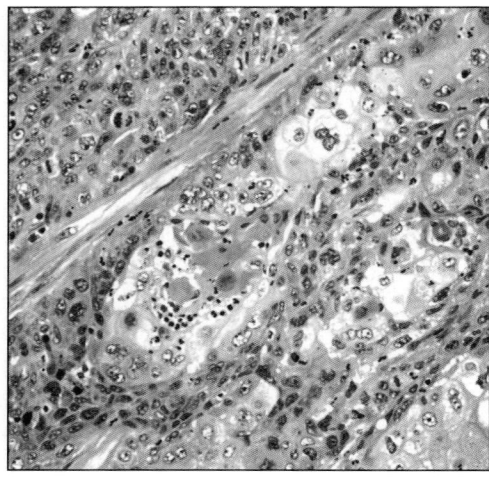

(Left) Squamous metaplasia of benign prostatic glands may be seen adjacent to an area of infarction, and in patients with prior TURP, hormonal, or radiation therapy. Areas of better squamous differentiation may be seen in squamous nests. Associated inflammation and resultant atypia may compound the diagnostic difficulty. *(Right)* Squamous metaplasia of benign prostatic glands is shown. The squamous epithelium has a reactive appearance and shows a distinct basal cell layer.

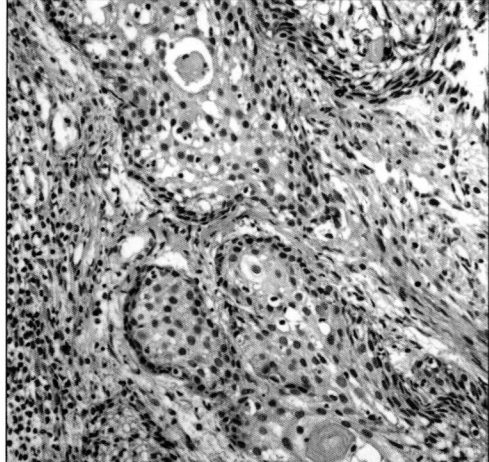
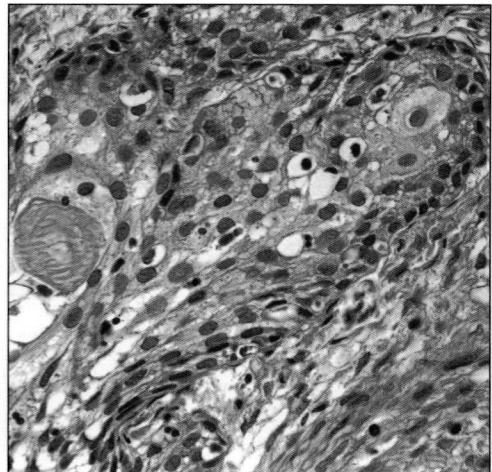

CARCINOMAS WITH SQUAMOUS DIFFERENTIATION

Differential Diagnosis and Immunohistochemistry

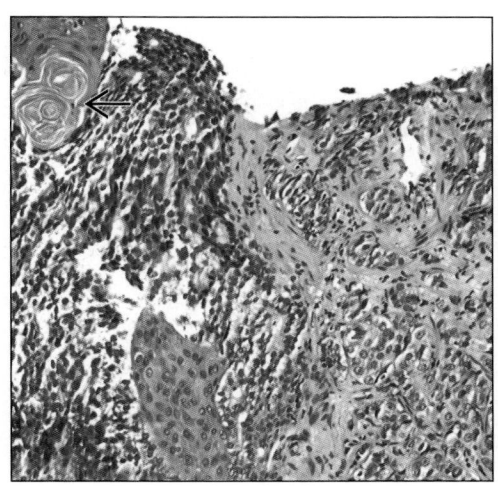
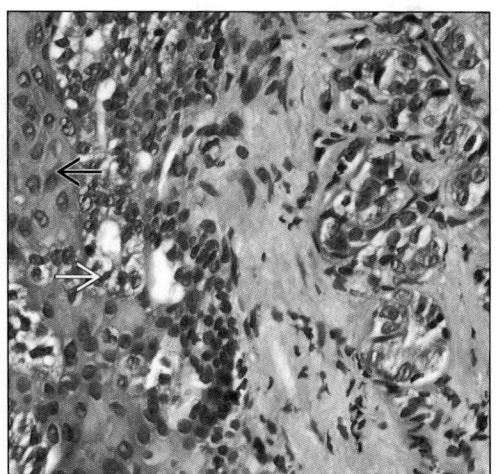

(Left) ASC of prostate in a needle biopsy shows nests of abrupt squamous differentiation, including keratin pearl ➡️ formation, present within cribriform Gleason score 9 prostate adenocarcinoma. *(Right)* ASC of the prostate shows squamous differentiation ➡️ within high-grade adenocarcinoma of prostate ➡️. There is a separate focus of conventional acinar carcinoma, which helps in the distinction from primary SCC, secondary SCC, or urothelial carcinoma with squamous differentiation.

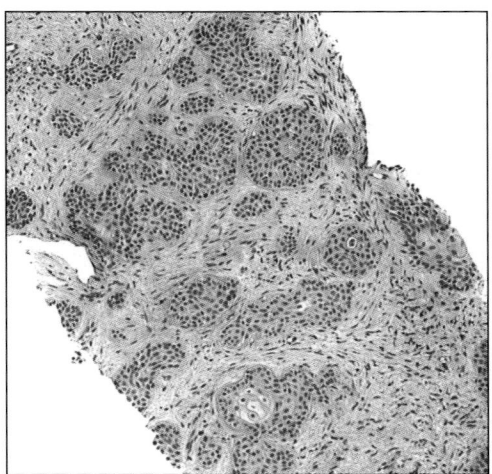
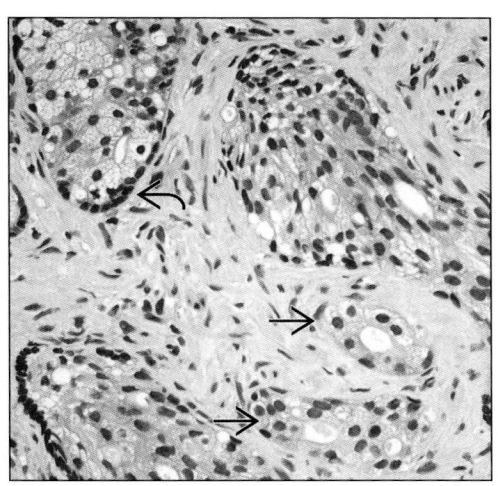

(Left) Needle core biopsy from a patient with prior radiation treatment for adenocarcinoma shows florid squamous metaplasia in benign prostatic epithelium. There is a maintenance of overall architecture and regular spacing between metaplastic glands arguing against an invasive process. *(Right)* Prostatic adenocarcinoma ➡️ adjacent to benign glands with squamous metaplasia. Benign glands show a distinct basal cell layer ➡️. Histology does not represent ASC of the prostate.

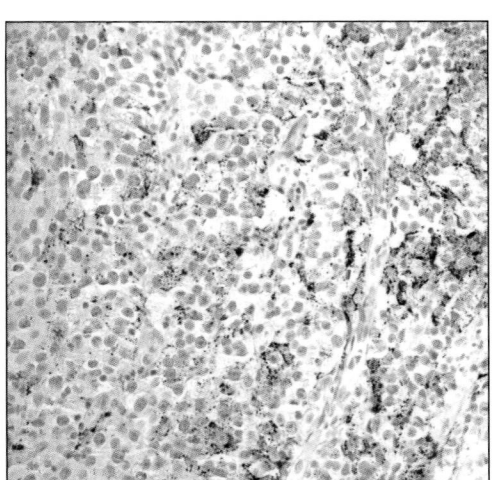
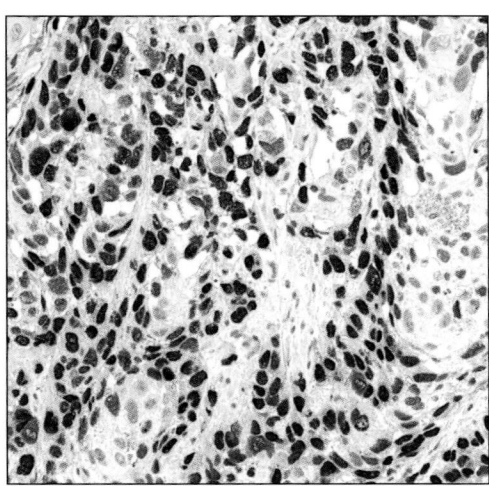

(Left) Poorly differentiated prostatic adenocarcinoma component of ASC shows patchy positivity with PSA immunostaining. PAP and PSMA may be alternatively used. *(Right)* Pure SCC of the prostate exhibits diffuse nuclear reactivity with p63. Both primary and secondary SCC involving the prostate are positive for p63. p63 immunoreactivity is not expected in poorly differentiated prostatic adenocarcinoma.

STROMAL TUMORS

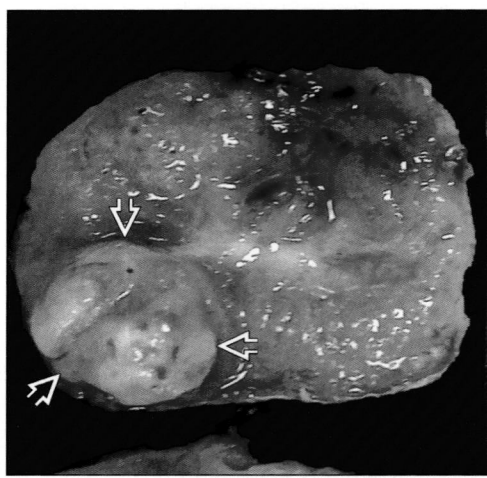

Cut section of prostate shows a PSS ⬌ involving the peripheral zone. Tumor is circumscribed, pale tan, and more solid in consistency than surrounding benign prostatic parenchyma.

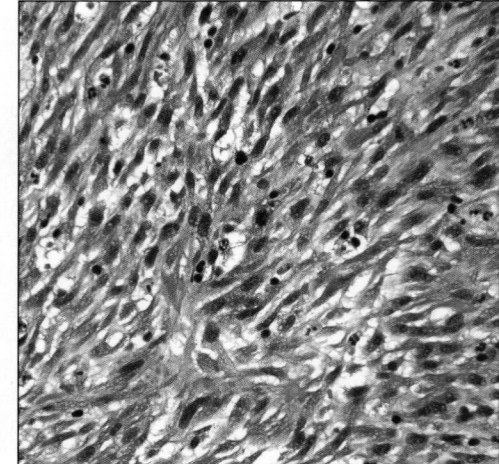

High-grade PSS shows nondescript growth of spindle cells with marked hypercellularity and pleomorphism. The histologic pattern is different from other sarcomas of distinctive histogenesis.

TERMINOLOGY

Abbreviations
- Prostatic stromal tumors of uncertain malignant potential (STUMP)
- Prostatic stromal sarcoma (PSS)

Synonyms
- Phyllodes tumor of prostate and atypical stromal hyperplasia preferred by other authors
- Prostatic stromal hyperplasia with atypia (PSHA)
- Phyllodes type of hyperplasia
- Phyllodes type of atypical hyperplasia
- Cystic epithelial stromal tumor
- Cystadenoleiomyofibroma
- Cystosarcoma phyllodes
- Sarcoma of specialized prostatic stroma

Definitions
- Controversy exists in terminology, definition, and pathology of stromal tumors
  - Neoplastic nature of at least a subset of STUMP, particularly those categorized as PSHA by other authors, is debated
- Tumors putatively derived from specialized stroma of prostate and include pure mesenchymal and mixed epithelial stromal (phyllodes) tumors
- Classified into STUMP and PSS in 2004 WHO classification of prostate tumors
  - Biphasic phyllodes tumors of prostate are categorized into STUMP and PSS based on degree of stromal atypia
- STUMP encompasses cellular spindle cell lesions of specialized prostatic stroma ± epithelial component
  - Lack significant cellular atypia, mitotic activity, necrosis, or extraprostatic growth
- PSS, low grade or high grade, is malignant cellular spindle cell lesion of specialized prostatic stroma with potential for local invasion or metastasis

ETIOLOGY/PATHOGENESIS

Origin
- PR is frequently expressed in STUMP and PSS supporting derivation from hormonally responsive mesenchyme of prostate
- Epithelial component of phyllodes pattern of STUMP and PSS expresses PSA and PAP confirming its prostatic acinar origin

Clonality
- Clonal but dissimilar loss of heterozygosity patterns observed in epithelial and stromal components of phyllodes tumor
- Both epithelial and stromal components of phyllodes tumor are neoplastic but suggested to have different clonal origins

CLINICAL ISSUES

Epidemiology
- Incidence
  - Rare, ~ 150 cases described in literature
  - Clinicopathologic characterization of these lesions mainly based on 3 major series published to date; largest series included 50 cases
- Age
  - Mean: 58 years old, range: 27-83 years
  - More than 1/2 of patients with PSS are younger than 50 years old
  - 1/5 of patients with STUMP are younger than 50 years old

Presentation
- Majority present with lower urinary tract symptoms (LUTS)
- Abnormal digital rectal examination (DRE), hematuria, hematospermia, acute urinary retention, secondary renal dysfunction may be present

STROMAL TUMORS

Key Facts

Terminology
- Tumors putatively derived from specialized stroma of prostate and include pure mesenchymal and mixed epithelial stromal (phyllodes) tumors
- Classified into STUMP and PSS in 2004 WHO classification of prostate tumors

Clinical Issues
- Mean: 58 years old, range: 27-83 years
- More than 1/2 of patients with PSS are younger than 50 years old
- Majority presents with lower urinary tract symptoms
- STUMP generally has good prognosis since mostly confined to prostate, but may recur, and uncommonly can adhere to adjacent organ
- PSS has high recurrence rate, locally aggressive, and can metastasize

Microscopic Pathology
- STUMP lacks significant cellular atypia, mitotic activity, necrosis, or extraprostatic growth
- 4 histologic patterns of STUMP, including degenerative atypia, hypercellular stroma, myxoid, and phyllodes-type
- PSS is characterized by stromal overgrowth, greater cellularity, pleomorphism, presence of increased mitosis, and necrosis
- Biphasic phyllodes tumor with sarcomatous stroma included in this group
- Stromal cells CD34(+) and PR(+)
- Epithelial component (phyllodes tumor) PSA/PAP(+)
- Main differentials include sarcomatoid carcinoma, BPH, smooth muscle tumors, GIST, solitary fibrous tumor, and seminal vesicle epithelial stromal tumor

---

- May be asymptomatic; lesion detected upon work-up for elevated serum PSA level

Natural History
- PSS suggested to rarely arise from STUMP but may arise de novo without prior STUMP

Treatment
- STUMP
  - Appropriate treatment approach currently unknown
  - Transurethral resection of prostate (TURP) to relieve LUTS
  - Additional sampling to rule out presence of higher grade lesion
  - Proposed recommendation for definitive resection to be based on patient age, treatment preference, and size or extent of lesion
  - Active surveillance proposed for elderly patients with limited lesion on biopsy and with no discernible mass on DRE or imaging studies
- PSS
  - Radical prostatectomy, cystoprostatectomy, or pelvic exenteration for locally aggressive tumors
  - Multimodal therapy, including chemotherapy for advanced and metastatic tumors may be of value
    - Complete remission reported in PSS metastatic to lung using anthracycline and alkylating agent-based regimen followed by metastasectomy

Prognosis
- STUMP
  - Generally has good prognosis since tumors are confined to prostate; they may recur
  - Has more rapid growth compared to nodules of benign prostatic hyperplasia (BPH)
  - Rarely may progress to PSS
    - STUMP is uncommonly seen in association with PSS, including in previous biopsies or resection of subsequent PSS
    - Progression to PSS in subset of STUMP with interglandular growth, particularly under those described as PSHA, is controversial
- PSS

- High recurrence rate, 65% of cases reported to recur in 1 series, with 2 years average time to 1st recurrence
- Locally aggressive and may directly invade seminal vesicle, urinary bladder, colon, pelvis, and perineum
- May metastasize, more frequently in high-grade PSS
  - Reported metastatic sites include lung (most common), bone, abdominal wall, and retroperitoneum

MACROSCOPIC FEATURES

General Features
- STUMP
  - Solid or partially cystic mass, the latter corresponding to phyllodes pattern of STUMP
  - Solid tumors are firm, white, tan, or yellow
  - Partially cystic tumors are multilobated, with variably sized cyst that may contain bloody, mucinous, or clear fluid
  - Most tumors arise from peripheral zone and transition zone, or may involve both zones
- PSS
  - Solid or partially cystic mass, the latter corresponding to phyllodes pattern of PSS
  - Solid tumors are gray, tan-yellow circumscribed or infiltrative mass
  - Solid-cystic mass of phyllodes pattern of PSS has relatively more evident solid component and may contain necrosis

Size
- STUMP: Range 0.7-15 cm
- PSS: Range 2-18 cm

MICROSCOPIC PATHOLOGY

Histologic Features
- STUMP
  - 4 histologic patterns

STROMAL TUMORS

- Pure mesenchymal: Degenerative atypia, hypercellular stroma, and myxoid patterns; may exhibit interglandular pattern of growth
- Phyllodes-type: Biphasic with both stromal and epithelial proliferation
- Admixture of different patterns may be seen
- Mitotic activity is absent to rare in all patterns
- Necrosis is absent
- Proliferation may be seen between benign normal glands
  - **Degenerative atypia**
    - Normal to mildly hypercellular stroma with scattered atypical degenerative-appearing cells surrounding benign prostatic glands
    - Atypical stromal cells contain enlarged, single or multiple pleomorphic nuclei with degenerate-type smudgy chromation
    - Most common pattern of STUMP (50%)
  - **Hypercellular stroma**
    - Moderately hypercellular, cytologically bland, fusiform stromal cells surrounding benign prostatic glands
    - Resembles florid mixed epithelial and stromal hyperplasia of BPH
    - In contrast to BPH, greater degree of cellularity and stromal cells have more eosinophilic cytoplasm
  - **Myxoid**
    - Extensive stromal overgrowth of stromal cells often embedded in myxoid stroma and often lacking benign glands
    - May resemble stromal-predominant BPH but lacks multinodularity
  - **Phyllodes-type growth**
    - Leaf-like growth with compressed slit-like pattern of benign glandular epithelium containing hypocellular fibrous stroma
    - Resembles benign phyllodes tumor of breast
    - Epithelial cells are low cuboidal to columnar and show distinct layer of basal cells
    - Spindle cells tend to be more cellular or condensed around cystic or glandular epithelium
- **PSS**
  - Stromal overgrowth with overt infiltration, greater cellularity, pleomorphism, increased mitoses, necrosis, and extraprostatic extension
    - Diagnosis of sarcoma based on presence of many or all of these features
  - Biphasic phyllodes tumor with sarcomatous stroma is included in this group
  - Sarcomatous growth: Spindled cells, ± epithelioid component
  - Spindled component: Herringbone, short fascicles, or patternless
  - Grading PSS as high grade or low grade, as proposed in AFIP fascicle, is preferred by authors
    - High-grade tumors based on increased cellularity, frequent mitoses, cytologic atypia, necrosis, and stromal overgrowth
    - Low-grade tumors are less atypical; prominent cellularity, appreciable mitoses, nuclear atypia,

necrosis, and extraprostatic spread indicate malignant nature
  - 3-tier grading system for phyllodes tumors has been proposed
  - Low grade
    - Low to moderate stromal cellularity
    - Absent or rare cytological atypia
    - Mitosis < 2/10 HPF; absent necrosis
    - Low or mildly hypercellular stroma lined by complete epithelium with frequent leaf-like pattern
  - Intermediate grade
    - Moderate to high stromal cellularity
    - Intermediate number of atypical cells with moderate to marked atypia
    - Mitosis 2-5/10 HPF; absent necrosis
  - High grade
    - Moderate to high cellularity, marked anaplasia
    - Mitosis > 5/10 HPF; necrosis may be present
    - High, markedly hypercellular stroma with scattered lining epithelium, infrequent leaf-like pattern
  - Recurrent tumor of PSS may show higher grade features than initial tumor

Predominant Pattern/Injury Type
- Neoplastic

Predominant Cell/Compartment Type
- Mesenchymal

Immunohistochemistry
- Stromal cells
  - Vimentin(+), CD34(+), PR(+)
  - Desmin, SMA, and actin-HHF-35 shows variable (±) reactivity
  - S100(-), CD117(-), ER mostly(-)
- Epithelial component (phyllodes tumor)
  - PAN-CK(AE1/AE3)(+), PSA/PAP(+)

DIFFERENTIAL DIAGNOSIS

Sarcomatoid Carcinoma
- May be associated with malignant glandular component
- May be associated with history of prostatic adenocarcinoma with radiation/hormone treatment
- Cytokeratin, HMCK(34βE12), CK5/6, and p63 positive in spindle cell component
- PSA/PAP positive in malignant glandular component

Benign Prostate Hyperplasia (BPH)
- STUMP with hypercellular stroma pattern mimics mixed epithelial stromal BPH
- STUMP with myxoid pattern mimics stromal predominant BPH
- Uncommon in younger patients
- Typical multinodular growth, unlike STUMP, which is often solitary
- Most commonly arises from transition zone, unlike STUMP, which may involve both transition and peripheral zones

STROMAL TUMORS

- In contrast to STUMP, stromal predominant BPH shows abundant stromal capillaries and may show condensation of stromal cells around vessels
- In contrast to STUMP with hypercellular stroma, glands of mixed epithelial stromal BPH are hyperplastic, and stromal cells are less eosinophilic

Smooth Muscle Tumors

- Includes leiomyoma and leiomyosarcoma of prostate
- Leiomyosarcoma is most common sarcoma involving adult prostate
- Leiomyosarcoma vary from those resembling smooth muscle cells with moderate atypia and increased mitotic activity to pleomorphic tumors
- Leiomyosarcoma may exhibit epithelioid features
- Leiomyoma may contain atypical bizarre nuclei, but nevertheless remain with benign clinical behavior
- May be PR positive similar to stromal tumors, thus not helpful in differential diagnosis
- May exhibit distinct fascicular growth characteristic of smooth muscle cells
- CD34 is usually negative, and desmin is strongly positive in smooth muscle tumors

Gastrointestinal Stromal Tumor (GIST)

- GIST from colorectal region may invade into prostate and may even present as intraprostatic mass
- CD34 positive similar to stromal tumors
- Diffusely and strongly positive for CD117 and DOG1

Solitary Fibrous Tumor

- Ropey collagen and thick-walled, irregular or hemangiopericytomatous blood vessels
- May arise primarily from prostate or from pelvis with secondary involvement of prostate
- About 1/2 of cases are malignant
- CD34 and bcl-2 positive

Seminal Vesicle Epithelial Stromal Tumor

- Histologically similar to phyllodes tumor of prostate
- Tumor is grossly and histologically intimately associated with seminal vesicle and often separated from prostatectomy specimen
- Unlike prostatic phyllodes tumor, epithelial component is PSA and PAP negative

DIAGNOSTIC CHECKLIST

Pathologic Interpretation Pearls

- Spindle cell proliferations of specialized prostatic stroma that span a spectrum from monophasic to biphasic (phyllodes-type) tumors
- Classified based on stromal cellularity, stromal overgrowth, cellular atypia, mitoses, necrosis, infiltrative growth, and extraprostatic extension
- Categorized based on histologic features
  - STUMP
    - Includes lesions of PSHA
  - PSS, low grade
  - PSS, high grade
- Positive for CD34 and PR; SMA and desmin variable

- Definitive categorization as PSS may not be possible in needle biopsies or transurethral resection specimens
  - In such cases, diagnostic terminology, such as "at least stromal tumor of unknown malignant potential," should be made
  - Definitive characterization be recommended only on basis of examination of additional tissue or from prostatectomy specimen, if performed

SELECTED REFERENCES

1. Egevad L et al: Atypical stromal hyperplasia of the prostate. Scand J Urol Nephrol. 42(5):484-7, 2008
2. Hossain D et al: Prostatic stromal hyperplasia with atypia: follow-up study of 18 cases. Arch Pathol Lab Med. 132(11):1729-33, 2008
3. Herawi M et al: Specialized stromal tumors of the prostate: a clinicopathologic study of 50 cases. Am J Surg Pathol. 30(6):694-704, 2006
4. Bostwick DG et al: Phyllodes tumor of the prostate: long-term followup study of 23 cases. J Urol. 172(3):894-9, 2004
5. McCarthy RP et al: Molecular genetic evidence for different clonal origins of epithelial and stromal components of phyllodes tumor of the prostate. Am J Pathol. 165(4):1395-400, 2004
6. Lam KC et al: Chemotherapy induced complete remission in malignant phyllodes tumor of the prostate metastasizing to the lung. J Urol. 168(3):1104-5, 2002
7. Watanabe M et al: Malignant phyllodes tumor of the prostate: retrospective review of specimens obtained by sequential transurethral resection. Pathol Int. 52(12):777-83, 2002
8. Schapmans S et al: Phyllodes tumor of the prostate. A case report and review of the literature. Eur Urol. 38(5):649-53, 2000
9. Tijare JR et al: Phyllodes type of atypical prostatic hyperplasia. J Urol. 162(3 Pt 1):803-4, 1999
10. Gaudin PB et al: Sarcomas and related proliferative lesions of specialized prostatic stroma: a clinicopathologic study of 22 cases. Am J Surg Pathol. 22(2):148-62, 1998
11. Kevwitch MK et al: Prostatic cystic epithelial-stromal tumors: a report of 2 new cases. J Urol. 149(4):860-4, 1993
12. Kerley SW et al: Giant cystosarcoma phyllodes of the prostate associated with adenocarcinoma. Arch Pathol Lab Med. 116(2):195-7, 1992
13. Young JF et al: Malignant phyllodes tumor of the prostate. A case report with immunohistochemical and ultrastructural studies. Arch Pathol Lab Med. 116(3):296-9, 1992
14. Yum M et al: Leiomyosarcoma arising in atypical fibromuscular hyperplasia (phyllodes tumor) of the prostate with distant metastasis. Cancer. 68(4):910-5, 1991
15. Lopez-Beltran A et al: Malignant phyllodes tumor of prostate. Urology. 35(2):164-7, 1990
16. Leong SS et al: Atypical stromal smooth muscle hyperplasia of prostate. Urology. 31(2):163-7, 1988
17. Attah EB et al: Atypical stromal hyperplasia of the prostate gland. Am J Clin Pathol. 67(4):324-7, 1977

STROMAL TUMORS

Microscopic Features of STUMP

(Left) Low-power magnification of STUMP in needle biopsy specimen shows cellular stroma without associated glands. There is no pleomorphism, and proliferation appears circumscribed in sampled tissue. *(Right)* Higher power magnification of STUMP shows mild nuclear atypia of stromal cells. Other features of malignancy, including nuclear anaplasia and mitotic activity, are lacking.

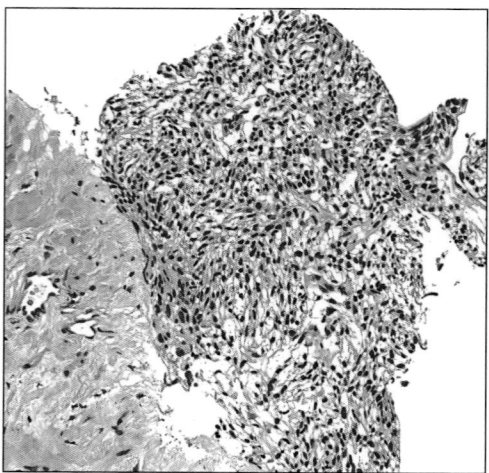
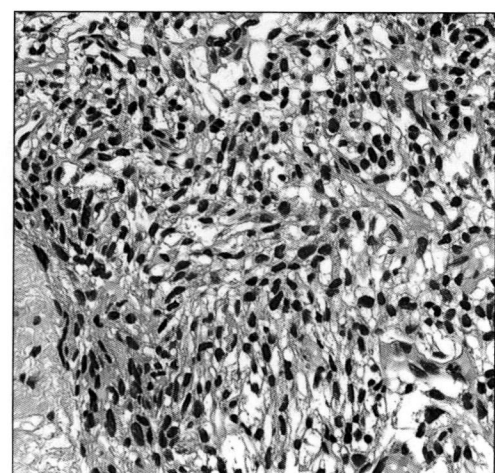

(Left) Low-power magnification of STUMP in needle biopsy specimen shows cellular spindle cell stroma focally with myxoid background ⟶. There is no evidence of necrosis. The spindle cells have nondescript patternless growth. *(Right)* Higher power magnification of STUMP shows cellular stromal cells surrounding a benign gland. The spindle cells have uniform nuclear contours and lack chromatin abnormalities and mitotic activity.

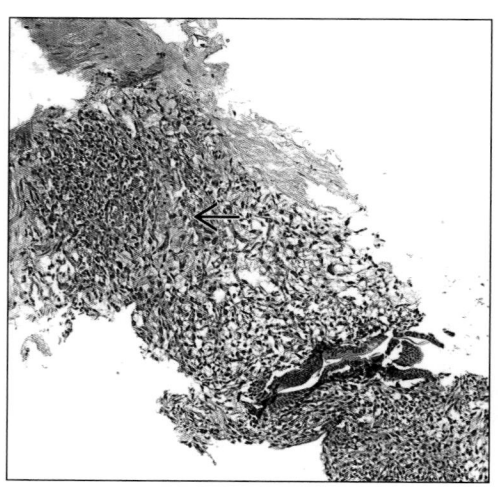
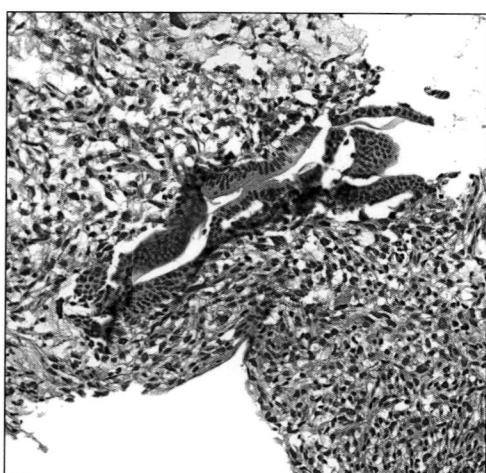

(Left) Low-power magnification of STUMP in needle biopsy specimen shows cellular stroma with atypical cells in between benign glands. There is marked stromal overgrowth. Necrosis and marked pleomorphism are lacking. *(Right)* Higher power magnification shows cellular atypia within stromal cells. There is no mitotic activity. Diagnosis of malignancy (PSS) is based on the accumulative assessment of multiple adverse pathologic features.

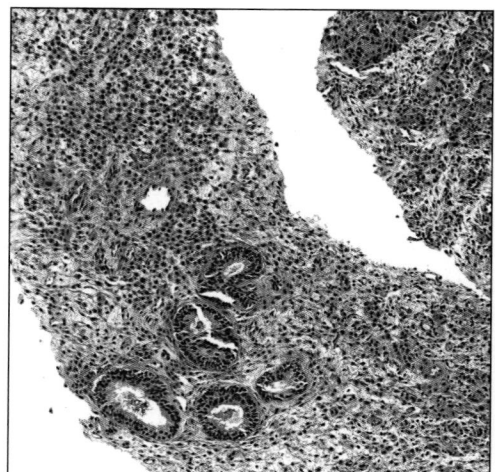
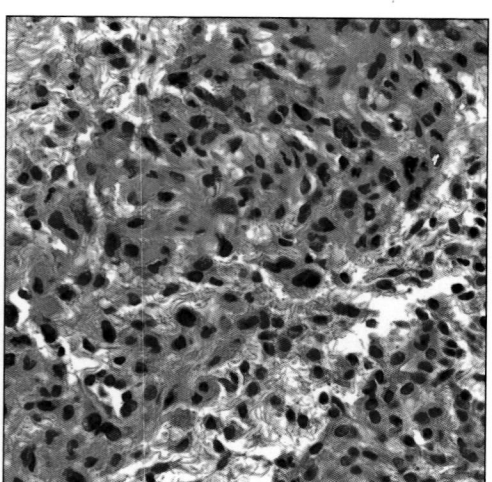

STROMAL TUMORS

Microscopic Features of PSS

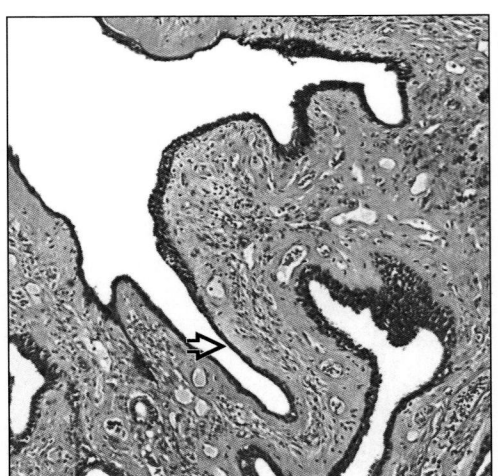

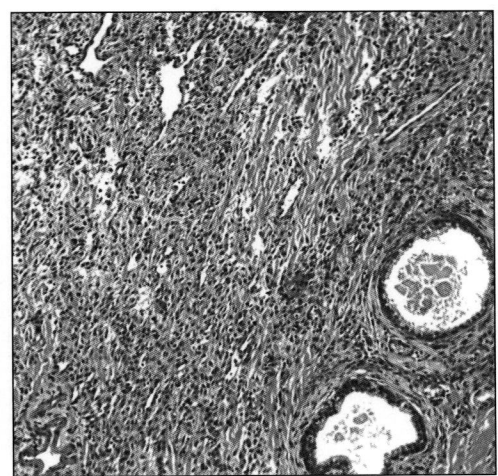

(Left) PSS, low grade, phyllodes pattern exhibits leaf-like growth ⇗ of epithelial glandular cells with an investing spindle cell stroma. Some of the cystic glands amid the stromal proliferation are compressed or slit-like in appearance. This epithelial component shows 2 cell types and is immunohistochemically positive for PSA. **(Right)** Low-power magnification of PSS, low grade, shows hypercellular tumor consisting of spindle cells seen infiltrating between benign-appearing glands.

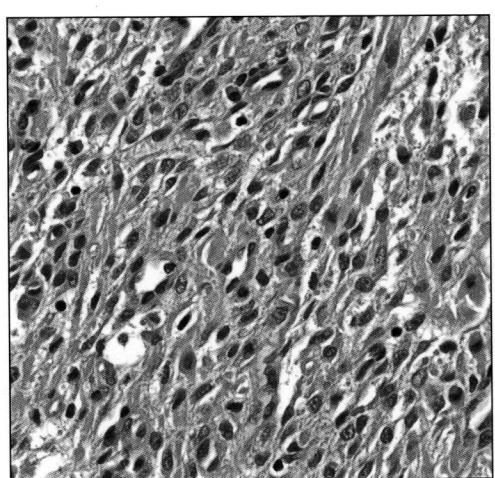

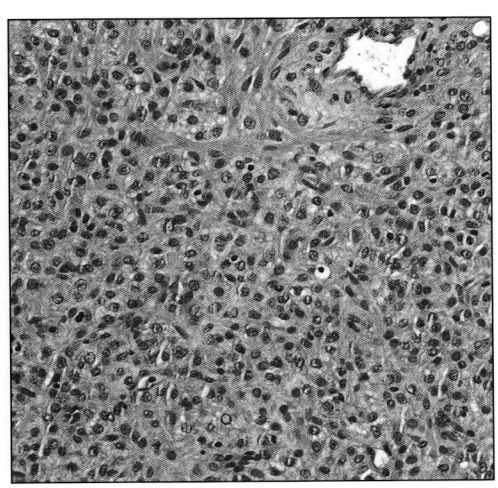

(Left) High-power magnification of PSS, low grade, shows fusiform spindle cells. No distinct growth pattern, such as fascicular, storiform, or herringbone, is seen in this tumor. Cytoplasm of spindle cells is compact and not fibrillar. **(Right)** PSS, low grade, consists of hypercellular sheets of epithelioid cells. There is moderate nuclear atypia. Differential diagnosis is with sarcomatoid carcinoma, solitary fibrous tumor, and GIST.

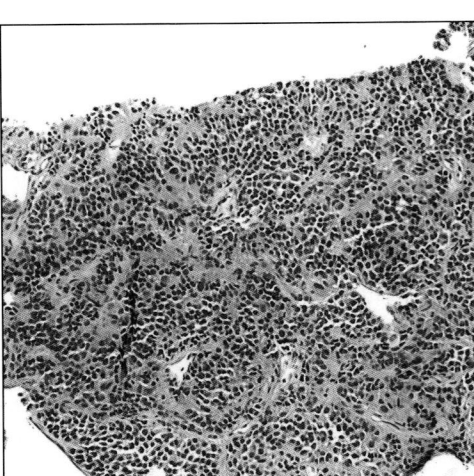

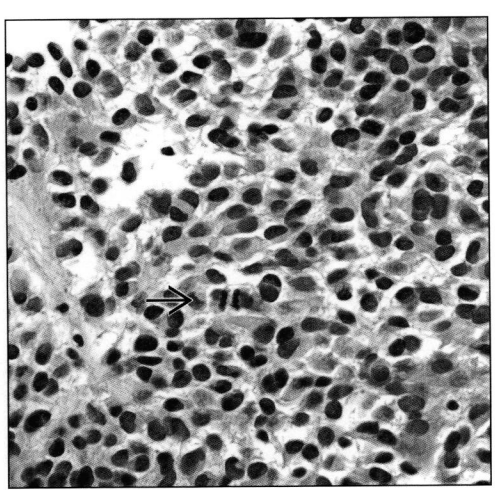

(Left) Low-power magnification of epithelioid PSS, high grade, encountered in needle biopsy. In such cases, differentials may include other "round cell tumors," such as small cell carcinoma, rhabdomyosarcoma, lymphoma, and melanoma. **(Right)** High-power view of epithelioid PSS, high grade, shows marked atypia and mitotic activity ⇨ in epithelioid cells. Approach to such malignant proliferations requires a judicious immunohistochemical panel.

STROMAL TUMORS

Microscopic and Immunohistochemical Features

(Left) PSS, high grade, in TURP associated with broad area of necrosis ⮕. Tumor is markedly hypercellular, consisting of atypical spindle cells. Presence of hypercellularity, pleomorphism, increased mitosis, and tumor-related necrosis are used for sarcoma designation. *(Right)* PSS, high grade, shows tumor-related necrosis characterized by tumor "ghost" cells and abrupt transition between necrosis and viable tumor cells.

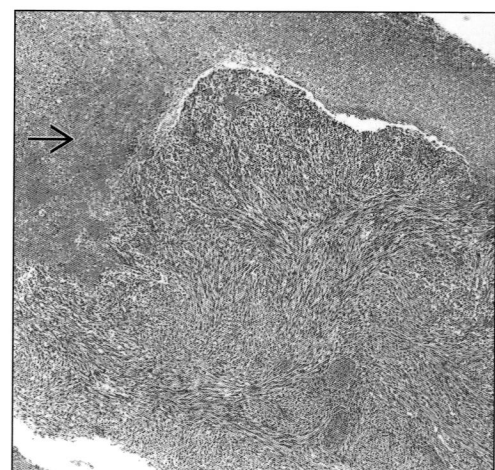 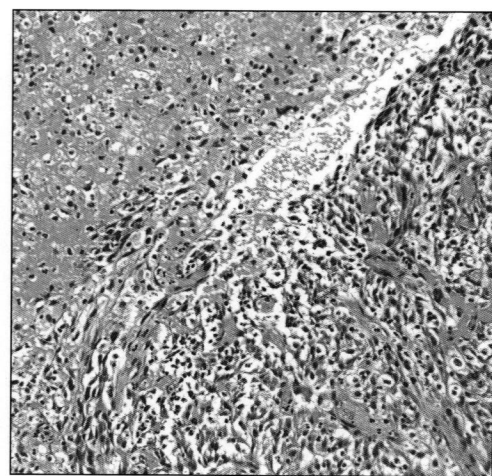

(Left) PSS, high grade, shows spindle cells with focal fascicular growth pattern. PSS may demonstrate variable architecture not distinctive of other sarcomas involving prostate, including leiomyosarcoma, malignant solitary fibrous tumor, and GIST. *(Right)* PSS, high grade, shows spindle cells with focal storiform pattern. Adequate sampling is necessary in order to assess features of malignancy, which may not be overt.

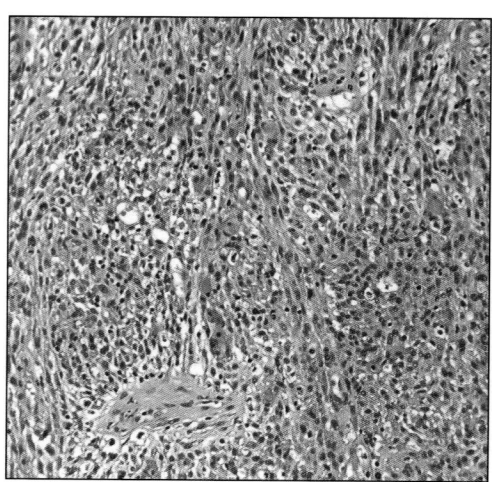 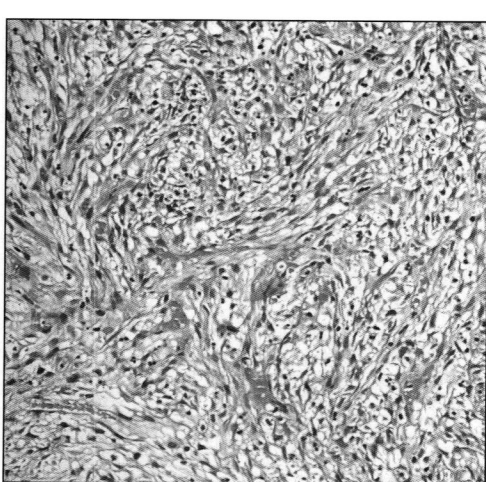

(Left) PSS, high grade, is shown with phyllodes pattern. The glandular component, by definition, is benign. Presence of phyllodes pattern does not influence classification of stromal tumors as benign or malignant. *(Right)* STUMP exhibits nuclear PR positivity, supporting derivation from the hormonally responsive specialized mesenchyme of the prostate. PR may also be expressed by smooth muscle tumors; hence, CD34 is more discriminatory.

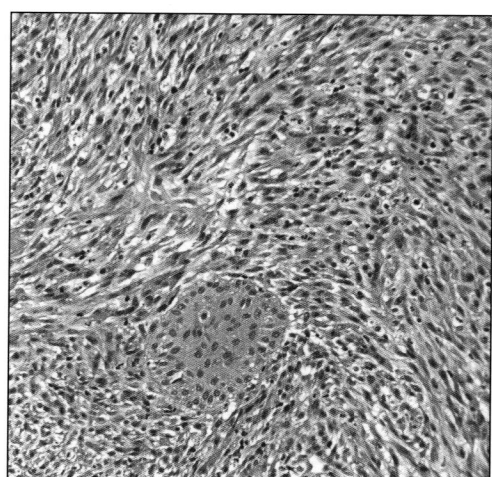 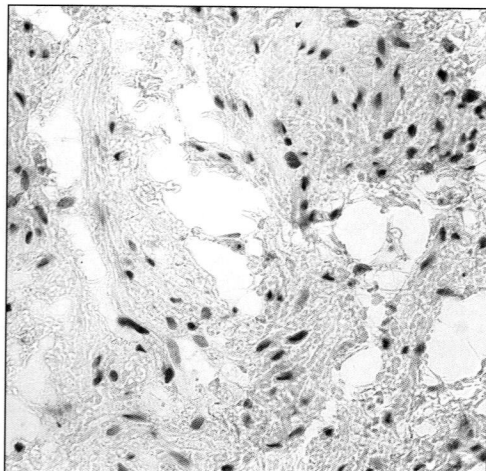

STROMAL TUMORS

Immunohistochemical Features and Differential Diagnosis

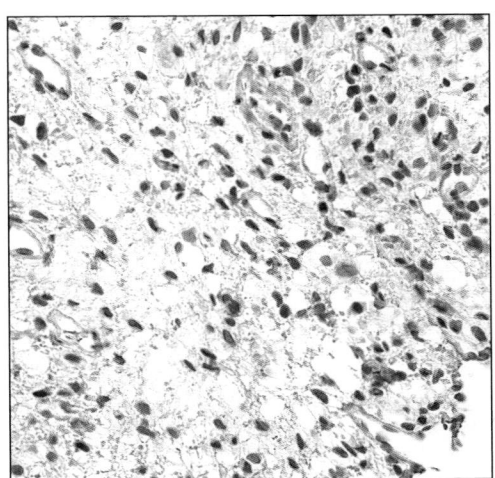
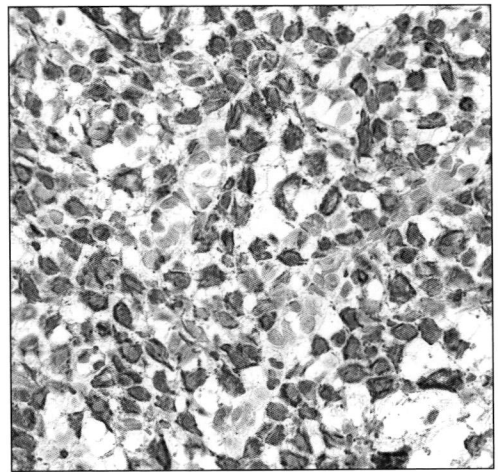

(Left) STUMP exhibits nuclear ER positivity. In contrast to PR, ER is rarely positive in stromal tumors. (Right) PSS, low grade, with epithelioid features shows diffuse staining with SMA. Stromal tumors show variable immunoreactivity to SMA. Thus, this stain is not helpful in distinguishing stromal neoplasms from smooth muscle tumors. It would be unusual for sarcomatoid carcinomas to express this degree of SMA positivity.

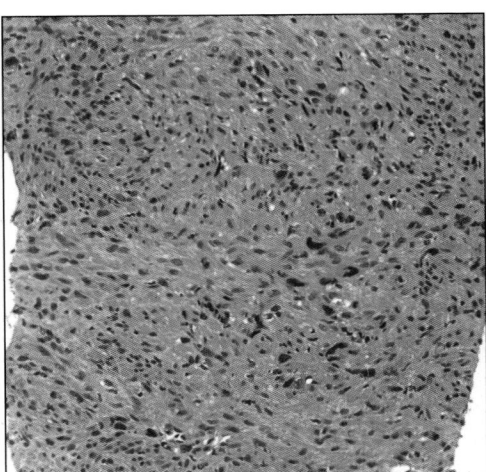
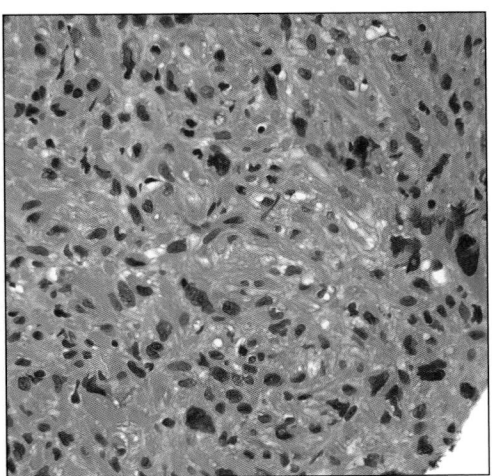

(Left) Leiomyosarcoma of prostate in needle biopsy shows marked cellular pleomorphism. Smooth muscle differentiation is suggested in this tumor based on presence of fascicular growth. Leiomyosarcoma is the most common sarcoma involving the adult prostate. (Right) Leiomyosarcoma, high grade, shows marked nuclear anaplasia in spindle cells. It shares smooth muscle actin, desmin, and PR positivity with stromal sarcoma but is negative for CD34.

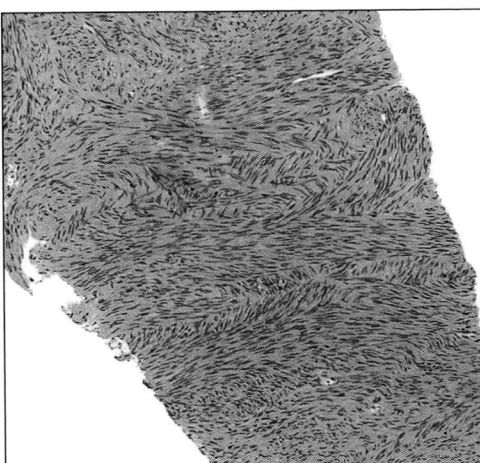
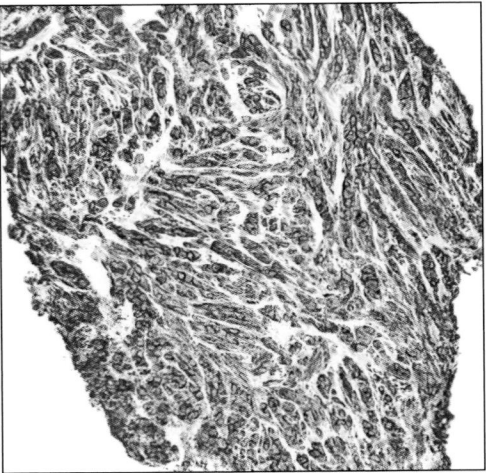

(Left) Cellular leiomyoma of prostate in needle biopsy shows fascicular growth of bland-appearing spindle cells reminiscent of smooth muscle bundles. Additional assessment of the tumor revealed lack of mitotic activity and necrosis. (Right) Spindle cell GIST involving prostate in needle biopsy shows diffuse CD117 positivity. GIST from colorectal region may invade into prostate and may even present as intraprostatic mass. In contrast, stromal tumors do not express CD117.

SECONDARY TUMORS OF THE PROSTATE

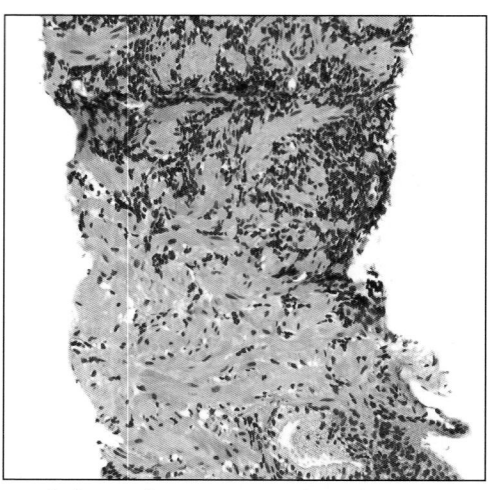

Needle biopsy shows prostate with involvement by B-cell CLL. Hematopoietic tumors are the most common secondary prostate malignancy. Metastatic tumors from distant sites may also involve the prostate.

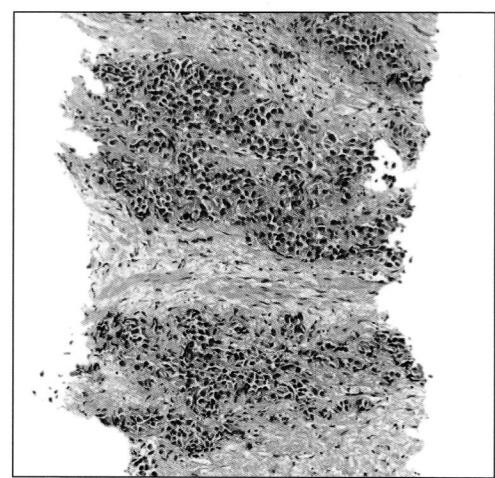

Needle biopsy shows high-grade urothelial carcinoma from the urinary bladder invading the prostate. Bladder carcinoma is the most common malignancy to invade the prostate via direct extension.

TERMINOLOGY

Definitions
- Neoplasms involving prostate through direct spread from adjacent organs or metastasis from distant sites

ETIOLOGY/PATHOGENESIS

Pattern of Spread
- Most distant metastases reach prostate through arterial (rather than venous) dissemination
- Direct prostate invasion of cancers arising from urinary bladder or colorectal region

Origin
- Distant metastases
  ○ Majority are hematopoietic tumors (58%)
    ▪ B-cell chronic lymphocytic leukemia (CLL) most common (11%)
  ○ Most common origin of distant solid tumor metastasis
    ▪ Lungs (49%), laryngotracheal (2%)
    ▪ Skin, including melanoma (24%)
    ▪ Pancreaticobiliary (9%), gastrointestinal tract (7%)
    ▪ Isolated cases from kidney, penis, thyroid, breast, and eye
- Direct tumor spread
  ○ Urinary bladder (85%)
  ○ Rectum (15%)

CLINICAL ISSUES

Epidemiology
- Incidence
  ○ Very rare, encountered in only 0.2% of male autopsies
  ○ Seen in 5.6% of male autopsies with malignancies
    ▪ 44% via direct spread
    ▪ 56% via distant metastasis
  ○ Seen in 0.2% of prostate resections and biopsies
    ▪ 93% via direct spread
    ▪ 7% via distant metastasis
- Age
  ○ Median: 66 years; range: 39-83 years

Presentation
- Distant metastases to prostate are mostly incidental autopsy findings of disseminated tumors
- Clinical presentation of distant metastasis to prostate prompting urologic work-up is very rare
  ○ Few reported examples presented with obstructive uropathy and inflammatory symptoms
- Metastasis to prostate as initial histologic diagnosis of malignancy seen in only 2% of cases
- In surgical pathology specimens, direct spread is more frequently encountered than distant metastasis

Treatment
- Supportive care
- May require surgical management as palliation for obstructive symptoms

Prognosis
- Extremely poor
- Involvement of prostate by metastasis indicates late or widely disseminated stage of tumor
- Distant metastasis to prostate is almost invariably associated with carcinomatosis to other organs
  ○ Mainly involves liver (90%), lungs (79%), kidneys (77%), adrenal glands (61%)

IMAGE FINDINGS

General Features
- Radiologic work-up helpful in investigating unknown primary origin

SECONDARY TUMORS OF THE PROSTATE

Key Facts

Terminology
- Neoplasms involving prostate through direct spread from adjacent organs or metastasis from distant sites

Clinical Issues
- Seen in 5.6% of male autopsies with malignancies and 0.2% of prostate resections and biopsies
- Mostly encountered as incidental autopsy findings
- Indicates late or widely disseminated stage of disease

Microscopic Pathology
- Hematopoietic tumors (58%) are most common
- B-cell CLL (11%) is most common secondary hematopoietic tumor
- Distant solid metastasis mostly originate from lungs (49%), skin (24%), and pancreaticobiliary (9%)

- Direct tumor spread predominantly from urinary bladder (85%) and rectum (15%)
- Differential diagnosis of poorly differentiated prostate vs. bladder urothelial and rectal cancers may be very difficult in limited sample (i.e., biopsy)
- Distinction important due to differing therapies (i.e., hormonal for prostate cancer, chemotherapy for bladder cancer, and radiotherapy for rectal cancer)
- Rarely, GIST from colorectal region may invade into prostate, and may even present as intraprostatic mass

Ancillary Tests
- Use of immunohistochemistry can be crucial in differential diagnosis of primary vs. secondary tumors of prostate

MACROSCOPIC FEATURES

General Features
- Variable gross features
- Prostate often enlarged and nodular; may be bulky
- Less commonly normal in size with microscopic tumor

MICROSCOPIC PATHOLOGY

Histologic Features
- Similar to primary tumors from organ of origin

Predominant Pattern/Injury Type
- Neoplastic

Predominant Cell/Compartment Type
- Metastatic tumor cell

ANCILLARY TESTS

Immunohistochemistry
- May be crucial in differential diagnosis of primary vs. secondary tumors of prostate
- Poorly differentiated carcinomas
  - Poorly differentiated prostate carcinomas
    - PSA (±) and PAP(±)
    - Negative for p63, HMCK, CDX-2, and β-catenin
    - CK7(+/-) and CK20(+/-)
    - Other (+) markers: P501S, PSMA, NKX3, pPSA
  - Poorly differentiated urothelial carcinoma
    - Positive for p63 and HMCK(34βE12)
    - Negative for PSA or PAP, CDX-2, and β-catenin
    - CK7(±) and CK20(±)
    - Other (+) markers: GATA3, thrombomodulin, CK5/6, uroplakin-3
    - AMACR also positive and is not helpful
  - Poorly differentiated rectal adenocarcinoma
    - Positive for CDX-2 and β-catenin (nuclear)
    - CK7(-) and CK20(+)
    - Negative for PSA or PAP, p63, and HMCK
- Lymphoma vs. poorly differentiated carcinomas

  - Malignant lymphoma
    - Positive for CD45, CD20, CD79-α, or CD3
    - Negative for PAN-CK(AE1/AE3)
  - Poorly differentiated carcinomas
    - Positive for PAN-CK(AE1/AE3)
    - Negative for CD45, CD20, CD79-α, and CD3
- Spindle cell tumors involving the prostate
  - Gastrointestinal stromal tumors (GIST)
    - Positive for CD117 (diffuse) and CD34
    - S100 negative; often negative for actin-sm and desmin
  - Primary prostatic mesenchymal tumors
    - Prostatic stromal tumors of unknown malignant potential (STUMP) and stromal sarcoma are positive for CD34 and PR
    - Smooth muscle tumors positive for actin-sm and desmin
    - SFT positive for CD34

DIFFERENTIAL DIAGNOSIS

Secondary Poorly Differentiated Carcinomas
- Distinction of poorly differentiated bladder urothelial and rectal cancers vs. prostate cancer may be very difficult in limited sample (i.e., biopsy)
- Distinction important due to differing therapy (i.e., hormonal for prostate cancer, chemotherapy for bladder cancer, and radiotherapy for rectal cancer)

Secondary Spindle Cell Neoplasms
- GIST from colorectal region may invade into prostate and may even present as intraprostatic mass

SELECTED REFERENCES
1. Bates AW et al: Secondary solid neoplasms of the prostate: a clinico-pathological series of 51 cases. Virchows Arch. 440(4):392-6, 2002
2. Zein TA et al: Secondary tumors of the prostate. J Urol. 133(4):615-6, 1985
3. Johnson DE et al: Secondary tumors of the prostate. J Urol. 112(4):507-8, 1974

Microscopic and Immunohistochemical Features

(Left) B-cell CLL involving the prostate shows monotonous small-sized lymphoid cells with regular round nuclei containing clumped chromatin. Lymphomas involving the prostate are often indolent and occur with concurrent lymphoma elsewhere. **(Right)** Mantle cell lymphoma in a TURP specimen shows monotonous small-sized lymphoid cells in the prostatic stroma. Involvement by lymphoma may be subtle and missed if there is no high index of suspicion for it.

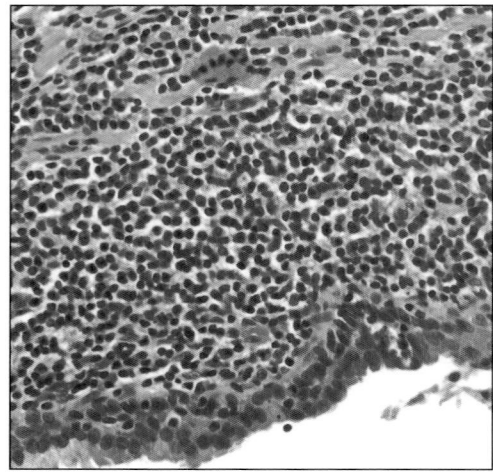 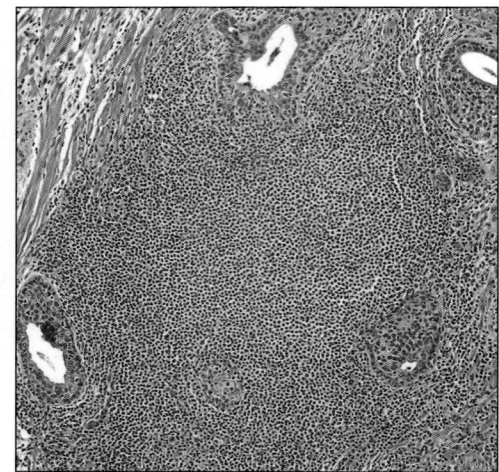

(Left) B-cell CLL in needle biopsy shows diffuse staining with CD20. These lymphoid cells also coexpress CD5 and CD23, typical for B-cell CLL. **(Right)** Needle biopsy of prostate with bladder urothelial carcinoma shows infiltrating poorly differentiated carcinoma cells. Differentiation between bladder urothelial carcinoma and high-grade prostate carcinoma can be very difficult. Distinction is important due to different treatment modalities particularly in tumors with high stage.

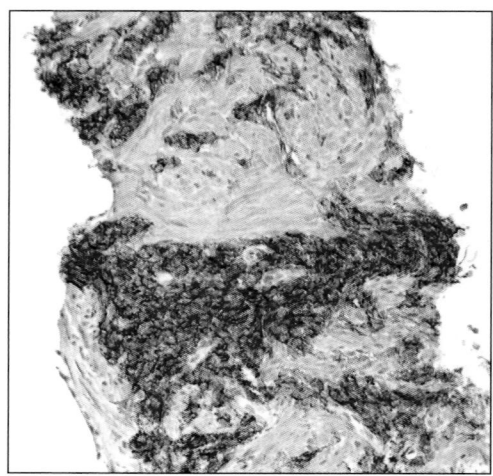 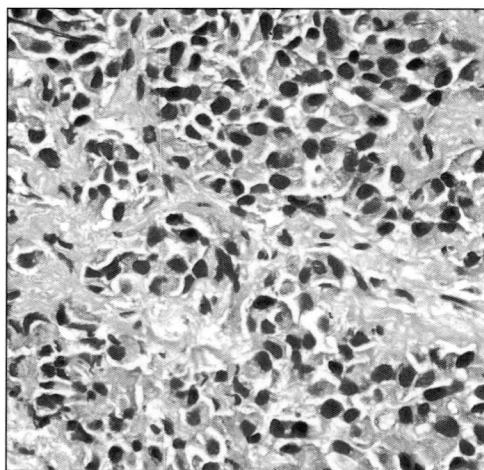

(Left) Invasive urothelial carcinoma seen in a TURP specimen. The tumor is high grade with tumor cell necrosis ➡ simulating a comedo-type prostate carcinoma. Direct extension of the prostatic stroma by bladder cancer denotes high-stage cancer (pT4). **(Right)** Bladder urothelial carcinoma shows diffuse AMACR positivity. AMACR is not useful in distinguishing urothelial carcinoma vs. prostate carcinoma, since both tumors will be positive with this stain.

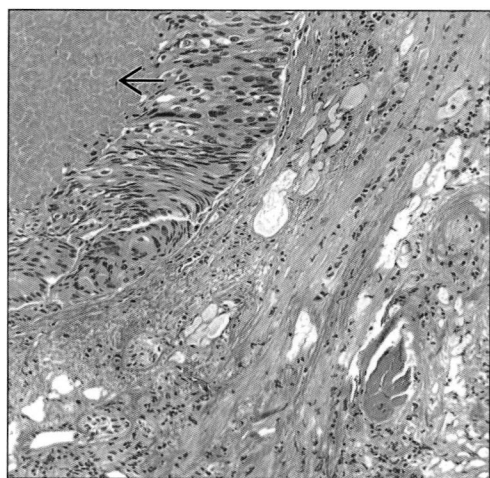 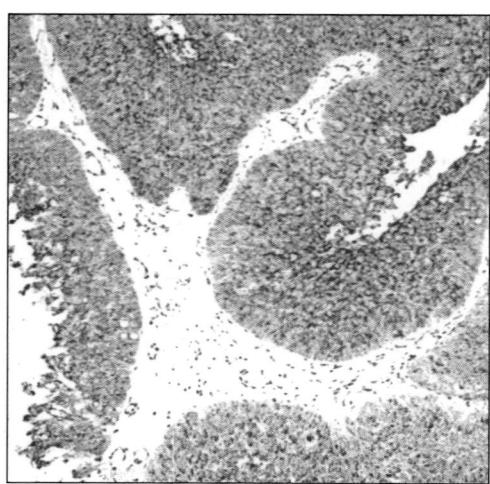

SECONDARY TUMORS OF THE PROSTATE

Microscopic and Immunohistochemical Features

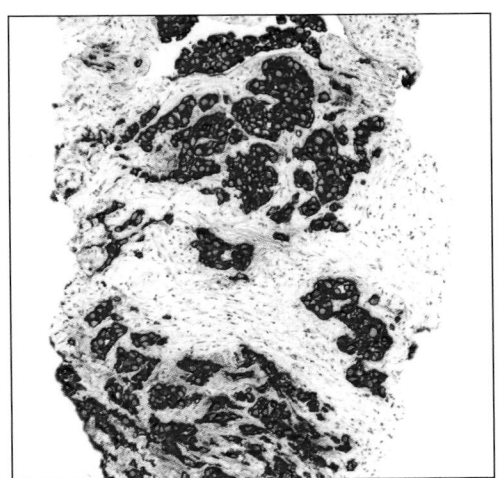

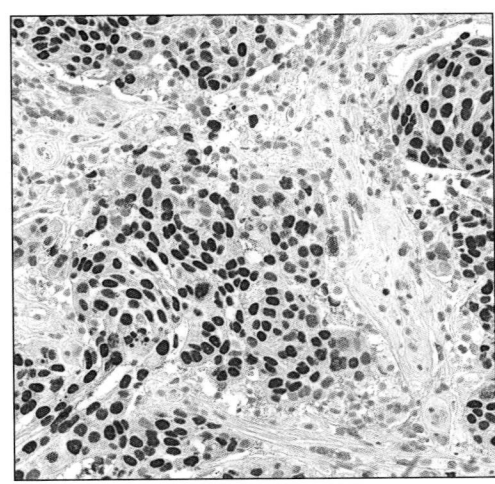

(Left) Bladder urothelial carcinoma involving the prostate in a needle biopsy shows diffuse positivity to CK7. Urothelial carcinomas are typically CK7(+) and CK20(±); however, these stains alone are not confirmatory in distinguishing from prostate carcinoma. (Right) p63 immunohistochemical stain shows diffuse nuclear positivity in urothelial carcinoma. p63 is useful in distinguishing urothelial carcinoma vs. prostate carcinoma, which is typically negative.

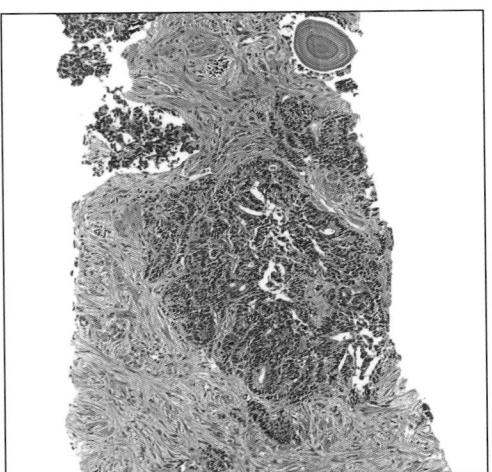

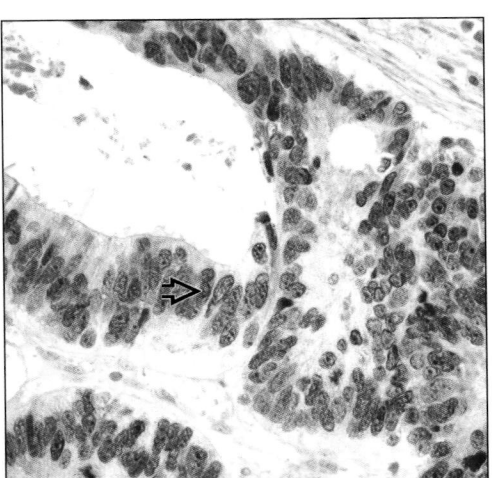

(Left) Prostate needle biopsy shows infiltrating moderately differentiated adenocarcinoma of colorectal primary invading the prostate. Prostate involvement by rectal adenocarcinoma denotes high-stage rectal cancer (pT4). (Right) CDX-2 ➡ immunohistochemical stain shows strong nuclear immunoreactivity in colonic adenocarcinoma. CDX-2 is helpful in distinguishing colonic carcinoma from prostate carcinoma, which is typically negative. PSA, PAP, and PSMA are also useful.

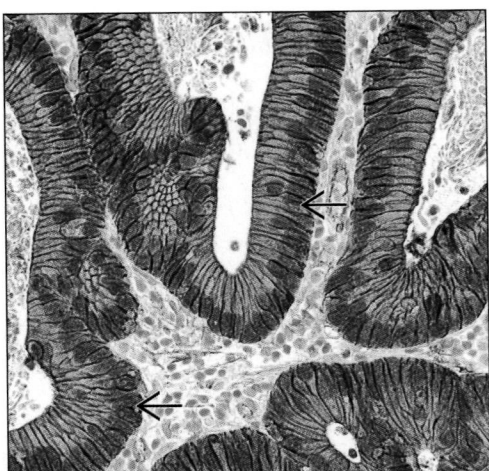

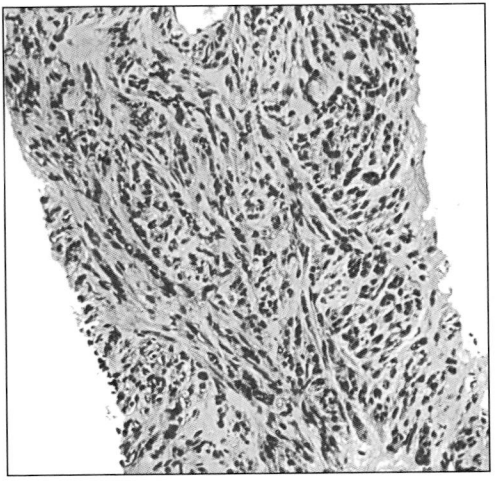

(Left) β-catenin stain shows nuclear positivity ➡ in colonic adenocarcinoma. In contrast to prostate carcinoma and primary bladder adenocarcinoma that may invade the prostate, colonic adenocarcinoma is commonly nuclear positive. (Right) GIST secondarily involving the prostate shows spindle cells mimicking primary prostatic sarcomas. GIST is strongly positive for CD117, in contrast to the common primary mesenchymal tumors of the prostate that are negative.

CYSTADENOMA AND EPITHELIAL STROMAL TUMOR

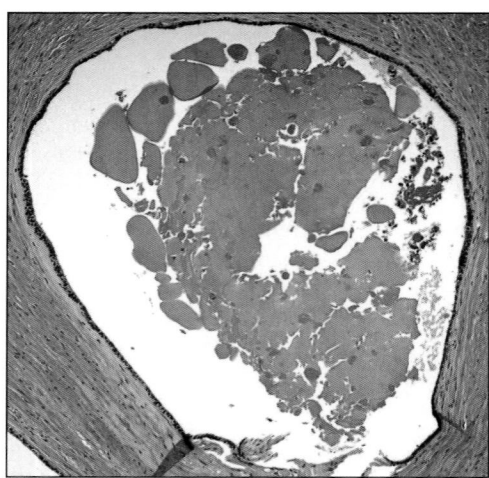

Seminal vesicle cystadenoma consists of cysts lined by single to few layers of epithelial cells and underlying fibromuscular stroma. The cyst lumen contains amorphous eosinophilic material.

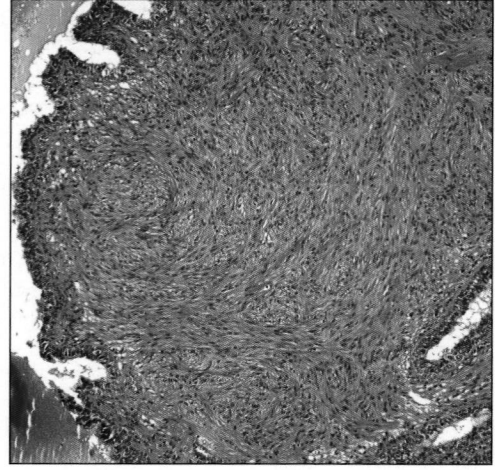

Seminal vesicle epithelial stromal tumor shows phyllodes-like growth pattern consisting of epithelium with investing cellular spindle cell stroma.

TERMINOLOGY

Synonyms
- Cystadenoma
  - Multilocular cyst
- Epithelial stromal tumors
  - Mesonephric hamartoma, fibroepithelial tumor, cystomyoma, mesenchymoma, phyllodes tumor, cystosarcoma phyllodes, müllerian adenosarcoma-like tumor

Definitions
- **Cystadenoma**
  - Benign cystic epithelial neoplasm of seminal vesicle
  - Tumor lacking significant stromal proliferation or containing only usual seminal vesicle-type stroma
- **Epithelial stromal tumor**
  - Seminal vesicle neoplasm with proliferation of both glandular and stromal elements
- Considerable overlap in literature with use of terminology regarding cystadenoma and low-grade epithelial stromal tumor
- Debatable whether cystadenoma is in same spectrum with low-grade epithelial stromal tumors that lack prominent stromal proliferation

ETIOLOGY/PATHOGENESIS

Developmental Anomaly
- No association with ureter or renal developmental anomalies, in contrast to nonneoplastic congenital seminal vesicle cysts, which have such an association

CLINICAL ISSUES

Epidemiology
- Incidence
  - Very rare

- Overall, < 25 reported tumors within spectrum of seminal vesicle cystadenoma and epithelial stromal tumors, including malignant cases
- Age
  - Mean: 51 years, range: 33-70 years

Presentation
- Obstructive symptoms most common
  - Acute urinary retention, decreased urine stream, hesitancy, frequency, dysuria, and nocturia
- Other symptoms include lower abdominal pain, painful ejaculation, constipation, fever
- Few cases are asymptomatic &/or detected as pelvic or rectal mass on physical examination

Laboratory Tests
- Normal serum PSA level
- Normal serum CA125 level (in contrast to seminal vesicle adenocarcinoma, which may have elevated level)

Treatment
- Tumor resection with vesiculectomy, prostatectomy, or cystoprostatectomy
- Systemic chemotherapy for malignant epithelial and stromal tumor, particularly if metastatic

Prognosis
- Cystadenoma has a benign course but may recur
- No metastasis reported in epithelial stromal tumors lacking high-grade features but may recur
- 2 reports of high-grade epithelial stromal tumors have demonstrated metastasis to lung with subsequent death in 1 patient

CYSTADENOMA AND EPITHELIAL STROMAL TUMOR

Key Facts

Clinical Issues
- Rare, < 25 reported tumors within spectrum of seminal vesicle cystadenoma and epithelial stromal tumors
- Obstructive symptoms most common presentation
- Cystadenoma and low-grade epithelial stromal tumors have benign course but may recur
- 2 reports of high-grade epithelial stromal tumors with metastasis

Microscopic Pathology
- Cystadenoma
  ○ Consists of multiple variably sized cystic and glandular formations lined by single to few layers of bland cuboidal to low columnar epithelial cells
  ○ Variable amount of stroma that resembles usual seminal vesicle fibromuscular stroma

- Epithelial stromal tumors
  ○ Consist of neoplastic proliferation of both glandular and stromal elements
  ○ May have broad leaf-like growth consisting of epithelium with investing spindle cell stroma (phyllodes-like growth)
  ○ Histologic spectrum of benign to malignant tumors defined by degree of atypicality of stromal component
  ○ Includes low-grade fibroadenoma/adenomyoma and high-grade epithelial stromal tumors
  ○ High-grade tumors contain frank sarcomatous areas, including marked stromal overgrowth, pleomorphism, frequent mitosis, and necrosis

Ancillary Tests
- Epithelial component PSA/PAP(-)

IMAGE FINDINGS

General Features
- CT and MR show multilocular cystic or solid-cystic pelvic mass centered in region of seminal vesicle between rectum and urinary bladder or prostate
- Tumor may appear more solid in malignant cases
- Large mass often compresses or displaces urinary bladder and prostate
- Imaging may be key to determine origin (seminal vesicle vs. prostate), particularly in biopsy specimens

MACROSCOPIC FEATURES

General Features
- Lobulated mass with glistening, smooth, tan surface and multilocular or solid-cystic cut surface
  ○ Cysts may contain gelatinous to serous fluid
  ○ Malignant tumors are relatively more solid, reflecting marked sarcomatous overgrowth
- Mass located at seminal vesicle bed; may be seen contiguous with identifiable seminal vesicle remnants
- May be completely separable from prostate or bladder in radical excision specimens
- Most reports detailing gross examination have described unilateral involvement

Size
- Range: 3-16 cm in largest dimension, mean: 8.9 cm

MICROSCOPIC PATHOLOGY

Histologic Features
- **Cystadenoma**
  ○ Multiple variably sized cystic and glandular formations
  ○ Lined by single to few layers of bland cuboidal to low columnar epithelial cells
  ○ Nuclei are round, regular, with inconspicuous nucleoli

  ○ Cysts and glands may contain homogeneous or amorphous eosinophilic material
  ○ Variable amount of stroma that resembles usual seminal vesicle fibromuscular stroma
- **Epithelial stromal tumors**
  ○ Consist of neoplastic proliferation of both glandular and stromal elements
  ○ May have broad, leaf-like growth consisting of epithelium with investing spindle cell stroma (phyllodes-like growth)
    ■ This architectural pattern may not be seen in all cases; therefore, term "epithelial stromal tumor" is preferred over "phyllodes tumor"
  ○ **Epithelial component**
    ■ Cysts and glands vary in size and shape, sometimes branching, distorted, or slit-like
    ■ Lining epithelium consists of single to few layers of cuboidal or low columnar cells, generally lacking marked atypia
    ■ Occasionally, 2 cell layers may be seen, consisting of inner layer of cuboidal or low columnar cells and basal layer of cuboidal or flattened cells
    ■ Focal cellular stratification may be present
    ■ Lipofuscin pigment may rarely be appreciated
  ○ **Stromal component**
    ■ Stroma composed of spindled cells with varying degree of cellularity
    ■ Tendency of spindle cells to be more cellular or condensed around cysts and glandular formations
    ■ Rare case with myomatous (adenomyoma) or myxomatous stroma with spindle cells
    ■ Less cellular areas may show pale basophilic stroma
  ○ Cysts and glands may contain homogeneous or amorphous eosinophilic materials, mucinous material, and rarely, eosinophilic crystalline debris
  ○ Blending of cystic tumor with seminal vesicle fibromuscular wall and lining epithelium, which contains lipofuscin pigment, may be present
  ○ Degree of atypia of stromal component helps in distinction between benign and malignant tumors and their stratification

CYSTADENOMA AND EPITHELIAL STROMAL TUMOR

- Epithelial stromal tumors classified into
  - **Fibroadenoma/Adenomyoma**
    - Hypocellular stroma with no cytologic atypia or mitosis
    - Epithelium consists of single to few layers of cuboidal to low columnar cells with no atypia or mitosis
    - Biphasic tumor containing benign myomatous stroma (adenomyoma) has been reported
  - **Low-grade epithelial stromal tumors**
    - Stroma is hypercellular and may show cytologic atypia and rare mitoses
    - Some authors classify tumors with marked stromal pleomorphism but with absent or rare mitotic activity and no necrosis as intermediate grade
  - **High-grade epithelial stromal tumors**
    - Demonstrate frank sarcomatous areas characterized by marked stromal overgrowth, pleomorphism, frequent mitoses, and necrosis
    - Atypical mitoses may be present
    - Marked stromal pleomorphism is characterized by spindle cells with large bizarre hyperchromatic or anaplastic nuclei
    - Although epithelial component may be atypical and exhibit stratification, there is no obvious carcinomatous change

Predominant Pattern/Injury Type
- Neoplastic

Predominant Cell/Compartment Type
- Epithelial, glandular
- Mesenchymal, spindle

ANCILLARY TESTS

Immunohistochemistry
- Epithelial component
  - PAN-CK(AE1/AE3)(+)
  - HMCK(34βE12)(+) may detect presence of basal cells
  - PSA/PAP(-)
  - CA125(-)
- Stromal component
  - Vimentin(+)
  - CD34(+)
  - Actin-sm and desmin (variable +)

Electron Microscopy
- Epithelial component
  - Cells contain intracytoplasmic tonofilaments
  - Microvilli within glandular lumens
  - Cells joined by desmosomes and junctional complexes
  - Does not show larger, irregular cytolysosomes containing lipid-like and electron-dense material seen in normal seminal vesicle epithelium
- Stromal component
  - Variable fibroblastic to myoblastic differentiation

DIFFERENTIAL DIAGNOSIS

Congenital or Developmental Seminal Vesicle Cysts
- Most are congential and associated with ipsilateral ectopic ureter and renal dysplasia or agenesis
- Acquired cysts may be due to genitourinary infection, prostate surgery, or ejaculatory duct lithiasis
- Cyst is usually unilocular but may be multilocular
- Easily evacuated by needle puncture
- Histologically resembles dilated seminal vesicle with attenuated epithelial lining
- Cyst contents may include spermatozoa debris, blood, or inflammatory cells

Phyllodes Tumor of Prostate
- Histologically similar to phyllodes-type epithelial stromal tumor of seminal vesicle
- Tumor is grossly and histologically intimately associated with prostatic parenchyma
- Glandular epithelial component PSA/PAP(+)

DIAGNOSTIC CHECKLIST

Pathologic Interpretation Pearls
- Seminal vesicle cystadenoma
  - Benign multilocular cyst lined by single to few layers of bland cuboidal or columnar cells lacking significant stromal proliferation
- Seminal vesicle epithelial and stromal tumor
  - Neoplasm consisting of mixed epithelial and stromal proliferation, sometimes exhibiting phyllodes-like growth, with varying stromal atypia ranging from benign to frank sarcomatous features

SELECTED REFERENCES

1. Lorber G et al: Seminal Vesicle Cystadenoma: A Rare Clinical Perspective. Eur Urol. Epub ahead of print, 2009
2. Monica B et al: Low grade epithelial stromal tumour of the seminal vesicle. World J Surg Oncol. 6:101, 2008
3. Son HJ et al: Phyllodes tumor of the seminal vesicle: case report and literature review. Pathol Int. 54(12):924-9, 2004
4. Abe H et al: Cystosarcoma phyllodes of the seminal vesicle. Int J Urol. 9(10):599-601, 2002
5. Baschinsky DY et al: Seminal vesicle cystadenoma: a case report and literature review. Urology. 51(5):840-5, 1998
6. Fain JS et al: Cystosarcoma phyllodes of the seminal vesicle. Cancer. 71(6):2055-61, 1993
7. Laurila P et al: Mullerian adenosarcomalike tumor of the seminal vesicle. A case report with immunohistochemical and ultrastructural observations. Arch Pathol Lab Med. 116(10):1072-6, 1992
8. Mazzucchelli L et al: Cystadenoma of the seminal vesicle: case report and literature review. J Urol. 147(6):1621-4, 1992
9. Mazur MT et al: Cystic epithelial-stromal tumor of the seminal vesicle. Am J Surg Pathol. 11(3):210-7, 1987
10. Damjanov I et al: Cystadenoma of seminal vesicles. J Urol. 111(6):808-9, 1974

CYSTADENOMA AND EPITHELIAL STROMAL TUMOR

Microscopic Features

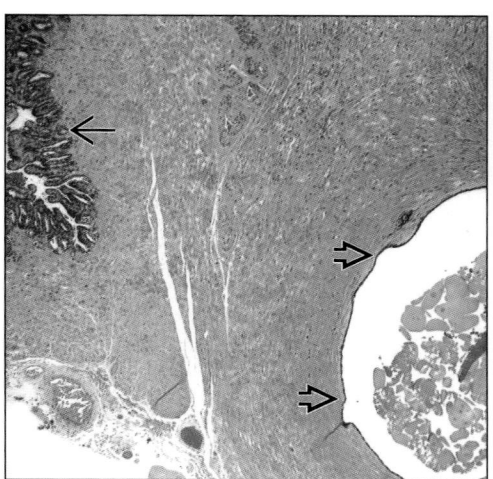
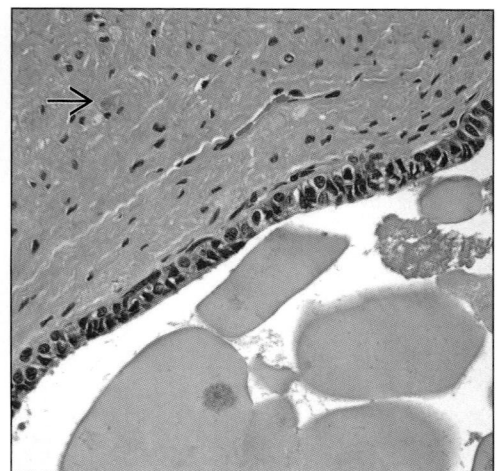

(Left) Cystadenoma contiguous with seminal vesicle fibromuscular wall is seen. Normal seminal vesicle glandular epithelium may be visible ➡, which contrasts with the adjacent cystadenoma ⊟ that shows simple lining epithelium with luminal eosinophilic material. (Right) Lining epithelium shows few layers of cuboidal cells with bland nuclei. The stroma is less cellular and is similar to the usual seminal vesicle fibromuscular stroma, which may contain dense hyaline bodies ➡.

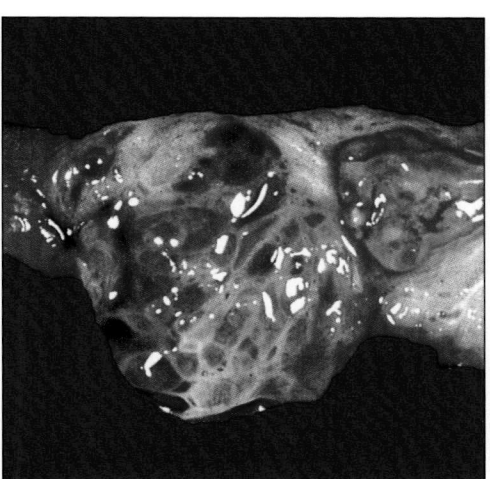
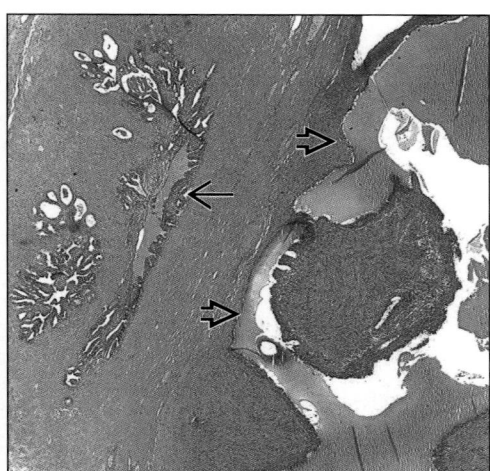

(Left) Gross photograph of seminal vesicle epithelial stromal tumor shows multicystic cut surface. (Courtesy E.C. Jones, MD.) (Right) An epithelial stromal tumor ⊟ contiguous with the seminal vesicle fibromuscular wall is seen. Normal seminal vesicle glandular epithelium is present ➡ adjacent to a dilated neoplastic cyst with polypoid growth, which contains more cellular stroma. Note the presence of eosinophilic material in the cystic lumen.

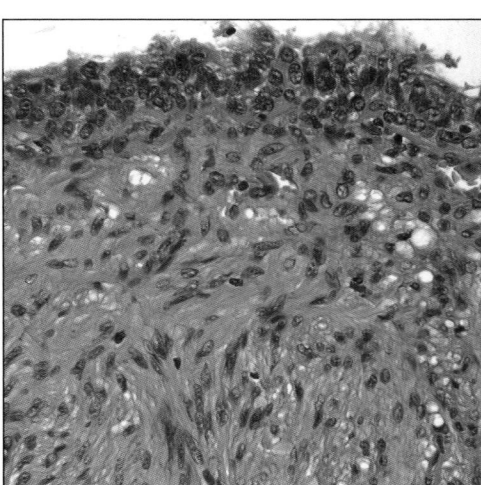
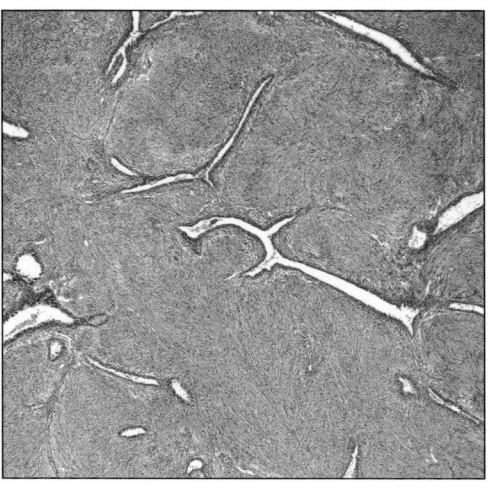

(Left) Low-grade epithelial stromal tumor shows few layers of bland polygonal cell epithelial lining and subjacent spindle cell stroma, lacking both cellular atypia and mitoses. (Right) Epithelial stromal tumor consists of several branching slit-like glands surrounded by a spindle cell stromal proliferation. The spindle cell stroma may vary in cellularity. The degree of stromal atypia defines the histologic (and biologic) spectrum of this tumor.

SEMINAL VESICLE ADENOCARCINOMA

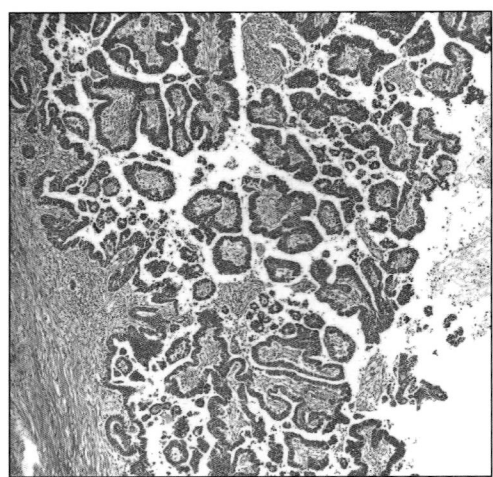

Seminal vesicle adenocarcinoma is shown with papillary architecture, which is the most recognized feature of this tumor. (Courtesy L. Egevad, MD, PhD.)

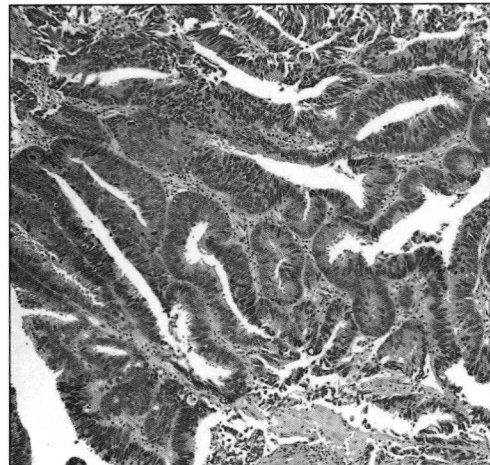

Seminal vesicle adenocarcinoma is shown with tubuloglandular formations. These malignant glands are lined by high-grade columnar cells. (Courtesy L. Egevad, MD, PhD.)

TERMINOLOGY

Synonyms
- Papillary adenocarcinoma of seminal vesicle

Definitions
- Malignant neoplasm of seminal vesicle glandular epithelial cell origin

CLINICAL ISSUES

Epidemiology
- Incidence
  - Rare; < 55 acceptable published cases
- Age
  - Mean: 63 years, range: 19-90 years
  - 1/5 of patients younger than 40 years

Presentation
- Bladder outlet obstruction
- Hematuria
- Hematospermia
- Pelvic or perineal pain
- Mostly palpable as nontender mass above or contiguous with prostate on digital rectal examination

Laboratory Tests
- Serum CA125 elevated
  - Can be useful in monitoring disease
- Serum PSA and PAP levels normal
- Serum CEA can be elevated

Natural History
- Manifests with advanced symptomatic disease

Treatment
- Mainstay is surgical resection with negative margin
- Adjuvant radiotherapy or androgen deprivation able to prolong survival in some patients

Prognosis
- Extremely poor
- Although ~ 1/2 of cases in recent reports are free of recurrence after 1 to 4 years
- Majority of patients with metastasis at time of diagnosis

IMAGE FINDINGS

General Features
- Computed tomography scan and transrectal ultrasound helpful in diagnosis
- Solid or partly cystic mass centered at seminal vesicle area between rectum and bladder or prostate

MACROSCOPIC FEATURES

General Features
- Usually large and invades adjacent bladder or rectum
- Irregular, firm, gray-white to brown tumor nodules
- May be partly cystic
- Bilateral involvement in 8% of cases

MICROSCOPIC PATHOLOGY

Histologic Features
- Variable histologic pattern
- Papillary architecture lined by columnar cells is most recognized feature
- Can be glandular or poorly differentiated tumor with solid, nested, or cord-like growth
- May have clear cells or "hobnail" morphology
  - Similar to clear cell adenocarcinoma of female genital tract
- Mucin production present, sometimes may be copious
- Desmoplasia seen around infiltrating glands
- Carcinoma in situ may be seen
  - Helpful in poorly differentiated cases

SEMINAL VESICLE ADENOCARCINOMA

Key Facts

Terminology
- Malignant neoplasm of seminal vesicle glandular epithelial cell origin

Clinical Issues
- Rare
- Mean age: 63 years; range: 19-90 years
- Presents mostly with bladder outlet obstruction
- Serum CA125 elevated, PSA and PAP normal
- Extremely poor prognosis

Macroscopic Features
- Usually large and invades adjacent bladder or rectum

Microscopic Pathology
- Papillary pattern lined by columnar cells
- Can be glandular or poorly differentiated tumor with solid, nested, or cord-like growths
- May have clear cells or "hobnail" morphology
- Mucin production present, sometimes copious
- Typically CA125(+), PSA/PAP(-), CK7(+)/CK20(-)

ANCILLARY TESTS

Immunohistochemistry
- CA125(+)
- PSA(-) and PAP(-)
- Typically CK7(+)/CK20(-)
- CEA variably (+)

DIFFERENTIAL DIAGNOSIS

Seminal Vesicle Cystadenoma
- Very rare benign tumor
- Cystically dilated glandular spaces with pale intraluminal secretions lined by few layers of cuboidal or columnar cells surrounded by spindle cell stroma
- Lacks cytologic atypia and invasive features

Prostate Adenocarcinoma
- Secondary involvement of seminal vesicle considerably more common than primary adenocarcinoma
- Ductal adenocarcinoma with papillary architecture mimics seminal vesicle adenocarcinoma
- Unusual to have cystic growth
- Stromal desmoplastic response not typical
- PSA/PAP(+), CA125(-)

Urinary Bladder Adenocarcinoma
- Correlation of clinical, radiologic, and gross findings critical

- CA125(-); most are CK7(+)/CK20(+)

Rectal Adenocarcinoma
- Correlation of clinical, radiologic, and gross findings critical
- Typically invasive intestinal-type glands with abundant necrosis ("dirty necrosis")
- CA125(-); most are CK7(-)/CK20(+)

DIAGNOSTIC CHECKLIST

Pathologic Interpretation Pearls
- Diagnosis requires careful clinical, radiologic, gross, and histologic correlation for adenocarcinoma, usually high-grade papillary, centered at seminal vesicle area

SELECTED REFERENCES

1. Egevad L et al: Primary seminal vesicle carcinoma detected at transurethral resection of prostate. Urology. 69(4):778, 2007
2. Thiel R et al: Primary adenocarcinoma of the seminal vesicles. J Urol. 168(5):1891-6, 2002
3. Ormsby AH et al: Primary seminal vesicle carcinoma: an immunohistochemical analysis of four cases. Mod Pathol. 13(1):46-51, 2000
4. Benson RC Jr et al: Carcinoma of the seminal vesicle. J Urol. 132(3):483-5, 1984

IMAGE GALLERY

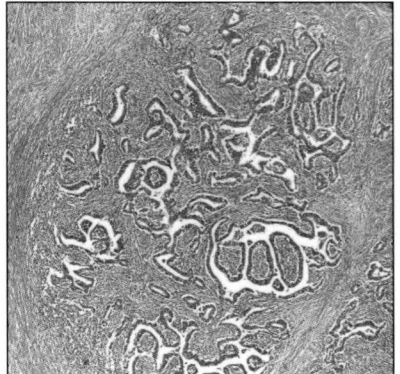 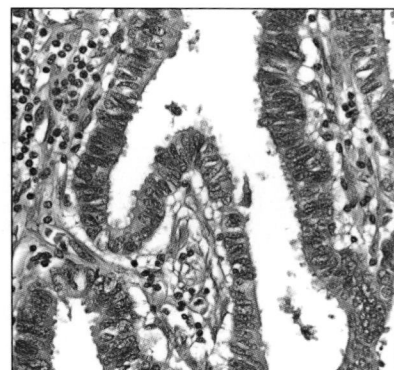 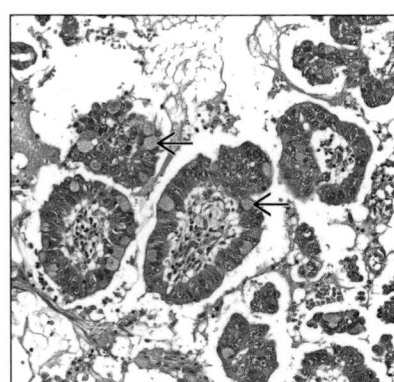

(Left) Seminal vesicle adenocarcinoma shows tubulopapillary formations with associated stromal fibrosis. *(Center)* Seminal vesical adenocarcinoma shows glands lined by columnar cells with high-grade hyperchromatic nuclei and can be difficult to distinguish from primary adenocarcinoma of rectum or bladder. *(Right)* Papillary projections can be complex and show detached fronds. Occasionally, intracellular mucin production ➔ can be seen. (Courtesy L. Egevad, MD, PhD.)

PROTOCOL FOR PROSTATE CANCER SPECIMENS

Prostate Gland: Needle Biopsy

Surgical Pathology Cancer Case Summary (Checklist)

Histologic Type

____ Adenocarcinoma (acinar, not otherwise specified)

____ Other (specify): _____

Histologic Grade

Gleason pattern

(If 3 patterns present, use most predominant pattern and worst pattern of remaining 2)

____ Not applicable

____ Cannot be determined

Primary (predominant) pattern

____ Grade 1

____ Grade 2

____ Grade 3

____ Grade 4

____ Grade 5

Secondary (worst remaining) pattern

____ Grade 1

____ Grade 2

____ Grade 3

____ Grade 4

____ Grade 5

Total Gleason score: _____

Tumor Quantitation

Number cores positive: _____

Total number of cores: _____

> **or**

Total number of cores: _____

> **and**

Total linear millimeters of carcinoma: _____ mm

Total linear millimeters of needle core tissue: _____ mm

> **or**

Number cores positive: _____

Total number of cores: _____

> **and**

Proportion (percent) of prostatic tissue involved by tumor: _____ %

> **and**

Total linear millimeters of carcinoma: _____ mm

Total linear millimeters of needle core tissue: _____ mm

*Proportion (percentage) of prostatic tissue involved by tumor for core with the greatest amount of tumor: _____ %

Periprostatic Fat Invasion (document if identified)

*____ Not identified

____ Present

Seminal Vesicle Invasion (document if identified)

*____ Not identified

____ Present

*Lymph-Vascular Invasion

*____ Not identified

*____ Present

*____ Indeterminate

PROTOCOL FOR PROSTATE CANCER SPECIMENS

*Perineural Invasion

* *____ Not identified
* *____ Present

*Additional Pathologic Findings (select all that apply)

* *____ None identified
* *____ High-grade prostatic intraepithelial neoplasia (PIN)
* *____ Atypical adenomatous hyperplasia (adenosis)
* *____ Inflammation (specify type): _____
* *____ Other (specify): _____

The Gleason grade and score and tumor extent measures should be documented for each positive specimen (container). The essential information in each specimen could be conveyed with a simple diagnostic line such as, "Adenocarcinoma, Gleason grade 3 + 4 = score of 7, in 1 of 2 cores, involving 20% of needle core tissue, and measuring 4 mm in length." * Data elements with asterisks are not required. However, these elements may be clinically important but are not yet validated or regularly used in patient management. Adapted with permission from College of American Pathologists, "Protocol for the Examination of Specimens from Patients with Carcinoma of the Prostate Gland." Web posting date October 2009, www.cap.org.

Prostate Gland: Transurethral Prostatic Resection (TUR), Enucleation Specimen (Subtotal Prostatectomy)

Surgical Pathology Cancer Case Summary (Checklist)

Procedure

____ Transurethral prostatic resection

____ Enucleation

____ Other (specify): _____

____ Not specified

Specimen Size

Weight: _____ g

Size (enucleation specimens only: _____ x _____ x _____ cm

Histologic Type

____ Adenocarcinoma (acinar, not otherwise specified)

____ Other (specify): _____

Histologic Grade

Gleason pattern

(If 3 patterns present, use most predominant pattern and worst pattern of remaining 2)

____ Not applicable

____ Cannot be determined

Primary (predominant pattern)

____ Grade 1

____ Grade 2

____ Grade 3

____ Grade 4

____ Grade 5

Secondary (worst remaining) pattern

____ Grade 1

____ Grade 2

____ Grade 3

____ Grade 4

____ Grade 5

Total Gleason score: _____

Tumor Quantitation: TUR Specimens

Proportion (percentage) of prostatic tissue involved by tumor: _____ %

____ Tumor incidental histologic finding in no more than 5% of tissue resected with Gleason score 2 to 6 (cT1a)

____ Tumor incidental histologic finding in more than 5% of tissue resected or Gleason score 7 to 10 (cT1b)

*Number of positive chips: _____

*Total number of chips: _____

PROTOCOL FOR PROSTATE CANCER SPECIMENS

Tumor Quantitation: Enucleation Specimens

Proportion (percent) of prostatic tissue involved by tumor: _____ %

*Tumor size (dominant nodule, if present)

    *Greatest dimension: _____ cm

    *Additional dimensions: _____ x _____ cm

Periprostatic Fat Invasion (document if identified)

*____ Not identified

____ Present

Seminal Vesicle Invasion (document if identified)

*____ Not identified

____ Present

*Lymph-Vascular Invasion

*____ Not identified

*____ Present

*____ Indeterminate

*Perineural Invasion

*____ Not identified

*____ Present

*Additional Pathologic Findings (select all that apply)

*____ None identified

*____ High-grade prostatic intraepithelial neoplasia (PIN)

*____ Atypical adenomatous hyperplasia (adenosis)

*____ Nodular prostatic hyperplasia

*____ Inflammation (specify type): _____

*____ Other (specify): _____

*Data elements with asterisks are not required. However, these elements may be clinically important but are not yet validated or regularly used in patient management.

Prostate Gland: Radical Prostatectomy

Surgical Pathology Cancer Case Summary (Checklist)

Procedure

____ Radical prostatectomy

____ Other (specify): _____

____ Not specified

Prostate Size

Weight: _____ g

Size: _____ x _____ x _____ cm

Lymph Node Sampling

____ No lymph nodes present

____ Pelvic lymph node dissection

Histologic Type

____ Adenocarcinoma (acinar, not otherwise specified)

____ Prostatic duct adenocarcinoma

____ Mucinous (colloid) adenocarcinoma

____ Signet ring cell carcinoma

____ Adenosquamous carcinoma

____ Small cell carcinoma

____ Sarcomatoid carcinoma

____ Undifferentiated carcinoma, not otherwise specified

____ Other (specify): _____

Histologic Grade

Gleason pattern

PROTOCOL FOR PROSTATE CANCER SPECIMENS

(If 3 patterns are present, record the most predominant and second most common patterns; the tertiary pattern should be recorded if higher than the primary and secondary patterns but it is not incorporated into the Gleason score)

____ Not applicable

____ Cannot be determined

Primary pattern

    ____ Grade 1

    ____ Grade 2

    ____ Grade 3

    ____ Grade 4

    ____ Grade 5

Secondary pattern

    ____ Grade 1

    ____ Grade 2

    ____ Grade 3

    ____ Grade 4

    ____ Grade 5

Tertiary pattern

    ____ Grade 3

    ____ Grade 4

    ____ Grade 5

    ____ Not applicable

Total Gleason score: _____

Tumor Quantitation

Proportion (percentage) of prostate involved by tumor: _____ %

  &/or

Tumor size (dominant nodule, if present)

  Greatest dimension: _____ mm

  Additional dimensions: _____ x _____ mm

Extraprostatic Extension (select all that apply)

____ Not identified

____ Present

  ____ Focal

    *Specify site(s): _____

  ____ Nonfocal (established, extensive)

    *Specify site(s): _____

____ Indeterminate

Seminal Vesicle Invasion (invasion of muscular wall required)

____ Not identified

____ Present

____ No seminal vesicle present

Margins (select all that apply)

____ Cannot be assessed

*____ Benign glands at surgical margin

____ Margins uninvolved by invasive carcinoma

____ Margin(s) involved by invasive carcinoma

  *____ Unifocal

  *____ Multifocal

  ____ Apical

  ____ Bladder neck

  ____ Lateral

  ____ Posterolateral (neurovascular bundle)

  ____ Posterior

  ____ Other(s) (specify): _____

PROTOCOL FOR PROSTATE CANCER SPECIMENS

Treatment Effect on Carcinoma (select all that apply)

____ Not identified

____ Radiation therapy effect present

____ Hormonal therapy effect present

____ Other therapy effect(s) present (specify): _____

Lymph-Vascular Invasion

____ Not identified

____ Present

____ Indeterminate

*Perineural Invasion

*____ Not identified

*____ Present

Pathologic Staging (pTNM)

TNM descriptors (required only if applicable) (select all that apply)

____ m (multiple)

____ r (recurrent)

____ y (post-treatment)

Primary tumor (pT)

____ Not identified

____ pT2: Organ confined

*____ pT2a: Unilateral, involving 1/2 of 1 slide or less

*____ pT2b: Unilateral, involving > 1/2 of 1 slide but not both sides

*____ pT2c: Bilateral disease

pT3: Extraprostatic extension

____ pT3a: Extraprostatic extension or microscopic invasion of bladder neck

____ pT3b: Seminal vesicle invasion

____ pT4: Invasion of rectum, levator muscles, &/or pelvic wall

Note: There is no pathologic T1 classification. Subdivision of pT2 disease is problematic and has not proven to be of prognostic significance.

Regional lymph nodes (pN)

____ pNX: Cannot be assessed

____ pN0: No regional lymph node metastasis

____ pN1: Metastasis in regional lymph node or nodes

Specify

Number examined: _____

Number involved: _____

Diameter of largest lymph node metastasis: _____ mm

Distant metastasis (pM)

____ Not applicable

____ pM1: Distant metastasis

____ pM1a: Nonregional lymph node(s)

____ pM1b: Bone(s)

____ pM1c: Other site(s) with or without bone disease

Note: When > 1 site of metastasis is present, the most advanced category is used. pM1c is most advanced.

*Additional Pathologic Findings (select all that apply)

*____ None identified

*____ High-grade prostatic intraepithelial neoplasia (PIN)

*____ Inflammation (specify type): _____

*____ Atypical adenomatous hyperplasia (adenosis)

*____ Nodular prostatic hyperplasia

*____ Other (specify): _____

*Ancillary Studies

*Specify: _____

PROTOCOL FOR PROSTATE CANCER SPECIMENS

*____ Not performed

*Data elements with asterisks are not required. However, these elements may be clinically important but are not yet validated or regularly used in patient management.

Anatomic Stage/Prognostic Groups

Group	T	N	M	PSA	Gleason
1	T1a-c	N0	M0	PSA < 10	Gleason ≤ 6
	T2a	N0	M0	PSA < 10	Gleason ≤ 6
	T1-2a	N0	M0	PSA < 20	Gleason X
IIA	T1a-c	N0	M0	PSA < 20	Gleason 7
	T1a-c	N0	M0	PSA ≥ 10 < 20	Gleason ≤ 6
	T2a	N0	M0	PSA < 20	Gleason ≤ 7
	T2b	N0	M0	PSA < 20	Gleason ≤ 7
	T2b	N0	M0	PSA X	Gleason X
IIB	T2c	N0	M0	Any PSA	Any Gleason
	T1-2	N0	M0	PSA ≥ 20	Any Gleason
	T1-2	N0	M0	Any PSA	Gleason ≥ 8
III	T3a-c	N0	M0	Any PSA	Any Gleason
IV	T4	N0	M0	Any PSA	Any Gleason
	Any T	N1	M0	Any PSA	Any Gleason
	Any T	Any N	M1	Any PSA	Any Gleason

Note: When either prostate specific antigen (PSA) or Gleason is not available, grouping should be determined by T stage &/or whichever of either the PSA or Gleason is available. Used with the permission of the American Joint Committee on Cancer (AJCC), Chicago, Illinois. The original source for this material is the AJCC Cancer Staging Manual, Seventh Edition (2010) published by Springer Science and Business Media LLC, www.springerlink.com.

IMMUNOHISTOCHEMISTRY, PROSTATE

Prostatic Adenocarcinoma and Its Mimics

Antibody	Adenocarcinoma	Seminal Vessel & Ejaculatory Duct	Nephrogenic Adenoma	Cowper Gland	Mesonephric Hyperplasia*	Stromal Sarcoma	Small Cell Carcinoma
PSA	+	-/+	-/weak +	-/+ (rare)	-	-	-
PAP	+	-/+	-/weak+	-	-	-	-
PSMA	+	-	-	-	-	-	-
CD57	+	-	-	-	-	-	-
AR	+	+	-	-	+	-	+/-
AMACR	+	-/NS	+/-	-	-	-	-/+ (47%)
HMCK(34βE12)	-	+ (basal cells)	-/+	+	-/+ (33%)	-	-
PAN-CK(AE1/AE3)	+	+	+	+	-/+	-	+ (dot-like)
Pax-2	-	+	+	ND	-	-	-
Actin-sm	-	-	-	+	-	-/+	-
Desmin	-	-	-	ND	-	-/+	-
MyoD1	-	-	-	-	-	-	-
Myogenin	-	-	-	-	-	-	-
CD99	-	-	-	-	ND	-	-/+
CD45(LCA)	-	-	-	-		-	-
ER	+/-	-	-	ND	-	-/+	-
PR	+/-	-	-	ND	-	+	-
CD34	-	-	-	-	-	+	-
p63	-	+ (basal cells)	-/+	+	+/-	-	-
CD117	-	-	-	-	-	-	-
Synaptophysin	V	-	-	-	-	-	+
Chromogranin	V	-	-	-	-	-	+
CD56	V	-	-	-	-	-	+
TTF-1	-	-	-	-	-	-	+

*ND = No Data, V = Variable, NS = Nonspecific staining in pigment. *Mesonephric remnants also positive for CD10, calretinin, and vimentin.*

Important Immunohistochemical Stains in Diagnosis of Prostate Carcinoma

Immunostain	Rationale for Use
Basal cell-associated markers HMCK(34βE12), CK5/6, p63, basal cell cocktail	Benign vs. malignant proliferation; complete absence of basal cell layer is defining criterion for invasive prostate carcinoma
Prostate carcinoma-associated marker AMACR (p504S)	Benign vs. malignant proliferation; absence of basal cell-associated markers favoring invasive prostate carcinoma
Epithelial lineage PAN-CK(AE1/AE3)	Identification of subtle infiltrating cells in post-treatment setting; in differential diagnosis of carcinoma vs. nonepithelial process or malignancy
Prostate lineage-specific marker PSA, PAP, PSMA	Prostatic vs. nonprostatic origin, e.g., Cowper gland, mesonephric remnant, nephrogenic adenoma, seminal vesicle vs. prostate cancer

Atypical Glandular Proliferations, Small Glands

Antibody	Benign Glands	Post-Atrophic Hyperplasia and Atrophy	Prostatic Adenocarcinoma	Basal Cell Hyperplasia	Outpouching of High-Grade PIN	AAH (Adenosis)
Basal cell-associated markers	+	+ (patchy)	-	+	+	-/+ (patchy)
AMACR	-/+ (rare)	-/+	+ (strong circumferential)	-	+	-/+

Single-Individual Cell Patterns

Antibody	Gleason Pattern 5 Prostate Carcinoma	Post-Treatment Carcinoma	Marked Inflammation	Granulomatous Prostatitis
PAN-CK(AE1/AE3)	+	+		-
Basal cell marker	-	-		-
AMACR	+	+/-		-

IMMUNOHISTOCHEMISTRY, PROSTATE

Select Large Glandular Proliferations

Antibody	Cribriform Gleason Patterns 3, 4, 5	Ductal Adenocarcinoma	High-Grade PIN	Carcinoma with Intraductal Growth	Squamous and Urothelial Metaplasia
Basal cell marker	-	-/+	+	+	+
AMACR	+	+	+/-	+	-

Benign Mimics of Prostate Carcinoma

Antibody	Seminal Vesicle Ejaculatory Duct	Cowper Gland	Mesonephric Remnants	Verumontanum Hyperplasia	Nephrogenic Adenoma
PSA/PAP	-/+	-/+	-	+/-	-/+
Basal cell marker	+ (basal cell)	+	-/+	+ (basal cell)	-/+
AMACR	-/NS	-	-	-	+/-

NS is nonspecific, frequently marks pigment. Mesonephric remnants are also positive for CD10, calretinin, and vimentin.

3

Prostate Immunohistochemical Features

(Left) HMCK(34βE12) highlights basal cells in benign prostatic acini. Secretory cells are negative. HMCK(34βE12) is a high molecular weight keratin that stains intermediate cytoplasmic keratin filaments present only in basal cells. *(Right)* p63 shows nuclear positivity in basal cells of benign prostatic acini. Secretory cells are negative. p63 is comparable to HMCK(34βE12) in sensitivity and specificity, although nuclear localization of p63 provides greater sensitivity.

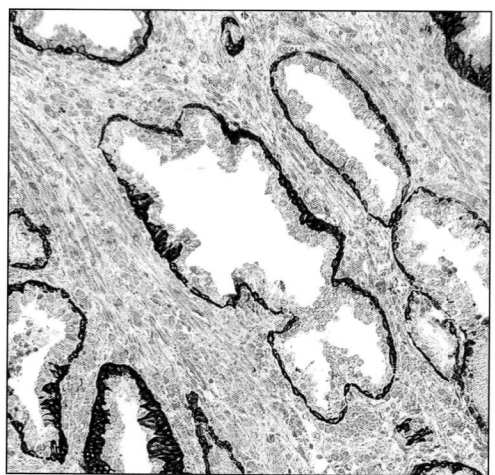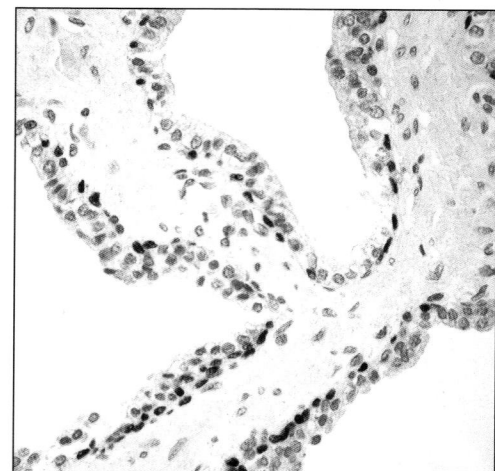

(Left) HMCK(34βE12) shows patchy basal cell positivity in AAH. *(Right)* Some foci of atrophy show patchy ➡ or negative ▷ p63 staining in occasional glands. The presence of basal cell staining argues against a malignant diagnosis. Diagnosis of carcinoma requires complete absence of basal cell marker staining in all atypical glands in the atypical focus. Comparison of staining reaction in another level, if available, would be helpful.

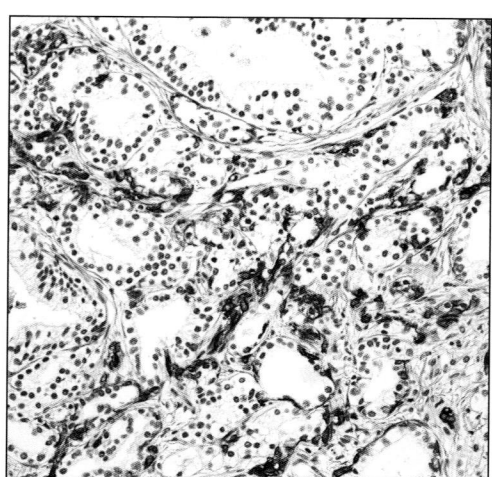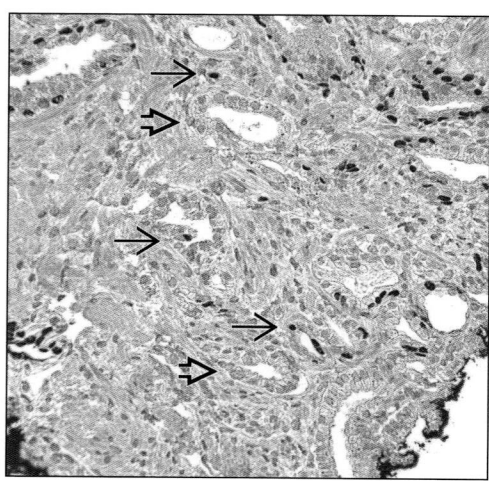

(Left) HMCK(34βE12) shows absent staining in a focus of atypical small acinar proliferation (ASAP) ➡. Adjacent benign acini show presence of HMCK(34βE12) staining ➡. *(Right)* p63 shows a rare basal cell in 1 gland of ASAP ▷. Other atypical glands are completely negative ➡. Adjacent benign glands ➡ show more consistent p63 positivity in basal cells. Diagnosis of carcinoma requires complete absence of basal cell markers in all atypical glands in suspicious foci.

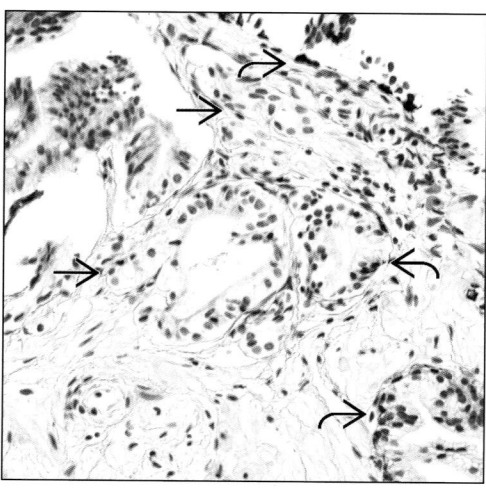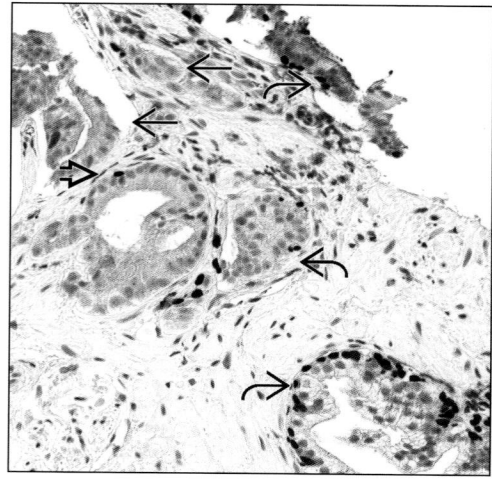

3

Prostate Immunohistochemical Features

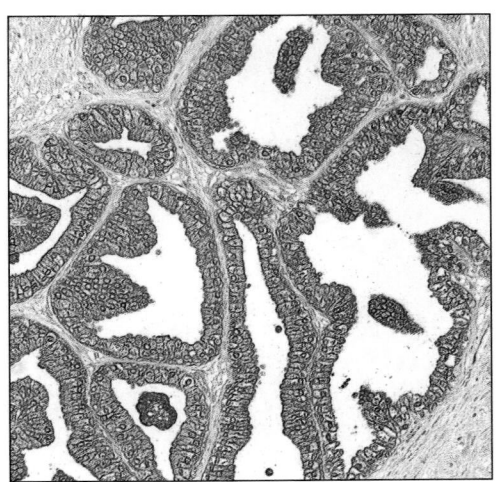

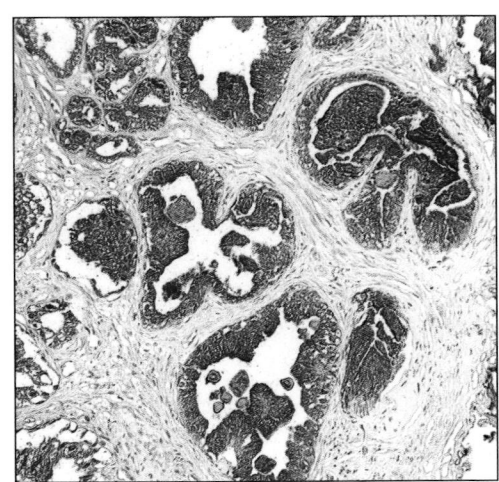

(Left) PSA shows cytoplasmic positivity in benign prostatic acini. PSA and PAP are used to confirm prostatic acinar cell origin and are useful in ruling out nonprostatic carcinoma mimics. Another use of PSA and PAP is in the differential diagnosis of unusual variants of prostate carcinoma (positive) vs. secondary tumors involving prostate, such as bladder or colonic adenocarcinomas (typically negative). (Right) PAP shows cytoplasmic positivity in benign prostatic acini.

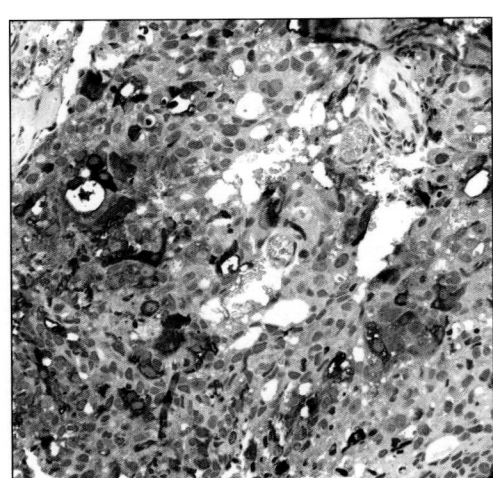

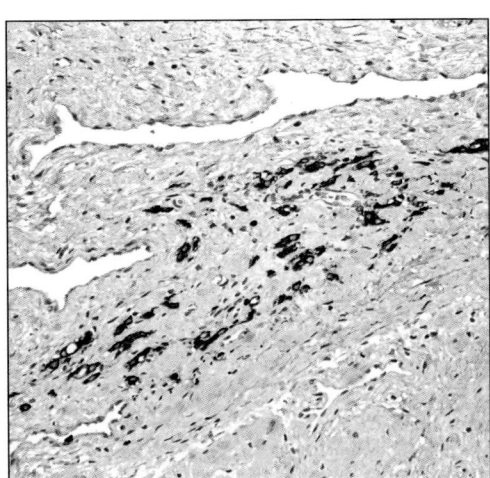

(Left) Metastatic prostate carcinoma shows PSA expression. A potential diagnostic pitfall with PSA is that expression may be weak and focal and rarely negative in such settings. (Right) PAN-CK(AE1/AE3) highlights residual prostate carcinoma with severe treatment effect after androgen ablation. Epithelial markers are more helpful in post-treatment setting than PSA (expression may be suppressed by therapy). PAN-CK(AE1/AE3) is also useful in distinguishing inflammation vs. carcinoma.

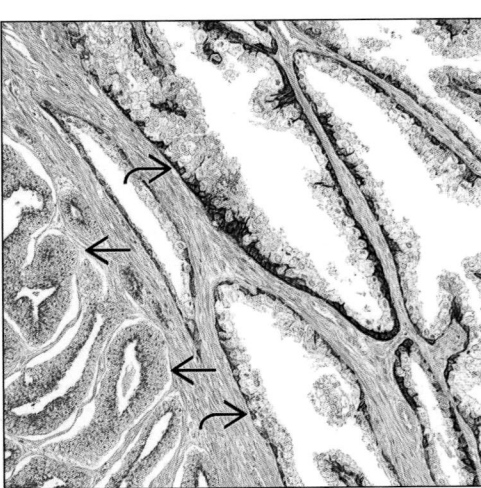

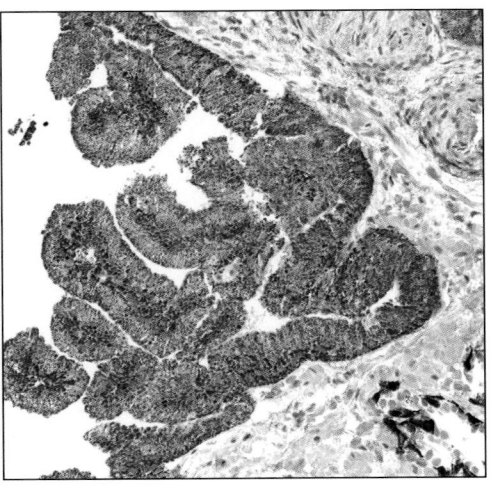

(Left) PIN cocktail combining AMACR (red) and basal cell markers (brown) shows malignant acini ➡ with strong AMACR expression and lacking basal cells. Benign glands ➡ are usually AMACR negative (rarely weak or focal) and show presence of basal cells. AMACR positivity in carcinoma should be strong, circumferential, with granular quality. (Right) PIN cocktail shows diffuse AMACR (red) positivity and lack of basal cell marker (brown) staining in ductal adenocarcinoma of prostate.

Prostate Immunohistochemical Features

(Left) PIN cocktail shows AMACR overexpression & lack of basal cell marker staining in a poorly differentiated carcinoma. **(Right)** Inadvertently sampled colonic mucosa in a prostate biopsy may show stronger AMACR positivity in adenomatous glands ➡. AMACR is not prostate specific & is not helpful in metastatic settings. Colonic adenocarcinoma & urothelial ca secondarily involving the prostate may express AMACR; positivity in nephrogenic adenoma is another pitfall.

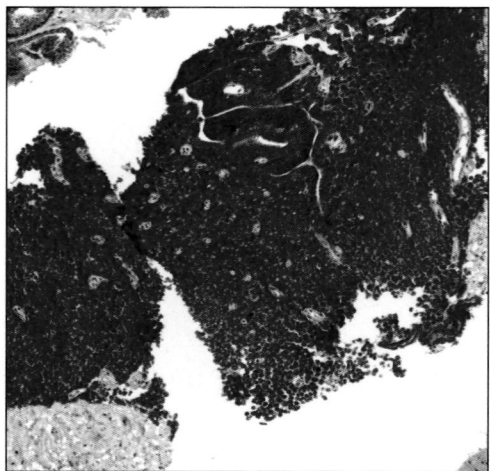
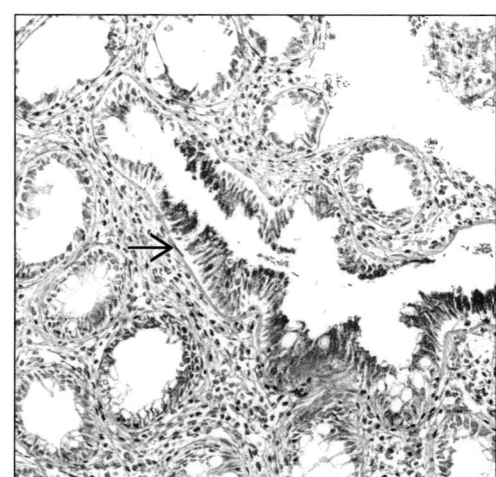

(Left) PIN cocktail in HGPIN shows AMACR overexpression in acinar cells and positivity for basal cell markers. **(Right)** PIN cocktail may rarely show aberrant nuclear p63 (brown) expression in prostate carcinoma ➡. AMACR (red) is weakly expressed by the neoplastic cells. Note more typical staining pattern in adjacent benign gland ➡. Aberrant p63 positivity in carcinoma is very rare and staining is nonbasal, more florid, and usually lacks HMCK(34βE12) coexpression.

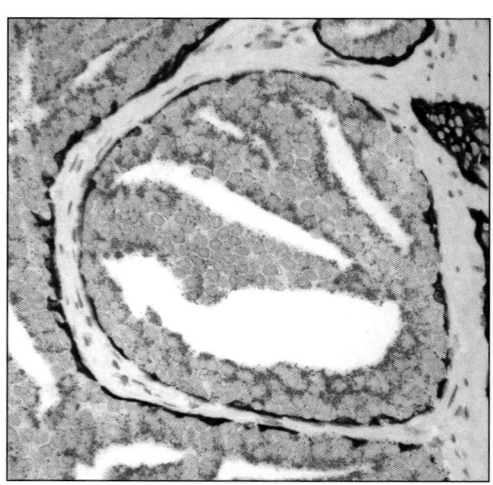
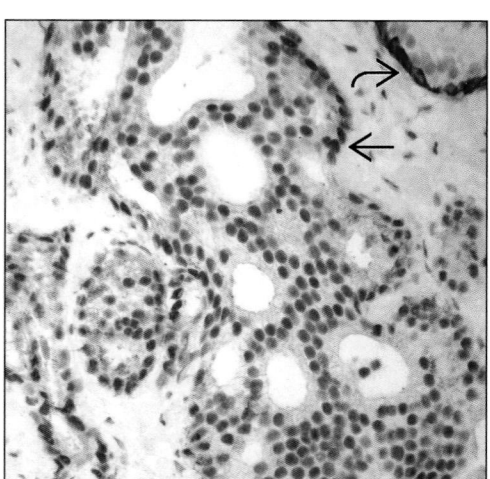

(Left) Focus of prostate carcinoma ➡ shows infiltrative small glands with rigid lumina, pale cytoplasm, and nuclear atypia adjacent to a benign gland ➡. **(Right)** PIN cocktail shows lack of basal cell markers (p63 and HMCK[34βE12]) staining in prostate carcinoma ➡ and basal cell marker positivity in benign glands ➡. AMACR is reported to be negative or weakly expressed in 5-25% of prostate carcinoma; awareness of this false-negative staining is important.

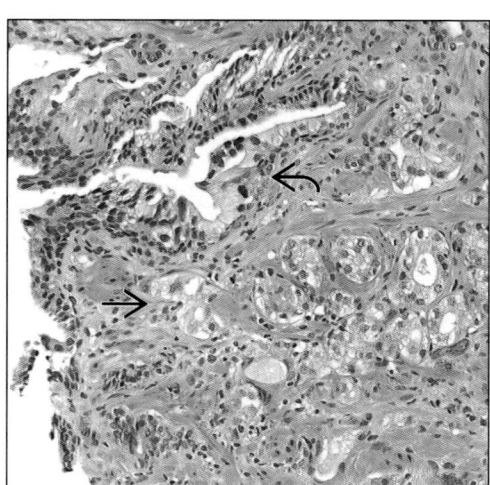
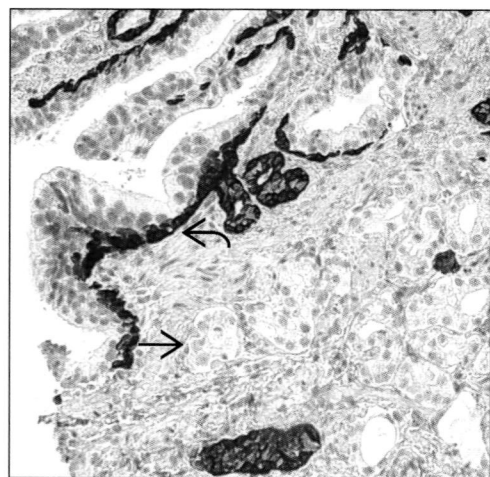

Prostate Immunohistochemical Features

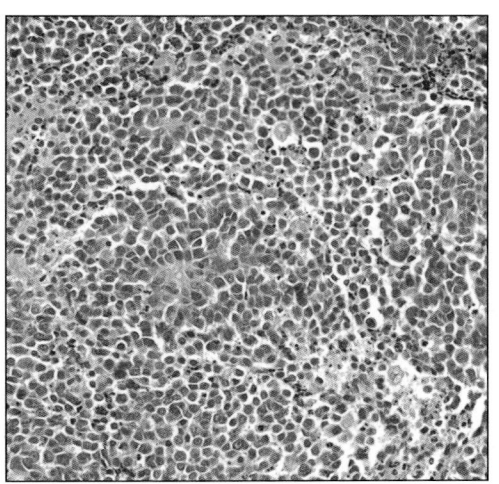

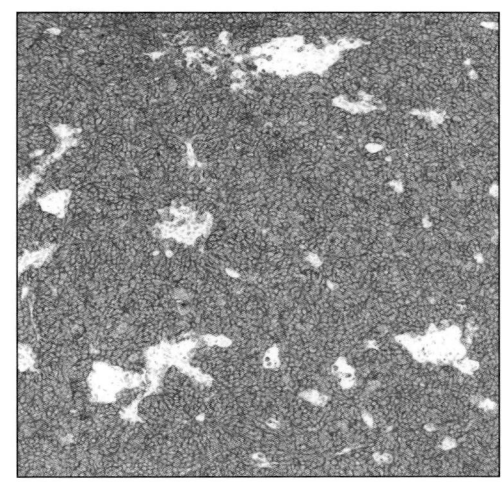

(Left) Small cell carcinoma of prostate shows undifferentiated small cells with abundant apoptosis. (Right) Small cell carcinoma (SCC) of prostate shows diffuse and strong synaptophysin expression. Synaptophysin may also be expressed by pure poorly differentiated adenocarcinoma. In contrast, SCC may also express other neuroendocrine markers, is more often negative or rarely weakly positive for PSA/PAP, may express TTF-1 (~ 50%), and may exhibit paranuclear dot-like PAN-CK staining.

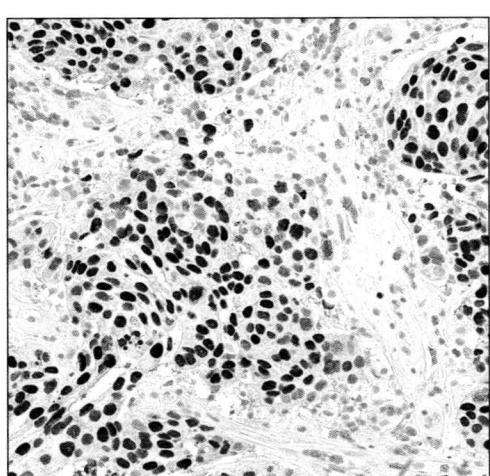

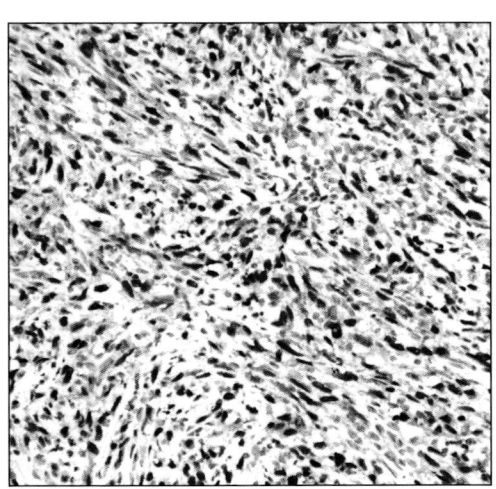

(Left) p63 shows diffuse nuclear positivity in urothelial carcinoma involving prostate. p63 is useful in the setting of poorly differentiated tumors to distinguish prostate carcinoma (negative) vs. urothelial carcinoma (positive). AMACR is not helpful in this setting, since AMACR is expressed by both prostate and urothelial carcinomas. (Right) p63 shows nuclear positivity in sarcomatoid carcinoma of prostate. p63 is often more intense in epithelioid than spindled cells.

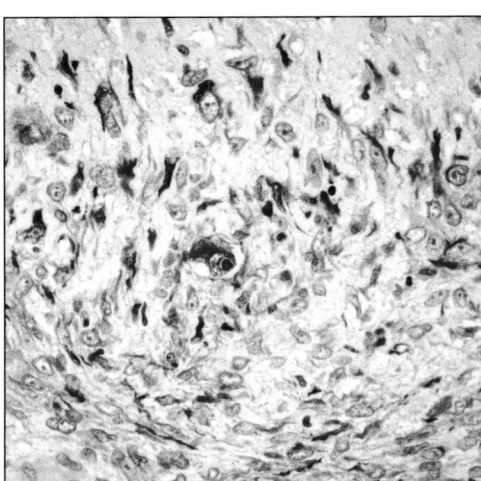

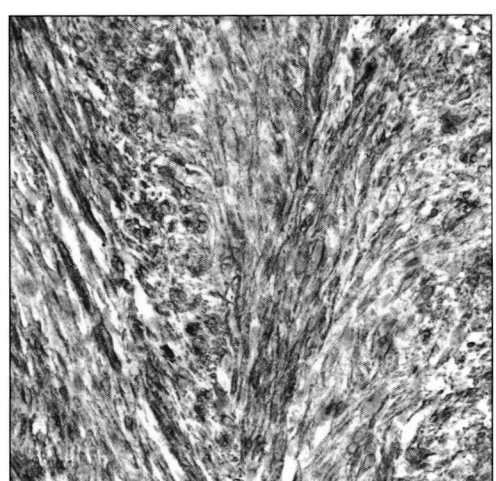

(Left) PAN-CK(AE1/AE3) shows cytoplasmic positivity in sarcomatoid carcinoma of the prostate. In contrast, stromal sarcoma and leiomyosarcoma are typically negative for AE1/AE3. Focal positivity may be seen in leiomyosarcoma but not diffuse positivity. (Right) Actin-sm shows diffuse positivity in leiomyosarcoma of prostate. Actin-sm is negative to focal in stromal sarcoma and sarcomatoid carcinoma. Positivity for p63 and PAN-CK(AE1/AE3) helps distinguish sarcomatoid carcinoma.

Testis and Paratesticular Structures

CLASSIFICATION OF TESTIS AND PARATESTIS TUMORS AND TUMOR-LIKE LESIONS

NONNEOPLASTIC LESIONS

Tumor-like Lesions
- Sertoli cell-only syndrome
- Infections
- Nonspecific granulomatous orchitis, granulomatous orchitis
- Tuberculous epididymo-orchitis
- Adrenal cortical rests
- Hematoma/hematocoele
- Sarcoidosis
- Cryptorchidism
- Leydig cell hyperplasia
- Sertoli cell nodule (Pick adenoma)
- Torsion/Infarct
- Testicular appendages and Walthard nests
- Malakoplakia
- Inflammatory pseudotumor
- Hyperplasia of rete testis
- Sperm granuloma
- Mesothelial hyperplasia
- Cysts (parenchymal, rete of tunics, epididymal)

NEOPLASMS

Germ Cell Tumors
- Precursor lesions
  ○ Intratubular germ cell neoplasia, unclassified
  ○ Intratubular germ cell neoplasia, classified
- Intratubular germ cell neoplasia with microinvasion
- Seminoma
  ○ With syncytiotrophoblastic cells
- Nonseminomatous germ cell tumor
  ○ Embryonal carcinoma
  ○ Yolk sac tumor
  ○ Choriocarcinoma and variants
    ▪ Monophasic
    ▪ Placental site trophoblastic tumor
  ○ Teratoma
    ▪ With secondary malignant component
    ▪ Monodermal variants
      – Carcinoid
      – Primitive neuroectodermal tumor
  ○ Epidermoid and dermoid cysts; pilomatricoma
- Specialized mixed germ cell tumors
  ○ Diffuse embryoma
  ○ Polyembryoma
- Spermatocytic seminoma
  ○ Sarcomatoid variant
- Regressed germ cell tumor
  ○ Scar only
  ○ Scar with intratubular germ cell neoplasia
  ○ Scar with minor residual germ cell tumor

Sex Cord/Gonadal Stromal Tumors
- Fibroma
- Leydig cell tumors
- Sertoli cell tumors
  ○ Sertoli tumor NOS
  ○ Sertoli, sclerosing
  ○ Large cell calcifying Sertoli cell tumor
  ○ Intratubular large cell hyalinizing
- Sertoli-Leydig
- Granulosa cell tumor
  ○ Adult
  ○ Juvenile
- Sex cord stromal tumor, mixed/unclassified
- Gonadoblastoma
- Tumors of adrenogenital syndrome

Hematopoietic Tumors
- Leukemia
- Lymphoma
- Plasmacytoma

Tumors of Rete Testis
- Adenomatous hyperplasia
- Adenoma
- Adenocarcinoma

Tumors of Paratesticular Structures
- Adenomatoid tumor
- Malignant mesothelioma
- Paratesticular multicystic mass of Wolffian origin

Ovarian-type Tumors
- Brenner tumor
- Mucinous cystadenocarcinoma
- Papillary serous carcinoma, müllerian subtype

Epididymal Tumors
- Adenomatoid tumor
- Papillary cystadenoma
- Rhabdomyoma
- Adenocarcinoma
- Melanotic neuroectodermal
- Mesothelioma

Spermatic Cord
- Aggressive angiomyxoma
- Angiomyofibroblastoma
- Embryonal rhabdomyosarcoma
  ○ Spindle cell
  ○ Alveolar
- Hemangioma
- Lipoma
- Liposarcoma
  ○ Well differentiated
  ○ Pleomorphic round cell
- Malignant fibrous histiocytoma
- Paraganglioma
- Vascular myxolipoma

Other
- Adenoid cystic carcinoma
- Angiosarcoma
- Chondrosarcoma
- Hemangioma
- Mesothelioma
- Ossified intratesticular mucinous osteosarcoma
- Melanotic neuroectodermal tumor (retinal anlage tumor)
- Leiomyosarcoma
- Desmoplastic small round cell tumor

Metastatic Tumors of Testis and Paratestis
- Prostate, lung, kidney, and other

4

CRYPTORCHIDISM

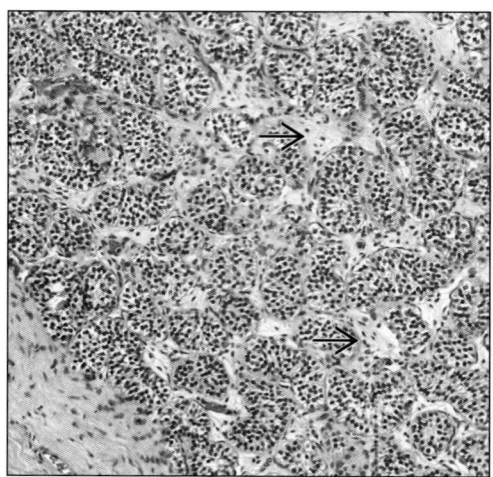

Low-power photomicrograph shows cryptorchid testis with crowded seminiferous tubules with no spermatogenesis and decreased tubular size. The interstitium is edematous ➡.

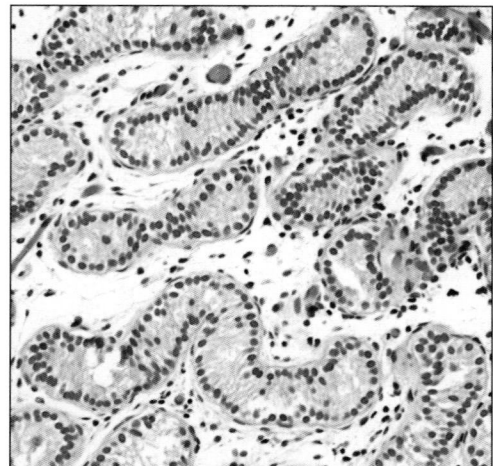

This photomicrograph from a cryptorchid testis shows seminiferous tubules with no spermatogenesis and marked interstitial edema. The tubules are lined by Sertoli cells only.

TERMINOLOGY

Synonyms
- Undescended testis

Definitions
- Greek word "crypto" (meaning hidden) and "orchid" (meaning testicle)
- 1 or both testes present outside scrotum with failure to descend into scrotum (empty scrotum)

ETIOLOGY/PATHOGENESIS

Developmental Anomaly
- Idiopathic
- Anomalies in anatomic development
- Defect in fetal androgens or excess maternal estrogen
- Possible common genetic abnormality causing undescended testis and predisposing to carcinoma of testis
- Associated with "congenital malformation syndromes," such as Prader-Willi syndrome, Noonan syndrome, cloacal exstrophy

Acquired Cryptorchidism
- Postoperative trapped testis
- Spontaneous ascent (idiopathic)

CLINICAL ISSUES

Epidemiology
- Incidence
  - Most common birth defect of male genitalia
  - 3% of full-term newborns have undescended testis (testes)
  - 1% of infants have incompletely descended testes 12 months after birth
  - More common in premature infants (30% of boys born at 30 weeks gestational age)
  - True cryptorchidism accounts for 25% of cases of empty scrotum

Presentation
- No particular symptoms; empty scrotal sac usually detected by parents
- About 2/3 unilateral and 1/3 bilateral
- 90% may be palpable in inguinal canal (10% in abdomen or nonexistent, truly hidden, or anorchia)
- May be found anywhere along "path of descent" from retroperitoneum to inguinal ring
- Rarely located outside of "path of descent" (ectopic), such as outside of inguinal canal, perineum, opposite scrotum, femoral canal, or under skin

Natural History
- Predisposition to testicular germ cell neoplasia
  - Cryptorchidism increases risk of testicular cancer by 4-10x
  - Most common tumor in undescended testis is seminoma
  - Contralateral testis is primary site in 20% of cases
  - Orchiopexy facilitates self examination and may decrease risk of germ cell tumor
- Infertility
  - Most common problem caused by cryptorchidism
  - Tubular fertility index (number of germ cells per cross-sectioned tubule) is most important factor
  - 75-85% of cryptorchid males have sperm count below normal
  - Location and size of cryptorchid testis have no influence on fertility
- Torsion
- Psychological

Treatment
- May receive hormone injection (β-HCG or testosterone) to try to bring testicle into scrotum
- If medical treatment is unsuccessful, early orchiopexy (about 1 year old) should be performed to prevent irreversible damage to testicle

CRYPTORCHIDISM

Key Facts

Terminology
- Testis present outside scrotum and cannot be moved into scrotum

Clinical Issues
- Most common birth defect of male genitalia
- 1% of infants have incompletely descended testes 12 months after birth
- Cryptorchidism increases risk of testicular cancer 4-10x
- Most common problem caused by cryptorchidism is infertility
- 90% can be palpable in inguinal canal (10% in abdomen or nonexistent, truly hidden, or anorchia)

Macroscopic Features
- Abnormal location and usually smaller-sized testis than normal or contralateral testis

Microscopic Pathology
- Type I (slight alterations): Tubular fertility index > 50; mean tubular diameter decreased by < 10%
- Type II (marked germinal hypoplasia): Tubular fertility index 30-50; mean tubular diameter 10-30% below normal
- Type III (severe germinal hypoplasia): Tubular fertility index < 30; mean tubular diameter > 30% below normal
- Testicular parenchyma can be hypoplastic or dysgenetic

Prognosis
- Most will descend into scrotum without any intervention during 1st year of life
- Medical or surgical correction are both effective
- About 5% of patients with undescended testicles do not have testicles at surgery (vanished or absent testis)

IMAGE FINDINGS

Ultrasonographic Findings
- "Snowstorm" pattern by ultrasonography if there is severe microlithiasis

MACROSCOPIC FEATURES

General Features
- Testicle in abnormal location and size is usually smaller than normal testis and comparatively smaller than contralateral testis

MICROSCOPIC PATHOLOGY

Histologic Features
- Type I (slight alterations): Tubular fertility index > 50; mean tubular diameter decreased by < 10%
  - Spermatogenesis present
- Type II (marked germinal hypoplasia): Tubular fertility index 30-50; mean tubular diameter 10-30% below normal
  - Spermatogonia irregularly distributed and grouped within a lobule
- Type III (severe germinal hypoplasia): Tubular fertility index < 30; mean tubular diameter more than 30% below normal
  - Giant spermatogonia with dark nuclei
  - Ring-shaped tubules and megatubules
  - Eosinophilic bodies or microliths
  - Focal granular changes in Sertoli cells
  - Absent spermatogenesis with Sertoli cells filling the tubules

- Thickening and hyalinization of tubular basement and interstitial edema
- Interstitial, particularly peritubular fibrosis evident at age of 1 year
- Interstitial (Leydig cells) cells usually spared and may show hyperplasia
- Pick adenoma (Sertoli cell nodule)
- Contralateral descended testis may show regressive changes
- Testicular parenchyma may be hypoplastic or dysgenetic
- Intratubular germ cell neoplasia (ITGCN) may be present

Predominant Pattern/Injury Type
- Tubular diameter decreased, ranges from slightly to severely
- Germ cell number decreased

DIAGNOSTIC CHECKLIST

Pathologic Interpretation Pearls
- Abnormal testis location and variable development and maturation of testicular parenchyma
- In biopsies and orchiectomy specimens, it is important to look for ITGCN
  - Sampling and immunohistochemistry may be necessary

SELECTED REFERENCES

1. Wood HM et al: Cryptorchidism and testicular cancer: separating fact from fiction. J Urol. 181(2):452-61, 2009
2. Walsh TJ et al: Prepubertal orchiopexy for cryptorchidism may be associated with lower risk of testicular cancer. J Urol. 178(4 Pt 1):1440-6; discussion 1446, 2007
3. Cendron M et al: Anatomical, morphological and volumetric analysis: a review of 759 cases of testicular maldescent. J Urol. 149(3):570-3, 1993

CRYPTORCHIDISM

Microscopic Features

(Left) This low-power photomicrograph shows cryptorchid testis with seminiferous tubules filled with primitive germ cells. The tubules are small, and there is marked interstitial edema. A few scattered Leydig cells are observed ➡. *(Right)* Cryptorchid testis shows seminiferous tubules filled with Sertoli cells and no spermatogenesis. The interstitium shows scattered chronic inflammatory cells. Adequate sampling is necessary in post pubertal specimens for ITGCN.

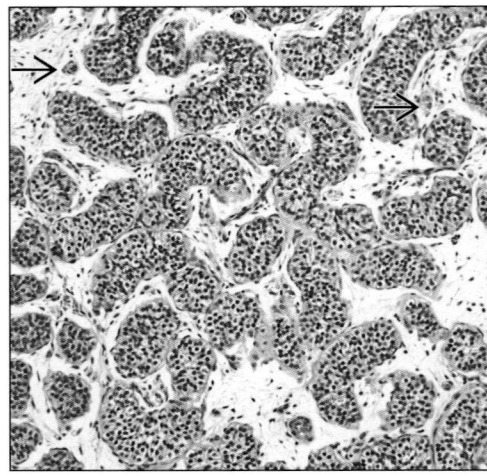
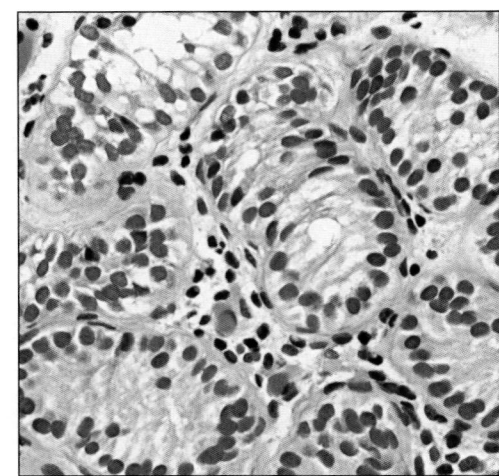

(Left) Cryptorchid testis shows seminiferous tubules with immature spermatogenesis with rare spermatogonia ➡ or clusters. There is interstitial fibrosis and scattered primitive Leydig cells ➡. *(Right)* Cryptorchid testis showing large spermatogonia ➡ with clear cytoplasm resemble those of ITGCN. Podoplanin(D2-40) and Oct3/4 immunostains are helpful to make the distinction. ITGCN is positive for these stains, but normal germ cells are negative.

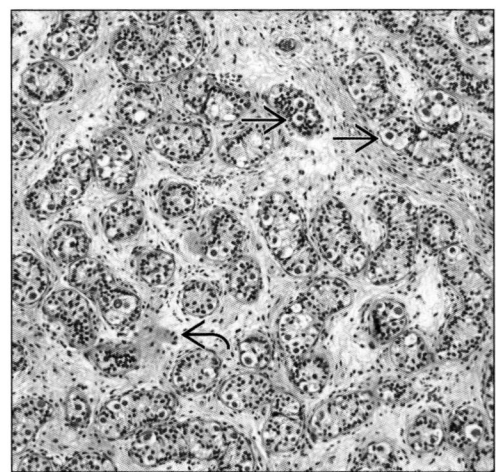
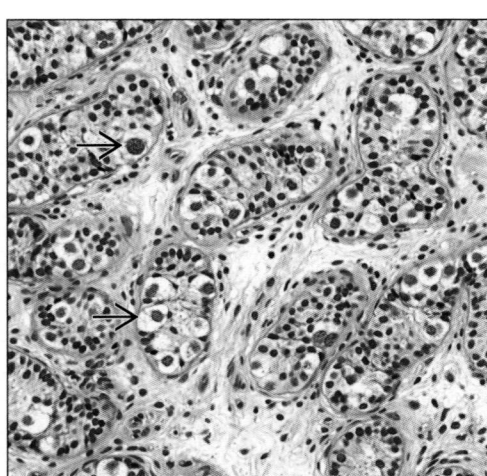

(Left) Cryptorchid testis shows seminiferous tubules with uneven maturation. Some tubules lack spermatogenesis ➡ and others have incomplete spermatogenesis ➡. Intratubular microlithiasis ➡ and Leydig cell hyperplasia ➡ are seen. *(Right)* Cryptorchid testis composed of seminiferous tubules with Sertoli cell only pattern ➡ and intratubular microlith ➡. There is peritubular fibrosis and chronic inflammatory cell infiltration in the interstitium ➡.

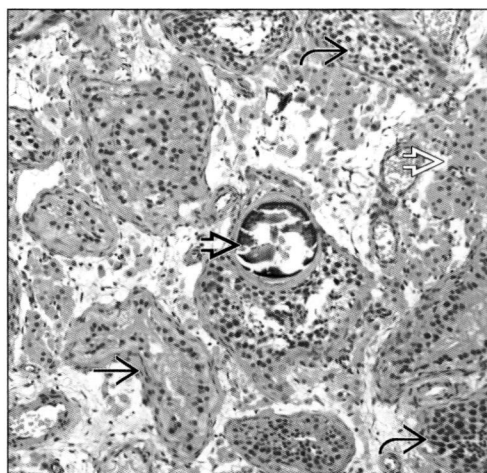
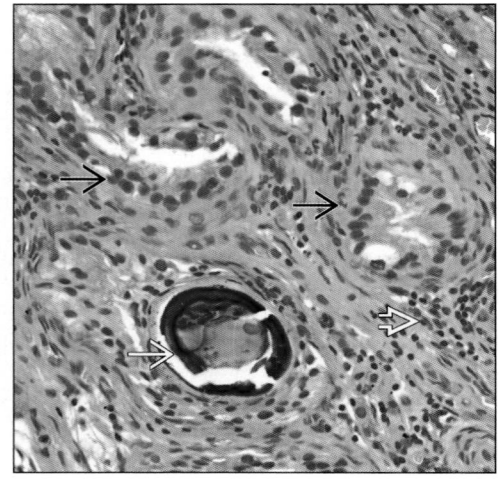

CRYPTORCHIDISM

Microscopic Features

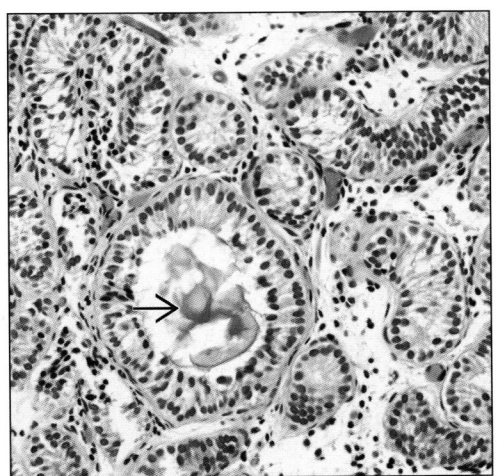

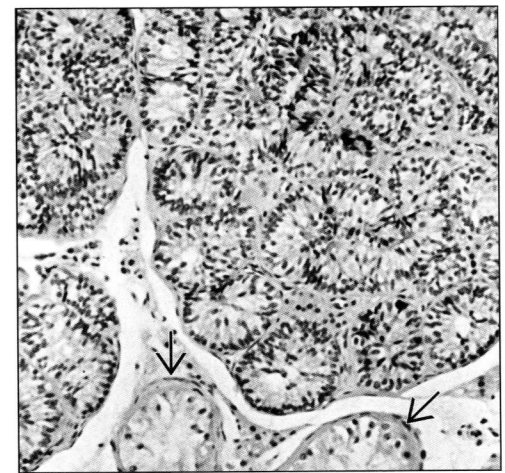

(Left) This is an example of cryptorchid testis with marked germinal hypoplasia and megatubules with eosinophilic bodies ➡. The interstitium shows edema and a few lymphocytes. *(Right)* This photomicrograph shows a Sertoli cell nodule (Pick adenoma) in a patient with cryptorchid testis. The nodule is small and well demarcated from the surrounding seminiferous tubules ➡. Formation of a nodule (adenoma) is the main difference from Sertoli cell-only pattern testis.

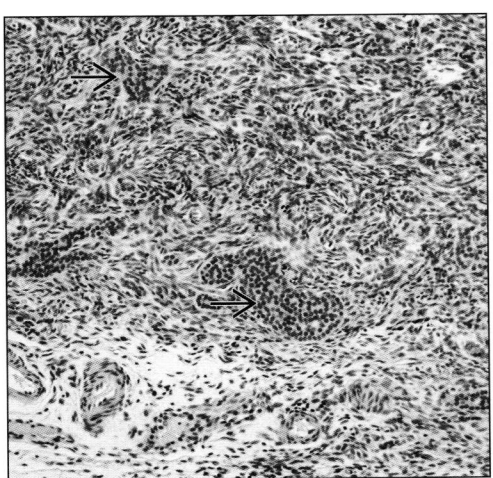

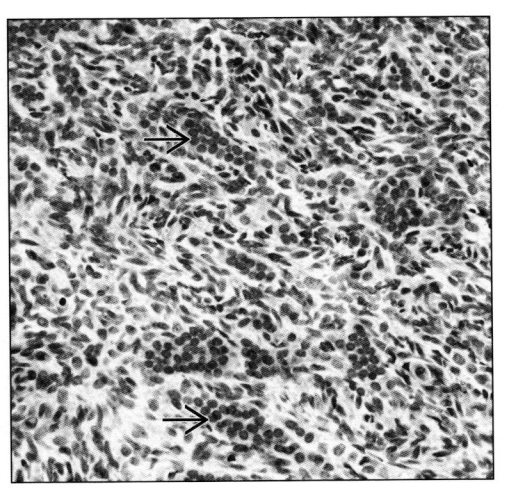

(Left) This low-power photomicrograph shows cryptorchid testis with marked dysgenetic features with nondescriptive undifferentiated sex cord stromal tissue and nests resembling that of immature seminiferous tubules ➡. *(Right)* Higher power view from cryptorchid testis shows undifferentiated sex cord stromal tissue and nests resembling immature seminiferous tubules ➡. The absence of a mass lesion on gross examination argues against a sex cord stromal neoplasm.

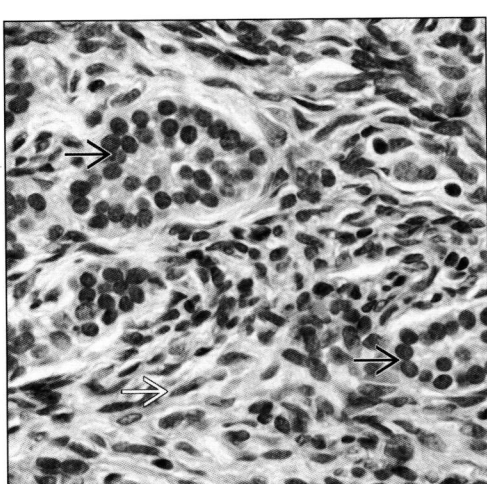

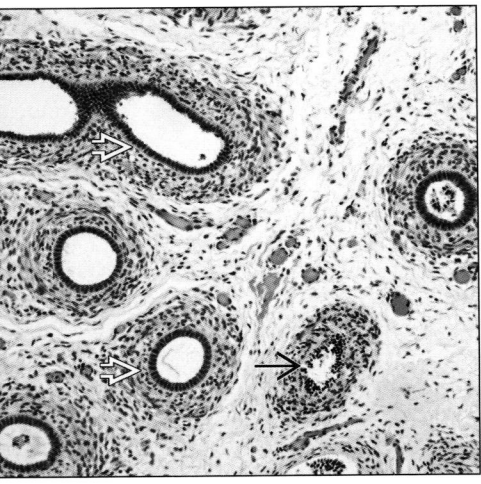

(Left) High-power view shows undifferentiated sex cord spindle cells with elongated nuclei ➡ and pale cytoplasm. Poorly formed tubules filled with round to ovoid cells resembling Sertoli cells in seminiferous tubules ➡ are also present. *(Right)* This photomicrograph from cryptorchid testis shows immature paratesticular tissue, including efferent ductules ➡ and epididymis ➡ surrounded by immature spindle cells with eosinophilic cytoplasm.

SERTOLI CELL-ONLY SYNDROME

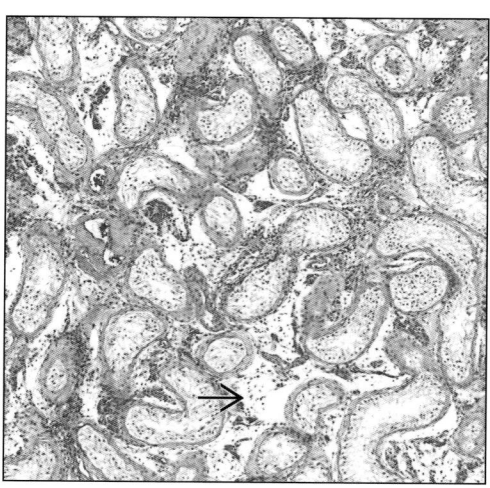

Sertoli cell-only syndrome shows smaller-sized seminiferous tubules containing Sertoli cells and lack of spermatogenesis. The tunica propria layer is thickened, and the interstitium is edematous ➡.

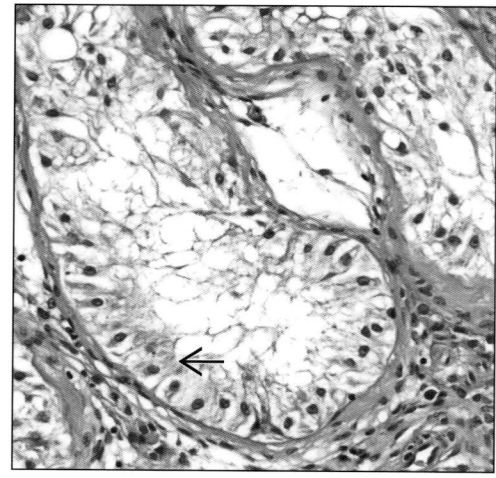

Sertoli cell-only syndrome shows columnar or pyramidal Sertoli cells with oval to round nuclei and abundant clear to eosinophilic cytoplasm ➡. No spermatogenesis is present.

TERMINOLOGY

Synonyms
- Germ cell aplasia
- Del Castillo syndrome (old term, now replaced by specific subtypes)

Definitions
- All azoospermias in which seminiferous tubules lack germ cells and contain Sertoli cells only

ETIOLOGY/PATHOGENESIS

Developmental Anomaly
- Sertoli cell-only syndrome with immature Sertoli cells caused by deficiency of both FSH and LH
- Sertoli cell-only syndrome with dysgenetic Sertoli cells has Sertoli cells that proceed to pubertal maturation but variably deviate from normal maturation
  - Associated with cryptorchidism, Y chromosome abnormalities, Klinefelter syndrome (47XXY), and idiopathic infertility
  - May be seen at edge of germ cell neoplasms
- Sertoli cell-only syndrome with mature Sertoli cells is thought to be due to failure of migration of germ cells

Environmental Exposure
- Sertoli cell-only syndrome with involuting Sertoli cells may be secondary to irradiation, cytotoxic therapy, hormonal therapy for prostate cancer, chemical/toxin exposure, and viral infection
- Sertoli cell-only syndrome with dedifferentiated Sertoli cells is associated with androgen deprivation therapy, estrogen treatment for transsexuality, and platinum chemotherapy agents

CLINICAL ISSUES

Epidemiology
- Age
  - Range: 20-40 years

Presentation
- Infertility, azoospermia, &/or hypogonadism
- 5-10% of infertility in men is due to Sertoli cell-only syndrome
- Well-developed secondary male sexual characteristics
- Normal virilization with no gynecomastia

Laboratory Tests
- Gonadotropins may be increased or decreased depending on type of syndrome
- Most common types (dysgenetic, adult, and involuting) have elevated FSH, normal or elevated LH, and normal or decreased testosterone
- Immature type has decreased FSH and LH beginning in childhood

Treatment
- No known effective treatment options
- Immature Sertoli cell type may be treated with hormone therapy to recover some degree of spermatogenesis
- Secondary Sertoli cell-only syndrome may be reversible after elimination of specific etiology

Prognosis
- Extensive fine-needle aspiration may recover some spermatozoa in some types

MACROSCOPIC FEATURES

General Features
- Testes are normal, small, or atrophic

SERTOLI CELL-ONLY SYNDROME

Key Facts

Terminology
- Germ cell aplasia
- All azoospermias in which seminiferous epithelium consists of only Sertoli cells

Clinical Issues
- Infertility, azoospermia, &/or hypogonadism
- Usually present between ages 20-40 years for evaluation of infertility
- 5-10% of infertile men are due to Sertoli cell-only syndrome
- Well-developed secondary male sexual characteristics
- Normal virilization with no gynecomastia
- Gonadotropins may be increased or decreased depending on type of syndrome

Macroscopic Features
- Testes are usually normal, smaller, or atrophic

Microscopic Pathology
- Seminiferous tubules contain only Sertoli cells and 5 histologic variants have been described
  - Immature Sertoli cells
  - Dysgenetic Sertoli cells
  - Adult Sertoli cells
  - Involuting Sertoli cells
  - Dedifferentiated Sertoli cells

Top Differential Diagnoses
- Intratubular germ cell neoplasia
- Maturation arrest or hypospermatogenesis
- Tubular hyalinization

MICROSCOPIC PATHOLOGY

Histologic Features
- Seminiferous tubules contain only Sertoli cells and 5 histologic variants have been described
  - Immature Sertoli cells
    - Immature prepubertal appearance with pseudostratification
    - Increased cellularity with small tubules often lacking lumina
  - Dysgenetic Sertoli cells
    - Morphology varies within and between tubules
    - Nuclei have mature and immature features
    - Hyalinized tubules are frequent
  - Adult Sertoli cells
    - Mature Sertoli cells with increased numbers
    - Small diameter tubules
  - Involuting Sertoli cells
    - Lobulated nuclei with irregular outlines
    - Seminiferous tubules have variable thickening of basement membrane
    - Leydig cells variably involuted
  - Dedifferentiated Sertoli cells
    - Immature Sertoli cells in otherwise mature tubules
    - Tubule wall thickened with increased elastic fibers and collagen
    - Markedly decreased tubular diameter

Predominant Pattern/Injury Type
- Developmental

Predominant Cell/Compartment Type
- Sertoli cell only; no germ cells at any stage of maturation

DIFFERENTIAL DIAGNOSIS

Intratubular Germ Cell Neoplasia
- Normal spermatogenesis may be present
- Concurrent invasive malignant germ cell tumor

- Atypical germ cells positive for Podoplanin(D2-40), PLAP, Oct3/4, SALL4, and CD117

Maturation Arrest or Hypospermatogenesis
- Presence of spermatogonia or maturating spermatocytes

Tubular Hyalinization
- Variable degree of hyalinized tubules
- Isolated tubules containing germ cells or Sertoli cells
- Caused by dysgenetic, ischemic, postinflammatory, obstructive etiologies

DIAGNOSTIC CHECKLIST

Clinically Relevant Pathologic Features
- Correlate hormone levels with morphology

Pathologic Interpretation Pearls
- Complete or near-complete absence of spermatogenesis with only Sertoli cells occupying tubular epithelium

SELECTED REFERENCES

1. Venkatachala S et al: Testicular biopsies--histomorphologic patterns in male infertility. Indian J Pathol Microbiol. 50(4):726-9, 2007
2. Bar-Shira Maymon B et al: Maturation phenotype of Sertoli cells in testicular biopsies of azoospermic men. Hum Reprod. 15(7):1537-42, 2000
3. Terada T et al: Morphological evidence for two types of idiopathic 'Sertoli-cell-only' syndrome. Int J Androl. 14(2):117-26, 1991
4. Nistal M et al: Sertoli cell types in the Sertoli-cell-only syndrome: relationships between Sertoli cell morphology and aetiology. Histopathology. 16(2):173-80, 1990
5. Christiansen P: Urinary gonadotrophins in the Sertoli-Cell-only syndrome. Acta Endocrinol (Copenh). 78(1):180-91, 1975

SERTOLI CELL-ONLY SYNDROME

Microscopic Features

(Left) Sertoli cell-only syndrome shows seminiferous tubules with thickened tunica propria layer and filled entirely by Sertoli cells with abundant pale eosinophilic cytoplasm. No germ cells are seen. Clusters of Leydig cells ⮕ are present. (Right) Seminiferous tubule is filled entirely by Sertoli cells, which have ovoid or elongated nuclei, prominent nucleoli ⮕ and abundant pale to eosinophilic cytoplasm. This appearance has been referred to as a "wind swept" appearance.

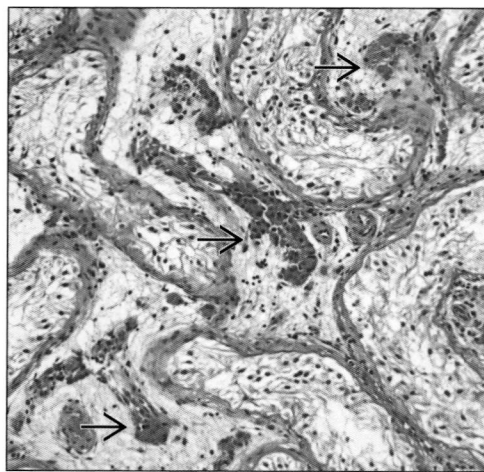
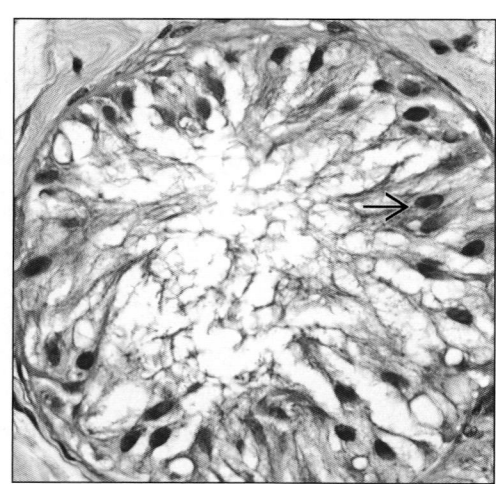

(Left) This low-power view of Sertoli cell-only syndrome shows atrophic seminiferous tubules; some are filled with only Sertoli cells ⮕ and others are entirely sclerotic ⮕. (Right) This photomicrograph shows seminiferous tubules filled entirely by Sertoli cells. Two tubules ⮕ have markedly thickened tunica propria. One tubule has normal thickness of tunica propria ⮕. Clusters of Leydig cells ⮕ are present within the interstitium.

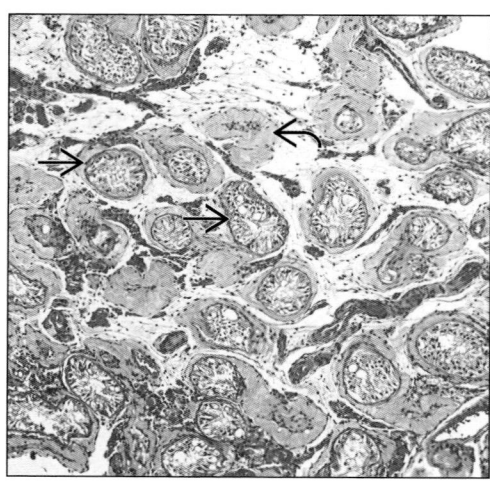
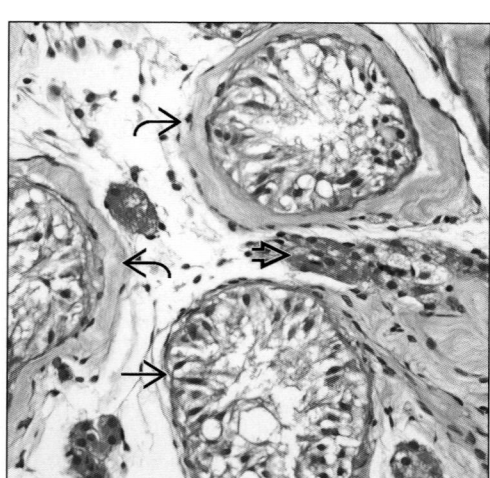

(Left) This high-power image shows Sertoli cells with ovoid or elongated nuclei, occasional prominent nucleoli ⮕, and abundant pale to eosinophilic cytoplasm. No germ cell component is present. In rare cases the nuclei may have prominent nucleoli, raising the possibility of ITGCN. The cell borders, however, are not well defined in most cases. (Right) This photomicrograph shows seminiferous tubules filled with Sertoli cell-only and surrounded by extensive Leydig cell hyperplasia.

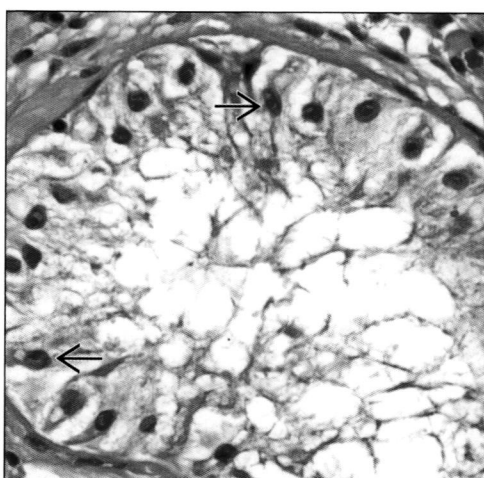
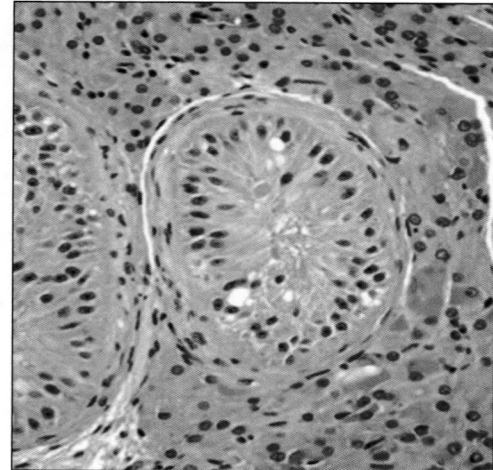

Microscopic Features and Differential Diagnoses

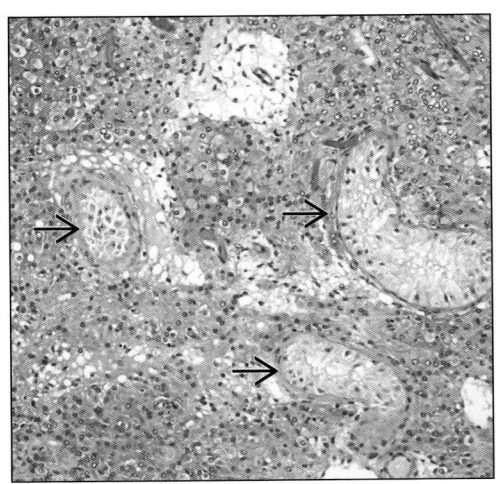

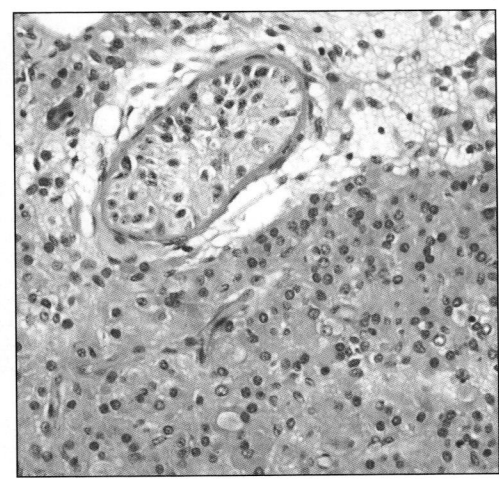

(Left) This image is from a testicular biopsy of a patient with Klinefelter syndrome. There is marked intersitial Leydig cell hyperplasia and few seminiferous tubules with Sertoli cells only ➡. No germ cells are seen in these tubules. *(Right)* High-power photomicrograph of testicular biopsy of a patient with Klinefelter syndrome shows intersitial Leydig cell hyperplasia and one seminiferous tubule filled with only Sertoli cells. No spermatogenesis is present.

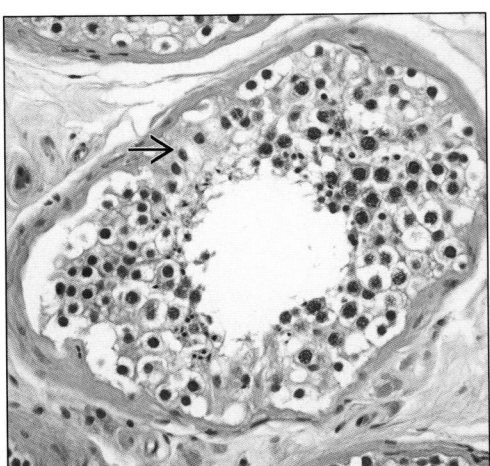

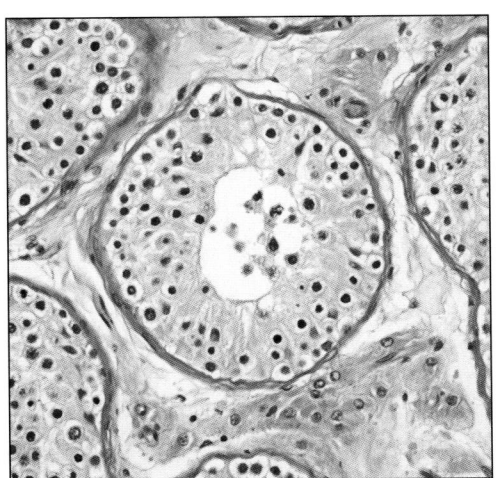

(Left) Normal seminiferous tubule with appropriate spermatogenesis is shown. Normally the Sertoli cells ➡ account for 8-10% of the cellularity within a tubule (germ cell/Sertoli cell ratio of 13:1), and there is an average 10-12 Sertoli cells per tubule. *(Right)* Maturation arrest shows spermatogonia and spermatocytes, but no mature forms, such as spermatids or spermatozoa, are present. This condition should be differentiated from Sertoli cell-only syndrome.

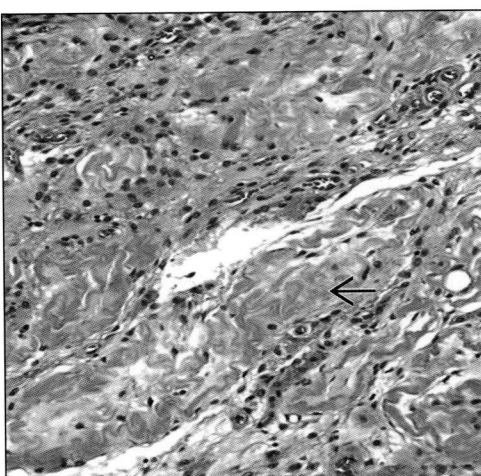

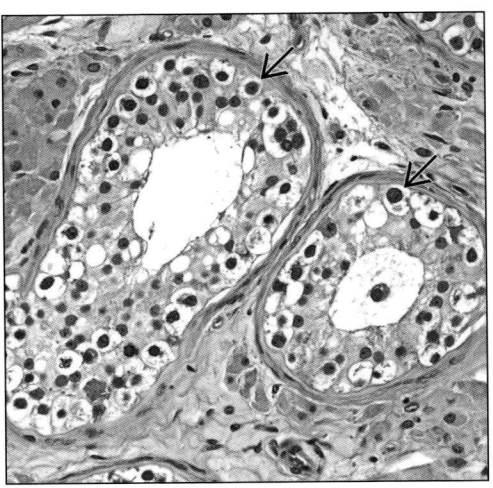

(Left) An example of a hyalinized seminiferous tubule is shown. The tubules are completely sclerotic with intratubular and peritubular hyalinization ➡. No germ cells or Sertoli cells are present. *(Right)* Intratubular germ cell neoplasia (ITGCN) is characterized by large atypical cells with clear cytoplasm situated at the periphery of the tubules ➡. ITGCN is commonly seen in association with germ cell tumors and positive for PLAP, Podoplanin(D2-40), Oct3/4, and CD117.

INFECTIONS

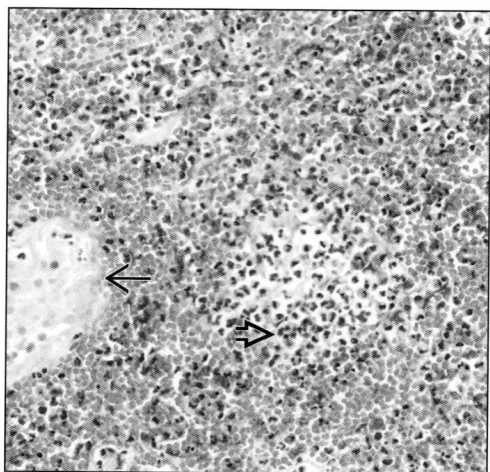

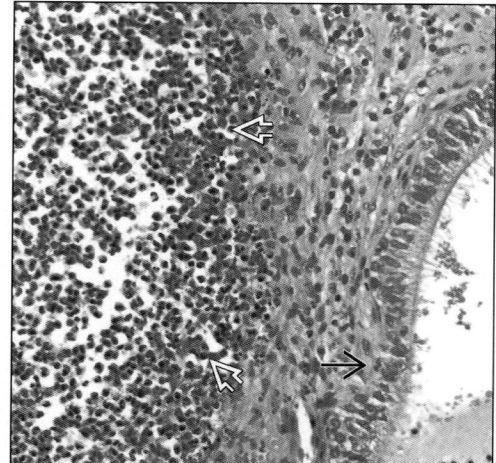

This image shows acute bacterial orchitis with acute inflammation and necrosis of seminiferous tubule ➡. Microabscesses ⧎ associated with lymphocytes and hemorrhage are seen in the interstitium.

Acute epididymitis with abscess formation ⧎ is adjacent to epididymal epithelium ➡. There is a localized acute suppurative inflammation extending to the epididymal epithelium and stroma.

TERMINOLOGY

Synonyms
- Orchitis, epididymitis, epididymo-orchitis

Definitions
- Inflammatory process of testis or epididymis due to microorganisms (bacteria, fungus, virus, etc.)

ETIOLOGY/PATHOGENESIS

Infectious Agents
- Bacteria
  - In younger men (< 35 years), sexually transmitted bacterial pathogens are most common cause
    - *Chlamydia trachomatis* antigen is detected in 30% of cases of epididymitis and 11-35% of cases of epididymo-orchitis
    - *Neisseria gonorrhoeae* is also common
  - In older men (> 35 years), urinary tract pathogens, such as *Escherichia coli*, are most common bacterial cause of epididymitis and secondary orchitis
  - Chronic orchitis with microabscesses can be due to many types of bacteria
  - Tertiary syphilis
  - *Brucella* associated with ingestion of raw milk and contact with animals
  - *Mycobacterium leprae*
  - Tuberculosis: *Mycobacterium tuberculosis*
- Virus
  - Mumps: Epididymo-orchitis occurs in 15-30% of adult cases of mumps but is rare before puberty
  - Coxsackie B
  - Uncommonly: Influenza, echovirus, Epstein-Barr virus, adenovirus, and others
- Fungus
  - Fungal orchitis is rare but may be caused by *Coccidioides*, *Histoplasma*, and *Cryptococcus*
- Parasites
  - Injury is secondary to vascular lesions
  - Main organisms are *Schistosoma*, filarial worms, *Leishmania*, *Toxoplasma*, *Echinococcus*, *Trichomonas*, *Entamoeba*

CLINICAL ISSUES

Presentation
- General
  - Painful mass or swelling
  - Fever and other systemic signs of infection
- Mumps orchitis occurs in 15-30% of adult cases but is rare before puberty
  - Bilateral in 15-30% of cases
  - Onset 4-8 days after parotiditis

Treatment
- Surgical approaches
  - Not indicated unless infarction occurs
- Drugs
  - Antibiotics, antifungal, or agents against parasites

Prognosis
- Pyogenic orchitis can cause testicular infarction
- Can cause oligospermia, or azoospermia if bilateral

MACROSCOPIC FEATURES

General Features
- General enlargement of testicle
- Mass lesion with pus, hemorrhagic cut surface

MICROSCOPIC PATHOLOGY

Histologic Features
- Variable mixed acute, chronic, or granulomatous inflammation
- Abscess formation and seminiferous tubule necrosis

INFECTIONS

Key Facts

Terminology
- Inflammatory process of testis or epididymis due to microorganisms (bacteria, fungus, virus, etc.)

Etiology/Pathogenesis
- Bacteria
- Virus
- Fungus
- Parasites

Macroscopic Features
- General enlargement of testicle
- Mass lesion with pus, hemorrhagic cut surface

Microscopic Pathology
- Variable mixed acute, chronic, or granulomatous inflammation
- Abscess formation and seminiferous tubule necrosis

- Acute bacterial orchitis causes abscesses with acute inflammation
  - Lepromatous leprosy causes granulomatous orchitis and usually has macrophages filled with acid-fast bacilli
  - Brucellosis has dense lymphohistiocytic inflammation with noncaseating granulomas
  - Chlamydia inflammation may involve urethra, epididymis, and testicular parenchyma
- Syphilitic orchitis is usually granulomatous and has abundant plasma cells
  - Interstitial inflammation with sclerotic tubules and endarteritis obliterans leading to fibrosis
  - Gummatous orchitis has well-delineated zones of necrosis with lymphocytes, plasma cells, and giant cells
- Mump orchitis characterized by intersitial edema, vascular congestion, inflammatory infiltrate consisting mainly of lymphocytes and plasma cells
- Fungal infection characterized by mixed inflammation ± necrosis

Predominant Pattern/Injury Type
- Infectious

Predominant Cell/Compartment Type
- Neutrophils, lymphocytes, plasma cells, histocytes/macrophages

DIFFERENTIAL DIAGNOSIS

Testicular Trauma or Torsion
- History and lack of fever

Sarcoidosis
- Noncaseating granulomatous inflammation
- Special stains negative for microorganisms

Seminoma or Other Germ Cell Neoplasm
- Seminoma may have intense sarcoid-like granulomatous reaction
- Presence of tumor cells

SELECTED REFERENCES

1. Trojian TH et al: Epididymitis and orchitis: an overview. Am Fam Physician. 79(7):583-7, 2009
2. Cunningham KA et al: Male genital tract chlamydial infection: implications for pathology and infertility. Biol Reprod. 79(2):180-9, 2008
3. Hviid A et al: Mumps. Lancet. 371(9616):932-44, 2008
4. Garthwaite MA et al: The implementation of European Association of Urology guidelines in the management of acute epididymo-orchitis. Ann R Coll Surg Engl. 89(8):799-803, 2007
5. Richens J: Genital manifestations of tropical diseases. Sex Transm Infect. 80(1):12-7, 2004

IMAGE GALLERY

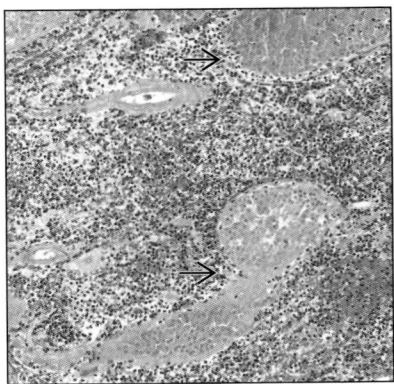 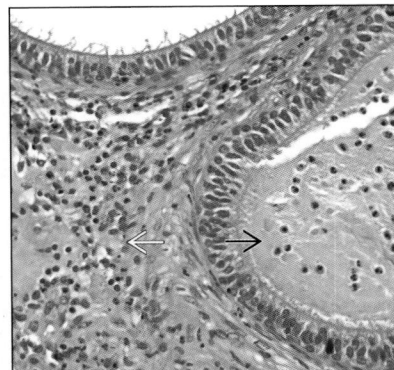 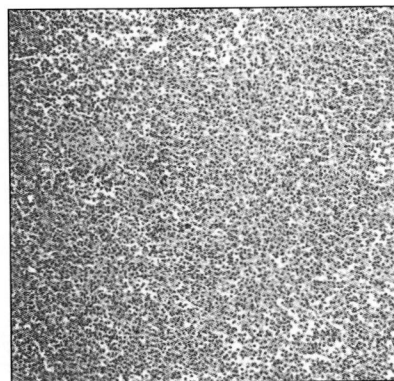

(Left) Interstitial acute inflammation and necrosis of seminiferous tubules ➡ is shown. Predominantly neutrophilic infiltration is seen with extensive hemorrhage. The tubules are totally necrotic with preservation of their architecture (ghost tubules). *(Center)* Hematoxylin & eosin shows acute epididymitis with neutrophilic infiltration within the lumen of epididymal gland ➡ and stroma ➡. *(Right)* Acute orchitis with abscess formation is seen.

NONSPECIFIC GRANULOMATOUS ORCHITIS

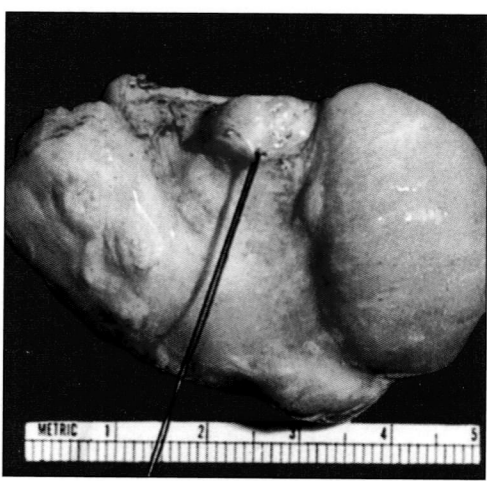

Nonspecific granulomatous orchitis is shown. Bivalved testis with ill-defined nodules variably involve the testis and paratestis. Due to the pseudotumorous firm consistency, malignancy is mimicked.

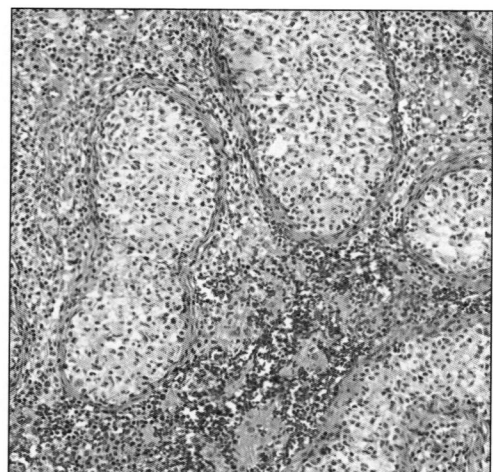

Typical features of early stage are characterized by intratubular histiocytic infiltration with a few lymphocytes, mimicking granulomas. Special stains for microorganisms are negative.

TERMINOLOGY

Definitions
- Mixed chronic and granulomatous orchitis with no specific etiology; may be autoimmune or post-traumatic reaction

ETIOLOGY/PATHOGENESIS

Unknown Causes
- Trauma, infection, extravasated sperm, and autoimmune disease have been postulated as possible pathogenetic mechanisms
  - May be associated with urinary tract infection, history of prostatectomy, and inguinal hernia repair
  - Autoimmune reaction to sperm antibodies
  - Vascular compromise with ischemia or infarction

CLINICAL ISSUES

Epidemiology
- Incidence
  - Rare; more common in African-Americans
- Age
  - Range: 29-79 years old (average: 55 years old)

Presentation
- Usually unilateral testicular enlargement (more common in right side) but can be bilateral
- May be accompanied by tenderness, fever, or heaviness
- Ipsilateral or contralateral hydrocele
- May be associated with gram-negative urinary tract infection

Treatment
- Symptomatic control or surgical resection
- In cases with bilateral involvement with 1 testis already removed, steroid treatment is optional

MACROSCOPIC FEATURES

General Features
- Unilateral, solid nodular enlargement of testis or thickened tunica layer
- Testis may be totally or partially involved
- Poorly defined nodules with variable, yellowish or tan-white, hard cut surface
- Epididymis and tunics may be involved concurrently

MICROSCOPIC PATHOLOGY

Histologic Features
- Early stage: Mainly intratubular infiltration of histiocytes with destruction of predominantly germ cells, but also Sertoli cells (lesser extent)
- Late stage: Tubular destruction and atrophy with extensive fibrosis
- Variable degree of intratubular aggregation of epithelioid histiocytes, plasma cells, and lymphocytes
- No well-formed granulomas or necrosis
- Giant cells and dystrophic calcification may be present
- May be associated with sperm granuloma

Predominant Pattern/Injury Type
- Inflammatory, chronic; inflammatory granulomatous

Predominant Cell/Compartment Type
- Histiocytes/macrophage

ANCILLARY TESTS

Histochemistry
- Gram stain
  - Reactivity: Negative
- Ziehl-Neelsen stain
  - Reactivity: Negative
- GMS (Gomori methenamine silver)
  - Reactivity: Negative

NONSPECIFIC GRANULOMATOUS ORCHITIS

Key Facts

Terminology
- Mixed chronic and granulomatous orchitis with no specific etiology

Clinical Issues
- Usually unilateral testicular enlargement
- May be accompanied by tenderness, fever, or heaviness

Microscopic Pathology
- Early stage: Mainly intratubular infiltration of histiocytes with destruction of predominantly germ cells, but also Sertoli cells (lesser extent)
- Late stage: Tubular destruction and atrophy with extensive fibrosis
- Intratubular aggregation of epithelioid histiocytes, plasma cells, and lymphocytes
- No well-formed granulomas or necrosis

DIFFERENTIAL DIAGNOSIS

Infectious Orchitis due to Specific Infections
- Syphilis may cause granulomatous orchitis, interstitial orchitis, or gummatous orchitis
  - Usually abundant plasma cells; Warthin-Starry stain may demonstrate spirochetal organisms
- Lepromatous leprosy
  - Early stage shows perivascular lymphocytic inflammation and interstitial macrophages filled with acid-fast bacilli
  - Late stage shows tubular atrophy, clustering of Leydig cells, endarteritis obliterans, fibrosis
- Brucellosis
  - Dense lymphohistiocytic inflammation with noncaseating granulomas in interstitium
- Tuberculosis
  - Necrotizing granulomatous inflammation with acid-fast bacilli

Sarcoidosis
- Confluent well-formed granulomas; systemic involvement and diagnosis of exclusion

Seminoma
- Clinical history; abnormal serum tumor markers; presence of tumor cells

Malignant Lymphoma
- Predominantly interstitial infiltrative pattern of uniform lymphoma cells

Sperm Granuloma
- Presence of sperm; positive AFB stain in sperm may be misinterpreted as mycobacteria

Malakoplakia
- Presence of Michaelis-Gutmann bodies (may be highlighted by von Kossa or iron stains)

SELECTED REFERENCES
1. Varma R et al: Acute syphilitic interstitial orchitis mimicking testicular malignancy in an HIV-1 infected man diagnosed by Treponema pallidum polymerase chain reaction. Int J STD AIDS. 20(1):65-6, 2009
2. Wegner HE et al: Granulomatous orchitis--an analysis of clinical presentation, pathological anatomic features and possible etiologic factors. Eur Urol. 26(1):56-60, 1994
3. Perimenis P et al: Idiopathic granulomatous orchitis. Eur Urol. 19(2):118-20, 1991
4. Sporer A et al: Granulomatous orchitis. Urology. 19(3):319-21, 1982
5. Akhtar M et al: Lepromatous leprosy presenting as orchitis. Am J Clin Pathol. 73(5):712-5, 1980
6. Kahn RI et al: Granulomatous disease of the testis. J Urol. 123(6):868-71, 1980
7. Elicker ER et al: Granulomatous orchitis. J Urol. 113(2):199-200, 1975

IMAGE GALLERY

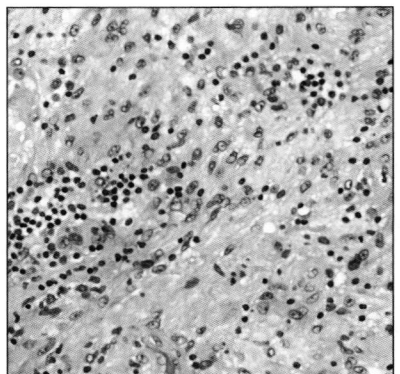 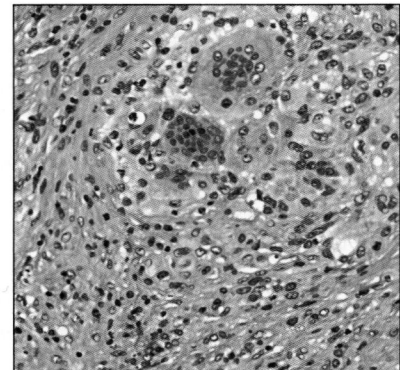 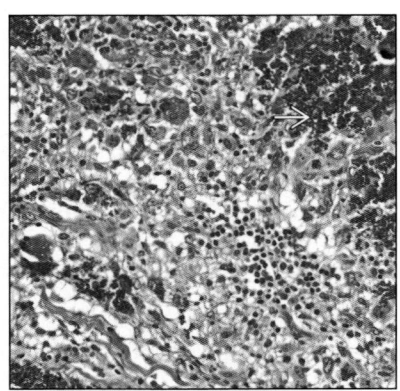

(Left) Late-stage nonspecific granulomatous orchitis with complete destruction of seminiferous tubules shows dense fibrosis and mixed inflammation with histiocytes and lymphocytes. (Center) Nonspecific granulomatous orchitis shows epithelioid histiocytes and a few multinucleated giant cells within the interstitium. (Right) This is an example of longstanding sperm granulomas with collections of histiocytes, lymphocytes, and sperm ➡.

TUBERCULOUS EPIDIDYMO-ORCHITIS

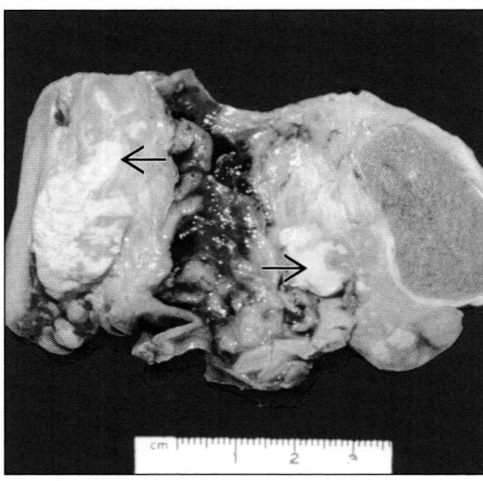

Gross photograph of a tuberculous epididymo-orchitis shows involvement of testis and epididymis by an irregular gray-white pseudotumorous mass with chalky white areas of necrosis →.

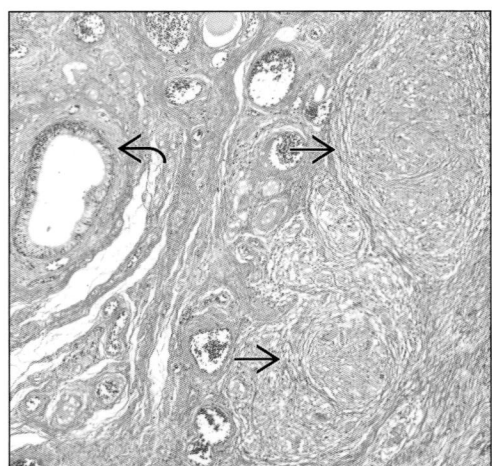

Several large epithelioid granulomas → are seen in the epididymis and surrounding paratesticular soft tissue →. Most testicular tuberculosis in adults starts with involvement of the epididymis.

TERMINOLOGY

Definitions
- Infection of testis and epididymis due to *Mycobacterium tuberculosis*

ETIOLOGY/PATHOGENESIS

Infectious Agents
- *Mycobacterium tuberculosis*
- Most cases of tuberculous epididymo-orchitis are associated with genitourinary tract involvement at other sites
- In adults, almost all are result of tuberculous prostatitis
- In children, > 1/2 of patients have advanced pulmonary tuberculosis and miliary spread

CLINICAL ISSUES

Epidemiology
- Incidence
  - High incidence in developing countries, immigrants, and immunocompromised patients
  - May be late manifestation of intravesical bacillus Calmette-Guérin (BCG) therapy
- Age
  - Affects any age but mainly adults (> 72% are older than 35 years)

Presentation
- Mild testicular enlargement and scrotal pain
- Associated with other constitutional symptoms of tuberculous infection
- Commonly associated with tuberculosis of lung and genitourinary tract
- Bilateral involvement (30%)
- Formation of abscess or sinus tract (50%)
- Secondary hydrocele (30%)

Treatment
- Surgical resection and systemic antituberculous therapy

Prognosis
- Excellent with modern antituberculous treatment

IMAGE FINDINGS

General Features
- Nonspecific heterogeneous or homogeneous mass of epididymis or testis on ultrasonography

MACROSCOPIC FEATURES

General Features
- Epididymis is almost always primary site of involvement with secondary spread to testis
- Irregular mass with foci of caseating necrosis
- When testis is involved, swollen and nodular
- Late stages: Extensive cystic change due to necrosis, associated hydronephrosis

MICROSCOPIC PATHOLOGY

Histologic Features
- Destruction of epididymis/tubules with caseating or noncaseating granulomatous inflammation in interstitium
- Multiple confluent granulomas with central caseating necrosis
- Aggregates of epithelioid cells with peripheral rim of lymphocytes
- Langhans giant cells (fusion of epithelioid cells with nuclei arranged in horseshoe-shaped pattern, often pointing toward necrosis)
- Schaumann (basophilic, shell-like crystals) and asteroid bodies may be present

TUBERCULOUS EPIDIDYMO-ORCHITIS

Key Facts

Terminology
- Infection of testis and epididymis due to *Mycobacterium tuberculosis*

Etiology/Pathogenesis
- *Mycobacterium tuberculosis*
- Most tuberculous epididymo-orchitis are associated with other genitourinary tract involvement

Clinical Issues
- Affects any age but mainly adults (> 72% are older than 35 years)
- Mild testicular enlargement and scrotal pain

Macroscopic Features
- Epididymis is almost always primary site of involvement with secondary spread to testis
- Irregular mass with foci of caseating necrosis

Microscopic Pathology
- Multiple confluent granulomas with central caseating necrosis
- Aggregates of epithelioid cells with peripheral rim of lymphocytes
- Destruction of seminiferous tubules and interstitium by caseating or noncaseating granulomatous inflammation
- Langhans giant cells may be present
- Late stage with fibroblastic response with scar formation

Ancillary Tests
- Acid-fast bacteria stain positive

- Late stage with fibroblastic response with scar formation

Predominant Pattern/Injury Type
- Infectious

Predominant Cell/Compartment Type
- Histiocytes/macrophages, lymphocytes, and plasma cells

ANCILLARY TESTS

Histochemistry
- Ziehl-Neelsen (acid-fast bacillus)
  - Reactivity: Positive

DIFFERENTIAL DIAGNOSIS

Nonspecific Granulomatous Orchitis
- Lack of necrosis or well-formed granuloma
- Predominantly intratubular location
- No involvement of epididymis
- Special stains negative for microorganisms; caution due to sperm staining with AFB

Seminoma with Extensive Granulomatous Inflammation
- Presence of large tumor cells
- Large cells positive for CD117, Podoplanin(D2-40), and Oct3/4
- Serum tumor markers (LDH and HCG) may be elevated

Malakoplakia
- Diffuse infiltrate of macrophages with granular eosinophilic cytoplasm; granulomas absent
- Presence of typical Michaelis-Gutmann bodies

Sperm Granuloma
- History of vasectomy is common
- Granulomatous inflammation with sperm
- No significant necrosis

Other Infectious Granulomatous Epididymo-orchitis
- Caused by fungi and parasites
- Organisms may be visualized with GMS or PAS stains
  - Correlation with microbiology cultures is essential

DIAGNOSTIC CHECKLIST

Pathologic Interpretation Pearls
- Confluent caseating granulomas

SELECTED REFERENCES

1. Jacob JT et al: Male genital tuberculosis. Lancet Infect Dis. 8(5):335-42, 2008
2. Wise GJ et al: An update on lower urinary tract tuberculosis. Curr Urol Rep. 9(4):305-13, 2008
3. Ramdial PK et al: Tuberculids as sentinel lesions of tuberculous epididymo-orchitis. J Cutan Pathol. 34(11):830-6, 2007
4. Muttarak M et al: Tuberculous epididymitis and epididymo-orchitis: sonographic appearances. AJR Am J Roentgenol. 176(6):1459-66, 2001
5. Chung JJ et al: Sonographic findings in tuberculous epididymitis and epididymo-orchitis. J Clin Ultrasound. 25(7):390-4, 1997
6. Kim SH et al: Tuberculous epididymitis and epididymo-orchitis: sonographic findings. J Urol. 150(1):81-4, 1993
7. Koyama Y et al: Tuberculous epididymo-orchitis. Urology. 31(5):419-21, 1988
8. Riehle RA Jr et al: Tuberculosis of testis. Urology. 20(1):43-6, 1982

Gross and Microscopic Features

(Left) Gross photograph shows tuberculous epididymo-orchitis with predominant involvement of the epididymis with focal extension into the testicular parenchyma ➡. Large areas of geographic necrosis ➡ are present. There is a secondary hydrocele ➡. (Right) This gross photograph shows tuberculous epididymo-orchitis with extensive involvement of both epididymis ➡ and testicular parenchyma ➡. There is prominent secondary hydrocele ➡.

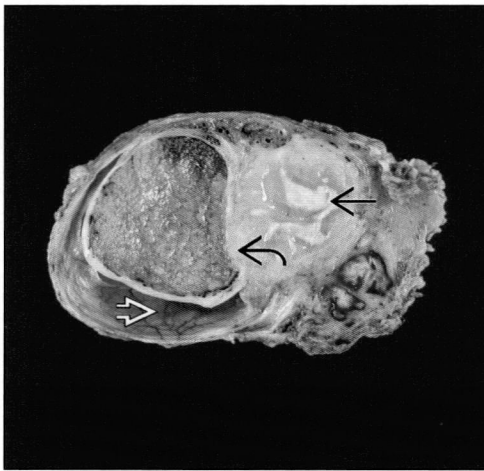
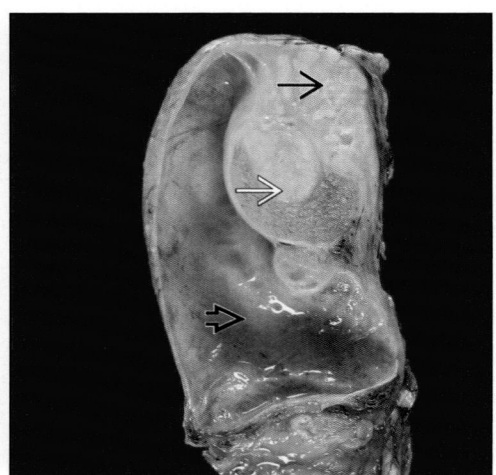

(Left) Gross photograph shows testicular tuberculosis with extensive involvement of the testicular parenchyma by irregular nodular discoloration ➡ due to poorly defined areas of granulomatous inflammation ➡ and areas of necrosis. (Right) Testicular tuberculosis shows necrotizing granulomas ➡ scattered within the interstitium. The confluent inflammation destroys the normal architecture and correlates with an inflammatory mass on gross examination and at microscopy ➡.

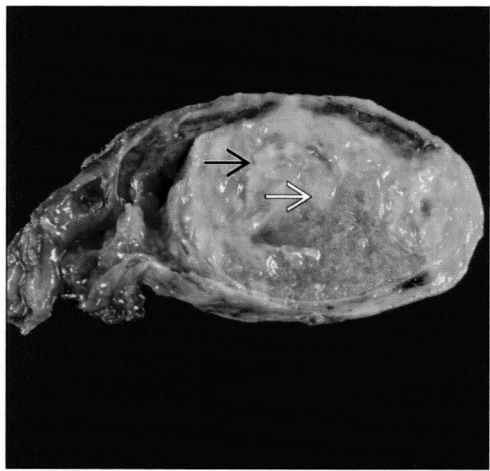
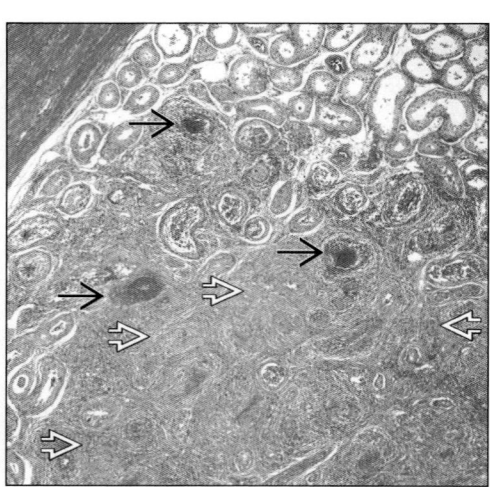

(Left) Well-formed caseating ➡ and noncaseating granulomas ➡ with epithelioid histiocytes are shown. Lymphocytes as well as neutrophils are seen in the interstitium. Also seen are uninvolved seminiferous tubules ➡. (Right) Testicular tuberculosis shows geographic necrosis ➡, palisading epithelioid histiocytes ➡, and peripheral rim of lymphocytes. The testicular parenchyma in this area is destroyed by necrosis and inflammation.

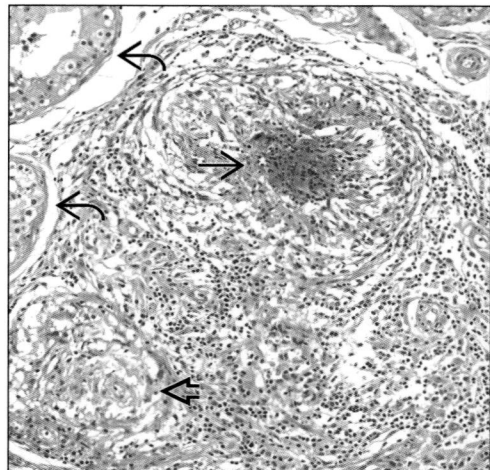
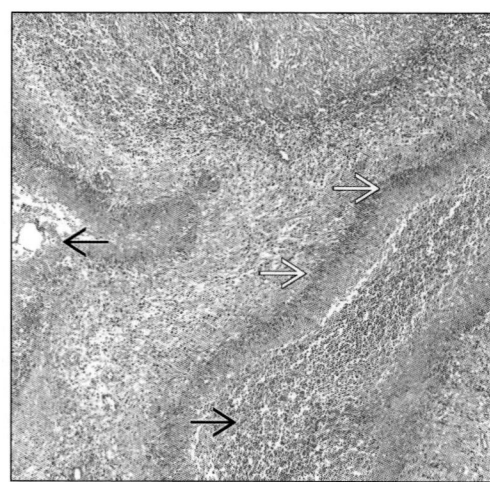

TUBERCULOUS EPIDIDYMO-ORCHITIS

Microscopic Features

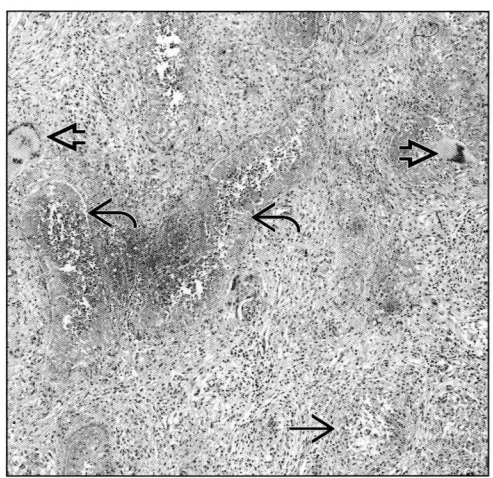
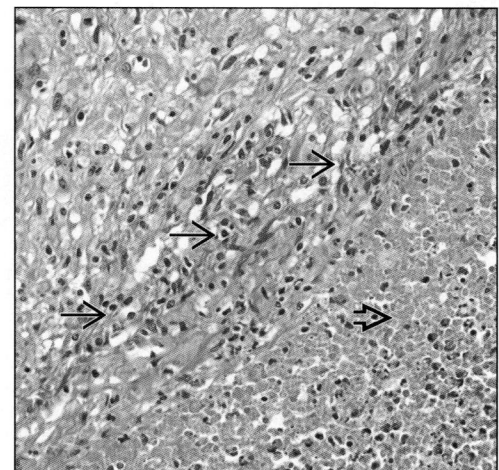

(Left) This image shows testicular tuberculosis with necrotizing granulomas ➡ and multinucleated Langhans giant cells ⮊ destroying the seminiferous tubules ➡. In contrast, the inflammatory infiltrate in nonspecific granulomatous orchitis is intratubular. **(Right)** High-power photomicrograph of testicular tuberculosis shows necrotizing granulomatous inflammation with epithelioid histiocytes ➡ and lymphocytes surrounding central caseating necrosis ⮊.

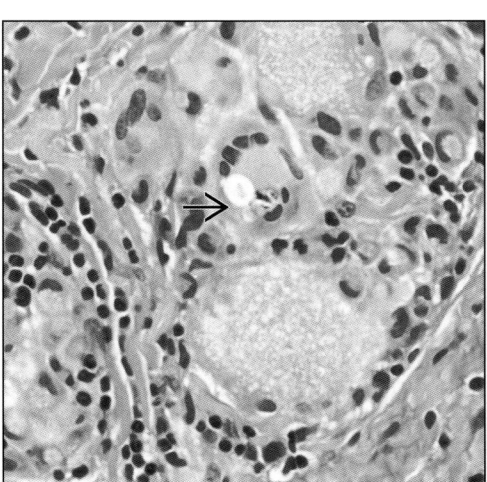
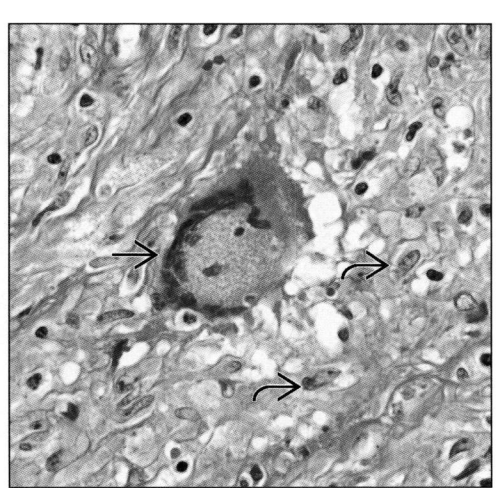

(Left) High-power photomicrograph shows a basophilic, shell-like structure (Schaumann body) ➡ in the cytoplasm of multinucleated giant cells of granuloma. This finding is not specific for tuberculosis and may occur in most other types of granulomatous disease. **(Right)** This image shows epithelioid histiocytes ➡ with a multinucleated Langhans giant cell with horseshoe-like arrangement of nuclei ➡. The hollow of the "horseshoe" most commonly points toward the area of caseation.

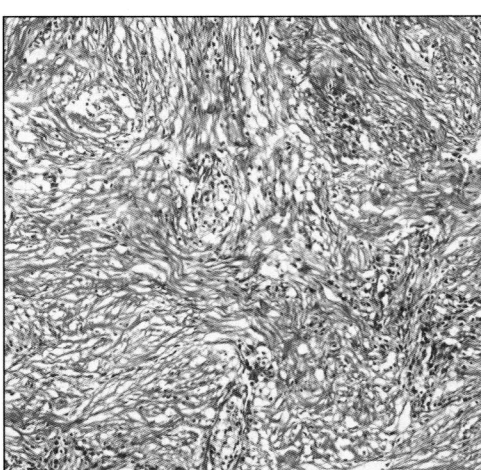
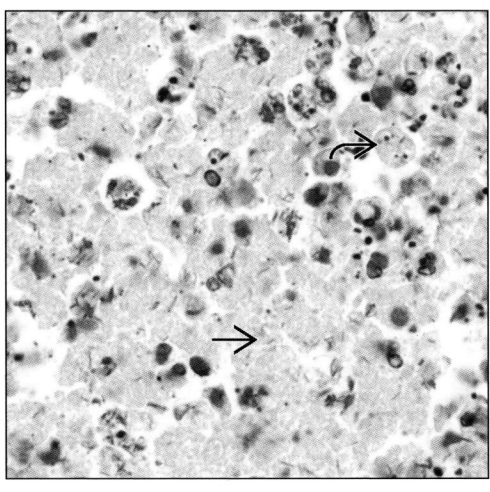

(Left) Fibroblastic response with scar formation is shown. There is no visible testicular parenchyma or granulomas. This may be seen at the periphery of the tuberculous epididymo-orchitis or healed tuberculosis after treatment. **(Right)** Ziehl-Neelsen technique shows acid-fast bacilli within the necrotic debris ➡ and in histiocytes ➡. Correlation with microbiology cultures is essential for speciating the type of tuberculous infection.

GENERAL CONCEPTS, GERM CELL TUMORS

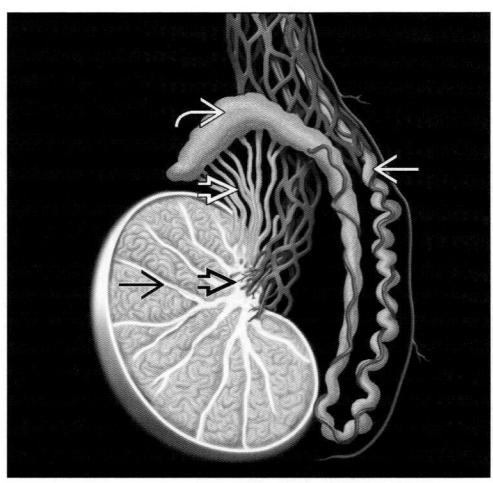

Schematic diagram of testis and paratestis is shown. The testicular parenchyma is separated by fibrous septae ➡, The tubules converge and exit to the rete testis ➡, efferent ducts ➡, epididymis ➡, and vas deferens ➡.

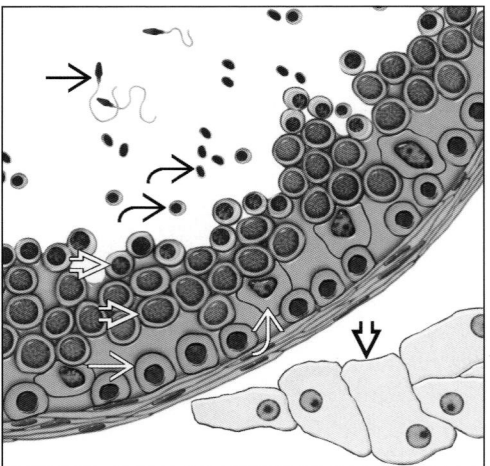

Schematic diagram shows seminiferous tubule with spermatogenesis (spermatogonia ➡, spermatocytes ➡, spermatids ➡, spermatozoa ➡). Sertoli cells ➡ and Leydig cells ➡ are also shown.

TERMINOLOGY

Synonyms
- Germ cell tumor (GCT), seminoma, nonseminomatous germ cell tumor (NSGCT), mixed germ cell tumor (MGCT)

Definitions
- Diverse group of tumors arising from totipotential germ cells with embryonic or extraembryonic differentiation

EPIDEMIOLOGY

Age Range
- Most GCTs occur between 20-50 years of age with peak incidence at 30 years
- Seminoma occurs at age ranging 35-45 years
- NSGCTs occur at age ranging 25-35 years (10 years younger than seminoma)

Ethnicity Relationship
- Incidence is higher in Western and Northern Europe, Australia/New Zealand, and North America (5.4-7.9 per 100,000)
- Incidence is lower in Africa, Caribbean, and Asia (2 per 100,000)

Incidence
- Estimated 8,400 new cases and 380 deaths from testicular cancer in USA in 2009 (American Cancer Society)
- Approximately 49,000 new cases and 9,000 deaths each year worldwide (2002 data)
- Worldwide incidence has more than doubled in last 40 years

Natural History
- Intratubular germ cell neoplasia (ITGCN) is a precursor to most GCTs except for spermatocytic seminoma and infantile germ cell tumors
- NSGCTs are more likely than seminoma to present with metastasis
- Choriocarcinoma often presents with early vascular dissemination to lung, liver, and bone
  - May present with choriocarcinoma syndrome (hemorrhagic metastasis)
- Metastasis of GCTs occurs in stepwise pattern of lymphatic spread through testicular mediastinum to retroperitoneal lymph nodes

ETIOLOGY/PATHOGENESIS

Cytogenetic Changes
- GCTs arising in prepubertal gonads (teratoma and yolk sac tumor) are usually diploid
- GCTs in postpubertal men typically have 1 or more copies of chromosome 12p (most commonly i[12p]), and other forms of 12p abnormalities and aneuploidy
- Approximately 80% of GCTs have at least 1 isochromosome 12 (i[12p])
- Other genetic changes in postpubertal men include loss of chromosome 11, 13, 18, and Y, and gains of 7, 8, and X
- Spermatocytic seminoma may be either diploid or aneuploid and may show loss of chromosome 9

Risk Factors
- Prior history of GCT
- Positive family history of GCT
- Cryptorchidism
- Testicular dysgenesis
- Klinefelter syndrome
- Infertility

CLINICAL IMPLICATIONS

Clinical Presentation

- Often unilateral painless testicular swelling or mass (bilaterality is rare: < 2%)
- Gynecomastia or exophthalmos may be presenting symptom (related to human chorionic gonadotropin [hCG] production)
- Approximately 10% may present with symptoms related to metastasis at initial presentation
- Elevation of serum tumor markers, including lactate dehydrogenase(LDH), α-fetoprotein(AFP), hCG

Laboratory Tests

- Elevated serum AFP usually seen in yolk sac tumor
- Highly elevated serum hCG suggests choriocarcinoma; borderline hCG elevation is not uncommon in seminoma and in germ cell tumors with syncytiotrophoblasts
- Serum levels of LDH, AFP, and hCG are incorporated into TNM staging

Treatment

- Treatment options depend on TNM stage and whether tumor is seminoma or NSGCT
  - Stage I seminoma
    - Radical inguinal orchiectomy followed by surveillance protocol (serum markers, chest radiographs, and CT scan), single-dose carboplatin adjuvant therapy, or radiation therapy
  - Stage I NSGCT
    - Radical inguinal orchiectomy followed by retroperitoneal lymph node dissection (RPLND), surveillance protocol, or cisplatin-based adjuvant chemotherapy
  - Stage II seminoma
    - Radical inguinal orchiectomy followed by radiation or cisplatin-based adjuvant therapy
  - Stage II NSGCT
    - Radical inguinal orchiectomy followed by RPLND, RPLND and chemotherapy, or chemotherapy and delayed RPLND
  - Stage III seminoma or NSGCT
    - Radical inguinal orchiectomy followed by multidrug chemotherapy

Prognosis

- Depends on histologic type, stage, and treatment
- Most types have favorable prognosis and respond well to chemotherapy &/or radiation therapy, as appropriate for tumor type
- Overall 95% survival rate in USA
- Morphologic prognostic factors
  - Lymphovascular invasion (pathologic stage at least pT2)
  - Proportion of embryonal carcinoma (> 80% poor prognosis)
  - Proportion of teratoma component (> 50% favorable prognosis)
  - Others: Tumor size (> 4 cm) and rete testis invasion (for seminoma)

Imaging Findings

- General Features
  - Testicular ultrasound may detect a testicular mass
  - Abdominopelvic computed tomographic (CT) scan may detect retroperitoneal lymph node metastasis
  - Chest radiograph and CT scan may detect lung metastasis
  - Magnetic resonance imaging (MR) may detect metastasis to bone and brain

MACROSCOPIC FINDINGS

Anatomic Features

- Testes are paired ovoid organ with average weight of 15-19 g and dimension of 2 x 3 x 4 cm
- Surrounded by thick capsule composed of 3 layers: Tunica vaginalis (outer layer), albuginea (middle), and vasculosa (inner)
- Posterior mediastinum contains blood vessels, lymphatics, and rete testis
- Fibrous septae divide testis into approximately 250 lobules: Seminiferous tubules and interstitium
- GCTs replace normal structures and present with tumoral pattern

General Features

- Testicular mass with variable appearance depending on histologic type and component

Specimen Handling

- Radical Resection
  - Orient specimen and ink appropriately, if necessary
  - Procure spermatic cord margin before specimen is opened/bivalved
  - Submit tumor entirely if small (< 2 cm)
  - For large tumors, at least 1 section per cm tumor
    - Section to include areas with different appearance
    - Section to include hemorrhagic and necrotic area (usually high-grade component, such as embryonal or choriocarcinoma)
    - More sections may be required in pure seminoma to rule out other germ cell components, especially if there are areas of hemorrhage and necrosis or serum AFP levels are elevated
    - Section to include rete testis and epididymis
    - Section to include uninvolved testicular parenchyma adjacent to tumor
    - At least 1 section of uninvolved testicular parenchyma away from tumor
- Subtotal Resection
  - Orient specimen and ink resection margins appropriately
  - Perpendicular section of tumor with margin for possible frozen section for margin and diagnosis
  - Sections usually include entire tumor
  - Section to include uninvolved testicular parenchyma

MICROSCOPIC FINDINGS

Normal Anatomy and Histology
- Histologic compartment of testis
  - Testis is composed of seminiferous tubules and interstitium
- Seminiferous tubules and spermatogenesis
  - Composed of Sertoli cells and germ cells in varying stages of differentiation or maturation
  - Germ cells mature from base to center of lumen and are divided into different stages based on their levels of maturation
    - Spermatogonia: Situated adjacent to basement membrane; small, round, dense nuclei with finely granular and vesicular chromatin and small nucleolus, clear or basophilic cytoplasm
    - Primary spermatocytes: More centrally located; largest cell type; variable nuclear appearance, clumped chromatin (spireme type), beaded cytoplasm
    - Secondary spermatocytes: More centrally located; smaller and fewer than primary spermatocytes; coarsely granular chromatin; no nucleoli
    - Spermatids: Located near lumen; small cells with darkly stained chromatin
    - Spermatozoa: Located in lumen; elongated eccentric nucleus with long cytoplasmic tail
  - Sertoli cells: Elongated pyramidal cells attached to basal lamina (10-12 Sertoli cells/tubules; germ cells:Sertoli cells ratio ~ 13:1)
- Interstitium is divided into intertubular and peritubular regions
  - Peritubular region contains basement membrane and thin lamina propria
  - Intertubular interstitium contains blood vessels, lymphatics, nerve, and Leydig cells

General Features
- World Health Organization (WHO) Histologic Classification of Testicular Germ Cell Tumors
  - Germ cell tumors
    - Intratubular germ cell neoplasia (ITGCN), unclassified
    - Other types
  - Tumors of 1 histologic type (pure forms)
    - Seminoma
    - Seminoma with syncytiotrophoblastic cells
    - Spermatocytic seminoma (SS)
    - Embryonal carcinoma (EC)
    - Yolk sac tumor (YST)
    - Trophoblastic tumors: Choriocarcinoma, monophasic choriocarcinoma, placental site trophoblastic tumor
    - Teratoma: Dermoid cyst, monodermal teratoma (carcinoid tumor), teratoma with somatic-type malignancies
  - Tumors of more than 1 histologic type (mixed forms; mixed NSGCT)

Cytologic Features
- Seminoma: Evenly spaced large uniform cells with no nuclear overlapping and distinct cell borders

- Embryonal carcinoma: Pleomorphic and anaplastic cells, nuclear overlapping and indistinct cell borders, prominent nucleoli, multiple nucleoli and nucleolar pleomorphism are frequent
- Yolk sac tumor: Cuboidal to flattened cells with indistinct cell borders, cytoplasmic vacuoles, and eosinophilic globules; polymorphic tumor cell population from epithelial-appearing to spindled
- Choriocarcinoma: 2 cell types: Large multinucleated cells with dense eosinophilic cytoplasm (syncytiotrophoblasts) and mononuclear cells with pale or clear cytoplasm (cytotrophoblasts) in hemorrhagic/necrotic background
- Teratoma: Multiple different types of tissues and cells

Predominant Pattern
- Tumoral/solid pattern (well- or ill-defined tumor mass)
  - Tumoral/solid pattern forms a mass with replacement of seminiferous tubules and interstitium
  - Hemorrhage and necrosis are not uncommon, particularly in NSGCTs
  - Entities typically displaying tumoral/solid pattern
    - Seminoma, NSGCTs, sex cord stromal tumor
- Interstitial pattern
  - Tumor cells infiltrate interstitium with relative preservation of seminiferous tubules
  - Distinct tumor nodule may not be grossly apparent
  - Entities typically displaying interstitial pattern
    - Intertubular seminoma, lymphoma, plasmacytoma and leukemia, metastatic carcinoma; infectious and inflammatory processes are also interstitial
- Intratubular pattern
  - Lesions predominantly seen within seminiferous tubules with relative preservation of interstitium
  - Distinct tumor nodule may not be seen grossly
  - Lesions typically with intratubular pattern
    - ITGCN or intratubular extension of germ cell tumor (e.g., intratubular seminoma, embryonal carcinoma, spermatocytic seminoma, etc.)
    - Intratubular extension of lymphoma, metastatic carcinoma, or idiopathic granulomatous orchitis

Predominant Cell Type
- Germ cells, seminomatous
- Germ cells, nonseminomatous

IMMUNOHISTOCHEMISTRY

Oct3/4
- POU-domain, octamer-binding transcription factor in neoplastic germ cells with pluripotent potential
- Positive in ITGCN, seminoma, and embryonal carcinoma (negative in spermatocytic seminoma, yolk sac tumor, and choriocarcinoma)

SALL4
- Zinc finger transcription factor in human embryonic stem cells
- Positive in all germ cell tumors (seminoma, YST, EC, choriocarcinoma, and immature teratoma)

Placenta-like Alkaline Phosphatase (PLAP)
- 120 kd membrane-bound enzyme present in placental syncytiotrophoblastic cells, germ cell tumors, and tumors of other tissue
- Positive in all germ cell tumors (seminoma, EC, YST, choriocarcinoma)
- Clinical utility has diminished due to availability of more specific and sensitive markers

CD117
- Receptor tyrosine kinase important for proliferation, survival, and differentiation of primordial germ cells
- Positive in ITGCN, seminoma, and spermatocytic seminoma

Podoplanin(D2-40)
- Monoclonal antibody against oncofetal membrane antigen (M2A) present in fetal germ cells, lymphatic endothelial cells, and mesothelial cells
- Positive for seminoma (diffuse membranous), ITGCN, and some EC (focal apical membrane)

CD30(BerH2)
- Member of tumor necrosis factor receptor superfamily limited to immune cells, decidual tissue, and human embryonal carcinoma
- Positive in embryonal carcinoma (membranous stain); may be focally positive in seminoma

SOX2
- Transcription factor expressed in embryonic stem cells
- Positive in embryonal carcinoma (nuclear)

α-fetoprotein (AFP)
- Fetal protein produced by fetal yolk sac and resembles albumin
- Positive in YST, variable in EC

Glypican-3
- Heparin sulfate proteoglycan involving embryonic cell growth and differentiation
- Positive in YST, syncytiotrophoblasts, and immature teratoma

Human Placental Lactogen (HPL)
- 22 kd cytoplasmic protein with homology to growth hormone
- Positive in choriocarcinoma (syncytiotrophoblastic cells) and placental site trophoblastic tumor

REPORTING CRITERIA

Key Elements
- Histologic type (seminoma vs. NSGCT)
- For germ cell tumors, report whether tumor is pure or mixed
- For mixed germ cell tumors, report percentage of each germ cell tumor component, beginning with predominant type, including seminoma
- Lymphovascular invasion (should state even in cases with no vascular invasion)
- Tumor size and rete testis invasion
- Presence of ITGCN
- Presence of syncytiotrophoblasts
- Margin status
- Involvement of adjacent structures

TNM TUMOR STAGING

Primary Tumor (pT)
- pTX: Primary tumor cannot be assessed
- pT0: No evidence of primary tumor (e.g., histologic scar in testis)
- pT1
  - Tumor limited to testis and epididymis without vascular/lymphatic invasion
  - Tumor may invade into tunica albuginea but not tunica vaginalis
- pT2
  - Tumor limited to testis and epididymis with vascular/lymphatic invasion or
  - Tumor extends through tunica albuginea with involvement of tunica vaginalis
- pT3: Tumor invades spermatic cord with or without vascular/lymphatic invasion
- pT4: Tumor invades scrotum with or without vascular/lymphatic invasion

Regional Lymph Node (pN)
- pNX: Regional lymph nodes cannot be assessed
- pN0: No regional lymph node metastasis
- pN1: Metastasis with lymph node mass ≤ 2 cm in greatest dimension; or multiple lymph nodes (≤ 5 lymph nodes), none > 2 cm in greatest dimension
- pN2: Metastasis with a lymph node mass, > 2 cm but ≤ 5 cm in greatest dimension; or > 5 lymph nodes, any 1 mass > 2 cm but ≤ 5 cm in greatest dimension; extranodal extension present
- pN3: Metastasis with a lymph node (nodes) mass > 5 cm in greatest dimension

Distant Metastasis (M)
- MX: Distant metastasis cannot be assessed
- M0: No distant metastasis
- M1a: Nonregional nodal or pulmonary metastasis
- M1b: Distant metastasis other than to nonregional lymph nodes and lungs

Serum Tumor Markers (S)
- SX: Marker studies not available or not performed
- S0: Marker study levels within normal limits
- S1: LDH < 1.5x upper normal limit and hCG < 5,000 mIu/mL and AFP < 1,000 ng/mL
- S2: LDH < 1.5-10x normal upper limit or hCG 5,000-50,000 mIu/mL or AFP < 1,000 ng/mL
- S3: LDH > 10x normal upper limit or hCG > 50,000 mIu/mL or AFP >10,000 ng/mL

SELECTED REFERENCES

1. Cao D et al: SALL4 is a novel sensitive and specific marker for metastatic germ cell tumors, with particular utility in detection of metastatic yolk sac tumors. Cancer. 115(12):2640-51, 2009

GENERAL CONCEPTS, GERM CELL TUMORS

Differential Histologic Features of Pure Malignant Germ Cell Neoplasms

	Classic Seminoma	Spermatocytic Seminoma	Embryonal Carcinoma	Yolk Sac Tumor	Choriocarcinoma
Growth pattern	Diffuse	Diffuse	Solid, glandular, papillary	Multiple patterns	Nodular
Lobular arrangement	Present	Uncommon	Variable	Absent	Variable
Fibrovascular septae	Present	Absent	Variable	Absent	Absent
Lymphocytes	Present	Absent	Variable	Variable	Absent
Granulomas	Present	Absent	Rare	Rare	Absent
Tumor cell nucleus	Polygonal/round	Polymorphous (3 cell types)	Very pleomorphic	Pleomorphic	2 cell populations
Nuclear chromatin	Fine	Variable	Coarse, vesicular	Fine	Variable
Nucleolus	Large, regular	Variable	Large, irregular	Usually small	Variable
Mitoses	Frequent	Infrequent	Brisk	Infrequent	Variable
Tumor cell spacing	Evenly spaced	Evenly spaced	Overlapping	Overlapping	Overlapping
Cell boundary	Distinct	Indistinct	Indistinct	Variable	Distinct
Cytoplasm	Abundant, clear	Scant, dense acidophilic	Amphophilic	Variable	Variable
Cytoplasmic content	Glycogen	-	-	Eosinophilic globules	-

2. Gopalan A et al: Testicular mixed germ cell tumors: a morphological and immunohistochemical study using stem cell markers, OCT3/4, SOX2 and GDF3, with emphasis on morphologically difficult-to-classify areas. Mod Pathol. 22(8):1066-74, 2009

3. Jemal A et al: Cancer statistics, 2009. CA Cancer J Clin. 59(4):225-49, 2009

4. Large MC et al: Retroperitoneal lymph node dissection: reassessment of modified templates. BJU Int. 104(9 Pt B):1369-75, 2009

5. Looijenga LH: Human testicular (non)seminomatous germ cell tumours: the clinical implications of recent pathobiological insights. J Pathol. 218(2):146-62, 2009

6. Mai PL et al: The International Testicular Cancer Linkage Consortium: A clinicopathologic descriptive analysis of 461 familial malignant testicular germ cell tumor kindred. Urol Oncol. Epub ahead of print, 2009

7. Tarin TV et al: Estimating the risk of cancer associated with imaging related radiation during surveillance for stage I testicular cancer using computerized tomography. J Urol. 181(2):627-32; discussion 632-3, 2009

8. Westermann DH et al: High-risk clinical stage I nonseminomatous germ cell tumors: the case for chemotherapy. World J Urol. 27(4):455-61, 2009

9. de Jong J et al: Differential expression of SOX17 and SOX2 in germ cells and stem cells has biological and clinical implications. J Pathol. 215(1):21-30, 2008

10. Fléchon A et al: Management of advanced germ-cell tumors of the testis. Nat Clin Pract Urol. 5(5):262-76, 2008

11. Heidenreich A et al: Postchemotherapy retroperitoneal lymph node dissection in advanced germ cell tumours of the testis. Eur Urol. 53(2):260-72, 2008

12. Hersmus R et al: New insights into type II germ cell tumor pathogenesis based on studies of patients with various forms of disorders of sex development (DSD). Mol Cell Endocrinol. 291(1-2):1-10, 2008

13. Ponti G et al: The impact of histopathologic diagnosis on the proper management of testis neoplasms. Nat Clin Pract Oncol. 5(10):619-22, 2008

14. Taskinen S et al: Testicular tumors in children and adolescents. J Pediatr Urol. 4(2):134-7, 2008

15. Ulbright TM: The most common, clinically significant misdiagnoses in testicular tumor pathology, and how to avoid them. Adv Anat Pathol. 15(1):18-27, 2008

16. Young RH: Testicular tumors--some new and a few perennial problems. Arch Pathol Lab Med. 132(4):548-64, 2008

17. Emerson RE et al: Morphological approach to tumours of the testis and paratestis. J Clin Pathol. 60(8):866-80, 2007

18. Karellas ME et al: ITGCN of the testis, contralateral testicular biopsy and bilateral testicular cancer. Urol Clin North Am. 34(2):119-25; abstract vii, 2007

19. Looijenga LH et al: Chromosomes and expression in human testicular germ-cell tumors: insight into their cell of origin and pathogenesis. Ann N Y Acad Sci. 1120:187-214, 2007

20. Rajpert-de Meyts E et al: From gonocytes to testicular cancer: the role of impaired gonadal development. Ann N Y Acad Sci. 1120:168-80, 2007

21. del Vecchio MT et al: Intratubular germ cell neoplasia of unclassified type. Anal Quant Cytol Histol. 28(3):157-70, 2006

22. Carver BS et al: Germ cell tumors of the testis. Ann Surg Oncol. 12(11):871-80, 2005

23. di Pietro A et al: Testicular germ cell tumours: the paradigm of chemo-sensitive solid tumours. Int J Biochem Cell Biol. 37(12):2437-56, 2005

24. Emerson RE et al: The use of immunohistochemistry in the differential diagnosis of tumors of the testis and paratestis. Semin Diagn Pathol. 22(1):33-50, 2005

25. Hentrich M et al: Management and outcome of bilateral testicular germ cell tumors: Twenty-five year experience in Munich. Acta Oncol. 44(6):529-36, 2005

26. Hoei-Hansen CE et al: Carcinoma in situ testis, the progenitor of testicular germ cell tumours: a clinical review. Ann Oncol. 16(6):863-8, 2005

27. Parkin DM et al: Global cancer statistics, 2002. CA Cancer J Clin. 55(2):74-108, 2005

28. Ulbright TM: Germ cell tumors of the gonads: a selective review emphasizing problems in differential diagnosis, newly appreciated, and controversial issues. Mod Pathol. 18 Suppl 2:S61-79, 2005

29. Dieckmann KP et al: Clinical epidemiology of testicular germ cell tumors. World J Urol. 22(1):2-14, 2004

30. Honecker F et al: New insights into the pathology and molecular biology of human germ cell tumors. World J Urol. 22(1):15-24, 2004

4

Microscopic Features

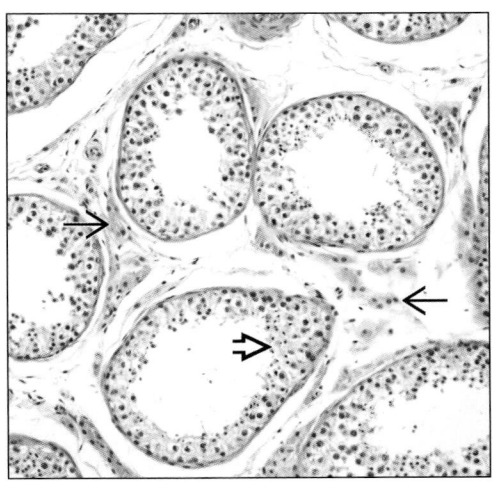
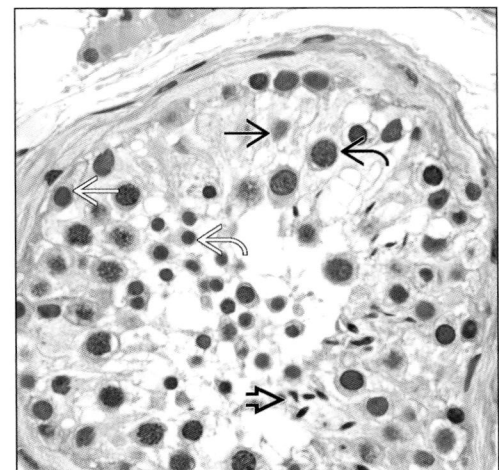

(Left) Low-power view of the testis shows seminiferous tubules with spermatogenesis ➾ and the interstitium. The tubules are surrounded by a delicate basement membrane and a thin lamina propria. Scattered Leydig cells ➾ are present within the interstitium. (Right) High-power view shows different stages of germ cells (spermatogonia ➾, primary spermatocytes ➾, spermatids ➾, and spermatozoans ➾) and Sertoli cell ➾ within seminiferous tubule.

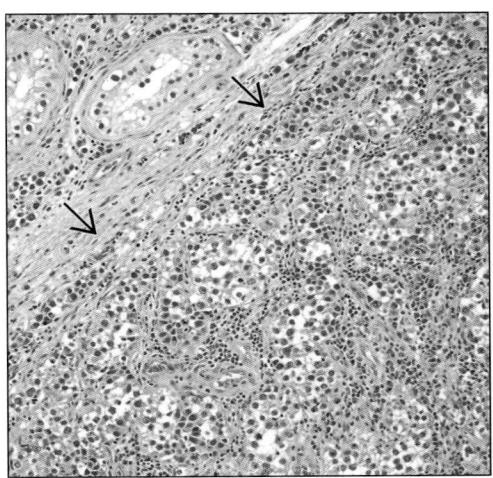
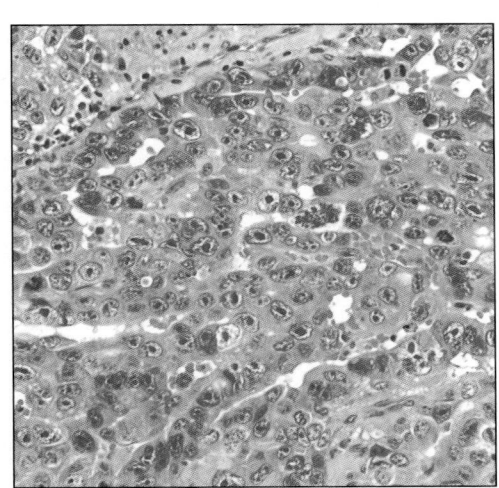

(Left) Testicular pathology may be approached as solid (tumoral), interstitial, and tubular patterns. This image shows the solid pattern ➾ of seminoma forming a nodule with total effacement of seminiferous tubules. Adjacent to the tumor, the tubules and interstitium are discernible. (Right) H&E shows solid (tumoral) growth in EC. The tumor completely replaces the seminiferous tubules and interstitium. The nuclear features in this case are essential for the diagnosis.

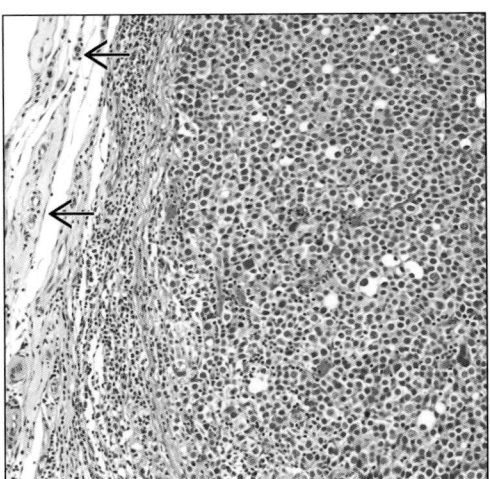
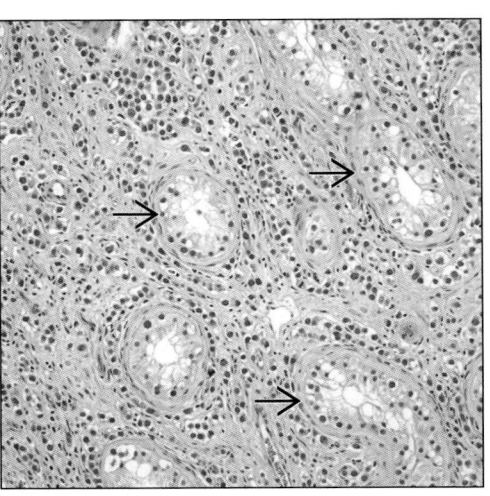

(Left) H&E shows solid (tumoral) pattern of spermatocytic seminoma. Spermatocytic seminoma cells replace the seminiferous tubules and interstitium, forming a well-circumscribed mass from the surrounding atrophic testis parenchyma ➾. (Right) H&E shows interstitial growth pattern of seminoma. The tumor cells infiltrate the interstitium with architectural preservation of the seminiferous tubules ➾ and interstitium. If this is the sole pattern, grossly, tumor may not be evident.

Microscopic Features

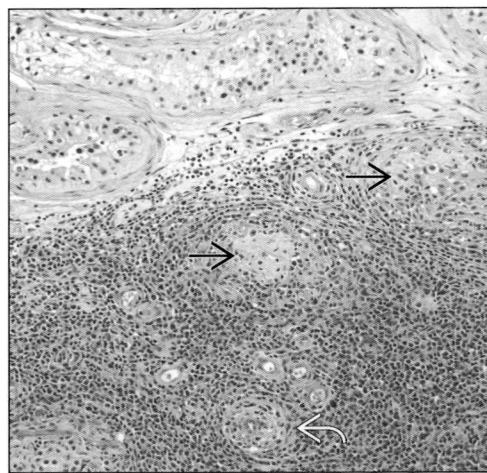 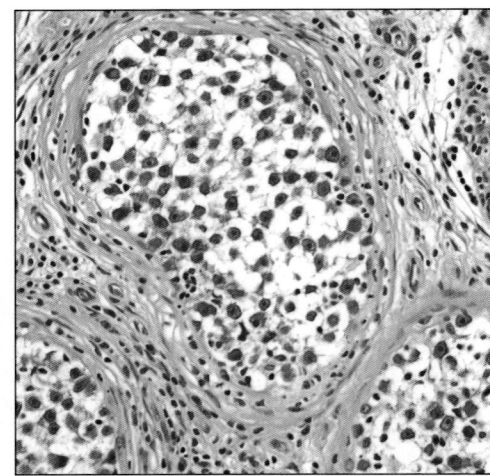

(Left) An interstitial growth pattern is characteristic of most lymphomas involving the testis. Tumor cells predominantly involve the interstitium with relative preservation of the tubules ➡. The tubular wall and lumen are focally involved ➡ and may occasionally be obliterated. *(Right)* H&E shows intratubular seminoma. In contrast to intratubular germ cell neoplasia, the tubules are completely filled, replaced, and expanded by large monotonous clonal seminoma cells.

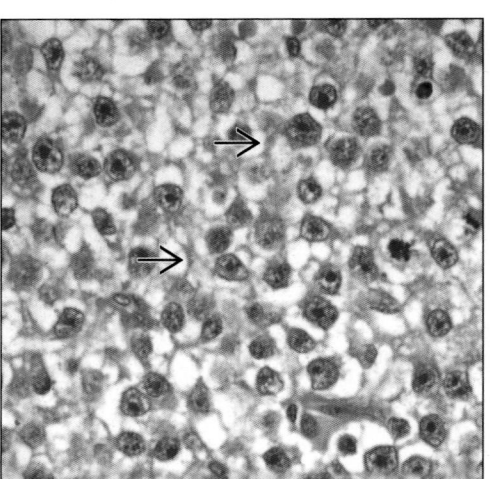 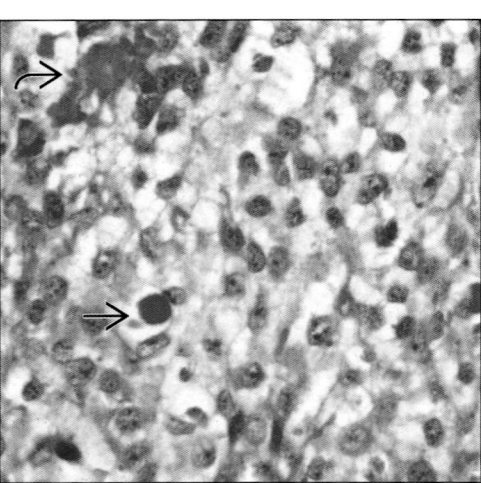

(Left) H&E shows seminoma with large uniform cells & prominent nucleoli. The cells are evenly spaced with abundant clear cytoplasm and distinct cell boundaries ➡. These cytologic features are diagnostic of seminoma. *(Right)* H&E shows YST with solid pattern. The cells are cuboidal or flattened with uneven cellular distribution and no distinct cell boundaries. Eosinophilic hyaline globules ➡ and basement membrane-like material ➡ are important clues to the diagnosis.

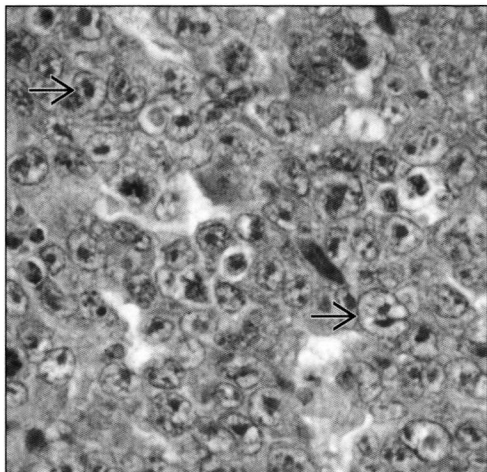 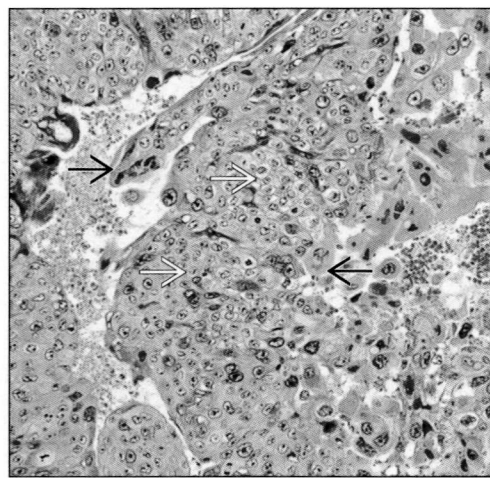

(Left) Anaplastic tumor cells and nuclear overlapping with indistinct cell boundaries are diagnostic features of embryonal carcinoma. The nucleoli ➡ are much more prominent and irregular than in seminoma. *(Right)* Diagnostic triad for choriocarcinoma includes hemorrhage and necrosis, 2 cell populations with multinucleated cells ➡ and mononuclear cells ➡, and spatial relationship with multinucleated cells wrapping around mononuclear cells, forming villous configurations.

Immunohistochemical Features

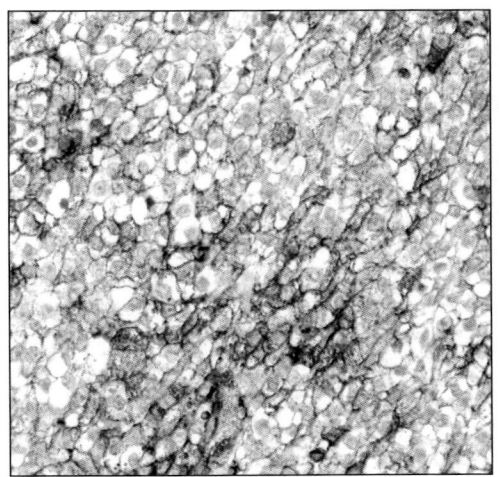
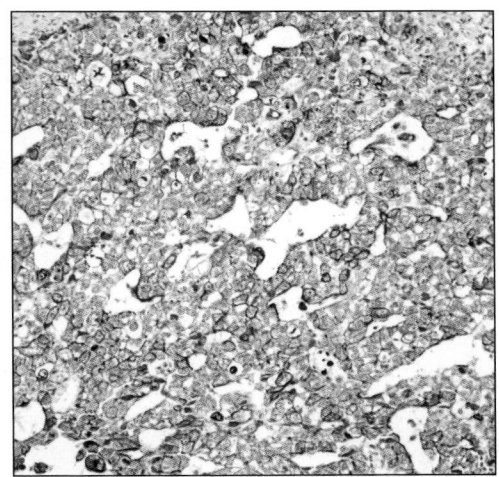

(Left) This image shows cytoplasmic and membranous staining of seminoma by PLAP. When the tumor has unusual features or is poorly preserved, immunostains with germ cell tumor markers (PLAP, Podoplanin, Oct3/4, and SALL4) may be necessary for the diagnosis. *(Right)* PAN-CK is helpful to distinguish seminoma from nonseminomatous tumors. Seminoma is often negative or focally weakly positive, but embryonal carcinoma (shown here) & other germ cell tumors are positive.

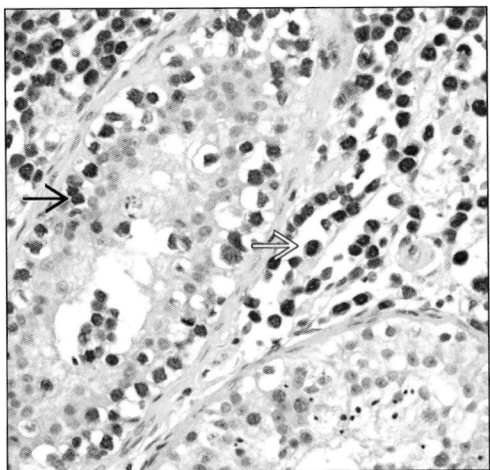
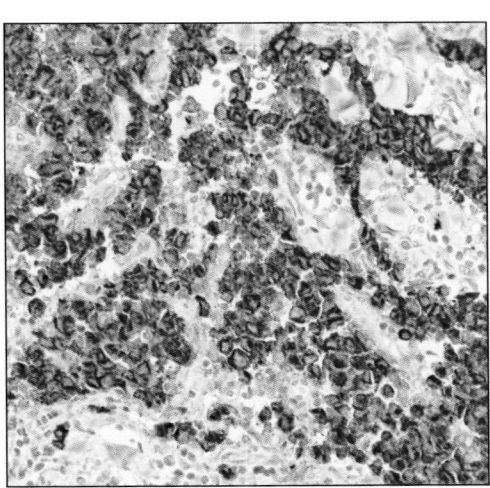

(Left) Oct3/4 immunostain shows intratubular germ cell neoplasia ⇨ and interstitial seminoma ➡. Nuclear staining and high sensitivity makes Oct3/4 a better marker than PLAP in diagnosing some germ cell tumor components. *(Right)* Strong membranous and cytoplasmic staining of seminoma with Podoplanin is shown. In addition to seminoma, EC is also positive for Podoplanin and Oct3/4, but YST and choriocarcinoma are usually negative. SALL4 is positive in YST and choriocarcinoma.

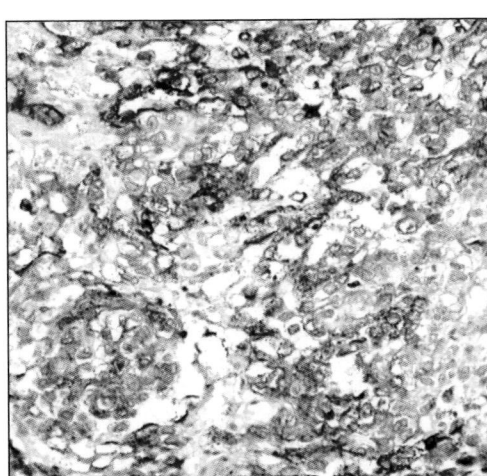
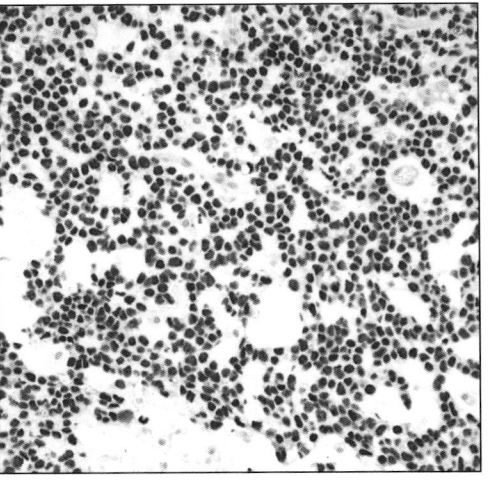

(Left) Besides AFP immunostaining, yolk sac tumor is strongly immunoreactive for Glypican-3, whereas other germ cell tumors are usually negative. Yolk sac tumors are negative for other germ cell tumor markers (PLAP, Podoplanin and Oct3/4). *(Right)* Yolk sac tumor shows strong positivity for SALL4 (nuclear). Since SALL4 is positive in all germ cell tumor components, it is useful in distinguishing germ cell tumors from nongerm cell tumors, particularly at metastatic sites.

INTRATUBULAR GERM CELL NEOPLASIA

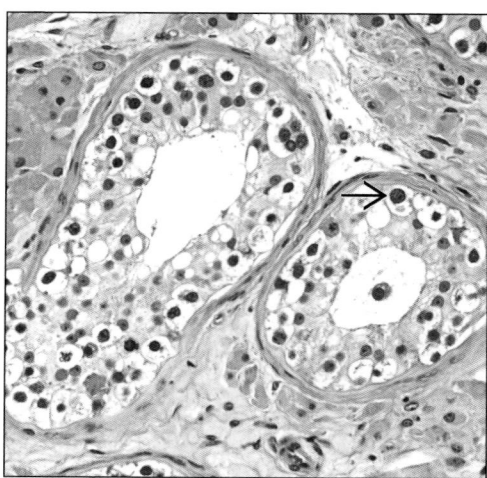

ITGCN is characterized by large atypical cells located along the periphery of the tubules ➡️. The cells have centrally located nuclei, prominent nucleoli, and abundant clear cytoplasm.

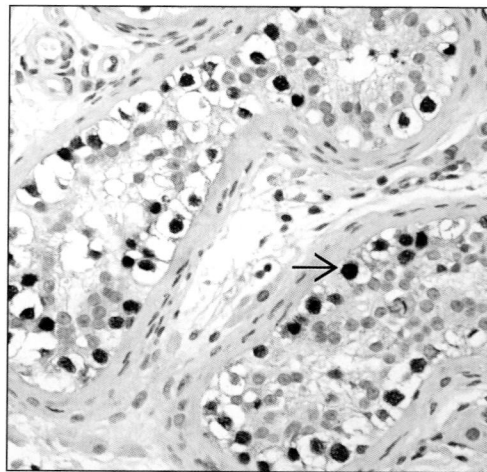

Immunohistochemical stain for Oct3/4 shows strong nuclear immunoreactivity in ITGCN cells ➡️ within the seminiferous tubules. Normal germ cells are negative.

TERMINOLOGY

Abbreviations
- Intratubular germ cell neoplasia (ITGCN)

Synonyms
- Carcinoma in situ; ITGCN, unclassified type

Definitions
- Proliferation of uncommitted neoplastic germ cells within seminiferous tubules; usually aligned at periphery of tubules

CLINICAL ISSUES

Epidemiology
- Incidence
  - Present in ipsilateral uninvolved testis in 80-95% of patients with malignant germ cell tumors
  - Present in contralateral testis in 5-8% of patients with malignant germ cell tumors

Presentation
- In cryptorchid testis or in association with malignant germ cell tumor
- Risk factors
  - Cryptorchidism
  - Microlithiasis
  - Gonadal dysgenesis with Y chromosome
  - Family history (1st-degree male relative)
  - Androgen insensitivity syndrome

Treatment
- Surgical approaches
  - Unilateral ITGCN usually managed by active surveillance or orchiectomy
  - Bilateral ITGCN may be treated by orchiectomy
- Radiation
  - May be used for bilateral ITGCN

Prognosis
- May progress to seminomatous or nonseminomatous germ cell tumors in about 50% of cases within 5 years

IMAGE FINDINGS

General Features
- Usually no abnormalities or microlithiasis on ultrasound

MACROSCOPIC FEATURES

General Features
- No demonstrable testicular mass; testis size may be normal or smaller

MICROSCOPIC PATHOLOGY

Histologic Features
- Intratubular proliferation of malignant germ cells distributed along periphery of tubules
- Seminiferous tubules may be atrophic, decreased in diameter, and may have thickened basement membrane
- Large atypical cells with prominent cell borders, centrally located nuclei with enlarged nuclei, evenly distributed chromatin, and prominent nucleoli
- Tumor cells with abundant clear to faintly eosinophilic cytoplasm
- Tubules with decreased or absent spermatogenesis
- May be associated with microlithiasis
- Pagetoid extension of ITGCN into rete testis may be seen; more frequent in nonseminomatous germ cell tumor than in seminoma

Cytologic Features
- Large atypical cells with abundant clear to faintly eosinophilic cytoplasm; mitoses may be seen

INTRATUBULAR GERM CELL NEOPLASIA

Key Facts

Terminology
- Proliferation of uncommitted neoplastic germ cells within seminiferous tubules

Clinical Issues
- Often present in association with malignant germ cell tumor

Microscopic Pathology
- Intratubular proliferation of malignant germ cells distributed along periphery of tubules or filling tubules completely (seminoma in situ)
- Large atypical cells with centrally located nuclei, thickened nuclear membrane, evenly distributed chromatin, and prominent nucleoli
- Tumor cells with abundant clear to faintly eosinophilic cytoplasm
- Pagetoid extension of ITGCN into rete testis may be seen; more frequent in nonseminomatous germ cell tumors than in seminoma

Ancillary Tests
- Positive for PLAP, CD117, Podoplanin(D2-40), Oct3/4
- Negative for cytokeratin, α-fetoprotein, CD30(BerH2) (may be positive in intratubular embryonal carcinoma)

Top Differential Diagnoses
- Normal spermatogonia
- Malignant lymphoma (intratubular)
- Metastatic carcinoma or melanoma (intratubular)
- ITGCN with microscopic invasive seminoma
- Spermatocytic seminoma (intratubular)

Predominant Pattern/Injury Type
- Intratubular growth pattern, no mass formation

Predominant Cell/Compartment Type
- Germ cells, uncommitted atypical germ cells, seminomatous/undifferentiated

ANCILLARY TESTS

Histochemistry
- PAS-diastase
  - Reactivity: Positive but sensitive to diastase
  - Staining pattern
    - Cytoplasmic

Immunohistochemistry
- Positive for CD117, Podoplanin(D2-40), Oct3/4, and PLAP
- Negative for cytokeratin, α-fetoprotein, and CD30(BerH2)

DIFFERENTIAL DIAGNOSIS

Normal Spermatogonia
- Usually accompanied by mixture of spermatogonia, spermatocytes, spermatids, and spermatozoa
- No tubular atrophy or thickening of peritubular tunica basement membrane
- Lacks prominent nucleoli
- Negative for CD117, Podoplanin(D2-40), Oct3/4, and PLAP

Malignant Lymphoma (Intratubular)
- Usually associated with diffuse interstitial infiltrative growth
- Positive for CD45(LCA), CD20, and CD3
- Negative for germ cell tumor markers

Metastatic Carcinoma or Melanoma (Intratubular)
- Metastatic carcinoma or melanoma may be intratubular; usually more pleomorphic with mitoses
- Metastatic carcinoma positive for pankeratin, EMA/MUC1, and tissue-specific markers (TTF-1, PSA, etc.)
- Melanoma positive for S100 and HMB-45

ITGCN with Microscopic Invasive Seminoma
- Lymphoplasmacytic infiltrate in interstitium
- Atypical tumor cells may be scattered among lymphocytes

Spermatocytic Seminoma (Intratubular)
- Abnormal cells packing seminiferous tubules
- Intratubular proliferation is pleomorphic
- Negative for germ cell tumor markers

DIAGNOSTIC CHECKLIST

Pathologic Interpretation Pearls
- Large atypical cells with clear cytoplasm in atrophic tubules with decreased or no spermatogenesis

SELECTED REFERENCES

1. Lau SK et al: Association of intratubular seminoma and intratubular embryonal carcinoma with invasive testicular germ cell tumors. Am J Surg Pathol. 31(7):1045-9, 2007
2. Balzer BL et al: Spontaneous regression of testicular germ cell tumors: an analysis of 42 cases. Am J Surg Pathol. 30(7):858-65, 2006
3. Berney DM et al: The association between intratubular seminoma and invasive germ cell tumors. Hum Pathol. 37(4):458-61, 2006
4. de Jong J et al: Diagnostic value of OCT3/4 for pre-invasive and invasive testicular germ cell tumours. J Pathol. 206(2):242-9, 2005
5. Jones TD et al: OCT4: A sensitive and specific biomarker for intratubular germ cell neoplasia of the testis. Clin Cancer Res. 10(24):8544-7, 2004
6. Rørth M et al: Carcinoma in situ in the testis. Scand J Urol Nephrol Suppl. (205):166-86, 2000

INTRATUBULAR GERM CELL NEOPLASIA

Microscopic Features

(Left) The smaller tubules ➡ exhibit large cells with abundant clear cytoplasm (ITGCN). The ITGCN cells are present at the periphery of tubules. The uninvolved tubules ➡ display active spermatogenesis with maturation sequelae of germ cells. *(Right)* High-power photomicrograph shows a seminiferous tubule with large ITGCN cells at the periphery of the tubule ➡ with centrally located nuclei, prominent nucleoli, and abundant clear cytoplasm.

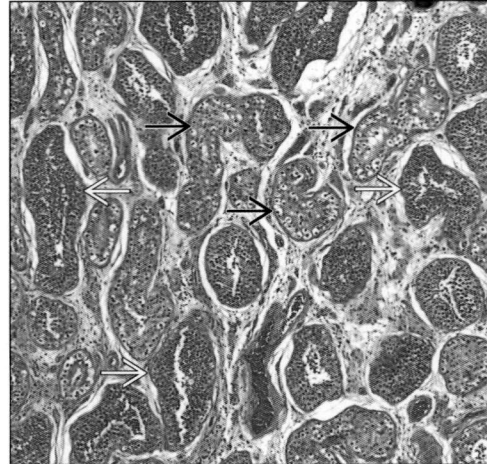
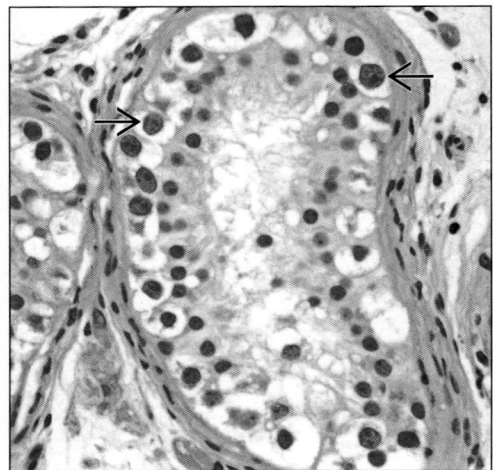

(Left) Hematoxylin & eosin stain shows the entire length of a seminiferous tubule containing ITGCN cells (large cells with clear cytoplasm and prominent nucleoli) along the periphery. *(Right)* High-power photomicrograph shows an atrophic tubule with prominent thickening of peritubular tunica basement membrane and large atypical cells ➡ at the periphery of the tubule.

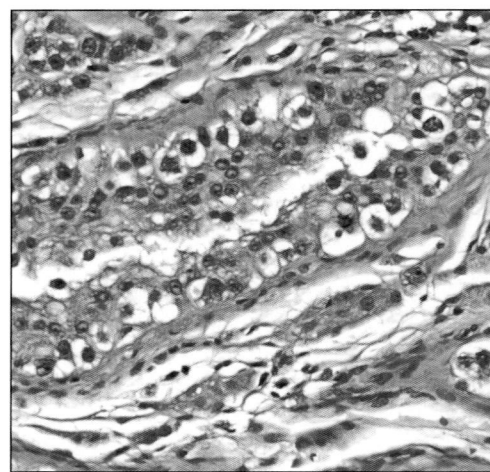
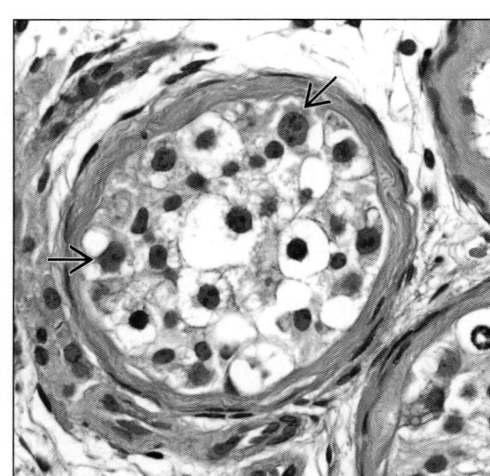

(Left) This image shows comparison of 1 tubule involved by ITGCN ➡ with adjacent seminiferous tubules with normal spermatogenesis ➡. Clusters of Leydig cells ➡ are seen within the interstitium. *(Right)* This photomicrograph shows ITGCN with intratubular calcification (microlithiasis) ➡. Microlithiasis is frequently observed in cryptorchid, ex-cryptorchid testes, tubules adjacent to germ cell tumors, and infertile patients. It is a useful clue to identify ITGCN.

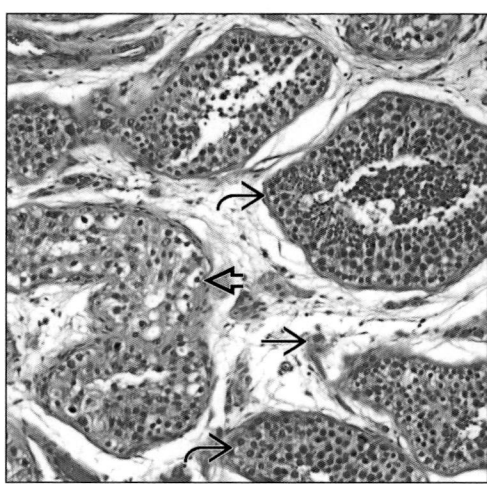
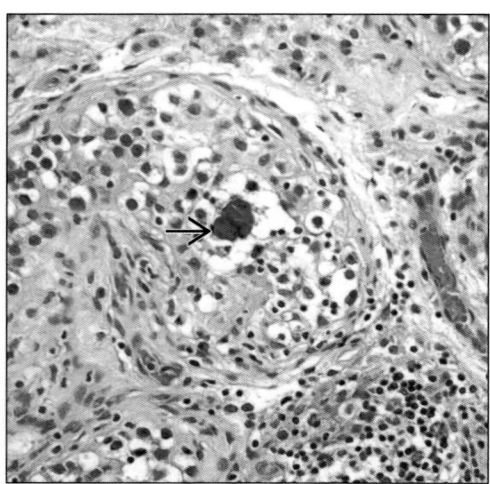

INTRATUBULAR GERM CELL NEOPLASIA

Microscopic Features

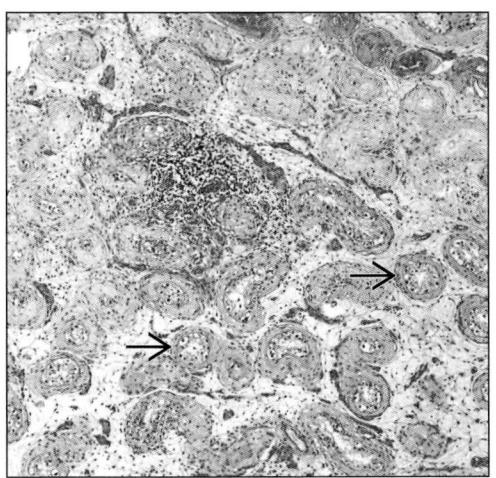

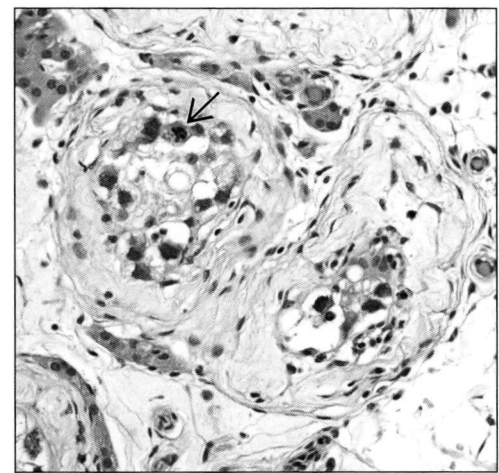

(Left) Low-power photomicrograph shows testis with diffuse tubular atrophy and marked thickening of tubular walls. Some tubules are completely sclerotic; others are involved by ITGCN ➡. In a cryptorchid testis, it is important to scrutinize lymphoid aggregates adjacent to ITGCN as such foci may contain microinvasive seminoma. (Right) High-power photomicrograph shows atrophic and sclerotic tubules involved by ITGCN. Note rare mitotic figure ➡.

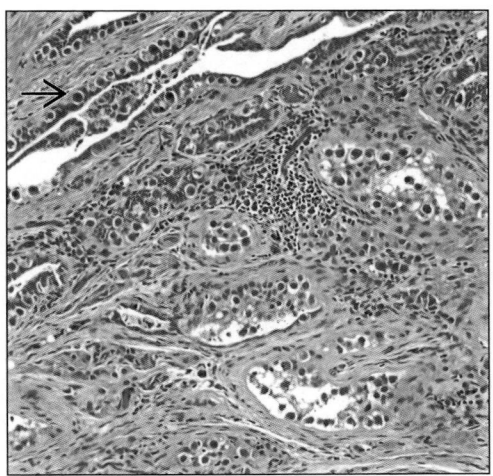

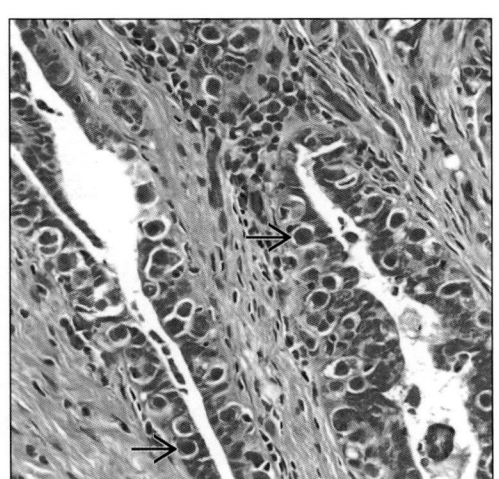

(Left) ITGCN cells involve several seminiferous tubules and extend to the rete testis in a pagetoid fashion ➡. This may occur in the absence of overt invasive seminoma. (Right) This high-power photomicrograph shows that rete testis is involved by pagetoid extension of ITGCN ➡. The stroma adjacent to the rete testis shows no invasive germ cell tumor component. Immunostains for CD117 and Oct3/4 may be useful.

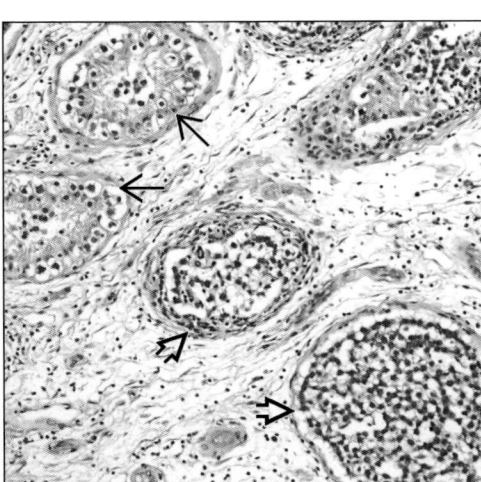

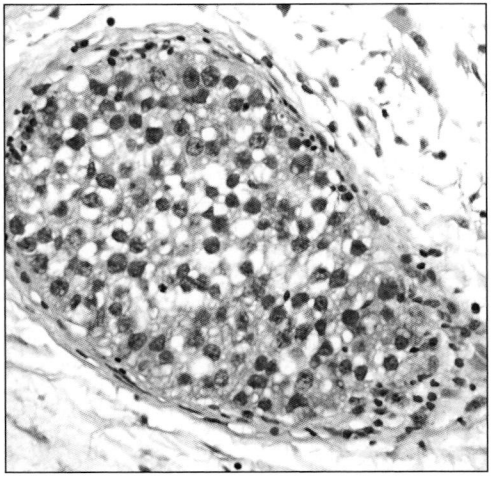

(Left) Two seminiferous tubules are involved by ITGCN ➡ and other tubules are filled and greatly expanded by cells of classic seminoma (intratubular seminoma) ➡. ITGCN is a precursor lesion for most germ cell tumors whereas intratubular seminoma represents extension of seminoma into seminiferous tubules. (Right) High-power photomicrograph shows an example of so-called intratubular seminoma. The seminiferous tubule is greatly distended by cells of classic seminoma.

Microscopic Features and Differential Diagnoses

(Left) This is an example of intratubular seminoma with microinvasive seminoma ⊡. Early invasive seminoma is almost always associated with lymphocytic response, a sign of invasion. Such foci may occur in a cryptorchid testis or in a testis containing a germ cell tumor in the vicinity or distant from such foci. *(Right)* This photomicrograph shows microinvasive seminoma ⊡ and multiple tubules involved by ITGCN ⊡. One normal tubule ⊡ with spermatogenesis is also present.

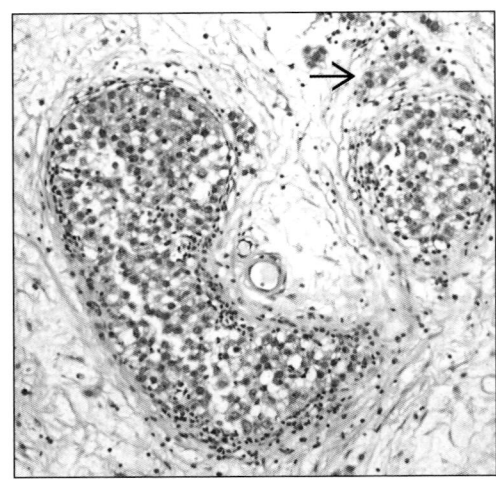 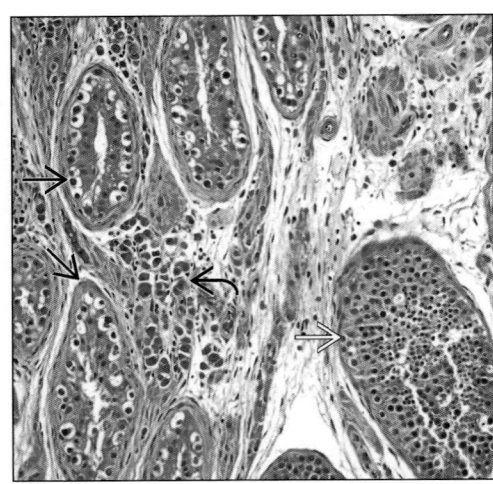

(Left) This is another example of intratubular seminoma with focal microinvasive seminoma ⊡. The cytology of the intratubular and invasive component is identical. *(Right)* This is an example of intratubular large B-cell lymphoma with large lymphoma cells and a few small lymphocytes. Elsewhere within the testis, typical diffuse interstitial large B-cell lymphoma was present. Immunohistochemical stains for CD45(LCA)(+) and Oct3/4(-) will help narrow the differential diagnosis.

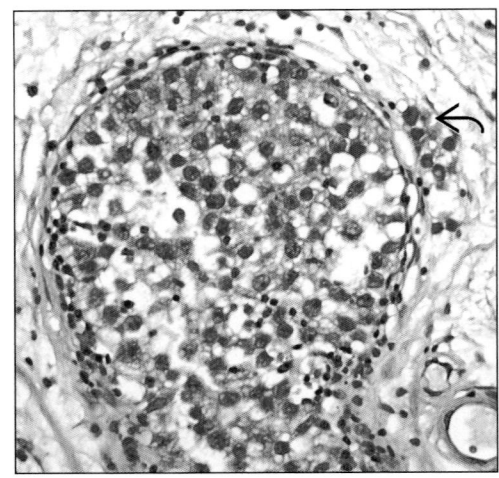 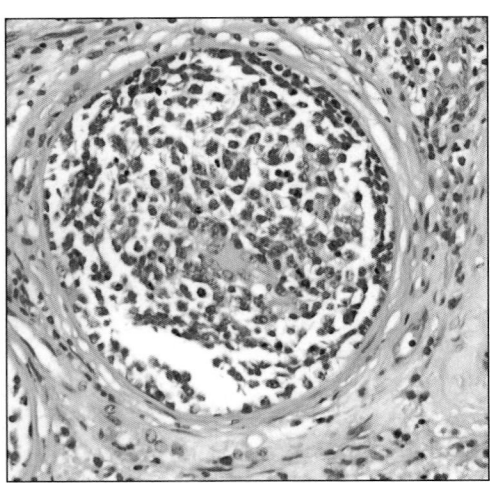

(Left) Metastatic high-grade prostate carcinoma can also have an intratubular growth pattern. The tumor cells are relatively uniform and have large nucleoli and prominent nucleoli. Invasive tumor cells are also present in the interstitium. *(Right)* Pagetoid extension of embryonal carcinoma in seminiferous tubules is shown. The tumor cells have crowded and overlapping nuclei, vesicular chromatin, and prominent nucleoli ⊡. Background nonneoplastic tubular elements ⊡ are present.

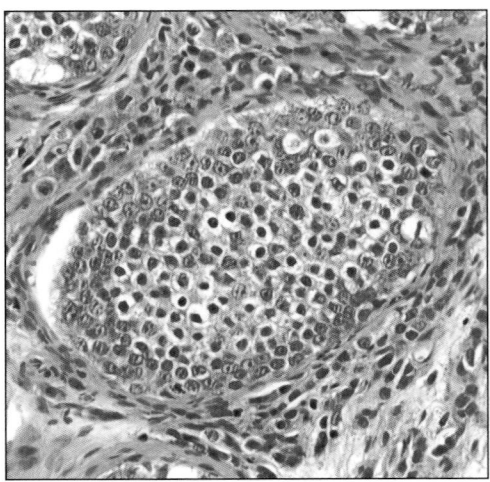 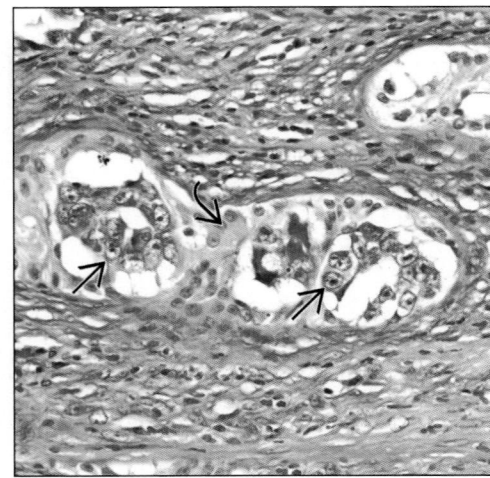

4

INTRATUBULAR GERM CELL NEOPLASIA

Immunohistochemical Features

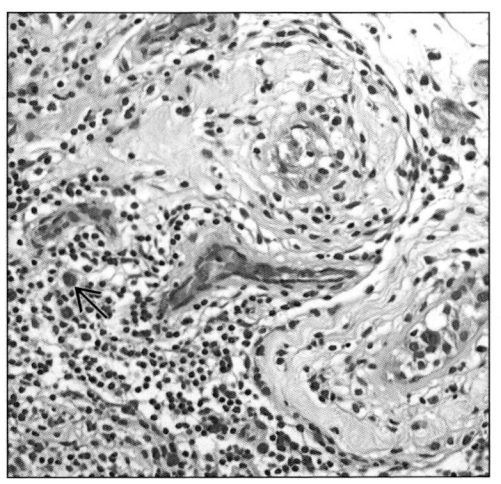

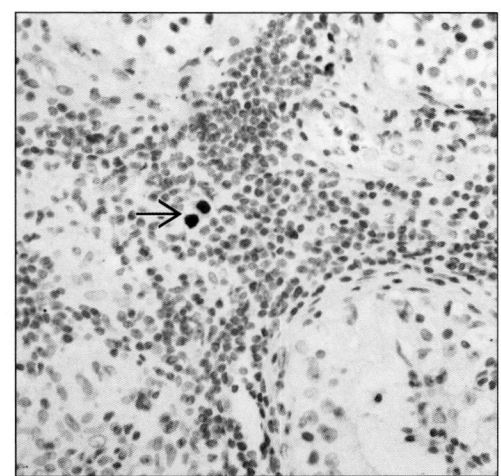

(Left) This photomicrograph focus shows intense chronic inflammation surrounding 2 atrophic seminiferous tubules with ITGCN. A single large atypical cell ⇒, suspicious for invasive seminoma, is present. *(Right)* This photomicrograph shows immunostain of Oct3/4. Two malignant cells exhibit intense nuclear staining for Oct3/4 ⇒, which is very helpful to identify and confirm the rare invasive tumor cells in the interstitium.

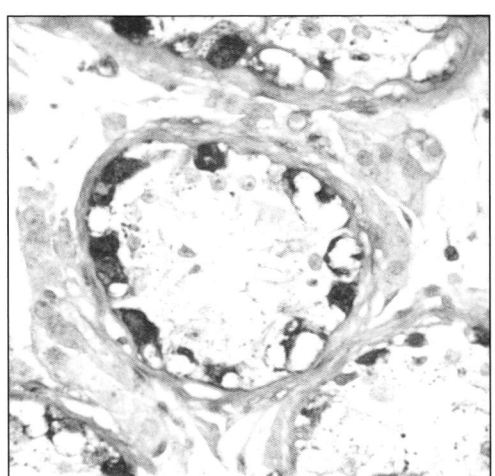

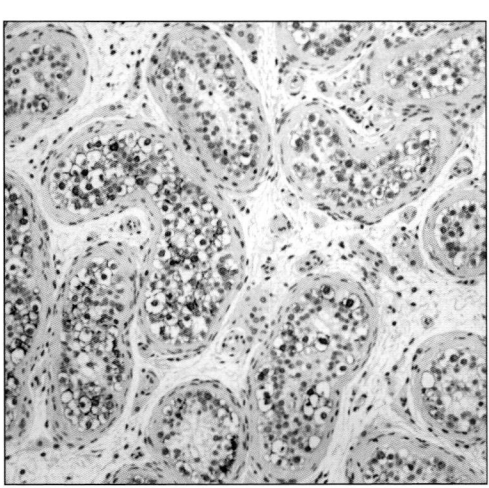

(Left) PAS stain without diastase shows strong cytoplasmic positivity in ITGCN cells, reflecting high content of cytoplasmic glycogen. This positivity is lost after diastase treatment. Sensitive and specific markers for ITGCN have minimized the use of PAS to confirm this finding in routine surgical pathology practice. *(Right)* Immunostain with PLAP highlights the tumor cells of ITGCN in a cytoplasmic membranous pattern.

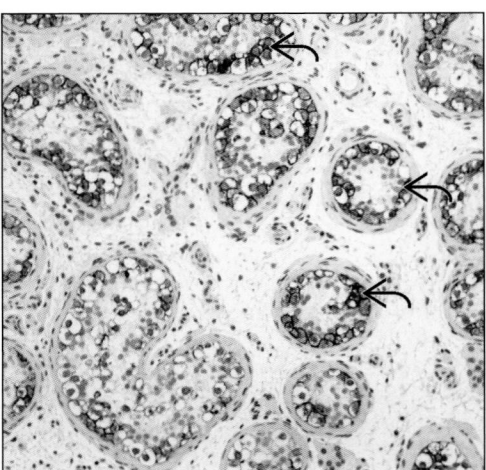

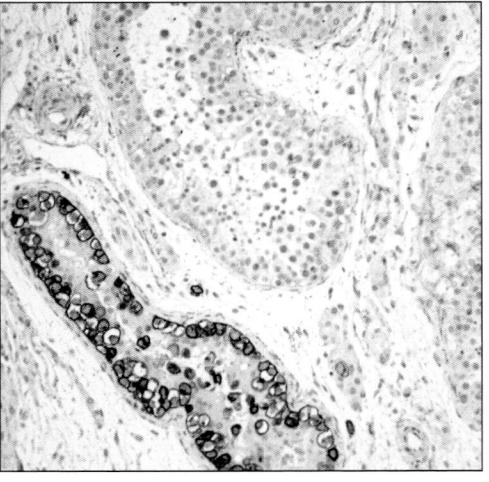

(Left) Podoplanin stains the cells of ITGCN in a cytoplasmic membranous pattern ⇒. Podoplanin also stains background lymphatic endothelial cells. It is positive in classic seminoma but not in other germ cell components. *(Right)* Immunostain with CD117 shows ITGCN with a cytoplasmic membranous staining pattern. The cells in the adjacent normal tubules are negative, although we have anecdotally seen CD117 positivity in nonneoplastic germ cells in testicular biopsies.

SEMINOMA

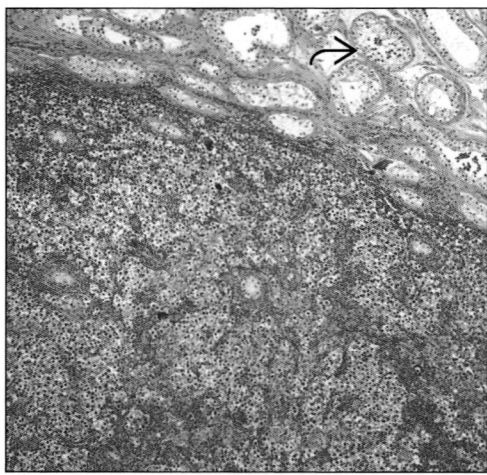

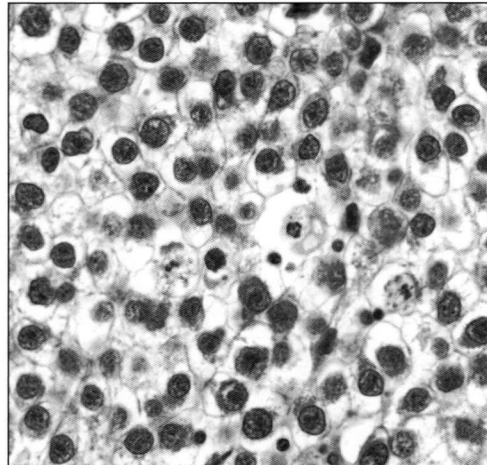

Low-power photomicrograph shows a well-defined classic seminoma surrounded by nonneoplastic seminiferous tubules ➚. Fibrovascular septae with small lymphocytic infiltrate divide the tumor into lobules.

High-power photomicrograph of classic seminoma shows tumor cells with large nuclei, prominent nucleoli, abundant clear cytoplasm, distinct cell membranes, and even distribution of tumor cells.

TERMINOLOGY

Synonyms
- Classic seminoma, typical seminoma
- Germinoma in extragonadal sites
- Dysgerminoma in females

Definitions
- Most common pure germ cell tumor composed of relatively uniform cells with abundant clear cytoplasm, well-defined cell borders, and nuclei with 1 or more prominent nucleoli

CLINICAL ISSUES

Epidemiology
- Incidence
  - 30-45% of testicular germ cell tumors
- Age
  - Most commonly in men 35-45 years old
  - Uncommon in men over 50 years and rare in children
  - Mean age 5-10 years older than nonseminomatous germ cell tumors

Presentation
- Most commonly painless testicular mass (70%)
- Other presentations
  - Scrotal pain (10%)
  - Symptoms of metastasis (10%)
  - Asymptomatic (4%)
  - Gynecomastia and exophthalmos (rare)
- Mostly unilateral and rarely bilateral (about 2%); bilaterality more common than in nonseminomatous germ cell tumors
- Spermatic cord involvement (rarer than in nonseminomatous germ cell tumors; < 5%)

Laboratory Tests
- Serum markers may be elevated

- Serum lactate dehydrogenase (LDH)
  - Human chorionic gonadotropin (hCG)
- α-fetoprotein (AFP) should be normal for pure seminoma
  - AFP elevation in patient with pure seminoma is clinically treated as nonseminomatous germ cell tumor

Treatment
- For patients with stage I seminoma, 3 options are available
  - Radical inguinal orchiectomy and surveillance with measurement of serum markers, chest x-ray, and CT
  - Radical inguinal orchiectomy with single dose carboplatin adjuvant therapy
  - Radical inguinal orchiectomy with radiation therapy
- For patients with stage II seminoma
  - Radical inguinal orchiectomy followed by radiation therapy to retroperitoneal and ipsilateral pelvic lymph nodes, or combination chemotherapy
- For patients with stage III seminoma
  - Radical inguinal orchiectomy followed by multidrug (bleomycin, etoposide, and cisplatin) chemotherapy

Prognosis
- Excellent prognosis with 98% cure rate for stage I or II seminoma
- Associated with pathologic stage, tumor size, rete testis invasion, and intertubular growth > 3 high-power fields
- Lymphovascular invasion is important prognostic factor in univariate analysis but not independent prognostic factor
- Concept of "anaplastic" seminoma (> 3 mitoses per high-power field) is not accepted as separate entity and not adverse prognostic factor

SEMINOMA

Key Facts

Terminology
- Most common pure germ cell tumor composed of relatively uniform cells with abundant clear cytoplasm, well-defined cell borders, and nuclei with 1 or more prominent nucleoli

Clinical Issues
- 30-45% of testicular germ cell tumors

Macroscopic Features
- Well circumscribed and homogeneous ± lobulation
- Gray-white, tan, creamy, fleshy or firm, often bulging cut surface

Microscopic Pathology
- Fibrous septae divide sheets or nests of tumor cells into lobules
- Tumor cells are evenly spread without nuclear overlap in well-fixed tissues
- Prominent cytoplasmic membranes (distinct cell boundary)
- Large round-polygonal tumor cells with abundant clear cytoplasm
- Lymphoplasmacytic infiltrate, occasionally extensive with germinal centers in fibrous septae
- Granulomatous inflammation in approximately 30%; can be extensive, which can create diagnostic difficulty in recognizing tumor cells

Ancillary Tests
- PAS positive with diastase sensitive
- (+) for Oct3/4 (nuclear), Podoplanin(D2-40), & PLAP
- (-) for cytokeratin (may be focal or weak), CD30(BerH2), & α-fetoprotein

MACROSCOPIC FEATURES

General Features
- Well circumscribed and homogeneous ± lobulation; 90% confined to testis
- Gray-white, tan, creamy, fleshy or firm, often bulging cut surface; usually no hemorrhage or necrosis
  - Tumors with hemorrhage and necrosis often indicate nonseminomatous germ cell components
- May have geographic infarct-type necrosis (usually large tumors)
- Punctate hemorrhage (usually in areas of syncytiotrophoblasts)
- Rare spermatic cord invasion (< 5%)

Size
- Average 5.0 cm (range 2.0-24 cm)

MICROSCOPIC PATHOLOGY

Histologic Features
- Main architectural growth patterns
  - Solid sheets or nests (most common)
  - Interstitial (in between seminiferous tubules; rare)
  - Tubular, alveolar, or pseudoglandular (rare)
  - Trabecular (rare)
  - Sclerotic (very rare)
- Fibrous septae divide sheets or nests of tumor cells into lobules
- Tumor cells are evenly spread without nuclear overlap in well-fixed tissues
- Lymphoplasmacytic infiltrate, occasionally extensive, with germinal centers in fibrous septae
- Granulomatous inflammation in approximately 30%; may be extensive, which can create diagnostic difficulty in recognizing tumor cells
- Fibrosis and sclerosis may be prominent (burnt-out seminoma when no tumor cells present)
- Hemorrhage and necrosis are rarely seen
- Syncytiotrophoblastic giant cells may be seen in areas of hemorrhage
- Intratubular germ cell neoplasia (ITGCN) in surrounding seminiferous tubules or pagetoid spread to rete testis

Cytologic Features
- Large round-polygonal tumor cells with abundant clear cytoplasm
- Prominent cytoplasmic membranes (distinct cell boundary)
- Relatively uniform, large central nuclei with 1-2 prominent nucleoli
- Mitotic figures range from rare to frequent
- Some tumors can have larger cells, high N:C ratio, and more mitoses (> 3/high-power field); known as "anaplastic seminoma"
- Rarely, tumor cells can have rhabdoid appearance with abundant eosinophilic cytoplasm and eccentrically located nuclei; often occurs in poorly fixed specimens

Predominant Pattern/Injury Type
- Neoplastic

Predominant Cell/Compartment Type
- Uncommitted large atypical malignant germ cells

ANCILLARY TESTS

Histochemistry
- Periodic acid-Schiff without diastase
  - Reactivity: Positive
  - Staining pattern
    - Cytoplasmic

Immunohistochemistry
- Positive for PLAP, Oct3/4, CD117, Podoplanin(D2-40), vimentin, SALL4
- Negative for cytokeratin (may be focal or weak), α-fetoprotein, HCG, inhibin-α, CD30, glypican-3

DIFFERENTIAL DIAGNOSIS

Embryonal Carcinoma, Solid Pattern
- Usually admixed with glandular, papillary, and solid growth patterns
- Marked cellular pleomorphism, vesicular nuclei, nuclear crowding with overlapping and indistinct cell border, irregularly shaped nucleoli, frequent mitoses or apoptoses
- Positive for cytokeratin and CD30(BerH2)

Yolk Sac Tumor, Solid Pattern
- Variable growth patterns, most commonly microcystic and reticular
- Schiller-Duval bodies, basement membrane deposition, and hyaline globules are characteristic, if present
- Positive for cytokeratin, α-fetoprotein, and glypican-3

Malignant Lymphoma
- Usually older age group, history of lymphoma, and frequent bilateral involvement
- Predominantly interstitial pattern of tumor cells between seminiferous tubules
- Cytokeratin and germ cell markers negative; CD45(LCA) and B- or T-cell markers positive (depending on type, B more common than T)
- Frequent spermatic cord involvement (> 40%)

Spermatocytic Seminoma
- Older age group (average: 56 years)
- No association with ITGCN; intratubular growth may be seen
- Presence of 3 distinct types of tumor cells
- Lack of lymphocytic infiltration or granulomatous inflammation; no fibrous septa
- PAS stain negative
- Negative for germ cell tumor markers (PLAP, Oct3/4, Podoplanin[D2-40]); CD117 may be positive

Monophasic Choriocarcinoma
- Extremely rare; primary or metastatic foci post-chemotherapy
- Mononucleated tumor cells of variable sizes
- More frequent hemorrhage and necrosis
- Positive for HCG and human placental lactogen (HPL)

Nonspecific Granulomatous Orchitis
- Mixed population of inflammatory cells
- Predominantly involves seminiferous tubules
- Need to differentiate from burnt out seminoma

Sertoli Cell Tumor
- Usually more prominent tubular or cystic growth
- Particularly for those with solid or sheets of clear cells
- Usually lack fibrous septae with lymphoplasmacytic and granulomatous inflammation
- Usually positive for α-inhibin and cytokeratin, negative for PLAP, Podoplanin(D2-40), and Oct3/4

DIAGNOSTIC CHECKLIST

Pathologic Interpretation Pearls
- Relatively uniform tumor cells with abundant clear cytoplasm, distinct cell boundaries, evenly spaced tumor cells without nuclear overlapping
- Fibrous septae with lymphoplasmacytic infiltrates and granulomatous reaction
- Diagnostically difficult patterns
  - Extensive granulomatous inflammation
  - Tubular or pseudoglandular pattern
  - Extensive sclerosis
  - Extensive features of regression
  - Interstitial growth pattern
  - ITGCN with microinvasion (microscopic invasion)
  - Poorly fixed; "seminoma with atypia"
    - Must look for ITGCN

REPORTING CONSIDERATIONS

Key Elements to Report
- General information
  - Laterality
  - Multifocality
  - Tumor size
- Histologic type (pure classic or with other germ cell components)
- Pathologic stage (pTNM)
  - Tumor extension
  - Regional lymph node status
  - Distant metastasis
- Rete testis invasion
- Margin status (spermatic cord and others)
- Venous/lymphatic vessel invasion
- Additional pathologic findings, if present

SELECTED REFERENCES

1. Young RH: Testicular tumors--some new and a few perennial problems. Arch Pathol Lab Med. 132(4):548-64, 2008
2. Valdevenito JP et al: Correlation between primary tumor pathologic features and presence of clinical metastasis at diagnosis of testicular seminoma. Urology. 70(4):777-80, 2007
3. Ulbright TM et al: Seminoma with tubular, microcystic, and related patterns: a study of 28 cases of unusual morphologic variants that often cause confusion with yolk sac tumor. Am J Surg Pathol. 29(4):500-5, 2005
4. Tickoo SK et al: Testicular seminoma: a clinicopathologic and immunohistochemical study of 105 cases with special reference to seminomas with atypical features. Int J Surg Pathol. 10(1):23-32, 2002
5. Warde P et al: Prognostic factors for relapse in stage I seminoma managed by surveillance: a pooled analysis. J Clin Oncol. 20(22):4448-52, 2002
6. Nazeer T et al: Histologically pure seminoma with elevated alpha-fetoprotein: a clinicopathologic study of ten cases. Oncol Rep. 5(6):1425-9, 1998
7. Cockburn AG et al: Poorly differentiated (anaplastic) seminoma of the testis. Cancer. 53(9):1991-4, 1984
8. Percarpio B et al: Anaplastic seminoma: an analysis of 77 patients. Cancer. 43(6):2510-3, 1979

SEMINOMA

Gross Features

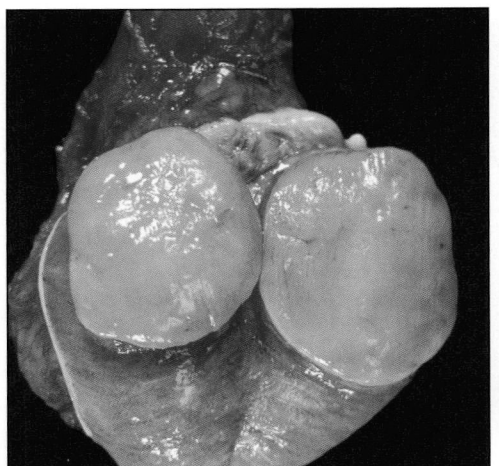

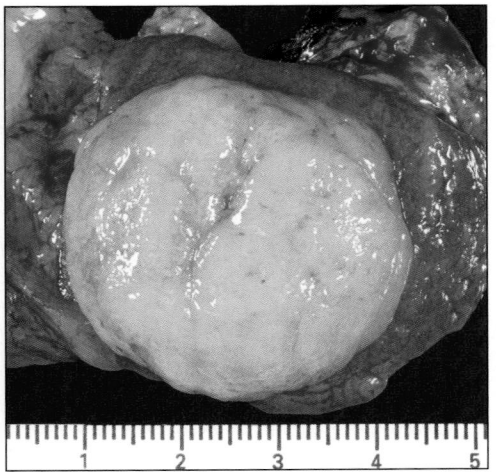

(Left) This gross photograph shows a classic seminoma. The tumor is a well-circumscribed, bulging mass with a tan fleshy homogeneous cut surface. No necrosis or hemorrhage is present. *(Right)* This photograph shows the typical gross appearance of a classic seminoma with a well-circumscribed mass with a tan fleshy homogeneous cut surface. No hemorrhage or necrosis is present.

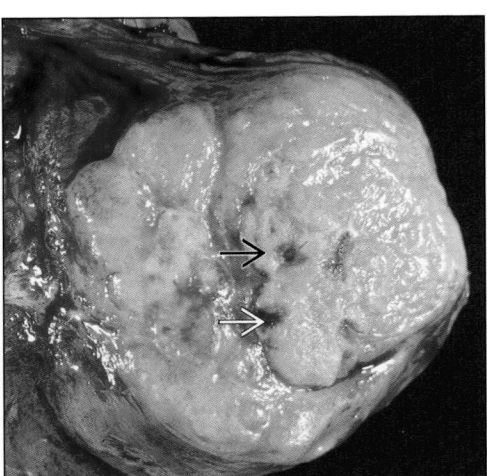

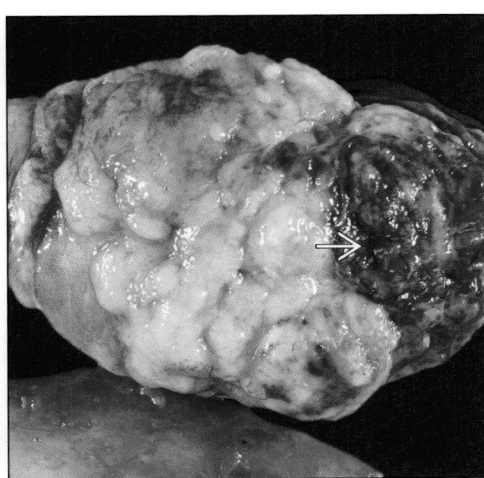

(Left) Cut surface of a large classic seminoma shows focal necrosis ➔ and hemorrhage ➔. Necrosis and hemorrhage are much more commonly seen in embryonal carcinoma or mixed germ cell tumor. *(Right)* This photograph shows a large classic seminoma involving almost the entire testis with a lobulated appearance. Focal hemorrhage and necrosis ➔ are present.

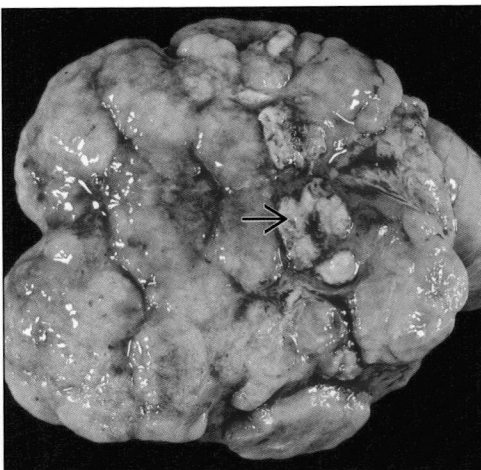

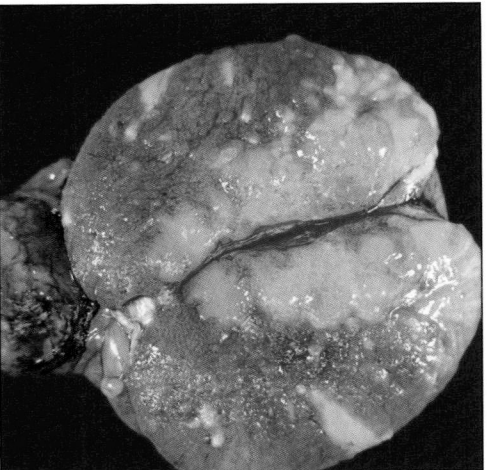

(Left) This classic seminoma shows prominent lobulation and focal necrosis ➔. Rete testis is also involved by tumor. *(Right)* Cut surface of a classic seminoma shows multifocal and interstitial infiltrative tumor pattern. There is no well-defined tumor nodule as seen in other examples. This appearance may be very similar to that of malignant lymphoma.

Microscopic Features

(Left) Touch preparation cytology of classic seminoma shows dimorphic population of large seminomatous cells ⇒ with relatively uniform round nuclei, prominent nucleoli, and small dark lymphocytes ➡. *(Right)* Diffuse sheets or nests of tumor cells are separated into lobules by fibrous septae containing small lymphocytes. The tumor cells in this example exhibit abundant eosinophilic cytoplasm.

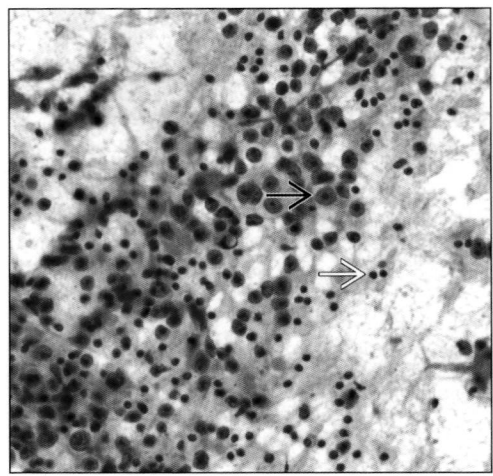
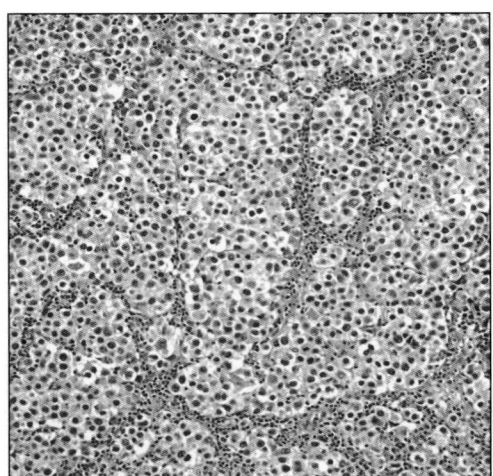

(Left) This high-power photomicrograph shows nests of uniform seminomatous cells ⇒ with abundant clear cytoplasm, centrally located nuclei, prominent nucleoli, and distinct cells membranes. Fibrovascular septae with small lymphocytes ⇒ are characteristic of seminoma. *(Right)* Solid sheets of clear seminomatous cells are separated by delicate fibrovascular septae with rare lymphocytes. The tumor cells are evenly distributed, and prominent cell boundaries are evident.

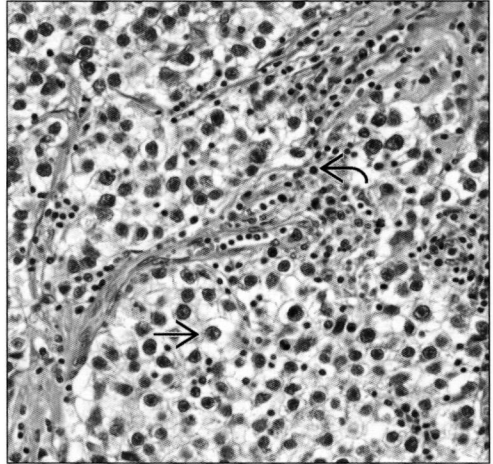
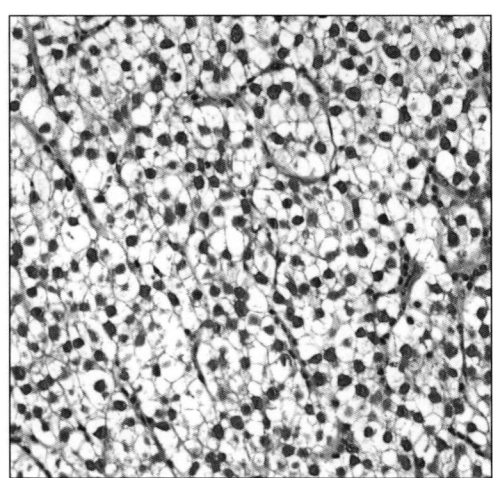

(Left) This image shows nests of seminomatous tumor cells ⇒ with extensive granulomas ⇒ and a lymphoid aggregate with germinal center ➡. The tumor cells contain abundant clear cytoplasm. *(Right)* This photomicrograph shows a classic seminoma with scattered large seminomatous germ cells ⇒ with extensive lymphoplasmacytic infiltrates and vessels with plump endothelial cells. In some cases, the tumor cells can be sparse and difficult to find.

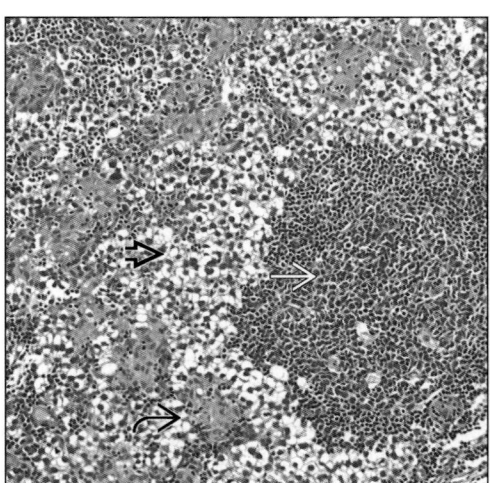
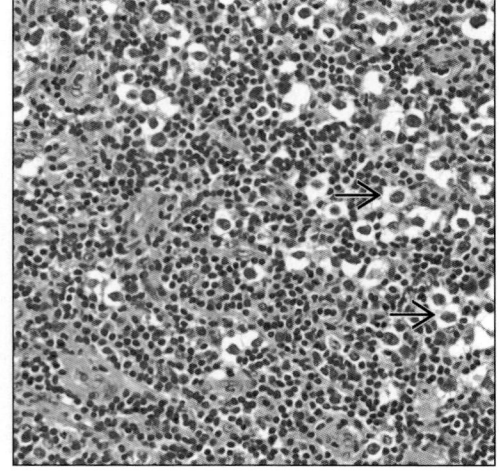

SEMINOMA

Microscopic Features

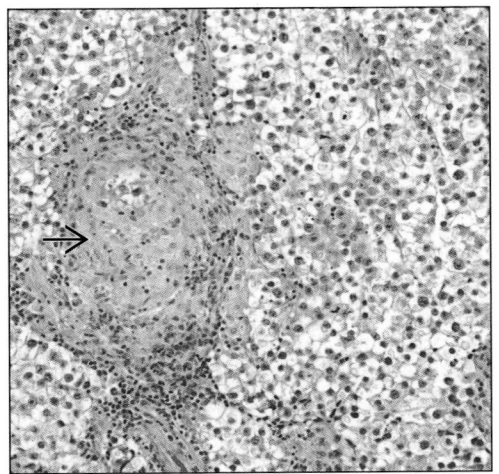

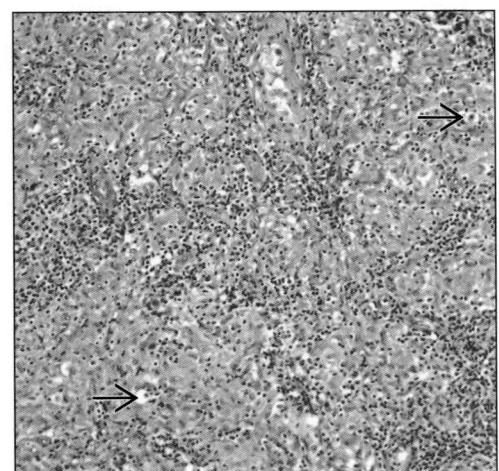

(Left) This image shows a classic seminoma with a large well-formed granuloma ⮕ surrounded by small lymphocytes. The tumor cells have abundant clear cytoplasm and prominent cytoplasmic membrane. *(Right)* A classic seminoma with confluent granulomatous inflammation is shown. Only rare tumor cells ⮕ may be seen. Elsewhere on the same slide, more characteristic tumor cells are present. In rare situations, immunostain with Oct3/4 might be helpful to identify the tumor cells.

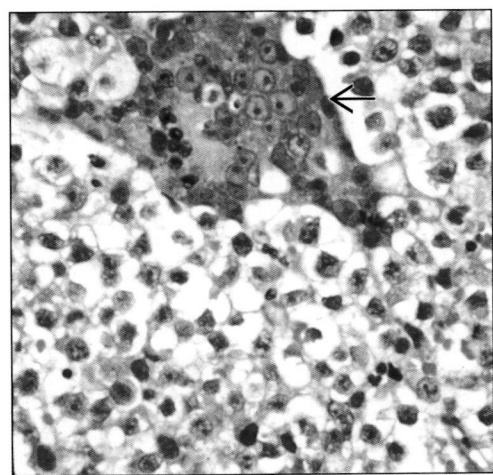

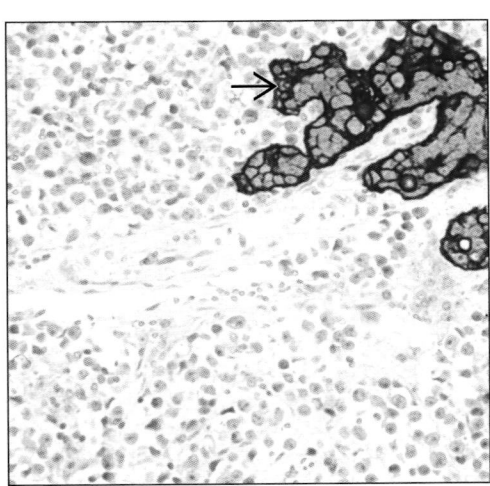

(Left) A classic seminoma with a multinucleated syncytiotrophoblastic giant cell ⮕ is shown. Approximately 30% of patients with pure seminoma have mild elevation of hCG (usually < 500 IU/mL). Presence of syncytiotrophoblast is not an adverse prognostic feature. *(Right)* Cytokeratin immunostain strongly highlights the syncytiotrophoblasts ⮕, whereas seminoma tumor cells are negative.

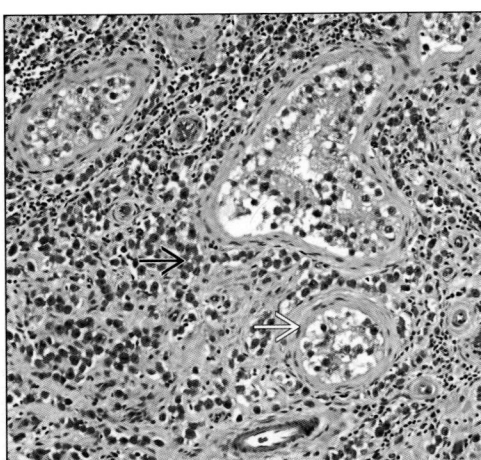

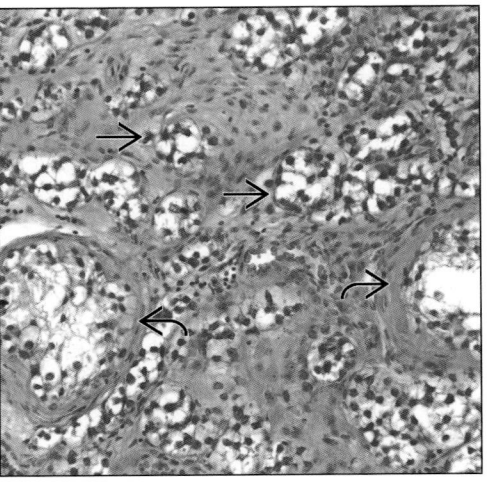

(Left) This photomicrograph shows interstitial infiltrative pattern of seminomatous tumor cells ⮕ in between the atrophic seminiferous tubules involved by intratumoral germ cell neoplasm ⮕. Also present are many small lymphocytes. *(Right)* Another example of interstitial growth of seminoma is shown. Small nests or clusters of seminoma cells ⮕ are present in between atrophic seminiferous tubules ⮕ and associated with dense fibrous stroma. This area may not be grossly evident.

Microscopic Features

(Left) This photomicrograph shows seminoma with tubular or pseudoglandular pattern. The cytologic features are those of classic seminoma with relatively uniform nuclei and clear cytoplasm. Also seen are fibrovascular septae with small lymphocytes ➜. *(Right)* This is a high-power photomicrograph of seminoma with tumor cells in tubular growth pattern. The tumor cells have characteristic cytologic features of seminoma with relatively uniform nuclei and abundant clear cytoplasm.

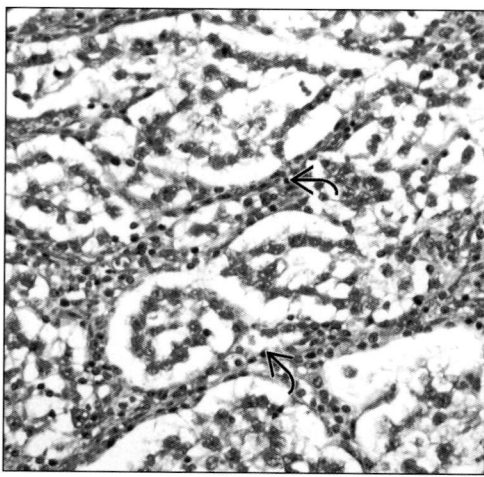
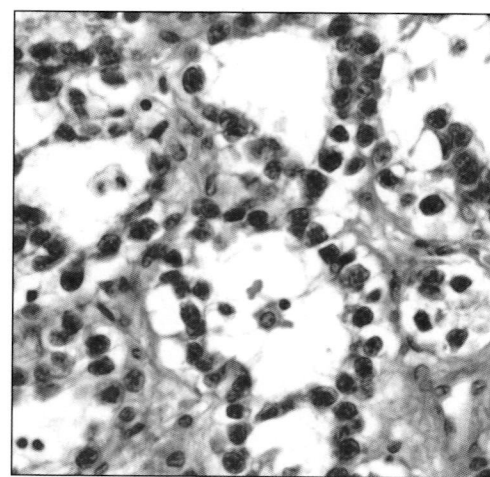

(Left) This low-power image shows a seminoma with dense sclerotic stroma, scattered tumor cells ➜, and small lymphocytes. In cases where tumor cells are difficult to identify by light microscopy, immunostain with Oct3/4 can be very helpful. *(Right)* High-power photomicrograph shows a classic seminoma with dense sclerotic stroma and scattered large seminomatous tumor cells ➜. Small lymphocytes and plasma cells ➜ are present.

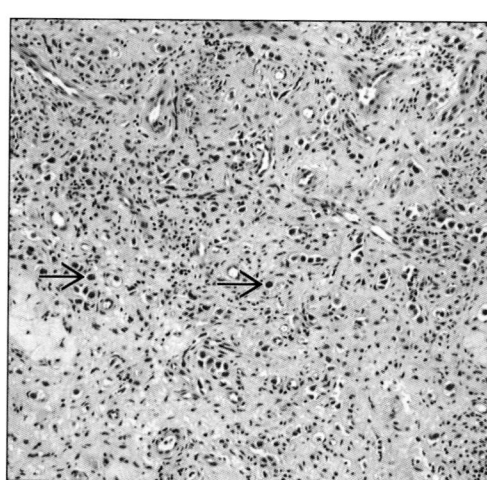
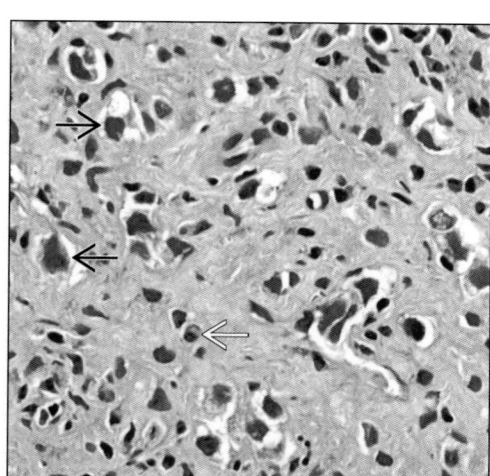

(Left) This photomicrograph shows a seminoma with cord-like or trabecular growth pattern. There is interstitial fibrosis and a lymphoplasmacytic infiltrate. *(Right)* This image shows a classic seminoma with trabecular or elongated tubular growth pattern and fibrovascular septae. The tumor cells have relatively uniform nuclei with prominent nucleoli and abundant clear cytoplasm.

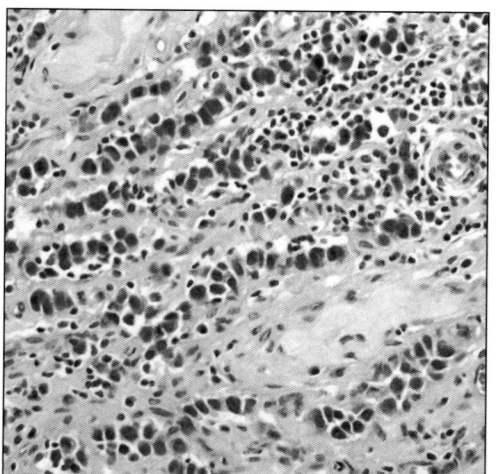
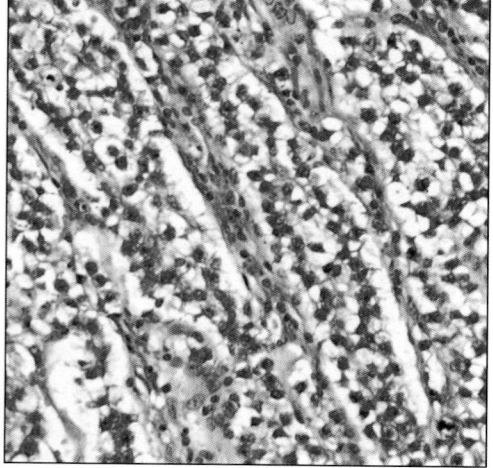

SEMINOMA

Microscopic Features

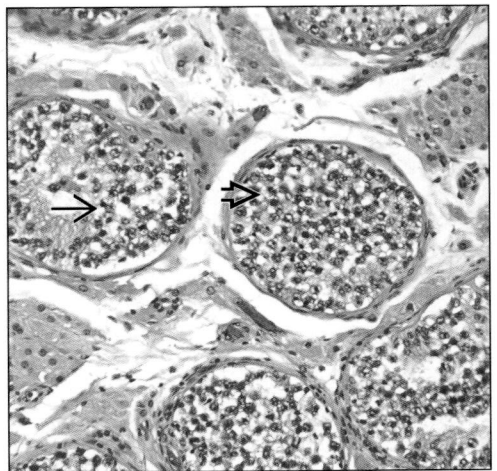

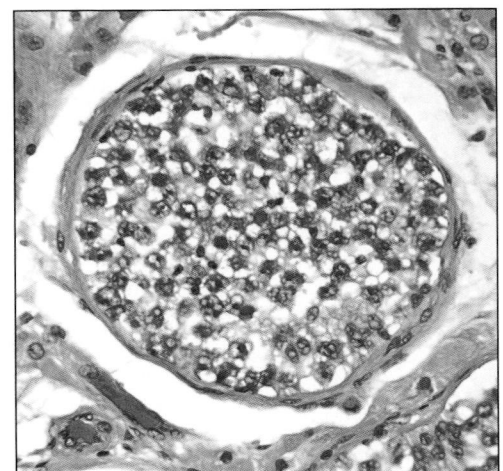

(Left) Intratubular seminoma is characterized by expansion of seminiferous tubules by monotonous seminomatous cells (complete ⇒ and partial →). This is often present away from the main tumor mass and is usually not grossly evident. *(Right)* High-power photomicrograph shows complete replacement of a seminiferous tubule by cells of classic seminoma. In contrast, ITGCN has similar atypical cells preferentially along the basement membrane.

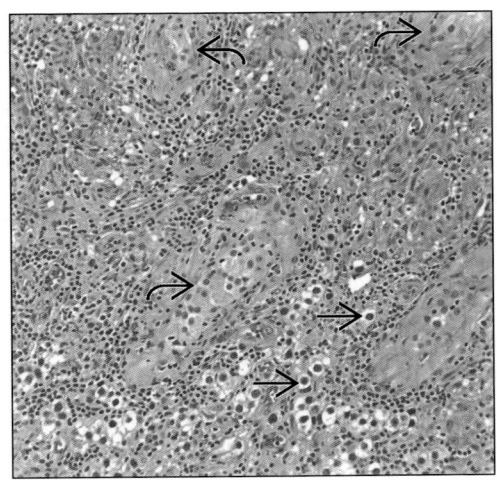

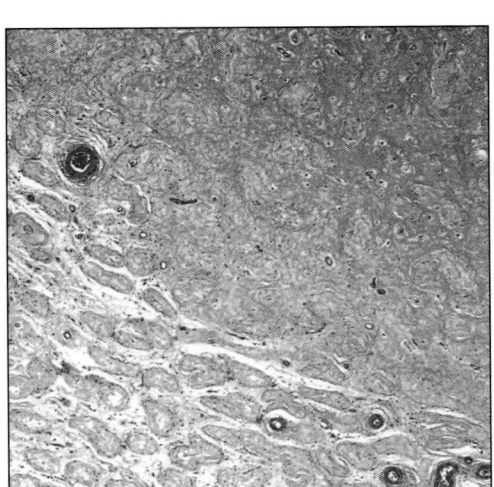

(Left) This image shows a classic seminoma with interstitial seminoma and extensive granulomatous inflammation and small lymphocytes. The tumor cells contain large round nuclei, prominent nucleoli, and prominent clear cytoplasm →. The seminiferous tubules ⇗ are preserved. *(Right)* This image shows an example of burnt-out germ cell tumor with diffuse interstitial fibrosis (scar) and small vessels. The seminiferous tubules are completely sclerotic with a ghost outline.

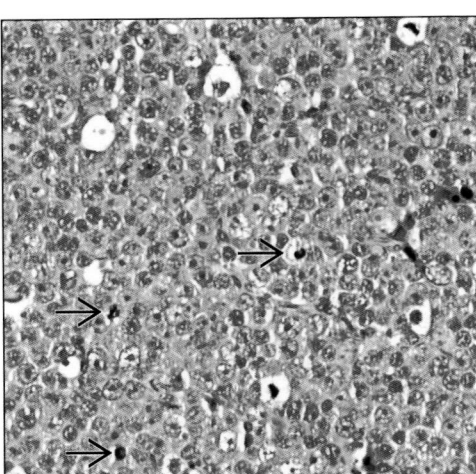

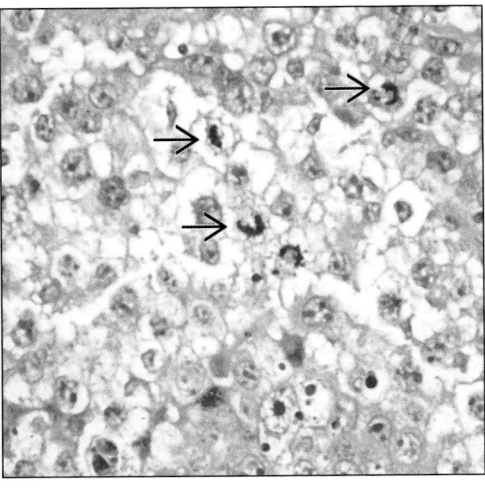

(Left) This is an example of so-called anaplastic seminoma. The tumor consists of solid tumor cells with larger nuclei, higher N:C ratio, and more cellular pleomorphism than typical seminoma. Frequent mitoses → are present. *(Right)* High-power view of a so-called anaplastic seminoma is characterized by large tumor cells with larger nuclei, more cellular pleomorphism than typical seminoma, and frequent mitoses →.

Microscopic and Immunohistochemical Features

(Left) An area of tumor cell necrosis (not common) is seen in this classic seminoma. The viable tumor cells have characteristic cytologic features of seminoma. *(Right)* This image shows sheets of seminomatous cells with rhabdoid appearance (abundant eosinophilic cytoplasm pushing the nucleus to the edge of the cell). Scattered in the background are many small lymphocytes.

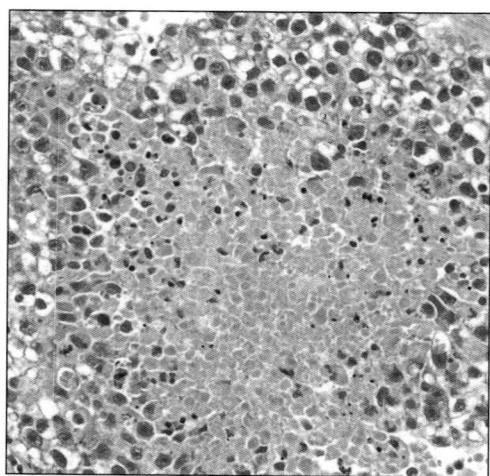
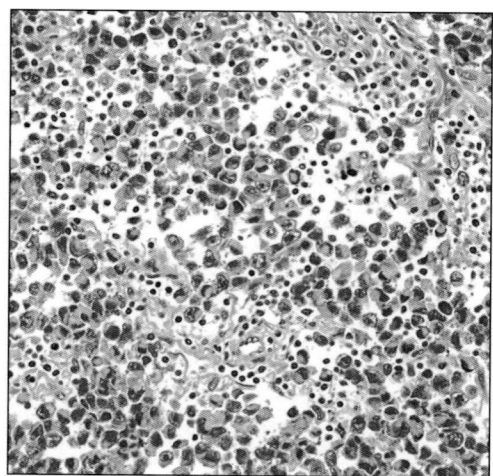

(Left) High-power photomicrograph of rete testis shows pagetoid spread of ITGCN. The tumor cells have large nuclei and abundant clear cytoplasm ➡. *(Right)* An example of rete testis ➡ extension by invasive seminoma is shown. The seminomatous tumor cells ➡ have large nuclei and abundant clear cytoplasm. Prominent lymphoid infiltrate is also present.

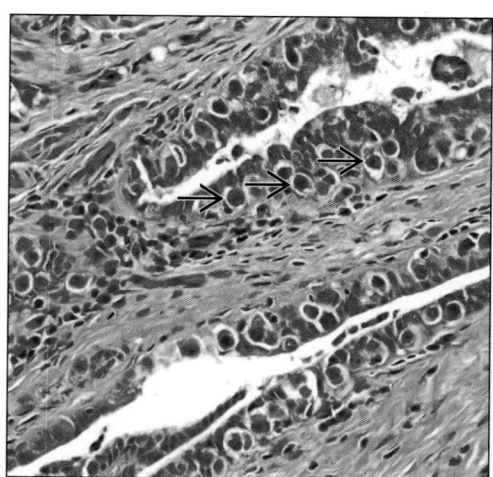
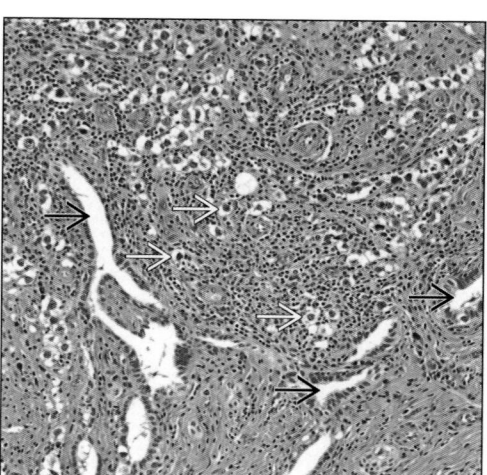

(Left) Oct3/4 stains the seminoma in strong nuclear pattern. Oct3/4 is a very useful marker for identification of seminoma and embryonal carcinoma, particularly in a metastatic setting. *(Right)* Podoplanin(D2-40) stains the seminoma with a strong cytoplasmic and membranous pattern.

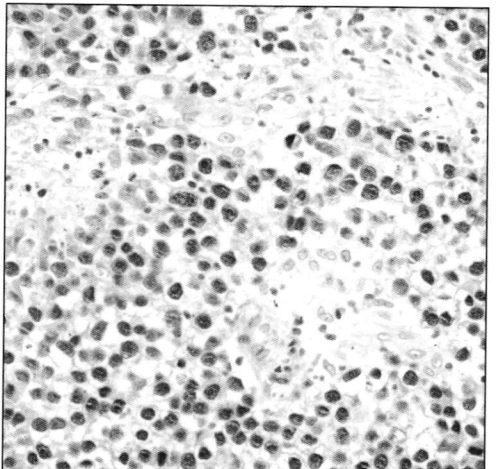
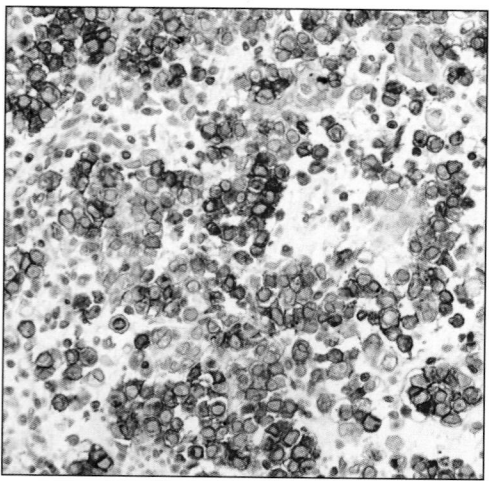

Microscopic Features and Differential Diagnoses

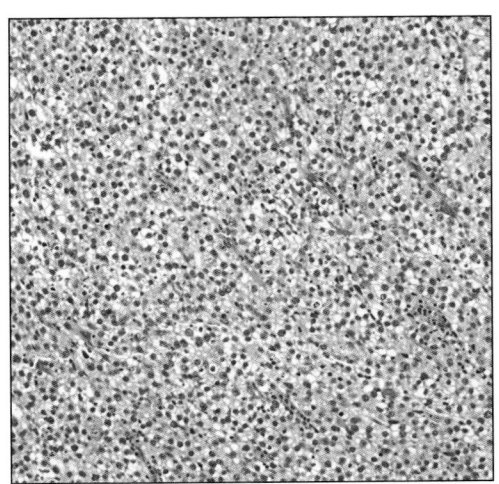

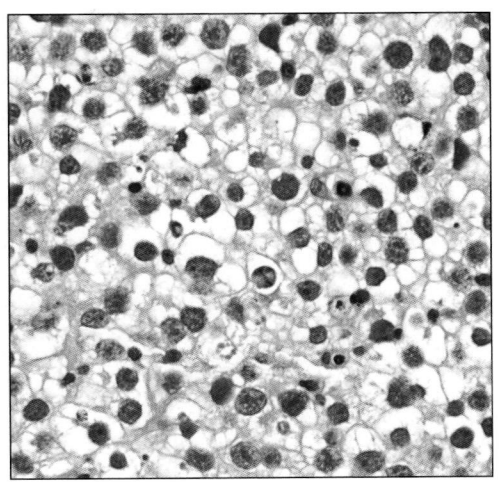

(Left) Low-power photomicrograph of classic seminoma shows solid growth pattern with no obvious fibrovascular septae and lymphoplasmacytic infiltrate. When this pattern is predominant, a number of differential diagnoses should be considered. *(Right)* High-power photomicrograph shows a classic seminoma with solid growth pattern. Note the relatively uniform and evenly distributed tumor cells with round nuclei, small nucleoli, and prominent cytoplasmic membrane boundaries.

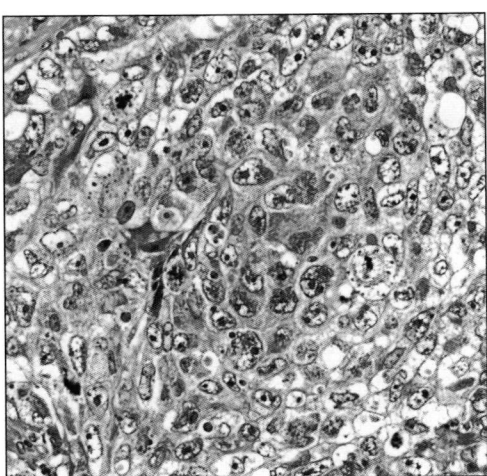

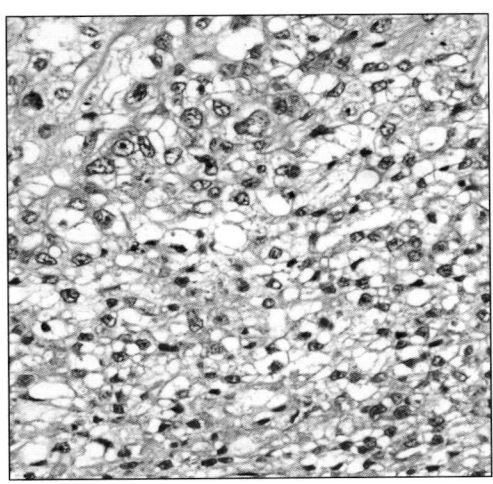

(Left) Solid embryonal carcinoma is composed of anaplastic tumor cells with nuclear overlapping. The tumor cells have coarse and vesicular chromatin nuclei, macro- and irregular nucleoli, and frequent mitoses and apoptotic bodies. *(Right)* An example of a yolk sac tumor with a solid growth pattern is shown. The cytologic features are moderately pleomorphic cells with abundant clear or eosinophilic cytoplasm, cytoplasmic vacuoles, and microcyst formation.

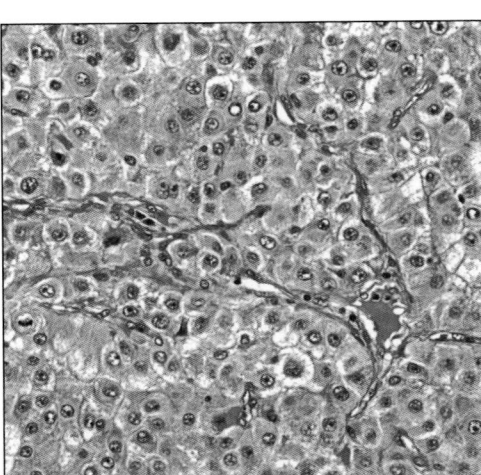

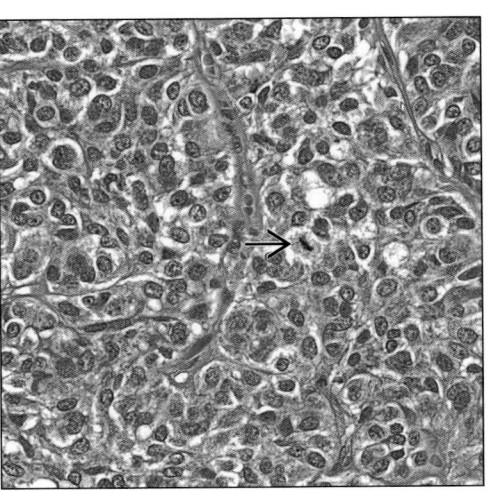

(Left) This high-power photomicrograph shows a monophasic choriocarcinoma with solid growth of mononucleated trophoblasts with round to ovoid nuclei and abundant eosinophilic to clear cytoplasm. *(Right)* A high-power photomicrograph of a solid Sertoli cell tumor is shown. The cytologic features show relatively uniform ovoid nuclei, prominent nucleoli, and abundant eosinophilic to clear cytoplasm. Rare mitoses may be seen ➡.

EMBRYONAL CARCINOMA

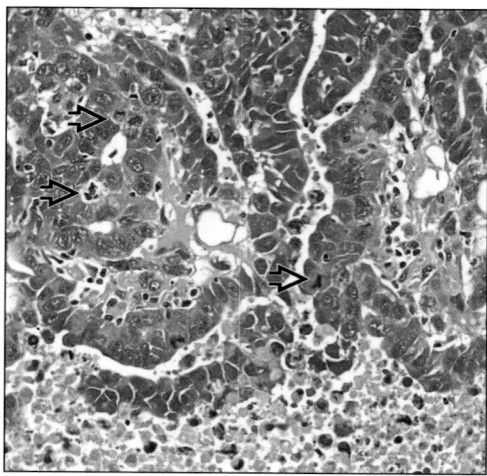

This image shows complex glandular growth of EC with highly pleomorphic cells with indistinct cell borders, overlapping nuclei, prominent nucleoli, and frequent mitoses ⊳. Tumor cell necrosis is also present.

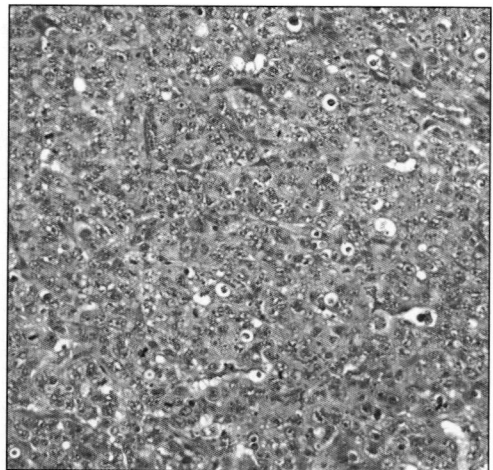

This solid EC shows sheets of large anaplastic cells with crowded nuclei, prominent nucleoli, and indistinct cell borders. In contrast, seminoma shows nonoverlapping cells with distinct cell borders.

TERMINOLOGY

Abbreviations
- Embryonal carcinoma (EC)

Definitions
- Germ cell tumor composed of undifferentiated cells of epithelial appearance with marked cytologic anaplasia and variety of growth patterns

CLINICAL ISSUES

Epidemiology
- Incidence
  - 2nd most common pure testicular germ cell neoplasm (< 5%)
  - More commonly seen as mixed with other germ cell tumor components
- Age
  - 15-35 years (10 years younger than patients with seminoma)
  - Does not occur in infants or children; rare after 5th decade

Presentation
- Testicular mass or swelling
- Symptoms of metastasis, such as back pain, dyspnea, and neurologic symptoms
- Serum α-fetoprotein and hCG may be elevated

Treatment
- Similar to other nonseminomatous germ cell tumors; depends mainly on clinical stage

Prognosis
- Poorest among all germ cell tumors
  - Cure rate > 95% for stage I, 70-85% for bulky stage II and stage III disease

IMAGE FINDINGS

General Features
- Ultrasonography may detect mass lesion (typically ill-defined and heterogeneous) in testis

MACROSCOPIC FEATURES

General Features
- Often poorly circumscribed mass
- Variegated cut surface with large areas of hemorrhage and necrosis

Size
- Variable (mean tumor: 2.5 cm); usually smaller than classic seminoma

MICROSCOPIC PATHOLOGY

Histologic Features
- Heterogeneous tumor with 3 main growth patterns: Solid, glandular, and papillary
- Appliqué pattern (central solid EC surrounded by peripheral degenerating tumor cells) may be seen
- Large cohesive, highly pleomorphic tumor cells with moderate amount of amphophilic cytoplasm and indistinct cell membranes
- Syncytial growth with nuclear overlapping with uneven cellular distribution, coarse or vesicular chromatin, prominent and irregular nucleoli
- Frequent mitoses and apoptoses
- Hemorrhage and necrosis are common
- Vascular invasion, rete testis, epididymis, and spermatic cord invasion more frequent than seminoma
- Intratubular germ cell neoplasia (ITGCN) and intratubular embryonal carcinoma with necrosis and calcification

EMBRYONAL CARCINOMA

Key Facts

Terminology
- Germ cell tumor composed of undifferentiated cells of epithelial appearance with marked cytologic anaplasia and variety of growth patterns

Clinical Issues
- 2nd most common pure testicular germ cell neoplasm (< 5%)
- Age ranges from 15-35 years (10 years younger than patients with seminoma)

Macroscopic Features
- Often poorly circumscribed mass with more frequent extension to rete testis, epididymis, or spermatic cord (20%) than seminoma
- Variegated cut surface with large areas of hemorrhage and necrosis

Microscopic Pathology
- Heterogeneous tumor with 3 main growth patterns: Solid, glandular, and papillary
- Large cohesive, highly pleomorphic tumor cells with moderate amount of amphophilic cytoplasm and indistinct cell membrane
- Nuclear overlapping with uneven cellular distribution, coarse or vesicular chromatin, and prominent and often irregularly shaped nucleoli
- Frequent mitoses and apoptoses
- Hemorrhage and necrosis common

Ancillary Tests
- Positive for cytokeratin, CD30(BerH2), Oct3/4, Podoplanin(D2-40), and PLAP

Predominant Pattern/Injury Type
- Neoplastic

Predominant Cell/Compartment Type
- Germ cells

ANCILLARY TESTS

Immunohistochemistry
- Positive for cytokeratin, CD30(BerH2), Oct3/4, PLAP, SALL4, SOX2; may be focally positive for HCG or α-fetoprotein
- Negative for EMA/MUC1, CK20, HMCK, and α-inhibin

DIFFERENTIAL DIAGNOSIS

Seminoma ("Anaplastic Seminoma")
- Sheets or lobules of tumor cells with less cytologic atypia and distinct cell borders; lymphoplasmacytic infiltrate or granulomas
- Positive for CD117 and Oct3/4; negative for CD30(BerH2); negative or only focally positive for cytokeratin

Anaplastic Spermatocytic Seminoma
- Older age; associated with classic area of spermatocytic seminoma
- Negative for CD30, cytokeratin, Podoplanin(D2-40), PLAP, and Oct3/4; positive for CD117

Yolk Sac Tumor (Solid or Papillary)
- Relatively bland tumor cells with more abundant cytoplasm and eosinophilic globules
- Positive for α-fetoprotein and glypican-3; negative for CD30(BerH2), Oct3/4, or Podoplanin(D2-40)

Metastatic Carcinoma
- Clinical history, older age; more frequently bilateral; lack of ITGCN
- Positive for EMA/MUC1 and tissue specific markers of metastatic origin

Malignant Lymphoma
- Older age and more frequently bilateral (40%)
- Diffuse & interstitial growth pattern; tumor cells less cohesive & pleomorphic than embryonal carcinoma
- Positive for leukocyte common antigen (LCA) and B cell markers

DIAGNOSTIC CHECKLIST

Pathologic Interpretation Pearls
- Epithelial growth patterns (solid, glandular, and papillary) and highly anaplastic cytologic features

REPORTING CONSIDERATIONS

Key Elements to Report
- Pure or mixed with other germ cell tumor components (if mixed, indicate relative percentage of each component)
- Status of lymphovascular invasion
- Rete testis, spermatic cord, and tunica invasion
- Spermatic cord margin status
- Pathologic stage (pTNM)

SELECTED REFERENCES

1. de Jong J et al: Differential expression of SOX17 and SOX2 in germ cells and stem cells has biological and clinical implications. J Pathol. 215(1):21-30, 2008
2. Berney DM et al: The frequency of intratubular embryonal carcinoma: implications for the pathogenesis of germ cell tumours. Histopathology. 45(2):155-61, 2004
3. Leroy X et al: CD30 and CD117 (c-kit) used in combination are useful for distinguishing embryonal carcinoma from seminoma. J Histochem Cytochem. 50(2):283-5, 2002
4. Moul JW et al: Percentage of embryonal carcinoma and of vascular invasion predicts pathological stage in clinical stage I nonseminomatous testicular cancer. Cancer Res. 54(2):362-4, 1994

EMBRYONAL CARCINOMA

Gross and Microscopic Features

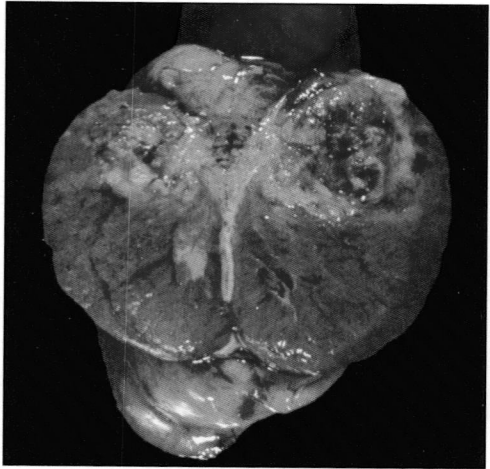
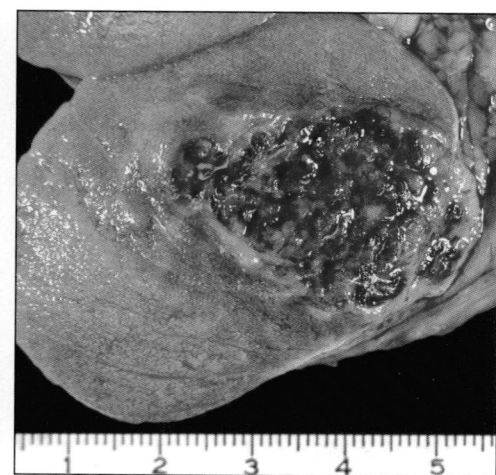

(Left) EC with a variegated cut surface, hemorrhage, and necrosis is shown. The tumor is poorly circumscribed. The rete testis and spermatic cord are more commonly involved in EC than in seminoma. *(Right)* This photo shows an EC with variegated, hemorrhagic, and necrotic appearance and poorly demarcated borders. Hemorrhage and necrosis in a germ cell tumor often contain EC and choriocarcinoma components, such that sections should be taken from these areas when identified grossly.

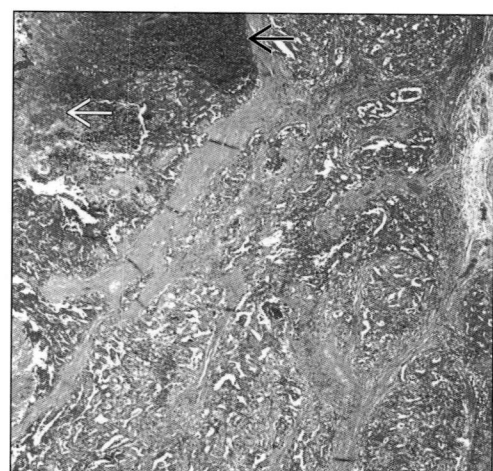
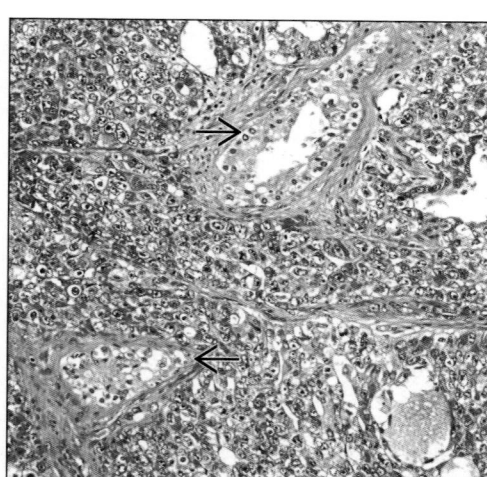

(Left) Low-power photomicrograph of EC shows areas of hemorrhage ⇒ and necrosis ⇒. EC usually has a heterogeneous growth appearance with multiple patterns in the same tumor, including areas of glandular, papillary, and solid patterns. *(Right)* At the periphery, EC may be present between the seminiferous tubules ⇒. The tumor has solid and glandular growth patterns with cohesive anaplastic tumor cells. Prominent nucleoli are readily apparent even under medium power.

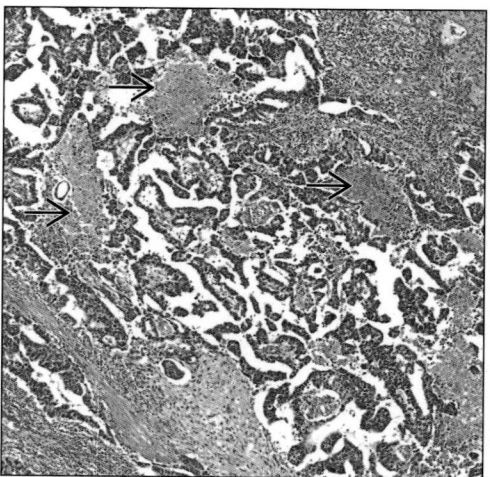
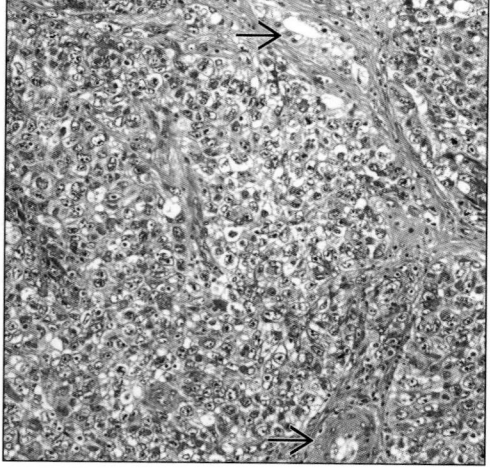

(Left) EC with papillary growth pattern and fibrovascular cores is shown. There are multiple foci of necrosis ⇒. Although yolk sac tumor may be papillary, it has a much lesser degree of cytologic atypia and necrosis. *(Right)* This image shows a solid EC with sheets of tumor cells divided by fibrous septa. Distinction from seminoma is based on cytologic features and absence of lymphocytic or granulomatous reaction. Also present are compressed atrophic seminiferous tubules ⇒.

EMBRYONAL CARCINOMA

Microscopic Features

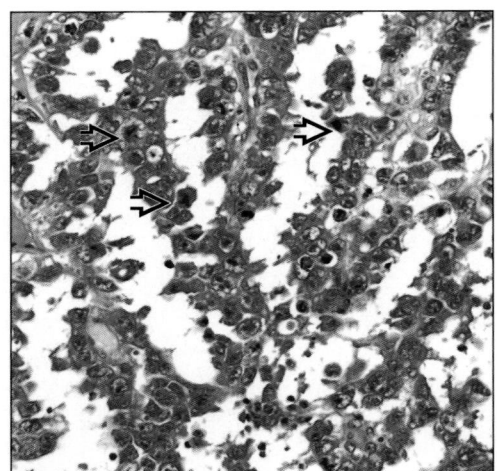

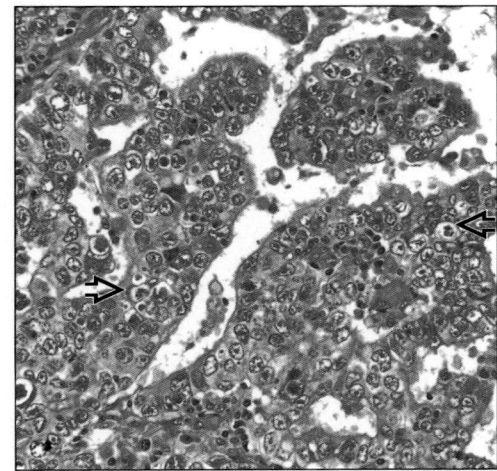

(Left) This EC has delicate papillae lined by highly pleomorphic tumor cells. The tumor cells exhibit nuclear overlapping, macronucleoli, and frequent mitoses ⧐. *(Right)* High-power photomicrograph shows papillary EC composed of cohesive anaplastic tumor cells with nuclear overlapping, uneven cellular distribution, large vesicular nuclei, macronucleoli, and frequent apoptoses ⧐. The cytoplasm is eosinophilic to amphophilic, and cell boundaries are indistinct.

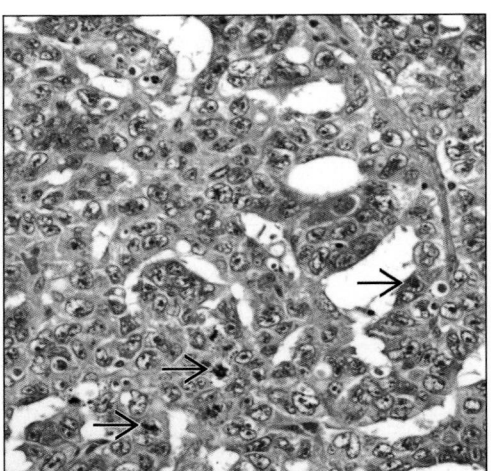

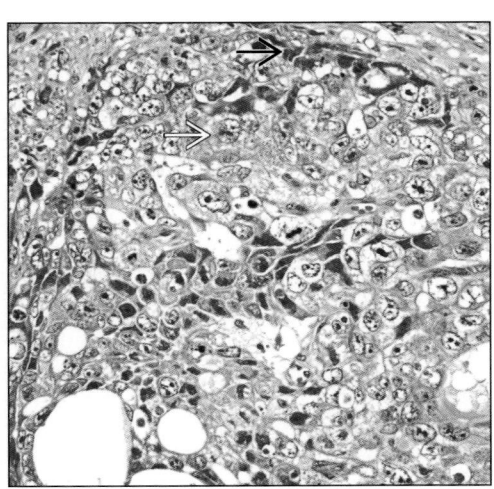

(Left) EC with complex glandular pattern is shown. It is composed of anaplastic tumor cells with overlapping nuclei, vesicular chromatin, and frequent mitoses ⧐. *(Right)* This is an example of EC with appliqué pattern. The central solid EC ⧐ is wrapped by degenerating cells ⧐, which may mimic "biphasic" pattern of choriocarcinoma. The lack of true syncytiotrophoblasts, hemorrhage, and villous configuration prevent the erroneous diagnosis of choriocarcinoma.

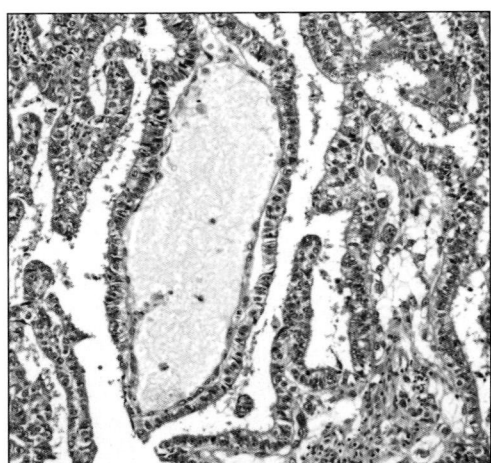

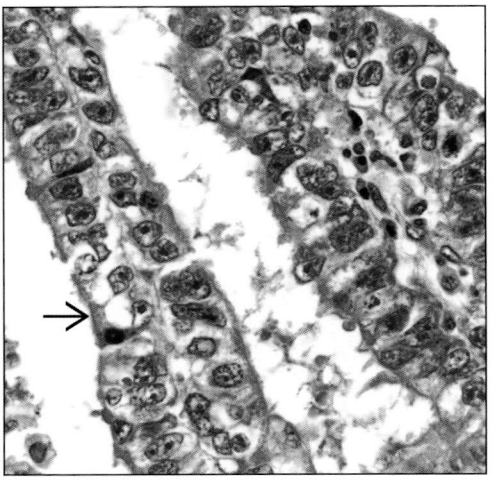

(Left) Papillary/glandular pattern of EC with columnar cells may mimic papillary YST, but YST has less pronounced cytologic atypia than EC. In difficult situations, immunostain with a panel of markers CD30 & Oct3/4 for EC, α-fetoprotein & glypican-3 for YST) may be helpful. *(Right)* High-power image shows glandular EC with columnar cells & a brush border ⧐ resembling YST with enteric/endometrioid pattern. Cytologic features are more pleomorphic than those of YST.

Microscopic Features

(Left) This image shows EC with cribriform glands surrounded by desmoplastic stroma and retraction artifact, mimicking lymphovascular invasion. This pattern may raise the possibility of metastatic carcinoma. *(Right)* EC with cribriform glandular pattern and central necrosis is shown. The artifactual space around the tumor nest should not be interpreted as vascular invasion. In difficult cases, vascular markers, such as CD31, may be used to resolve the issue.

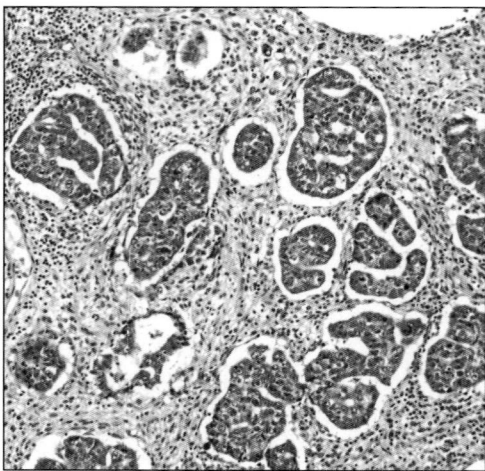 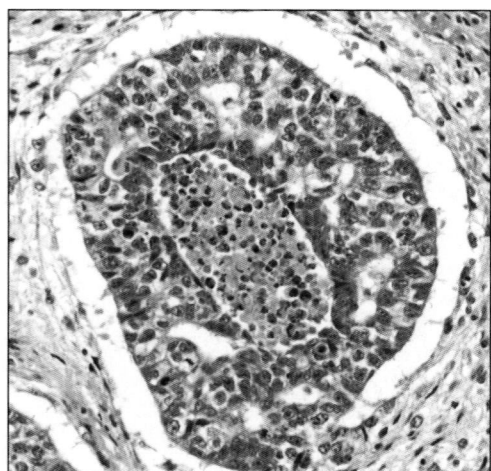

(Left) EC with multifocal vascular invasion ➡ is shown. Features that confirm vascular invasion include peritumoral location ➡, tumor conforming to the shape of the vessels, and intravascular growth based on plump endothelial-lined spaces or attachment to the vascular wall. Vascular lymphatic invasion is an adverse prognostic factor and determines pathologic stage. *(Right)* Complex glandular growth of EC is shown with areas of hemorrhage and necrosis, a common finding in this tumor.

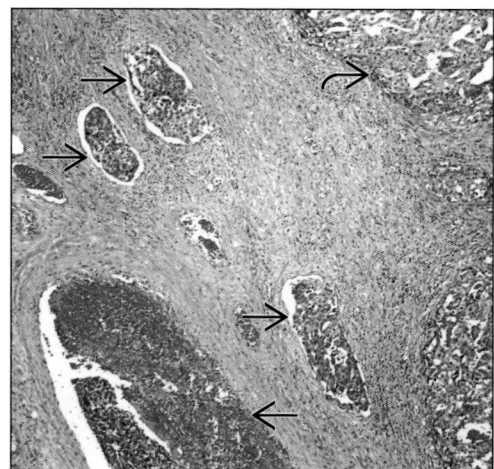 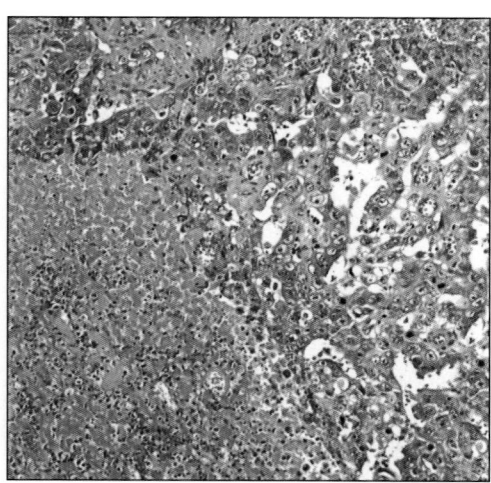

(Left) Intratubular EC may be seen within or at the edge of the tumor. Markedly atypical cells of EC within the seminiferous tubules, often with central comedo necrosis ➡, may be present. Necrotic tumor cell debris is often seen ➡. *(Right)* This photomicrograph shows intratubular EC with anaplastic tumor cells ➡ partially replacing the cellular constituents of the seminiferous tubules ➡. The intratubular EC cells are identical to that of invasive EC cells.

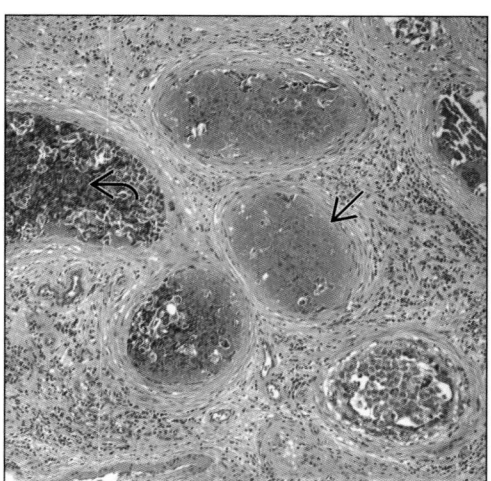 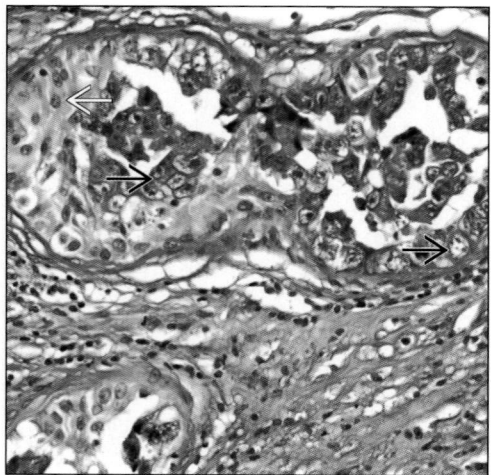

4

EMBRYONAL CARCINOMA

Microscopic and Immunohistochemical Features

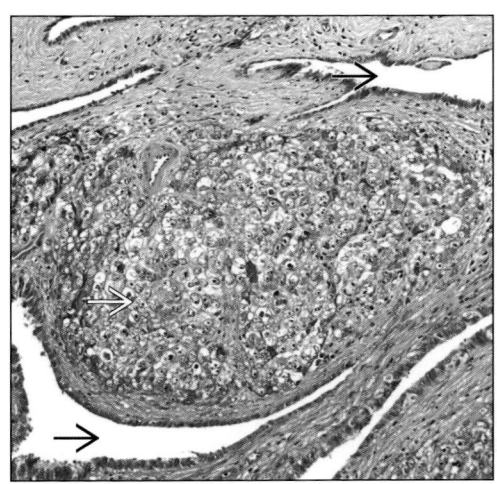

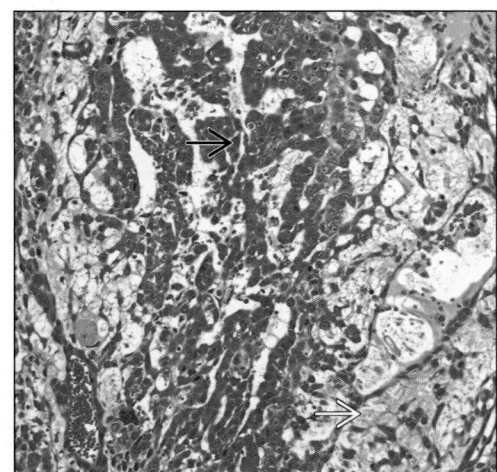

(Left) Invasion of rete testis ⇨ by solid EC ➡ is shown. In contrast to seminoma, EC invading into the rete testis is not an independent adverse prognostic factor. **(Right)** EC ➡ admixed with YST ➡ is a frequent finding of mixed germ cell tumor. The YST component is often seen at the edge of EC tumor cell nests. YST tumor cells may be deceptively benign with cuboidal or flattened cells. The relative percentage of the different germ cell components must be specified.

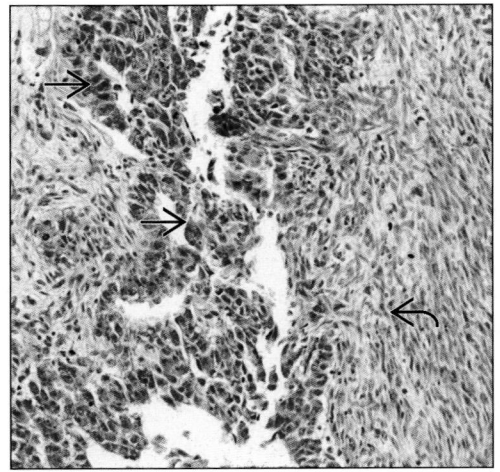

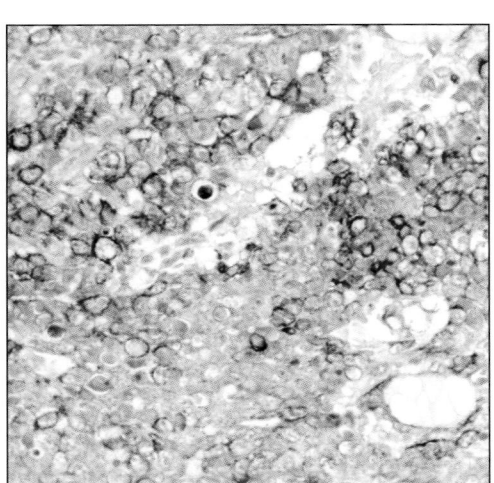

(Left) Image shows papillary EC ➡ associated with cellular, spindled, & undifferentiated stroma with high mitoses (immature teratoma component) ⇨. This combination is also a common finding in mixed germ cell tumors. **(Right)** EC is often diffusely positive for PAN-CK, whereas seminoma is typically negative or only focally weakly positive. Thus, in any situation when EC & seminoma is a serious differential diagnosis, cytokeratin & CD30(BerH2) may be used for this purpose.

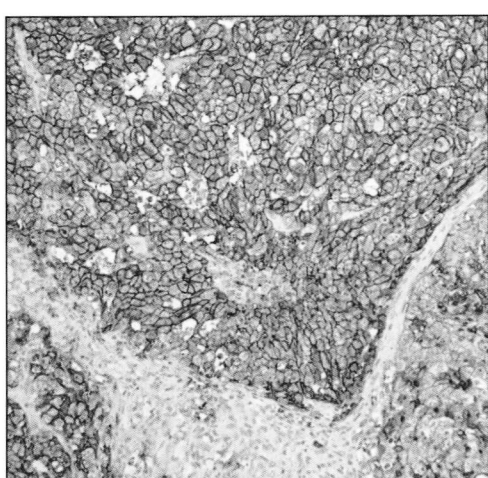

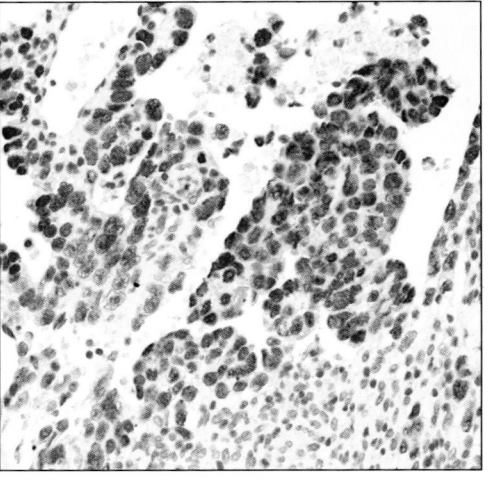

(Left) The tumor cells of EC are strongly positive for CD30(BerH2) with membranous staining pattern. Such positivity with CD30(BerH2) is not seen in yolk sac tumor or seminoma. **(Right)** The tumor cells of EC are positive for Oct3/4 in a nuclear pattern, similar to seminoma. The tumor cells of YST and choriocarcinoma are typically negative for Oct3/4. A combination of cytokeratin, Oct3/4, and CD30(BerH2) is diagnostic of EC in the appropriate histologic context.

YOLK SAC TUMOR

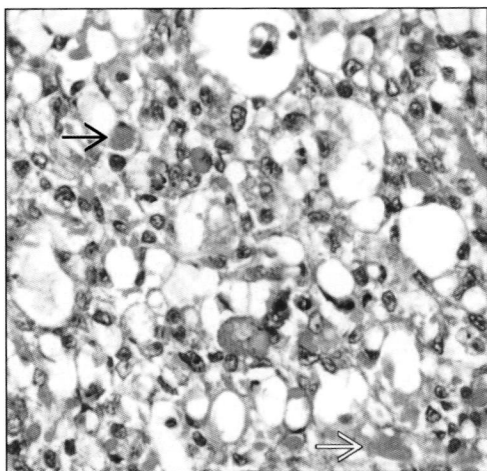

H&E shows microcystic and reticular YST patterns in which tumor cells contain vacuolated cytoplasm, intercellular eosinophilic globules ➔, & extracellular pink basement membrane-like material ➔.

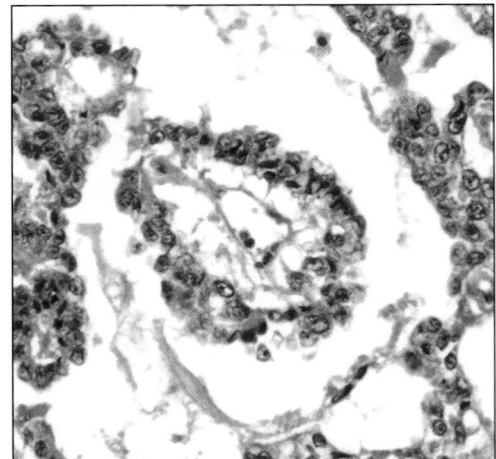

This image shows a Schiller-Duval body in YST, which is characterized by a central vessel surrounded by a layer of tumor cells, a hollow space, and another layer of similar or more flattened cells.

TERMINOLOGY

Abbreviations
- Yolk sac tumor (YST)

Synonyms
- Endodermal sinus tumor (EST)

Definitions
- Germ cell tumor characterized by variety of growth patterns that recapitulate yolk sac, allantois, and extraembryonic mesenchyme

CLINICAL ISSUES

Epidemiology
- Incidence
  - Pure YST is most common testicular tumor of infants and young children
    - Accounts for 75% of all childhood testicular neoplasms
    - No association with cryptorchidism or other germ cell tumor components
  - Pure YST is extremely rare in adult testes
    - At extragonadal sites, especially mediastinum, pure YST may be seen
  - YST is frequent component of mixed germ cell tumors (in ~ 40%) in adults
- Age
  - Mean age: 16-18 months for pure YST
  - Mean age: 25-35 years for adult YST
    - 10 years younger than patients with seminoma

Presentation
- Nonsymptomatic, rapid testicular enlargement
- Approximately 90% of patients with childhood YST have clinical stage I disease
- Presence of YST in adult patients with mixed germ cell tumor is frequently associated with lower stage presentation

Laboratory Tests
- More than 95% patients have elevated serum α-fetoprotein (AFP)
- Test for serum AFP is valuable tool in diagnosis and monitoring effectiveness of therapy

Treatment
- For infants and children with pure YST
  - Radical inguinal orchiectomy for stage I tumor with close follow-up protocol (surveillance)
  - Cisplatin-based therapy for relapse on surveillance, advanced stage disease, or metastasis
- For adult YST (usually mixed with other germ cell tumor)
  - Similar to other nonseminomatous germ cell tumor based on clinical stage
  - Radical inguinal orchiectomy ± retroperitoneal lymph node dissection
  - Cisplatin-based chemotherapy for metastatic disease

Prognosis
- Prognosis associated with clinical stage, lymphovascular invasion, degree of serum AFP elevation
- Children have better prognosis than adults

IMAGE FINDINGS

General Features
- Ultrasonography may detect scrotal mass

MACROSCOPIC FEATURES

General Features
- Nonencapsulated, gray-white, soft or firm, homogeneous mass
- Typical myxoid or gelatinous cut surface
- Hemorrhage and necrosis may be present
- Tumors in adults are typically more heterogeneous

YOLK SAC TUMOR

Key Facts

Terminology
- Germ cell tumor characterized by variety of growth patterns that recapitulate yolk sac, allantois, and extraembryonic mesenchyme

Clinical Issues
- Most common germ cell tumor of infants and young children
- No association with cryptorchidism
- Pure form rare in adults: Usually present as component of mixed germ cell tumors

Microscopic Pathology
- YST has multiple growth patterns with 1 dominant pattern or more frequently mixed patterns
  - Reticular or microcystic pattern most frequent (80%)
  - Other common patterns include endodermal sinus, solid, papillary, and glandular
- Relatively uniform cells with clear or vacuolated to lightly eosinophilic cytoplasm
- Bland cuboidal, columnar to flattened, or spindle cells
- Presence of small, spherical, intracellular or extracellular hyaline globules
- Prominent basement membrane deposition

Ancillary Tests
- Positive for cytokeratin, AFP, PLAP (variable), SALL4, glypican-3
- Negative for CD30(BerH2), Podoplanin(D2-40), Oct3/4, hCG, inhibin-α
  - Podoplanin(D2-40) and Oct3/4 are positive in seminoma and embryonal carcinoma

Size
- Range: 2-6 cm

MICROSCOPIC PATHOLOGY

Histologic Features
- YST frequently has multiple growth patterns with 1 dominant pattern
  - Microcystic or reticular pattern most frequent (80%)
    - Anastomosing thin cords forming round or irregular spaces or tubules of variable size
    - Characteristic intracellular vacuoles and merging of cells create sieve-like appearance
    - Nuclei are irregularly shaped (round, columnar, stellate, triangular) and are often pushed to edge of cells
  - Endodermal sinus pattern
    - Composed of numerous Schiller-Duval bodies (resembling fetal glomeruli) with central fibrovascular core
    - Fibrovascular core is lined by cuboidal to columnar tumor cells, which are surrounded by cystic spaces and more flattened layer of tumor cells
    - Labyrinthine spaces or perivascular arrangement of tumor cells are common
  - Solid pattern
    - Solid sheets of polygonal tumor cells with pale eosinophilic or clear cytoplasm, which lack fibrovascular septae, lymphocytes, or granulomas
    - May be confused with seminoma, embryonal carcinoma, and monophasic areas of choriocarcinoma
    - Tumor cells with random pleomorphism; slightly greater atypia than seminoma but less than embryonal carcinoma
  - Papillary and tubulopapillary
    - Papillae ± central fibrovascular cores
    - Tumor cells are often cuboidal and low columnar with "hobnail" appearance
  - Polyvesicular vitelline pattern
    - Large constricted vesicles lined by flattened to cuboidal cells
    - Often associated with abundant myxoid or loosely fibrous stroma
  - Glandular-alveolar pattern
    - Simple round to complex branching glands with intervening myxoid stroma
  - Parietal pattern
    - Epithelial cells surrounded by pink bands of basement membrane material
  - Enteric or endometrioid pattern
    - Glandular pattern with columnar cells, cytoplasmic clearing, subnuclear vacuoles, and smooth luminal surface
  - Hepatoid pattern
    - Sheets of tumor cells with abundant eosinophilic cytoplasm and eosinophilic globules
  - Spindled cell or sarcomatoid pattern
    - Composed of spindle (or sarcomatoid) cells with myxoid stroma
  - Myxomatous pattern
    - Epithelioid to spindle cells dispersed in paucicellular light blue myxoid stroma
    - Frequently under-recognized due to innocuous appearance
  - Macrocystic pattern
    - Large cystic spaces due to coalescence of microcysts lined by flattened tumor cells
  - Mixed pattern
    - Mixture of any of above growth patterns
- Intra- and extracellular PAS-positive hyaline globules
  - More commonly seen in microcystic and reticular, solid, and hepatoid patterns

Cytologic Features
- Relatively uniform epithelioid cells with clear or vacuolated to pale eosinophilic cytoplasm
- Bland cuboidal, columnar to flattened, or frankly spindled cells
- Minimal to mild nuclear pleomorphism
- Nuclear overlapping with indistinct cell borders

YOLK SAC TUMOR

Predominant Pattern/Injury Type
- Neoplastic

Predominant Cell/Compartment Type
- Germ cell

ANCILLARY TESTS

Histochemistry
- PAS-diastase
  - Reactivity: Positive
  - Staining pattern
    - Hyaline globules

Immunohistochemistry
- Positive for cytokeratin, AFP, glypican-3, PLAP (variable), SALL4
- Negative for CD30(BerH2), Podoplanin(D2-40), Oct3/4, CD117, hCG, inhibin-α

DIFFERENTIAL DIAGNOSIS

Leydig Cell Tumor (Microcystic)
- Well-circumscribed mass; solid growth with uniform cells and more prominent eosinophilic cytoplasm
- Positive for inhibin and calretinin; negative for AFP, SALL4, and glypican-3

Embryonal Carcinoma
- Marked cytologic anaplasia, nuclear crowding, frequent mitoses and necrosis
- Solid pattern is more common
- Positive for CD30(BerH2) and Oct3/4; negative for AFP and glypican-3

Seminoma (Tubular)
- Tubular growth pattern accompanied by more typical solid areas with lobules separated by fibrous septa, lymphoplasmacytic infiltrate and granulomas
- Distinct cell boundaries with no nuclear overlapping and abundant clear cytoplasm
- Tumor cells are larger and more uniform than yolk sac tumor
- Positive for CD117, Podoplanin(D2-40), and Oct3/4; negative for cytokeratin, AFP, and glypican-3

Rete Testis Hyperplasia ± Hyaline Globules
- May occur in association with germ cell tumor or without neoplasia in testis
- Retiform proliferation of bland cuboidal cells with or without intracellular hyaline globules
- Lack of cytologic atypia or mitotic figures
- Spermatozoa may be seen in some cases
- Positive for EMA/MUC1; negative for germ cell markers (SALL4, AFP, and glypican-3)

DIAGNOSTIC CHECKLIST

Pathologic Interpretation Pearls
- Multiple different growth patterns
- Microcystic and reticular patterns are common

- Basement membrane deposition and hyaline globules
- Schiller-Duval bodies

REPORTING CONSIDERATIONS

Key Elements to Report
- Pathologic stage
- Presence of lymphovascular invasion
- Involvement of rete testis, epididymis, spermatic cord, and tunica
- Status of spermatic cord margin
- Pathology of uninvolved testicular parenchyma

SELECTED REFERENCES

1. Cao D et al: SALL4 Is a Novel Diagnostic Marker for Testicular Germ Cell Tumors. Am J Surg Pathol. Epub ahead of print, 2009
2. Wang F et al: Diagnostic Utility of SALL4 in Extragonadal Yolk Sac Tumors: An Immunohistochemical Study of 59 Cases With Comparison to Placental-like Alkaline Phosphatase, Alpha-fetoprotein, and Glypican-3. Am J Surg Pathol. Epub ahead of print, 2009
3. McLean TW et al: Pediatric genitourinary tumors. Curr Opin Oncol. 20(3):315-20, 2008
4. Ulbright TM: The most common, clinically significant misdiagnoses in testicular tumor pathology, and how to avoid them. Adv Anat Pathol. 15(1):18-27, 2008
5. Oottamasathien S et al: Testicular tumours in children: a single-institutional experience. BJU Int. 99(5):1123-6, 2007
6. Ota S et al: Oncofetal protein glypican-3 in testicular germ-cell tumor. Virchows Arch. 449(3):308-14, 2006
7. Zynger DL et al: Glypican 3: a novel marker in testicular germ cell tumors. Am J Surg Pathol. 30(12):1570-5, 2006
8. Sesterhenn IA et al: Pathology of germ cell tumors of the testis. Cancer Control. 11(6):374-87, 2004
9. Ciftci AO et al: Testicular tumors in children. J Pediatr Surg. 36(12):1796-801, 2001
10. Medica M et al: Adult testicular pure yolk sac tumor. Urol Int. 67(1):94-6, 2001
11. Foster RS et al: Clinical stage I pure yolk sac tumor of the testis in adults has different clinical behavior than juvenile yolk sac tumor. J Urol. 164(6):1943-4, 2000
12. Horie Y et al: Hepatoid variant of yolk sac tumor of the testis. Pathol Int. 50(9):754-8, 2000
13. Billings SD et al: Microcystic Leydig cell tumors mimicking yolk sac tumor: a report of four cases. Am J Surg Pathol. 23(5):546-51, 1999
14. Ulbright TM et al: Rete testis hyperplasia with hyaline globule formation. A lesion simulating yolk sac tumor. Am J Surg Pathol. 15(1):66-74, 1991

Gross Features

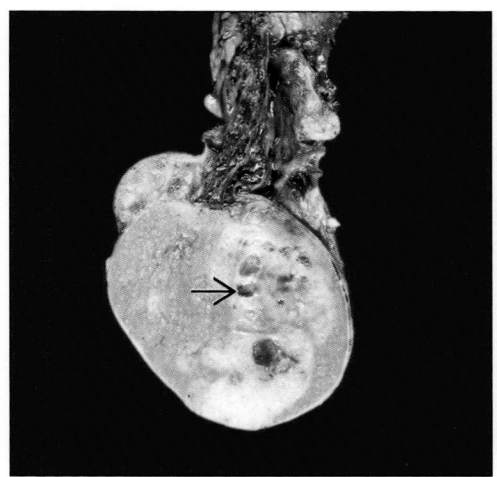

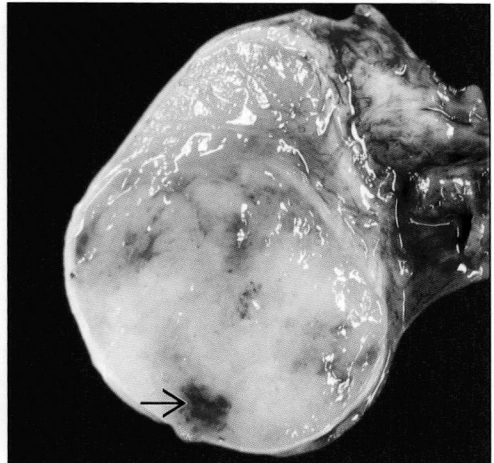

(Left) YST forms an ill-defined mass with poorly defined borders with the surrounding testicular parenchyma. The tumor has a white-tan appearance with focal cystic and hemorrhagic changes ➡. *(Right)* Large YST with relatively homogeneous, white, mucoid cut surface is shown. Focal hemorrhage is present ➡. A gelatinous or myxoid appearance is common in pediatric yolk sac tumors that are histologically pure.

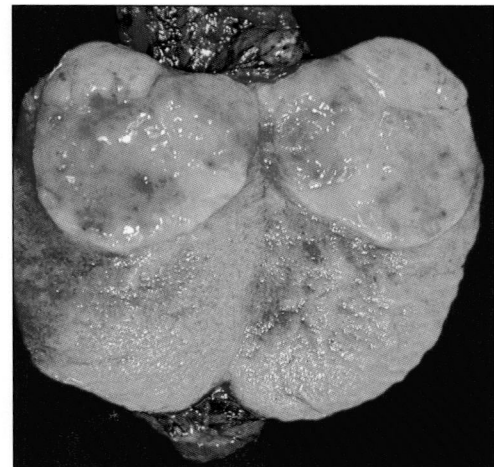

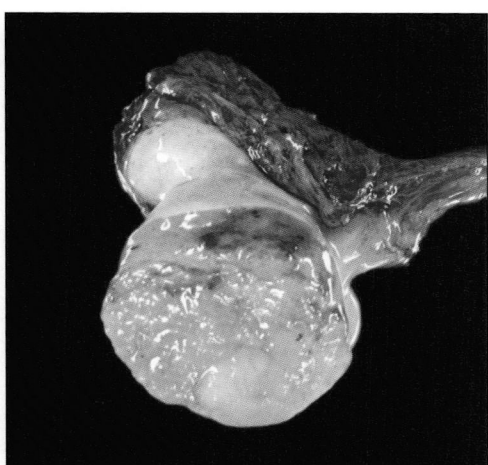

(Left) This is an adult pure YST, which has a homogeneous, mucoid cut surface. The finding of a pure yolk sac tumor in adults is extraordinarily rare. The relatively homogeneous appearance is in keeping with a pure histology under microscopy. (Courtesy Z. Qu, MD, PhD.) *(Right)* This photo shows a YST in a child. It has a bulging, white, myxoid, and yellow cut surface. Pure YST is the most common testicular tumor of infants and young children.

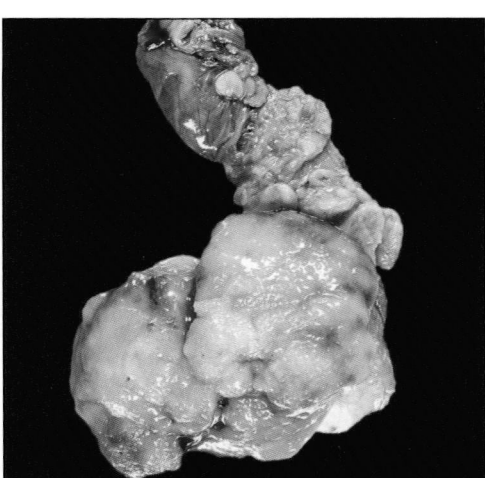

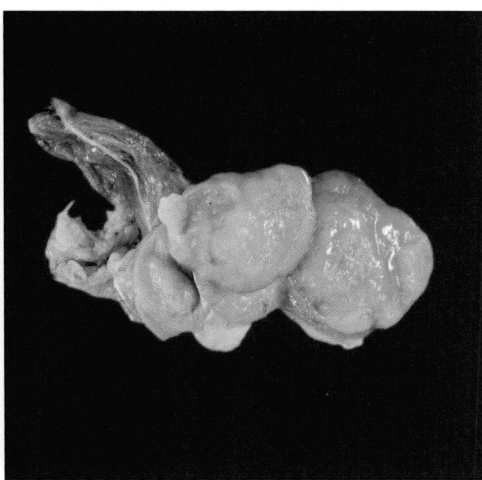

(Left) YST in a child with a white and yellow myxoid cut surface is shown. The tumor involves the spermatic cord. Most pediatric yolk sac tumors present with low clinical stage. *(Right)* Another gross photograph of YST in a child shows a relatively homogeneous, yellow, myxoid cut surface. No hemorrhage or necrosis is present.

Microscopic Features

(Left) This image shows microcystic or reticular pattern of YST with tumor cells forming microcysts and a meshwork of spaces. Some cells contain intracytoplasmic vacuoles ⇨ resembling lipoblasts. Eosinophilic globules ➡, which are a hallmark of YST, are present. *(Right)* Macrocystic YST results when multiple microcysts coalesce. YST shows a spectrum of cytoplasmic features that vary from flattened ⇨ to cuboidal ⇨ to columnar.

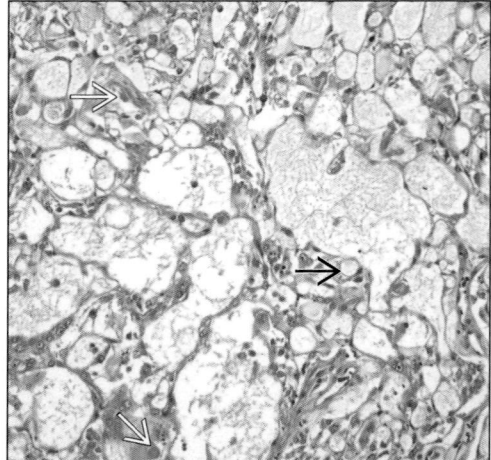
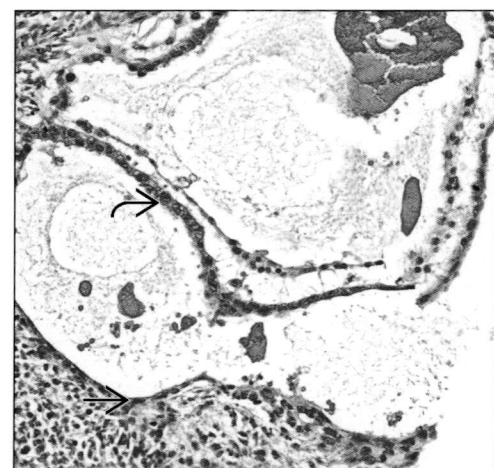

(Left) Microcystic and reticular pattern of YST with abundant extracellular eosinophilic material is shown. The tumor cells vary in size and shape and are distinct from embryonal carcinoma cells, which show obvious nuclear atypia. In contrast, seminoma cells show abundant clear cytoplasm with well-defined cell borders. *(Right)* Low-power photomicrograph shows microcystic and reticular pattern of YST with abundant eosinophilic (colloid-like) material.

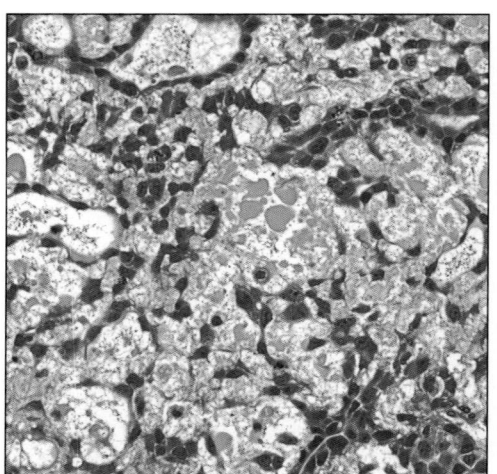
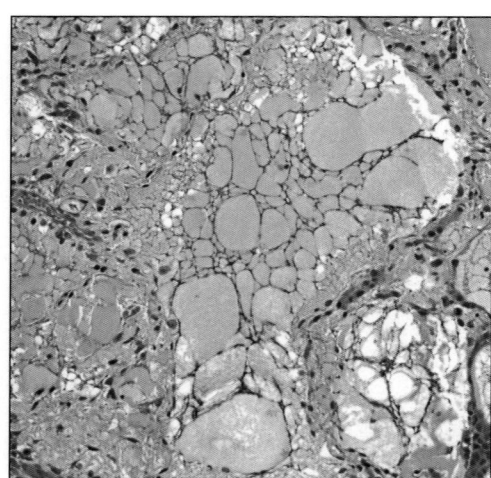

(Left) YST with typical endodermal sinus pattern is shown. Multiple Schiller-Duval bodies ⇨, which are sectioned in variable planes, are distributed amidst a loose, myxoid stroma. A central blood vessel with a mantle of cells surrounded by space and another cellular layer are typical of this pattern. *(Right)* This image shows endodermal sinus pattern of YST with a Schiller-Duval body ⇨. The tumor cells are often unevenly distributed within edematous and myxoid stroma.

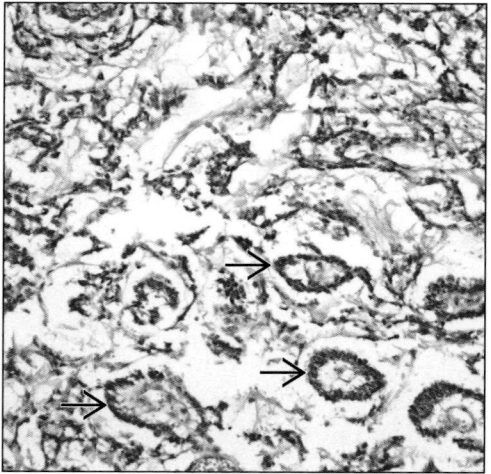
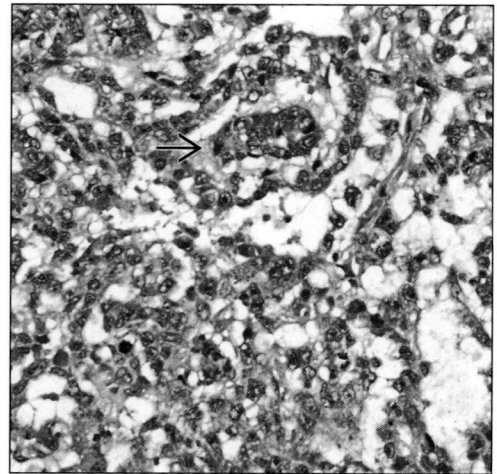

Microscopic Features

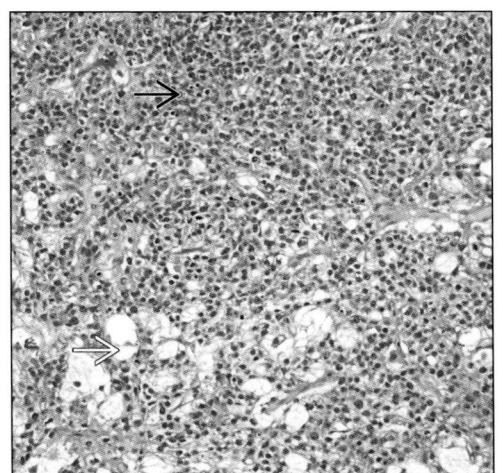
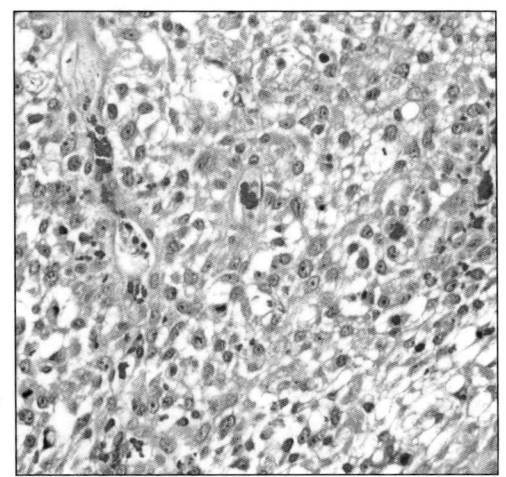

(Left) *Solid (upper ⇨) and microcystic (lower ➡) growth pattens of YST are shown. The tumor cells are relatively uniform with ovoid to round nuclei and abundant pale eosinophilic cytoplasm.* *(Right)* *Solid growth patten of YST is shown. The cells contain abundant pale eosinophilic to clear cytoplasm, similar to that of seminoma, although an inflammatory infiltrate is absent. Distinction is possible based on the presence of multiple concurrent patterns elsewhere.*

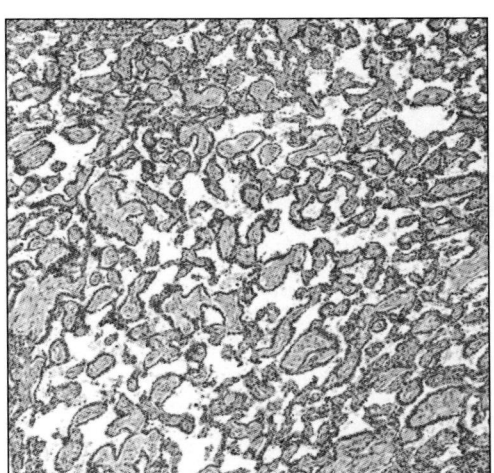
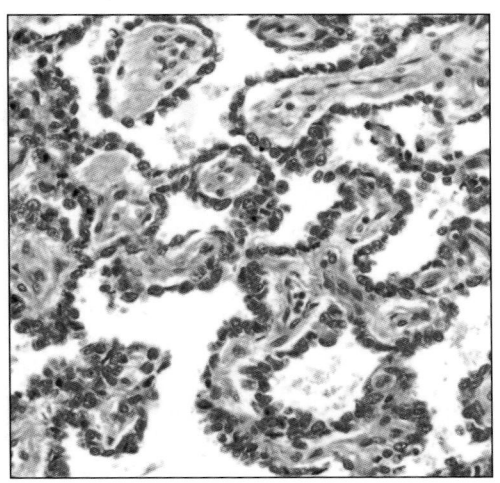

(Left) *Low-power photomicrograph shows a YST with exuberant papillary growth pattern and central fibrovascular cores. The appearance of tumor cells is relatively low grade.* *(Right)* *High-power image shows papillary YST with central fibrovascular core lined by relatively uniform cuboidal to "hobnail" tumor cells. The bland cytologic features of this tumor are distinct from those of embryonal carcinoma with papillary growth, which have distinct high-grade nuclear atypia.*

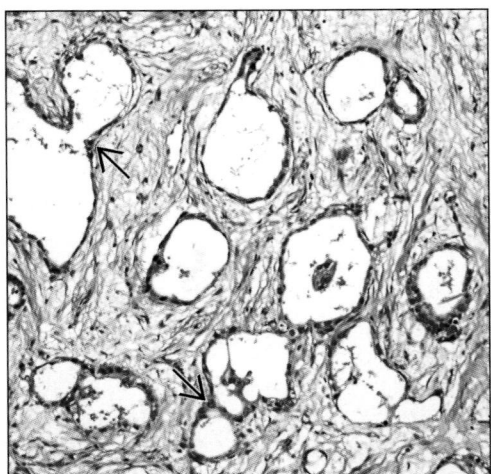
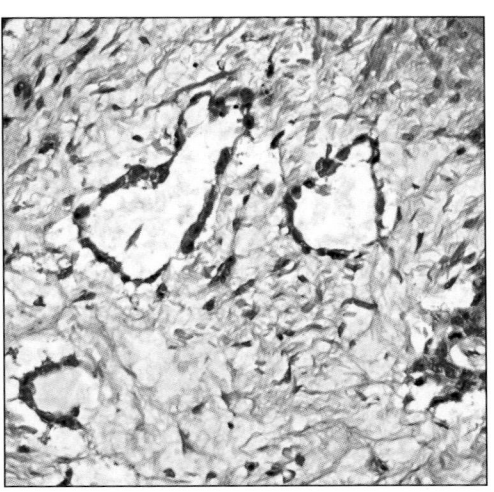

(Left) *This photomicrograph show polyvesicular vitelline pattern of YST. It is composed of irregularly shaped cysts with central to eccentric constriction ⇨ and loose myxoid stroma. The tumor cells are flattened and distributed in a variably cellular mesenchyme.*
(Right) *Polyvesicular vitelline pattern of YST shows irregularly shaped cysts lined by flattened to cuboidal epithelium. The vesicles recapitulate embryonic subdivision of the primary yolk sac into the secondary yolk sac.*

YOLK SAC TUMOR

Microscopic Features

(Left) A glandular growth pattern of YST with myxoid stroma is shown. The tumor cells are relatively uniform, a feature that is different from the glandular pattern in embryonal carcinoma or metastatic carcinoma. *(Right)* This images show glandular and reticular growth pattern of YST with prominent myxoid stroma. A combination of multiple patterns within the same tumor is a key distinguishing feature in YST and is also helpful in diagnosis at extragonadal sites.

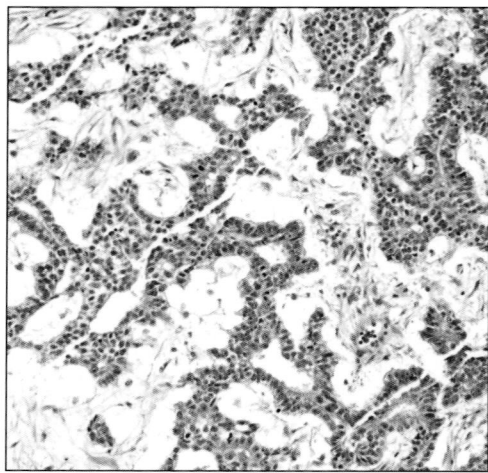
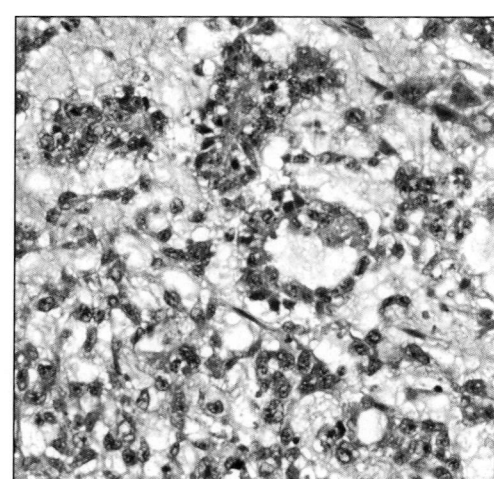

(Left) Parietal pattern of YST is composed of tumor cells surrounded by abundant bands of pink basement membrane-like material. This pattern is typically associated with microcystic or reticular pattern YST. *(Right)* High-power view of parietal pattern of YST shows tumor cells surrounded by dense pink-staining basement membrane-like material, which represents recapitulation of the parietal layer of the embryonic yolk sac of the rodent; it is usually negative for AFP.

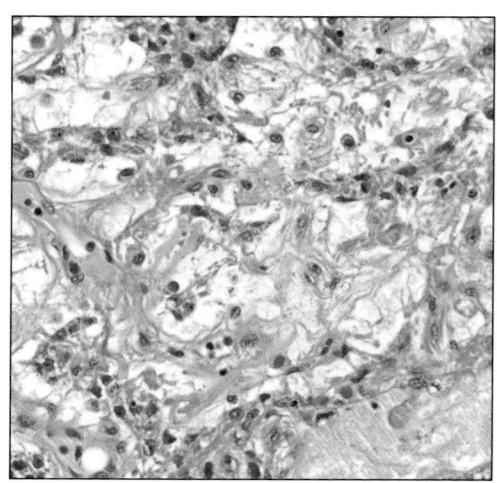
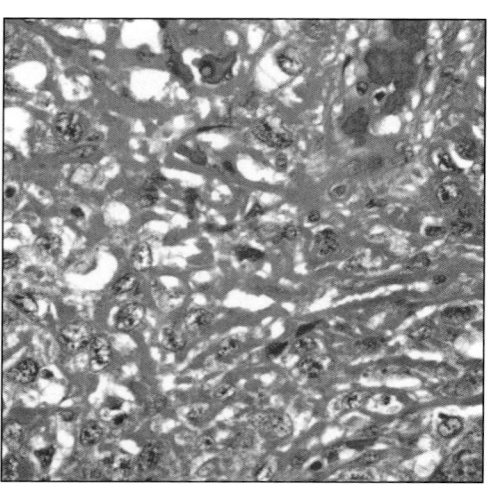

(Left) Enteric (endometrioid) pattern of YST with columnar cells and subnuclear vacuoles is shown. Also note the focal presence of pink basement membrane-like material ➡. *(Right)* Enteric (endometrioid) pattern of YST has tall columnar cells and subnuclear vacuoles ➡ resembling secretory phase endometrial glands. Although embryonal carcinoma may rarely demonstrate this pattern, cytologic features are discriminatory. Note that the luminal surface is smooth.

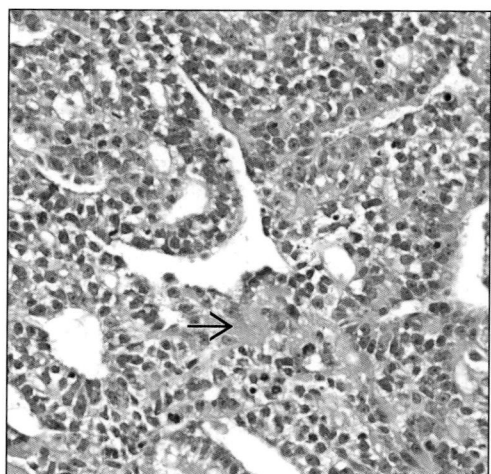
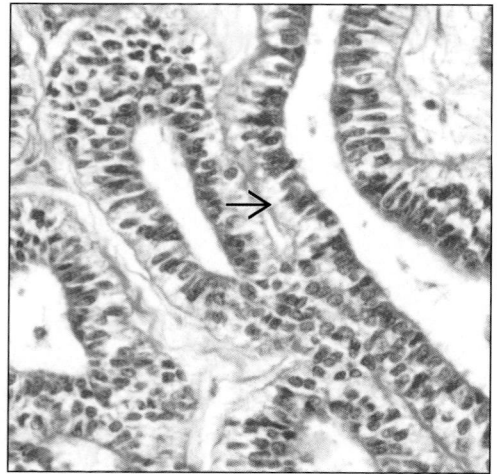

YOLK SAC TUMOR

Microscopic and Immunohistochemical Features

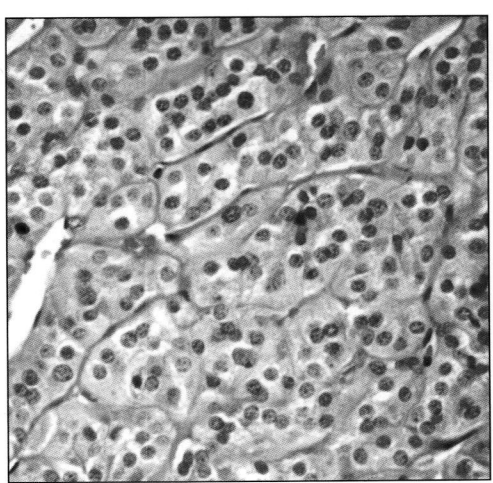
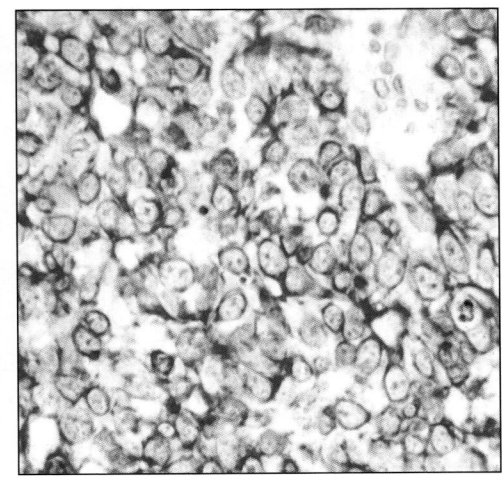

(Left) Hepatoid pattern of YST has solid sheets of tumor cells containing abundant pink cytoplasm and thin fibrovascular septae with sinusoidal arrangement. The cells are intensely AFP positive. The tumor cells may occasionally demonstrate a bile canalicular pattern, although bile production is not present. Hyaline globules are commonly seen in this pattern. *(Right)* The tumor cells of YST are strongly positive for cytokeratin, a feature distinguishing it from seminoma.

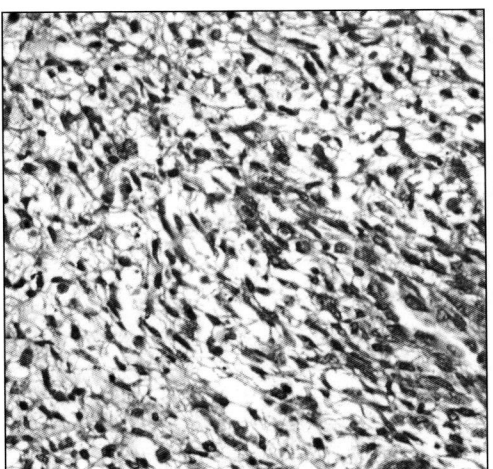
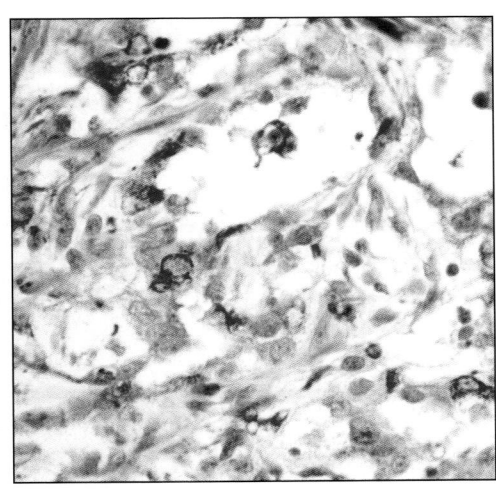

(Left) An example of spindle cell (sarcomatoid) area of a YST in an myxoid background is shown. Such foci are often seen in continuity with other classic patterns. Occasionally this pattern may predominate after chemotherapy. Cytokeratin positivity is retained and, along with history of germ cell tumor, is diagnostic for YST. *(Right)* AFP staining in YST is often quite variable, ranging between 55-100% in different studies. The staining may be focal and weak in some cases.

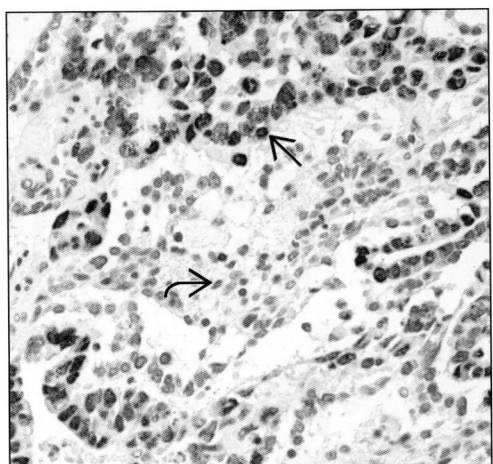
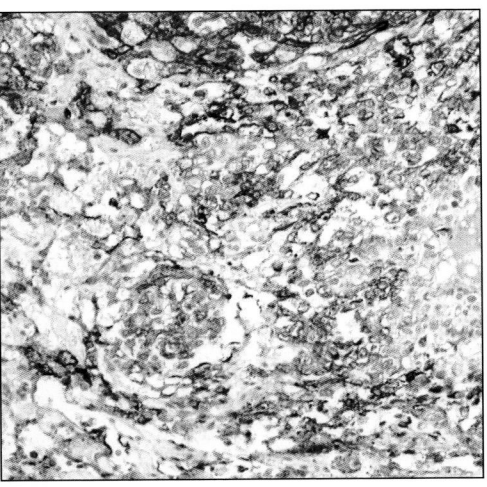

(Left) Mixed germ cell tumor with YST and embryonal carcinoma with differential staining for Oct3/4 ➔ is shown. The tumor cells of YST are negative, but embryonal carcinoma cells ➔ are positive (nuclear). *(Right)* The tumor cells of YST are positive for glypican-3. Seminoma and embryonal carcinoma are typically negative for glypican-3, although syncytiotrophoblasts and rarely choriocarcinoma and teratoma may be positive.

CHORIOCARCINOMA AND VARIANTS

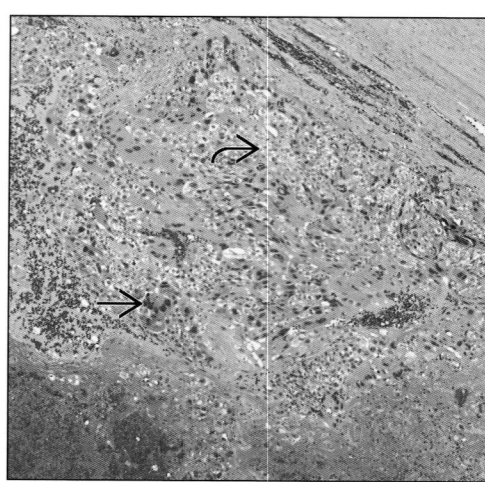

This photomicrograph shows the features of CC with large areas of hemorrhage and necrosis, and 2 types of cells, i.e., syncytiotrophoblasts ⇨ and cytotrophoblasts ⇨.

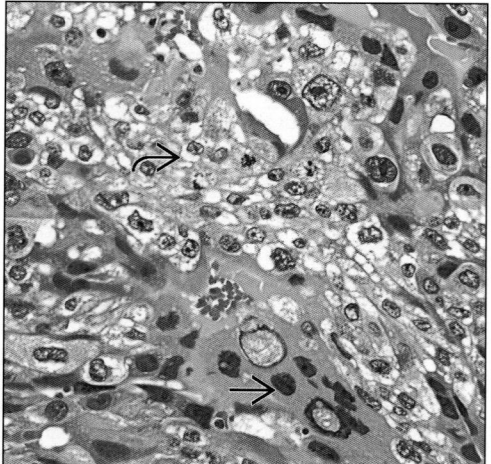

CC shows close spatial relationship of cytotrophoblasts ⇨ with clear cytoplasm and multinucleated syncytiotrophoblasts ⇨ with abundant eosinophilic cytoplasm and smudged nuclei.

TERMINOLOGY

Abbreviations
- Choriocarcinoma (CC)

Synonyms
- Trophoblastic tumor

Definitions
- Germ cell tumor composed of admixture of mononucleate cytotrophoblastic and multinucleate syncytiotrophoblastic cells
- Monophasic choriocarcinoma (rare, lacks syncytiotrophoblasts)
- Placental site trophoblastic tumor (extremely rare; tumor of intermediate trophoblasts)

CLINICAL ISSUES

Epidemiology
- Incidence
  - Pure choriocarcinoma accounts for < 1% of germ cell tumors
  - Usually mixed with other germ cell tumor components (8% of mixed germ cell tumors)
- Age
  - 25-30 years

Presentation
- Testicular mass (often small)
- Symptoms due to hematogenous metastasis (hemoptysis, central nervous system dysfunction, hematemesis, melena, hypotension, anemia)
  - May present with metastasis with subsequent detection of primary
- May have gynecomastia or hyperthyroidism

Laboratory Tests
- Patients typically have very high circulating human chorionic gonadotropin (hCG) (usually > 100,000 mIU/mL)

Treatment
- Radical orchiectomy and systemic chemotherapy

Prognosis
- Worse prognosis than other germ cell tumors, if pure
- Level of hCG correlates with prognosis, reflecting tumor burden

IMAGE FINDINGS

General Features
- Similar to other nonseminomatous germ cell tumors, but mass is usually small or inapparent in pure CC

MACROSCOPIC FEATURES

General Features
- For pure tumors
  - Hemorrhagic and necrotic mass with blood clot; ill-defined gray to tan tissue at periphery
  - Primary site may be totally regressed with "burnt-out" focus

Size
- Variable (may be quite small)

MICROSCOPIC PATHOLOGY

Key Descriptors
- Predominant Pattern/Injury Type
  - Neoplastic
- Predominant Cell/Compartment Type
  - Mononucleated cytotrophoblasts and multinucleated syncytiotrophoblasts

CHORIOCARCINOMA AND VARIANTS

Key Facts

Terminology

- Germ cell tumor composed of mixture of mononucleate trophoblastic cells and multinucleate syncytiotrophoblasts

Clinical Issues

- Pure choriocarcinoma comprises < 1% of germ cell tumor
- Known for early hematogenous metastasis to lung, liver, and brain
- Patients typically have very high circulating human chorionic gonadotropin (hCG) (usually > 100,000 mIU/mL)

Macroscopic Features

- Hemorrhagic and necrotic mass with blood clot; ill-defined gray to tan tissue at periphery

Microscopic Pathology

- Classic choriocarcinoma consists of mixture of cytotrophoblasts and multinucleate syncytiotrophoblasts
- Syncytiotrophoblasts wrapping around mononuclear cytotrophoblastic cells and forming villous configuration
- Significant hemorrhage and necrosis
- Intratubular germ cell neoplasia (ITGCN) in adjacent testis

Ancillary Tests

- Positive for cytokeratin, HCG, HPL, EMA/MUC1 (only for syncytiotrophoblast), and SALL4
- Negative for vimentin, CD30(BerH2), Podoplanin(D2-40), Oct3/4, and inhibin

---

- Histologic Features
  - Classic choriocarcinoma consists of mixture of cytotrophoblasts and multinucleate syncytiotrophoblasts
    - Cytotrophoblasts are round or polygonal cells with prominent cell borders, clear cytoplasm, and usually single bland nucleus
    - Syncytiotrophoblasts are large multinucleate cells, often degenerate appearing, with abundant eosinophilic and vacuolated cytoplasm
    - These 2 cell populations exhibit spatial relationship with syncytiotrophoblasts wrapping around mononuclear cytotrophoblastic cells
    - Villous configuration is occasionally seen and is typical for choriocarcinoma
  - Monophasic choriocarcinoma, a variant of choriocarcinoma, is usually seen in metastatic sites following chemotherapy
    - Composed of predominantly mononucleate squamoid-appearing cytotrophoblasts with rare mitoses
  - Placental site trophoblastic tumor (PSTT), another rare variant of choriocarcinoma has been reported
    - Composed of intermediate trophoblasts with smudged, hyperchromatic nuclei and moderate amount of eosinophilic to amphophilic cytoplasm
  - Significant hemorrhage and necrosis
  - Intratubular germ cell neoplasia (ITGCN) in adjacent testis

ANCILLARY TESTS

Immunohistochemistry

- Positive for cytokeratin, HCG, HPL, EMA/MUC1 and glypican-3 (only for syncytiotrophoblasts), CEA, and SALL4
- Negative for vimentin, CD30(BerH2), Podoplanin(D2-40), Oct3/4, and inhibin

DIFFERENTIAL DIAGNOSIS

Hemorrhage Due to Nonneoplastic Process

- Appropriate clinical history (testicular torsion, trauma)
- Coagulative necrosis with ghost outlines of seminiferous tubules

Other Germ Cell Tumor with Syncytiotrophoblasts, Particularly Seminoma

- Histologic features of other germ cell components
- Lack of diagnostic triad for CC
  - Hemorrhagic and necrotic background
  - 2 cell population with spatial relationship
  - Classic or vague villous configuration

DIAGNOSTIC CHECKLIST

Clinically Relevant Pathologic Features

- May present with disseminated metastases without overt testicular mass
- Production of hCG by tumor may lead to serum hCG elevation resulting in gynecomastia and thyrotoxicosis

Pathologic Interpretation Pearls

- 2 cell types; frequent hemorrhage and necrosis
- Large multinucleate giant cells surrounding cytotrophoblasts with villous configuration

SELECTED REFERENCES

1. Ulbright TM: The most common, clinically significant misdiagnoses in testicular tumor pathology, and how to avoid them. Adv Anat Pathol. 15(1):18-27, 2008
2. Ulbright TM et al: Trophoblastic tumors of the testis other than classic choriocarcinoma: "monophasic" choriocarcinoma and placental site trophoblastic tumor: a report of two cases. Am J Surg Pathol. 21(3):282-8, 1997
3. Ulbright TM et al: Choriocarcinoma-like lesions in patients with testicular germ cell tumors. Two histologic variants. Am J Surg Pathol. 12(7):531-41, 1988
4. Manivel JC et al: Intermediate trophoblast in germ cell neoplasms. Am J Surg Pathol. 11(9):693-701, 1987

CHORIOCARCINOMA AND VARIANTS

Gross and Microscopic Features

(Left) Gross photograph of CC shows typical hemorrhagic cut surface. There are nodules of blood clot and tumor with cystic degenerative changes. *(Courtesy T. Ulbright, MD.)* *(Right)* Low-power photomicrograph shows CC with a central zone of hemorrhage and necrosis surrounded by a mixture of mononucleate cytotrophoblasts and multinucleate syncytiotrophoblasts. Gross or microscopic hemorrhage should always raise the possibility of a CC component.

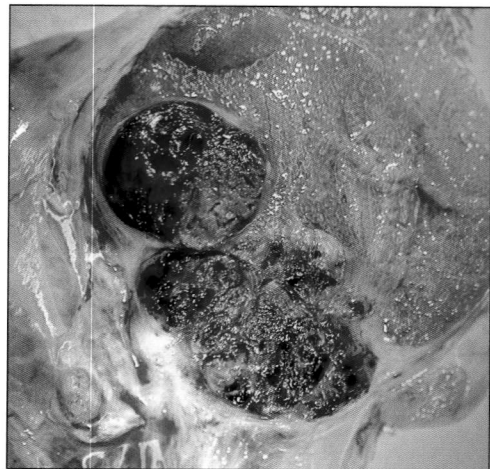 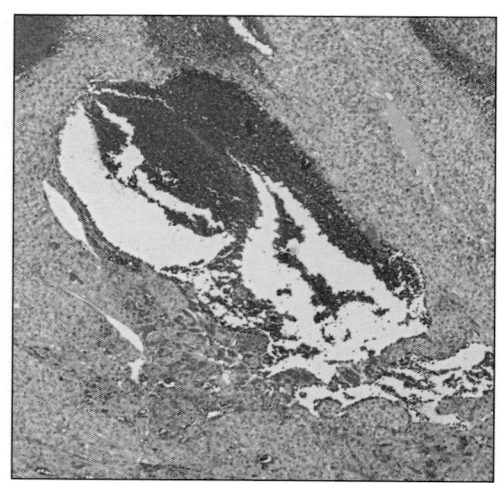

(Left) CC with typical syncytiotrophoblasts invading blood vessels is shown here. Fibrinoid necrosis and hemorrhage are present. Sheets of cytotrophoblasts are at the periphery of the hemorrhagic and necrotic zone. *(Right)* This photomicrograph shows necrotic tumor with ghost outlines of multinucleate syncytiotrophoblasts ⇨ and cytotrophoblasts ⇨. Necrosis and hemorrhage are a prominent feature of a CC.

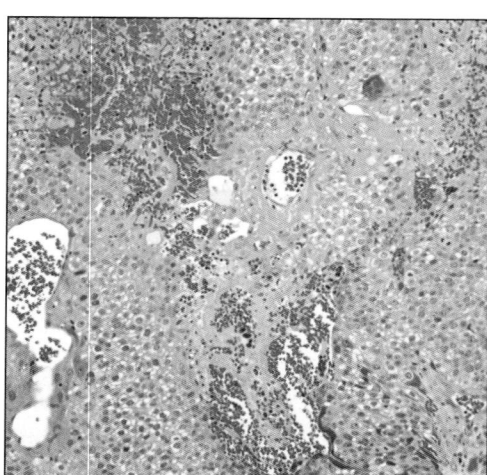 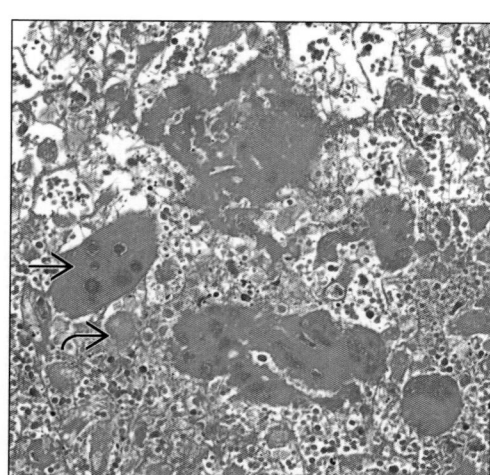

(Left) High-power photomicrograph shows CC with a central zone of hemorrhage and necrosis surrounded by multinucleate syncytiotrophoblasts ⇨ with dark staining or smudged nuclei. *(Right)* High-power view of CC shows a central zone of hemorrhage. Pale cytotrophoblasts ⇨ are surrounded by multinucleate syncytiotrophoblasts ⇨ with dense eosinophilic cytoplasm. The close relationship of the 2 distinctive cell types is characteristic of CC.

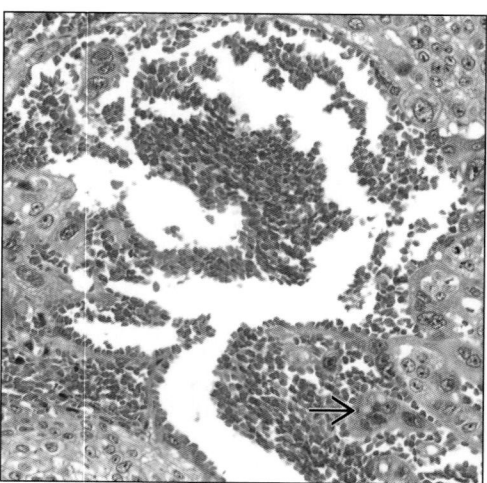 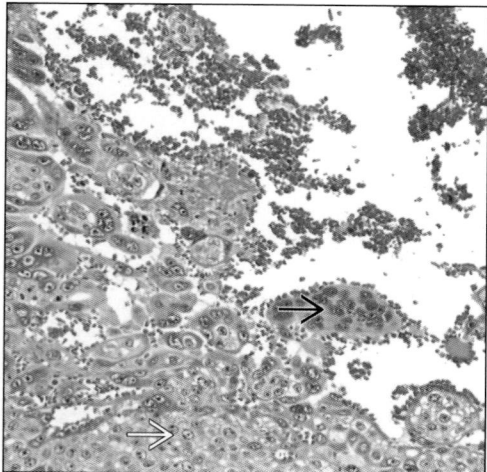

Microscopic Features

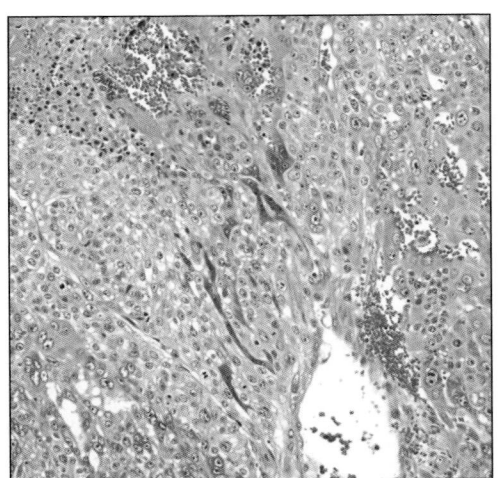
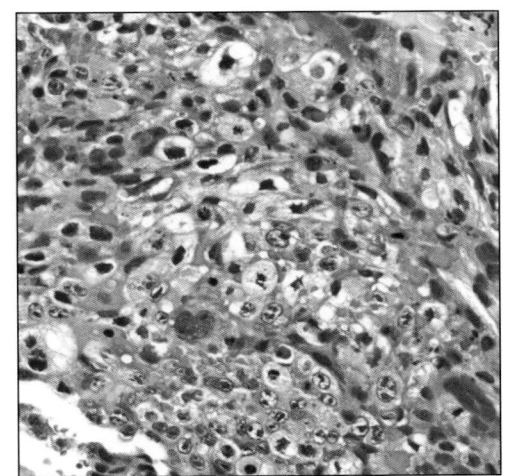

(Left) Intimate admixture of mononucleate cytotrophoblasts with clear cytoplasm and a few multinucleate syncytiotrophoblasts is typical for CC. Fibrinoid necrosis and hemorrhage are present. *(Right)* This photomicrograph shows intimate admixture of mononucleate cytotrophoblasts with clear cytoplasm and a few multinucleate syncytiotrophoblasts with dense eosinophilic cytoplasm and smudged nuclei.

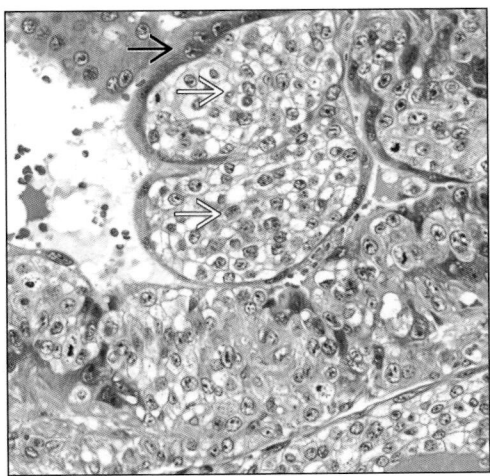
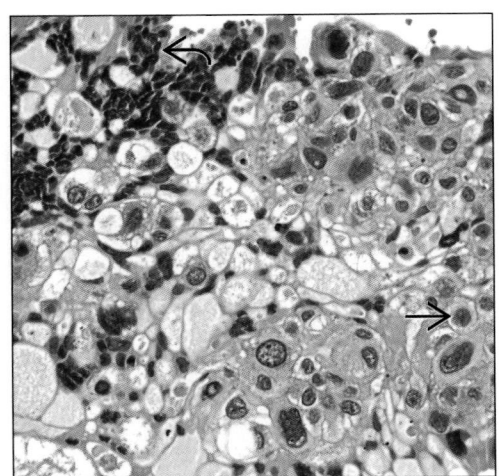

(Left) This photomicrograph shows syncytiotrophoblastic ➡ "capping" of nests of cytotrophoblasts ➡, a feature reminiscent of immature placental villi. *(Right)* Cytotrophoblasts ➡ have open chromatin and clear cytoplasm, and syncytiotrophoblasts ➡ are multinucleate with eosinophilic cytoplasm. Syncytiotrophoblasts associated with other germ cell tumors are often misdiagnosed as choriocarcinoma.

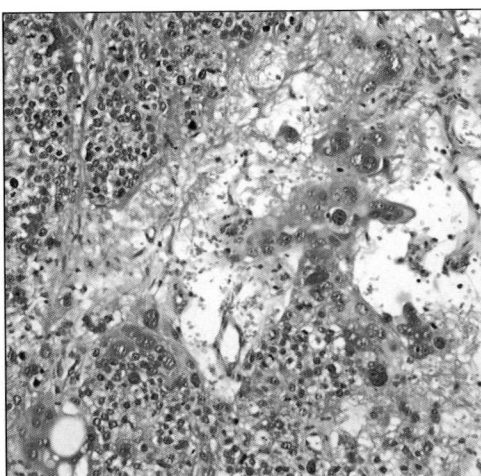
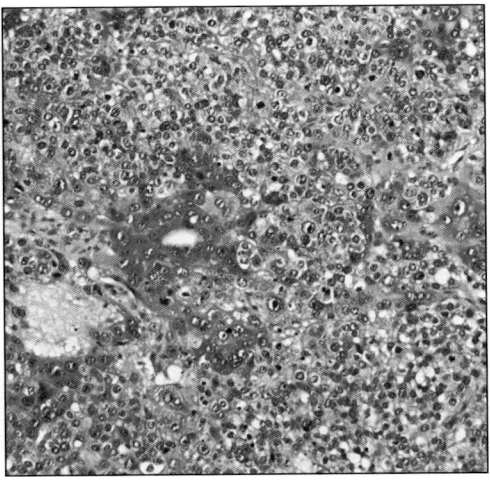

(Left) CC in which the 2 cell types (syncytiotrophoblasts and cytotrophoblasts) are present but do not show the typical biphasic pattern. Syncytiotrophoblasts are more commonly seen at the periphery in most CC, as in this case. *(Right)* CC demonstrates a spectrum of malignant trophoblastic cells from relatively small to large mononucleate cells, as well as multinucleate syncytiotrophoblastic tumor cells. The arrangement of cytotrophoblasts is in sheets.

Microscopic and Immunohistochemical Features

(Left) High-power photomicrograph shows nests of cytotrophoblasts with relatively uniform round to ovoid nuclei, vesicular nuclei, prominent nucleoli, clear to pale eosinophilic cytoplasm, and a distinct cytoplasmic membrane. *(Right)* This high-power photomicrograph shows several syncytiotrophoblasts ➡ with multiple irregular hyperchromatic and smudged nuclei, dense eosinophilic or amphophilic cytoplasm. Also present are mononucleate cytotrophoblasts ➡.

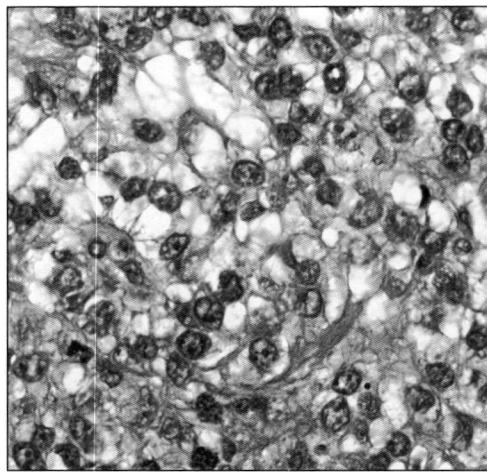 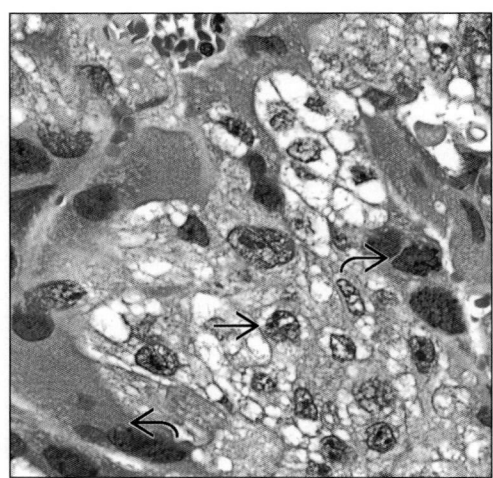

(Left) An example of "monophasic" CC with sheets of relatively uniform mononucleate cytotrophoblasts with eosinophilic cytoplasm is shown. Syncytiotrophoblasts are not seen in this image, although elsewhere they were present. *(Right)* This is a lung metastatic "monophasic" CC in a patient with testicular mixed germ cell tumor after chemotherapy. The tumor is composed of sheets of cytotrophoblasts with clear to eosinophilic cells resembling that of a non-small cell carcinoma of lung.

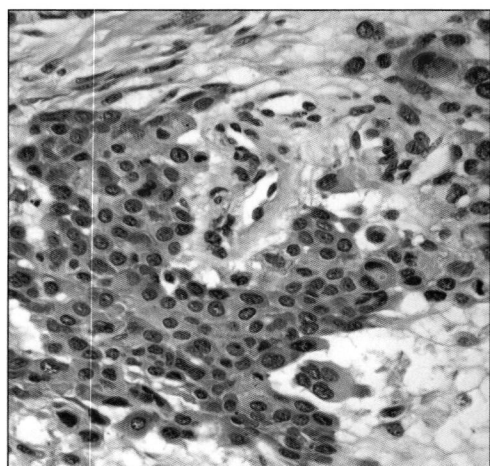 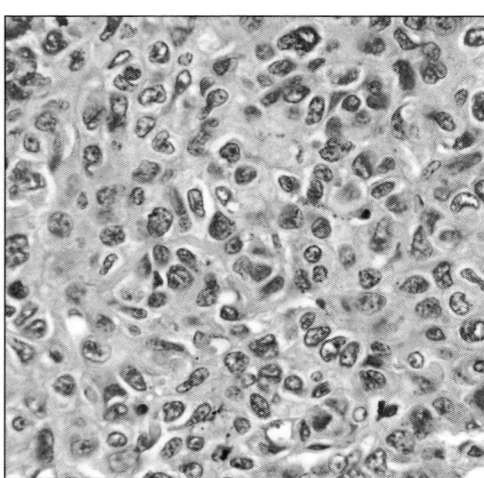

(Left) The tumor cells of "monophasic" choriocarcinoma are diffusely positive for β-hCG. Immunohistochemistry is necessary to confirm CC when syncytiotrophoblasts are scant to absent. When this morphology is encountered, the differential diagnosis includes other germ cell tumor components but most closely resembles a solid yolk sac tumor. *(Right)* This is a high-power view of "monophasic" choriocarcinoma, which is diffusely positive for HPL.

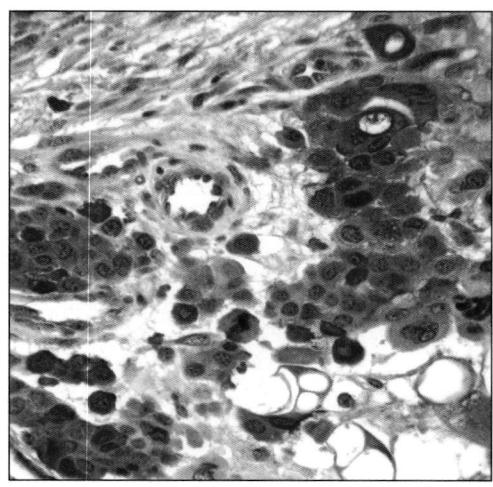 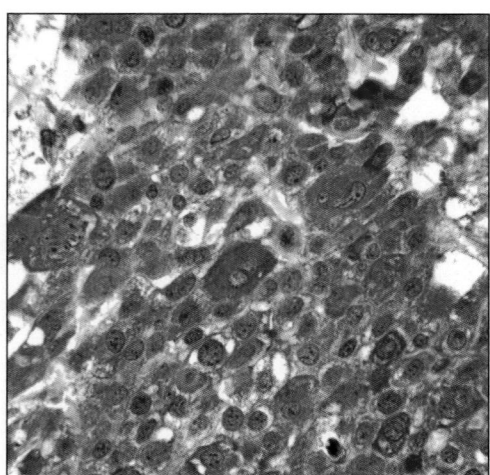

CHORIOCARCINOMA AND VARIANTS

Microscopic and Immunohistochemical Features

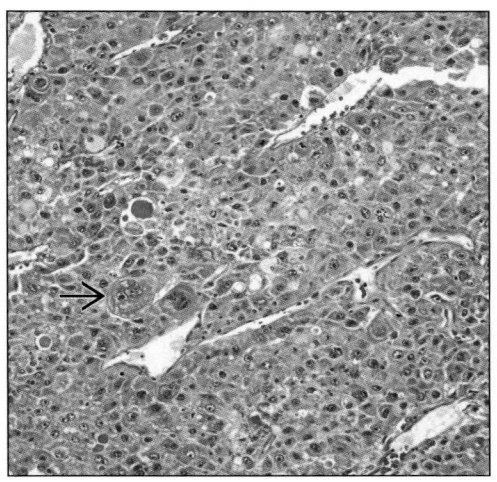

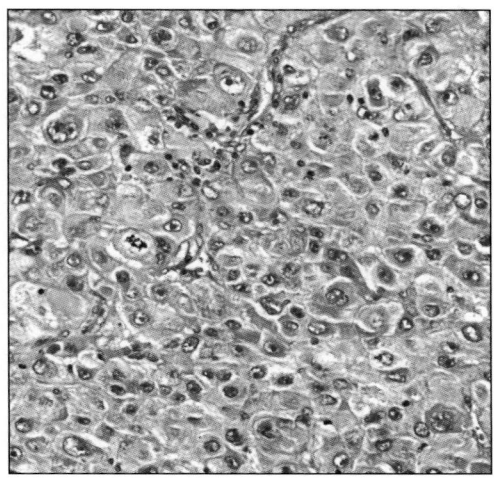

(Left) This is an example of "monophasic" choriocarcinoma with sheets of mononucleate epithelioid tumor cells with round to ovoid nuclei and abundant pale eosinophilic cytoplasm. Rare, scattered syncytiotrophoblasts ➡ are seen. *(Right)* High-power photomicrograph shows a "monophasic" choriocarcinoma with sheets of mononucleated epithelioid or "squamoid" tumor cells with round to ovoid nuclei, prominent nucleoli, and abundant pale eosinophilic cytoplasm.

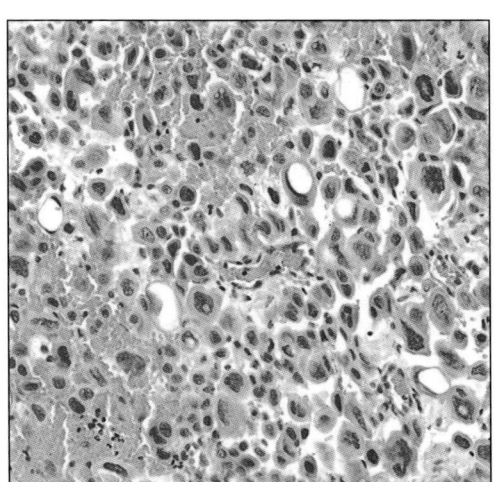

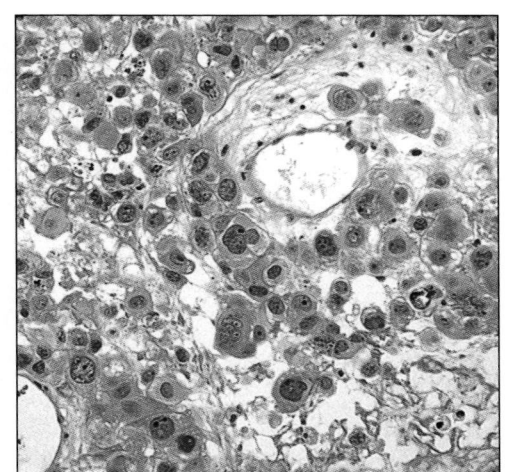

(Left) Placental site trophoblastic tumor (PSTT) is composed of intermediate trophoblastic cells that are large and mononucleate with abundant, dense eosinophilic cytoplasm. The nuclei are irregularly shaped and have smudged chromatin. *(Right)* High-power view of PSTT shows an intermediate trophoblastic proliferation. Some of the tumor cells are larger with multiple nuclei or multilobation. Tumor cells may extend into blood vessels and are strongly HPL positive.

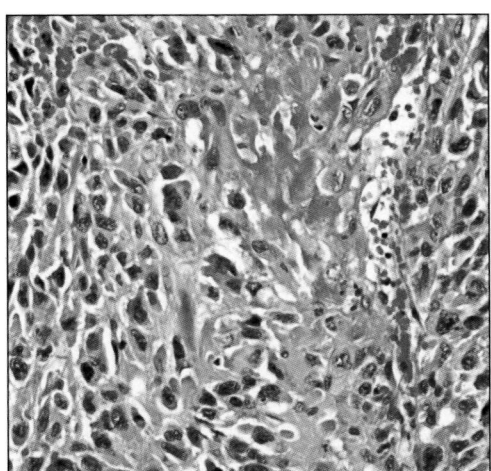

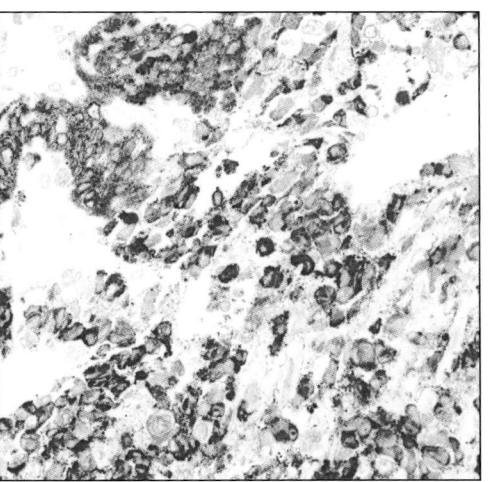

(Left) PSTT is composed of atypical mononucleate intermediate trophoblastic cells and perivascular fibrinoid necrosis. The tumor may have sheet-like growth or may be interstitial (between seminiferous tubules) in location. Syncytiotrophoblasts are lacking. Occasional foci of hemorrhage may be present, but necrosis is uncommon. *(Right)* The intermediate trophoblastic tumor cells of a PSTT are diffusely positive for β-hCG. These tumors are also strongly positive for HPL.

TERATOMA

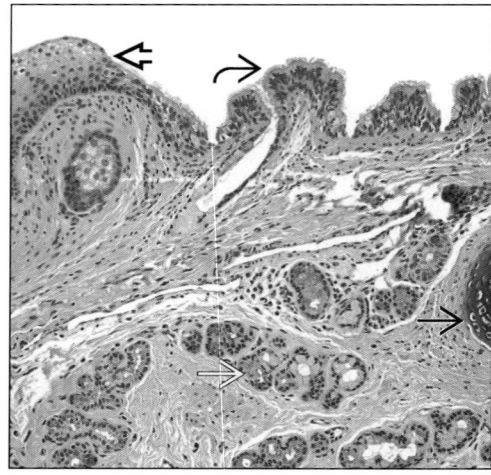

This mature teratoma shows squamous ⊳ and respiratory epithelium ⇗, seromucinous glands ⇥, and cartilage ⇥. Virtually all somatic tissue types may be seen in a teratoma.

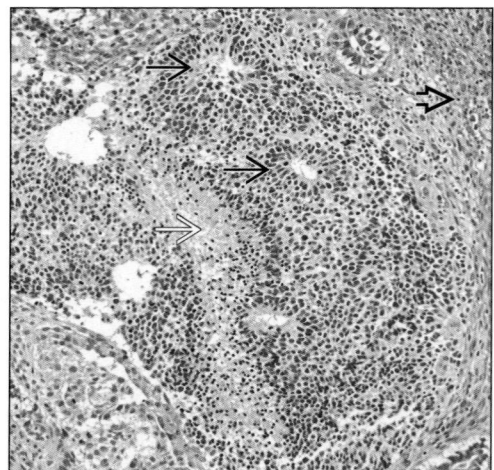

Immature teratoma shows neuroectodermal cells and neural tube-like structures ⇥. Focal necrosis ⇥ and cellular spindle immature mesenchymal tissue ⊳ are also present.

TERMINOLOGY

Synonyms
- Mature teratoma, immature teratoma

Definitions
- Tumors with > 1 somatic tissue of different germinal layers (ectoderm, mesoderm, or endoderm)

ETIOLOGY/PATHOGENESIS

Genetics
- Pediatric teratomas are diploid
- Adult teratomas are often aneuploid (hypotriploid)

CLINICAL ISSUES

Epidemiology
- Incidence
  - Pure form constitutes 4-9% of all testicular tumors
    - 2nd most common childhood germ cell tumor after yolk sac tumor in infants and young children
    - Pure teratoma in adults is extremely rare
  - Frequently mixed with other germ cell tumor types (approximately 50%)
- Age
  - Occurs in 2 distinct age groups: Pediatric (< 4 years of age) and adults (2nd to 4th decades)

Presentation
- Painless firm testicular mass

Treatment
- For teratoma in prepubertal children, orchiectomy without lymph node dissection
- For teratoma in adults, regardless of maturation, at least orchiectomy with close follow-up

Prognosis
- Prepubertal teratomas are almost always benign
- Adult teratomas are considered malignant because of relatively high recurrence or metastasis (22-37%)

IMAGE FINDINGS

General Features
- Solid and cystic testicular mass by ultrasound

MACROSCOPIC FEATURES

General Features
- Often well-circumscribed, nodular and firm mass with heterogeneous cut surface with solid and cystic areas
- Cysts filled with clear, white, flaky, gelatinous or mucoid material
- Mature tissue with hair, cartilage, bone, or teeth may be seen

Size
- Variable

MICROSCOPIC PATHOLOGY

Histologic Features
- Mature teratoma
  - Composed of mixture of elements of ectoderm, endoderm, and mesoderm
    - Ectoderm: Epidermis, neuronal tissue
    - Endoderm: Gastrointestinal or respiratory mucosa, other seromucous glands
    - Mesoderm: Bone, cartilage, muscle
  - Most common components are different types of epithelia, cartilage, or nerve
  - Respiratory and gastrointestinal epithelium, muscle, and cartilage are more commonly seen in testis than in ovary

TERATOMA

Key Facts

Terminology
- Tumors with somatic tissue of different germinal layers (ectoderm, mesoderm, or endoderm)

Clinical Issues
- 2nd most common childhood germ cell tumor in infants and young children
- Pure teratoma rare in adult and is often present mixed with other germ cell tumor

Macroscopic Features
- Often well-circumscribed, nodular and firm mass with heterogeneous cut surface with solid and cystic areas

Microscopic Pathology
- Mature teratoma
  - Composed of mixture of elements of ectoderm, endoderm, and mesoderm
  - Most common components are different types of epithelium, cartilage, or nerve
- Immature teratoma
  - Undifferentiated spindle cell component or primitive neuroectodermal tissue
- Stromal overgrowth with foci of embryonal rhabdomyosarcoma, Wilms tumor-like elements, or angiosarcoma
- Carcinomatous transformation with invasive growth

Top Differential Diagnoses
- Primary or metastatic sarcoma
- Mixed germ cell tumor
- Metastatic carcinoma

  - Pancreatic, dental, renal, and thyroid tissue are less commonly seen in testis than in ovary
- Immature teratoma
  - Primitive mesoderm: Undifferentiated spindle cell component (most common immature element in testis)
  - Primitive endoderm and primitive neuroectoderm (resembling neural tube and embryonic nervous system)
  - Blastomatous tissue (resembling blastema and embryonic tubules of developing lung or kidney), embryonic rhabdomyoblastic tissue
  - Teratoma with secondary malignant (somatic type) transformation
    - Sarcomatous transformation of teratoma: Foci of embryonal rhabdomyosarcoma, Wilms tumor-like element, or angiosarcoma
    - Carcinomatous elements in teratoma (such as squamous cell carcinoma, adenocarcinoma) with invasive growth
    - When histology of malignant component forms pure nodule of substantial size (> 1 field of 4x objective)

Cytologic Features
- Highly variable and depends on tissue type and maturity

Predominant Pattern/Injury Type
- Neoplastic

Predominant Cell/Compartment Type
- Variable tumor cells from > 1 germ cell layer

ANCILLARY TESTS

Immunohistochemistry
- Highly variable and depends on component of teratoma (rarely necessary in clinical practice)
  - Cytokeratin, CEA, and EMA/MUC1: Positive in epithelial tissue or carcinoma of teratomatous type
  - Vimentin: Positive in mesenchymal tissue
  - Germ cell markers: HCG (syncytiotrophoblastic cells), AFP (enteric and hepatoid tissue), PLAP (may be glandular tissue)
  - Other tissue specific markers for different type of tissues

DIFFERENTIAL DIAGNOSIS

Primary or Metastatic Sarcoma
- Usually involves the paratesticular structures, more homogeneous population of pleomorphic spindle cells

Metastatic Carcinoma
- Older age, clinical history, and pure carcinomatous component

Splenogonadal Fusion
- Rare congenital anomaly with fusion of spleen and testis

Adrenal Heterotopia
- Usually present in spermatic cord, epididymis, or rete testis

Mature Dermoid and Epidermoid Cysts
- Lack of intratubular germ cell neoplasia (ITGCN)

DIAGNOSTIC CHECKLIST

Pathologic Interpretation Pearls
- Multiple mature &/or immature tissue components of > 1 germ layer

SELECTED REFERENCES

1. Ulbright TM: Gonadal teratomas: a review and speculation. Adv Anat Pathol. 11(1):10-23, 2004

Gross Features

(Left) This mature teratoma shows a predominantly cystic mass with chalky keratin debris ⇨. Solid mucoid and gelatinous components ⇨ are also present, and these frequently correlate microscopically with immature teratomatous components. Uninvolved testis is pushed to 1 side ⇨. *(Right)* Mature teratoma with cystic ⇨ and solid ⇨ components is shown. The cyst is lined by whitish gray tissue, which coincided microscopically with mucosal-type tissue.

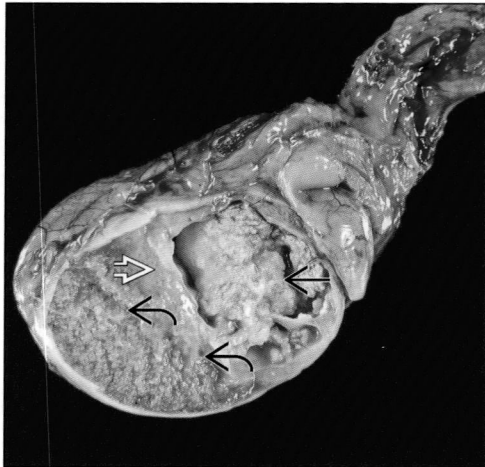
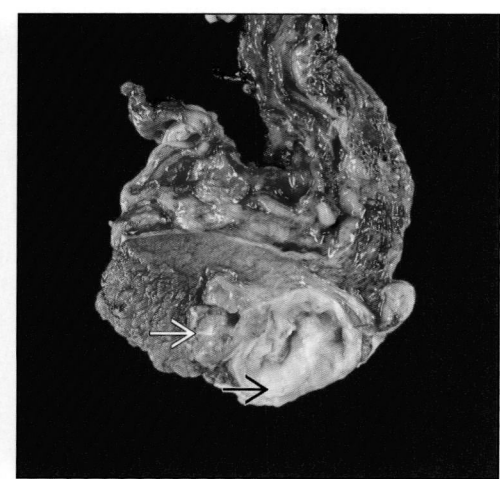

(Left) Mature teratoma with both solid ⇨ and cystic ⇨ components is shown. The cystic component contains chalky keratinous material. The solid areas are mucoid and gelatinous microscopically coinciding with glandular tissue component. *(Right)* This is a partial orchiectomy specimen from a child with mature teratoma. The tumor is well demarcated and has a cystic cavity containing mucoid material. Immature uninvolved testicular parenchyma ⇨ is seen at the periphery.

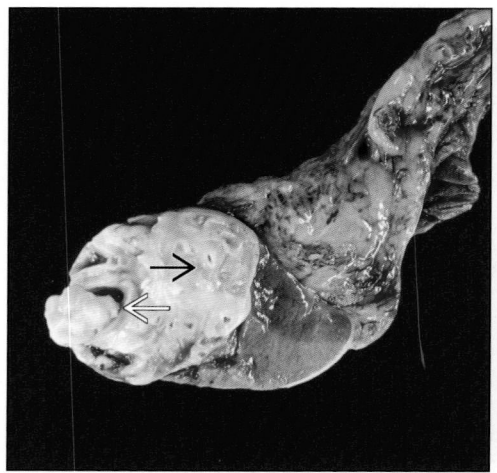
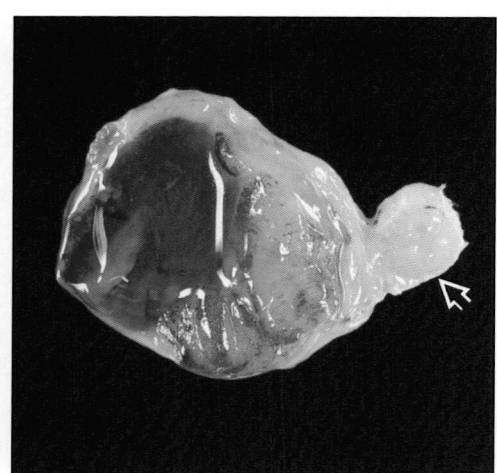

(Left) This immature teratoma is composed of multiple variably sized cysts and intervening whitish-gray solid areas, corresponding to cellular spindle mesenchymal tissue and glandular tissue microscopically. There is focal hemorrhage ⇨. *(Right)* This germ cell tumor shows a gelatinous to mucoid appearance ⇨ and firm solid gray-whitish areas. Histologically, both mature and immature components were present. Involvement of the spermatic cord is rare in pure teratomas.

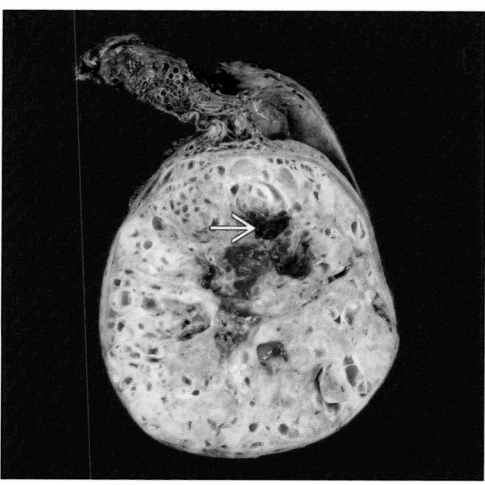
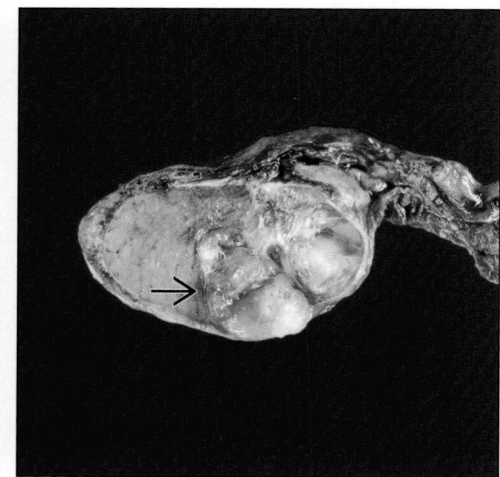

Microscopic Features

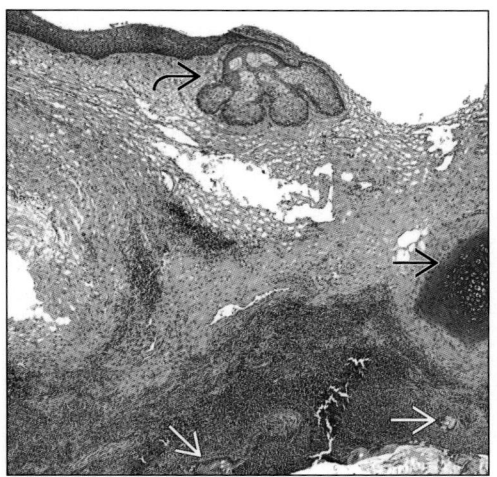

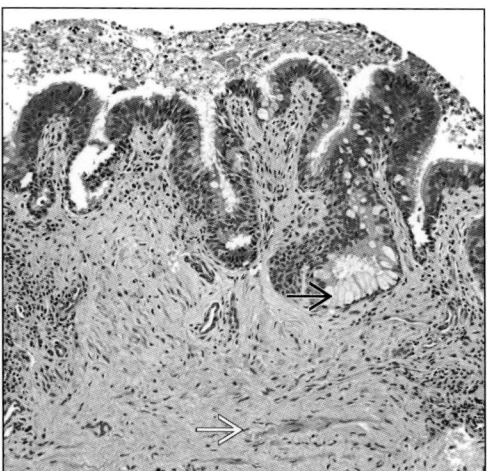

(Left) Mature teratoma shows skin and adnexal structure, including pilosebaceous units ➡, cartilage ➡, and focal intestinal epithelium with abundant lymphoid stroma ➡. *(Right)* Mature teratoma is shown with ciliated respiratory epithelium. Focally, goblet cells ➡ are present in the lining mucosa. There are scattered smooth muscle bundles in the wall of the cyst ➡. A smooth muscle wall of variable thickness lining cystic spaces is frequently present in teratomas.

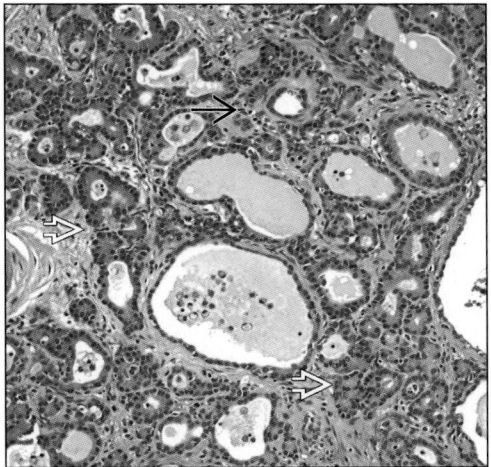

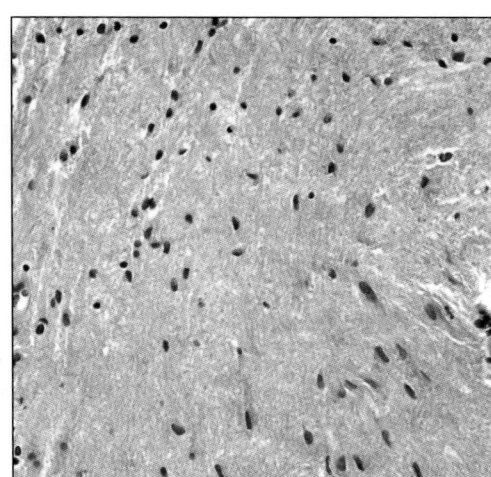

(Left) This mature teratoma shows ductal and glandular epithelium of pancreatic ➡ and gastric type ➡. The dilated glands are lined by attenuated flat epithelium and contain mucinous secretions. Pancreatic tissue is more commonly present in ovarian rather than testicular teratomas. *(Right)* Mature teratoma with mature glial tissue is shown. In adjacent areas (not shown), other mature teratomatous components, including bone, cartilage, glands, and squamous epithelium, were seen.

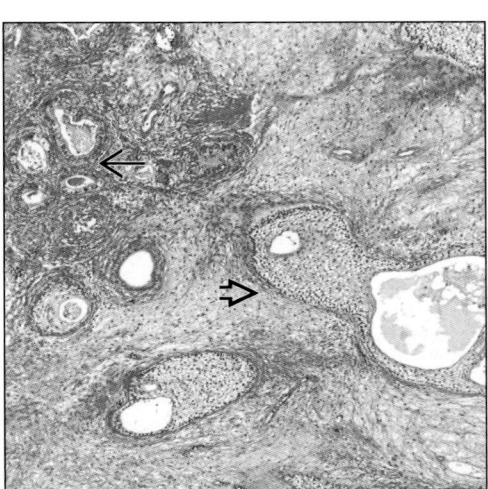

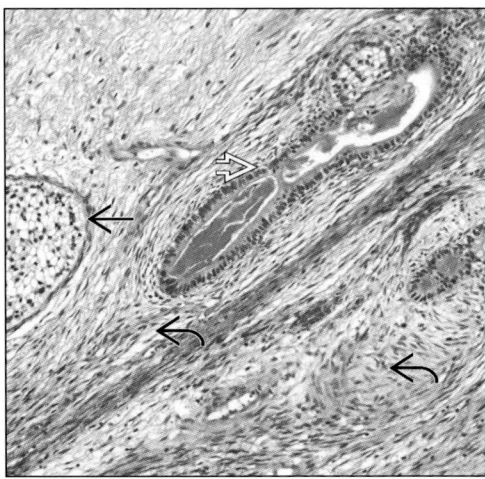

(Left) This mature teratoma has multiple somatic tissue components, including squamous ➡ and glandular epithelium ➡, and nondescriptive loose mesenchymal tissue component. Respiratory and gastrointestinal epithelium are the most frequent endodermal components in mature teratoma. *(Right)* This mature teratoma is composed of squamous epithelium ➡, glandular epithelium ➡, and immature loosely arranged spindle cell mesenchymal tissue ➡.

Microscopic Features

(Left) This teratoma is composed of an admixture of mature components, including squamous epithelium ➡ & cystic glandular tissue ➡. Surrounding the mature components is a circumferential rim of immature cellular spindle mesenchymal tissue ➡. *(Right)* Immature teratoma shows immature glandular epithelium ➡ surrounded by cellular spindle cell mesenchymal tissue ➡ around the glands. The immature spindle component often encircles the glandular & squamous components.

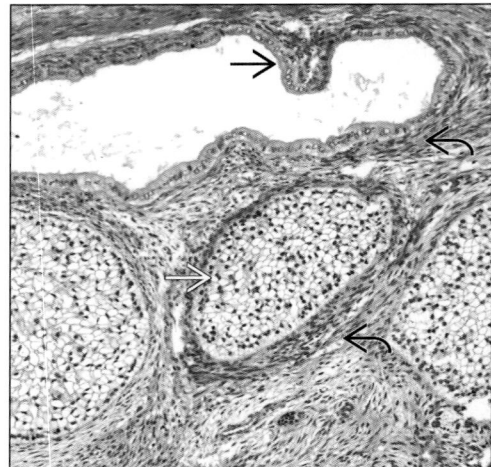
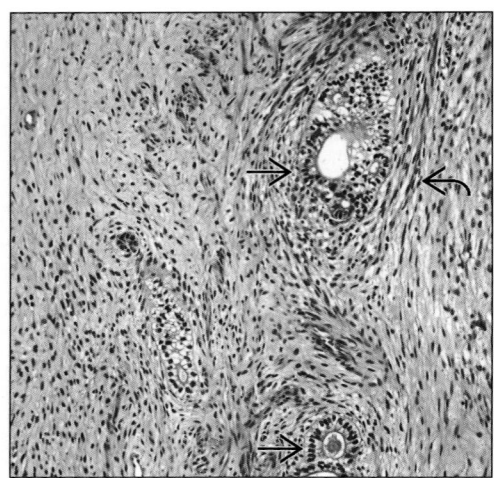

(Left) This image shows immature teratoma with glandular tissue surrounded by cellular spindle mesenchymal component with frequent mitoses ➡. This is the most common pattern of immature teratoma in the testis. *(Right)* Immature teratoma shows mature squamous epithelium on the top and immature cellular spindle cells with frequent mitoses ➡. It is rare for this immature component to show sarcomatous overgrowth, as it is frequently interspersed with squamous or glandular tissue.

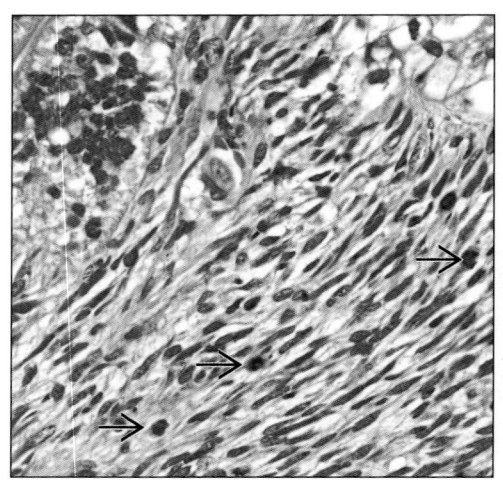
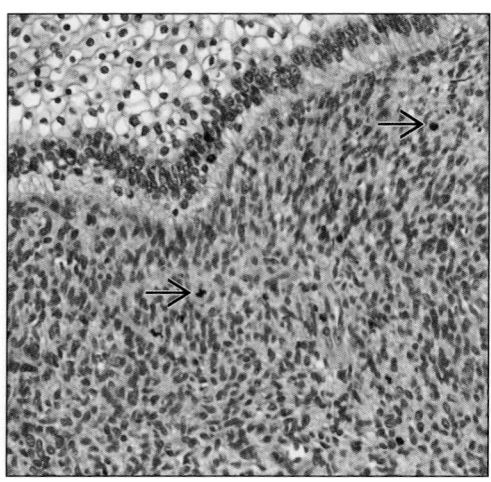

(Left) An immature teratoma shows cellular spindle cell mesenchymal tissue ➡ admixed with immature primitive neuroectodermal tissue composed of small round cells forming rosettes ➡. *(Right)* Primitive neuroectodermal tumor component is composed of hypercellular blue cells with poorly formed rosettes ➡. In order to designate a secondary malignant transformation of a primitive neuroectodermal tumor in an immature teratoma, growth exceeding 1 low power field is required.

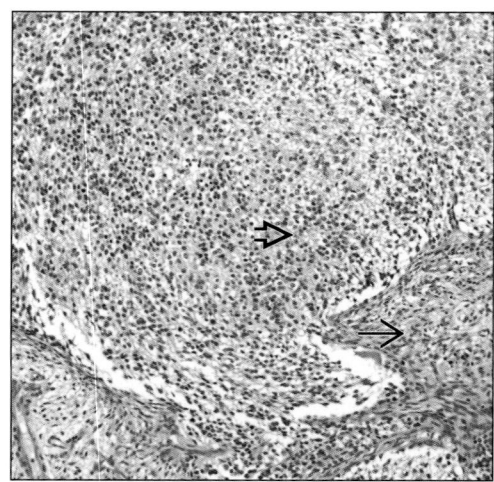
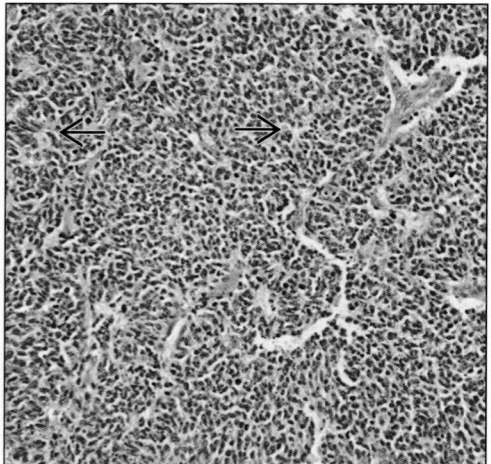

Microscopic Features and Differential Diagnoses

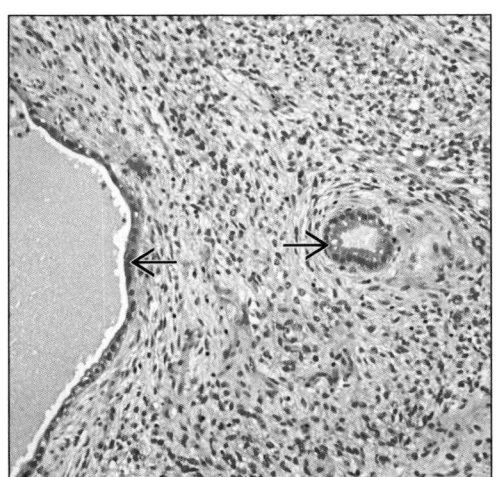

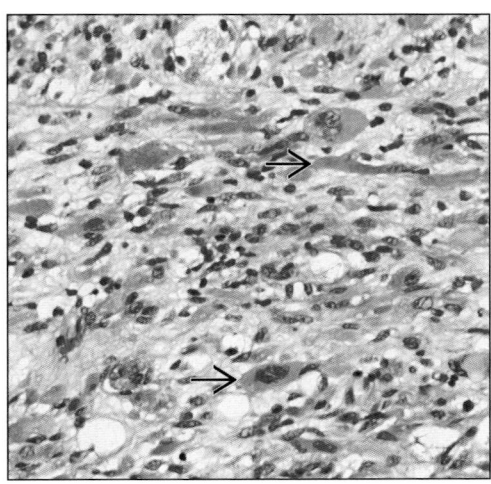

(Left) This image shows immature teratoma with benign glandular components ⊟ and cellular embryonal rhabdomyoblasts. To designate the tumor as rhabdomyosarcoma, pure stromal overgrowth (> 1 low-power field) is required. *(Right)* High-power photomicrograph shows an embryonal rhabdomyosarcoma with rhabdomyoblastic cells containing abundant pink cytoplasm. Tadpole cells ⊟ with vague cross striation are seen. These cells are positive for MYOD1 and myogenin.

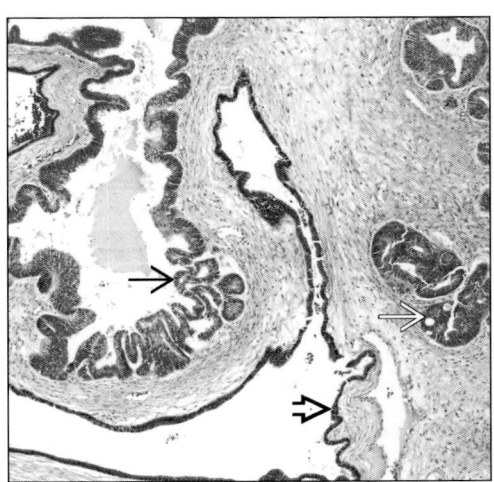

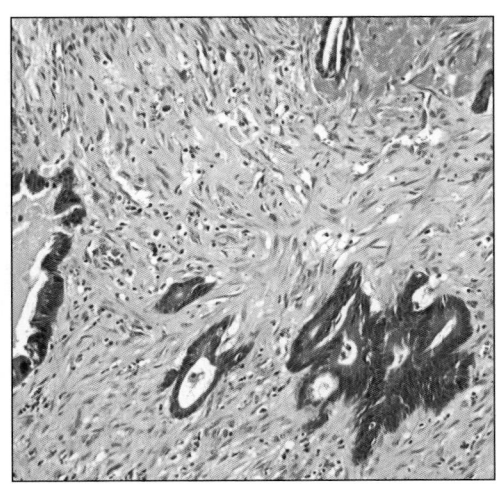

(Left) Secondary malignant transformation (adenocarcinoma) in a germ cell tumor (immature teratoma) is shown. There are infiltrative malignant glands ⊟ with abnormal cytology ⊟ and dilated gland lined by bland epithelium ⊟ (teratoma). *(Right)* Adenocarcinoma of somatic type shows irregular and cribriform glands, destructive invasive growth, and desmoplastic stroma. For carcinomatous transformation in a teratoma, true invasive growth is necessary for the diagnosis.

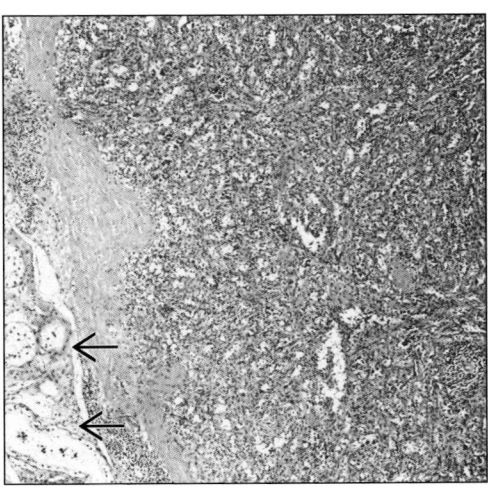

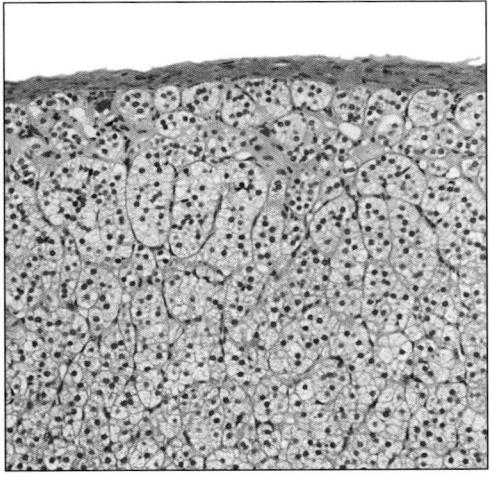

(Left) This photomicrograph shows splenogonadal fusion, a rare congenital anomaly in which there is fusion of the splenic and gonadal anlagen. This is not considered to be a teratoma. Seminiferous tubules are present ⊟. *(Right)* This is an example of ectopic adrenal tissue within the epididymis. It may occur anywhere along the route of descent of testis from the abdomen to the scrotum. It should not be considered a teratoma. Typically lesions are small, < 5 mm in size.

EPIDERMOID AND DERMOID CYSTS

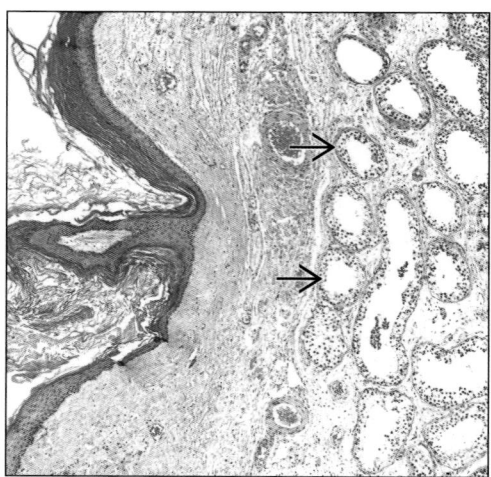

Unilocular epidermoid cyst is lined by keratinizing squamous epithelium and luminal keratin debris with no skin adnexal structures. The cyst is well demarcated from surrounding seminiferous tubules ➡.

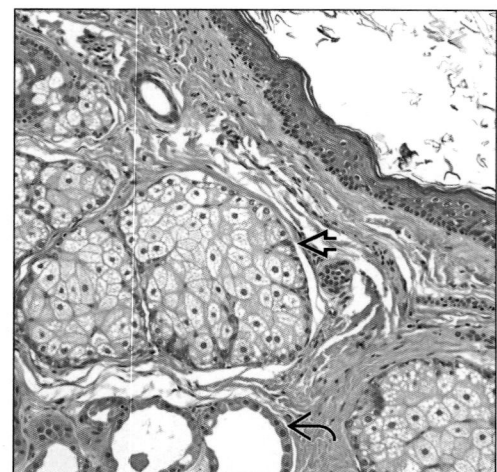

Dermoid cyst is characterized by keratinizing squamous epithelium and adnexal structures with well-organized sebaceous ⬅ and apocrine ➡ glands. No ITGCN was present in the surrounding seminiferous tubules.

TERMINOLOGY

Definitions
- Specialized benign form of testicular cyst with keratinizing squamous lining without skin adnexal structures (epidermoid cyst)
- Specialized benign form of monodermal cystic teratoma with keratinizing squamous lining and skin adnexal structures (dermoid cyst)

ETIOLOGY/PATHOGENESIS

Pathogenesis
- Pathogenesis of epidermoid cyst is still controversial
  - Some consider it as nonteratogenic, either from epithelial inclusion or from metaplastic mesothelium
  - Others suggest that it is teratomatous because of loss of heterozygosity for certain chromosomal loci
- Dermoid cyst is considered a specialized form of teratoma
  - Different from mature teratoma; believed to be derived from nontransformed germ cells and is unrelated to intratubular germ cell neoplasia (ITGCN)

CLINICAL ISSUES

Epidemiology
- Incidence
  - < 1% of testicular tumors
  - Dermoid cyst more rare than epidermoid cyst
- Age
  - Range: 10-40 years

Presentation
- Painless or painful palpable testicular enlargement over several years

- May be incidental finding

Laboratory Tests
- Serum tumor markers (LDH, AFP, and hCG) are not elevated

Treatment
- Surgical approaches
  - Cured by resection
  - May be amenable to partial orchiectomy

Prognosis
- Benign behavior

IMAGE FINDINGS

General Features
- Intratesticular hypoechoic cystic mass with "onion ring" appearance on ultrasound due to laminated keratin

MACROSCOPIC FEATURES

General Features
- Intraparenchymal, well-defined fibrous-walled cystic lesion containing degenerating keratin debris ± adnexal structures (dermoid vs. epidermoid cyst)

MICROSCOPIC PATHOLOGY

Histologic Features
- Epidermoid cyst
  - Usually unilocular cyst with keratinized squamous epithelial lining containing a granular cell layer without skin adnexal structures
  - Cystic wall may be calcified or ossified
- Dermoid cyst
  - Usually unilocular cyst filled with keratin debris or hair

EPIDERMOID AND DERMOID CYSTS

Key Facts

Terminology

- Specialized benign form of testicular cyst with keratinizing squamous lining without skin adnexal structures (epidermoid cyst)
- Specialized benign form of monodermal cystic teratoma with keratinizing squamous lining and skin adnexal structures (dermoid cyst)

Clinical Issues

- < 1% of testicular tumors
- Dermoid cyst more rare than epidermoid cyst
- Painless testicular enlargement over several years
- Cured by surgical resection

Macroscopic Features

- Unilocular intraparenchymal cystic lesion containing keratin debris

Microscopic Pathology

- Epidermoid cyst: Unilocular cyst with keratinized squamous epithelial lining containing granular cell layer, no skin adnexal structures
- Dermoid cyst: Usually unilocular cyst lined by epidermis and dermis containing skin adnexal structures (hair follicle, sebaceous, apocrine or eccrine glands)
- Other noncutaneous elements (such as ciliated epithelium, small bowel mucosa and submucosa) may be seen but maintain organoid arrangement
- Lipogranulomatous reaction to cyst contents may be seen
- Uninvolved testis has normal spermatogenesis with no significant atrophy or "dysgenetic features"

- o Lined by epidermis and dermis containing skin adnexal structures (hair follicle, sebaceous, apocrine or eccrine glands)
- o Orderly arrangement of pilosebaceous units to epidermal surface resembling that of skin
- o Other noncutaneous elements (such as ciliated epithelium, small bowel mucosa and submucosa) may be seen, but maintain organoid arrangement
- o Cystic wall with smooth muscle bundles may be present; cartilage, fibrous tissue, and neuroglia have rarely been reported
- o Lipogranulomatous reaction to cyst contents may be seen
- o "Pilomatrixoma" as variant of dermoid cyst has been reported
- o Uninvolved testis has normal spermatogenesis with no significant atrophy or "dysgenetic features"
- Lack of intratubular germ cell neoplasia (ITGCN)
- No other somatic tissue or malignant germ cell elements

Cytologic Features

- Mature keratinizing squamous epithelial cells (both dermoid and epidermoid) and skin adnexal structures (dermoid)

Predominant Pattern/Injury Type

- Cystic

Predominant Cell/Compartment Type

- Epithelial, squamous, skin adnexal tissue

ANCILLARY TESTS

Immunohistochemistry

- Cytokeratin may rarely be necessary to demonstrate squamous epithelium in ruptured or calcified/ossified lesion
- Immunostain with germ cell markers (CD117, Oct3/4, Podoplanin[D2-40]) to rule out presence of ITGCN

Cytogenetics

- Isochromosome 12p abnormality is absent

DIFFERENTIAL DIAGNOSIS

Mature Cystic Teratoma

- Presence of other teratomatous components and presence of ITGCN
- Uninvolved testis shows pronounced widespread atrophy or "dysgenetic features"
- No lipogranulomatous reaction

DIAGNOSTIC CHECKLIST

Clinically Relevant Pathologic Features

- Meticulous sampling and evaluation of background testis to rule out ITGCN or other germ cell tumor component

Pathologic Interpretation Pearls

- Benign, mature, squamous-lined cyst with granular cell layer and keratin material; without (epidermoid cyst) and with skin adnexal structures (dermoid cyst)

SELECTED REFERENCES

1. Ulbright TM: The most common, clinically significant misdiagnoses in testicular tumor pathology, and how to avoid them. Adv Anat Pathol. 15(1):18-27, 2008
2. Ulbright TM et al: Dermoid cyst of the testis: a study of five postpubertal cases, including a pilomatrixoma-like variant, with evidence supporting its separate classification from mature testicular teratoma. Am J Surg Pathol. 25(6):788-93, 2001
3. Garrett JE et al: Cystic testicular lesions in the pediatric population. J Urol. 163(3):928-36, 2000
4. Simmonds PD et al: Primary pure teratoma of the testis. J Urol. 155(3):939-42, 1996
5. Leibovitch I et al: Adult primary pure teratoma of the testis. The Indiana experience. Cancer. 75(9):2244-50, 1995

EPIDERMOID AND DERMOID CYSTS

Gross and Microscopic Features

(Left) This well-defined unilocular cyst ➡ bulging from the testicular surface is a testicular epidermoid cyst. The inner surface is smooth and lacks a solid component. The background testis is unremarkable. *(Right)* This gross photograph shows a large, well-circumscribed testicular dermoid cyst ➡ with a collection of granular, chalky keratin, and sebaceous material. The surrounding testicular parenchyma is unremarkable.

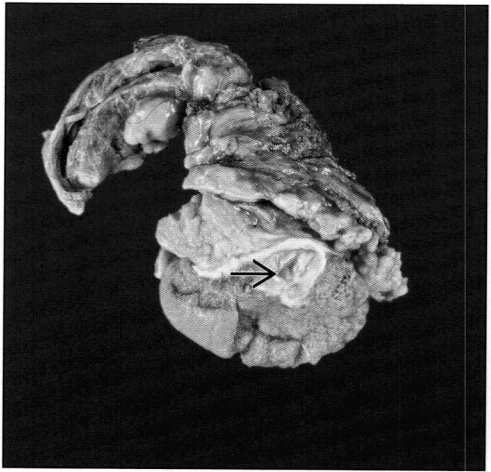
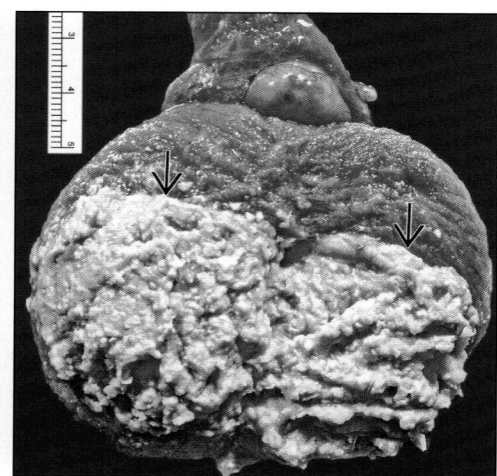

(Left) A testicular epidermoid cyst is composed of a unilocular cystic structure lined by keratinizing squamous epithelium and keratin debris. Note that there are no skin adnexal structures. ITGCN is not present in the surrounding testicular parenchyma. *(Right)* This epidermoid cyst shows that a part of cyst wall is lined by mature squamous epithelium with a granular cell layer ➡. There is laminated keratinous material on the luminal surface. No skin adnexal structures are seen.

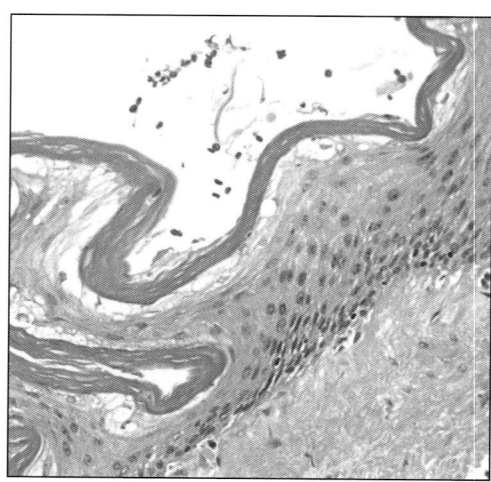
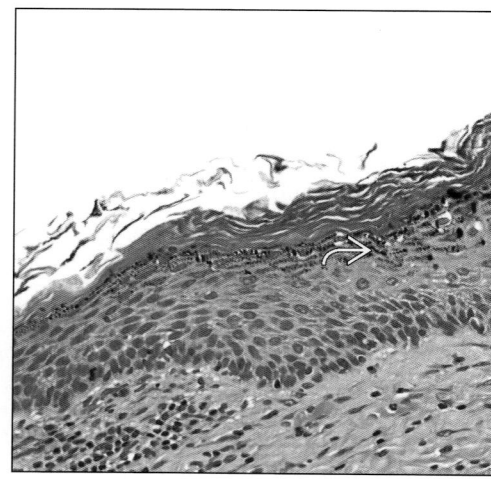

(Left) Low-power photomicrograph of dermoid cyst shows the interface of cyst wall and testicular parenchyma. Rare adnexal structures were present (not shown). The background testis ➡ lacks ITGCN. *(Right)* This dermoid cyst shows well-organized keratinizing squamous epithelium, pilosebaceous units, and adipose tissue. Ciliated epithelium or cartilage may be present, but these elements must maintain an organoid pattern. Haphazard presence of these structures indicates a mature teratoma.

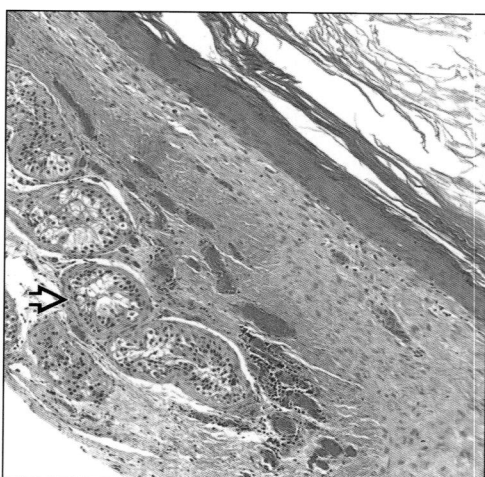
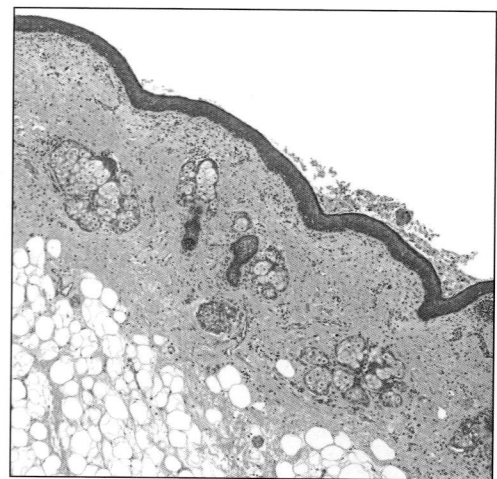

EPIDERMOID AND DERMOID CYSTS

Microscopic Features

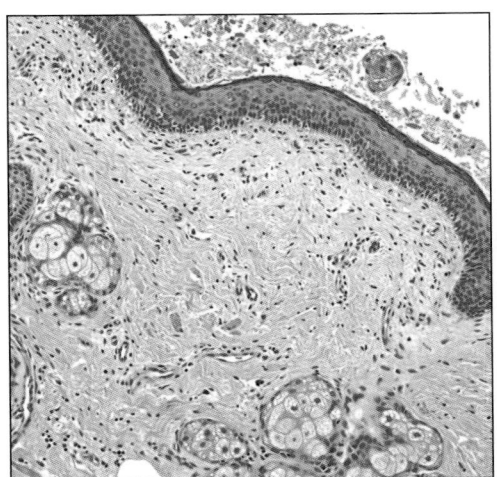 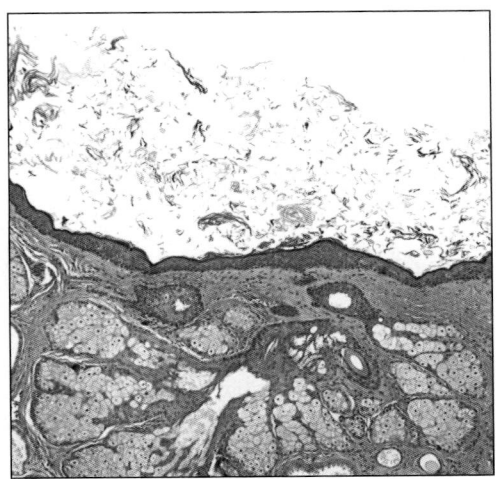

(Left) Dermoid cyst is lined by keratinizing squamous epithelium and contains keratin debris in the lumen. The cyst wall contains sebaceous glands and fibrous tissue. In the adjacent seminiferous tubules, there was no ITGCN. *(Right)* This example of dermoid cyst shows extensive but organoid pilosebaceous units in the fibrotic cystic wall. Grossly, this lesion had grumous "cheesy" material within the cyst corresponding to the keratin material.

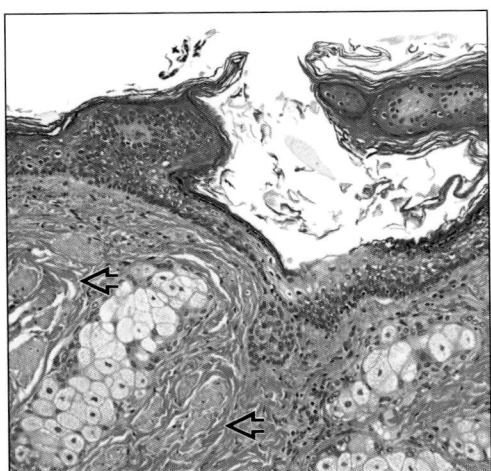 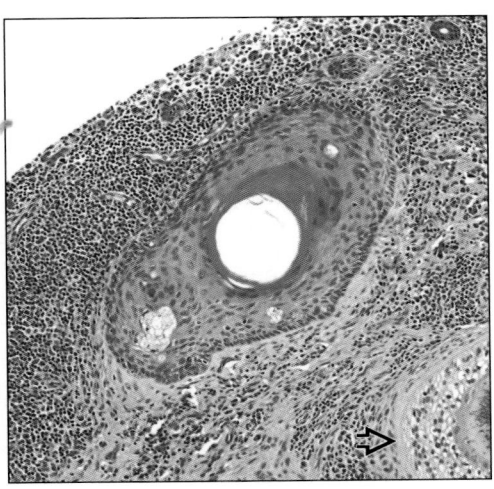

(Left) The squamous epithelium of dermoid cysts may be variably hyperplastic with scattered granular layer. In the cyst wall, there are skin adnexal structures and smooth muscle bundles ⊵. *(Right)* A dermoid cyst is shown in which the lining epithelium is denuded and associated with extensive chronic inflammation and granulation tissue. The diagnosis of dermoid cyst is tenable due to the presence of adnexal structures in the cyst wall with a pilosebaceous unit ⊵.

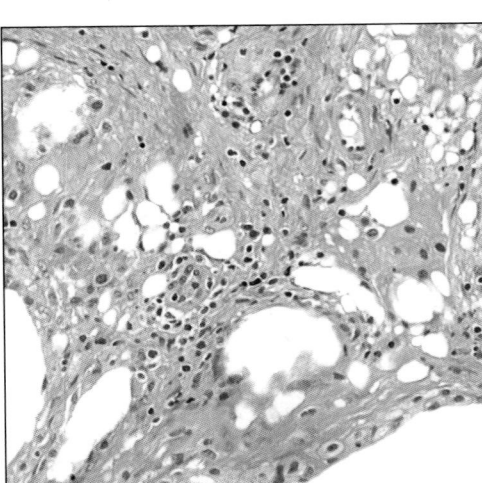 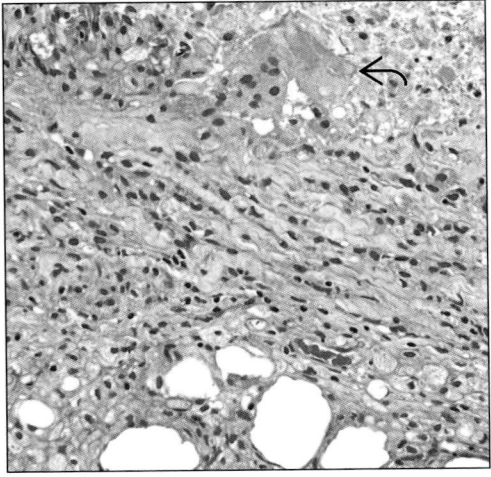

(Left) This dermoid cyst shows florid lipogranulomatous reaction adjacent to the cyst wall. In other sections, giant cells containing keratinous debris are present (not shown). Lipogranulomatous reaction is usually not seen in teratomatous lesions. *(Right)* This dermoid cyst required multiple sections to identify keratin debris ⊵ within a lipogranulomatous reaction as well as rare adnexal structures (not shown). Lipogranulomatous reaction is a characteristic finding in dermoid cysts.

MIXED GERM CELL TUMORS

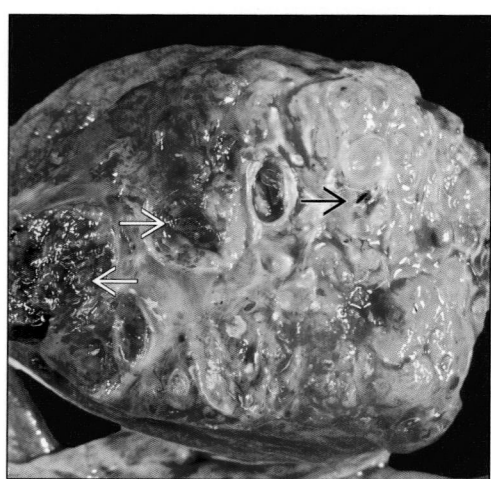

Large MGCT with a variegated cut surface replaces the testicular parenchyma. The tumor is predominantly teratoma ➡; other areas are solid, hemorrhagic, and necrotic EC and YST components ➡.

A MGCT composed of variable germ cell tumor components includes mature teratoma (including cartilage, bone, and squamous nest ➡), immature teratoma ➡, EC ➡, and YST ➡.

TERMINOLOGY

Abbreviations
- Mixed germ cell tumor (MGCT), mixed nonseminomatous germ cell tumor (MNSGCT)

Synonyms
- Mixed nonseminomatous germ cell tumor

Definitions
- Germ cell tumor composed of > 1 histologic type of germ cell tumor, including seminoma

CLINICAL ISSUES

Epidemiology
- Incidence
  ○ 2nd most common germ cell tumor after seminoma
  ○ Accounts for 30-40% of all testicular germ cell tumors
- Age
  ○ Range: 20-40 years (10 years younger than seminoma)
  ○ Rarely seen in prepubertal children and older adults (> 50 years)

Presentation
- Testicular mass or swelling ± pain

Treatment
- Similar to pure nonseminomatous germ cell tumor and depends on clinical stage
- Radical inguinal orchiectomy ± retroperitoneal lymph node dissection or adjuvant therapy

Prognosis
- Depends on clinical stage, proportion of embryonal carcinoma (unfavorable) and mature teratoma (favorable) component, and lymphovascular invasion
- Cure rate > 95% for stage I and stage II disease
- Cure rate approximately 70-85% for stage III disease

IMAGE FINDINGS

Radiographic Findings
- Heterogeneous testicular mass on ultrasound examination
- May be accompanied by retroperitoneal lymph node enlargement

MACROSCOPIC FEATURES

General Features
- Variegated cystic and solid mass with hemorrhage and necrosis
- Seminomatous germ cell component with solid white and gray areas
- Nonseminomatous component with granular and firm areas with hemorrhage, necrosis, and cystic areas
- Teratoma with bone, cartilage, and skin elements

Sections to Be Submitted
- Multiple sections of different areas of tumor and at least 1 section per cm tumor
- Should include necrotic and hemorrhagic areas

Size
- Variable, often large bulky mass

MICROSCOPIC PATHOLOGY

Histologic Features
- Variable combination and percentage of all germ cell tumor components
- Embryonal carcinoma (EC) and teratoma (T) are most common (26%)
- Other combinations include
  ○ EC and seminoma (S) (16%)
  ○ EC, yolk sac tumor (YST), and T (11%)

MIXED GERM CELL TUMORS

Key Facts

Terminology
- Germ cell tumor composed of > 1 histologic type of germ cell tumor, including seminoma

Clinical Issues
- Accounts for 30-40% of all testicular germ cell tumors
- Depends on clinical stage, proportion of embryonal carcinoma component, and lymphovascular invasion

Macroscopic Features
- Variegated cystic and solid mass with hemorrhage and necrosis

Microscopic Pathology
- Variable combination and percentage of all germ cell tumor components
- Embryonal carcinoma (EC) and teratoma (T) are most common (26%)

- Other combinations include teratoma and EC, teratoma with EC and yolk sac tumor (YST)
- Areas of necrosis and hemorrhage are common
- Rare special variants include polyembryoma and diffuse embryoma

Ancillary Tests
- Immunoprofile reflects histologic component of different germ cell tumors
- 1st-line germ cell markers: Oct3/4, CD30(BerH2), PLAP, cytokeratin

Top Differential Diagnoses
- Pure germ cell tumor, such as EC, YST, or teratoma, and metastatic carcinoma

---

- o EC, T, and choriocarcinoma (CC) (7%)
- o EC, T, and S (6%)
- o T and S (6%)
- o EC and YST (4%)
- o EC and CC (4%)
- o Other combinations may occur (16%)
- Areas of necrosis and hemorrhage are common
- Rare variants include polyembryoma and diffuse embryoma
  - o Polyembryoma is composed of entirely or predominantly embryoid bodies with embryonic disc, yolk sac, and surrounded by myxoid stroma
  - o Diffuse embryoma is characterized by intimately admixture of EC and YST with YST wrapping around EC component

Cytologic Features
- Reflects histologic composition of each component

Predominant Pattern/Injury Type
- Neoplastic

Predominant Cell/Compartment Type
- > 1 type of germ cell tumor component

ANCILLARY TESTS

Immunohistochemistry
- Immunoprofile reflects histologic component of different germ cell tumors
- 1st-line germ cell markers: Oct3/4, PLAP, Podoplanin(D2-40), CD30(BerH2), α-fetoprotein, HCG, cytokeratin
- Other germ cell markers: CD117, glypican-3, SALL4, NANOG

DIFFERENTIAL DIAGNOSIS

Pure Germ Cell Tumor
- Such as embryonal carcinoma, yolk sac tumor, or teratoma

- Multiple sections are required to demonstrate different germ cell tumor components

Metastatic Carcinoma
- Old age, history, and bilaterality
- Interstitial pattern is frequently seen in metastatic carcinoma
- Positive for EMA/MUC1; negative for germ cell tumor markers

DIAGNOSTIC CHECKLIST

Pathologic Interpretation Pearls
- Mixture of different histologic components of germ cell neoplasm

REPORTING CONSIDERATIONS

Key Elements to Report
- Specific histologic types and percentage of each component
- Lymphovascular invasion
- Involvement of rete testis, epididymis, spermatic cord, and tunica
- Pathology of uninvolved testicular parenchyma

SELECTED REFERENCES

1. Berney DM et al: Malignant germ cell tumours in the elderly: a histopathological review of 50 cases in men aged 60 years or over. Mod Pathol. 21(1):54-9, 2008
2. Mosharafa AA et al: Histology in mixed germ cell tumors. Is there a favorite pairing? J Urol. 171(4):1471-3, 2004
3. Sesterhenn IA et al: Pathology of germ cell tumors of the testis. Cancer Control. 11(6):374-87, 2004
4. Ayala AG et al: Testicular tumors: clinically relevant histological findings. Semin Urol Oncol. 16(2):72-81, 1998

MIXED GERM CELL TUMORS

Gross and Microscopic Features

(Left) MGCT usually shows an irregular mass with variegated cut surface. Creamy gray lobulated areas suggest seminoma ➡, mucoid areas suggest teratoma ➡, and hemorrhagic brown areas suggest EC ➡. Gross appearances are not absolutely specific for histologic subtype. *(Right)* MGCT with typical variegated cut surface is shown. The cystic mucoid areas represent mature teratoma ➡, the tan fleshy area represents seminoma ➡, and hemorrhagic and necrotic areas represent EC ➡.

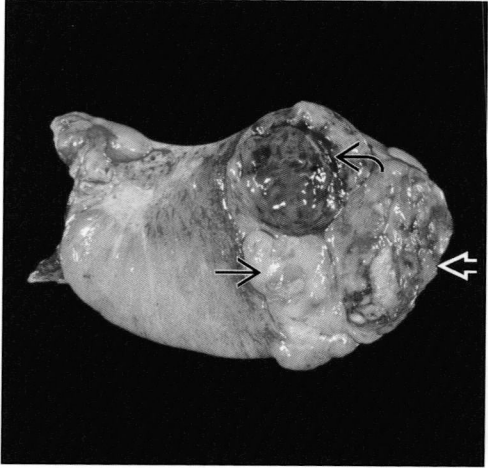
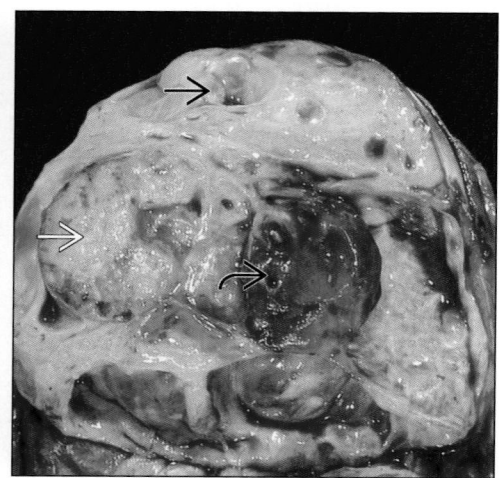

(Left) This MGCT is composed of cystic and solid areas with hemorrhage and extensive necrosis. There is a gelatinous cystic area of teratoma component ➡, and the hemorrhagic and necrotic areas were EC and EST components on microscopy. *(Right)* Teratomatous component of a MGCT includes cartilage, bone, and immature cellular spindle mesenchymal tissue ➡. Focal glandular epithelium ➡ is also present. In other areas (not shown), EC and YST components were present.

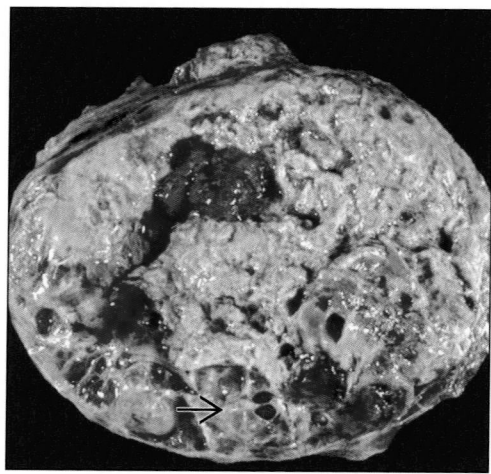
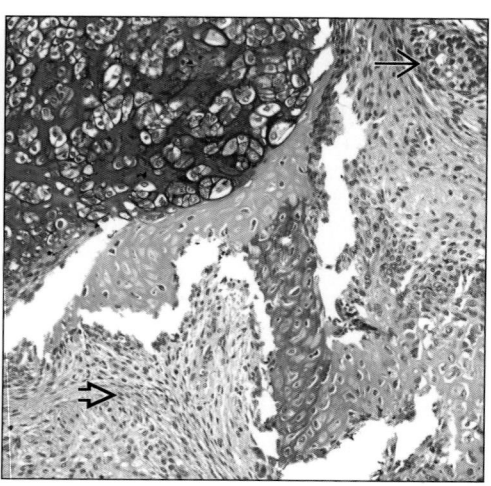

(Left) MGCT shows glandular embryonal carcinoma component and myxoid areas of more bland-appearing yolk sac tumor elements characterized by spindled cells with low nuclear grade. This component is often underdiagnosed. *(Right)* Image of MGCT shows intimate admixture of papillary and glandular histology of EC ➡ and microcystic or reticular morphology of YST ➡. This is 1 of the most common combinations of MGCT. Immunostaining is rarely necessary in such settings.

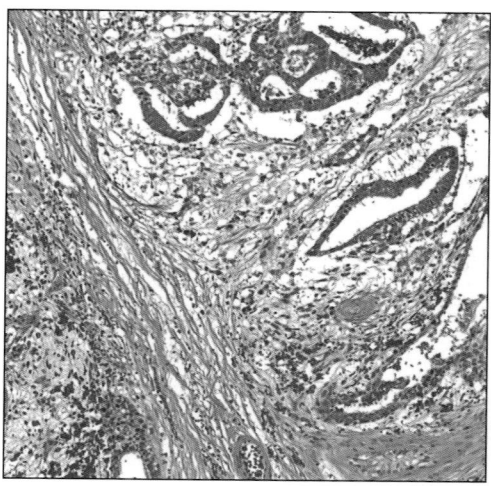
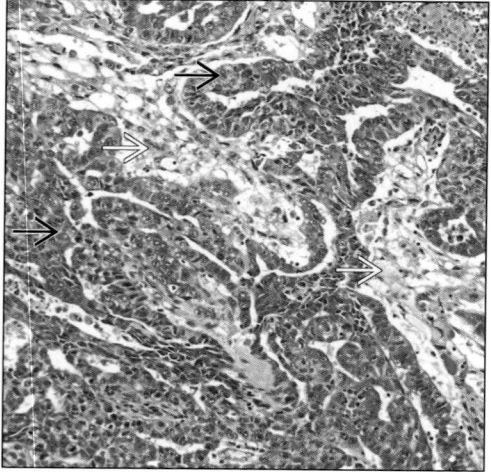

4

Microscopic Features

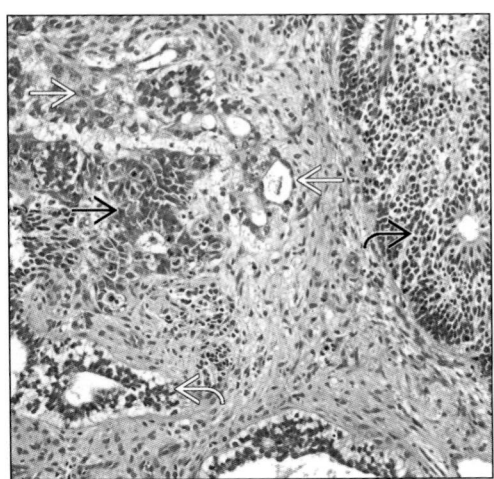
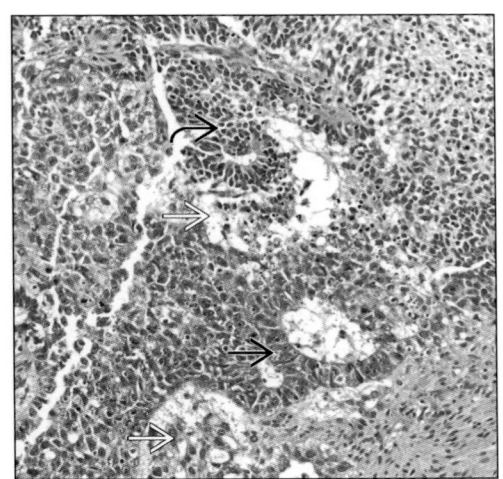

(Left) This area of MGCT has a variety of germ cell tumor components, including EC with cohesive pleomorphic cells ⮕, reticular pattern of YST with bland-appearing cuboidal to flattened cells ⮕, teratomatous glands ⮕, and primitive neuroepithelial tissue ⮕. *(Right)* MGCT shows components of glandular EC with cohesive, pleomorphic cells and nuclear overlapping ⮕, microcystic and reticular YST ⮕, and immature neuroepithelial tissue with neurotubule formation ⮕.

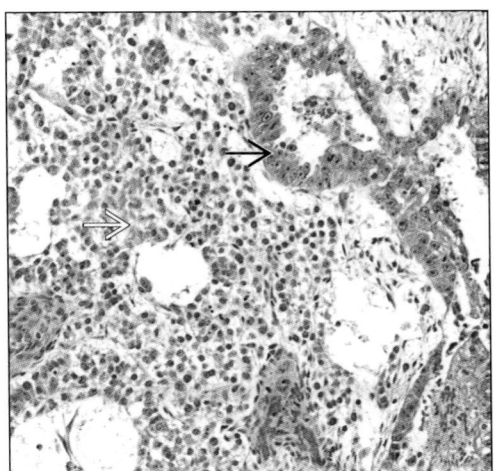
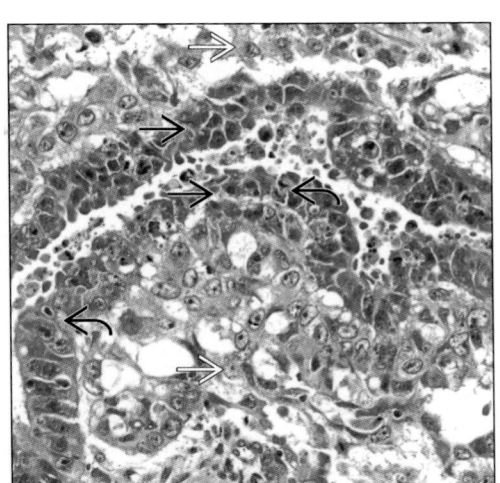

(Left) MGCT with EC and YST is shown. Glandular EC component ⮕ with markedly atypical cells contrasts with solid and cystic YST component composed of relatively bland-appearing nuclei with pale cytoplasm and ill-defined cell boundaries ⮕. *(Right)* High-power photomicrograph shows a MGCT with a so-called double-layered EC ⮕ with cohesive, pleomorphic cells, numerous mitoses, and apoptosis ⮕. Microcystic and reticular patterns of YST ⮕ surround EC.

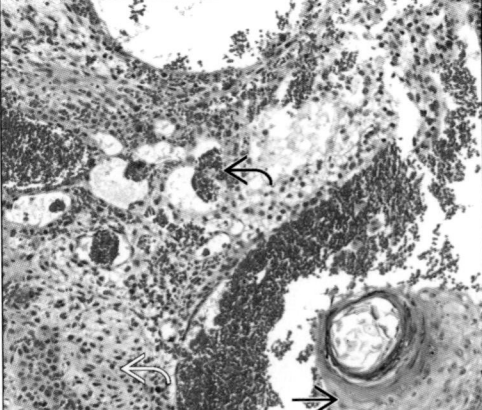
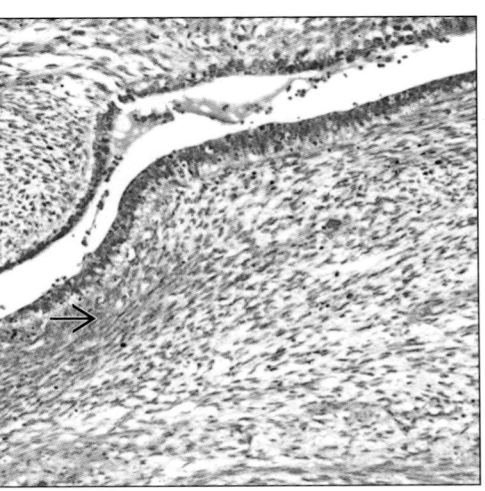

(Left) This MGCT shows microcystic ⮕ and solid YST ⮕, admixed with mature teratoma with keratinizing squamous epithelial nests ⮕. The tumor cells of YST are sometimes deceptively bland and are frequently underdiagnosed. *(Right)* This image shows teratomatous component of MGCT with immature stratified glandular epithelium and surrounded by immature cellular spindled mesenchymal tissue ⮕. In other areas (not shown), EC and YST components were also present.

MIXED GERM CELL TUMORS

Microscopic Features

(Left) A MGCT composed of EC ⇨ and seminoma ⇨ is shown. The 2 tumor types are contrasted from one another by the marked nuclear atypia and hyperchromasia of EC vs. the more monotonous appearance of seminoma. *(Right)* High-power photomicrograph of MGCT shows EC ⇨ admixed with seminoma ⇨. Seminoma cells are evenly spaced with abundant clear cytoplasm. EC cells are more cohesive with overlapping nuclei and marked nuclear pleomorphism.

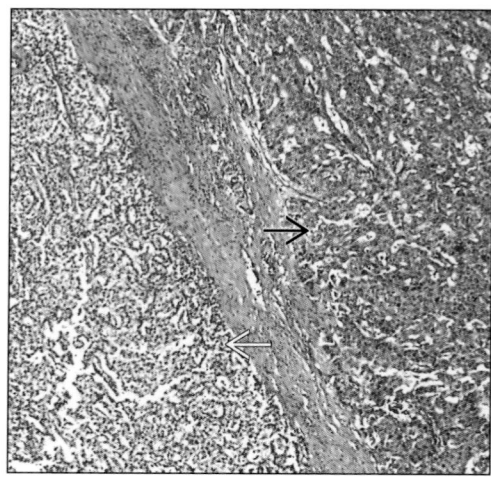
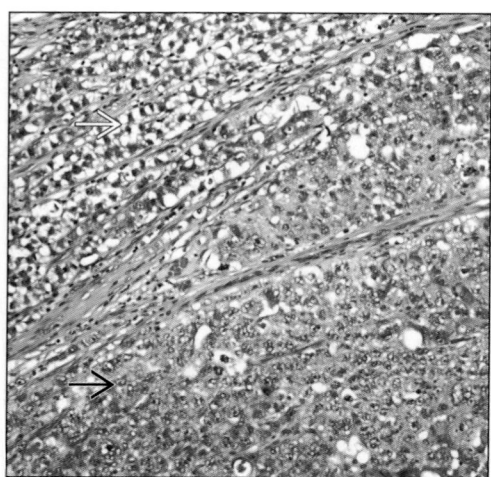

(Left) MGCT is composed of reticular pattern of YST ⇨, cellular spindled mesenchymal tissue of immature teratoma ⇨, and mature squamous epithelial tissue ⇨ (teratoma). This histologic combination accounts for approximately 10% of MGCT. *(Right)* This area of MGCT shows YST ⇨ with scattered syncytiotrophoblastic giant cells ⇨ and hemorrhage. The levels of serum hCG and α-fetoprotein are often good indicators of the different germ cell tumor components that may be present.

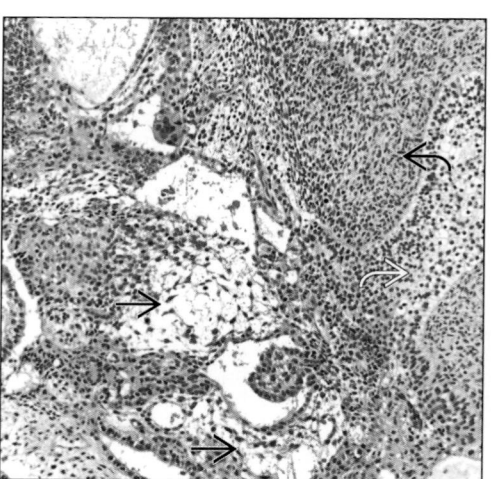
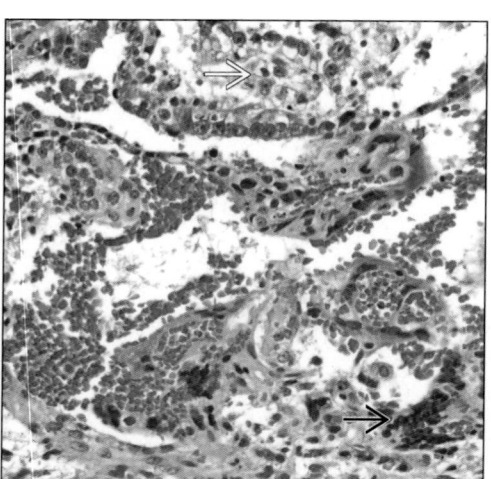

(Left) This MGCT shows a significant choriocarcinomatous component characterized by cytotrophoblasts ⇨ with clear cytoplasm surrounded by a layer of multinucleated syncytiotrophoblasts ⇨. Hemorrhage and necrosis ⇨ are present. *(Right)* MGCT with vascular-lymphatic invasion is shown. Nests of EC tumor cells are attached to the vascular wall and conform to the shape of the spaces. Vascular invasion status is a significant prognostic factor and determinant of pathologic stage.

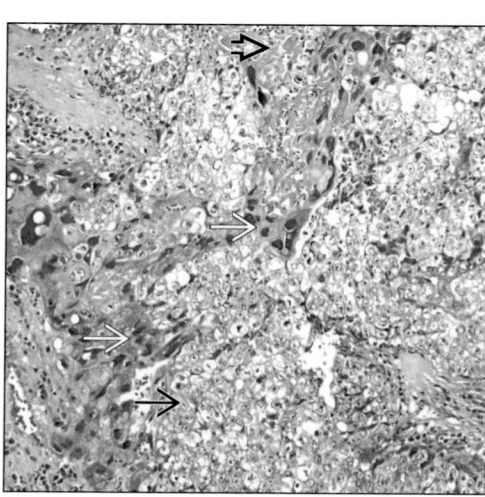
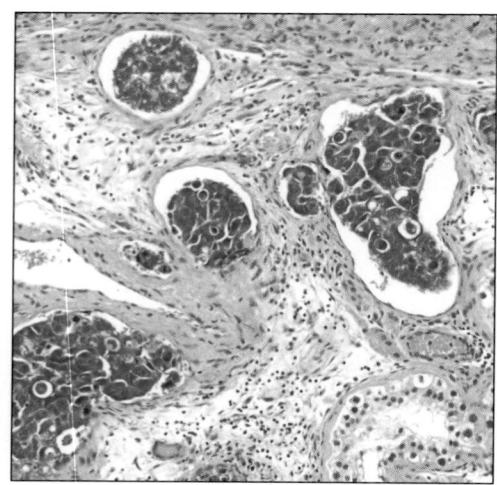

MIXED GERM CELL TUMORS

Microscopic and Immunohistochemical Features

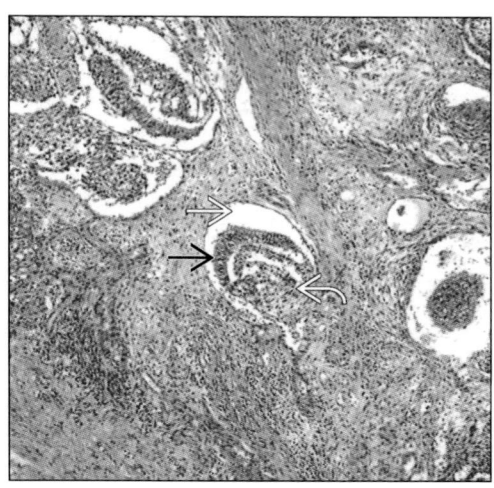
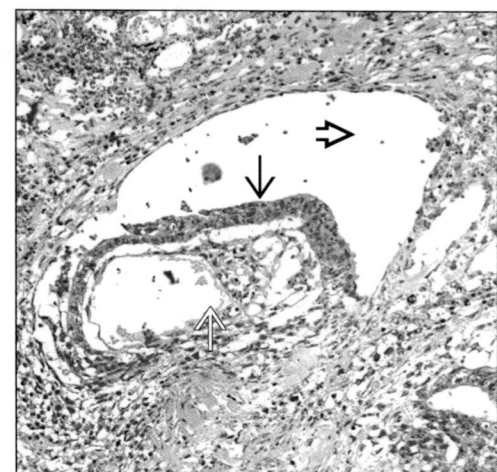

(Left) Polyembryoma, a special type of MGCT, is composed exclusively or predominantly of embryoid bodies in a myxoid stroma. The embryoid body is characterized by a central embryonic disc ➡, amniotic sac ➡, and yolk sac ➡. *(Right)* High-power photograph of an embryoid body is shown. The central embryonic disc is composed of primitive atypical cells of EC ➡, an amniotic-like cavity ➡, and a yolk sac component with microcystic and reticular patterns ➡.

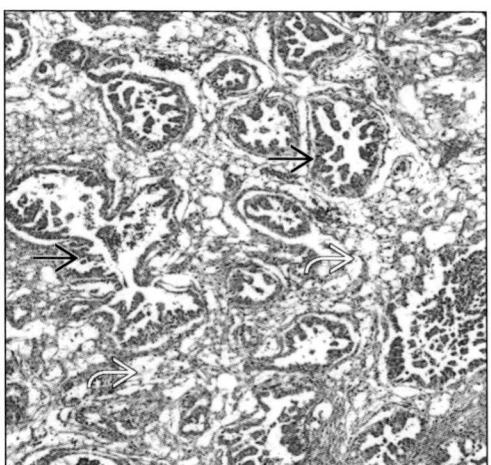
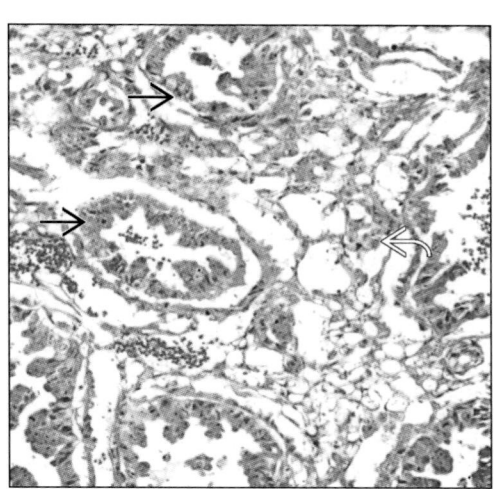

(Left) Diffuse embryoma, the other special MGCT type, is composed of equal amounts of papillary EC ➡ and microcystic and reticular patterns of YST ➡. The EC component exhibits complex papillary infolding with a stellate lumen. *(Right)* Diffuse embryoma exhibits close proximity of EC ➡ and YST ➡ components in a specialized arrangement. This tumor shows a diffuse, orderly admixture of circular patterns of atypical EC component surrounded by relatively bland YST component.

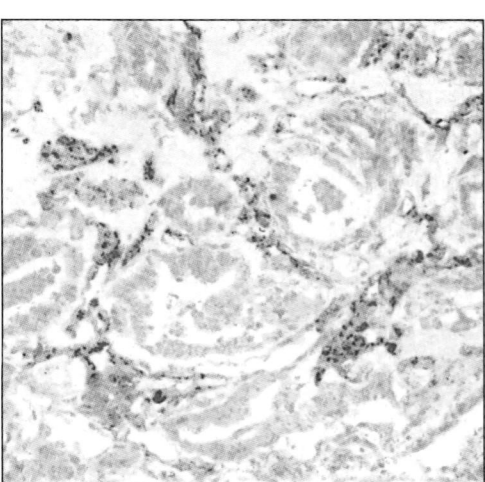
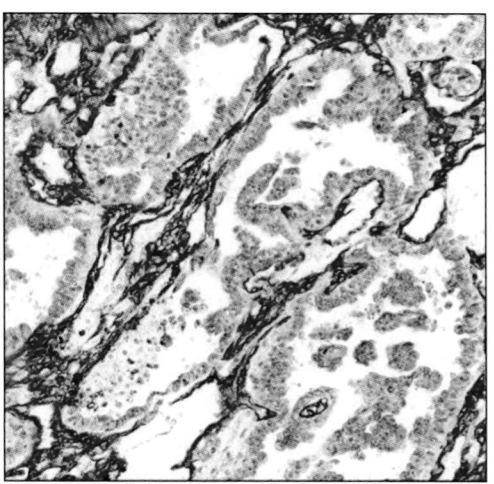

(Left) Positive α-fetoprotein immunoreactivity highlights the YST component of a diffuse embryoma. The EC component is negative. *(Right)* Cytokeratin immunostain shows strong immunoreactivity for YST but significantly weaker staining in EC (differential staining pattern). Immunohistochemistry is usually not necessary for the histologic diagnosis of germ cell tumors; however, it may be useful in situations when there is ambiguous histology or work-up for a metastasis.

SPERMATOCYTIC SEMINOMA

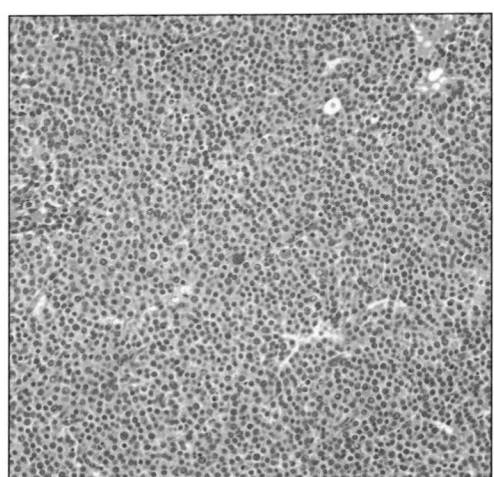

Low-power view of diffuse growth pattern of spermatocytic seminoma reveals no fibrovascular septae and no lymphocytic or granulomatous inflammation, typical features of classic seminoma.

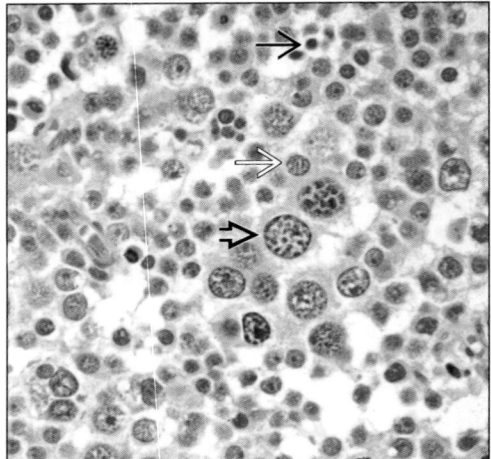

This high-power photomicrograph shows the characteristic 3 cell types in SS: Small lymphocyte-like cells ⇛ with darkly stained nuclei, intermediate ⇒ and giant cells with "spireme-type" chromatin ⇟.

TERMINOLOGY

Abbreviations
- Spermatocytic seminoma (SS)

Definitions
- Germ cell tumor recapitulating spermatogenic sequence composed of 3 cell types of variable sizes, ranging from 6-100 μm

ETIOLOGY/PATHOGENESIS

Cytogenetic Changes
- Diploid or near hypodiploid, different from that of seminoma
- Chromosomal numerical changes (most commonly gain of chromosome 9)

CLINICAL ISSUES

Epidemiology
- Incidence
  - Extremely rare; only 2 major series reported
  - Bilaterality (up to 9%) is more common than in seminoma
  - Occurs only in testis; no ovarian counterpart, no extragonadal primary tumors
  - No race predilection as in other germ cell tumors
  - Not associated with cryptorchidism
- Age
  - Range: 25-87 years (average: 53.6 years)
  - Rare under 30 years

Presentation
- Painless testicular swelling and mass
- Serum tumor markers are not elevated

Treatment
- Radical inguinal orchiectomy alone is curative

- Postoperative prophylactic radiation or chemotherapy do not offer additional benefit and not routinely recommended

Prognosis
- Excellent prognosis with rare malignant behavior (less than 1%)
- Sarcomatoid transformation is rare, but when present is associated with distant metastasis and death

MACROSCOPIC FEATURES

General Features
- Well-circumscribed, soft mass with mucoid or gelatinous bulging cut surface
- Lobulation, cystic change, and focal hemorrhage or necrosis may be seen

Size
- Range: 2-20 cm (average: 7.0 cm)

MICROSCOPIC PATHOLOGY

Histologic Features
- Diffuse or solid sheet-like pattern with scant fibrous or edematous stroma is most common finding
- Other rarer patterns include pseudoglandular, microcystic, trabeculae, nests, or single cells
- Polymorphous cell population with 3 distinct cell types is hallmark of spermatocytic seminoma
  - Small lymphocyte-like cells: 6- 8 μm; densely hyperchromatic nuclei and scant amount of eosinophilic to basophilic cytoplasm
  - Intermediate cells: 15-20 μm; most common cell type; round nuclei, finely granular chromatin, moderate amount of cytoplasm
  - Giant cells: 50-100 μm; least common cell type; distinctive filamentous or "spireme-type" chromatin

SPERMATOCYTIC SEMINOMA

Key Facts

Terminology
- Germ cell tumor composed of 3 cell types of variable sizes ranging from 6-100 μm

Clinical Issues
- Extremely rare
- Age range: 25-87 years

Macroscopic Features
- Well-circumscribed, soft, friable, tan-gray mass with mucoid or gelatinous, bulging cut surface

Microscopic Pathology
- Diffuse or solid sheet pattern with scant fibrous or edematous stroma is most common finding
- Rare growth patterns include pseudoglandular, microcystic, trabeculae, nests, or single cells

- Polymorphous cell population is hallmark of spermatocytic seminoma
- Small lymphocyte-like cells: 6-8 μm; densely hyperchromatic nuclei and scant amount of eosinophilic to basophilic cytoplasm
- Intermediate cells: 15-20 μm; most common cell type; round nuclei, finely granular chromatin, moderate amount of cytoplasm
- Giant cells: 50-100 μm; least common cell type; distinctive filamentous or "spireme-type" chromatin

Ancillary Tests
- Negative for most germ cell-associated markers (Oct3/4, Podoplanin(D2-40), PLAP, α-fetoprotein, glypican-3, HCG, and CD30[BerH2])

- Lack cytoplasmic glycogen, fibrovascular septae, lymphoplasmacytic infiltrate, or granulomatous inflammation
- Intratubular growth of spermatocytic seminoma is rarely seen and is characterized by large, highly atypical cells expanding tubules
- Tumor typically lacks association with intratubular germ cell neoplasia (ITGCN)
- Anaplastic spermatocytic seminoma is characterized by predominantly monomorphous intermediate-sized cells with prominent nucleoli (significance of designation as anaplastic is debated)
- Sarcomatous transformation may rarely occur (6%) in spermatocytic seminoma
  - Characterized by undifferentiated primitive spindle cell sarcoma associated SS; rhabdomyoblastic differentiation has been reported

Cytologic Features
- 3 distinct cell types with small, intermediate, and giant cells

ANCILLARY TESTS

Histochemistry
- PAS-diastase
  - Reactivity: Negative

Immunohistochemistry
- Negative for most germ cell-associated markers (PLAP, α-fetoprotein, Oct3/4, HCG, Podoplanin(D2-40), glypican-3, and CD30[BerH2])
- Negative for cytokeratin and vimentin
- May be positive for SALL4 and CD117

DIFFERENTIAL DIAGNOSIS

Classic Seminoma
- Relatively monotonous cell population
- Fibrovascular septa, lymphoplasmacytic and granulomatous inflammation

- Positive for germ cell-associated markers (Oct3/4, PLAP, Podoplanin(D2-40), CD117, SALL4)

Embryonal Carcinoma (Solid Pattern)
- Greater extent of cytologic anaplasia
- Variation of growth patterns with solid, glandular, and papillary growth
- Positive for cytokeratin and germ cell-associated markers (Oct3/4, Podoplanin(D2-40), PLAP, SALL4, and CD30[BerH2])

Malignant Lymphoma
- Typical interstitial growth pattern
- Lack of 3 distinct cell types and giant cells
- Positive for CD45(LCA), and CD20 or CD3, as appropriate

DIAGNOSTIC CHECKLIST

Pathologic Interpretation Pearls
- Polymorphous cell population with 3 distinct cell types, including small lymphocytic, intermediate, and large giant cells
- Lack of fibrovascular septa and lymphoplasmacytic infiltrates or granulomas

SELECTED REFERENCES

1. Bahrami A et al: An overview of testicular germ cell tumors. Arch Pathol Lab Med. 131(8):1267-80, 2007
2. Bomeisl PE et al: Spermatocytic seminoma. J Urol. 177(2):734, 2007
3. Chung PW et al: Spermatocytic seminoma: a review. Eur Urol. 45(4):495-8, 2004
4. Verdorfer I et al: Molecular cytogenetic analysis of human spermatocytic seminomas. J Pathol. 204(3):277-81, 2004
5. Albores-Saavedra J et al: Anaplastic variant of spermatocytic seminoma. Hum Pathol. 27(7):650-5, 1996
6. Eble JN: Spermatocytic seminoma. Hum Pathol. 25(10):1035-42, 1994

SPERMATOCYTIC SEMINOMA

Gross and Microscopic Features

(Left) SS has a bulging, nodular, soft, tan-gray, mucoid cut surface. Classic seminoma, spermatocytic seminoma, and lymphoma may have a similar gross appearance, but they differ in age, frequency of bilaterality, and spermatic cord involvement. *(Right)* Low-power photomicrograph of SS shows cystic spaces due to accumulation of edema fluid and lack of stroma. The edematous fluid and lack of cell cohesion are helpful features of this tumor in making the distinction from seminoma.

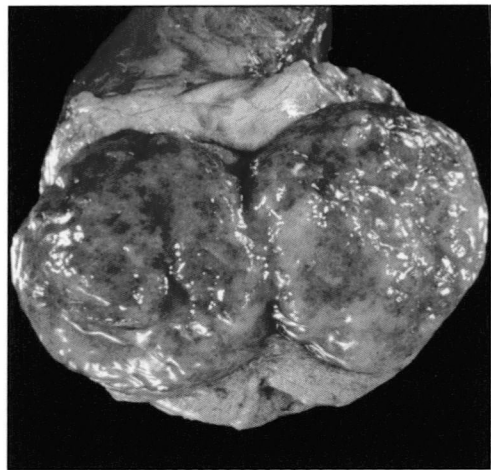
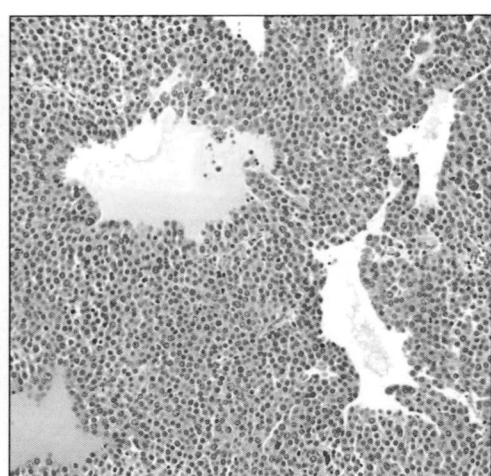

(Left) Cellular polymorphism is the hallmark of SS. The most common cell type is the intermediate-sized cell. There are few small cells ⇨ and giant cells ⇨ in this example. Mitoses ⇨ may be brisk in some cases. *(Right)* This photomicrograph shows the cytologic features of the 3 cell types in SS: Small lymphocyte-like cells ⇨, intermediate ⇨ and giant cells ⇨. Mitoses ⇨ are also seen. This degree of cellular polymorphism would be most unusual in classic seminoma.

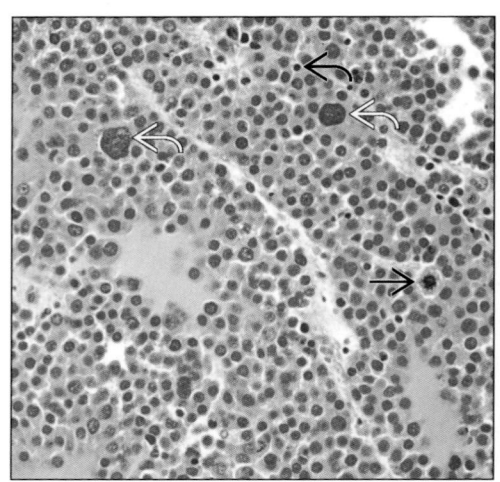
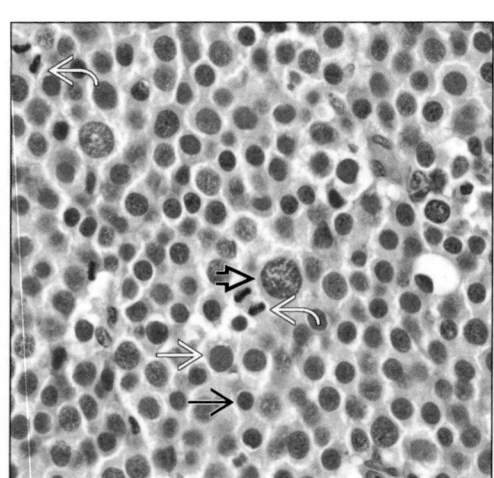

(Left) SS with extensive intercellular edema is shown. This results in a cystic and mucoid gross appearance. This pseudoglandular or cystic histology raises the possibility of other testicular tumors. *(Right)* Occasional fibrous bands separate diffuse sheets of SS into lobules. There are no lymphocytic infiltrates or granulomas, features that are different from classic seminoma. The tumor cells do not show distinct cell boundaries and lack abundant clear cytoplasm.

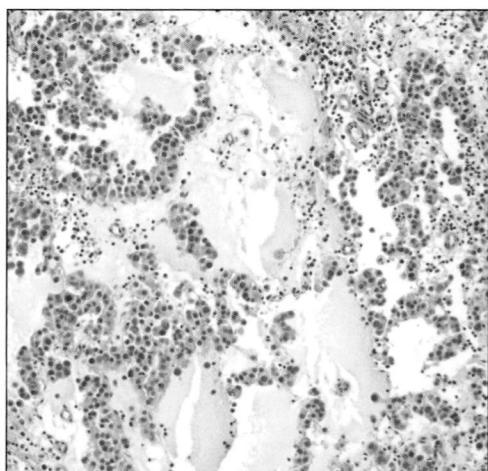
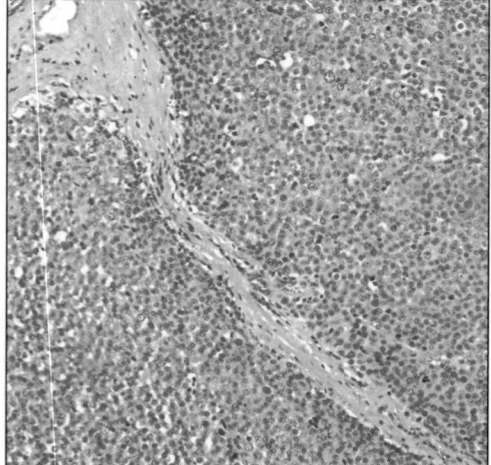

Microscopic Features

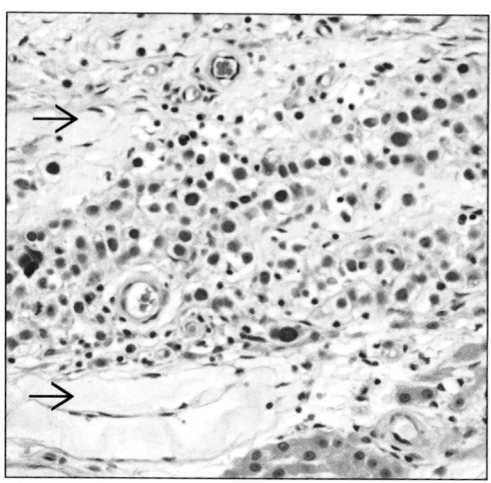
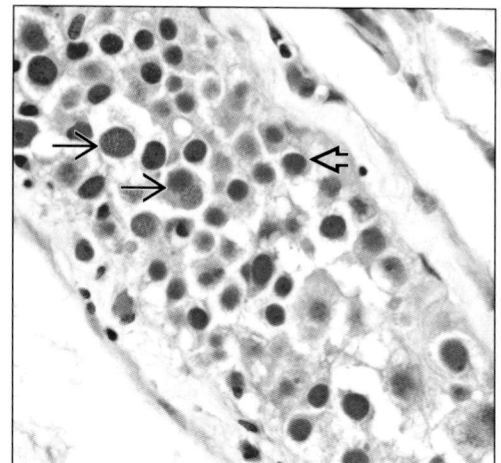

(Left) At the periphery of SS, an interstitial pattern between seminiferous tubules ➡ may be seen. Lymphocytic infiltrate, a feature seen in early invasive seminoma, is not present. *(Right)* Intratubular SS is characterized by a polymorphic cell population with large atypical cells ➡ filling the lumen of a seminiferous tubule with few preserved germ cells ➡. This pattern is different from that of ITGCN in which neoplastic cells are typically located at the periphery.

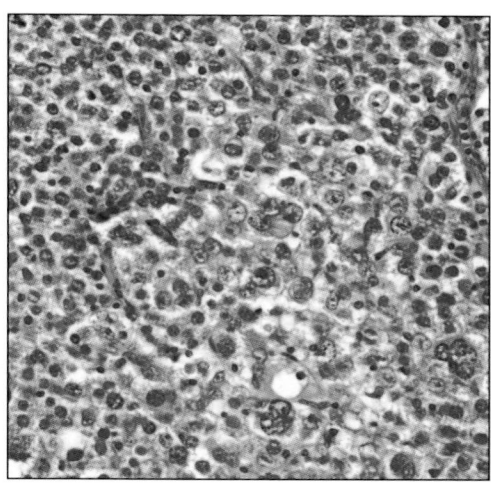
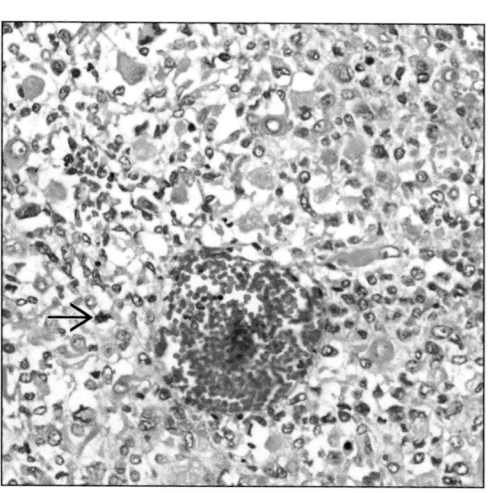

(Left) So-called anaplastic SS is characterized by proliferation of predominantly intermediate cells with coarse chromatin and prominent nucleoli. Embryonal carcinoma and classic seminoma are the main differential diagnoses raised by this histology. *(Right)* This is an example of rhabdomyoblastic sarcomatous transformation of SS. There is a proliferation of atypical spindle cells with abundant pink cytoplasm and frequent mitoses ➡. In other areas, a classic SS histology was seen.

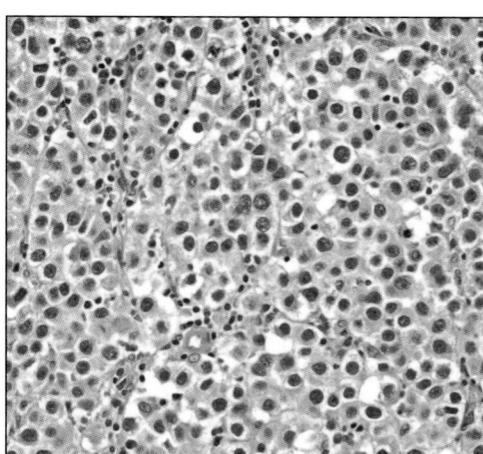
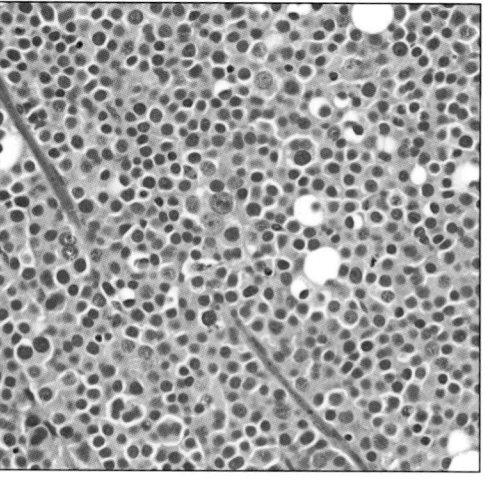

(Left) Classic seminoma, as in this picture, is the major differential diagnosis of SS. In addition to the fibrovascular septae with small lymphocytes, the tumor cells have a uniform monomorphous population and contain eosinophilic and clear cytoplasm, as well as more distinct cell membranes. *(Right)* Compared with classic seminoma, this SS has a polymorphous population of 3 cell types and lacks the features of fibrovascular septa, lymphocytes, and granulomas.

CARCINOID TUMOR

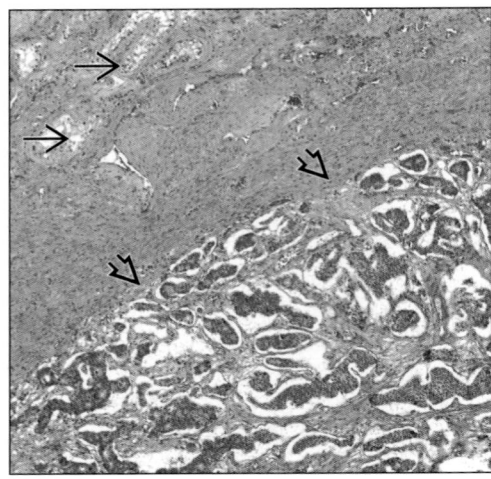

Testicular carcinoid tumor ⇨ shows a well-circumscribed nodule demarcated from the adjacent seminiferous tubules ⇨. The tumor has nested, trabecular, and insular growth patterns.

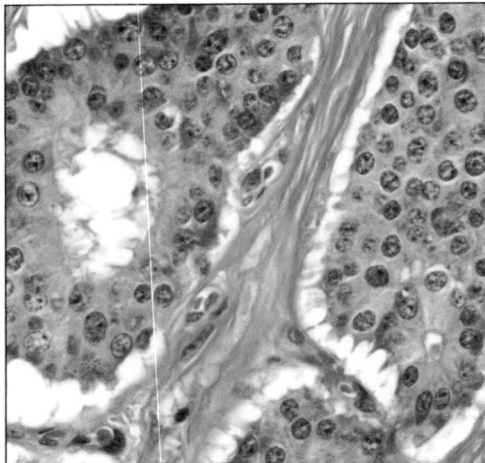

High-power view shows a carcinoid tumor with relatively uniform cells, round to ovoid nuclei, "salt and pepper" chromatin, and abundant eosinophilic and granular cytoplasm.

TERMINOLOGY

Synonyms
- Well-differentiated neuroendocrine carcinoma

Definitions
- Well-differentiated tumor with neuroendocrine differentiation, which may occur as pure tumor, as component associated with teratoma or metastatic to testis

ETIOLOGY/PATHOGENESIS

Pathogenesis
- Considered to be a monodermal form of teratoma

CLINICAL ISSUES

Epidemiology
- Incidence
  - Extremely rare
  - Majority (70%) are pure carcinoid &/or associated with a teratoma (20%)
  - Rare cases of metastatic carcinoid (10%) from lung or gastrointestinal tract have been reported
- Age
  - Range 10-83 years (average: 46 years); primary carcinoid: 44 years; metastasis: 61 years; carcinoid within teratoma: 38 years
  - In general, occurs in older age group than most other types of germ cell tumor

Presentation
- Testicular enlargement ± pain
- Equally distributed in left and right sides
- May be associated with hydrocele (10%)
- Carcinoid syndrome may occur (12%)

Laboratory Tests
- 5-hydroxyindoleacetic acid (5-HIAA) or metabolite of serotonin may be elevated

Treatment
- Surgical approaches
  - Surgical excision is preferred therapy
  - Other therapies (somatostatin analogues, interferon-α) may be used for symptom control
  - Chemotherapy and radiotherapy usually ineffective
  - Receptor-targeted radiotherapy shows encouraging preliminary results

Prognosis
- Prognosis is excellent for patients with localized testicular carcinoid
- Tumor size and presence of carcinoid syndrome correlates with metastatic potential
- Neither tumor necrosis nor local tumor invasion (vascular invasion or tunica invasion, etc.) correlate with adverse prognosis
- Late metastasis may occur, and all patients with carcinoid tumors require long-term follow-up and urine 5-HIAA measurement

IMAGE FINDINGS

General Features
- Well-circumscribed hypervascular mass on ultrasonography
- CT, MR, and nuclear imaging techniques (1-meta-iodobenzylguanidine and somatostatin receptor scintigraphy) are used to exclude metastasis

CARCINOID TUMOR

Key Facts

Terminology
- Well-differentiated tumor of testis with neuroendocrine differentiation

Clinical Issues
- Majority (70%) are pure carcinoid &/or associated with teratoma (20%)
- Testicular enlargement ± pain
- Prognosis is excellent for patients with localized testicular carcinoid

Macroscopic Features
- Pure carcinoid tumors are usually solid, well-circumscribed mass with pale yellow to brown cut surface
- Cystic component usually indicate teratoma

Microscopic Pathology
- Growth patterns: Insular, solid nests, trabecular, or acinar
- Delicate fibrous to hyalinized stroma
- Tumor cells with round nuclei, coarse or "salt and pepper" chromatin
- Usually monotonous tumor cells with occasional large cells
- Abundant eosinophilic, granular cytoplasm
- Teratomatous component may be seen in some cases (25%)

Ancillary Tests
- Positive for cytokeratin, synpatophysin, chromogranin, and CD56

MACROSCOPIC FEATURES

General Features
- Pure carcinoid tumor is usually solid, well-circumscribed mass with pale yellow to brown cut surface
- Cystic component usually indicates associated teratoma

Size
- Variable range from 0.1-11 cm (mean: 3.5 cm) for pure carcinoid tumor
- Carcinoid tumor associated with teratoma is usually smaller than those occurring in pure form

MICROSCOPIC PATHOLOGY

Histologic Features
- Growth patterns: Insular, solid, nests, trabecular, or acinar
- Delicate fibrous to hyalinized stroma
- Predominantly monotonous tumor cells with occasional interspersed larger cells
- Abundant eosinophilic, granular cytoplasm
- Tumor cells with round nuclei, peripheral palisading, inconspicuous nucleoli, and coarse or "salt and pepper" chromatin
- Teratomatous component may be seen in some cases (20%)
- Intratubular germ cell neoplasia (ITGCN) is extraordinarily rare in tumors not associated with teratoma
- Other than tumor size (which has been correlated with malignant outcome), there are no other reliable histologic features predictive of malignancy

ANCILLARY TESTS

Immunohistochemistry
- Positive for cytokeratin, synpatophysin, chromogranin, and CD56
- Also positive for hormones, including serotonin, substance-P, gastrin, VIP
- Negative for germ cell tumor markers (PLAP, Podoplanin(D2-40), Oct3/4, SALL4) and sex cord tumor markers (inhibin, calretinin, Melan-A[MART-1])

DIFFERENTIAL DIAGNOSIS

Metastatic Carcinoid
- Clinical history and imaging finding of tumor occurring in locations where carcinoid is known
- Presence of teratoma favors primary carcinoid
- Lymphovascular invasion, bilaterality and multifocal involvement favors metastasis

Leydig or Sertoli Cell Tumor
- Less distinct insular or nested arrangement
- Lack of characteristic "salt and pepper" chromatin and presence of nucleoli
- Positive for inhibin and calretinin

DIAGNOSTIC CHECKLIST

Pathologic Interpretation Pearls
- Insular and nested patterns, "salt and pepper" chromatin and nuclear palisading at periphery of tumor cell nests

SELECTED REFERENCES

1. Abbosh PH et al: Germ cell origin of testicular carcinoid tumors. Clin Cancer Res. 14(5):1393-6, 2008
2. Merino J et al: Pure testicular carcinoid associated with intratubular germ cell neoplasia. J Clin Pathol. 58(12):1331-3, 2005
3. Ulbright TM et al: Carcinoid tumor of the testis. Am J Clin Pathol. 121(2):297; author reply 298, 2004
4. Reyes A et al: Neuroendocrine carcinomas (carcinoid tumor) of the testis. A clinicopathologic and immunohistochemical study of ten cases. Am J Clin Pathol. 120(2):182-7, 2003

CARCINOID TUMOR

Microscopic Features

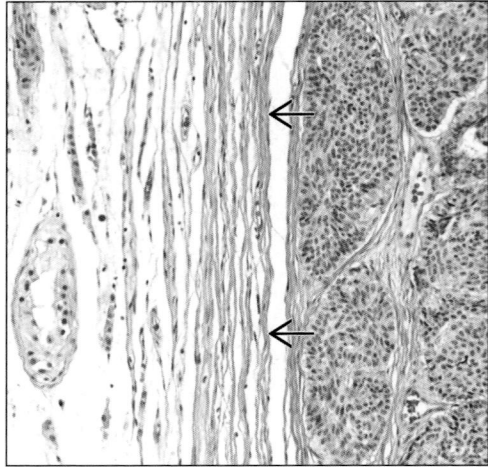
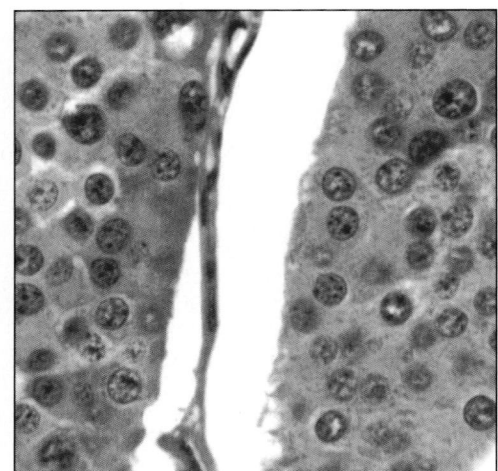

(Left) Testicular carcinoid tumor is well demarcated from the uninvolved testicular parenchyma by thin fibrous tissue ➡. The tumor shows neuroendocrine features with uniform cells forming nests. *(Right)* High-power photomicrograph shows classic cytology of carcinoid tumor with relatively uniform nuclei, "salt and pepper" chromatin, and abundant eosinophilic and granular cytoplasm. No mitosis or necrosis is seen.

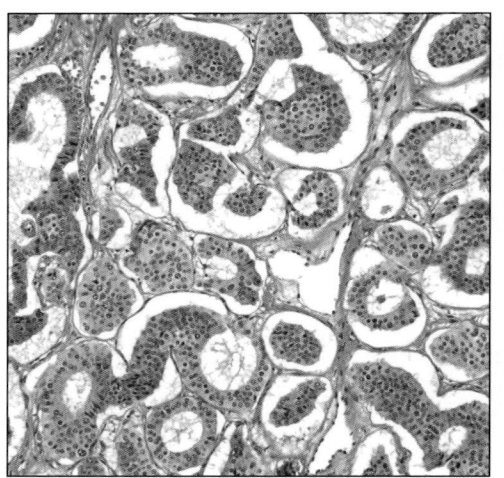
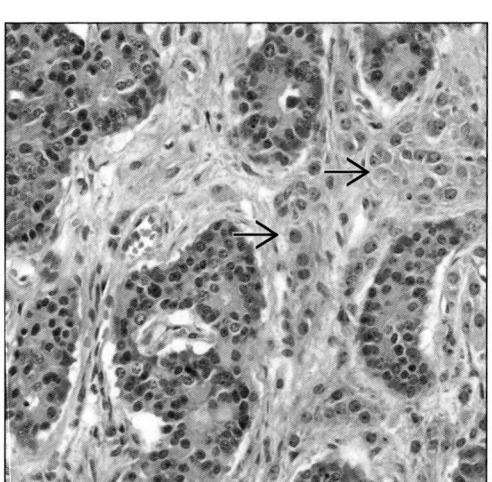

(Left) Testicular carcinoid tumor shows nested and insular growth patterns with delicate fibrous stroma. Artifactual retraction spaces are prominent in this carcinoid tumor. *(Right)* In the stroma of this carcinoid tumor, there are scattered Leydig cells ➡, indicating infiltrative growth of the tumor at the periphery. Notice the monotony of the tumor cells and peripheral nuclear palisading.

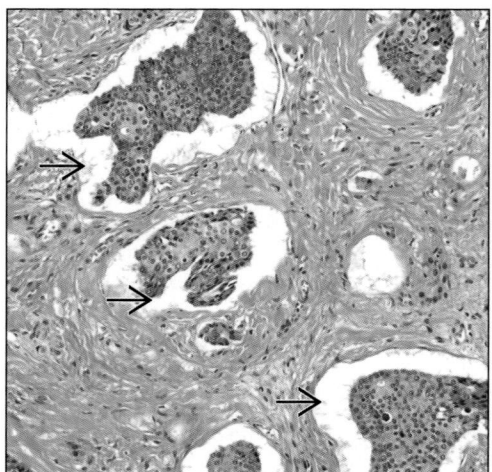
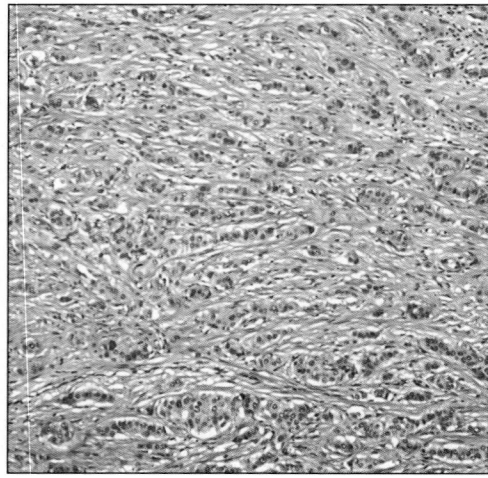

(Left) Solid nests of tumor cells are surrounded by prominent hyalinized fibrous stroma. Peritumoral artifactual spaces ➡ as seen in this case are 1 of the helpful features to make the diagnosis of carcinoid. *(Right)* This carcinoid tumor shows cords of tumor cells with dense hyalinized stroma. The differential diagnoses include Sertoli cell or Leydig cell tumor, metastatic carcinoma, or cellular adenomatoid tumor. Neuroendocrine markers are required to make a definitive diagnosis.

CARCINOID TUMOR

Immunohistochemical Features and Differential Diagnoses

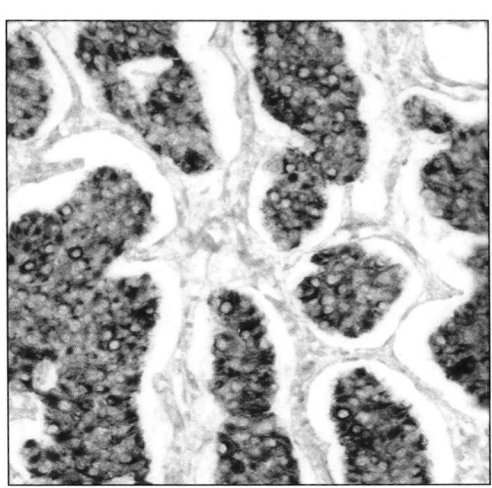
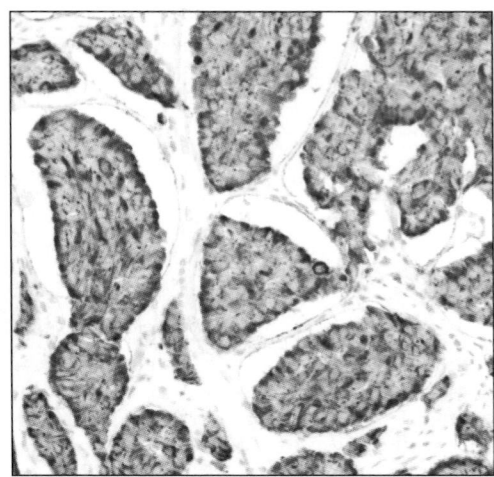

(Left) This image shows strong and diffuse immunoreactivity with PAN-CK(AE1/AE3) within a carcinoid tumor. Although sex cord stromal tumor may be positive for cytokeratin, the positivity is usually less intense and diffuse. *(Right)* Immunohistochemical stain with chromogranin shows diffuse cytoplasmic positivity within the tumor cells, further supporting the diagnosis of carcinoid tumor. Distinct from sex cord stromal tumors, carcinoid tumors are negative for inhibin and calretinin.

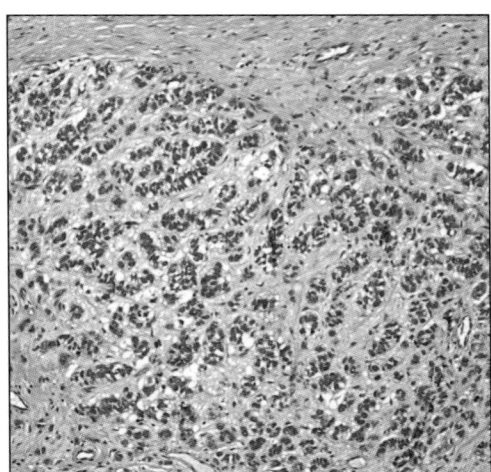
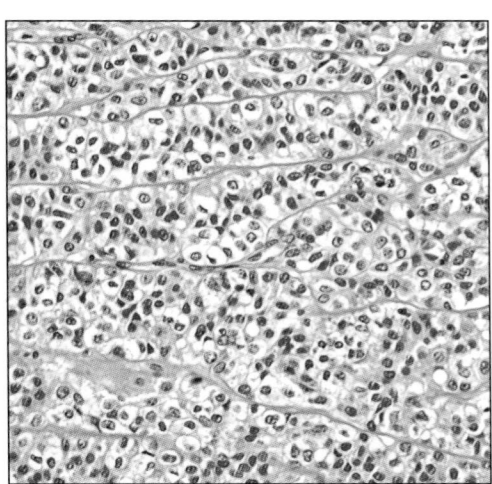

(Left) This Sertoli cell tumor shows nested growth and dense stroma, similar to that of a carcinoid tumor. Unlike carcinoid tumor, the tumor cells are positive for inhibin and negative for neuroendocrine markers. *(Right)* This image shows diffuse and trabecular growth of Sertoli cell tumor. In contrast to carcinoid tumor, the nucleoli are prominent and nuclei lack a "salt and pepper" appearance. Prominent clear cytoplasm also favors Sertoli cell tumor.

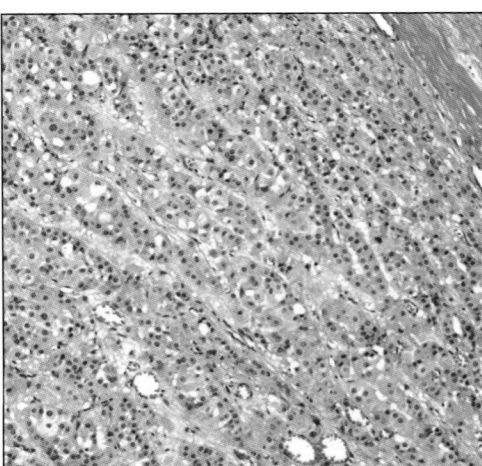
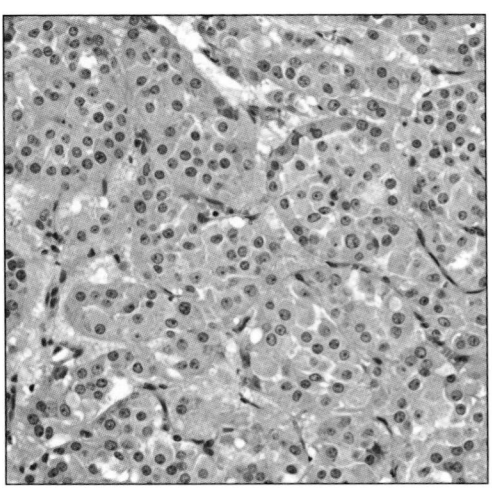

(Left) The nested and trabecular growth patterns of this Leydig cell tumor are similar to that of a carcinoid tumor. Immunohistochemical stains with inhibin and neuroendocrine markers are helpful in making a definitive diagnosis. *(Right)* Although the cytoplasmic features of this Leydig cell tumor are similar to those of a carcinoid tumor, the prominent nucleoli and lack of "salt and pepper" chromatin favor the diagnosis of Leydig cell tumor.

GENERAL CONCEPTS, SEX CORD/GONADAL STROMAL TUMORS

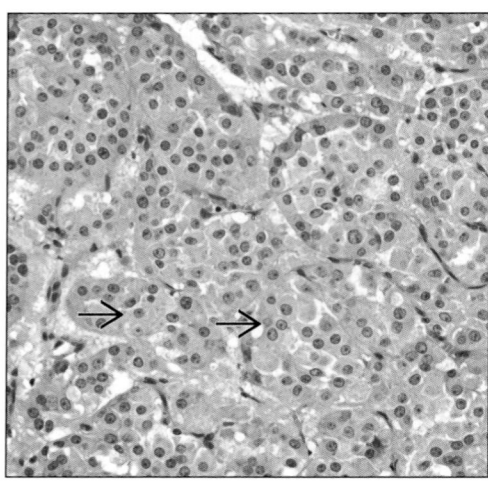

Leydig cell tumor with solid and nested growth patterns is shown. The tumor cells are uniform, round, and have prominent nucleoli ➔ and abundant eosinophilic/granular cytoplasm.

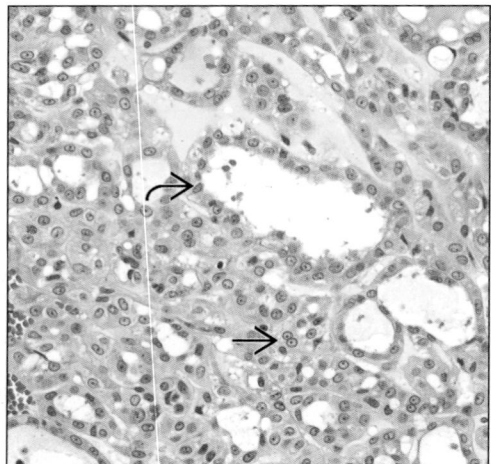

Sertoli cell tumor with tubular ⇗ pattern is shown. The tumor cells have ovoid to round nuclei with occasional prominent nucleoli ➔ and pale eosinophilic cytoplasm.

TERMINOLOGY

Definitions
- Neoplasms that have features of Leydig (interstitial) cells, Sertoli cells, granulosa cells, or rarely, theca cells
- Sex cord stromal tumor (SCST) may be of mixed classifiable sex cord stromal cells (mixed SCST) or unclassifiable sex cord stromal cell (unclassified SCST)
- Cases of mixed germ cell and SCST reported (gonadoblastoma and unclassified type)

EPIDEMIOLOGY

Incidence
- 4-6% of adult testicular neoplasms
- 30% of testicular tumors in infants and children
- Unlike germ cell tumors, there is no racial difference in frequency

ETIOLOGY/PATHOGENESIS

Histogenesis
- Poorly understood in general
- May relate to disruption of hypothalamic-pituitary-testicular axis and hormonal disturbance
- No definitive association with cryptorchidism
- Specific types of sex cord stromal tumor may be associated with genetic syndromes; e.g., large cell calcifying Sertoli cell tumor in Peutz-Jeghers syndrome and testicular feminization syndrome for Sertoli cell tumors
- Although testicular granulosa cell or theca cell tumors have been reported, no granulosa or theca cells are present in normal testis

CLINICAL IMPLICATIONS

Presentation
- Painless mass (rarely painful)
- Asymptomatic or hormone-related symptoms
- Infants with Leydig cell tumor usually present with isosexual pseudoprecocity
- Some types may cause gynecomastia or impotence

Treatment
- Surgical approaches
  - Orchiectomy is curative; staging work-up required
  - Testis sparing resection possible

Prognosis
- Approximately 10% of adult-type SCSTs are malignant and may metastasize
- Metastasis is the only reliable criterion for malignancy; histologic factors alone may not predict malignancy
- Features that may be associated with disease progression include
  - Nuclear pleomorphism, frequent and abnormal mitosis (> 4/10 high-power fields), necrosis
  - Infiltrative growth, large size (> 5 cm), extension to paratesticular tissue, and vascular invasion
- Tumors occurring in infants and children are almost always benign with rare exceptions

Clinical Presentation
- Painless testicular swelling or mass
- Symptomatology of hormonal disturbance or genetic syndrome

MACROSCOPIC FINDINGS

General Features
- Size
  - Range from microscopic to several cm (malignant forms usually larger, > 5 cm)

Specimen Handling

- Total Resection
  - Procure cord margin before cutting into testis
  - Small tumors may be entirely embedded
  - Submit at least 1 section/cm tumor
    - Sections to include: Tumor with adjacent parenchyma
    - Sections to include: Rete testis, epididymis, and spermatic cord
    - At least 2 sections of grossly normal parenchyma
- Subtotal Resection
  - Ink resection margin 1st
  - Take perpendicular sections of tumor with margin
  - Submit entire tumor, if appropriate
  - Sections to include: Normal parenchyma

MICROSCOPIC FINDINGS

Normal Histology

- Interstitial (Leydig) cells
  - Present in interstitium as single cells or in clusters
  - They may be also present in tunica albuginea, rete testis, epididymis, and spermatic cord (ectopic Leydig cells)
  - Leydig cells have uniform, round nuclei, prominent nucleoli, and abundant eosinophilic cytoplasm
  - Intracytoplasmic lipofuscin pigment may be seen, particularly in older men
  - Reinke crystalloids (better demonstrated with trichrome stains)
  - Immunoreactive with vimentin, inhibin, and calretinin, but not cytokeratin (may be focally and weakly positive)
- Seminiferous tubules and Sertoli cells
  - Sertoli cells are located within seminiferous tubules and comprise approximately 10-15% of cells within tubules (germ cell:Sertoli cell ratio is ~ 13:1)
  - Located 1 or 2 cells away from basement membrane of tubules
  - Pyramidal shaped-cells with round to ovoid nuclei, finely granular chromatin, often prominent nucleoli
  - Cytoplasm is eosinophilic and granular with fine vacuoles
  - Immunoreactive with vimentin, Cam5.2, CK19, inhibin, and calretinin
- Granulosa cells
  - Probably represent precursor Sertoli cells in fetal seminiferous tubules
  - These cells are cuboidal or columnar in shape and rest on tubular basement membrane
  - Not found in normal adult testis
- Undifferentiated sex cord stromal cells
  - Present early in fetal gonadal development
  - Primitive cells with potential for elaboration of steroid hormones
  - Not found in normal adult testis

General Features

- World Health Organization (WHO) Histologic Classification of sex cord stromal tumors of testis
  - Leydig cell tumor (LCT)
  - Malignant LCT
  - Sertoli cell tumor (SCT)
    - SCT, lipid-rich variant
    - Sclerosing SCT
    - Large cell calcifying SCT
  - Malignant SCT
  - Granulosa cell tumor (GCT)
    - Adult type GCT
    - Juvenile GCT
  - Tumor of thecoma/fibroma group
    - Thecoma
    - Fibroma
  - Sex cord/gonadal stromal tumor (SCST), mixed/unclassified type
    - Incompletely differentiated SCST
    - SCSTs, mixed forms
    - Malignant SCSTs
  - Tumors containing both germ cell and sex cord/gonadal stromal elements
    - Gonadoblastoma
    - Germ cell sex cord/gonadal stromal tumors, unclassified

Cytologic Features

- Depends on tumor types

Predominant Pattern

- Solid or nested pattern
  - Usually seen in LCTs, GCTs, unclassified SCST, fibroma-thecoma
- Pseudoglandular, trabecular, or tubular
  - Usually seen in SCTs, may be seen in LCTs, GCTs
- Mixed growth patterns
  - Often seen in unclassified or mixed SCSTs, or less commonly in LCTs or SCTs

Predominant Cell Type

- LCT
  - Round to polygonal cells with abundant eosinophilic cytoplasm, lipofuscin pigment, and often prominent nucleoli
- SCT
  - Uniform cuboidal or columnar cells with moderate pale to light eosinophilic cytoplasm and cytoplasmic vacuoles
- GCT
  - Uniform round, ovoid, or carrot-shaped cells with scant, lightly staining cytoplasm and characteristic nuclear grooves
- Fibroma-thecoma
  - Uniform spindle cells with scant cytoplasm
- Incomplete or undifferentiated SCSTs
  - Mixture of epithelioid cells with vesicular nuclei, prominent nucleoli, and nondescript undifferentiated spindle cells

IMMUNOHISTOCHEMISTRY

Inhibin

- 32 kD dimeric glycoprotein composed of α and β subunit

GENERAL CONCEPTS, SEX CORD/GONADAL STROMAL TUMORS

Immunohistochemistry of Sex Cord Stromal Tumor

	Inhibin	Calretinin	Keratin	Vimentin	S100	Actin-sm	Melan-A
Leydig cell tumor	+	+	-/+	+	-/+	-	+
Sertoli cell tumor, NOS	+/-	+/-	+	+	+/-	-/+	-
Granulosa cell tumor	+	+	-/+	+	+/-	-/+	-
Sex cord-stromal tumor, NOS	+/-	+/-	-/+	+	+	+	+/-

- Produced by ovarian granulosa cells and testicular Sertoli and Leydig cells
- Immunoreactive with LCT, SCT, large cell calcifying SCT, and GCT

Calretinin
- 29 kD intracellular calcium-binding protein expressed in a variety of tumors, including mesothelioma
- Immunoreactive with LCT, SCT, and SCST, NOS

PAN-CK(AE1/AE3)
- SCT usually positive, LCT usually negative or focally positive; positive in mixed unclassified SCST

Vimentin
- Most SCSTs usually positive for vimentin

S100
- SCT usually positive, LCT may be positive (more nuclear positivity and weak cytoplasmic)
- Large cell calcifying Sertoli cell tumor is frequently positive

Actin-sm
- Positive in unclassified SCST, myofibroblastic differentiation

Melan-A(MART-1)
- All sex cord stromal tumors may be positive for Melan-A(MART-1); most frequently expressed in Leydig cell tumors

WT1
- Present in normal granulosa cells, expressed by a majority of sex cord stromal tumors

CD99
- Present in normal granulosa cells, expressed by a majority of sex cord stromal tumors, including adult and juvenile granulosa cell tumors and Sertoli-Leydig cell tumors (focal)

DIFFERENTIAL DIAGNOSIS

Germ Cell Tumors
- Usually more heterogeneous with different growth pattern; tumor cells more pleomorphic with increased mitoses
- Frequent hemorrhage and necrosis
- Negative for inhibin and calretinin; positive for germ cell markers (Oct3/4, SALL4)

Metastatic Carcinoma or Melanoma
- Older age and clinical history
- Tumor cells have greater pleomorphism and more frequent mitoses
- Interstitial growth pattern and frequent vascular-lymphatic invasion
- Negative for inhibin and calretinin; positive for tissue-specific markers

Lymphoma/Leukemia
- Diffuse and interstitial infiltration of tumor cells
- Positive for LCA or B-cell and T-cell markers; negative for inhibin and calretinin

Adenomatoid Tumor (Cellular)
- Rarely intratesticular
- More prominent stroma and cytoplasmic vacuoles
- Depending on cytology and architecture, may mimic Leydig cell tumor or Sertoli cell tumor
- Negative for inhibin; positive for Podoplanin(D2-40), CK5/6, calretinin, WT1 (calretinin and WT1 staining overlap with sex cord stromal tumor)

SELECTED REFERENCES

1. Acar C et al: Current treatment of testicular sex cord-stromal tumors: critical review. Urology. 73(6):1165-71, 2009
2. Passman C et al: Testicular lesions other than germ cell tumours: feasibility of testis-sparing surgery. BJU Int. 103(4):488-91, 2009
3. Irving JA et al: Granulosa cell tumors of the ovary with a pseudopapillary pattern: a study of 14 cases of an unusual morphologic variant emphasizing their distinction from transitional cell neoplasms and other papillary ovarian tumors. Am J Surg Pathol. 32(4):581-6, 2008
4. Al-Agha OM et al: An in-depth look at Leydig cell tumor of the testis. Arch Pathol Lab Med. 131(2):311-7, 2007
5. Michal M et al: Mixed germ cell sex cord-stromal tumours of the testis. Virchows Arch. 451(6):1095-6, 2007
6. Verdorfer I et al: Sertoli-Leydig cell tumours of the ovary and testis: a CGH and FISH study. Virchows Arch. 450(3):267-71, 2007
7. Michal M et al: Mixed germ cell sex cord-stromal tumors of the testis and ovary. Morphological, immunohistochemical, and molecular genetic study of seven cases. Virchows Arch. 448(5):612-22, 2006
8. Young RH: Sex cord-stromal tumors of the ovary and testis: their similarities and differences with consideration of selected problems. Mod Pathol. 18 Suppl 2:S81-98, 2005
9. Henley JD et al: Malignant Sertoli cell tumors of the testis: a study of 13 examples of a neoplasm frequently misinterpreted as seminoma. Am J Surg Pathol. 26(5):541-50, 2002
10. Ulbright TM et al: Leydig cell tumors of the testis with unusual features: adipose differentiation, calcification with ossification, and spindle-shaped tumor cells. Am J Surg Pathol. 26(11):1424-33, 2002

4

Microscopic Features

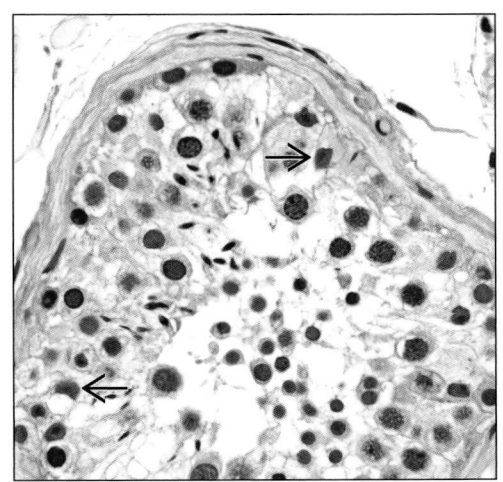

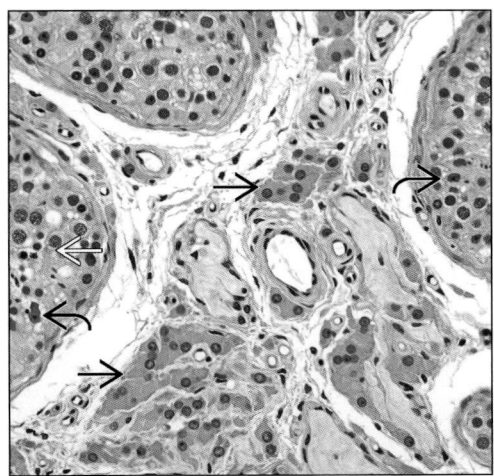

(Left) This image shows a seminiferous tubule with germ cells in different stages of spermatogenesis. The Sertoli cells ➡ have a pyramidal shape and abundant, pale eosinophilic cytoplasm with prominent nucleoli. *(Right)* This image shows seminiferous tubules with spermatogenesis ➡ and Sertoli cells ➡. The interstitium contains several clusters of Leydig cells ➡ with abundant eosinophilic cytoplasm and round, central nuclei with occasional prominent nucleoli.

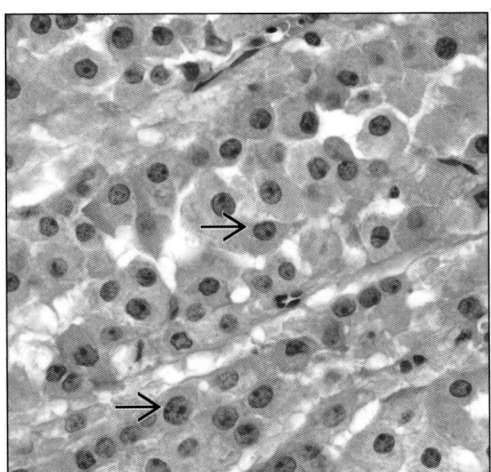

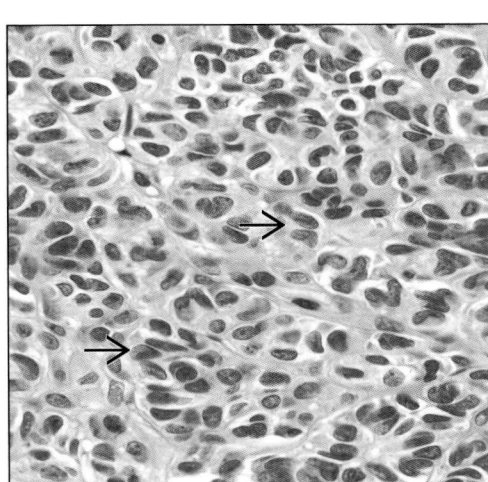

(Left) A typical LCT shows solid sheets and trabeculae of tumor cells with voluminous eosinophilic cytoplasm, round nuclei, and prominent nucleoli ➡. *(Right)* This unclassified SCST is composed of short, oval to spindled tumor cells with nuclear grooves ➡ and moderate cytoplasm. The morphology may suggest granulosa cell differentiation, and the vaguely nested pattern may resemble Sertoli cell tumor.

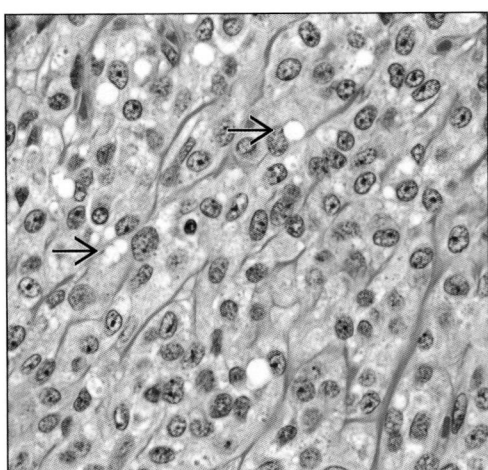

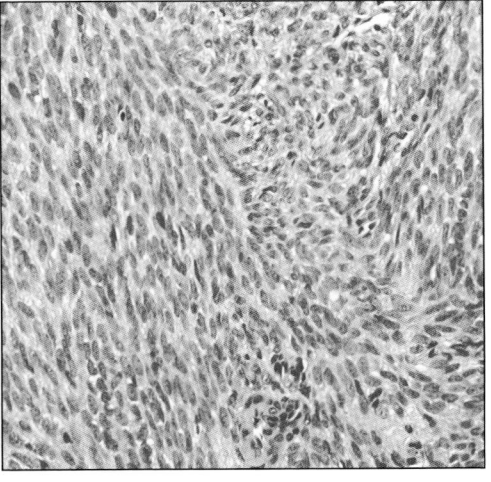

(Left) The solid pattern of SCT may resemble LCT, but the nuclei are slightly irregular and have coarsely granular chromatin, pale eosinophilic cytoplasm with vacuoles ➡. SCT is usually positive for cytokeratin, whereas LCT is often negative or weakly positive. *(Right)* Fibroma-thecoma shows fascicles of spindle cells with scant cytoplasm. Although rare, these may occur in the testis or paratestis. The tumor may be diagnosed as unclassified sex cord stromal tumor by some.

Microscopic and Immunohistochemical Features

(Left) LCT with adverse histologic features is shown. The tumor has solid growth and invades through the tunica. Although there are no reliable histologic criteria to predict malignant behavior, invasive growth and high cellularity, as seen here, may often result in clinical metastasis. *(Right)* This LCT shows significant cytologic atypia and frequent mitoses ➡. A combination of adverse features is predictive of malignancy.

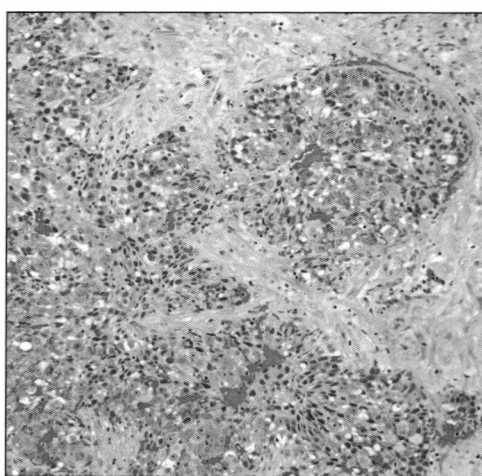
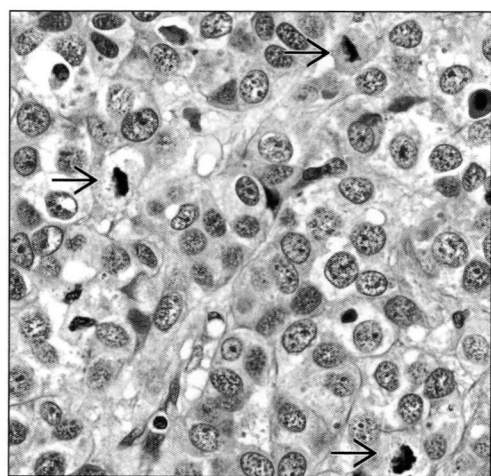

(Left) SCT with adverse histologic feature is shown. There are large geographical areas of necrosis ➡. Features that are associated with malignancy include invasive growth, vascular invasion, nuclear pleomorphism, increased mitoses (> 4/10 HPFs), and necrosis. *(Right)* In this SCT, there is marked nuclear pleomorphism and frequent mitoses ➡. The cells contain clear cytoplasm and cytoplasmic vacuoles ➡, features that are suggestive of SCT.

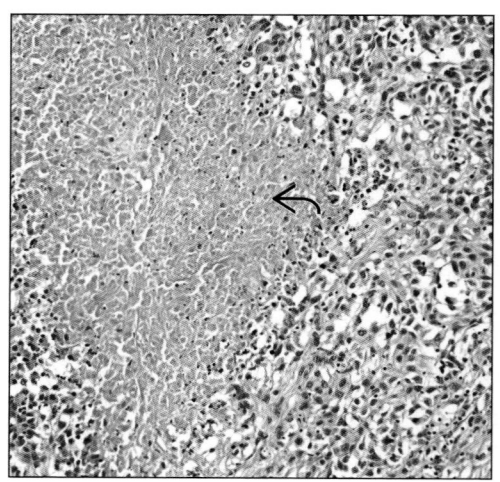
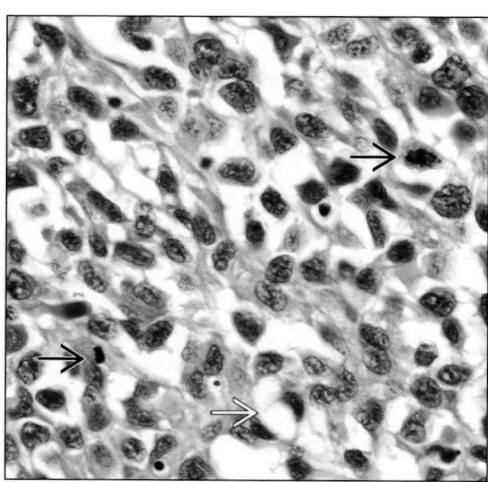

(Left) LCT shows strong positivity for inhibin. Inhibin is one of the most reliable markers for the diagnosis of sex cord stromal tumor of testis. Other markers include Melan-A(MART-1), WT1, calretinin, and CD99. *(Right)* Inhibin immunostaining in a GCT is shown. Among sex cord stromal tumors, cytokeratin positivity is most typical in SCT; it is often negative to weak in LCT and variable in GCT.

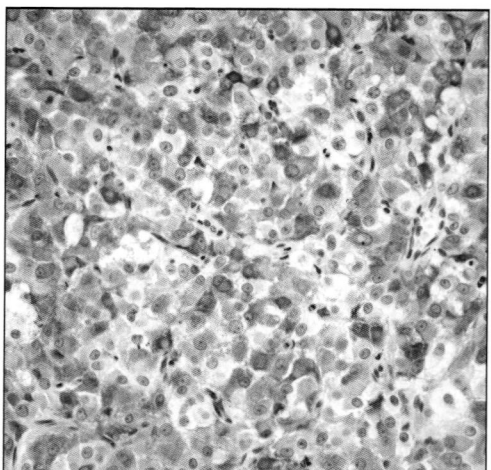
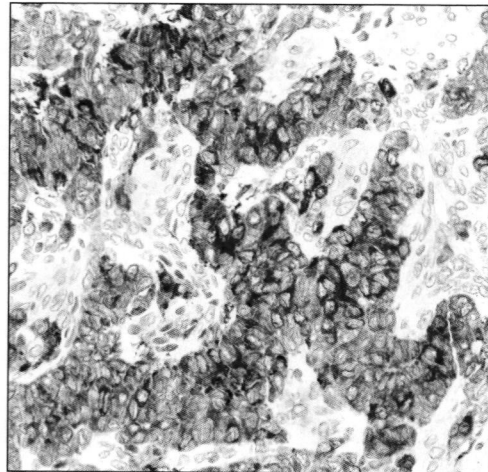

Differential Diagnoses

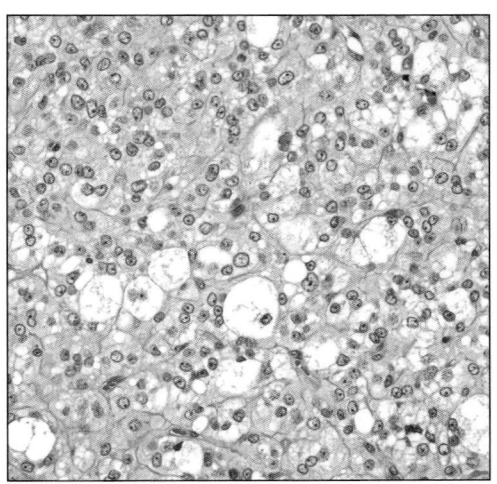

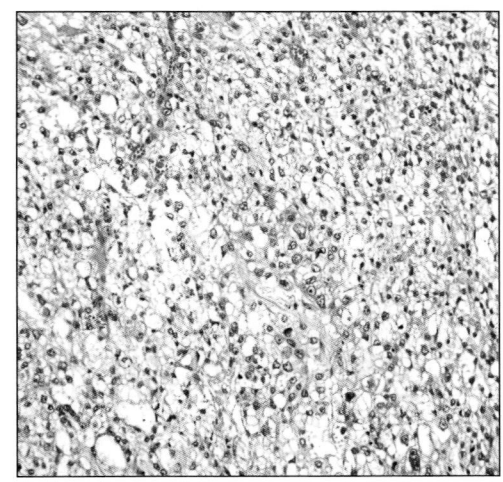

(Left) This LCT shows prominent cytoplasmic vacuoles and microcystic appearance, which resembles a yolk sac tumor. Multiple patterns, hyaline globules, basement membrane deposition, or Schiller-Duval bodies, as seen in yolk sac tumor, are not present. *(Right)* Yolk sac tumor with microcystic and solid growth patterns may mimic a LCT or SCT. α-fetoprotein, glypican-3, and SALL4 are positive, and inhibin and calretinin are negative in yolk sac tumor.

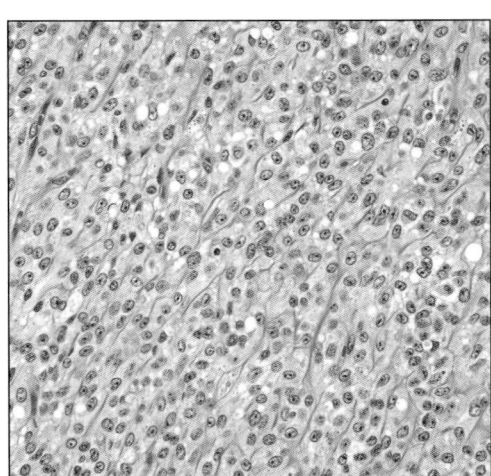

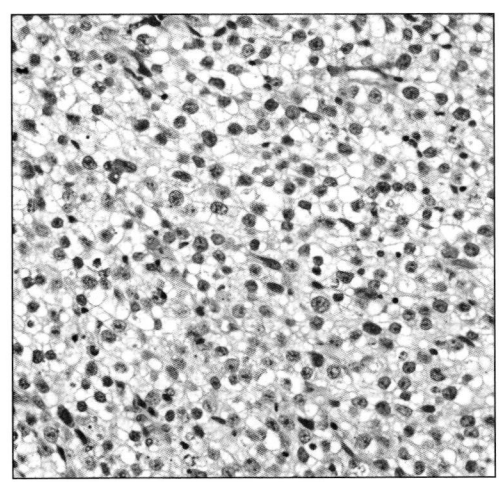

(Left) This image shows a solid SCT with delicate fibrous septae. The tumor cells are relatively uniform, with prominent nucleoli and pale eosinophilic cytoplasm with cytoplasmic vacuoles, superficially resembling a seminoma. *(Right)* This classic seminoma shows tumor cells with clear and pale eosinophilic cytoplasm. When there is a paucity of lymphocytes and fibrous septae, seminoma may resemble a solid pattern that is seen in SCT or LCT.

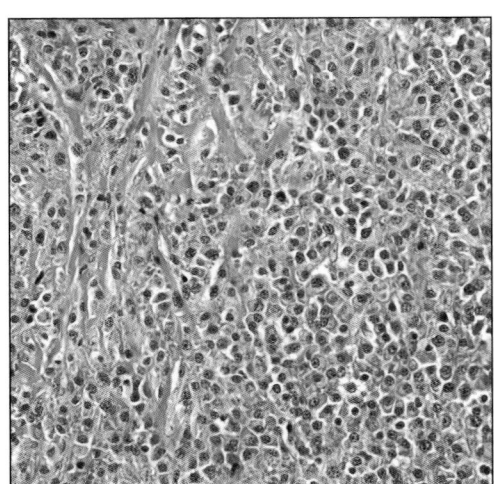

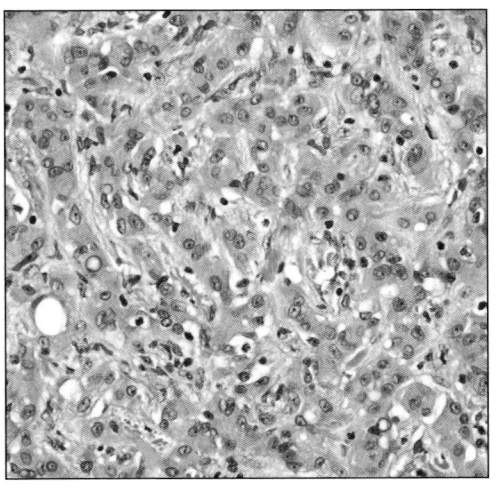

(Left) This plasmacytoma has a vaguely nested appearance, which may resemble a LCT. Closer examination shows that the tumor cells have plasmacytoid nuclear features and perinuclear halos. Inhibin and calretinin are negative. *(Right)* Cellular adenomatoid tumor may mimic a LCT. The tumor cells contain abundant eosinophilic cytoplasm and prominent nucleoli. Cytokeratin and Podoplanin are strongly positive, and inhibin is negative in this paratesticular tumor.

LEYDIG CELL TUMORS

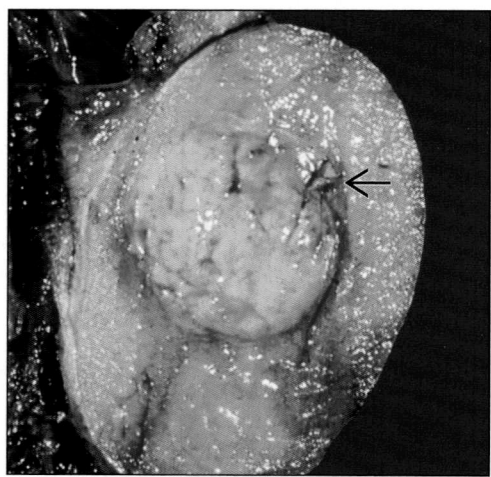

LCT is often a well-circumscribed mass with a homogeneous yellow-tan cut surface. Focal cystic change ⇲ is present. Hemorrhage or necrosis is lacking. LCT often do not replace the entire testis.

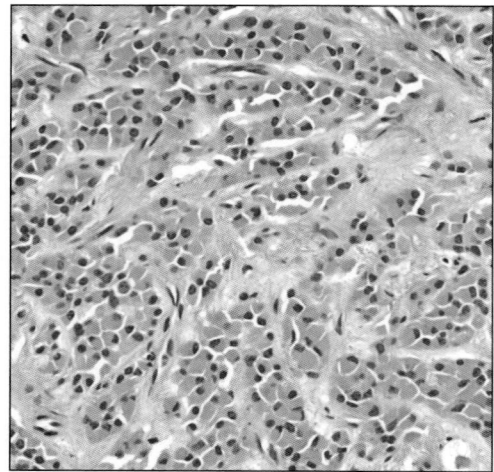

LCT is composed of broad cords of tumor cells separated by paucicellular and edematous fibrous stroma. The tumor cells have uniform, round to ovoid nuclei and abundant eosinophilic cytoplasm.

TERMINOLOGY

Abbreviations
- Leydig cell tumor (LCT)

Synonyms
- Interstitial cell tumor

Definitions
- Pure testicular stromal tumor composed of cells that recapitulate normal interstitial Leydig cells

CLINICAL ISSUES

Epidemiology
- Incidence
  - Most common type of sex cord stromal tumor (1-3% of testicular neoplasms)
- Age
  - Occurs in any age with 2 peaks: 5-10 & 30-35 years

Presentation
- Testicular enlargement, usually painless, decreased libido (20%), gynecomastia (15%), undescended testis (10%), or precocious puberty
- May produce testosterone, androstenedione, and dehydroepiandrosterone
- May be associated with cryptorchidism, testicular atrophy, infertility
- Bilaterality in 3% of cases

Treatment
- Surgical approaches
  - Orchiectomy is curative in majority of tumors; baseline staging work-up is required
  - Retroperitoneal lymph node dissection may be required in older patients and those with tumors with unfavorable histology
  - Testis-sparing surgery possible for young men

Prognosis
- Majority have benign behavior
- Approximately 10% malignant and may metastasize

MACROSCOPIC FEATURES

General Features
- Well-circumscribed, intraparenchymal mass with golden-brown to yellow, or gray-white homogeneous cut surface
- Focal hemorrhage or necrosis may be seen (25%)
- Most confined within testis; extratesticular extension possible (10%)

Size
- Range: 1-10 cm (average: 3 cm)

MICROSCOPIC PATHOLOGY

Histologic Features
- Growth patterns: Solid (most common), insular, tubular, ribbon-like, and pseudofollicular
- Large, round or polygonal cells with well-defined cell borders, eosinophilic or vacuolated cytoplasm
- Relatively uniform round or ovoid nuclei, prominent nucleoli; focal nuclear pleomorphism (including endocrine-type), binucleated, or multinucleated cells may be seen
- Cytoplasmic vacuoles or foamy cytoplasm (lipid content), lipofuscin (15%), and Reinke crystals (30-40%) may be seen
- Frequent fibrous, hyalinized, edematous or myxoid stroma
- Other uncommon features: Fatty metaplasia; spindle, clear cell, or microcystic changes; myxoid degeneration; calcification or ossification; and rhabdoid features

LEYDIG CELL TUMORS

Key Facts

Terminology
- Pure testicular stromal tumor composed of cells that recapitulate normal interstitial Leydig cells

Clinical Issues
- Most common type of sex cord stromal tumor (1-3% of testicular neoplasms)
- Majority have benign behavior; 10% malignant

Macroscopic Features
- Well-circumscribed, intraparenchymal nodule with golden-brown to yellow, or gray-white homogeneous cut surface

Microscopic Pathology
- Growth patterns: Solid (most common), insular, tubular, ribbon-like, and pseudofollicular

- Large, round or polygonal cells with well-defined cell borders, eosinophilic or vacuolated cytoplasm
- Relatively uniform round or ovoid nuclei, prominent nucleoli; focal nuclear pleomorphism, binucleated or multinucleated cells may be seen
- Cytoplasmic vacuoles or foamy cytoplasm (lipid content), lipofuscin (15%), and Reinke crystals (30-40%) may be seen
- Other uncommon features: Fatty metaplasia; spindle, clear cell, or microcystic changes; myxoid degeneration; calcification or ossification; and rhabdoid features

Ancillary Tests
- Positive for inhibin-α, calretinin, Melan-A(MART-1), and vimentin (strong and diffuse)

- Features that tend to be seen more often in malignant tumors: Large tumor size (> 5 cm), infiltrative margins, vascular invasion, nuclear atypia, necrosis, high mitotic rate (> 3/10 high-power fields)

Cytologic Features
- Large, round or polygonal cells with prominent nucleoli, abundant eosinophilic cytoplasm, and well-defined cell borders

Predominant Pattern/Injury Type
- Diffuse and solid neoplastic growth

Predominant Cell/Compartment Type
- Sex cord stromal cells

ANCILLARY TESTS

Immunohistochemistry
- Positive for inhibin-α, calretinin, Melan-A(MART-1), WT1, androgenic hormones (P450scc, 3β-HSD, etc.), and vimentin (strong and diffuse)
- Negative for cytokeratin (rarely focally positive), S100 (usually negative), PLAP, HMB-45, Podoplanin(D2-40), Oct3/4, SALL4

DIFFERENTIAL DIAGNOSIS

Malignant Lymphoma
- Older age, frequent bilaterality, interstitial growth, malignant cytologic features, "onion skin" appearance of seminiferous tubule involvement
- Positive for CD45(LCA), and usually B-cell marker positive; negative for inhibin-α, calretinin, Melan-A(MART-1)

Large Cell Calcifying Sertoli Cell Tumor
- More calcification, high bilaterality (40%), intratubular growth of tumor cells, nests or cords of growth

Testicular Tumors of Adrenogenital Syndrome
- Multinodular, bilaterality, pleomorphism, pigmentation, and hyalinized fibrous stroma, interstitial growth pattern with entrapped seminiferous tubules

Ectopic Leydig Cells Mimicking Extratesticular Extension
- Cytologically bland Leydig cell proliferation in extratesticular locations (tunica albuginea, epididymis, spermatic cord)
- Intraneural, perineural, perivascular locations

Leydig Cell Hyperplasia
- Small size (< 0.5 cm), multifocal, shows interstitial growth with intervening seminiferous tubules

Other Lesions with Eosinophilic Cytoplasm
- Malakoplakia, hepatoid yolk sac tumor, carcinoid tumor, and metastatic malignant melanoma

DIAGNOSTIC CHECKLIST

Pathologic Interpretation Pearls
- Well-defined solid tumoral growth of relatively bland-looking uniform cells with eosinophilic cytoplasm
- Metastasis is only criterion for malignancy

SELECTED REFERENCES

1. Jou P et al: Leydig cell tumor of the testis. J Urol. 181(5):2299-300, 2009
2. Ulbright TM et al: Leydig cell tumors of the testis with unusual features: adipose differentiation, calcification with ossification, and spindle-shaped tumor cells. Am J Surg Pathol. 26(11):1424-33, 2002

LEYDIG CELL TUMORS

Gross and Microscopic Features

(Left) A well-circumscribed LCT is shown with solid, homogeneous, yellow-tan cut surface. There is no hemorrhage or necrosis. The tumor is confined within the testis without extratesticular extension. *(Right)* Low-power image of LCT shows a nodular pattern of tumor cells with fibrous septae. Even at this low power, the eosinophophilic cytoplasm of the tumor is appreciated. The tumor is demarcated from the seminiferous tubules ➡, which lack intratubular germ cell neoplasia.

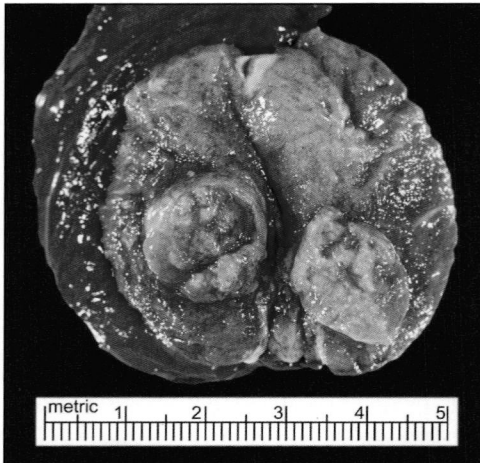
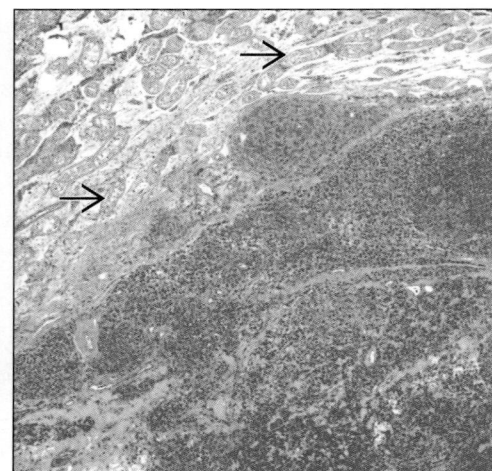

(Left) LCT with uniform, oval to round tumor cells is shown. The cells are uniform and have abundant eosinophilic cytoplasm with distinct cell boundaries. Nucleoli ➡ are prominent. The tumor is vaguely divided into lobules by delicate sinusoidal vessels. There is absence of pleomorphism, necrosis, or mitosis. *(Right)* Touch preparation imprint cytology of LCT shows uniform round nuclei, prominent nucleoli, and abundant eosinophilic cytoplasm. The background lacks tumor diathesis.

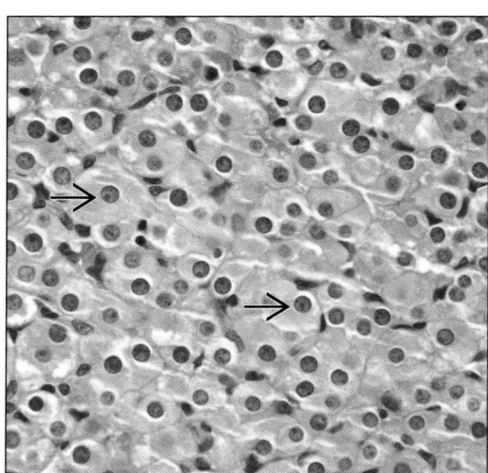
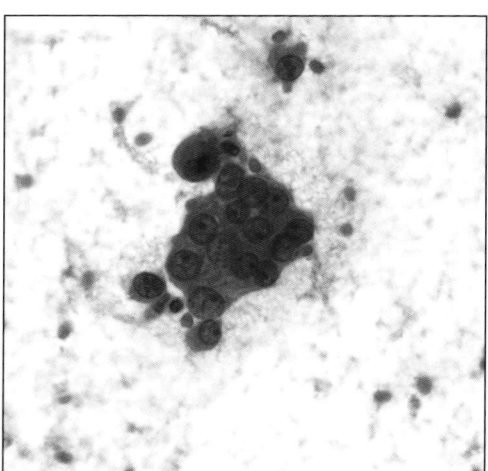

(Left) Lower power photomicrograph of an LCT shows nests and cords of tumor cells separated by sclerotic and myxoid stroma. *(Right)* An example of alveolar pattern of LCT is shown, which is characterized by abundant delicate fibrovascular network. This may have superficial resemblance to a seminoma, but the tumor cells contain abundant eosinophilic (not clear) cytoplasm and lack lymphocytic infiltrate or granulomas within the fibrous septae. Absence of adjacent ITGCN is helpful.

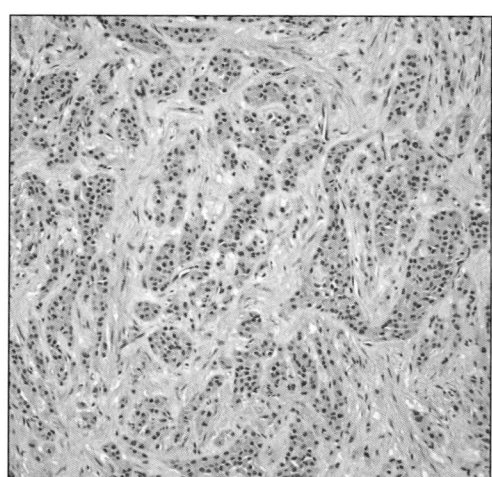
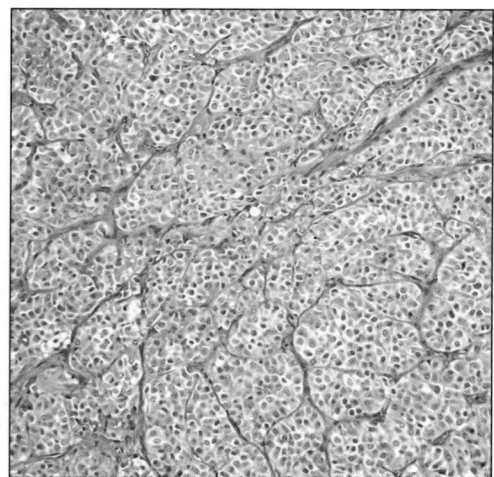

LEYDIG CELL TUMORS

Microscopic Features

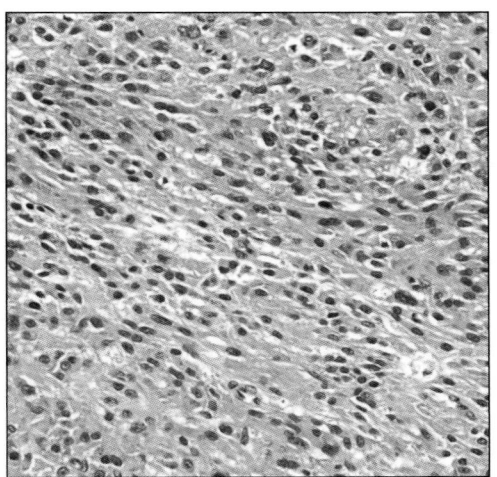

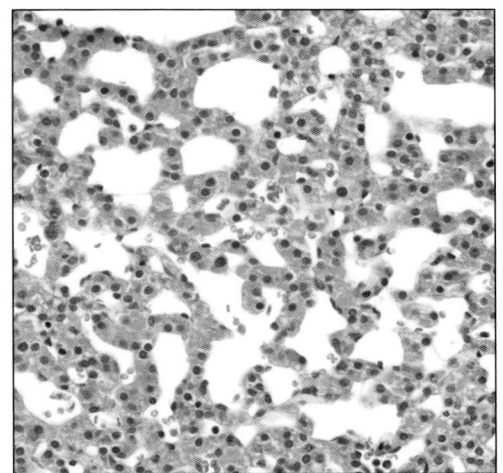

(Left) LCT may have an area of vaguely fascicular arrangement of spindle cells containing abundant eosinophilic cytoplasm. The differential diagnosis from an unclassified sex cord stromal tumor may be a problem. In this case, areas of more typical LCT component were present. (Right) An example of LCT with tubular or pseudoglandular pattern is shown. The individual tumor cell morphology is that of a typical LCT. The tumor cells are uniform and contain abundant eosinophilic cytoplasm.

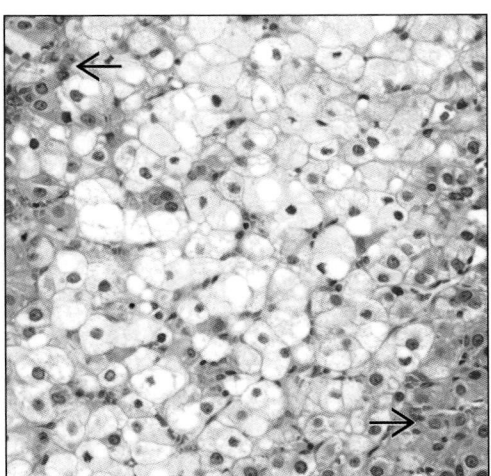

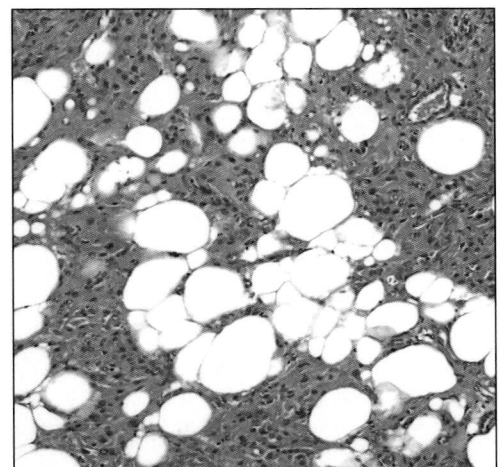

(Left) LCT may have prominent clear cells and abundant anastomosing capillary network resembling that of the zona fasciculata of the adrenal cortex. Typical features of LCT are seen in adjacent areas ➔. (Right) Intermediate-power photomicrograph of LCT with adipose tissue component is shown. The histogenesis of the fatty component is unclear. It may be either a metaplastic or an infiltrative process. This finding does not have any clinical significance.

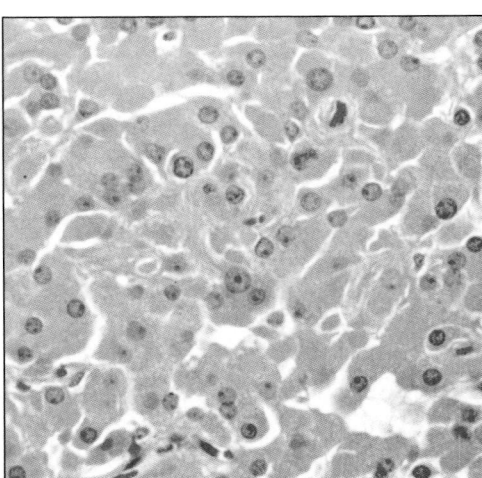

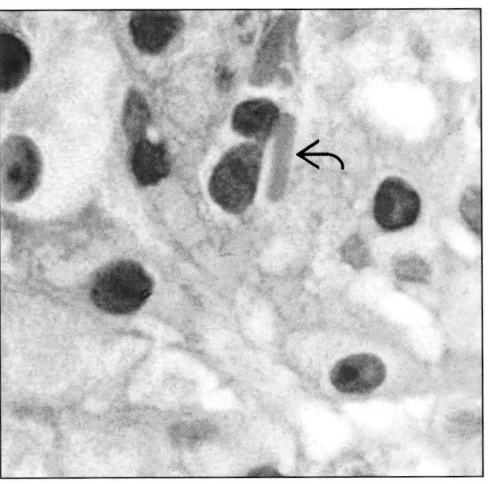

(Left) Oncocytic LCT is characterized by uniform round nuclei, prominent nucleoli, and voluminous pink cytoplasm. Mitoses, nuclear pleomorphism, and necrosis are lacking. The differential diagnosis includes other oncocytic tumors, including testicular tumor of adrenogenital syndrome and large cell calcifying Sertoli cell tumor. (Right) LCT with rod-shaped intracytoplasmic Reinke crystalloids ➔ is shown, a feature in approximately 30% of LCT. The finding is typically focal.

LEYDIG CELL TUMORS

Microscopic Features

(Left) LCT with ossification and calcification is shown. The tumor cells are arranged in cords and trabeculae with fibrous tissue. The differential diagnosis from a large cell calcifying Sertoli cell tumor (LCCSCT) may be difficult. Bilaterality, association with syndromes, and strong keratin positivity are helpful features for LCCSCT. *(Right)* LCT with intracytoplasmic lipofuscin pigment ⇒ is shown. Mild degree of nuclear irregularity and prominent nucleoli ⇒ are present.

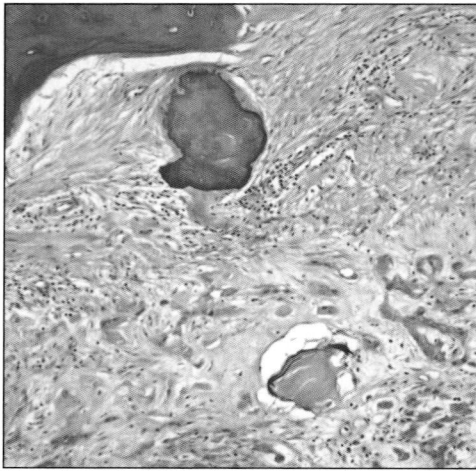
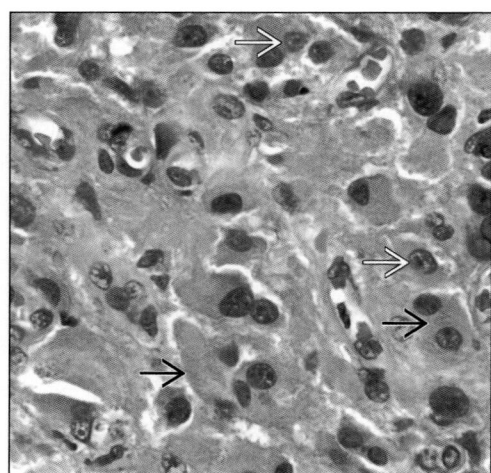

(Left) LCT with "rhabdoid features" shows tumor cells with voluminous eosinophilic cytoplasm, eccentrically located nuclei, and prominent nucleoli. Besides other more common oncocytic tumors, the differential diagnoses include malignant melanoma and plasmacytoma. *(Right)* The tumor cells in this LCT with rhabdoid features are strongly positive for inhibin and negative for cytokeratin. Other useful markers include Melan-A(MART-1), WT1, and calretinin.

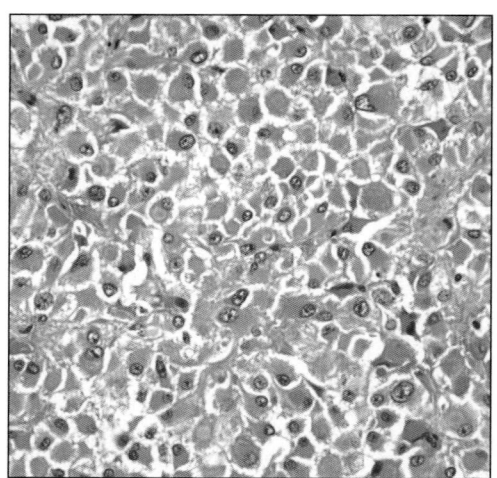
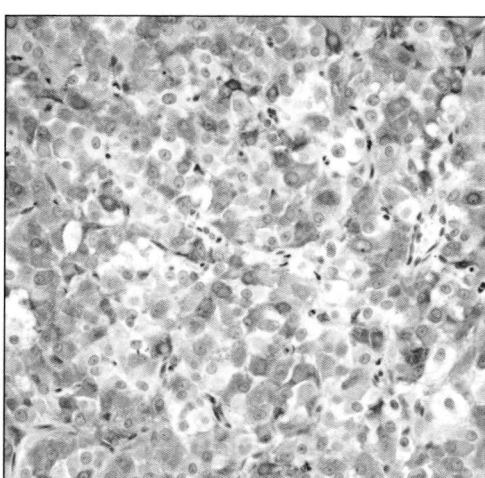

(Left) This image shows an area of typical LCT ⇒ juxtaposed with an area of LCT with histologically malignant features, such as increased cellularity, high N:C ratio, frequent mitoses and apoptoses ⇒. Approximately 10% of LCT are malignant. *(Right)* A malignant LCT with several mitoses ⇒ is shown. Features seen more commonly in tumors with malignant outcome include capsular or vascular invasion, mitoses > 3/10 high-power fields, significant pleomorphism, and necrosis.

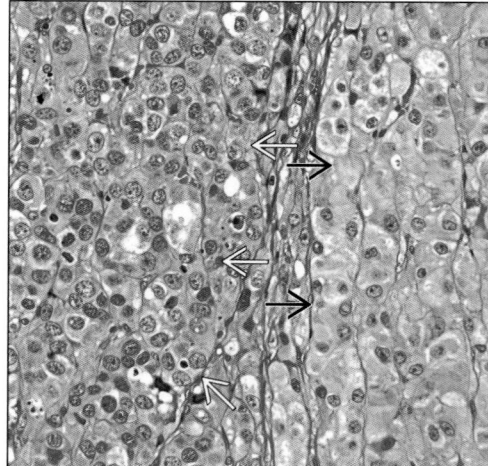
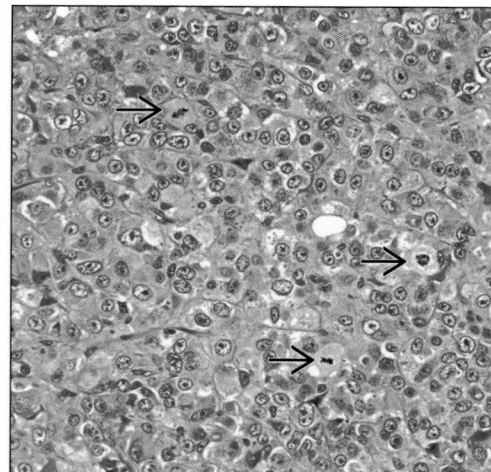

LEYDIG CELL TUMORS

Microscopic and Immunohistochemical Features

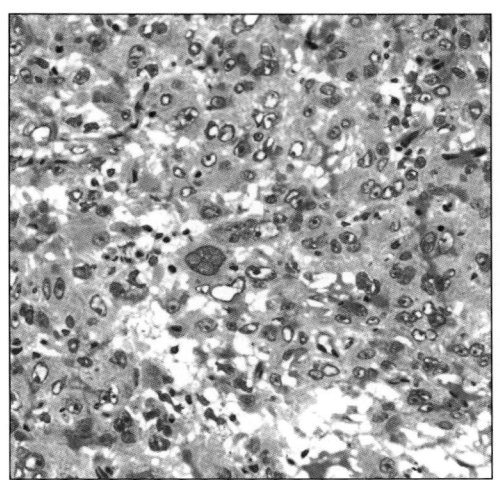
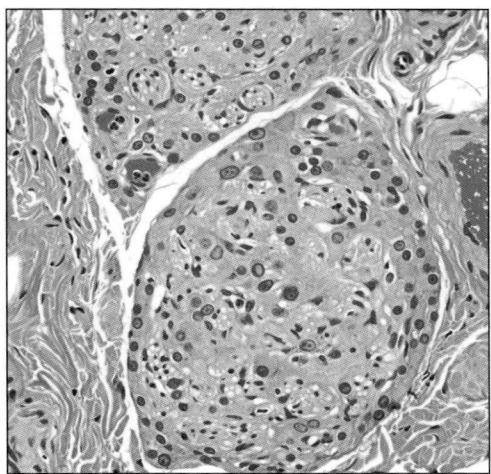

(Left) An example of a LCT with cytologic atypia on frozen section is shown. There is marked nuclear pleomorphism and occasional multinucleation, raising the suspicion for a malignant germ cell tumor or metastatic carcinoma. (Right) Ectopic Leydig cells in a nerve within the spermatic cord is shown. This finding is very common and usually very focal and subtle but may raise the suspicion of perineural invasion by LCT or even metastatic prostate carcinoma.

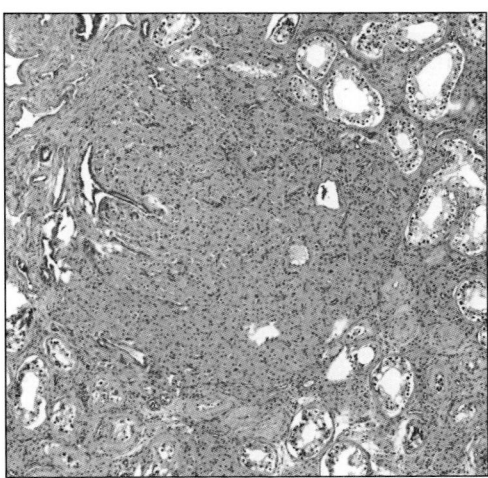
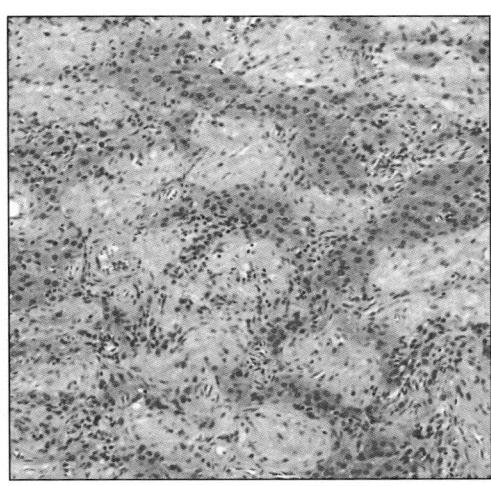

(Left) This low-power photomicrograph shows a small focus (< 0.5 cm) of nodular Leydig cell hyperplasia with extension of Leydig cells into the surrounding interstitium. (Right) Leydig cell hyperplasia with interstitial pattern is shown with proliferation of Leydig cells between atrophic hyalinized seminiferous tubules. In general, Leydig cell hyperplasia does not form a gross tumor mass, and the hyperplastic nodule does not exceed 5 mm.

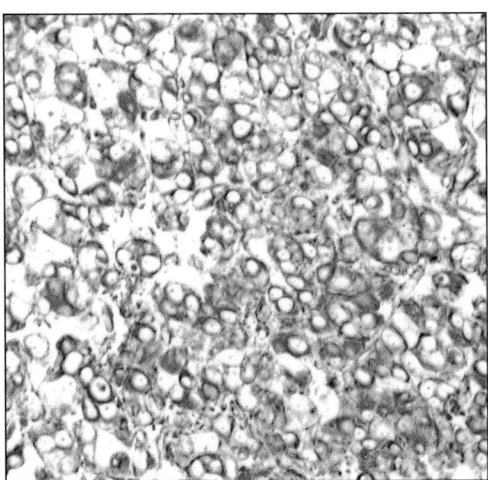
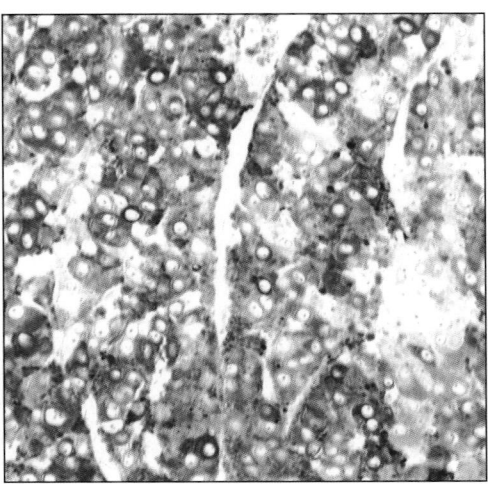

(Left) The tumor cells of LCT are diffusely positive for vimentin. All sex cord stromal tumors are positive for vimentin. Cytokeratin, however, is negative or focal or weakly positive in LCT. (Right) Leydig cell tumors show diffuse cytoplasmic positivity for α-inhibin. Other useful markers include Melan-A(MART-1), calretinin, and WT1. Androgenic hormones may be positive but are rarely necessary in clinical practice.

SERTOLI CELL TUMORS

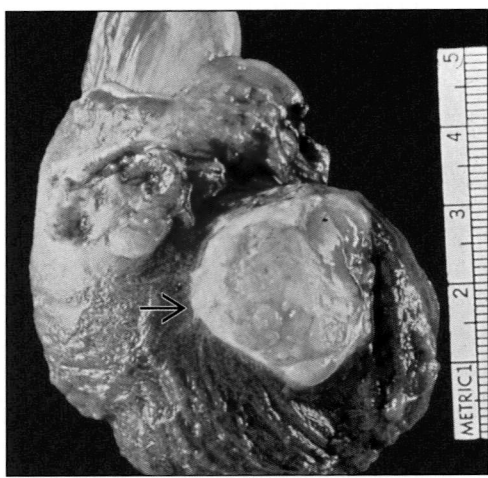

A well-circumscribed SCT ⇨ with a tan-white firm cut surface is shown. The gross finding is different from Leydig cell tumor, which usually is tan-brown to yellow due to high lipid content.

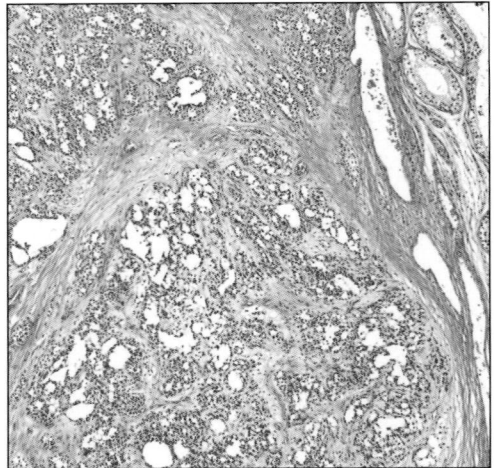

Low-power image shows a well-circumscribed SCT with a lobular growth pattern, tubular and microcystic architecture, and hyalinized stroma. Tubular differentiation is the hallmark of this neoplasm.

TERMINOLOGY

Abbreviations
- Sertoli cell tumor (SCT)

Synonyms
- Androblastoma, arrhenoblastoma

Definitions
- Pure sex cord stromal tumor that shows variety of architectural patterns, including solid growth, but which shows at least focal tubular differentiation

CLINICAL ISSUES

Epidemiology
- Incidence
  - < 1% of testicular tumors; most are sporadic
  - In patients with undescended testes, Peutz-Jeghers syndrome, Carney syndrome, androgen insensitivity, and testicular feminization syndromes
- Age
  - No known age predilection (average: 45 years)
  - Up to 30% occur in 1st decade of life

Presentation
- Slowly enlarging testicular mass
- Hormone-related symptoms are unusual; may present with hyperestrinism (gynecomastia)
- Most unilateral but bilateral cases have been reported

Treatment
- Surgical approaches
  - Surgical resection is often curative (radiation and chemotherapy have little effect)
  - Small size may be treated with partial orchiectomy

Prognosis
- Up to 10% may be malignant
- Excellent prognosis unless metastasis occurs

MACROSCOPIC FEATURES

General Features
- Usually small well-circumscribed, homogeneous gray-white to yellow, firm mass
- May be lobulated with focal cystic changes or hemorrhage

Size
- Range: 1-10 cm (average: 3.5 cm)

MICROSCOPIC PATHOLOGY

Histologic Features
- Growth patterns: Tubules, microcystic, cords, nests, solid sheets and rarely spindled (sarcomatoid)
  - Most common pattern is tubules, which are hollow, round, solid, or elongated
- Uniform cuboidal or columnar cells with moderate pale to lightly eosinophilic cytoplasm, often with prominent cytoplasmic vacuoles
- Bland round to ovoid nuclei, occasional centrally located nucleoli, and rare mitoses
- May have paucicellular, hyalinized, or vascular fibrous stroma; lymphoid aggregates may be present
- May have clear cells arranged in nests by fibrous septa and lymphoid infiltrates resembling that of seminoma
- Entrapped germ cells within Sertoli cell tumor (usually at periphery) may mimic mixed germ cell sex cord stromal tumor
- Some tumors may have abundant cytoplasmic lipid (lipid-rich variant)
- Features seen more often in tumors with malignant outcome include
  - Large size (≥ 5 cm), lymphovascular invasion, and extratesticular extension
  - Marked nuclear pleomorphism, increased mitoses (> 5/10 high power fields), and necrosis
- Sclerosing Sertoli cell tumor

SERTOLI CELL TUMORS

Key Facts

Terminology
- Pure sex cord stromal tumor composed of cells resembling Sertoli cells

Clinical Issues
- < 1% of testicular tumors; most are sporadic
- All ages (average: 45 years)
- Slowly enlarging testicular mass

Macroscopic Features
- Small, well-circumscribed, homogeneous gray-white to yellow, firm mass

Microscopic Pathology
- Growth patterns: Tubules, microcystic, solid cords and nests, and rarely spindle (sarcomatoid)
- Most common pattern is tubules surrounded by basement membrane

- Uniform cuboidal or columnar cells with moderate pale to lightly eosinophilic cytoplasm, often prominent cytoplasmic vacuoles
- Bland round to ovoid nuclei, occasional centrally located nucleoli, and rare mitoses
- Charcot-Böttcher filaments (perinuclear arrays of filaments) are considered pathognomonic of Sertoli cell differentiation
- May have paucicellular, hyalinized, vascular fibrous stroma, or lymphoid aggregates

Ancillary Tests
- Positive for PAN-CK(AE1/AE3), EMA/MUC1, vimentin, α-inhibin, Melan-A(MART-1), WT1, CD99, calretinin, S100 (weak), synaptophysin
- Negative for PLAP, Podoplanin(D2-40), Oct3/4, SALL4, α-fetoprotein, CD30(BerH2), HCG

---

o Variant of Sertoli cell tumor characterized by markedly sclerotic fibrous stroma containing cords, solid or hollow tubules, and nests of Sertoli cells
o Usually contains entrapped nonneoplastic tubules

Cytologic Features
- Cuboidal to columnar cells, pale to eosinophilic cytoplasm, round to ovoid nuclei, and variably centrally located nucleoli

Predominant Pattern/Injury Type
- Tubular-glandular pattern or solid sheets, rarely spindle cell sarcomatoid pattern

Predominant Cell/Compartment Type
- Uniform, bland, oval to round cells

ANCILLARY TESTS

Immunohistochemistry
- Positive for PAN-CK(AE1/AE3), EMA/MUC1, vimentin, α-inhibin, Melan-A(MART-1), WT1, CD99, calretinin, S100 (weak), synaptophysin
- Negative for PLAP, Podoplanin(D2-40), Oct3/4, SALL4, α-fetoprotein, CD30(BerH2), HCG

Electron Microscopy
- Charcot-Böttcher filaments (perinuclear arrays of filaments) are pathognomonic of Sertoli cell differentiation

DIFFERENTIAL DIAGNOSIS

Seminoma (Tubular)
- Classic seminoma areas comprised of large tumor cells with abundant clear cytoplasm, prominent nucleoli, and lymphoid infiltrate; granulomas
- Positive for Oct3/4, Podoplanin(D2-40), CD117, PLAP; negative for inhibin, calretinin, and cytokeratin

Leydig Cell Tumor
- Usually solid growth with large cells containing abundant eosinophilic cytoplasm
- Yellow to brown gross appearance, lack of tubular differentiation, and negative for cytokeratin

Adenomatoid Tumor
- Location usually in paratesticular site or epididymis
- Negative for inhibin

Rete Testis Carcinoma or Metastatic Carcinoma
- Greater cytologic anaplasia and desmoplastic stroma
- Dysplastic rete testis epithelium or history of extratesticular carcinoma

Sertoli Cell Nodule
- Microscopic to small size (< 0.5 cm)
- Tubules with thickened basement membranes and hyaline bodies lined by immature Sertoli cells

DIAGNOSTIC CHECKLIST

Pathologic Interpretation Pearls
- Tubular pattern, range of cytologic features and cytoplasmic characteristics, cytokeratin and inhibin positive

SELECTED REFERENCES

1. Adayener C et al: Sertoli cell tumor of the testis: a case with late metastasis. Int Urol Nephrol. 40(4):1005-8, 2008
2. Talon I et al: Sertoli cell tumor of the testis in children: reevaluation of a rarely encountered tumor. J Pediatr Hematol Oncol. 27(9):491-4, 2005
3. Henley JD et al: Malignant Sertoli cell tumors of the testis: a study of 13 examples of a neoplasm frequently misinterpreted as seminoma. Am J Surg Pathol. 26(5):541-50, 2002
4. Young RH et al: Sertoli cell tumors of the testis, not otherwise specified: a clinicopathologic analysis of 60 cases. Am J Surg Pathol. 22(6):709-21, 1998

SERTOLI CELL TUMORS

Gross and Microscopic Features

(Left) An encapsulated SCT with a tan-white and gelatinous cut surface is shown. There are cystic changes ⮑ and focal hemorrhage ⮑. The tumor is confined within the testis. Massive replacement of the testis is uncommon. *(Right)* High-power photomicrograph of SCT shows uniform cuboidal or ovoid tumor cells arranged in elongated and hollow tubules separated by a delicate fibrous stroma. The amount of cytoplasm varies between tumors and in different areas of the tumor.

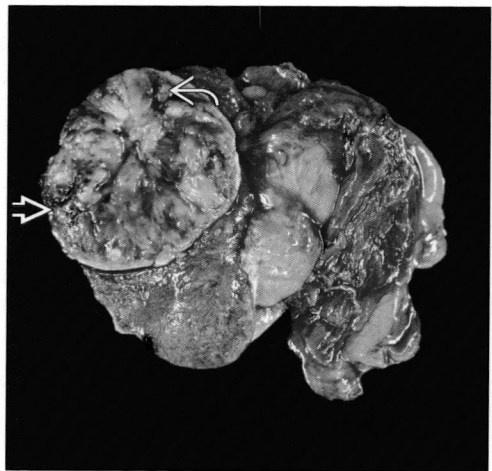
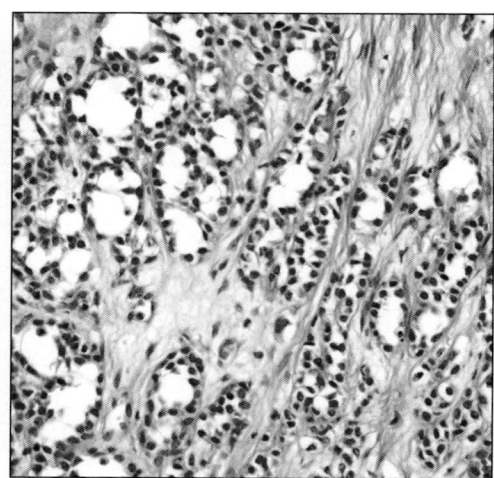

(Left) SCT typically have tubules ⮑, microcysts ⮑, and cords ⮑ lined by bland ovoid to round tumor cells with scant clear to eosinophilic cytoplasm. There is no nuclear pleomorphism, tumor necrosis, or mitotic activity. *(Right)* High-power photomicrograph of SCT shows tubules ⮑, microcysts ⮑, and cords lined by bland ovoid to elongated tumor cells with clear to pale eosinophilic cytoplasm or cytoplasm with fine vacuolization ⮑.

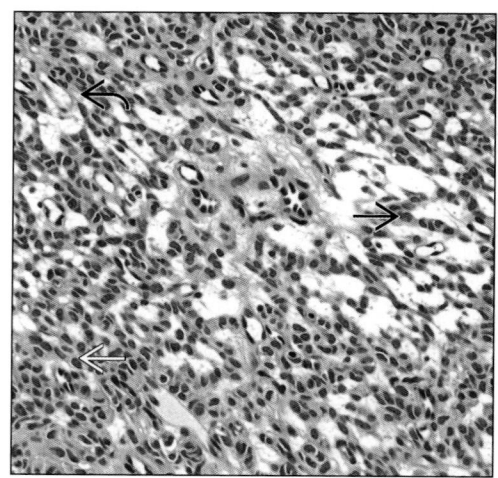
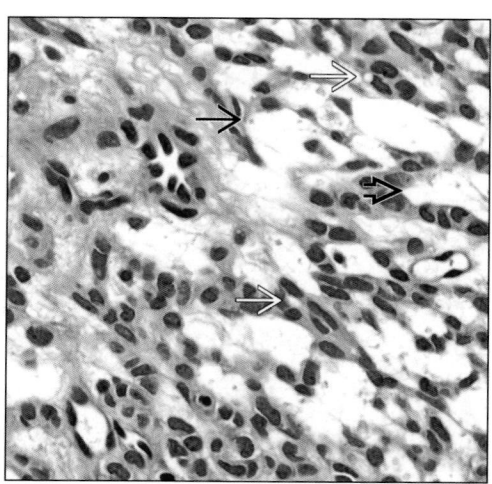

(Left) Microcystic ⮑ and tubular ⮑ patterns of SCT may superficially resemble that of a yolk sac tumor. SCT may rarely have lymphoid infiltrates, raising the differential diagnosis of seminoma with tubular growth pattern. *(Right)* SCTs are known to exhibit numerous architectural patterns. A high-power photomicrograph of SCT demonstrates tubules ⮑ and cords ⮑. The amount of stroma may vary and prominent areas of hyalinization are not uncommon.

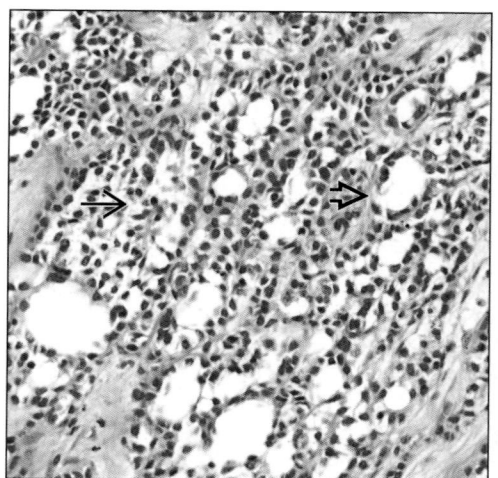
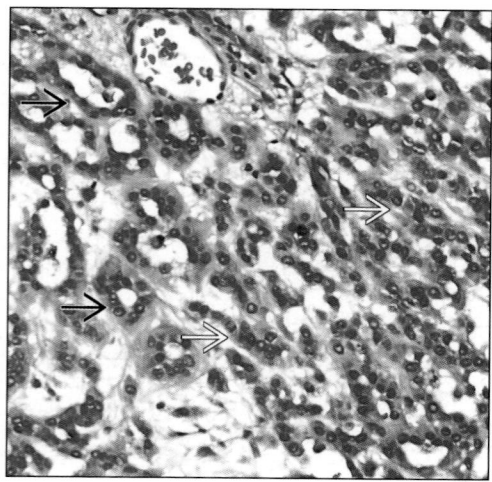

SERTOLI CELL TUMORS

Microscopic Features

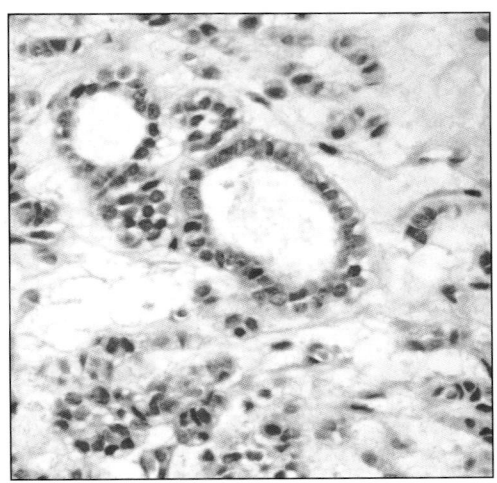

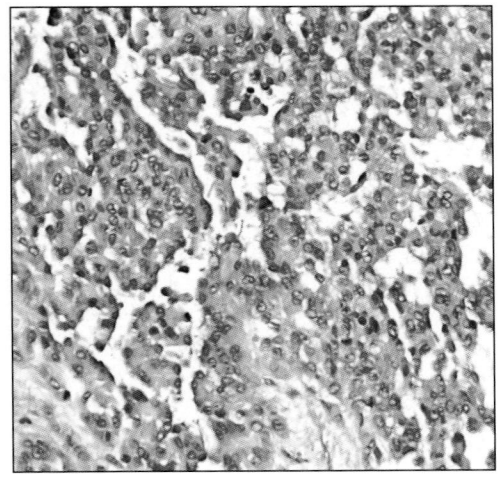

(Left) This SCT shows tubules of differing sizes lined by a single layer of monotonous cuboidal cells with clear cytoplasm. The background stroma is edematous and myxoid. Tubules lined by clear cells are 1 of the most helpful diagnostic features of SCT. (Right) This is an example of SCT with a focal retiform growth pattern characterized by irregularly elongated branching channels lined by bland cuboidal to flattened tumor cells.

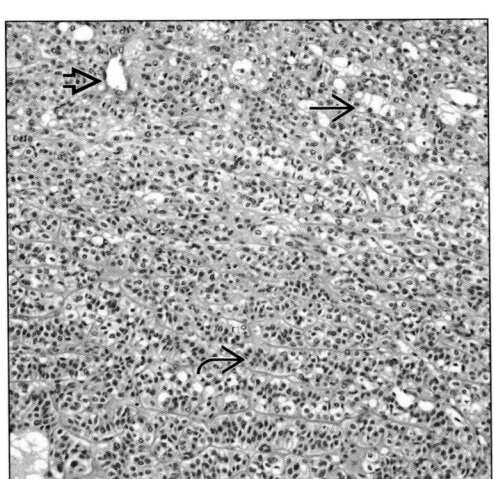

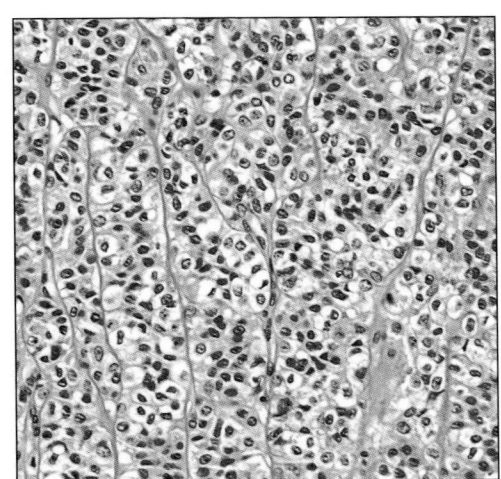

(Left) Low-power image of a SCT shows solid ➡, tubular ➡, and microcytic ➡ areas. Although the tumor is fairly cellular, there is no significant cytologic atypia, increased mitoses, or necrosis. (Right) SCT shows a solid tubular growth pattern with thin fibrous septae. The cells have bland, ovoid nuclei and abundant clear cytoplasm with vacuolization. Some SCT may have a variety of cytoplasmic features, including clear cells, eosinophilic cells, and lipid-rich cells.

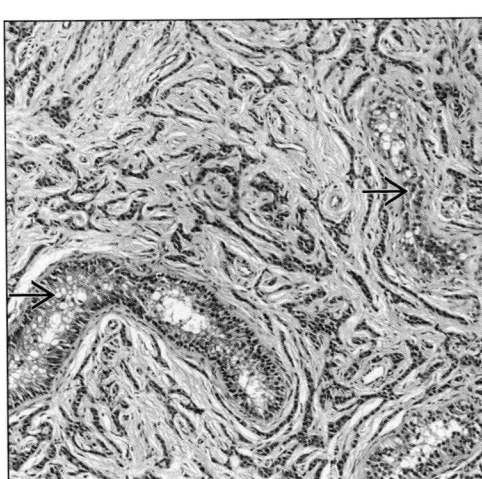

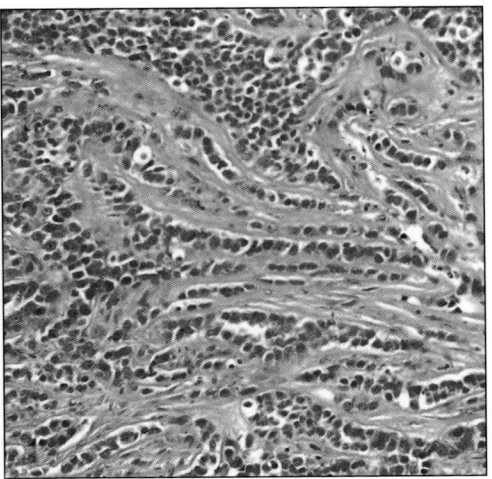

(Left) Low-power photomicrograph of a sclerosing SCT shows cord-like growth of tumor cells within a dense sclerotic stroma. Compressed entrapped seminiferous tubules are present ➡ and are more frequent with this variant of Sertoli cell tumor. (Right) Sclerosing SCT with a cord-like growth pattern and dense sclerotic stroma is shown. To date, metastasis has not been reported in the sclerosing variant of SCT. Carcinoid tumor and adenomatoid tumor are in the differential.

Microscopic Features

(Left) SCT is composed of cords of tumor cells embedded in a paucicellular hyalinized fibrous stroma. The blood vessels show hyalinization of the wall ⇥ and perivascular edema ➍. *(Right)* This SCT has small and markedly dilated follicles lined by bland cuboidal or flattened tumor cells. Because of follicular features, juvenile granulosa cell tumor (JGCT) may be in the differential diagnosis. However, JGCT occurs almost exclusively in children younger than 6 months.

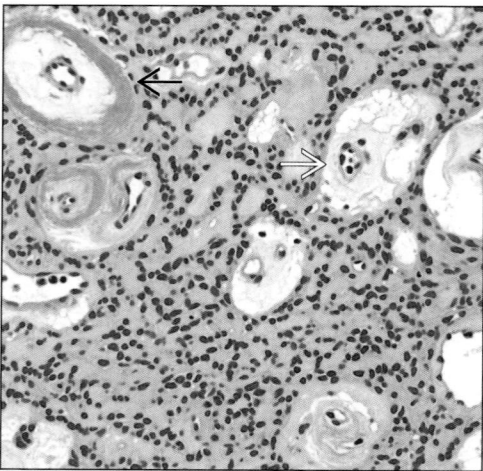
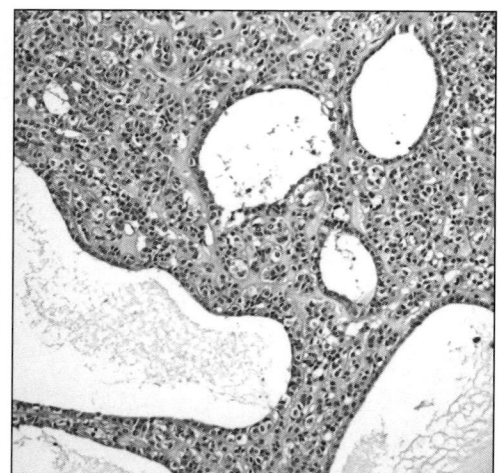

(Left) SCT can have diffuse, sheet-like and nested growth and is composed of cells with clear to eosinophilic cytoplasm, which may mimic a Leydig cell tumor. However, in other areas, classic SCT with tubules was seen. *(Right)* SCT with prominent spindle cells (sarcomatoid growth) is shown. There is moderate clear to pale eosinophilic cytoplasm. The chief differential diagnosis is an unclassified sex cord stromal tumor. In this case, there were areas of classic SCT.

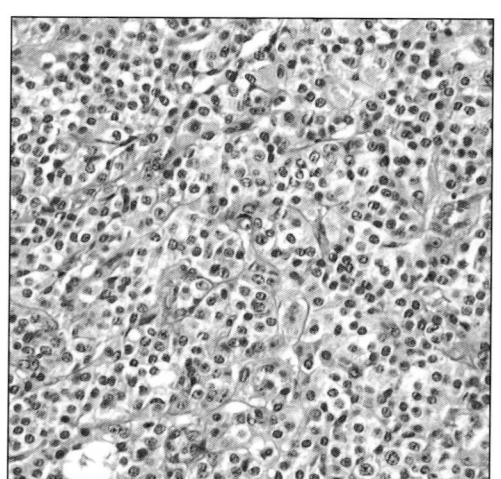
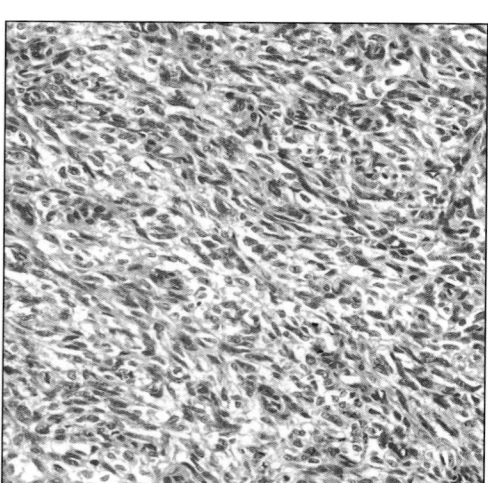

(Left) This SCT shows a solid growth pattern interspersed with variable collagenized stroma. The lobular appearance superficially resembles a seminoma; however, the cytologic features are key in the distinction. *(Right)* SCT can have tubules ⇥ and microcysts ⇥ of variable sizes with prominent myxoid stroma, which may resemble a yolk sac tumor. However, the nuclear features are relatively bland, and there is absence of hyaline globules or basement membrane material.

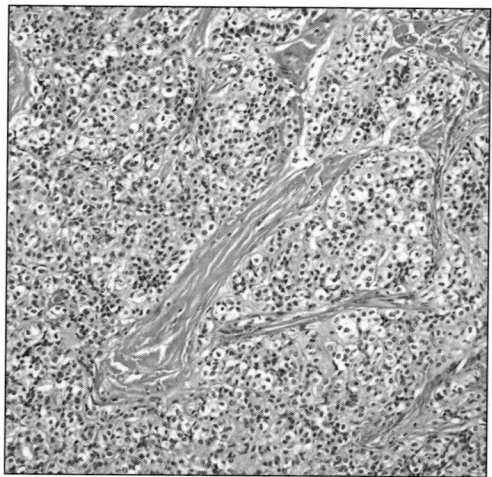
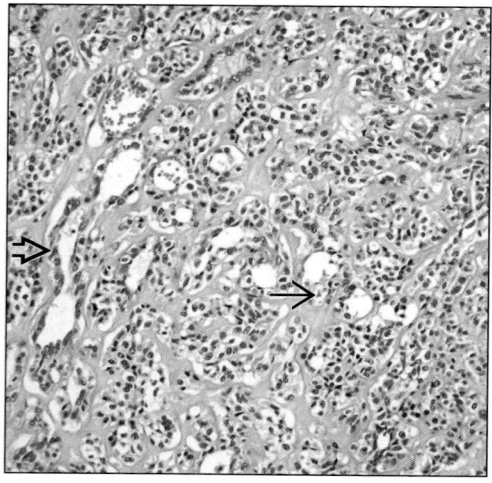

SERTOLI CELL TUMORS

Microscopic and Immunohistochemical Features

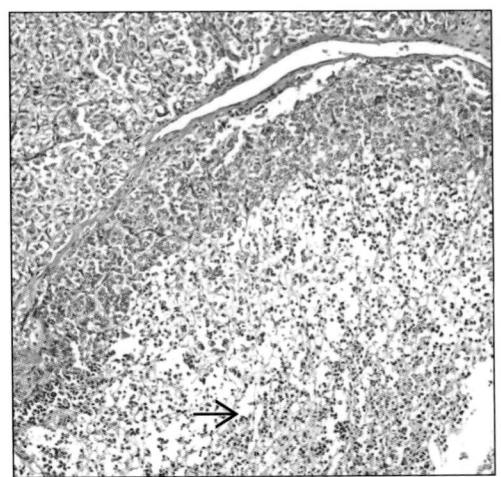

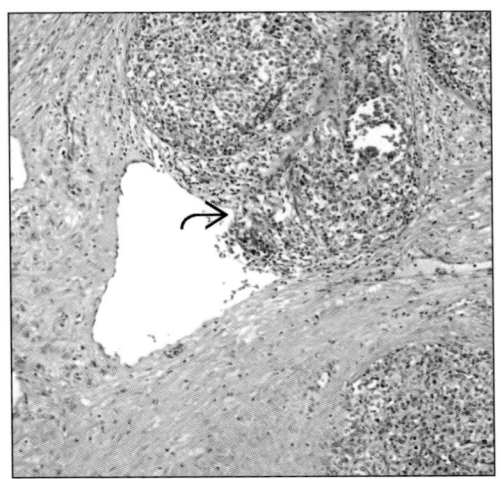

(Left) SCT with a malignant outcome shows solid sheets of tumor cells with hypercellularity, increased N:C ratio, and a large area of necrosis ➡. There is no single diagnostic criterion for malignant SCT. Features that are seen more often in malignant SCT include pleomorphism, increased mitoses, necrosis, vascular invasion, and infiltrative growth pattern. *(Right)* A malignant SCT is composed of solid tumor nodules seen outside of the testis with focal vascular invasion ➡.

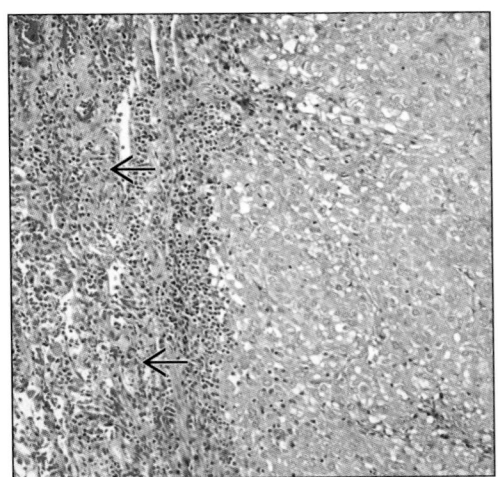

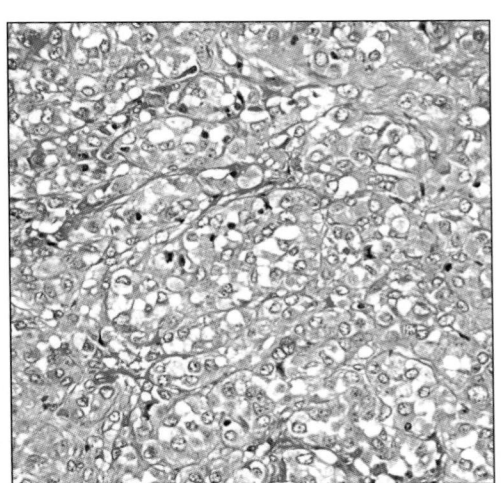

(Left) Metastatic SCT nodule to the lung ➡ is composed of sheets of epithelioid cells with pale eosinophilic cytoplasm. The tumor in the testis showed more obvious Sertoli cell features. *(Right)* Metastatic SCT to the lung shows a solid tubular growth pattern with large tumor cells, prominent nucleoli, and abundant eosinophilic cytoplasm separated by delicate fibrovascular septa. Clinical history and immunoreactivity with inhibin and cytokeratin are helpful in making the diagnosis.

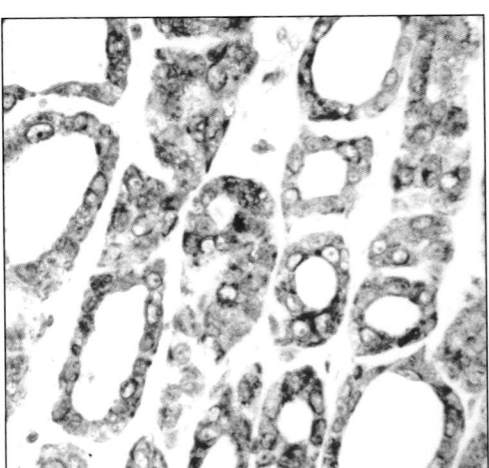

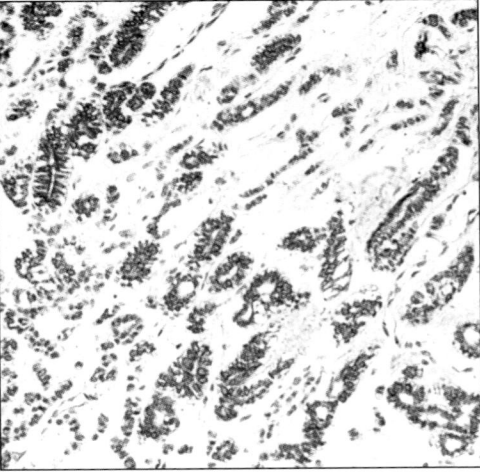

(Left) The tumor cells in this tubular SCT are strongly positive for inhibin. Positive immunoreactivity with inhibin, calretinin, WT1, CD99, and Melan-A(MART-1) are very helpful in establishing sex cord stromal cell differentiation. *(Right)* Tumor cells of SCT are strongly positive for PAN-CK(AE1/AE3), a helpful feature for the diagnosis of SCT. In contrast, Leydig cell tumors and granulosa cell tumors are often weakly or focally positive or negative for cytokeratin.

LARGE CELL CALCIFYING SERTOLI CELL TUMOR

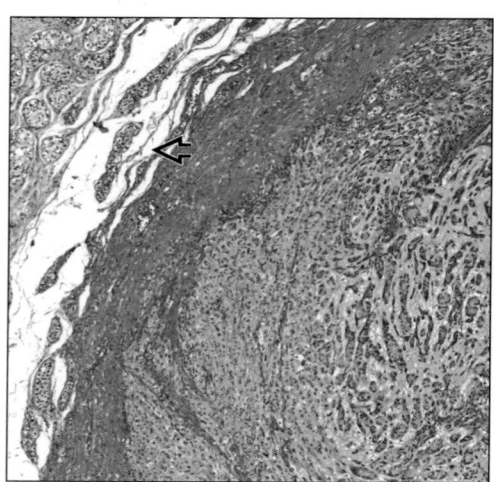

A well-circumscribed LCCSCT is demarcated from the adjacent testis ⊳ by a thick fibrous capsule. The tumor is composed of cords and nests of tumor cells with hyalinized or myxoid stroma.

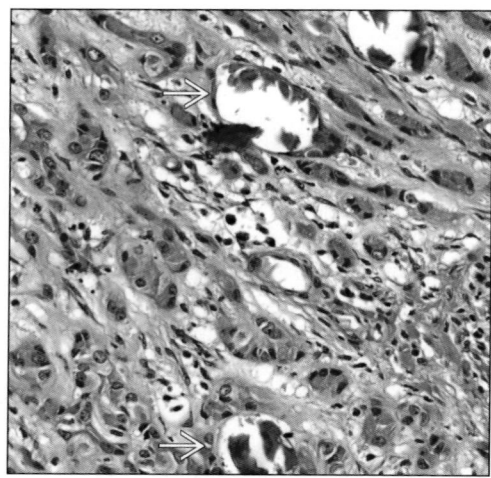

A LCCSCT is shown with cords of large epithelioid cells containing abundant eosinophilic cytoplasm. The hallmark of this tumor is the presence of scattered calcifications ➔.

TERMINOLOGY

Abbreviations
- Large cell calcifying Sertoli cell tumor (LCCSCT)

Definitions
- Variant of Sertoli cell tumor with large epithelioid cells and peculiar calcifications, often associated with clinical syndromes

CLINICAL ISSUES

Epidemiology
- Incidence
  - Extremely rare, < 60 have been reported
- Age
  - Range: 1.5-48 years (average: 16 years)

Presentation
- Slowly enlarging, painless testicular mass
- Sporadic (60%) or as a component of Carney and Peutz-Jeghers syndromes
- Some patients may have gynecomastia or precocious puberty
- Acromegaly or gigantism may be seen due to associated pituitary adenoma
- Association with cardiac myxoma or sudden death
- May be associated with adrenocortical hyperplasia, hypercortisolemia, or testicular Leydig cell tumor
- High frequency of bilaterality (40%) and multifocality (60%)
- Intratubular LCCSCT is a variant of LCCSCT occurring in boys with Peutz-Jeghers syndrome; often estrogenic, bilateral and multifocal; always benign
- Malignant form: Mean age: 39 years; more often unilateral and solitary compared to benign tumors

Treatment
- Surgical approaches

- Orchiectomy is usually curative; long-term follow-up is necessary

Prognosis
- Excellent, but some (20%) may have malignant behavior

IMAGE FINDINGS

Radiographic Findings
- Ultrasound may detect testicular mass with brightly echogenic area (calcification)

MACROSCOPIC FEATURES

General Features
- Well-circumscribed, white-tan or yellow mass associated with granular or gritty calcifications

Size
- Usually smaller than 4 cm

MICROSCOPIC PATHOLOGY

Histologic Features
- Common growth patterns include nests, cords, trabeculae, or solid tubules
- Large polygonal cells with abundant eosinophilic, "ground-glass," or finely granular cytoplasm
- Tumor cells have vesicular nuclei and prominent nucleoli
- Calcifications are a hallmark; large, wavy laminated nodules, sometimes small psammoma bodies and rare ossification
- Fibrous or myxohyaline stroma
- May have marked neutrophilic infiltration
- Intratubular large cell calcifying Sertoli cell tumor
  - Distinct morphologic variant of LCCSCT

LARGE CELL CALCIFYING SERTOLI CELL TUMOR

Key Facts

Terminology
- Variant of Sertoli cell tumor with large epithelioid cells and peculiar calcifications, often associated with clinical syndromes

Clinical Issues
- Extremely rare; only ~ 50 cases have been reported
- Range: 1.5-48 years (average: 16 years)
- Sporadic (60%) or as a component of Carney and Peutz-Jeghers syndromes

Macroscopic Features
- Well-circumscribed white-tan or yellow mass associated with granular or gritty calcification
- Usually smaller than 4 cm

Microscopic Pathology
- Common growth patterns include nests, cords or trabeculae, or solid tubules
- Large polygonal cells with abundant eosinophilic, "ground-glass," or finely granular cytoplasm
- Tumor cells: Vesicular nuclei & prominent nucleoli
- Fibrous or myxohyaline stroma with marked calcifications
- May have marked neutrophilic infiltration
- Some have intratubular growth

Ancillary Tests
- Positive for vimentin, inhibin-α, NSE, S100, desmin, actin-sm
- Negative for cytokeratin (can be focally positive), α-fetoprotein, HCG, PLAP, Podoplanin, and Oct3/4

- o Abnormal large seminiferous tubules filled with Sertoli cells and peritubular basement membrane material with psammoma body-type calcification
- o Sertoli cells often have abundant pale to eosinophilic, vacuolated cytoplasm with fibrillar quality; bland nuclei and no mitosis
- Features seen more often in malignant tumors: size > 4 cm, ≥ 4 mitoses/10 high-power fields, marked cytologic atypia, necrosis, angiolymphatic invasion

Predominant Pattern/Injury Type
- Neoplastic with nests or cords arrangement and calcifications

Predominant Cell/Compartment Type
- Large polygonal cells, superficially resemble Leydig cells

ANCILLARY TESTS

Immunohistochemistry
- Positive for vimentin, Melan-A(MART-1), inhibin-α, NSE, S100, desmin, actin-sm
- Negative for cytokeratin (may be focally positive), α-fetoprotein, HCG, PLAP, Podoplanin(D2-40), and Oct3/4

DIFFERENTIAL DIAGNOSIS

Leydig Cell Tumor
- Usually lacks calcification and has a more solid growth pattern, although it may be rarely ossified
- No intratubular growth and bilaterally is less common
- Usually sporadic with no syndromic association

Tumor of Adrenogenital Syndrome
- Solid growth pattern is more frequent with no intratubular component
- Frequently present between entrapped tubules; lacks calcification

- Prominent fibrous bands and spotty nuclear atypia are common

Sertoli Cell Tumor
- Large epithelioid cells with eosinophilic cytoplasm are distinctly uncommon
- Calcification or neutrophilic infiltration is absent; uncommonly bilateral

DIAGNOSTIC CHECKLIST

Pathologic Interpretation Pearls
- Large cells, calcifications, nests and cords formation, neutrophilic stromal infiltrate
- Tumors with malignant outcome occur in older age group, are unilateral, and less frequently associated with syndromes
- Extratesticular extension, size > 4 cm, frequent mitoses (≥ 4 mitoses/10 hpf), necrosis and vascular invasion are associated with malignant outcome

SELECTED REFERENCES

1. Halat SK et al: Large cell calcifying Sertoli cell tumor of testis. J Urol. 177(6):2338, 2007
2. Ulbright TM et al: Intratubular large cell hyalinizing sertoli cell neoplasia of the testis: a report of 8 cases of a distinctive lesion of the Peutz-Jeghers syndrome. Am J Surg Pathol. 31(6):827-35, 2007
3. Tanaka Y et al: A case of large cell calcifying Sertoli cell tumor in a child with a history of nasal myxoid tumor in infancy. Pathol Int. 49(5):471-6, 1999
4. Kratzer SS et al: Large cell calcifying Sertoli cell tumor of the testis: contrasting features of six malignant and six benign tumors and a review of the literature. Am J Surg Pathol. 21(11):1271-80, 1997
5. Nogales FF et al: Malignant large cell calcifying Sertoli cell tumor of the testis. J Urol. 153(6):1935-7, 1995
6. Plata C et al: Large cell calcifying Sertoli cell tumour of the testis. Histopathology. 26(3):255-9, 1995
7. Tetu B et al: Large cell calcifying Sertoli cell tumor of the testis. A clinicopathologic, immunohistochemical, and ultrastructural study of two cases. Am J Clin Pathol. 96(6):717-22, 1991

4

LARGE CELL CALCIFYING SERTOLI CELL TUMOR

Microscopic Features

(Left) LCCSCT shows cords or tubules of large cells embedded in a fibromyxoid stroma. Multiple scattered calcifications are present. When one sees scattered calcifications in a sex cord stromal tumor, LCCSCT should be the top diagnostic consideration. *(Right)* LCCSCT shows nests of large epithelioid cells with abundant eosinophilic cytoplasm and psammoma body-type calcifications ⮞. Within the myxoid stroma, there are numerous neutrophils ➔.

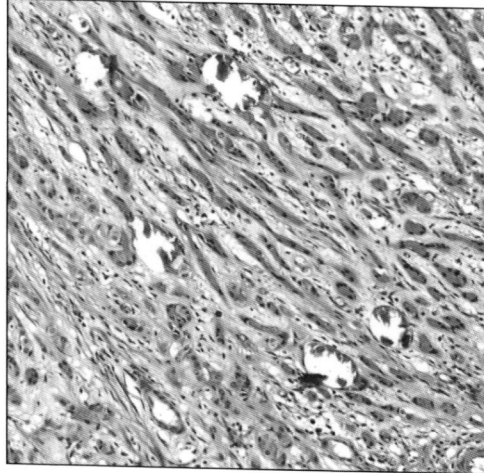
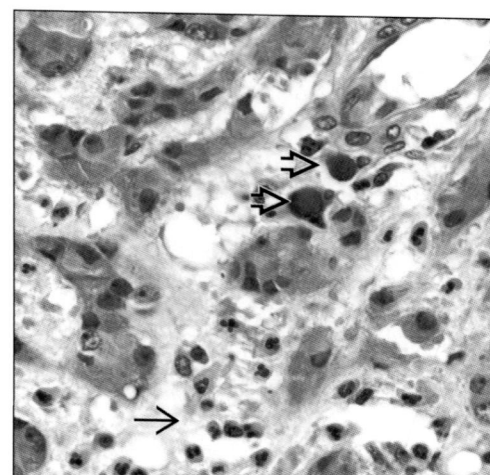

(Left) LCCSCT is seen arranged singly or in groups of large epithelioid cells, surrounded by large areas of calcifications, which are often intercellular. A calcified or ossified Leydig cell tumor should also be included in the differential diagnosis. However, bilaterality and syndrome association favor the diagnosis of LCCSCT. *(Right)* LCCSCT is shown with nests of large epithelioid cells with abundant eosinophilic cytoplasm. A large area of calcification is seen in the loose fibromyxoid stroma.

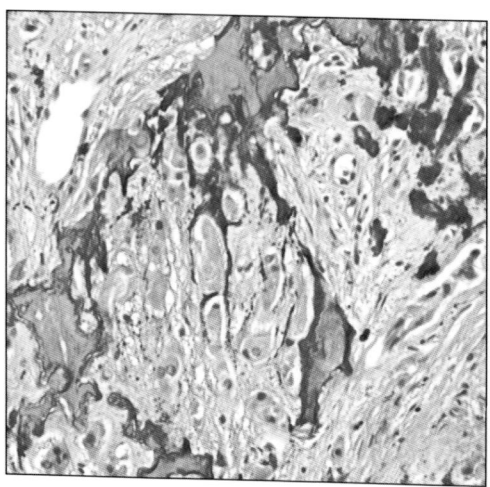
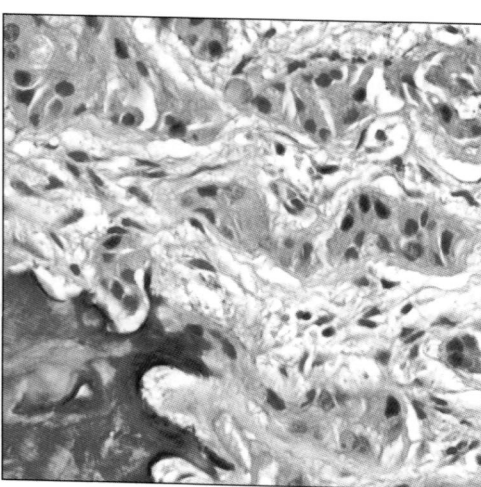

(Left) LCCSCT shows cords and small nests of large epithelioid cells embedded in a fibrous background with dense neutrophilic infiltrate and a psammoma body ⮞. A neutrophilic background is an important diagnostic feature. *(Right)* Cords and trabeculae of large epithelioid cells embedded in a fibromyxoid background is typical for LCCSCT. A large area of calcification ➔ is present. There is marked morphologic overlap with Leydig cell tumor, which does not have an intratubular component.

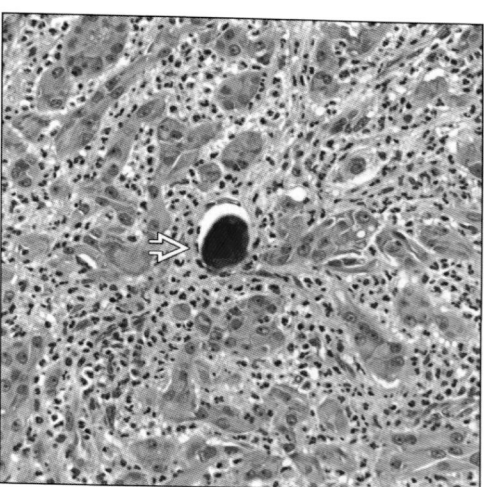
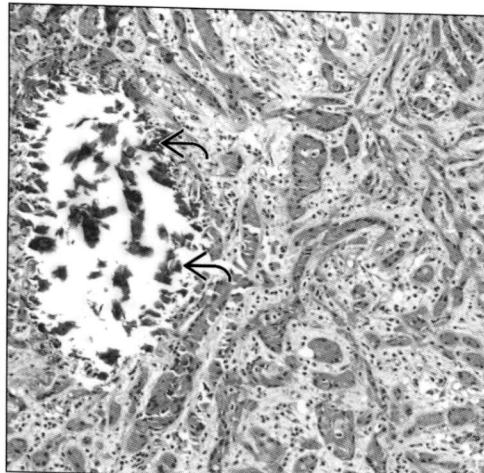

LARGE CELL CALCIFYING SERTOLI CELL TUMOR

Microscopic Features and Differential Diagnoses

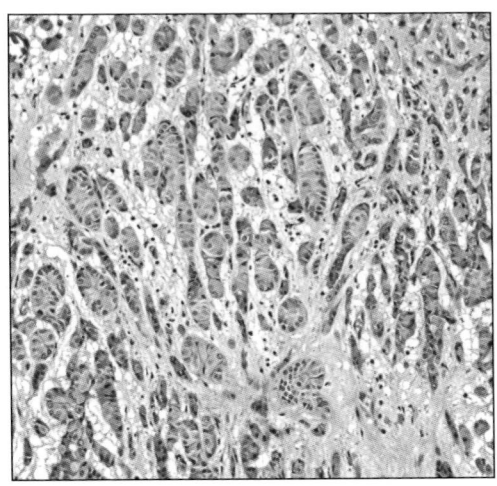

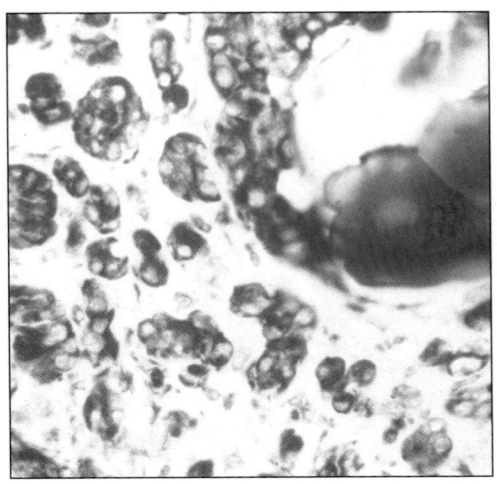

(Left) LCCSCT shows solid tubules and trabeculae of large epithelioid cells with abundant eosinophilic cytoplasm. In the absence of prominent calcification, Leydig cell tumor and testicular tumor of adrenogenital syndrome are in the differential. *(Right)* Similar to other sex cord stromal cell tumors, the tumor cells in a LCCSCT are strongly positive for inhibin by immunohistochemistry. S100 and keratin positivity are more common compared to Leydig cell tumor.

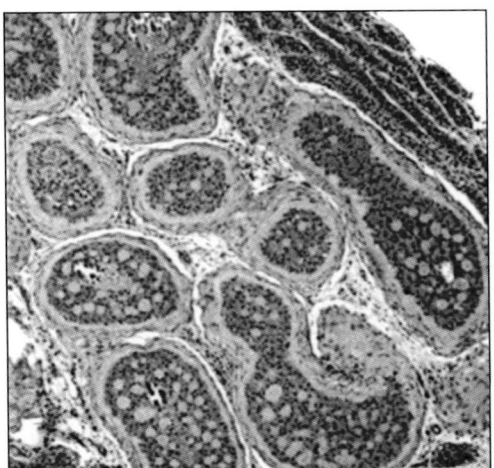

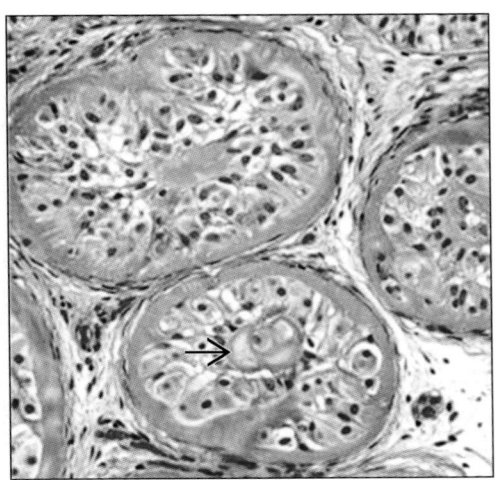

(Left) Testicular tumor occurring in a patient with Peutz-Jeghers syndrome is shown. There is prominent expansion and intratubular growth of cells resembling Sertoli cells and associated with peritubular and intratubular hyalinization. *(Right)* Testicular tumor in a patient with Peutz-Jeghers syndrome is shown. The cytoplasm tumor cells have a fibrillary quality with uniform nuclei and nucleoli. Note the prominent peritubular and intratubular hyalinization and dystrophic calcification ⊡.

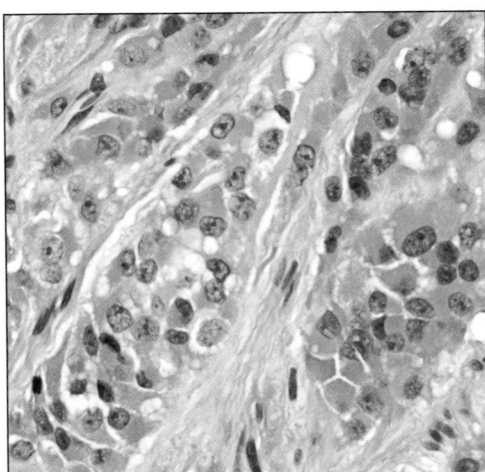

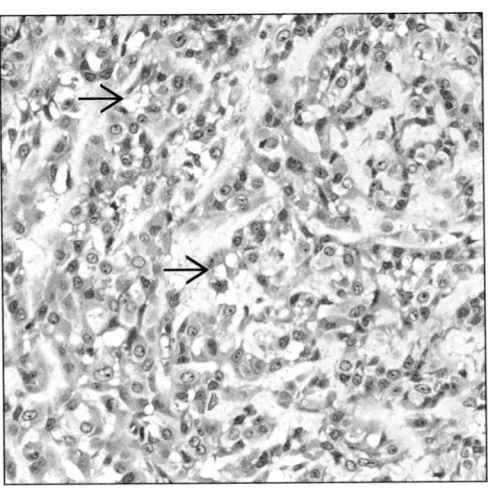

(Left) High-power photomicrograph of a Leydig cell tumor shows cords and nests of large epithelioid tumor cells with abundant eosinophilic cytoplasm. There are no calcifications or neutrophilic infiltrates, which are often seen in a LCCSCT. *(Right)* A Sertoli cell tumor is composed of nests of tumor cells with eosinophilic cytoplasm and myxoid stroma. There are cytoplasmic vacuoles ⊡. Bilaterality and multifocality are rare in Sertoli cell tumors, compared to LCCSCT.

GRANULOSA CELL TUMOR

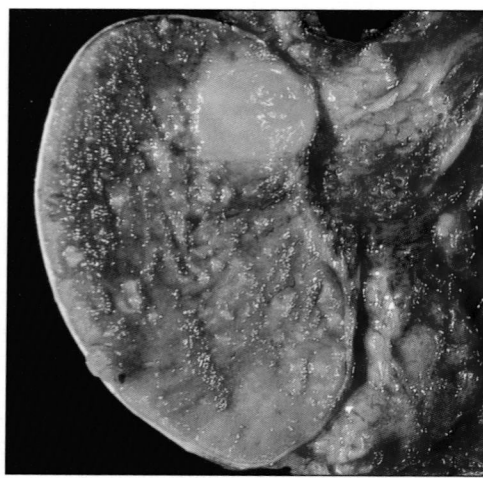

A GCT shows a well-circumscribed, homogeneous, tan-white nodule. The tumor is small and like many sex cord stromal tumors, does not extensively involve the testis. Hemorrhage and necrosis are lacking.

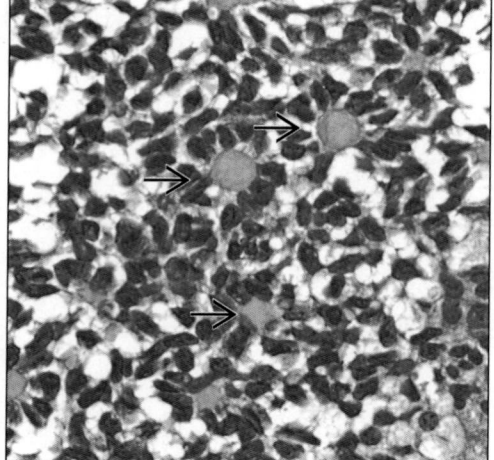

A GCT shows typical Call-Exner bodies ⇨ characterized by central eosinophilic material and palisading tumor cells resulting in a rosette appearance. The tumor cells have scant cytoplasm.

TERMINOLOGY

Abbreviations
- Granulosa cell tumor (GCT)

Definitions
- Sex cord stromal tumor of testis occurring in adults and resembling its counterpart of ovarian granulosa cell tumor

CLINICAL ISSUES

Epidemiology
- Incidence
  - Extremely rare; fewer than 2 dozen cases have been documented
- Age
  - Range: 16-76 years (mean: 44 years)
  - Juvenile GCT occurs in 1st few months of life

Presentation
- Painless testicular mass
- May be associated with gynecomastia (about 25%)

Treatment
- Surgical approaches
  - Curable by surgical resection in most cases
  - May be managed by partial orchiectomy

Prognosis
- Most have indolent clinical course but have malignant potential
- Metastasis has been reported (20% of cases)
- Long-term follow-up is recommended for all patients

MACROSCOPIC FEATURES

General Features
- Well-circumscribed, sometimes encapsulated, homogeneous yellow to gray firm mass
- ± small cysts
- Hemorrhage or necrosis is unusual

Size
- Range: 2-10 cm (average: 5 cm)

MICROSCOPIC PATHOLOGY

Histologic Features
- Growth patterns: Microfollicular (most common), solid, trabecular, insular, macrofollicular, gyriform, or cystic
- Presence of Call-Exner bodies (eosinophilic material surrounded by palisading granulosa cells)
- Relatively uniform round or ovoid cells (carrot-shaped) with scant, lightly staining cytoplasm
- Elongated or angular nuclei with grooves (coffee bean-shaped) with 1 or 2 peripherally located nucleoli
- Focal cytologic atypia and rare mitoses; mitoses may be high with varying degree of nuclear pleomorphism
- May intermingle with seminiferous tubules and infiltrate tunica albuginea
- Some show focal theca cell differentiation or have smooth muscle or osteoid differentiation
- Rare hemorrhage, necrosis, or angiolymphatic invasion
- Features seen more often in tumors with malignant outcome: Large size (> 7 cm), frequent mitoses (> 4/10 HPFs), hemorrhage, necrosis, lymphovascular invasion

Predominant Pattern/Injury Type
- Solid and microfollicular

Predominant Cell/Compartment Type
- Sex cord stromal cells of granulosa cell type

GRANULOSA CELL TUMOR

Key Facts

Terminology
- Testicular tumor of granulosa cell differentiation resembling analogous ovarian counterpart

Clinical Issues
- Extremely rare; fewer than 2 dozen cases have been well documented
- Range: 16-76 years (average: 44 years)

Macroscopic Features
- Well-circumscribed, sometimes encapsulated, homogeneous yellow to gray firm mass

Microscopic Pathology
- Growth patterns: Microfollicular (most common), solid, trabecular, insular, macrofollicular, gyriform, or cystic

- Presence of Call-Exner bodies (eosinophilic materials surrounded by palisading granulosa cells)
- Relatively uniform round or ovoid cells (carrot-shaped) with scant, lightly staining cytoplasm
- Elongated or angular nuclei with groove (coffee bean-shaped) with 1 or 2 peripherally located nucleoli
- Some show focal theca cell differentiation or have smooth muscle or osteoid differentiation
- Features seen more often in malignant tumor: Large size (> 7 cm), hemorrhage, necrosis, lymphovascular invasion

Ancillary Tests
- Positive for vimentin, inhibin, calretinin, SMA, CD56, and focally positive for PAN-CK(AE1/AE3)
- Negative for PLAP, Podoplanin(D2-40), Oct3/4, AFP, HCG, CD30(BerH2)

ANCILLARY TESTS

Immunohistochemistry
- Positive for inhibin, Melan-A(MART-1), calretinin, actin-sm, CD56, CD99, vimentin; focally positive for PAN-CK(AE1/AE3)
- Negative for PLAP, Podoplanin(D2-40), Oct3/4, SALL4, AFP, HCG, CD30(BerH2)

DIFFERENTIAL DIAGNOSIS

Malignant Lymphoma
- Interstitial growth of discohesive lymphoid cells
- Frequently bilateral with spermatic cord involvement
- Old age presentation
- Positive for CD45(LCA) and frequently for B-cell markers; negative for PAN-CK(AE1/AE3) and inhibin-α

Small Cell Carcinoma
- Frequent mitoses or apoptoses
- Positive for neuroendocrine markers (synaptophysin and chromogranin) and negative for inhibin-α

Carcinoid Tumor
- Typical organoid, insular, or trabecular growth patterns
- Diffusely positive for neuroendocrine markers, strong and diffuse PAN-CK(AE1/AE3) positive and negative for inhibin-α

Sertoli Cell Tumor
- More prominent well-formed tubules, cords, and nests
- Abundant clear or eosinophilic cytoplasm with large vesicular nuclei and prominent centrally located nucleoli
- Positive for PAN-CK(AE1/AE3)

Leydig Cell Tumor
- Solid growth with fine fibrous or fibromyxoid septa
- Abundant eosinophilic cytoplasm, often round nuclei and prominent nucleoli

Mixed Germ Cell and Sex Cord Stromal Tumor (Gonadoblastoma or Unclassified)
- Prominent rounded nests with large seminoma-like cells
- Spindle cell or round cell unclassified stromal component or differentiated stromal component, including granulosa cell
- Positive for germ cell markers (Oct3/4, CD117, Podoplanin[D2-40]) and sex cord stromal markers (inhibin, Melan-A(MART-1), CD99)

Unclassified/Mixed Sex Cord Stromal Tumor
- Spindle cell or round cell unclassified stromal component ± differentiated stromal component, including granulosa cell component

DIAGNOSTIC CHECKLIST

Pathologic Interpretation Pearls
- Carrot-shaped cells with nuclear grooves and Call-Exner bodies resembling ovarian counterpart

SELECTED REFERENCES

1. Hammerich KH et al: Malignant advanced granulosa cell tumor of the adult testis: case report and review of the literature. Hum Pathol. 39(5):701-9, 2008
2. Suppiah A et al: Adult granulosa cell tumour of the testis and bony metastasis. A report of the first case of granulosa cell tumour of the testicle metastasising to bone. Urol Int. 75(1):91-3, 2005
3. Guzzo T et al: Granulosa cell tumor of the contralateral testis in a man with a history of cryptorchism. Urol Int. 72(1):85-7, 2004
4. Wang BY et al: Gonadal tumor with granulosa cell tumor features in an adult testis. Ann Diagn Pathol. 6(1):56-60, 2002
5. Al-Bozom IA et al: Granulosa cell tumor of the adult type: a case report and review of the literature of a very rare testicular tumor. Arch Pathol Lab Med. 124(10):1525-8, 2000

GRANULOSA CELL TUMOR

Gross and Microscopic Features

(Left) A well-circumscribed AGCT with adjacent uninvolved testicular seminiferous tubules ➡️ is shown. The tumor is arranged in solid nests, trabeculae, and micro- and macrofollicles. *(Right)* GCT with gyriform, trabecular, macro- and microfollicular growth patterns is shown. The entire tumor should have similar cytologic features to be designated as GCT, as tumors may contain other sex cord stromal elements, justifying the classification of a mixed sex cord stromal tumor.

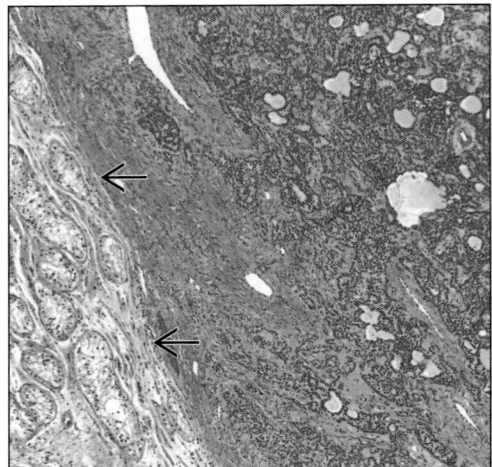
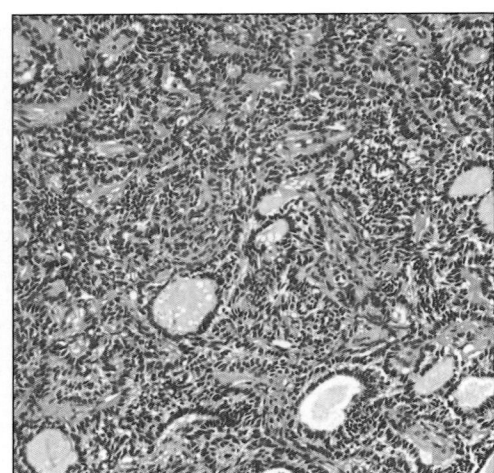

(Left) GCT shows diffuse growth pattern and focal palisading. The tumor is composed of carrot-shaped spindle cells with scant pale staining cytoplasm. No pleomorphism or necrosis is seen. When these cells predominate, unclassified sex cord stromal tumor should be included in the differential diagnosis. *(Right)* The tumor cells of a GCT have angulated nuclei, pale staining chromatin, and clear to lightly eosinophilic cytoplasm. Occasional nuclear grooves ➡️ are present.

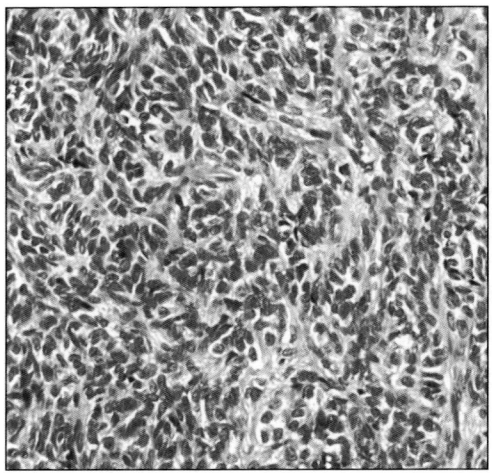
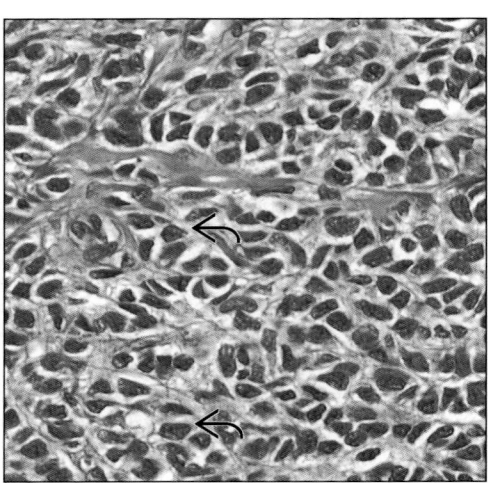

(Left) High-power photomicrograph of GCT shows macrofollicles ➡️ with eosinophilic amorphous edematous fluid and microfollicles with central eosinophilic material (Call-Exner body ➡️). *(Right)* High-power view of GCT shows sheets of tumor cells and a Call-Exner body ➡️. The tumor cells have elongated or angulated nuclei with occasional nuclear grooves ➡️ and scant cytoplasm. GCT is positive for sex cord stromal markers, including inhibin, Melan-A(MART-1), CD99, and WT1.

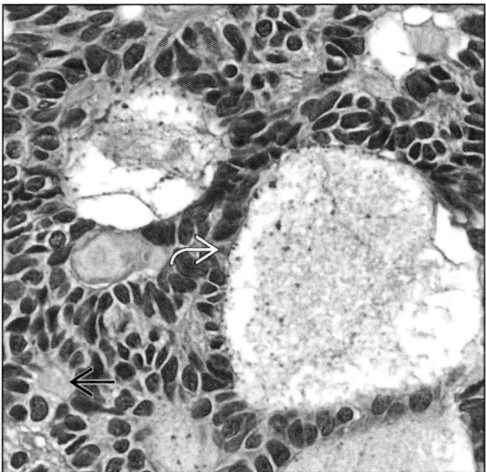
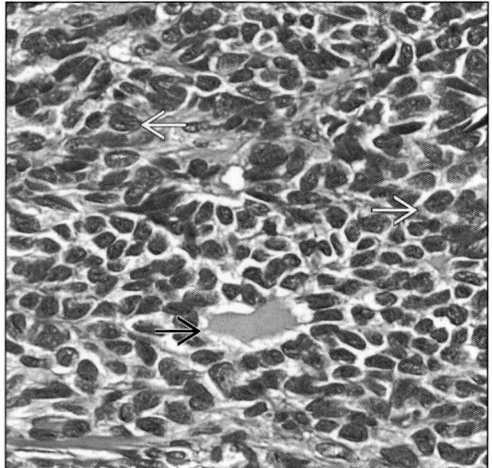

GRANULOSA CELL TUMOR

Microscopic and Immunohistochemical Features

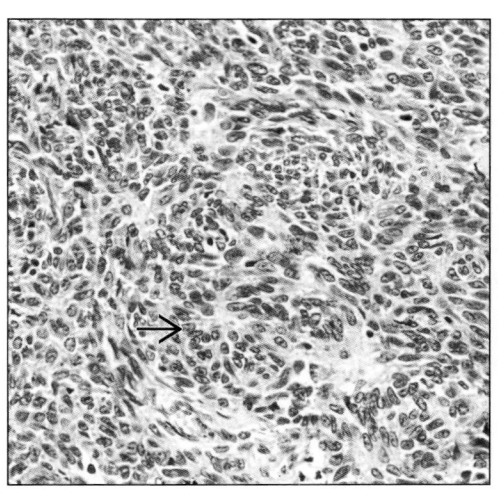

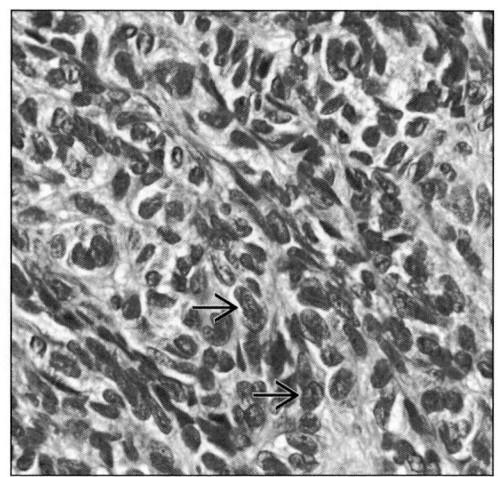

(Left) Some GCTs show a more prominent spindle cell appearance (pseudosarcomatous appearance). Vague follicular differentiation with rosette appearance ⊡ is discernible. *(Right)* GCT with pseudosarcomatous appearance is shown. Random cellular pleomorphism and crowding are evident. The cells are carrot-shaped with occasional nuclear grooves ⊡, which are characteristic cytologic features of GCT.

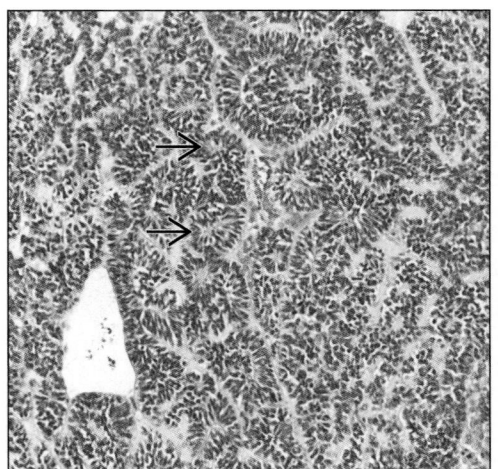

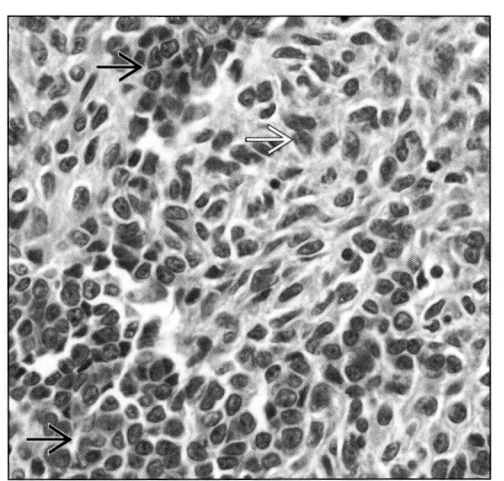

(Left) GCT shows epithelial growth pattern with nests or trabeculae composed of elongated hyperchromatic tumor cells. Although small follicular arrangement ⊡ is present, no well-defined Call-Exner bodies are seen. *(Right)* GCT shows nests ⊡ of tumor cells with ovoid to round nuclei, small nucleoli, and occasional nuclear grooves ⊡. Mitotic rate is generally low in these tumors and rarely a prominent fibrothecomatous pattern may be present.

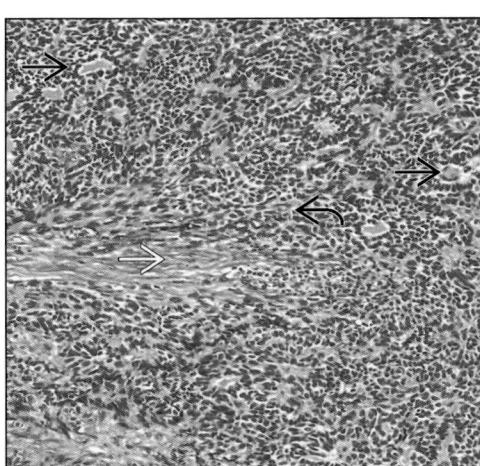

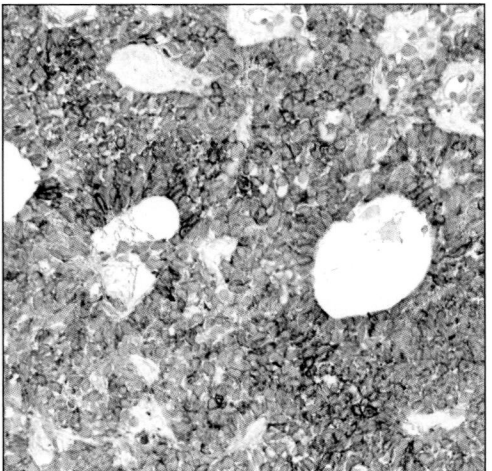

(Left) GCT has numerous microfollicles (Call-Exner bodies ⊡) intermingled with spindle cells ⊡ and spindle cells with possible myogenic differentiation ⊡ showing fibrillar cytoplasm. *(Right)* Tumor cells of GCT are diffusely positive for inhibin-α, a diagnostic immunostain for all sex cord stromal tumors. GCT is positive for sex cord stromal markers, including inhibin, Melan-A(MART-1), calretinin, CD99, and WT1. EMA/MUC1 and CK7 are usually negative.

JUVENILE GRANULOSA CELL TUMOR

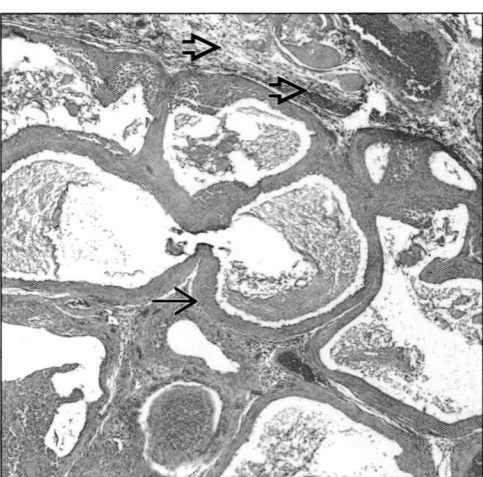

JGCT, which is relatively well circumscribed from the surrounding testis ⊵, is composed of multicystic follicular spaces lined by multilayers of granulosa cells ⊳ containing basophilic fluid.

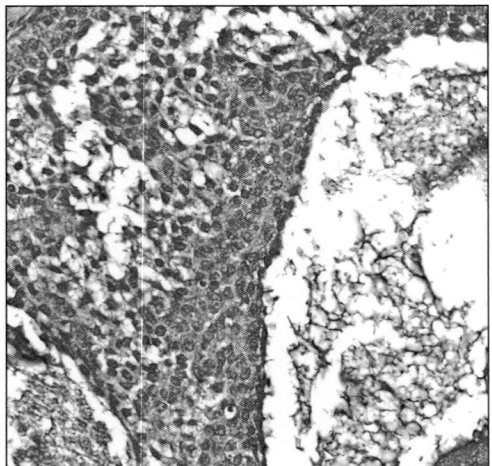

JGCT has solid and follicular areas composed of cells with uniform round to oval nuclei and moderate cytoplasm. Prominent extracellular and intraluminal basophilic mucinous material is present.

TERMINOLOGY

Abbreviations
- Juvenile granulosa cell tumor (JGCT)

Definitions
- Testicular tumor that is multicystic and composed of multiple follicles lined by granulosa and theca-like cells occurring predominantly in infants

CLINICAL ISSUES

Epidemiology
- Incidence
  - Extremely rare in testis
  - Most common testicular tumor in infants
  - 6.6% of all prepubertal testicular tumors
- Age
  - Infants younger than 2 years (most younger than 6 months)
  - Rarely occurs in adults

Presentation
- Painless scrotal or abdominal mass
- Associations
  - Undescended testes
  - Gonadal dysgenesis with chromosomal abnormality affecting Y chromosome or 45X/46XY mosaicism (Denys-Drash syndrome)
- Contralateral testis is often undescended
- No known presentation with gynecomastia or endocrine disorders

Treatment
- Surgical approaches
  - Orchiectomy is curative
  - Partial orchiectomy (testis sparing) may be option

Prognosis
- Clinically benign

- Malignant behavior or metastasis has not been reported

IMAGE FINDINGS

General Features
- Complex, multiseptated, hypoechoic mass on ultrasonography

MACROSCOPIC FEATURES

General Features
- Well-circumscribed or partially encapsulated multicystic mass with solid yellow and papillary areas

Size
- Range: 0.8-6.0 cm

MICROSCOPIC PATHOLOGY

Histologic Features
- Multiple irregular cystic areas interspersed with solid areas
- Variably sized follicles lined by oval to round cells arranged in single or multiple layers with outer layers resembling theca cells
- Granulosa cells have round to ovoid nuclei, inconspicuous nucleoli, and scanty to vacuolated cytoplasm
- Mitotic activity is usually evident and often prominent
- Theca-like cells are elongated and have scant cytoplasm
- Basophilic to faintly eosinophilic fluid within follicles
- Call-Exner bodies and nuclear grooves that are often seen in adult GCT are absent
- Sarcomatoid transformation has not been reported, in contrast to ovarian counterpart

JUVENILE GRANULOSA CELL TUMOR

Key Facts

Terminology
- Testicular tumor that is multicystic and composed of multiple follicles lined by granulosa and theca-like cells

Clinical Issues
- Rare, but is most common congenital testicular neoplasm (6.6 % of all prepubertal testicular tumors)
- Infants younger than 2 years old; most common testis tumor in infants < 6 months

Macroscopic Features
- Well-circumscribed or partially encapsulated multicystic mass with solid yellow and papillary areas

Microscopic Pathology
- Multiple irregular cystic areas interspersed with solid areas

- Variably sized follicles lined by bland-looking oval round cells arranged in single or multiple layers with outer layers resembling theca cells
- Granulosa cells have round to ovoid nuclei, inconspicuous nucleoli, scanty, vacuolated cytoplasm
- Mitotic activity is usually evident and often prominent
- Basophilic to faintly eosinophilic fluid within follicles
- Call-Exner bodies and nuclear grooves, often seen in adult GCT are absent

Ancillary Tests
- Positive for Cam5.2, vimentin, S100; focal actin-sm, inhibin-α, CD99
- Negative for EMA/MUC1, cytokeratin, α-fetoprotein, PLAP, Podoplanin(D2-40), Oct3/4, SALL4, glypican-3, CD45(LCA)

Predominant Pattern/Injury Type
- Cystic and solid growth pattern

Predominant Cell/Compartment Type
- Sex cord stromal cell tumor

ANCILLARY TESTS

Immunohistochemistry
- Positive for Cam5.2, vimentin, S100; focally positive for actin-sm, desmin, inhibin-α, and CD99
- Negative for EMA/MUC1, cytokeratin, α-fetoprotein, Podoplanin(D2-40), Oct3/4, glypican-3, SALL4, CD45(LCA)

DIFFERENTIAL DIAGNOSIS

Yolk Sac Tumor
- Occurs more commonly in older age group (> 1 year)
- Variety of patterns, including microcystic and reticular, within the same tumor
- Cysts are lined by single layer of cells with greater atypia
- Presence of intracellular or extracellular eosinophilic hyaline globules and Schiller-Duval bodies
- Positive for germ cell markers (α-fetoprotein, SALL4, glypican-3) and cytokeratin
- Negative for S100 and inhibin-α

Sex Cord Stromal Tumor, Unclassified
- Variable morphologic patterns with biphasic epithelioid and spindle cell components
- Lack of cystic follicles

Rhabdomyosarcoma
- More typically in paratesticular location
- Lacks follicle formation; small round blue cells with rhabdomyoblasts
- Positive for desmin, MYOD1, and myogenin

DIAGNOSTIC CHECKLIST

Pathologic Interpretation Pearls
- Variably sized follicles lined by round to ovoid cells; occurs in patients < 6 months of age

SELECTED REFERENCES

1. Dudani R et al: Juvenile granulosa cell tumor of testis: case report and review of literature. Am J Perinatol. 25(4):229-31, 2008
2. Alexiev BA et al: Testicular juvenile granulosa cell tumor in a newborn: case report and review of the literature. Int J Surg Pathol. 15(3):321-5, 2007
3. Shukla AR et al: Juvenile granulosa cell tumor of the testis:: contemporary clinical management and pathological diagnosis. J Urol. 171(5):1900-2, 2004
4. Fagin R et al: Juvenile granulosa cell tumor of the testis. Urology. 62(2):351, 2003
5. Chan YF et al: Juvenile granulosa cell tumor of the testis: report of two cases in newborns. J Pediatr Surg. 32(5):752-3, 1997
6. Perez-Atayde AR et al: Juvenile granulosa cell tumor of the infantile testis. Evidence of a dual epithelial-smooth muscle differentiation. Am J Surg Pathol. 20(1):72-9, 1996
7. Groisman GM et al: Juvenile granulosa cell tumor of the testis: a comparative immunohistochemical study with normal infantile gonads. Pediatr Pathol. 13(4):389-400, 1993
8. May D et al: Juvenile granulosa cell tumor of an intraabdominal testis. Pediatr Radiol. 22(7):507-8, 1992
9. Nistal M et al: Juvenile granulosa cell tumor of the testis. Arch Pathol Lab Med. 112(11):1129-32, 1988
10. Lawrence WD et al: Juvenile granulosa cell tumor of the infantile testis. A report of 14 cases. Am J Surg Pathol. 9(2):87-94, 1985
11. Young RH et al: Juvenile granulosa cell tumor--another neoplasm associated with abnormal chromosomes and ambiguous genitalia. A report of three cases. Am J Surg Pathol. 9(10):737-43, 1985

Microscopic Features

(Left) JGCT is composed of cystic/follicular structures ➡ and solid tumor components. The follicular/cystic lumen is filled with basophilic secretion characteristic of JGCT. *(Right)* JGCT is composed of follicular and solid components of tumor with fibrous stroma. The follicular lumen is filled with basophilic secretion. Also seen is spindle theca-like cells in the stroma ➡. Separated from the tumor by a thin fibrous tissue are immature seminiferous tubules ➡.

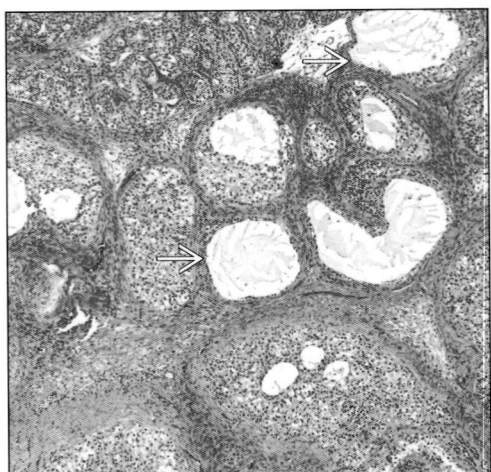
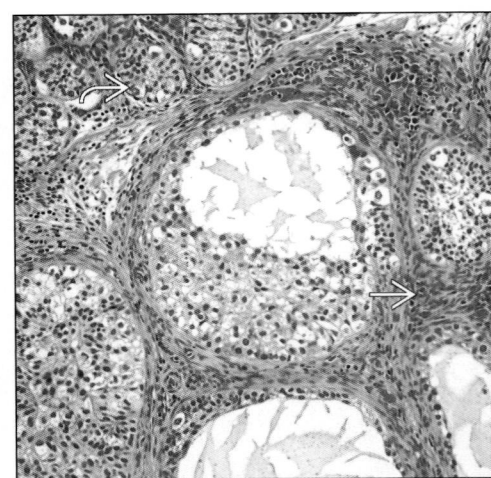

(Left) JGCT with mixed solid and follicular patterns is shown. The tumor cells in both areas are similar and have round to ovoid nuclei, inconspicuous nucleoli, and eosinophilic to vacuolated cytoplasm. Mitotic activity is variable and frequently brisk. *(Right)* High-power photomicrograph of JGCT shows a follicle lined by uniform tumor cells with oval to round nuclei and moderate amounts of pale eosinophilic and vacuolated cytoplasm. The basophilic material is positive for mucicarmine.

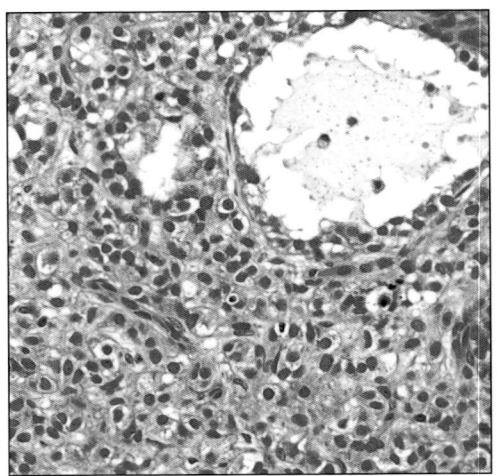
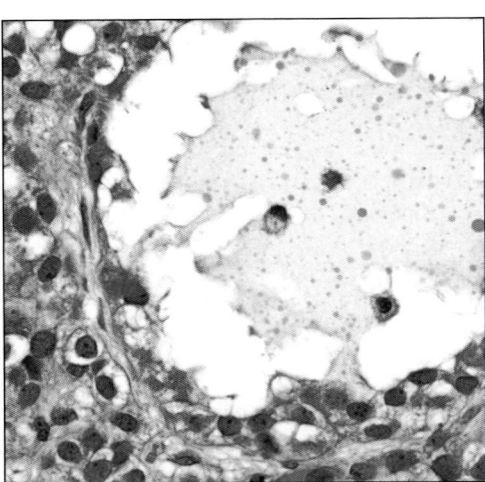

(Left) The solid area in a JGCT is shown. Medium- to large-sized tumor cells are arranged in sheets. The nuclei lack nuclear grooves and have numerous mitoses ➡. There is abundant clear to eosinophilic and vacuolated cytoplasm. *(Right)* A solid area of JGCT is shown with relatively uniform tumor cells with moderate amounts of pale eosinophilic and vacuolated cytoplasm, a feature that is not typically seen in adult GCT. Call-Exner-like structures and nuclear grooves are not present.

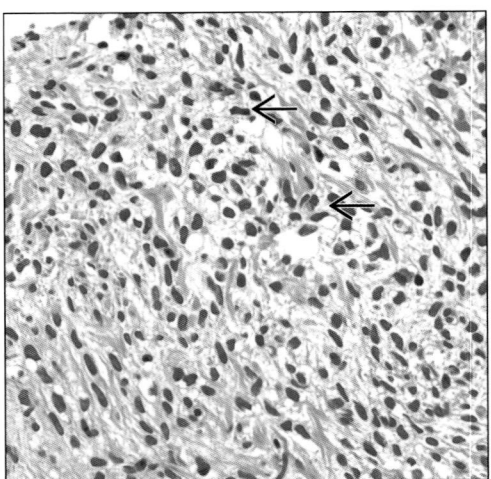
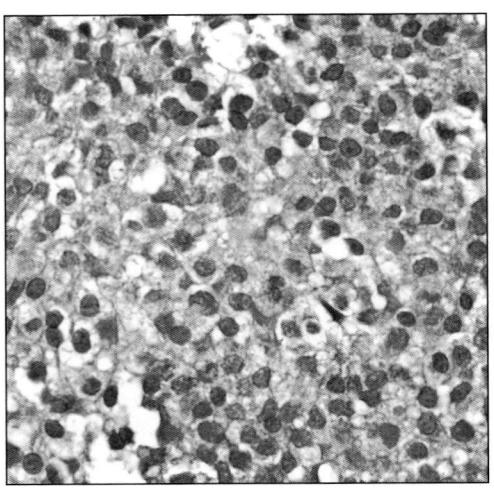

JUVENILE GRANULOSA CELL TUMOR

Microscopic Features

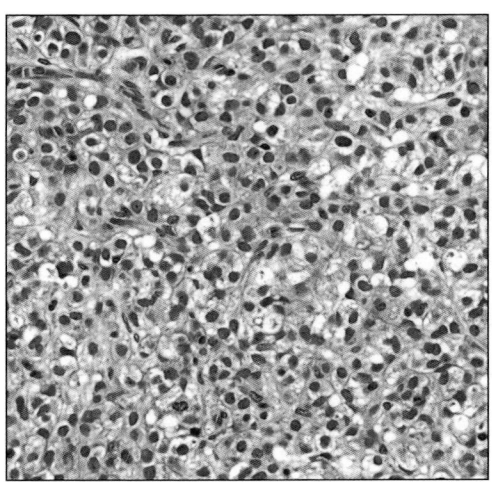
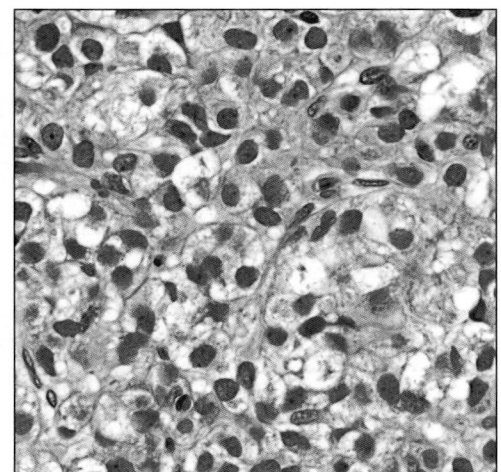

(Left) The solid area of JGCT shows uniform tumor cells. Nuclear pleomorphism or necrosis is not seen. *(Right)* High-power photomicrograph of JGCT shows tumor cells that are relatively uniform with ovoid to round nuclei, occasional small nucleoli, and abundant pale eosinophilic and vacuolated cytoplasm. Mitotic activity may be brisk. The cells of JGCT are not carrot-shaped and lack nuclear grooves. Solid areas may be interspersed by areas with prominent hyalinization.

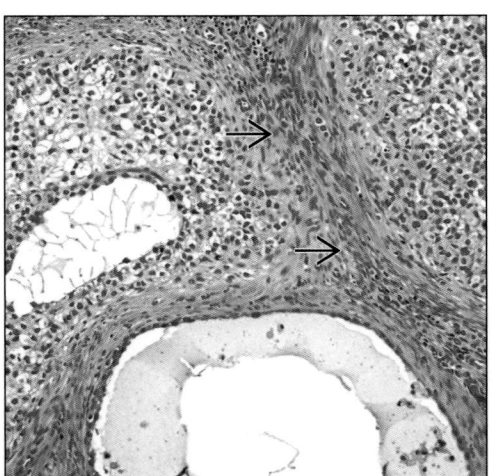
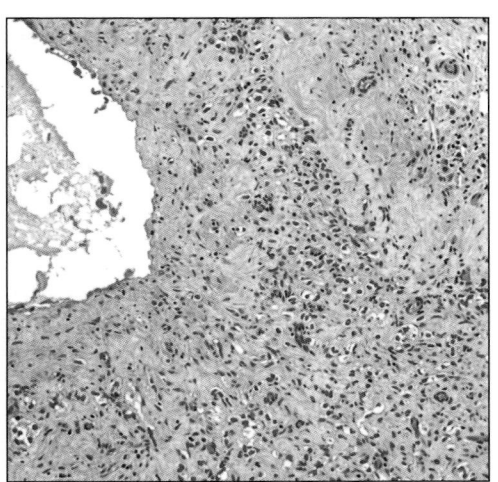

(Left) The tumor cells in both cystic/follicular and solid areas of JGCT are similar. Cellular theca-like spindle cells ➡ are seen in the stroma. When myxoid areas are prominent, the resemblance to reticular pattern of yolk sac tumor may be marked. *(Right)* The cystic and solid components of JGCT show degeneration and fibrosis with paucity of tumor cells and stromal collagenization in the solid area.

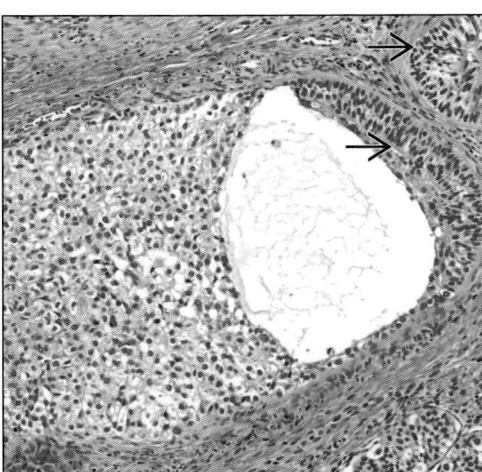
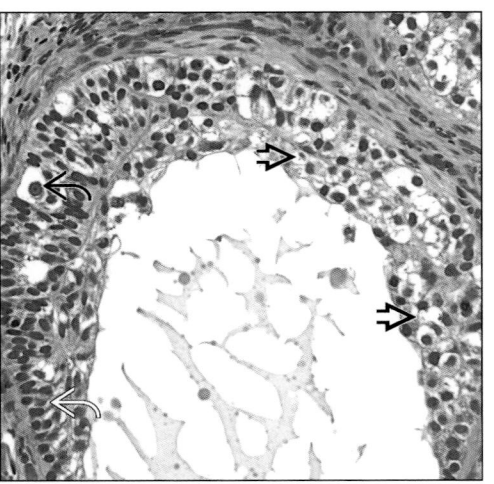

(Left) A large cystic follicle is partially involved by JGCT. Residual immature seminiferous tubules lined by Sertoli cells ➡ are seen at the periphery. Basophilic secretions, a hallmark of the tumor, are a helpful feature. *(Right)* High-power photomicrograph shows a large cystic follicle partially involved by JGCT cells ➡. Residual seminiferous tubule contains Sertoli cells ➡ and immature germ cells with large nuclei ➡. There is absence of intratubular germ cell neoplasia.

TESTICULAR "TUMOR" OF ADRENOGENITAL SYNDROME

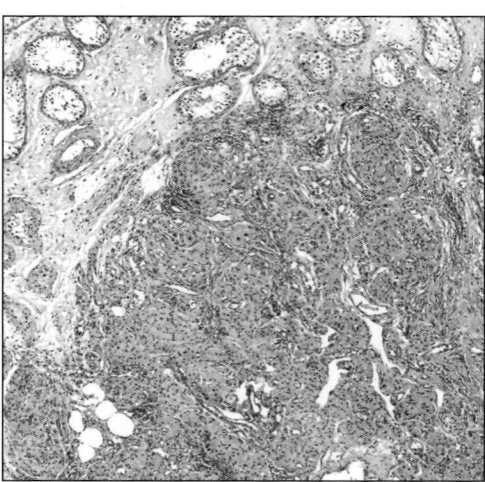

TTAGS shows a well-circumscribed nodule composed of cells with abundant eosinophilic cytoplasm similar to that of a Leydig cell tumor. (Courtesy R. H. Young, MD.)

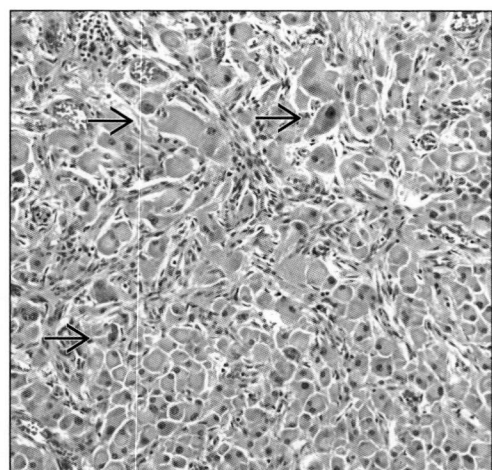

This TTAGS is composed of large polygonal cells with abundant eosinophilic cytoplasm. Random cells show nuclear pleomorphism ➡. Multifocality and bilaterality are common. (Courtesy R. H. Young, MD.)

TERMINOLOGY

Abbreviations
- Testicular "tumor" of adrenogenital syndrome (TTAGS)

Synonyms
- Congenital adrenal hyperplasia

Definitions
- Benign bilateral testicular lesions in patients with congenital adrenal hyperplasia leading to growth of adrenal-like cells in testis that resemble Leydig cell tumor
- Bilaterality, multifocality, and response to medical treatment argue against this being a neoplastic lesion

ETIOLOGY/PATHOGENESIS

Developmental Anomaly
- 21-hydroxylase deficiency (most common)
- Other associated conditions
  - 11-hydroxylase deficiency
  - Cushing disease
  - Addison disease
  - Idiopathic enzyme defect
- Cellular origin uncertain; hilar pluripotential cells, adrenal cortical rest cells, Leydig cells are possible candidates

CLINICAL ISSUES

Epidemiology
- Incidence
  - Rare; a few dozen cases reported
- Age
  - Children to early adult (average: 22.5 years)

Presentation
- Bilateral orchialgia (92%)
- Testicular masses (2/3 palpable)
- Symptoms related to steroid hormone deficiency
  - Salt-losing form of adrenal disorder in 2/3 and non-salt-losing form in 1/3
- Isosexual precocious puberty

Laboratory Tests
- Steroid hormone evaluation (increased ACTH)
- Tumor markers (AFP, hCG, LDH) to exclude possible germ cell tumor

Treatment
- Drugs
  - Exogenous high-dose corticosteroids are mainstay of medical treatment (pain control and regression of tumor)
- Surgical approaches
  - Tumor enucleation or partial orchiectomy for persistently painful masses and steroid unresponsive lesions in setting of bilaterality
  - Radical orchiectomy is generally not indicated

Prognosis
- Benign lesion, symptoms relieved by steroid therapy or surgery
- Very rarely associated with seminoma, and 1 reported case of malignant transformation

IMAGE FINDINGS

Ultrasonographic Findings
- Bilateral hypoechoic intraparenchymal infiltrative nodules with variable vascularity

MACROSCOPIC FEATURES

General Features
- Well-circumscribed but not encapsulated, dark brown, lobulated mass with fibrous septa

TESTICULAR "TUMOR" OF ADRENOGENITAL SYNDROME

Key Facts

Terminology
- Benign bilateral testicular tumor in patients with congenital adrenal hyperplasia leading to growth of adrenal-like cells in testis that resembles Leydig cell tumor

Clinical Issues
- Age: Children to early adult (average: 22.5 years)
- Presentation
  - Bilateral orchialgia (92%)
  - Testicular masses (2/3 palpable)
- Exogenous high-dose corticosteroids are standard medical treatment (pain control, regression of tumor)

Macroscopic Features
- Well-circumscribed but not encapsulated, dark brown, lobulated mass with fibrous septa
- Often bilateral (83%), frequently multiple nodules

Microscopic Pathology
- Sheets, nests, cords, nodules, or diffuse proliferation of large cells separated by band of fibrous tissue
- Polyhedral or polygonal cells resembling Leydig cells
- Abundant eosinophilic cytoplasm with lipofuscin pigment
- Centrally located nuclei and prominent nucleoli
- Frequent nuclear pleomorphism, but no or rare mitoses
- Lack of Reinke crystalloid material

Ancillary Tests
- Positive for vimentin, inhibin, Melan-A(MART-1), and synaptophysin

---

- Often bilateral (83%), frequently multiple nodules
- Most commonly present in hilar region (86%)

Size
- Range: 0.5-10 cm
- Larger size tumor usually seen in older patients

MICROSCOPIC PATHOLOGY

Histologic Features
- Sheets, nests, cords, nodules, or diffuse proliferation of large cells separated by bands of fibrous tissue
- Polyhedral or polygonal cells resembling Leydig cells
- Abundant eosinophilic cytoplasm with lipofuscin pigment, which may be prominent and diffuse
- Centrally located nuclei and prominent nucleoli
- Frequent nuclear pleomorphism but no or rare mitoses
- Crystalloids of Reinke are absent
- May have adipocytic metaplasia and lymphoid aggregates
- Extensive fibrosis may be present
- Atrophic or sclerotic seminiferous tubules present within lesion
- Myelolipomatous component has been reported

Predominant Pattern/Injury Type
- Neoplastic vs. hyperplastic

Predominant Cell/Compartment Type
- Cells of unknown histogenesis resembling Leydig cells but without Reinke crystalloids may arise from pluripotential hilar cells

ANCILLARY TESTS

Immunohistochemistry
- Positive for vimentin, inhibin, Melan-A(MART-1), and synaptophysin
- Negative for cytokeratin

DIFFERENTIAL DIAGNOSIS

Leydig Cell Tumor
- Usually nonsymptomatic and unilateral
- Nuclear pleomorphism, fibrosis, lymphoid aggregates, and lipofuscin pigment less common
- Reinke crystals present in about 1/3 of tumors

Leydig Cell Hyperplasia
- Small nodules (< 0.5 cm)
- Crystalloids of Reinke are present

Large Cell Calcifying Sertoli Cell Tumor
- Intratubular growth and calcification
- Syndromic association with Carney complex and Peutz-Jeghers syndrome

Steroid Cell Nodules with Other Adrenal Diseases
- Patients with bilateral adrenalectomy and rapidly growing pituitary adenoma
- Patients with Carney complex (not large cell calcifying Sertoli cell tumor)
- Clinical correlation important

DIAGNOSTIC CHECKLIST

Pathologic Interpretation Pearls
- Fibrosis, synaptophysin expression, and nuclear pleomorphism are characteristic of TTAGS
- Correlate with steroid hormone levels

SELECTED REFERENCES

1. Ashley RA et al: Clinical and pathological features associated with the testicular tumor of the adrenogenital syndrome. J Urol. 177(2):546-9; discussion 549, 2007
2. Rutgers JL et al: The testicular "tumor" of the adrenogenital syndrome. A report of six cases and review of the literature on testicular masses in patients with adrenocortical disorders. Am J Surg Pathol. 12(7):503-13, 1988

TESTICULAR "TUMOR" OF ADRENOGENITAL SYNDROME

Microscopic Features

(Left) This TTAGS shows nests of polygonal cells with abundant eosinophilic cytoplasm separated by broad bands of collagenous stroma. Viewed in isolation, the similarity with Leydig cell tumor is marked. *(Right)* This photomicrograph shows nodules of eosinophilic cells with dense hyalinization with dilated vascular channels. There is spotty nuclear pleomorphism ➡. Reinke crystals are absent in these tumors.

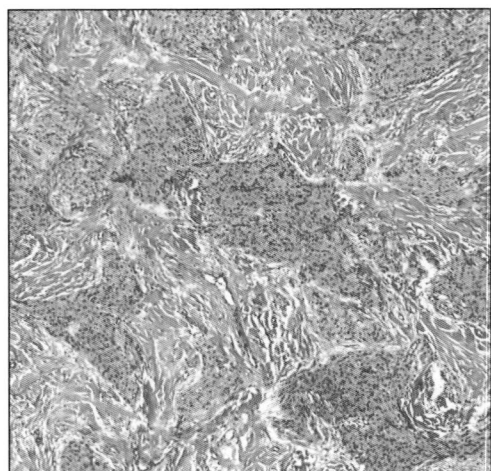 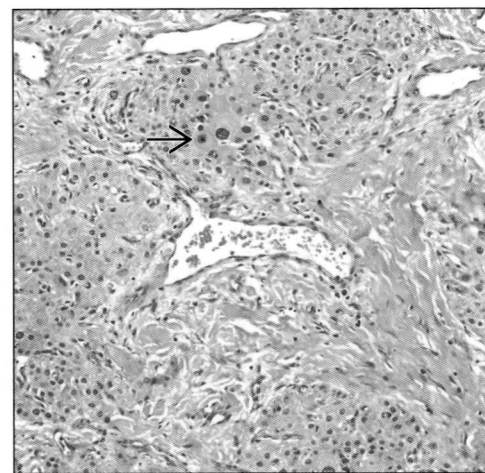

(Left) This photomicrograph shows the cytologic features of TTAGS. The tumor cells are polygonal and have round to ovoid nuclei, prominent nucleoli, and characteristic abundant eosinophilic and granular cytoplasm. Lipofuscin pigment ➡ is seen in some cells. *(Right)* TTAGS with clusters of tumor cells amidst prominent vascularity and stromal fibrosis is shown. The tumor cells ➡ are distinguished by their round to ovoid nuclei, prominent nucleoli, and abundant eosinophilic cytoplasm.

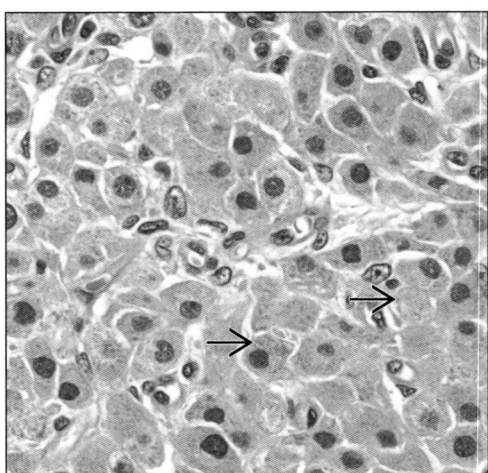 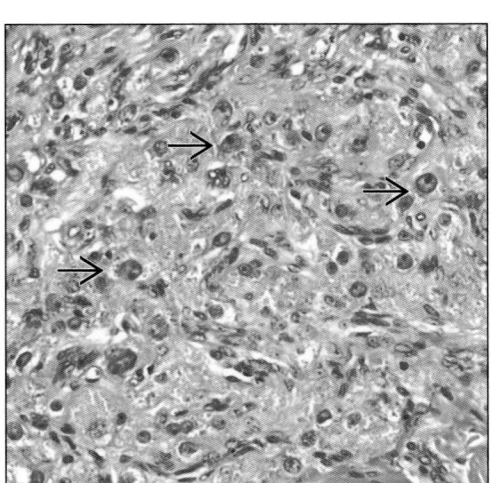

(Left) TTAGS shows marked nuclear pleomorphism, prominent nucleoli, and lipofuscin pigment. The atypia is usually random in nature, typical of "endocrine atypia." Lipofuscin is more common in TTAGS than in Leydig cell tumors. *(Right)* Photomicrograph of TTAGS shows nuclear pleomorphism, irregular nuclear contours, and prominent nucleoli. The tumor cells are separated in this case by edematous stroma. There is intracytoplasmic lipofuscin ➡ and absence of Reinke crystals.

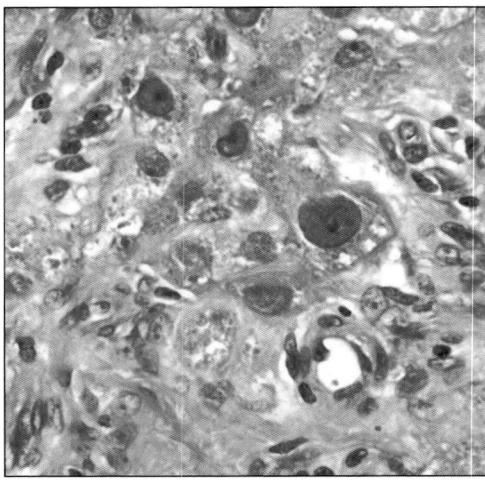 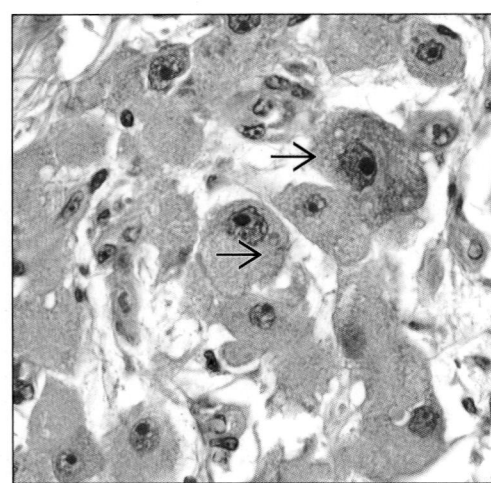

Microscopic Features

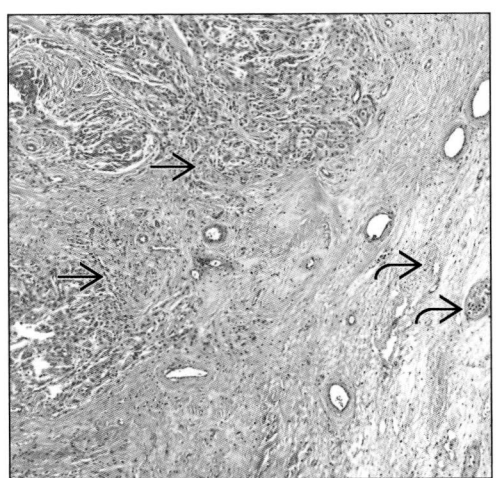
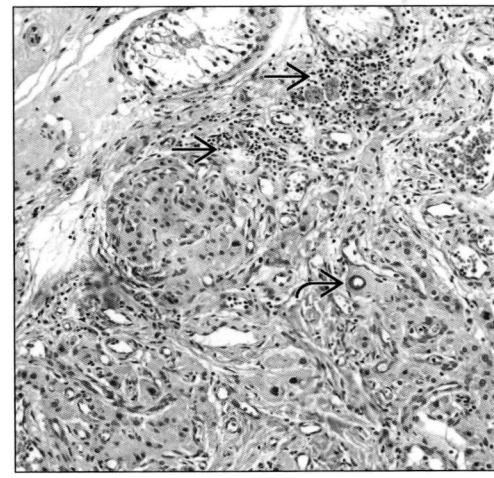

(Left) Low-power view of a TTAGS with dense fibrosis at the periphery of the tumor shows a mild lymphocytic infiltrate ➡. Atrophic and hyalinized seminiferous tubules ⇨ are seen outside the confines of the lesion. *(Right)* At the periphery of a TTAGS, nests or clusters of tumor cells are surrounded by fibrous stroma and foci of lymphoid infiltrates ➡. Nuclear pleomorphism ⇨ is evident. The adjacent seminiferous tubules show lack of spermatogenesis.

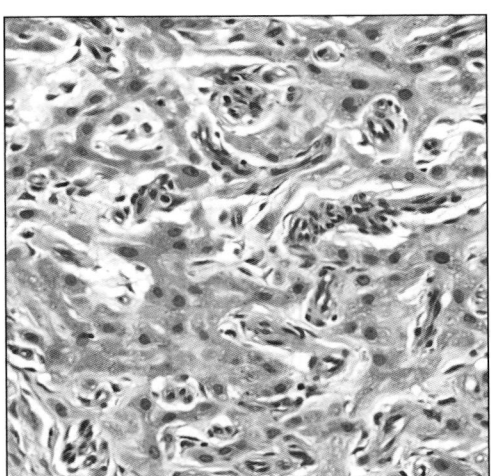
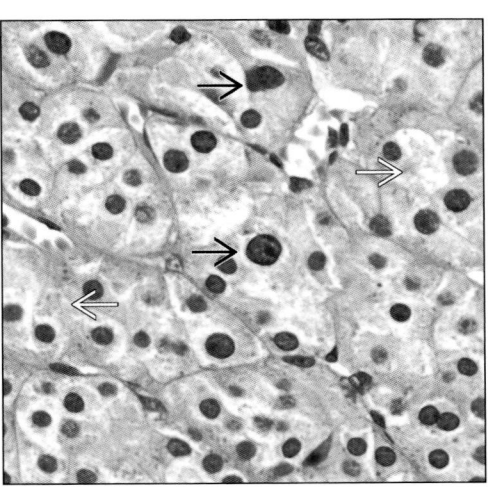

(Left) High-power photomicrograph of TTAGS shows irregularly branching cords of tumor cells separated by a fibromyxoid stroma with prominent vascularity. In this particular example, the cell borders are not well preserved. *(Right)* In this example, the TTAGS shows prominent nested arrangement with delicate fibrovascular septae. The cells have a slightly "clear" appearance with spotty nuclear pleomorphism ⇨ and prominent nucleoli. Lipofuscin pigment ➡ is also discernible.

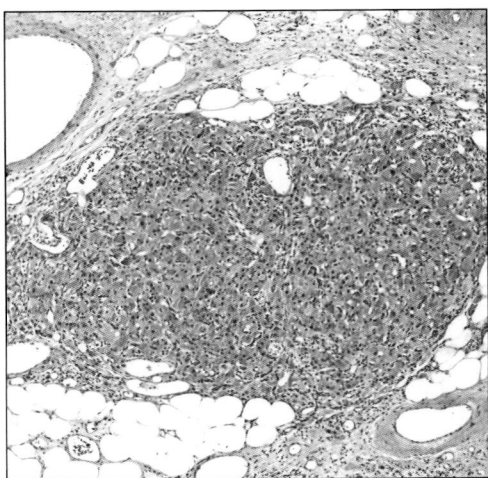
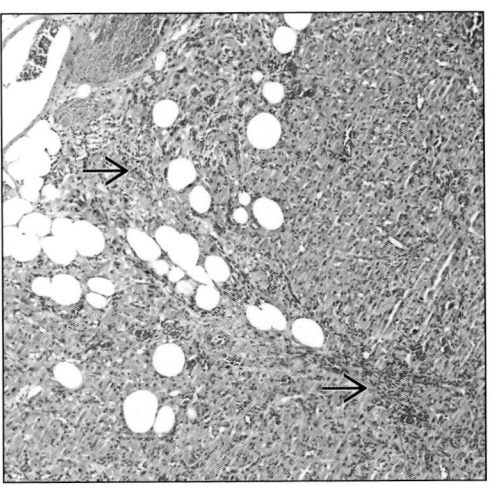

(Left) This photomicrograph shows a nodule of TTAGS with adipocytic metaplasia at the periphery as well as within the nodule. This finding is more common in TTAGS than in Leydig cell tumor but by itself is not discriminatory. *(Right)* This photomicrograph of TTAGS shows sheets of tumor cells with adipocytic metaplasia within the nodule. A lymphoid infiltrate ➡ is also present within the fibrous septa.

SEX CORD STROMAL TUMOR, MIXED/UNCLASSIFIED

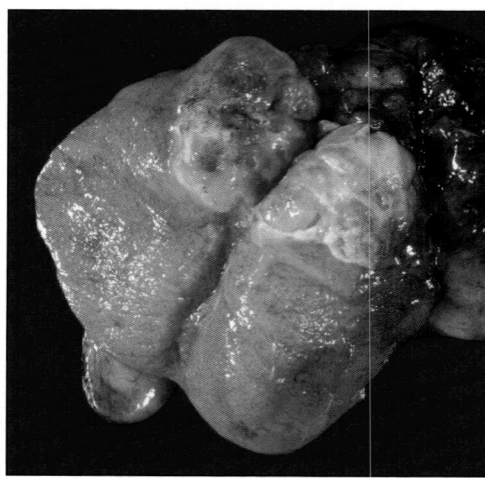

Gross photograph shows a well-circumscribed unclassified SCST. It has heterogeneous, soft, tan nodular areas with dense white fibrotic septae. SCSTs frequently do not replace the entire testis.

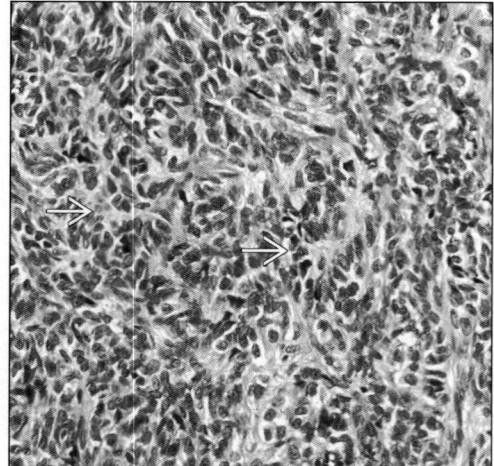

Unclassified SCST is shown with cellular proliferation of ovoid or elongated cells with scant, pale cytoplasm. No obvious differentiation is present. Vague rosette formation ➡ is seen.

TERMINOLOGY

Abbreviations
- Sex cord stromal tumor (SCST), Leydig cell tumor (LCT), Sertoli cell tumor (SCT), granulosa cell tumor (GCT)

Definitions
- Group of SCSTs with mixture of recognizable cell types or composed of incomplete or undifferentiated sex cord stromal cells

CLINICAL ISSUES

Epidemiology
- Incidence
  - Extremely rare (< 1% of testicular neoplasms)
- Age
  - All ages
  - More commonly seen in children (30% < 1 year old)

Presentation
- Painless testicular enlargement
- 15% associated with gynecomastia

Treatment
- Surgical approaches
  - Surgical resection is usually curative
  - Testis sparing partial orchiectomy may be possible
  - Radical orchiectomy with retroperitoneal lymph node dissection may be required for patients with clinical evidence of metastasis or high-risk pathologic features

Prognosis
- Almost always benign in prepubertal children
- May be malignant in adults (20%)

MACROSCOPIC FEATURES

General Features
- Well-circumscribed, lobulated, white-yellow, nodular mass; similar to other SCST with no unique gross features
- Cystic areas may be seen
- Hemorrhage and necrosis are uncommon

MICROSCOPIC PATHOLOGY

Histologic Features
- Mixture of recognizable SCST components (Leydig cell, Sertoli cell, or granulosa cell, rarely theca cells)
- Mixture of undifferentiated or unclassifiable epithelioid and spindle cell components
- Epithelioid component
  - Solid or hollow tubules, irregular aggregates, or anastomosing trabeculae (SCT)
  - Round to ovoid cells with eosinophilic, amphophilic, or vacuolated cytoplasm and prominent nucleoli (LCT)
  - Oval round cells with nuclear grooves, Call-Exner-like bodies (GCT)
  - Mixture of above mentioned recognizable SCST
  - Unclassified epithelioid cells with vesicular nuclei, occasional prominent nucleoli, rare mitotic figures
  - Signet ring cell SCST has been reported
- Undifferentiated spindle cell component
  - Usually hypercellular spindle cells merged with fibrous stroma
  - Spindle cells may form fascicles
  - Spindle cells may have nuclear grooves
  - Cellular pleomorphism and mitotic figures are variable
  - Has been reported as a variant of granulosa cell tumor because of its immunohistochemical similarities

SEX CORD STROMAL TUMOR, MIXED/UNCLASSIFIED

Key Facts

Terminology
- Group of SCST with mixture of recognizable types
- SCST with incomplete differentiation or undifferentiated spindle cells or mixed spindle and epithelioid cells

Clinical Issues
- Extremely rare (< 1% of testicular neoplasms)

Macroscopic Features
- Well-circumscribed, lobulated, white-yellow nodule

Microscopic Pathology
- Mixture of growth patterns and mixture of recognizable SCST components (LCT, SCT, or GCT)
- Mixture of epithelioid and undifferentiated spindle cell components

- Epithelioid component forms solid or hollow tubules, irregular aggregates, or anastomosing trabeculae
- Round to ovoid cells with eosinophilic, amphophilic, or vacuolated cytoplasm
- Undifferentiated stromal cell component is usually hypercellular spindle cells and merged with fibrous stroma
- Features that are seen more often in malignant tumors: Invasive growth, angiolymphatic invasion, nuclear atypia, mitotically active, and areas of necrosis

Ancillary Tests
- Positive for vimentin, desmin, actin-sm, S100, CD99, cytokeratin (may be focal), inhibin and calcitonin (focal)

- Features that are more commonly associated with malignant outcome: Invasive growth pattern, angiolymphatic invasion, nuclear atypia, mitotically active, and areas of necrosis

Predominant Pattern/Injury Type
- Neoplastic; diffuse spindle cells, mixed epithelioid and spindle cells, or combined form of known SCSTs

Predominant Cell/Compartment Type
- Sex cord stromal cells

ANCILLARY TESTS

Immunohistochemistry
- Positive for vimentin, desmin, actin-sm, S100, CD99, cytokeratin (may be focal), inhibin and calcitonin (focal)
- Negative for PLAP, Oct3/4, Podoplanin(D2-40), SALL4, HMB-45

DIFFERENTIAL DIAGNOSIS

Metastatic Melanoma
- Interstitial growth pattern and greater cytologic atypia
- Positive for S100 and HMB-45

Sarcoma, NOS
- Greater pleomorphism, mitotic activity, and necrosis
- Involves paratesticular structures, not primarily intraparenchymal

Mixed Germ Cell Tumor with Prominent Immature Teratoma Component
- High cellularity and increased mitoses
- Presence of various other germ cell tumor components
- Immature teratoma component positive for cytokeratin and CD34; negative for inhibin and calretinin

Adult Granulosa Cell Tumor
- More homogeneous neoplasm with well-formed Call-Exner bodies
- Immunohistochemical overlap with SCST

Sertoli Cell Tumor
- Usually demonstrates tubular morphology and is composed of single cell type population
- Sarcomatoid variant of SCT may be challenging but has more classic SCT present

DIAGNOSTIC CHECKLIST

Pathologic Interpretation Pearls
- Purely undifferentiated spindle cell or mixed spindle and epithelioid proliferation or > 1 known SCST component

SELECTED REFERENCES

1. Tarjàn M et al: Unclassified sex cord/gonadal stromal testis tumor with predominance of spindle cells. APMIS. 114(6):465-9, 2006
2. Ulbright TM et al: Sex cord-stromal tumors of the testis with entrapped germ cells: a lesion mimicking unclassified mixed germ cell sex cord-stromal tumors. Am J Surg Pathol. 24(4):535-42, 2000
3. Iczkowski KA et al: Inhibin A is a sensitive and specific marker for testicular sex cord-stromal tumors. Mod Pathol. 11(8):774-9, 1998
4. McCluggage WG et al: Immunohistochemical study of testicular sex cord-stromal tumors, including staining with anti-inhibin antibody. Am J Surg Pathol. 22(5):615-9, 1998
5. Renshaw AA et al: Immunohistochemistry of unclassified sex cord-stromal tumors of the testis with a predominance of spindle cells. Mod Pathol. 10(7):693-700, 1997
6. Goswitz JJ et al: Testicular sex cord-stromal tumors in children: clinicopathologic study of sixteen children with review of the literature. Pediatr Pathol Lab Med. 16(3):451-70, 1996
7. Düe W et al: Testicular sex cord stromal tumour with granulosa cell differentiation: detection of steroid hormone receptors as a possible basis for tumour development and therapeutic management. J Clin Pathol. 43(9):732-7, 1990

SEX CORD STROMAL TUMOR, MIXED/UNCLASSIFIED

Microscopic Features

(Left) *A well-circumscribed unclassified SCST composed of cellular spindle cells with focal condensation. Note the relationship to the tunica* ⊡ *and uninvolved testicular parenchyma* ➡. *(Right)* *This photomicrograph shows an area of epithelial component in a mixed SCST with prominent microcystic and tubular patterns and cords of cells resembling those of Sertoli cell tumor. Other areas of the tumor had undifferentiated spindle cells, hence categorization as mixed/ unclassified.*

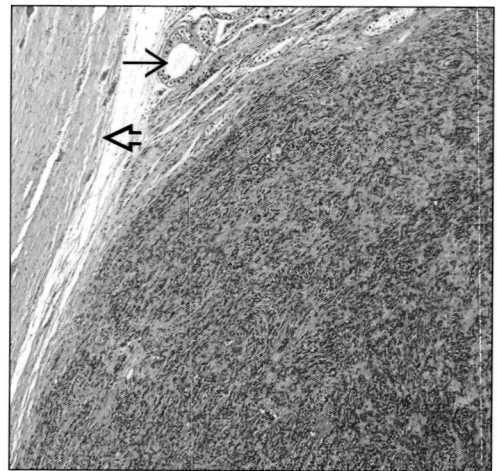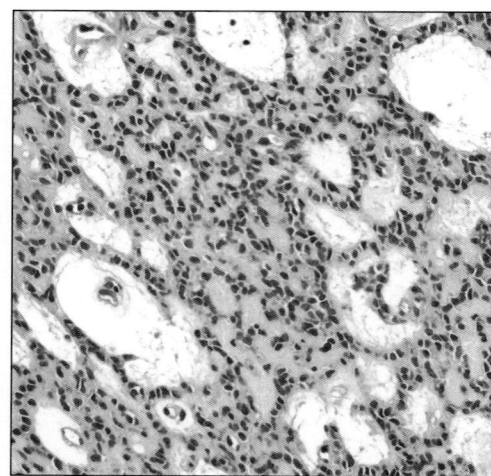

(Left) *Low-power photomicrograph of a mixed SCST shows poorly formed or compressed tubules of SCT* ➡ *and a microscopic area of LCT with oval, round cells with abundant eosinophilic cytoplasm* ⊡. *(Right)* *Higher power photomicrograph a mixed SCST shows nests and poorly formed tubules* ➡ *lined by cells with ovoid or elongated nuclei and scant pale cytoplasm and clusters of Leydig cells* ➡ *with abundant eosinophilic cytoplasm and prominent nucleoli.*

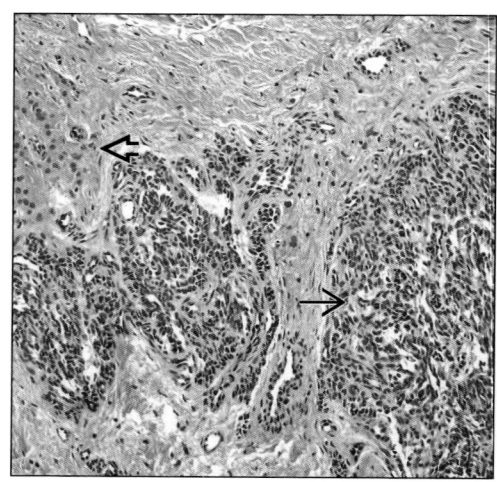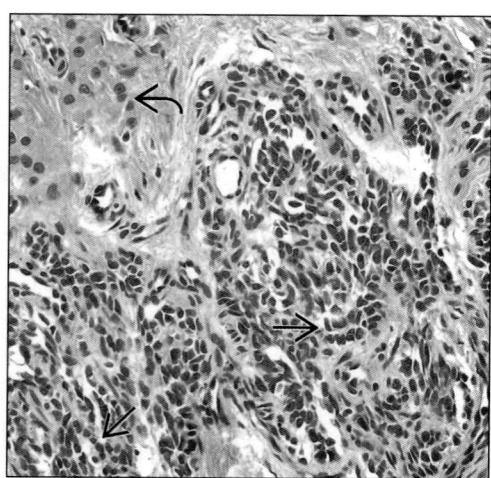

(Left) *An encapsulated unclassified SCST is shown. The tumor is composed of sheets of tumor cells with short spindle to ovoid nuclei and moderately abundant pale eosinophilic cytoplasm. No pleomorphism or necrosis is seen. (Right) High-power photomicrograph shows epithelioid cells with variable amounts of pale eosinophilic cytoplasm and indistinct cell boundaries. There is noticeable cellular pleomorphism* ➡ *and occasional nuclear grooves* ➡.

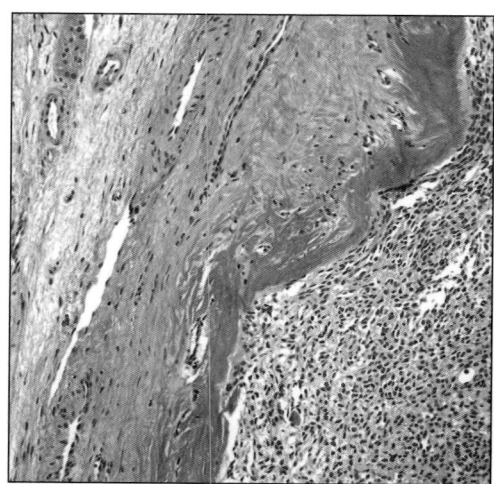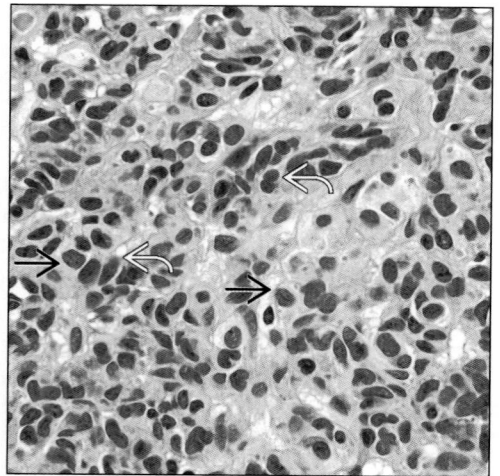

SEX CORD STROMAL TUMOR, MIXED/UNCLASSIFIED

Microscopic and Immunohistochemical Features

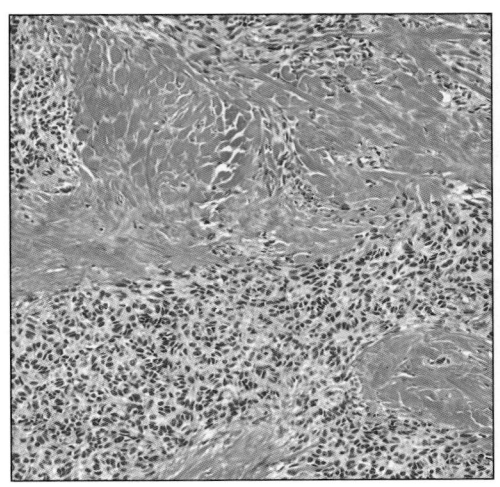

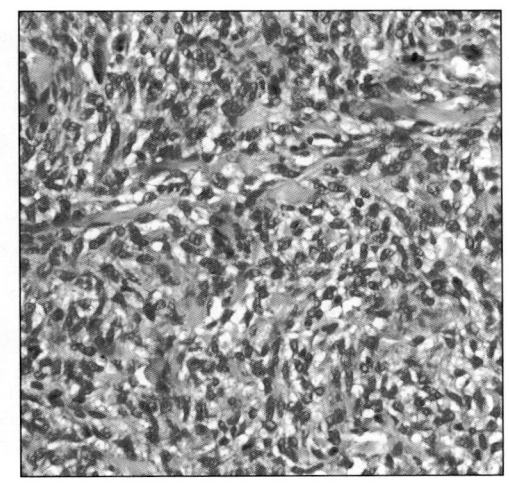

(Left) Unclassified SCST is shown with spindle-shaped tumor cells divided into lobules by paucicellular collagenized fibrous stroma. There is no specific line of differentiation. *(Right)* Unclassified SCST with cellular proliferation of cells with clear to pale eosinophilic cytoplasm is similar to smooth muscle or myofibroblastic cells. These cells were positive for inhibin and calretinin indicating SCST. In contrast to intratesticular sarcomas, which are rare, anaplasia is not common.

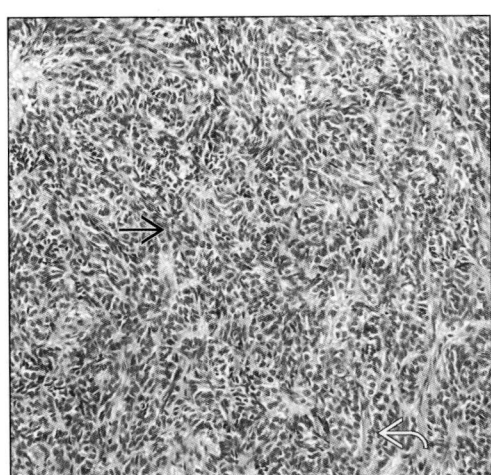

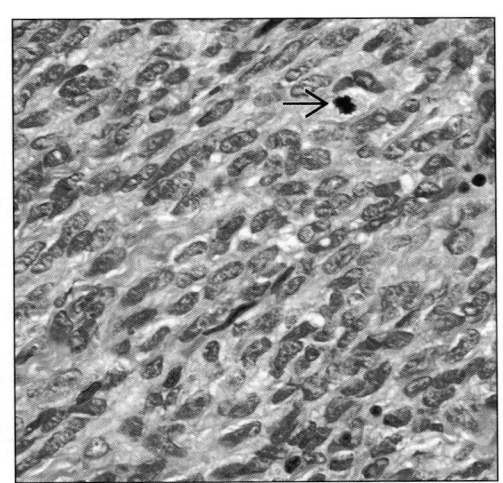

(Left) This photomicrograph of unclassified SCST shows compact growth of ovoid or spindle cells with focal, vague cord ⊡ or tubule ⊡ formation and focal storiform pattern. Tumor necrosis and pleomorphism are absent. *(Right)* Undifferentiated spindle cells of unclassified SCST have moderate nuclear pleomorphism and occasional mitoses ⊡. Unclassified SCST is regarded as being potentially malignant except for small and cytologically innocuous tumors and those occurring in children.

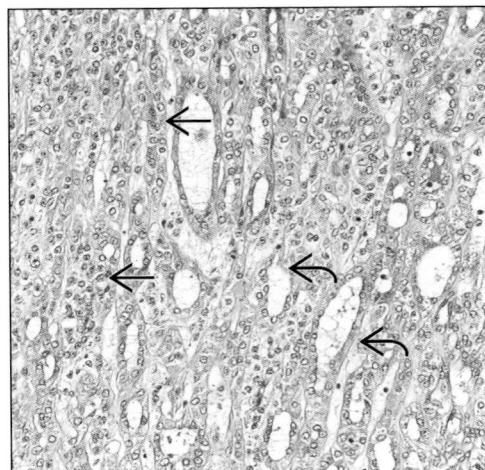

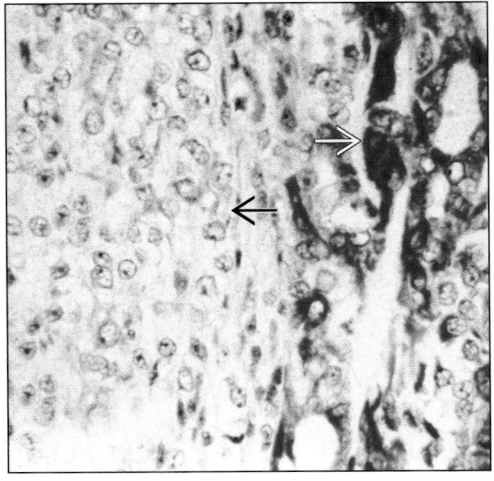

(Left) Mixed SCST is shown with solid growth of Leydig cell ⊡ and Sertoli cell differentiation with tubule formation ⊡. This combination of sex cord stromal tumor histology is distinctly rare in the testis. *(Right)* The mixed SCST with Leydig cell ⊡ and Sertoli cell differentiation ⊡ may be supported by their differential immunohistochemical staining intensity with cytokeratin. The Sertoli cell component stains much stronger than the Leydig cell component.

GONADOBLASTOMA

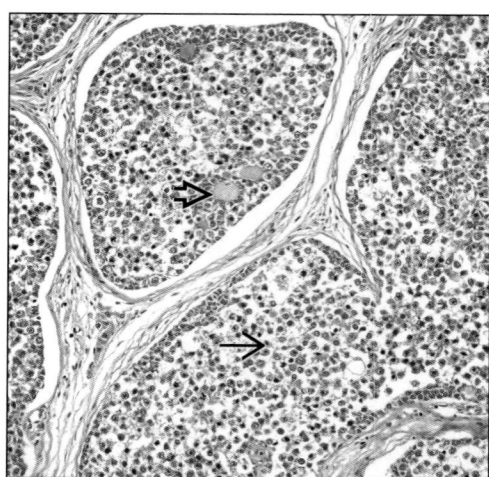

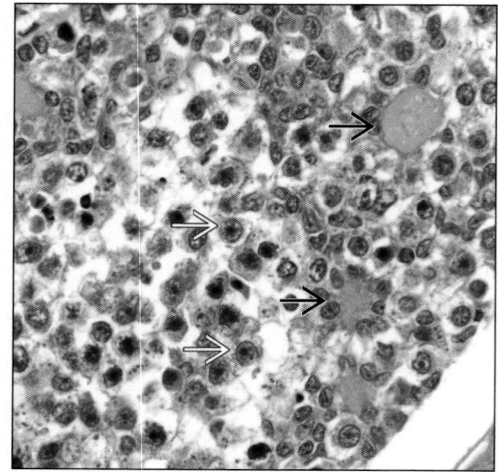

Gonadoblastoma is characterized by nests containing large seminomatous germ cells ⇥, located in the center and sex cord stromal cells forming Call-Exner-like structures ⇲ at the periphery of the nests.

Gonadoblastoma shows smaller sex cord stromal cells forming Call-Exner body-like structures ⇥ and large seminomatous cells with abundant clear cytoplasm and prominent nucleoli ⇥.

TERMINOLOGY

Synonyms
- Mixed germ cell and sex cord stromal cell tumor

Definitions
- Tumor composed of mixture of seminomatous germ cells and immature sex cord tumor elements resembling Sertoli or granulosa cell tumors

CLINICAL ISSUES

Epidemiology
- Incidence
  - Extremely rare
  - Occurs usually in patients with abnormal, dysgenetic gonads
- Age
  - Younger than 20 years old
- Gender
  - 20% phenotypically male, 80% phenotypically female (during early embryonic development, immature bi-potential gonads fail to differentiate along male pathway)
  - XY gonadal dysgenesis or X0-XY mosaicism may be seen

Presentation
- Cryptorchidism, hypospadias or other ambiguous genitalia, and gynecomastia

Treatment
- Surgical approaches
  - Bilateral gonadectomy is recommended and curative

Prognosis
- Excellent if no associated invasive germ cell or malignant sex cord stromal tumor components

MACROSCOPIC FEATURES

General Features
- Gray to yellow-brown mass with a soft, fleshy or firm and gritty cut surface
- Streak gonads with incidental findings in very small-sized tumors
- Invasive malignant germ cell tumor component, usually seminoma, results in larger tumors

Size
- Range: Microscopic focus to 8 cm

MICROSCOPIC PATHOLOGY

Histologic Features
- Nests of tumor cells composed of mixture of 2 types of cells (seminomatous germ cells and sex cord stromal cells)
- Germ cells are large and round with vacuolated or clear cytoplasm, central nuclei with fine chromatin and prominent nucleoli
- Sex cord stromal cells are usually immature Sertoli cells or granulosa cells, but rarely cells resemble Leydig cells or luteinizing theca-like cells
- Sex cord stromal cells are located at periphery of nests
- Small round to oval sex cord derivative cells form Call-Exner bodies with central eosinophilic hyaline material
- Marked hyalinization or calcification present within nests or stroma
- Adjacent seminiferous tubules with intratubular germ cell neoplasia may be seen
- Overgrowth of malignant germ cell tumor (usually seminoma) may obliterate gonadoblastomatous foci

Predominant Pattern/Injury Type
- Neoplastic; nests of tumor cells with germ cells and sex cord stromal tumor

GONADOBLASTOMA

Key Facts

Terminology
- Tumor composed of mixture of seminomatous cells and immature sex cord tumor resembling Sertoli or granulosa cell tumors

Clinical Issues
- Extremely rare
- Occurs usually in patients with abnormal, dysgenetic gonads

Microscopic Pathology
- Nests of tumor cells composed of mixture of 2 types of cells (seminomatous germ cells and sex cord stromal cells)
- Germ cells are large and round with vacuolated or clear cytoplasm, fine chromatin, and inconspicuous nucleoli

- Sex cord stromal cells are usually immature Sertoli cells or granulosa cells, but rarely cells resembling Leydig cells or lutein-like cells
- Small round to oval sex cord derivative forming Call-Exner bodies with central eosinophilic hyaline material
- Marked hyalinization or calcification present within nests or stroma
- Adjacent seminiferous tubules with intratubular germ cell neoplasia may be seen
- Overgrowth of malignant germ cell tumor (usually seminoma) may obliterate gonadoblastomatous foci

Ancillary Tests
- Germ cells (+) for PLAP, Podoplanin, Oct3/4, CD117
- Stromal cells (+) for inhibin, calretinin, vimentin, and may be positive for cytokeratin

Predominant Cell/Compartment Type
- Mixed germ cells and sex cord stromal cells

ANCILLARY TESTS

Immunohistochemistry
- Germ cells positive for PLAP, Podoplanin(D2-40), Oct3/4, SALL4, CD117
- Gonadal stromal cells positive for inhibin, calretinin, Melan-A(MART-1), vimentin; may be positive for cytokeratin

DIFFERENTIAL DIAGNOSIS

Unclassified Mixed Germ Cell and Sex Cord Stromal Tumors
- Occurs in patients with normal gonads and without cytogenetic abnormalities (normal XY chromosomes)
- Diffuse growth with no well-defined nodules
- Some authors argue about existence of this entity and classify this lesion under unclassified sex cord stromal tumor with entrapped germ cells

Seminoma (Classic)
- No dysgenetic gonad; lack of sex cord stromal tumor component or gonadoblastoma in background; often larger tumor size and older age (35-45 years)

Unclassified Sex Cord Stromal Tumors
- No germ cell tumor components

Sex Cord Stromal Tumor with Annular Tubules
- Extremely rare in testis; associated with androgen insensitivity syndrome or Peutz-Jeghers syndrome; lack of germ cell tumor component

Intratubular Germ Cell Neoplasia
- Often associated with invasive malignant germ cell tumor; lack of sex cord stromal tumor component

Sertoli Cell Nodule
- No germ cell component or hyaline nodules

Sertoli Cell Nodule with Intratubular Germ Cell Neoplasia
- Associated gonad is not dysgenetic; seminoma-like cells are not uniformly distributed throughout tumor

DIAGNOSTIC CHECKLIST

Pathologic Interpretation Pearls
- Dysgenetic gonad; well-defined nested growth with hyaline nodules and basement membrane; 2 cell populations with germ cells and sex cord stromal cells

SELECTED REFERENCES

1. Ng SB et al: Gonadoblastoma-associated mixed germ cell tumour in 46,XY complete gonadal dysgenesis (Swyer syndrome): analysis of Y chromosomal genotype and OCT3/4 and TSPY expression profile. Histopathology. 52(5):644-6, 2008
2. Kersemaekers AM et al: Identification of germ cells at risk for neoplastic transformation in gonadoblastoma: an immunohistochemical study for OCT3/4 and TSPY. Hum Pathol. 36(5):512-21, 2005
3. Hussong J et al: Gonadoblastoma: immunohistochemical localization of Müllerian-inhibiting substance, inhibin, WT-1, and p53. Mod Pathol. 10(11):1101-5, 1997
4. Jørgensen N et al: Heterogeneity of gonadoblastoma germ cells: similarities with immature germ cells, spermatogonia and testicular carcinoma in situ cells. Histopathology. 30(2):177-86, 1997
5. Roth LM et al: Gonadoblastoma. Immunohistochemical and ultrastructural observations. Int J Gynecol Pathol. 8(1):72-81, 1989
6. Scully RE: Gonadoblastoma. A review of 74 cases. Cancer. 25(6):1340-56, 1970

GONADOBLASTOMA

Microscopic Features

(Left) Low-power view shows a well-circumscribed gonadoblastoma ➡ in the background of a streak dysgenetic gonad with epididymis ➡ and fallopian tube ➡. The tumor is cellular and shows vague nodular configuration. *(Right)* Gonadoblastoma is composed of an intimate mixture of large seminomatous germ cells with large round nuclei and abundant clear cytoplasm ➡ and sex cord stromal cells forming Call-Exner body-like structures ➡. Focal scattered calcifications are present ➡.

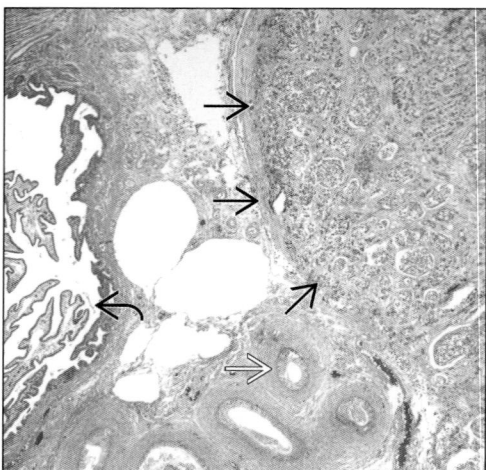
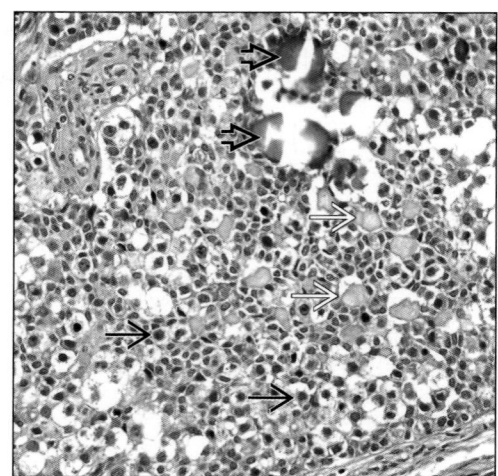

(Left) A gonadoblastoma shows nests of cellular proliferation of seminomatous germ cells with clear cytoplasm ➡ and sex-cord stromal cells with lesser amount of cytoplasm. Call-Exner body-like structures ➡ and large area of calcification (top) are present. *(Right)* High-power view of gonadoblastoma shows intimate admixture of seminomatous germ cells with prominent nucleoli and abundant clear cytoplasm ➡ and sex cord stromal cells forming a Call-Exner body-like structure ➡.

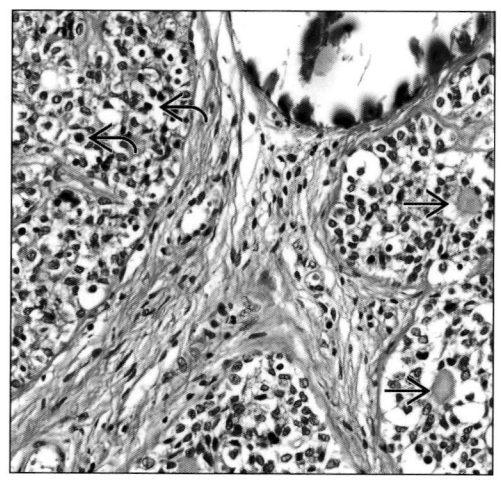
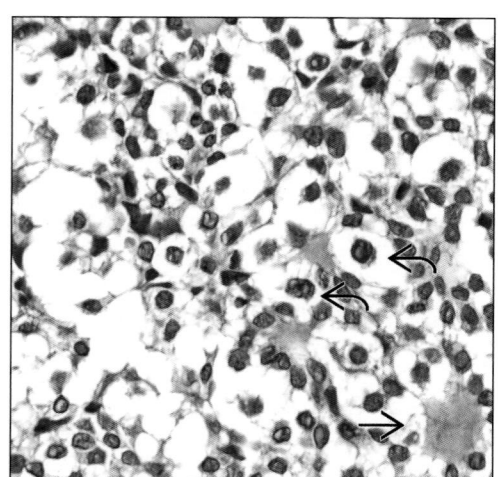

(Left) This image shows gonadoblastoma ➡ with adjacent intratubular germ cell neoplasia characterized by large cells with abundant clear cytoplasm ➡ and tubules containing only Sertoli cells ➡. Gonadoblastoma with characteristic low-power features is seen on the left. *(Right)* The adjacent seminiferous tubule in a case of gonadoblastoma may show Sertoli cell only ➡, while others tubules have extensive involvement by intratubular germ cell neoplasia ➡.

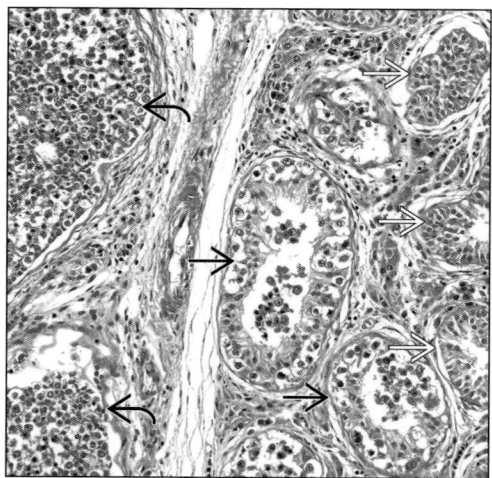
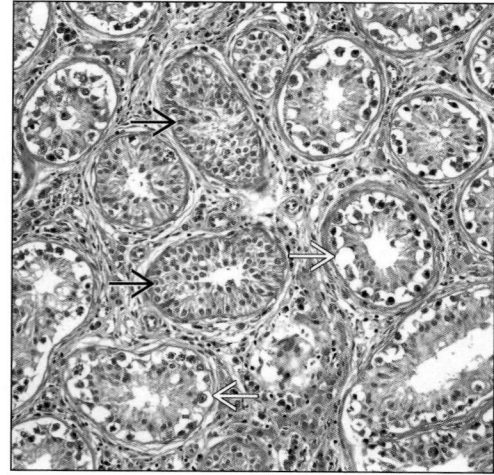

GONADOBLASTOMA

Microscopic Features

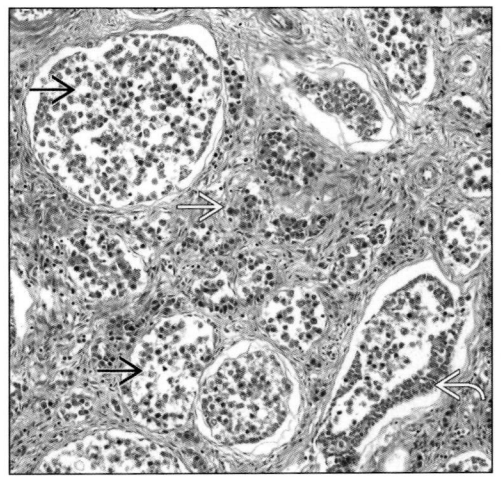

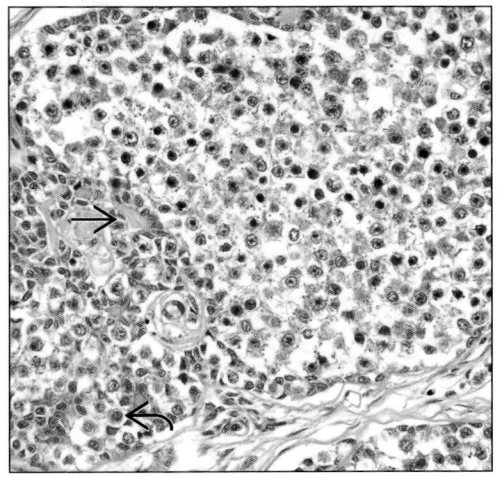

(Left) Gonadoblastoma with intratubular seminomatous overgrowth ⮕ coexists with microscopic foci of invasive seminoma associated with lymphocytes ⮕. Focal Call-Exner-like structures are seen at the periphery ⮕ of some tumor nests. *(Right)* One large nest of gonadoblastoma is composed of overgrowth of seminomatous germ cells with prominent nucleolus, abundant clear cytoplasm, and distinct cell boundary and area with mixture of germ cells ⮕ and sex cord stromal cells ⮕.

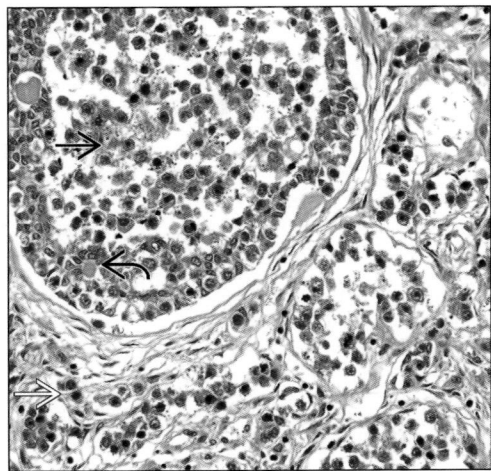

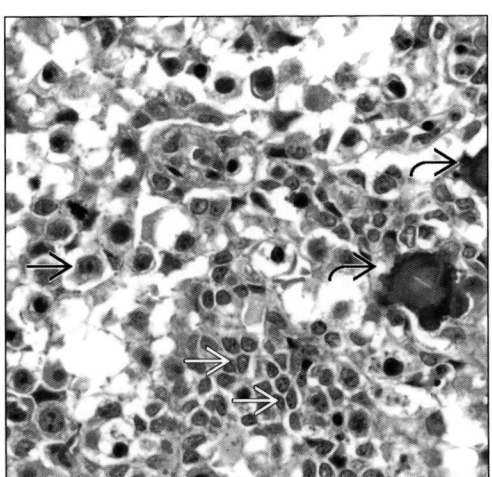

(Left) Gonadoblastoma with intratubular seminoma overgrowth ⮕ and microscopic foci of invasive seminoma ⮕ is shown. Focal Call-Exner-like structures ⮕ are still present at the periphery of the large tumor nest. *(Right)* High-power photomicrograph shows a gonadoblastoma composed of intratubular large seminoma tumor cells ⮕ with prominent nucleoli and abundant clear cytoplasm and clusters of smaller angulated sex cord stromal cells ⮕ and calcifications ⮕.

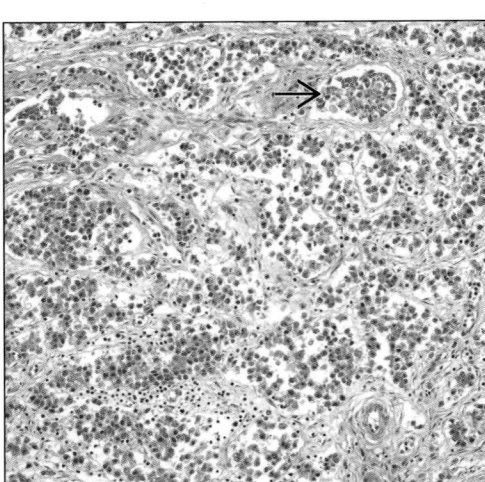

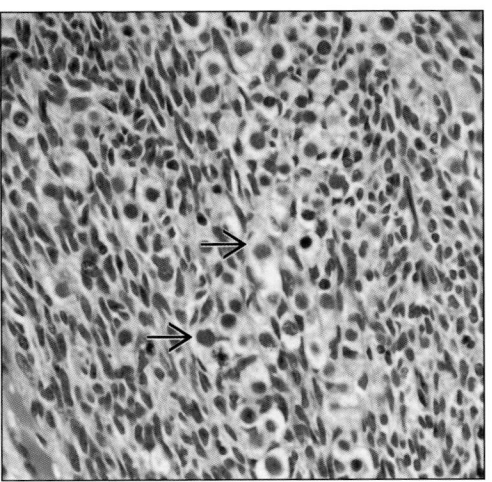

(Left) This photomicrograph shows overgrowth of invasive seminoma composed of nests of tumor cells within the fibrous stroma and scattered lymphocytic infiltrate and a small focus of gonadoblastoma ⮕. *(Right)* A mixed germ cell-sex cord stromal tumor shows unclassified sex cord elements and scattered large round cells ⮕, reminiscent of uncommitted germ cell tumor cells. Some authors classify this tumor under unclassified sex cord stromal tumor with entrapped germ cells.

LYMPHOMA/LEUKEMIA/PLASMACYTOMA

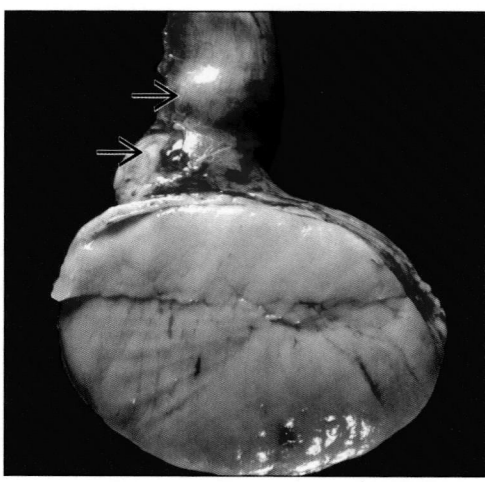

Malignant lymphoma involves the testis with a homogeneous, tan-cream, bulging cut surface. The testicular parenchyma is replaced, and there is extension to the epididymis and spermatic cord ➡.

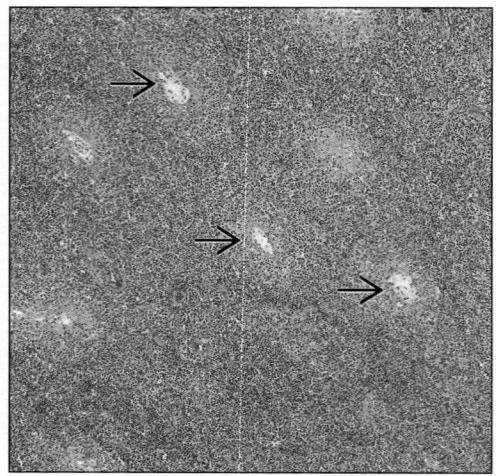

Testicular lymphoma with a diffuse interstitial infiltration of round blue cells with preserved but significantly effaced or atrophic seminiferous tubules ➡.

TERMINOLOGY

Synonyms
- Malignant lymphoreticular neoplasms

Definitions
- Lymphoma and plasmacytoma involve testis or paratesticular structures as either primary neoplasms or as secondary tumors due to systemic spread
- Leukemic involvement represents secondary spread to testis or paratesticular structures (testis is one of common sanctuary sites)

CLINICAL ISSUES

Epidemiology
- Incidence
  - Malignant lymphoma accounts for 2-5% of all testicular neoplasms
    - Secondary involvement is more common than primary lymphoma
  - Primary plasmacytoma of testis is extremely rare (only handful of cases have been reported)
    - Secondary plasmacytoma occurs in 2% of patients with multiple myeloma at autopsy (clinically usually occult)
  - Frequent finding in patients with leukemia (at autopsy)
    - 40-65% of patients with acute leukemia have leukemic infiltrate
    - 20-35% of patients with chronic leukemia have leukemic infiltrate
- Age
  - Lymphoma and plasmacytoma: Average age 56-60 years in different studies
    - 50% of testis tumors in patients over 60 years are lymphomas
  - Leukemic infiltrates usually occur in children

Presentation
- Testicular mass or enlargement
- Systemic symptoms may occur, such as fever, night sweats, weight loss
- Frequent bilaterality (20-38%); majority are metachronous
- Testicular lymphoma has predilection for widespread association with unusual sites, including CNS, Waldeyer ring, skin, and lung lymphoma

Treatment
- Radical orchiectomy is often performed in older-aged patients with primary testicular lymphoma or plasmacytoma
- Adjuvant therapy
  - Similar to that of nodal or other extranodal lymphomas
  - Doxorubicin- and rituximab-based chemotherapy with prophylactic intrathecal chemotherapy and radiation to contralateral testis

Prognosis
- Generally poor for adult testicular lymphoma
- The 5- and 10-year overall survival is 37-48% and 19-27%, respectively, for all testicular lymphoma
- Prognostic factors include age, stage, epididymal or spermatic cord involvement, and histologic sclerosis
- Secondary lymphoma involvement in children often have excellent prognosis by chemotherapy alone
- Primary testicular plasmacytoma has favorable prognosis compared to multiple myeloma
- Leukemic involvement is predictive of subsequent systemic relapse

IMAGE FINDINGS

General Features
- Similar to and indistinguishable from testicular germ cell tumor on ultrasonography

LYMPHOMA/LEUKEMIA/PLASMACYTOMA

Key Facts

Terminology
- Lymphoma and plasmacytoma of testis or paratesticular structures of either primary or secondary due to systemic spread
- Leukemic infiltrates, secondary (testis is one of common sanctuary sites)

Clinical Issues
- Malignant lymphoma accounts for 2-5% of all testicular neoplasms

Macroscopic Features
- Lymphoma and plasmacytoma: Partial or complete replacement of testicular parenchyma by diffuse or lobulated mass
- Fleshy, creamy colored, tan, pale yellow or slightly pink homogeneous cut surface

- Leukemia: No gross abnormalities and usually found by testicular biopsy

Microscopic Pathology
- Most common type of primary lymphoma is diffuse large B-cell lymphoma
- Diffuse interstitial pattern is most frequent finding
- Tumoral and intratubular replacement also occurs
- Effacement and infiltration of seminiferous tubules by lymphoma may be seen
- Other lymphomas include primary MALT lymphomas, follicular lymphomas, T-cell lymphomas, and Burkitt lymphoma
- Plasmacytoma is characterized by sheets of variably differentiated, monomorphic neoplastic plasma cells
- Leukemia (including granulocytic sarcoma) is similar to that of lymphoma microscopically

---

- More frequent spermatic cord involvement than germ cell tumors
- There may be no imaging abnormalities or testicular enlargement in leukemic patients

MACROSCOPIC FEATURES

General Features
- Lymphoma and plasmacytoma
  - Partial or complete replacement of testicular parenchyma by diffuse or lobulated mass
  - Fleshy, cream-colored, tan, pale yellow, or slightly pink homogeneous cut surface; similar to that of seminoma or spermatocytic seminoma
  - Focal hemorrhage and necrosis may be seen
  - Frequent epididymis (50%) or spermatic cord involvement
- Testicular leukemia
  - Usually no gross abnormalities with detection on surveillance biopsy
  - May rarely result in palpable mass, induration, or testicular enlargement

Size
- Lymphoma and plasmacytoma: Mean 6 cm

MICROSCOPIC PATHOLOGY

Histologic Features
- Malignant lymphoma
  - Diffuse interstitial pattern is most frequent finding: Relative preservation of tubules
  - Tumoral (sheet-like) and intratubular growth may occur
  - Effacement and infiltration of seminiferous tubules by lymphoma ("onion skin" with reticulin stain) may be seen
  - Variable sclerosis: Presence of sclerosis is associated with more favorable prognosis
  - Most common type of primary lymphoma is diffuse large B-cell lymphoma (70-90%)

- Composed of sheets of large atypical lymphoid cells of variable morphology (noncleaved, cleaved, multilobated, or immunoblastic)
- Most belong to nongerminal center B-cell-like large cell lymphoma (CD10 and bcl-6 negative and MUM1 positive)
  - Other lymphomas include primary MALT lymphomas, follicular lymphomas, T-cell lymphomas, CD30(BerH2) positive anaplastic large cell lymphoma, Burkitt lymphoma (children), and rarely Hodgkin disease
    - Features similar to that of nodal or other extranodal locations
- Plasmacytoma/myeloma
  - Composed of sheets of variably differentiated, monomorphic neoplastic plasma cells
- Leukemia (include granulocytic sarcoma)
  - Similar to that of lymphoma microscopically and may be misdiagnosed as lymphoma
  - Tumor cells usually have smaller, more evenly dispersed chromatin and less prominent nucleoli than that of lymphoma
  - Often prominent vessel wall invasion
  - Rare seminiferous tubule invasion

ANCILLARY TESTS

Immunohistochemistry
- Positive for CD45(LCA), most are positive for CD20, CD79a
- May also be positive for bcl-2, CD10 (follicular)
- Plasmacytomas are positive for CD138 and monoclonal κ or λ light chain
- Leukemias are positive for lysozyme, MPO, CD117, CD68

DIFFERENTIAL DIAGNOSIS

Seminoma, Classic or Spermatocytic
- Younger age; bilaterality and spermatic cord invasion less frequent

LYMPHOMA/LEUKEMIA/PLASMACYTOMA

- Usually diffuse tumoral pattern; interstitial pattern less prominent and commonly at periphery only
- Tumor cells are more monotonous with abundant clear cytoplasm and distinct cell boundaries compared to those of lymphoma
- Presence of intratubular germ cell neoplasia (ITGCN)
- Positive for germ cell markers (PLAP, Podoplanin(D2-40), Oct3/4, and SALL4); negative for CD45(LCA), CD20, and CD3

Embryonal Carcinoma
- Younger age (25-35 years) and less frequently bilateral
- Hemorrhage and necrosis are more common
- Cohesive and epithelial growth patterns with solid, papillary and tubular arrangements
- Anaplastic tumor cells with more numerous mitoses and irregular and prominent nucleoli
- Presence of ITGCN
- Positive for germ cell markers (PLAP, Podoplanin(D2-40), Oct3/4, and SALL4)
- Positivity for CD30 represents a pitfall, as both embryonal carcinoma and CD30(BerH2)-positive anaplastic large cell lymphoma are positive

Chronic Orchitis
- Cellular infiltrate is usually more patchy and lacks cytologic atypia
- Heterogeneous population of cells with lymphocytes, plasma cells, histiocytes, and neutrophils

Metastatic Tumors
- Clinical history of malignancy elsewhere
- Cohesive growth pattern in carcinoma
- Melanoma cells may be diffuse and discohesive, similar to that of lymphoma/plasmacytoma
- Positive for epithelial markers (cytokeratin, EMA/MUC1, etc.) in carcinoma
- Positive for S100, HMB-45, Melan-A(MART-1) in malignant melanoma
- Negative for lymphoma markers

Leydig Cell Tumor
- Neoplastic tumor cells have more abundant granular cytoplasm, lesser degree of cytologic atypia, and no or few mitoses
- Expansile mass without destruction of seminiferous tubules
- Positive for inhibin and calretinin; negative for lymphoma markers

DIAGNOSTIC CHECKLIST

Pathologic Interpretation Pearls
- Presence of bilaterality and extensive involvement of testicular parenchyma with epididymal or spermatic cord involvement in older patients should raise strong possibility of malignant lymphoma
- Histologic interstitial growth pattern is typical and shared by metastatic carcinoma and orchitis; interstitial pattern in seminoma is extremely rare
- Leukemic involvement may or may not result in a mass and is frequently diagnosed by biopsy

- Malignant lymphoma along with spermatocytic seminoma and metastatic tumors represents triad of testicular tumors occurring in patients > 50-60 years of age

STAGING

According to Ann Arbor Staging System Proposed for Hodgkin Lymphoma
- Staging evaluation includes: Physical, complete hematologic, and biochemical examination, testicular ultrasound, CT scan, bone marrow biopsy, CSF examination, brain MR
- Staging subclassification system
  - Stage I: Involves unilateral testis only
  - Stage II: Involves bilateral testis and its regional lymph node (below diaphragm)
  - Stage III: Involves testis and lymph nodes of both sides of diaphragm or spleen
  - Stage IV: Disseminated (multifocal) involvement of 1 or more extralymphatic sites

SELECTED REFERENCES

1. Verma N et al: Testicular lymphoma: an update for clinicians. Am J Med Sci. 336(4):336-41, 2008
2. Vitolo U et al: Primary testicular lymphoma. Crit Rev Oncol Hematol. 65(2):183-9, 2008
3. Bacon CM et al: Primary follicular lymphoma of the testis and epididymis in adults. Am J Surg Pathol. 31(7):1050-8, 2007
4. Vural F et al: Primary testicular lymphoma. J Natl Med Assoc. 99(11):1277-82, 2007
5. Al-Abbadi MA et al: Primary testicular diffuse large B-cell lymphoma belongs to the nongerminal center B-cell-like subgroup: A study of 18 cases. Mod Pathol. 19(12):1521-7, 2006
6. Darby S et al: Localised non-Hodgkin lymphoma of the testis: the Sheffield Lymphoma Group experience. Int J Oncol. 26(4):1093-9, 2005
7. Constantinou J et al: Testicular granulocytic sarcoma, a source of diagnostic confusion. Urology. 64(4):807-9, 2004
8. Miyoshi I et al: Granulocytic sarcoma of the testis. Br J Haematol. 124(6):695, 2004
9. Lagrange JL et al: Non-Hodgkin's lymphoma of the testis: a retrospective study of 84 patients treated in the French anticancer centres. Ann Oncol. 12(9):1313-9, 2001
10. Vega F et al: Primary paratesticular lymphoma: a report of 2 cases and review of literature. Arch Pathol Lab Med. 125(3):428-32, 2001
11. Tondini C et al: Diffuse large-cell lymphoma of the testis. J Clin Oncol. 17(9):2854-8, 1999
12. Ferry JA et al: Granulocytic sarcoma of the testis: a report of two cases of a neoplasm prone to misinterpretation. Mod Pathol. 10(4):320-5, 1997
13. Ferry JA et al: Testicular and epididymal plasmacytoma: a report of 7 cases, including three that were the initial manifestation of plasma cell myeloma. Am J Surg Pathol. 21(5):590-8, 1997
14. Ferry JA et al: Malignant lymphoma of the testis, epididymis, and spermatic cord. A clinicopathologic study of 69 cases with immunophenotypic analysis. Am J Surg Pathol. 18(4):376-90, 1994

LYMPHOMA/LEUKEMIA/PLASMACYTOMA

Gross and Microscopic Features

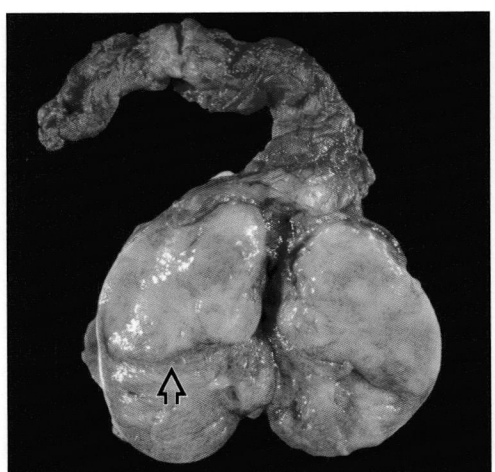
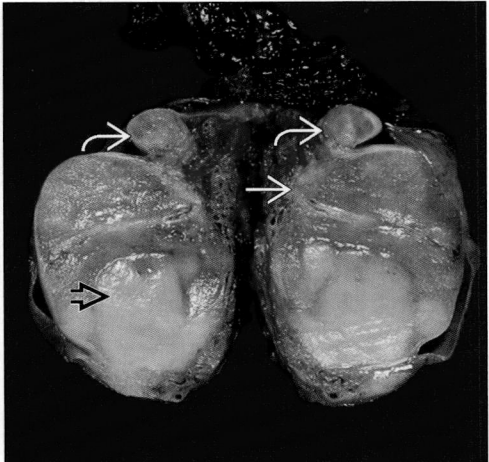

(Left) Malignant lymphoma ⊃ partially involves the testis and demonstrates sharp demarcation from the testicular parenchyma. It is relatively homogeneous, tan-white with a bulging cut surface and similar to seminoma or spermatocytic seminoma. *(Right)* Lymphoma is seen involving the testis ⊃, rete testis ➡, and epididymis ➡. Although it has a gross appearance similar to that of seminoma, involvement of paratesticular structures suggests greater likelihood of lymphoma.

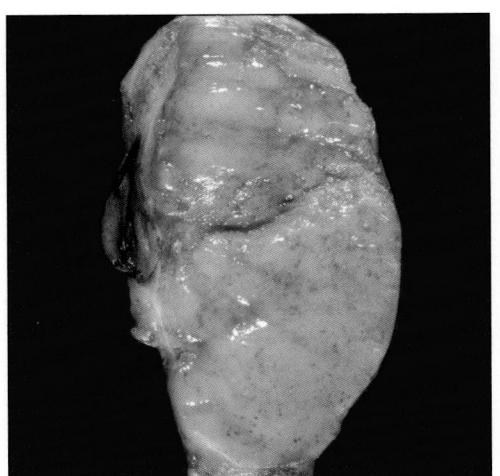
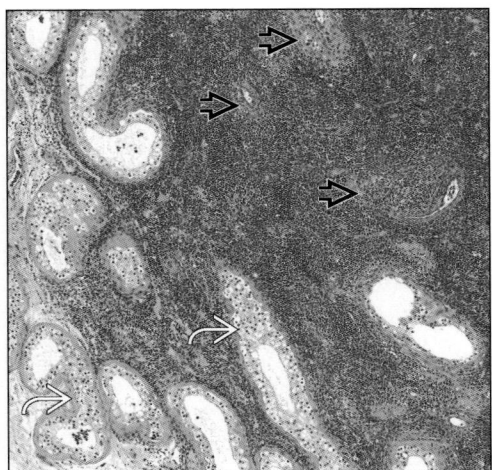

(Left) This testis is completely replaced by malignant lymphoma. It has a homogeneous, tan-white, bulging cut surface. Hemorrhage or necrosis is not present, & there is vague nodularity. *(Right)* Testicular lymphoma is seen with diffuse interstitial infiltration by lymphoma cells. The tubules within the tumor are atrophic or hyalinized ⊃, while some ➡ show thickening of the basement membrane. Metastatic Merkel cell carcinoma is another rare round blue cell tumor involving the testis.

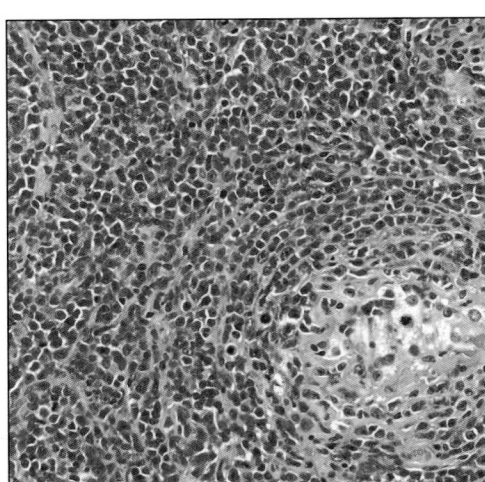
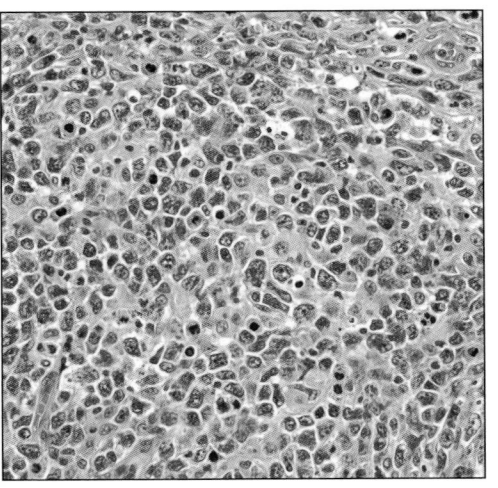

(Left) Closer scrutiny of cytologic features shows that the interstitial infiltrate of lymphoma cells has a prominent concentric peritubular "onion skin" arrangement around seminiferous tubules. The tubular wall is heavily infiltrated by lymphoma cells. *(Right)* In contrast to seminoma, this large B-cell lymphoma shows greater pleomorphism, uneven cellular distribution, and indistinct cell boundaries with lesser amounts of cytoplasm. Fibrous septae are absent.

Microscopic Features

(Left) High-power photomicrograph of lymphoma shows diffuse interstitial infiltration of large, cleaved and noncleaved discohesive tumor cells, infiltrating the thickened wall ⮞ of seminiferous tubules ("onion skin" pattern). *(Right)* Reticulin stain of testicular lymphoma shows typical "onion skin" appearance around the seminiferous tubules. Reticulin staining is rarely required in clinical practice, as immunophenotyping has more diagnostic, prognostic, and therapeutic relevance.

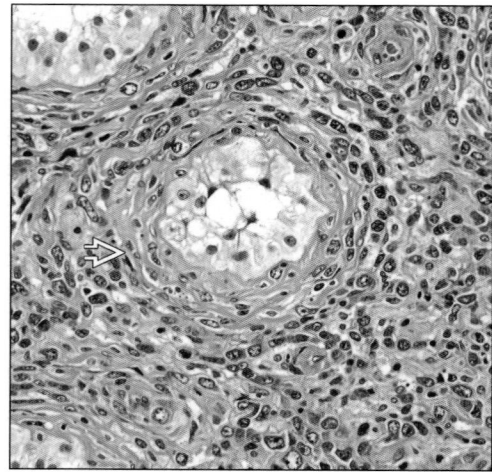

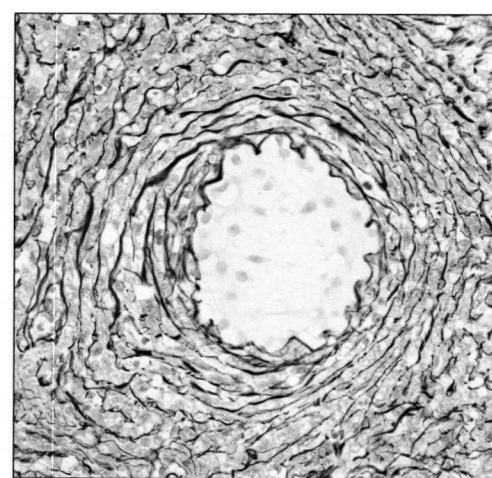

(Left) This photomicrograph shows partial to complete destruction of seminiferous tubules ⮞ by infiltrating lymphoma cells. Early sclerosis of the interstitium is seen ⮞. *(Right)* This photomicrograph shows a large B-cell lymphoma with significant sclerosis in the interstitium ⮞. The histologic finding of sclerosis in testicular lymphoma is 1 of the features associated with a favorable prognosis; other prognostic factors include age and stage of disease.

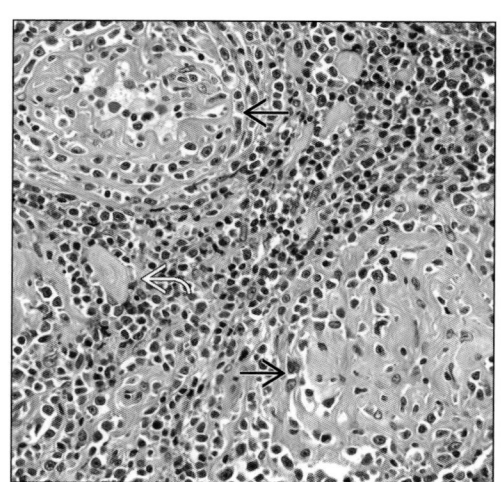

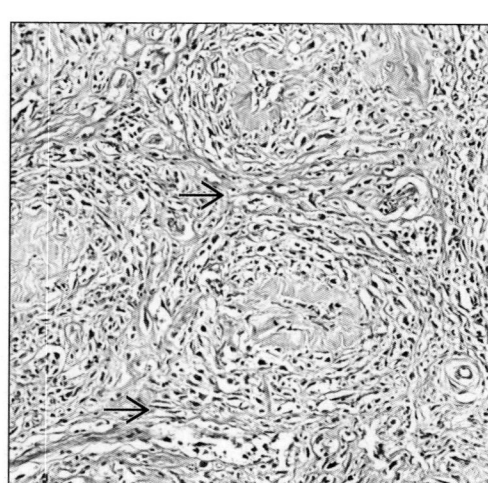

(Left) Seminiferous tubules involved by lymphoma cells (intratubular growth) may be easily confused with intratubular seminoma or embryonal carcinoma. In problematic cases, germ cell markers (Podoplanin(D2-40), Oct3/4, SALL4) and lymphoma markers will be discriminatory. *(Right)* Intratubular growth of lymphoma by anaplastic tumor cells with numerous mitoses ⮞ and frequent apoptoses ⮞; it should be noted that CD30(BerH2) staining is seen in embryonal carcinoma and anaplastic lymphoma.

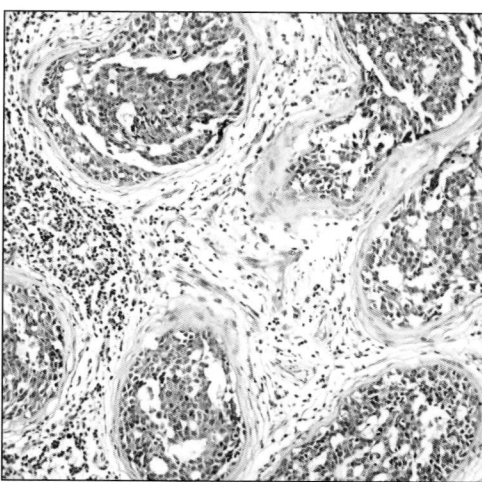

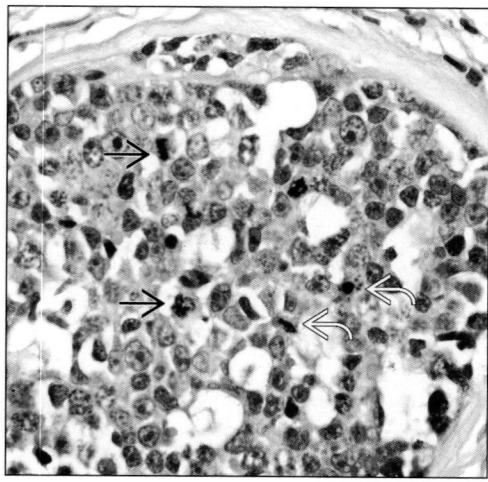

Microscopic and Gross Features

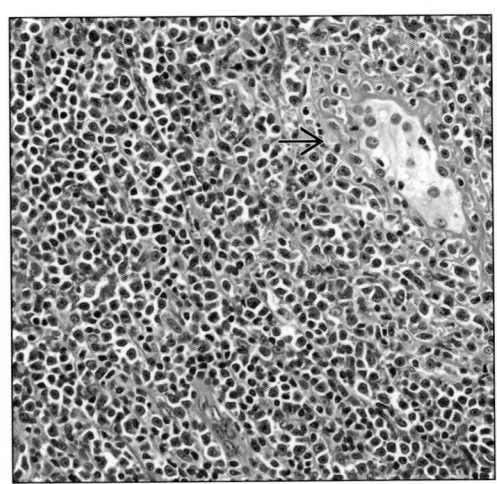

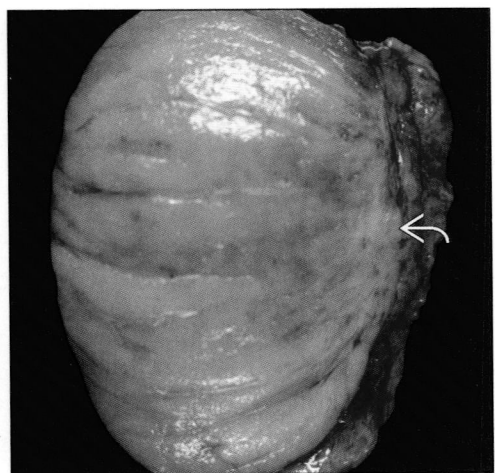

(Left) H&E shows interstitial infiltration of large cleaved & noncleaved lymphoma cells and a residual tubule focally infiltrated by lymphoma cells ➡. Interstitial growth in germ cell tumors is rare and occurs at the periphery. *(Right)* Gross photograph shows Burkitt lymphoma involving the entire testis & rete testis ➡. The tumor is homogeneous, tan-gray with lobulation and a bulging cut surface. Hemorrhage or necrosis is not present. It may involve the pediatric population and is known for rapid growth.

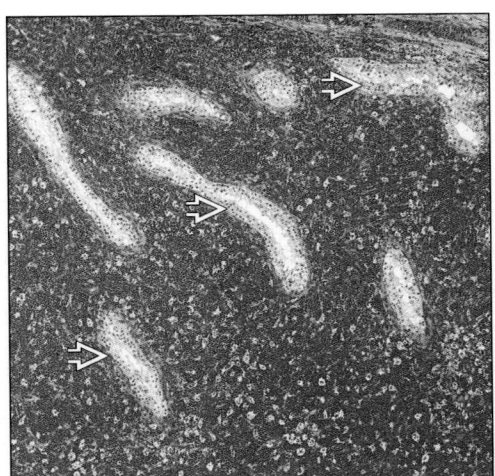

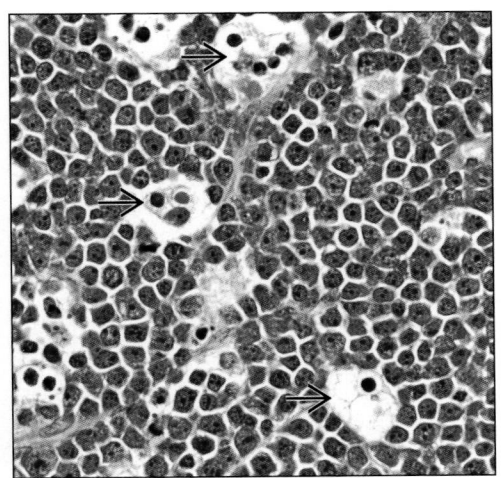

(Left) H&E shows Burkitt lymphoma of testis in a child. It is characterized by a diffuse interstitial infiltration of highly cellular lymphoid cells with a "starry sky" appearance. Note the relatively intact seminiferous tubules ➡. *(Right)* High-power photomicrograph of Burkitt lymphoma shows monotonous tumor cells with hyperchromatic nuclei and scant cytoplasm. Tingible body macrophages engulfing cell debris ➡ create the "starry sky" appearance.

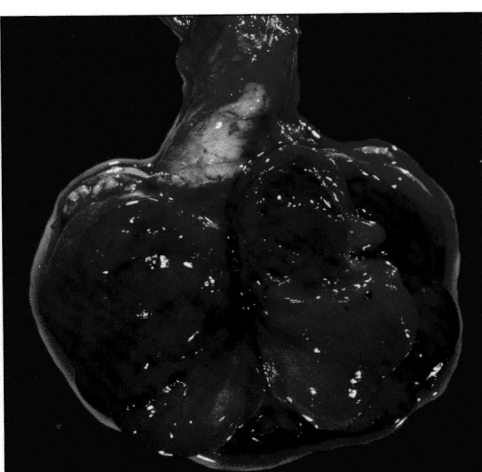

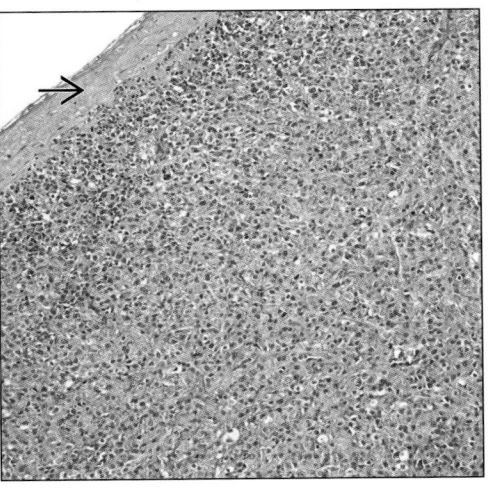

(Left) Testicular plasmacytoma with extensive hemorrhage. Most plasmacytomas show a soft, tan to gray-white cut surface, similar to seminoma. Extensive hemorrhage may occur and obscure the typical features of the tumor, as seen in this case. *(Right)* This is a low-power view of a plasmacytoma with sheets of atypical plasma cells. The tunica vaginalis and albuginea ➡ are intact. The differential diagnosis includes non-Hodgkin lymphoma and spermatocytic seminoma.

Microscopic Features

(Left) Plasmacytoma shows atypical tumor cells with eccentric round to oval nuclei, abundant eosinophilic cytoplasm, & perinuclear clearing (halo) ➡. Other differential diagnoses include rhabdoid type of Leydig cell tumor & chronic orchitis. (Right) H&E shows involvement of the rete testis ➡ by lymphoma. In contrast to seminoma, which may exhibit pagetoid growth, the tumor cells are more pleomorphic, unevenly distributed with nuclear overlapping and indistinct boundaries.

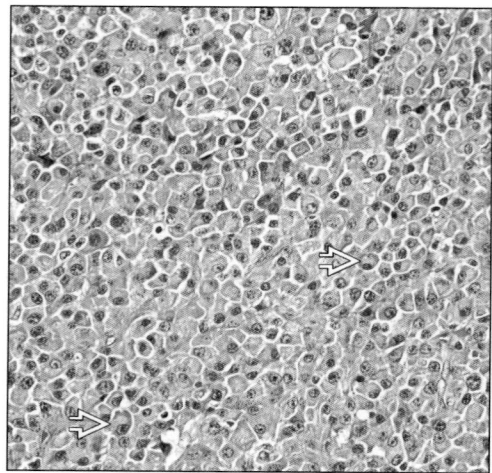
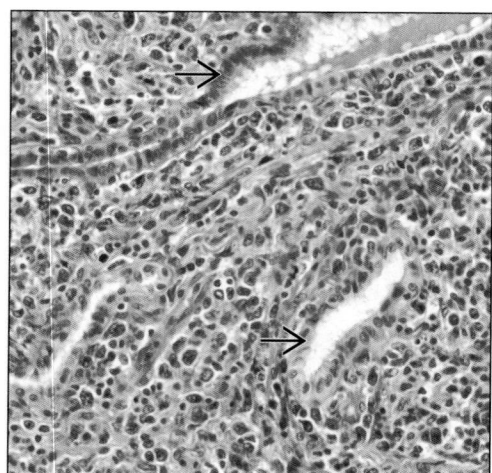

(Left) H&E shows a core biopsy of testicular leukemia. The testicular parenchyma is diffusely infiltrated by a highly cellular proliferation of tumor cells. The residual outline of a seminiferous tubule with "onion skinning" is present ➡. (Right) High-power view shows leukemic cells with relatively small nuclei, fine chromatin, and scant cytoplasm. Crush artifact of nuclei is present. Leukemic involvement of the testis is frequently misdiagnosed as malignant lymphoma and requires clinical correlation.

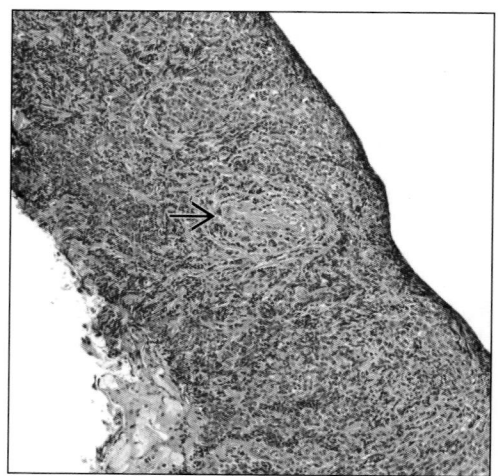
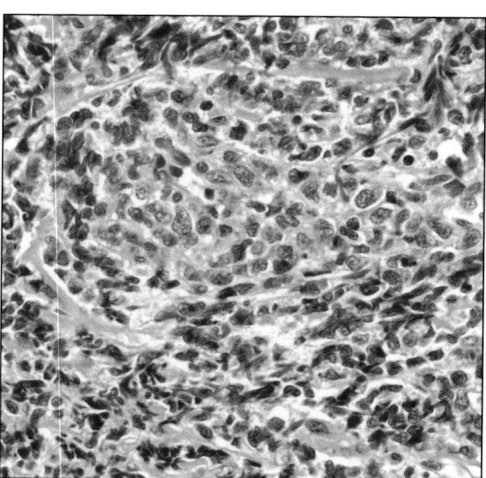

(Left) Another example of leukemic involvement of the testis is shown with the residual outline of a seminiferous tubule ➡. The testis is 1 of the sanctuary sites of leukemic patients, and a biopsy may be performed to diagnose relapse. (Right) High-power view shows leukemic cells with interstitial ➡ and intratubular ➡ infiltration by tumor cells with abundant pale eosinophilic cytoplasm. The intratubular involvement superficially resembles that of granulomatous inflammation.

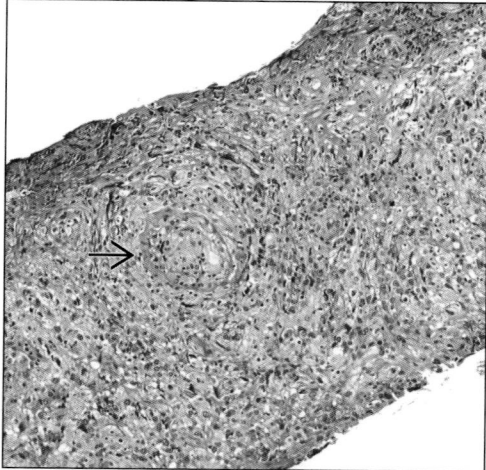
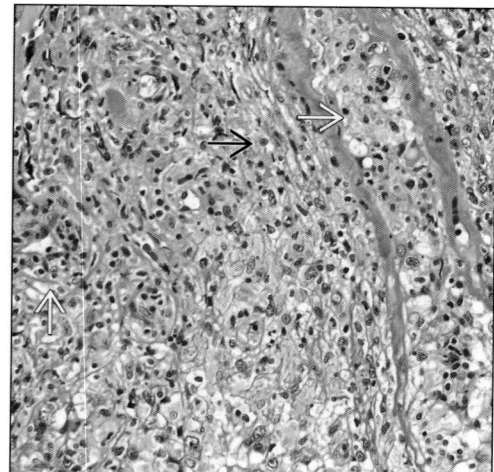

LYMPHOMA/LEUKEMIA/PLASMACYTOMA

Differential Diagnoses and Immunohistochemical Features

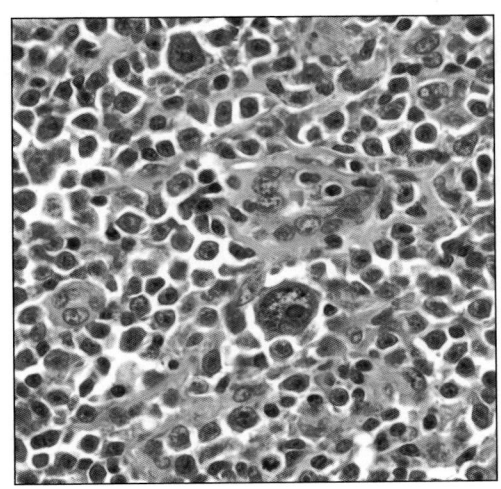
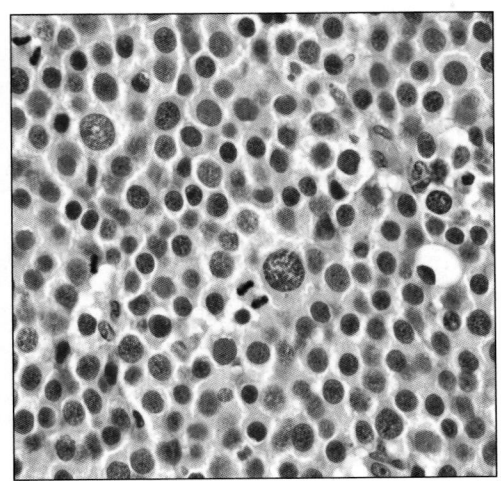

(Left) Diffuse large B-cell lymphoma shows occasional large giant cells that mimic spermatocytic seminoma. Both entities occur in older men; however, spermatocytic seminoma is distinct & shows cells with typical "spireme" chromatin. *(Right)* High-power view shows spermatocytic seminoma. The key features distinguishing it from a lymphoma include 3 different cell populations: Uniform round nuclei, fine or granular spireme-type chromatin, & more abundant cytoplasm.

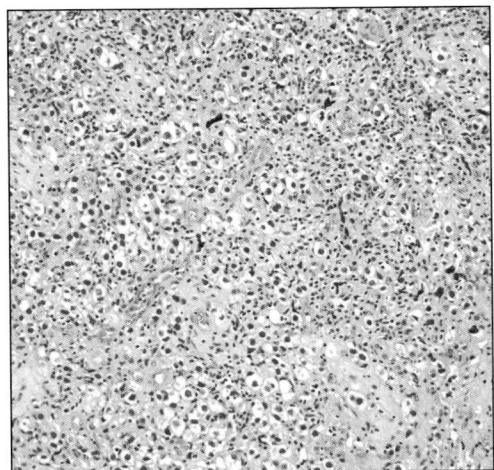
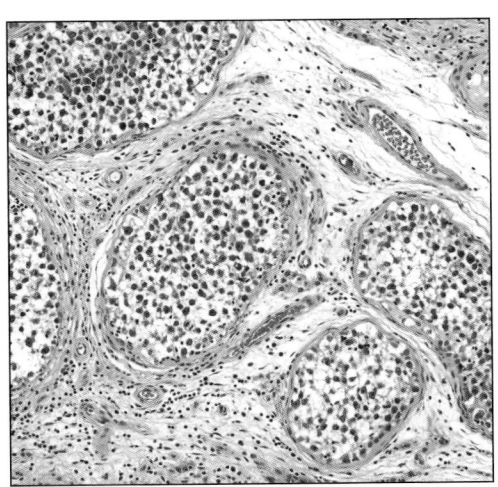

(Left) A classic seminoma with an interstitial infiltrative pattern may simulate a malignant lymphoma. Helpful clues for the diagnosis for seminoma are 2 cell populations: Large tumor cells with abundant clear cytoplasm and scattered small lymphocytes. *(Right)* This intratubular seminoma may be similar to intratubular lymphoma. In contrast to lymphoma, the seminoma cells are evenly distributed and have abundant clear cytoplasm and distinct cell boundaries.

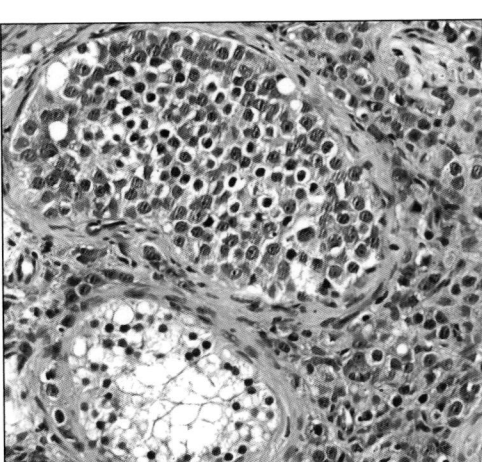
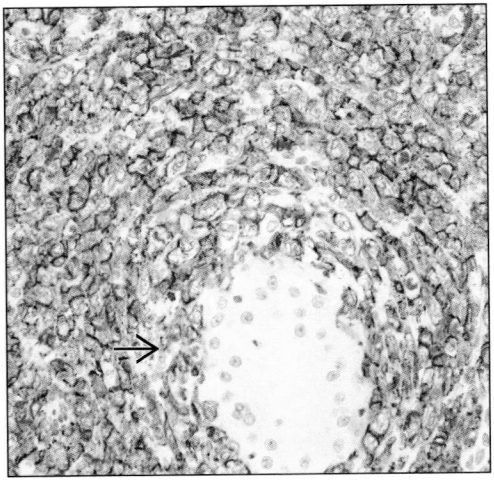

(Left) This is an example of metastatic high-grade prostate carcinoma with intratubular and interstitial growth patterns, similar to that of a large cell lymphoma. Clinical history and immunostains are critical for the correct diagnosis. *(Right)* This photomicrograph shows the immunostain of a large B-cell lymphoma with strong membranous staining by CD20. The tumor cells are seen in both the interstitium and the wall of a thickened seminiferous tubule ➡.

ADENOMATOID TUMOR

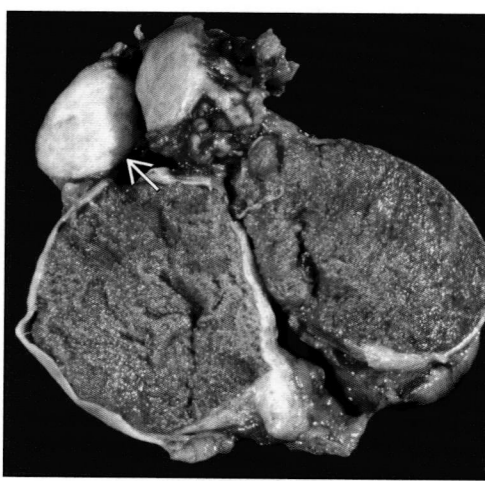

Adenomatoid tumor, the most common adnexal tumor, presents as a well-demarcated white-tan firm mass ➡ in the epididymis. It lacks hemorrhage, necrosis, or gross infiltrative characteristics.

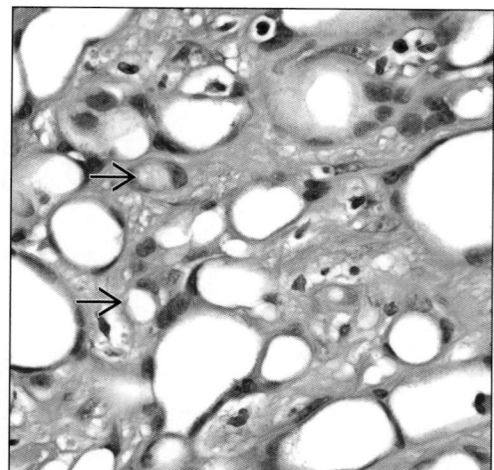

Adenomatoid tumor is composed of gland-like spaces lined by flattened cells. A few isolated cells with cytoplasmic vacuoles mimic signet ring cells ➡. A variety of patterns are usually present.

TERMINOLOGY

Definitions
- Benign paratesticular tumor of mesothelial cell origin, which has a variety of growth patterns, including glands, cysts, tubules, cords, or isolated cells

CLINICAL ISSUES

Epidemiology
- Incidence
  - Most common tumor of testicular adnexa
- Age
  - Range: 18-79 years (average: 36 years)

Presentation
- Usually asymptomatic, small and solid intrascrotal mass
- Most commonly occurs in head of epididymis, although it may occur in tunica vaginalis, albuginea, and rete testis
- Tumors may rarely be intratesticular and involve parietal tunica or spermatic cord

Treatment
- Surgical approaches
  - Surgical excision is curative

Prognosis
- Benign clinical course

MACROSCOPIC FEATURES

General Features
- Small, well-circumscribed, white-tan, homogeneous, firm mass
- No hemorrhage or necrosis

Size
- < 5 cm (majority < 2 cm)

MICROSCOPIC PATHOLOGY

Histologic Features
- Well-circumscribed, unencapsulated mass
- Tubules; gland-like, irregular cystic spaces or channels
- Nests and cords; true solid pattern rare
- Cuboidal, flat, or ovoid cells with round nuclei and abundant dense cytoplasm with vacuoles
- May show signet ring cell appearance
- May be cellular or infarcted
- Intervening fibrous stroma ± smooth muscle fibers
- Lymphoid aggregates may be prominent within or at periphery of tumor
- Rare tumors may be infarcted
  - Surrounding inflammation and reactive myofibroblastic proliferation may simulate invasion

Cytologic Features
- Eosinophilic, vacuolated, signet ring

Predominant Pattern/Injury Type
- Nests, cords, gland-like, tubular, cystic, and plexiform

Predominant Cell/Compartment Type
- Cuboidal to flat to ovoid with uniform cytology

ANCILLARY TESTS

Histochemistry
- PAS-diastase
  - Reactivity: Negative
- Mucicarmine
  - Reactivity: Negative

ADENOMATOID TUMOR

Key Facts

Terminology

- Benign paratesticular tumor of mesothelial cell origin, which has a variety of growth patterns, including glands, cysts, tubules, cords, or isolated cells

Clinical Issues

- Most common tumor of testicular adnexa (32%)
- Usually asymptomatic, small and solid intrascrotal/extratesticular adnexal mass
- Most commonly in epididymis, also in tunica vaginalis, albuginea, and rete testis

Macroscopic Features

- Small well-circumscribed white tan, homogeneous firm mass
- < 5 cm (majority < 2 cm)

Microscopic Pathology

- Well-circumscribed, nonencapsulated tumor mass
- Channels, gland-like or irregular cystic spaces, and nests and cords
- Cuboidal to flat or ovoid cells with round nuclei, abundant dense cytoplasm with vacuoles
- May show signet ring cell appearance
- Intervening fibrous stroma ± smooth muscle
- Lymphoid aggregates may be prominent within or at periphery of tumor

Ancillary Tests

- Positive for cytokeratin, calretinin, Podoplanin(D2-40), CK5/6, thrombomodulin, WT1
- Negative for CEA, CD15, FXVIIIAg, S100, CD31, CD34, FLI-1(vascular markers)

Immunohistochemistry

- Positive for cytokeratin, calretinin, Podoplanin(D2-40), CK5/6, thrombomodulin, WT1
- Negative for CEA, CD15, MOC-31, EpCAM/BER-EP4/CD326, FXVIIIAg, S100, CD31, CD34, FLI-1

DIFFERENTIAL DIAGNOSIS

Sex Cord Stromal Tumor

- Usually intraparenchymal tumor
- Positive for inhibin and Melan-A(MART-1)
- Negative for cytokeratin

Malignant Mesothelioma

- Larger tumor, destructive and infiltrative growth
- Greater cytologic atypia

Metastatic Signet Ring Cell Carcinoma

- Clinical history and older age
- Infiltrative growth, greater cytologic atypia, frequent mitoses
- Positive for CEA, CD15, EpCAM/BER-EP4/CD326, and MOC-31; negative for calretinin and Podoplanin(D2-40)

Epithelioid Hemangioma/Hemangioendothelioma

- Vasoformative lesion composed of vacuolated cells
- Positive for vascular markers (CD31, CD34, FLI-1); negative or weakly/focally positive for cytokeratin

Germ Cell Tumors (Particularly Yolk Sac Tumor)

- Intraparenchymal mass with heterogeneous appearance
- Obvious malignant cytologic features
- Positive for Oct3/4, SALL4, and CD30(BerH2); negative for calretinin

Leiomyosarcoma or Leiomyoma (vs. Leiomyomatous Adenomatoid Tumor)

- More compact cellular spindle cell proliferation with cytologic atypia and increased mitoses
- Lack of tubules or cystic spaces
- Negative or focally positive for cytokeratin

Liposarcoma

- Presence of lipoblasts and variable cells with adipocytic quality

DIAGNOSTIC CHECKLIST

Pathologic Interpretation Pearls

- Adenomatoid tumor may show a variety of patterns mimicking signet ring cell carcinoma, vascular tumor, and sex cord stromal tumor
- Paratesticular location and excellent circumscription are key in distinction of histologic differential diagnosis with malignant outcome

SELECTED REFERENCES

1. Pacheco AJ et al: Intraparenchymatous adenomatoid tumor dependent on the rete testis: A case report and review of literature. Indian J Urol. 25(1):126-8, 2009
2. Amin MB: Selected other problematic testicular and paratesticular lesions: rete testis neoplasms and pseudotumors, mesothelial lesions and secondary tumors. Mod Pathol. 18 Suppl 2:S131-45, 2005
3. Skinnider BF et al: Infarcted adenomatoid tumor: a report of five cases of a facet of a benign neoplasm that may cause diagnostic difficulty. Am J Surg Pathol. 28(1):77-83, 2004
4. Williams SB et al: Adenomatoid tumor of the testes. Urology. 63(4):779-81, 2004
5. Delahunt B et al: Immunohistochemical evidence for mesothelial origin of paratesticular adenomatoid tumour. Histopathology. 36(2):109-15, 2000
6. Samad AA et al: Adenomatoid tumor of intratesticular localization. Eur Urol. 30(1):127-8, 1996
7. Horstman WG et al: Adenomatoid tumor of testicle. Urology. 40(4):359-61, 1992

ADENOMATOID TUMOR

Microscopic and Gross Features

(Left) Adenomatoid tumor is characterized by irregularly shaped gland-like structures in a fibromyxoid stroma. The tumor cells are cuboidal to flattened and contain vacuolated cytoplasm ⊟. *(Right)* Adenomatoid tumor shows gland-like spaces of variable sizes lined by ovoid to cuboidal tumor cells with occasional prominent nucleoli ⊟ and vacuolated cytoplasm ⊟. Also seen are microcysts ⊟ lined by flattened lining cells. The amount of stroma is variable and often prominent.

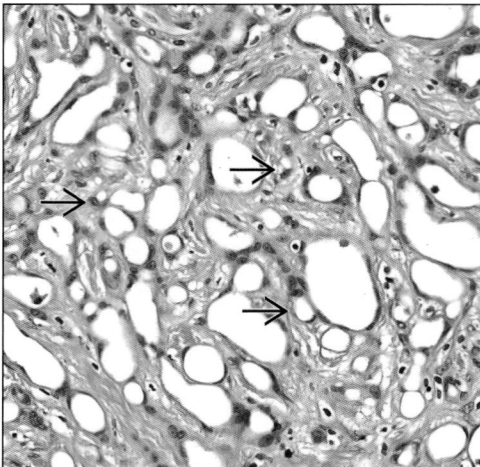
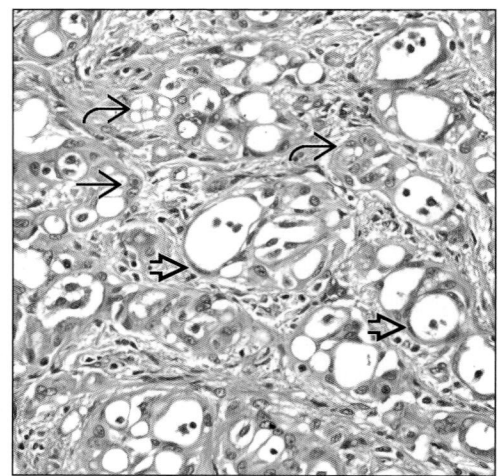

(Left) A small, well-circumscribed intraparenchymal adenomatoid tumor ⊟ is shown. The tumor has a homogeneous, firm, tan-white cut surface. The main differential diagnosis based on gross examination is a sex cord stromal tumor, which it may often microscopically resemble. *(Right)* This image shows a well-circumscribed, intraparenchymal adenomatoid tumor with irregular tubules in a fibrous stroma. Atrophic ⊟ seminiferous tubules are present.

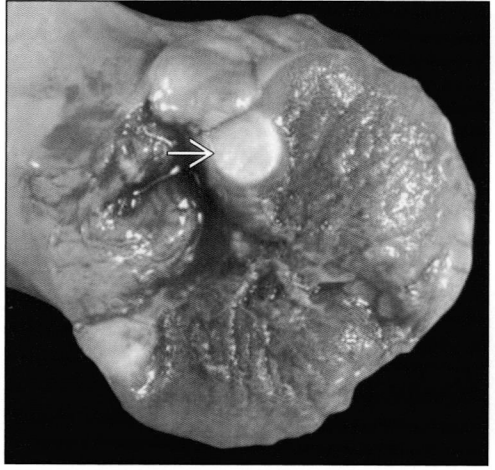
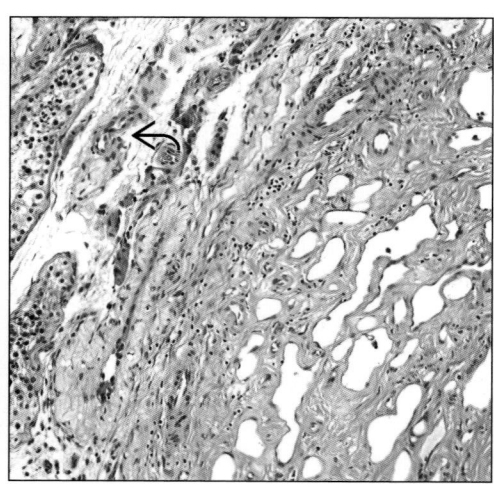

(Left) Adenomatoid tumor involving the rete testis ⊟ is shown. The tumor ⊟ shows variably sized tubules lined by cuboidal to flattened cells and accompanying dense, hyalinized, collagenous stroma. Also present are scattered lymphoid infiltrates ⊟. *(Right)* On high-power magnification, this adenomatoid tumor has dilated tubules ⊟ and irregular solid nests ⊟ infiltrating large bundles of hyalinized collagen. Occasional cells show a signet ring cell appearance.

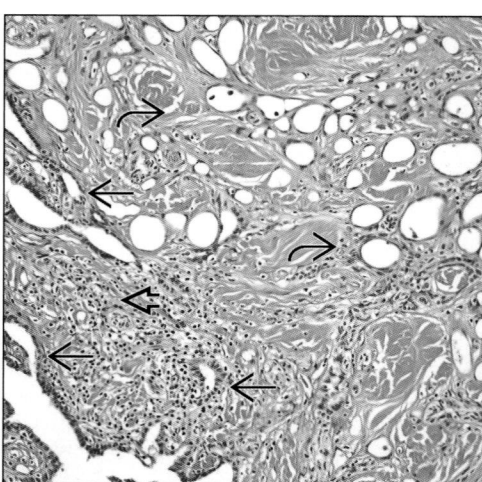
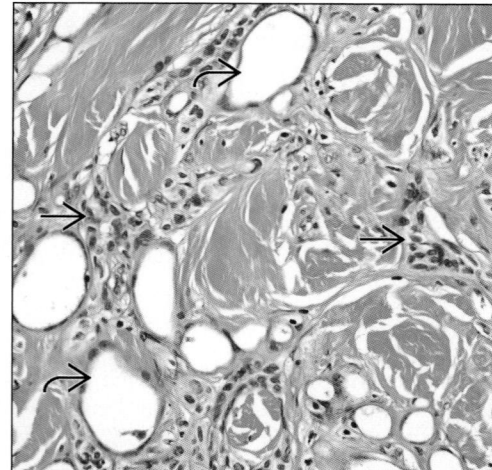

ADENOMATOID TUMOR

Microscopic Features

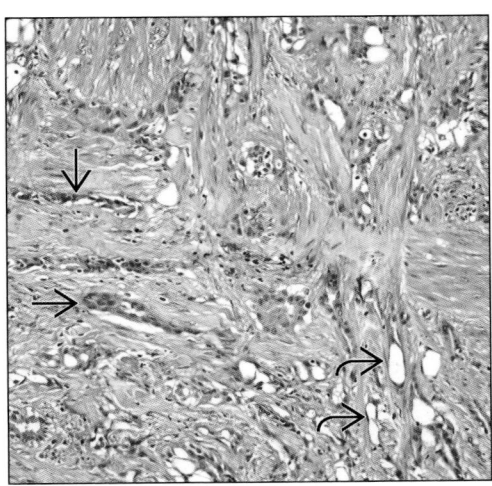

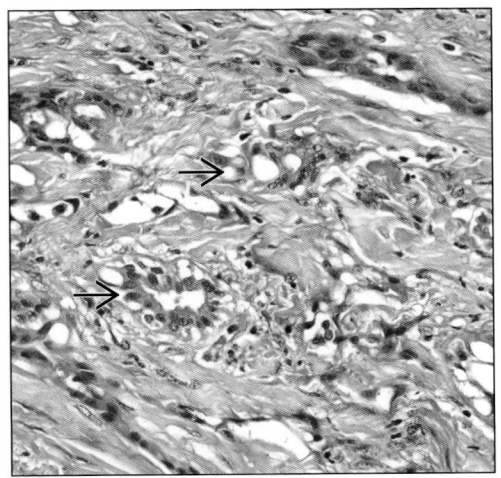

(Left) This adenomatoid tumor shows solid tubules ⮕ and gland-like spaces ⮕ lined by flattened to cuboidal cells in the background of dense fibrocollagenous stroma, mimicking an infiltrating adenocarcinoma. *(Right)* Adenomatoid tumor shows tubules ⮕ resembling an adenocarcinoma. The cytologic atypia is minimal and lacks significant mitotic activity or desmoplastic stromal response. The gross appearance of a circumscribed neoplasm is important for diagnosis.

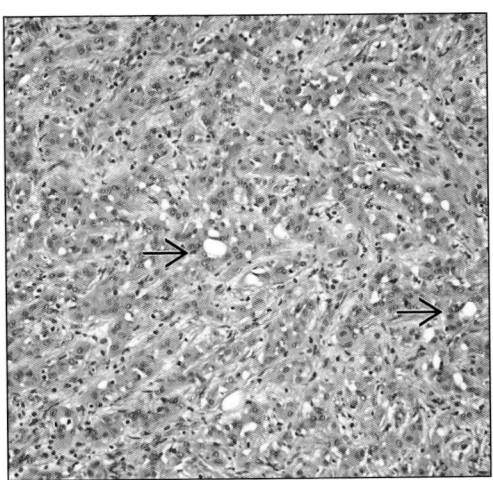

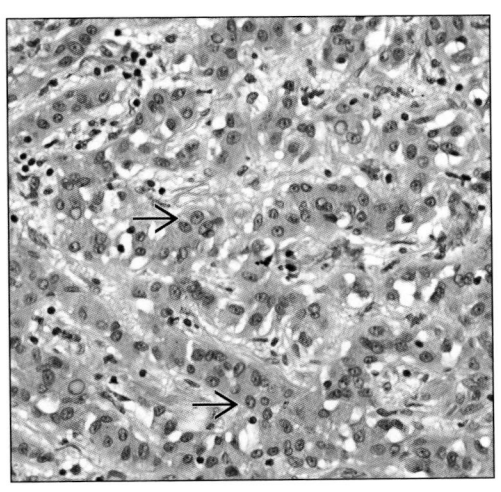

(Left) Cellular adenomatoid tumor shows solid sheets and trabeculae of tumor cells within a dense fibrous stroma. There is focal tubular formation ⮕. *(Right)* High-power photomicrograph shows trabeculae of adenomatoid tumor with epithelioid tumor cells with prominent nucleoli ⮕ in a dense fibrous stroma, resembling a Leydig cell tumor or mesothelioma. Lack of significant cytologic atypia and positivity for calretinin and Podoplanin(D2-40) favor the diagnosis of adenomatoid tumor.

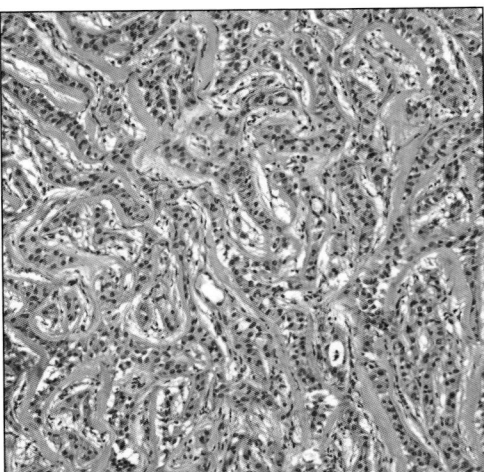

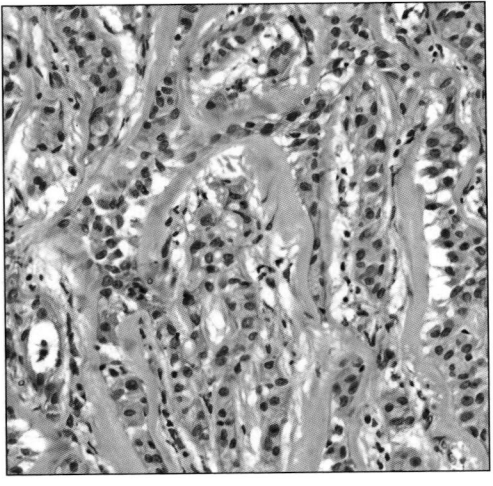

(Left) This adenomatoid tumor shows cords and trabeculae of cells within a hyalinized stroma. Because of the extensive epithelial configuration, a misdiagnosis of carcinoma may be rendered in an older patient during frozen section evaluation. *(Right)* Distinct from carcinoma, the tumor cells in this cellular adenomatoid tumor are relatively uniform, and no mitoses are present. The differential diagnosis also includes a sex cord stromal tumor.

MALIGNANT MESOTHELIOMA

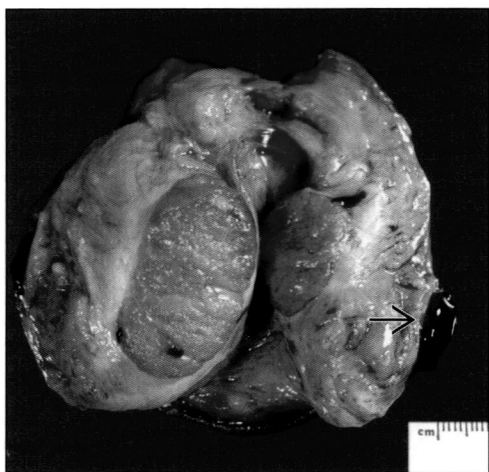

Malignant mesothelioma demonstrates a large paratesticular mass with nodular appearance, hemorrhage ➡, and necrosis encasing the testis and replacing the tunica around the testis.

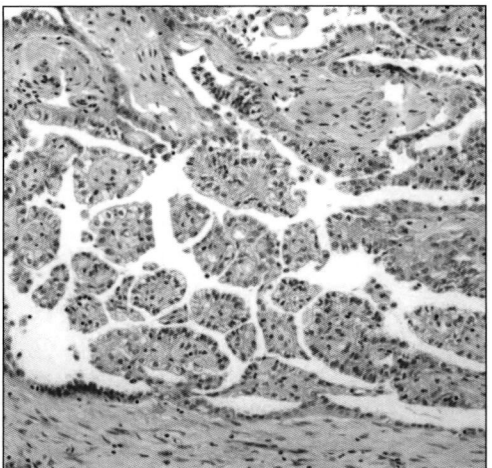

Malignant mesothelioma with papillary growth is shown. Papillary mesothelial hyperplasia is the main differential diagnosis. In this case, formation of mass lesion and areas of tunica invasion were seen.

TERMINOLOGY

Synonyms
- Mesothelioma

Definitions
- Malignant tumor arising from mesothelial cells in tunica vaginalis

ETIOLOGY/PATHOGENESIS

Pathogenesis
- Asbestos exposure is only known risk factor (associated with < 50% of cases in testicular mesothelioma)

CLINICAL ISSUES

Epidemiology
- Incidence
  - Rare, but 2nd most common paratesticular malignancy after soft tissue sarcoma
- Age
  - Range: 6-90 years old (average: 54 years)
  - 10% of cases occur in patients younger than 25 years old

Presentation
- Paratesticular mass or associated with hydrocele
- May be incidental finding during hernia repair

Treatment
- Surgical approaches
  - Surgical resection is choice of therapy
  - Adjuvant chemotherapy has been proved to have limited effect

Prognosis
- Variable depending on clinical stage

MACROSCOPIC FEATURES

General Features
- Variable, often diffuse thickening of tunica vaginalis with multiple friable nodules or excrescences
- Tumor may invade tunica albuginea, testis, epididymis, and spermatic cord

MICROSCOPIC PATHOLOGY

Histologic Features
- Majority are pure epithelial type (60-70%) or biphasic (30-40%)
- Rare sarcomatoid or desmoplastic types may also occur
- Papillary, tubulopapillary, glandular (well differentiated), or solid growth patterns (poorly differentiated)
- Round or cuboidal cells with mild or moderate cellular pleomorphism and often prominent nucleoli
- Dense chromatin with variable mitotic activity
- Foam cells or psammoma bodies may be present
- Cytologic atypia or mesothelial proliferation alone may not be diagnostic for malignant mesothelioma
- Invasion beyond tunica is key diagnostic criterion

Predominant Pattern/Injury Type
- Solid, papillary and tubulopapillary

Predominant Cell/Compartment Type
- Cuboidal or oval round, relatively uniform cells with prominent nucleolus

ANCILLARY TESTS

Immunohistochemistry
- Positive for (PAN-CK)AE1/AE3, EMA/MUC1, vimentin, calretinin, Podoplanin(D2-40), CK5/6, thrombomodulin, mesothelin, WT1

4

MALIGNANT MESOTHELIOMA

Key Facts

Terminology
- Malignant tumor originating from mesothelial cells of tunica vaginalis

Clinical Issues
- Rare, but 2nd most common paratesticular malignancies after soft tissue sarcoma
- < 50% reported cases associated with asbestos exposure
- Age range: 6-90 years old (average: 54 years)
- Paratesticular mass or associated with hydrocele; may be incidental finding during hernia repair

Microscopic Pathology
- Majority are pure epithelial type (60-70%) or biphasic (30-40%)
- Rare sarcomatoid or desmoplastic type occur as well

- Papillary, tubulopapillary, glandular (well differentiated) or solid growth patterns (poorly differentiated)
- Round or cuboidal cells with mild or moderate cellular pleomorphism and often prominent nucleoli
- Dense hyperchromatic chromatin and frequent mitoses
- Foam cells, psammoma bodies may be seen
- Invasion is key diagnostic criterion

Ancillary Tests
- Positive for PAN-CK(AE1/AE3), EMA/MUC1, vimentin, calretinin, Podoplanin(D2-40), CK5/6, thrombomodulin, mesothelin, and WT1
- Negative for CEA, TAG72, CD15, EpCAM/BER-EP4/CD326

- Negative for CEA, TAG72, CD15, EpCAM/BER-EP4/CD326, desmin (frequent)

DIFFERENTIAL DIAGNOSIS

Adenocarcinoma of Rete Testis
- More striking nuclear pleomorphism, significant desmoplasia, transition from rete testis epithelium
- Negative for calretinin, Podoplanin(D2-40), or CK5/6

Metastatic Carcinoma
- Clinical history of carcinoma elsewhere, usually greater cytologic atypia
- Negative for calretinin or Podoplanin(D2-40)

Embryonal Carcinoma
- Marked cytologic anaplasia, intratesticular mass, younger age
- Positive for CD30(BerH2), PLAP, Podoplanin(D2-40), SALL4, and Oct3/4

Primary or Metastatic Sarcoma vs. Sarcomatoid Mesothelioma
- High-grade spindle cells with greater cytologic atypia
- Epicenter in spermatic cord

Serous Carcinoma of Rete Testis/Epidydimis
- Morphologically, may be very similar with histology of high-grade adenocarcinoma
- Positive for CD15, CA125, CEA; usually negative for calretinin, Podoplanin(D2-40), or CK5/6

Adenomatoid Tumor
- Often asymptomatic, small size and well circumscribed, commonly seen in epididymis
- Bland cytologic features, no necrosis, no or few mitoses

Mesothelial Hyperplasia
- Overall less cytologic atypia and lack of architectural complexity and true invasion
- May be extremely difficult to distinguish from mesothelioma in small biopsy

- Desmin is more frequently positive in mesothelial hyperplasia than mesothelioma

DIAGNOSTIC CHECKLIST

Pathologic Interpretation Pearls
- Tubulopapillary, papillary, biphasic, or rarely sarcomatous tumor with epicenter in tunica vaginalis
- Tumor demonstrates invasive characteristics and mesothelial derivation by immunohistochemistry

SELECTED REFERENCES

1. Al-Qahtani M et al: Malignant mesothelioma of the tunica vaginalis. Can J Urol. 14(2):3514-7, 2007
2. Frias-Kletecka MC et al: Mesothelioma of the tunica vaginalis. J Urol. 178(4 Pt 1):1489, 2007
3. Schure PJ et al: Mesothelioma of the tunica vaginalis testis: a rare malignancy mimicking more common inguino-scrotal masses. J Surg Oncol. 94(2):162-4; discussion 161, 2006
4. Tolhurst SR et al: Well-differentiated papillary mesothelioma occurring in the tunica vaginalis of the testis with contralateral atypical mesothelial hyperplasia. Urol Oncol. 24(1):36-9, 2006
5. Winstanley AM et al: The immunohistochemical profile of malignant mesotheliomas of the tunica vaginalis: a study of 20 cases. Am J Surg Pathol. 30(1):1-6, 2006
6. Amin MB: Selected other problematic testicular and paratesticular lesions: rete testis neoplasms and pseudotumors, mesothelial lesions and secondary tumors. Mod Pathol. 18 Suppl 2:S131-45, 2005
7. Perez-Ordonez B et al: Mesothelial lesions of the paratesticular region. Semin Diagn Pathol. 17(4):294-306, 2000
8. Plas E et al: Malignant mesothelioma of the tunica vaginalis testis: review of the literature and assessment of prognostic parameters. Cancer. 83(12):2437-46, 1998
9. Jones MA et al: Malignant mesothelioma of the tunica vaginalis. A clinicopathologic analysis of 11 cases with review of the literature. Am J Surg Pathol. 19(7):815-25, 1995

MALIGNANT MESOTHELIOMA

Microscopic Features

(Left) Papillary mesothelioma with exophytic growth is shown. The main differential diagnosis is papillary mesothelial hyperplasia. Mesothelioma is usually large and shows a more complex growth pattern. However, the most important finding in mesothelioma is invasion. *(Right)* This is a papillary mesothelioma arising from the tunica vaginalis. The differential diagnoses includes ovarian-type papillary serous carcinoma.

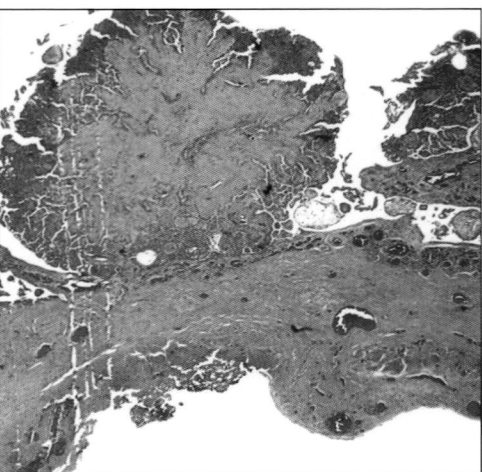
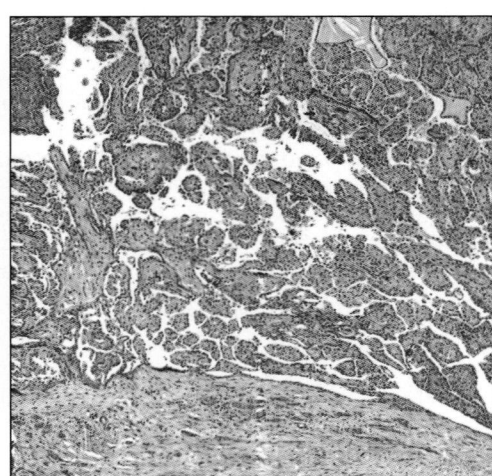

(Left) Papillary mesothelioma shows complex papillae lined by relatively uniform mesothelial cells. Grossly the tumor was large and encased the testis. Relationship with the tunica is important when other differential diagnoses are concerned. *(Right)* Mesothelioma shows partly solid ➡ and well-formed glandular spaces ➡ lined by relatively uniform neoplastic cells with prominent nucleoli. In contrast to most adenocarcinoma, there is lack of significant cytologic atypia.

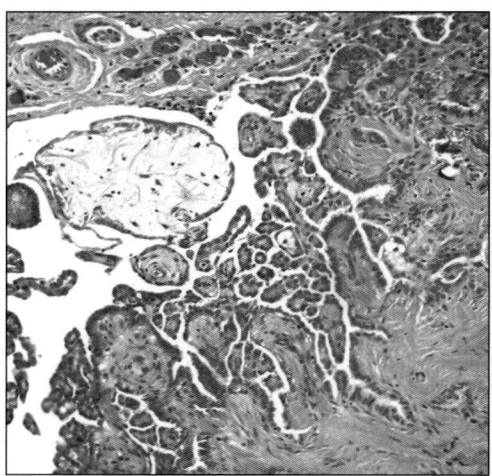
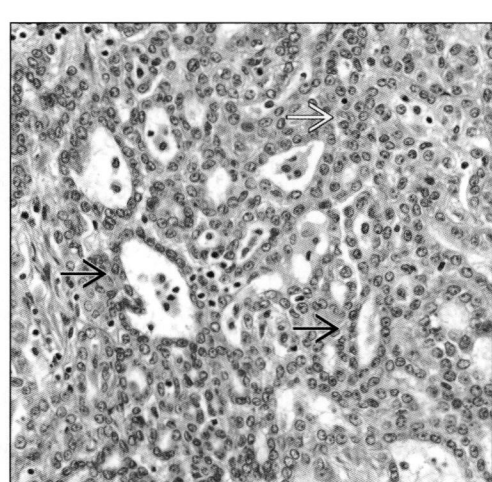

(Left) This area of mesothelioma shows exophytic papillary and endophytic invasive growth of tumor cells. The tumor cells lining the papillae are relatively uniform. The nuclei of the invasive component are larger ➡ and have prominent nucleoli. *(Right)* Mesothelioma is composed of solid sheets of tumor cells with poor evidence of glandular differentiation ➡. Metastatic prostate carcinoma is in the differential diagnosis, although the latter is centered in the rete.

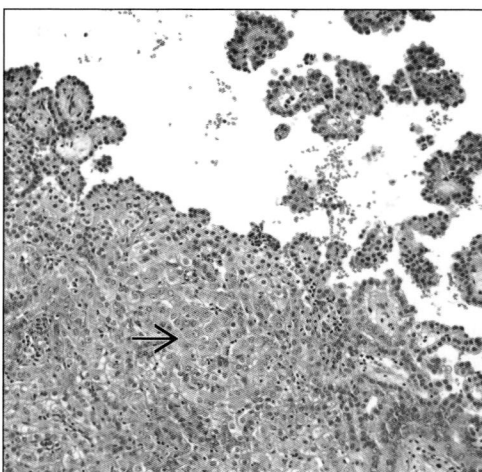
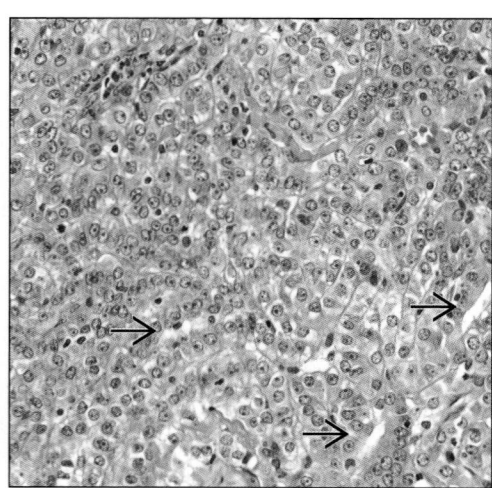

MALIGNANT MESOTHELIOMA

Microscopic Features

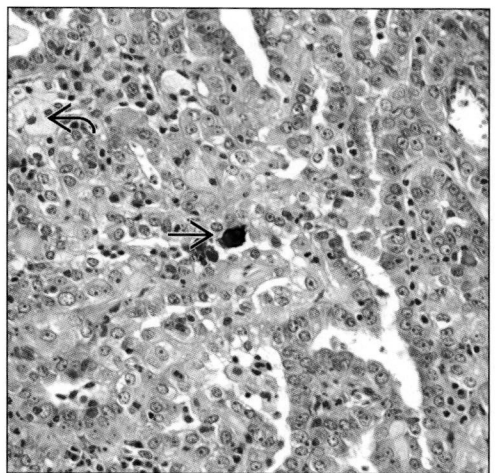

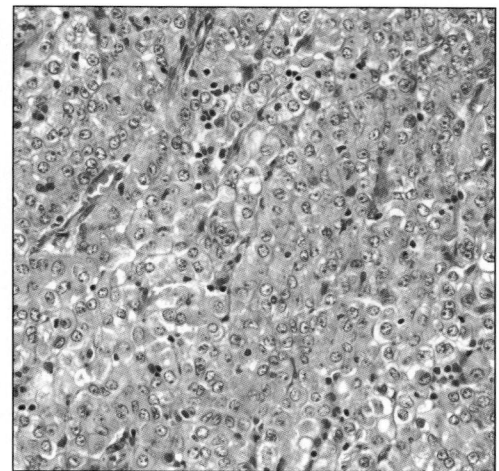

(Left) Mesothelioma shows irregular anastomosing tubules and papillae lined by relatively uniform tumor cells with vesicular chromatin and prominent nucleoli. Psammoma body-type calcification is present ➡. A few foam cells ➘ are seen. *(Right)* Poorly differentiated mesothelioma with solid growth pattern is shown. Mesotheliomas demonstrate a range of architecture ranging from papillary to tubular to glandular and solid with or without spindled (sarcomatoid) biphasic growth.

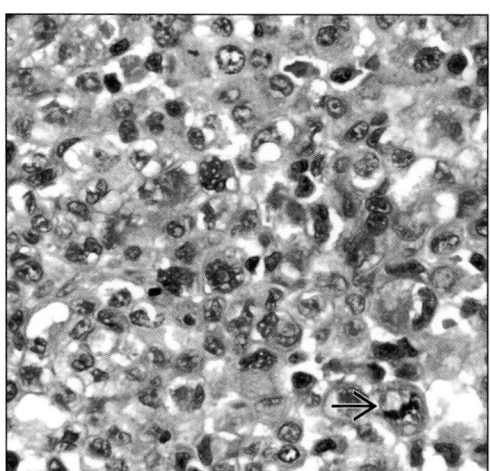

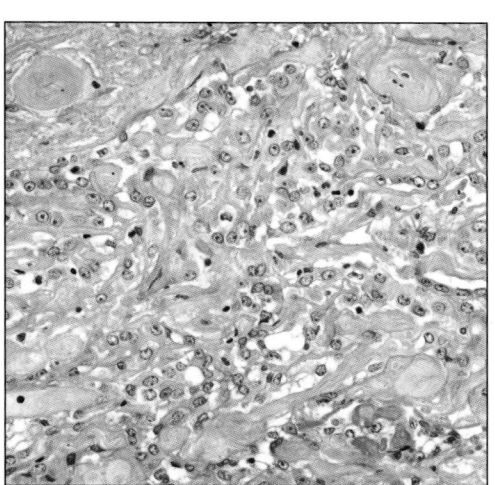

(Left) Although uncommon, mesothelioma can have marked nuclear pleomorphism, coarse chromatin, & increased mitoses ➡. Immunostains with a mesothelioma-associated panel (including calretinin, Podoplanin(D2-40), CK5/6, CEA, or CD15) are mandatory. *(Right)* Mesothelioma with invasion into the tunica is shown. The hyalinized stroma & irregular anastomosing channels lined by uniform tumor cells are superficially reminiscent to that of adenomatoid tumor.

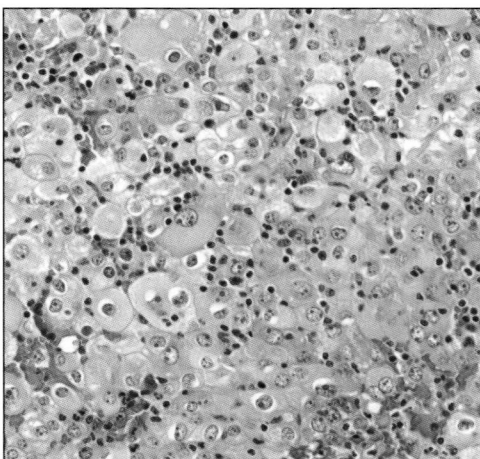

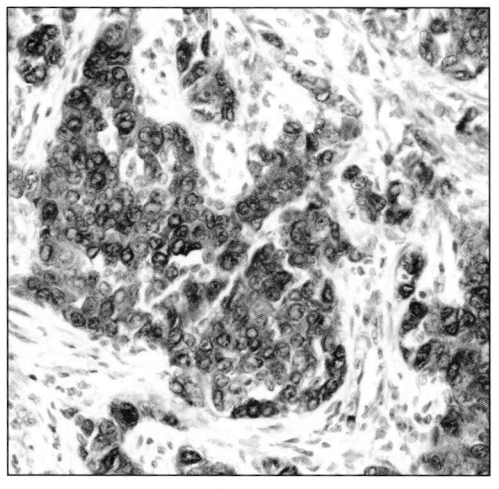

(Left) This mesothelioma is composed of sheets of large epithelioid cells with abundant eosinophilic cytoplasm and prominent nucleoli, which may be referred to as deciduoid or histiocytoid variant of mesothelioma. *(Right)* Mesothelioma is strongly positive (nuclear and cytoplasmic) for calretinin. A number of other markers (Podoplanin(D2-40), CK5/6, WT1) are available for detection of mesothelial differentiation and are helpful to differentiate from carcinoma.

ADENOCARCINOMA OF RETE TESTIS/EPIDIDYMIS

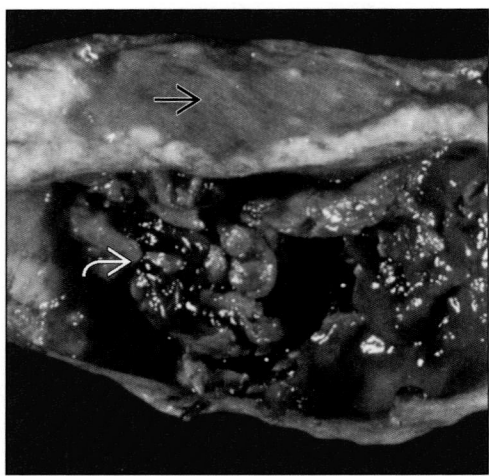

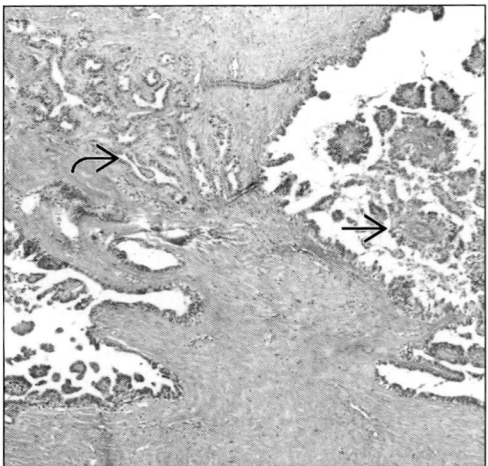

Carcinoma of rete testis with large hemorrhagic and cystic neoplasm in the hilum ➡ is shown. The testicular parenchyma is uninvolved ➡. Precise location of the mass is the key to determining the primary.

Carcinoma of the rete testis shows a transition from normal-appearing rete ➡ to a complex intracystic papillary architecture with abnormal cytology ➡. Infiltrative growth was seen elsewhere.

TERMINOLOGY

Definitions
- Primary carcinoma with glandular differentiation arising from rete testis or epididymis
- Carcinomas occurring at either site may be morphologically indistinguishable
- Criteria for rete testis adenocarcinoma include
  - Absence of similar extrascrotal tumor (ruling out metastasis)
  - Tumor centered in hilum
  - Tumor incompatible with other testicular or paratesticular tumor
  - Papillary serous carcinoma and mesothelioma ruled out by immunohistochemistry

CLINICAL ISSUES

Epidemiology
- Incidence
  - Extremely rare; only handful of cases reported
- Age
  - Range: 20-90 years (majority > 60 years)

Presentation
- Large solid scrotal mass associated with pain
- About 25% are associated with hydrocele, inguinal hernia, or fistula

Treatment
- Surgical resection is treatment of choice
- Chemotherapy/radiation therapy in advanced and metastatic disease

Prognosis
- Generally poor when locally advanced or when distant metastasis occurs

IMAGE FINDINGS

General Features
- Large heterogeneous mass by ultrasonography

MACROSCOPIC FEATURES

General Features
- White to gray firm, rubbery, nonencapsulated infiltrative mass
- Hilar location (rete carcinoma) and epididymal location (epididymal carcinoma)

Size
- Range: 1-10 cm

MICROSCOPIC PATHOLOGY

Histologic Features
- Solid, papillary or tubulopapillary growth with range of differentiation
- Invasive growth with desmoplasia
- Morphologic transition from nonneoplastic rete or epididymis to adenocarcinoma, including in situ changes
- Nuclear stratification, moderate to marked nuclear pleomorphism with mitoses, apoptosis, and necrosis
- Intracytoplasmic or extracellular mucin may be seen; signet ring cells may be seen
- Sarcomatoid carcinoma has been reported

Predominant Pattern/Injury Type
- Neoplastic/gland forming

Predominant Cell/Compartment Type
- Tubular, papillary, tubulopapillary and solid patterns with columnar and cuboidal cells

ADENOCARCINOMA OF RETE TESTIS/EPIDIDYMIS

Key Facts

Terminology
- Carcinoma with glandular differentiation arising from rete testis or epididymis

Clinical Issues
- Very rare
- Age range: 20-90 years (majority > 60 years)
- Large solid scrotal mass with pain

Macroscopic Features
- Located in hilum of testis or epididymal area, white to gray firm mass with hemorrhage or necrosis

Microscopic Pathology
- Solid, papillary, tubulopapillary, or tubular growth patterns with different degree of differentiation
- Invasive into surrounding tissue with desmoplasia

- Morphologic transition from nonneoplastic rete or epididymis to adenocarcinoma
- Nuclear stratification, moderate to marked nuclear pleomorphism, frequent mitoses, apoptosis, and necrosis
- Intracytoplasmic or extracellular mucin may be seen

Ancillary Tests
- Positive for cytokeratin, CEA, MOC-31, CD15, EpCAM/BER-EP4/CD326, EMA/MUC1, and CK7
- Negative for PLAP, Oct3/4, SALL4, CD30(BerH2), α-fetoprotein, HCG, calretinin, inhibin, and CK5/6

Top Differential Diagnoses
- Malignant mesothelioma
- Metastatic carcinoma
- Tumors of müllerian origin

ANCILLARY TESTS

Histochemistry
- PAS-diastase
  - Reactivity: Positive
  - Staining pattern
    - Diffuse cytoplasmic
- Mucicarmine and Alcian blue
  - Reactivity: Positive (usually)
  - Staining pattern
    - Diffuse cytoplasmic

Immunohistochemistry
- Positive for cytokeratin, CEA, EMA/MUC1, MOC-31, CD15, EpCAM/BER-EP4/CD326, and CK7
- Negative for PLAP, Podoplanin(D2-40), Oct3/4, SALL4, CD30(BerH2), α-fetoprotein, HCG, calretinin, inhibin, and CK5/6

DIFFERENTIAL DIAGNOSIS

Malignant Mesothelioma
- Epicenter in tunica vaginalis
- Histologic transition from mesothelial lining
- Positive for calretinin, Podoplanin(D2-40), CK5/6; negative for MOC-31, CEA, CD15, EpCAM/BER-EP4/CD326

Metastatic Carcinoma
- History of carcinoma elsewhere, usually small size, lack of histologic transition from rete testis or epididymis
- Frequent vascular-lymphatic invasion and interstitial growth

Tumors of Müllerian Origin
- Lack of histologic transition from rete or epididymis, epicenter in tunica
- Papillary serous, endometrioid, clear cell or mucinous morphology
- Borderline tumor may be seen

Embryonal Carcinoma
- Commonly seen in younger age group (25-35 years)
- More pronounced pleomorphism
- Frequently associated with other germ cell tumor components and ITGCN
- Positive for germ cell markers (PLAP, Podoplanin(D2-40), Oct3/4, SALL4, and CD30[BerH2]); negative for EMA/MUC1

Rete Testis Hyperplasia
- Expands preexisting rete epithelium
- Intracytoplasmic and extracellular hyaline globules
- No cytologic atypia or invasive growth
- No desmoplastic reaction

Cystadenoma of Epididymis
- Frequently associated with von Hippel-Lindau syndrome
- Usually occurs in young adults and frequently bilateral
- Small size with well-defined boundary
- Tumor cells have abundant clear cytoplasm and lack significant cytologic atypia

DIAGNOSTIC CHECKLIST

Pathologic Interpretation Pearls
- Gland-forming carcinoma with histologic transition from rete or epididymal epithelium, epicenter either in hilum of testis or epididymis

SELECTED REFERENCES

1. Sogni F et al: Primary adenocarcinoma of the rete testis: diagnostic problems and therapeutic dilemmas. Scand J Urol Nephrol. 42(1):83-5, 2008
2. Nakagawa T et al: Primary adenocarcinoma of the rete testis with preceding diagnosis of pulmonary metastases. Int J Urol. 13(12):1532-5, 2006
3. Amin MB: Selected other problematic testicular and paratesticular lesions: rete testis neoplasms and pseudotumors, mesothelial lesions and secondary tumors. Mod Pathol. 18 Suppl 2:S131-45, 2005

ADENOCARCINOMA OF RETE TESTIS/EPIDIDYMIS

Microscopic Features

(Left) Carcinoma of rete testis with infiltrating malignant glands ➡ and dense desmoplasia shows a close relationship to dysplastic and in situ carcinoma ➡ of the rete, a diagnostic feature of rete testis carcinoma. *(Right)* In situ adenocarcinoma shows stratified glandular epithelium with secondary lumina formation and nuclear atypia with mitoses ➡. In the absence of in situ changes, metastatic carcinoma, mesothelioma, and papillary serous carcinoma are important differentials.

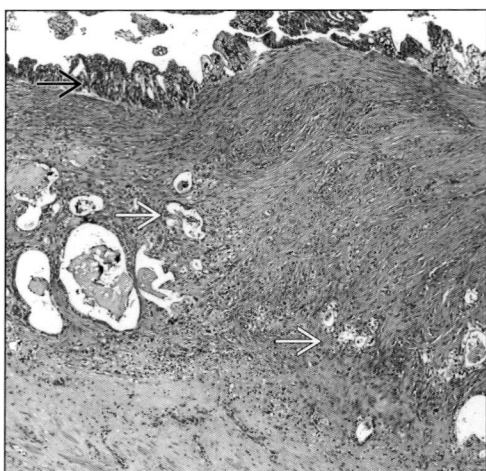
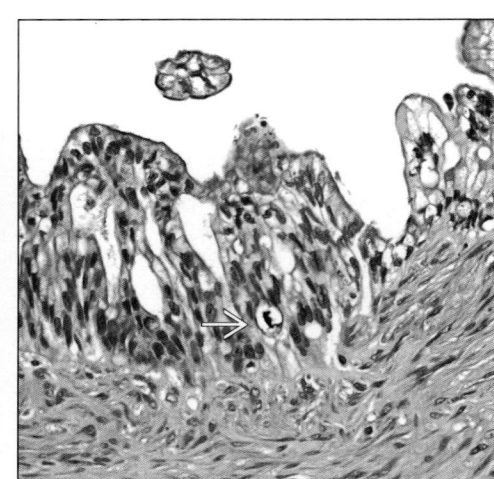

(Left) Carcinoma of rete testis shows nests of tumor cells with focal glandular lumina and infiltrative growth ➡. The key diagnostic features include histologic transition ➡ and epicenter in the rete epithelium. *(Right)* Although unequivocal histologic transition from epididymis ➡ was not demonstrated, this tumor was diagnosed as primary epididymal carcinoma ➡ based on its location in the epididymis and lack of primary tumor elsewhere despite an extensive work-up.

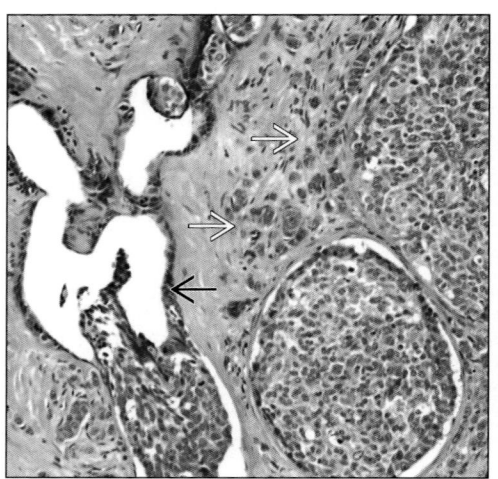
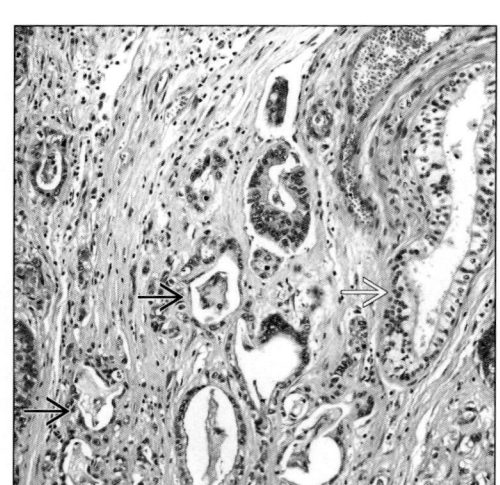

(Left) This photomicrograph shows infiltrating adenocarcinoma ➡ in the epididymis with irregular and variable-sized glands and prominent desmoplasia. The carcinoma infiltrates between normal epididymal glands ➡. *(Right)* Infiltrating adenocarcinoma of the epididymis shows small poorly formed glands ➡ and tumor cell nests ➡ in a desmoplastic stroma. Determination of the location in the epididymis and ruling out a primary elsewhere are important to determine the diagnosis.

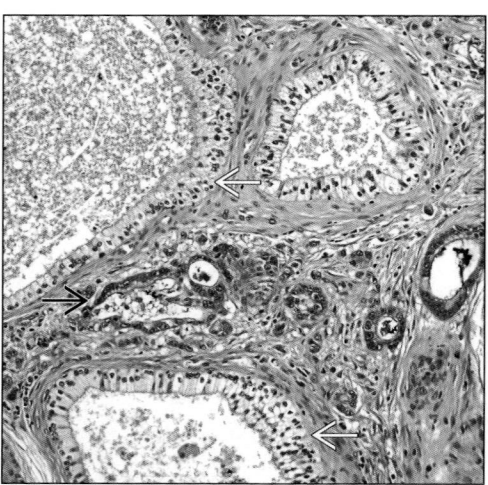
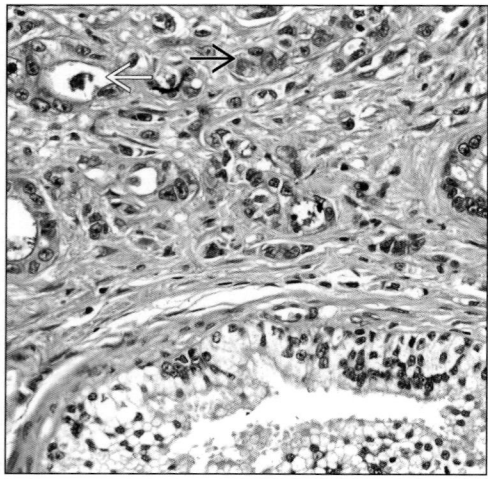

Microscopic Features and Differential Diagnoses

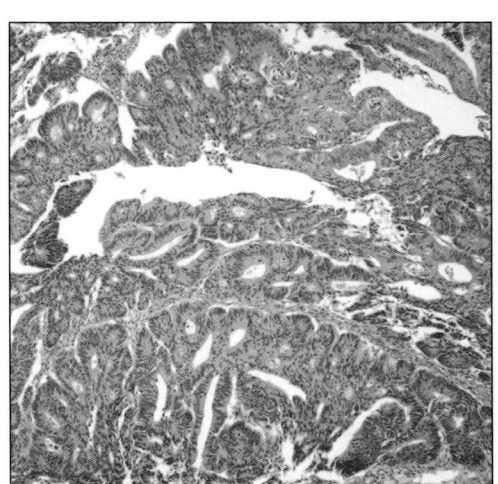

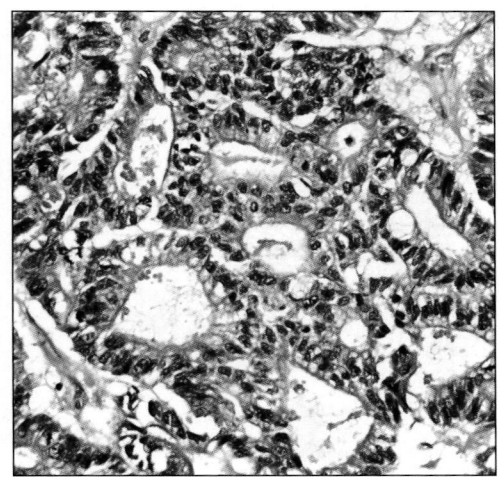

(Left) This epididymal adenocarcinoma is morphologically indistinguishable from a colonic adenocarcinoma. In this case, an extensive work-up disclosed no tumor elsewhere, and the tumor was located in the epididymis. *(Right)* This area shows well-differentiated adenocarcinoma of the epididymis with back-to-back glandular components. To make a diagnosis of a primary rete testis or epididymal adenocarcinoma, clinicopathologic correlation is mandatory.

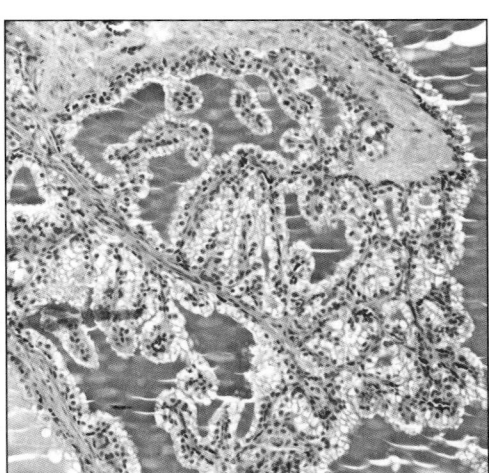

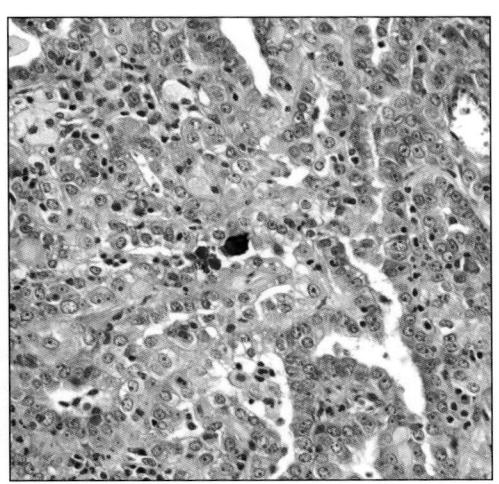

(Left) Papillary adenoma of the epididymis is characterized by papillary proliferation confined to the epididymis. The tumor cells are bland and have abundant clear cytoplasm. This tumor is frequently associated with von Hippel-Lindau syndrome. *(Right)* A papillary mesothelioma may mimic a carcinoma of rete testis/epididymis. Immunostains with epithelial and mesothelial markers are helpful in making the diagnosis, as is determining the epicenter of the neoplasm.

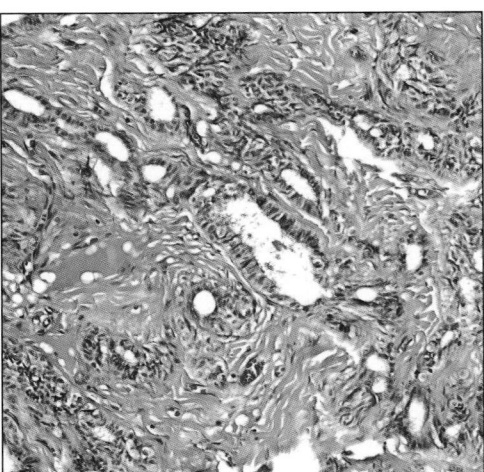

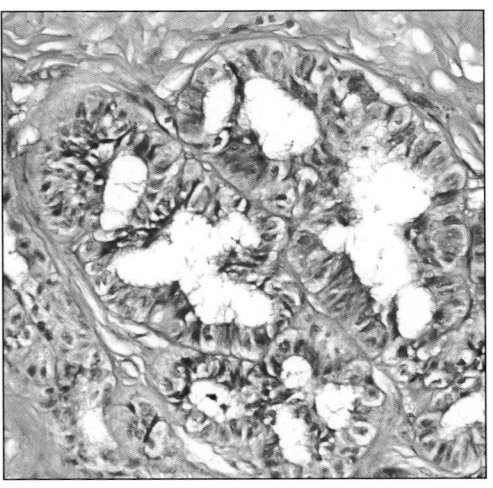

(Left) Rete testis hyperplasia is characterized by proliferation of rete epithelium within dense fibromuscular stroma. There is no cytologic atypia, desmoplastic reaction, or invasive growth. *(Right)* Rete testis hyperplasia shows glandular proliferation of rete epithelium with focal stratification and nuclear enlargement. There may be marked expansion within the rete testis of epithelium, lacking cytologic atypia and containing intracytoplasmic and extracellular hyaline globules.

PAPILLARY SEROUS CARCINOMA, MULLERIAN SUBTYPE

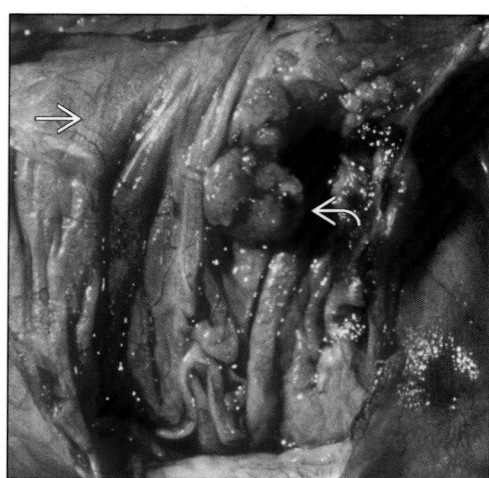

Gross image of a serous papillary tumor of borderline malignancy is shown. There is a large cystic component with a smooth wall ➡ interspersed with nodular and papillary excrescences ➡.

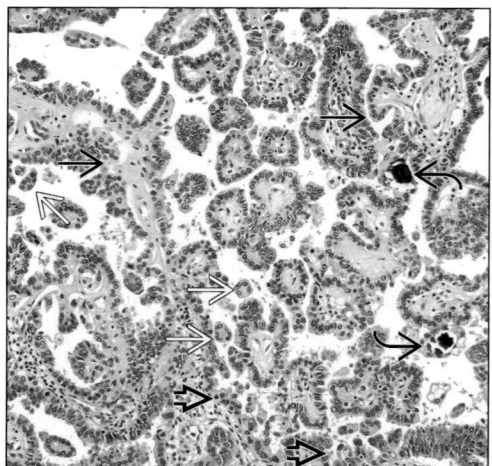

Papillary serous borderline tumor shows polypoid excrescences ➡, micropapillae ➡, stratified cells with budding ➡, and psammoma bodies ➡. There is no stromal invasion.

TERMINOLOGY

Synonyms
- Ovarian-type (müllerian-type) epithelial tumors

Definitions
- Paratesticular homolog of ovarian malignant müllerian-type epithelial neoplasm with serous differentiation
- Borderline serous tumor may also occur in testis

ETIOLOGY/PATHOGENESIS

Pathogenesis Remains Speculative
- 2 possible theories
  - Müllerian metaplasia of tunica vaginalis or rarely intratesticular mesothelial inclusions
  - Müllerian rests in paratesticular soft tissue or of appendix testis

CLINICAL ISSUES

Epidemiology
- Incidence
  - Extremely rare; < 40 well-documented cases reported
- Age
  - Range for patients with borderline tumors: 14-77 years (mean: 56 years)
  - Range for patients with invasive tumors: 16-42 years (mean: 31 years)

Presentation
- Dull pain, swelling, palpable mass, hydrocele
- Mass located at testiculoepididymal groove, paratesticular soft tissues, rete testis, and tunica vaginalis

Laboratory Tests
- CA125 is elevated in some patients

Treatment
- Radical orchiectomy
- Chemotherapy or radiotherapy for locally advanced or metastatic disease

Prognosis
- Borderline tumors are cured by radical orchiectomy
- Invasive carcinomas may recur or metastasize

MACROSCOPIC FEATURES

General Features
- Borderline tumors are typically cystic with papillary excrescences
- Serous carcinomas are usually firm, gritty masses with indistinct margins, may have solid or cystic component
- Mucinous tumors are predominantly cystic ± solid masses containing mucinous material
- May be associated with hydrocele

MICROSCOPIC PATHOLOGY

Histologic Features
- Histologic range includes serous borderline tumor, borderline tumor with microinvasion, and carcinoma
- Borderline tumors exhibit papillae with fibrovascular cores lined by stratified epithelium with varying atypia and mitotic activity
- Invasive clusters and papillae are lined by serous cuboidal or columnar cells with eosinophilic cytoplasm
- Cytologic atypia ranges from bland to anaplastic
- Micropapillary pattern with small clusters or nests of cells surrounded by lacunar spaces may be present
- Psammoma bodies, ciliated and "hobnail" cells are clues to serous differentiation

PAPILLARY SEROUS CARCINOMA, MULLERIAN SUBTYPE

Key Facts

Terminology

- Malignant müllerian-type epithelial neoplasms with serous differentiation, identical to ovarian counterpart
- Borderline serous tumor may also occur in testis

Clinical Issues

- Extremely rare, < 40 well-documented cases reported
- Range for patients with borderline tumors: 14-77 years (mean: 56 years)
- Range for patients with invasive tumors: 16-42 years (mean 31 years)

Macroscopic Features

- Serous carcinomas are usually firm, gritty masses with indistinct margins

Microscopic Pathology

- Invasive papillae lined by serous cuboidal or columnar cells with eosinophilic cytoplasm
- Cytologic atypia can range from bland to frankly anaplastic
- Micropapillary pattern with small clusters or nests of cells surrounded by lacunar spaces
- Abundant psammoma bodies are common
- Mucinous, endometrioid, Brenner, and clear cell-type invasive carcinoma as well as borderline tumor have rarely been reported

Ancillary Tests

- Positive staining for CK7, CA125, S100, EMA/MUC1, EpCAM/BER-EP4/CD326, CD15, TAG72, CEA

- Mucinous, endometrioid, Brenner, and clear cell-type invasive carcinoma as well as borderline tumors have been reported

Cytologic Features

- Bland to high grade

ANCILLARY TESTS

Immunohistochemistry

- Positive staining for CK7, WT1, CA125, EMA/MUC1, EpCAM/BER-EP4/CD326, CD15, TAG72, CEA, and S100
- May rarely be positive for PLAP and vimentin
- Negative for mesothelial-associated markers, such as Podoplanin(D2-40), CK5/6, and calretinin; negative for CK20

DIFFERENTIAL DIAGNOSIS

Papillary Cystadenoma of Epididymis

- Often associated with von Hippel-Lindau disease
- Well circumscribed, golden yellow, solid and cystic
- Little or no atypia, no mitotic activity or stratification
- Tends to have more clear cells and may resemble renal cell carcinoma

Malignant Mesothelioma

- Diffuse thickening of tunica vaginalis with multiple solid nodules
- Transition from normal to hyperplastic to atypical mesothelium and invasive growth
- Positive staining for Podoplanin(D2-40) and calretinin

Carcinoma of Rete Testis or Epididymis

- Usually tubular, tubulocystic, or tubulopapillary high-grade adenocarcinomas
- Tumor epicenter in rete or epididymis determines primary site
- Histologic transition from rete or epididymal lining
- Often contains clear tumor cell component

- CD10 positive; negative for WT1, CA125, and mesothelioma-associated markers

Metastatic Adenocarcinoma

- Clinical history of malignancy elsewhere
- Metastatic tumors usually small in size, often bilateral
- Positive for tissue specific markers (TTF-1 for lung, PSA for prostate)
- Except for metastatic prostate cancer, most metastases have greater pleomorphism and less prominent papillary growth

DIAGNOSTIC CHECKLIST

Pathologic Interpretation Pearls

- Papillary growth, psammoma bodies and epicenter of mass in tunica vaginalis (strong resemblance to ovarian counterpart)
- Metastatic carcinoma and malignant mesothelioma must be ruled out

SELECTED REFERENCES

1. Kurian RR et al: Paratesticular papillary serous cystadenocarcinoma--a case report. Indian J Pathol Microbiol. 49(1):36-7, 2006
2. Amin MB: Selected other problematic testicular and paratesticular lesions: rete testis neoplasms and pseudotumors, mesothelial lesions and secondary tumors. Mod Pathol. 18 Suppl 2:S131-45, 2005
3. Guarch R et al: Papillary serous carcinoma of ovarian type of the testis with borderline differentiation. Histopathology. 46(5):588-90, 2005
4. Ulbright TM et al: Primary mucinous tumors of the testis and paratestis: a report of nine cases. Am J Surg Pathol. 27(9):1221-8, 2003
5. Henley JD et al: Miscellaneous rare paratesticular tumors. Semin Diagn Pathol. 17(4):319-39, 2000
6. Jones MA et al: Paratesticular serous papillary carcinoma. A report of six cases. Am J Surg Pathol. 19(12):1359-65, 1995

PAPILLARY SEROUS CARCINOMA, MULLERIAN SUBTYPE

Microscopic Features

(Left) Low-power photomicrograph of papillary serous carcinoma of paratestis shows focal invasion into the underlying tunica ⇨ with accompanying desmoplastic reaction. Examination of cytologic features is essential in the differential diagnosis with mesothelioma. *(Right)* Papillary serous carcinoma of the paratestis arising from tunica vaginalis is composed of small papillae lined by uniform tumor cells with eosinophilic cytoplasm. *(Courtesy R. Young, MD.)*

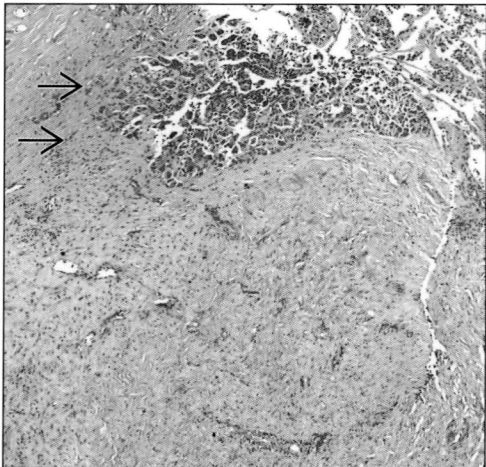
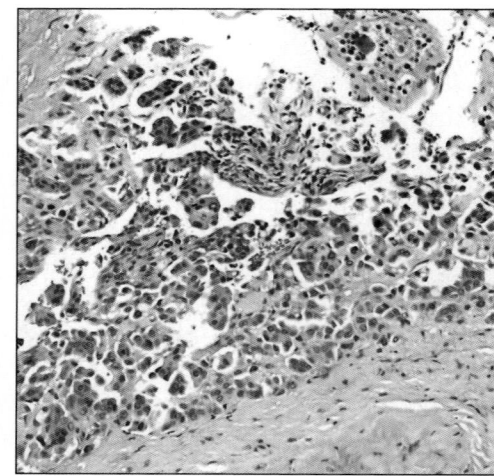

(Left) Complex growth of a borderline serous tumor demonstrates pseudostratified atypical cuboidal to columnar epithelium-associated psammoma bodies. The contours of the glandular structures are smooth, arguing against invasive serous adenocarcinoma. *(Right)* High-power photomicrograph of borderline serous tumor shows an area with relatively bland nuclei and abundant cytoplasm. The main differential diagnosis is with a mesothelioma at the well-differentiated end of the spectrum.

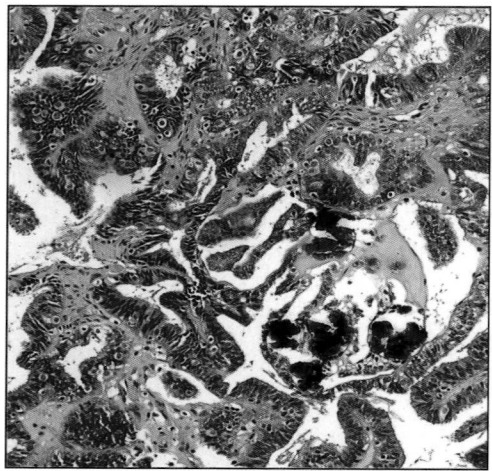
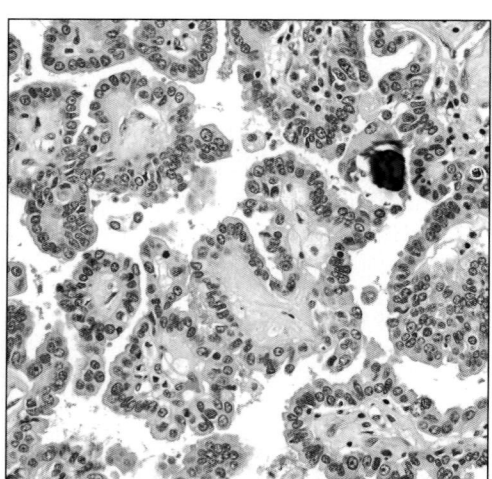

(Left) Invasive serous carcinoma shows small clusters of tumor cells surrounded by lacunar spaces, a characteristic feature of ovarian-type papillary serous carcinoma. *(Courtesy R. Young, MD.)* *(Right)* Invasive serous carcinoma (micropapillary features) is composed of clusters of tumor cells with eosinophilic cytoplasm in lacunar spaces ⇨. This micropapillary pattern has been described in carcinomas of lung, bladder, and other locations such that metastases should be ruled out.

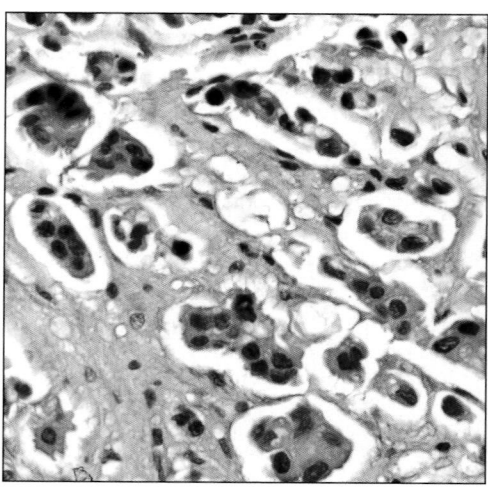
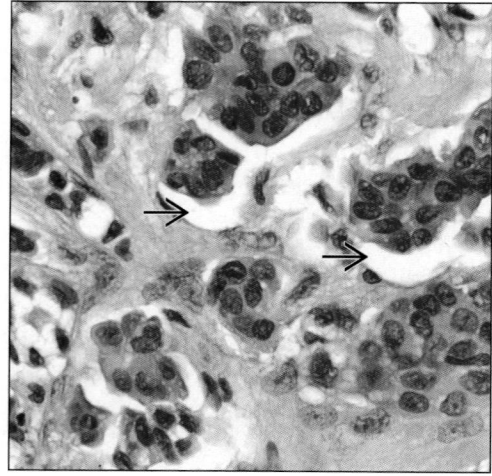

Microscopic Features and Differential Diagnosis

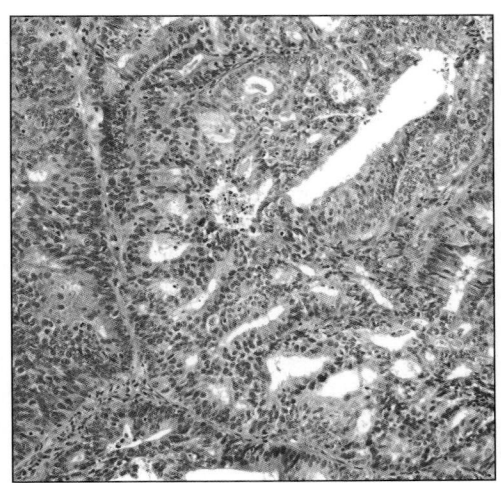

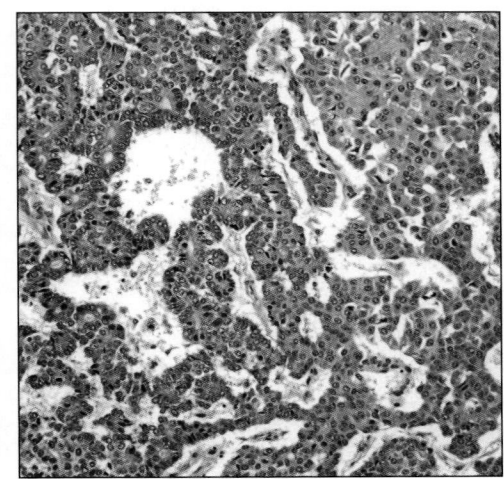

(Left) Endometrioid adenocarcinoma arising from the tunica vaginalis is shown. Large confluent cribriform glands are lined by stratified columnar cells, resembling its female counterpart: Endometrioid carcinoma of the uterus or ovary. *(Right)* Endometrioid carcinoma shows complex tubuloglandular architecture. The differential diagnosis includes carcinomas arising from the rete testis and epididymis as well as metastases, and hence correlation with gross and clinical history is important.

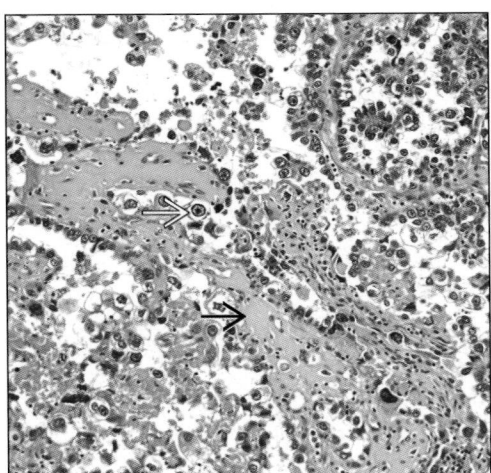

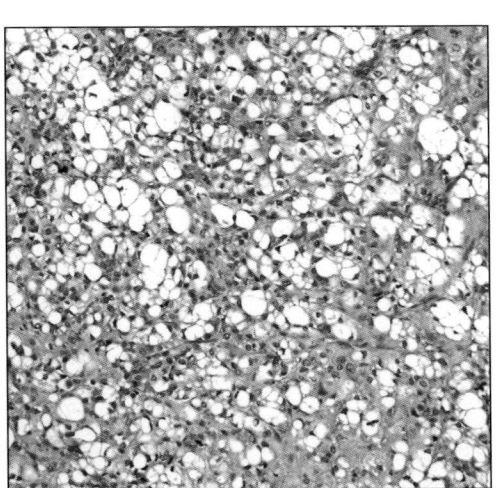

(Left) Clear cell carcinoma shows high-grade nuclear features with abundant clear cytoplasm and prominent nucleoli ➡. Papillary growth and deposition of basement membrane-like material ➡ are seen. Like its ovarian counterpart, a range of growth patterns, including papillary, tubular, and solid architecture, may be seen. *(Right)* Clear cell carcinoma with solid growth is shown. Rete or epididymal carcinomas may show clear cell change as well.

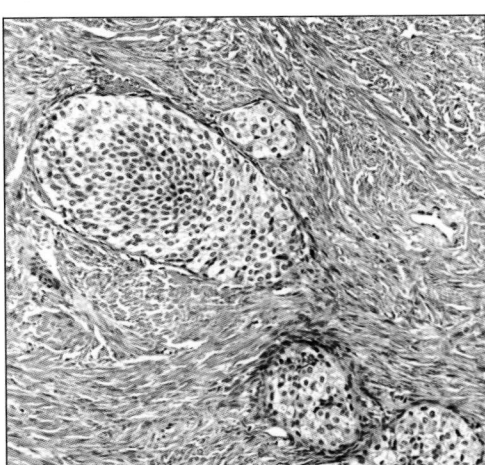

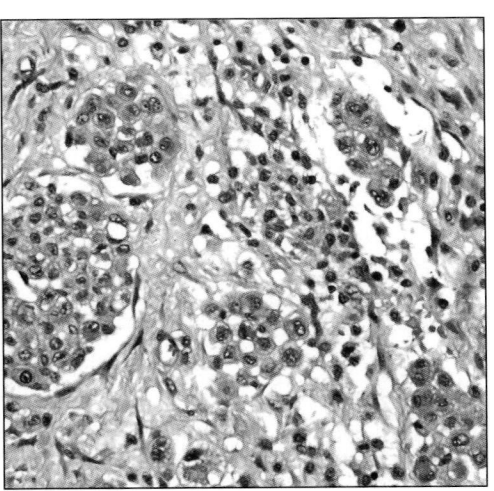

(Left) Brenner tumor of epididymis is characterized by nests of well-differentiated neoplastic urothelium surrounded by dense fibrous stroma. There is no significant cytologic atypia. *(Right)* This is an image of paratesticular mesothelioma, which is 1 of the major differential diagnoses of müllerian-type papillary serous carcinoma. Immunohistochemistry with a panel of mesothelial- and adenocarcinoma-associated markers is often necessary to make a definitive diagnosis.

LIPOSARCOMA

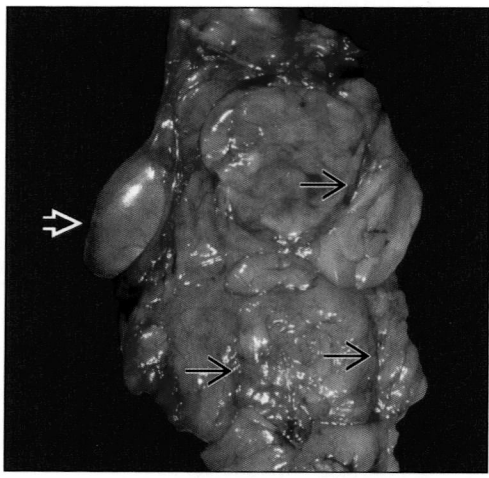

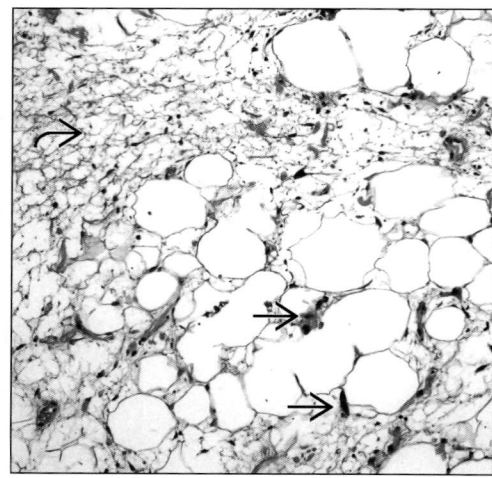

Bulky paratesticular mass with multilobulation due to fibrous bands ➡ and golden yellow appearance suggests an adipocytic tumor. Uninvolved testis ⬛➤ is pushed to 1 side.

Lipoma-like WDL shows mature adipocytes of variable size and shape with fibrous bands ➡ and scattered atypical stromal cells ➡. Typical lipoblasts are not seen in this image.

TERMINOLOGY

Synonyms
- Atypical lipomatous tumor (ALT), well-differentiated liposarcoma (WDL)

Definitions
- Malignant neoplasm showing adipocytic differentiation

CLINICAL ISSUES

Epidemiology
- Incidence
  - Rare, but is most common sarcoma in paratesticular tissue in adults
- Age
  - Range: 41-87 years old (average: 63 years old)

Presentation
- Large scrotal mass
- Usually involves spermatic cord, testicular tunica, or epididymis

Treatment
- Surgical approaches
  - Surgical resection is usually curative

Prognosis
- Favorable with complete excision
- Unfavorable with dedifferentiation or metastasis
- Local recurrence may occur

IMAGE FINDINGS

General Features
- Large hyperechoic mass by ultrasonography
- CT and MR are more specific as they may detect fat component

MACROSCOPIC FEATURES

General Features
- Soft homogeneous multilobular yellow to tan mass
- May be mistaken for lipoma except for its large size and fibrous bands
- Fleshy white to tan-gray firm areas with hemorrhage or necrosis indicate dedifferentiation

Size
- Range: 3-30 cm (average: 12 cm)

MICROSCOPIC PATHOLOGY

Histologic Features
- Mature adipose tissue of variable cellularity with variable fibrous bands
- Marked variation in adipocyte size and shape
- Lipoblasts should be present but may be few in numbers
- Atypical cells with large, hyperchromatic nuclei
- Dedifferentiated components, such as high-grade fibrosarcoma or pleomorphic sarcoma, may be seen
- May have areas of low-grade leiomyosarcomatous differentiation, which does not affect prognosis
- Myxoid variant of liposarcoma has rarely been reported

Predominant Pattern/Injury Type
- Lipomatous, sclerotic, or inflammatory

Predominant Cell/Compartment Type
- Mature adipose tissue and atypical pleomorphic nonlipogenic cells

ANCILLARY TESTS

Immunohistochemistry
- Positive for S100, CDK4, mdm2

LIPOSARCOMA

Key Facts

Terminology
- Malignant neoplasm showing adipocytic differentiation

Clinical Issues
- Rare, but is most common sarcoma in paratesticular tissue in adults
- Range: 41-87 years old (average: 63 years old)
- Large scrotal mass

Macroscopic Features
- Soft, homogeneous, multilobular, yellow to ivory mass
- May mistaken for lipoma except for its large size and fibrous bands
- Fleshy white tan to tan-gray firm areas with hemorrhage or necrosis indicating dedifferentiation

Microscopic Pathology
- Mature adipose tissue of variable cellularity and fibrous tissue
- Marked variation in adipocyte size and shape
- Atypical cells with large, hyperchromatic nuclei
- Lipoblasts with multivacuolated or univacuolated cytoplasm should be present but should be difficult to identify

Ancillary Tests
- Positive for S100, CDK4, mdm2

Top Differential Diagnoses
- Lipoma
- Adenomatoid tumor
- Sclerosing lipogranuloma

- Negative for HMB-45, actin-sm, desmin, MYOD1, or myogenin

DIFFERENTIAL DIAGNOSIS

Lipoma
- Usually small size
- Uniform adipocytes with no irregular fibrous bands
- Lack of atypical cells or lipoblasts

Adenomatoid Tumor
- Small, well-circumscribed nodule
- Cytoplasmic vacuoles rather than true lipogenic differentiation
- Positive for calretinin, WT1

Rhabdomyosarcoma
- Occurs in children or young adults
- Composed of primitive cells and rhabdomyoblasts
- Lack of lipogenic differentiation
- Positive for desmin, MYOD1, myogenin

High-Grade Undifferentiated Sarcoma (Malignant Fibrous Histiocytoma)
- Lack of typical areas of well-differentiated liposarcoma
- No prior history of well-differentiated liposarcoma

Leiomyoma or Leiomyosarcoma
- Uniform spindle cells with eosinophilic cytoplasm
- Smooth muscle differentiation, including fascicles
- Lack of lipogenic differentiation
- Strong and uniformly positive for actin-sm and desmin

Sclerosing Lipogranuloma
- Histiocytes, giant cells, and granulomatous reaction due to exogenous lipid
- Abundant inflammatory cells and absent lipoblasts

DIAGNOSTIC CHECKLIST

Pathologic Interpretation Pearls
- Presence of well-differentiated adipocytic mass-forming lesion in inguinal canal warrants serious consideration for liposarcoma

SELECTED REFERENCES

1. Fitzgerald S et al: Paratesticular liposarcoma. J Urol. 181(1):331-2, 2009
2. Ghosh A et al: Unusual presentation of dedifferentiated liposarcoma as paratesticular mass. Indian J Pathol Microbiol. 51(1):42-4, 2008
3. Dotan ZA et al: Adult genitourinary sarcoma: the 25-year Memorial Sloan-Kettering experience. J Urol. 176(5):2033-8; discussion 2038-9, 2006
4. Ozkara H et al: Recurrent paratesticular myxoid liposarcoma in a young man. J Urol. 171(1):343, 2004
5. Montgomery E et al: Paratesticular liposarcoma: a clinicopathologic study. Am J Surg Pathol. 27(1):40-7, 2003
6. Folpe AL et al: Lipoleiomyosarcoma (well-differentiated liposarcoma with leiomyosarcomatous differentiation): a clinicopathologic study of nine cases including one with dedifferentiation. Am J Surg Pathol. 26(6):742-9, 2002
7. Laurino L et al: Well-differentiated liposarcoma (atypical lipomatous tumors). Semin Diagn Pathol. 18(4):258-62, 2001
8. Kitamura K et al: Liposarcoma developing in the paratesticular region: report of a case. Surg Today. 26(10):842-5, 1996
9. Rao CR et al: Adult paratesticular sarcomas: a report of eight cases. J Surg Oncol. 56(2):89-93, 1994
10. Sønksen J et al: Liposarcoma of the spermatic cord. Case report. Scand J Urol Nephrol. 25(3):239-40, 1991

LIPOSARCOMA

Gross and Microscopic Features

(Left) Dedifferentiated liposarcoma shows nodular and fleshy white firm areas with hemorrhage. In other areas (not shown), there was yellow lobulated tissue of WDL. Close gross examination and sampling of yellow areas is key to recognize WDL in a high-grade paratesticular sarcoma. *(Right)* WDL ➔ with dedifferentiation ➔ is shown. In addition to typical WDL histology, there is an expansile area with highly atypical spindle cells of the dedifferentiated component.

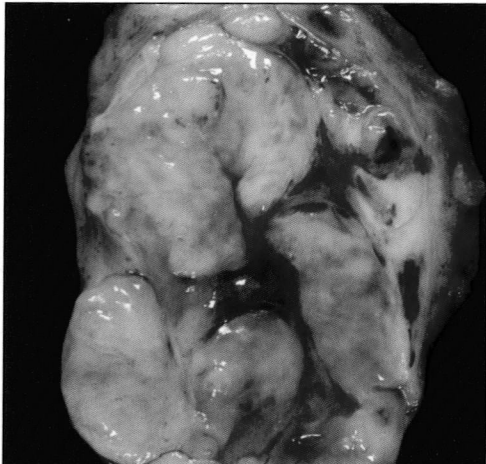
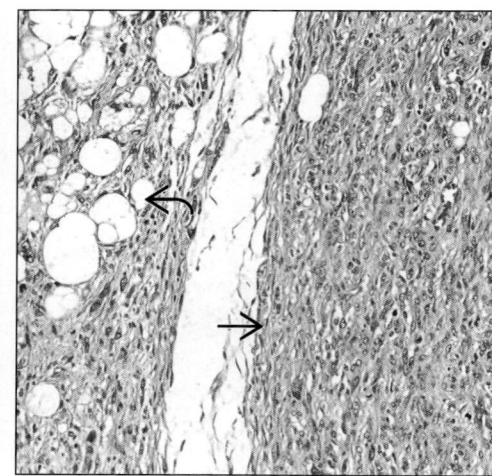

(Left) WDL shows irregularly shaped adipocytes, intervening loose fibrous tissue, and scattered atypical stromal cells. The tumor contrasts itself from a lipoma by large size, variation in size of adipocytes, and by presence of atypical stromal cells. *(Right)* Lipoma-like subtype of WDL is shown. There is a significant variation in size and shape of adipocytes, increased fibrous tissue between adipocytes, and scattered atypical stromal cells ➔. A multivacuolated lipoblast ➔ is present.

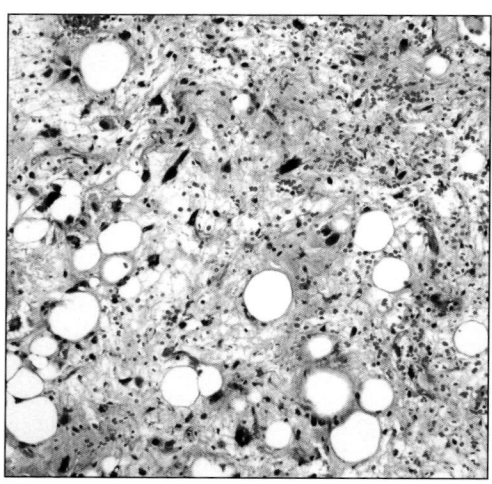
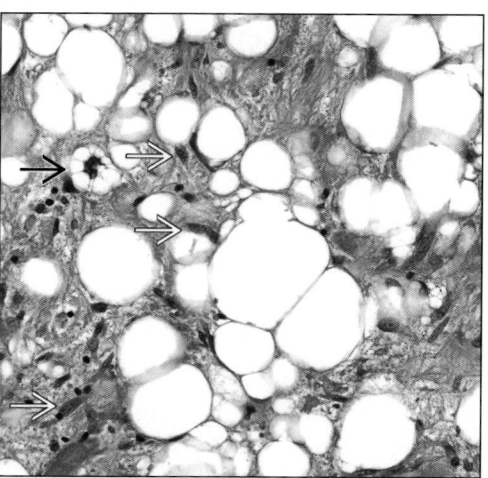

(Left) Sclerosing variant of WDL shows sheets of dense mature collagen and fibrous tissue with irregularly sized and shaped adipocytes and scattered atypical stromal cells ➔. Sclerosing liposarcomas are more common in the inguinal region compared to other sites. *(Right)* WDL, sclerosing type shows irregular-sized adipocytes scattered in dense collagenous stroma and accompanied by markedly atypical stromal cells ➔. Atypical stromal cells are not present in sclerosing lipogranuloma.

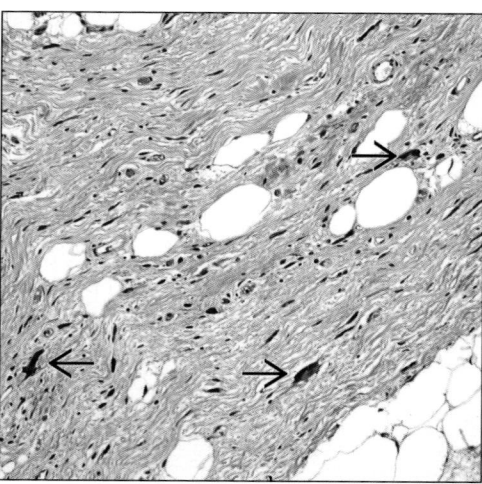
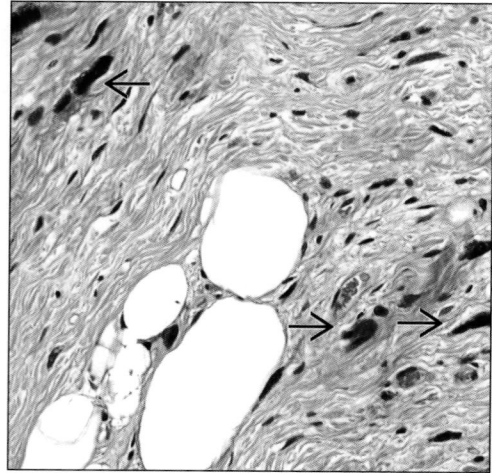

Microscopic Features and Differential Diagnoses

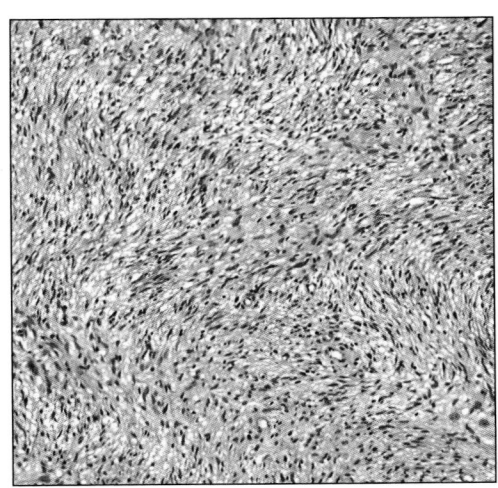 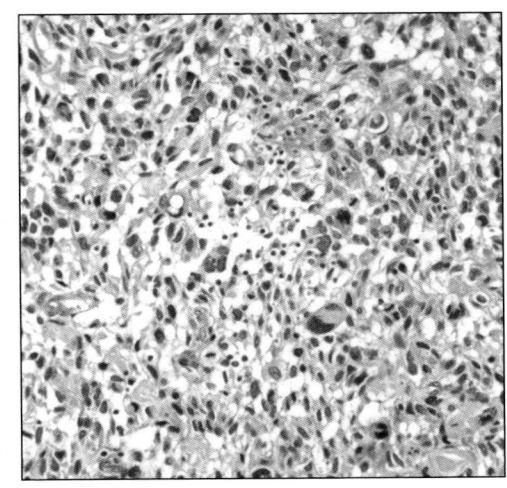

(Left) Dedifferentiated liposarcoma shows cellular spindle cell nonlipogenic tumor of high grade. In other areas of this tumor, lipoma-like WDL was seen. *(Right)* Dedifferentiated liposarcoma shows pleomorphic spindle to round cells with numerous mitoses, resembling malignant fibrous histiocytoma. To make a diagnosis of dedifferentiated liposarcoma, areas of WDL/prior history at the same site is required. Since this impacts prognosis, evaluating WDLs for high-grade areas is crucial.

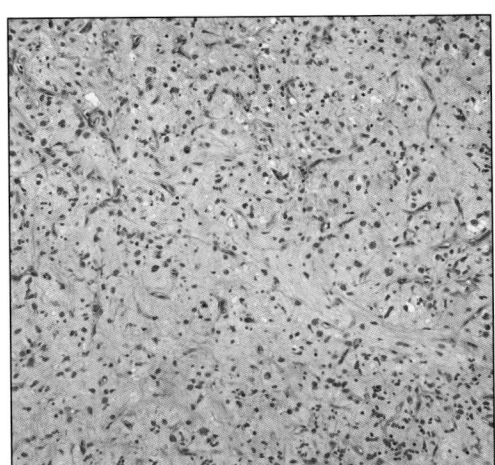 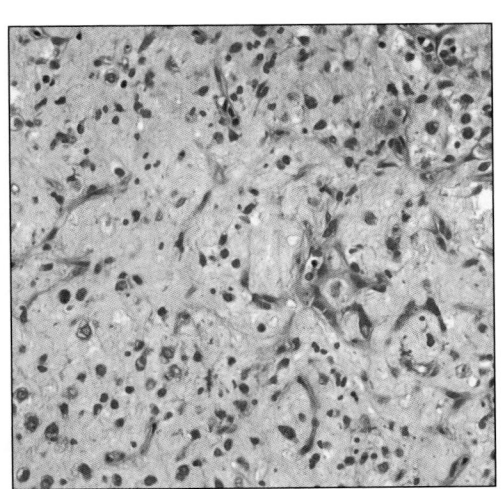

(Left) Myxoid liposarcoma shows myxoid stroma and characteristic "chicken wire" thin arborizing vasculature. At low power, myxoid malignant fibrous histiocytoma, embryonal rhabdomyosarcoma, and aggressive angiomyxoma are in the differential diagnosis. *(Right)* Arborizing and plexiform vasculature of capillary vessels and relatively bland cells in a myxoid stroma are characteristic of myxoid liposarcoma. Multivacuolated lipoblasts may/may not be present.

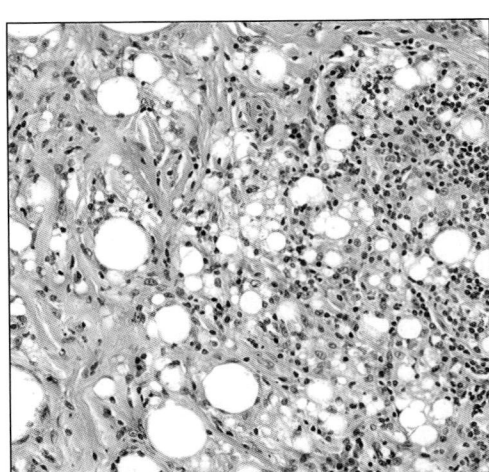 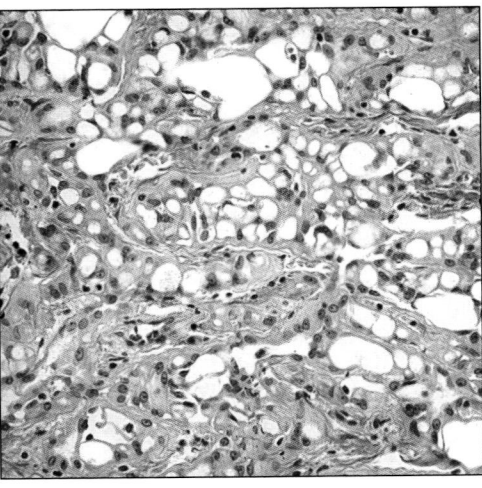

(Left) Sclerosing lipogranuloma is shown. Although there is a variation in size and shape of the adipose tissue with fibrous bands, the presence of an inflammatory infiltrate and absence of atypical stromal cells helps rule out WDL. *(Right)* Adenomatoid tumor with "adipocytic" morphology is shown. These tumors are very rarely massive lesions and tend to be primarily paratesticular rather than centered in the spermatic cord or inguinal canal.

MELANOTIC NEUROECTODERMAL TUMOR

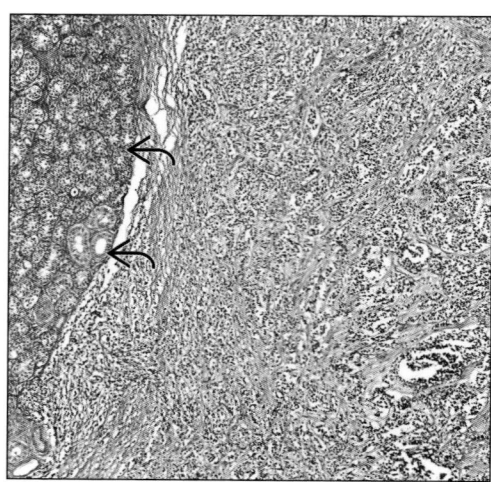

Melanotic neuroectodermal tumor shows a paratesticular cellular tumor, which is well demarcated from the adjacent testis ⤳. It is characterized by sheets of small blue cells in a fibrous background.

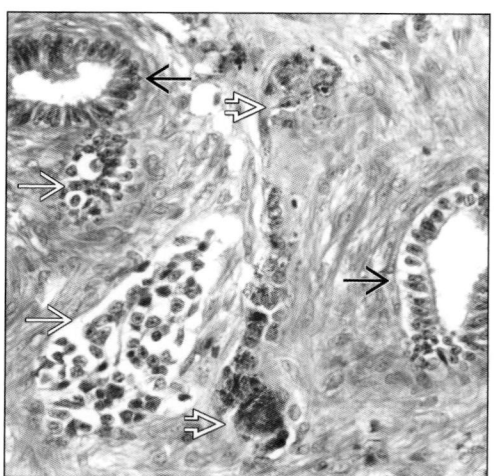

High-power image shows a melanotic neuroectodermal tumor involving epididymis ⇨. There are clusters of small blue cells ➔ and large epithelioid cells with brown pigment ➱.

TERMINOLOGY

Synonyms
- Retinal anlage tumor, melanotic progonoma, melanotic hamartoma

Definitions
- Rare paratesticular (usually epididymal) tumor of neural crest origin in infants and young children

CLINICAL ISSUES

Epidemiology
- Incidence
  - Extremely rare
  - < 1 dozen cases reported in testis or epididymis (more common in jaw)
- Age
  - Range: 4 months to 8 years (80% younger than 1 year old)

Presentation
- Firm mass in epididymis; may be associated with hydrocele

Laboratory Tests
- Mild elevation of serum α-fetoprotein, urine vanillylmandelic acid (VMA), and homovanillic acid in some cases

Treatment
- Surgical resection, occasionally with adjuvant therapy (chemotherapy or radiotherapy)

Prognosis
- Generally behaves in benign fashion with rare recurrence and metastasis

MACROSCOPIC FEATURES

General Features
- Round to oval homogeneous white-gray to bluish firm nodule
- May show dark brown or black areas due to pigmentation
- Closely apposed to, but usually does not involve, testicular parenchyma

Size
- Usually < 4 cm

MICROSCOPIC PATHOLOGY

Histologic Features
- Distinct biphasic tumor composed of 2 types of cells
  - Small neuroblast-like round cells with scant cytoplasm forming sheets or irregularly shaped nests
  - Large polygonal epithelioid cells with abundant eosinophilic cytoplasm, large vesicular nuclei, small nucleoli, and variable amounts of melanin deposits
- Large cells may form nests, cords, and gland-like structures
- Typically prominent fibrous and hyalinized stroma

Predominant Pattern/Injury Type
- Biphasic with sheets of small round cells and large polygonal cells with melanin pigment

Predominant Cell/Compartment Type
- 2 cell components: Small cells, and large cells with melanin pigment

MELANOTIC NEUROECTODERMAL TUMOR

Key Facts

Terminology

- Congenital melanocarcinoma, retinal anlage tumor, melanotic progonoma, melanotic hamartoma
- Rare paratesticular (usually epididymis) tumor of neural crest origin in infants and young children

Clinical Issues

- Extremely rare; < 1 dozen cases reported involving testis or epididymis
- Range: 4 months to 8 years (80% < 1 year old)
- Firm mass in epididymis; may be associated with hydrocele

Macroscopic Features

- Round to oval homogeneous white-gray to bluish firm nodule; may show areas of dark pigmentation

Microscopic Pathology

- Distinct biphasic tumor composed of 2 types of cells
  - Small neuroblast-like round cells with scant cytoplasm forming sheets or irregularly shaped nests
  - Large polygonal epithelioid cells with abundant eosinophilic cytoplasm, large vesicular nuclei, small nucleoli, and variable amounts of melanin deposits
- Large cells may form nests, cords, and gland-like structures
- Typically prominent fibrous and hyalinized stroma

Ancillary Tests

- Large cells positive for cytokeratin, vimentin, HMB-45, and S100
- Small cells positive for CD56, NSE, and synaptophysin; negative for keratin

---

ANCILLARY TESTS

Immunohistochemistry

- Large cells positive for cytokeratin, vimentin, HMB-45 and S100 (less common), synaptophysin, NSE, GFAP, and desmin; CD99 rarely positive
- Small cells positive for CD56, NSE, and synaptophysin; negative for cytokeratin

DIFFERENTIAL DIAGNOSIS

Desmoplastic Small Round Cell Tumor

- Occurs in older age patients
- Tumor consists of only a small cell population and has more prominent desmoplasia
- Lack of large cells with melanin pigment
- Positive for cytokeratin and desmin

Embryonal Rhabdomyosarcoma

- Tumor with rhabdomyoblasts in varying stages of differentiation
- Small cells with minimal cytoplasm to fusiform cells with abundant cytoplasm and spindle cells with fibrillary background (so-called leiomyomatous rhabdomyosarcoma)
- Positive for desmin, MYOD1, and myogenin

Malignant Lymphoma/Leukemia

- Diffuse interstitial infiltrative pattern and relatively uniform cell population
- Primarily testicular parenchymal involvement with secondary extension into paratesticular tissues
- Positive for leukocyte common antigen CD45(LCA) and B- or T-cell related markers (depending on immunophenotype)

Metastatic Melanoma

- Occurs in older age patients and in those with history of primary tumor
- Prominent nucleoli, pseudonuclear inclusions, and numerous mitoses
- Most cells positive for melanocytic markers

Neuroblastoma

- Rare in paratesticular location
- Uniform 1 cell population
- CD99 and FLI-1 positive

DIAGNOSTIC CHECKLIST

Pathologic Interpretation Pearls

- Tumor composed of 2 distinct cell populations with small round cells and large epithelioid cells containing melanin
- Age (usually < 1 year) and gross circumscription are important for diagnosis

SELECTED REFERENCES

1. Chaudhary A et al: Melanotic neuroectodermal tumor of infancy: 2 decades of clinical experience with 18 patients. J Oral Maxillofac Surg. 67(1):47-51, 2009
2. Kruse-Lösler B et al: Melanotic neuroectodermal tumor of infancy: systematic review of the literature and presentation of a case. Oral Surg Oral Med Oral Pathol Oral Radiol Endod. 102(2):204-16, 2006
3. Desai S et al: Recurrent melanotic neuroectodermal tumour of infancy of the epididymis and testis: a case report. Indian J Pathol Microbiol. 48(3):363-4, 2005
4. Kobayashi T et al: Melanotic neuroectodermal tumor of infancy in the epididymis. Case report and literature review. Urol Int. 57(4):262-5, 1996
5. Calabrese F et al: Melanotic neuroectodermal tumor of the epididymis in infancy: case report and review of the literature. Urology. 46(3):415-8, 1995
6. Diamond DA et al: Melanotic neuroectodermal tumor of infancy: an important mimicker of paratesticular rhabdomyosarcoma. J Urol. 147(3):673-5, 1992
7. Pettinato G et al: Melanotic neuroectodermal tumor of infancy. A reexamination of a histogenetic problem based on immunohistochemical, flow cytometric, and ultrastructural study of 10 cases. Am J Surg Pathol. 15(3):233-45, 1991
8. Johnson RE et al: Melanotic neuroectodermal tumor of infancy. A review of seven cases. Cancer. 52(4):661-6, 1983

MELANOTIC NEUROECTODERMAL TUMOR

Microscopic Features

(Left) This image shows a melanotic neuroectodermal tumor involving efferent ductules of the rete testis. There are large cells forming clusters ⇥ and scattered small blue cells ⇥ in a dense fibrous stroma. *(Right)* Melanotic neuroectodermal tumor involves efferent ductules of the rete testis ⇥. The tumor is composed of the characteristic cellular components of small blue cells ⇲ and large epithelioid cells with brown pigment ⇥ amidst a dense fibrous stroma.

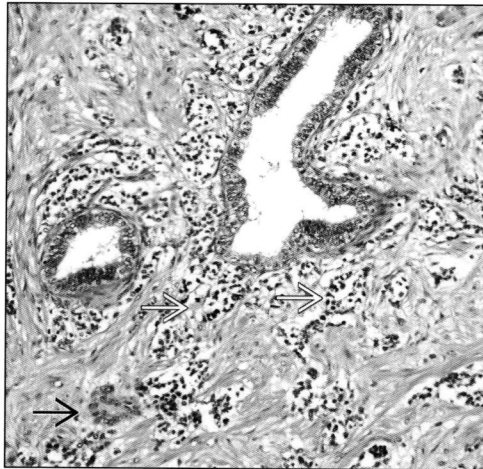
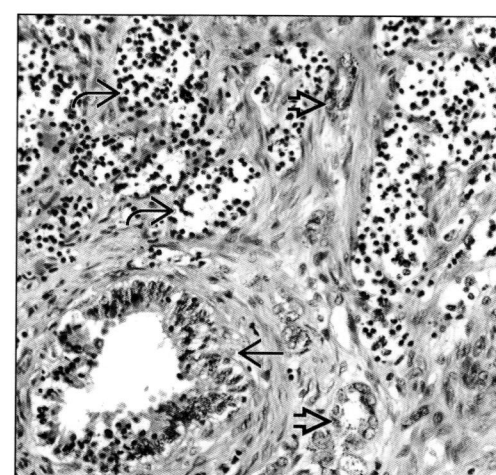

(Left) Melanotic neuroectodermal tumor shows nests of small blue cells ⇥ within artifactual spaces, and large epithelioid cells with melanin pigment ⇥. The fibrous stromal response is a typical feature of the tumor. *(Right)* Typical biphasic appearance of melanotic neuroectodermal tumor is shown here. On the right is a sheet of small blue cells with hyperchromatic nuclei ⇥, and on the left are epithelioid cells ⇲ with melanin pigment and glandular formation.

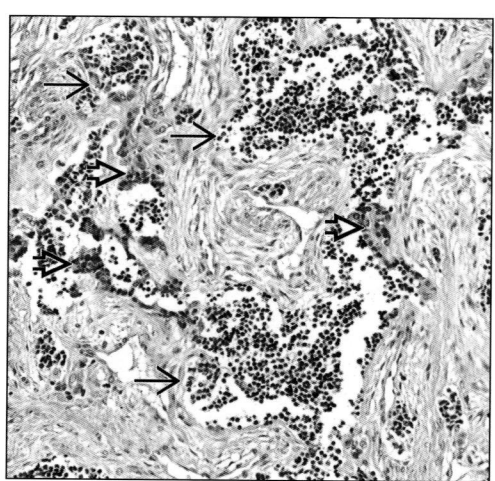
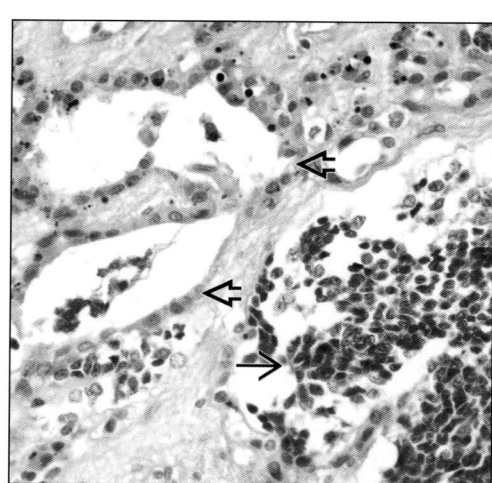

(Left) High-power photomicrograph shows a biphasic tumor composed of clusters of large epithelioid cells ⇥ and nests of small blue cells ⇥. The degree of melanin may vary and may occasionally be inconspicuous. *(Right)* High-power view of melanotic neuroectodermal tumor shows nests of large epithelioid cells with vesicular nuclei, prominent nucleoli, and coarse melanin pigment ⇥. Also seen are scattered small blue cells ⇥ and dense fibrous stroma.

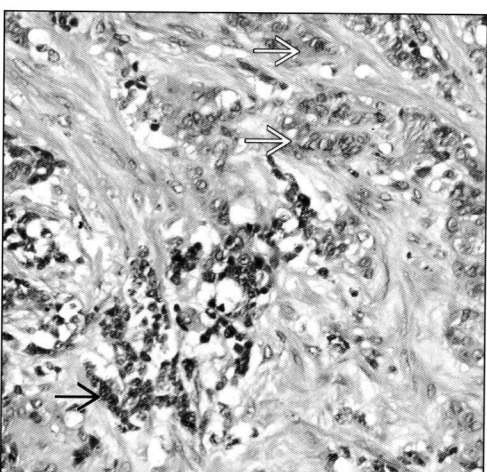
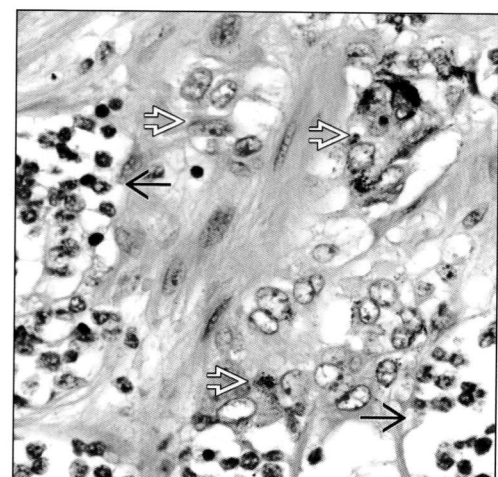

Testis and Paratesticular Structures

MELANOTIC NEUROECTODERMAL TUMOR

Microscopic Features and Differential Diagnosis

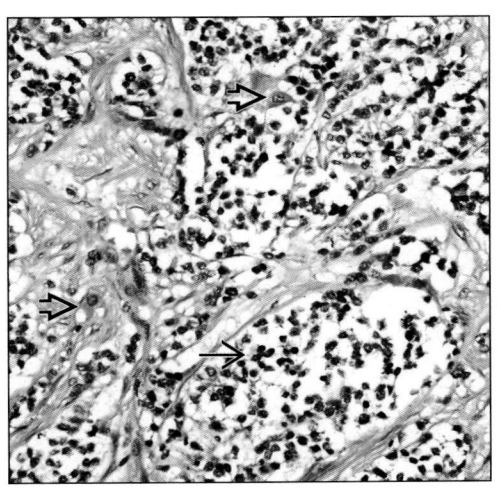

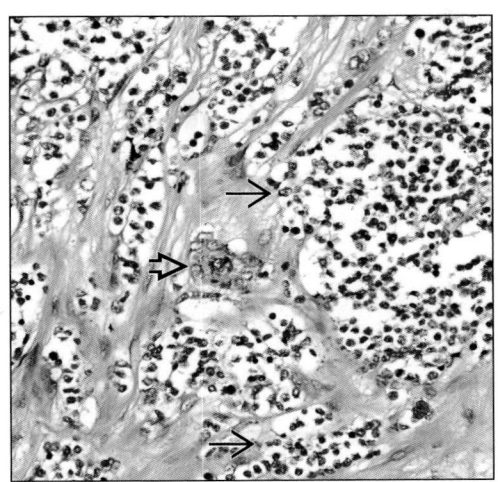

(Left) Melanotic neuroectodermal tumor shows nests of small blue cells ⊃ surrounded by delicate fibrous septae. A few large epithelioid cells ⊅ are present. In this situation, the differential diagnosis from other small blue cell tumors in children may be difficult. (Right) Irregular nests and sheets of small blue cells ⊃ separated by dense fibrous stroma and large epithelioid cells ⊅ containing melanin pigment are diagnostic components for melanotic neuroectodermal tumor.

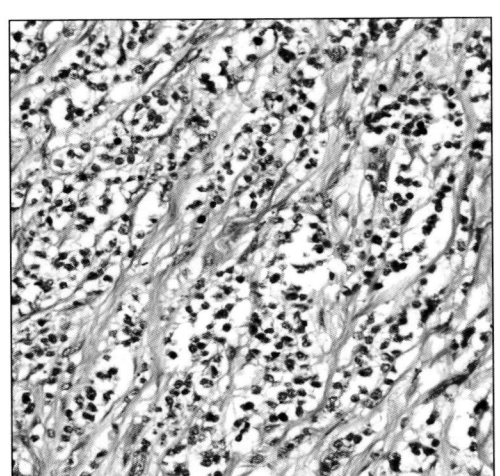

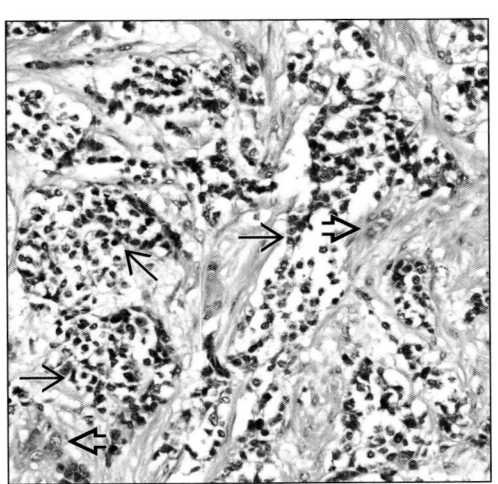

(Left) This area of a melanotic neuroectodermal tumor shows nests and sheets of small blue cells separated by delicate fibrous septae with pseudoglandular formation. In other areas, the other diagnostic component of large epithelioid cells with melanin pigment was observed. (Right) Cellular nests of small neuroblastoma-like blue cells ⊃ are admixed with a few large epithelioid cells ⊅. Homer Wright rosettes are not seen in this tumor and help in the differential diagnosis.

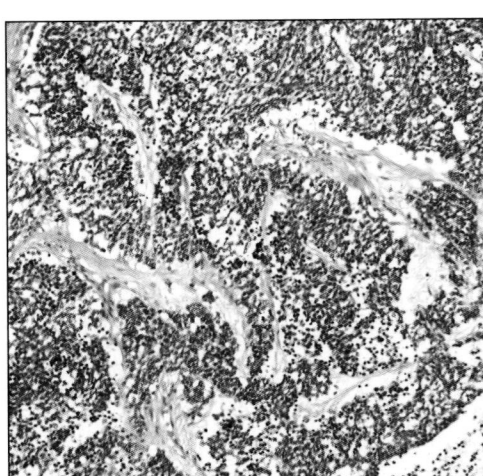

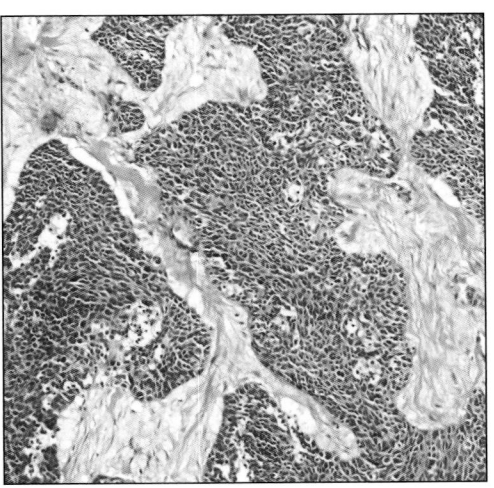

(Left) This area of melanotic neuroectodermal tumor exhibits sheets of cellular small blue cells within dense stroma, similar to those of a desmoplastic round cell tumor or other small blue cell tumors, such as Ewing sarcoma or neuroblastoma. (Right) Desmoplastic round cell tumor has a similar appearance to that of a melanocytic neuroectoderma tumor. Age, identification of large epithelioid cells with melanin pigment, and typical immunostaining profile allow the distinction.

4

163

EMBRYONAL RHABDOMYOSARCOMA

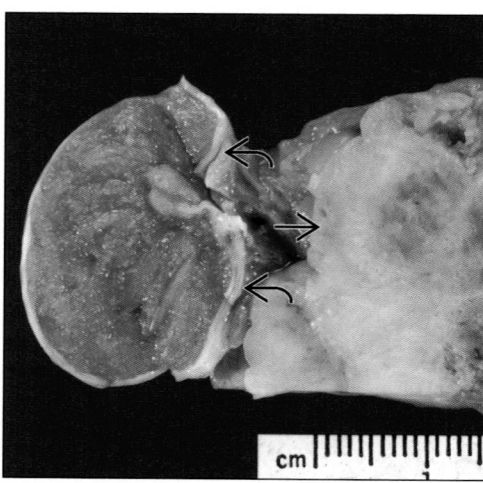

Paratesticular embryonal rhabdomyosarcoma with a tan-white, gelatinous cut surface ➡, and lacking necrosis or hemorrhage. The adjacent testicular parenchyma ➡ is uninvolved.

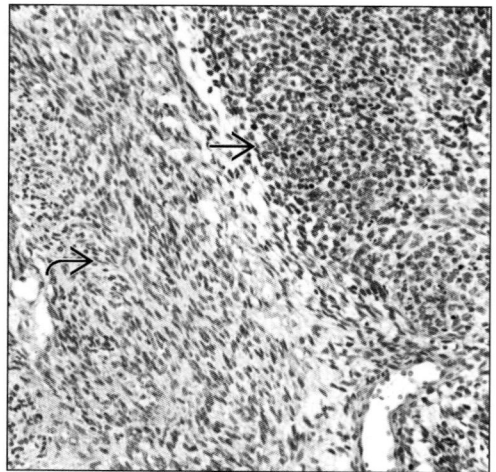

Embryonal rhabdomyosarcoma, NOS, shows alternating cellular primitive ovoid small cells ➡ and less cellular myxoid ➡ areas composed of short spindle cells, characteristic of this tumor.

TERMINOLOGY

Synonyms
- Embryonal rhabdomyosarcoma, NOS; spindle leiomyomatous rhabdomyosarcoma

Definitions
- Malignant neoplasm with skeletal muscle differentiation that recapitulates embryogenesis of skeletal muscle and encompasses spindle cell and anaplastic variants

CLINICAL ISSUES

Epidemiology
- Incidence
  - Most common sarcoma in children
  - Paratesticular location is 1 of more common sites of rhabdomyosarcoma (4% of all)
- Age
  - Range: 7-36 years
  - 60% of cases occur in 1st 2 decades

Presentation
- Paratesticular mass in young patients
- Gradual enlargement of scrotal sac with no acute onset symptoms
- Transillumination may be positive when lesion is associated with hydrocele
- May be clinically confused with epididymitis due to hydrocele
- May spread to paraaortic or paracaval lymph nodes and to bone and lung

Treatment
- Usually multimodal, surgical resection ± radiotherapy or chemotherapy

Prognosis
- Favorable prognosis in general with surgery, chemotherapy, and radiation therapy
- Prognosis associated with histologic type, age, tumor size and stage, and adequacy of resection
  - Embryonal, NOS, and spindle cell variants have excellent prognosis compared to anaplastic variant
  - Alveolar and pleomorphic types generally have poor prognosis and occur in adults
  - Paratesticular rhabdomyosarcoma has significantly better prognosis than tumors occurring elsewhere in genitourinary tract
  - Patients > 10 years of age and tumors > 5 cm have worse prognosis

MACROSCOPIC FEATURES

General Features
- Well-circumscribed paratesticular mass
- Often multinodular with gelatinous, gray-white cut surface
- Patchy areas of necrosis, hemorrhage, or cystic change may be seen

Size
- Range: 1-18 cm (average range: 4-6 cm)

MICROSCOPIC PATHOLOGY

Histologic Features
- Mixture of primitive and variable proportion of well-differentiated rhabdomyosarcomatous component
- Alternating cellular and less cellular myxoid areas (embryonal rhabdomyosarcoma, NOS)
- Spindle cells with fascicular pattern, mimicking leiomyosarcoma (spindle leiomyomatous rhabdomyosarcoma)

4

EMBRYONAL RHABDOMYOSARCOMA

Key Facts

Terminology

- Malignant neoplasm with skeletal muscle differentiation that recapitulates embryogenesis of skeletal muscle and encompasses spindle cell and anaplastic variants

Clinical Issues

- Range: 7-36 years
- Paratesticular location is 1 of more common sites of rhabdomyosarcoma (4% of all)

Macroscopic Features

- Well-circumscribed large paratesticular mass (average 4-6 cm)
- Often multinodular with gelatinous, gray-white cut surface

Microscopic Pathology

- Mixture of primitive and variable proportion of well-differentiated rhabdomyosarcomatous component
- Alternating cellular and less cellular myxoid areas (embryonal rhabdomyosarcoma, NOS)
- Spindle cells with fascicular pattern, mimicking leiomyosarcoma (spindle leiomyomatous rhabdomyosarcoma)
- Primitive cells (blue cells) with small round to oval hyperchromatic cells or spindle cells
- Differentiating rhabdomyosarcoma cells with eosinophilic cytoplasm, fibrillary material, or cross striation

Ancillary Tests

- Positive for desmin, actin-HHF-35, myoglobin, MYOD1, myogenin, and vimentin

---

- Primitive cells (blue cells) with small round to oval hyperchromatic cells or spindle cells
- Differentiating rhabdomyosarcoma cells with eosinophilic cytoplasm, fibrillary material, or cross striation
- Diffuse anaplasia with atypical mitoses (anaplastic variant of embryonal rhabdomyosarcoma) may be seen
- Alveolar, pleomorphic, or botryoid types of rhabdomyosarcoma are extremely rare in paratesticular area

Predominant Pattern/Injury Type

- Myxoid spindle cell tumor with cellular and less cellular areas or interlacing fascicles of spindle cells

Predominant Cell/Compartment Type

- Small round or spindle cells with dense eosinophilic cytoplasm (rhabdomyoblasts) and may show cross striation

ANCILLARY TESTS

Immunohistochemistry

- Positive for desmin, actin-HHF-35, myoglobin, MYOD1, myogenin, and vimentin
- Negative for S100 and cytokeratin

DIFFERENTIAL DIAGNOSIS

Leiomyosarcoma

- Occurs in older age group
- Uniform fascicular spindle cells with eosinophilic cytoplasm
- Diffusely positive for actin-sm and desmin; negative for myoglobin, MYOD1, and myogenin

Dedifferentiated Liposarcoma

- History of well-differentiated liposarcoma (atypical lipomatous tumor)
- Tumor with areas of atypical lipomatous component
- No skeletal muscle differentiation

- mdm2, CDK4 positive

Malignant Lymphoma/Leukemia

- Relatively uniform tumor cells and lack of cells with abundant eosinophilic cytoplasm
- Primarily testicular involvement with paratesticular extension
- Positive for CD45(LCA) and CD20

Other Small Blue Cell Tumors

- Uniform small cell proliferation with lack of spindle cells and cells with eosinophilic cytoplasm
- Lack alternating cellular and myxoid areas
- Negative for desmin, myoglobin, MYOD1, and myogenin

DIAGNOSTIC CHECKLIST

Pathologic Interpretation Pearls

- Myxoid spindle cell tumor with cellular and less cellular areas containing pink (rhabdomyoblastic) cells; interlacing fascicles with spindle cells resembling leiomyosarcoma

SELECTED REFERENCES

1. Kishore B et al: A rare case of paratesticular pleomorphic rhabdomyosarcoma diagnosed by fine needle aspiration: a case report. Diagn Cytopathol. 38(2):121-6, 2010
2. Reeves HM et al: Paratesticular rhabdomyosarcoma. J Urol. 182(4):1578-9, 2009
3. Rypens F et al: Paratesticular rhabdomyosarcoma presenting as thickening of the tunica vaginalis. Pediatr Radiol. 39(9):1010-2, 2009
4. Wu HY et al: Genitourinary rhabdomyosarcoma: Which treatment, how much, and when? J Pediatr Urol. Epub ahead of print, 2009
5. Sugita Y et al: Testicular and paratesticular tumours in children: 30 years' experience. Aust N Z J Surg. 69(7):505-8, 1999
6. Stewart LH et al: Thirty-year review of intrascrotal rhabdomyosarcoma. Br J Urol. 68(4):418-20, 1991

EMBRYONAL RHABDOMYOSARCOMA

Gross and Microscopic Features

(Left) Paratesticular embryonal rhabdomyosarcoma has a homogeneous, tan-white, gelatinous cut surface ➡. No necrosis or hemorrhage is seen. The testis ➡ is compressed but not involved. *(Right)* Gross photograph of a paratesticular rhabdomyosarcoma shows a homogeneous, fish-flesh appearance. A circumscribed, myxoid paratesticular mass in the child is most likely to be a rhabdomyosarcoma unless proved otherwise. (Courtesy H. Zhou, MD.)

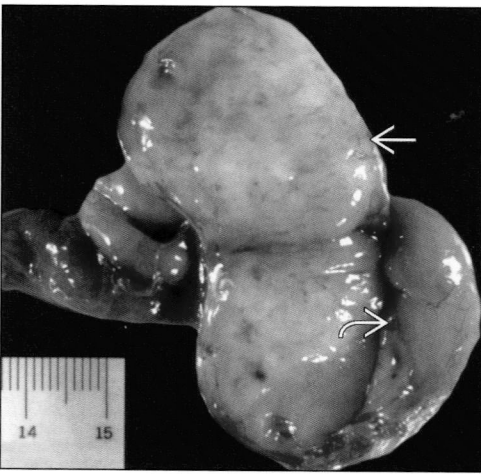
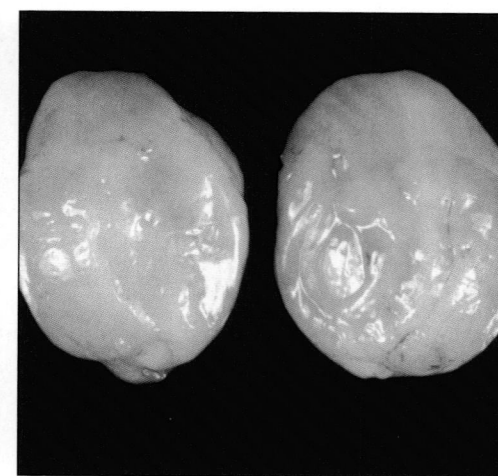

(Left) Embryonal rhabdomyosarcoma shows small, primitive, ovoid cells ➡ and numerous large elongated and ovoid cells with dense eosinophilic fibrillar cytoplasm (rhabdomyoblasts) ➡. *(Right)* Embryonal rhabdomyosarcoma of spindle leiomyomatous type is shown. The tumor cells are arranged in a fascicular pattern, mimicking leiomyosarcoma. In children and young adults, the spindle cell variant of embryonal rhabdomyosarcoma should be considered with appropriate support by immunostains.

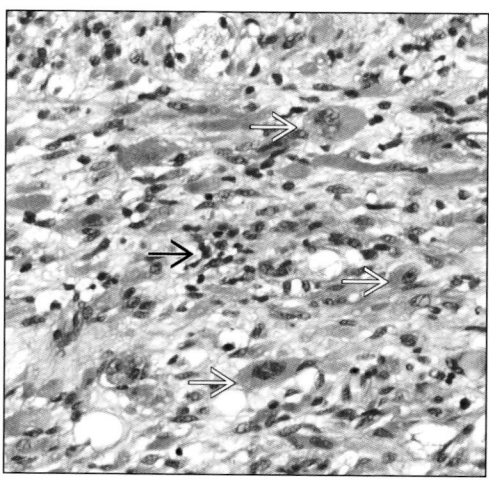
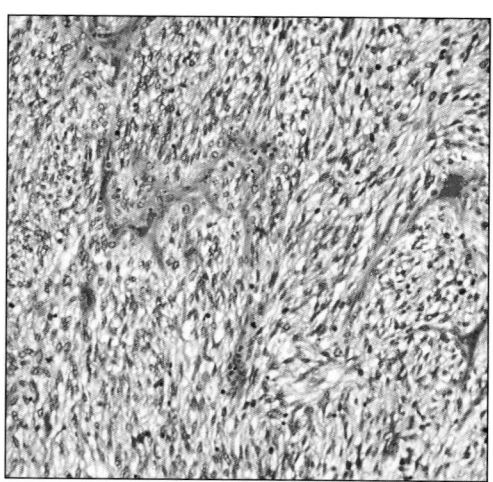

(Left) Leiomyomatous rhabdomyosarcoma shows relatively uniform spindle cells arranged in an irregular fascicular pattern, superficially resembling leiomyosarcoma. A panel of immunostains (myoglobin, myogenin, and MYOD1) is helpful to make the correct diagnosis. *(Right)* Spindle leiomyomatous rhabdomyosarcoma shows spindle tumor cells and a mitotic figure ➡. Occasionally, there may be prominent collagen with cells arranged in a storiform or whorled pattern (collagen-rich form).

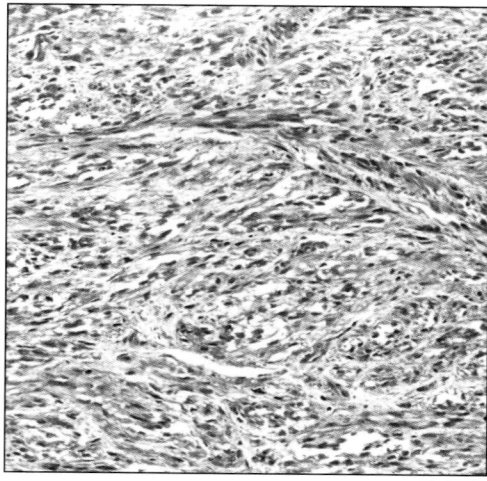
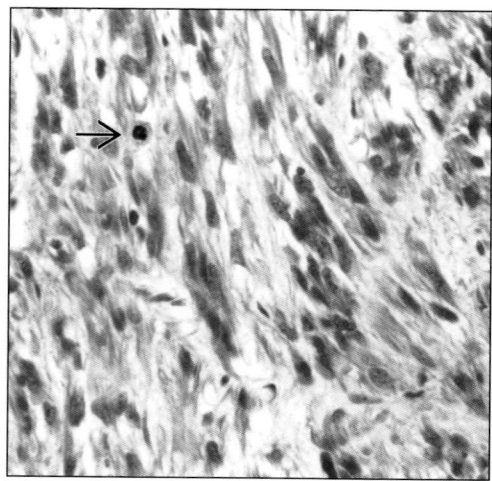

EMBRYONAL RHABDOMYOSARCOMA

Microscopic and Immunohistochemical Features

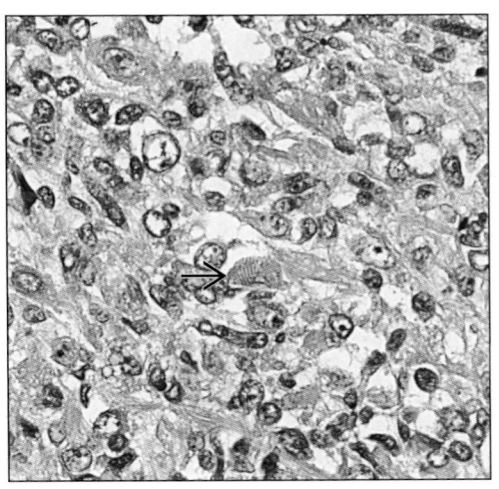

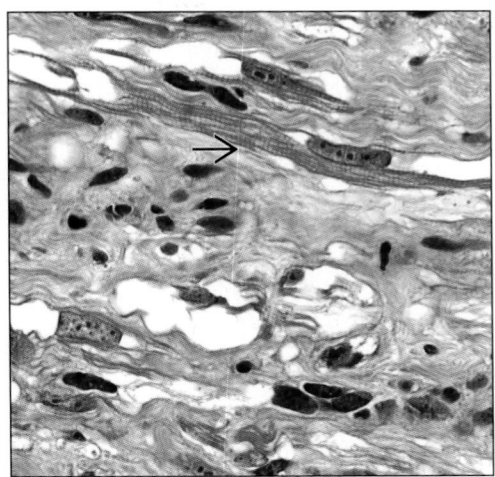

(Left) Embryonal rhabdomyosarcoma shows well-differentiated rhabdomyoblasts with prominent cross striations ➡️. Manipulation of the condenser of the microscope is often helpful to appreciate cross striations. *(Right)* High-power photomicrograph of embryonal rhabdomyosarcoma shows well-differentiated rhabdomyoblasts (strap cells) with abundant eosinophilic cytoplasm & cross striations ➡️. The stroma is fibromyxoid.

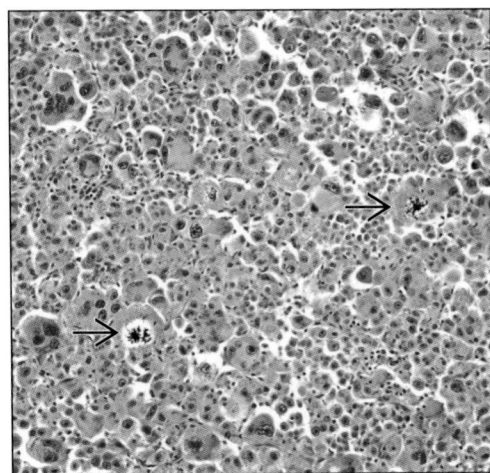

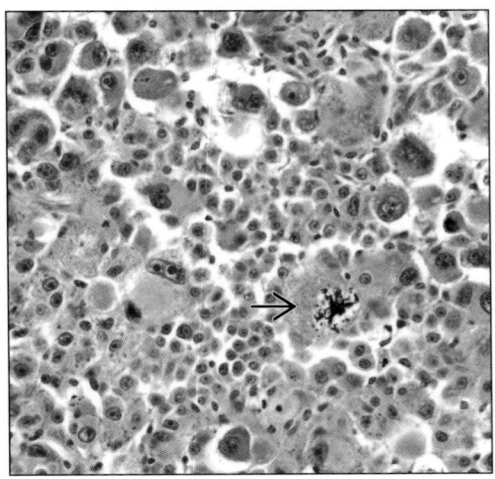

(Left) Anaplastic embryonal rhabdomyosarcoma shows diffuse anaplasia and multiple atypical mitoses ➡️. In other areas, the histology of a classic embryonal rhabdomyosarcoma was seen. It is rare in this location and behaves more aggressively. *(Right)* Higher power of anaplastic variant of embryonal rhabdomyosarcoma shows diffuse anaplasia with atypical mitosis ➡️. It is similar to pleomorphic rhabdomyosarcoma but occurs in children and has more rhabdomyoblasts.

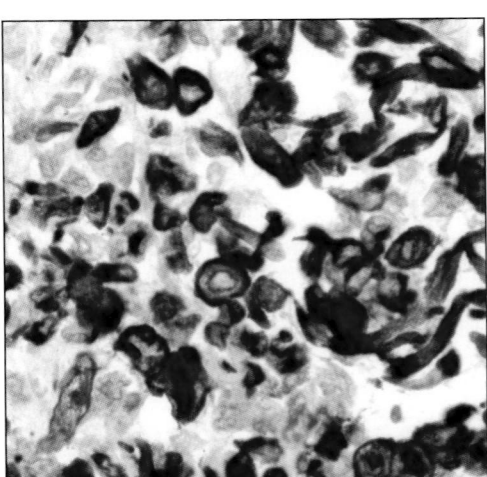

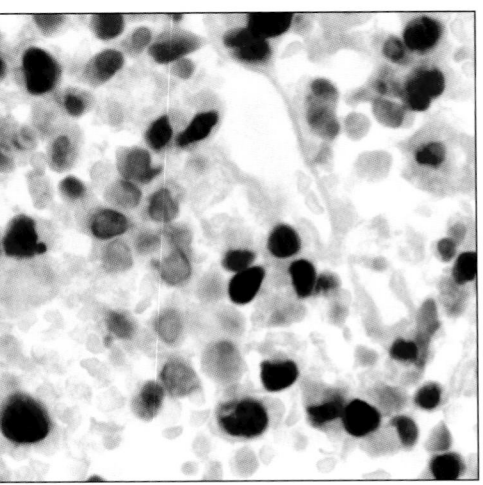

(Left) Immunohistochemical stain of rhabdomyosarcoma shows diffuse strong staining with desmin. Virtually all rhabdomyosarcomas are also positive for actin-HHF-35. *(Right)* Immunohistochemical stain of a embryonal rhabdomyosarcoma shows strong nuclear positivity of tumor cells for MYOD1, which is a specific marker for rhabdomyosarcomatous differentiation. Nonspecific cytoplasmic positivity for MYOD1 may also be seen in other tumors and has no diagnostic significance.

OTHER SARCOMAS

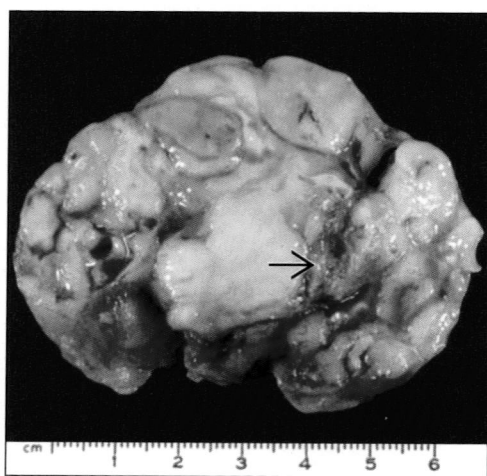

Large, multinodular, tan paratesticular leiomyosarcoma with focal hemorrhage and necrosis ➡. The major differential diagnosis is a dedifferentiated liposarcoma in this location in adults.

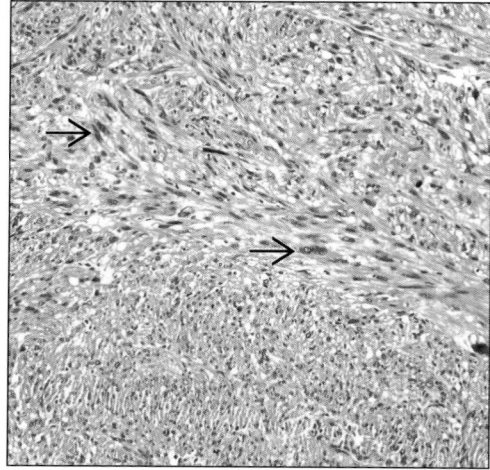

Leiomyosarcoma is composed of a cellular spindle cell proliferation with bundles or fascicles. Cytologic atypia ➡ is evident. The main differential diagnosis is with leiomyomatous rhabdomyosarcoma.

TERMINOLOGY

Synonyms
- Malignant mesenchymal tumors

Definitions
- Malignant soft tissue tumors of paratesticular tissue origin other than the more commonly occurring liposarcoma (adults) or rhabdomyosarcoma (children, young adults)

CLINICAL ISSUES

Epidemiology
- Incidence
  ○ Rare; < 1% of all soft tissue sarcomas
- Age
  ○ Range: 16-84 years (average: 55 years)

Site
- Spermatic cord (most common), tunics, and epididymis

Presentation
- Paratesticular mass

Treatment
- Surgical approaches
  ○ Resection ± radiation or chemotherapy

Prognosis
- Local recurrence or metastasis; prognostic factors include histologic type, tumor grade, and stage at presentation

IMAGE FINDINGS

General Features
- Nonspecific hyperechoic mass by ultrasonography

MACROSCOPIC FEATURES

General Features
- Similar to those occurring in more common sites
- Bulky mass with overall circumscription, tan-white, fleshy cut surface with hemorrhage or necrosis

MICROSCOPIC PATHOLOGY

Histologic Features
- Liposarcoma is most common paratesticular sarcoma in adults
- Rhabdomyosarcoma is most common paratesticular sarcoma in children
- Leiomyosarcoma is 2nd most common sarcoma in adults
  ○ Characterized by fascicles of spindle cells with eosinophilic fibrillar cytoplasm, hyperchromatic blunt-ended nuclei, and paranuclear vacuoles
  ○ May have prominent myxoid areas, pleomorphic component, inflammatory background, or epithelioid cells
- Desmoplastic small round cell tumor
  ○ Similar to those occurring in abdomen or pelvis
  ○ Characterized by epithelial-type nested growth of small blue cells in prominent desmoplastic stroma
- Other sarcomas are much less common
  ○ Malignant fibrous histiocytoma (MFH) and fibrosarcoma are diagnosis of exclusion
  ○ Malignant peripheral nerve sheath tumor (MPNST), osteosarcoma, Kaposi sarcoma, and angiosarcoma have been reported

ANCILLARY TESTS

Immunohistochemistry
- Immunoprofile similar to that of sarcomas in other more common locations

OTHER SARCOMAS

Key Facts

Terminology
- Malignant soft tissue tumors of paratesticular tissue origin other than the more commonly occurring liposarcoma or rhabdomyosarcoma

Clinical Issues
- Range: 16-84 years (average: 55 years)
- Spermatic cord, testicular tunica, and epididymis
- Local recurrence or metastasis; prognostic factors include histologic type, tumor grade, and stage at presentation

Macroscopic Features
- Bulky mass with overall circumscription, tan-white, fleshy cut surface with hemorrhage or necrosis

Microscopic Pathology
- Liposarcoma is most common paratesticular sarcoma in adults
- Rhabdomyosarcoma is most common paratesticular sarcoma in children
- Leiomyosarcoma is 2nd most common sarcoma in adults
- Desmoplastic small round cell tumor may occur in this location and is similar to abdominal/pelvic counterpart
- Other sarcomas (MFH, fibrosarcoma, MPNST, etc.) are much less common

---

- o Leiomyosarcoma is positive for actin-sm, actin-HHF-35, and desmin; may be positive for CD34 and keratin
- o Desmoplastic small round cell tumor is positive for cytokeratin, EMA/MUC1, vimentin, desmin, and neuroendocrine markers (NSE, chromogranin, and synaptophysin)
- o Malignant fibrous histiocytoma is positive for CD68; may be focally positive for actin-sm, cytokeratin
- o Fibrosarcoma positive for actin-sm and vimentin

DIFFERENTIAL DIAGNOSIS

Rhabdomyosarcoma
- Primitive and well-differentiated tumor with rhabdomyoblasts
- Positive for MYOD1, myogenin, and desmin
- Embryonal rhabdomyosarcoma mimics sarcomas with round blue cell undifferentiated morphology
- Embryonal rhabdomyosarcoma (spindle cell leiomyomatous histology) mimics leiomyosarcoma

Sarcoma Arising in Teratoma
- Presence of mature or immature teratoma component
- Epicenter in testis parenchyma

Sex Cord Stromal Tumor, Mixed/Unclassified
- Predominantly intratesticular mass; rarely paratesticular
- Sex cord stromal differentiation in form of tubules or Call-Exner bodies may occur in background of predominantly spindle cell histology
- Cytologic features less atypical with infrequent mitoses and usually no necrosis
- Positive for inhibin, calretinin, WT1, CD99, and variably for keratin and actin-sm

Metastatic Sarcomatoid Carcinoma
- Biphasic histology may be present
- Clinical history is important

Other Benign Soft Tissue Tumors
- Lipoma, leiomyoma, neurofibroma, granular cell tumor, angiomyofibroblastoma-like tumor, calcifying fibrous tumor, cellular angiofibroma, superficial angiomyxoma, aggressive angiomyxoma
- Usually small size, often well circumscribed, bland cytologic features and incidental findings
- Aggressive angiomyxoma is rarely reported to be large

DIAGNOSTIC CHECKLIST

Pathologic Interpretation Pearls
- There are several differential diagnostic considerations in malignant paratesticular spindle cell tumors besides the more common leiomyosarcoma (adults) and rhabdomyosarcoma (children)
- Besides distinctive sarcoma types, sex cord stromal tumor, teratoma arising in sarcoma, and sarcomatoid carcinoma should be in differential diagnosis

SELECTED REFERENCES

1. Fitzgerald S et al: Paratesticular liposarcoma. J Urol. 181(1):331-2, 2009
2. Korkes F et al: Paratesticular sarcomas in Brazil. Urol Int. 82(4):448-52, 2009
3. Dotan ZA et al: Adult genitourinary sarcoma: the 25-year Memorial Sloan-Kettering experience. J Urol. 176(5):2033-8; discussion 2038-9, 2006
4. Ozkan B et al: Adult paratesticular myxofibrosarcoma: report of a rare entity and review of the literature. Int Urol Nephrol. 38(1):5-7, 2006
5. Montgomery E et al: Paratesticular liposarcoma: a clinicopathologic study. Am J Surg Pathol. 27(1):40-7, 2003
6. Ferrari A et al: Paratesticular rhabdomyosarcoma: report from the Italian and German Cooperative Group. J Clin Oncol. 20(2):449-55, 2002
7. Fisher C et al: Leiomyosarcoma of the paratesticular region: a clinicopathologic study. Am J Surg Pathol. 25(9):1143-9, 2001

Gross and Microscopic Features

(Left) Low-power photomicrograph shows a hypercellular leiomyosarcoma involving paratesticular tissue. The tumor is well circumscribed and separated from the rete testis ➡. *(Right)* Leiomyosarcoma shows a fascicular growth pattern and nuclear pleomorphism ➡. The cytoplasm is eosinophilic and fibrillar, indicating myogenic differentiation. When this type of spindle cell tumor occurs in children or young adults, spindle leiomyomatous rhabdomyosarcoma should be excluded.

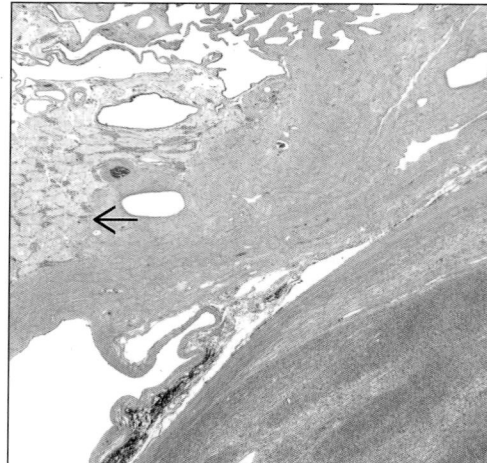
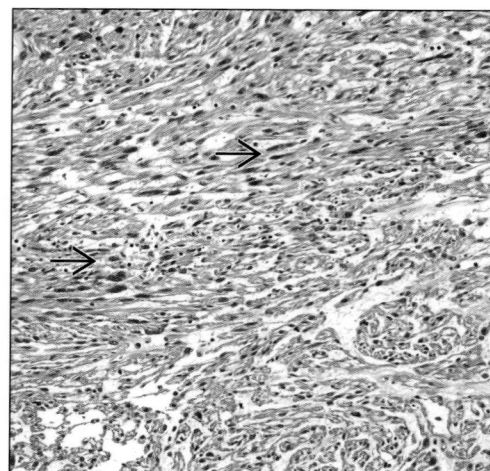

(Left) Leiomyosarcoma at high-power magnification exhibits pleomorphic spindle cells with abundant, fibrillary eosinophilic cytoplasm and occasional mitoses ➡. The nuclei are typically cigar-shaped. *(Right)* Leiomyosarcoma is shown with scattered pleomorphic nuclei ➡ and fibrillary eosinophilic cytoplasm. There are prominent cytoplasmic vacuoles ➡. The age of the patient and immunohistochemistry are important in the distinction from rhabdomyosarcoma with leiomyomatous histology.

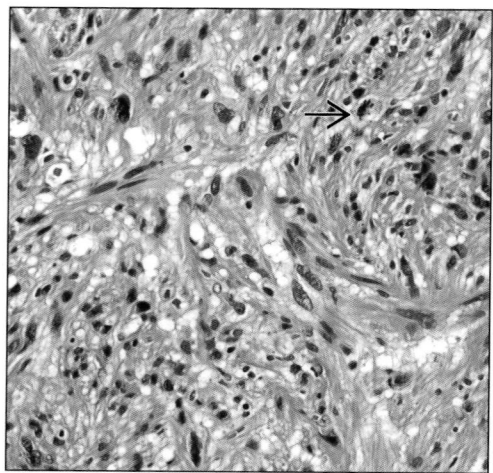
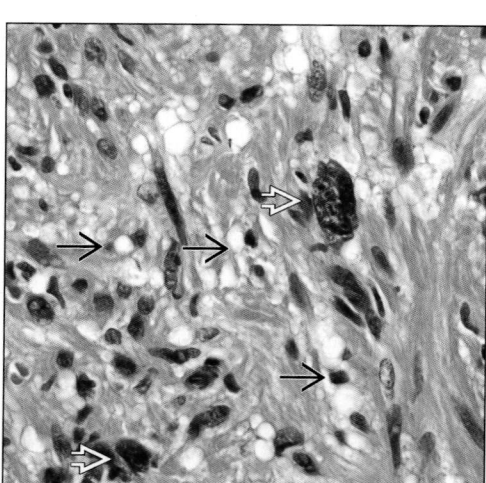

(Left) Malignant peripheral nerve sheath tumor (MPNST) is an extremely rare tumor in the paratesticular location. There are alternating hypo- ➡ and hypercellular ➡ spindle cell areas. *(Right)* MPNST shows hypercellular elongated ovoid tumor cells with fine nuclear chromatin. Mitoses are frequently seen ➡. There is vague palisading of nuclei. The tumor cells were focally positive for S100 and negative for muscle markers, supporting the diagnosis of MPNST.

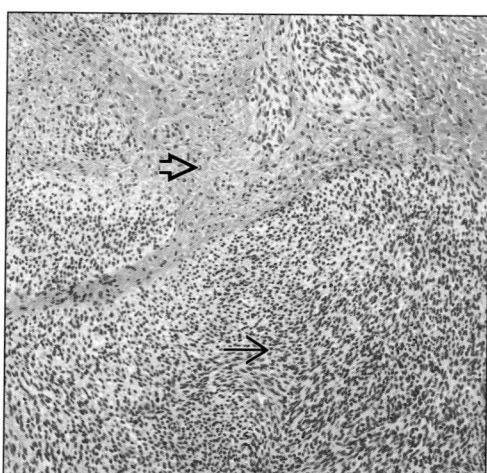
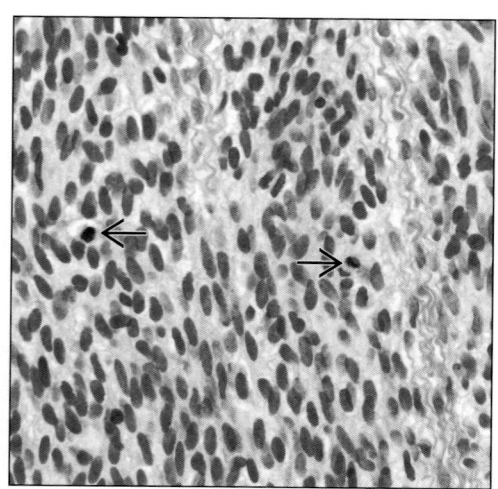

4

OTHER SARCOMAS

Microscopic Features

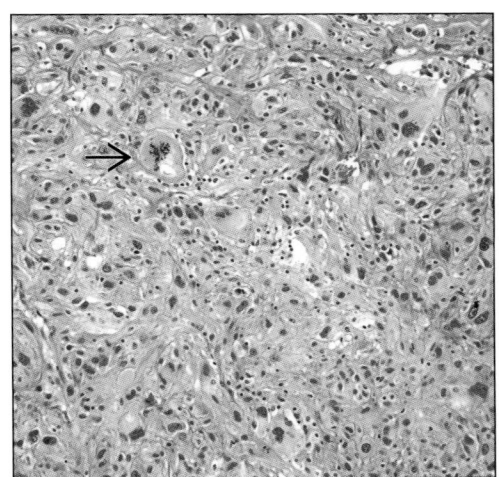 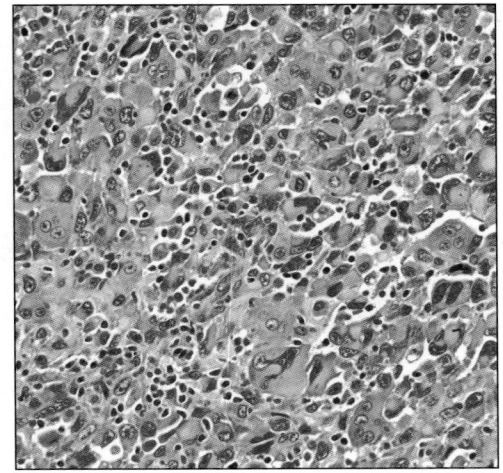

(Left) Malignant fibrous histiocytoma (MFH) with marked cytologic atypia and atypical mitoses ⊞. The diagnosis of MFH is made only after exclusion of other pleomorphic high-grade sarcomas, i.e., dedifferentiated liposarcoma, rhabdomyosarcoma, leiomyosarcoma & MPNST, & sarcomatoid carcinoma using an appropriate panel of immunostains. *(Right)* This is another example of MFH with numerous bizarre tumor giant cells. There are scattered inflammatory cells as well.

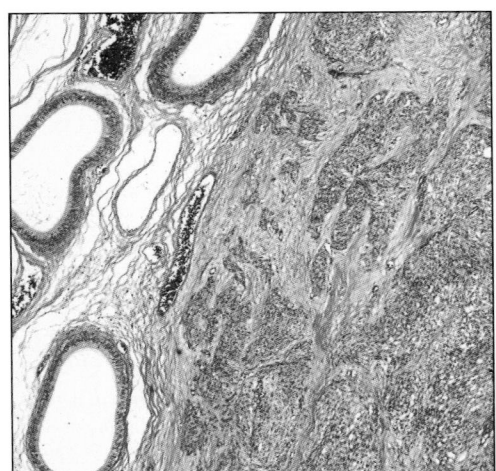 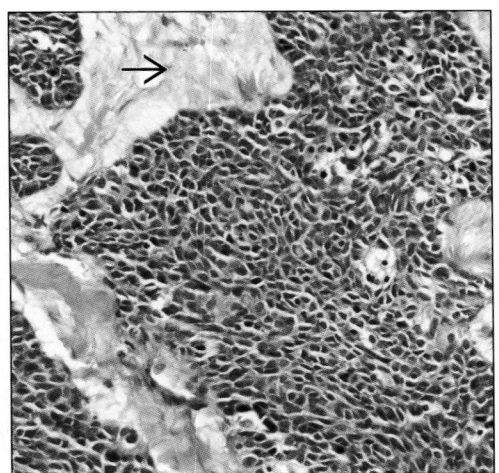

(Left) Desmoplastic small round cell tumor is seen involving the epididymis. It is characterized by nests of small blue cells surrounded by desmoplastic stroma. The tumor cells are positive for both epithelial markers and desmin, a diagnostic immunohistochemical panel. *(Right)* Desmoplastic small round cell tumor shows nests of small blue cells with scant cytoplasm, finely stippled chromatin, and inconspicuous nucleoli. Note also the prominent myxoid stroma in the background ⊞.

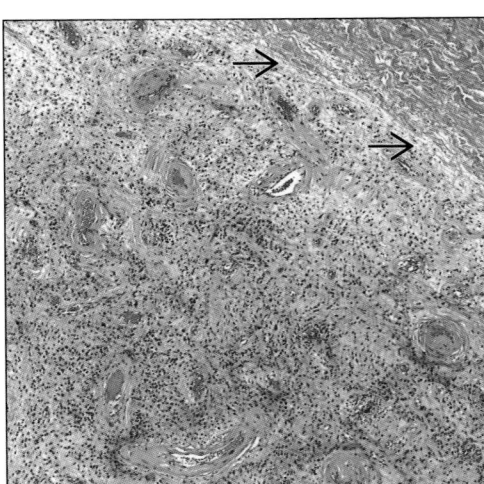 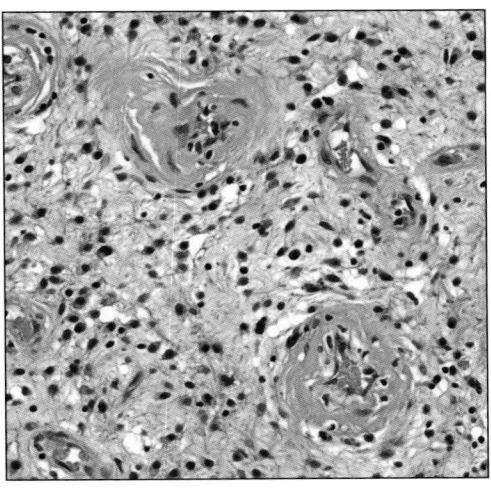

(Left) Angiomyofibro-blastoma-like tumor is seen with a well-circumscribed border from uninvolved paratesticular tissue ⊞. There are abundant vascular channels with perivascular hyalinization. This is a rare benign tumor of the paratesticular region & should be differentiated from sarcoma. *(Right)* Angiomyofibroblastoma-like tumor shows vessels with perivascular hyalinization & ovoid tumor cell proliferation in between, with no cytologic atypia or mitosis.

METASTATIC TUMORS, TESTIS AND PARATESTICULAR STRUCTURES

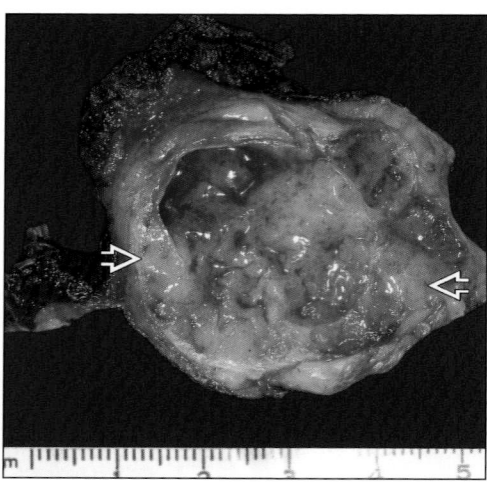

Metastatic prostatic carcinoma ⊡ *is shown extensively involving the testis. The tumor is composed of a tan-pink, soft mass with focal cystic changes. This gross finding mimics a primary germ cell tumor.*

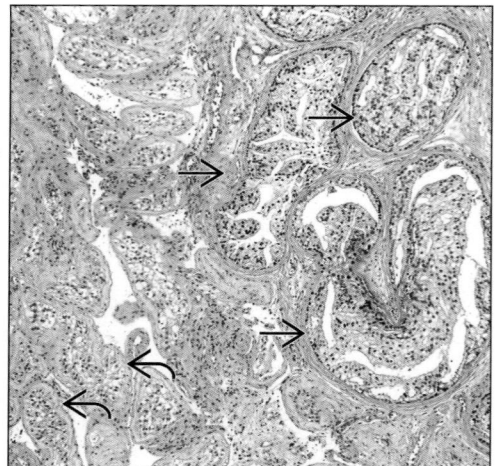

Metastatic prostate adenocarcinoma shows a cribriform growth pattern of tumor cells with abundant clear cytoplasm ⊡. *The uninvolved tubules are atrophic* ⊡ *with no spermatogenesis.*

TERMINOLOGY

Synonyms
- Secondary tumors of testis

Definitions
- Tumors secondarily involving testis and paratesticular structures by hematogenous metastasis or intraperitoneal spread from distant sites; excludes hematopoietic tumors

CLINICAL ISSUES

Epidemiology
- Incidence
  ○ Metastases are rarer in testis than in ovary
  ○ Occur in 0.68% of patients with solid organ malignancy in autopsy studies; incidence is higher in autopsy studies than in clinical practice
- Age
  ○ Majority are > 50 years old

Presentation
- Nonsymptomatic or incidental finding during hormonal ablation orchiectomy or autopsy for metastatic prostate cancer
- Symptomatic metastasis
  ○ Very rare; occurs in patients with advanced stage
  ○ In symptomatic metastasis, tumor is usually solitary and unilateral (> 90%)
- May present very rarely as carcinoma of unknown primary and mimic primary testicular and paratesticular tumors
- Rare metastasis to primary testicular germ cell tumor (tumor to tumor metastasis) is known to occur

Treatment
- Surgical resection for palliative pain control
- Adjuvant therapy based on primary site and histology

Prognosis
- Generally poor prognosis

IMAGE FINDINGS

General Features
- Radiologic studies are helpful in defining local extent of disease and primary site of tumor

MACROSCOPIC FEATURES

General Features
- Localized mass, multiple nodules, or diffuse enlargement of testis with no grossly apparent mass
- Usually unilateral and solitary (> 90%)

MICROSCOPIC PATHOLOGY

Histologic Features
- Histologic features recapitulate their site of origin
  ○ Metastatic carcinomas are most common
    ■ Most common primary sites include prostate, lung, kidney, and gastrointestinal tract
    ■ Less common and rare sites include esophagus, bladder, pancreas
  ○ Metastatic melanoma to testis has been reported
  ○ Extremely rare for sarcoma metastasis
  ○ Secondary involvement of testis by hematopoietic neoplasms is common
- Histology not typical of germ cell tumor or sex cord stromal tumor
  ○ Interstitial infiltrative growth pattern between seminiferous tubules
  ○ Discrete tumoral mass, nodules, or extensive infiltration of parenchyma
  ○ Intratubular growth pattern is rare and may mimic a primary tumor
  ○ Prominent vascular invasion (~ 70%)

METASTATIC TUMORS, TESTIS AND PARATESTICULAR STRUCTURES

Key Facts

Terminology

- Tumors secondarily involving testis and paratesticular structures by hematogenous metastasis or intraperitoneal spread from distant sites; excludes hematopoietic tumors

Clinical Issues

- Metastatic tumors are more rare in testis and occur in 0.68% of patients in autopsy studies
- Majority are > 50 years old
- Generally has poor prognosis

Macroscopic Features

- Localized mass, multiple nodules, or diffuse enlargement of testis with no grossly apparent mass
- Usually unilateral and solitary (> 90%)

Microscopic Pathology

- Histologic features recapitulate their site of origin
- Metastatic carcinomas are most common; prostate, lung, kidney, and gastrointestinal tract are frequent sites
- Histology not typical of germ cell tumor or sex cord stromal tumor
- Interstitial infiltrative growth pattern between seminiferous tubules
- Prominent lymphovascular invasion

Ancillary Tests

- Panel of stains should be based on differential diagnosis generated from clinical history, imaging, and histopathology

---

Predominant Pattern/Injury Type

- Neoplastic

ANCILLARY TESTS

Immunohistochemistry

- Useful in distinction of primary vs. metastases
- Unlike germ cell tumors, EMA/MUC1, HMCK(34βE12) are positive in non-germ cell tumor epithelial malignancies
- Panel of stains should be based on differential diagnoses generated from clinical history, imaging, and histopathology

DIFFERENTIAL DIAGNOSIS

Primary Testicular Germ Cell Tumor

- Usually younger age at presentation
- Incidence of bilaterality and multifocality is low
- Diffuse rather than interstitial growth pattern
- Positive for germ cell markers (Oct3/4, SALL4, etc.)
- Usually negative for EMA/MUC1 and HMCK(34βE12)

Primary Testicular Sex Cord Stromal Tumor

- Cytologically more banal-appearing tumor cells
- Leydig cell tumor may mimic malignant melanoma; Sertoli cell tumor may mimic carcinoma
- Positive for inhibin and calretinin; weakly positive or negative for cytokeratin
- EMA/MUC1 usually negative

Rete/Epididymal Carcinoma

- Lack of clinical history of malignancy elsewhere
- Histologic transition from rete testis or epididymal epithelium is key feature
- Epicenter of mass in rete or epididymis

Malignant Mesothelioma

- Usually extensively and diffusely involves tunica
- Positive for mesothelial-associated markers (calretinin, Podoplanin(D2-40), WT1, CK5/6)

Malignant Lymphoma

- Interstitial growth pattern of round blue cells
- Relative preservation of seminiferous tubules; rarely intratubular growth
- Positive for lymphoid markers; negative for cytokeratin and neuroendocrine markers

Ovarian-Type (Müllerian) Carcinoma

- Lack of clinical history of malignancy elsewhere
- Immunostains, including WT1 and CA125

DIAGNOSTIC CHECKLIST

Pathologic Interpretation Pearls

- Multifocality, bilaterality, interstitial growth, vascular-lymphatic invasion, and unusual histology for testis or paratesticular structures should raise possibility of metastasis
- In paratestis, malignant mesothelioma, primary rete testis/epididymal carcinoma, and ovarian-type carcinoma should always be in differential diagnosis with metastatic carcinoma

SELECTED REFERENCES

1. Gillen S et al: Testicular metastasis from adenocarcinoma of the esophagus. Ann Thorac Surg. 87(3):957-9, 2009
2. Ulbright TM et al: Metastatic carcinoma to the testis: a clinicopathologic analysis of 26 nonincidental cases with emphasis on deceptive features. Am J Surg Pathol. 32(11):1683-93, 2008
3. Dutt N et al: Secondary neoplasms of the male genital tract with different patterns of involvement in adults and children. Histopathology. 37(4):323-31, 2000
4. Ro JY et al: Lung carcinoma with metastasis to testicular seminoma. Cancer. 66(2):347-53, 1990
5. Ro JY et al: Merkel cell carcinoma metastatic to the testis. Am J Clin Pathol. 94(4):384-9, 1990

METASTATIC TUMORS, TESTIS AND PARATESTICULAR STRUCTURES

Gross and Microscopic Features

(Left) Metastatic carcinoma from the lung is shown with a small solitary nodule ⮞ in an atrophic testis. An intraparenchymal, well-circumscribed, white-tan nodule is present. Grossly, this tumor mimics a sex cord stromal tumor. *(Right)* Metastatic poorly differentiated lung carcinoma with an interstitial ⮞ growth pattern and tumor cells is seen involving seminiferous tubules ⮞ (intratubular growth). The tumor does not resemble any of the known germ cell tumor components.

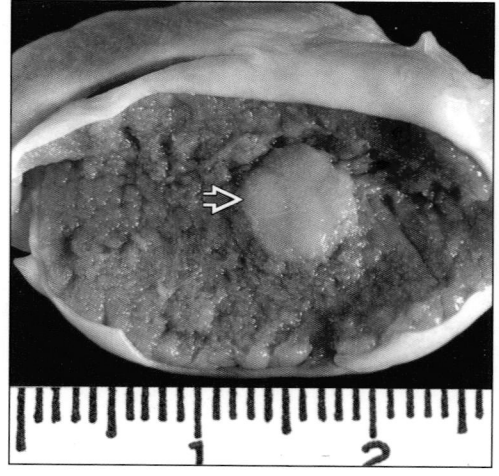
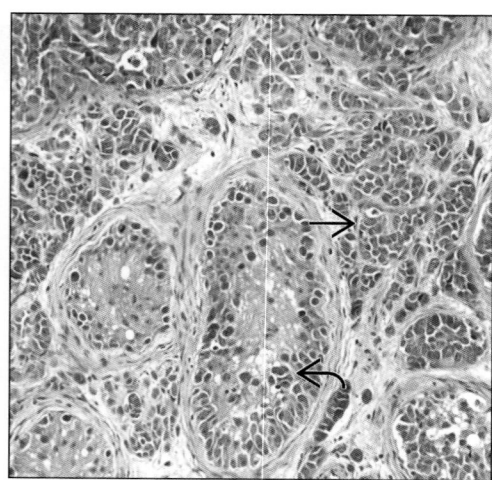

(Left) This image shows metastatic clear cell renal cell carcinoma adjacent to the rete testis ⮞. The tumor is composed of sheets of clear cells with a prominent thin sinusoidal vascular network. *(Right)* Metastatic clear cell renal cell carcinoma shows a distinct fibrovascular-supporting network between tumor cells containing abundant clear cytoplasm. It may mimic a seminoma but has a greater degree of nuclear pleomorphism and lacks a lymphoid infiltrate.

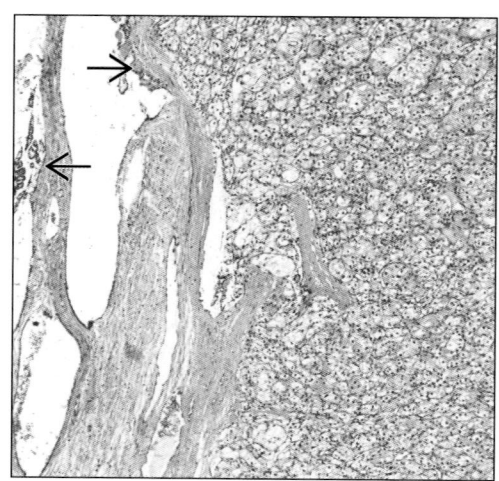
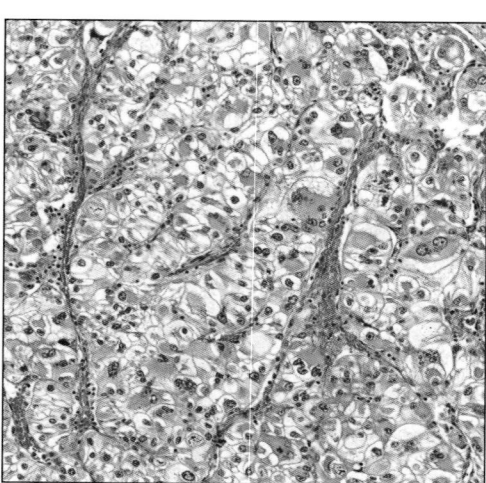

(Left) Metastatic prostate carcinoma of ductal type shows complex cribriform and papillary growth patterns. Ductal-type prostate carcinoma has been reported to have predilection for testicular metastasis and may mimic an embryonal carcinoma. *(Right)* Metastatic prostate carcinoma is shown with intratubular ⮞ and interstitial ⮞ growth patterns in the testis. The tumor cells within and surrounding the tubules are similar and have relatively uniform cells with prominent nucleoli.

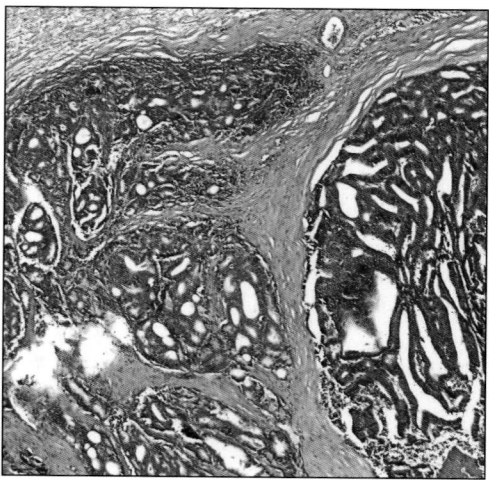
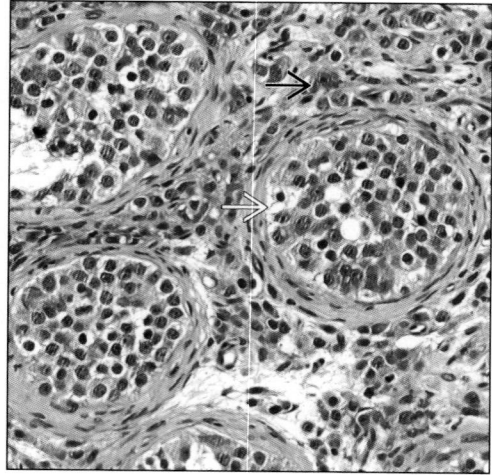

Microscopic Features

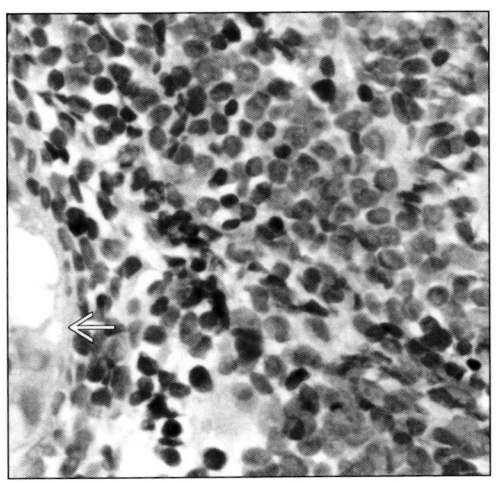 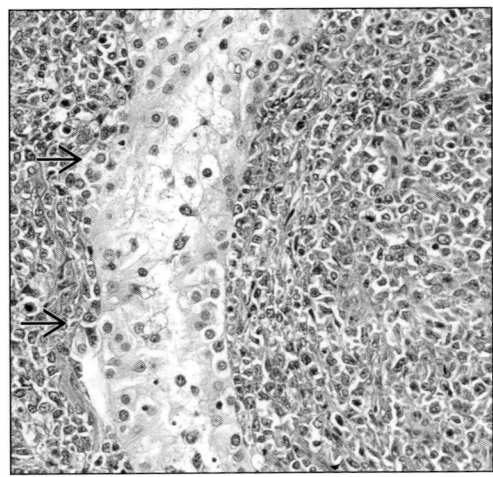

(Left) In this metastatic Merkel cell carcinoma to the testis, the tumor is composed of sheets of small blue cells with fine chromatin and scant cytoplasm. Malignant lymphoma is a major differential diagnosis. The tumor cells spare the seminiferous tubules ➡. Immunohistochemistry showed dot-like cytokeratin positivity. **(Right)** In this large B-cell lymphoma involving the testis, the tumor has a diffuse interstitial pattern and spares the seminiferous tubules ➡.

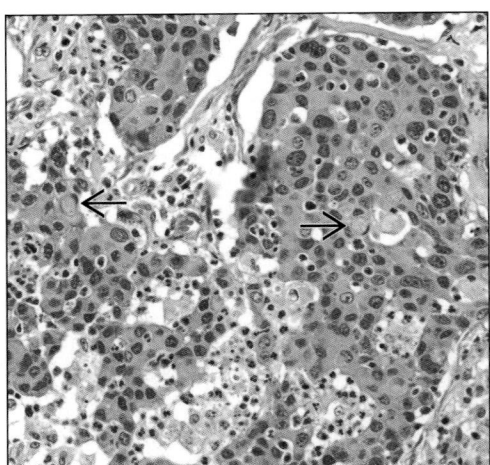 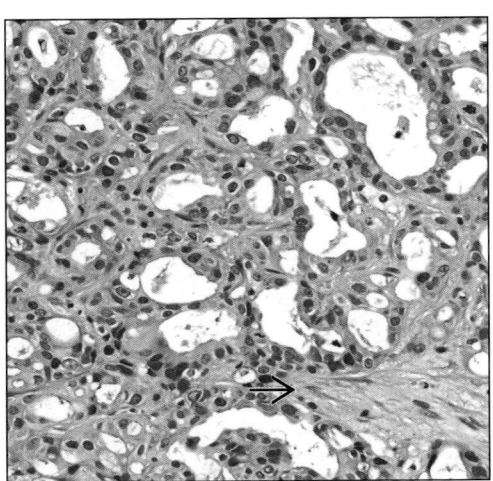

(Left) Poorly differentiated cecal adenocarcinoma metastatic to the testis is shown. Tumor cells are pleomorphic and rare cells show intracytoplasmic mucin ➡. Typical enteric histology is not evident. **(Right)** In this pancreatic adenocarcinoma metastatic to the paratestis, the tumor is composed of glands of variable size and shape with desmoplastic stroma ➡. These features may be seen in a primary rete testis/epididymal carcinoma, and clinicopathologic correlation is mandatory.

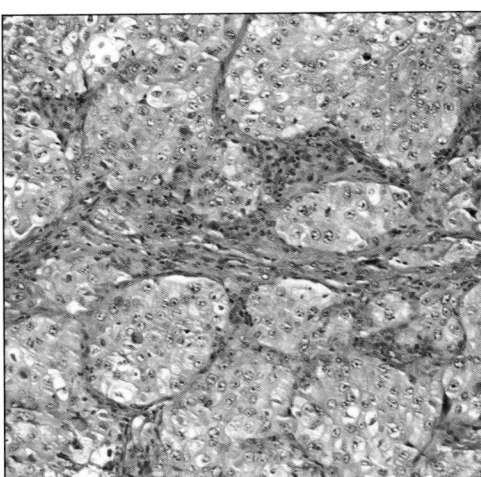 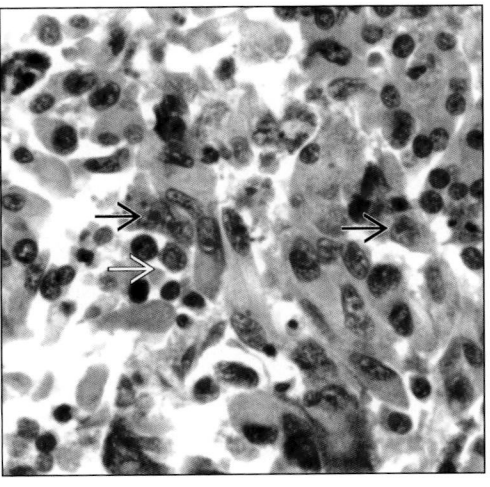

(Left) Metastatic urothelial carcinoma to the testis shows tumor cell nests, which may resemble embryonal carcinoma or seminoma. The patient's age, clinical history of urothelial carcinoma, and appropriate immunohistochemistry should be helpful to confirm the diagnosis. **(Right)** Metastatic melanoma to the testis shows pleomorphic tumor cells with characteristic macronucleoli ➡, pseudonuclear inclusions ➡, and abundant finely granular melanin pigment.

PROTOCOL FOR TESTIS CANCER SPECIMENS

Testis: Radical Orchiectomy

Surgical Pathology Cancer Case Summary (Checklist)

Serum Tumor Markers (select all that apply)

(See serum tumor markers [S] classification)

*____ Unknown

*____ Serum marker studies within normal limits

*____ α-fetoprotein (AFP) elevation

*____ β-subunit of human chorionic gonadotropin (β-hCG) elevation

*____ Lactate dehydrogenase (LDH) elevation

Specimen Laterality

____ Right

____ Left

____ Both

____ Not specified

Tumor Focality

____ Unifocal

____ Multifocal

Tumor Size

Greatest dimension of main tumor mass: _____ cm

*Additional dimensions: _____ x _____ cm

Greatest dimensions of additional tumor nodules: _____ cm, _____ cm, etc.

____ Cannot be determined (see comment)

Macroscopic Extent of Tumor (select all that apply)

____ Confined to the testis

____ Invades hilar soft tissues

____ Invades tunica vaginalis (perforates mesothelium)

____ Invades epididymis

____ Invades spermatic cord

____ Other (specify): _____

Histologic Type (select all that apply)

____ Intratubular germ cell neoplasia, unclassified only

____ Seminoma, classic type

____ Seminoma with associated scar

____ Seminoma with syncytiotrophoblastic cells

____ Mixed germ cell tumor (specify components and approximate percentages)

    _____

    _____

____ Embryonal carcinoma

____ Yolk sac tumor

____ Choriocarcinoma, biphasic

____ Choriocarcinoma, monophasic

____ Placental site trophoblastic tumor

____ Teratoma

____ Teratoma with a secondary somatic-type malignant component (specify type): _____

____ Monodermal teratoma, carcinoid

____ Monodermal teratoma, primitive neuroectodermal tumor

____ Monodermal teratoma, other (specify): _____

____ Spermatocytic seminoma

____ Spermatocytic seminoma with a sarcomatous component

____ Mixed germ cell-sex cord stromal tumor, gonadoblastoma

____ Mixed germ cell-sex cord stromal tumor, others (specify): _____

PROTOCOL FOR TESTIS CANCER SPECIMENS

____ Testicular scar

    ____ Scar only

    ____ Scar with intratubular germ cell neoplasia

____ Sex cord-stromal tumor

    ____ Leydig cell tumor

    ____ Sertoli cell tumor

      ____ Classic

      ____ Sclerosing

      ____ Large cell calcifying

    ____ Granulosa cell tumor

      ____ Adult-type

      ____ Juvenile-type

    ____ Mixed, with components (specify components and approximate percentages)

      _____

      _____

    ____ Unclassified

____ Malignant neoplasm, type cannot be determined

____ Other (specify): _____

Margins

Spermatic cord margin

____ Cannot be assessed

____ Uninvolved by tumor

____ Involved by tumor

Other margin(s)

____ Cannot be assessed

____ Uninvolved by tumor (specify): _____

____ Not applicable

Microscopic Tumor Extension (select all that apply)

*____ Rete testis

*____ Epididymis

*____ Hilar fat

____ Spermatic cord

____ Tunica vaginalis (perforates mesothelium)

____ Scrotal wall

____ None of the above

Lymph-Vascular Invasion

____ Absent

____ Present

____ Indeterminate

Pathologic Staging (pTNM)

TNM descriptors (required only if applicable) (select all that apply)

____ m (multiple)

____ r (recurrent

____ y (post-treatment)

Primary tumor (pT)

____ pTX: Cannot be assessed

____ pT0: No evidence of primary tumor

____ pTis: Intratubular germ cell neoplasia (carcinoma in situ)

____ pT1: Tumor limited to the testis and epididymis without vascular/lymphatic invasion; tumor may invade tunica albuginea gut not tunica vaginalis

____ pT2: Tumor limited to the testis and epididymis with vascular/lymphatic invasion, or tumor extending through the tunica albuginea with involvement of the tunica vaginalis

____ pT3: Tumor invades the spermatic cord with or without vascular/lymphatic invasion

____ pT4: Tumor invades the scrotum with or without vascular/lymphatic invasion

PROTOCOL FOR TESTIS CANCER SPECIMENS

Regional lymph nodes (pN)

____ pNX: Cannot be assessed

____ pN0: No regional lymph node metastasis

____ PN1: Metastasis with a lymph node mass ≤ 2 cm in greatest dimension, or ≤ 5 positive nodes, none > 2 cm in greatest dimension

____ PN2: Metastasis with a lymph node mass >2 cm but not > 5 cm in greatest dimension; or > 5 nodes positive, none > 5 cm; or evidence of extranodal extension of tumor

____ pN3: Metastasis with a lymph node mass > 5 cm in greatest dimension

Specify: Number examined: _____

Number involved: _____

Distant metastasis (pM)

____ Not applicable

____ pM1: Distant metastasis present

____ pM1a: Nonregional nodal or pulmonary metastasis

____ pM1b: Distant metastasis other than to nonregional lymph nodes and lung

*Specify site(s), if known: _____

*Serum Tumor Markers (S)

*____ SX: Serum marker studies not available or performed

*____ S0: Serum marker study levels within normal limits

*____ S1: LDH < 1.5 X N† and HCG < 5,000 mIU/mL and AFP < 1000 ng/mL

*____ S2: LDH 1.5-10 X N or HCG 5,000-50,000 mIU/mL or AFP 1,000-10,000 ng/mL

*____ S3: LDH > 10 X N or HCG > 50,000 mIU/mL or AFP > 10,000 ng/mL

†N indicates the upper limit of normal for the LDH assay

*Additional Pathologic Findings (select all that apply)

*____ None identified

*____ Intratubular germ cell neoplasia

*____ Hemosiderin-laden macrophages

*____ Atrophy

*____ Other (specify): _____

* Data elements with asterisks are not required. However, these elements may be clinically important but are not yet validated or regularly used in patient management. Adapted with permission from College of American Pathologists, "Protocol for the Examination of Specimens from Patients with Malignant Germ Cell and Sex Cord-Stromal Tumors of the Testis." Web posting date October 2009, www.cap.org.

Testis: Retroperitoneal Lymphadenectomy

Surgical Pathology Cancer Case Summary (Checklist)

*Pre-lymphadenectomy Treatment

*____ Chemo/radiation therapy

*____ No chemo/radiation therapy

*____ Unknown

*Serum Tumor Markers (select all that apply)

*____ Unknown

*____ Serum marker studies within normal limits

*____ α-fetoprotein (AFP) elevation

*____ β subunit of human chorionic gonadotropin (β-hCG) elevation

*____ Lactate dehydrogenase (LDH) elevation

*Specimen Site(s)

*Specify: _____

*Number of Nodal Groups Present

*Specify: _____

*____ Cannot be determined

Size of Largest Metastatic Deposit in Lymph Node

Greatest dimension: _____ cm

*Additional dimensions: _____ x _____ cm

PROTOCOL FOR TESTIS CANCER SPECIMENS

Histologic Viability of Tumor (if applicable)

_____ Viable teratoma present

_____ Viable nonteratomatous tumor present

_____ No viable tumor present

Histologic Type of Metastatic Tumor

_____ Seminoma, classic type

_____ Seminoma with syncytiotrophoblastic cells

_____ Mixed germ cell tumor (specify components and approximate percentages)

_____

_____

_____ Embryonal carcinoma

_____ Yolk sac tumor

_____ Choriocarcinoma, biphasic

_____ Choriocarcinoma, monophasic

_____ Cystic trophoblastic tumor

_____ Placental site trophoblastic tumor

_____ Teratoma

_____ Teratoma with a secondary somatic-type malignant component (specify type): _____

_____ Monodermal teratoma (specify type): _____

_____ Spermatocytic seminoma

_____ Malignant neoplasm, type cannot be determined

_____ Other (specify): _____

Regional Lymph Nodes (pN)

_____ pNX: Cannot be assessed

_____ pN0: No regional lymph node metastasis

_____ PN1: Metastasis with a lymph node mass < 2 cm in greatest dimension, or ≤ 5 positive nodes, none > 2 cm in greatest dimension

_____ PN2: Metastasis with a lymph node mass > 2 cm but not > 5 cm in greatest dimension, or > 5 nodes positive, none > 5 cm; or evidence of extranodal extension of tumor

_____ pN3: Metastasis in a lymph node > 5 cm in greatest dimension

Specify: Total number examined: _____

Total number involved: _____

Nonregional Lymph Node Metastasis (M1a)

_____ Not applicable

_____ Not identified

_____ Present

* Data elements with asterisks are not required. However, these elements may be clinically important but are not yet validated or regularly used in patient management.

Anatomic Stage/Prognostic Groups

Group	Tumor	Node	Metastasis	Serum Tumor Markers
Stage 0	pTis	N0	M0	S0
Stage I	pT1-4	N0	M0	SX
Stage 1A	pT1	N0	M0	S0
Stage IB	pT2	N0	M0	S0
	pT3	N0	M0	S0
	pT4	N0	M0	S0
Stage IS	Any pT/TX	N0	M0	S1-3 (post-orchiectomy)
Stage II	Any pT/TX	N1, N2, N3	M0	SX
Stage IIA	Any pT/TX	N1	M0	S0
	Any pT/TX	N1	M0	S1
Stage IIB	Any pT/TX	N2	M0	S0
	Any pT/TX	N2	M0	S1
Stage IIC	Any pT/TX	N3	M0	S0
	Any pT/TX	N3	M0	S1
Stage IIIB	Any pT/TX	N1, N2, N3	M0	S2

PROTOCOL FOR TESTIS CANCER SPECIMENS

	Any pT/TX	Any N	M1a	S2
Stage IIIC	Any pT/TX	N1, N2, N3	M0	S3
	Any pT/TX	Any N	M1a	S3
	Any T	Any N	M1b	Any S

Used with the permission of the American Joint Committee on Cancer (AJCC), Chicago, Illinois. The original source for this material is the AJCC Cancer Staging Manual, Seventh Edition (2010) published by Springer Science and Business Media LLC, www.springerlink.com.

IMMUNOHISTOCHEMISTRY, TESTIS

Tumors with Diffuse Arrangement and Pale and Clear Cytoplasm

Antibody	Classic Seminoma	Spermatocytic Seminoma	Embryonal Carcinoma	Yolk Sac Tumor	Sertoli Cell Tumor	Lymphoma	Renal Cell Carcinoma	Melanoma
CD117	+	+	-	V	-	-/+	V	V
Oct3/4	+	-	+	-	-	-	-	-
CD30(BerH2)	-/+ (rare focal cells)	-	+	-	-	V	ND	-
α-fetoprotein	-	-	-	+	-	ND	-	-
Glypican-3	-	-	-	+	-	-	-	-
PAN-CK(AE1/AE3)	-	-	+	+	+/-	-	+	-
CK7	V	ND	+	-/+	-	ND	V	-
EMA/MUC1	-	-	+	-/+	V	-	+	-
Inhibin	- (+STC)	ND	-	-	+	-	-	-
CD45(LCA)	-	-	-	-	-	+	-	-
S100	-	-	-	-	-	-	-	+
RCC	-	ND	V	-	-	-	+	-

V = Variable, ND = No Data, STC = Syncytiotrophoblast

Tumors with Glandular/Tubular Pattern

Antibody	Embryonal Carcinoma	Seminoma	Yolk Sac Tumor	Sertoli Cell Tumor	Rete Testis Tumor	Metastatic Adenocarcinoma
Oct3/4	+	+	-	-	-	-
CD30(BerH2)	+	-/+ (rare focal cells)	Rare +	-	-	V
CD117	-	+	-	-	-	V
Inhibin	-	-	-	+	-	-
EMA/MUC1	-	-	+	-/+	V	+
SALL4	+	+	+	-	-	-
α-fetoprotein	-	-	+	-	-	-
Calretinin	-	-	-	+	+	-/+
Chromogranin	-	-	-	+	-	-
Glypican-3	-	-	+	-	-	- (+ in hepatocellular carcinoma)

Tumors with Microcystic Pattern

Antibody	Yolk Sac Tumor	Seminoma	Leydig Cell Tumor	Sertoli Cell Tumor	Paratesticular Adenomatoid Tumor
α-fetoprotein	+	-	-	-	-
PAN-CK(AE1/AE3)	+	+ (rare)	-/+	+/-	+
Oct3/4	-	+	-	-	-
CD117	-	+	-	-	V
Inhibin	-	-	+	+	-
Melan-A(MART-1)	-	-	+	+	-
Calretinin	-	-	+	+	+
WT1	-	-	+	+	+

Tumors with Oxyphilic Cytoplasm

Antibody	Leydig Cell Tumor	Large Cell Calcifying Sertoli Cell	Sertoli Cell Tumor, NOS	Carcinoid	Plasmacytoma
Inhibin	+	+	V	-	-
PLAP	-	-	-	-	-
PAN-CK(AE1/AE3)	-/+	-/+	+/-	+	-
Vimentin	+	+	V	V	V
S100	V	+	V	V	V
Synaptophysin	V	ND	V	+	-

V = Variable, ND = No Data.

IMMUNOHISTOCHEMISTRY, TESTIS

Intratubular Atypical Cells: Pseudo-ITGCN vs. ITGCN

Antibody	ITGCN	Pseudo-ITGCN
CD117	+	+
Oct3/4	+	-
Podoplanin(D2-40)	+	-
SALL4	+	-
PAN-CK(AE1/AE3)	-	-

Metastatic Poorly Differentiated Carcinoma in a Young Adult Man vs. Germ Cell

Antibody	Germ Cell Tumor	Metastatic Carcinoma
SALL4	+	-
Oct3/4	+	-
EMA/MUC1	-	+
S100	-	Melanoma
WT1	-	Mesothelioma, müllerian, sex cord stromal tumors
CD45(LCA)	-	Lymphoma

Paratesticular Tumors with Glandular/Tubular Pattern

Antibody	Metastatic Adenocarcinoma	Müllerian Epithelial Tumors	Sertoliform Cystadenoma of Rete Testis	Adenomatoid Tumor	Rete Adenocarcinoma	Mesothelioma	Paratesticular Sertoli Cell Tumor
PAN-CK(AE1/AE3)	+	+	+/-	+	+	-	+
CD30(BerH2)	-	-/+	-	-	-	-	-
ER	-/+	+	-	-	-	-	-
PR	-/+	+	-	-	-	-	-
CK7	+/-	+	+/-	-/+	+	-/+	-
Vimentin	-/+	-/+	-	-	-	-	+
Calretinin	-	-	-	+	-	+	+
WT1	-	+	-	+	-	+	+
Podoplanin(D2-40)	-	-	-	+	-	+	-

Paratesticular Papillary Tumors

Antibody	Müllerian Papillary Serous Carcinoma	Mesothelioma	Prostatic Adenocarcinoma
ER, PR	+	-	+/-
CK7	+	-/+	-
Calretinin	-	+	-
MOC-31	-	-	-
CD15	+	-	-
CK5/6	-	+	-
Podoplanin(D2-40)	-	+	-
PSA, PAP	-	-	+

Paratesticular Tumors with Spindle Cell Morphology

Antibody	Leiomyosarcoma	Sarcomatoid Carcinoma	Melanoma	Mesothelioma	Unclassified Sex Cord Stromal Tumor
PAN-CK(AE1/AE3)	-/+	+/-	-	+	-/+
Inhibin	-	-	-	-	V
S100	-	-	+	-	+
Actin-sm	+	-/+	-	-/+	+
Calretinin	-	-	-	+	V
Melan-A(MART-1)	-	-	+	-	V

V = Variable, ND = No Data

IMMUNOHISTOCHEMISTRY, TESTIS

Testicular Tumors vs. Metastasis

Müllerian	Mesothelial	Epithelial	Germ Cell	Sex Cord
CA125	Calretinin	EMA/MUC1	Oct3/4	Inhibin
WT1	HMCK(34βE12)	CEA	PLAP	S100
ER, PR	Podoplanin(D2-40)	CD15	SALL4	Calretinin
	Thrombomodulin	CK7	CD30	WT1
	Mesothelin	CK20	CD117	CD99
	WT1	PSA (prostate)	Podoplanin(D2-40)	Actin-sm
	CK5/6	TTF-1 (lung and thyroid)		
		CDX2 (colorectal)		

Microscopic and Immunohistochemical Features

(Left) H&E shows intratubular germ cell neoplasia (ITGCN) composed of large atypical cells ⊟ situated at the periphery of an atrophic seminiferous tubule. The atypical cells have abundant clear cytoplasm and enlarged nuclei with prominent nucleoli. *(Right)* The tumor cells ⊟ of ITGCN are highlighted by strong nuclear staining by Oct3/4. The nonneoplastic germ cells in adjacent seminiferous tubule ⊟ are negative. Immunostaining is useful in small biopsies in high-risk patients.

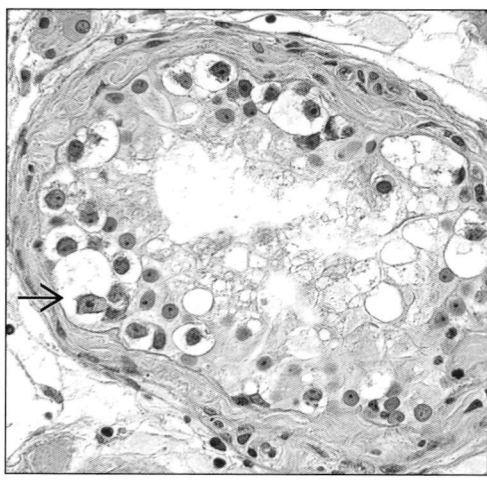
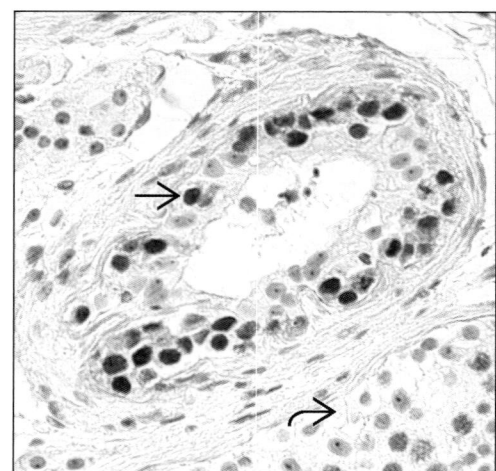

(Left) This is an example of classic seminoma with nests of seminomatous tumor cells separated by fibrous septae containing small lymphocytes. *(Right)* This image shows strong positive nuclear staining of seminoma cells by Oct3/4. The small lymphocytes are negative. Oct3/4 is a useful marker for seminoma and embryonal carcinoma. It is also useful in metastatic setting or extragonadal germ cell tumors. Being a nuclear stain, it tends to be more reliable and easy to interpret.

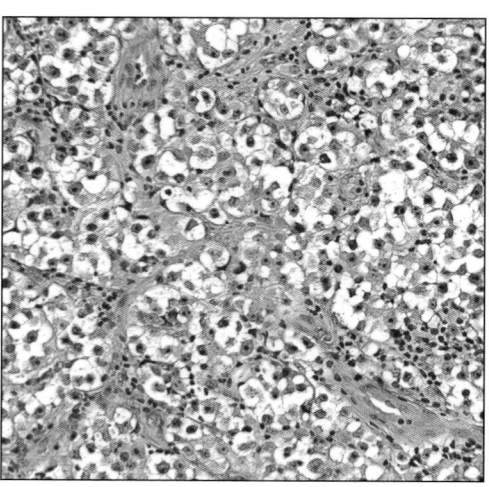
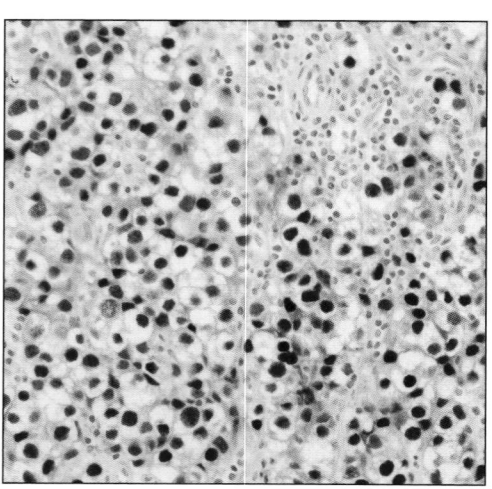

(Left) This image shows strong membranous staining of classic seminoma by CD117. It is also a sensitive marker for intratubular germ cell neoplasia. Embryonal carcinoma is negative and yolk sac tumor may show rare and focal weak staining. *(Right)* This photomicrograph shows strong membranous and cytoplasmic staining of seminoma by Podoplanin(D2-40). Podoplanin(D2-40) is an antibody against oncofetal protein M2A , which also stains lymphatic endothelial cells and mesothelial cells.

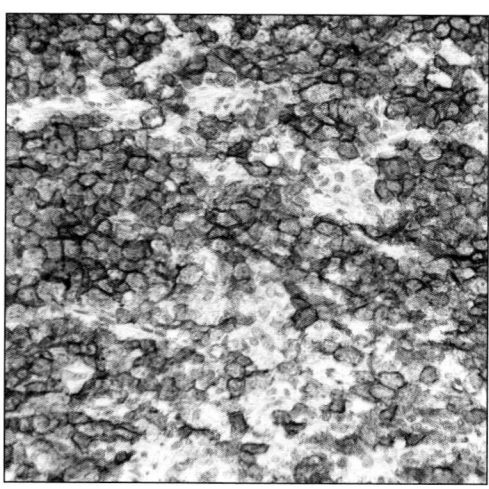
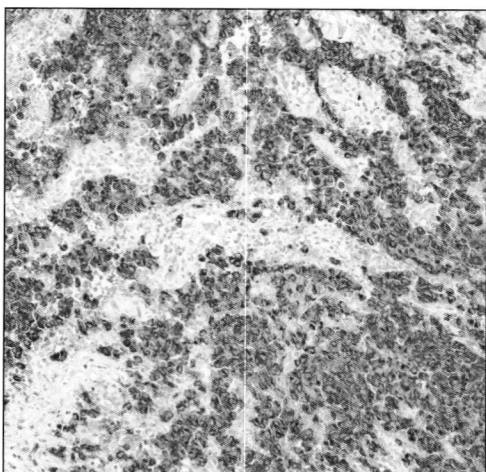

Microscopic and Immunohistochemical Features

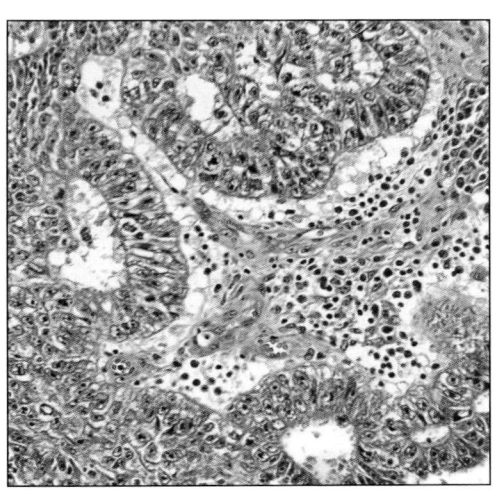

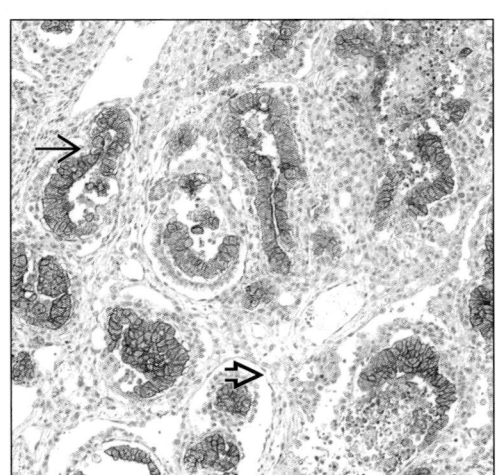

(Left) This image shows embryonal carcinoma with prominent glandular pattern. Important differential diagnoses include YST and metastatic carcinoma. *(Right)* Embryonal carcinoma shows membranous staining for CD30(BerH2) ➡; the surrounding yolk cell tumor component is negative ⇨. Germ cell tumors are typically EMA/MUC1(-) compared to visceral epithelial malignancies. CD30(BerH2) also stains anaplastic large cell (Ki-1) lymphoma and hence should be used in a panel.

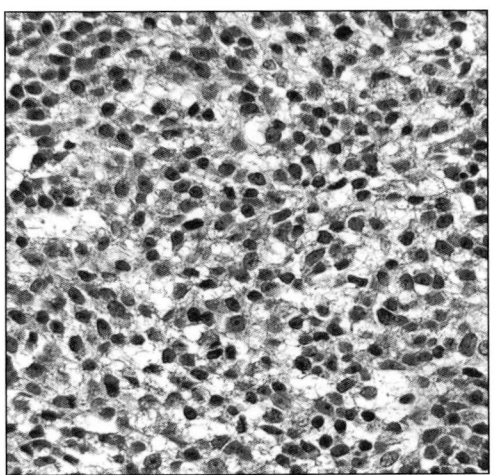

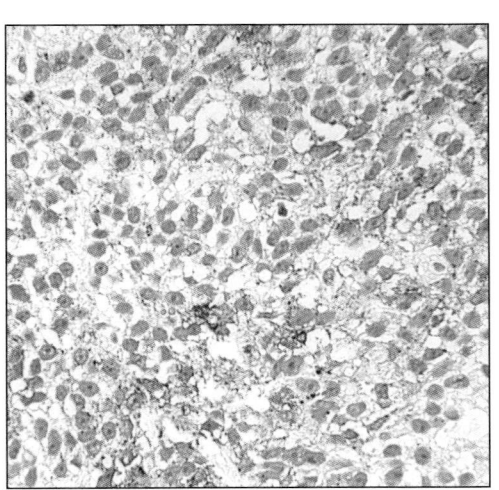

(Left) This is an example of yolk sac tumor with solid growth pattern. When predominant, the morphologic differential diagnoses would include seminoma, embryonal carcinoma, monophasic choriocarcinoma, and solid Leydig cell and Sertoli cell tumors. *(Right)* Positive membranous and cytoplasmic staining of the solid yolk sac tumor for glypican-3 is shown. Other germ cell tumor components are negative for glypican-3 except in syncytiotrophoblasts and rarely in immature teratoma.

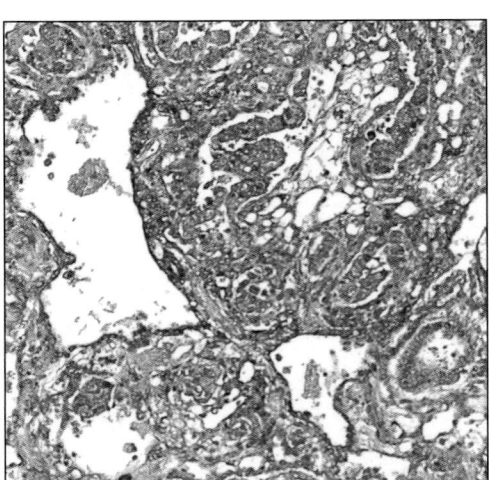

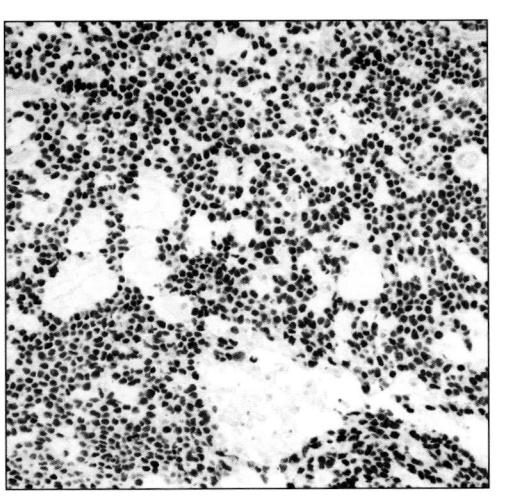

(Left) This image shows strong positive immunostaining of yolk sac tumor by α-fetoprotein is a time-honored marker, but it stains only 55-78% of YST and staining is often blotchy, frequently with nonspecific background staining. *(Right)* Strong nuclear staining of yolk sac tumor by SALL4 is shown, a zinc finger transcription factor expressed in human embryonic stem cells. SALL4 stains all germ cell tumor components and appears to be the most sensitive marker for yolk sac tumor.

Microscopic and Immunohistochemical Features

(Left) Choriocarcinoma (CC) shows prominent hemorrhage with intimate admixture of mononucleated cytotrophoblasts and multinucleated syncytiotrophoblasts. Presence of syncytiotrophoblasts with other germ cell components may be overdiagnosed as CC. *(Right)* Choriocarcinoma shows strong cytoplasmic staining of mononucleated and multinucleated trophoblasts by β-HCG. Syncytiotrophoblasts are positive for cytokeratin and glypican-3.

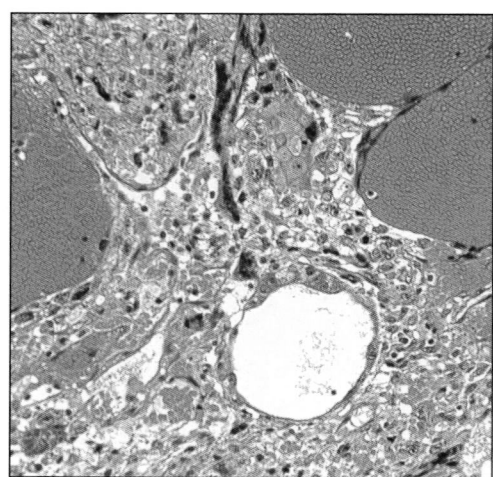
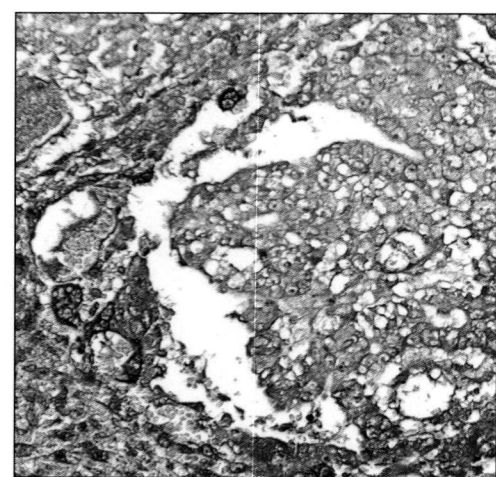

(Left) This image shows one of the most frequent combinations of mixed germ cell tumor, i.e., embryonal carcinoma ➡ and yolk sac tumor ➤. Yolk sac tumor can be quite inconspicuous on H&E sections and is frequently underdiagnosed due to subtle histology of its variant pattern. *(Right)* This photomicrograph shows Oct3/4 immunostaining of mixed germ cell tumor with embryonal carcinoma (EC) and yolk sac tumor (YST) components. Oct3/4 selectively stains EC ➡ but not YST ➤.

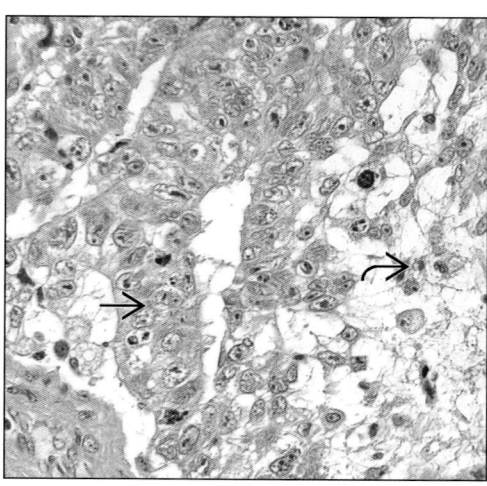
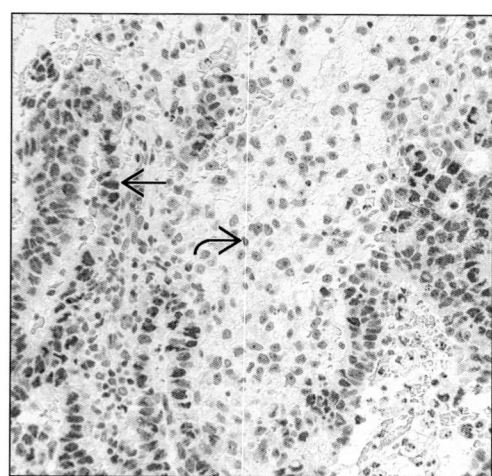

(Left) This image shows glypican-3 immunostaining in a mixed germ cell tumor with embryonal carcinoma (EC) and yolk sac tumor (YST) components. Glypican selectively stains YST, but the EC component is negative. *(Right)* This image shows embryonal carcinoma and yolk sac tumor stained by PAN-CK(AE1/AE3). The differential staining in intensity is a helpful feature to identify the relative composition of EC and YST as the staining in YST ➡ is much stronger than in the EC component ➤.

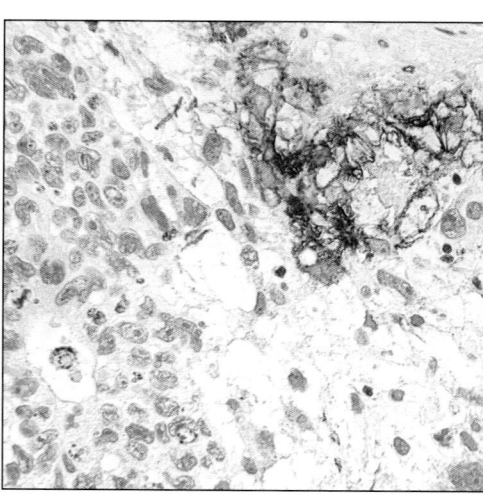
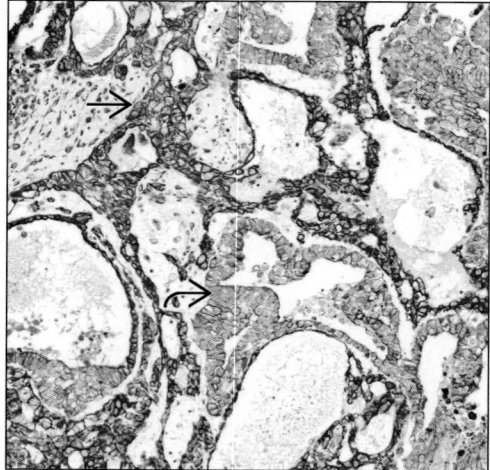

Penis and Scrotum

CLASSIFICATION OF PENIS TUMORS & TUMOR-LIKE LESIONS

NONNEOPLASTIC LESIONS

Tumor-like/Inflammatory Lesions
- HPV-associated lesions
- Lichen sclerosus et atrophicus
- Lipogranuloma
- Scrotal calcinosis
- Inflammatory pseudotumor
- Lentiginous melanosis
- Papillomatosis of glans corona
- Penile cyst
- Pseudoepitheliomatous keratotic and micaceous balanitis
- Verruciform xanthoma
- Syphilis
- Granuloma inguinale
- Lymphogranuloma venereum
- Molluscum contagiosum
- Chancroid
- Bacillary angiomatosis
- Peyronie disease
- Tancho nodules
- Fournier gangrene
- Wegener granulomatosis
- Squamous hyperplasia
- Other (sarcoidosis, Crohn disease, amyloidosis, sebaceous hyperplasia)

NEOPLASMS

Benign Tumors
- Papilloma
- Condyloma acuminatum
- Giant condyloma
- Nevi and melanocytic proliferations
- Hemangioma
- Glomus tumor
- Angiokeratoma
- Fibrous histiocytoma
- Neurofibroma
- Granular cell tumor
- Myointimoma
- Leiomyoma

Premalignant Lesions
- Bowen disease
- Bowenoid papulosis
- Penile intraepithelial neoplasia (PeIN)
- Erythroplasia of Queyrat

Malignant Epithelial Tumors
- Squamous cell carcinoma, usual type
- Squamous cell carcinoma variants
  - Pseudohyperplastic carcinoma
  - Warty carcinoma
  - Verrucous carcinoma
  - Basaloid carcinoma
  - Sarcomatoid carcinoma
  - Carcinoma cuniculatum
  - Adenosquamous (mucoepidermoid)
  - Papillary carcinoma NOS
  - Pseudoglandular (acantholytic, adenoid)
  - Mixed carcinoma (hybrid)
- Paget disease
- Basal cell carcinoma
- Clear cell carcinoma

Malignant Mesenchymal Tumors
- Kaposi sarcoma
- Leiomyosarcoma
- Angiosarcoma
- Rhabdomyosarcoma
- Proximal type epithelioid sarcoma

Other Malignant Tumors
- Melanoma
- Lymphoma

Metastatic Tumors
- Bladder
- Kidney
- Prostate
- Testis
- Colon

HPV-ASSOCIATED LESIONS

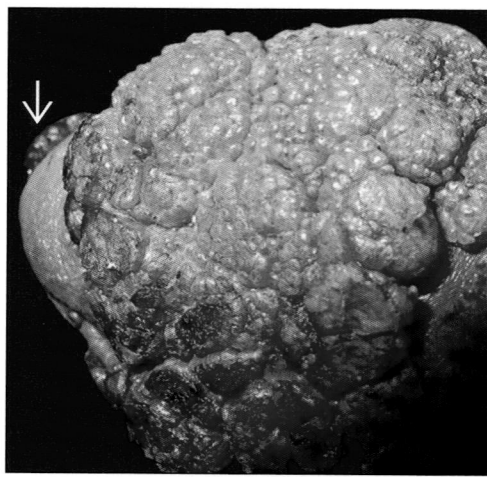

Exophytic tumoral multicentric ➡ growth with a "cobblestone" and cauliflower-like appearance replaces most of distal penis, which corresponds to a giant condyloma.

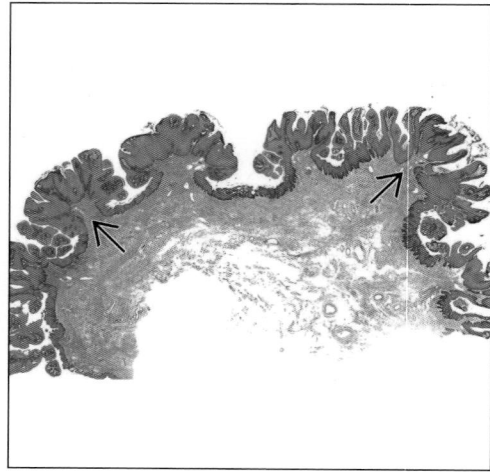

Condyloma acuminatum shows an exophytic papillomatous growth, regular and broad pushing tumor base, and easily recognizable fibrovascular cores ⇨.

TERMINOLOGY

Abbreviations
- Human papillomavirus (HPV)

Synonyms
- Genital wart, benign or typical condyloma (condyloma acuminatum)
- Buschke-Löwenstein tumor (giant condyloma)

Definitions
- Exophytic and verruciform nonmalignant epithelial lesions

ETIOLOGY/PATHOGENESIS

Infectious Agents
- Evidence of HPV infection found in most cases
- Low-risk serotypes (6, 11) predominate
- Incidence of HPV-6 is higher than HPV-11
- Other serotypes identified include 16, 18, 30-32, 42-44, and 51-55

CLINICAL ISSUES

Epidemiology
- Incidence
  - Condyloma acuminatum
    - Very common in sexually active young males
  - Giant condyloma
    - Very unusual
- Age
  - Condyloma acuminatum
    - Prevalence is higher in 2nd to 3rd decades of life
  - Giant condyloma
    - Patients tend to be older than those with condyloma acuminatum

Site
- Predilection for anogenital area
- Condyloma acuminatum
  - Glans is most frequently affected site, followed by foreskin, meatus urethralis, and penile shaft
- Giant condyloma
  - Tend to affect foreskin and coronal sulcus

Presentation
- Clinically may be confused with molluscum contagiosum, Fordyce spots, or condyloma latum
- Diagnosis is straightforward on histological grounds

Treatment
- For small tumors: Cryosurgery, electrofulguration, laser ablation, and topical treatments
- For medium-sized and large tumors: Surgical excision
- Giant condyloma: Wide local excision

Prognosis
- Malignant transformation is rare in condyloma acuminatum
- Giant condyloma has tendency to locally recur
- Giant condyloma often harbors carcinomatous foci
- Increased risk for anogenital cancers

MACROSCOPIC FEATURES

General Features
- Papillary cauliflower-like exophytic tumor
- Size ranges from few mm to several cm
- Average size of giant condylomata is 5-10 cm

MICROSCOPIC PATHOLOGY

Histologic Features
- Arborescent papillae with prominent fibrovascular cores
- Variable parakeratosis and orthokeratosis

HPV-ASSOCIATED LESIONS

Key Facts

Terminology
- Synonyms include condyloma acuminatum and giant condyloma
- Exophytic and verruciform nonmalignant epithelial tumors
- Clear predilection for anogenital area
- Condyloma acuminatum is relatively common and giant condyloma is very unusual

Etiology/Pathogenesis
- Evidence of HPV infection found in most cases
- Low-risk HPV serotypes (6, 11) predominates

Macroscopic Features
- Papillary cauliflower-like exophytic tumor
- Size range: Few mm to several cm

Microscopic Pathology
- Arborescent papillae with prominent fibrovascular cores
- Papillomatosis, acanthosis, hyper- and parakeratosis in variable degrees
- Broad and sharply defined tumoral base
- Conspicuous koilocytosis
- Morphological features in giant condyloma are more prominent
- Giant condyloma presents endophytic pattern of growth

Top Differential Diagnoses
- Warty, papillary, and verrucous carcinomas
- Condyloma with malignization
- Papillomatosis of glans corona

- Conspicuous surface koilocytosis
- Typical koilocytes exhibit perinuclear vacuolization, wrinkled and hyperchromatic nuclei with frequent binucleation
- Sharply defined base that is broad and pushing
- Morphological features in giant condyloma are more prominent
- Giant condyloma presents characteristic and evident endophytic pattern of growth
- Cutaneous fistulae can sometimes be observed with giant condyloma

DIFFERENTIAL DIAGNOSIS

Warty Carcinoma
- Affects older patients
- Higher cytologic grade and nuclear atypia
- Koilocytes frequently show pleomorphism
- More abundant mitoses
- Jagged and irregular tumor base
- Stromal invasion
- Presence of high-risk HPV
- Usually positive for p16 overexpression

Papillary Carcinoma, NOS
- Papillomatosis with acanthosis and hyperkeratosis
- Complex papillae with irregular fibrovascular cores
- Cytologic atypia ranges from mild to moderate
- No koilocytosis
- Jagged and irregular tumor base
- Lack of evidence of HPV infection in most of cases
- Negative for p16 overexpression

Verrucous Carcinoma
- Acanthosis with papillomatosis and hyperkeratosis
- Minimal cytologic atypia
- Absence of koilocytosis
- Inconspicuous or absent fibrovascular cores
- Broad and pushing tumor base
- Not associated with HPV infection
- Negative for p16 overexpression

Condyloma with Malignization
- Giant condyloma may harbor foci of SCC
- Malignant transformation is extremely rare in condyloma acuminatum
- Usual SCC is most commonly associated subtype
- In some cases, warty carcinoma represents malignant component
- Malignant foci tend to be located in deep portions
- Generous sampling of giant condylomata should be done in order to rule out minute foci of malignancy

Papillomatosis of Glans Corona
- Synonyms: Pearly penile papules/hirsutoid papilloma
- Very common (about 1/3 of normal males)
- Associated with marked sexual activity
- Located in dorsal aspect of glans corona
- Lesions are uniform and arranged in 2-3 rows
- Histologically small fibroepithelial papillomas

DIAGNOSTIC CHECKLIST

Pathologic Interpretation Pearls
- Giant condyloma should be extensively sampled as it may harbor foci of high-grade dysplasia or invasive carcinoma
- In penile pathology, verrucous carcinoma and giant condyloma are not synonymous

SELECTED REFERENCES

1. Giuliano AR et al: Epidemiology of human papillomavirus infection in men, cancers other than cervical and benign conditions. Vaccine. 26 Suppl 10:K17-28, 2008
2. Nordenvall C et al: Cancer risk among patients with condylomata acuminata. Int J Cancer. 119(4):888-93, 2006
3. el Mejjad A et al: [Giant condyloma acuminata -- Buschke Lowenstein tumor (report of 3 cases).] Prog Urol. 13(3):513-7, 2003
4. Buechner SA: Common skin disorders of the penis. BJU Int. 90(5):498-506, 2002

HPV-ASSOCIATED LESIONS

Microscopic Features

(Left) In condyloma acuminatum, tumor base ➡ is broad and sharply defined, fibrovascular cores are prominent ➡ and surface koilocytosis ➡ and parakeratosis ➡ are easily found. *(Right)* Condyloma acuminatum is characterized by papillomatosis and prominent fibrovascular cores ➡, epithelium is acanthotic and exhibits squamous maturation, koilocytes ➡ are easily found, and parakeratosis ➡ is common.

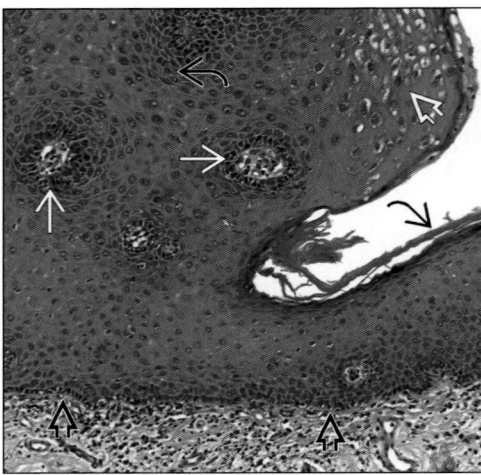
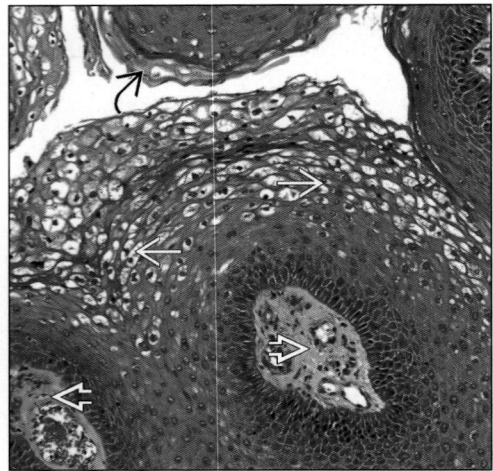

(Left) Papillomatosis with evident fibrovascular cores ➡, surface koilocytosis ➡, and absence of evident nuclear atypias are pathognomonic findings of condyloma acuminatum. *(Right)* Giant condyloma is characterized by marked acanthosis and an endophytic pattern of growth with bulbous extension of the base, prominent fibrovascular cores ➡, and clear areas ➡, which correspond to koilocytosis at higher power.

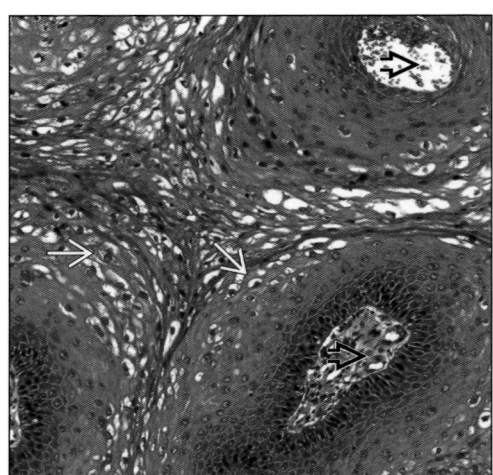
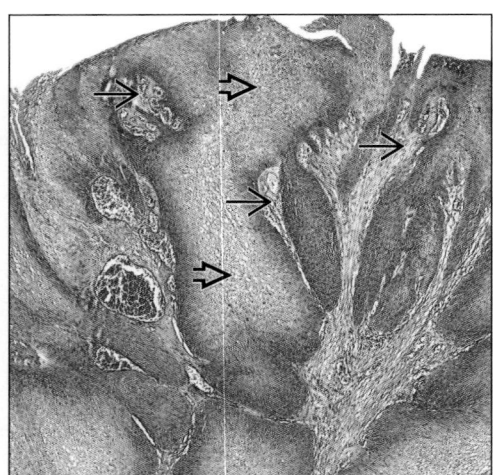

(Left) In both condyloma acuminatum and giant condyloma, koilocytes are easily found, subtle nuclear atypia may be present in cells of the basal layer ➡, especially in the latter, and a thin parakeratotic layer ➡ is commonly observed. *(Right)* Koilocytes are characterized by clear perinuclear halos ➡ and wrinkled and hyperchromatic nuclei, cytoplasm is eosinophilic, cellular borders are distinctive, and binucleation is common.

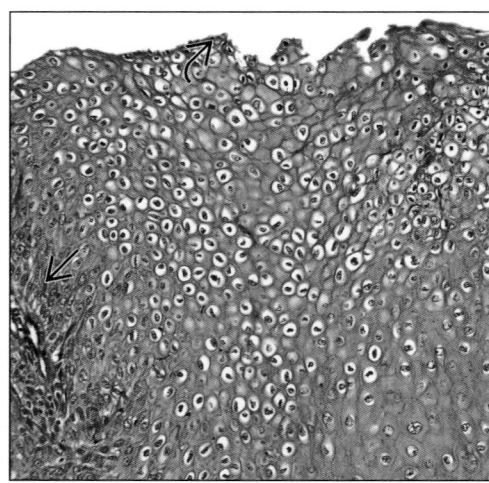
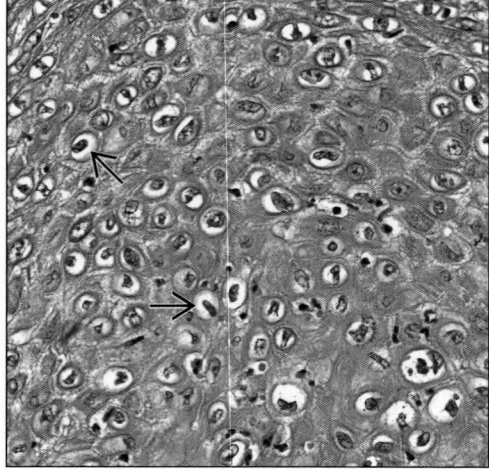

HPV-ASSOCIATED LESIONS

Microscopic Features and Differential Diagnosis

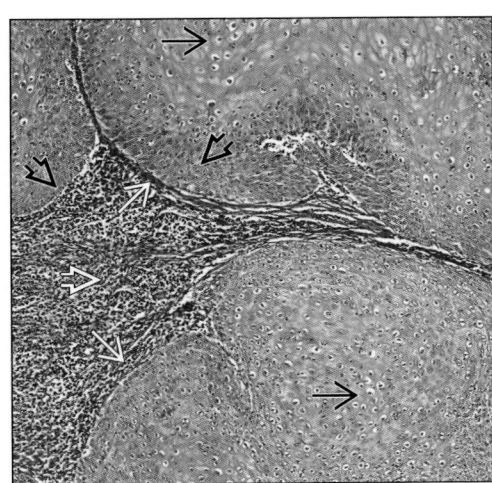

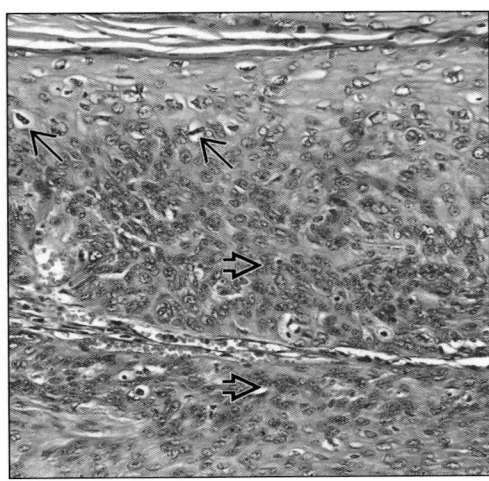

(Left) The front base of giant condyloma shows broad, pushing, smooth borders ➡, koilocytes ➡, which are easily found throughout the lesion, basal cells ⇨ with slight nuclear atypia, and a prominent stromal reaction ➡. *(Right)* In giant condyloma, koilocytes ➡ are readily found, nuclear atypia is restricted to the basal region only ⇨, and basal cells are more pleomorphic when compared to condyloma acuminatum, although frankly malignant changes are absent.

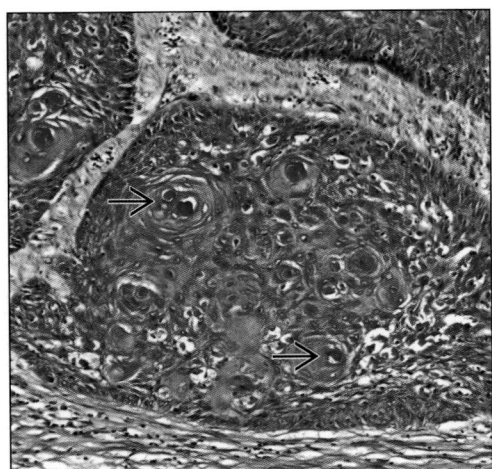

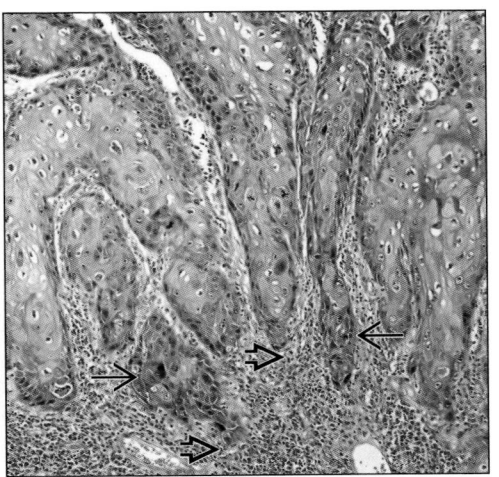

(Left) Giant condyloma with foci of well-differentiated usual SCC in which neoplastic cells of tumor nests show mild but obvious nuclear atypia and clear-cut squamous differentiation ➡. *(Right)* Warty carcinoma shows papillomatosis, acanthosis, conspicuous koilocytosis, moderate to marked nuclear atypia ➡ throughout the tumor, prominent fibrovascular cores, and an irregular and jagged base ⇨.

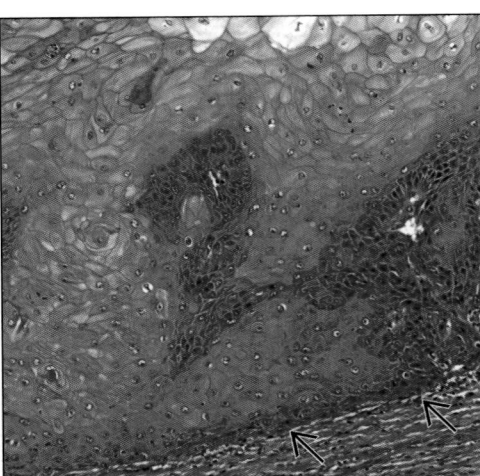

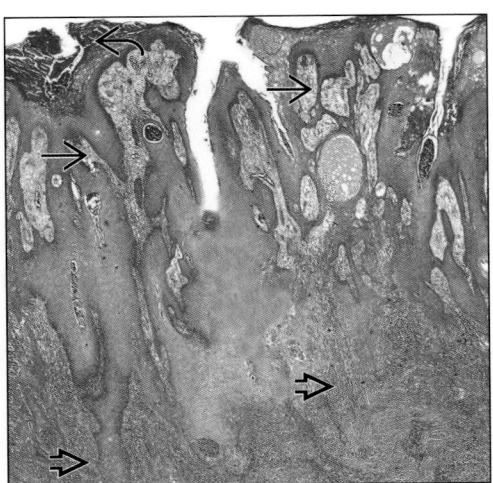

(Left) In verrucous carcinoma, papillomatosis and acanthosis are prominent, koilocytes are absent, neoplastic cells exhibit subtle but distinct nuclear atypia, tumor base ➡ is broad and pushing, and fibrovascular cores are inconspicuous or absent. *(Right)* Papillary carcinoma is characterized by complex papillae with blunt or sharp tips, irregular fibrovascular cores ➡, and parakeratosis ➡. Note the jagged tumor base ⇨ and no koilocytosis.

LICHEN SCLEROSUS ET ATROPHICUS

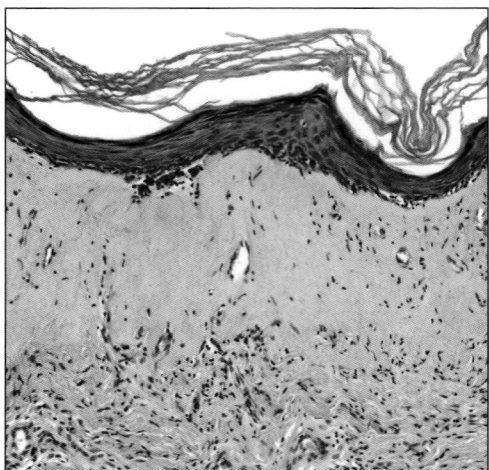

Note the atrophic epidermis associated with vacuolar alteration of the basal layer and a thick hyalinized connective tissue band in the papillary dermis in this case of lichen sclerosus.

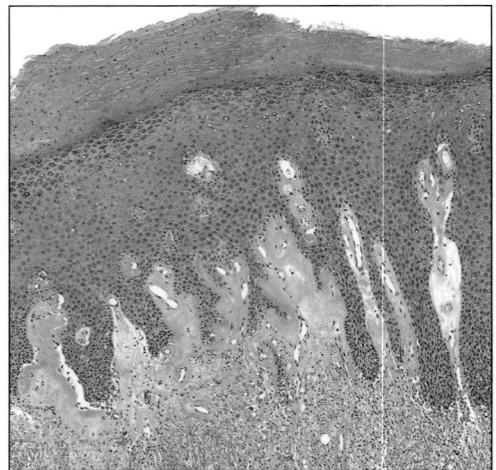

Lichen sclerosus with hyperplastic epithelium is seen. This is a frequent finding in longstanding lesions. In other areas, the epidermis may be atrophic.

TERMINOLOGY

Synonyms
- Lichen sclerosus (LS), balanitis xerotica obliterans

Definitions
- Interface vacuolar/lichenoid dermatitis with thickened papillary dermis/lamina propria showing band-like hyalinization (sclerosis)

ETIOLOGY/PATHOGENESIS

Pathogenesis
- Unknown

CLINICAL ISSUES

Presentation
- Early lesions appear as pink or purple macules that become papules
- Purpura and telangiectases are common
- Well-established lesions appear as white-gray, irregular geographic, and atrophic areas
- Erosion, ulceration may be present
- Elevated hyperkeratotic foci may also be seen
- Advanced cases may result in acquired phimosis or paraphimosis
- Lesions usually affect inner aspect of foreskin, glans, and perimeatal region
- Lesions tend to be broad and multifocal

Treatment
- Medical
- Circumcision (if only/predominantly affecting foreskin)

Prognosis
- Chronic condition

- Associated with squamous cell carcinoma (SCC) in minority of cases (approximately 9% of affected patients will develop penile SCC)

MACROSCOPIC FEATURES

Sections to Be Submitted
- When dealing with large specimen (such as circumcision), it is important to extensively sample thick, hyperkeratotic areas

MICROSCOPIC PATHOLOGY

Histologic Features
- Atrophic epithelium (early lesions)
  - Frequently intermixed with hyperplastic areas (chronic lesions)
- Vacuolar alteration of basal layer
- Thickened lamina propria/dermis with classic band-like hyalinization/sclerosis
- Telangiectasias within band of sclerosis
- Scattered melanophages in superficial dermis/lamina propria
- Band-like lymphoid infiltrate underneath band of sclerosis (well-established lesions)
  - Early lesions show more superficial lymphoid infiltrate underneath epithelium without well-formed sclerotic band
- Late lesions are sclerotic with minimal inflammation
- Sometimes prominent edema of papillary dermis/ lamina propria
- Dermal-epidermal clefting or blisters may be seen secondary to marked basal cell vacuolar alteration
- Minority of cases of chronic LS may be associated with atypical foci in epithelium (differentiated, non-HPV-related, PeIN)
- Minority of cases of LS will evolve to SCC
  - Most common types of SCC associated with LS are well-differentiated keratinizing SCC (usually HPV

LICHEN SCLEROSUS ET ATROPHICUS

Key Facts

Terminology
- Synonyms
  - Lichen sclerosus (LS); balanitis xerotica obliterans

Clinical Issues
- White atrophic patches affecting glans, coronal sulcus, &/or foreskin

Microscopic Pathology
- Hallmark of lesion is hyalinized/sclerotic band underneath epithelium
- Interface vacuolar alteration of basal layer
- Atrophic epithelium (often associated with at least focal hyperplastic areas)
- Variable degree of lymphoid infiltrate underneath sclerotic band

---

unrelated), such as pseudohyperplastic SCC and verrucous carcinoma

Predominant Pattern/Injury Type
- Interface dermatitis with sclerosis

Predominant Cell/Compartment Type
- Epithelium and superficial dermis/lamina propria

DIFFERENTIAL DIAGNOSIS

Lichen Planus
- Denser and more superficial band-like lymphoid infiltrate obscuring dermal-epidermal junction
- Absence of classic hyalinized band in superficial dermis/lamina propria
- Wedge-shaped hypergranulosis

DIAGNOSTIC CHECKLIST

Clinically Relevant Pathologic Features
- Hyperplastic areas as seen in longstanding lesions may be associated with differentiated PeIN

Pathologic Interpretation Pearls
- Hallmark of LS is hyalinized (sclerotic) band in lamina propria/papillary dermis
  - Early lesions do not show classical band-like area of sclerosis/hyalinization

- Thickened basement membrane and hyalinization around superficial blood vessels are a clue for diagnosis of early lichen sclerosus

SELECTED REFERENCES

1. Innocenzi D et al: Penile lichen sclerosus: Correlation between histopathologic features and risk of cancer. Acta Dermatovenerol Croat. 14(4):225-9, 2006
2. Cubilla AL et al: Pseudohyperplastic squamous cell carcinoma of the penis associated with lichen sclerosus. An extremely well-differentiated, nonverruciform neoplasm that preferentially affects the foreskin and is frequently misdiagnosed: a report of 10 cases of a distinctive clinicopathologic entity. Am J Surg Pathol. 28(7):895-900, 2004
3. Velazquez EF et al: Lichen sclerosus in 68 patients with squamous cell carcinoma of the penis: frequent atypias and correlation with special carcinoma variants suggests a precancerous role. Am J Surg Pathol. 27(11):1448-53, 2003
4. Micali G et al: Lichen sclerosus of the glans is significantly associated with penile carcinoma. Sex Transm Infect. 77(3):226, 2001
5. Nasca MR et al: Penile cancer among patients with genital lichen sclerosus. J Am Acad Dermatol. 41(6):911-4, 1999

IMAGE GALLERY

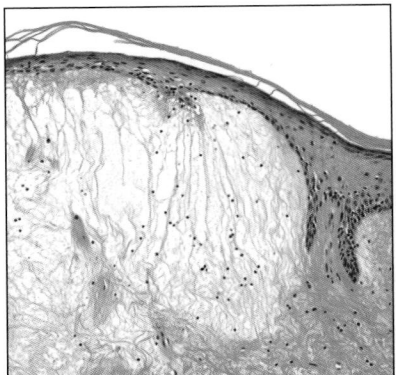 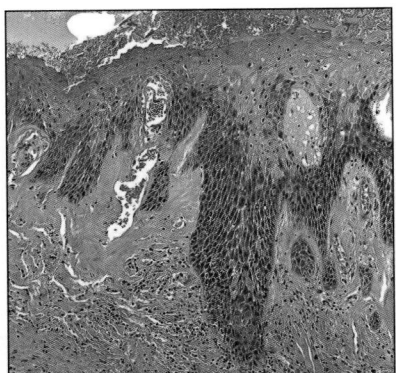 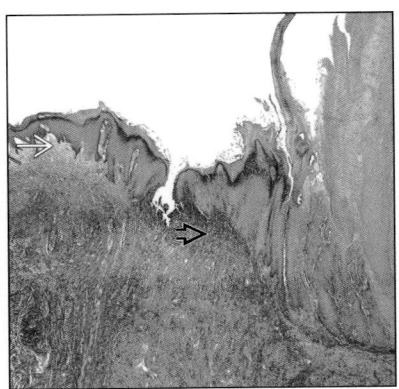

(Left) Some cases of lichen sclerosus show prominent papillary dermal edema. Note also the atrophic epidermis. *(Center)* Lichen sclerosus associated with hyperplastic squamous epithelium with atypia (differentiated, non-HPV-related, PeIN, and lichen sclerosus) is shown. Such changes are usually seen adjacent to moderately to well-differentiated invasive squamous cell carcinomas. *(Right)* Low-power view shows lichen sclerosus ➡ with hyperplastic and mild atypical changes (differentiated, non-HPV-related, PeIN) adjacent to a verrucous carcinoma ➡.

SQUAMOUS HYPERPLASIA

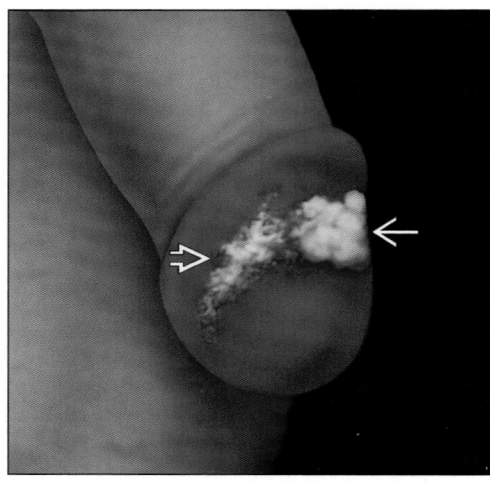

Squamous hyperplasia typically presents as whitish pearly areas ⇒ with irregular borders merging with an adjacent in situ or invasive component ➡.

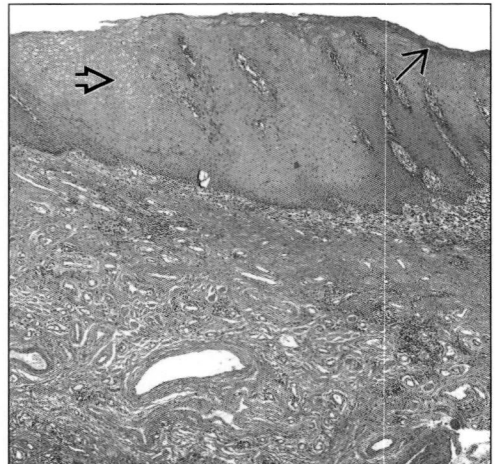

Squamous hyperplasia is characterized by acanthosis ⇒, retained epithelial maturation, absence of cytologic atypia, hyperkeratosis ⇒, and a flat surface.

TERMINOLOGY

Abbreviations
- Squamous hyperplasia (SH), squamous cell carcinoma (SCC), penile intraepithelial neoplasia (PeIN)

Definitions
- Thickening of mucosal squamous epithelium without cytologic atypia

ETIOLOGY/PATHOGENESIS

Pathogenesis
- Unknown
- Reactive condition rather than specific entity
- Most common epithelial change associated with penile cancer
- Almost all keratinizing SCC have associated SH
- May be associated with reactive inflammatory conditions

CLINICAL ISSUES

Site
- SH may affect any penile mucosal compartment

Presentation
- Usually found in continuity or slightly distant from in situ or invasive SCC
- Distinction between SH and normal mucosa may be subtle
- Inapparent lesions may be better visualized with acetic acid (peniscopy)
- Clinically, it may be difficult to distinguish from PeIN
- Micaceous balanitis and penile horn are clinically florid forms of SH with prominent hyperkeratosis

Treatment
- Benign epithelial change and usually no treatment is required

Prognosis
- May be precursor lesion of HPV-unrelated variants of SCC, but more studies are required to confirm this hypothesis

MACROSCOPIC FEATURES

General Features
- Whitish areas with irregular borders
- Slightly raised areas with pearly appearance

MICROSCOPIC PATHOLOGY

Histologic Features
- Acanthosis with orthokeratotic hyperkeratosis
- Normal epithelial maturation
- Chronic inflammation may be present
- Absence of cytologic atypia
- Absent koilocytosis
- Minimal to absent parakeratosis
- Absent intraepithelial keratin whorls (pearls)
- Associated with lichen sclerosus in some cases
- Frequently associated with differentiated PeIN
- Usually found in association with usual, papillary, and verrucous SCC (HPV-unrelated variants of SCC)
- Rarely present adjacent to condylomatous (warty) and basaloid SCC
- Merging of SH with PeIN &/or invasive SCC is common finding

Histological Subtypes
- Flat
  - Most common subtype
  - Nonatypical acanthosis
  - Hyperkeratosis with orthokeratosis

SQUAMOUS HYPERPLASIA

Key Facts

Terminology

- Thickening of mucosal squamous epithelium without atypia
- Most common epithelial alteration associated with penile cancer
- Frequently associated with differentiated PeIN
- Found in association with usual, papillary, and verrucous SCC (HPV-unrelated variants of SCC)

Macroscopic Features

- Whitish areas with irregular borders

Microscopic Pathology

- Acanthosis with hyperkeratosis
- Normal maturation with no atypias
- Parakeratosis is uncommon
- Koilocytes are absent

- Merging of SH with PeIN &/or invasive SCC is common finding
- Flat squamous hyperplasia is most common pattern
- Other subtypes include papillary, pseudoepitheliomatous, and verrucous
- Mixed forms represent about 1/3 of cases

Top Differential Diagnoses

- Differentiated PeIN
- Warty PeIN
- Basaloid PeIN
- Warty/basaloid PeIN
- Pseudohyperplastic SCC
- Verruciform xanthoma
- Warty, papillary, and verrucous carcinomas

---

  o Linear interface between basal layer and stroma
- Papillary
  o Represents minority of cases
  o Serrated appearance on low-power view
  o Jagged interface with underlying stroma
  o Nonatypical acanthosis with short hyperkeratotic papillae
- Pseudoepitheliomatous
  o Unusual pattern of SH
  o Acanthosis
  o Downward elongated proliferation of rete ridges that appear detached from epithelium
  o Regular epithelial nests with peripheral palisading
  o Stromal reaction is not prominent
  o Typically associated with papillary SH
- Verrucous
  o Present adjacent to verrucous carcinoma
  o Marked acanthosis with no atypia
  o Hyperkeratosis with hypergranulosis
  o Slight papillomatosis
- Mixed
  o 2nd most common type
  o Presence of mixed areas of flat and papillary SH

DIFFERENTIAL DIAGNOSIS

Differentiated PeIN

- Acanthosis, parakeratosis
- Aberrant keratinization with cytologic atypia
- Retained squamous maturation

Warty/Basaloid PeIN

- Acanthosis with parakeratosis
- Cytologic atypia with loss of squamous maturation
- Monotonous population of small cells with scant cytoplasm throughout epithelium in basaloid variant
- Pleomorphic cells with conspicuous koilocytosis and spiky surface in warty variant
- Detection of HPV in high proportion of cases
- Immunohistochemical overexpression of p16

Pseudohyperplastic SCC

- SCC simulating pseudoepitheliomatous hyperplasia
- Preferential foreskin location
- Minimal cytologic atypia
- Irregular epithelial nests
- Extension into lamina propria and superficial tissues
- Prominent stromal reaction
- Clinically forms mass lesion

Verruciform Xanthoma

- Exophytic lesion with acanthosis and hyperkeratosis
- "Xanthoma" cells (foamy histocytes) in lamina propria

Verruciform SCC

- Includes warty, papillary, and verrucous carcinomas
- Evidence of destructive stromal invasion
- Diagnosis may be difficult in small biopsies

DIAGNOSTIC CHECKLIST

Pathologic Interpretation Pearls

- Thickened squamous epithelium with hyperkeratosis and without cytologic atypia

SELECTED REFERENCES

1. Velazquez EF et al: Epithelial abnormalities and precancerous lesions of anterior urethra in patients with penile carcinoma: a report of 89 cases. Mod Pathol. 18(7):917-23, 2005
2. Cubilla AL et al: Epithelial lesions associated with invasive penile squamous cell carcinoma: a pathologic study of 288 cases. Int J Surg Pathol. 12(4):351-64, 2004
3. Velazquez EF et al: Lichen sclerosus in 68 patients with squamous cell carcinoma of the penis: frequent atypias and correlation with special carcinoma variants suggests a precancerous role. Am J Surg Pathol. 27(11):1448-53, 2003
4. Cubilla AL et al: Morphological features of epithelial abnormalities and precancerous lesions of the penis. Scand J Urol Nephrol Suppl. (205):215-9, 2000

SQUAMOUS HYPERPLASIA

Microscopic Features

(Left) Squamous hyperplasia, noted as a thickening of the squamous mucosa ➡, is frequently found in association with either in situ ➡ or invasive ➡ penile squamous cell carcinomas and can extend into the distal urethra ➡. **(Right)** In flat squamous hyperplasia, the interface between the epithelium and lamina propria is regular and straight ➡, surface is flat ➡, acanthosis is prominent but no cytologic atypia is seen, and hyperkeratosis ➡ is commonly found.

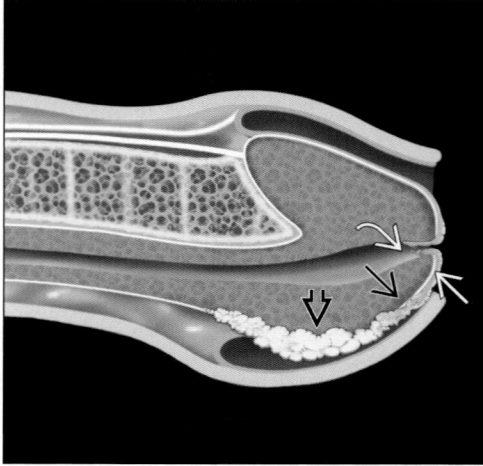
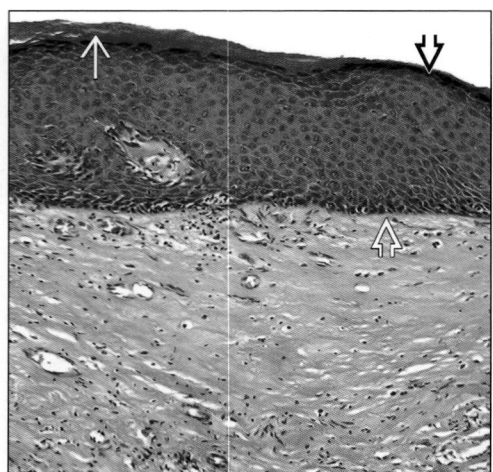

(Left) SH depicts hyperkeratosis ➡, usually associated with hypergranulosis ➡, rete ridges ➡ slightly elongated with regular borders, no evidence of stromal invasion, and a mild to moderate chronic inflammatory infiltrate ➡. **(Right)** Papillary squamous hyperplasia is shown with short papillae ➡ and downward ("pseudoepitheliomatous") proliferation of rete ridges ➡, which may be prominent enough to raise the differential diagnosis of SCC.

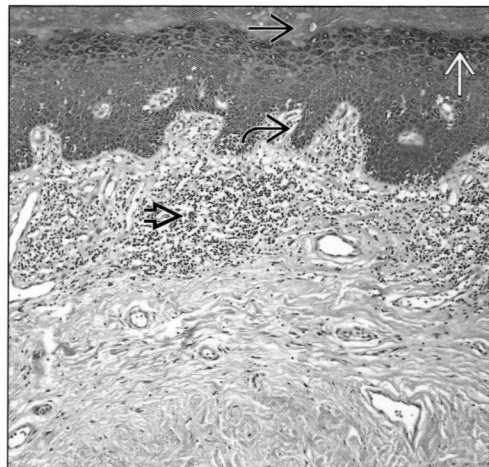
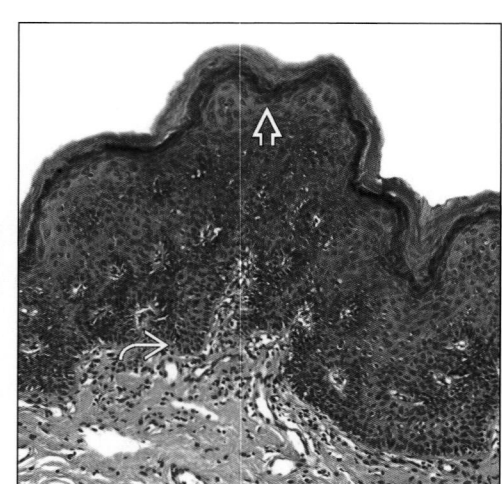

(Left) SH with prominent orthokeratotic hyperkeratosis ➡ and hypergranulosis ➡, retained epithelial maturation with no cytologic atypia, slightly elongated rete ridges ➡, and changes of lichen sclerosus in the submucosa ➡ with a mild inflammatory infiltrate.
(Right) SH associated with lichen sclerosus with evident acanthosis and hyperkeratosis in the epithelium and dense subepithelial sclerosis ➡ with a band-like chronic inflammatory infiltrate ➡.

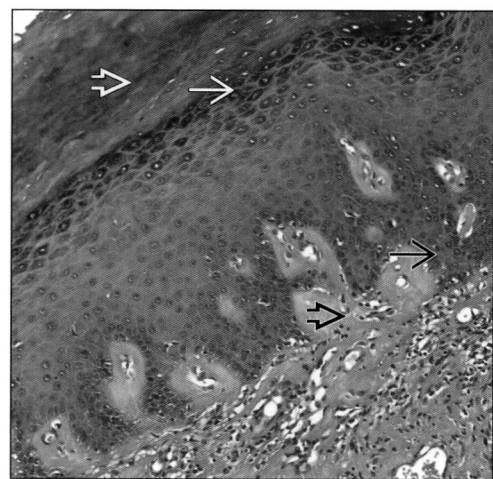
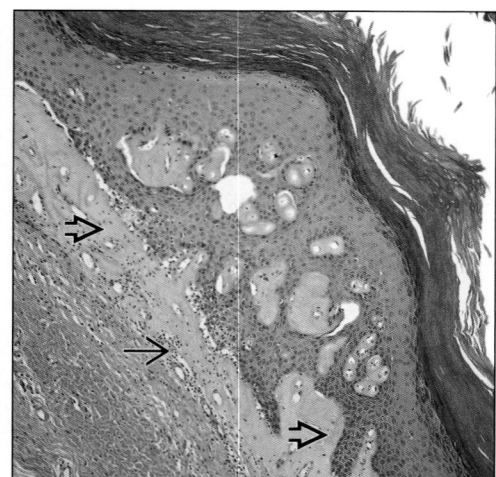

SQUAMOUS HYPERPLASIA

Differential Diagnosis

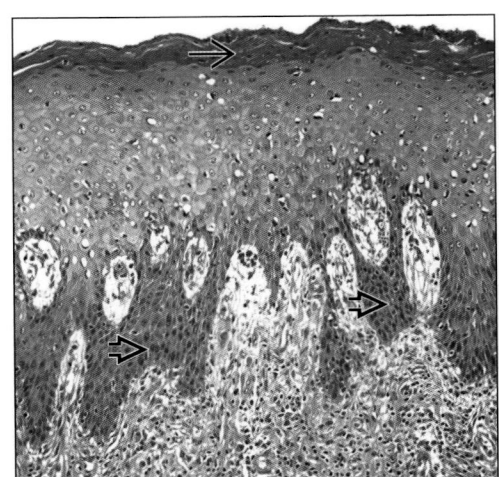
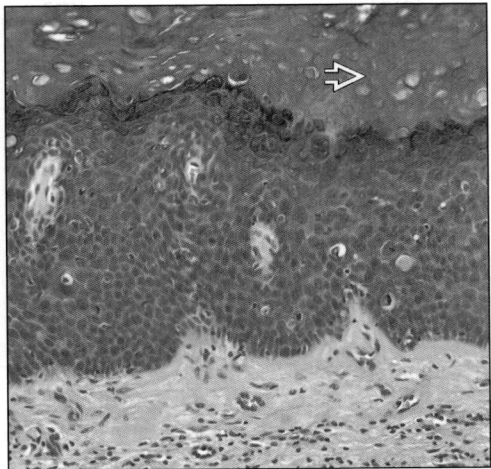

(Left) In differentiated PeIN, cytologic atypia is observed throughout the entire epithelium, although it is more prominent in the basal layer ➡. Parakeratosis ➡ is a common finding. (Right) In basaloid PeIN, the entire epithelium is replaced by a monotonous population of small to intermediate-sized cells with scant cytoplasm and indistinct cellular borders. Note also a prominent hyperkeratosis ➡.

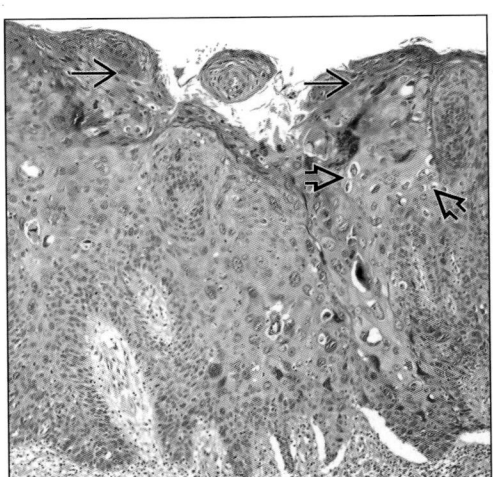
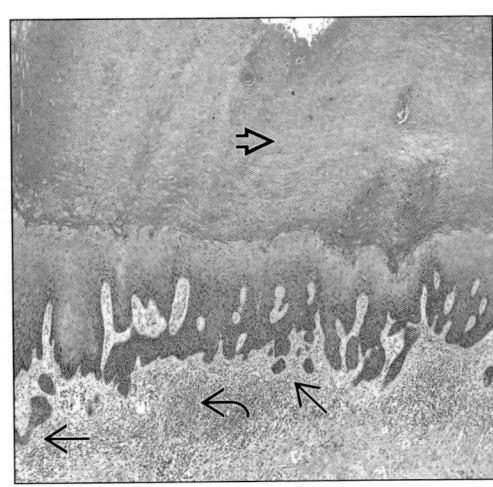

(Left) In warty PeIN, pleomorphic cells are seen throughout the entire epithelium, koilocytes ➡ are easily identified, surface is spiky, and parakeratosis ➡ is common. (Right) Pseudohyperplastic carcinoma shows acanthosis, slight cytological atypia, prominent hyperkeratosis ➡, with irregular neoplastic nests ➡ at tumor base extending into the lamina propria and a moderate stromal reaction ➡.

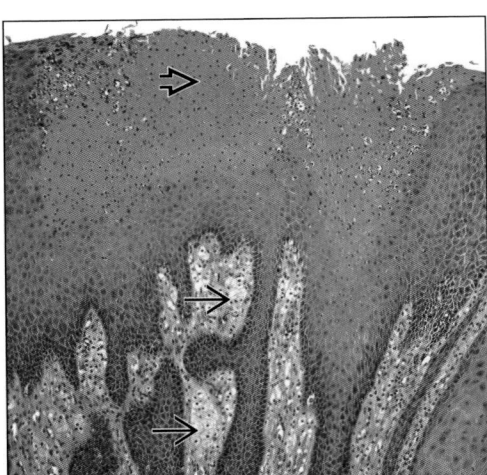
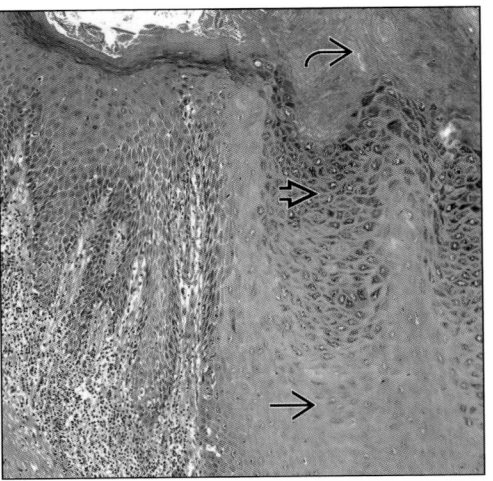

(Left) Verruciform xanthoma is characterized by prominent acanthosis, hyperkeratosis ➡, papillomatosis, absence of cytologic atypia, and foamy cells ➡ present in lamina propria between rete ridges. (Right) Some verruciform lesions showing acanthosis ➡, hypergranulosis ➡, and hyperkeratosis ➡ are sometimes difficult to classify. The differential diagnosis between verrucous SH and verrucous carcinoma is not always possible, especially in superficial biopsies.

LIPOGRANULOMA

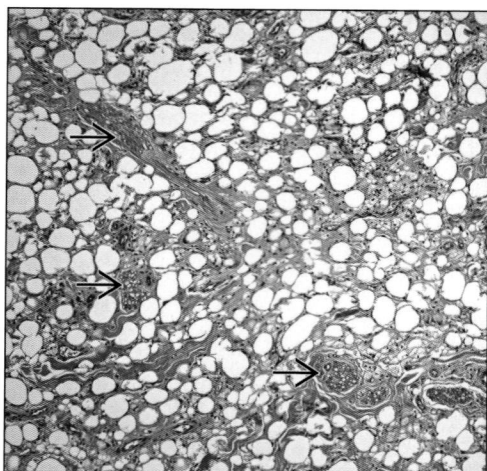

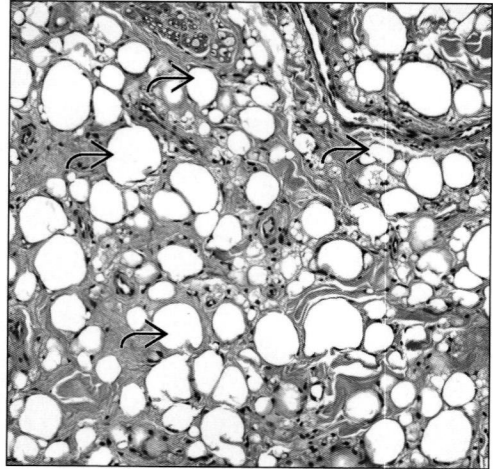

Sclerosing lipogranuloma of the scrotum is seen. Numerous lipid vacuoles of different sizes are apparent in the dermis and dartos. Note the dartos smooth muscle bundles ➡ in the background.

Higher power view of a case of sclerosing lipogranuloma shows numerous vacuoles ➡ of different size embedded in a sclerotic stroma.

TERMINOLOGY

Synonyms
- Paraffinoma

Definitions
- Foreign body histiocytic/granulomatous and sclerotic reaction to oil-based substances

ETIOLOGY/PATHOGENESIS

Etiology
- Most cases are secondary to injection of oil-based substances, such as paraffin, silicone, or oil
- Less frequently secondary to topical application of oil-based substances
- Rarely, they may also be related to cold weather or trauma

Pathogenesis
- T-cell-mediated immune reaction appears to be important in its pathogenesis

CLINICAL ISSUES

Epidemiology
- Age
  - Usually patients younger than 40 years old

Site
- May affect penis &/or scrotum

Presentation
- Indurated and sometimes tender plaque or mass that varies in size from a few cm to massive replacement of genital area
- Biopsy is necessary to exclude neoplasm, especially if there is no history of injection of exogenous material

MACROSCOPIC FEATURES

General Features
- Specimen usually consists of firm, yellow to gray-white pieces of tissue with solid or multicystic appearance

MICROSCOPIC PATHOLOGY

Histologic Features
- Numerous lipid vacuoles of variable size embedded in sclerotic stroma
- Infiltrate of foamy histiocytes admixed with variable number of multinucleate giant cells
- Lymphoid cells and eosinophils are usually present
- Inflammatory infiltrate may be nodular or interspersed in sclerotic stroma
- Inflammatory infiltrate varies from mild to marked
- If necessary, sections from frozen tissue showing positive staining with oil red O may be helpful

Predominant Pattern/Injury Type
- Sclerotic and vacuolar

Predominant Cell/Compartment Type
- Hematopoietic, histiocytic

ANCILLARY TESTS

Immunohistochemistry
- Immunohistochemical studies have shown expression of lysozyme, α-1-antitrypsin, α-1-antichymotrypsin, and CD68 by multinucleated giant cells and epithelioid histiocytes
- Most of the lymphocytes infiltrating lesions are CD3(+) T cells associated with some S100(+) dendritic cells

LIPOGRANULOMA

Key Facts

Terminology
- Synonym: Paraffinoma

Etiology/Pathogenesis
- Most frequently secondary to injection of oil-based substances

Microscopic Pathology
- Numerous lipid vacuoles of variable size embedded in sclerotic stroma

- Mixed cell inflammatory infiltrate, including histiocytes, multinucleate giant cells, lymphoid cells, and eosinophils

Ancillary Tests
- Immunohistochemical studies have shown expression of CD68 by multinucleate giant cells and epithelioid histiocytes
- If necessary, sections from frozen tissue showing positive staining with oil red O may be helpful

DIFFERENTIAL DIAGNOSIS

Liposarcoma
- Lobulated, bulky neoplasm in paratesticular soft tissue
- Well-differentiated or sclerosing type
- Presence of bizarre atypical cells
- If present, identification of lipoblasts may be helpful
- Absence of foreign body giant cell reaction and foamy histiocytes

Metastatic Carcinoma with Signet Ring or Clear Cell Changes
- Immunohistochemistry for keratin is positive in carcinoma and negative in lipogranuloma
- Atypical nuclei indented by intracytoplasmic mucin

Adenomatoid Tumor
- Benign mesothelial tumor
- Characterized by cystic and slit-like spaces lined by flattened or cuboidal cells
- Immunohistochemistry shows positivity with keratin and calretinin

Lymphangioma
- Benign proliferation of dilated lymphatic vessels
- If necessary, vascular markers (CD31, FVIIIRAg) may help to clarify diagnosis

DIAGNOSTIC CHECKLIST

Clinically Relevant Pathologic Features
- Clinical correlation with injection of exogenous material is important to confirm diagnosis

Pathologic Interpretation Pearls
- Numerous vacuoles of different sizes in dermis/lamina propria and dartos
- At low power, they resemble adipose cells or lipoblasts
- Intimately associated at higher power; many are within histiocytes and multinucleated giant cells
- Sclerotic background with variable numbers of lymphoid cells and eosinophils
- Diagnosis usually not difficult, especially when there is good clinical history

SELECTED REFERENCES

1. Ohtsuki Y et al: Three cases of sclerosing lipogranuloma: an immunohistochemical study. Med Mol Morphol. 40(2):108-11, 2007
2. Watanabe K et al: Immunohistochemical profile of primary sclerosing lipogranuloma of the scrotum: report of five cases. Pathol Int. 45(11):854-9, 1995
3. Oertel YC et al: Sclerosing lipogranuloma of male genitalia. Review of 23 cases. Arch Pathol Lab Med. 101(6):321-6, 1977

IMAGE GALLERY

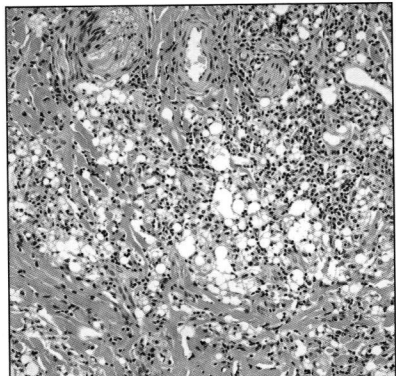 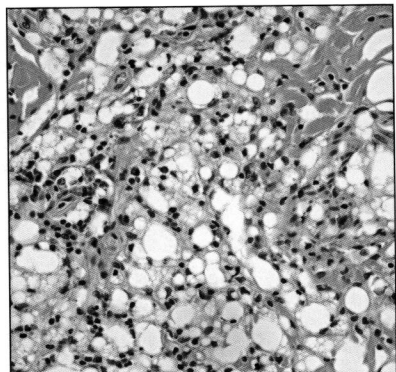 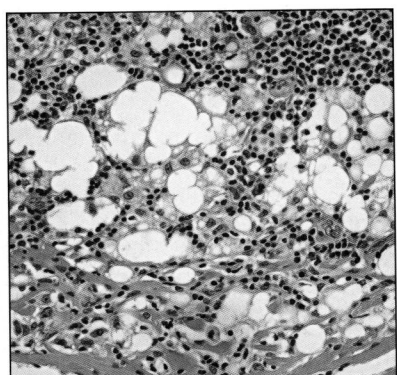

(Left) Sclerosing lipogranuloma of the penis is seen. Numerous vacuoles of different sizes are dispersed in a sclerotic stroma. The lymphocytic-rich inflammatory infiltrate is prominent in this case. *(Center)* In this case of sclerosing lipogranuloma, note the different sizes of the vacuoles and the mixed cell infiltrate with lymphoid cells and scattered eosinophils. *(Right)* High-power view shows that many of the vacuoles appear to be inside histiocytes. The inflammatory response is rich in histiocytes, including multinucleate giant cells.

SCROTAL CALCINOSIS

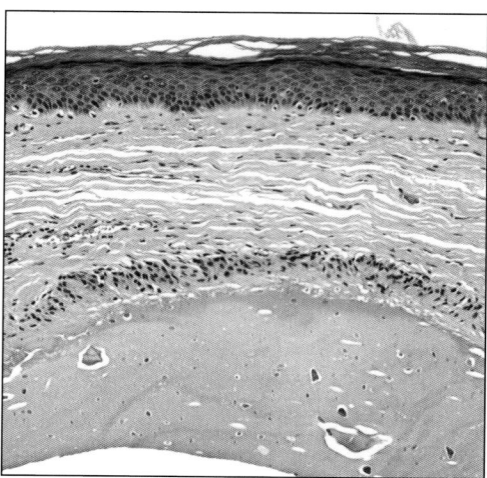

Underneath a normal epidermis there is a nodular basophilic homogeneous deposit surrounded by palisading histiocytic response.

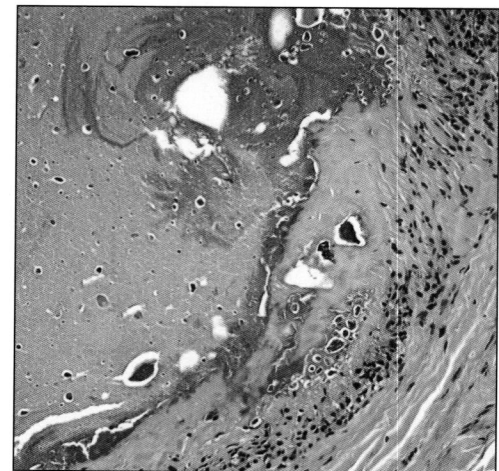

Within the dermis, there are purple deposits of calcified material surrounded by a granulomatous response.

TERMINOLOGY

Synonyms
- Idiopathic calcinosis of scrotum

Definitions
- Benign, uncommon condition characterized by presence of single or multiple calcified nodules in scrotal skin

ETIOLOGY/PATHOGENESIS

Etiology
- Originally considered idiopathic condition
- Now accepted that majority of cases develop from dystrophic calcification of cyst contents

CLINICAL ISSUES

Epidemiology
- Incidence
  ○ Uncommon
- Age
  ○ Children and young adults

Site
- Scrotal skin

Presentation
- Single or multiple hard, marble-like nodules affecting scrotal skin
- Nodules vary in size from a few millimeters to a few centimeters
- Usually start to appear in childhood or early adult life
- Over time, nodules increase in number and size
- Nodules may break down and discharge a chalky material
- Rarely, lesions may be polypoid
- Usually asymptomatic

Treatment
- Symptomatic single or grouped nodules can be excised surgically

Prognosis
- Benign condition
- Slow progression throughout life
- Lesions remain discrete and do not become confluent

IMAGE FINDINGS

Radiographic Findings
- Radiologic studies show calcified nodules

MICROSCOPIC PATHOLOGY

Histologic Features
- Granular and globular deposition of basophilic calcified material
- Histiocytic/giant cell granulomatous inflammatory response may be associated with deposits
- Process is located within dermis and may extend to dartos
- Early lesions start out as cysts, but they lose their cyst walls as they age and calcify
- Histologic remnants of preexisting epidermoid cyst or, even more rarely, partially cystic adnexal tumor (e.g., syringoma) may be identified
- Calcified material is positive with Von Kossa stain

Predominant Pattern/Injury Type
- Calcification

Predominant Cell/Compartment Type
- Dermis

SCROTAL CALCINOSIS

Key Facts

Etiology/Pathogenesis
- Formerly considered an idiopathic process
- Most cases represent ruptured and calcified cysts with eventual destruction of cyst wall

Clinical Issues
- Hard calcified nodules appear on skin of scrotum during childhood or early adult life

Microscopic Pathology
- Basophilic homogeneous deposits within dermis and upper part of dartos
- Usually surrounded by palisading histiocytes
- Remnants of cystic lesion may be identified

Ancillary Tests
- Calcified material is positive with von Kossa stain

DIFFERENTIAL DIAGNOSIS

Nodular Amyloidosis
- Eosinophilic (noncalcified) nodular deposits within dermis
- Usually associated with plasma cell-rich infiltrate
- Foreign body giant cell reaction may be present
- Amyloid deposits are positive for crystal violet and Congo red stains
  - Green birefringence under polarized light when stained with Congo red
- von Kossa negative

DIAGNOSTIC CHECKLIST

Clinically Relevant Pathologic Features
- Lesions slowly progress throughout life
  - They slowly increase in number and size
- Nodules are mobile and do not attach to underlying structures

Pathologic Interpretation Pearls
- Globular and granular purple deposits within dermis surrounded by giant cell granulomatous reaction
- Sometimes remnants of cystic lesion can be identified
- Very distinctive appearance with almost no histologic differential diagnosis

SELECTED REFERENCES

1. Gi N et al: Idiopathic scrotal calcinosis - a pedunculated rare variant. J Plast Reconstr Aesthet Surg. 61(4):466-7, 2008
2. Parlakgumus A et al: Scrotal calcinosis due to resorption of cyst walls: a case report. J Med Case Reports. 2(1):375, 2008
3. Shah V et al: Scrotal calcinosis results from calcification of cysts derived from hair follicles: a series of 20 cases evaluating the spectrum of changes resulting in scrotal calcinosis. Am J Dermatopathol. 29(2):172-5, 2007
4. Ito A et al: Dystrophic scrotal calcinosis originating from benign eccrine epithelial cysts. Br J Dermatol. 144(1):146-50, 2001
5. Saad AG et al: Scrotal calcinosis: is it idiopathic? Urology. 57(2):365, 2001
6. Dini M et al: Should scrotal calcinosis still be termed idiopathic? Am J Dermatopathol. 20(4):399-402, 1998
7. Polk P et al: Polypoid scrotal calcinosis: an uncommon variant of scrotal calcinosis. South Med J. 89(9):896-7, 1996
8. Dave AJ: Scrotal calcinosis. J Am Acad Dermatol. 23(1):150-1, 1990
9. Song DH et al: Idiopathic calcinosis of the scrotum: histopathologic observations of fifty-one nodules. J Am Acad Dermatol. 19(6):1095-101, 1988
10. Moskovitz B et al: Idiopathic calcinosis of scrotum. Eur Urol. 13(1-2):130-1, 1987
11. Sarma DP et al: Scrotal calcinosis: calcification of epidermal cysts. J Surg Oncol. 27(2):76-9, 1984
12. Bhawan J et al: The so-called idiopathic scrotal calcinosis. Arch Dermatol. 119(9):709, 1983

IMAGE GALLERY

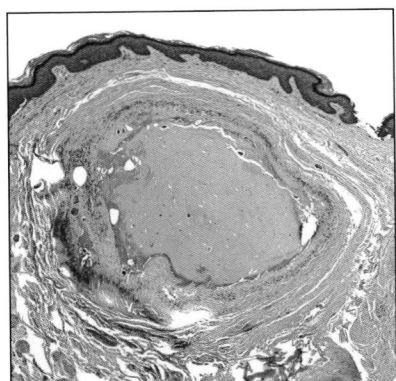
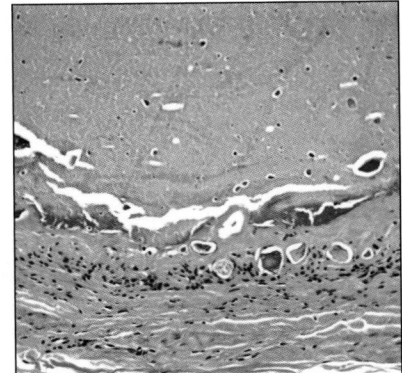
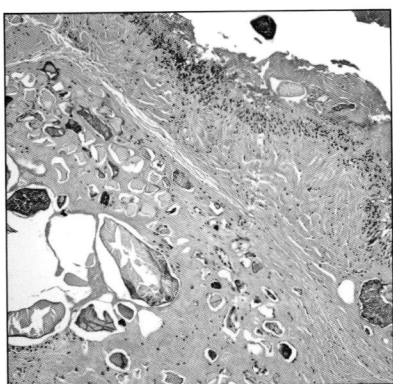

(Left) Low-power view highlights the calcific deposits within the dermis and upper part of the dartos. *(Center)* Histiocytes forming a palisade are usually seen at the periphery of the calcified deposits. *(Right)* Homogeneous granular and globular pink and purple material is seen within the dermis.

PENILE INTRAEPITHELIAL NEOPLASIA (PEIN)

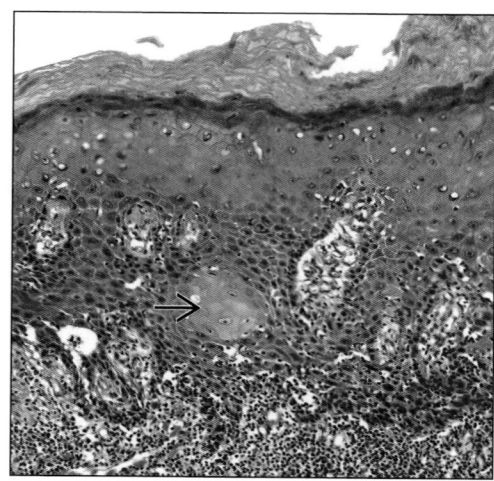

Note the enlarged keratinocytes with abundant eosinophilic cytoplasm throughout most of the epithelium in differentiated PeIN. Characteristic keratin pearl formation is present ➡.

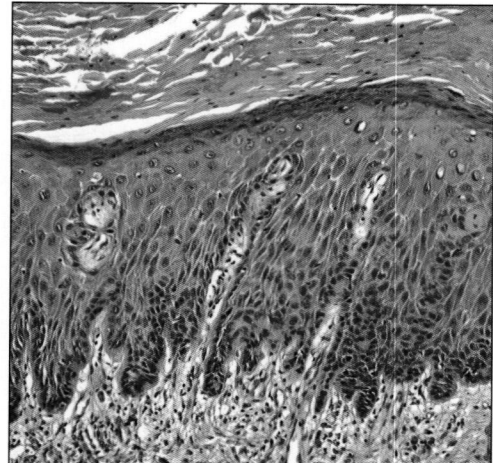

Acanthotic epithelium with subtle abnormal maturation and hyperchromatic atypical basilar cells are features of differentiated PeIN. Parakeratosis is seen on the surface.

TERMINOLOGY

Abbreviations
- Penile intraepithelial neoplasia (PeIN)

Synonyms
- Erythroplasia of Queyrat, Bowen disease, squamous cell carcinoma in situ, squamous intraepithelial lesion (SIL)

Definitions
- PeIN is considered intraepithelial (in situ) precursor lesion of invasive SCC

ETIOLOGY/PATHOGENESIS

Pathogenesis
- Basaloid, warty and warty/basaloid (undifferentiated) PeIN are HPV-related (especially HPV-16)
- Differentiated (simplex) PeIN is unrelated to HPV
- Lichen sclerosus may be implicated in pathogenesis of differentiated PeIN

CLINICAL ISSUES

Epidemiology
- Incidence
  - Real incidence is unknown
  - 2/3 associated with invasive SCC
  - When invasive SCC is associated with PeIN, 65% are differentiated PeIN and 35% are undifferentiated PeIN
- Age
  - 5th and 6th decades

Presentation
- Differentiated PeIN
  - Seen in older patients, frequently affects foreskin
  - Usually arises in setting of chronic scarring, inflammatory dermatosis, especially lichen sclerosus
- Warty/basaloid PeIN
  - Seen in younger patients; usually affects glans, perimeatal region
  - Usually not associated with lichen sclerosus
  - Patients may have history of condyloma

Treatment
- Surgery, locally destructive treatments

Prognosis
- Since most studies on PeIN are retrospective analyses of lesions associated with invasive SCCs, real prognosis of PeIN remains unknown

MACROSCOPIC FEATURES

General Features
- Gross appearance of PeIN is heterogeneous
- Gross appearance does not allow distinction between different types
- Uni- or multifocal
- Sharp or ill-defined borders
- Flat to slightly elevated hyperkeratotic or even papillary lesions
- Pearly white, moist, erythematous, dark brown/black
- Macules, papules, or plaques
- Differentiated PeIN usually arises in background of lichen sclerosus

MICROSCOPIC PATHOLOGY

Histologic Features
- Differentiated (simplex) PeIN (HPV-unrelated)
  - Thickened epithelium
  - Elongated and anastomosing rete ridges
  - Atypical basal cells with hyperchromatic nuclei

PENILE INTRAEPITHELIAL NEOPLASIA (PEIN)

Key Facts

Terminology
- Most warty/basaloid PeIN replace most or entire thickness of epithelium and represent carcinoma in situ
- Low-grade warty/basaloid PeIN (atypical cells replacing only lower part of epithelium) is exceptional
- Differentiated (simplex) PeIN is considered a high-grade lesion

Microscopic Pathology
- Differentiated (simplex) PeIN
  - Elongated and anastomosing rete ridges
  - Atypical basal cells with hyperchromatic nuclei
  - Subtle abnormal maturation (large eosinophilic keratinocytes)
  - Whorling and keratin pearl formation

- Usually associated with lichen sclerosus
- Basaloid PeIN
  - Basaloid cells replace most to full thickness of epithelium
  - Prominent apoptosis and mitosis
- Warty PeIN
  - Pleomorphic cells with koilocytic changes replace most to full thickness of epithelium
  - Undulated/spiky surface
- Warty-basaloid PeIN
  - Pleomorphic cells with koilocytic changes seen on upper epidermis
  - Basaloid cells replace lower epidermis
  - Usually undulated/spiky surface

  - Subtle abnormal maturation (enlarged keratinocytes with abundant eosinophilic cytoplasm)
  - Whorling and keratin pearl formation (usually in deep rete ridges)
  - Prominent intercellular bridges (spongiosis and sometimes acantholysis)
  - Parakeratosis is frequent
  - Absence of koilocytosis
  - Usually associated with lichen sclerosus
  - Preferential association with HPV-unrelated variants of invasive SCC (usual type, verrucous carcinoma, pseudohyperplastic SCC)
- HPV-related
  - Warty PeIN
    - Undulating/spiky surface with atypical parakeratosis
    - Pleomorphic cells with koilocytic changes (multinucleation, nuclei with irregular contours, perinuclear halo and dyskeratosis) replace epithelium
    - Mitoses tend to be numerous
  - Basaloid PeIN
    - Epithelium replaced by monotonous population of small immature cells with high nuclear/cytoplasmic ratios
    - Apoptosis and mitotic figures are numerous
  - Mixed PeIN (warty-basaloid)
    - Combined features of basaloid and warty types of PeIN
    - Lower part of epithelium is replaced by small cells with high nuclear/cytoplasmic ratio
    - Upper portion of epithelium shows features of warty PeIN
    - Surface often slightly undulated/papillary
    - Mitosis and apoptosis are prominent
    - Warty/basaloid PeIN is usually seen adjacent to HPV-related variants of invasive SCC (basaloid and warty types)

Predominant Pattern/Injury Type
- Dysplasia

Predominant Cell/Compartment Type
- Epithelial, squamous

DIFFERENTIAL DIAGNOSIS

Differentiated PeIN
- Squamous hyperplasia/lichen simplex chronicus
  - Reactive condition
  - Basilar atypia and abnormal maturation are not seen

Warty/Basaloid PeIN
- Condyloma
  - Koilocytosis confined to upper epithelium
  - Absence of nuclear pleomorphism
  - Mitoses are scant and confined to lower epithelium
- Bowenoid papulosis
  - Indistinguishable from warty/basaloid PeIN on histology alone
  - Clinical correlation is essential for this diagnosis

DIAGNOSTIC CHECKLIST

Pathologic Interpretation Pearls
- Differentiated PeIN: At low power, atypia seems to be present only in lower levels of epidermis
  - At higher power, it is more clear that there is subtle but abnormal maturation in all levels of epithelium
- Warty/basaloid PeIN PeIN is HPV-related and p16 may be useful morphologic surrogate

SELECTED REFERENCES

1. Sideri M et al: Squamous vulvar intraepithelial neoplasia: 2004 modified terminology, ISSVD Vulvar Oncology Subcommittee. J Reprod Med. 50(11):807-10, 2005
2. Cubilla AL et al: Epithelial lesions associated with invasive penile squamous cell carcinoma: a pathologic study of 288 cases. Int J Surg Pathol. 12(4):351-64, 2004

5

PENILE INTRAEPITHELIAL NEOPLASIA (PEIN)

Differentiated PeIN

(Left) Note the elongated rete-ridges and atypical basilar cells. Abnormal maturation ➜, spongiosis, keratin pearl formation, and parakeratosis is also appreciated. *(Right)* There are enlarged keratinocytes with plump vesicular nuclei and abundant eosinophilic cytoplasm. Atypia in the basilar/parabasal layer is easily recognized. Parakeratosis is seen on the surface.

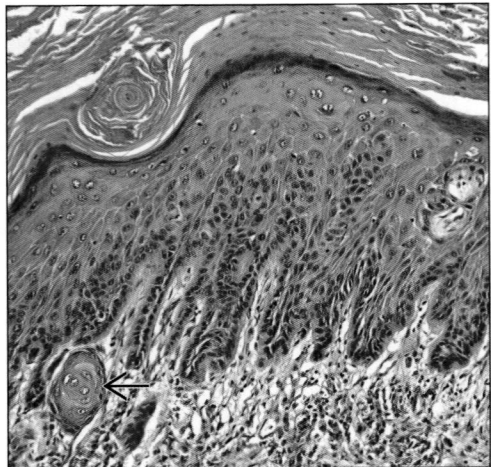
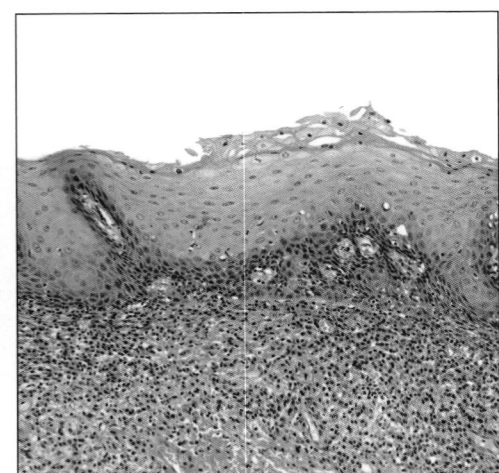

(Left) There is a markedly thickened epithelium with atypical basal and parabasal cells in this example of differentiated PeIN arising in a background of lichen sclerosus. *(Right)* The abnormal maturation is easily appreciated in this example. Some of the cells show marked atypia ➜. There is also a thickened basement membrane and hyalinization of the upper lamina propria corresponding to associated lichen sclerosus.

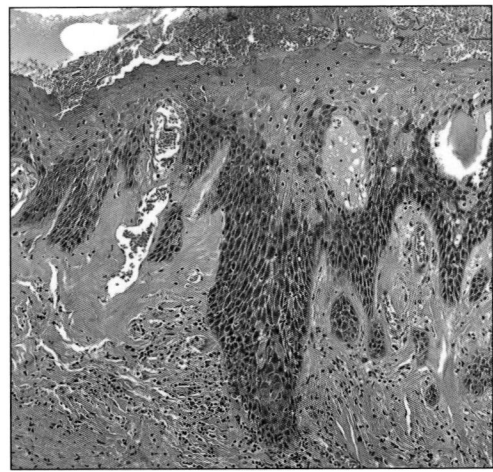
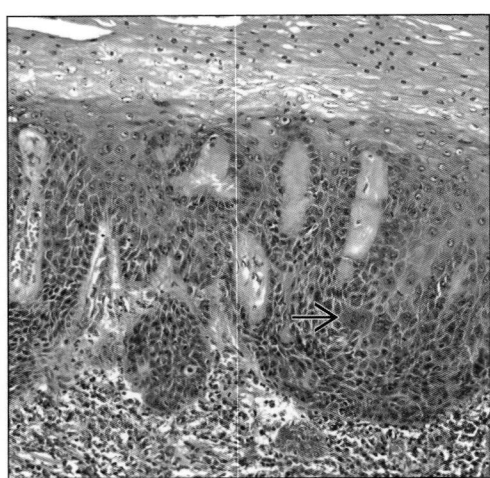

(Left) Differentiated PeIN ➔ is seen adjacent to an invasive SCC ➤. Note the characteristic elongation of the rete ridges and basilar hyperchromasia. In spite of the apparently subtle cytologic changes, juxtaposition to carcinoma argues for its premalignant potential. *(Right)* Differentiated PeIN ➔ is shown adjacent to an invasive SCC ➤. Note the elongation of the rete ridges and subtle abnormal maturation of the epithelium. Cytologic atypia is minimal.

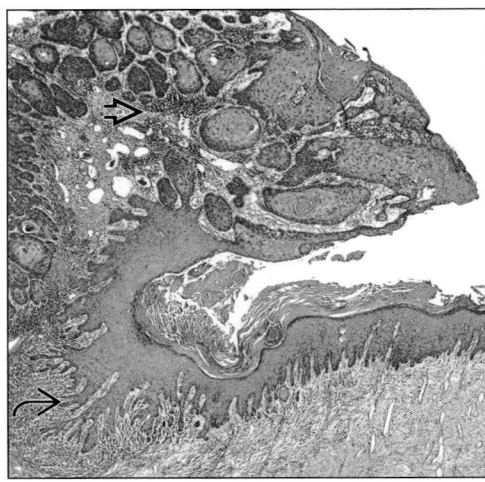
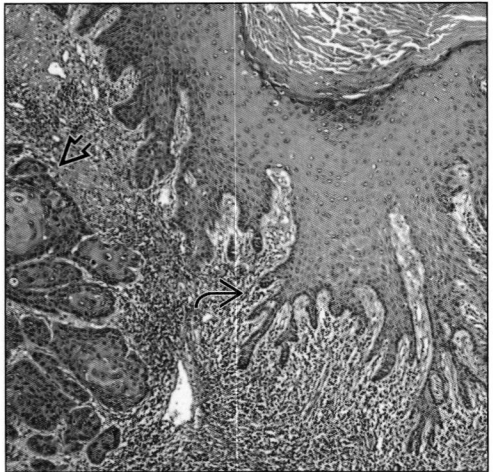

PENILE INTRAEPITHELIAL NEOPLASIA (PEIN)

Warty, Basaloid, and Warty/Basaloid PeIN

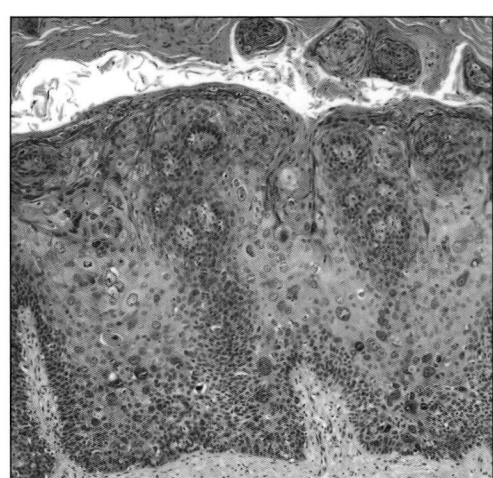 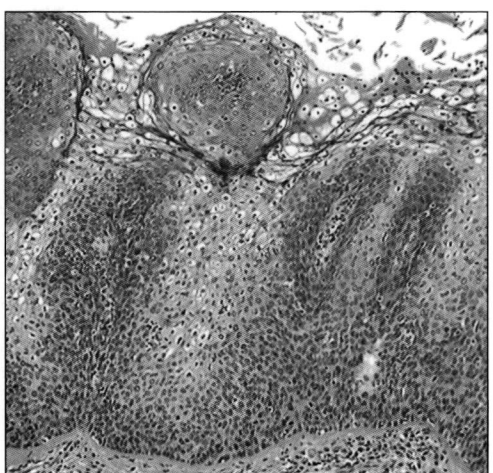

(**Left**) The epithelium is replaced by large pleomorphic and hyperchromatic nuclei in this example of warty PeIN. Irregular nuclear contours, bi- and multinucleation, and numerous mitoses are easily identified. (**Right**) There is full thickness replacement of the epidermis by atypical cells. The lower part of the epidermis is replaced by small basaloid cells, and the upper part is replaced by larger cells showing koilocytotic changes. These features characterize PeIN of warty-basaloid type.

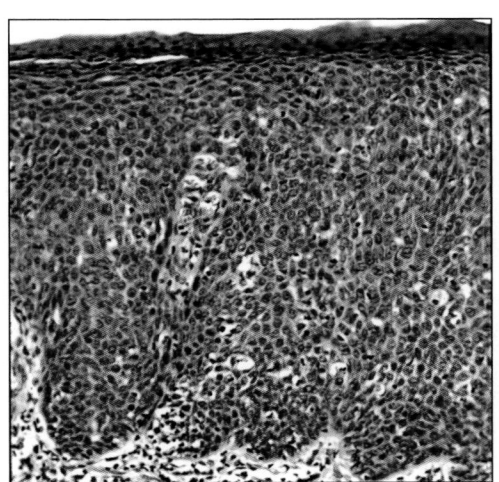 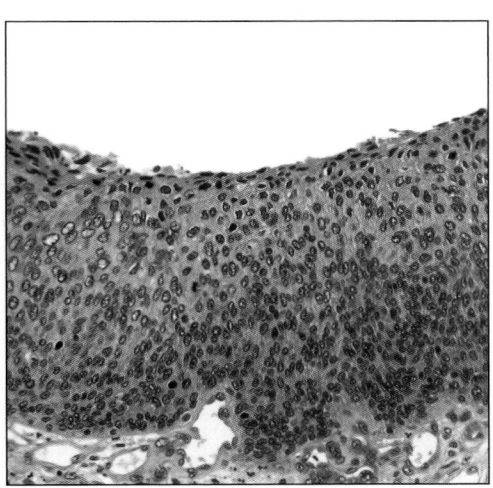

(**Left**) Proliferation of small round cells with high nuclear/cytoplasmic ratios and hyperchromatic nuclei replacing the entire thickness of the epithelium is seen in this case of basaloid PeIN. (**Right**) The epithelium is completely replaced by atypical cells with basaloid features. Numerous mitoses and apoptotic bodies are seen. The diagnosis of carcinoma in situ is easily achieved in high-grade basaloid PeIN.

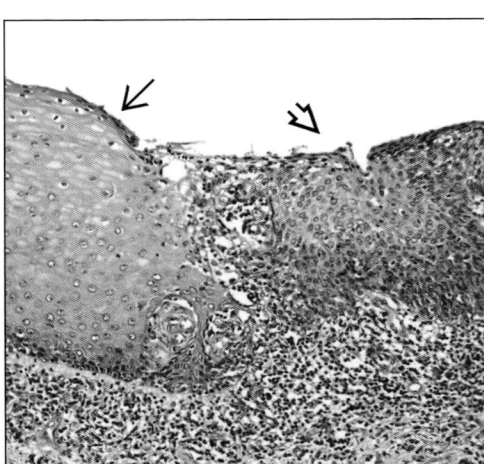 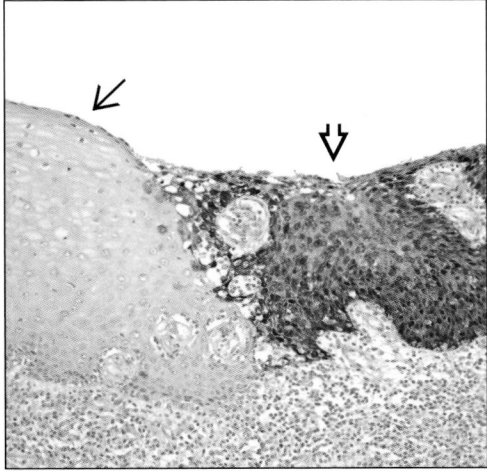

(**Left**) This picture illustrates a sharp demarcation between the basaloid PeIN ⊵ and hyperplastic squamous epithelium ➡. (**Right**) Immunohistochemistry with p16 (surrogate marker for oncogenic HPV) is strongly positive in the area of basaloid PeIN ⊵. The hyperplastic epithelium is negative ➡.

BOWENOID PAPULOSIS

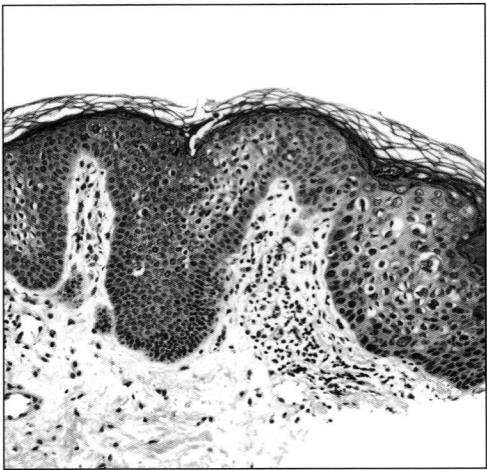

Patchy foci of atypia are present throughout the epidermis. Atypical cells vary from small basaloid to larger and more pleomorphic cells with koilocytic-like changes.

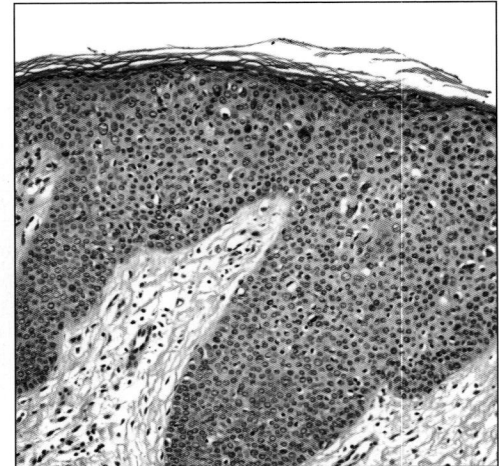

There is full thickness atypia of the squamous epithelium with preserved maturation and koilocytic change.

TERMINOLOGY

Abbreviations
- Bowenoid papulosis (BP)

Definitions
- Multifocal HPV-related papular condition affecting anogenital region in young adults
- Lesions exhibit spectrum of changes from dysplasia to in situ carcinoma; usually associated with favorable prognosis

ETIOLOGY/PATHOGENESIS

Etiology
- Related to high-risk types of HPV, especially type 16
- Other types of HPV (18, 31, 32, 33, 34, 35, 39, 42, 48, 51, 52, 53, and 54) have also been implicated
- Usually transmitted via sexual contact

Pathogenesis
- Oncogenic HPV elaborate proteins that interfere with normal cellular homeostasis

CLINICAL ISSUES

Epidemiology
- Incidence
  - Unknown and probably underestimated
  - Immunosuppression, including HIV infection, greatly increases risk for bowenoid papulosis
- Age
  - Mean: 31 years

Presentation
- Young, sexually active adults with solitary or more often multiple soft papules or macules with flat surface
  - Surface may be verruciform
- Lesions are often small, red, brown, or flesh-colored

- Usually affect skin of shaft
- May also affect epithelium of glans, coronal sulcus, or foreskin
- May be pruritic or painful
- Usually asymptomatic
- Lesions in immunosuppressed patients tend to be more widespread

Treatment
- Usually may be treated with locally destructive modalities
  - Important to remember that BP may be multifocal and has malignant potential: Follow-up is advised

Prognosis
- Most BP lesions run benign course with spontaneous regression occurring within several months
- Some lesions (especially in older or immunocompromised patients) last longer or never regress at all
- Minority of lesions evolve to invasive squamous cell carcinoma (SCC)

MICROSCOPIC PATHOLOGY

Histologic Features
- Proliferation of atypical cells with high nuclear/cytoplasmic ratio (basaloid cells) that may be scattered throughout epidermis, often with preserved maturation
- Koilocytic-like changes are also seen in most cases
- Range of atypia from scattered atypical cells to low-grade dysplasia to full thickness atypia of the squamous epithelium
- Most lesions are indistinguishable from squamous cell carcinoma in situ (SCCIS)
- Morphological features are similar to HPV-related penile intraepithelial neoplasia (PeIN)
- Variable increased pigmentation of basal layer

BOWENOID PAPULOSIS

Key Facts

Etiology/Pathogenesis
• Most often related to HPV 16

Clinical Issues
• Often multifocal
• Benign-looking papules
• Usually affecting skin of shaft of young adults
• May also affect glans and coronal sulcus

Microscopic Pathology
• Proliferation of atypical basaloid and koilocytic cells as scattered single units or involving full thickness of epithelium
• Most cases are indistinguishable from SCCIS

Top Differential Diagnoses
• Squamous cell carcinoma in situ (SCCIS)
• Treated condyloma

Predominant Pattern/Injury Type
• Dysplasia

Predominant Cell/Compartment Type
• Epithelial, squamous

DIFFERENTIAL DIAGNOSIS

Squamous Cell Carcinoma In Situ (SCCIS)
• Despite clinically benign-looking appearance of BP, histopathologic findings reveal features that may be identical to those of SCCIS
• Clinical correlation is crucial to make the distinction

Treated Flat Condyloma
• Changes secondary to podophyllin application
• Prominent degenerative changes that tend to be focal
• Pallor of epithelium, nuclear enlargement, necrotic keratinocytes
• Increase in number of mitotic figures (metaphase arrest)
• Atypical mitoses should not be seen
• Clinical correlation is necessary to make correct diagnosis

DIAGNOSTIC CHECKLIST

Pathologic Interpretation Pearls
• BP is clinicopathological diagnosis

• Histologically, most cases are indistinguishable from SCCIS
• Histopathological features similar to warty/basaloid PeIN
• Presence of only scattered atypical cells or more patchy pattern of full thickness squamous dysplasia may suggest BP
• Clinical correlation is crucial to make distinction

SELECTED REFERENCES

1. Liu H et al: Expression of p16 and hTERT protein is associated with the presence of high-risk human papillomavirus in Bowenoid papulosis. J Cutan Pathol. 33(8):551-8, 2006
2. Cubilla AL et al: Epithelial lesions associated with invasive penile squamous cell carcinoma: a pathologic study of 288 cases. Int J Surg Pathol. 12(4):351-64, 2004
3. Wade TR et al: The effects of resin of podophyllin on condyloma acuminatum. Am J Dermatopathol. 6(2):109-22, 1984
4. Eisen RF et al: Spontaneous regression of bowenoid papulosis of the penis. Cutis. 32(3):269-72, 1983
5. Wade TR et al: Bowenoid papulosis. JAMA. 246(7):732-3, 1981
6. Wade TR et al: Bowenoid papulosis of the genitalia. Arch Dermatol. 115(3):306-8, 1979
7. Wade TR et al: Bowenoid papulosis of the penis. Cancer. 42(4):1890-903, 1978

IMAGE GALLERY

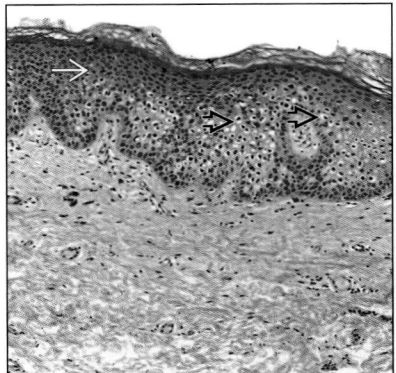 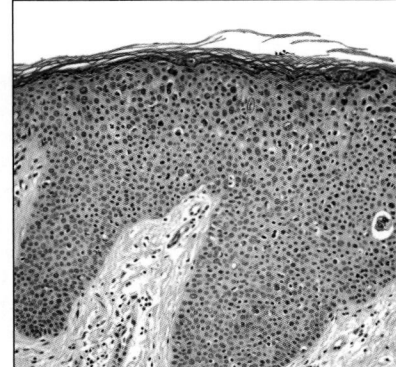 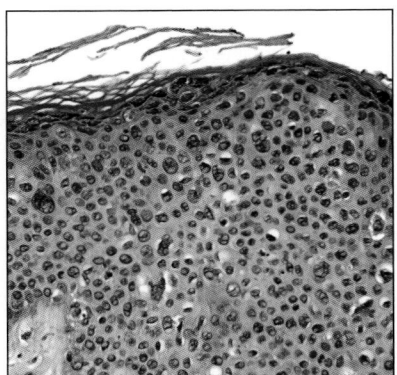

(Left) BP is seen with preserved maturation and scattered full thickness atypia. Dyskeratotic and apoptotic keratinocytes ➡ and koilocytic changes ⊵ are present. *(Center)* The changes are indistinguishable from those seen in squamous carcinoma in situ (HPV-related PeIN). *(Right)* This higher power view shows basaloid and pleomorphic cells replacing the epidermis.

SQUAMOUS CELL CARCINOMA, GENERAL CONCEPTS

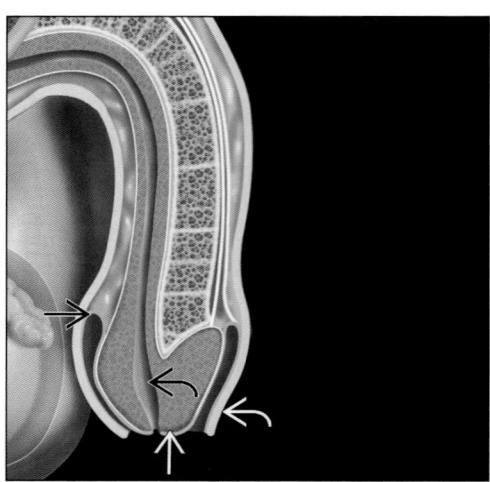

Distal penis includes the glans ➡️ (mostly composed of corpus spongiosum and containing the penile urethra ➡️), coronal sulcus ➡️, and foreskin ➡️ with an inner mucosal and an outer skin surface.

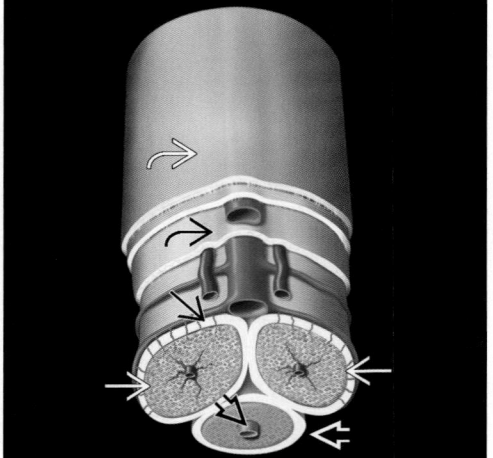

Transverse section of penile shaft depicts both dorsal corpora cavernosa ➡️, ventral corpus spongiosum ➡️ with penile urethra ➡️, tunica albuginea ➡️, penile fascia ➡️, and skin ➡️.

TERMINOLOGY

Abbreviations
- Squamous cell carcinoma (SCC)

Definitions
- Malignant epithelial neoplasia showing keratinocytic differentiation

ANATOMY AND HISTOLOGY

Anatomical Considerations
- Penile anatomical regions are glans, foreskin, and shaft
- Glans is distal, most cone-shaped region, formed by corpus spongiosum (CS) covered by squamous mucosa
  - Distal urethra opens up into meatus, a ventrally located slit-like orifice in glans
  - Glans corona separates glans from coronal sulcus
- Coronal sulcus is cul-de-sac between glans and foreskin
- Foreskin covers glans and presents mucosal (inner) and cutaneous (outer) surface
  - Frenulum connects foreskin to ventral portion of glans corona
- Penile shaft is composed mainly by ventral column of corpus spongiosum and 2 dorsal columns of corpora cavernosa
- Penile root anchors penis to perineal membrane and pubic arc

Histological Features
- Glans, coronal sulcus, and inner foreskin are covered by nonkeratinized squamous epithelium overlying loose lamina propria
- Penile erectile tissues comprising 2 corpora cavernosa (CC) and CS surrounding penile urethra form body of penile shaft
  - Irregular vascular spaces with intermingling elastic connective tissue form penile erectile tissues
  - Vascular spaces of CS are more widely spaced and irregular when compared with CC
  - CC present more densely packed vascular spaces with less intervening stroma
  - Tunica albuginea composed of dense connective tissue encompasses both CC and separates them from CS
  - CS is also covered by tunica albuginea
- Outer foreskin and shaft are covered by skin
- Bundles of dartos muscle extend underneath dermis throughout shaft and foreskin

EPIDEMIOLOGY

Age Range
- Most frequent in 6th to 7th decades
- Average age is 58 years

Incidence
- SCC represents most common malignant tumor of penis
- Wide range of geographical variation
  - Low incidence in USA and Europe
  - High incidence in South America, Africa, Asia

Natural History
- Local invasion of penile anatomical levels
- Extension to adjacent tissues
  - Scrotum, perineum, prostate
- Metastasis to inguinal lymph nodes
  - Sentinel node(s), superficial and deep nodes
- Metastasis to pelvic lymph nodes
- Systemic dissemination (nonregional lymph nodes, visceral, and bone involvement)
- Liver is most common site of metastatic dissemination followed by lungs and heart
- Systemic dissemination presents in up to 1/3 of patients in high-risk regions

SQUAMOUS CELL CARCINOMA, GENERAL CONCEPTS

ETIOLOGY/PATHOGENESIS

HPV-Related
- 30-40% of all SCC are HPV-related
- High-risk HPV predominates
  - HPV-16 is most common genotype encountered
  - HPV-18 is 2nd most common type
  - Other reported genotypes include 45, 52, and 74
- Low-risk HPV infection is uncommon
  - Low-risk HPV reported are genotypes 6 and 11
- Striking correlation of HPV presence and tumor morphology
  - Basaloid and condylomatous (warty) SCC are HPV-related in most cases
  - HPV incidence is low in usual, sarcomatoid, and papillary SCC

HPV-Unrelated
- Verrucous, pseudohyperplastic, and cuniculatum SCC are typically HPV-negative tumors
- Chronic inflammatory conditions (such as lichen sclerosus) are common in these cases

Risk Factors
- Phimosis is major risk factor for penile cancer
- Lack of neonatal circumcision
- HPV infection (especially by high-risk genotypes)
- History of genital warts
- Poor hygiene
- Smoking
- Treatment with psoralen and ultraviolet A (PUVA) therapy

CLINICAL IMPLICATIONS

Clinical Presentation
- Most penile SCCs originate from squamous mucosal surface of distal penis (glans, coronal sulcus, &/or foreskin)
  - Glans is most common affected site followed by inner foreskin and coronal sulcus
  - About 1/2 of penile carcinomas affect multiple anatomic compartments
- SCC of penile shaft are exceedingly rare
- Presence of painless tumoral mass is most frequent clinical presentation
- Ulceration may be present
- Urinary obstruction secondary to urethral tumoral extension is uncommon
- Phimosis is found in 50% of cases

MACROSCOPIC FINDINGS

General Features
- Patterns of growth include superficial spreading, vertical, verruciform, and multicentric
  - **Superficial spreading**
    - Broad horizontal/superficial extension with involvement of 1 or more anatomical compartments
    - Extensive in situ component with tumoral invasion usually confined to lamina propria
  - **Vertical growth**
    - Deeply infiltrative tumor with frank invasion of corpus spongiosum or corpus cavernosum
  - **Verruciform**
    - Exophytic cauliflower-like tumor mass usually invading only superficial anatomical levels
  - **Multicentric**
    - Presence of 2 or more independent foci of SCC
- Mixed/combinations of any of aforementioned patterns may be seen
- Superficial spreading tumors show intermediate risk for inguinal metastasis
- Vertical growth tumors show higher rate of nodal involvement and poor outcome
- Verruciform tumors may reach large sizes but tend to be localized and metastatic rate is low
- In multicentric tumors, foci should be separately evaluated

Specimen Handling
- Wide local excision specimen
  - Fix in 10% buffered formalin, preferably overnight
  - Measure and describe specimen, identifying and describing tumor
  - Photograph or diagram specimen
  - Ink entire surgical margin of specimen
  - Section specimen transverse to longest axis
  - Submit tumor entirely if < 3-4 cm and section at least 1 per cm, including grossly apparent deepest penetration and all margins (if not entirely submitted)
- Circumcision specimen for tumor
  - Lightly stretch and pin specimen to flat surface
  - Fix in 10% buffered formalin, preferably overnight
  - Measure and describe specimen, identifying and describing tumor
  - Photograph or diagram specimen
  - Ink mucosal and cutaneous margins of resection with different colors
  - Section specimen transversally to its longest axis
  - Label each section from 1-12 clockwise
  - Submit entirely if < 3-4 cm, section at least 1 per cm, including grossly apparent deepest penetration and all margins (if not entirely submitted)
- Partial/total penectomy specimen
  - Fix entire specimen in 10% buffered formalin, preferably overnight
  - When fixed, section specimen in 2 halves using meatus and anterior urethra as a guide
  - Do **not** probe urethra
  - If foreskin is not affected by tumor, separate leaving 3 mm margin from coronal sulcus and include as circumcision specimen
  - If foreskin is affected by tumor, do **not** remove
  - Photograph or diagram specimen, focusing on tumor invasion of anatomic levels
  - Section each 1/2 longitudinally to longest axis, at 3-5 mm intervals
  - Photograph (or diagram) and submit entirely section, depicting deepest anatomic level infiltrated by tumor

SQUAMOUS CELL CARCINOMA, GENERAL CONCEPTS

TNM Staging for Penile Carcinoma (2009)

Stage	Description
Primary Tumor (T)	
Tx	Primary tumor cannot be assessed
T0	No evidence of primary tumor
Tis	Carcinoma in situ
Ta	Noninvasive verrucous carcinoma
T1a	Tumor invades subepithelial connective tissue without vascular invasion and is not poorly differentiated
T1b	Tumor invades subepithelial connective tissue with vascular invasion or is poorly differentiated
T2	Tumor invades corpus spongiosum or cavernosum
T3	Tumor invades urethra
T4	Tumor invades other adjacent structures
Regional Lymph Nodes (N)	
Clinical Stage Definition	
cNx	Regional lymph nodes cannot be assessed
cN0	No palpable or visibly enlarged inguinal lymph nodes
cN1	Palpable mobile unilateral inguinal lymph node
cN2	Palpable mobile multiple or bilateral inguinal lymph nodes
cN3	Unilateral or bilateral palpable fixed inguinal nodal mass or pelvic lymphadenopathy
Pathologic Stage Definition	
pNx	Regional lymph nodes cannot be assessed
pN0	No regional lymph node metastasis
pN1	Metastasis in a single inguinal lymph node
pN2	Metastasis in multiple or bilateral inguinal lymph nodes
pN3	Unilateral or bilateral extranodal extension of lymph node metastasis or pelvic lymph node(s)
Distant Metastasis (M)	
M0	No distant metastasis
M1	Distant metastasis

Anatomic Stage/Prognostic Groups (2009)

Stage	T	N	M
0	Tis	N0	M0
	Ta	N0	M0
I	T1a	N0	M0
II	T1b	N0	M0
	T2	N0	M0
	T3	N0	M0
IIIa	T1-T3	N1	M0
IIIb	T1-T3	N2	M0
IV	T4	Any N	M0
	Any T	N3	M0
	Any T	Any N	M1

- Ultrasound, TAC, PET scan, and MR may be useful and dynamic sentinel lymph node biopsy may be indicated

SELECTED REFERENCES

1. Chaux A et al: Histologic Grade in Penile Squamous Cell Carcinoma: Visual Estimation Versus Digital Measurement of Proportions of Grades, Adverse Prognosis With any Proportion of Grade 3 and Correlation of a Gleason-like System With Nodal Metastasis. Am J Surg Pathol. 33(7):1042-1048, 2009
2. Chaux A et al: The Prognostic Index: A Useful Pathologic Guide for Prediction of Nodal Metastases and Survival in Penile Squamous Cell Carcinoma. Am J Surg Pathol. 33(7):1049-1057, 2009
3. Cubilla AL: The role of pathologic prognostic factors in squamous cell carcinoma of the penis. World J Urol. 27(2):169-77, 2009

SQUAMOUS CELL CARCINOMA, GENERAL CONCEPTS

Gross Features and Patterns of Growth

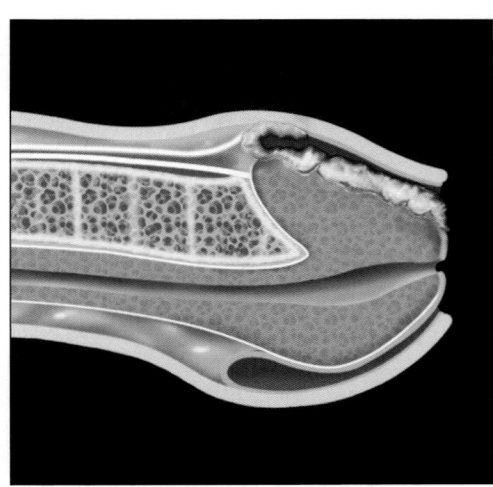

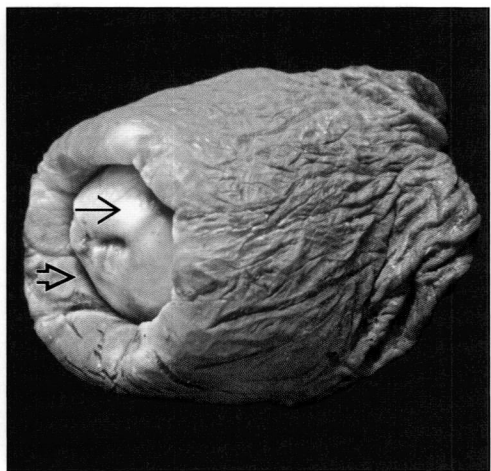

(Left) Superficial spreading pattern of growth is characterized by a horizontal dissemination of tumor mass along the squamous mucosa of glans, coronal sulcus, and even inner foreskin with minimal infiltration of deeper tissues. *(Right)* Predominantly in situ penile SCC with isolated foci of infiltration in lamina propria depicts a superficial spreading pattern of growth characterized by whitish and irregular areas extensively affecting glans ⇒ and extending to foreskin ⇒.

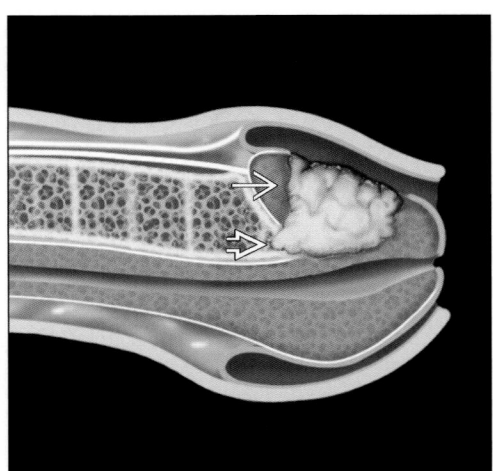

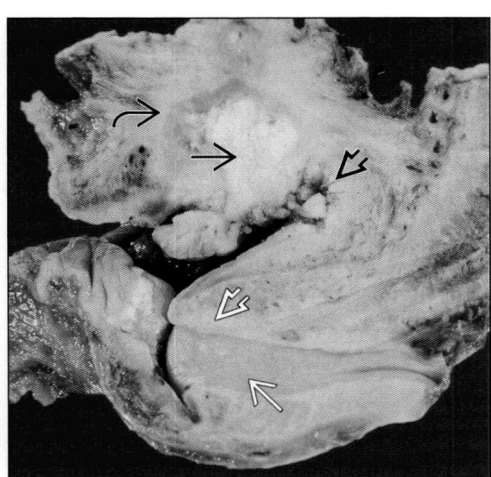

(Left) Tumors with vertical pattern of growth usually show an ulcerated surface and invade deep into penile erectile tissues, either corpus spongiosum ⇒ or cavernosum ⇒, and typically correspond to SCC variants, such as high-grade usual, basaloid, or sarcomatoid carcinomas. *(Right)* High-grade usual SCC ⇒ located in foreskin ⇒ and extending to coronal sulcus ⇒ with a vertical growth pattern is shown invading into deep preputial levels and sparing glans ⇒ and distal urethra ⇒.

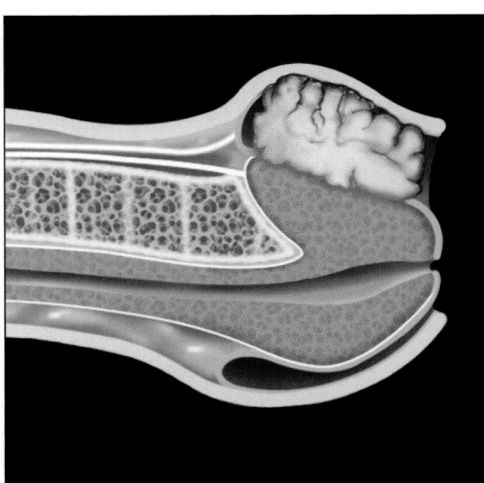

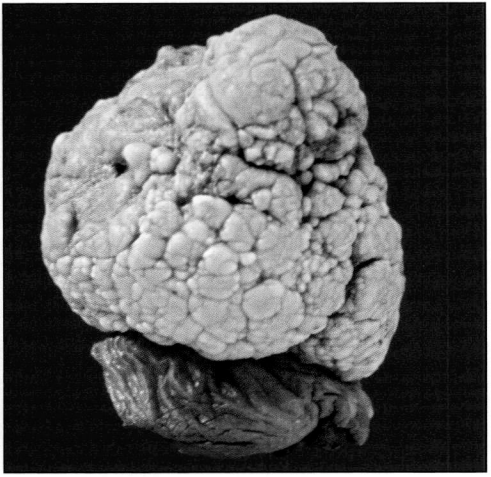

(Left) Penile verruciform tumors include warty, papillary, and verrucous carcinoma and are characterized by an exophytic papillomatous pattern of growth, infiltration up to lamina propria, or corpus spongiosum, and are associated with a good prognosis. *(Right)* Verruciform tumor corresponding to a warty carcinoma entirely replacing glans and coronal sulcus in which, notwithstanding its large size, tumor invasion was limited to superficial corpus spongiosum.

SQUAMOUS CELL CARCINOMA, GENERAL CONCEPTS

Gross and Microscopic Features

(Left) Exophytic cauliflower-like tumor with a verruciform pattern of growth, histologically corresponds to a warty carcinoma, located in the foreskin and extending up to the coronal sulcus ⇒ without affecting the glans ⊇. *(Right)* Highly aggressive penile SCC histologically corresponds to a sarcomatoid carcinoma, with extensive areas of necrosis and hemorrhage located in glans and deeply infiltrates the corpora cavernosa ⇒ and perforates the tunica albuginea ⊇.

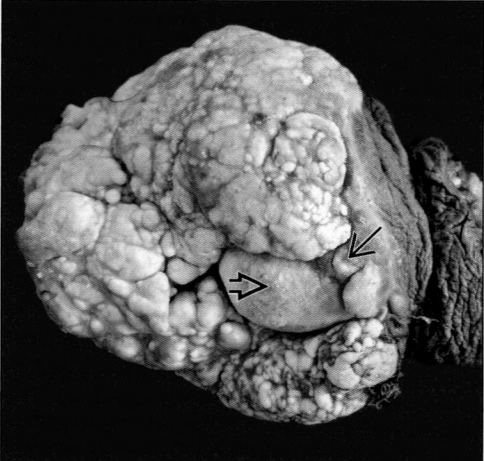
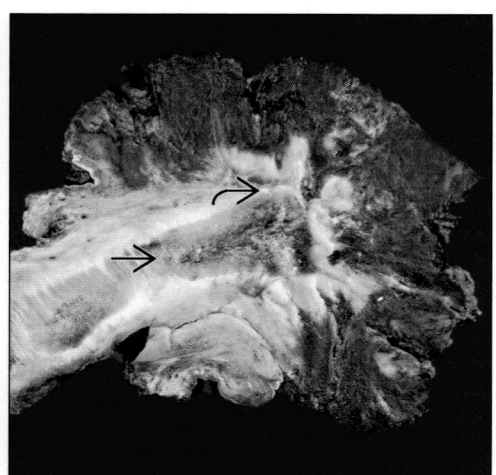

(Left) Circumcision specimen shows an exophytic tumor ⊇ located in the inner foreskin mucosa ⇒ corresponding to a well-differentiated usual SCC with superficial infiltration of preputial tissues. *(Right)* In well-differentiated (grade 1) usual SCC, neoplastic cells in tumoral nests are almost indistinguishable from their normal counterparts, except for minimal basal/parabasal atypia, prominent keratinization ⊇, and infiltration of penile tissues with surrounding stromal reaction.

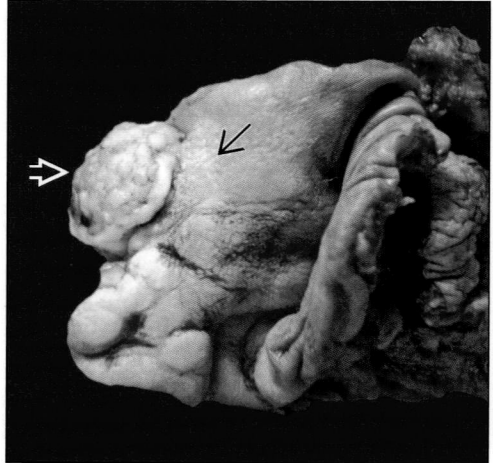
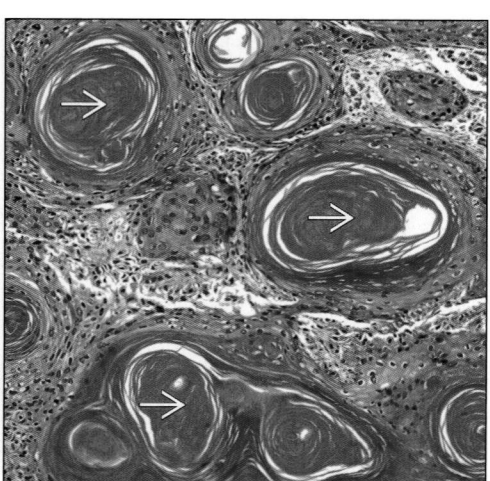

(Left) In moderately differentiated (grade 2) usual SCC, cytologic atypia is more evident and pleomorphic cells are easily recognized; cytoplasm is ample and eosinophilic and epithelial maturation with keratinization ⊇ is retained. *(Right)* Solid tumoral nests composed of highly pleomorphic neoplastic cells with anaplastic features ⇒ and ample eosinophilic cytoplasm indicate some degree of squamous differentiation and characterize poorly differentiated (grade 3) usual SCC.

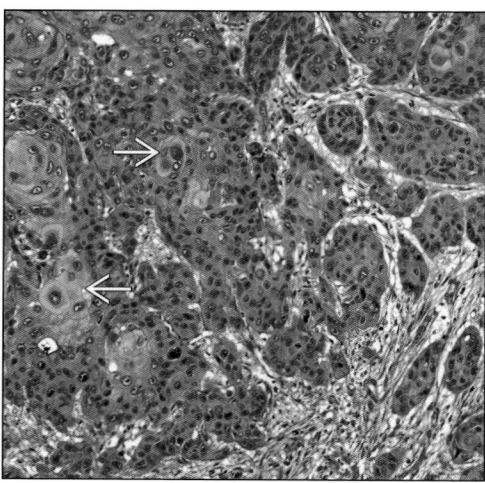
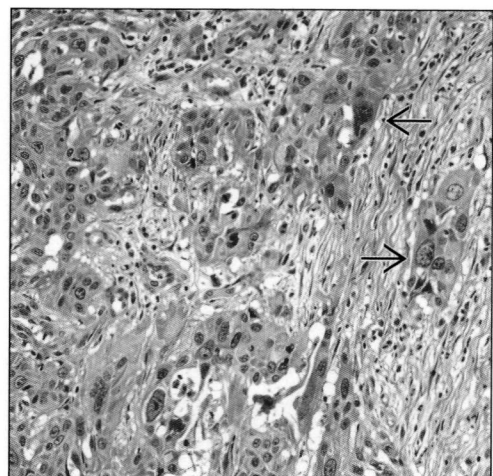

SQUAMOUS CELL CARCINOMA, GENERAL CONCEPTS

Microscopic Features

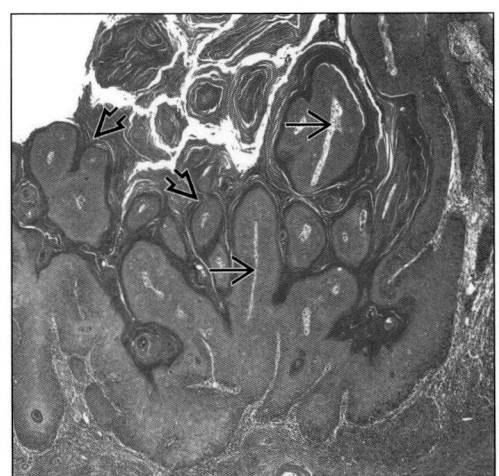
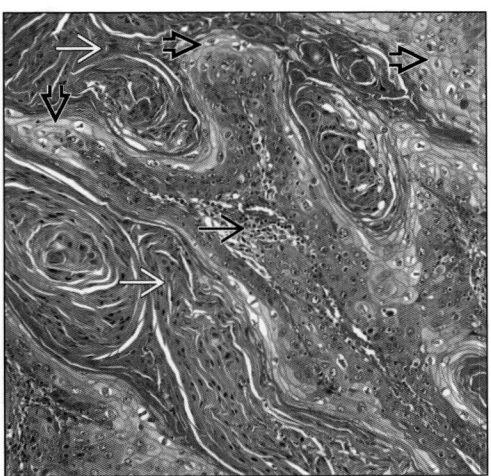

(Left) Warty (condylomatous) carcinoma is a verruciform tumor characterized by acanthosis, papillomatosis, and hyperkeratosis, with straight and spiky parakeratotic papillae ➡, prominent and constant fibrovascular cores ➡, and irregular and jagged tumor base. *(Right)* The papillae in warty carcinoma are elongated and spiky, show evident fibrovascular cores ➡, mild to moderate acanthosis, and parakeratotic hyperkeratosis ➡, and koilocytic changes ➡ are easily found.

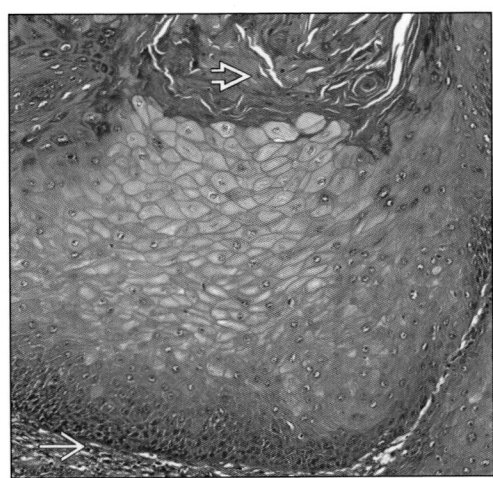
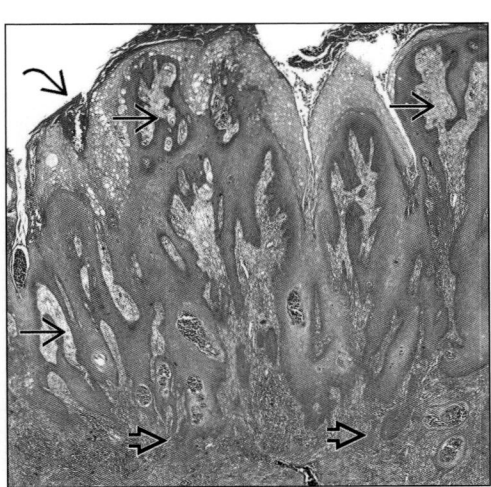

(Left) Verrucous carcinoma is characterized by papillomatosis, moderate to marked acanthosis, minimal cytological atypia, prominent hyperkeratosis ➡ with absent or inconspicuous fibrovascular cores, and a broad, pushing tumor base ➡. *(Right)* In papillary carcinoma, papillae are complex and fibrovascular cores ➡ are irregular, tips are blunt, round, or spiky, hyperkeratosis ➡ is commonly found, and the tumor base is irregular and jagged ➡ with prominent stromal reaction.

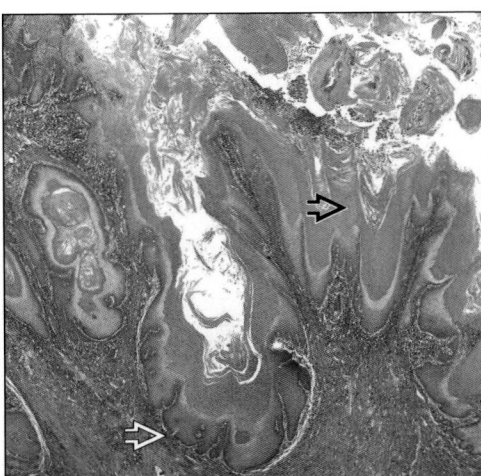
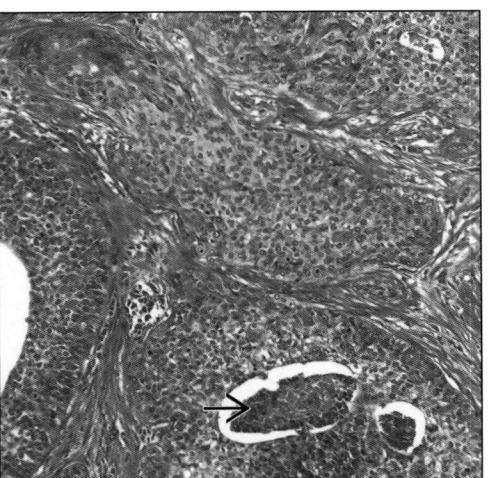

(Left) Carcinoma cuniculatum, a rare verruciform tumor, shows prominent acanthosis, papillomatosis and hyperkeratosis ➡, broad and pushing tumor base ➡, and a deeply infiltrating endophytic pattern of growth. *(Right)* Basaloid carcinoma is characterized by highly infiltrative tumor nests, with frequent central necrosis ➡, composed of a monotonous population of small to intermediate-sized cells with scant cytoplasm, abundant mitoses, and indistinct borders.

SQUAMOUS CELL CARCINOMA, GENERAL CONCEPTS

Microscopic Features

(Left) Basaloid carcinomas may be composed of irregular tumor nests and greater nuclear pleomorphism but should not be confused with high-grade usual SCC, which is characterized by tumor cells with ample eosinophilic cytoplasm, distinctive borders, and intercellular bridges. *(Right)* Adenosquamous carcinoma is a biphasic SCC variant characterized by the presence of a solid high-grade squamous component ⇨ intermingled with areas showing glandular differentiation ➨.

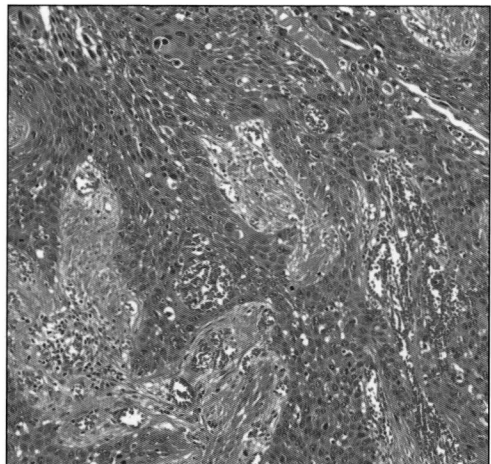
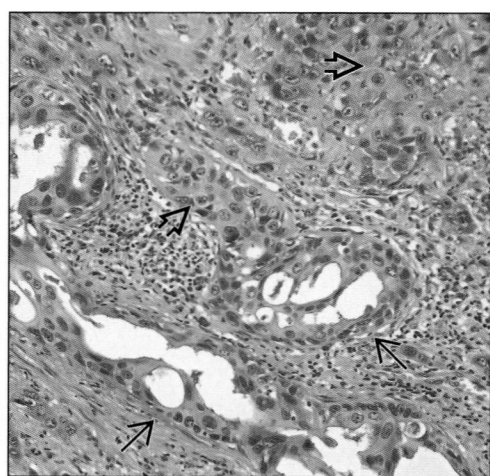

(Left) In pseudoglandular SCC, solid tumor nests exhibit extensive central necrosis, intracytoplasmic vacuoles ➩, and acantholysis ➨, resulting in an appearance resembling glandular lumina. *(Right)* Pseudohyperplastic carcinoma, which may be difficult to distinguish from pseudoepitheliomatous hyperplasia, exhibits acanthosis and hyperkeratosis ⇨, downward proliferation of irregular epithelial nests ➨ with infiltration of lamina propria, and prominent stromal reaction.

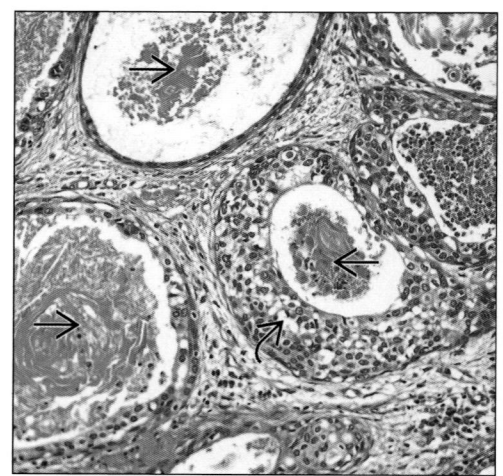
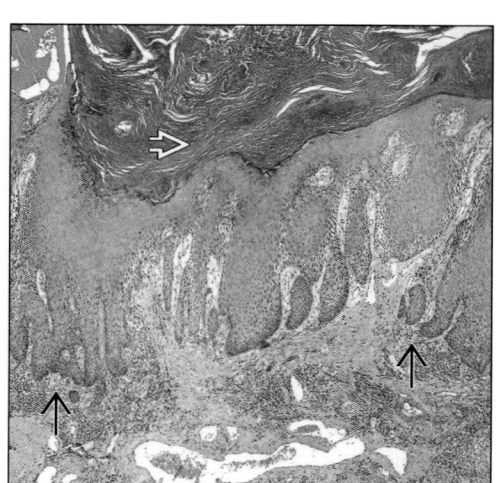

(Left) Warty/basaloid carcinoma is a mixed SCC in which koilocytes ➨, typical of warty carcinomas, are mingled with basaloid cells ➨ either in superficial condylomatous papillae, frequently exhibiting parakeratosis ⇨, or in deeply infiltrative nests. *(Right)* Sarcomatoid carcinoma is a highly aggressive SCC variant composed of a predominant spindle cell component, with marked nuclear atypia and abundant mitoses ➨ resembling leiomyosarcoma or fibrosarcoma.

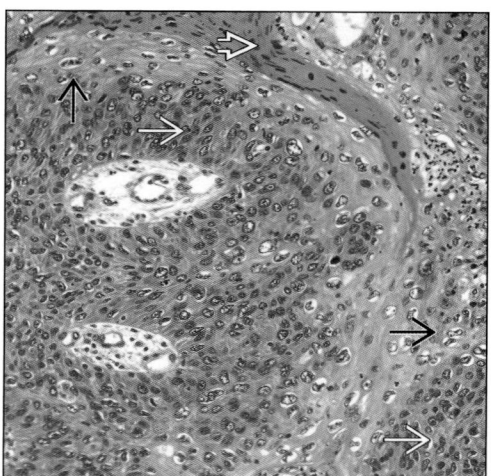
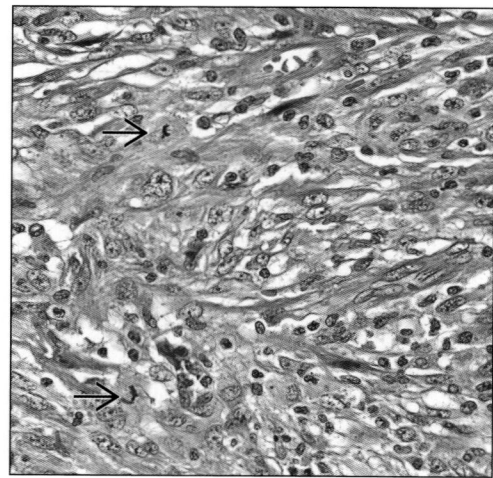

SQUAMOUS CELL CARCINOMA, GENERAL CONCEPTS

Microscopic Features

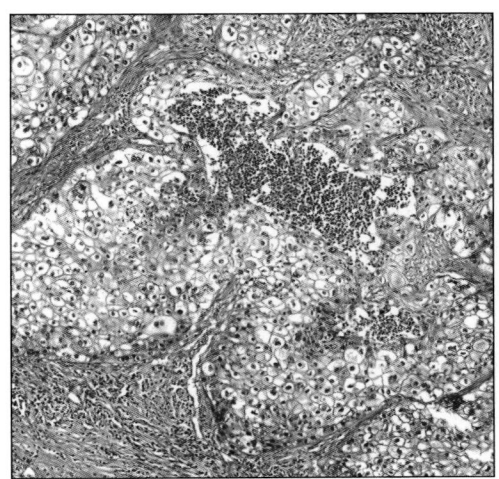

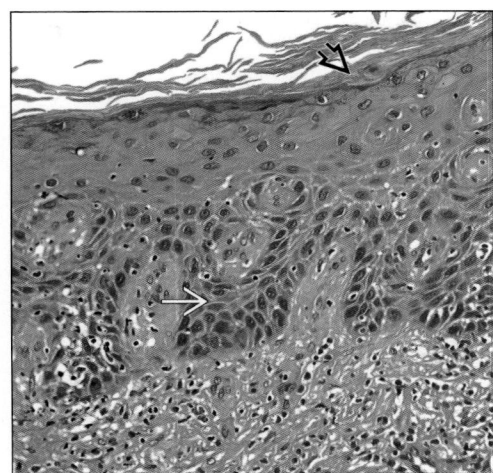

(Left) It is not unusual to find focal clear cell changes in an otherwise typical SCC, although in rare occasions this morphological aspect, usually due to abundant glycogen, may be the predominant histology and may be confused with clear cell carcinoma. *(Right)* Differentiated PeIN, frequently associated with keratinizing SCC variants, is characterized by atypical squamous cells, more prominent at bottom layers ➡, with a tendency to epithelial maturation and parakeratosis ➪.

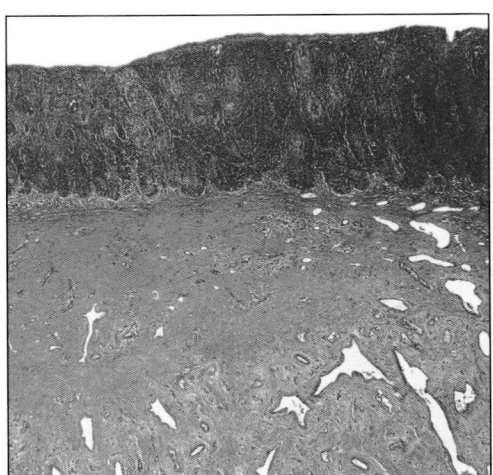

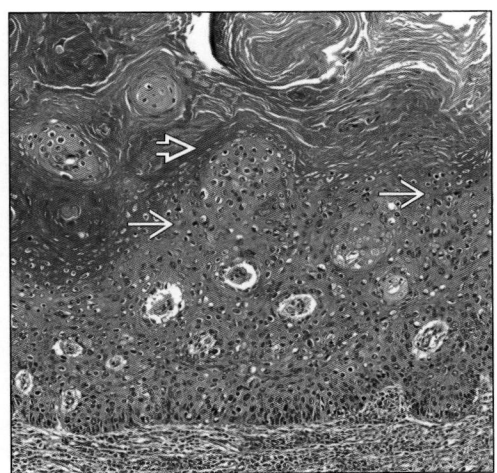

(Left) Basaloid PeIN, found in association with warty/basaloid tumors, is characterized by replacement of the epithelium by a monotonous population of small to intermediate-sized cells with high nuclear/cytoplasmic ratio, indistinct borders, abundant mitoses, and flat surface. *(Right)* Warty PeIN, usually found adjacent to invasive carcinomas with warty/basaloid features, is characterized by acanthosis, a spiky and parakeratotic surface ➡, and conspicuous koilocytosis ➡.

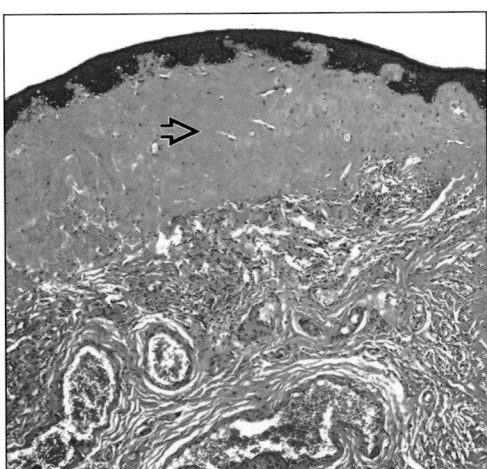

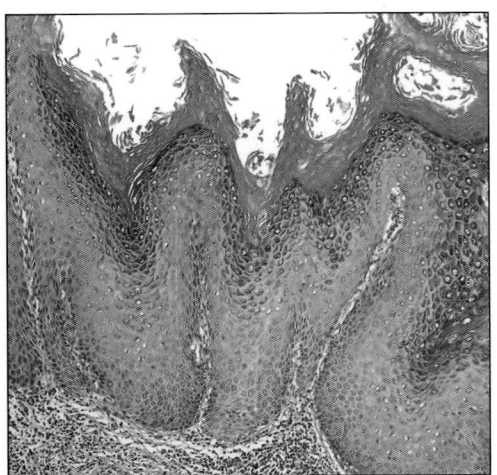

(Left) In lichen sclerosus, a dense area of collagenization ➪ is observed underneath the squamous epithelium, which shows atrophic, hyperplastic, or atypical changes. *(Right)* Well-differentiated verrucoid lesions are often difficult to classify, especially in small biopsies, and the differential includes verrucous squamous hyperplasia and verrucous carcinoma, the latter characterized by a clinically exophytic and large lesion when compared with the former.

SQUAMOUS CELL CARCINOMA, USUAL TYPE

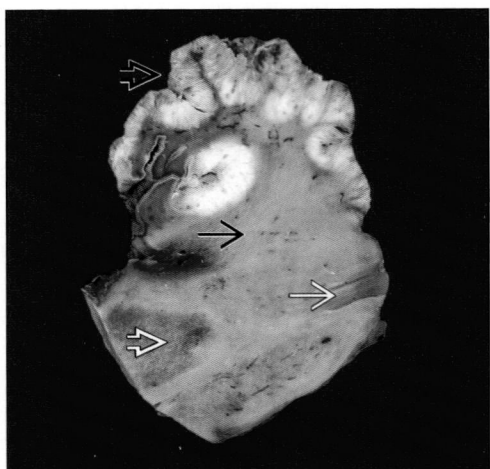

Gross photograph of a penile SCC ⊟ with an exo-endophytic pattern of growth invades up to the corpus spongiosum ⮕ of glans but spares urethra ⮕ and corpus cavernosum ⮕.

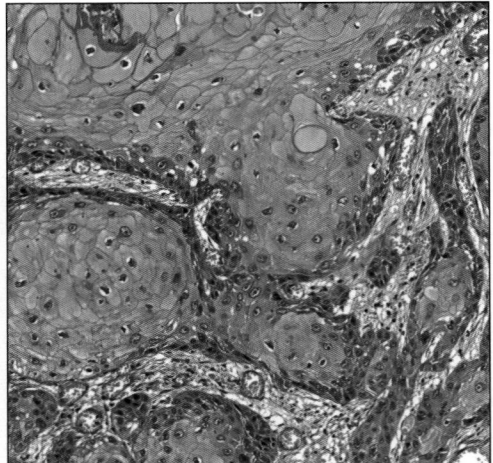

Tumor nests of well-differentiated usual SCC are composed of neoplastic cells with ample, eosinophilic and keratinized cytoplasm, distinctive cellular borders, and retained epithelial maturation.

TERMINOLOGY

Abbreviations
- Squamous cell carcinoma (SCC)

Synonyms
- Conventional/typical SCC
- Epidermoid carcinoma
- SCC, not otherwise specified (NOS)

Definitions
- Invasive carcinoma with features of keratinization (intracellular keratin pearls and intracellular bridges)

ETIOLOGY/PATHOGENESIS

Infectious Agents
- Human papillomavirus (HPV) infection in about 1/4 of cases

CLINICAL ISSUES

Epidemiology
- Incidence
  - Most common histologic subtype of penile SCC (60-65%)
- Age
  - Average: 58 years

Presentation
- Solid tumoral mass usually affecting glans
- Ulceration, pain, bleeding, or erythema may be seen

Treatment
- Primary treatment is surgical
- Penile-preserving therapy in low-grade superficial tumors
- Radiotherapy as adjuvant or neoadjuvant therapy
- Chemotherapy for advanced cases (irresectable primary tumor &/or regional involvement)
- Inguinal lymphadenectomy according to risk group

Prognosis
- Most important prognostic factors include
  - Histologic grade
  - Anatomic level of infiltration (pathologic stage)
  - Vascular, lymphatic, and perineural invasion
- Recurrences in 1/4 of cases
- Inguinal nodal metastases in 1/3 of patients

MACROSCOPIC FEATURES

General Features
- Most tumors affect glans
- Tumors exclusive of foreskin are less common
- Superficial spreading is predominant pattern of growth
- Gross features are nondistinctive
- Average size is 2-4.8 cm

MICROSCOPIC PATHOLOGY

Histologic Features
- Evident squamous differentiation (keratinization)
- Most are well to moderately differentiated
  - Pure grade 1 or 3 tumors are very rare
- More than 1 histologic grade in about 1/2 of cases
  - Only highest grade is considered for tumor grading
- Focal areas of spindle, trabecular, solid, or clear cells in some cases
- Evident stromal reaction
  - Mainly lymphocytes and plasma cells
- Vascular and perineural invasion in about 1/3 of cases
- Extension to distal urethra in almost 1/2 of cases
- Squamous hyperplasia (SH) and differentiated penile intraepithelial neoplasia (PeIN) commonly found in adjacent areas
- Basaloid and warty PeIN rarely found

SQUAMOUS CELL CARCINOMA, USUAL TYPE

Key Facts

Etiology/Pathogenesis
- HPV infection in about 1/4 of cases

Macroscopic Features
- Glans frequently affected
- Superficial pattern of growth in most cases
- Gross features are nondistinctive

Microscopic Pathology
- Most common histological subtype of penile SCC
- Keratinization evident in most cases
- Mostly well-to-moderately differentiated
  - Pure grade 1 or 3 is very rare
- Heterogeneous tumors in about 1/2 of all cases
  - Focal presence of anaplastic cells is enough for grade 3
- Frequent invasion of penile erectile tissues

- Frequent extension to multiple compartments
- SH and differentiated PeIN commonly found
- Most important prognostic factors
  - Histologic grade
  - Anatomical level of infiltration
  - Vascular invasion
  - Perineural invasion
- Inguinal nodal metastases in 1/3 of patients

Top Differential Diagnoses
- Pseudoepitheliomatous hyperplasia
- Pseudohyperplastic carcinoma
- Urothelial carcinoma of distal urethra
- High-grade SCC
- Mixed SCC
- Metastatic SCC to penis

- Lichen sclerosus in almost 1/2 of patients

Anatomic Extension
- Frequent invasion of penile erectile tissues
- Extension up to lamina propria very rare
- Extension to multiple compartments is common

DIFFERENTIAL DIAGNOSIS

Pseudoepitheliomatous Hyperplasia
- Pseudoinfiltrative pattern of growth
- Epithelial nests orderly disposed
- No cytologic atypia
- Peripheral palisading
- No stromal reaction

Pseudohyperplastic Carcinoma
- Extreme squamous differentiation
- Irregular tumor nests
- Inconspicuous peripheral palisading
- Prominent stromal reaction
- Multicentricity is common
- Lichen sclerosus frequently found

Urothelial Carcinoma of Distal Urethra
- Clinical antecedents of urothelial carcinoma
- Urothelial carcinoma in situ in adjacent areas
- No associated squamous changes (SH, PeIN)
- CK20 and uroplakin-3 positive urothelial carcinoma and negative in SCC

Mixed SCC
- Foci of usual SCC intermingled with other subtypes
- Mostly with verrucous carcinoma
- Uncommon with HPV-related tumors

High-Grade SCC
- Sarcomatoid carcinoma usually shows foci of usual SCC
- Pleomorphic basaloid carcinoma can be confused with solid high-grade SCC
  - Cytoplasm is scant and basophilic in basaloid carcinoma

- Cytoplasm is more ample and eosinophilic in high-grade SCC

Metastatic SCC to Penis
- Most penile secondary tumors are of genitourinary origin
  - Prostatic adenocarcinomas and bladder urothelial carcinoma
  - May exhibit prominent squamous differentiation
- Tumor located in penile shaft
- Tumor nests located mainly in vascular spaces of penile erectile tissues
  - Squamous mucosa covering glans, coronal sulcus, or inner foreskin is usually unaffected
- Clinical antecedent of primary malignancy elsewhere
- Priapism in 1/3 to 1/2 of patients

SELECTED REFERENCES

1. Chaux A et al: Histologic Grade in Penile Squamous Cell Carcinoma: Visual Estimation Versus Digital Measurement of Proportions of Grades, Adverse Prognosis With any Proportion of Grade 3 and Correlation of a Gleason-like System With Nodal Metastasis. Am J Surg Pathol. 33(7):1042-1048, 2009
2. Chaux A et al: The Prognostic Index: A Useful Pathologic Guide for Prediction of Nodal Metastases and Survival in Penile Squamous Cell Carcinoma. Am J Surg Pathol. 33(7):1049-1057, 2009
3. Guimarães GC et al: Penile squamous cell carcinoma clinicopathological features, nodal metastasis and outcome in 333 cases. J Urol. 182(2):528-34; discussion 534, 2009
4. Velazquez EF et al: Epithelial abnormalities and precancerous lesions of anterior urethra in patients with penile carcinoma: a report of 89 cases. Mod Pathol. 18(7):917-23, 2005
5. Cubilla AL et al: Histologic classification of penile carcinoma and its relation to outcome in 61 patients with primary resection. Int J Surg Pathol. 9(2):111-20, 2001

SQUAMOUS CELL CARCINOMA, USUAL TYPE

Gross and Microscopic Features

(Left) Gross photograph of a usual SCC is shown affecting multiple anatomic compartments and extending through glans ➡, coronal sulcus ➡, and foreskin ➡ but sparing distal urethra ➡, tunica albuginea ➡, and corpus cavernosum ➡. *(Right)* Usual squamous cell carcinoma tends to affect multiple anatomical compartments and extend through glans, coronal sulcus, and inner foreskin, although invading only superficial anatomical levels, a pattern named "superficial spreading."

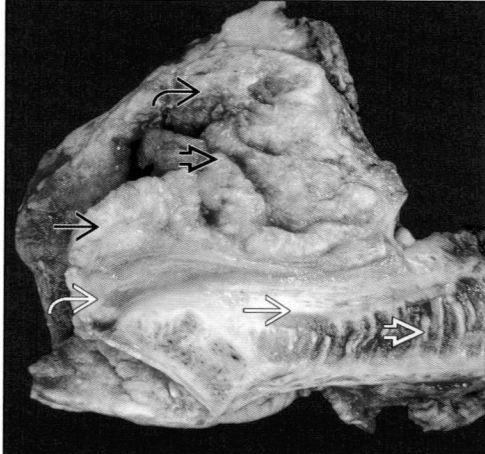
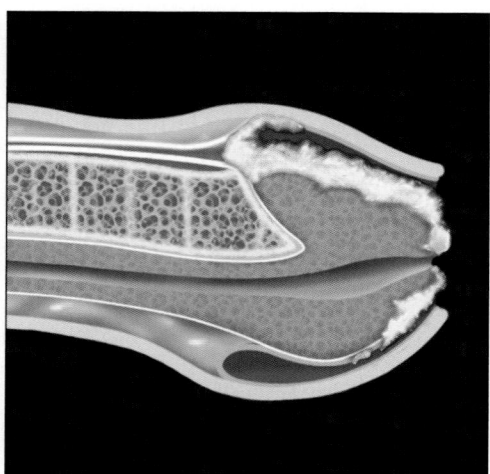

(Left) Tumor nests of grade 1 usual SCC show retained epithelial maturation, extensive keratinization with prominent keratin pearl formation ➡, and minimal cytologic atypia limited to basal/parabasal layers. *(Right)* In grade 2 usual SCC, nuclear atypia is more evident and extensive, but neoplastic cells still exhibit features of squamous differentiation with ample eosinophilic cytoplasm, distinctive cellular borders, and foci of keratinization ➡.

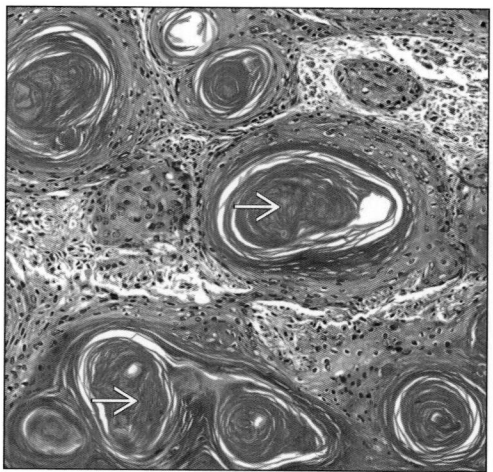
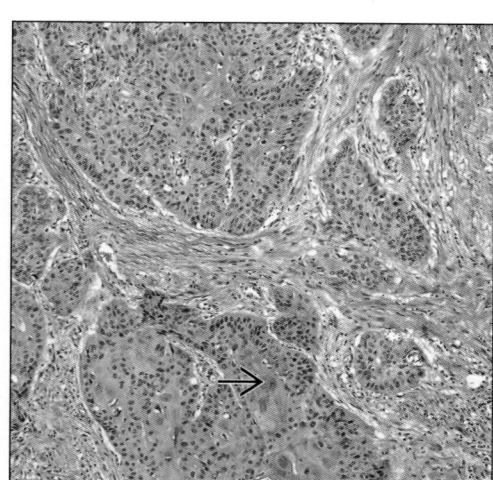

(Left) In grade 3 usual SCC, there is high-grade nuclear atypia and only minimal evidence of squamous differentiation ➡, but cells retain the morphological features of squamous differentiation with ample, eosinophilic cytoplasm and distinctive cellular borders. *(Right)* Presence of focal areas of anaplastic cells ➡, with nuclear pleomorphism, coarse chromatin, irregular nucleolema and evident nucleoli, in an otherwise low-grade usual SCC is sufficient to grade the tumor as grade 3.

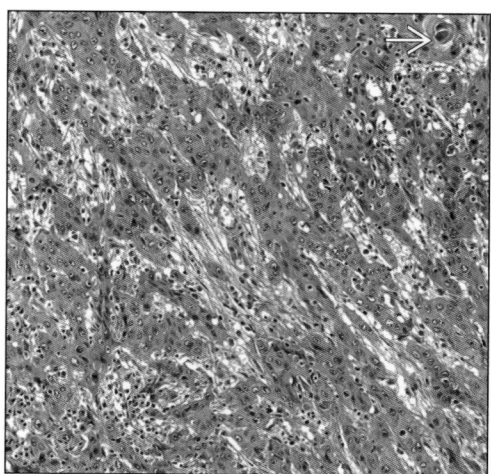
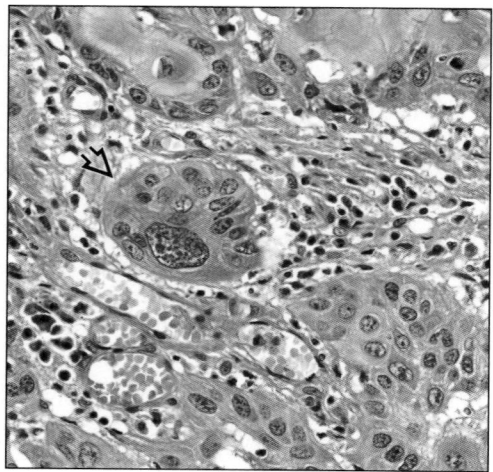

SQUAMOUS CELL CARCINOMA, USUAL TYPE

Microscopic Features

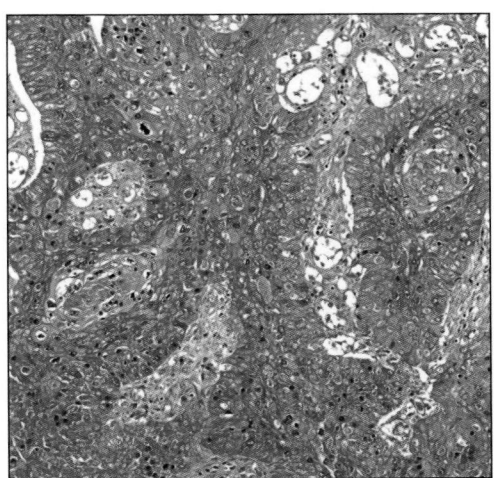

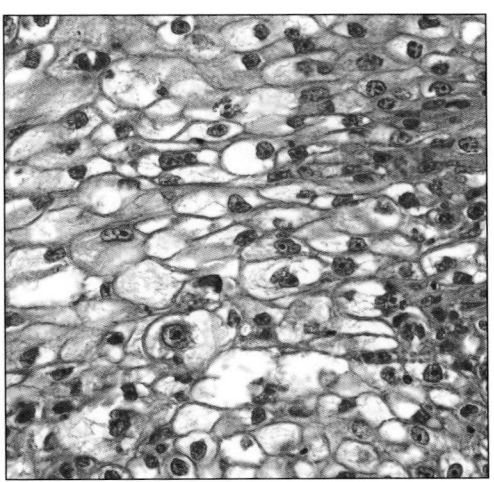

(Left) Tumor necrosis is a common feature of high-grade carcinomas, and it is characterized by neoplastic cells with diffuse cytoplasmic eosinophilia, retained cell shape, and pyknotic to absent nuclei, intermingled with viable cells. *(Right)* Clear cells, showing ample and pale cytoplasm, distinctive cellular borders, and nuclear pleomorphism ranging from mild to moderate, may be observed in some cases of usual SCC, but they are usually focal and not prominent.

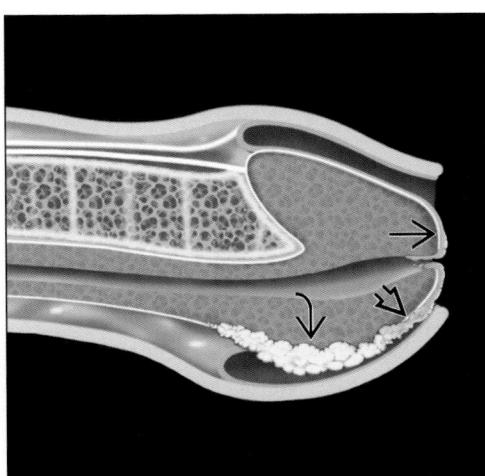

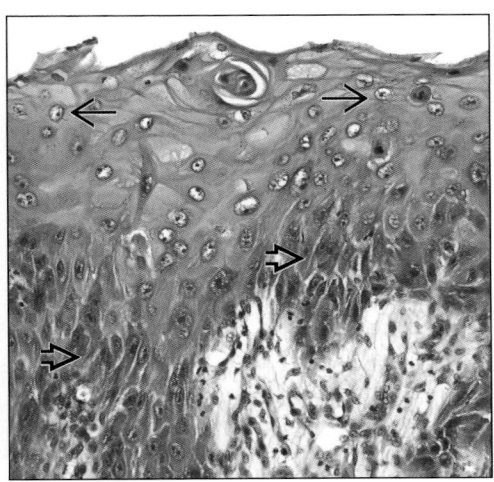

(Left) Most invasive usual SCC ⇒ are topographically associated with areas of squamous hyperplasia ⇒ and penile intraepithelial neoplasia ⇒, either adjacent or in continuity with the main tumor mass. *(Right)* Differentiated PeIN is commonly found in areas adjacent to the invasive component, and it is characterized by atypical cells ⇒ distributed throughout the entire epithelium ⇒ with retained squamous differentiation and slight to moderate parakeratosis.

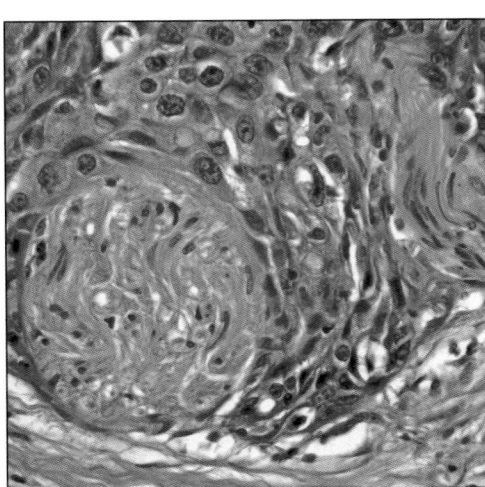

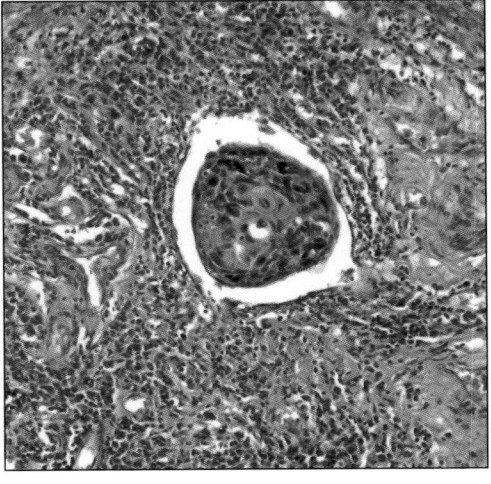

(Left) Perineural invasion, an important pathological prognostic factor, is accurately defined as invasion of perineural space by neoplastic cells and not just extension of the tumor along nerve bundles (nerve entrapment). *(Right)* Vascular invasion, another important prognostic factor, is characterized by presence of tumor emboli within vascular spaces, either within or in the periphery of the tumor, and can affect nutritional vessels as well as the penile erectile tissues.

PSEUDOHYPERPLASTIC CARCINOMA

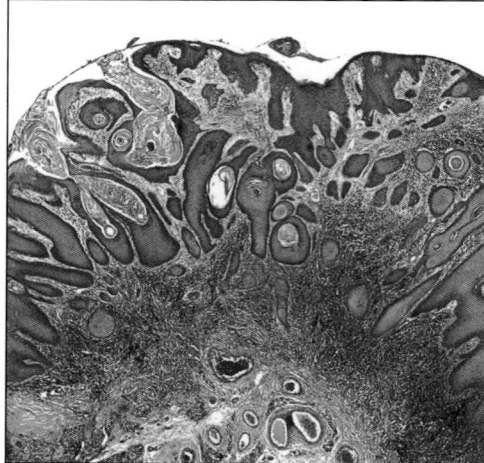

Well-differentiated pseudohyperplastic SCC is seen with flat to polypoid surface and downward proliferation of irregular nests. The differential diagnosis is with pseudoepitheliomatous hyperplasia.

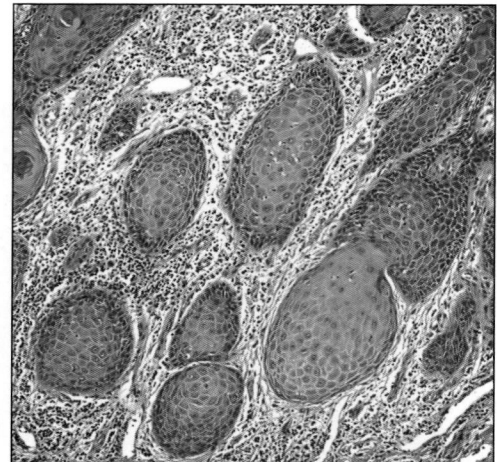

Appreciation of infiltrative tongues of well-differentiated tumor that invade the subepithelial connective tissue helps distinguish pseudohyperplastic carcinoma from a pseudoneoplastic lesion.

TERMINOLOGY

Abbreviations
- Squamous cell carcinoma (SCC)

Synonyms
- Pseudohyperplastic squamous cell carcinoma

Definitions
- Nonverruciform low-grade SCC preferentially affecting foreskin of older patients and strongly associated with lichen sclerosus (LS)

ETIOLOGY/PATHOGENESIS

Pathogenesis
- Unknown
- Probably unrelated to HPV
- Strong association with LS

CLINICAL ISSUES

Epidemiology
- Incidence
  - Only a few cases reported in literature
- Age
  - 8th decade

Site
- Foreskin

Presentation
- Nonverruciform hyperkeratotic tumor
- Usually affecting foreskin
- Often multicentric
- Other concurrent tumor pattern may be verrucous carcinoma
- Slowly growing lesions usually arising in background of LS

Treatment
- Surgical

Prognosis
- Excellent
- Minority of cases may recur showing higher grade areas

MACROSCOPIC FEATURES

General Features
- Hyperkeratotic flat or slightly elevated, nonverruciform tumors usually affecting foreskin
- Often multicentric
- Background of lichen sclerosus

Sections to Be Submitted
- Due to multicentricity, careful examination of margins is advised

Size
- Mean size is 2 cm

MICROSCOPIC PATHOLOGY

Histologic Features
- Extremely well-differentiated tumor
- May be confined to subepithelial connective tissue or infiltrate dartos in foreskin
- Downward proliferation of keratinizing nests of squamous cells
- Horn-pearl formation within infiltrating nests
- Occasional individual cell keratinization and mild atypia of basal cells
- Lack of koilocytosis
- Flat or slightly elevated surface
- Variable club-shaped and uneven/jagged infiltrative borders

PSEUDOHYPERPLASTIC CARCINOMA

Key Facts

Etiology/Pathogenesis
- Strong association with lichen sclerosus

Macroscopic Features
- Foreskin location
- Multicentricity
- Tumor with flat or slightly elevated hyperkeratotic surface

Microscopic Pathology
- Extremely well-differentiated carcinoma
- Flat or slightly elevated surface
- Background of LS

Top Differential Diagnoses
- Verrucous carcinoma
- Pseudoepitheliomatous hyperplasia

- Asymmetrical infiltrative nests surrounded by reactive fibrous stroma
- Inflammation is usually mild
- Adjacent epithelium shows LS with hyperplasia; may show differentiated PeIN

Predominant Pattern/Injury Type
- Squamous

Predominant Cell/Compartment Type
- Epithelial, biphasic or mixed

DIFFERENTIAL DIAGNOSIS

Verrucous Carcinoma
- Verruciform growth pattern with papillary architecture
- Elongated, broad, bulbous projections with pushing base

Pseudoepitheliomatous Hyperplasia
- Difficult differential diagnosis, especially in small biopsy specimens
- Limited to subepithelial connective tissue
- Infiltration of dartos or corpus spongiosum is not seen in hyperplasia
- Downward proliferation is more organized with elongated rete ridges
- Keratinization (keratin pearls) is less frequent
- Inflammation tends to be more prominent

DIAGNOSTIC CHECKLIST

Clinically Relevant Pathologic Features
- Often multicentric

Pathologic Interpretation Pearls
- It mimics pseudoepitheliomatous hyperplasia but deeper and more disorganized
  - Clinically, presence of a mass favors carcinoma
- Pseudohyperplastic SCC is seen in elderly with longstanding LS
- Extreme caution is advised before making diagnosis of pseudohyperplastic SCC in young patients, especially in absence of LS

SELECTED REFERENCES

1. Velazquez EF et al: Penile squamous cell carcinoma: anatomic, pathologic and viral studies in Paraguay (1993-2007). Anal Quant Cytol Histol. 29(4):185-98, 2007
2. Cubilla AL et al: Pseudohyperplastic squamous cell carcinoma of the penis associated with lichen sclerosus. An extremely well-differentiated, nonverruciform neoplasm that preferentially affects the foreskin and is frequently misdiagnosed: a report of 10 cases of a distinctive clinicopathologic entity. Am J Surg Pathol. 28(7):895-900, 2004

IMAGE GALLERY

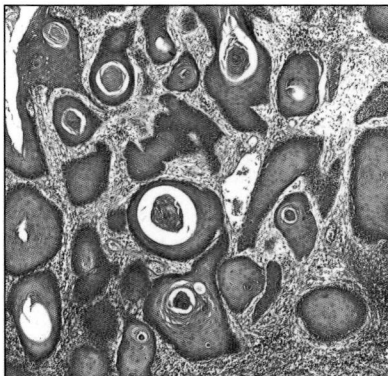 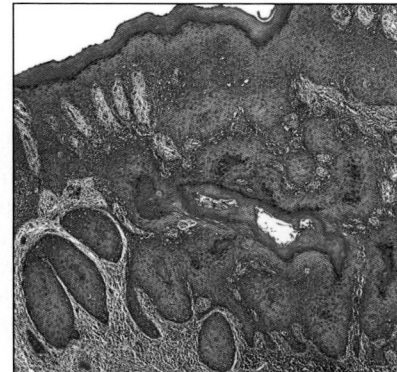 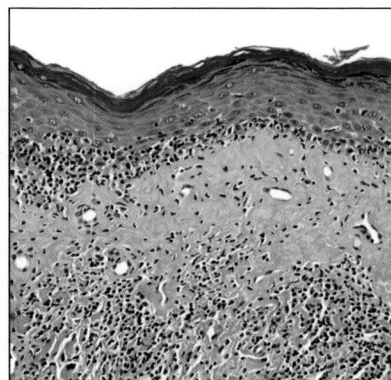

(Left) H&E of pseudohyperplastic SCC shows deep invasion by well-differentiated nests of varying size and shape help identify this lesion as a carcinoma. Pseudocysts are present due to keratin accumulation. *(Center)* Broad areas with pushing borders may also be present. Size of the lesion, overall complexity of architecture, and depth of penetration are important clues for malignancy. *(Right)* This picture illustrates classical features of lichen sclerosus. Pseudohyperplastic carcinoma classically arises in a background of longstanding lichen sclerosus.

WARTY CARCINOMA

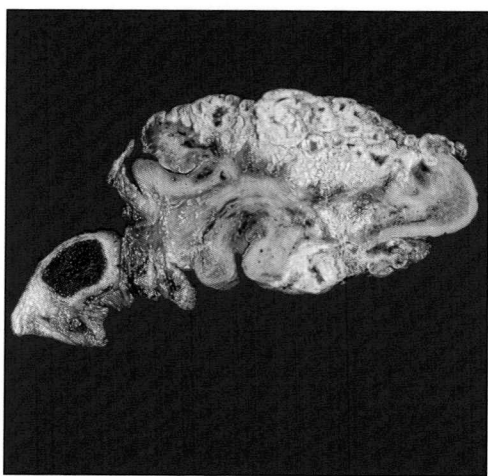

Cut section of a partial penectomy specimen shows a cauliflower, complex, papillomatous neoplasm deeply invading into corpus spongiosum, a warty (condylomatous) carcinoma.

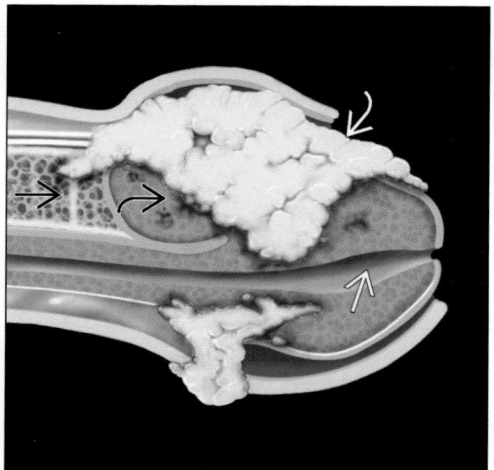

Diagram shows a warty carcinoma infiltrating the corpus spongiosum. Carcinoma ➽, corpus spongiosum ➽, corpus cavernosum ➽, and urethra ➽ are shown.

TERMINOLOGY

Abbreviations
- Warty carcinoma (WC)

Synonyms
- Condylomatous carcinoma

Definitions
- Tumor related to human papilloma virus (HPV)
  ○ Shares some gross and microscopic characteristics with condyloma
  ○ Definitive malignant histology and metastatic potential

ETIOLOGY/PATHOGENESIS

Etiology
- HPV-related in majority of cases (most cases associated with HPV-16)

Pathogenesis
- HPV oncoproteins E6 and E7 appear crucial in process of carcinogenesis
- E6 interferes with p53 pathway, causing suppression of p53 normal inhibitory function of cell cycle
- E7 targets retinoblastoma protein (pRB) interfering with p16/cyclin-D1/rb pathway

CLINICAL ISSUES

Epidemiology
- Incidence
  ○ 5-10% of penile squamous cell carcinoma
- Age
  ○ 50-55 years old

Presentation
- Slow-growing verruciform/papillary tumor usually affecting glans
- Coronal sulcus &/or foreskin may also be affected
- ± cobblestone appearance

Treatment
- Surgical

Prognosis
- Intermediate between that of other types of low-grade verruciform tumors (verrucous and papillary) and squamous cell carcinoma of usual type
- It may be associated with inguinal nodal metastasis
- Deeper tumors and higher histologic grade are associated with worse prognosis

MACROSCOPIC FEATURES

General Features
- Verrucous exo- to endophytic cauliflower-like tumor
- Usually affects more than 1 anatomical compartment (glans, coronal sulcus, and foreskin)
- Cut sections show papillomatous surface
- Deep borders usually penetrate into corpora spongiosa &/or cavernosa

Size
- 5 cm in average diameter

MICROSCOPIC PATHOLOGY

Histologic Features
- Often long and undulating papillae with prominent central fibrovascular core
- Sometimes rounded, arborescent papillae
- Atypical parakeratosis containing large nuclei is frequent

WARTY CARCINOMA

Key Facts

Terminology
- Condylomatous carcinoma

Etiology/Pathogenesis
- HPV-related tumor

Clinical Issues
- Papillomatous tumor with cobblestone appearance usually affecting glans

Macroscopic Features
- Usually large, cauliflower-like tumor
- Exo- to endophytic neoplasm
- Papillomatous surface
- Variable (pushing or infiltrative) deep border
- Usually infiltrates corpus spongiosum

Microscopic Pathology
- Low-power view shows classical clear and dark pattern
- Arborescent papillae
- Pleomorphic tumor
- Numerous mitoses
- Koilocytosis throughout neoplasm
- Variable (bulbous or infiltrative) deep borders
- Clear cell changes may be prominent

Top Differential Diagnoses
- Condyloma acuminatum (including giant condyloma)
- Verrucous carcinoma
- Papillary carcinoma
- Adnexal carcinomas
- Metastatic renal cell carcinoma

- Mixture of basaloid (lower epithelial layers) and koilocytotic cells (upper epithelial layers) gives classic light and dark low-power pattern
- Cells with enlarged nuclei with irregular contours, binucleation, multinucleation, clear perinuclear halo, and dyskeratosis are prominent (koilocytotic cells)
- Koilocytosis is present throughout tumor and not restricted to surface
- Cellular anaplasia may be marked
- Clear cell changes may be diffuse and prominent
- Numerous mitotic figures (including atypical ones) are frequent
- Variable deep borders: Pushing &/or jagged
- Deep endophytic growth pattern may be seen
- Intraepithelial abscesses may be prominent
- Adjacent epithelium shows penile intraepithelial neoplasia (PeIN) of warty/basaloid-type
- p16 is positive in majority of cases

Predominant Pattern/Injury Type
- Papillary

Predominant Cell/Compartment Type
- Epithelial, squamous

DIFFERENTIAL DIAGNOSIS

Giant Condyloma
- No nuclear anaplasia or invasion is present
- Benign extremely well-differentiated lesion with bulbous base
- Koilocytosis confined to surface

Verrucous Carcinoma
- Extremely well-differentiated lesion with bulbous base
- Lack of koilocytosis

Papillary Carcinoma
- Well-differentiated tumor with jagged infiltrative base
- Lack of koilocytosis

Clear Cell Carcinoma
- Tumor of sweat gland origin

- Affects inner portion of foreskin
- Exophytic but not papillomatous tumor
- Clear tumoral cells with intracytoplasmic PAS-D(+) material; CEA positive
- High metastatic potential

Metastatic Carcinomas with Clear Cell Features
- Usually not connected to overlying epithelium
- Lack of papillomatous surface
- No true koilocytic changes

Mixed Warty-Basaloid Carcinoma
- WC admixed with foci of basaloid carcinoma
- Important to recognize because basaloid component has worse prognosis

DIAGNOSTIC CHECKLIST

Clinically Relevant Pathologic Features
- Most frequent penile carcinoma seen in HIV-positive patients

Pathologic Interpretation Pearls
- Clear and dark low-power pattern
- Arborescent undulating papillae
- Koilocytosis with atypical features throughout

SELECTED REFERENCES

1. Liegl B et al: Penile clear cell carcinoma: a report of 5 cases of a distinct entity. Am J Surg Pathol. 28(11):1513-7, 2004
2. Bezerra AL et al: Clinicopathologic features and human papillomavirus dna prevalence of warty and squamous cell carcinoma of the penis. Am J Surg Pathol. 25(5):673-8, 2001
3. Cubilla AL et al: Warty (condylomatous) squamous cell carcinoma of the penis: a report of 11 cases and proposed classification of 'verruciform' penile tumors. Am J Surg Pathol. 24(4):505-12, 2000

WARTY CARCINOMA

Microscopic Features

(Left) Low-power view of warty carcinoma illustrates condylomatous arborescent papillae with prominent fibrovascular core. Note the dark (base) and clear (top) pattern. *(Right)* Another case of warty carcinoma shows long and undulating papillae. As seen at low power, the key differential diagnosis is papillary carcinoma, NOS, although the dark and clear pattern is a helpful feature.

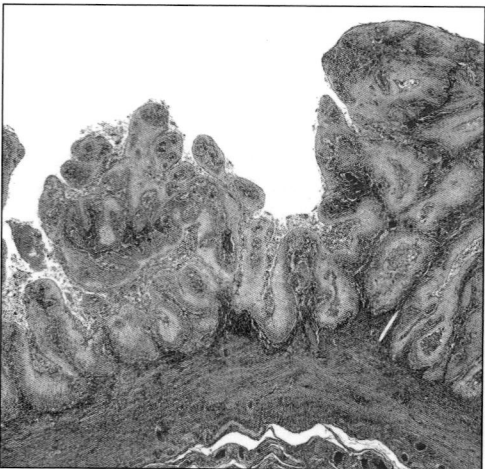
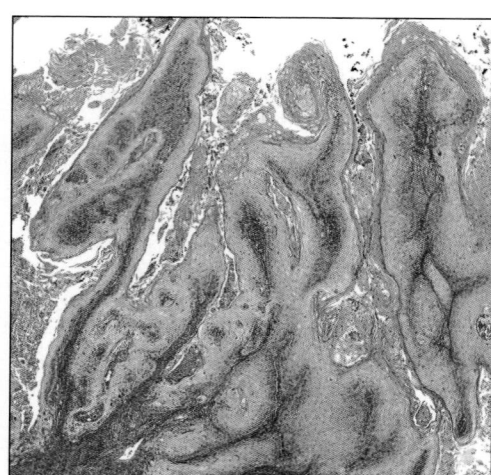

(Left) Higher power view shows the papillae with prominent koilocytosis. There is marked parakeratosis ⊟ and aberrant keratinization ⊡. *(Right)* Higher power view of warty carcinoma highlights the clear (koilocytic cells) ⊟ and dark (basaloid cells) pattern ⊡. The tumor stromal interface shows irregular jagged areas.

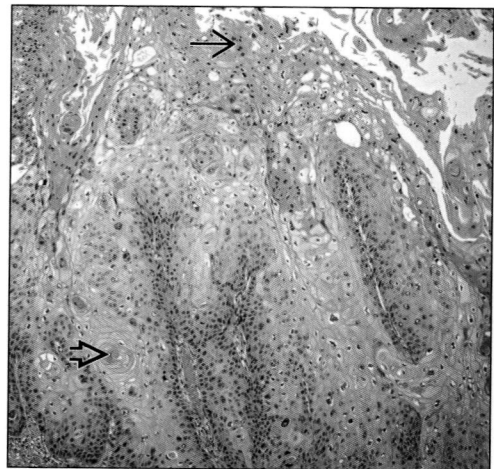
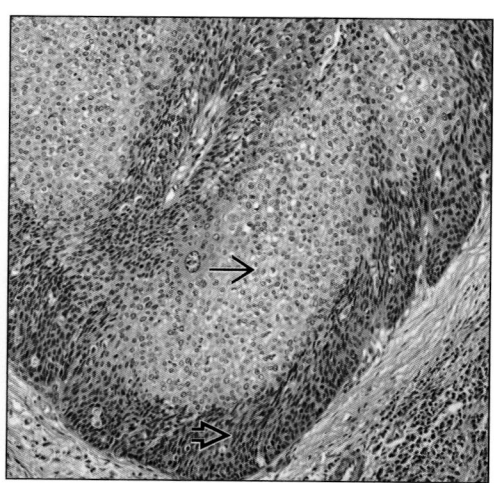

(Left) Koilocytosis is seen throughout the neoplasm. Note the obvious pleomorphic features of the neoplastic cells that are distributed randomly throughout. *(Right)* Well-differentiated warty carcinoma is shown with markedly atypical koilocytic changes that also affect the deeper portions of the tumor. The tumor-stromal interface is irregular and signifies destructive invasion, a feature that is not expected in a giant condyloma.

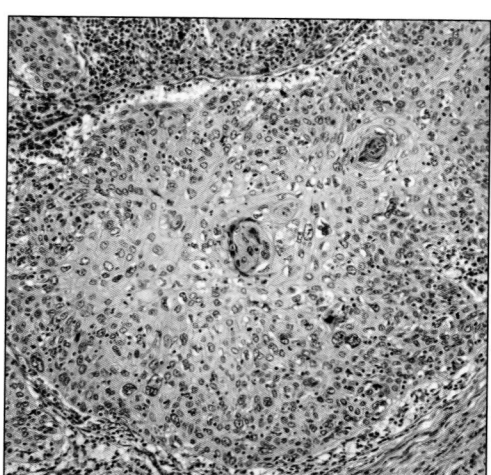
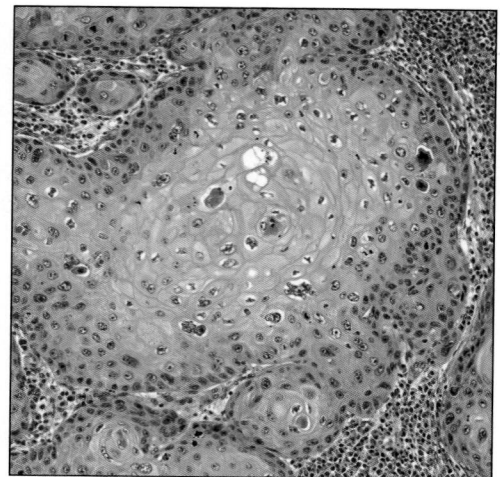

WARTY CARCINOMA

Microscopic Features

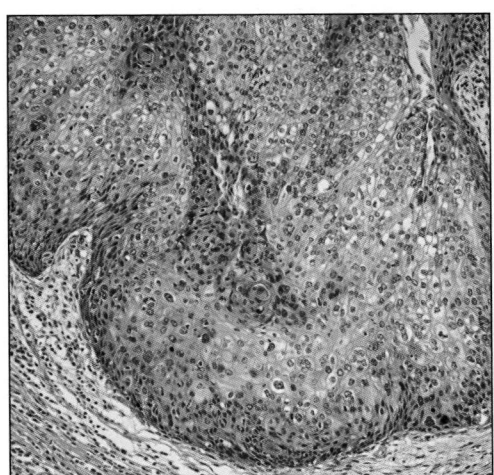

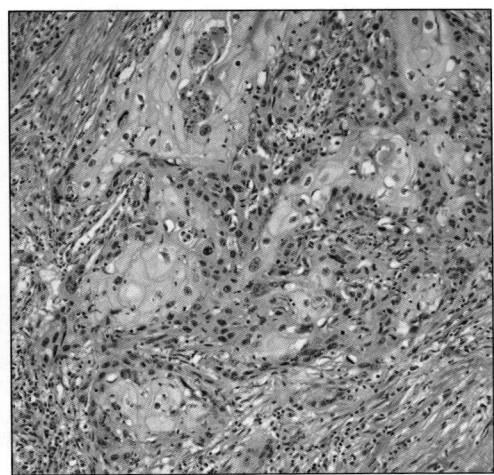

(Left) Warty carcinoma is shown with round pushing borders. Note the marked atypical koilocytic changes throughout the lesion. Although there may be some features reminiscent of condyloma, warty carcinoma clearly demonstrates malignant cytologic and architectural features. (Right) Warty carcinoma with infiltrative and jagged deep borders is seen. In contrast to conventional invasive carcinoma, warty carcinoma shows atypical koilocytic changes.

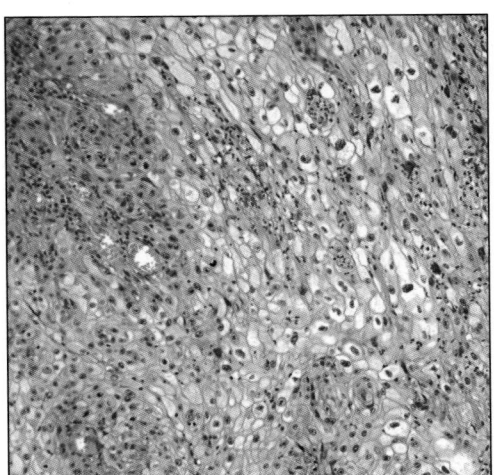

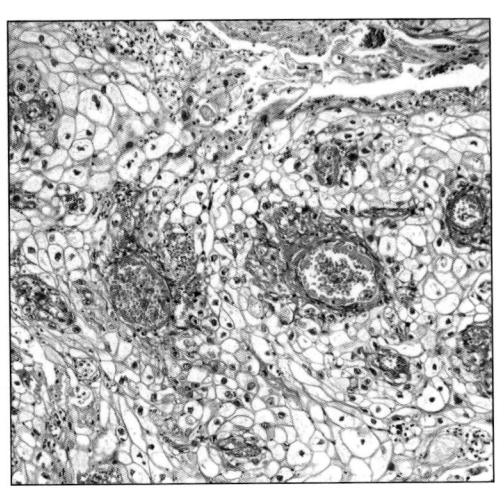

(Left) Warty carcinoma with focal clear cell changes is seen. In other foci of the tumor, typical cytoarchitectural features were present. (Right) Warty carcinoma with prominent clear cell features is seen. In spite of the prominent clear cell change, the neoplastic cells have a distinct squamous cell character, which helps distinguishing WC from metastatic carcinoma with clear cell features.

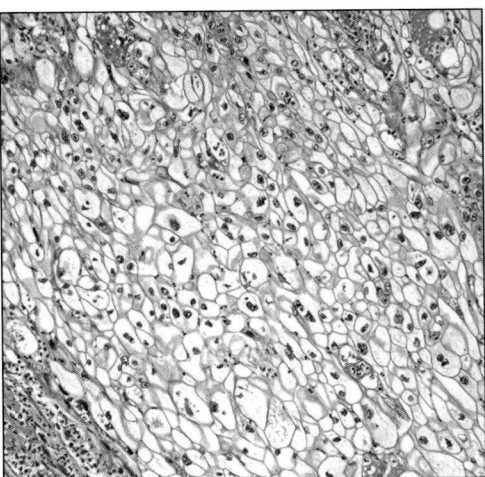

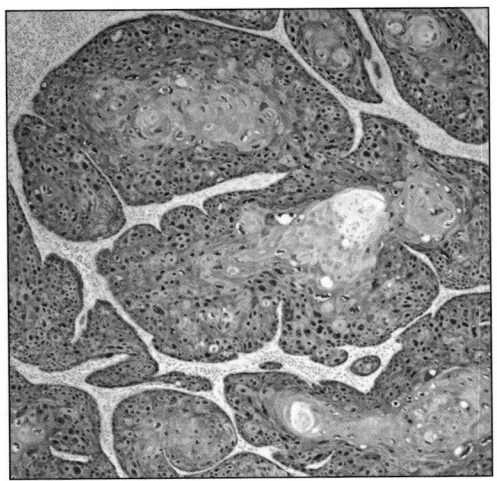

(Left) Prominent clear cell features are seen in this warty carcinoma. In contrast to other carcinomas with clear cell features that may affect the penis, the tumor has a distinct squamous cell appearance with well-defined cell borders. Other typical areas demonstrating intracellular keratin, keratin pearls, or intercellular bridges were also present. (Right) Immunohistochemistry with p16 shows diffuse positivity supporting the association of warty carcinoma with high-risk HPV.

VERRUCOUS CARCINOMA

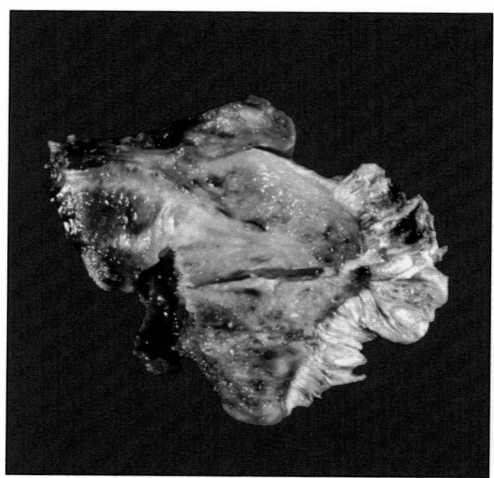

Cut section of a partial penectomy specimen shows a verruciform tumor with sharp bulbous base confined to the lamina propria.

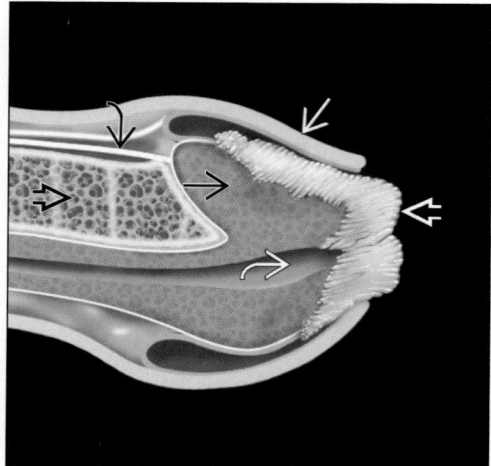

Graphic of a verrucous carcinoma (yellow) highlights the papillary, spiky surface and well-demarcated base. Note the VC ➡, corpus spongiosum ➡, foreskin ➡, albuginea ➡, corpus cavernosum ➡, and urethra ➡.

TERMINOLOGY

Abbreviations
• Verrucous carcinoma (VC)

Synonyms
• Well-differentiated squamous cell carcinoma

Definitions
• Extremely well-differentiated verruciform squamous cell carcinoma with bulbous deep borders and lack of koilocytosis

ETIOLOGY/PATHOGENESIS

Unknown Pathogenesis
• Likely HPV-unrelated
• Some cases are associated with lichen sclerosus
• Tumor suppressor gene *TP53* and its functional protein product p53 are believed to be involved in HPV-unrelated pathway of carcinogenesis

CLINICAL ISSUES

Epidemiology
• Incidence
  ○ Rare; approximately 4% of all penile carcinoma
• Age
  ○ Mean is 62 years

Site
• Glans &/or foreskin
• May be multicentric and affect more than 1 anatomic site

Presentation
• Exophytic white-gray neoplasm
• 1-3 cm in diameter
• May affect glans, coronal sulcus, &/or foreskin

• Unicentric tumors are more frequent
• Multicentric tumors may occur

Treatment
• Surgical

Prognosis
• Pure VCs have excellent prognosis
• Tumors may recur but almost never metastasize
• Sporadic reports of sarcomatoid transformation after radiation therapy

MACROSCOPIC FEATURES

General Features
• Exophytic white-gray neoplasms with papillary, sometimes spiky surface
• Cut sections reveal broad base between tumor and stroma
• Tumors are usually confined to lamina propria
• Involvement of deeper structures is less frequent
• Irregular jagged borders or foci of necrosis are not features of pure verrucous carcinoma

Size
• Average: 2 cm in diameter

MICROSCOPIC PATHOLOGY

Histologic Features
• Extremely well-differentiated neoplasm
• Thick acanthotic papillae with slender fibrovascular cores
• Papillae are separated by prominent keratin craters
• Orthokeratosis with presence of granular layer
• Parakeratosis may be occasional
• Absence of koilocytosis
• Pushing, club-shaped deep borders

VERRUCOUS CARCINOMA

Key Facts

Clinical Issues
- Unicentric tumors are more frequent
- Multicentric tumors may occur
- Some cases may be associated with longstanding lichen sclerosus

Macroscopic Features
- Exophytic papillary tumor
- Broad and pushing base
- Usually confined to lamina propria
- Rarely affects superficial corpus spongiosum

Microscopic Pathology
- Acanthotic papillae
- Slender fibrovascular cores
- Prominent (orange) keratin craters between papillae
- Lack of koilocytosis

- Extremely well differentiated
- Epithelium of papillae and keratin predominate over fibrovascular core
- Pushing, club-shaped base
- Higher grade areas &/or infiltrative borders are not features of pure VC and raise possibility of hybrid (mixed) VC

Top Differential Diagnoses
- Condyloma acuminatum/giant condyloma
- Warty (condylomatous) carcinoma
- Papillary carcinoma, NOS
- Mixed VC/SCC of usual type
- Carcinoma cuniculatum

- Adjacent epithelium often shows verrucous squamous hyperplasia &/or differentiated penile intraepithelial neoplasia (differentiated PeIN)
- Some cases associated with background of lichen sclerosus

Predominant Pattern/Injury Type
- Papillary

Predominant Cell/Compartment Type
- Epithelial, squamous

DIFFERENTIAL DIAGNOSIS

Giant Condyloma
- More rounded, arborescent papillae
- Koilocytosis on surface

Warty Carcinoma
- Higher histological grade
- Prominent koilocytosis throughout neoplasm
- May have infiltrative deep borders

Papillary Carcinoma
- Well to moderately differentiated
- Infiltrative borders

Mixed (Hybrid) Verrucous Carcinoma
- VC admixed with foci of SCC of usual type
- Focal infiltrative, jagged borders
- Focal higher grade areas
- Prognosis is not as good as pure verrucous carcinoma
- 25% of cases associated with lymph node metastasis

Carcinoma Cuniculatum
- Hybrid (mixed) VC
- Characteristic burrowing pattern
- Focal higher grade areas
- Focal jagged borders

DIAGNOSTIC CHECKLIST

Pathologic Interpretation Pearls
- If entire lesion is not sampled, recommended diagnosis is "well-differentiated squamous cell carcinoma, verrucous histology"
  - Acknowledges likelihood of unsampled moderately or poorly differentiated invasive conventional carcinoma in definitive excision
- Acanthotic papillae with thin fibrovascular cores
- Piling up of keratin between papillae (keratin craters) is characteristic
- Epithelium and keratin predominate over fibrovascular cores
- Keratin within craters tends to have orange color
- Extremely well-differentiated tumor from top to bottom
- Club-shaped pushing base

SELECTED REFERENCES

1. Chaux A et al: Comparison of Subtypes of Penile Squamous Cell Carcinoma From High and Low Incidence Geographical Regions. Int J Surg Pathol. Epub ahead of print, 2009
2. Stankiewicz E et al: HPV infection and immunochemical detection of cell-cycle markers in verrucous carcinoma of the penis. Mod Pathol. 22(9):1160-8, 2009
3. Velazquez EF et al: Penile squamous cell carcinoma: anatomic, pathologic and viral studies in Paraguay (1993-2007). Anal Quant Cytol Histol. 29(4):185-98, 2007
4. Velazquez EF et al: Lichen sclerosus in 68 patients with squamous cell carcinoma of the penis: frequent atypias and correlation with special carcinoma variants suggests a precancerous role. Am J Surg Pathol. 27(11):1448-53, 2003
5. Fukunaga M et al: Penile verrucous carcinoma with anaplastic transformation following radiotherapy. A case report with human papillomavirus typing and flow cytometric DNA studies. Am J Surg Pathol. 18(5):501-5, 1994

VERRUCOUS CARCINOMA

Microscopic Features

(Left) Low-power view of a verrucous carcinoma illustrates the thick acanthotic papillae, thin fibrovascular cores, and the classic piling up of keratin between papillae. *(Right)* Note the abundant orange keratin ⮥ and bulbous base typical of verrucous carcinoma. The acanthotic epithelium and abundant keratin are much more prominent than the thin fibrovascular cores.

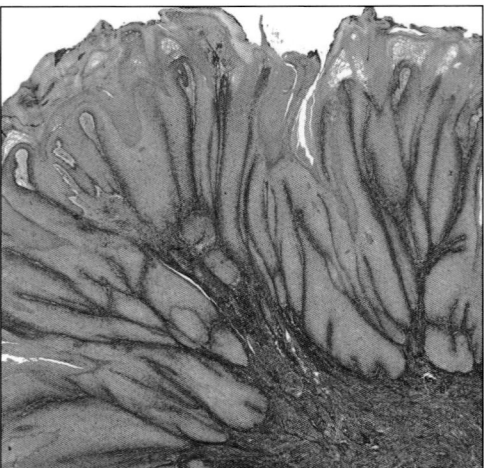 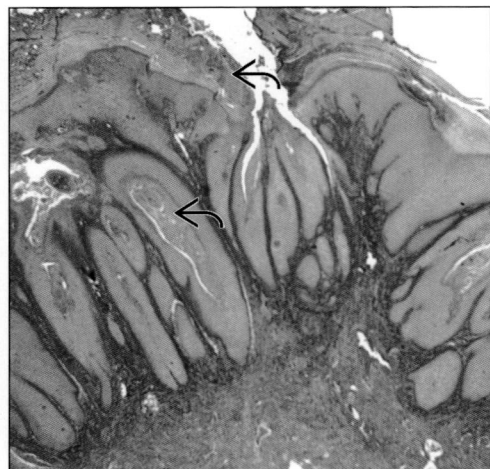

(Left) Verrucous carcinoma shows extremely well-differentiated endophytic bulbous borders. *(Right)* Abundant keratin-filled craters are usually seen in verrucous carcinoma. In a superficial biopsy specimen in which the entire architecture cannot be appreciated, the diagnosis of malignancy can be challenging. Clinicopathologic correlation with the size of the lesion &/or additional sampling is necessary.

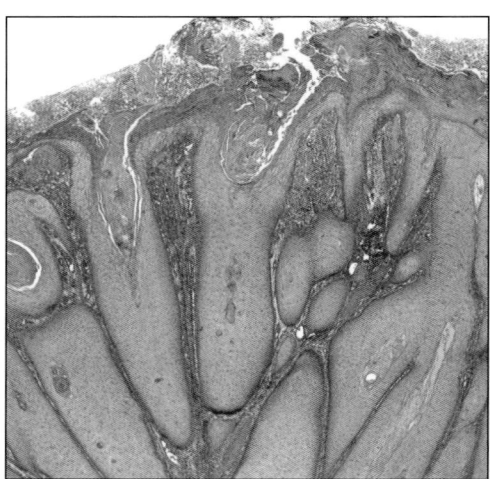 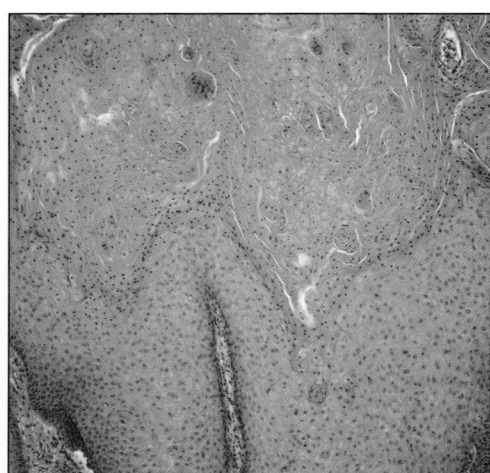

(Left) Extremely well-differentiated tumor with craters containing abundant (orange) keratin material ⮥ in this case of verrucous carcinoma. *(Right)* Note the club-shaped bulbous deep borders. Pure verrucous carcinoma is extremely well-differentiated, including its deep portion. The bulbous base is a key differentiating feature from pseudoepitheliomatous hyperplasia, which has narrow elongated rete ridges. The absence of koilocytic atypia helps distinguish it from a giant condyloma.

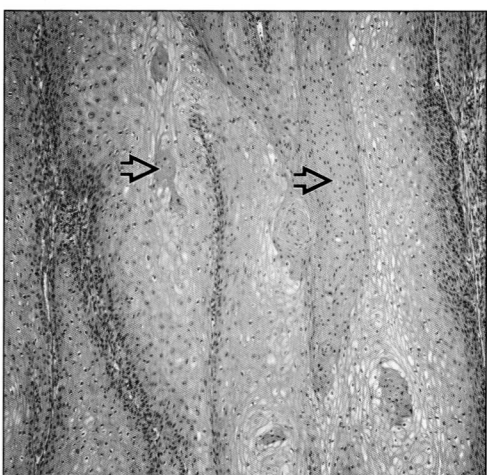 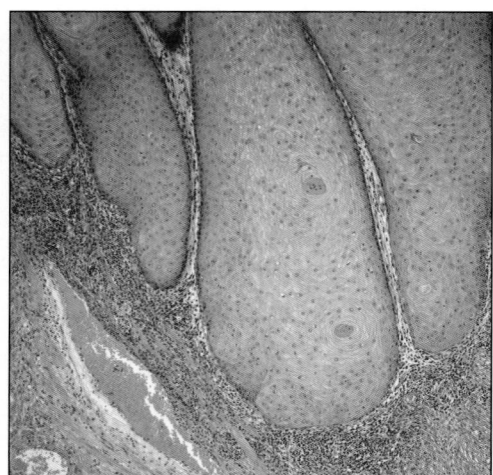

VERRUCOUS CARCINOMA

Differential Diagnosis

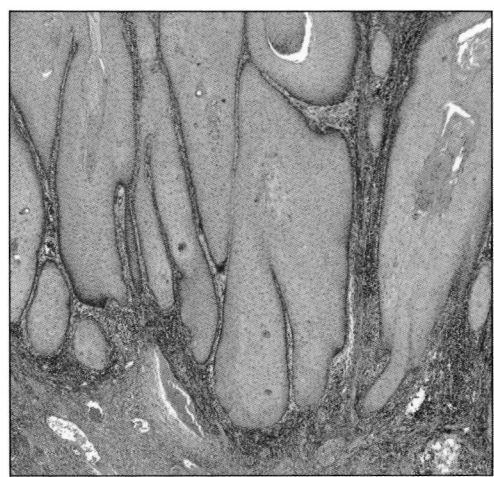

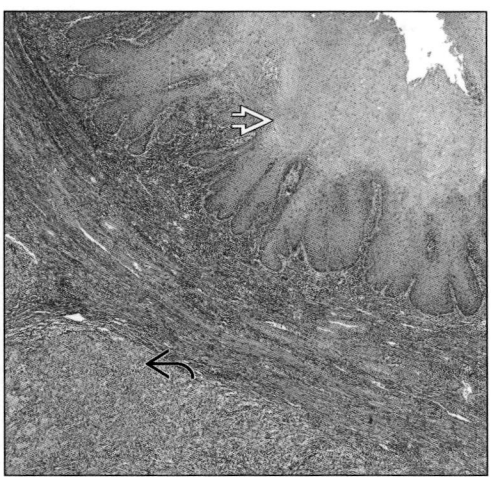

(Left) Deep borders are bulbous and club-shaped in this case of pure verrucous carcinoma. *(Right)* Hybrid (mixed) VC shows areas of classic VC ➡ associated with poorly differentiated areas ➡. If the entire lesion is not sampled, the recommended diagnosis is "well-differentiated squamous cell carcinoma, verrucous histology." This acknowledges the likelihood that there may be unsampled moderately or poorly differentiated invasive conventional carcinoma in the definitive excision.

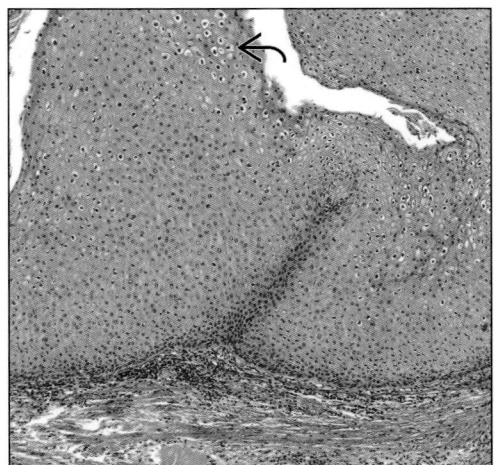

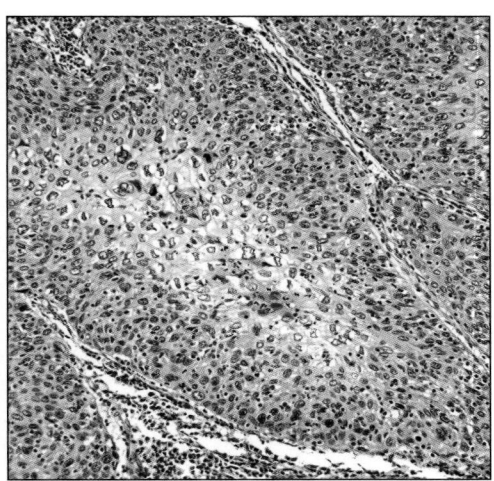

(Left) In this case of condyloma acuminatum, the lesion has some features reminiscent of verrucous carcinoma; however, there is koilocytosis on the surface ➡. *(Right)* Atypical koilocytic changes are seen throughout the tumor in this case of warty carcinoma. In addition to malignant cytologic features, this neoplasm demonstrates conventional destructive invasion at the base.

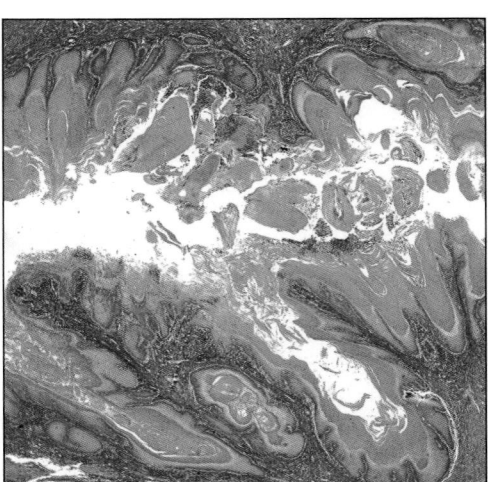

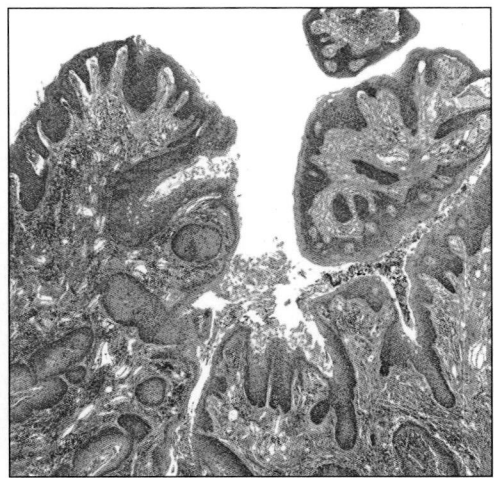

(Left) In this case of carcinoma cuniculatum, the bulk of the tumor has features of verrucous carcinoma. The hallmark of the lesion is an endophytic and complex burrowing pattern. *(Right)* Papillary carcinoma, NOS, shows arborescent papillae. Fibrovascular cores are more prominent than in VC. Papillary carcinoma, NOS, is less well differentiated than VC and shows infiltrative deep borders. It is distinguished from warty carcinoma by lack of atypical koilocytic changes.

BASALOID CARCINOMA

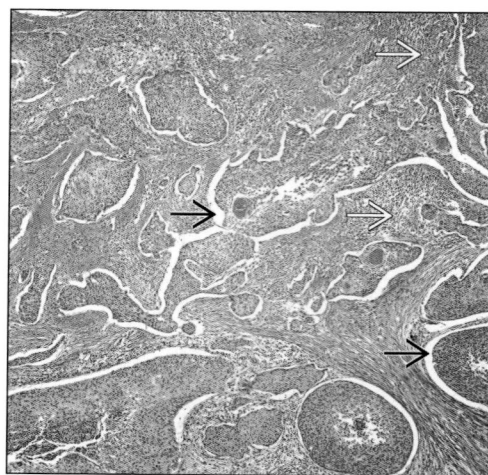

Low-power view of basaloid carcinoma depicts the typical highly infiltrative pattern of nests composed of poorly differentiated cells with retraction artifact ➡ and intense stromal reaction ➡.

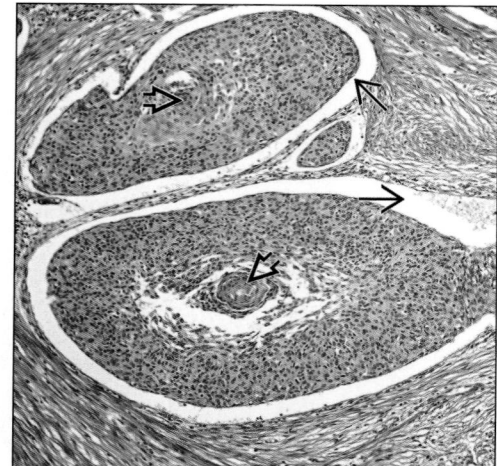

Basaloid SCC nests of poorly differentiated carcinoma are seen with retraction spaces ➡ and central, abrupt foci of keratinization ➡. Keratinization is typically focal in the majority of cases.

TERMINOLOGY

Synonyms
- Basaloid squamous cell carcinoma (SCC)

Definitions
- Aggressive variant of nonkeratinizing SCC composed of small to intermediate-sized basaloid cells

ETIOLOGY/PATHOGENESIS

Infectious Agents
- Most cases are associated with human papillomavirus (HPV)
- Serotype 16 is most common

CLINICAL ISSUES

Epidemiology
- Incidence
  - 10-14% of all penile SCC
- Age
  - Average = 52-54 years at presentation

Presentation
- Large, ulcerated, nonexophytic mass
- 1/2 to 2/3 of patients have positive inguinal nodes at diagnosis

Treatment
- Surgical approaches
  - Deep tumors are treated with total penectomy and bilateral groin dissection
  - Tumors confined to superficial corpus spongiosum may be treated with partial penectomy
- Adjuvant therapy
  - Chemotherapy for advanced cases
- Radiation
  - Selected cases with superficial erectile tissue invasion

Prognosis
- Local recurrence seen in 1/3 of cases
- Regional metastases present in > 1/2 of patients
- High cancer-specific mortality

MACROSCOPIC FEATURES

General Features
- Unicentric tumor
- Usually affects glans
- May extend to coronal sulcus and foreskin
- Exclusive foreskin location is uncommon
- Deeply invasive solid tumor
- Vertical growth pattern
- Tan-gray color often showing minute yellow dot-like areas of punctate necrosis
- Invasion of corpus cavernosum seen in many cases

MICROSCOPIC PATHOLOGY

Histologic Features
- Nests of infiltrative basaloid cells with variable intervening stroma
- Tumoral nests are frequently surrounded by retraction artifact
- Inconspicuous to absent peripheral palisading
- Central necrosis (comedonecrosis) commonly found in nests
- Focal and abrupt central keratinization may be seen in some nests
- Neoplastic cells are small to medium-sized and round to oval
- High nuclear:cytoplasmic ratio (blue cells)
- Mild to moderate nuclear pleomorphism; overall monomorphous appearance
- Numerous mitoses and prominent apoptosis are characteristic
  - "Starry sky" pattern is common

BASALOID CARCINOMA

Key Facts

Etiology/Pathogenesis
- HPV is detected in most cases
- Serotype 16 is most common

Clinical Issues
- Represents 10-14% of all penile SCC
- Up to 2/3 of patients have positive inguinal nodes at diagnosis

Macroscopic Features
- Usually affecting the glans
- Vertical growth pattern
- Deeply invasive into deep anatomical structures

Microscopic Pathology
- Closely packed nests of basaloid cells
- Central necrosis and keratin debris
- Focal and abrupt central keratinization

- Peripheral clefting between tumor nests and stroma
- Peripheral palisading is inconspicuous
- Scant intervening stroma
- Tumoral cells show high nuclear:cytoplasmic ratio
- Numerous mitoses and prominent apoptosis
- Sometimes "starry sky" pattern
- Spindle and pleomorphic cells in some cases
- PeIN of basaloid type frequently found in adjacent areas

Top Differential Diagnoses
- Usual type of SCC with a nesting pattern
- Warty/basaloid carcinoma
- Urothelial carcinoma of distal urethra
- Cutaneous basal cell carcinoma
- Small cell neuroendocrine carcinoma

- Adenoid cystic-like morphology secondary to extensive acantholysis is rare but may predominate
- Clear cell changes and spindle cell features may be seen in rare cases
- Perineural invasion seen in 1/2 of cases
- Extension to distal urethra present in 2/3 of cases
- Basaloid type of penile intraepithelial neoplasia (PeIN) is frequently found in adjacent areas

Predominant Cell/Compartment Type
- Epithelial, basaloid

DIFFERENTIAL DIAGNOSIS

Usual SCC with a Nesting Pattern
- Predominantly composed of large cells with ample eosinophilic cytoplasm (pink cells)
- Higher nuclear pleomorphism

Warty/Basaloid (Mixed) Carcinoma
- Mixed SCC variant composed of admixture of warty and basaloid carcinomas
- Mixed verruciform-vertical patterns of growth
- Frequently warty and basaloid areas are intimately admixed
- Less frequently, warty and basaloid areas are separate
- Any of the morphological components may predominate
- Poor prognosis (similar to basaloid carcinoma)

Urothelial Carcinoma of Distal Urethra
- Previous or concurrent history of urinary tract urothelial carcinoma
- Urothelial features usually recognizable with more pleomorphic cells
- Usually associated with urothelial carcinoma in situ
- Frequent association with squamous &/or glandular differentiation
- Immunohistochemical positivity for uroplakin-3 and thrombomodulin

Cutaneous Basal Cell Carcinoma
- Preferential penile shaft location
- Less pleomorphic neoplastic cells
- Peripheral palisading and myxoid stromal changes

Small Cell Neuroendocrine Carcinoma
- Extremely rare
- May be difficult to differentiate from basaloid carcinoma on morphology alone
- Immunohistochemical stains for neuroendocrine markers may be necessary

DIAGNOSTIC CHECKLIST

Pathologic Interpretation Pearls
- Neoplastic cells are small round and blue (basaloid cells)
- Arranged in solid nests frequently showing comedonecrosis or abrupt central keratinization
- Peripheral clefting seen between tumor and stroma

SELECTED REFERENCES

1. Guimarães GC et al: Penile squamous cell carcinoma clinicopathological features, nodal metastasis and outcome in 333 cases. J Urol. 182(2):528-34; discussion 534, 2009
2. Rubin MA et al: Detection and typing of human papillomavirus DNA in penile carcinoma: evidence for multiple independent pathways of penile carcinogenesis. Am J Pathol. 159(4):1211-8, 2001
3. Cubilla AL et al: Basaloid squamous cell carcinoma: a distinctive human papilloma virus-related penile neoplasm: a report of 20 cases. Am J Surg Pathol. 22(6):755-61, 1998
4. Gregoire L et al: Preferential association of human papillomavirus with high-grade histologic variants of penile-invasive squamous cell carcinoma. J Natl Cancer Inst. 87(22):1705-9, 1995

BASALOID CARCINOMA

Microscopic Features

(Left) Tumor nests of basaloid carcinoma extensively infiltrate penile parenchyma. There is central comedonecrosis ⊟ and focal vascular lymphatic invasion ⊟. Peripheral palisading is inconspicuous. This carcinoma is frequently associated with vertical growth pattern of penile carcinoma. *(Right)* A tumor nest of basaloid carcinoma with central necrosis is seen containing keratin debris ⊟. The retraction artifact ⊟ surrounding the tumor nest is a common feature.

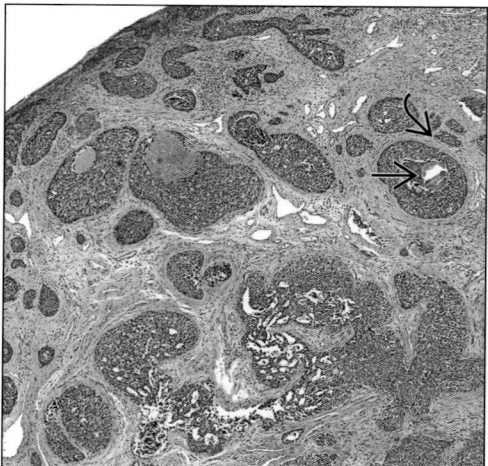
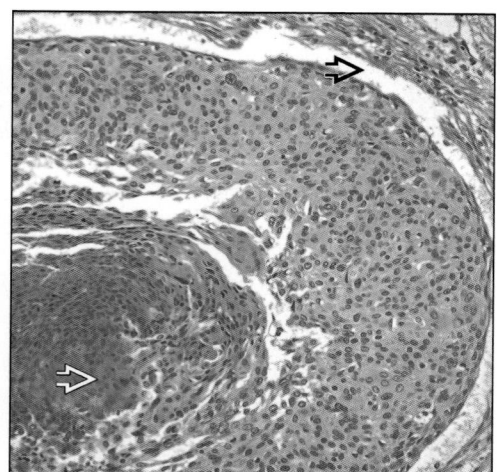

(Left) Neoplastic cells of basaloid carcinomas show moderate nuclear pleomorphism, indistinct cellular borders, and nonkeratinized cytoplasm. The cell population is monotonous and fairly uniform. There is an abundance of mitotic figures ⊟ which, on low power, may impart a "starry sky" appearance. *(Right)* Focally, more pleomorphic and solid patterns may also be observed with greater degree of nuclear atypia and irregularly shaped tumor nests.

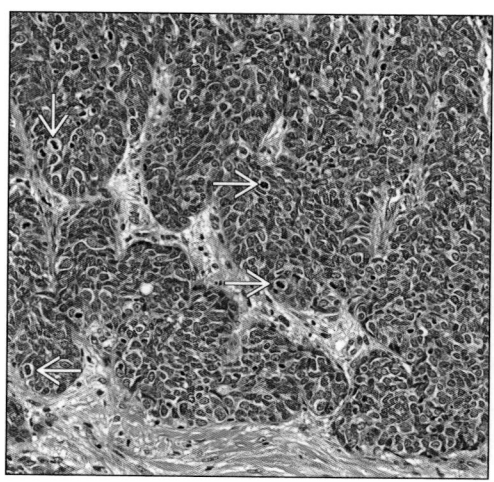
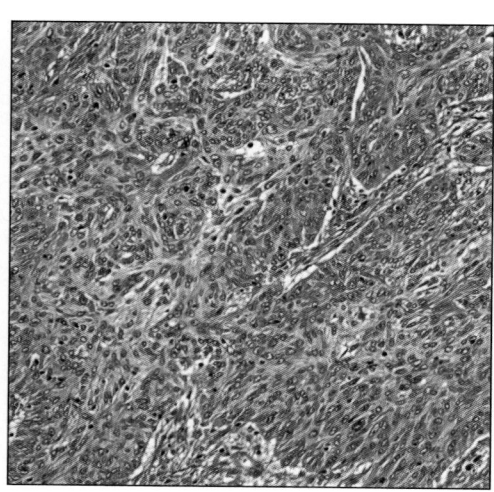

(Left) In this case of basaloid carcinoma, there are areas with greater pleomorphism and spindle cell morphology. Cytoplasm retains typical basaloid features with lack of keratinization, high nuclear:cytoplasmic ratios, and indistinct cellular borders. *(Right)* Basaloid (HPV-associated) PeIN is frequently found adjacent to the invasive component. The entire epithelium is replaced by a monotonous population of basaloid cells. Parakeratosis ⊟ is a common finding.

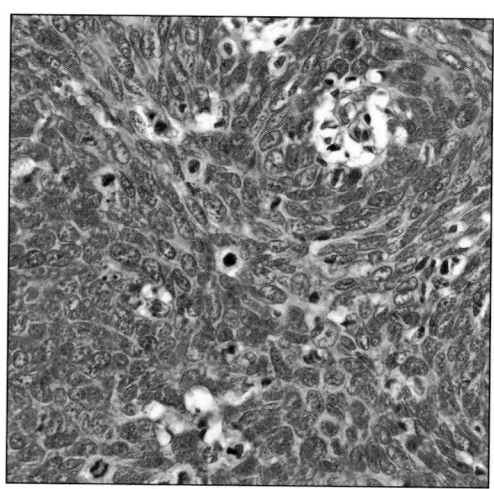
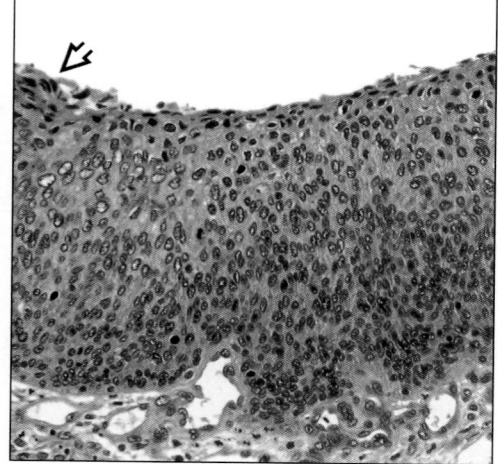

BASALOID CARCINOMA

Microscopic Features and Differential Diagnosis

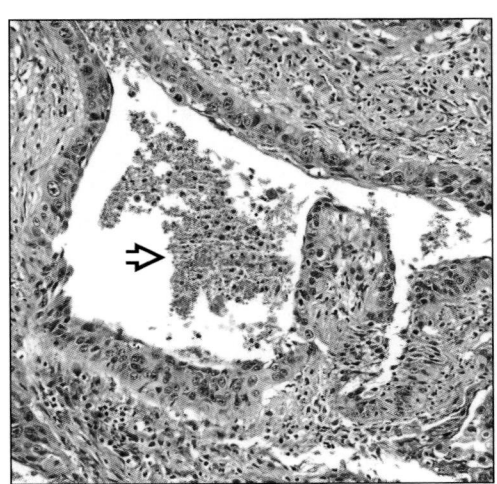

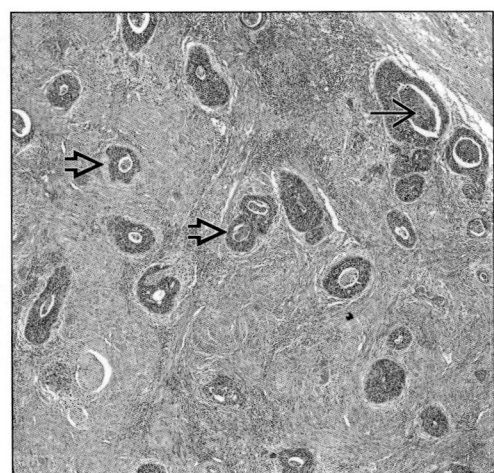

(Left) Tumor nests with extensive central necrosis ⊟ simulate pseudoglandular structures. When these features predominate throughout the tumor, the diagnosis of pseudoglandular (acantholytic) carcinoma is appropriate. *(Right)* An adenoid cystic-like appearance may focally be observed, with highly infiltrative small and regular tumor nests ⊟ and central necrosis → simulating glandular lumina. A poorly differentiated urothelial carcinoma is also in the differential diagnosis.

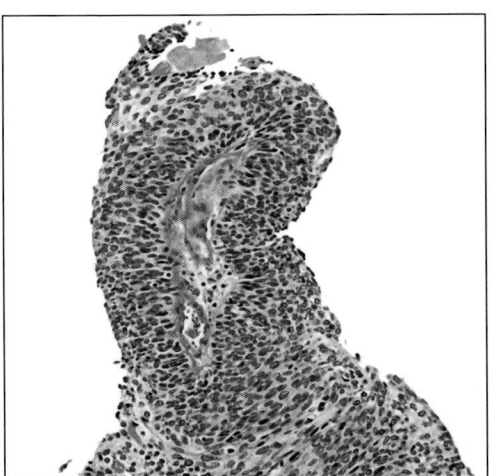

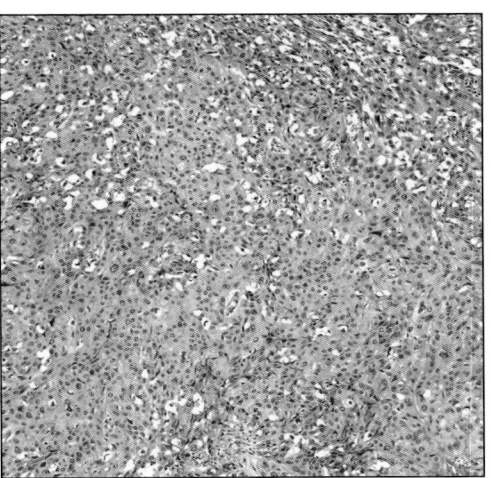

(Left) In extremely rare cases, basaloid carcinomas show an exophytic papillary pattern of growth. Papillae are lined by typical basaloid cells. This variant of basaloid carcinoma should be distinguished from urothelial carcinoma. *(Right)* High-grade usual SCC with a predominantly solid pattern of growth may simulate basaloid carcinoma. However, the neoplastic cells are typically more pleomorphic and retain squamous features, with ample and keratinized (eosinophilic) cytoplasm.

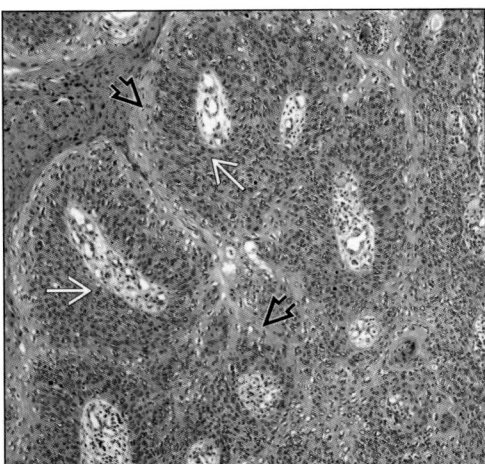

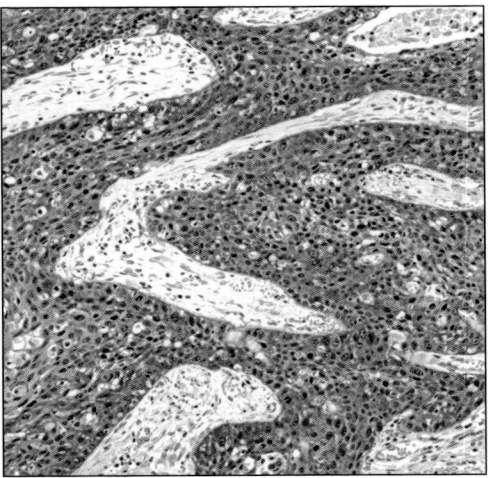

(Left) Warty/basaloid carcinoma is a mixed subtype of penile SCC with condylomatous papillae and tumor nests lined by pleomorphic koilocytes in the surface/periphery ⊟ and basaloid cells in the deep/central areas ➡. *(Right)* In basaloid carcinomas, the neoplastic cells typically show strong and diffuse immunoreactivity for p16 over-expression.

SARCOMATOID CARCINOMA, PENIS

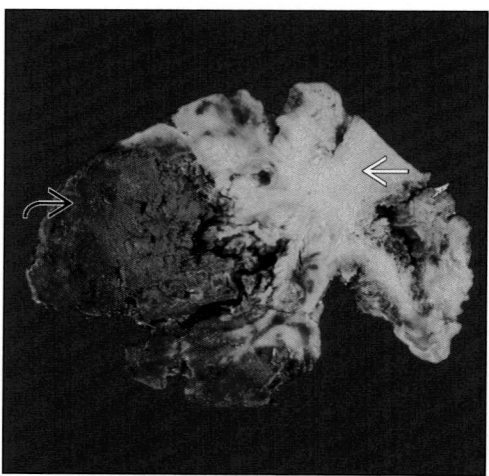

Partial penectomy specimen shows a large and hemorrhagic, deeply invasive tumor ⇗ arising from the distal portion of the organ. The tumor extensively invades the corpora cavernosa ➡.

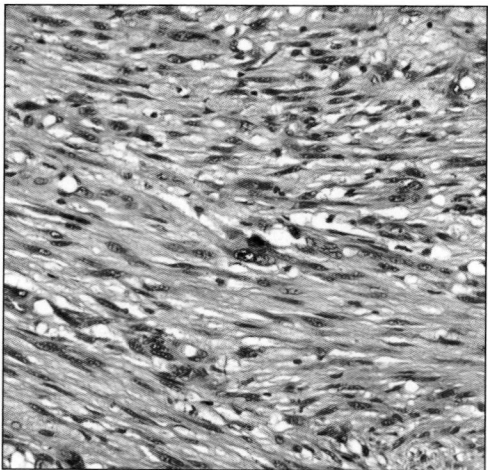

This sarcomatoid carcinoma is predominantly composed of fascicles of atypical spindle cells with pleomorphic nuclei and mitoses.

TERMINOLOGY

Abbreviations
- Sarcomatoid squamous cell carcinoma (SCC)

Synonyms
- Spindle cell carcinoma, carcinosarcoma, metaplastic carcinoma

Definitions
- Undifferentiated carcinoma arising from squamous epithelium composed of malignant spindle cells

ETIOLOGY/PATHOGENESIS

Pathogenesis
- Uncertain
- HPV association unknown; unlikely

CLINICAL ISSUES

Epidemiology
- Incidence
  ○ Approximately 4% of penile SCCs
- Age
  ○ Mean is 60 years

Site
- Glans, often extending to coronal sulcus and foreskin

Presentation
- Large, polypoid, and ulcerated mass deeply invading corpora spongiosum and cavernosa

Treatment
- Surgical or multimodal

Prognosis
- Usually associated with lymph node metastasis
- Poor prognosis

MACROSCOPIC FEATURES

General Features
- Large, polypoid, and ulcerated mass affecting glans, coronal sulcus, &/or foreskin
- Cut surface shows solid white/gray to hemorrhagic deeply invasive neoplasm
- Usually invades corpora spongiosum and cavernosa
- Smaller satellite nodules may be present away from main mass

MICROSCOPIC PATHOLOGY

Histologic Features
- Predominantly composed of patternless atypical spindle cells or those in interlacing fascicles
- May resemble fibrosarcoma or leiomyosarcoma
- Pleomorphic giant cells mimicking malignant fibrous histiocytoma may be seen
- Myxoid changes may be prominent
- May have pseudovascular pattern mimicking angiosarcoma
- Foci of bone and cartilaginous heterologous differentiation may be observed
- Mitotic figures are numerous and necrosis may be prominent
- Lymphovascular and perineural invasion are common findings
- SCC in situ &/or clear-cut squamous invasive component may be focally present

Margins
- Large main tumor or smaller satellite nodules may involve surgical margin

Predominant Pattern/Injury Type
- Sarcomatoid

SARCOMATOID CARCINOMA, PENIS

Key Facts

Terminology
- Synonyms
  - Spindle cell carcinoma, carcinosarcoma

Macroscopic Features
- Large polypoid mass usually affecting glans, coronal sulcus, and foreskin
- Deeply invading into corpora spongiosa and cavernosa
- Separate satellite nodules may be present

Microscopic Pathology
- Predominantly composed of atypical spindle cells disposed in interlacing fascicles
- Myxoid changes may be marked
- Pseudovascular spaces may be prominent mimicking angiosarcoma

- Carcinoma in situ or clear-cut invasive SCC may be only very focally present

Ancillary Tests
- Immunohistochemical studies are often necessary to make diagnosis
  - Spindle cells are positive for vimentin, cytokeratins, and p63
  - Cytokeratin expression (especially PAN-CK[AE1/AE3] and Cam5.2) by spindle cells may be only focal
  - PAN-CK(AE1/AE3) and HMCK(34βE12) tend to be more diffusely expressed by spindle cells

Top Differential Diagnoses
- Spindle cell melanoma
- Sarcoma

Predominant Cell/Compartment Type
- Epithelial, squamous with predominant spindle cell component

ANCILLARY TESTS

Immunohistochemistry
- Immunohistochemical studies are often necessary to make correct diagnosis
- Spindle cells are positive for vimentin, cytokeratins, and p63
- Cytokeratin expression (especially PAN-CK[AE1/AE3] and Cam5.2) by spindle cells may be only focal
- PAN-CK(AE1/AE3) and HMCK(34βE12) tend to be more diffusely expressed by spindle cells
- Smooth muscle actin is usually negative
- Desmin is negative
- S100 is negative

DIFFERENTIAL DIAGNOSIS

Spindle Cell Melanoma
- Recognition of associated melanoma in situ is helpful
- Immunohistochemistry may be necessary
  - S100 positive (may be only positive melanocytic marker)
  - Other melanocytic markers, such as Melan-A (MART-1) and tyrosinase, are usually negative in spindle cell melanoma
  - Cytokeratins and p63 are negative

Sarcomas
- Usually located deep within corpora spongiosum or cavernosa with no connection to surface epithelium
- Absence of clear-cut squamous differentiation
- Immunohistochemistry may be necessary
  - Negative for cytokeratins and p63
  - Positive for mesenchymal markers depending on histogenesis
    - Leiomyosarcoma: Positive for SMA, desmin, calponin
    - Angiosarcoma: Positive for CD31, FLI-1, CD34

DIAGNOSTIC CHECKLIST

Pathologic Interpretation Pearls
- Sarcomatoid carcinoma may be almost entirely composed of spindle cells closely mimicking sarcoma
- Malignant spindle cell neoplasm arising from distal portion of penis that is related to surface epithelium is more likely to be carcinoma than sarcoma or melanoma
- PAN-CK(AE1/AE3) and Cam5.2 may be negative or only focally positive in the spindle cells
- PAN-CK(AE1/AE3) and HMCK(34βE12) tend to be more commonly positive

SELECTED REFERENCES

1. Chaux A et al: Comparison of morphologic features and outcome of resected recurrent and nonrecurrent squamous cell carcinoma of the penis: a study of 81 cases. Am J Surg Pathol. 33(9):1299-306, 2009
2. Velazquez EF et al: Penile squamous cell carcinoma: anatomic, pathologic and viral studies in Paraguay (1993-2007). Anal Quant Cytol Histol. 29(4):185-98, 2007
3. Katona TM et al: Soft tissue tumors of the penis: a review. Anal Quant Cytol Histol. 28(4):193-206, 2006
4. Sánchez-Ortiz R et al: Melanoma of the penis, scrotum and male urethra: a 40-year single institution experience. J Urol. 173(6):1958-65, 2005
5. Velazquez EF et al: Sarcomatoid carcinoma of the penis: a clinicopathologic study of 15 cases. Am J Surg Pathol. 29(9):1152-8, 2005
6. Lont AP et al: Sarcomatoid squamous cell carcinoma of the penis: a clinical and pathological study of 5 cases. J Urol. 172(3):932-5, 2004

5

SARCOMATOID CARCINOMA, PENIS

Diagrammatic and Microscopic Features

(Left) Schematic representation shows a large and hemorrhagic sarcomatoid carcinoma ⮡ deeply invading the corpora cavernosa ➡. (Right) Sarcomatoid carcinoma predominantly composed of fascicles of spindle cells mimics a sarcoma. In the absence of a recognizable epithelial component, a sarcoma is in the differential diagnosis. Detailed morphologic evaluation and immunohistochemistry are helpful.

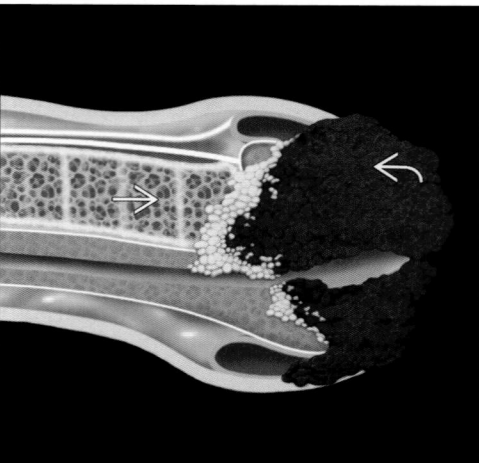
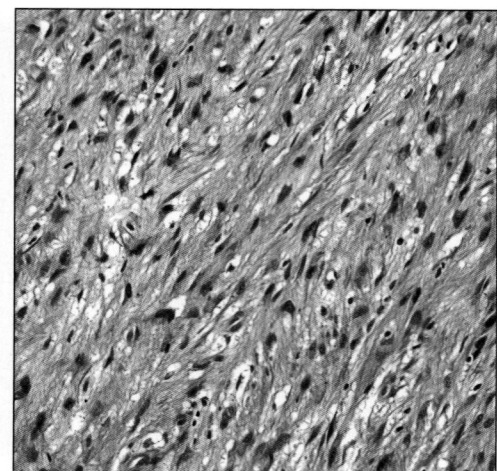

(Left) A storiform pattern is observed in this case of sarcomatoid carcinoma. Note the nuclear pleomorphism and scattered multinucleated giant cells. (Right) Sarcomatoid carcinoma shows prominent myxoid changes. Some tumors may be predominantly myxomatous. In the absence of an associated invasive SCC, the diagnosis can be done with the help of immunohistochemistry (keratin and p63 expression with negative muscle markers), previous history of SCC, or associated squamous cell carcinoma in situ (SCCIS).

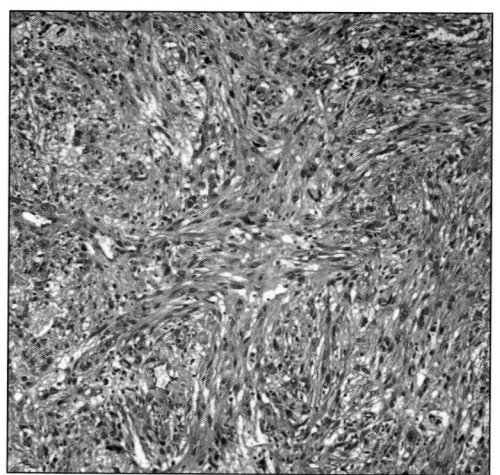
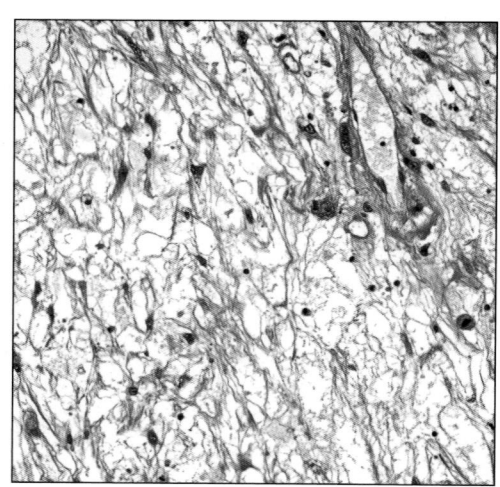

(Left) Low-power view illustrates an ulcerated tumor ⮡ corresponding to a sarcomatoid carcinoma with pseudovascular features affecting the foreskin. The nonulcerated epithelium shows squamous hyperplasia ⮢. (Right) Sarcomatoid carcinoma with pseudovascular features (angiosarcomatoid SCC) is predominantly composed of interanastomotic channels mimicking an angiosarcoma. The formation of such spaces is secondary to acantholysis.

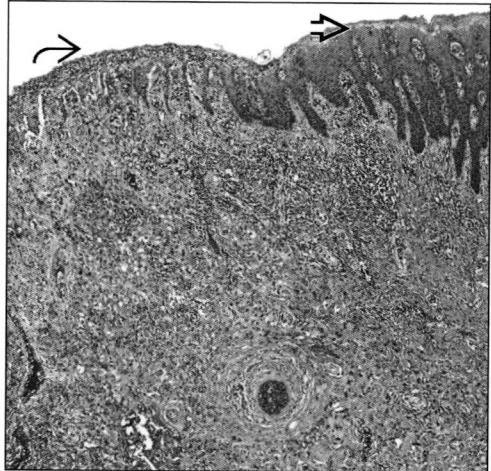
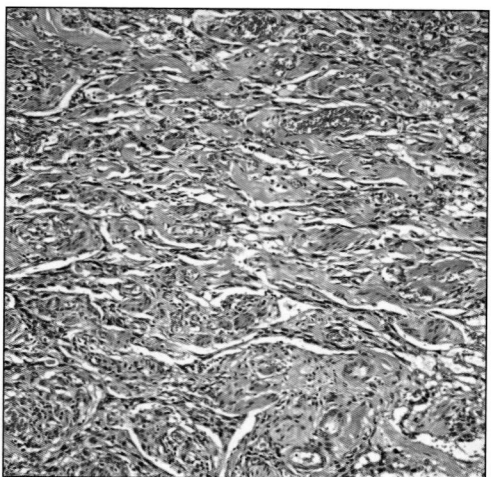

Microscopic and Immunohistochemical Features

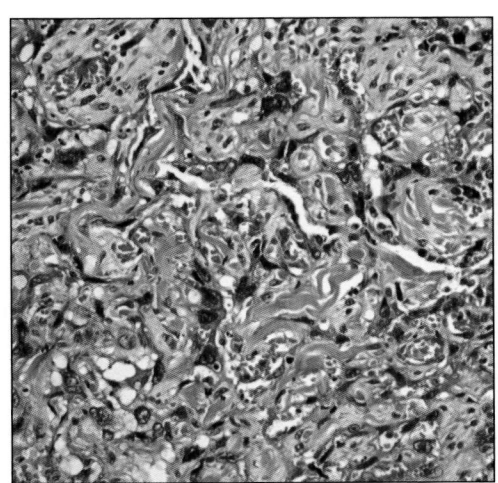

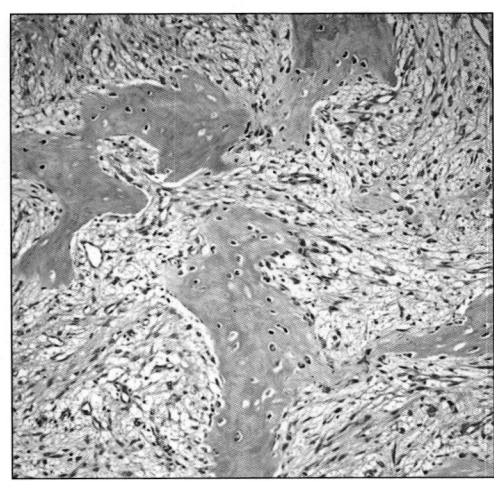

(Left) Sarcomatoid carcinoma with prominent pseudovascular spaces lined by large, atypical cells with pleomorphic nuclei can mimic angiosarcoma. Vascular markers (e.g., CD31) are negative in carcinomas. *(Right)* Foci of heterologous bone formation (osteosarcomatous differentiation) may be seen. A tumor with sarcomatous histology affecting the distal penis is more likely to represent sarcomatoid carcinoma than true sarcoma.

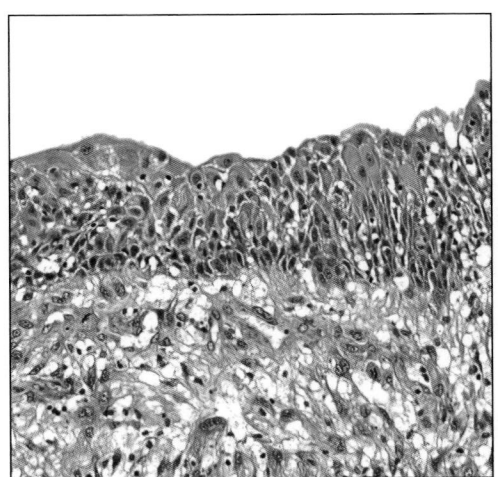

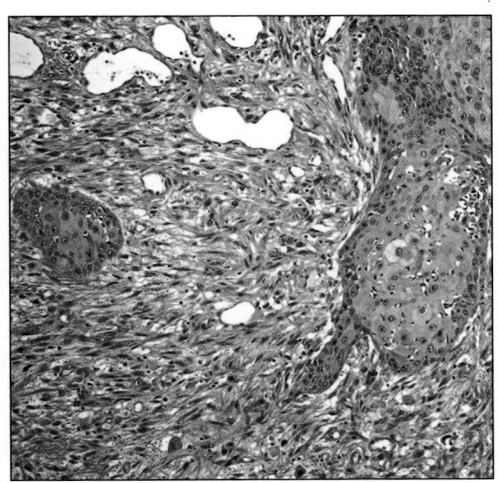

(Left) SCC in situ may be only focally present in cases of sarcomatoid carcinoma. Strict criteria should be used to recognize SCCIS, as reactive changes may mimic dysplasia and overdiagnosis may result in misdiagnosis of the underlying tumor as a carcinoma. *(Right)* Clear-cut foci of invasive SCC are seen admixed with malignant spindle cells in this sarcomatoid carcinoma. Tumors may be almost entirely composed of spindle cells and such squamous foci may be very difficult to identify.

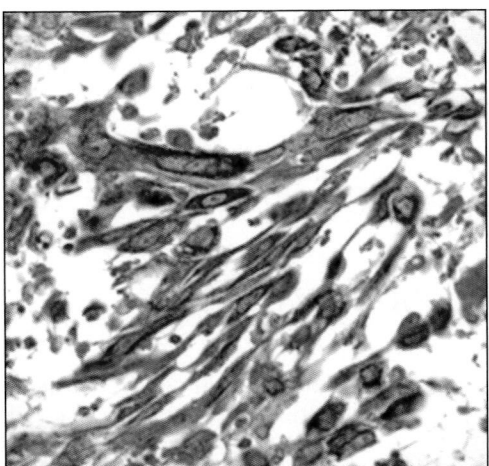

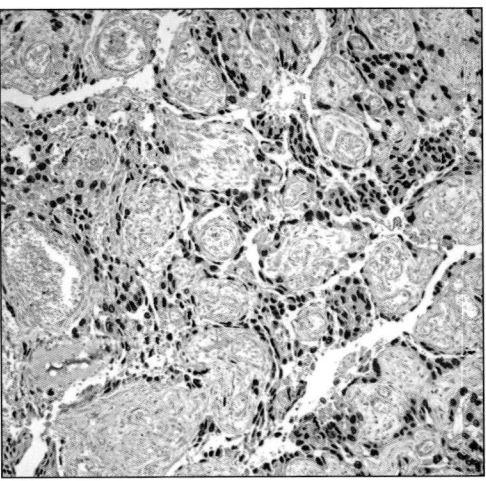

(Left) HMCK(34βE12) expression confirms the epithelial nature of this tumor. Expression of different cytokeratins and p63 is supportive of a diagnosis of sarcomatoid carcinoma. Muscle markers, including smooth muscle actin, should be negative or rarely focally positive. *(Right)* Diffuse p63 nuclear expression by the neoplastic cells in a case of sarcomatoid carcinoma with pseudovascular features (angiosarcomatoid carcinoma) supports the epithelial nature of this tumor.

CARCINOMA CUNICULATUM

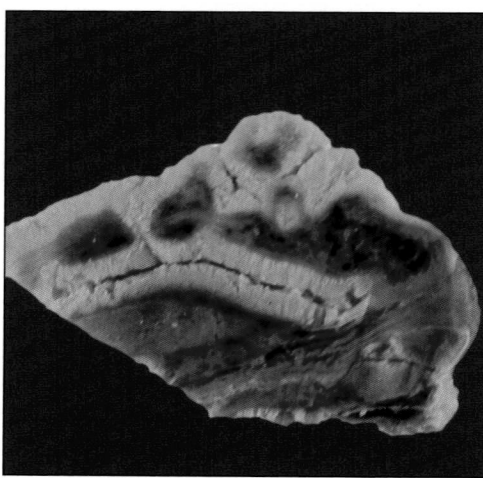

Cut section of a partial penectomy specimen shows a carcinoma cuniculatum. Note the deep tumoral invagination following the tunica albuginea and involving the corpus cavernosum.

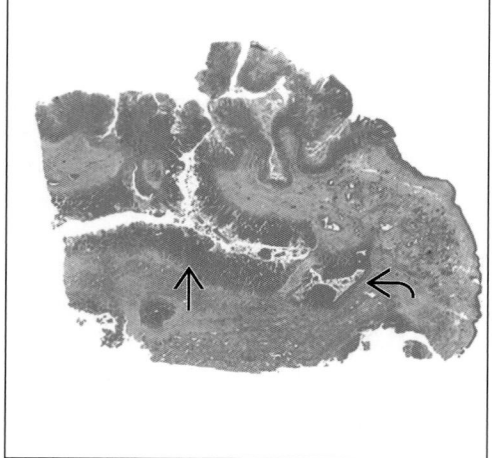

Low-power view of a cut section shows carcinoma cuniculatum. Note the endophytic burrowing channels ➡ and the deep pseudocystic space filled with keratin ➡.

TERMINOLOGY

Abbreviations
- Carcinoma cuniculatum (CC)

Synonyms
- Squamous cell carcinoma, hybrid verrucous carcinoma

Definitions
- Distinct variant of verrucous carcinoma characterized by deep burrowing growth pattern mimicking rabbit burrows (cuniculi)
- Represents hybrid (mixed) verrucous carcinoma with unique growth pattern

ETIOLOGY/PATHOGENESIS

Pathogenesis
- Unknown
- Likely not HPV-related

CLINICAL ISSUES

Epidemiology
- Incidence
  - Very rare
  - Few cases described in literature
- Age
  - Mean: 77 years

Site
- Usually affects glans and extends to coronal sulcus and foreskin

Presentation
- Large, papillomatous tumors with "cobblestone" appearance

Treatment
- Surgery

Prognosis
- Good prognosis
- No reported metastases

MACROSCOPIC FEATURES

General Features
- Large, papillomatous lesion
- "Cobblestone" and sometimes spiky appearance
- Usually affects glans and extends to coronal sulcus and foreskin
- Cut sections reveal hallmark of neoplasm: Deeply endophytic tumoral invaginations mimicking rabbit burrows
- Neoplastic invaginations invade through lamina propria and corpus spongiosum to involve tunica albuginea and corpora cavernosa
  - Deep and narrow complex tumor invaginations connect to surface through sinus tracts
- Deeply invasive keratin-filled pseudocysts or crypts are frequently seen
- Similar to plantar epithelioma cuniculatum originally described by Aird in 1954

Size
- Usually large tumors affecting several anatomic compartments of penis
- Average = 6.3 cm

MICROSCOPIC PATHOLOGY

Histologic Features
- Deep invaginations form interanastomosing channels and pseudocystic structures filled with keratin
- Interanastomosing channels and pseudocystic structures are lined by well-differentiated squamous cell carcinoma
- Bulk of lesion has features of verrucous carcinoma

CARCINOMA CUNICULATUM

Key Facts

Macroscopic Features
- Large exoendophytic tumor with "cobblestone" appearance
- Affects several anatomical compartments (glans, coronal sulcus, and foreskin)
- Hallmark of lesion is seen upon sectioning: Deep endophytic and interanastomosing pattern mimicking rabbit burrows

Microscopic Pathology
- In most cases, carcinoma cuniculatum is hybrid (mixed) verrucous carcinoma with peculiar deep growth pattern
- Most of lesion is extremely well-differentiated (verrucous carcinoma)
- Interanastomotic channels contain abundant keratin
- Sinus tracts are commonly seen

- Focal higher grade areas and infiltrative pattern are common (SCC of usual type)

Top Differential Diagnoses
- Verrucous carcinoma
  - Lack higher grade areas and jagged borders
  - Lack classic burrowing pattern
- Warty carcinoma
  - Prominent atypical koilocytosis
- Papillary carcinoma
  - Lack classic burrowing pattern
- Giant condyloma
  - Benign lesion with koilocytosis on surface

- Extremely well-differentiated squamous cell carcinoma
- Acanthotic papillae with thin fibrovascular cores
- Piling up of keratin among papillae
- Bulbous deep borders
- Lack of koilocytosis
- Usually minor component showing features of SCC of usual type
  - Focal higher grade areas
  - Focal infiltrative borders

Predominant Pattern/Injury Type
- Squamous

Predominant Cell/Compartment Type
- Epithelial, squamous

DIFFERENTIAL DIAGNOSIS

Verrucous Carcinoma
- Extremely well-differentiated verruciform tumor
- Lacks classic burrowing pattern
- Lack of focal higher grade areas
- Lack of infiltrative pattern

Warty Carcinoma
- Prominent koilocytosis with malignant nuclear features
- Higher grade areas frequently with destructive invasion
- Lacks prominent burrowing pattern

Papillary Carcinoma
- Well-differentiated verruciform lesion
- Irregular jagged borders
- Lacks classic burrowing pattern

Condyloma Acuminatum/Giant Condyloma
- Koilocytosis is seen on surface
- Lacks prominent burrowing pattern
- Lacks higher grade areas
- Lacks infiltrative pattern

DIAGNOSTIC CHECKLIST

Pathologic Interpretation Pearls
- Bulk of tumor is identical to verrucous carcinoma
- Well-differentiated tumor
- Acanthotic papillae separated by abundant keratin
- Deep pushing borders
- Hallmark of lesion is deep and complex burrowing pattern
- Interanastomosing channels are lined by well-differentiated squamous cell carcinoma and contain abundant keratin
- Sinus tract formation is characteristic
- Focally, higher grade areas and jagged borders are frequent

SELECTED REFERENCES

1. Chaux A et al: Comparison of morphologic features and outcome of resected recurrent and nonrecurrent squamous cell carcinoma of the penis: a study of 81 cases. Am J Surg Pathol. 33(9):1299-306, 2009
2. Barreto JE et al: Carcinoma cuniculatum: a distinctive variant of penile squamous cell carcinoma: report of 7 cases. Am J Surg Pathol. 31(1):71-5, 2007
3. Rai VM et al: Ulceroproliferative growth on the heel: epithelioma cuniculatum. Dermatol Online J. 12(4):8, 2006
4. Steffen C: Dermatopathology in historical perspective: epithelioma cuniculatum (Aird). Am J Dermatopathol. 28(5):451-61, 2006
5. Cubilla AL et al: Warty (condylomatous) squamous cell carcinoma of the penis: a report of 11 cases and proposed classification of 'verruciform' penile tumors. Am J Surg Pathol. 24(4):505-12, 2000
6. Ho J et al: An ulcerating verrucous plaque on the foot. Verrucous carcinoma (epithelioma cuniculatum). Arch Dermatol. 136(4):547-8, 550-1, 2000
7. Seehafer JR et al: Epithelioma cuniculatum: verrucous carcinoma of the foot. Cutis. 23(3):287-90, 1979
8. Aird I et al: Epithelioma cuniculatum: a variety of squamous carcinoma peculiar to the foot. Br J Surg. 42(173):245-50, 1954

CARCINOMA CUNICULATUM

Microscopic Features

(Left) The bulk of carcinoma cuniculatum has features of a verrucous carcinoma. Note the acanthotic papillae with prominent piling up of orange keratin ➤ between them. *(Right)* In most areas, carcinoma cuniculatum is indistinguishable from verrucous carcinoma. Note the deep, elongated, broad bulbous projections ➤ at the base of the tumor.

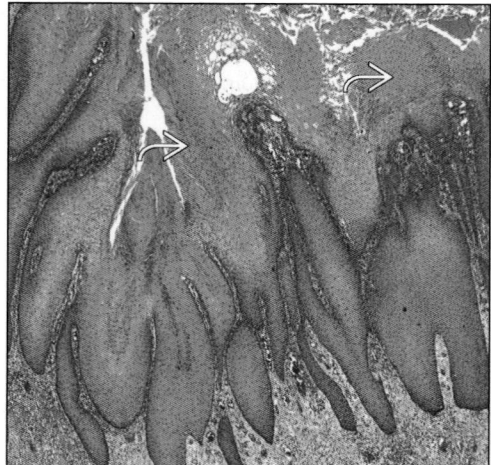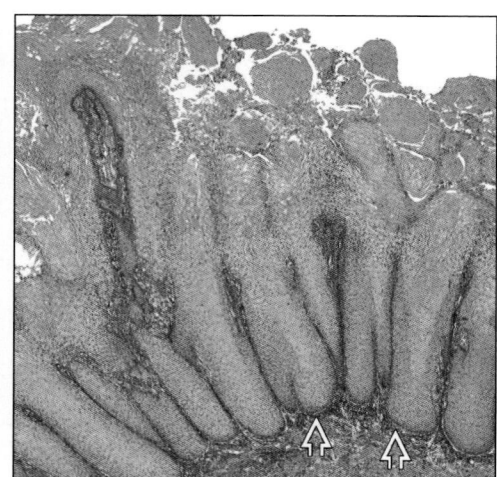

(Left) Bulbous deep borders and wide craters filled with abundant keratin ➤ are characteristic of the lesion. In a superficial biopsy, the presence of a well-differentiated epithelium with wide craters should raise the possibility of a verrucous carcinoma or carcinoma cuniculatum. Clinicopathologic correlation is necessary in such settings. *(Right)* Note the verruciform papillae with abundant interspersed orange keratin in this case of carcinoma cuniculatum.

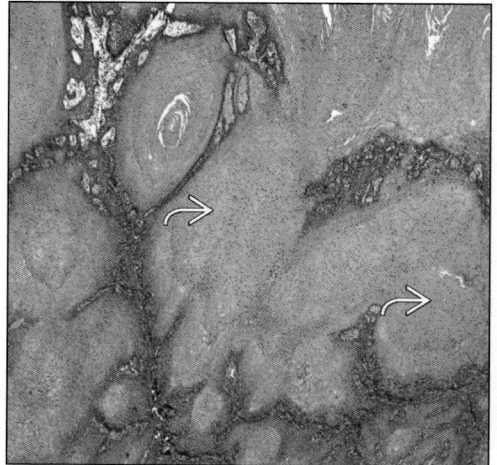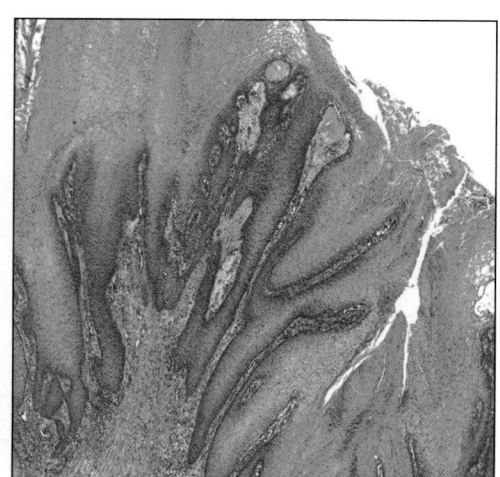

(Left) Complex tumor shows numerous irregular fistulae toward the surface. *(Right)* Sinus tracts communicating with the tumor surface are a frequent finding and a hallmark of this lesion. Note the opening of a sinus tract to the surface ➤.

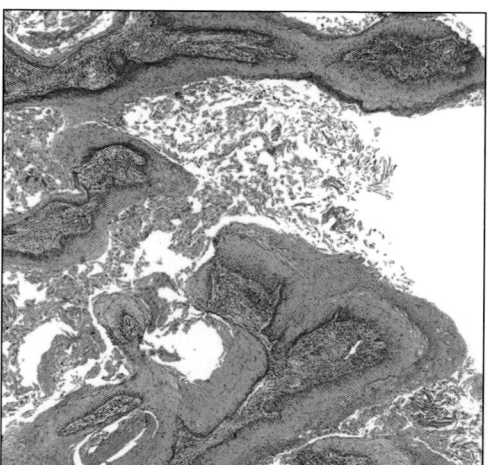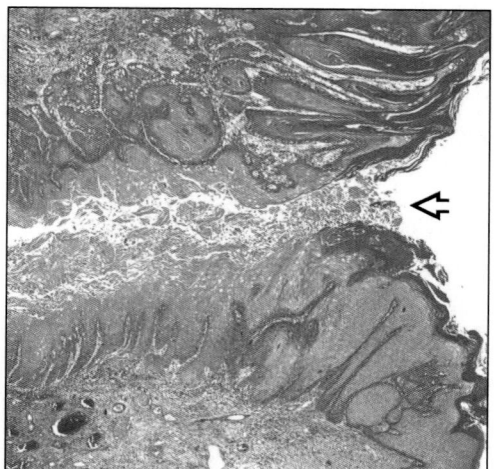

CARCINOMA CUNICULATUM

Microscopic Features

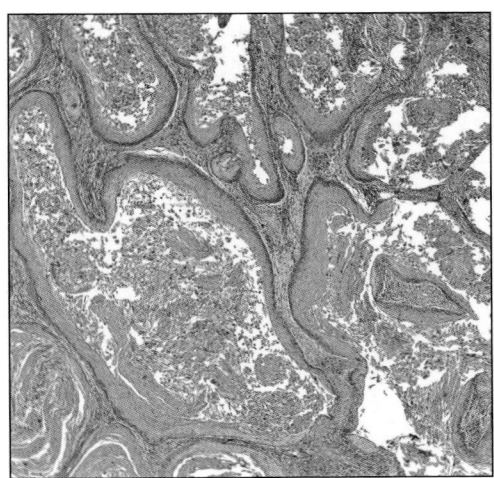
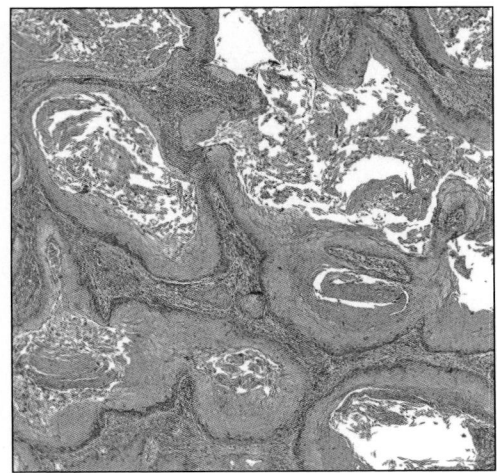

(Left) Interanastomotic pattern showing complex channels filled with keratin is characteristic of the lesion. *(Right)* Interanastomosing and complex endophytic pattern is characteristic of carcinoma cuniculatum. The acanthotic epithelium is well differentiated and shows overall maintenance of polarity. Note the abundance of keratin within the endophytic channels.

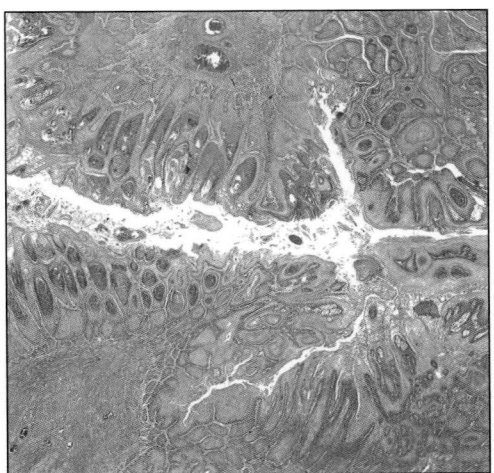
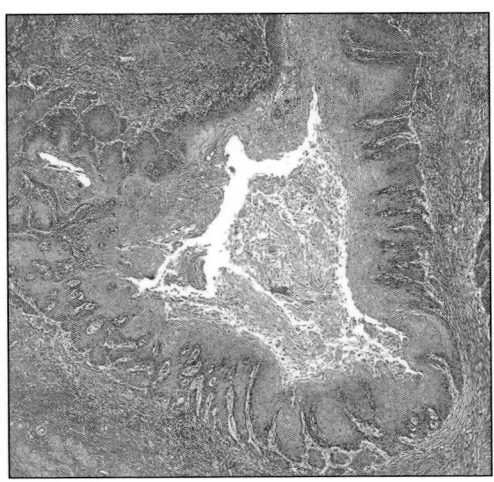

(Left) Low-power view of carcinoma cuniculatum highlights the interanastomotic and complex pattern of this lesion. The deep burrowing pattern of well-differentiated epithelium mimicking rabbit burrows is the diagnostic hallmark. *(Right)* Carcinoma cuniculatum. Deep tumoral invaginations may mimic cysts in some sections. This feature may be appreciated even at the macroscopic level. Note the orderly and well-differentiated nature of the epithelium.

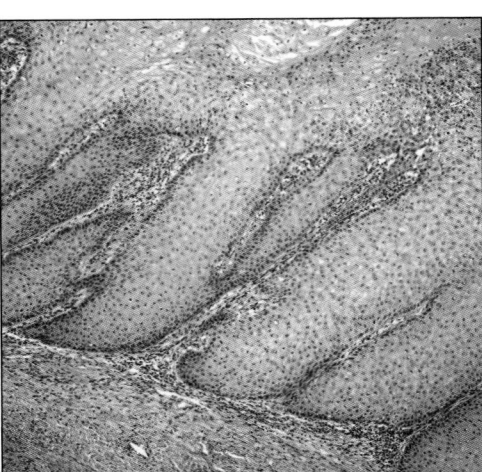
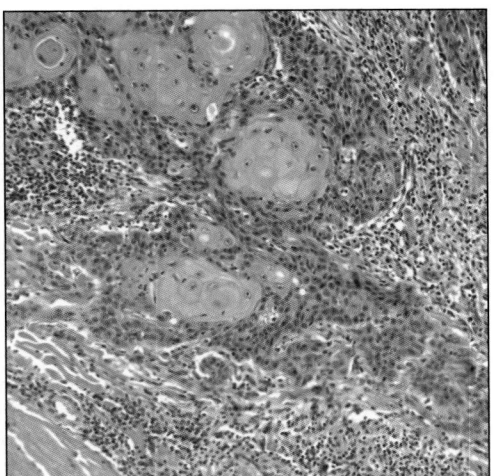

(Left) The bulk of carcinoma cuniculatum is well differentiated. Note the sharp pushing borders similar to verrucous carcinoma. *(Right)* Higher grade areas and jagged borders are frequently a minor component of carcinoma cuniculatum. This feature clearly contrasts this tumor from verrucous carcinoma and underscores the importance of generous sampling.

MIXED CARCINOMA

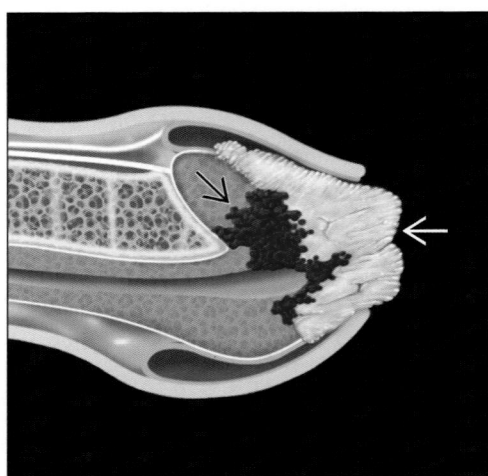

Diagram of a mixed penile tumor depicts a low-grade superficial exophytic tumor ➡, corresponding to a verrucous carcinoma, and a focus of deeply infiltrating high-grade usual SCC ➲.

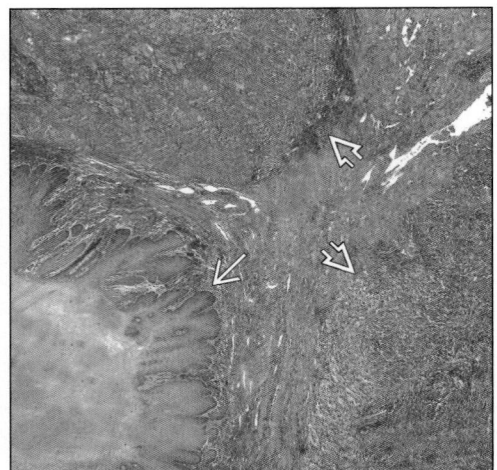

Hybrid verrucous carcinoma shows concomitant presence of low-grade verrucous carcinoma with its typical bulbous tumor base ➡ intermingled with solid nests of a high-grade usual SCC ➲.

TERMINOLOGY

Abbreviations
- Squamous cell carcinoma (SCC)

Definitions
- Coexistence of 2 or more histologic subtypes
- 20% or more of at least 1 of the histologic components

CLINICAL ISSUES

Epidemiology
- Incidence
  - Represents 1/3 of all penile SCC
- Age
  - Mean age: 56 years old

Site
- Glans is most frequently affected site
- Foreskin location is uncommon

Treatment
- Depends mainly on local extent and histologic grade of tumor
- Surgical approach should be considered for tumors invading beyond lamina propria
- Groin dissection should be performed based on risk group stratification

Prognosis
- Related to higher grade component
- Clinical behavior is variable in concordance with histologic picture and relative proportion of different components
- Local and regional recurrences may occur
- Inguinal nodal involvement is rarely seen
- Cancer-specific mortality rate is low

MACROSCOPIC FEATURES

General Features
- Gross appearance is variable
- Mixed patterns of growth are common
- Verruciform and superficial spreading patterns correspond to low-grade tumors
- Vertical growth pattern is observed in high-grade tumors
- Multicentricity is not uncommon
- Average tumor size: 4.1 cm

MICROSCOPIC PATHOLOGY

Histologic Features
- Most frequent patterns include mixture of human papillomavirus (HPV)-related histologic subtypes
- Mixtures of usual SCC with other HPV-related and unrelated variants are also common
- Histologic grade distribution is variable and depends on subtypes present
- Vascular invasion, perineural invasion, and extension to distal urethra may be seen in about 1/3 of cases
- Mixtures of differentiated, basaloid, &/or warty penile intraepithelial neoplasia (PeIN) may be identified in adjacent overlying mucosa
- Warty/basaloid carcinoma
  - Typical warty areas admixed with basaloid foci
  - Most frequently observed mixed SCC
  - Warty pattern may be superficial and basaloid histology is present in deeply invasive tumor
  - Warty and basaloid areas may occasionally be randomly intermingled
  - Condylomatous papillae may be composed of both clear warty and small basaloid cells
  - HPV and p16 positivity is present in most cases
  - Approximately 1/2 of cases are associated with presence of typical condylomata
  - Clinically it behaves as basaloid SCC

MIXED CARCINOMA

Key Facts

Terminology
- 20% or more of at least 1 of the histological components

Macroscopic Features
- Glans is most frequently affected site
- Mixed patterns of growth are common
- Verruciform and superficial spreading patterns correspond to low-grade tumors
- Vertical growth pattern is observed in high-grade tumors

Microscopic Pathology
- Coexistence of 2 or more histological subtypes
- Represents 1/3 of all penile SCC
- Histological grade distribution is variegated and depends on subtypes admixed

- Warty/basaloid is most frequent mixed SCC
- Hybrid verrucous represents 2nd most common type of mixed SCC
- Other patterns include usual-warty, usual-basaloid, and usual-papillary
- Mixtures of differentiated and undifferentiated PeIN can also be identified
- Focal areas of usual SCC are observed in > 1/2 of sarcomatoid carcinoma cases
- Rare mixtures include adeno-basaloid SCC, mucoepidermoid SCC, and polymorphic variants

Top Differential Diagnoses
- Pure SCC variants
- Basaloid carcinomas
- Sarcomatoid carcinomas

- Usual-verrucous carcinoma
  - Represents approximately 1/4 of all mixed carcinomas
  - Also known as hybrid verrucous carcinoma
  - Admixture of usual SCC and verrucous carcinoma
  - Verrucous carcinoma is always low grade
  - Usual SCC may be well, moderately well, or poorly differentiated
  - Biological behavior is dictated by highest histologic grade
  - Even small foci of high-grade tumor impart metastatic potential, which is not the case in pure verrucous carcinoma
  - Pure verrucous SCC may locally recur as hybrid verrucous carcinoma (probably not sampled usual SCC in primary)
- SCC with mixed sarcomatoid features
  - At least focal areas of usual SCC are observed in > 1/2 of sarcomatoid carcinomas
  - In some cases, typical areas of verrucous, papillary, and basaloid may be present
  - Regardless of presence of other histologic subtypes, all of these tumors are considered sarcomatoid carcinoma
- Other mixed patterns
  - Mixed usual-warty SCCs are unusual mixed penile carcinomas
  - Mixtures of basaloid SCC with usual SCC are also unusual
  - Papillary SCC admixed with usual SCC may be seen in minority of cases
  - Other mixtures include adeno-basaloid SCC, mucoepidermoid SCC, and polymorphic variants

Anatomical Extension
- Many tumors invade penile erectile tissues, either corpus spongiosum (44%) or cavernosum (56%)
- Tumors limited to lamina propria are exceedingly rare

DIFFERENTIAL DIAGNOSIS

Pure SCC Variants
- Tumors should be adequately sampled in order to identify minor mixed areas
- Strict criteria should be applied in histologic subtyping
- High grade areas and variants may have random distribution
- Special attention should be paid in separating hybrid verrucous carcinoma from pure verrucous carcinoma
- Mixed SCC with basaloid component behaves clinically as basaloid SCC

Basaloid Carcinoma
- Mixed forms in which basaloid cells are present should be properly recognized
- Biological behavior of mixed SCC with basaloid features is expected to be similar to pure basaloid carcinoma

Sarcomatoid Carcinoma
- In sarcomatoid carcinoma, presence of other intermingled SCC variants is not unusual
- Sarcomatoid carcinoma is clinically aggressive regardless of presence and extension of other morphological components

SELECTED REFERENCES

1. Chaux A et al: Comparison of morphologic features and outcome of resected recurrent and nonrecurrent squamous cell carcinoma of the penis: a study of 81 cases. Am J Surg Pathol. 33(9):1299-306, 2009
2. Guimarães GC et al: Penile squamous cell carcinoma clinicopathological features, nodal metastasis and outcome in 333 cases. J Urol. 182(2):528-34; discussion 534, 2009
3. Cubilla AL et al: Histologic classification of penile carcinoma and its relation to outcome in 61 patients with primary resection. Int J Surg Pathol. 9(2):111-20, 2001
4. Kato N et al: Penile hybrid verrucous-squamous carcinoma associated with a superficial inguinal lymph node metastasis. Am J Dermatopathol. 22(4):339-43, 2000

MIXED CARCINOMA

Microscopic Features

(Left) Warty/basaloid carcinomas are composed of a mixed cell population of pleomorphic cells with koilocytic changes at surface ⮞ and small basaloid cells at papillae base ➡. *(Right)* Deep infiltrative nests of warty/basaloid carcinomas show a mixed population with a variable proportion of larger cells with koilocytotic atypia ⮞ intermingled with smaller basaloid cells ➡.

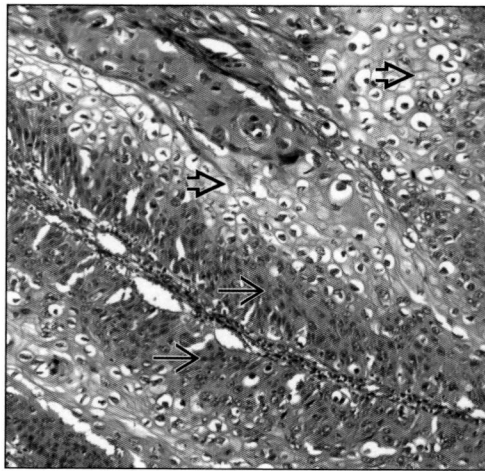
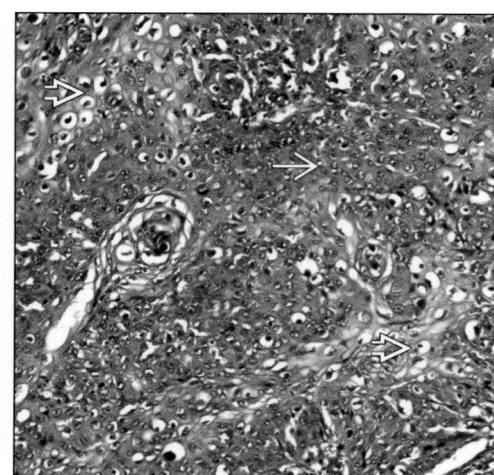

(Left) In warty/basaloid carcinoma, it is common to find associated areas of warty/basaloid PeIN in which epithelium is replaced by basaloid cells in the lower 2/3 ⮞ and by pleomorphic koilocytes on the surface ➡. *(Right)* Exophytic superficial area of a hybrid verrucous carcinoma in which the verrucous component, with its extreme squamous differentiation, broad tumor base, and chronic inflammatory desmoplastic reaction, is readily observed.

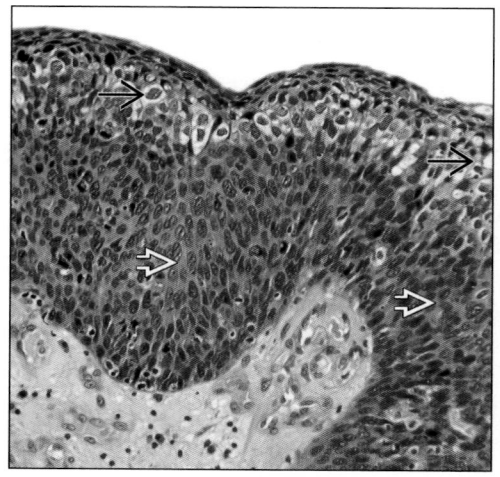
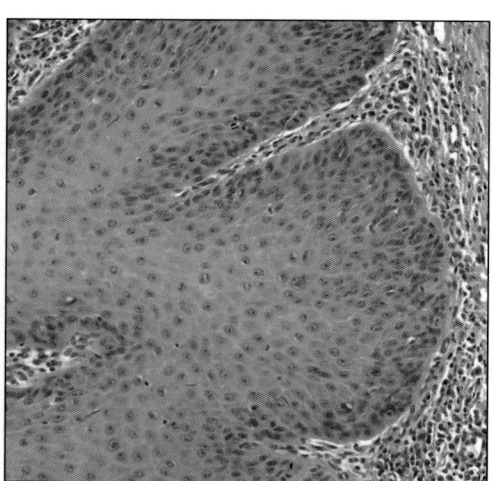

(Left) Infiltrative portion of a hybrid verrucous carcinoma with its usual carcinoma component shows solid nests with moderate nuclear pleomorphism and foci of keratin pearl formation ➡, corresponding to a grade 2 usual SCC, located beneath the verrucous component. *(Right)* Deeply infiltrative portion of a hybrid verrucous carcinoma shows foci of poorly differentiated (grade 3) usual SCC composed of pleomorphic cells with ample and keratinized cytoplasm.

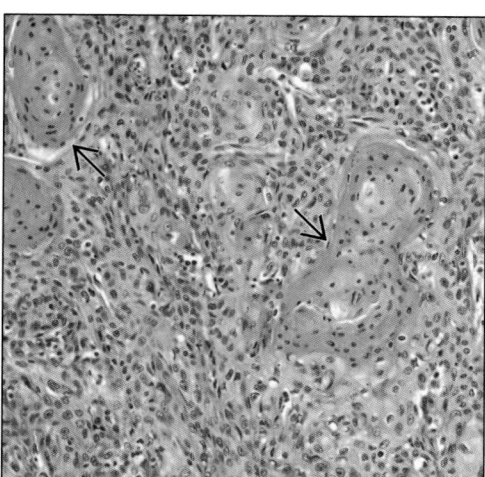
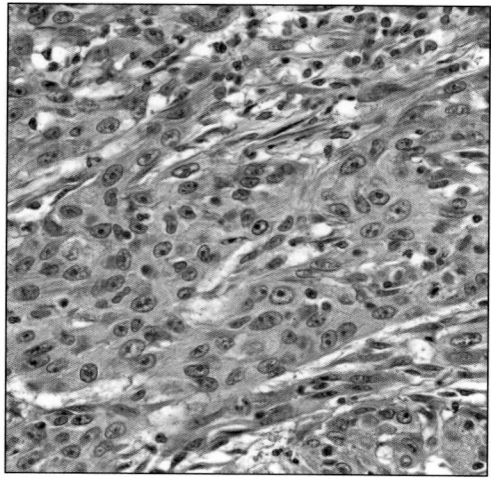

MIXED CARCINOMA

Microscopic Features and Differential Diagnosis

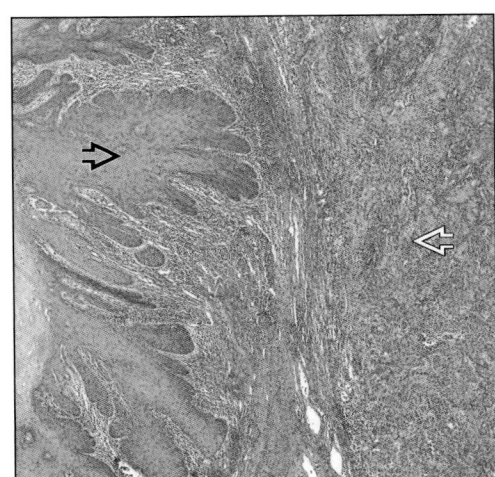

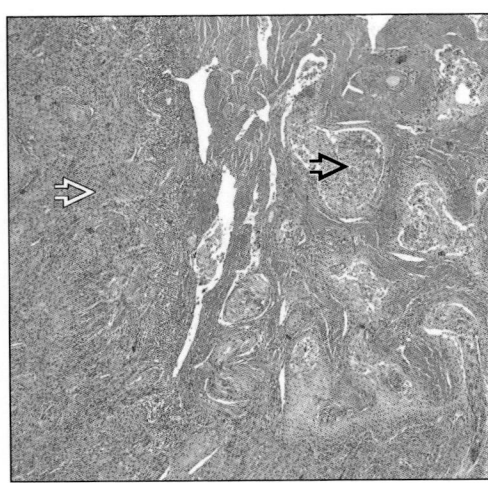

(Left) Hybrid verrucous carcinoma with extremely well-differentiated areas corresponds to the verrucous carcinoma component ⊳, and poorly differentiated foci corresponds to the high-grade SCC of usual type ⊳. *(Right)* Hybrid verrucous carcinoma shows solid areas of high-grade usual SCC ⊳ intermingled with highly infiltrative tumor nests having extensive central necrosis ⊳.

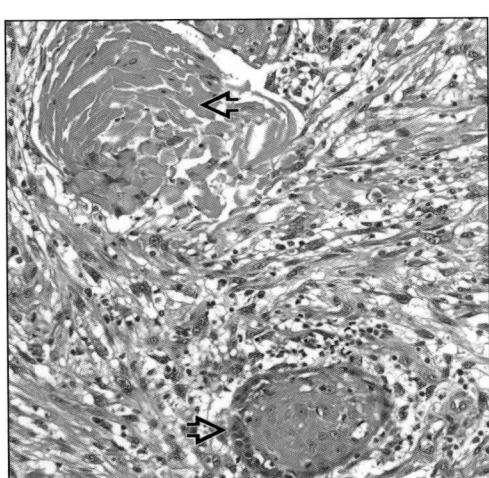

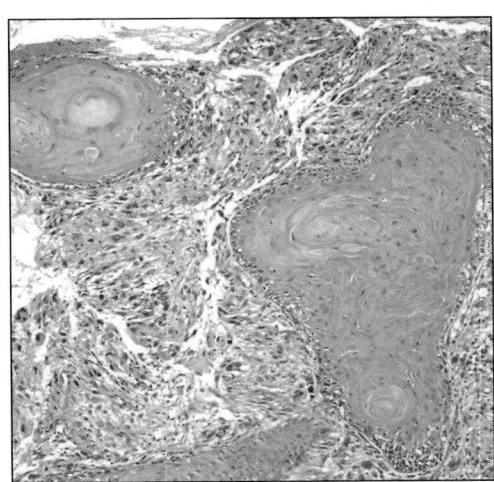

(Left) Isolated foci of squamous differentiation ⊳ are commonly observed in sarcomatoid carcinomas imprinting a biphasic appearance to the tumor although in most cases the spindle cell component usually predominates. *(Right)* The presence of well-differentiated atypical squamous nests surrounded by pleomorphic spindle cells helps identify the malignant spindle cell component as being sarcomatoid carcinoma over a high-grade sarcoma.

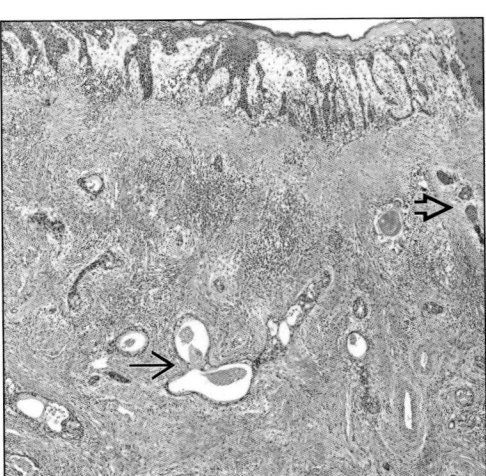

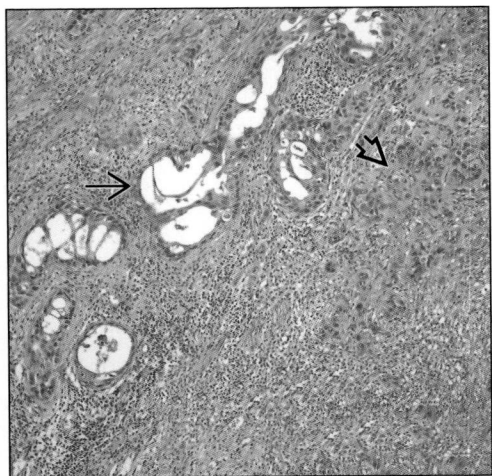

(Left) Adenosquamous carcinoma is a deeply infiltrative SCC variant in which foci of squamous ⊳ and glandular → differentiation coexist. *(Right)* Adenosquamous carcinoma shows the typical biphasic pattern in which irregularly shaped high-grade solid neoplastic nests of usual SCC ⊳ are juxtaposed with areas of glandular differentiation →.

PAPILLARY CARCINOMA

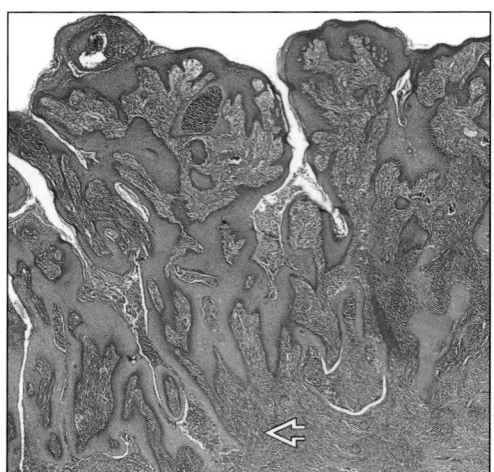

Low-power view of papillary SCC depicts the typical papillomatous pattern of growth with irregular and complex papillae and jagged tumor-stroma interface ➡ with a prominent stromal reaction.

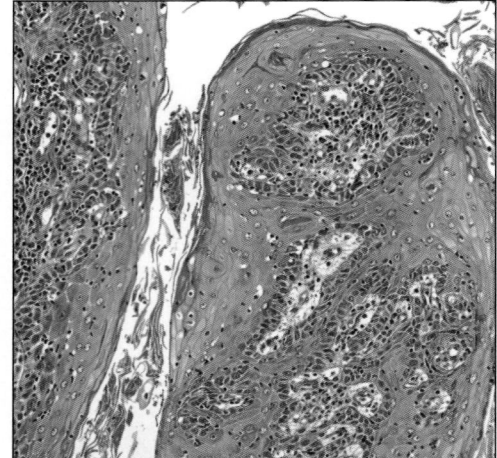

Histological features of the papillae include presence of mild acanthosis with moderate cytologic atypia, slight hyper- and parakeratosis, and no koilocytic changes in the epithelium.

TERMINOLOGY

Abbreviations
- Squamous cell carcinoma (SCC)

Synonyms
- Papillary carcinoma, NOS

Definitions
- Low-grade malignant epithelial tumor with typical exophytic pattern of growth
- Diagnosis is made only after exclusion of other verruciform tumors
- Represents 5-15% of all penile SCC
- Accounts for 27-53% of all verruciform tumors

ETIOLOGY/PATHOGENESIS

Etiologic Factors
- Etiology unknown but frequently associated with lichen sclerosus
- Evidence of human papillomavirus (HPV) infection found in minority of cases

CLINICAL ISSUES

Epidemiology
- Age
  - Average age is 63 years (range from 43-85 years)

Presentation
- Granular and firm cauliflower-like exophytic tumor

Treatment
- Partial penectomy as primary treatment
- Inguinal lymphadenectomy according to risk group stratification

Prognosis
- Less aggressive than usual SCC

  - Recurrence rate of about 1/10, usually due to insufficient surgery
  - Inguinal metastases are found in about 1/10 of patients
  - Cancer-specific mortality rate very low
- Similar to other verruciform tumors in biological behavior

MACROSCOPIC FEATURES

General Features
- Tumors present exophytic verruciform pattern of growth
  - Glans is most frequently affected anatomical compartment
  - Foreskin exclusively affected in minority of cases
- Extension to multiple anatomical compartments in up to 50% of cases
- Average size = 4.5-5.8 cm
- Cut surface depicts serrated tumoral base
- Poorly defined tumor-stroma interface
- Invasion of penile erectile tissues is common

Anatomical Extension
- Most tumors (65%) invade up to corpus spongiosum or dartos
- Tumors limited to lamina propria are uncommon
- Invasion of deep corpus cavernosum is unusual

MICROSCOPIC PATHOLOGY

Histologic Features
- Papillomatous pattern of growth
- Mild to moderate acanthosis
- Hyperkeratosis with parakeratosis
- Papillae are architecturally complex and can be short or elongated
  - Tips of papillae may be blunt or spiky
  - Central fibrovascular cores may be noted

PAPILLARY CARCINOMA

Key Facts

Terminology
- Represents 5-15% of all penile SCC
- Accounts for 27-53% of all verruciform tumors

Etiology/Pathogenesis
- Evidence of HPV infection found in minority of cases

Clinical Issues
- Inguinal metastases are found in 0-12% of patients
- Cancer-specific mortality rate of 0-6%
- Less aggressive than usual SCC

Macroscopic Features
- Exophytic verruciform pattern of growth
- Glans is most frequently affected compartment
- Extension to multiple compartments

Microscopic Pathology
- Papillae are architecturally complex
- Tips of papillae can be blunt or spiky
- Well- to moderately well-differentiated
- High-grade areas unusual; absent koilocytotic atypia
- Tumoral base irregular and jagged
- Squamous hyperplasia, differentiated PeIN, and lichen sclerosus are frequently found

Top Differential Diagnoses
- Warty (condylomatous) carcinoma
- Verrucous carcinoma
- Carcinoma cuniculatum
- Mixed usual-verrucous carcinoma
- Giant condyloma

- Areas of intraepithelial keratin pearls are not uncommon
- Most tumors are well- to moderately well-differentiated SCC
  - High-grade areas are unusual and focal
- No koilocytotic atypia
- Tumoral base irregular and jagged; destructive stromal invasion
- Invasive nests at tumoral front surrounded by reactive stroma
- Microabscesses, acantholysis, and clear cell changes may be focally observed
- Vascular and perineural invasion may be observed in small subset of cases
- Extension to distal urethra is uncommon
- Presence in most cases of associated lesions in adjacent areas
  - Differentiated penile intraepithelial neoplasia (PeIN) and squamous hyperplasia commonly observed
  - Lichen sclerosus frequently found

DIFFERENTIAL DIAGNOSIS

Warty (Condylomatous) Carcinoma
- More pleomorphic neoplastic cells
- Conspicuous koilocytotic atypia
- Prominent fibrovascular cores
- Jagged and irregular tumoral base
- High-risk HPV infection detected in most cases
- Immunohistochemistry for p16 positive in most cases

Verrucous Carcinoma
- Less pleomorphic neoplastic cells
- Broad tumoral base with pushing borders
- Fibrovascular cores absent or very inconspicuous
- Koilocytic changes are absent
- Invasion up to lamina propria or superficial corpus spongiosum
- Consistently HPV negative

Carcinoma Cuniculatum
- Less pleomorphic neoplastic cells

- Broad tumoral base with pushing borders
- Absence of koilocytosis
- Deep invasion of erectile tissues, usually corpus cavernosum
- Presence of cysts and sinus-like tracts connecting tumoral surface with deeper invaded areas
- Consistently HPV negative

Mixed Usual-Verrucous Carcinoma
- a.k.a. hybrid verrucous carcinoma
- Mixed pattern of growth, usually verruciform with vertical growth
- Well-differentiated areas intermingled with more pleomorphic foci of neoplastic cells
- Irregular tumoral base due to presence of usual SCC
- Usual SCC component is frequently of high histological grade

Giant Condyloma
- Condylomatous papillae, similar to warty carcinomas
- Prominent fibrovascular cores
- Conspicuous koilocytic changes
- Absence of pleomorphic or clearly malignant cells
- Broad tumoral base with pushing borders
- Low-risk HPV infection detected in most of cases

SELECTED REFERENCES

1. Guimarães GC et al: Penile squamous cell carcinoma clinicopathological features, nodal metastasis and outcome in 333 cases. J Urol. 182(2):528-34; discussion 534, 2009
2. Cubilla AL et al: Histologic classification of penile carcinoma and its relation to outcome in 61 patients with primary resection. Int J Surg Pathol. 9(2):111-20, 2001
3. Cubilla AL et al: Warty (condylomatous) squamous cell carcinoma of the penis: a report of 11 cases and proposed classification of 'verruciform' penile tumors. Am J Surg Pathol. 24(4):505-12, 2000
4. Gregoire L et al: Preferential association of human papillomavirus with high-grade histologic variants of penile-invasive squamous cell carcinoma. J Natl Cancer Inst. 87(22):1705-9, 1995

PAPILLARY CARCINOMA

Microscopic Features

(Left) Diagnostic clues include presence of papillomatosis with irregularly shaped papillae and occasional superficial clear cell changes ⊳, not to be confused with koilocytes, more or less prominent fibrovascular cores, and jagged tumor base. *(Right)* Papillae, which may be short or elongated, depict a complex architecture, fibrovascular cores ⊳ are irregular and, on low-power view, the histologic picture may simulate condylomatous features resembling those of warty carcinoma.

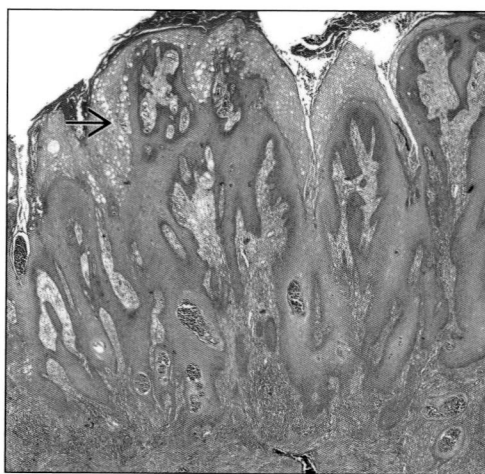
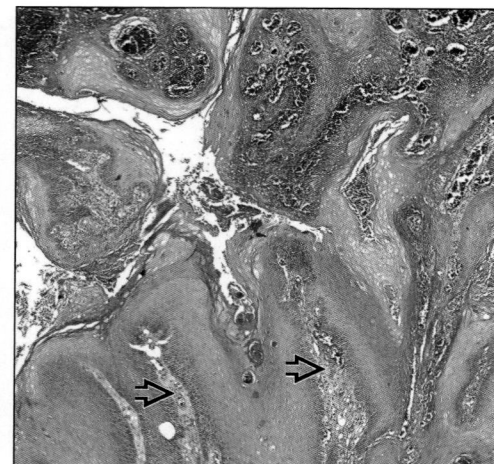

(Left) Papillae usually show mild acanthosis with parakeratosis ⊳ and neoplastic cells are well to moderately differentiated with easily recognized cytologic atypia and retained squamous maturation. *(Right)* Base of the papillae shows irregular nests of neoplastic cells with mild to moderate atypia, ample and acidophilic cytoplasm, distinctive cellular borders, and retained epithelial maturation.

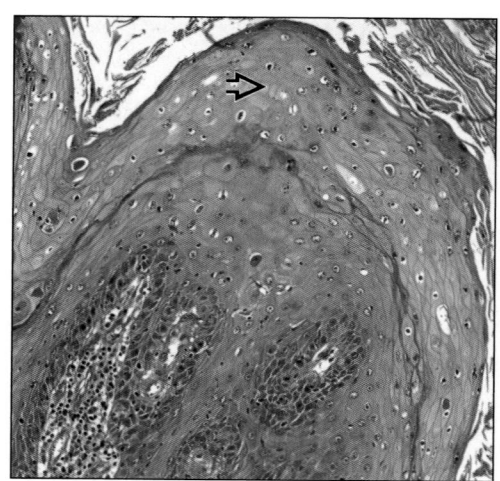
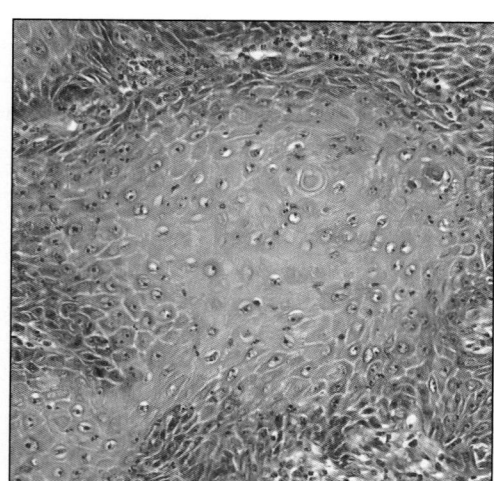

(Left) Front of invasion of papillary SCC with irregular nests of neoplastic cells imparts a jagged aspect to the tumoral base and an intense stromal reaction ⊳. *(Right)* Differentiated PeIN (low-grade intraepithelial lesion) ⊳, associated with underlying lichen sclerosus ⊳, is a common finding in papillary carcinoma.

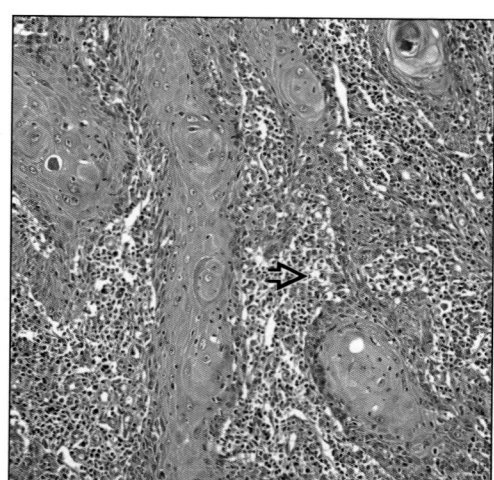
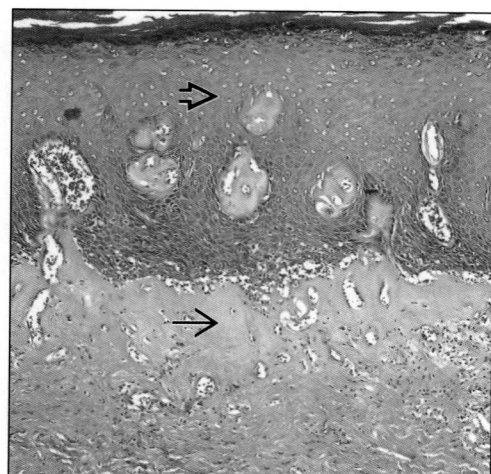

PAPILLARY CARCINOMA

Differential Diagnosis

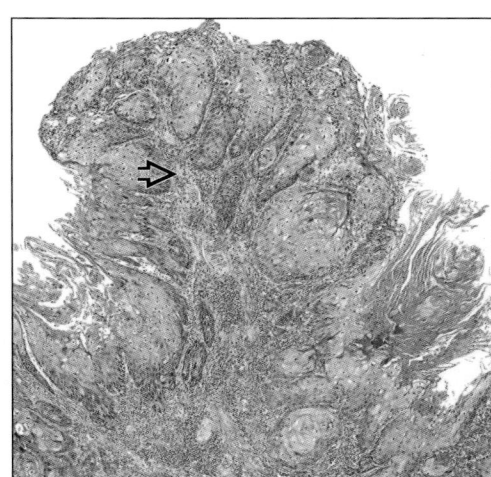

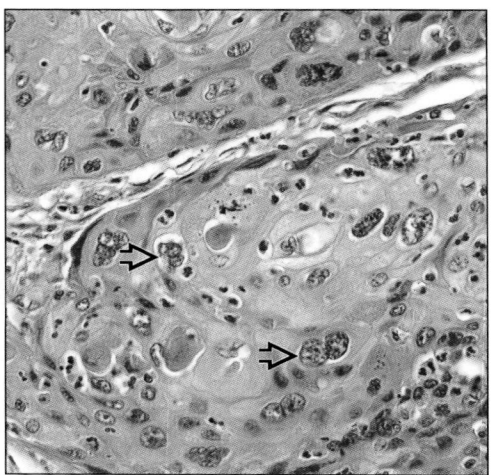

(Left) Warty carcinoma also shows a papillomatous pattern of growth and may be easily confused with papillary carcinoma, but fibrovascular cores ⊳ are consistently present in the former and most of the papillae are elongated and spiky. *(Right)* Warty carcinoma is defined by neoplastic cells with koilocytic atypia ⊳, sharing with papillary carcinoma a papillomatous architecture, keratinizing epithelium, and destructive stromal invasion.

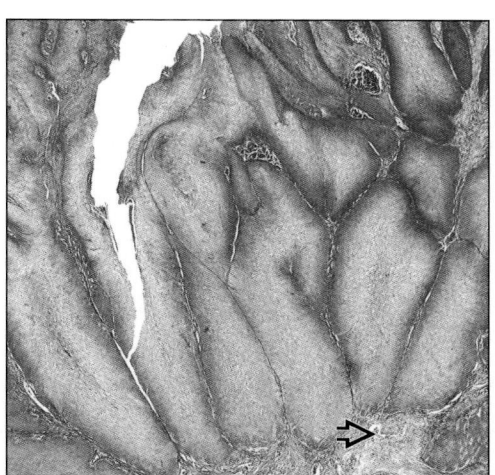

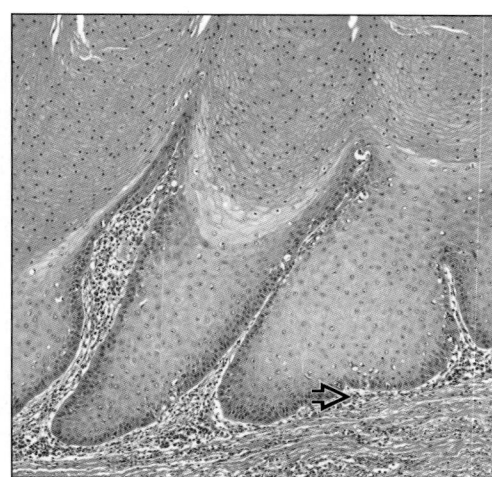

(Left) In giant condyloma, a verruciform tumor that may be confused with papillary carcinoma, koilocytes are easily found, although marked cytologic atypia is absent and tumoral front ⊳ is broad and pushing. *(Right)* In verrucous carcinoma, the tumor front ⊳ is broad and pushing, fibrovascular cores are inconspicuous or absent, and neoplastic cells are extremely well differentiated.

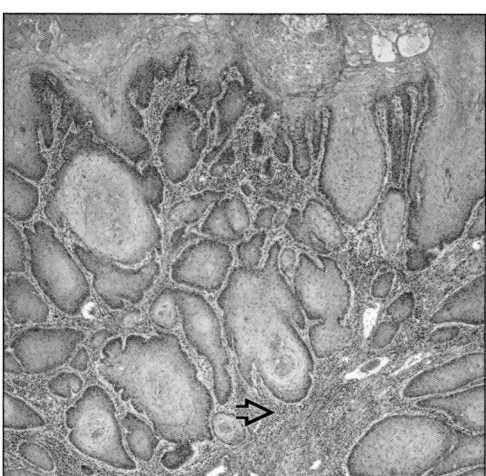

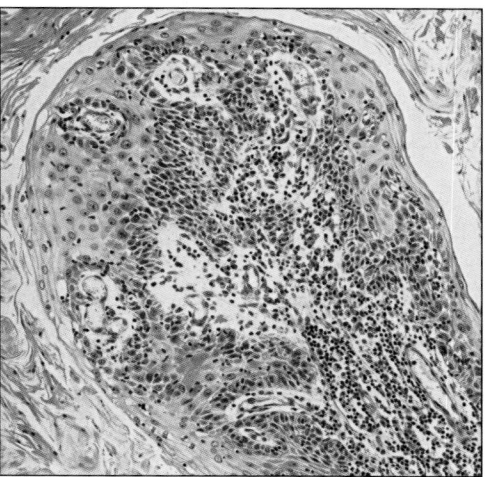

(Left) Carcinoma cuniculatum shows cytologic and architectural features similar to those of verrucous carcinoma but with extensive infiltration of deep anatomical levels ⊳ and formation of sinus tracks and cyst-like structures, findings that are absent in papillary carcinomas. *(Right)* Papillary carcinoma usually does not show overexpression of p16, a cell cycle-related protein that is used as surrogate for high-risk HPV infection.

PAGET DISEASE

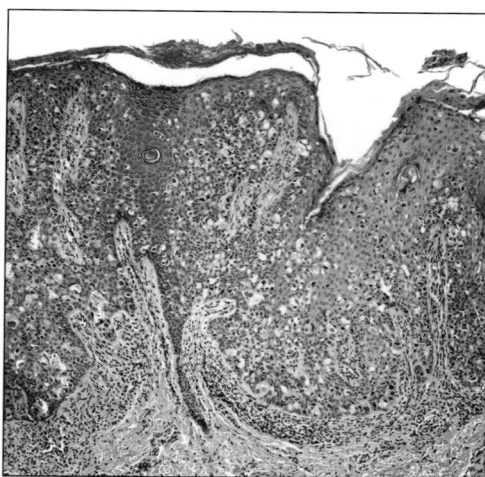

Primary Paget disease of the penis is shown. There is an intraepithelial proliferation of large atypical cells with pale cytoplasm.

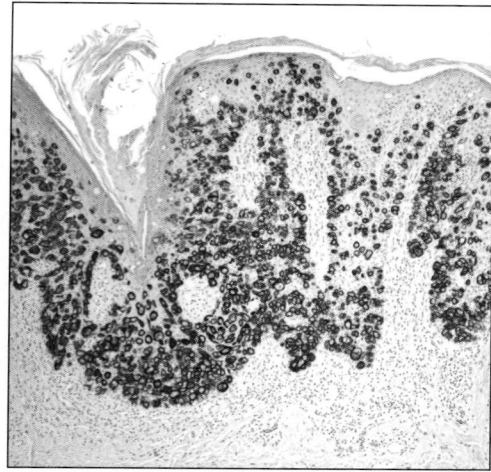

In this case of primary Paget disease of the penis, immunohistochemistry with CK7 highlights the neoplastic cells in all levels of the epidermis.

TERMINOLOGY

Synonyms
- Extramammary Paget disease (EMPD)

Definitions
- Adenocarcinoma involving epidermis and commonly extending to epithelium of eccrine glands &/or hair follicles (adenocarcinoma in situ)
- May involve dermis in minority of cases

ETIOLOGY/PATHOGENESIS

Pathogenesis
- Uncertain
- Cases limited to epidermis are postulated to originate from intraepidermal portion of sweat glands or from intraepidermal stem cells
- Heterogeneous condition; can be classified as primary (cutaneous origin) and secondary (extracutaneous origin)
  - Rarely, primary EMPD is associated with underlying sweat gland adenocarcinoma
  - Secondary EMPD may represent extension from urethral, bladder, or anal/rectal carcinoma

CLINICAL ISSUES

Epidemiology
- Age
  - 6th or 7th decade

Site
- Skin regions rich in apocrine glands, such as anogenital area
- Primary EMPD
  - Scrotum and perineum with extension to adjacent areas are most frequent sites in primary lesions

- Primary EMPD exclusively affecting penis is more rare
- Primary Paget disease of penis may extend to urethral epithelium
- Secondary EMPD
  - Secondary Paget disease tends to affect glans and especially perimeatal region
  - May also affect perianal area extending to perineum and scrotum

Presentation
- Circinate or annular moist erythematous scaly patches or plaques
- Gray-white eczematous patches are also common
- Hypopigmented macules, ulceration, crusting, or palpable tumor may be present
- Pruritus is frequent
- Bleeding, oozing, tenderness or burning sensation can occur
- EMPD may mimic eczema
- Lesions may be multifocal

Treatment
- Complete surgical excision is treatment of choice for primary EMPD
- Treatment in secondary lesions will depend on associated carcinoma

Prognosis
- Primary EMPD confined to epidermis and epithelium of adnexal structures (in situ carcinoma) has good prognosis when completely excised
- Patients require long-term follow-up because of multifocal nature of condition and high recurrence rate
- Dermal invasion is associated with worse prognosis
- Prognosis in secondary Paget disease is related to underlying carcinoma and is usually poor

PAGET DISEASE

Key Facts

Terminology
- Extramammary Paget disease (EMPD)

Clinical Issues
- Erythematous patches or plaques with sharply defined borders
- May clinically mimic chronic eczema

Microscopic Pathology
- Round large pale cells in all levels of epidermis arranged as single units or confluent aggregates
- Round vesicular nuclei with prominent nucleoli
- Abundant clear cytoplasm
- Absence of intercellular bridges
- Paget cells often extend to adnexal structures
- Flattened basal keratinocytes

Ancillary Tests
- Paget cells positive for mucin
- Primary EMPD positive for CK7 and negative for CK20
- Secondary EMPD has more variable immunohistochemical profile
  - Secondary EMPD associated with urothelial carcinoma positive for CK7 and CK20
  - Secondary EMPD associated with anal/rectal carcinoma positive for CK20 and negative for CK7

Top Differential Diagnoses
- Melanoma in situ
- Squamous cell carcinoma in situ
- Clear cell papulosis
- Benign mucinous metaplasia of penis

MACROSCOPIC FEATURES

General Features
- Erythematous patches or plaques with sharply defined borders

Sections to Be Submitted
- Important to carefully evaluate margins because neoplastic cells may extend beyond clinical borders

Size
- Lesions a few mm in size to lesions that broadly involve entire anogenital area
- Focal or multicentric

MICROSCOPIC PATHOLOGY

Histologic Features
- Intraepithelial proliferation of large round atypical cells (Paget cells)
- Epithelium varied from hyperplastic to atrophic
- Epithelium may be eroded or ulcerated
- Cytoplasm of neoplastic cells is abundant and pale or vacuolated
- Melanin pigment may be present within cytoplasm of Paget cells
- Intercellular bridges not appreciated between Paget cells on light microscopy
- Nuclei are large and vesicular
- Nucleoli prominent
- Mitoses may be numerous
- Early lesions show only scattered single Paget cells in epidermis
- As lesions evolve, Paget cells are more numerous and are arranged as single cells and confluent aggregates
- Paget cells compress squamous cells
- Flattened basal keratinocytes lying between neoplastic cells and underlying dermis are observed
- Neoplastic cells often extend to epithelium of adnexal structures

- Neoplastic cells may form true intraepidermal glandular lumina
- Dermal mixed cell infiltrate is usually present
- Dermal involvement by tumoral cells may occur

Predominant Pattern/Injury Type
- Adenocarcinoma

Predominant Cell/Compartment Type
- Paget cells

ANCILLARY TESTS

Histochemistry
- Mucicarmine
  - Reactivity: Positive
  - Staining pattern
    - Cytoplasmic

Immunohistochemistry
- Primary EMPD is positive for CEA, low molecular weight cytokeratins (especially CK7 and Cam5.2), EMA/MUC1, and GCDFP-15
- Primary EMPD is negative for CK20
- Primary EMPD is negative for melanocytic markers, such as S100, Melan-A(MART-1), tyrosinase, and HMB-45
- Immunohistochemical expression profile of secondary EMPD is related to associated carcinoma
  - Secondary EMPD associated with urothelial carcinoma
    - Usually expresses both CK7 and CK20
    - Also expresses uroplakin-3
    - Negative for CEA
  - EMPD secondary to anal/rectal carcinomas
    - Expresses CK20 and CEA
    - CDX-2 expression would be another indicator of associated anal/rectal malignancy
    - CK7 usually negative
    - GCDFP-15 negative

PAGET DISEASE

DIFFERENTIAL DIAGNOSIS

Melanoma In Situ
- Melanoma cells are present in all levels of epidermis, including basal layer
- No flattened basal cells are seen between melanoma cells and dermis
- Presence of melanin pigment in neoplastic cells does not indicate melanoma diagnosis
- Melanoma invades dermis much more frequently than Paget disease
- Immunohistochemical expression of melanocytic markers, such as S100, Melan-A(MART-1), and HMB-45

Squamous Cell Carcinoma In Situ with Pagetoid Pattern
- Presence of intercellular bridges among neoplastic cells
- Positive for HMCK(34βE12)
- Positive for p63
- Negative for mucicarmine
- Negative for CEA, GCDFP-15
- Negative for CK7 and CK20

Clear Cell Papulosis
- Young children
- More often Asian
- Small macules or papules
- Lower part of trunk
- Predominantly milk line location
- Clear cells with pagetoid features in lower part of epidermis
- PAN-CK(AE1/AE3) and CEA positive

Benign Mucinous Metaplasia of Penis
- Elderly patients
- Prepuce or glans
- Benign mucin containing cells in squamous epithelium
- Usually associated with chronic inflammatory conditions

Pagetoid Dyskeratosis
- Reactive process
- Intertriginous and genital area
- Lesional cells are keratinocytes showing early keratinization

Pagetoid Reticulosis
- Rare variant of cutaneous T-cell lymphoma
- Exclusive epidermal infiltration by medium to large sized T cells with abundant pale cytoplasm
- T cells are CD45(LCA) and CD3 positive
- T cells may be either CD4 or CD8 positive, or double negative
- T cell gene rearrangement can be demonstrated

Merkel Cell Carcinoma
- Sometimes may have prominent epidermotropic component
- Small round blue cells with scarce cytoplasm
- Not true glandular formation
- Characteristic dot-like pattern with CK20 and PAN-CK(AE1/AE3)

- In a minority of cases may coexpress CK7
- Positive expression of neuroendocrine markers, such as chromogranin and synaptophysin

DIAGNOSTIC CHECKLIST

Clinically Relevant Pathologic Features
- Tissue distribution
  - Important to distinguish in situ lesions, in which Paget cells are confined within epidermis and epithelium of adnexal structures, from tumors showing dermal invasion
  - Important to recognize EMPD associated with underlying sweat gland carcinoma
  - Important clinically to rule out secondary EMPD

Pathologic Interpretation Pearls
- Large round cells with abundant pale cytoplasm in all levels of epidermis (Paget cells)
- Sometimes true glandular formation by these neoplastic cell in epidermis
- Flattened basal keratinocytes lying between Paget cells and underlying basement membrane
- Presence of melanin does not rule out Paget disease

SELECTED REFERENCES

1. Wang Z et al: Penile and scrotal Paget's disease: 130 Chinese patients with long-term follow-up. BJU Int. 102(4):485-8, 2008
2. Liegl B et al: Mammary and extramammary Paget's disease: an immunohistochemical study of 83 cases. Histopathology. 50(4):439-47, 2007
3. Henning JS: Extramammary Paget's disease of the penis and scrotum. J Drugs Dermatol. 5(7):652-4, 2006
4. De Nisi MC et al: Usefulness of CDX2 in the diagnosis of extramammary Paget disease associated with malignancies of intestinal type. Br J Dermatol. 153(3):677-9, 2005
5. Yang WJ et al: Extramammary Paget's disease of penis and scrotum. Urology. 65(5):972-5, 2005
6. Salamanca J et al: Paget's disease of the glans penis secondary to transitional cell carcinoma of the bladder: a report of two cases and review of the literature. J Cutan Pathol. 31(4):341-5, 2004
7. Brown HM et al: Uroplakin-III to distinguish primary vulvar Paget disease from Paget disease secondary to urothelial carcinoma. Hum Pathol. 33(5):545-8, 2002
8. van Randenborgh H et al: Extramammary Paget's disease of penis and scrotum. J Urol. 168(6):2540-1, 2002
9. Kuan SF et al: Differential expression of mucin genes in mammary and extramammary Paget's disease. Am J Surg Pathol. 25(12):1469-77, 2001
10. Ohnishi T et al: The use of cytokeratins 7 and 20 in the diagnosis of primary and secondary extramammary Paget's disease. Br J Dermatol. 142(2):243-7, 2000
11. Val-Bernal JF et al: Benign mucinous metaplasia of the penis. A lesion resembling extramammary Paget's disease. J Cutan Pathol. 27(2):76-9, 2000
12. Val-Bernal JF et al: Pagetoid dyskeratosis of the prepuce. An incidental histologic finding resembling extramammary Paget's disease. J Cutan Pathol. 27(8):387-91, 2000
13. Lee JY: Clear cell papulosis: a unique disorder in early childhood characterized by white macules in milk-line distribution. Pediatr Dermatol. 15(4):328-9, 1998

PAGET DISEASE

Microscopic, Histochemical and Immunohistochemical

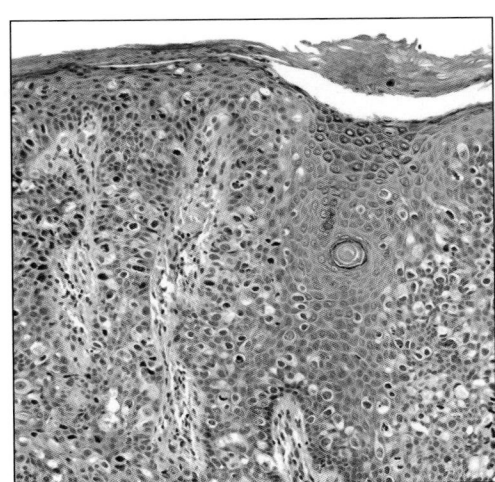
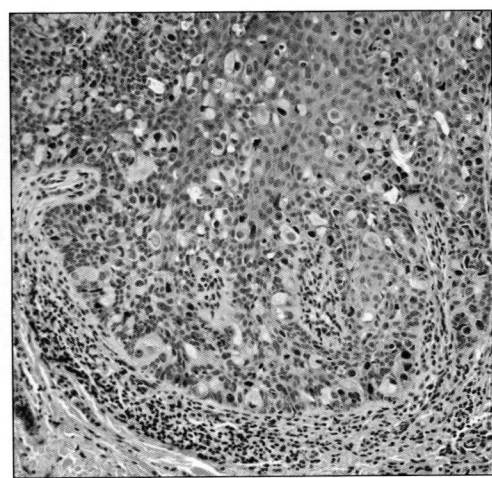

(Left) Note the numerous Paget cells in all levels of the epidermis in this case of extramammary Paget disease. The epidermis is hyperplastic. *(Right)* Paget cells are large round to oval and show ample pale cytoplasm.

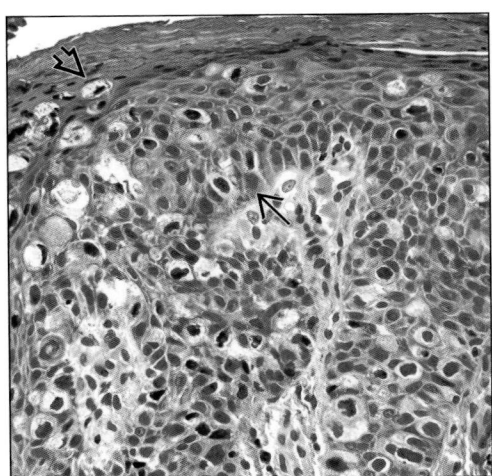
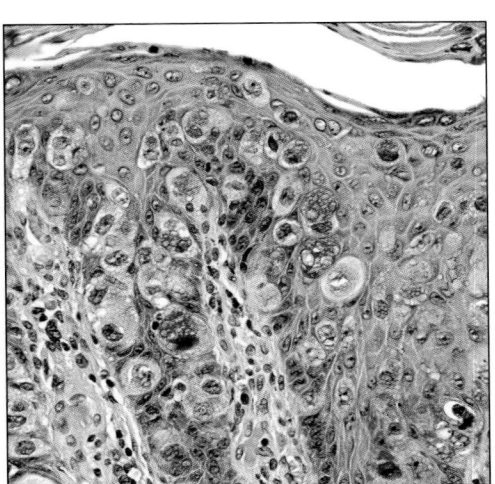

(Left) Numerous Paget cells ⮐ arranged as confluent single units are seen in all levels of the epidermis, including the cornified layer ➡. Note the flattened basal keratinocytes. *(Right)* Red positive staining of the cytoplasm is seen with mucicarmine in cases of EMPD.

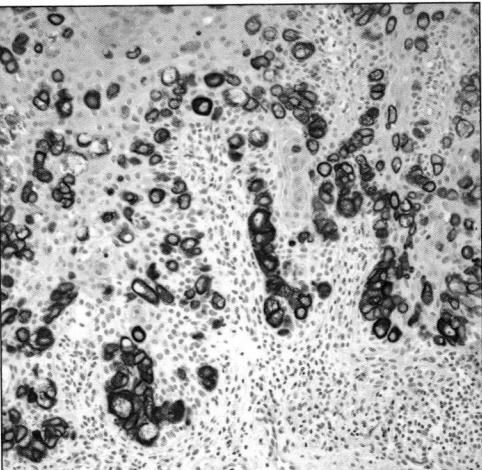
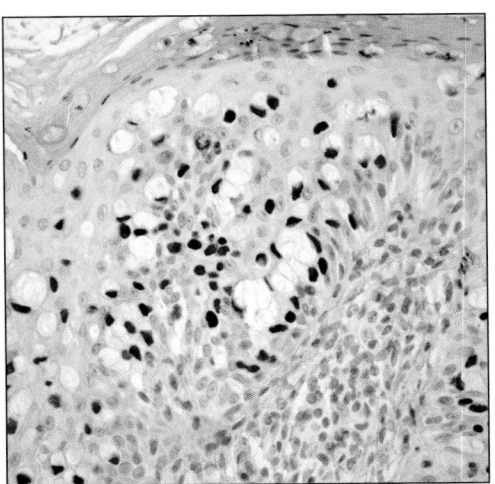

(Left) Note the CK20 expression by the neoplastic cells in this case of EMPD secondary to rectal/anal carcinoma. *(Right)* EMPD secondary to anal/rectal carcinoma. CDX-2 expression by the Paget cells would be another strong indicator of an associated synchronous or metachronous anal/rectal malignancy.

KAPOSI SARCOMA

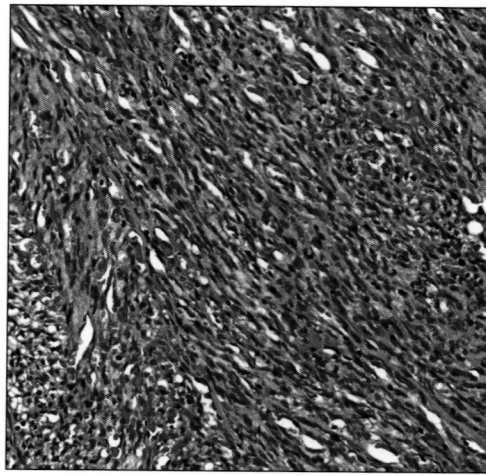

A well-established lesion of Kaposi sarcoma shows the characteristic honeycomb-like network of slit-like vascular spaces filled with erythrocytes separating the spindle cells.

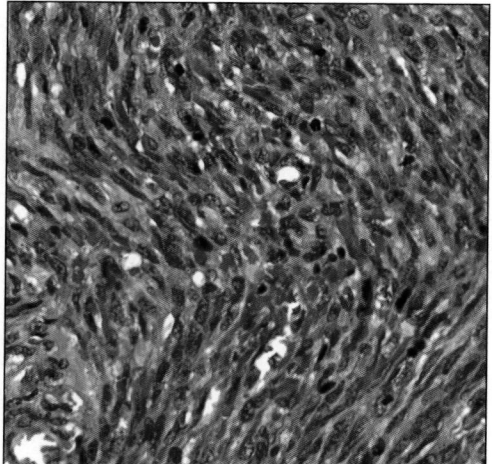

Monomorphic spindle cells in ill-defined fascicles and arcs intimately admixed with slit-like vascular channels containing erythrocytes are a classic feature of Kaposi sarcoma.

TERMINOLOGY

Abbreviations
- Kaposi sarcoma (KS)

Definitions
- Virus-associated vascular tumor

ETIOLOGY/PATHOGENESIS

Etiology
- Human herpes virus-8 (KSHV/HHV-8)
- Unclear whether KS represents true neoplasia or reactive condition

Pathogenesis
- Proliferating cell in KS appears to be lymphatic in origin
- KS can be classified into 4 main groups
  - Classic, endemic/African, AIDS-associated, and iatrogenic/transplantation-associated KS

CLINICAL ISSUES

Epidemiology
- Incidence
  - Penile and urogenital KS usually affects HIV(+) patients
    - Incidence has decreased with advent of antiretroviral therapy
  - May also be seen in patients affected by other forms of immunosuppression
  - Classic and endemic forms of KS affecting penis are extremely rare
- Age
  - AIDS-related KS and endemic forms affect younger patients
  - Classic KS and transplant-related KS tend to affect older patients

Site
- Most common location is the glans
- May also affect coronal sulcus, foreskin, and skin of shaft

Presentation
- From ill-defined erythematous macules to violaceous plaques and nodules
- Frequently multifocal
- Tends to affect penis in setting of multiple disseminated lesions, especially in AIDS patients

Treatment
- Irradiation &/or chemotherapy

Prognosis
- Variable and usually dependent on different interrelated factors, such as immunologic host status and stage of disease
  - AIDS-related KS runs more rapid evolution than classical form

MACROSCOPIC FEATURES

General Features
- Specimen received are usually punch or incisional/excisional biopsies

MICROSCOPIC PATHOLOGY

Histologic Features
- Patch stage
  - Subtle proliferation of slit-like &/or angulated/jagged vessels separating collagen bundles within dermis
  - Adnexal structures and preexisting vessels may protrude within newly formed vessels (promontory sign)

KAPOSI SARCOMA

Key Facts

Etiology/Pathogenesis
- HHV-8

Microscopic Pathology
- Early lesions are subtle and may start with proliferation of vessels around dermal sweat glands
- Well-established lesions show characteristic honeycomb-like network of blood-filled spaces/slits closely associated with spindle cell component

Ancillary Tests
- Immunohistochemistry for HHV-8 is helpful to confirm diagnosis
- Positive for FVIIIRAg, CD31, CD34, & Podoplanin

Top Differential Diagnoses
- Angioma
- Angiosarcoma
- Fibrosarcoma
- Sarcomatoid carcinoma

- o Extravasated red blood cells, siderophages, and patchy dermal infiltrate of lymphoid cells and plasma cells
- Plaque stage
  - o Vascular proliferation diffusely involves dermis and may extend to subcutis
  - o Relatively bland spindle cell component appears at this stage
  - o PAS-D(+) hyaline globules may be seen intra- and extracellularly
- Nodular stage
  - o Spindle cell proliferation becomes confluent to form well-defined nodules
    - Spindle cells are devoid of significant pleomorphism
  - o Fascicles and arcs of spindle cells intersect one another and are intimately admixed/separated by slit-like spaces containing erythrocytes
  - o Dilated blood vessels, inflammatory cells, and siderophages are often seen at periphery of nodules

DIFFERENTIAL DIAGNOSIS

Angioma
- Jagged vascular pattern among collagen bundles, promontory sign, and patchy infiltrate with plasma cells and siderophages is more characteristic of KS

Angiosarcoma
- Usually more pleomorphic cells lining vascular spaces

Fibrosarcoma
- Does not have slit-like spaces containing erythrocytes among spindle cells

Sarcomatoid Carcinoma
- Biphasic tumor, or may be positive for keratins (especially PAN-CK[AE1/AE3] and HMCK[34βE12]) and p63

DIAGNOSTIC CHECKLIST

Pathologic Interpretation Pearls
- Low-power view in early lesions shows slender cords of cells amongst collagen bundles that may mimic histiocytes or stromal cells
  - o Only closer view will reveal luminal differentiation or connection with preexisting blood vessels

SELECTED REFERENCES

1. Katona TM et al: Soft tissue tumors of the penis: a review. Anal Quant Cytol Histol. 28(4):193-206, 2006
2. Carroll PA et al: Kaposi's sarcoma-associated herpesvirus infection of blood endothelial cells induces lymphatic differentiation. Virology. 328(1):7-18, 2004
3. Micali G et al: Primary classic Kaposi's sarcoma of the penis: report of a case and review. J Eur Acad Dermatol Venereol. 17(3):320-3, 2003
4. Lowe FC et al: Kaposi's sarcoma of the penis in patients with acquired immunodeficiency syndrome. J Urol. 142(6):1475-7, 1989

IMAGE GALLERY

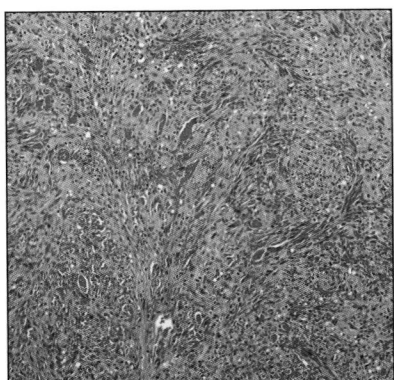 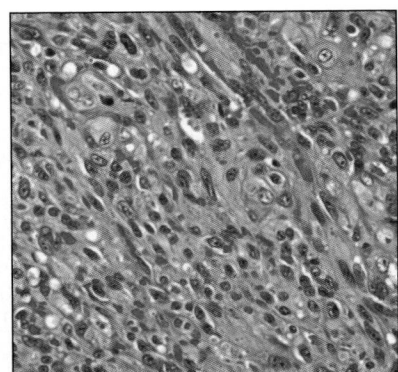 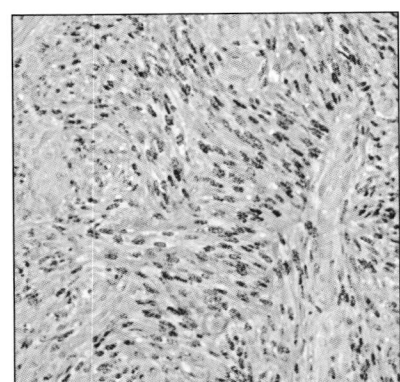

(Left) Low-power view in a well-established nodular lesion of Kaposi sarcoma shows a network of slit-like and slightly dilated vessels filled with red blood cells and a proliferation of relatively bland spindle cells. *(Center)* On transverse sections, the spindle cells appear more rounded and epithelioid. Note the slit-like vessels intimately admixed with the spindle cells. *(Right)* Immunohistochemical analysis with KSHV/HHV8 shows nuclear expression in Kaposi sarcoma.

MYOINTIMOMA

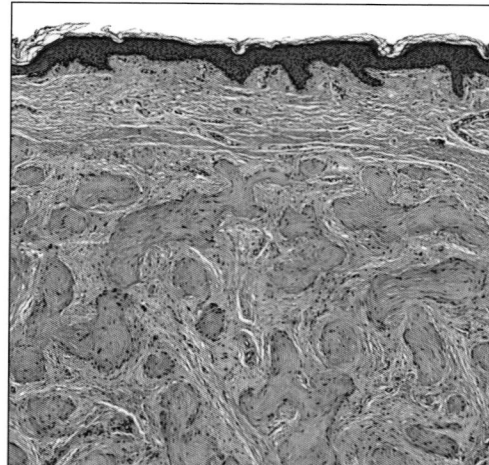

Penile myointimoma of the corpus spongiosum has a distinctive low-power serpiginous or nodular growth pattern secondary to extension along preexisting vascular channels.

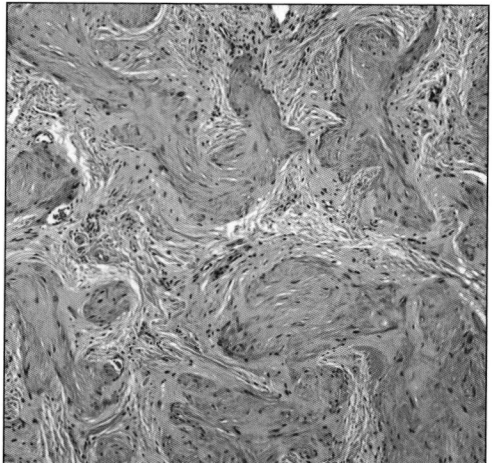

The lesional cells have a spindled myofibroblastic appearance and an associated fibrous and myxoid stroma. They expand the vascular spaces with atrophy of the vessel walls and loss of the lumen.

TERMINOLOGY

Definitions
- Benign myointimal proliferation occurring exclusively in corpus spongiosum of glans penis

CLINICAL ISSUES

Epidemiology
- Incidence
  - Rare tumor with few reported case series
- Age
  - Affects children and adults

Presentation
- Small palpable nodular lesion on glans penis

Treatment
- Simple conservative excision

Prognosis
- Benign
  - No recurrences reported
    - Even if incompletely excised
  - May regress in some cases

MACROSCOPIC FEATURES

Size
- Typically 0.5-2 cm

MICROSCOPIC PATHOLOGY

Histologic Features
- Plexiform or multinodular growth
  - Pure intravascular growth
  - Extension within preexisting vascular network of corpus spongiosum
- Individual cells have myofibroblast morphology
  - Spindled cell population
  - Elongated tapered cytoplasmic processes
    - Some multipolar
  - Fine nuclear chromatin
  - Pinpoint nucleoli common
  - Eosinophilic cytoplasm
  - No significant nuclear atypia
- Associated myxoid and fibrous stroma is characteristic
- Surrounding collarette of residual smooth muscle generally present at periphery
  - Centrally, no residual vessel wall is seen
- Intracytoplasmic juxtanuclear vacuoles are common

ANCILLARY TESTS

Immunohistochemistry
- Express smooth muscle markers
  - Actin-HHF-35
  - Muscle specific actin
  - Calponin
- Desmin highlights residual native smooth muscle of vessel walls
  - Seen best at periphery of lesion
  - Lesional spindled cells are desmin negative
- S100 negative
- CD31 and CD34 highlight residual endothelial cells at periphery

DIFFERENTIAL DIAGNOSIS

Intravascular Fasciitis
- Intravascular myofibroblastic proliferation
  - Extends within vessels creating similar multinodular/plexiform growth pattern
- Intralesional inflammatory cells are common
- Expansion of vascular spaces is common
- Admixed osteoclast-like giant cells are common

MYOINTIMOMA

Key Facts

Terminology
- Distinctive myointimal proliferation arising within corpus spongiosum of glans penis

Clinical Issues
- Small palpable nodular lesion on glans penis
- Simple conservative excision
- Benign, nonrecurring
- Rare tumor with few reported case series
- Affects children and adults

Microscopic Pathology
- Plexiform or multinodular growth
- Pure intravascular growth with extension along vessels of corpus spongiosum
- Individual cells have myofibroblast morphology

- Associated myxoid and fibrous stroma is characteristic
- Surrounding collarette of residual smooth muscle generally present at periphery
- Intracytoplasmic juxtanuclear vacuoles are common

Ancillary Tests
- Express actin-sm
- Desmin highlights residual native smooth muscle of vessel walls

Top Differential Diagnoses
- Intravascular fasciitis
- Plexiform fibrohistiocytic tumor
- Myofibroma
- Leiomyoma
- Epithelioid hemangioendothelioma

Plexiform Fibrohistiocytic Tumor
- Similar plexiform/nodular growth
- Not described in penis
- Not intravascular
- Dimorphic morphology
  - Fascicles of spindled myofibroblasts
    - Express actin-sm
  - Nodules of histiocytic cells with scattered osteoclast-type giant cells

Myofibroma
- Often have classic biphasic appearance
  - Myoid nodules are similar in morphology to myointimoma cells
  - Hemangiopericytoma-like foci often admixed
- Myoid predominant myofibromas do occur
- May involve vessels
  - Not exclusively confined to vascular lumina as in myointimoma
- Generally more cellular and more fascicular than myointimoma

Leiomyoma
- Intersecting fascicular architecture
- Not typically multinodular/plexiform
- Lesional cells express desmin
- Not typically myxoid
  - More eosinophilic appearance

Epithelioid Hemangioendothelioma
- Morphologically similar
  - Similar myxoid stroma
  - Usually more epithelioid but may be spindled
  - Intraluminal vacuoles common
- Rare in children
- Very uncommon in penis
  - Epithelioid hemangioma is more common in penis
    - However, less morphologic overlap with myointimoma
- Immunoreactivity for CD31 and CD34 in spindled/epithelioid cell population

Nerve Sheath Tumors
- May have multinodular/plexiform growth pattern
  - Neurofibroma
  - Schwannoma
  - Nerve sheath myxoma
- Usually have less condensed myxoid matrix
- Diffuse nuclear reactivity for S100
- Not common in penis

DIAGNOSTIC CHECKLIST

Clinically Relevant Pathologic Features
- This benign lesion does not require reexcision if transected

Pathologic Interpretation Pearls
- Anatomic site should alert pathologists to possibility of this diagnosis

SELECTED REFERENCES

1. Turner BM et al: Penile myointimoma. J Cutan Pathol. 36(7):817-9, 2009
2. McKenney JK et al: Penile myointimoma in children and adolescents: a clinicopathologic study of 5 cases supporting a distinct entity. Am J Surg Pathol. 31(10):1622-6, 2007
3. Vardar E et al: Myointimoma of the glans penis. Pathol Int. 57(3):158-61, 2007
4. Robbins JB et al: Penile nodule in a 54-year-old man: a case of a myointimoma. J Am Acad Dermatol. 53(6):1084-6, 2005
5. Fetsch et al: Mesenchymal tumours. In Eble JN et al (eds): Pathology & Genetics of Tumours of the Urinary System and Male Genital Organs. Lyon: IARC Press. 294, 2004
6. Fetsch JF et al: A distinctive myointimal proliferation ('myointimoma') involving the corpus spongiosum of the glans penis: a clinicopathologic and immunohistochemical analysis of 10 cases. Am J Surg Pathol. 24(11):1524-30, 2000

Microscopic Features

(Left) This low-power photomicrograph of a glans penis excision, which often include the overlying skin, highlights the small size of the lesion and its location within the corpus spongiosum. *(Right)* Myointimoma is characterized by this plexiform growth pattern, which is secondary to extension down the preexisting vascular spaces of the corpus spongiosum. This distinctive architecture is a requisite feature.

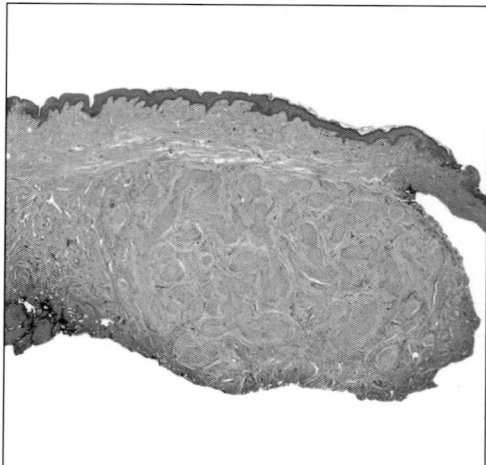
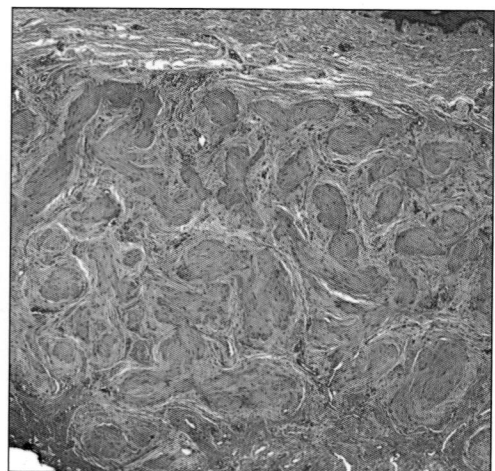

(Left) The nodular/plexiform growth pattern is distinctive of myointimoma. Preexisting vascular spaces are not easily identifiable in central areas of the lesion. The surrounding stroma has reactive myxoid changes, which is common. *(Right)* There is very little morphologic heterogeneity described for myointimoma. All reported cases have a similar serpiginous growth that distinguishes myointimoma from myofibroma, which may have a similar appearance on high-power examination.

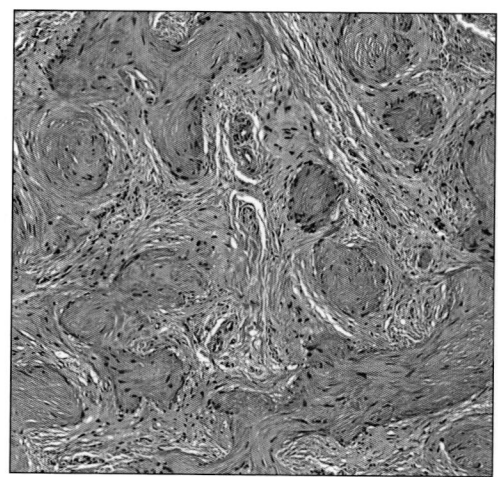
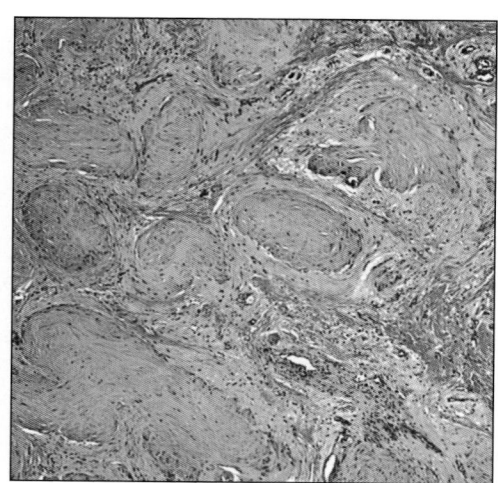

(Left) A nodule of myofibroblast-like cells expand the preexisting vascular space in a myointimoma. With expansion, the native vessel wall may become inapparent. *(Right)* Juxtanuclear intracytoplasmic vacuoles are common in myointimoma ➡. This histologic feature may cause diagnostic confusion with vascular lesions, such as epithelioid hemangioendothelioma.

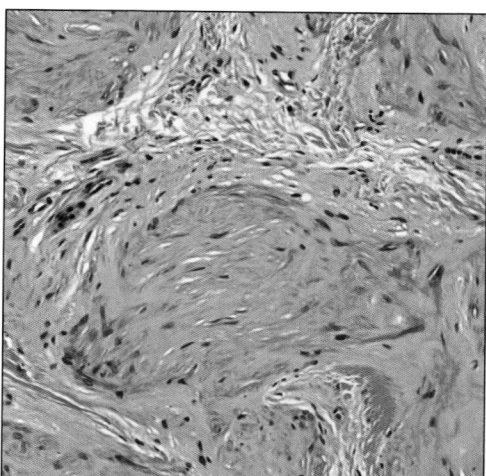
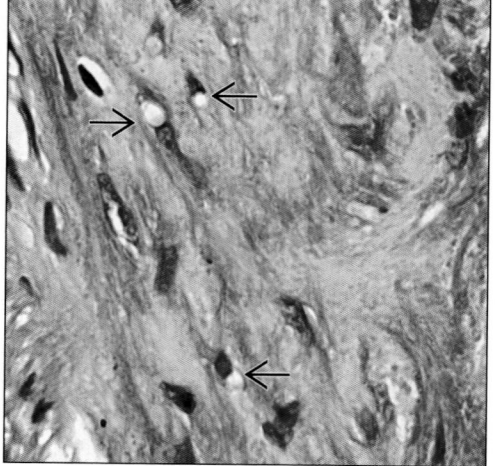

MYOINTIMOMA

Microscopic Features

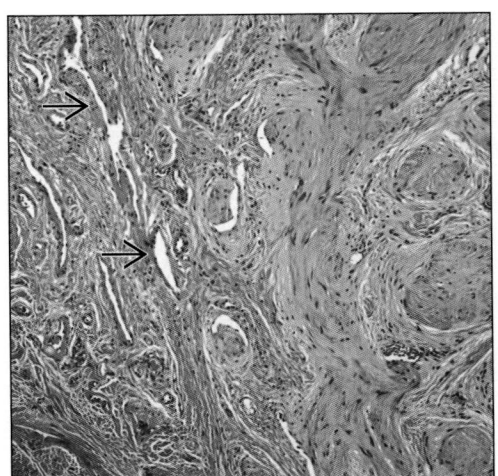
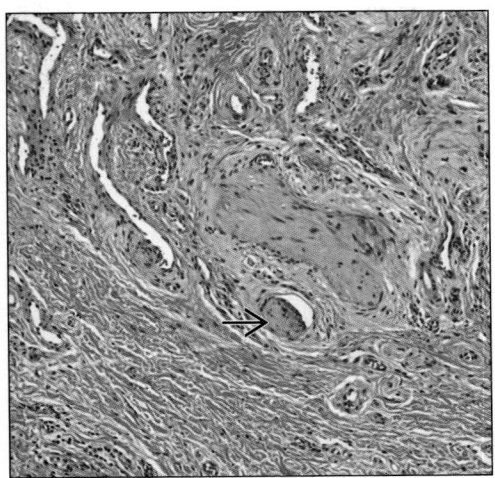

(Left) The periphery of myointimoma commonly shows features that aid in the differential diagnosis. This picture highlights the junction of a myointimoma with normal vessels of the corpus spongiosum ⊡. *(Right)* In these peripheral transition areas, there is partial filling of small vessel lumina by the lesional spindled cells with associated myxoid stroma ⊡. Residual endothelial cells and smooth muscle collarettes are common in these foci.

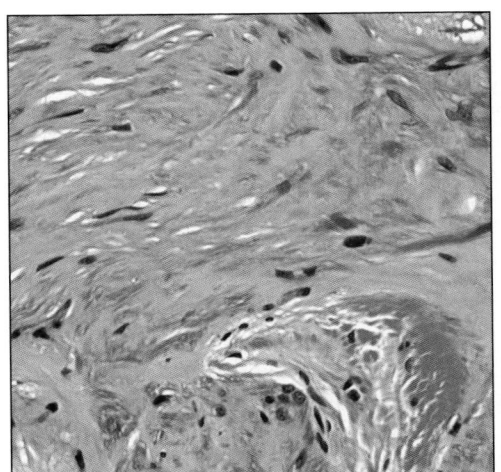
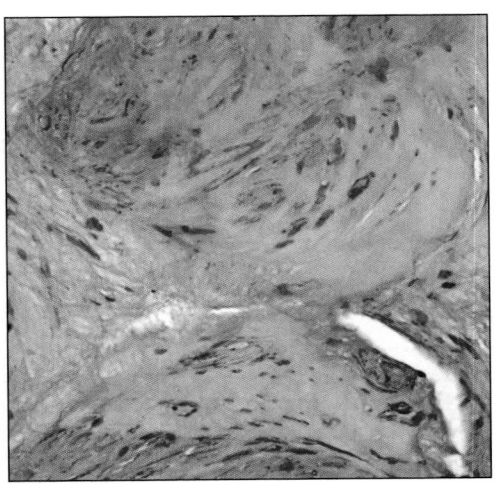

(Left) The lesional spindled cells of myointimoma are associated with a dense fibrous and myxoid stroma. They have tapered nuclei and elongated cytoplasmic processes. No significant nuclear atypia is seen. *(Right)* Smooth muscle actin highlights the lesional spindled cells of myointimoma; calponin shows similar findings. Desmin is not coexpressed by this population, an immunophenotype typical of myofibroblasts.

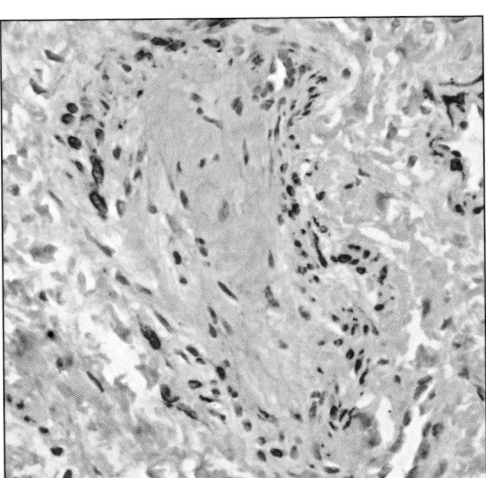
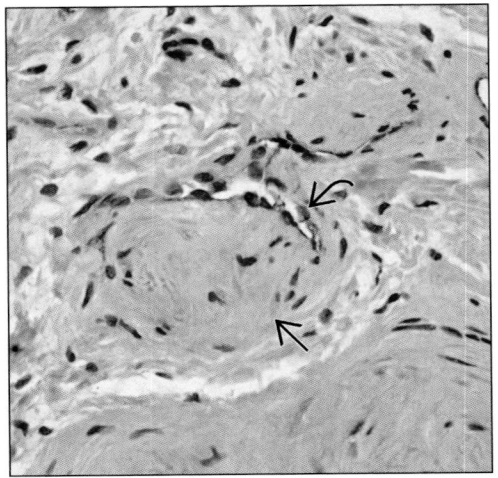

(Left) Desmin immunohistochemistry highlights a residual collarette of native smooth muscle within the preexisting vessel wall in a myointimoma. This feature is seen best at the periphery of the lesion because the collarettes become atrophied and inapparent centrally. *(Right)* A CD31 immunostain highlights the residual endothelial cells ⊡ that are compressed by the expanding myointimal proliferation ⊡. These are often inapparent centrally, as the lumina are obliterated.

METASTATIC TUMORS, PENIS

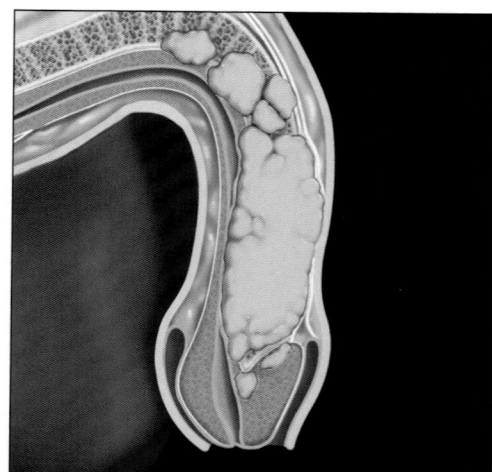

Diagram of a secondary prostatic adenosquamous carcinoma shows multiple deep-seated metastatic nodules mainly located in corpora cavernosa of the penile shaft without affecting the glans surface.

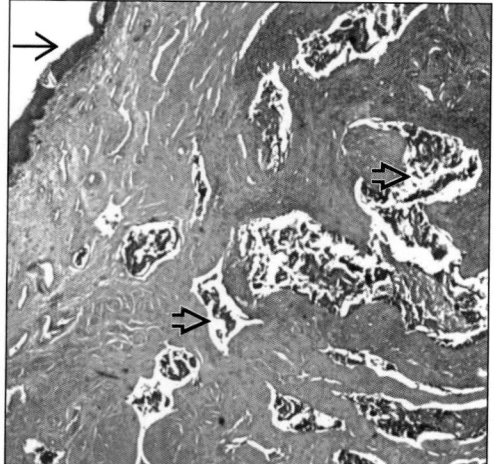

Metastatic adenocarcinoma from sigmoid colon extensively involving vascular spaces of penile erectile tissues ⊳ but with no involvement of penile shaft skin ⇨.

TERMINOLOGY

Definitions
- Secondary involvement of penis by malignancy with predilection for erectile tissues of corpora cavernosa

ETIOLOGY/PATHOGENESIS

Routes of Spread
- Mostly by retrograde venous or lymphatic spread
- Arterial spread, direct extension from regional sites, and secondary embolization

CLINICAL ISSUES

Site
- Predilection for erectile tissues of corpora cavernosa
- Among tumors metastatic to penis, genitourinary (GU) tumors are most common, although only a minority of GU tumors metastasize to penis
  - Bladder urothelial carcinoma and prostatic adenocarcinomas account for most primary tumors
  - Other GU primary sites include kidney (renal cell carcinoma) and testis (seminoma)
- Among gastrointestinal tumors, colonic (sigmoid and rectal) adenocarcinomas are most common
  - Pancreatic, gastric, and esophageal primaries have also been rarely reported
- Rare primary sites include melanoma, lung, thyroid gland, among others
- Malignant lymphomas may also secondarily affect penis due to systemic dissemination
- Range of sarcomas, including chondrosarcoma, synovial sarcoma, and angiosarcoma have been reported

Presentation
- Clinical history of primary tumor often available

- Very rarely penile metastasis is initial manifestation of disease
- 1/3 are detected concurrently with primary
- Common symptoms include difficulty in urination, dysuria, &/or urinary retention
- Priapism ("malignant priapism") occurs in about 1/2 of cases due to massive erectile tissue involvement
- Painless mass is not an infrequent clinical finding

Treatment
- Multidisciplinary approach is required

Prognosis
- Poor prognosis related to pathologic stage of primary
- Even with combined multimodal therapy, survival is poor (mean: 9 months)

IMAGE FINDINGS

General Features
- CT, MR, and ultrasound ± fine needle aspiration
- Cavernosography is also useful but has relatively high complication rate

MACROSCOPIC FEATURES

General Features
- Corpora cavernosa are most frequently involved
- Corpus spongiosum and glans are rarely involved
- Skin of shaft and foreskin are rarely involved

MICROSCOPIC PATHOLOGY

Histologic Features
- Tumor cells mainly in vascular spaces of penile erectile tissues
- Involvement may be extensive, proximal to distal corpora cavernosa

METASTATIC TUMORS, PENIS

Key Facts

Terminology
- GU tumors are most common primary sites
- Bladder urothelial carcinomas and prostatic adenocarcinomas account for most of cases

Macroscopic Features
- Corpora cavernosa are most frequent anatomic site affected
- Glans and foreskin are rarely involved

Microscopic Pathology
- Tumor cells mainly in vascular spaces of penile erectile tissues
- Histological subtypes rarely found as primary penile tumors

Top Differential Diagnoses
- Primary squamous cell carcinoma
- Primary penile sarcoma
- Urothelial carcinoma of urethra

- Histologic picture is consistent with morphology of primary tumor
- Pagetoid spread to urethra may be present in some urothelial carcinomas
- Perineural and vascular invasion are common findings
- Penile parenchymal involvement is rare and secondary to extensive vascular involvement

Cytologic Features
- Identification of "cercariform" cells in aspiration cytology permits diagnosis of metastatic urothelial carcinoma

DIFFERENTIAL DIAGNOSIS

Primary Squamous Cell Carcinoma
- Glans affected in most cases and in situ changes in surface epithelium are commonly present
- Corpora cavernosa involvement is secondary to invasion of consecutive anatomic levels

Primary Penile Sarcoma
- Often considered in differential diagnosis as mucosa/skin is uninvolved
- Predilection for deep erectile tissues and parenchyma
- Histology and immunohistochemistry typical of primary sarcoma
- Metastatic sarcomas are vanishingly rare

Urothelial Carcinoma of Urethra
- Urothelial carcinoma in situ or papillary urothelial carcinoma involving urethra
- Secondary involvement of penile tissues, including corpus spongiosum
- Immunohistochemistry for urothelial markers (uroplakin-3, thrombomodulin)

DIAGNOSTIC CHECKLIST

Pathologic Interpretation Pearls
- Nonsquamous histology, multicentricity, and prominent vascular erectile tissue venous invasion

SELECTED REFERENCES

1. Chaux A et al: Metastatic Tumors to the Penis: A Report of 17 Cases and Review of the Literature. Int J Surg Pathol. Epub ahead of print, 2010
2. da Cunha Santos G et al: Penile metastasis of urothelial carcinoma diagnosed by fine-needle aspiration. Cytojournal. 6:10, 2009
3. Cherian J et al: Secondary penile tumours revisited. Int Semin Surg Oncol. 3:33, 2006
4. Bates AW et al: Secondary tumours of the penis. J R Soc Med. 95(3):162-3, 2002
5. Perez LM et al: Penile metastasis secondary to supraglottic squamous cell carcinoma: review of the literature. J Urol. 147(1):157-60, 1992

IMAGE GALLERY

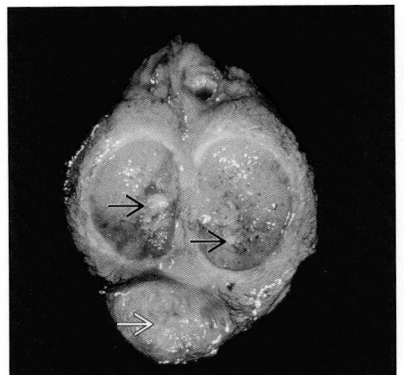 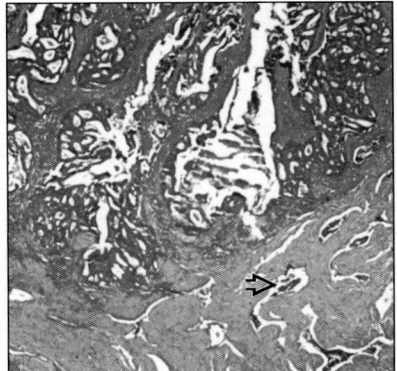 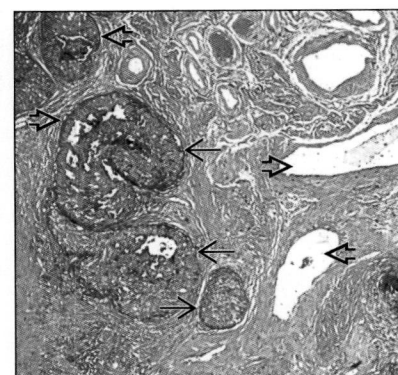

(Left) Transverse section shows extensive involvement of both corpora ⇨ as well as periurethral tissue ➡. *(Center)* Metastatic colonic adenocarcinoma extensively involves vascular spaces of erectile tissues with smaller tumor nests ⇥ in vascular lymphatic spaces. *(Right)* Urothelial carcinoma metastatic to the penis is shown with predilection of tumor nests ⇨ for vascular spaces ⇥ of the corpus cavernosum.

PROTOCOL FOR SPECIMENS OF PRIMARY PENILE CANCER

Penis: Incisional Biopsy, Excisional Biopsy, Partial Penectomy, Total Penectomy, Circumcision

Surgical Pathology Cancer Case Summary (Checklist)

Procedure

____ Incisional biopsy

____ Excisional biopsy

____ Partial penectomy

____ Total penectomy

____ Circumcision

____ Other (specify): _____

____ Not specified

Foreskin (Presence and Type) (select all that apply)

____ Present (uncircumcised)

*____ Short

*____ Medium

*____ Long

*____ Phimotic

____ Not identified (circumcised)

____ Cannot be determined

Lymphadenectomy

____ Not applicable

____ Sentinel node biopsy

____ Inguinal (superficial and deep)

____ External iliac

____ Pelvic nodes

____ Other (specify): _____

Lymph Node Sampling

Number of involved lymph nodes: _____

Total number of lymph nodes examined: _____

Specimen Size

Specify: _____ x _____ cm

Tumor Site (if multiple sites are involved, select all that apply)

____ Glans

____ Foreskin mucosal surface

____ Foreskin skin surface

____ Coronal sulcus (balanopreputial sulcus)

____ Skin of the shaft

____ Penile urethra

Tumor Size

Greatest dimension: _____ cm

*Additional dimensions: _____ x _____ cm

*Tumor Focality

*____ Unicentric

*____ Multicentric

*Tumor Macroscopic Features (select all that apply)

*____ Flat

*____ Ulcerated

*____ Polypoid

*____ Verruciform

*____ Necrosis

PROTOCOL FOR SPECIMENS OF PRIMARY PENILE CANCER

*____ Hemorrhage

*____ Other (specify): _____

Tumor Deep Borders (select all that apply)

*____ Pushing (broadly base)

*____ Infiltrative (jagged)

*____ Other (specify): _____

Macroscopic Extent of Tumor (select all that apply)

*In the glans

   *____ Tumor involves lamina propria

   *____ Tumor involves corpus spongiosum

   *____ Tumor involves tunica albuginea

   *____ Tumor involves corpus cavernosum

   *____ Tumor involves distal (penile) urethra

   *____ Not applicable

*In the foreskin

   *____ Tumor involves lamina propria

   *____ Tumor involves dartos

   *____ Tumor involves preputial skin

   *____ Not applicable

*In the shaft

   *____ Tumor involves skin

   *____ Tumor involves dartos

   *____ Tumor involves Buck fascia

   *____ Tumor involves corpus spongiosum

   *____ Tumor involves corpus cavernosum

   *____ Tumor involves proximal urethra

   *____ Not applicable

Macroscopic Assessment of Resection Margins (select all that apply)

____ Cannot be assessed

____ Grossly uninvolved

____ Grossly involved (specify for penectomy or circumcision specimen below)

For penectomy specimens

   ____ Urethral

   ____ Periurethral tissues (lamina propria, corpus spongiosum, Buck fascia)

   ____ Corpora cavernosa

   ____ Buck fascia at penile shaft

   ____ Skin

____ Other (specify): _____

For circumcision specimens

   ____ Coronal sulcus margin

   ____ Cutaneous margin

Histologic Type (select all that apply)

____ Squamous cell carcinoma (SCC)

   ____ Usual (keratinizing)

   ____ Basaloid

   ____ Verrucous

   *____ Cuniculatum

   *____ Papillary, not otherwise specified (NOS)

   ____ Sarcomatoid

   *____ Pseudohyperplastic

   *____ Acantholytic (pseudoglandular)

   *____ Mixed SCCs

   ____ Adenosquamous

PROTOCOL FOR SPECIMENS OF PRIMARY PENILE CANCER

_____ Primary neuroendocrine carcinoma

_____ Paget disease

_____ Adnexal carcinoma (specify type): _____

_____ Clear cell carcinoma

_____ Carcinoma, type cannot be determined

_____ Other (specify): _____

Histologic Grade

_____ Not applicable

_____ GX: Cannot be assessed

_____ G1: Well differentiated

_____ G2: Moderately differentiated

_____ G3: Poorly differentiated

Microscopic Tumor Extension (select all that apply)

Anatomical levels

In the glans

_____ Tumor involves lamina propria

_____ Tumor involves corpus spongiosum

_____ Tumor involves tunica albuginea

_____ Tumor involves corpus cavernosum

_____ Not applicable

In the coronal sulcus

_____ Tumor involves lamina propria

_____ Tumor involves dartos

_____ Tumor involves Buck fascia

_____ Not applicable

In the foreskin

_____ Tumor involves lamina propria

_____ Tumor involves dartos

_____ Tumor involves preputial skin

_____ Not applicable

In the shaft

_____ Tumor involves skin

_____ Tumor involves dartos

_____ Tumor involves Buck fascia

_____ Tumor involves corpus spongiosum

_____ Tumor involves corpus cavernosum

_____ Not applicable

Other extension

_____ Penile (distal) urethra

_____ Proximal urethra

_____ Prostate

_____ Scrotum

_____ Regional skin (pubis, inguinal)

*Tumor Thickness/Depth

*Specify: _____ mm

Margins of Resection (select all that apply)

_____ Cannot be assessed

_____ Histologically uninvolved

_____ Histologically involved (specify for penectomy or circumcision specimens below)

For penectomy specimens

_____ Urethral

_____ Periurethral tissues (lamina propria, corpus spongiosum, Buck fascia)

_____ Corpus cavernosum

PROTOCOL FOR SPECIMENS OF PRIMARY PENILE CANCER

____ Buck fascia at penile shaft

____ Skin

____ Other (specify): _____

For circumcision specimens

____ Coronal sulcus margin

____ Cutaneous margin

Lymph-Vascular Invasion

____ Not identified

____ Present

____ Indeterminate

Perineural Invasion

____ Not identified

____ Present

____ Indeterminate

Pathologic Staging (pTNM)

TNM descriptors (required only if applicable) (select all that apply)

____ m (multiple primary tumors)

____ r (recurrent)

____ y (posttreatment)

Primary tumor (pT)

____ pTX: Primary tumor cannot be assessed

____ pT0: No evidence of primary tumor

____ pTis: Carcinoma in situ

____ pTa: Noninvasive verrucous carcinoma†

____ pT1a: Tumor invades subepithelial connective tissue without lymph vascular invasion and is not poorly differentiated (i.e., grade 3-4)

____ pT1b: Tumor invades subepithelial connective tissue with lymph vascular invasion or is poorly differentiated

____ pT2: Tumor invades corpus spongiosum or cavernosum

____ pT3: Tumor invades urethra

____ pT4: Tumor invades other adjacent structures

†Broad pushing penetration (invasion) is permitted, but destructive invasion argues against this diagnosis.

Regional lymph nodes (pN)

____ pNX: Regional lymph nodes cannot be assessed

____ pN0: No regional lymph node metastasis

____ pN1: Metastasis in a single inguinal lymph node

____ pN2: Metastasis in multiple or bilateral inguinal lymph nodes

____ pN3: Extranodal extension of lymph node metastasis or pelvic lymph node(s) unilateral or bilateral

Distant metastasis (pM)

____ Not applicable

____ pM1: Distant metastasis†

†Lymph node metastasis outside of the true pelvis in addition to visceral or bone sites

*Additional Pathologic Findings (select all that apply)

*____ None identified

*____ Penile intraepithelial neoplasia (PeIN)

   *____ Differentiated (simplex)

   *____ Warty

   *____ Basaloid

   *____ Mixed (warty/basaloid)

   *____ Other (specify): _____

   *____ Focal

   *____ Multifocal

   *____ Margins uninvolved

   *____ Margins involved (specify margin): _____

*____ Lichen sclerosus

PROTOCOL FOR SPECIMENS OF PRIMARY PENILE CANCER

*___ Squamous hyperplasia

*___ Condyloma acuminatum

*___ Other (specify): _____

*Ancillary Studies

*Specify: _____

*___ Not performed

*Data elements with asterisks are not required. However, these elements may be clinically important but are not yet validated or regularly used in patient management. Adapted with permission from College of American Pathologists, "Protocol for the Examination of Specimens from Patients with Carcinoma of the Penis." Under development.

Anatomic Stage/Prognostic Groups

Group	Tumor	Node	Metastasis
Stage 0	Tis	N0	M0
	Ta	N0	M0
Stage I	T1a	N0	M0
Stage II	T1b	N0	M0
	T2	N0	M0
	T3	N0	M0
Stage IIIA	T1-3	N1	M0
Stage IIIB	T1-3	N1	M0
Stage IV	T4	Any N	M0
	Any T	N3	M0
	Any T	Any N	M1

Used with the permission of the American Joint Committee on Cancer (AJCC), Chicago, Illinois. The original source for this material is the AJCC Cancer Staging Manual, Seventh Edition (2010) published by Springer Science and Business Media LLC, www.springerlink.com.

IMMUNOHISTOCHEMISTRY, PENIS

Extramammary Paget Disease (EMPD)

Antibody	Primary EMPD	2° EMPD Associated with Urothelial Carcinoma	2° EMPD Associated with Anal/Rectal Carcinoma	Melanoma in situ	Squamous Cell Carcinoma in situ
CEA	+	-	+	-	-
CK7	+	+	-	-	-
Cam5.2	+	-	+/-	-	-/+
EMA/MUC1	+	-	+/-	-	-
GCDFP-15	+	-	-	-	-
CK20	-	+	+	-	-
S100	-	-	-	+	-
Melan-A(MART-1)	-	-	-	+	-
Tyrosinase	-	-	-	+	-
HMB-45	-	-	-	+	-
Uroplakin-3	-	+	-	-	-
CDX-2	-	-	+	-	-

HPV-associated Lesions

Antibody	Warty Carcinoma	Papillary Carcinoma NOS	Verrucous Carcinoma	Condyloma with Malignant Change
p16	+	-	-	-/+

Spindle Cell Lesions

Antibody	Sarcomatoid Carcinoma	Leiomyosarcoma	Angiosarcoma	Spindle Cell Melanoma
S100	-	-	-	+
Actin-sm	-/+	+	-	-
Desmin	-	+	-	-
Calponin	-	+	-	-
PAN-CK(AE1/AE3)	+/-	-/+ (focal)	-	-
Cam5.2	+/-	-	-	-
HMCK(34βE12)	+	-	-	-
p63	+	-	-	-
Vimentin	+	+	+	+
FVIIIRAg	-	-	+	-
FLI-1	-	-	+	-
CD31	-	-	+	-
CD34	-	-	+	-

Microscopic and Immunohistochemical Features

(Left) H&E shows the surface component of a warty-basaloid squamous cell carcinoma. The papillary surface of the tumor is lined by small basaloid cells at the center and larger pink cells with koilocytic changes at the periphery. Penile warty carcinoma, basaloid carcinoma, and mixed warty-basaloid carcinomas are usually associated with HPV. *(Right)* p16 immunohistochemical stain is strongly positive in this warty-basaloid squamous cell carcinoma, supporting its HPV-related etiopathogenesis.

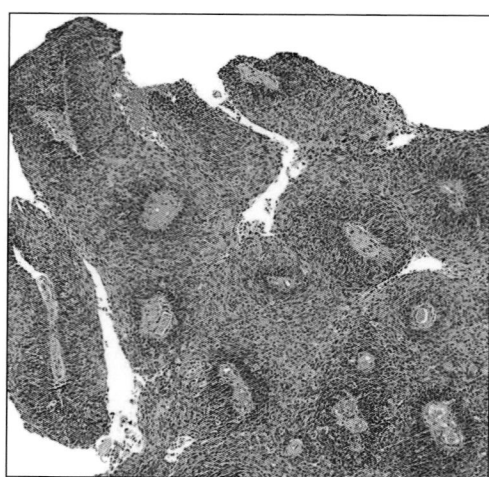
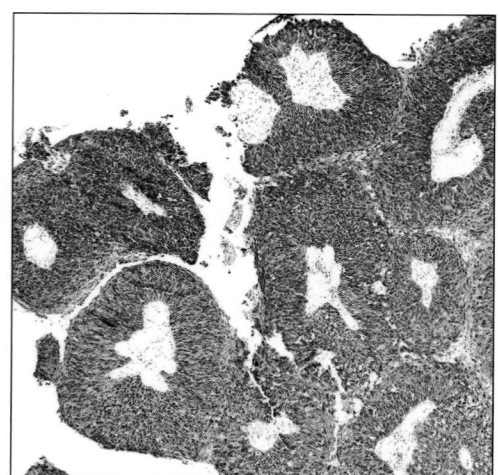

(Left) Sarcomatoid squamous cell carcinoma shows a predominant spindle cell component ⇒ and a focal but distinct component of invasive squamous cell carcinoma ⧐. Biphasic histology, presence of squamous cell carcinoma in situ, and previous history of squamous cell carcinoma support sarcomatoid differentiation. *(Right)* The focal positivity for PAN-CK in the spindle cell component of sarcomatoid carcinoma is further supportive of the diagnosis of sarcomatoid differentiation.

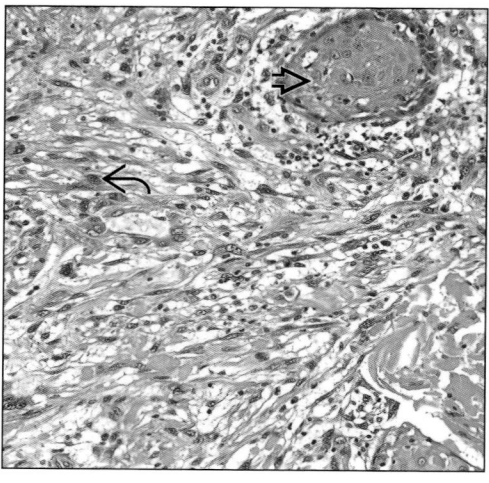
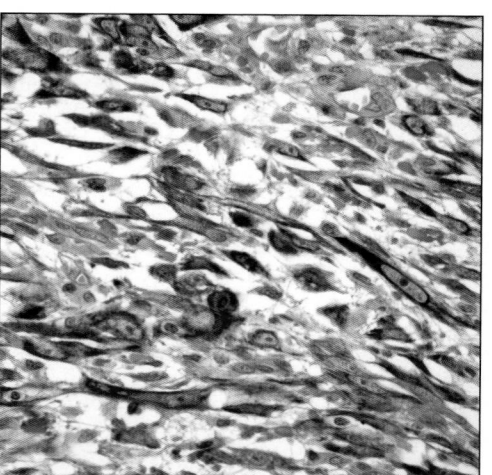

(Left) Kaposi sarcoma shows interlacing fascicles of spindle cells associated with slit-like vascular spaces. Leiomyosarcoma and sarcomatoid carcinoma are other spindle cell malignancies that more commonly involve the penis. *(Right)* The diagnosis of Kaposi sarcoma is supported by positive nuclear immunostaining for HHV8. Leiomyosarcoma is typically positive for actin-sm and desmin; cytokeratin may be aberrantly expressed, although usually focal.

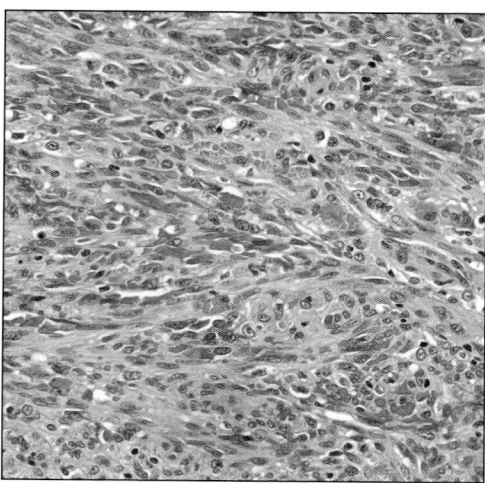
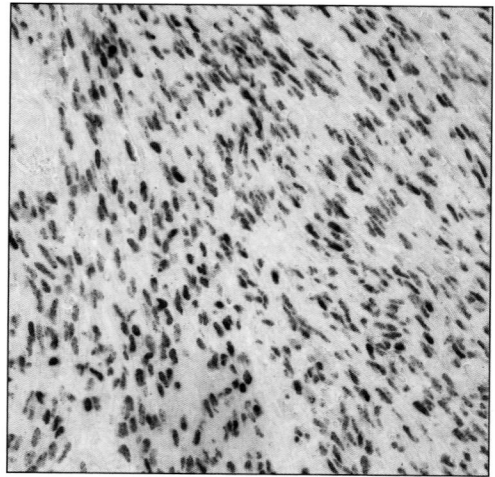

Antibody List   6-2

ANTIBODY LIST

Antibodies Discussed

Antibody Symbol	Antibody Description	Clones/Alternative Names
α-fetoprotein	α 1-fetoprotein	Z5A06, alpha1-fetoprotein, AFP, Clone C3,
β-catenin	beta-catenin	BETA CATENIN, BETA-CATENIN-MEMBRANE
κ light chain	kappa light chain	KAPPA
λ light chain	Lambda light chain	LAMBDA
34bE12	cytokeratin -high molecular weight (34bE12- CK 1, 5, 10, 14)	MA-903, 34BE12, 34βE12, high molecular weight keratin
Actin-HHF-35	actin-muscle (HHF35)	ACTIN-HHF35, MSA, muscle-specific actin (HHF35)
Actin-sm	actin-smooth muscle	ACTIN-SM, SMA, α SMA, ASM-1, CGA7, 1A4, HUC1-1
AE1	cytokeratin 10/14/15/16/19 (AE1)	
AE3	cytokeratin 01/02/03/04/05/06/07/08 (AE3)	cytokeratin
AE1/AE3	AE1/AE3	AE1_AE3
ALK1	anaplastic lymphoma kinase-1	ALK, ALKC
AMACR	alpha-methylacyl-CoA racemase (AMACR)	13H4, P504S
Androgen receptor	androgen receptor	AR441, F39.4.1, AR-N20, ANDROGEN RE
Bcl-2	B-cell CLL/lymphoma 2	ONCL2, BCL2/100/D5, 124, 124.3, BCL-2
CA125	CA 125	OV185:1, CA 125, OC125
CA15-3	CA 15-3	
CA9	carbonic anhydrase IX	CAIX, ab1508, M75, NB100-417
Caldesmon	caldesmon	
Calponin	calponin	N3, 26A11, CALP, CALPONIN
Calretinin	calretinin	Calretinin (mesothelial), CALRETININ, DAK-CALRET, 5A5, CAL 3F5, DC8, AB149
CD10	CD10, neutral endopeptidase, CALLA	NCL-270, CALLA, neprilysin, neutral endopeptidase, NEP
CD117	CD 117 (C-Kit)	C-19 (C-KIT), C-Kit, 104D2, 2E4, C-KIT, A4502, (C-KIT [CARBOXY TERMINUS], H300 (CD117 [AMINO TERMINUS]), CMA-767
CD138	CD138 (syndecan)	syndecan, B-B4, SYNDECAN, AM411-10M, MI15
CD15	CD15	Alpha 13 fucosyltransferase FucT antibody, EC 2.4.1. antibody, ELAM 1 ligand, fucosyltransferase antibody, ELAM ligand fucosyltransferase antibody, ELFT antibody, FCT3A antibody, 3C4, LEU-M1, TU9, VIM-D5, MY1, CBD1, MMA, 3CD1, C3D1 (CD15 [Leu-M1])
CD163	CD 163 (macrophage hemoglobin savenging system)	10D6, HEMOGLOBIN SCAVENGER RECEPTOR
CD1a	CD 1a (T cell surface glycoprotein)	JPM30, CD1A, O10, NA1/34
CD20	CD20 (membrane spanning 4-domains of B lymphocytes)	membrane spanning 4-domains, MS4A1, FB1, B1, L26 (CD20 [L26, B-cell])
CD3	CD 3 (T cell receptor)	F7238, A0452, CD3-P, CD3-M, SP7, PS1
CD30(BerH2)	CD 30 (tumor necrosis factor receptor SF8)	TNFRSF8, tumor necrosis factor receptor SF8
CD31	CD 31(PECAM-1, platelet endothelial cell adhesion molecule)	PECAM-1, platelet endothelial cell adhesion molecule, JC/70, JC/70A (PLATELET-ENDOTHELIAL CELL ADHESION MOLECULE)
CD34	CD 34 (hematopoetic progenitor cell antigen)	MY10, IOM34, QBEND10, 8G12, 1309, HPCA-1, HPCA, NU-4A1, TUK4, clone 581, BI-3C5
CD4	CD 4 (T cell surface glycoprotein, L3T4, T helper cells)	CD04, IF6, 1290, 4B12, 1F6
CD44	CD 44 (cell adhesion receptor for hyaluronic acid HCAM)	HCAM, CD44H, B-F24, A3D8, 2C5, CD44S, F10-44.2, 156-3C11, DF1485, BBA10, VFF-14, CD44V10, CD44V3, 3G5, CD44V3-10-P, CD44V3-10, 3D2, CD44V4_5, CD44V5, VFF-8, VFF-7, 2F10, VFF-18, CD44V6, CD44V7, VFF-9, CD44V7_8, VFF-17
CD45(LCA)	CD 45 (leukocyte common antigen, LCA)	PD7/26, 1.22/4.14, T29/33, CD45RB, RP2/18, PD7, 2D1, 2B11+PD7/26, LCA
CD5	CD 5 (T cell surface glycoprotein LEU1, T1)	CD 05, LEU1, T1, NCL-CD5, 4C7, 54/B4, 54/F6
CD56	CD 56 (NCAM (neural cellular adhesion molecule)	NCAM-1, MAB 735, ERIC-1, 25-KD11, 123C3, 24-MB2, BC56C04, 1B6 (NCAM), 14-MAB735, NCC-LU-243, MOC-1, LEU-19
CD57	CD 57 (Beta-1,3-glucuronyltransferase 1 (glucuronosyltransferase P), B3GAT1, LEU 7, NK1, HNK 1	LEU-7, HNK-1, TB01
CD68	CD 68 (cytoplasmic granule protein of monocytes, macrophages	PG-M1, KP-1, LN5

ANTIBODY LIST

CD7	CD 7 (T cell antigen precursor Leu 9)	CD 07, LEU 9 TP41, GP 40, Tp40, 272, CD7-272
CD8	CD 8 (T cell co-receptor antigen, Leu 2, T cytotoxic cells)	CD08, M7103, C8/144, C8/144B
CD99	CD 99 (cell surface glycoprotein for migration, T cell adhesion, MIC2)	CD99-MEMB, CD 99, MIC2, 12E7, HBA71, O13, P30/32MIC2, M3601
CDK4	cyclin dependant kinase 4	C-22, DCS-31
CDX-2	caudal type homeobox transcription factor 2	AMT28, 7C7/D4, CDX-2-88
CEA	carcinoembryonic antigen, monoclonal	CEA-M, CEA-B18, CEA-D14, CEA-GOLD 1, T84.6, CEA-GOLD 2, CEA 11, CEA-GOLD 3, CEA 27, CEA-GOLD 4, CEA-GOLD 5, T84.1, A5B7, CEJ065, IL-7, T84.66, TF3H8-1, 0062, D14, alpha-7, PARLAM 1, ZC23, CEM010, A115, COL-1, AF4, 11-7, 12.140.10, M773, CEA-M431_31, CEJO65
Chromogranin-A	chromogranin A	PHE-5, PHE5, E001, DAK-A3, LK2H10
CK14	cytokeratin 14	LL002, CK 14
CK17	cytokeratin 17	CK 17, E3
CK18	cytokeratin 18	M9, DC-10, CY-90, CK 18, KS18.04
CK19	cytokeratin 19	BA17, RCK108, LP2K, B170, A53-BA2, CK 19, KS19.1, 170.2.14
CK20	cytokeratin 20	CK 20, KS20.8,
CK5	cytokeratin 5	CK 05, XM26, RCK103, 34BEH12
CK5/6	cytokeratin 5/6	CK 05_06, D5/16 B4
CK7	cytokeratin 7	CK 7, K72.7, KS7.18, OVTL 12/30, LDS-68, CK 07
CAM5.2	cytokeratin 8/18	CK8/18/CAM5.2, CAM 5.2, cytokeratin LMW, 5D3, Zym5.2, KER 10.11, NCL-5D3, K8.8, 4.1.18, TS1, C-51, M20, CK 08, 35BH11 (Cytokeratin 8, LMW [35bH11]), MA-902 (Cytokeratin 8, LMW [35bH11])
HMCK(34βE12)	cytokeratin-HMW, not otherwise specified	CK-HMW, CK-HMW-NOS, HMWCK, 34bE12
PAN-CK(AE1/AE3)	cytokeratin-pan (AE1/AE3/LP34)	KERATIN-PAN, MAK-6, K576, LU-5, KL-1 (CYTOKERATIN 1,2,5-8,11,14,16-18), KC-8, MNF 116 (CYTOKERATIN 5,6,8,10,17,18)
Claudin-7	claudin 7	
COX-2	COX-2	Cyclooxygenase-2, CYCLOOXYGENASE-2 (PROSTAGLANDIN H SYNTHASE), CX229, CLONE 33, COX-2-P
Cyclin-D1	cyclin D1	Bcl-1 (Cyclin D1), A-12, PRAD1, AM29, DCS-6, SP4, 5D4, D1GM, P2D11F11
Desmin	desmin	M760, DE-R-11, D33, DE5, DE-U-10, ZC18
DOG1	DOG1	DOG1 (TMEM16A), DOG 1.1
E-cadherin	epithelial calcium dependent adhesion molecule	36B5, ECH-6, ECCD-2, CDH1, 5H9, E-CADHERIN, NCH 38, EPITHELIAL-CADHERIN, 4A2 C7, E9, 67A4, HECD-1, SC-8426
EMA/MUC1	epithelial membrane antigen	EMA, GP1.4, MUC1, MAM6, CA15.3, 214D4, MC5, E29, LICR-LON-M8, BC3, DF3, VU3D1, MUSEII (MUC1 [MAMMARY TYPE APOMUCIN]), RD-1(MUC1 [MAMMARY TYPE APOMUCIN]), MA695 (MUC1 [MAMMARY TYPE APOMUCIN]), MA552, PS2P446, 115D8, MUC01, Mucin 1, cell surface associated
EpCAM/BER-EP4/CD326	epithelial cell adhesion molecule	AUA1, VU-1D9, EPITH SPECIFIC ANTIGEN(EPCAM, EGP40), EPCAM GENE:GA733-2,EPCAMEPCAMEPCAM EPCAM, C10, HEA125, EpCAM, CD326, BER-EP4, Ber-Ep4 (epithelial antigen)
ERP	estrogen receptor protein	1D5, ER (estrogen receptor), 6F11, SP1, 15D, H222, TE111, ER1D5, NCLER611, NCL-ER-LH2
ERP-α	estrogen receptor protein α	ER-ALPHA,
ERP-β	estrogen receptor protein β	ER-BETA, 14C8, 57/3, PPG5/10
FLI-1	Friend leukemia virus integration 1	EWSR2, GI146-222, SC356, FLK-1, FLT-1
FSH	follicle stimulating hormone	beta-FSH
FVIIIRAg	factor -VIII-related-antigen	FVIIIRAG, F8/86, von Willebrand factor
GATA3	endothelial transcription factor 3	GATA-3
GCDFP-15	gross cystic fluid protein 15	SABP, GPIP4, Gp17, 23A3, BRST-2, D6 (GROSS CYSTIC DISEASE FLUID PROTEIN)
GFAP	glial fibrillary acidic protein	6F2, M761, GA-51, GFP-8A
GH	growth hormone	HGH

Glypican-3	glypican 3	1G12, GPC3
GST-α	glutathione S transferase alpha	GST-A
HBME-1	mesothelioma antibody	
h-caldesmon	h-caldesmon	High molecular weight caldesmon, H-CD
HCG	human chorionic gonadotropin	
HCG-β	human chorionic gonadotropin beta subunit	HCG-BETA, HCG (b-chorionic gonadotropin)
HER2	v-erb-b2 erythroblastic leukemia viral gene protein, human epidermal growth factor receptor 2	c-erb-B2, HER2/neu, NEU, HER-2, NCL-CBE1, 10A7, 9G6.10, SP3, 4B5, Epidermal Growth Factor Receptor 2, P185, 9G6.20, A0485, C-ERBB-2, CB11, ERBB-2, 3B5, TAB250, HERCEPTEST, E2-4001, HER-2_NEU,
HHV8	human herpes virus 8	Kaposi sarcoma associated herpes virus, KSHV, HUMAN HERPESVIRUS-8 LATENT NUCLEAR ANTIGEN-1, 13B10, LNA-1
HIF-1-α	hypoxia inducible factor 1 α	HIF-1ALPHA
HMB-45	HMB-45	HMB45 (melanosome)
HPL	human placental lactogen	
HPV	human papilloma virus	
Inhibin	inhibin	R1
Inhibin-α	inhibin α	Inhibin-alpha
Insulin	insulin	HB125
Ki-67	Ki-67 (MIB-1)	KI-67, MMI, KI88, IVAK-2, MIB1
Ksp-cadherin	Kidney-specific cadherin	
Laminin	laminin	LAMININ-4C7, 4C12.8, LAM-89
LF	lactoferrin	
LH	luteinizing hormone	beta-LH
Melan-A (Mart-1)	mart-1 clone of Melan A	MART-1, MELAN-A, melan-A,
mdm2	murine double minute oncogene (mdm2)	HUMAN HOMOLOG OF MURINE DOUBLE MINUTE 2, HDM2, MURINE DOUBLE MINUTE 2, IF2, 2A10, 1B10, SMP14, MDM-2,
melan-A103	melan-A103	MELAN-A103, A103, MELAN-A CLONE A103
Mesothelin	mesothelin	5B2,
met	met protooncogene	8F11, Hepatocyte growth factor receptor (C-MET), C-28, C-MET
MITF	microphthalmia-associated transcription factor	34CA5, D5, C5+D5
MK	neurite growth promoting factor 2	G2a, MIDKINE, Midkine
MOC-31	lung cancer marker	HUMAN EPITHELIAL RELATED ANTIGEN,
MPO	myeloperoxidase	
MSH6	mut S homolog 6	clone 44, GRBP.P1, DNA mismatch repair protein MSH6 antibody, G/T mismatch binding protein antibody, GTBP antibody, GTMBP antibody, HNPCC 5 antibody, HNPCC5 antibody, HSAP antibody, MSH 6 antibody, mutS (E. coli) homolog 6 antibody
MT	metallothionein	METALLOTHIO, CLONE E9
myc	myelocytomatosis viral oncogene	C-MYC, c-myc, 9E10, 9E11, 1-262
MYOD1	myogenic differentiation 1	5.8A, 5.2F
Myogenin	myogenin	F5D, MYF3, MYF4, MYOGENIN, LO26
Myosin	myosin	
NANOG	embryonic stem cell specific homeobox protein	NANOG (AF1997)
Neuroblastoma	neuroblastoma	NB84
NFP	neurofilament H/M phosphorylated protein	TPNFP-1A3, Neurofilament protein, SMI31, SMI32, SMI33, TA-51, 2F11,
NSE	neuron specific enolase	BSS/H14
p16	cyclin dependent kinase 4 inhibitor A	Cyclin dependent kinase inhibitor p16 antibody, INK4, INK4a, MLM, MTS1, multiple tumor suppressor 1 antibody, p12, p14, p16, p16 γ, p16 INK4, p16 INK4a, INK4 p19, TP16, P16_INK4A, E6H4, sc1661, JC8, ZJ11, G175-405, F-12, DCS-50, 6H12, 16P07, 16P04
P501S	prostein	

ANTIBODY LIST

p53	p53 tumor suppressor gene protein	DO7, 21N, BP53-12-1, AB6, CM1, PAB1801, DO1, BP53-11, PAB240, RSP53, MU195, PAB1801, nuclear p53, P53
p63	tumor protein p63	P63- P53 HOMOLOGOUS NULCEAR PROTEIN;DELTA-N-P63, 4A4, P63, H-137, 7JUL
PAP	prostatic acid phosphatase	PSAP, PASE/4LJ, PAP-P
Parafibromin		
Parvalbumin	parafibromin	2H1, PA-235
pax-2	paired box gene 2	PAX2, Z-RX2
pax-5	paired box gene 5	PAX5 (BSAP)
pax-8	paired box gene 8	
PLAP	placental alkaline phosphatase	228M, 8A9
PNA	peanut agglutinin	
Podoplanin(D2-40)	podoplanin	D2-40 clone, D2-40, M2A, PODOPLANIN, gp36, AGGRUS,GLYCOPROTEIN 36 KD, glycoprotein 36, gp 36,GP 38, GP 40, HT1A 1, HT1A1, hT1α1, hT1α2, lung type I cell membrane associated glycoprotein isoform a, OTS 8, PA2.26, PA2.26 antigen,PDPN, T1 α, T1 ALPHA GENE, T1A, TIA 2, TIA2
POU5F1	octamer-binding transcription factor-3	OCT3, OCT4, POU5F1 (OCT3/4), C-10
pPSA	pro prostate specific antigen	proPSA, PS2P446
PRP	progesterone receptor protein	PR, 10A9, PGR-1A6, KD68, PGR-ICA, PRP-P, PRI, 1A6, 1AR, HPRA3, PGR-636, 636, PR88, NCL-PGR
PSA	prostate specific antigen	PSA-M, PSA, ER-PR8, PSA-P, F5
PSMA	prostate surface membrane antigen	pro 232, 1G8
pVHL	von Hippel-Landau tumor suppressor protein	Ig33, pVHL
RCC	renal cell carcinoma	66.4C2, PN-15, RCC, renal cell carcinoma marker, RCC MA
Reg4	regenerating islet family 4	Regenerating islet-derived family member 4, Reg IV
S100	S100 polyclonal	S-100, A6, 15E2E2, Z311, 4C4.9
SAA1	serum amyloid A 1	
SALL4	sal-like protein 4	
SCC	small cell carcinoma	F2H7C
Serotonin	serotonin	5-HT, 5HT-H209
SNF5	SNF5	BAF47/SNF5, INI1
Somatostatin	somatostatin	
SOX2	SRY (sex-determining region Y)-box 2 protein	SOX2 (AB5603)
Synaptophysin	synaptophysin	SVP38, SY38, SNP-88
TFE3	transcription factor E3	
TFEB	transcription factor EB	
Thrombomodulin	thrombomodulin	1009,15C8
TTF-1	transcription termination factor	8G7G3/1, SPT-24, SC-13040
Tyrosinase	tyrosinase	NCL-TYROS, T311
ULEX-1	ulex euroopeaus agglutinin-01	UEA-1 (Ulex Europeaus Agglutinin-1),
Uroplakin-3	uroplakin 3	AU 1, Uroplakin III
VEGF	vascular endothelial growth factor	VEGF (Vascular Endothelial Growth Factor), JH121,26503.11, VPF, VPF/VEGF, VEGF-A, VEGF-C, RP 077, VEGFR-1, RP 076, VEGFR-2, 9D9, VEGFR-3, FLT-4
Villin	villin	1D2C3
Vimentin	vimentin	43BE8, 3B4, V10, V9, VIM-3B4, RPN1102
VIP	vasoactive intestinal peptide	
WT1	Wilms tumor gene-01	6F-H2, C-19, WT1

INDEX

INDEX

INDEX

INDEX

INDEX

INDEX

INDEX

INDEX

INDEX

INDEX

INDEX

T

INDEX

INDEX